Principles of **Medicine in Africa**

Third Edition

For students of medicine, and those who practise in the front line of medicine in Africa, this fully revised edition combines classical internal medicine with a rich understanding of the major influences on health and disease in Africa. It puts disease into the context of family and culture and is not afraid to address the effects of inequality on health and the problems of limited resources for health care. There is a much expanded section on non-communicable diseases as well as comprehensive accounts of HIV/AIDS, malaria, tuberculosis and other major infections in the continent.

Forward looking and evidence based, this new edition reflects the emergence of new diseases and health risks in the region. Compiled by the foremost international authorities, this is the one essential text for the medical student, medical officer, or post-graduate student wanting the most complete and up-to-date reference book on medicine in Africa.

Eldryd Parry has unrivalled experience of medicine in Africa, having worked in Ghana, Ethiopia and Nigeria, where he was both Professor and Dean of Medicine. He is now Visiting Professor and Honorary Fellow at the London School of Hygiene and Tropical Medicine, and Chairman of the Tropical Health Education Trust. He was awarded the OBE for services to medical education.

Richard Godfrey was, from 1990 to 1993, Professor of Medicine at Moi University in Kenya, and has had overseas consultancies in Kenya and Zambia. Until 2002 he was Consultant Physician and Honorary Senior Lecturer at Southampton University Hospitals, and at present works with Medical Emergency Relief International in programmes concerned with tuberculosis in sub-Saharan Africa.

David Mabey worked as a clinician at the Medical Research Council Laboratories, Gambia from 1978 to 1986. He has been Honorary Consultant Physician, at the Hospital for Tropical Diseases, London, since 1986 and is head of the Clinical Research Unit at the London School of Hygiene & Tropical Medicine. He has published approximately 150 papers in peer-reviewed journals mostly on HIV, other sexually transmitted infections and trachoma.

Geoffrey Gill has worked extensively in Africa and has published widely on chronic disease care in the tropics. He is Reader in the departments of Medicine and Tropical Medicine at the University of Liverpool.

Principles of **Medicine in Africa**

Third Edition

Edited by

Eldryd Parry
London School of Hygiene and Tropical Medicine, and THET, the Tropical Health and Education Trust, London, UK

Richard Godfrey
Medical Emergency Relief International (Merlin) and formerly Southampton University Hospitals Trust, Southampton, UK

David Mabey
London School of Hygiene and Tropical Medicine, London, UK

Geoffrey Gill
Liverpool School of Tropical Medicine, Liverpool, UK

CAMBRIDGE
UNIVERSITY PRESS

PUBLISHED BY THE PRESS SYNDICATE OF THE UNIVERSITY OF CAMBRIDGE
The Pitt Building, Trumpington Street, Cambridge, United Kingdom

CAMBRIDGE UNIVERSITY PRESS
The Edinburgh Building, Cambridge CB2 2RU, UK
40 West 20th Street, New York, NY 10011–4211, USA
477 Williamstown Road, Port Melbourne, VIC 3207, Australia
Ruiz de Alarcón 13, 28014 Madrid, Spain
Dock House, The Waterfront, Cape Town 8001, South Africa

http://www.cambridge.org

First published 2004

Printed in Singapore by Tien Wah Press (Pte) Ltd.

Typeface Utopia (*Adobe*) 8.5/12pt. *System* QuarkXPress® [SE]

A catalogue record for this book is available from the British Library

ISBN 0 521 80616 X hardback
Cambridge low-price edition 0 521 534380

Contents

Contributors

Ade Adebajo
Academic Rheumatology Group
Division of Molecular and Genetic Medicine
University of Sheffield
Royal Halamshire Hospital
Beech Hill Road
Sheffield S10 2RX
UK

George Alberti
Royal College of Physicians
11 St Andrews Place
London NW1 4LE
UK

Sylvester Anemana
Ministry of Health
Northern Region
PO Box 99
Tamale
Ghana

Ann Ashworth
London School of Hygiene and Tropical Medicine
49–51 Bedford Square
London WC1B 3DP
UK

Kingsley Asiedu
Communicable Diseases Control,
Prevention and Eradication
WHO
Avenue Appia 20
Geneva 27, 1211
Switzerland

Robin Bailey
Medical Research Council Laboratories
PO Box 273
Banjul
The Gambia

Guy Baily
Department of HIV/GU Medicine
Ambrose King Centre
Royal London Hospital
Whitechapel
London E1 1BB
UK

Imelda Bates
Liverpool School of Tropical Medicine
Pembroke Place
Liverpool L3 5QA
UK

George Bedu-Addo
Komfo Anokye Teaching Hospital
PO Box 1934
Kumasi
Ghana

Martin Boeree
Margrietstraat 6
6862 GP Oosterberk
Netherlands

Ruairi Brugha
Health Policy Unit
London School of Hygiene and Tropical Medicine
Keppel Street
London WC1E 7HT
UK

Anthony Bryceson
The Bull's House
3 Rousham Road
Tackley
Kidlington
Oxon OX5 3BB
UK

Donald Bundy
The Human Development Network
The World Bank
1818H Street
Washington DC 20433
USA

Tom Burns
St George's Hospital Medical School
Cranmer Terrace
London SW17 0RE
UK

Anthony Butterworth
Biomedical Research and Training Institute
PO Box CY 1753
Causeway
Harare
Zimbabwe

Francesco Cappuccio
Department of Community Health Sciences
St George's Hospital Medical School
Cranmer Terrace
London SW17 0RE
UK

J. M. Chakaya
Mbagathi District Hospital
Nairobi
Kenya

Peter Cleland
Department of Neurology
Sunderland Royal Hospital
Kayall Road
Sunderland SR4 7TP
UK

Ed Cooper
Department of Paediatrics
Newham Hospital
London, UK

Kevin M. De Cock
Centers for Disease Control and Prevention, KEMRI
Mbagathi Road
Off Mbagathi Way
Nairobi
Kenya

Phillip Debenham
Royal Children's Hospital
Flemington Road
Parkville
Victoria 3051
Australia

Tom Doherty
Department of Infectious and Tropical Diseases
London School of Hygiene and Tropical Medicine
Keppel Street
London WC1E 7HT
UK

Lesley J. Drake
Scientific Coordinating Centre for the Partnership for Child Development
Department of Infectious Disease Epidemiology
Imperial College School of Medicine
St. Mary's Campus
Norfolk Place
London W2 1PG
UK

Trevor Duke
Centre for International Child Health
University of Melbourne Department of Paediatrics
Royal Childrens' Hospital
Flemington Road
Parkville 3051
Victoria
Australia

John Eastwood
Department of Renal Medicine
St George's Hospital Medical School
Cranmer Terrace
London SW17 0RE
UK

Richard Edwards
Evidence for Population Health Unit
School of Epidemiology and Health Sciences
The Medical School
University of Manchester
Oxford Road
Manchester M13 9PT
UK

Alison M. Elliott
Medical Research Council Programme on AIDS in Uganda
c/o Uganda Viral Research Institute
PO Box 49
Entebbe
Uganda

Carlton Evans
Hospital for Tropical Diseases
Mortimer Market Centre
Capper Street
London WC1E 6AU
UK

Jeremy J Farrar
Oxford University Clinical Research Unit
Hospital for Tropical Diseases
190 Ben Ham Tu, Quan 5
Ho Chi Minh City
Vietnam

Daniel Fekade
Department of Medicine
Addis Ababa University
PO Box 1176
Addis Ababa
Ethiopia

Alan Fleming
Kilmersdon Common Farmhouse
Common Lane
Holcombe
Somerset BA3 5QB
UK

Allen Foster
Department of Infectious and Tropical Diseases
London School of Hygiene and Tropical Medicine
CRU Room 2486
Keppel Street
London WC1E 7HT
UK

Susan Foster
School of Public Health
Boston University
Boston MA
USA

Karen L. Frame
Mbarara University Medical School
PO Box 1410
Mbarara
Uganda

Juergen Freers
Department of Medicine
Makerere University
PO Box 7072
Kampala
Uganda

Geoffrey Gill
Department of Medicine
Walton Hospital
Liverpool L9 lAE
UK

Richard Godfrey
Medical Emergency Relief International
5–13 Trinity Street,
London SE1 1DB
UK

Melita Gordon
29 Crimicar Street
Sheffield S10 4FA
UK

Stephen Gordon
29 Crimicar Street
Sheffield S10 4FA
UK

Alison D. Grant
Department of Infectious and Tropical Diseases
London School of Hygiene and Tropical Medicine
Keppel Street
London WC1E 7HT
UK

Brian Greenwood
Clinical Research Unit
Department of Infectious and Tropical Diseases
London School of Hygiene and Tropical Medicine
Keppel St
London WC1E 7HT
UK

Heiner Grosskurth
Department of Infectious and Tropical Diseases
London School of Hygiene and Tropical Medicine
Keppel Street
London WC1E 7HT
UK

James Hakim
Department of Medicine
University of Zimbabwe
PO Box A176
Harare
Zimbabwe

Andy Hall
Department of Infectious and Tropical Diseases
London School of Hygiene and Tropical Medicine
Keppel St
London WC1E 7HT
UK

Nicola J. Hargreaves
Lilongwe Central Hospital
PO Box 149
Lilongwe
Malawi

Anthony D. Harries
c/o British High Commission
PO Box 30042
Lilongwe
Malawi

Yvonne Hart
Radcliffe Infirmary
Oxford OX3 9DU
UK

Rod J. Hay
St Johns Institute of Dermatology
Guy's, King's and St Thomas' School of Medicine
St Thomas's Hospital
London SE1 7EH
UK

Tim Healing
Medical Emergency Relief International
5–13 Trinity Street
London SE1 1DB
UK

Ken Huddle
Department of Medicine
Chris Wani Baragwanath Hospital
PO Bertsham
Johannesburg 2013
South Africa

Harry F. Hull
Global Polio Eradication Initiative
WHO
Avenue Appia 20
Geneva 27
CH-1211 Switzerland

Assan Jaye
MRC Laboratories
PO Box 273
Fajara
The Gambia
West Africa

Pontiano Kaleebu
Medical Research Council Programme on AIDs in Uganda
c/o Uganda Viral Research Institute
PO Box 49
Entebbe
Uganda

Elly T. Katabira
Department of Medicine
Makerere University
PO Box 7072
Kampala
Uganda

Patrick J. Kelly
Biomedical Research and Training Institute
PO Box CY 1753
Causeway
Harare
Zimbabwe

Paul Kelly
Department of Adult and Paediatric Gastroenterology
St Bartholomew's and the Royal London School of Medicine and Dentistry
Turner Street
London E1 2AD
UK

Richard Laing
School of Public Health
Boston University
641 Huntingdon Avenue
Boston
MA 02115
USA

Richard Laugharne
Mental Health Research Group
Peninsula Medical School
Wonford House Hospital
Exeter EX2 5AF
UK

Christopher Lavy
Beit/CVRE Hospital
Malawi Against Polio
PO Box 256
Malawi
Central Africa

Ruth Leekassa
ALERT
PO Box 165
Addis Ababa
Ethiopia

Diana Lockwood
Department of Infectious and Tropical Diseases
London School of Hygiene and Tropical Medicine
Keppel Street
London WC1E 7HT
UK

David Mabey
Clinical Research Unit
Department of Infectious and Tropical Diseases
London School of Hygiene and Tropical Medicine
Keppel Street
London WC1E 7HT
UK

Julie Makani
Department of Internal Medicine
Muhimbili University College Hospital
PO Box 65001
Dar-es-salaam
Tanzania

Kevin Marsh
Wellcome Collaborative Research Laboratories
PO Box 230
Bofa Road
Kilifil
Kenya

Lawrence H. Marum
Centers for Disease Control and Prevention
PO Box 30137
Nairobi
Kenya

Philippe Mayaud
Clinical Research Unit
Department of Infectious and Tropical Diseases
London School of Hygiene and Tropical Medicine
Keppel Street
London WC1E 7HT
UK

Jean-Claude Mbanya
Endocrine and Diabetes Unit
Faculty of Medicine and Biomedical Sciences
BP 8046
Yaounde
Cameroon

Edward Mbidde
Uganda Cancer Institute
Makerere University Medical School
Makerere University
PO Box 3935
Kampala
Uganda

Clara Menendez
Unidad de Epidemiologia & Bioestadistia
Hospital Clinic
Barcelona University
Vilaroth 170
E-08036 Barcelona
Spain

Anne Merriman
Hospice Africa Uganda
PO Box 7757
Kampala
Uganda

Kim Mulholland
Centre for International Child Health
Royal Children's Hospital
Flemington Road
Parkville Vic 3051
Australia

Ian E. Murdoch
Department of Infectious and Tropical Diseases
London School of Hygiene and Tropical Medicine
Keppel Street
London WC1E 7HT
UK

Michael E. Murdoch
7 The Brow
Chalfont St Giles
Bucks HP8 41D
UK

Harriet Myanja-Kizza
Department of Medicine
Makerere University
PO Box 7072
Kampala
Uganda

Ben Naafs
Gracht 15
Munnekeburen 8485KN
Netherlands

Francis Ndowa
Reproductive Health Research Unit
World Health Organization
20 Avenue Appia
Geneva 27
CH-1211 Switzerland

Peter Newman
Department of Neurology
Middlesbrough General Hospital
Ayresome Green Lane
Middlesbrough TS5 5AZ
UK

Charles R. J. C. Newton
Kenya Medical Research Institute and
Wellcome Trust Research Laboratories
Kilifi
Kenya

Ramou Njie
Medical Research Council Laboratories
PO Box 273
Fajara
The Gambia
West Africa

Chukwuedu Nwokolo
University of Ibadan
PMB 5116
Ibadan
OYO State
Nigeria

Yaw Osei
School of Medical Sciences
Kwame Nkrumah University of Science and Technology
Kumasi
Ghana

John Ouma
Division of Vector Borne Diseases
PO Box 20750
Nairobi
Kenya

Ayo Palmer
Royal Victoria Hospital
Banjul
The Gambia
West Africa

Philippe Parola
Unité des Rickettsies
Faculté de Médecine
CNRS UMR 6020
WHO Collaborative Center for Rickettsial Reference and Research
Marseille
France

Eldryd Parry
THET, Tropical Health and Education Trust
24 Eversholt Street
London NW1 1AD
UK

Michael Pelly
Department of Medicine
Chelsea and Westminster Hospital
369 Fulham Road
London SW10 9NH
UK

Jacob Plange-Rhule
Department of Medicine
Komfo Anokye Teaching Hospital
PO Box 1934
Kumasi
Ghana

Andrew Prentice
Public Health Nutrition Unit
London School of Hygiene and Tropical Medicine
49–51 Bedford Square
London WC1B 3DP
UK

Martin Prevett
Wessex Neurological Centre
Southampton General Hospital;
Southampton S016 6YD
UK

Didier Raoult
Unité des Rickettsies
Université de la Mediterranée
Faculté de Médecine
27 Boulevard Jean Moulin
Marseille cedex 5
13385 France

John Richens
Academic Department of Sexually Transmitted Diseases
University College London
Mortimer Market Centre
Capper Street
London WC1E 6AU

Susan E. Robertson
Vaccines and Biologicals
World Health Organization
Geneva
Switzerland

Lance Saker
Department of Epidemiology and Public Health
University of Newcastle
Newcastle-upon-Tyne
UK

Felix M. Salaniponi
National Tuberculosis Control Programme
Community Health Science Unit
Private Bag 65
Lilongwe
Malawi

Gisela Schneider
C/o Dr Robin Bailey
Medical Research Council Laboratories
PO Box 273
Banjul
The Gambia
West Africa

Anthony Scott
London School of Hygiene and Tropical Medicine
Keppel Street
London WC1E 7HT
UK

August Stich
Medical Mission Institute
Unit of Tropical Medicine and Epidemic Control
Hermann-Schell – Str. 7
Würzburg
D-97074 Germany

Giorgio Tamburlini
Unit for Health Services Research and International Health
Department of Paediatrics
Institute of Child Health IRCCS Burlo Garofolo
Via dell'Istria 65/1
34137 Trieste
Italy

Jan ter Meulen
Institute of Virology
Philipps University
Robert Voch Strasse 17
35037 Marburg
Germany

Sara Thomas
Infectious Disease Epidemiology Unit
London School of Hygiene and Tropical Medicine
Keppel St
London WC1E 7HT
UK

Mohammed Tikly
Department of Rheumatology
Chris Hani Baragwanath Hospital
PO Bertsham
Johannesburg 2013
South Africa

Charles Todd
Delegation of the European Commission to Zimbabwe
6th Floor Construction House
101 Union Avenue
PO Box 4252
Harare
Zimbabwe

Edemariam Tsega
Department of Internal Medicine
Montreal
Canada

Nigel Unwin
Departments of Diabetes and Epidemiology and Public Health
University of Newcastle
Newcastle-upon-Tyne
UK

Tjip van der Werf
Klooslaan 28
9721 XN Groningen
Netherlands

Richard Walker
Department of Medicine for the Elderly
North Tyneside General Hospital
Rake Lane
North Shields
Tyne and Wear NE29 8NH
UK

David Warrell
Nuffield Department of Clinical Medicine
John Radcliffe Hospital
Oxford OX3 9DU
UK

Martin Weber
Department of Child and Adolescent Health
World Health Organization
Avenue Appia 20
Geneva 27
CH-1211 Switzerland

Edwin Were
Department of Reproductive Health
Moi University
PO Box 4606
Eldoret
Kenya

Hilton C. Whittle
Medical Research Council Laboratories
PO Box 273
Fajara
The Gambia
West Africa

Christopher Whitty
Department of Infectious and Tropical Diseases
London School of Hygiene and Tropical Medicine
Keppel Street
London WC1E 7HT
UK

David Wilkinson
South Australian Centre for Rural and Remote Health
University of South Australia
Nicholson Avenue
Whyalla Norrie
South Australia 5608
Australia

Nomsa F. Wilkinson
South Australian Centre for Rural and Remote Health
University of South Australia
Nicholson Avenue
Whyalla Norrie
South Australia 5608
Australia

Peter A. Winstanley
Department of Pharmacology and Therapeutics
University of Liverpool Medical School
Ashton Street
Liverpool L69 3GE
UK

John Ziegler
USCF Cancer Risk Program
Box 0808
UCSF
San Francisco
CA 94143-0808
USA

Ed Zijlstra
Department of Medicine
College of Medicine
Private Bag 360
Chichiri
Blantyre 3
Malawi

Isaac Zulu
Department of Medicine
University of Zambia School of Medicine
University Teaching Hospital
PO Box 50110
Lusaka
Zambia

Preface

It is nearly 20 years since the second edition of this book. We have followed the pattern of the earlier editions and so we have put the medicine of Africa into its rural and urban context, we have emphasized basic mechanisms of disease, and we have tried to be practical and relevant for those who are at the front line of health care.

Our team of contributors represents many countries and writes from a wide African clinical, community or scientific experience. The book will be essential for undergraduate and postgraduate students of medicine in Africa, for health officers and clinical officers, for district medical officers, for teaching hospital doctors and indeed for all who are interested in, and who want to learn about, the practice and problems of medicine in Africa today.

HIV/AIDS dominates practice in many hospitals. It presents in so many ways that classical clinical method, which our book seeks to emphasize, is as important as ever, particularly in places where investigations are limited. We have therefore given HIV the prominence it deserves in a new section devoted to major infectious diseases.

Medicine in Africa is changing in other ways, too, and so we have new chapters on refugees, disability, palliative care and district health care. There is more paediatrics and a new secton on non-communicable disease. It has not been easy to strike the right balance between the ideal in investigation and treatment and what, realistically, is available in hospitals and health centres with limited resources. We have therefore given simple measures, while at the same time briefly describing more advanced methods, always centred on the patient and based as fully as possible on sound evidence.

As much is yet to be learned about the medicine of Africa, we want our book to help those who do their research, whether clinical studies, fieldwork or more sophisticated laboratory work. They will find in each chapter a generous list of references, which should also be useful for medical students in their project work.

Many people have helped in the preparation of this third edition. The Parthenon Trust gave a generous grant towards colour illustrations: John Eyers, deputy librarian at the London School of Hygiene and Tropical Medicine, has freely shared his expertise in finding relevant references: Adriana Falcinelli, Medical Illustration and Photographic Services, Southampton General Hospital did many of the illustrations: Ruth Brassington of the Wellcome Tropical Resource provided illustrations and colleagues with friends, too many to number, have encouraged and advised us. Mary Sanders has been a model of patience with our piles of typescript, and Richard Barling and his team at the Cambridge University Press have shown their confidence in the book throughout. We are grateful to them all. We have had explicit permission to use for teaching the photographs of people: where this has not been given or is uncertain, the individual's eyes have been blacked out.

Part I

Health and disease

1

Progress, problems and urban change

We start this book positively. Structures and changes in health services across Africa give grounds for much hope. More doctors and nurses are being trained in their own countries, and there are numerous examples of high-quality schemes to enable better access to basic health-care. Medical schools incorporate community aspects of health care increasingly in their curricula, and include periods of work often in communities away from the teaching hospitals during undergraduate training. Many faculties now train nurses, technicians and public health workers alongside doctors. Several African medical schools have forged links with schools in industrialized countries, with great mutual benefit. Through these links, imaginative developments have benefited local populations sometimes directly, for instance, through reliable provision of drugs to rural patients with chronic conditions such as diabetes and epilepsy in the Gondar region of Ethiopia.

On a larger scale, some of the WHO's recent disease control programmes backed by funding from major donors have been outstandingly successful (Table 1.1).

Table 1.1. Achievements in health care during the past two decades

Health Service provision
Excellent primary health care in some countries
Larger numbers of dedicated skilled health workers at all levels
New groups of health workers trained for specific tasks (e.g. nurse anaesthetists)
Carefully designed relevant national health plans
Disease control
Successful immunization policies and programmes
neonatal tetanus, polio, measles (some areas)
Reduction of parasitic disease
onchocerciasis control programme
impregnated bed nets in malaria
guinea worm control programme

Threats to health

The achievements in Table 1.1 are greatly overshadowed by many adverse influences on the health of Africans at the beginning of the third millennium, some of them catastrophic in their effects. The rest of this short opening chapter deals with some of them.

The HIV pandemic

Since the publication of the second edition of this book in 1984, the picture of health across almost the whole of Africa has been changed radically by the HIV/AIDS pandemic (Buvé et al., 2002). The catastrophic spread of the HIV virus, faster in Africa than anywhere else in the world, leaves in its wake not only individual human tragedy but also huge social and economic problems. It is, so often, the wage earner who dies. Grandmothers bury their children and try to raise their grandchildren. New orphanages cannot keep up with demand. Numbers of street children increase in the towns and cities, and are beginning in some places to breed a second generation of homeless infants. Whole villages in Uganda have disappeared. A vivid illustration of the impact of HIV on health services comes from the teaching hospital in Eldoret, Kenya. Between 1990 and 1992 the two adult medical wards experienced 80 deaths annually, the mean age at death being 52. In the year 2000 there were 1200 deaths on these same wards, with a mean age at death of 38 (J.Mamlin, personal communication). Concurrently with this enormous increase in hospital mortality, there is an added and progressive erosion of manpower amongst health workers, themselves victims of the combined effects of tuberculosis and HIV. A study from Malawi in 1999 showed that 2 per cent of health workers mostly aged 35–44 died in a single year (Harries et al., 2002).

The HIV-positive rate in young woman attending antenatal clinics in 2001 was 24 per cent in Nairobi, 55 per cent in Harare, and over 60 per cent in Kwa-Zulu. At the end of 2000, there were approximately 36.1 million HIV-infected people in the world, of whom 25.3 million lived in sub-Saharan Africa (UNAIDS/WHO, 2001). In many countries there has been a sharp drop in life expectancy, typically from the upper 50s to 35–40 years.

Despite improved access to cheaper antiretroviral drugs in some parts of Africa, the size of the problem, and the inability of most sufferers to pay, means that drug treatment will hardly scratch the surface of the pandemic. With the possibility of an effective vaccine still distant, hope rests in universal and open health education on all aspects of HIV prevention. It has been calculated that, in terms of value for money, prevention is 28 times more effective than use of antiretroviral drugs at present (Marseille et al., 2002).

Unfortunately, the AIDS pandemic is not the only calamity threatening the health of Africans at the present time. Some of the threats are obvious and dramatic, others insidious and far reaching. Table 1.2 lists a selection.

Amongst these many adverse influences on health in many parts of Africa, some call for special comment. The first must be the constant drain of corruption, which sustains a deeply divided society. Extremes of affluence and dire poverty exist alongside each other in every city. Bribery is established so deeply that it is discussed openly in the media and apparently accepted by many sections of society. Sustainable economic development is difficult to achieve against this background.

The adverse effect of commodity price fixing without guarantee by affluent nations also undermines the economic development of many countries. Economies have been restructured (often with concomitant destruction of natural resources) to increase production of crops such as coffee and cocoa, but without guarantee of market or price. Throughout the last three decades, prices paid to the producers of raw coffee, tea and cocoa have fallen in real terms and the trend, if anything, accelerates. In 2002 world coffee prices fell by 40 per cent in 6 months.

Debt relief is much heralded at the time of publication of this edition, but the amount of relief remains small and the conditions for receiving it, although understandable,

Table 1.2. Threats to health in Africa, 2002 (excluding HIV)

Climatic variation and El Nino effects
Recurrent drought in central southern Africa 1995–1998 and 2001–2002
Widespread famine reported in Zambia, Zimbabwe and Malawi
Floods in Mozambique 2000
Cyclone in Madagascar 2001
Economic disadvantage
World trade barriers
National debt
Commodity price fixing, without guarantees
Plunder of fish stocks by Japanese, Polish and Spanish factory trawlers
Negative economic growth (average −1.2% for sub-Saharan Africa 1980–1991)
Declining public expenditure on health (average 1.7% GNP 1990–2000)
Subordinate position of women
Corruption and violence
Urban crime and violence increasing
Worst genocide since World War II in Rwanda 1998
Wars in Sudan, Uganda and Congo continue, with potential flash points in many countries
Arms sales continue unchecked
Tobacco advertising increasing steadily, as manufacturers are denied advertising rights in western countries
Donated drugs, vehicles, medical equipment misused
Lack of transparency and accountability
Widespread informal charges in health care
Failed medical intervention
Access to medical care inadequate, particularly for rural people
Expanded programme of immunization (EPI) not sustainable in many countries
Tuberculosis incidence increasing (Chapter 17)
Trypanosomiasis reappearing (Chapter 33)
Resistance to anti-malarials now widespread (Chapter 15)
Urbanization (see detailed section below)
Poverty
Inadequate housing
Increased accidents and violence
Increased disease prevalence
Population pressure
High fertility rates
Degradation of pasture by overgrazing
Encourages Urban migration

are restrictive and overly bureaucratic. There remains doubt that relief of debt will actually make much difference for the people who most need it.

Urbanization

Urbanization underlies much of the increasing poverty, poor living conditions, and ill health of modern Africa. Its causes and effects are therefore analysed in some detail.

The movement of people from rural to urban areas is not new. It is a process that has been going on in various parts of the world for centuries. The so-called 'Industrial Revolution' in Victorian Britain led to massive rural–urban migration, with depopulation and deskilling of the countryside, as well as the consequences of over-crowded urban squalor in towns. Urbanization in Africa has been proceeding for several decades, but in the last 10 years, the process has become more rapid, and the social and health consequences more serious and diverse. African urbanization is also now linked strongly to the adverse adoption of western lifestyles; including reduced exercise and increased body weight, tobacco and alcohol abuse and poor quality diets. Together, urbanization and westernization (sometimes referred to jokingly as 'coca-colonization'), contribute to the process of 'epidemiological transition' (Harpham, 1997).

The size and extent of the problem

In 1990 it was estimated that one-third of Africa's population lived in towns. The population has risen steadily since and is now over 50 per cent. By 2010 about two-thirds of the continent's population will be urbanized (Marsella, 1995; Stephens, 1996). There is evidence that rates of rural–urban migration in Africa are amongst the highest in the world, and the health consequences more significant (Marsella, 1995).

The reasons for urban drift

There is no single cause for rural–urban migration, and in individual cases the reasons are often multi-factorial. Some important factors are as follows:
- drought and farming failure
- low income and high aspirations
- industrialization and mining
- war and civil disturbance
- 'pull' effects from urban relatives
- desire for better education
- dissatisfaction with 'traditional' lifestyles

Some of the factors – such as aspirations for employment and enhanced living standards and education are based frequently on misconceptions or out-of-date information. Apart from the mining towns and cities of central and southern Africa, industrialization is an uncommon factor favouring urban migration – unlike in western societies (Marsella, 1995). A major issue is probably the increasing dissatisfaction with, and rejection of, traditional rural African values and lifestyles (particularly by the young). The problem may escalate, as once one young member of a family moves to the town or city, there are powerful 'pull' factors on the rest of the family (especially spouses, children and siblings).

Social effects of migration

Urban migration brings massive changes in lifestyle compared with the rural pattern. Buses and taxis are used for transport, instead of walking. Alcohol and tobacco use increases, and the quality of diet deteriorates (often with commercial 'junk-food' availability). Despite family size tending to fall, housing usually is poor and small, with consequent overcrowding. Family or traditional values and rules tend to be abandoned – the mother often will go out to work in urban areas, and the system of authority, whether within families or by village heads, disintegrates.

Standards of housing are very variable, as shown in Fig. 1.1, and it is wrong to consider all urban Africans as living in squalor. Nevertheless, the 'first-stop' for many migrants from rural areas is often a 'shanty town' (see Fig. 1.1), with no sanitation or running water, and rudimentary shelter. The highest aspirations may be to obtain a tiny semi-permanent 'matchbox', hopefully with water and electricity (Fig. 1.1).

Adverse health effects of the urban environment

There are some health advantages of urbanization. Even in the poorest urban environment, snake bite, for example, will be much less frequent than in the country. Soil-transmitted helminths tend to be encountered less frequently, and if there is piped water and adequate sanitation, water-borne infections such as typhoid and cholera are reduced in prevalence. However, as already mentioned, a very large number of urban-dwellers are in poor-quality shacks with no adequate sanitation or water supplies. Here, they are at least as prone to water-borne infective disease as in rural areas, and in addition suffer the diseases of overcrowding (e.g. tuberculosis and other respiratory infections), as well as the longer-term chronic

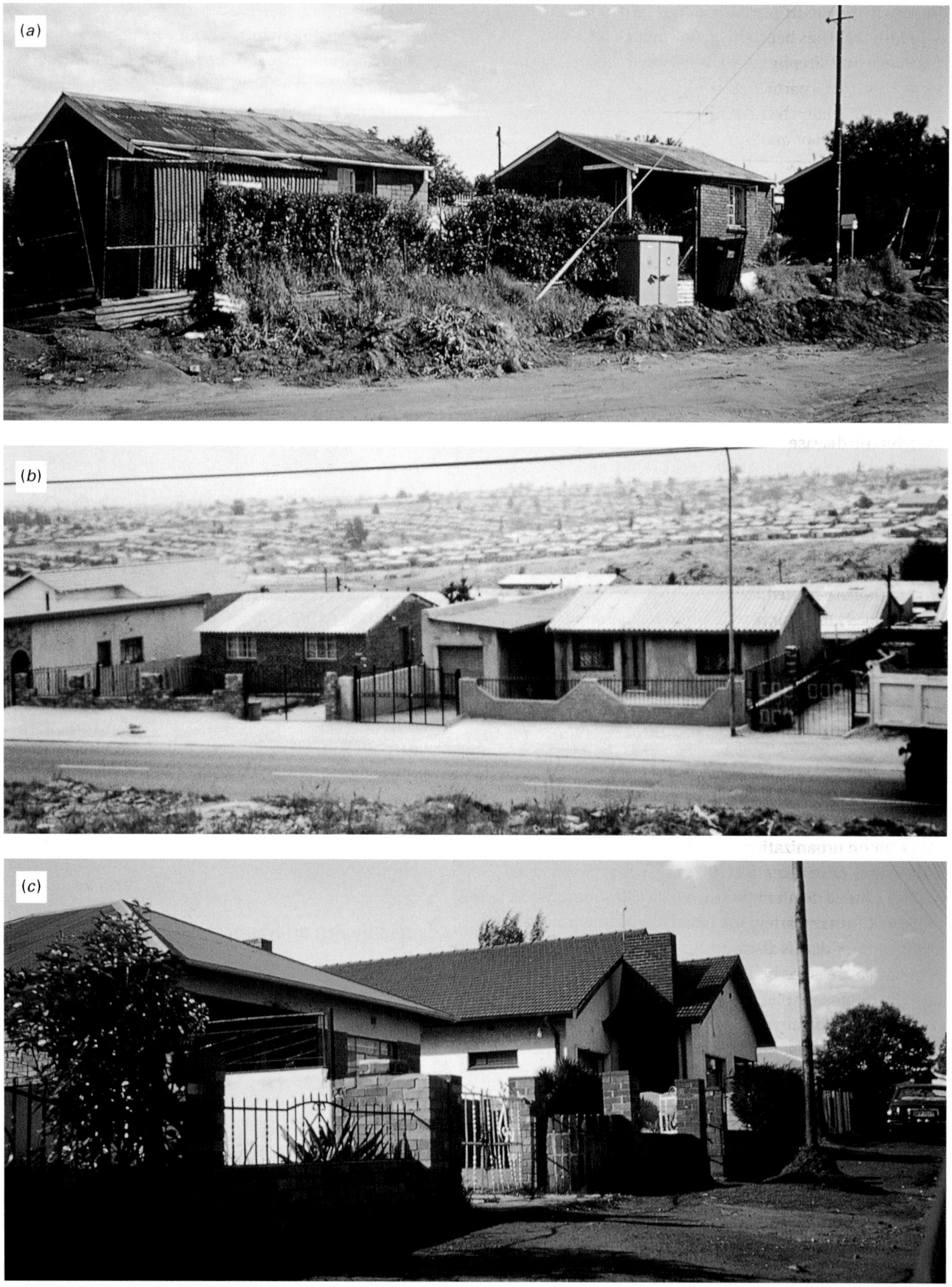
(a)
(b)
(c)

diseases of 'transition' (e.g. diabetes, hypertension, etc., see below). This has been termed the 'double-burden' of urban-dwelling (Stephens, 1996), and explains why urban mortality is high – particularly in shanty areas. A study from Accra in Ghana has shown that mortality there is five times higher in poor quality housing areas (McGranahan et al., 1999).

The range of diseases with known significantly increased prevalence in urbanized populations is diverse, with the following being an important, but not exhaustive, selection:

- respiratory infections
- chronic obstructive pulmonary disease
- obesity
- sexually transmitted disease
- burns in childhood
- road traffic accidents
- psychiatric disease
- asthma
- diabetes
- hypertension

Psychiatric disease is a rapidly increasing problem (Marsella, 1995), and traffic accidents are the leading cause of trauma-related urban hospitalization in Kenya, a situation likely to be similar throughout Africa (Odero, 1997).

The diseases of transition

Of particular concern, however, are the classical diseases of transition – the chronic non-communicable diseases (NCDs) of obesity, hypertension, diabetes and asthma. Table 1.3 shows some of the marked rises in prevalence that occur on urbanization. In the last 10 years, circulatory diseases have taken over from infective disease as the leading cause of death in urban Ghana (McGranahan et al., 1999). Coronary artery disease, until recently rare in sub-Saharan Africa, is also emerging now as a growing problem. The reasons behind the growth of NCDs in urban areas are complex and multi-factorial. They include radical dietary change, equally radical exercise reduction, and for asthma, increased allergen challenge. All will be discussed in much more detail in the specific chapters later in this book (see chapters 70, 71, 72, 75). For the moment, this brief review of the adverse health effects of urbanization has emphasized the difficulties and dangers of rural–urban migration. Sadly, it is a process which seems unlikely to be halted in the foreseeable future.

Table 1.3. Rural–urban differences in major chronic non-communicable diseases

Disease	Rural (%)	Urban (%)	Country	Reference
1. Obesity	2	30	Gambia	Prentice (2000)
2. Hypertension	18	26	Tanzania	Edwards et al. (2000)
3. Diabetes	1.7	5.9	Tanzania	Aspray et al. (2000)
4. Asthma*	13	23	Kenya	Ng'ang'a et al. (1998)

Notes:
* Childhood asthma detected by exercise challenge.

References

Aspray TJ, Mugusi F, Rashid S et al. (2000). Rural and urban differences in diabetes prevalence in Tanzania: the role of obesity, physical inactivity and urban living. *Trans Roy Soc Trop Med Hyg*; **94**: 537–644.

Buvé A, Bishikwabo-Nsaharza K, Mutangadura G. (2000). The spread and effect of HIV-1 infection in sub-Saharan Africa. *Lancet*; **359**: 2011–2017.

Edwards R, Unwin N, Mugusi F et al. (2000). Hypertension prevalence and care in an urban and rural area of Tanzania. *J Hypertens*; **18**: 145–152.

Harpham T. (1997). Urbanisation and health in transition. *Lancet*; **349**: sm11–14.

Harries AD, Hargreaves NJ, Gausi F et al. (2002). Preventing tuberculosis among health workers in Malawi. *Bull Wld Hlth Org*; **80**: 526–531.

McGranaham G, Lewin S, Fransen T et al. (1999). *Environmental Change and Human Health in Countries of Africa, the Caribbean and the Pacific*. Stockholm, Sweden: Environmental Institute.

Marseille E, Hofmann PB, Kahn JG. (2002). HIV prevention before HAART in sub-Saharan Africa. *Lancet*; **359**: 1851–1856.

Marsella AJ. (1995). Urbanisation, mental health and psychosocial well-being: some historical perspectives and considerations. In *Urbanisation and Mental Health in Developing Countries*, eds T. Harpham & I. Blue. Aldershot, UK: Publ Avebury.

Fig. 1.1. Three very different types of housing from Soweto, arguably the archetypal African township. (*a*) At the lower end of the scale is a peripheral 'shanty'; (*b*) in the mid-range is a standard 'Soweto matchbox' – permanent but tiny; (*c*) 'Millionaire's Row' where the successful businessmen and politicians live.

Ng'ang'a LW, Odhiambo JA, Mungai MW et al. (1998). Prevalence of exercise induced bronchospasm in Kenyan school children: an urban–rural comparison. *Thorax*; **53**: 919–926.

Odero W. (1997). Kenya: road traffic accidents. *Lancet*; **349**: sm13.

Prentice AM. (2000). Urban obesity in the Gambia. *Obes Pract*; **2**: 2–5.

Stephens C. (1996). Urbanisation: the implications for health. *Africa Hlth*; **18**: 14–15.

UNAIDS/WHO. (2001). AIDS epidemic update. UNAIDS/01.74E – WHO/CDS/CSR/NCS/2001.2 Geneva: UNAIDS/WHO.

People and their environment

2

A good clinical history includes information about a patient's home and life, work, culture and much else. Such information, which is supremely important in clinical practice in Africa today, is the basis of this chapter. It can therefore be used to guide clinical method so that the many factors that influence the cause and evolution of disease, and which affect the response of patients to their illness, are not forgotten. The approach to the patient is framed by four questions.

Why should this patient	WHO?
from this place	WHERE?
present in this way	HOW?
at this time?	WHEN?

Why should this patient . . . ?

The family – man, woman and children

When you see a patient, a man, a woman, or a child, ask yourself whether the symptoms, the patient's approach to their disease, and the effects of their disease on their home and family are distinctive just because it is a man, or just because it is a woman or a child who is ill. If your patient is a less-educated woman, both her lack of education and the fact that she is a woman could have delayed her seeking medical help (Needham & Foster, 2001).

Will the children be deprived of, for example, extra clothes if the woman is unable, on account of illness, to make a little money through petty trading?

Will the family be impoverished if the man is sick?

Will the mother have to stay at home and so lose this precious spending money if the child is sick? Some poor village families in the eastern states of Nigeria, who have at least one child with sickle cell disease, are further impoverished by the children's repeated sickle cell crises. Mother has to be at home and cannot trade, and father and mother together use any spare cash for clinical care and medicines (C. Nwokolo, 2001, personal communication). In Togo, whole families are distressed by having a sickle cell child (Assimadi et al., 2000).

- Consider the effects on the rest of the family if one member is sick.

Orphans

In this era of AIDS, the children of some families who have lost father, mother, uncles and aunts, may depend, with the other family orphans, on an old grandmother and may be deprived severely. AIDS has left many children as orphans. They present great problems now and their lack of mother and father may bring added and different problems as they grow into adulthood.

- If your patient is an AIDS orphan, mobilize whatever support you can for the patient and the family (Dabis et al., 2002).

Old people

Although the catastrophe of AIDS has cut the life expectancy sharply in Africa, so that the years gained through better health care and economic progress largely have been lost for the population as a whole, the already older population, uninfected by HIV, will provide a larger proportion of older people in the years ahead. The study of the health of older people in Africa is just beginning, and there is much to learn if health services are to adapt to meet the needs of these traditionally respected and valued members of the community.

People at home

When there is no piped water, when the nearest all weather road is some hours' walk away and when evening light is given by small tin lamps with a kerosene wick, it is hard for any family to be able to provide an environment which promotes health. Habits may be so entrenched that they are not easy to change. While education of mothers is often a powerful factor in keeping a family healthy, their environment may dominate their ability to change. In a semi-arid area of Tanzania, a programme was designed with the community to get children's faces washed: clean faces increased only from 9 per cent to 33 per cent (Lynch et al., 1994). Clean faces were more common significantly in those who had less than a 2-hour round trip to get water and in those with a metal roof to their house.

- Find out how your patient lives before you give advice about practices to promote health at home.

Poverty

There is plenty of evidence from all over the world that poverty is bad for health: poor farming families are particularly vulnerable. The poor are disadvantaged throughout Africa:

- unable to find the costs of travel and lodging;
- unable to pay registration or card fees at a hospital;
- unable to pay for prescribed treatment;
- unable to find money for supplemental feeding;
- unable to buy food when stocks are low in the hungry season;
- unable to improve a simple home.

The list of disadvantages is very long. Thus, for example, poverty can be desperately serious for nutrition: in the hungry season in an Ethiopian community the stocks of food of the poor were 6.5 times smaller than those of better-off families (Pastore et al., 1993) (Fig. 2.1).

Nevertheless, poor but healthy families can break out of poverty quicker than unhealthy ones, and their resilience and fortitude in adversity frequently is an example for all.

- Healthcare staff should take the lead in every effort to relieve poverty and to find ways to make all necessary services available to the poor.

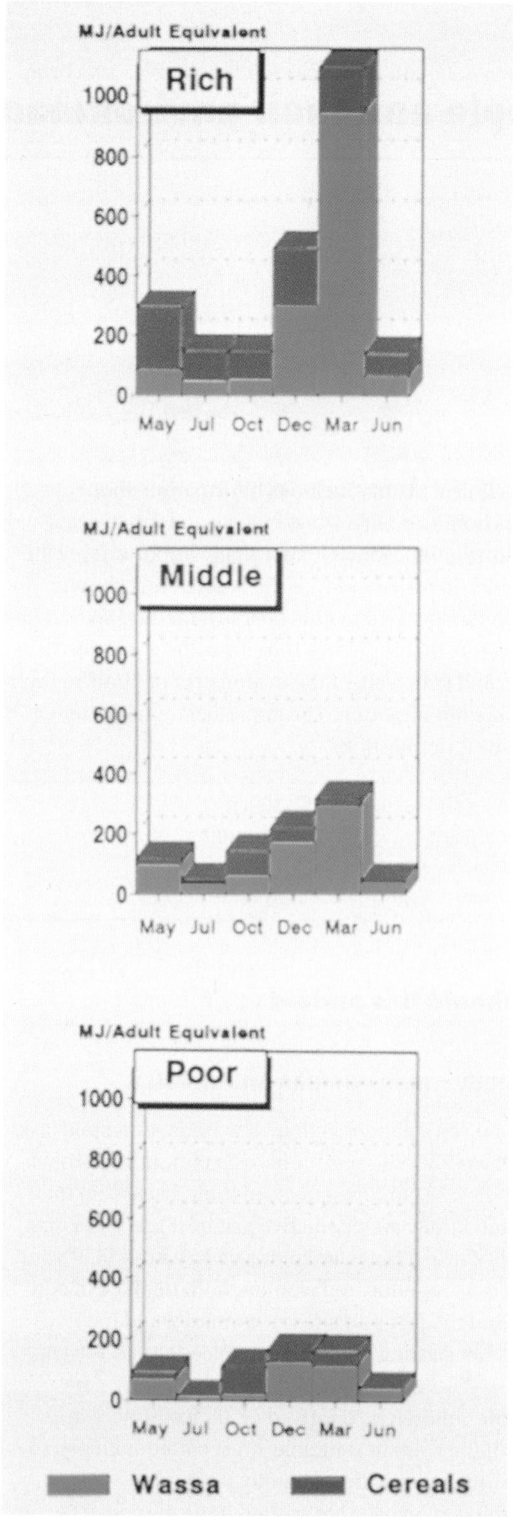

Fig. 2.1. Household energy stocks at different seasons in rich, middle income and poor families. (Adapted with permission from Pastore et al., 1993.)

Customs, culture, health and disease

Although more and more people are on the move to the towns, although the transistor radio is everywhere, and although travel by road and international aid have transformed some formerly remote places, throughout Africa cultural traditions continue to shape people's beliefs about the causes and significance of disease, how they respond to illness in themselves or in the family, and what remedies, practices or foods they will resort to in order to regain health.

In many places an adversary may be thought to be responsible for an illness, in other circumstances a malign spiritual force may be held responsible, while sometimes the individuals themselves are thought, rightly or wrongly, to have brought the illness on themselves. In each instance the remedy and the action will differ according to the local beliefs and practices.

- Whatever your role in the health team, get to grips with the local culture: do not dismiss ways in which it does not promote health, but rather try to understand them and then seek change.

Cultural beliefs and practices

While cultural beliefs and practices are at their most distinct in rural communities, they are beginning to lose their hold on those who have moved to cities and so are confronted by a bewildering array of ideas, advertisements, education and opportunities for health care. Some conditions carry a deep stigma, for example AIDS, leprosy with its depigmented patches and thus vitiligo, or any patch of depigmented skin, and of course epilepsy.

Example – Epilepsy (Chapter 74)

In diverse cultures all over Africa a profound and isolating stigma defines the individual who has had a seizure. This is not helped in those countries where the psychiatric service is also responsible for the care of epilepsy. The result is that the individual may have few opportunities for employment, may find it difficult to be accepted as a normal person and may even become an outcast (Billington,1968).

- Do all you can to educate and to change the attitudes of the community and of your patient's family about any disease that carries a social stigma.
- Do not consider treatment alone to be adequate, but work with the health team, through the community leaders, to rehabilitate and to find useful work for any patient with disease that carries a stigma.

Practices derived from beliefs

Strongly held beliefs about the cause of disease lead to carefully preserved practices, some of which may be harmful: an obvious example is mud applied to the umbilical stump, which can lead to neonatal tetanus. Some practices, however, may be beneficial.

- Identify the practices in your area that are harmful, or which delay recovery, and work with the health team to start to change them. Make this work continuous because ancient beliefs will not be changed quickly.

Example – Peripartum cardiac failure (PPCF) (Chapter 76, p. 866)

Traditional beliefs among Hausa women in northern Nigeria lead them to heat the body in the puerperium (Fig. 2.2) to protect them from *sanyi* (cold), which is thought to

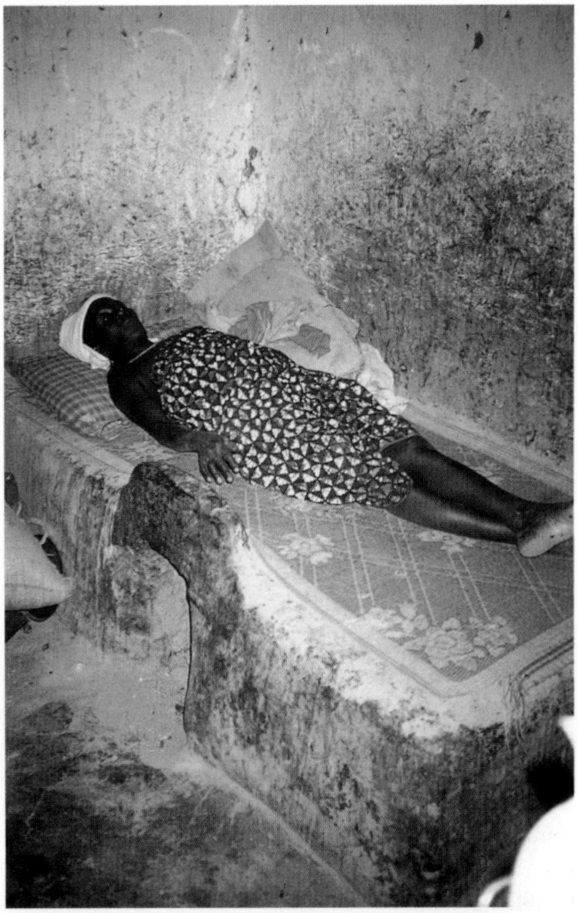

Fig. 2.2. A mother lying on a hot bed in her home, a traditional practice of women around Zaria, Nigeria: note the fire under the bed (copyright EHO Parry).

be responsible for disease. These mothers also take an excess of a sodium-rich rock salt (*kanwa*) to promote the flow of breast milk. Their habits contribute to the pathogenesis of this remarkable syndrome, but, despite orthodox clinical care and advice, most of the mothers who have had PPCF hold their traditional beliefs so deeply that they teach them to their daughters (Ford et al., 1998).

Practices to prevent disease

This example of PPCF shows how much people are prepared to do in order to prevent disease, based on what they think its cause to be.

Practices for the treatment of disease

These practices may involve a traditional practitioner or may be used in the home by the family of the sick person. Such home-prepared remedies may have significant toxic effects, which are as widely different as the remedies themselves, whether it be the excessive purgation of *Kosso* (Ethiopian highlands), the hepatic or renal damage caused by some traditional remedies, or the uterine rupture caused by a Kenyan plant which has oxytoxic properties. There may be distinctive habits in cooking or in use of food, for example, in the diluting of a cereal pap for a sick child, so that the child is deprived of essential energy from the pap.

- Define the traditional remedies used in your area: be alert to their possible toxic effects.

Health-seeking behaviour, traditional and orthodox medical practice

In many places those who are ill first consult a traditional practitioner and then wait for the given remedies to be effective. This can delay diagnosis and treatment critically, whether in rural Kenya (Scott et al., 2000) or in urban Zambia (Needham et al., 2001).

When user charges were introduced in Uganda, the health centres could use money taken in charges to buy, for example, drugs, dressings and the services of a cleaner. Few went to traditional healers because they received a good service from the health centres and were charged fairly for it. Then user fees were abolished. The health centres had no cash flow, their service became worse and worse, fewer people attended them, and more returned to traditional care, which they thought would be better.

Traditional healer

The work of the traditional healer is described in relation to mental health in Chapter 88 and to cancer in Chapter 90. In Burkina Faso, the Expanded Programme of Immunization (EPI) was understood and welcomed because the methods used were so similar to those that had been used by the traditional healers – a little scarification with some of the healing 'medicine' applied at the same place (Samuelsen, 2001).

Treatment – acceptable or not?

Amputation can be considered a desperate measure, which is feared because it destroys a person's identity: it can thus be rejected even when it is essential. Similarly, caesarean section is not considered by some west African women as normal and so is refused (Dumont et al., 2001; Okonofua, 2001). Unacceptable side effects of drugs often deter people from sticking to a prescribed course of treatment. Beliefs within a culture and experience through an illness may make forms of treatment, normal and routine in orthodox medicine, strange and unacceptable.

- Listen to your patients, find out what they feel, be sensitive to their culture and do not embark on any treatment that they will not accept.

Treatment – but for how long?

Many people cannot understand the need for taking drugs regularly. They often think that they are well as soon as their urgent symptoms are over, for example, the acute pain of a sickle cell crisis, or the need for prolonged treatment in tuberculosis. Some will give away drugs to another member of the family who is sick, or sell them in a market, or take them all at once. Since much traditional medicine involves a single dose, the continued treatment demanded by 'modern' medicine is hard to understand.

- Take time to explain to your patients the reason for long-term treatment and encourage them when they are seen at a follow-up clinic or in the home.

Treatment that causes local pain

Scarifications at the site of pain or of an obvious mass or pulsation, for example, over the pulmonary artery in children with early severe rheumatic heart disease, are common and often important to the family. If the scarring is old and healed, it shows that the symptoms are not recent. Scarification may also be responsible for transmission of hepatitis B and C viruses.

The widespread demand for a painful injection may depend on the belief that powerful treatment is expected to cause pain. Far too many unnecessary injections are given: these waste resources and allow the demand for injections to go unchecked.

- Educate your community and all the members of the health team about the use and the need for injections, and do not give them unnecessarily.

The perceived burden of disease

It may be all too easy to look at a man's hydrocoele in northern Ghana and advise him to have an operation, and yet he needs reassurance as much as surgery because the cultural burden of the deformity caused by the hydrocoele is considerable (Gyapong et al., 2000), as is that of the swellings of the legs due to filariasis in coastal Kenya (Amuyunzu, 1997). For young men in the highlands of Ethiopia, marriage is their most significant social achievement, but for those with spastic legs and uncertain gait due to lathyrism, the prospects of marriage were shattered, while many others were divorced (Getahun et al., 1998).

- When a patient presents with advanced or deforming disease, think beyond the advanced physical signs and try to find out his fears and worries and how he is coping in the community.

Work, employment and occupations

The people of tropical and subtropical Africa are still overwhelmingly rural, but the supposed opportunities for urban employment and the imagined riches of the city are causing a steady flow of people off the land and into the overcrowded cities. The diseases of the farmer and of the agricultural community still inhibit rural prosperity: these are considered below.

Hazards of employment and of industrial work

The growth of industry has not been matched by measures to protect the health of industrial workers, particularly in small-scale industry and in the informal business sector in many countries.

- Lead poisoning is a potential hazard and can lead to anaemia, which was found in 48 per cent of lead smelters and 12.5 per cent of petrol pump attendants, but surprisingly not in informal workers with cars in Accra (Ankrah et al., 1996).
- Industrial lung disease in South Africa has been shown to be a serious problem by the national Surveillance of Work-related and Occupational Respiratory Diseases in South Africa – SORDSA (Esterhuizen et al., 2001a): pneumoconiosis and other dust-related diseases are still a major health problem (Table 77.1): silicosis is increasing (Murray et al., 1996) and is a significant risk factor for tuberculosis in HIV-positive and HIV-negative men (Corbett et al., 2000). Many workers are being exposed excessively, chiefly in the paper and pulp industry, health care, and the chemical and food industries, to substances which have clinical effects after a short latent period. For example, isocyanates in spray paints and latex were found important in provoking occupational asthma (Esterhuizen et al., 2001b).
- Workers on big commercial farms are always vulnerable. In South Africa, they can be seriously undernourished, have a high rate of alcoholism and of head injury (London et al., 1998), while in Ethiopia chronic non-blinding onchocerciasis on a large coffee plantation led to absenteeism (Workneh et al., 1993).

Hazards and traditional occupations

Traditional methods in a wide variety of occupations may lead to significant symptoms and morbidity. For example, men and women in coastal Nigeria who dried their fish catches by burning firewood had defective lung function and many respiratory symptoms (Peters et al., 1999), and grindstone cutters north of Kano, Nigeria, who worked in small funnels in the ground, were exposed continuously to dust rich in silica particles. Nearly 40 per cent were found to have silicosis (Warrell et al., 1975) (Fig. 2.3).

- Take a careful history about a man's or a woman's work and, if there is a curious clinical picture, consider whether this may be due to occupational exposure to a toxic substance.

The vulnerable subsistence farmer

Injury and disease in a subsistence farmer and the subsequent incapacity can be disastrous, because the poorest may have no alternative source of income (Oladepo et al., 1997). If the incapacity is at a season when farming activity is high, the economic effects on the farmer may be even more disastrous (Fig. 2.4).

1. *Bites* Snake bite. The carpet viper, *Echis ocellatus*, is a particular scourge in the savannah, as it bites farmers just as they prepare the land for planting (Fig. 2.5).
2. *Injuries* can prevent effective farming (Fig. 2.6): for example, in the Ashanti Region of Ghana, machete wounds are important. Where injuries are common, find out why and then plan a programme to prevent them.

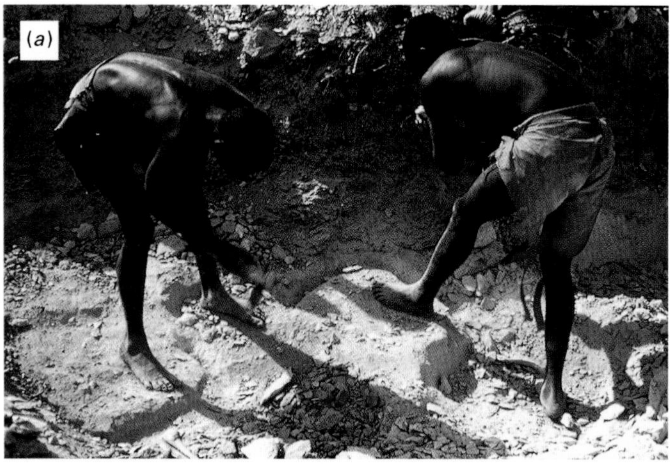

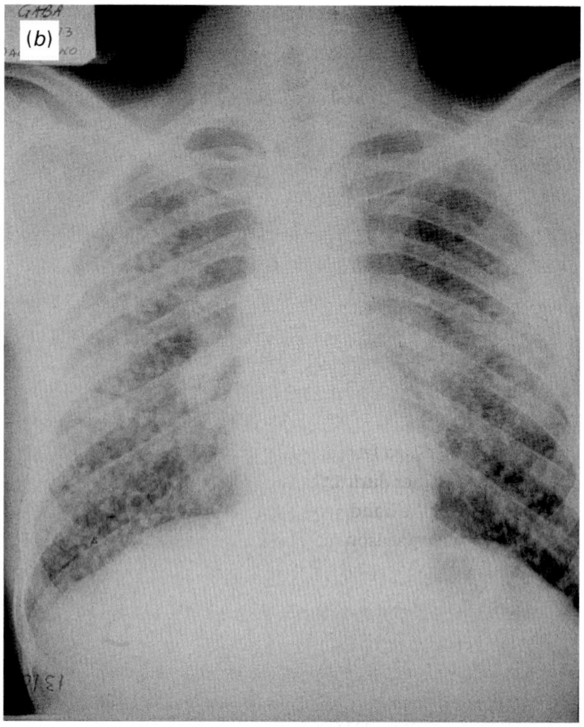

Fig. 2.3. (*a*) Cutting grinding stones in northern Nigeria. (*b*) Chest radiograph of a stone cutter to show military mottling of silicosis.

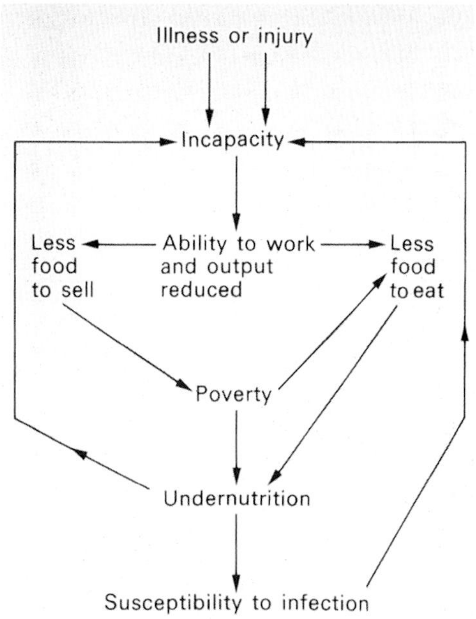

Fig. 2.4. The cycle of injury and poverty in a rural family when the farmer is ill or injured.

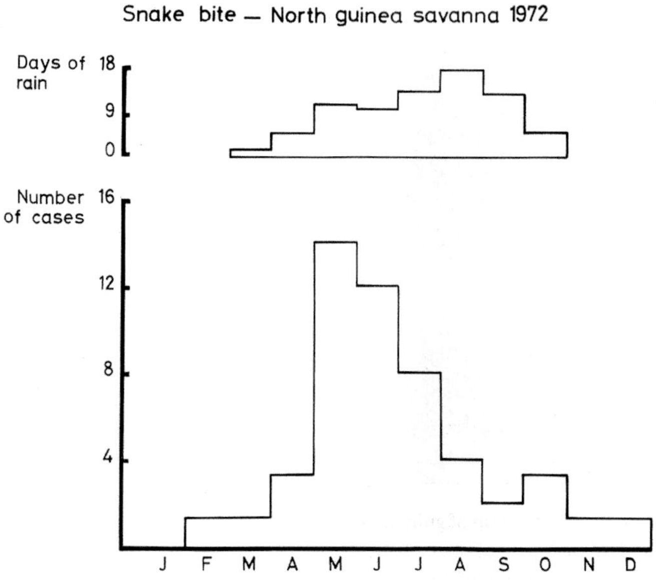

Fig. 2.5. The vulnerable farmer: snake bite in the guinea savannah of Nigeria when farming activity is high. (Adapted from Warrell et al., 1976.)

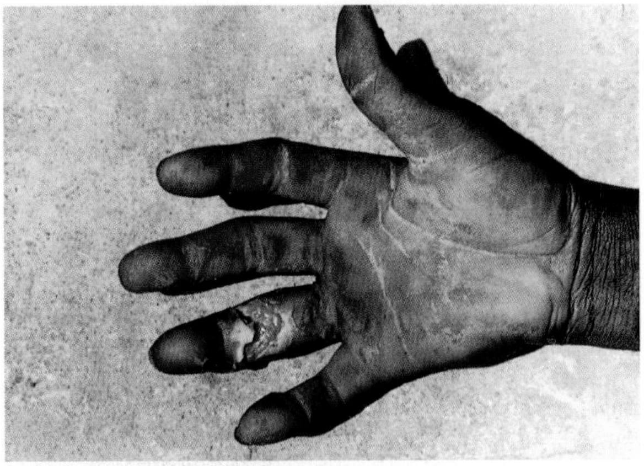

Fig. 2.6. The disabled farmer: soft tissue injuries like this can be crippling to a farmer during the rainy season: note the very thick cornified skin of the hand, which can crack when the humidity falls during the dry season (copyright EHO Parry).

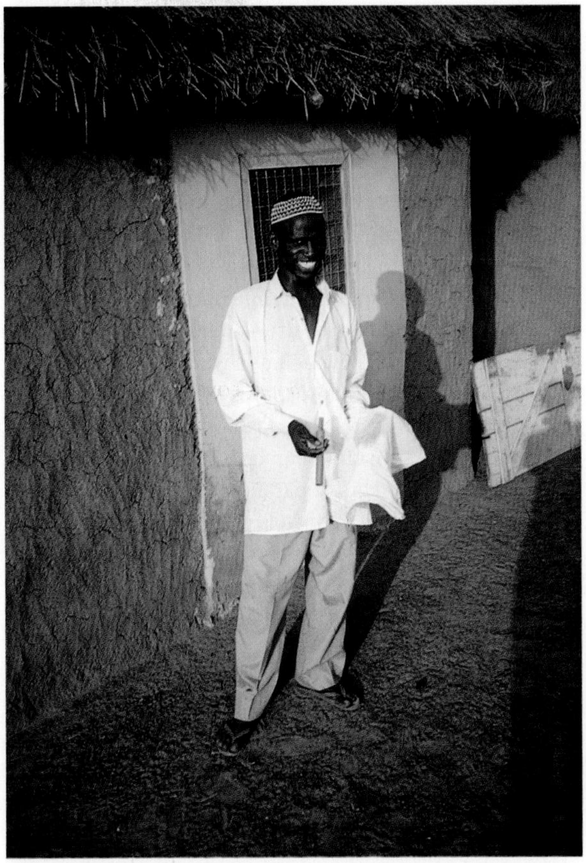

Fig. 2.8. Prevention of guinea worm: a health worker in the Northern Region of Ghana holds a micropore filter cloth for stored water in his left hand and a small tube with its own micropore filter. This can be used for sucking up standing surface water without fear of swallowing *Cyclops* (copyright EHO Parry).

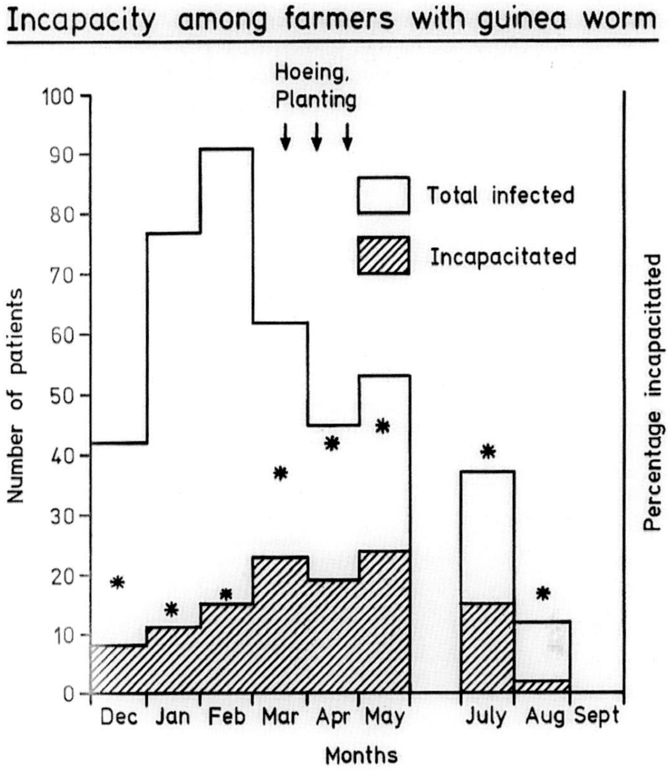

Fig. 2.7. Guinea worm: incapacity in a village. (Asterisks indicate percentage incapacitated.)

A small injury can become infected and lead to a tropical ulcer if it is not cleaned and dressed early.

3. *Infections* Guinea worm: before the eradication campaign (Fig. 2.7), and in areas where it is still prevalent, guinea worm can devastate agricultural output, (Adewale et al., 1997). This can reduce the family's income so that the children become malnourished (Tayeh & Cairncross, 1996) (Fig. 2.8).
4. *Nutrition* When food is short in the hungry season, farmers have a significant energy deficit: the poorest and their children have the greatest changes of weight and so are potentially most vulnerable (Pastore et al., 1993) (Fig. 2.9).
5. *Poisoning* Careless or untutored use of organophosphate fertilizers is an increasing risk, as farmers struggle to increase the yield of their crops. This is also a risk to their children, who may accidentally swallow the fertilizer.
6. *Hidden disability* Farmers in the rain forest or derived savannah who have dermal onchocerciasis may be disabled and may sleep badly as a result of their unforgiving itch, which can affect up to 40 per cent of people over the age of 20 (Murdoch et al., 2002).

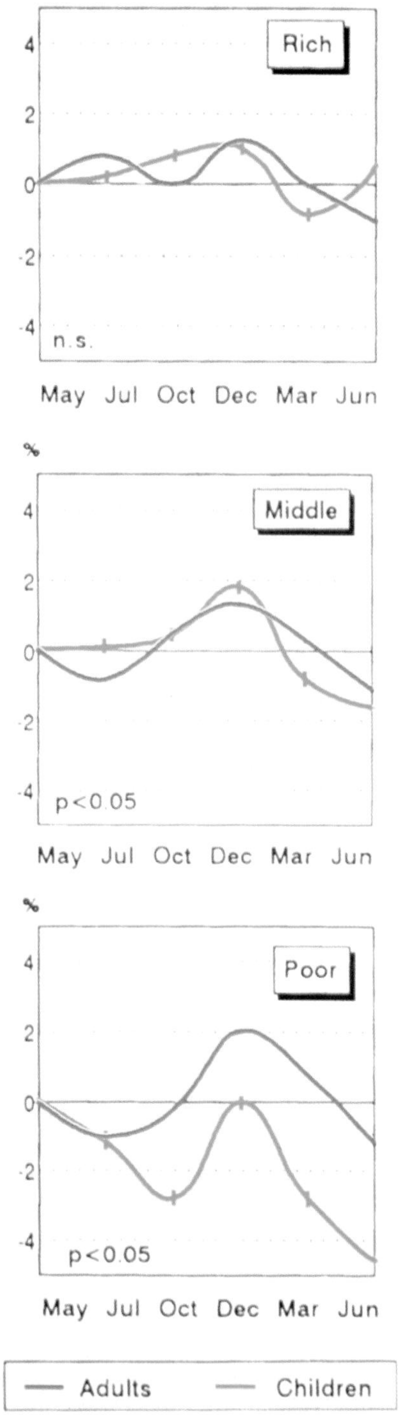

Fig. 2.9. The effect of poverty on weight change in children and adults of a southern Ethiopian farming community; the poor are particularly vulnerable in the hungry season. Note severe hungry season in second year due to previous year's poor harvest. (Adapted from Pastore et al., 1993.)

A fit farmer, who is not disabled, can contribute to the family's needs, therefore:

- Identify the common causes of incapacity and disability among the farmers, male and female, in your area, and find methods to reduce them and their impact.
- Study any possible seasonal changes in disability and disease. The Box considers injuries to farmers.

Injuries to the farmer

Study the problem and use the results for prevention. Find answers, at least, to these questions –

1. the time of day the injuries occur
2. the season of the year when they are most prevalent
3. whether the injuries are related to hunger or fatigue
4. whether the injuries are associated with any particular activity
5. the tool or other cause of the injury
6. the immediate treatment given
7. the days of work lost.

Habits

Alcohol

Every society has its customs or its prohibitions about the use of alcohol (Saungweme et al., 1999). At least 50 per cent of the sorghum crop may be used for a traditional brew; the matoke staple of Uganda provides a potent distilled *waragi*, which may be drunk relentlessly by village men so that they are incapacitated wholly some time after midday. The welfare and prosperity of the community is at risk if alcohol is used in this fashion.

Alcoholic excess in cities can be just as bad, particularly among migrant workers, separated from their families and perhaps confined in hostels or in crowded rented rooms. Drinking bouts on a Friday night are followed commonly by violence and trauma. Another hazard is a lung abscess because the victim aspirates vomit.

- Learn how alcohol is used in your area, and work with the district health team and the community if it is a significant problem.
- Is alcohol given to workers as a reward?
- When taking a history, be ready to probe to find out the volume the individual drinks: the heavy drinker rarely admits the true volume.

Tobacco and smoking

While tobacco is an important export crop from central Africa, it is promoted unashamedly by the international tobacco giants, who care nothing for the health of those to whom they seek to sell their cigarettes. They know full well that this wretched catalyst of ill health and disease will reap its fearful harvest of preventable disease, and yet they continue to advertise more and more in Africa.

- Promote campaigns to enable people to stop smoking and to ban advertisements for cigarettes.

Drugs and the use of khat (Cha'at)

Hard drugs spare no continent, but they do not yet have the hold in Africa that they do in some industrialized countries. In the Horn of Africa, however, the green leaves of khat (*Catha edulis*), which contain cathinone, are widely used, chiefly but not exclusively among younger men. Khat is addictive, has amphetamine-like stimulant properties, raises systolic and diastolic blood pressures and can cause serious psychosis. These effects can incapacitate men for meaningful work before the afternoon (Widler et al., 1994; Belew et al., 2000).

Why should this patient *from this place . . .* ?

Home and shelter

The quality of the home is very important but, equally important, the access to health care from the home. Housing, access, poverty, education – these are all interwoven, but there are particular problems associated with poor housing.

Quality of housing

Poor housing can promote the transmission of disease, and makes people potentially vulnerable to a range of diseases, for example, childhood malaria (Koram et al., 1995). If housing can be improved, as was pioneered in a programme among poor rural people in northern Malawi, the burden of disease among children under 5 can be significantly reduced (Wolff et al., 2001).

The numerous disadvantages include:

- overcrowding, which favours the aerosol spread of meningococci and streptococci, or, for example, the spread of the body louse, and thus of typhus, relapsing fever and trench fever;
- a large household can be a risk factor for injury (personal unpublished data) and for childhood mortality (Schellenberg et al., 2001);
- the absence of an adequate pit latrine, so that an unprotected well can be contaminated easily by organisms such as *V.cholerae*. But solar disinfection of drinking water, even in a difficult environment, can reduce childhood diarrhoea and morbidity significantly (Conroy et al., 1996);
- the absence of a constant supply of water, so that washing of clothes, of the body and of the face is limited, so that impetigo and pyogenic skin infections can flourish;
- the transmission of zoonoses in homes where animals are brought inside overnight;
- the inevitable hazard of burns from an unprotected fire under the cooking pot, whether from the fire or a boiling pot. Small children and those who have seizures, both of whom can upset the pot so easily, are at particular risk;
- inner-city children, crowded together in homes in a bad state of repair, whose parents are poor and poorly educated, have been found in Nigeria and South Africa to have raised blood lead levels, high enough to call for action (von Schirnding et al., 1991);
- a woman who cooks for the family inside the hut, and who thus is exposed constantly to smoke, can develop chronic bronchitis and even, less commonly, cor pulmonale.

Although better housing can protect against some of these hazards, it can have its own problems, such as the indoor use of a kerosene stove, which is a risk factor for asthma (Venn et al., 2001).

Action

As people who have bad housing face such a range of risks, and as they frequently have no voice:

- consider the hazards of poor housing when you plan the care of patients at home.
- be at the forefront of action to improve the way in which poorer people have to live.

Access to health care

Those who live far from a health facility are disadvantaged. Distance is bad for disease. Access may be impossible during the rains, the fare on a bus may be too great, the burden of being away from work and a means of livelihood too demanding, while the prospect of having to pay scarce and precious cash for care is altogether too much. In Kenya, among children with severe malaria, the admission rates of those who lived more than 25 km from a district hospital, were only one-fifth the rate of those living within 5 km of the hospital (Schellenberg et al., 1998).

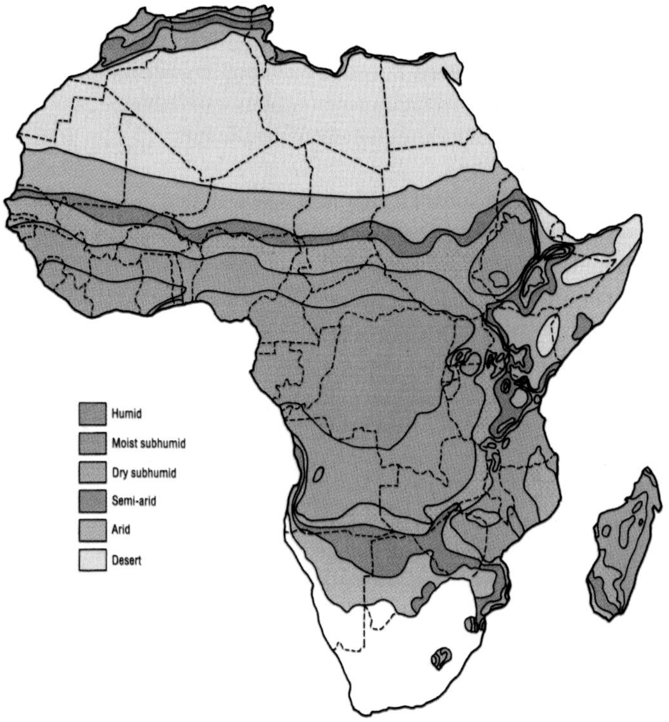

Fig. 2.10. The climatic and geographical zones of Africa. (Reproduced from *Atlas of African Agriculture*. Rome Food and Agriculture Organization, Rome, 1986, p. 46.)

Action

If long-term care is to succeed for those who live far from a hospital:

- Arrange follow-up care at their nearest health centre: train the health centre staff in this care. Wherever possible, try to enable those who travel far to recover the cost

The map of Africa

The continent of Africa has an area of 30 289 000 km^2 and an estimated population of about 650 million. Almost 80 per cent of Africa lies within the tropics (Fig. 2.10).

About 22 per cent of the people live in semi-arid grassland or savannah areas, where the rainfall is in the range 250–500 mm per year, and 42 per cent live in areas where the annual rainfall is in the range 500–1500 mm. These wetter areas include scrub and sudan savannah and much of the rain forest. Narrow coastal belts in West Africa and places in the Congo basin have a much greater rainfall. The rainfall, which is less than 250 mm in one-third of the continent and more than 1000 mm in a further third, is seasonal and changes from year to year, so that harvests may be poor, especially where the rains do not reach the required minimum (Fig. 2.11).

Water

All over Africa water, whether from rain, river or well, dominates life and profoundly determines health. People settle where there is water, but may be forced to abandon settlements if the very presence of water allows vectors to thrive and transmit the agents of diseases such as onchocerciasis and sleeping sickness.

Gastrointestinal infections can be dramatically reduced if there is clean pipe-borne water. Dirty septic skins cannot be kept clean without regular generous washing. No health outpost can be established without an adequate water supply. Whatever the area of Africa, water supply is fundamental for health and its lack or variation may affect health significantly.

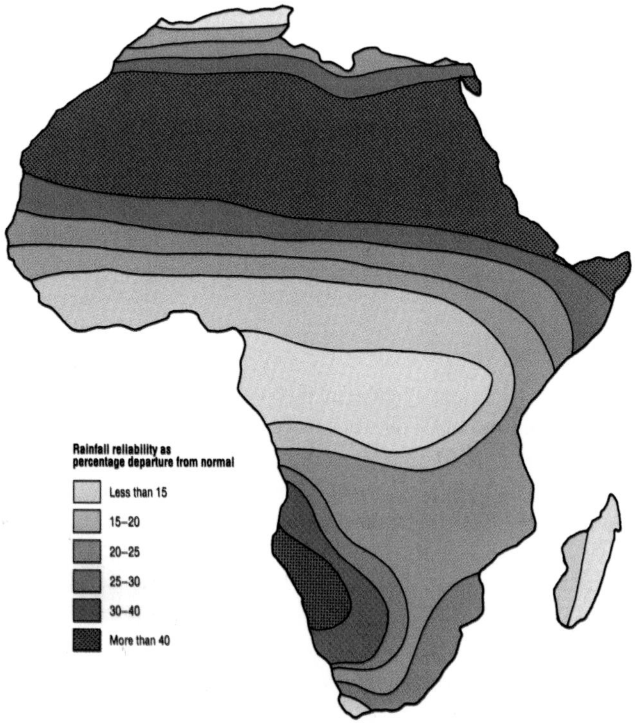

Fig. 2.11. Rainfall: its reliability in Africa and therefore the areas which are vulnerable to drought. Nearly two-thirds of the continent has a high or very high risk of drought. (Reproduced from *Atlas of African Agriculture*. Rome Food and Agriculture Organization, Rome, 1986, p. 47.)

Table 2.1. Food values of major African staples

	Amount per 100 g					
Staple	Water (ml)	Energy (J)	Carbohydrate	Fat	Protein	Remarks
Whole grains						
Wheat	13	1450	70	2.0	11.5 (8–15)	When milled to produce white flour, less fibre (1.0 mg from 2.0 mg), B vitamins and iron
Millet	11	1490	73	2.5	10.0 (6–14)	Good quality vegetable protein
Sorghum	12	1490	71	3.4	10.4 (8–14)	Calcium and iron high
Maize	12	1520	71	4.5	10.0	Tryptophan low. Vitamin B low if milled
Tef	11	1450	73	2.2	8.5	Iron 90 mg
Rice	12	1490	77	1.5	8.0	Thiamine low if milled. Iron 1–2 mg
Roots and bananas						
Cassava (fresh)	60	643	37	0.2	0.7	Protein low. Hydrocyanic acid in cuticle. Vitamin C 30 mg
Yam (fresh)	73	437	24	0.2	2.0	Water high, protein low. Vitamin C adequate (10 mg)
Potato Irish	80	315	17	–	2.0	Vitamin C 20 mg
Sweet	70	479	26	0.3	1.5	Vitamin C 30 mg
Plaintain (matoke)	67	538	31	0.2	1.0	Vitamin C high (30 mg)
Bread						
White bread	37.3 g	1002 (235 kcal)	49.3	1.9	8.4	Fibre (Southgate method) 3.8 g

Source: Adapted, with permission, from: Platt BS (1975) and Latham MC (1965).

Geographical regions

In general, the food zones follow the geographic zones of Africa, on account of the restriction of soils and climate, or as a result of local conditions and customs. Cultivation of their staple food, to provide the essential energy for daily needs, is the first agricultural task of rural and subsistence people. The composition of major traditional staples is shown in Table 2.1, where it includes the new staple of white bread, which is marketed and eaten so widely now.

All over the continent, among poorer people, festivals and celebrations are immensely important culturally and it is at these that more expensive foods are eaten: culture rather than need determines diet at such times (Table 2.2).

Mediterranean zone

Durum wheat and bread wheat are the staples of Egypt, Algeria, Tunisia and Morocco. In the rest of Africa, apart from South Africa, the crop is only grown in small areas usually under irrigation, but bread wheat, which has to be imported, is now being eaten more and more throughout Africa, and in some places bread has become a cheap staple during the 'hungry season'.

The grain is milled into a flour and in the process much of the outer coat and germ is lost. White flour, which can be stored better and is more popular, contains fewer vitamins of the B group and micronutrients, and less protein and fibre, than brown flour (Table 2.1).

Savannah

The savannah occupies over one-third of the area of Africa, over 40 per cent of the African tropics, and is the home for about 60 per cent of the population. The climate of the savannah is the typical climate of tropical Africa. In its vast areas, whether derived, guinea, or scrub savannah, temperature, rainfall, and therefore seasons change far more than in the rain forest. Since the savannah stretches from the rain forest to the desert and from highlands to the coast, its climate also varies, modified by the often very hot, dry season when water is scarce, and by altitude. People move during the slack, dry season when there is little farming (Fig.2.21), while pastoral nomads move over large areas to find pasture for their flocks and herds.

Farmers' work is highly seasonal: they harvest mainly protein-rich grains, cash crops in cotton and groundnuts, and sheanuts from their trees. For much of the year, therefore, they are far less exposed to vectors and organisms

Table 2.2. Food values of protein and other African foods

Staple	Amount per 100 g					Remarks
	Water (ml)	Energy (J)	Carbohydrate	Fat	Protein	
Animal protein						
Human milk	87	320	7	4.6	1.3	Iron low; vitamins A and B depend on mother's diet
Cow's milk	88	270	4.7	3.6	3.3	
Eggs	74	664	0.5	11.5	13	
Meat (beef)	66	848	0	14	19	Riboflavin, nicotinamide, and iron present
Chicken	73	584	–	7.0	19	
Fish (dried)	20	1300	0	6.3	63	Calcium, iron, and nicotinamide present
Vegetable protein						
Groundnut (fresh)	45	1390	12	25	15	Fat high: useful source of nicotinamide and tryptophan
Winged Bean (*psophocarpus tetragonolobus*)	14	1700	32	16	33	
Cowpea (*Vigna unguiculata*)	10	1430	60	1.5	22	Useful source of thiamine, nicotinamide, iron, and calcium
Black bean (*Lablab niger*)	8	1470	65	1.0	21	
Green leaves	91	120	4	0.3	2	Vitamin A 100 I.U./100 g, iron and calcium, vitamin C 50 mg/100 g
Palm oil	0	3780	0	100	0	Energy high. Vitamin A 200 000 I.U./100 g

Source: Adapted, with permission, from: Platt BS (1975) and Latham MC (1965).

associated with their work than forest dwellers, except where there is a local microclimate, for example, an irrigated area where *S. haematobium* is established, or woodlands where *Glossina* spp. (tsetse fly) can find shade from intense sunshine.

Water is scarce and is drawn from wells or dams, or from pools when there is rain. Hookworm infection is less common and severe than it is in the forest because the soil gets so dry that the larvae cannot survive.

The savannah is the great cereal-producing area of Africa. Grains are a concentrated food containing much less water than root crops. They are easier to store and transport and also have greater commercial possibilities. Millet, sorghum, and maize are the main cereals (Figs. 2.12, 2.13).

Millet

There are two main species of millet:

1. the west African sahel Pearl Millet (*Pennisetum* spp.), which is well suited to the dry parts of the savannah because it has a short growing season: it is grown over 14 m hectares (Fig. 2.12)
2. the east and central African variety Finger Millet (*Eleusine caracana*), which probably originated in the highlands of Ethiopia and Uganda, where it has been grown for thousands of years and was, in times of famine, priceless because its grains can be stored for years without damage from insects. But it demands intense labour for weeding, handling the harvest and in processing the grain.

Sorghum (*Sorghum bicolor*)

Widely known as guinea corn, sorghum has a longer growing season and can be grown in less arid areas than millet, over 18 m hectares in Africa. Storage in mud containers is quite efficient and losses due to fungal contaminants and insects are lower in drier savannah areas.

Although sorghum and millet have a low yield per hectare compared with the other staples, they are still the major staple of Africa, providing a valuable food, which has an adequate and well-balanced protein content and a high iron and calcium content (Table 2.1 and Fig. 2.13). The grain is ground roughly, so that few nutrients are lost, and is eaten as a ball (Hausa *fura,* millet) or paste (*tuwon dawa,* sorghum) with a sauce of groundnuts, oils, and vegetables. In non-Muslim areas part of the crop may be fermented to produce beer: sometimes as much as 50 per cent is used in this way.

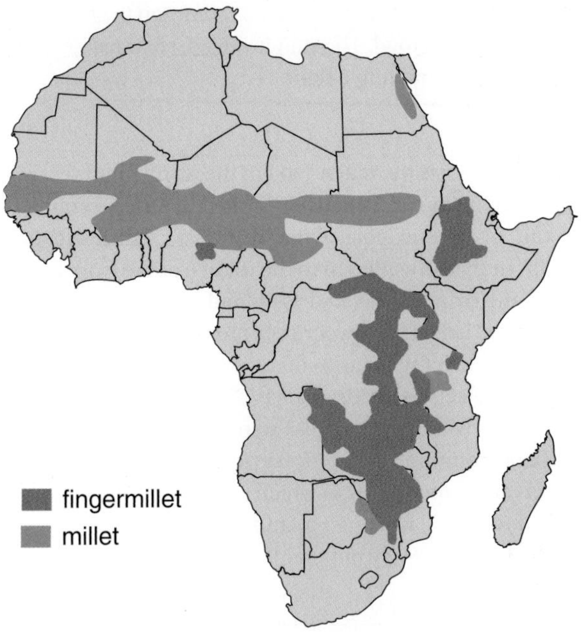

Fig. 2.12. Millet in Africa: Finger millet (brown) is dominantly distributed in a north south belt in the east, while Pearl millet (orange) is in a band across the west African savannah and sahel. (Adapted from Board on Science and Technology, *Lost Crops of Africa*, Vol 1, *Grains*. Washington, National Academy Press, 1996, pp. 42, 80.)

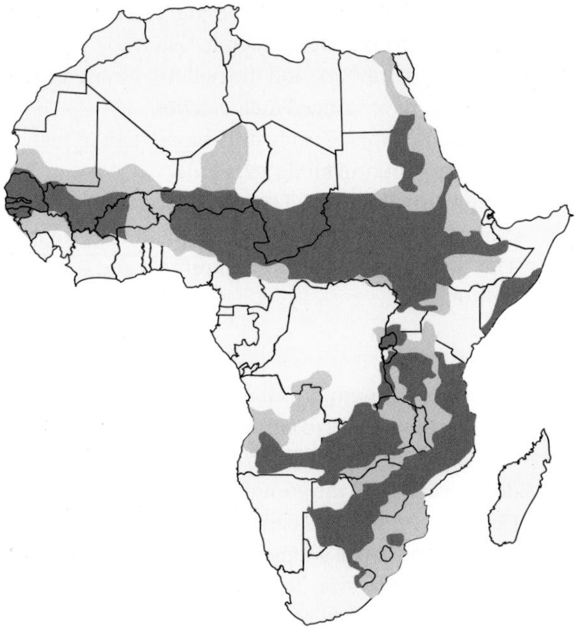

Fig. 2.13. Sorghum in Africa. (Adapted from Board on Science and Technology, *Lost Crops of Africa*, Vol 1, *Grains*. Washington, National Academy Press, 1996, p. 131.)

Those who live in the millet and sorghum zone have adequate protein in the food, and kwashiorkor is less common than in the forest areas where roots are the staples. In the savannah there may be significant seasonal shortages of food (Fig. 2.23).

Maize

This is the staple of the savannah of East Africa and most of southern Africa. It is also grown in areas of derived savannah. As a food, it is limited by the composition of its main protein, zein, which contains only small amounts of the essential amino acids lysine and tryptophan (Table 2.1). Deficiency of this amino acid, combined with a relative shortage of nicotinic acid, leads to pellagra. The area under maize is increasing: it gives a high yield per hectare, grows in warm, fairly dry, areas, matures rapidly, and is resistant to damage by birds. If the new breeds, containing higher amounts of lysine and tryptophan, are successful, the crop will have great potential.

Food is prepared by grinding the grain and cooking it into a stiff paste, which is eaten with a sauce. Unfortunately, the use of highly milled maize meal, deficient in protein and B vitamins, is becoming increasingly popular, so that the peri-urban migrant and the poor may be at risk of pellagra. As with millet and sorghum, much of the crop may be used to produce maize beer.

Rainforest

Rain falls for most of the year in coastal West Africa, the Congo basin, and eastern Madagascar. The humidity is high, the mean temperature varies little, and there are no extremes of heat or cold. In the West African coastal strip the population is dense. Water is generally not scarce and is obtainable from pools, rivers and streams. Farmers work throughout the year and harvest mainly low-protein root crops, but coffee, cocoa and palm kernels are important sources of cash in some areas. Farmers are therefore continuously exposed to micro-organisms, which thrive in a hot, wet climate, e.g. hookworm, and to anopheline mosquitoes and other vectors. As few cattle are reared and root crops or plantains supplemented by maize are the staples, malnutrition is always a threat.

These crops are very efficient producers of carbohydrate but yield little protein (Table 3.6). Milk and meat production is severely limited by trypanosomiasis in cattle, and fish remains the major source of animal protein. Coastal fishermen can get much protein from their catch, but the plunder of their fish stock by European factory trawlers, and the pollution from relentless oil drilling, have savaged their catches.

As the rainfall is more evenly distributed than in the savannah, the supply of food varies little.

The staple usually is boiled into a thick paste and eaten with a sauce of palm oil, leaves, and, sometimes, groundnuts. This 'soup' is a major source of protein and micronutrients.

Cassava

This is the most economic of all tropical root crops to produce. The root is easy to cultivate and gives high yields even in unproductive soils. The root can be stored for a considerable period in the ground. Cassava contains less than 1 per cent protein and considerably less iron and B vitamins than the cereal grains. The leaves, which are used in the soup, however, are rich in protein and micronutrients. The plant contains linamarin: on hydrolysis this yields hydrocyanic acid, which is responsible for *konzo*. It is, therefore, essential to peel the root before it is sliced or pulped. The pulp is fermented and dried to produce cassava flour or *gari*; the slices are dried and ground to produce a flour. *Gari* stores reasonably well, is exceptionally easy to use, and is exported in appreciable quantities to the markets of the savannah.

Yam

Yams require a fertile soil and the farmers usually reserve their best land for the crop. The tubers also grow extremely well in the derived savannah of West Africa. The area under cultivation is decreasing but the food is prized so that, in some areas, it is now a more expensive prestige food. Yam must be handled carefully, both in production and storage, as bruised tubers rot easily.

Yam yields considerably fewer calories per hectare than cassava because in some areas up to a quarter of the crop may be used as seed. The tuber contains 2 per cent protein, twice as much as cassava. It is either boiled and pounded or sliced and fried in oil.

Plantain

This crop requires a high rainfall and rich soil. As a staple, it is particularly important in the Congo basin, and in Uganda, where it is the *matoke* staple: it is also widely grown in the wetter parts of the forest zone of West Africa. The fruit is mainly carbohydrate. It contains adequate amounts of vitamins A and C but is particularly low in protein, calcium and iron. The water content is high and it is difficult to eat enough to provide adequate protein and energy, so that malnutrition is common in children weaned on this food. The fruit is boiled, steamed, fried, or dried and ground into a flour.

Rice

Although rice is the major food of the world, until recently cultivation has been relatively limited in Africa, confined to the very humid areas of the West Coast, which stretches south from GuineaBissau to the middle of the Ivory Coast. Here, the crop is cultivated as upland rice, i.e. without irrigation. Irrigated or wet rice is more widespread and is grown both in the swamps of the coast and in various irrigation projects in the drier areas (Fig. 2.14).

In areas where the crop is a staple the rice is harvested by hand pounding; this process preserves much of the outer layers and the germ which contain protein and micronutrients. By contrast, imported milled or white rice, which is already popular in the cities, is deficient in

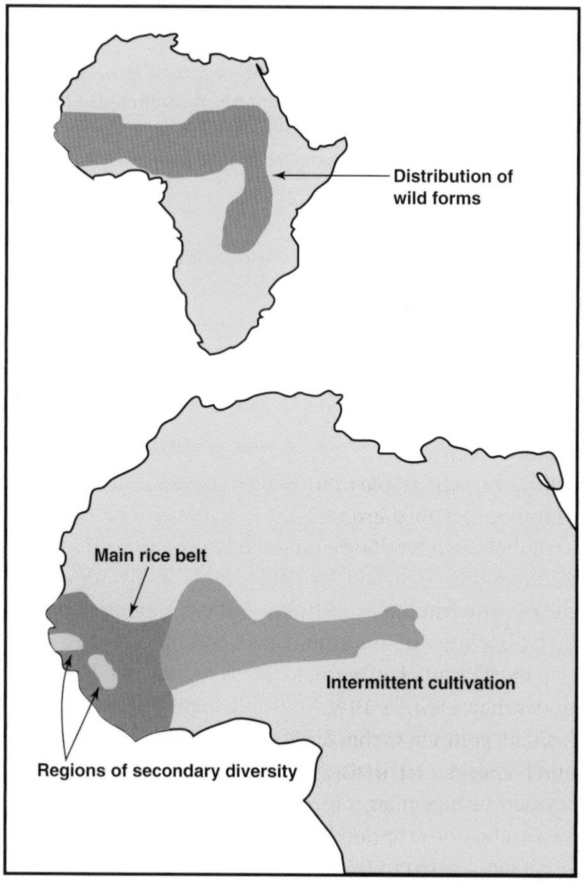

Fig. 2.14. Rice in Africa. Wild rice, upland rice and patterns of cultivation and areas of cultivation. (Adapted from Board on Science and Technology, *Lost Crops of Africa*, Vol 1, *Grains*. Washington, National Academy Press, 1996.)

protein and thiamine. Rice is now an important food, together with white bread, in urban areas of West Africa. Much of this demand has been met by imported rice, and inevitably imported wheat, which has proved politically easier than the encouragement of local production by import and price control.

Minor staples

Cocoyam and sweet potatoes, although widely cultivated in Africa, are only used as a staple by a few small groups, or as a supplement during their season in the savannah and in the forest.

Desert and semidesert

Desert or very arid areas of Africa, where the rainfall is less than 250 mm per year, cover one-quarter of the continent and are occupied by about 20 per cent of its inhabitants. In countries which are classified as semi-arid, 65 per cent of the total area is, on average, very arid or desert. The desert and semi-desert areas of the Sahara, Namib, Kalahari, and parts of the Horn of Africa (Ethiopia, Djibouti, Somalia, and Kenya) merge into the savannah and have much in common with it. Deforestation, overgrazing and climatic changes are extending the boundaries of the semi-arid areas: Lake Chad is becoming smaller rapidly. There are dramatic changes in temperature by day and night. In deserts water is the dominant problem, except at the rare oases, but more commonly at protected boreholes: these allow easy transmission of disease because people have intimate contact with animals and water; the surrounding pasture is denuded and trees are cut. The scattered people have scant medical care.

Dates are the staple of the Sahara, where barley is grown on the northern fringes. Some millet is grown on areas bordering the Sudan savannah.

Highlands

The highlands, which are relatively densely populated, are the home for 10–15 per cent of the population (Fig. 2.15). In contrast to the savannah, the lower temperatures and higher rainfall in the highlands modify the pattern of disease: in particular, it is too cold in most places for the malarial parasite to develop in the mosquito, typically in the Ethiopian high plateau, the mountains beside the Rift Valley in Kenya, the Ruwenzori, much of Rwanda and Burundi, and the great peaks of East Africa. When highlanders move to the lowlands, they are vulnerable to malaria.

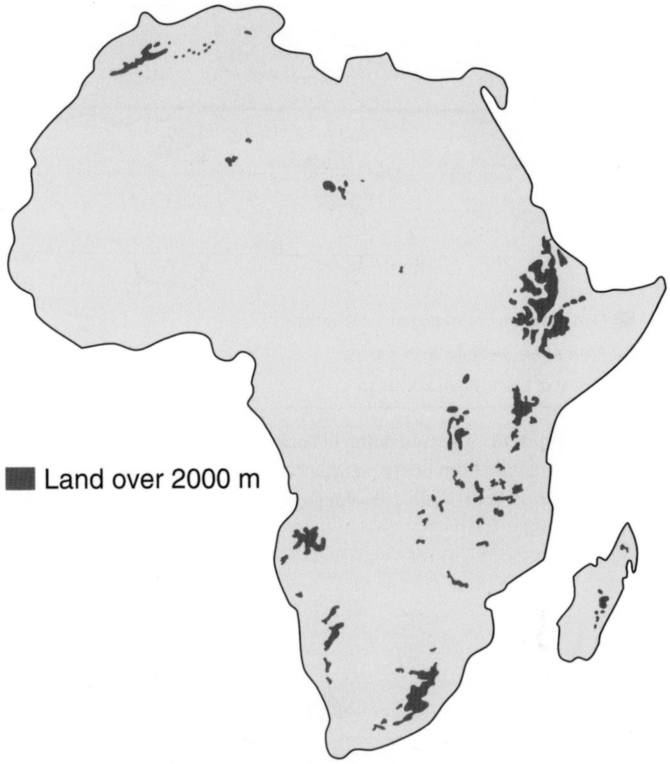

Fig. 2.15. Highlands of Africa: land over 2000 m.

Cereals grow well: in the highlands of Ethiopia, *Tef*, a fine grass (*Eragrostis tef*), is much valued as the true grain for making the *injera* staple. In south-west Ethiopia, the Gurage people have formed a cultural complex based upon *Ensete edulis*, a banana plant whose roots are eaten. *Fonio* or acha *(Digitaria exilis)*, can be grown on thin, rocky soil and was once widespread in the western Sudan, but now only survives as a supplemental staple in the highlands of the Jos plateau in Nigeria, Fouta Djallon in Guinea, and Bamenda in Cameroon (Fig. 2.16).

Focal distribution of disease

Throughout Africa, the distribution of infectious diseases depends on the environmental and climatic demands of the infecting micro-organism. The distribution of other conditions depends on a range of variables, for example, occupational lung disease depends primarily on the geology of the region, whether as a result of a small local industry, for example, grindstone cutters (Warrell et al., 1975) or an extensive gold mining seam in South Africa, while non-filarial elephantiasis depends on the constituents of the soil.

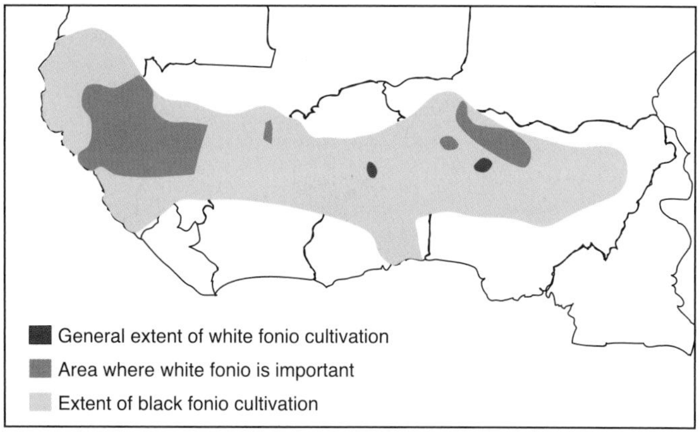

Fig. 2.16. The cultivation of Fonio or *Acha* in West Africa. (Adapted from Board on Science and Technology, *Lost Crops of Africa*, Vol 1, *Grains*. Washington, National Academy Press, 1996 p. 62.)

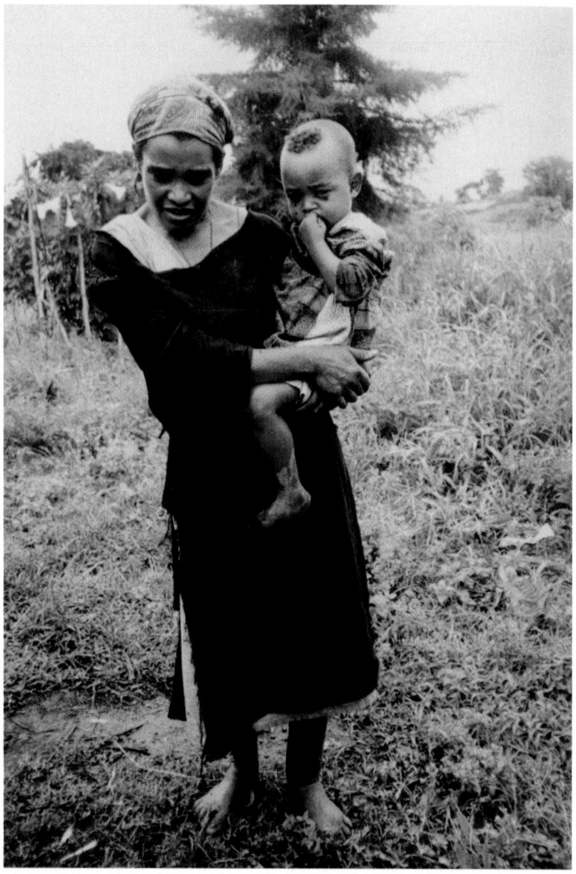

Fig. 2.17. Podoconiosis; woman near Shebe, SW Ethiopia, with early lymphoedema of the left leg (copyright, EHO Parry).

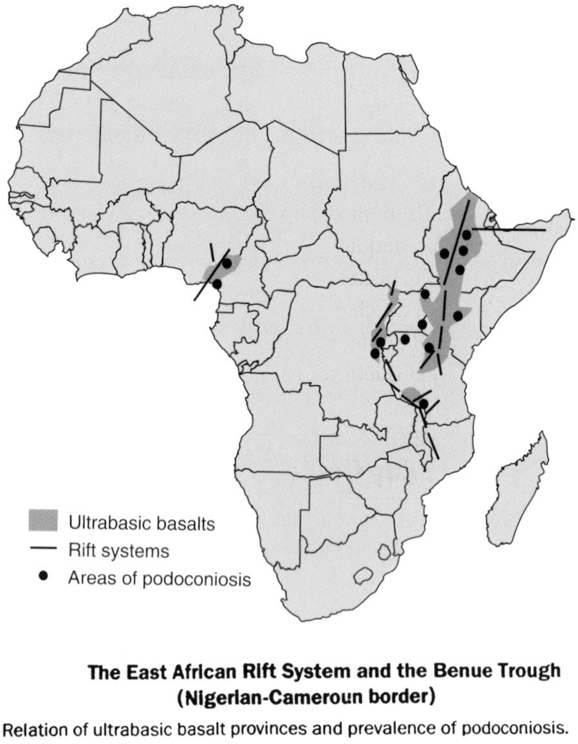

Ultrabasic basalts
Rift systems
Areas of podoconiosis
The East African Rift System and the Benue Trough
(Nigerian-Cameroun border)
Relation of ultrabasic basalt provinces and prevalence of podoconiosis.

Fig. 2.18. Distribution of podoconiosis in Africa. (By courtesy of Dr John Ziegler.)

Example – non-filarial elephantiasis

This condition is also known as Price's disease. Ernest Price, a leprosy surgeon working in Ethiopia, was doing rural clinics in the highlands and found to his surprise that there were many people with elephantiasis in some villages and yet there were none in other villages. It had been thought that the cases were all due to Bancroftian filariasis, but Price argued that this was most improbable because the cases were outside the known geographical distribution of the parasite with its mosquito vector.

What could be responsible for the filarial swelling? Price discovered that the condition was only found in areas where the soil was originally volcanic and was rich in silicates and alumina. He then showed that:

- the lymphatics had been fibrosed:
- traces of silica and its adjuvant alumina were found by mass spectroscopy in the inguinal lymph nodes.

He argued that the condition, which he called podoconiosis (a term derived from Greek words meaning *foot* and *dust*), was caused by particles of soil, which penetrated the skin of bare foot farmers. It could therefore be prevented by people wearing rubber boots (Price, 1978) (Figs. 2.17 and 2.18).

Effects of the climate of Africa on people

Water shortage and excessive heat affect health in several ways. The pattern and amount of rainfall determine whether people endure a hungry season or even famine. Excessive heat can be dangerous to anyone, particularly the unacclimatized, those forced to be active in such heat, or those with inadequate water. Although the desert and arid areas are the hottest and driest, the high ambient temperatures of much of the continent make it essential for people to get enough water to replace their fluid losses when they sweat (Elebute, 1969).

Water and body fluids

Estimated needs

The volume of water needed by a man of about 60 kg in hospital in Lagos and Accra, which are representative of the more humid areas of Africa, but not of the hotter drier places, has been determined as follows:

insensible loss	1700 ml
urine	1500 ml
	3200, less 200 ml for endogenous water.

The total sodium needed is 130 mmol (renal loss 114 mmol, sweat 16 mmol), and total potassium needed is 47 mmol. Thus, a patient who is unable to drink can have his 24-hour needs met by:

dextrose 5 per cent	2 litres
Ringer lactate	1 litre (Na 130, K 6, Ca 4, Cl 111, HCO_3 27 mmol/1) with 3 g KCl

In practice, isotonic sodium chloride is often used instead of Ringer lactate because it is generally available and because such maintenance fluid therapy commonly is only necessary for a short time, except in the unconscious. If the ambient temperature is very high, around 40 °C, more than 3 litres/24 h may be needed.

Korle Bu fluid

This fluid is an excellent basic infusion fluid, and is two-thirds 5 per cent dextrose with one-third Ringer lactate. Its advantages are:

(a) it provides Na throughout 24 hours;

(b) it makes parenteral therapy simple as it alone is used.

Precautions

Whatever fluid is used, it is essential to monitor its volume, to give additional fluid if there are other sources of loss and to monitor the output of urine. If signs of pulmonary congestion develop, stop all intravenous fluid and give frusemide 80 mg at once, together with the emergency measures needed in pulmonary oedema. Add Vitamin C, 100 mg ampoule, and a standard ampoule of a vitamin B multiple preparation, once every 24 hours to the intravenous fluid.

Heat gain and heat loss

Conduction, convection and radiation

There are three physical methods by which the body gains or loses heat (Fig. 2.19).

(a) Heat is lost by conduction if there is a gradient of temperature from body to air; if other compensatory mechanisms do not operate, heat is gained if the temperature gradient is reversed.

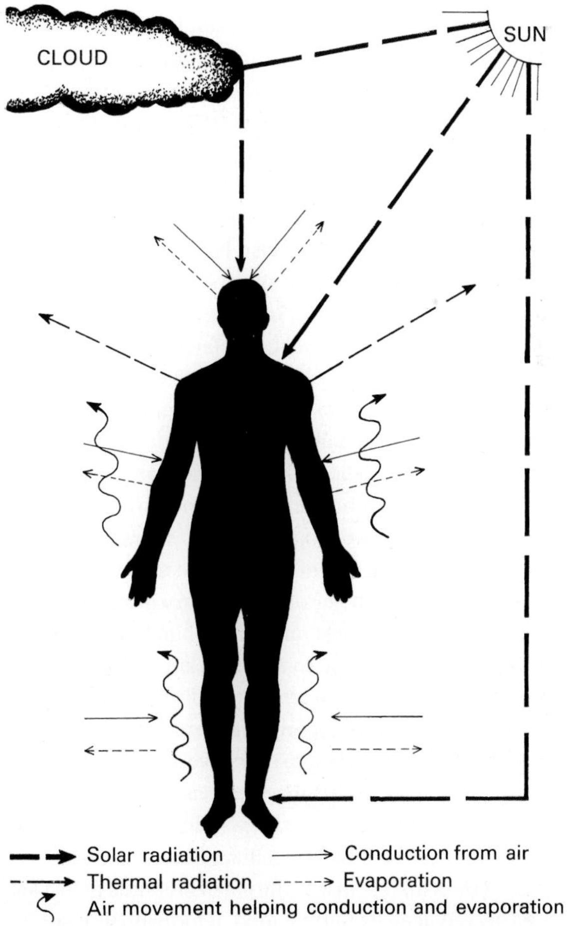

Fig. 2.19. Methods of heat gain and loss in arid conditions. (Adapted and modified from Cloudesley-Thompson, 1977.)

(b) Movement of air encourages heat and water loss from the skin because air heated by the body moves away and unheated air takes its place, increasing heat loss by convection.

(c) Radiation is the transfer of energy between two bodies at different temperatures. It can be a means of heat loss, but, because of solar radiation, in the tropics it is more often a source of heat gain. In very hot climates, 54.4 kJ per square metre per minute of heat from solar radiation strike the body. Some heat is reflected, and so about 17.5 kJ per square metre per minute are absorbed if the area of exposed skin is not great. Therefore, in an hour an individual may gain about 1050 kJ for every square metre of skin exposed, which must be lost primarily by evaporation of sweat.

Methods for losing heat

Vasodilatation and small changes to lose heat

When only small adjustments are needed to lose heat, an increased skin blood flow due to vasodilatation raises the skin temperature and increases loss of heat by radiation and convection. Arteriolar dilatation leads to a rise of pulse pressure and, because the diastolic pressure falls, to a rise in cardiac output. A clothed individual, however, does not lose heat in this way at 29.5 °C and above.

Sweat and large changes to lose heat

The normal insensible loss of sweat is 30 g/h, but 70 g/h can be lost in tropical Africa. In order to lose heat, the body must evaporate its sweat. The latent heat of vaporization of water at body temperature is 2.43 kJ/g; therefore, 72.9 kJ are needed to evaporate 30 ml sweat and about 2410 kJ to evaporate a litre of sweat.

Sweating causes sodium chloride and water to be lost; although sweat is hypotonic (Na 58.4 mmol/l; Cl 45.4 mmol/1) excessive sweating can lead to sodium and water depletion. The rate of evaporation of sweat from the skin and the efficiency of cooling vary inversely with the humidity. Sweat is lost only when there is a humidity gradient from body to air, so that the skin is always wet in a hot, wet climate (high relative humidity).

Throughout Africa, sweating leads primarily to excessive water loss, rather than to excessive sodium loss, because people are acclimatized to heat and therefore secrete sweat which contains little sodium. Loss of water affects extracellular and intracellular fluid: it is easily replaced by drinking, just as the small amounts of lost salt are easily replaced by normal food. If individuals lose much water, however, they may become confused and thus fail to understand their need to drink.

Those at risk of water depletion are:

- the sick, especially those with fever and tachypnoea (acute respiratory infection);
- the aged;
- infants;
- the confused, who do not drink water, from whatever cause.

Although farmers or heavy manual labourers sweat abundantly, they are usually fit and can anticipate the water they will need.

Acute salt and water depletion

Very heavy work in a very hot place, for example, a miner in a gold or copper mine, or a soldier doing harsh training, causes many litres of sweat, and thus sodium also, to be lost – acute water and salt depletion.

Symptoms

Confusion, vomiting, and muscle cramps: the victim may aggravate his deficiency by drinking water alone.

Similarly, the unacclimatized traveller to Africa may develop acute salt and water depletion because his sweat contains more sodium chloride than the indigene's. His extracellular fluid volume falls (because salt is a dominant constituent of it) and he may become hypovolaemic, hypotensive and confused. His need is not for water, but initially is for isotonic saline to restore his ECF volume.

Production of heat

In addition to climatic effects, heat may be gained, or its loss impaired, by other methods.

Metabolic heat production

Heat is gained after feeding.

Fat and lean people

Fat does not conduct heat as readily as water (its thermal conductivity is about 80–90 per cent less). A thick layer of fat slows the conduction of heat from the core of the body to the skin, so that a fat individual is less able to lose heat than one who is thin. The lean build of the desert nomads is ideal because they must be able to lose heat when the ambient temperature is high.

Clothes

Clothes may profoundly affect loss of heat, and the most suitable clothes differ in hot and wet and hot and dry places as the following examples show.

Hot and dry climate

Example – walking in the desert. A man walking at midday at 5 kph at an ambient temperature of 40 °C produces 1130 kJ/h. As solar radiation produces 1000 kJ/h/m^2, he will overheat unless he is able to evaporate about 880 g of water; similarly, unless he drinks at least this volume, he will become dehydrated.

Clothes do not interfere with evaporation of sweat unless the sweat rate is very high or they are made of fabric which is unusually impermeable to water vapour. They reduce heat gain from solar radiation and from hot winds. The colour of the clothes is far less important than the cover they give to areas where the sun strikes most – head, neck, and shoulders.

The Indigo robe of the Tuareg, similar to the long black robe of the Bedouin, absorbs more heat than white robes and its convective heat loss is also greater, but it nevertheless allows an inward flow of heat about three times that of a white robe. Beneath the robe the movement of air allows a much greater convective heat loss, so that the skin is not hotter whether a white or a black robe is worn (Shkolnik et al., 1980).

Hot and wet (humid) climate

Example – West African coast. As temperatures are lower in the forest than in the desert, an individual gets less hot and so needs less water, but he feels hotter and less comfortable because the evaporation of sweat is less efficient.

Clothes, ideally made of cotton, must be freely permeable to water vapour and should hang loosely to encourage ventilation, movement of air and evaporation of sweat.

Acclimatization

Acclimatization and heat load

People who live in hot places can withstand greater heat than those who move into them and who must therefore become acclimatized.

During acclimatization

(a) The rate of sweating increases greatly during the first 3 weeks.
(b) The sodium chloride content of sweat falls substantially.

After acclimatization

(a) Sweat contains very little sodium chloride.
(b) Peripheral vasodilatation, at a given body temperature, is greater.
(c) Body temperature and heart rate rise less after physical work.
(d) Postural hypotension and shifts of blood volume, which are excessive in unacclimatized people, making them liable to syncope, are less in the acclimatized.

Ability to acclimatize

(a) Those who live in hot countries lose ability to withstand heat after a stay in a temperate country.
(b) Age. Younger people acclimatize better than older people.
(c) Sex. There is little evidence to contrast men and women. During pregnancy many women tolerate heat loads badly.

Heat exhaustion syndrome

Those at risk are the unacclimatized or the ill. Over a few days the victim has a vague headache and feels tired and unwell, he sweats and so his body temperature remains normal. Gradually, if nothing is done, confusion, a falling arterial pressure, and a rising body temperature, may usher in heatstroke.

Heatstroke

Heatstroke occurs when an excessive heat load strikes someone; it is not a natural disease but a foreseeable and preventable incident. Those at risk are:

- travellers to hot places, who are unacclimatized (particularly older people);
- heavy manual workers in mines and in the developing industries of the hotter parts of Africa;
- army recruits during vigorous training.

Risk is greater if there is:

- lack of fluid to drink before or during activity;
- lack of sleep;
- any recent illness.

Prevention

Heatstroke can be prevented if those liable to excessive heat loads are carefully watched, are given plenty of water, and wear sensible clothes, and if those at risk avoid excessive heat and exercise.

Aged people or those who are ill among the pilgrims of the Hajj are vulnerable, and medical teams at Mecca should be aware of the potential mortality among such people, particularly when the Hajj falls in the hot season.

The patient with a very high fever due to an infection can present a similar problem, particularly if he is confused or unconscious and has had a long and hot journey to hospital.

Symptoms and signs

A mild confusional state with irrelevant speech and irrational behaviour are early symptoms; thirst, dizziness, psychotic behaviour, impaired consciousness and fits follow. Sweating, hypotension, tachycardia, and a rectal temperature of over 40 °C are common signs (Khogali & Weiner, 1980).

Investigations

Evidence of widespread tissue injury and disseminated intravascular coagulation may be found, such as: kidney – protein and casts in the urine and a raised blood urea; liver – a high serum bilirubin and raised enzymes; blood – prolonged prothrombin time, low fibrinogen levels and thrombocytopenia; skeletal muscle – raised levels of enzymes derived from muscles (creatine phosphokinase), and heart – raised myocardial enzymes.

The serum sodium, chloride, urea, creatinine, and osmolality are raised: the serum potassium and bicarbonate are usually low, and there is lactic acidosis with a raised serum lactate (Costrini et al., 1979).

Diagnosis

Suspect heatstroke in anyone who becomes disoriented or unconscious during exercise in a hot place, particularly a recent immigrant or one previously ill.

- Remember that a severe infection may present in the same way.

Treatment

Urgent action is essential as recovery depends partly upon the speed with which treatment is begun. The principles are:

- Cool the patient quickly.

Wet skin and warm air

If the skin can be kept at 32 °C, an active circulation is maintained in the skin so that core blood is cooled in its vessels. Such vasodilatation prevents shivering. A bed has been devised on which the patient can be sprayed with tap water at 15 °C and blown with warm air at 30–35 °C: it is a net suspended over a bath, and this makes nursing and the disposal of faeces or vomitus simpler. This method can lower body temperature by 2 °C in 6 minutes (Wiener & Kogali, 1980).

Immersion

Less satisfactory, the classical and familiar method of immersion in ice-cold water causes intense vasoconstriction so that heat is not lost through dilated surface veins: if the skin temperature falls to 28 °C, violent shivering can occur, which increases heat production.

- Restore extracellular fluid volume and correct hypokalaemia.
- Prevent fits.
- Manage predisposing condition.

Prognosis

Fits and prolonged unconsciousness make the prognosis bad.

Other disorders related to climate

Urinary tract calculi and water shortage

The relationship between water shortage and stone is not simple, as geographical variations in the prevalence of stone in the dry hot areas of Africa demonstrate that some other factor may be responsible: from Rwanda it has been suggested that something in the diet (possibly rubidium) also helps stones to form. Urinary tract stone, particularly in the bladder and often in children, is a recognized hazard in Sudan (Abboud et al., 1989) and in the countries of the Sahel, but the stones are still largely calcium oxalate based (Balla et al., 1998).

Hypothermia

This is a risk in cold countries and in Africa among those who are vulnerable.

Environment

During the cold nights of December–January in the southern savannah and Sahel of West Africa the temperature falls dramatically. Similarly, at the higher altitudes in Ethiopia, Kenya, Rwanda, Burundi and Botswana, cold nights can also be a potential hazard.

Those vulnerable

- The malnourished, particularly those with severe protein malnutrition, or those with so little subcutaneous fat that they lose heat easily – for example, a wasted patient with HIV.
- Adults with severe tuberculosis.
- The aged.
- Vagrants. In Uganda one-third of a group of hypothermic patients were chronically poorly nourished vagrants who had been sleeping out.

- Alcoholics.
- Those treated with phenothiazines, already vulnerable because of the factors listed here.

Clinical problem

The diagnosis is typical: a partially conscious wasted person who is cold – rectal temperature around 30–32 °C – and who is brought to hospital after being found exposed at the roadside. Hypoglycaemia is common and may aggravate the stupor. Pancreatitis is a recognized complication and may not be clinically evident (Sadikali et al., 1974).

Management

The principles of management are:

- to raise the body temperature. Wrap the patient in warmed blankets, close windows and, if available, use an electric fire to warm the room.
- to correct hypoglycaemia. Give 50 ml of 50 per cent dextrose intravenously.
- to treat any primary disease.
- to rehabilitate. This can be very difficult, but it may be made easier by the treatment of a chronic disease such as tuberculosis. If the patient has had phenothiazines, stop them.

Prognosis

This is very bad indeed: about half the patients die.

Effects of climate on agents of disease

Although climatic change may in future affect the distribution of disease profoundly and the vulnerability of the people of Africa to vector-borne disease, and although the patterns of rainfall appear to be changing in some areas, this subject is beyond the scope of this chapter.

Climate, and its changes in the different seasons of the year in Africa, can modify the pattern of disease profoundly in an area, not only because it determines what people do, but more fundamentally because it affects micro-organisms. There is a delicate balance between the host, the invader and the climate in Africa: some examples are given below.

Vectors

Vectors are either free-flying or wingless. The distinction is important because it helps to explain why the spread of some diseases depends on the movement of people, while others depend more on the vectors' movements. Free-flying vectors can spread disease among settled people: wingless vectors require the movement of people for the diseases, which they transmit to be widely spread.

Vectors can only transmit disease if they can survive and breed successfully. Climate is critical and Table 2.3 shows how such vectors depend on temperature and rainfall.

It is not enough, however, to think of the survival of vectors solely in terms of the broad climatic regions of Africa and the temperatures within these regions. There are also microclimates or limited areas where the climate is different enough from that of the surrounding region to allow particular vectors to flourish. Such areas can modify the local distribution of disease greatly within a region, as the following examples show.

Simulium spp. and onchocerciasis

The development of infective larvae of *Onchocerca volvulus* within the fly *Simulium damnosum or S. naevi* depends largely on external temperature, which is optimal at 24 °C between latitudes 10° and 12° N. Larvae do not develop at 18 °C. The breeding of the fly within these latitudes varies greatly from place to place. In the savannah, breeding is impossible during the dry season. It begins as soon as the rains start, when water flows rapidly in small rocky streams. Flies are most dense around the fast-flowing streams in the savannah and people who live near them are more likely to get onchocerciasis than those who live further away.

Glossina spp. and sleeping sickness

Trypanosoma gambiense can only multiply in tsetse flies at temperatures of 24 °C and above: 25–30 °C is the optimum. Extreme dryness or much wetness are lethal to the flies – a relative humidity of around 40 per cent is required. Temperatures of 35 °C and above are also lethal and few flies survive 40 °C. As such temperatures are common in the savannah during the dry season, foci of sleeping sickness will only be found in those places where the flies can survive because they are protected by shade trees and near water.

Phlebotomus spp. and kala-azar

In Kenya microfoci of kala-azar occur in groups of homesteads closely associated with low, eroded and shaded termite hills at the edges of patches of *Acacia* scrub, where the young men sit in the evening and are bitten by the vector *P. martini* which breeds in the termite hills. In southern and eastern Sudan, the *Acacia – Balanites* woodland is the critical environment and the mean annual maximum daily temperature and the soil type are

Table 2.3. Effects of climate on some vectors and agents of disease

Wet	Vector	Dry
Daily temperature varies Rainy season prolonged		Daily temperature varies considerably Rainy season short
Development of *Plasmodium* in mosquito depends on temperature (Table 2.4)	*Anopheles* Malaria	Low and seasonal rainfall prevents continuous intense endemicity of malaria
Breeding of *Aedes aegypti* needs water; virus matures in only 4 days at 37 °C, but at 18 °C it needs 36 days	*Aedes* Yellow fever	Transmission is possible only during the rains
Fly breeds in overgrown shaded marshy streams which flow slowly and have a layer of mud and decaying vegetation	*Chrysops* Loiasis	These conditions do not exist in the savannah
Trypanosoma can only develop in *Glossina* at temperatures of 24 °C and above (25–30 °C optimum) Few survive if very wet. Relative humidity 40–60% needed	*Glossina* spp. Trypanosomiasis	Temperatures of 35 °C and dryness are lethal; shade trees near streams and rivers essential
Optimum temperature is 20–25 °C in a wet place	*Ratflea* Plague	Greater temperature and dryness are unfavourable
This crustacean needs water and a temperature of 24 °C for successful breeding. Excessive rains wash *Cyclops* away and make ponds turbid, so transmission of disease stops during rainy season of forest zone	*Cyclops* Guinea worm	Less intense rains in savannah allow surface water to be collected and drunk, so transmission greatest during early rainy season
Few female flies survive to third blood meal in humid forest areas, i.e. maturation of larvae from microfilariae is impossible. Development of infective larvae from microfilariae in *S. damnosum* depends on external temperature	*Simulium* spp. Onchocerciasis	Infection is commonest between latitudes 10° and 12° N where female flies survive well
	Pathogens	
	Spirochaetal diseases	
Common in areas where annual rainfall more than 1250 mm; open infections and papillomatous lesions common and larger during the rainy season	*T. pallidum pertenue* Yaws	This is not a problem in the savannah, which is too dry
Increased incidence during the rainy season	*Borrelia vincenti* Tropical ulcer	
Worse during the rainy season	*T. pallidum pallidum* Endemic syphilis	Lesions regress or disappear during dry season
	Other bacterial diseases	
Increased incidence of pyoderma and its complications during the rainy season. More common in wet areas. Is surface drying of hot soil lethal?	*Streptococcus pyogenes* Pyoderma *Clostridium tetani* Tetanus *Neisseria meningitidis* Meningitis	Epidemics during the warmer dry season abruptly halted by rains. There is a negative correlation between absolute humidity and meningococcal meningitis

Table 2.3 (*cont.*)

Wet	Vector	Dry
	Nematodes	
Both infections commoner in areas where annual rainfall more than 1250 mm; larvae develop most rapidly at 26–32 °C	*Necator americanus* Hookworm infection	Only derived savannah and some parts of the guinea savannah have rainfall as great as this
	Strongyloides stercoralis Strongyloidiasis	Ova and larvae readily killed when surface soil dried by winds and sun
The relationship between climate and *Schistosoma* spp. and its snail intermediate hosts is complex	**Trematodes** *Schistosoma* spp.	

Table 2.4. Temperature and the time taken (days) for development of the malarial parasite within the mosquito

	Mean ambient temperature and days			
Species of parasite	30 °C	24 °C	20 °C	26 °C
P. vivax	7	9	16	
P. falciparum	9	11	20	
P. malariae	15	21	30	
P. ovale				15

the most important ecological determinants of *P. orientalis* (Thomson et al., 1999).

Parasites

The best example of a parasite, which depends very largely on climate for its breeding, is the malarial parasite. Table 2.4 shows the effect of varying temperatures on the number of days necessary for the parasite to develop within the mosquito host.

The result of this can be seen in the distribution of malaria within Africa and of diseases linked with malaria, such as Burkitt's lymphoma. Wherever there is a sufficiently low mean temperature, endemic malaria cannot occur unless there is a microclimate, for example, the inside of a hut: Garnham (1945), in a classic paper, described a catastrophic outbreak in the Kenyan highlands where the temperature inside a hut was 2–3 °C higher than that outside.

Viruses and bacteria

When a patient is seen, or a community is identified with an infection, consider how its transmission, eradication and treatment may be affected by changes in climate.

Examples:

Group B arbovirus – yellow fever

The virus can mature in the mosquito vector in 4 days at an ambient temperature of 37 °C, but it takes 36 days at 18 °C. Epidemics of yellow fever are therefore more likely to occur when the temperature is high enough for rapid multiplication and transmission.

Treponema pallidum pertenue – yaws

As the spirochaete needs a place where the rainfall is not less than 1250 mm and where the mean temperature is not less than 24 °C, yaws was a major problem in the humid forest and derived savannah zones of west Africa before mass penicillin treatment was given. It is still present in parts of Ghana and Benin.

Movement of people

Urban movement

All over Africa, the urban stampede continues. The effects have been described and emphasized in Chapter 1. The urban migrant, away from the restraint of a traditional society, is vulnerable in many ways. City life is becoming increasingly precarious and violent and, although young and hopeful adolescents continue to swell the slums of Africa's rapidly growing cities, they are more and more vulnerable, particularly in this era of HIV infection. In their villages they were constrained by the presence of their family and the village hierarchy, but now their apparent 'freedom' knows no limits and they lack any brake on their behaviour and activity. For example, in the slums of the cities, they become both sexually active at a younger age and have more sexual partners than in a rural environment (Buvé et al., 2002). The urban migrant may enjoy support from members of their family but the closeness of family support is lost. The vulnerable and sick migrant also suffers because the health infrastructure is often stretched so far that it cannot function efficiently.

- Always find out from your patient where they have come from and for how long they have been at their present address.

Rural movement

Small rural movements

These are typically seasonal and are considered below.

Large rural movements

These arise on account of:

- Population pressure in poor farming country.

- Drought and famine

This sort of movement creates appalling problems for these internally displaced people (IDP), who move because they have no alternative as they have no resources.

They often move to a town in an area that is unfamiliar, or even hostile, to them and their culture, where they become begging urban migrants. The dignity and independence of these dispossessed people is lost: they become dependent wholly on others, forced to live in shelter camps (Chapter 4).

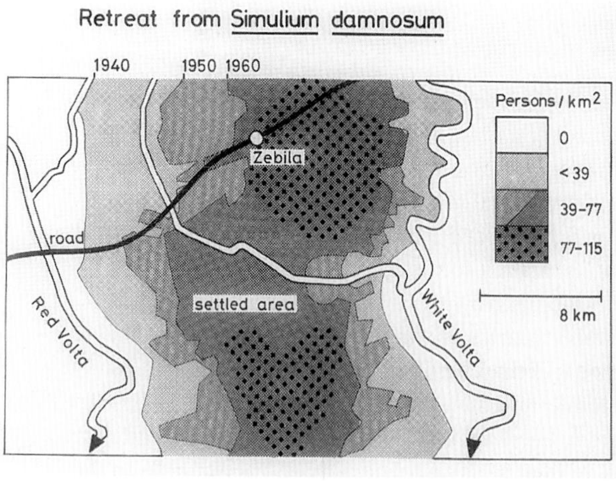

Fig. 2.20. Movement of people and abandonment of agricultural land by people incapacitated by onchocerciasis in Northern Ghana. (Data from Onchocerciasis, Volta Basin Project, WHO, 1973.)

- War and disorder (Chapter 4)

Not only are the refugees caught in a web of difficulty and deprivation, but the economy of the country where they take refuge can be affected seriously. Thus there can be huge pressures on the health service and on the supplies of food, as happened when over a million people crossed from Mozambique into Malawi.

- Return of people displaced by conflict

A different hazard is illustrated by the experience of people who returned to Soroti and its region in eastern Uganda after a period of conflict. They began to restock their cattle, which they had taken with them when they left. But the cattle came from the focus in S.E. Uganda of sleeping sickness (*Trypanosoma b rhodesiense*). Before long, there was an outbreak of sleeping sickness in Soroti, with its focus around the cattle market (Fevrè et al., 2001).

- Resettlement of people displaced by development

This produces a rural–rural migration, often hazardous to health on account of the peculiar health risks of development schemes. Dams and hydroelectric schemes can displace people and change the ecology of the area, and small dams or irrigation systems can lead to microfoci of new infections, for example, malaria (Ghebreyesus et al., 1999), schistosomiasis or soil-transmitted helminths.

Effects of movement on people

(a) Psychological trauma in losing their home. The movement of people from a traditional home to a strange one can be very traumatic so that they have no motive to farm and develop.
(b) Infection. They frequently have no immunity to diseases prevalent in the area to which they go. The classic example is highlanders moving into a malarious area, but any forced resettlement may expose people to new infections.
(c) Nutritional deficiency if they move to an area where the food is unfamiliar or if they have been unable to plant crops and gather their harvest in their first year.
(d) Loss of farming land or other sources of income. Historically, sleeping sickness and onchocerciasis are examples. The ravages of onchocerciasis depopulated large areas in the Volta river system of Ghana and Burkina Faso and many people sought new homes away from places where *Simulium damnosum* flourished. The area of good land farmed therefore fell and people had to move out of the area (Fig. 2.20); thus the Onchocerciasis Control Programme was needed badly.

Why should this patient from this place present in this way?

This is the immediate clinical problem: the necessary careful enquiring clinical approach can be understood from the following case summaries.

Examples

Fever in a migrant to Kampala from western Uganda

A woman aged 28 moved from Fort Portal district to join members of her family in Kampala. As an urban migrant she was potentially socially and psychologically vulnerable, but she was well supported by members of her family.

Why the high fever? The Fort Portal district has areas that have very little malaria: could this fever therefore, be the presenting symptom of malaria in a non-immune adult? It was: a blood film showed abundant ring forms of *P. falciparum*.

It was only when the question 'where has she come from?' was asked, that the first lead to the correct diagnosis was given.

Fever and abdominal pain in a laboratory assistant

A 21 year old woman had had vague abdominal pain, which she had never had before. She was admitted to a medical ward in the hospital where she worked, but gave no more symptoms to the young intern who saw her. He thought that she had a little free fluid in the abdomen, which he could not explain and he did not consider the need to go further into her history.

Why should this young woman have this pain?

She later said that she had had amenorrhoea for 2 months and that the pain had started suddenly.

A peritoneal tap drew blood: her ruptured ectopic gestation was safely dealt with.

Drowsiness in a 15-year-old schoolboy

The boy, the son of a professional father, was at a boarding school. He was seen in the casualty department of a large hospital accompanied by a friend, who believed the boy had had treatment for diabetes.

The blood glucose was 22.8 mmol/l and he had ketonuria. The school did not supply insulin and he had used all he had taken for his school term.

These examples show that answers to the questions *who*? and *where*? can be very important in the vast range of clinical problems in Africa. Further suggestions are given below.

Those with new symptoms who are seen for the first time

- Is the person particularly vulnerable? For example, a woman widowed by war, an AIDS orphan adolescent, or a prisoner.
- Is the school child about to sit important examinations?
- Has the aged grandmother been feeding the infant while mother is out at work?
- Are these symptoms the first evidence of HIV in a young adult?

Those who are known to have a disease

- Has the patient taken the prescribed medication?
- Has a well-recognized complication of the primary disease developed?
- Are the drugs that are being taken by the patient active or are they fake and inactive? (Taylor et al., 2001.)
- Has the patient, whose disease may have well-recognized complications in a body system, now developed symptoms of a new disease in the same system?
- Has the patient developed complications of treatment?

Why should this patient, from this place present in this way at this time? or The effects of seasons on health and disease

Seasons are very important in the ecology of health and disease in Africa, not only because of the effects of climate on micro-organisms, but also because of the relationship between seasons and food supply, food prices, work and disease, and the efficiency of the health services during the rainy season.

- Study the health and disease of the people in the area where you work, identify how they are affected by seasonal changes and who is potentially vulnerable at different times of year.

Seasons, food and work

Movement of people to find work during the slack farming season

When work is slack on farms and the harvest has been gathered and stored, men move to find seasonal work wherever they can, but they return again when the

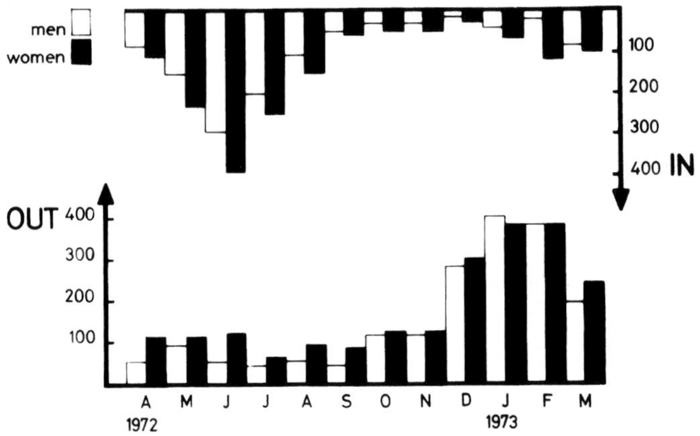

Fig. 2.21. Movement of people out of a savannah village during the dry season, when farming is slack and travel is easy, and the return just before the rainy season in readiness for the farming season. (Adapted from Molyneux & Grammiccia, 1980.)

farming season is imminent. Such movement, shown in Fig. 2.21 from a major study of malaria in northern Nigeria, may be even more pronounced now that motor transport makes long distance travel in search of work so much easier. But the less enterprising and the more vulnerable are left in their village and may lack the support of the younger and fitter members of the family.

Food supply

Food is short before harvest; both in quantity so that there is less available energy, and in essential nutrients, for example, folic acid derived from freshly harvested vegetables. Pregnant mothers and their babies, with lower birthweights, are inevitably affected but they lose less weight if they are given a food supplement (Ceesay et al., 1997); see Fig. 3.13. Animals also suffer, because not only does overgrazing shave off the grass, so that grass cover is almost lost in the dry season, but the grass itself is deficient in protein during the dry season (Figs 2.22(*a*) and (*b*).

Food prices

As the supply of food becomes short, so food prices rise. The poorest people are most at risk. The very people whose nutrition is probably only marginally adequate when supplies are adequate, are vulnerable as prices rise, and are impotent victims if there is a critical shortage of food when traders drive prices up and up (Fig. 2.23). In recent years, in many countries, but not uniformly throughout any country, more and more families are coming to depend on a regular supply of money sent as remittances from relations in rich countries. These people are protected therefore from the effects of this seasonal rise in food prices.

Food storage

The granaries are filled again after harvest, but if the harvest is poor, stocks of grain are soon exhausted. The poor have the smallest stocks (Fig. 2.1). If the methods of storage are poor, and the poorer, smaller farmers have less efficient stores, grain is blackened by fungal attack or devoured by rodents. During the rains before the next harvest, *Aspergillus* can produce significant concentrations of aflatoxin, which is found in highest concentration in food that has been longest in store. *Claviceps* contamination may lead to ergot poisoning.

- Assess the food security of the people in your area.
- On field visits, look at the structural state of the granaries and the level of stored grain in them.
- Get help from your colleagues in the agricultural service.

Agricultural work

The rainy season demands periods of intense work, chiefly from men, but in some areas also from women if they work on the farm. Undernutrition (shown by a low Body Mass Index – BMI) and disease reduce work and activity as measured by energy expenditure (Alemu & Lindtjorn, 1995).

Pregnant women who were active in the rice fields were shown to lose weight during the rains, as do any farmers at this season when work is at its most arduous, and food is scarce and costly. This is bad enough but, if the next year's harvest fails, the people are already hungry and will be unable to make up their need from the harvest. So they will be in dire need.

In 25 per cent of farmers the body weight shifts from the normal range of nutritional status into the category of chronic energy deficiency, so that they become true 'seasonal casualties' (Ferro-Luzzi et al., 1994).

Domestic work

Unlike the work of men, the work of women and their need for energy from food continue throughout the year. In some cultures they do much farming and so are as vulnerable to the demands of farming as are men (Fig. 2.24),

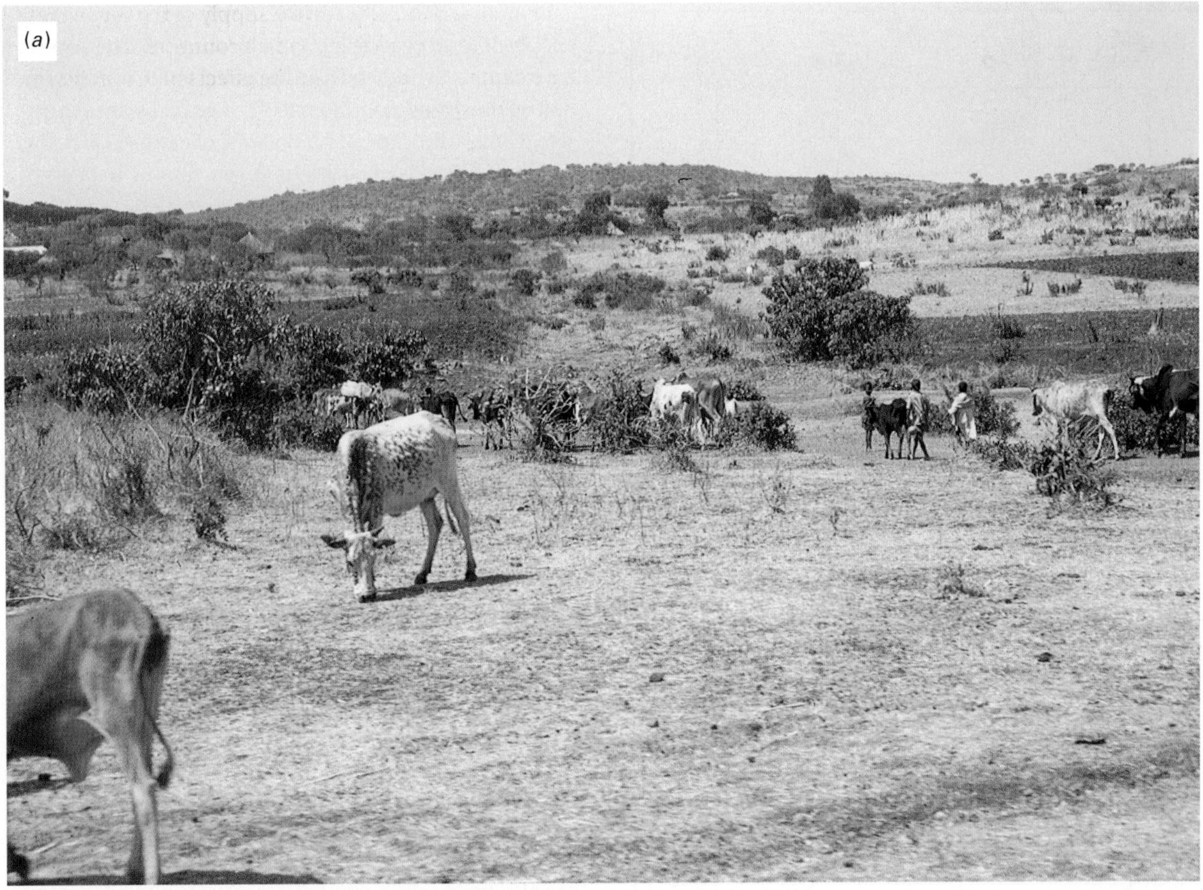

Fig. 2.22. (*a*) Overgrazing and poor cattle (copyright EHO Parry). (*b*) (bottom right) Lack of protein in grass during the dry season, when overgrazing is worst. (Adapted from Gill, 1991.)

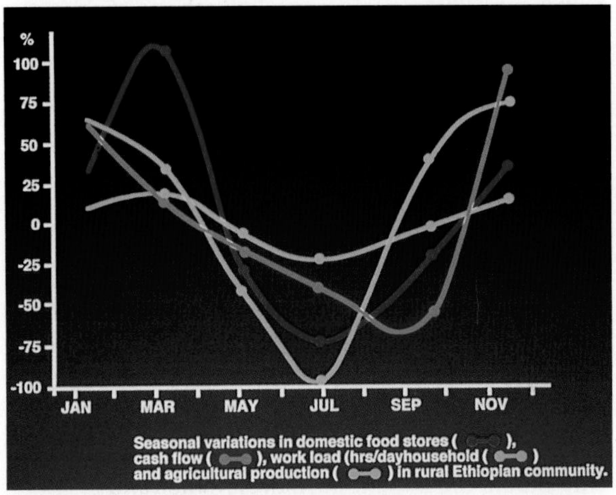

Fig. 2.23. Seasonal variations in domestic food stores, cash flow, work load (hours/day/household) and agricultural production in a rural Ethiopian community. (Adapted from Ferro-Luzzi, 1990.)

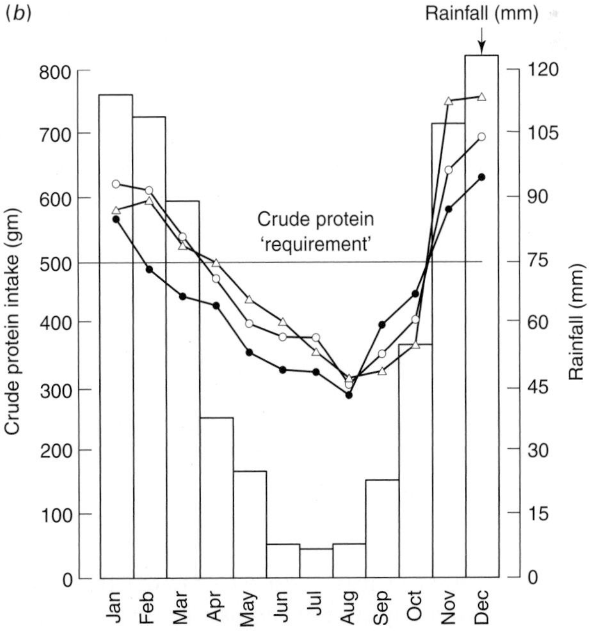

Fig. 2.22(*b*). Season, rainfall and crude protein intake from three different types of pasture in Southern Africa.

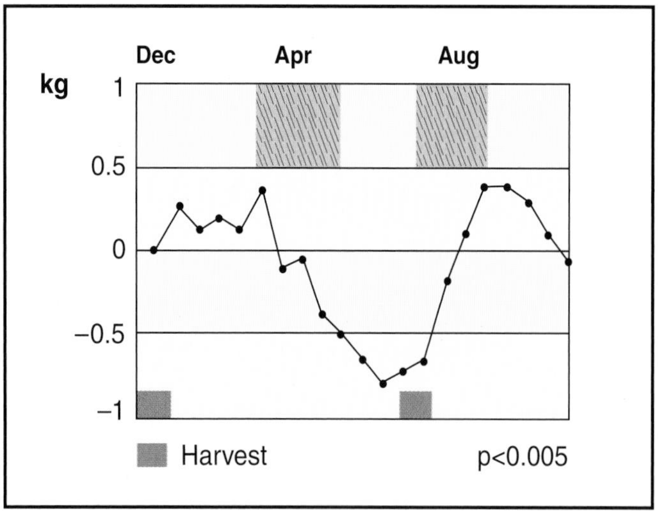

Fig. 2.24. Rural women in Benin. Effect of activity and seasons on body weight. (Adapted from Schultink et al., 1990.)

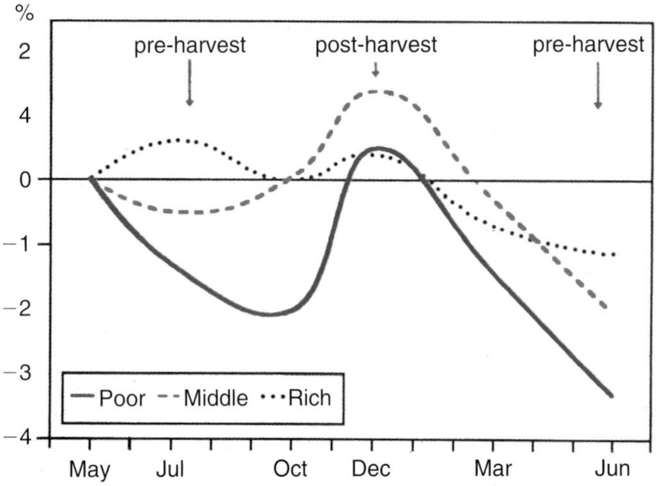

Fig. 2.25. Cumulative changes of weight by seasons in a southern Ethiopian farming community according to socioeconomic level. (Compare Fig. 2.9, p. 16.) (Adapted from Pastore et al., 1993.)

but in others they do little, for example, the Sidamo women of Ethiopia whose farming only accounts for 5 per cent of their total energy expenditure (Ferro-Luzzi et al., 1990).

Nutrition

The scarcity and increased cost of food toward the end of the dry season may cause under-nutrition and unmask kwashiorkor. Children and adults lose weight, but it is the poor who suffer most (Fig. 2.25).

Vitamin C (Fig. 3.28) and folate deficiency vary with the supply of fresh vegetables and root crops all over Africa: for example, in arid areas of Tanzania, folate is deficient during the dry season when fresh vegetables are expensive. Those who depend on the milk of cattle, like Samburu nomads of northern Kenya, may be in near-famine conditions for 4 months during the dry season when their only food is 2 litres of milk daily.

The hungry season is a grim reality: food is scarce, prices are high, stocks are exhausted and energy demands are high. Some of its impact is shown in Table 2.5.

- Recognize the hungry season and how some people, particularly the poorest, become vulnerable and develop a significant energy deficiency on account of the demands of their work.

Seasonal deficiencies and intoxications

One of the best examples is *Konzo*, which is both a deficiency and an intoxication. The disease is characterized by an acute *paraparesis*, which, in from about 70–90 per cent of reported cases, develops overnight.

It is classically related to seasonal lack of adequate food, of essential amino acids in protein food and of an appropriately prepared source of energy. *Konzo*, which has also been called *mantakassa*, was described first in cassava growing areas of Congo: it has also been studied in Mozambique and Tanzania, and reported in Angola and the Central African Republic.

Who is affected?

Women and children are the chief victims, as they potentially are more malnourished initially and also because the best food is first eaten by the men (see, for example, Table 3.15) so that the women have to eat the less well-prepared food.

Where do they live?

All the outbreaks have been reported from cassava-growing areas, but in northern Tanzania, families who lived close to Lake Victoria who supplemented their cassava with fish were spared, while those in villages away from the lake had many cases (Howlett et al., 1992).

Why should the patient have these symptoms?

The acute paraparesis is attributed to the neurotoxic effects of cyanide. The cassava tuber contains potentially toxic cyanogenic glycosides, chiefly linamarin. These are

Table 2.5. The hungry season: changes among different groups of people in 4 African countries

Fat-free mass significantly less than post-harvest	Benin	Rural women	Schultink et al. (1993)
Profound loss of fat – partially offset by dietary supplements	Gambia	Subsistence farming women	Lawrence et al. (1987)
Birthweight and weight gain in pregnancy increased significantly by supplementing high energy groundnut biscuits 4.3 mJ/day	Gambia	Chronically under-nourished village women	Ceesay et al. (1997)
Greater seasonal loss of weight if low socio-economic status	Southern Ethiopia	Subsistence farmers	Branca et al. (1993)
Less food available, loss of weight, activity unchanged	Southern Ethiopia	Rural women	Ferro-Luzzi (1990)
Food stocks of poor families 6.5 times smaller than richer families	Southern Ethiopia	Village people	Pastore et al. (1993)
Vitamin A,C,B group and iron, protein intake significantly lower	Kenyan highlands	Rural lactating women	Kigutha et al. (1995)

broken down during processing to acetone cyanohydrin, which spontaneously yields hydrogen cyanide (HCN). Women who prepare the cassava know well how to process the root properly but, when there is no other food, they are forced to give their children and to retain for themselves roots that have not been adequately processed (Banea et al., 1992). The HCN is detoxified by SH-groups to thiocyanate; urinary levels of thiocyanate have always been found to be much higher in cases of *konzo* than in controls. The Tanzanian lakeside people ate fish which contains cysteine and other sulphur-containing amino acids, as do beans, which thus supply the SH-groups so that cyanides can be detoxified into thiocyanate. Similarly, savannah villages in Congo, described as former Zaire (Banea-Mayambu et al., 1997), had many more cases than forest villages because the forest people added maize to their cassava, so that less cassava was consumed there.

When did the outbreaks occur?

War and drought, with the resulting inevitably devastated farming, have led to outbreaks (Cliff et al., 1997). Repeated failure of the rains led to dwindling supplies of food. There was little else to eat except bitter cassava and, because food was so short, this had to be eaten before it had been adequately prepared, so that there were acute cases of konzo at that time (Fig. 2.26). Normally, the cassava root is peeled and then is allowed to dry in the sun or is kept in water. Days later it is used, when the cyanogens have been leached out so that it is 'safe'. But in the villages where the outbreaks occurred, the bitter cassava was eaten on the first day.

Drought

Seasonal disease, hazards and seasonal activities

Drought is the ultimate result of a seasonal failure of the rains. If food supplies are quickly exhausted, the little food that is available goes first to the men, so that women and children are particularly vulnerable. They are further disadvantaged in the forced migration which follows, with its inevitable social disruption (Chapter 4).

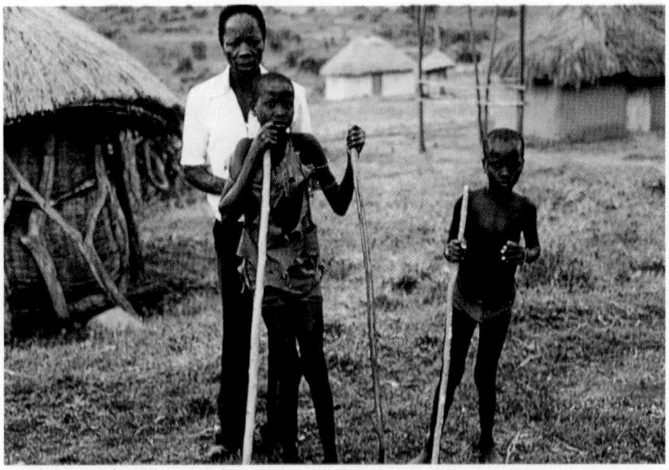

Fig. 2.26. Boys with spastic paraparesis caused by *konzo* in a Tanzanian village. (By courtesy of Dr William Howlett.)

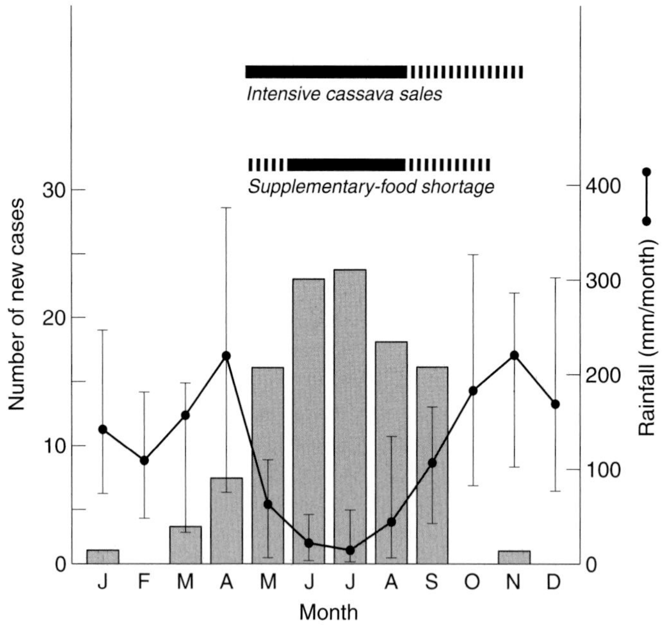

Fig. 2.27. Konzo: note that, in the dry season, the cases (bars) are at their peak, which is when there is a shortage of supplementary food and there are intensive sales of cassava. (Adapted from Tylleskar et al., 1991.)

The need to eat poorly stored or alternative food

Drought forces people to eat:

- poorly prepared food, as in the example of *konzo* (Fig. 2.27).
- contaminated food, where there are abundant fungi, which might be discarded in a time of plenty. Farmers in the Ethiopian highlands noticed that wild oats (*Avena abyssinica*) were growing instead of barley in their harvest, and that the grains were large and purplish-black, infected with the ergot fungus, *Claviceps purpurea.* Those who had other grain did not eat these grains, but poor people had no other food so that many died from ergot-induced gangrene (Demeke et al., 1979).
- food which, when taken in excess, can lead to intoxication. For example, the drought-resistant grass pea or chickling vetch, *Lathyrus sativus,* contains a neurotoxin, ß-oxalylaminoalanine (Getahun et al., 2002). When Ethiopian highlanders were forced by drought to use the pea for about one-third of their daily diet, an epidemic of neuro-lathyrism (sudden spastic paraparesis broke out among them, chiefly affecting boys aged 10–14. In this latest epidemic illiteracy was an important risk factor.

Seasonal changes in transmission of infection

In addition to specific climatic factors, which enable an organism to multiply, the complex relationship between people, their environment, and the infecting organism and its vector, is often significantly affected by seasonal change.

Thus:

1. Contact between human–vector or human–intermediate host is increased.
2. People become more susceptible to the pathogen.
3. The pathogen spreads more easily and so reaches more people.

There is often more than one reason for a change of disease by season, as some of the examples given below demonstrate. Further examples are shown in Table 2.6.

Vectors and intermediate hosts

Free-flying vector

Mosquitoes and yellow fever

A low seasonal rainfall, as in places with a long dry season, makes continuous transmission of this arbovirus disease impossible because mosquitoes cannot breed.

Intermediate host

Cyclops and guinea-worm

Guinea-worm infection differs between the guinea savannah and the forest belt of West Africa. The torrential rainy season of the forest washes away the crustacean *Cyclops* from the surface water, so infected water is not regularly drunk at this time and transmission decreases. The early rains of the savannah, however, fill surface pools from which people, accustomed to draw their water laboriously from distant wells, gladly collect water. These pools are a common habitat of *Cyclops.* Villagers in such areas recognize that guinea-worm infection usually becomes evident when the rainy season begins, a year after infected water was drunk; this is the time taken for the adult worm to mature. Now that the villagers have learnt the mode of transmission of guinea worm, and have been provided with micropore filters for drinking (Fig. 2.8), thanks to major campaigns to eradicate the parasite, the incidence of new infections has fallen.

Snails and schistosomiasis

In East Africa many seasonal variations have been found of which the following are a few. The very hot season of

Table 2.6. Examples of seasonal changes in disease

Rainy season
Dependent on flourishing of vector l intermediate host

Mosquito
Yellow fever – *Aedes* spp.

Malaria – Anopheles spp.
Sudan, arid NE: flourishes if/when short rains fall (Theander, (1998)

Cyclops
Guinea worm–variable in season, dependent on severity of rains.
Ghana, north: (Scott, 1969). south: (Belcher, et al., 1975).
Nigeria, southern (Kale, 1977)

Dependent on interruption of transmission of infections spread by aerosol
Neisseria meningitidis Abrupt fall with rains (Greenwood, 1999); see 'Dry season' below.

Dependent on easy transmission of micro-organisms in food/water/soil
Protozoa
Amoebiasis (Bray & Harris, 1977)
Bacteria
Vibrio cholerae. Outbreaks associated with rains: many reports, including –
Madagascar (Champetier de Ribes et al., 2000)
Nigeria, Ibadan (Lawoyin et al., 1999)
Tanzania (Mhalu et al., 1987)
Organisms responsible for gastroenteritis
Faecal coliforms. Gambia (Barrell & Rowland, 1979)
Helminths
Hookworm, Gambia (Knight & Merrett, 1981)

Dependent on flourishing of, or implantation of, micro-organisms on ? wet skin
Tropical ulcer
Nigeria, sudan savannah (Thomson, 1956, a classic paper by a hospital doctor)
Zambia, in children (Gernaat et al., 1998)
Zimbabwe (Tumwine et al., 1989)
Buruli ulcer
Uganda (Revill & Barker, 1972)

Infections – fungal
Gambia (Porter, 1980)
– Bacterial
Malawi (Kristensen, 1991)

Miscellaneous conditions or diseases
Acute glomerulonephritis, associated with infected scabies
Senegal (Dieng et al., 1998)
Ethiopia (Tewodros et al, 1992)
Cardiac failure. following hottest period of year, Nigeria, guinea savannah (Parry et al., 1977)
Blood pressure in puerperal women Nigeria, guinea savannah, (Davidson & Parry, 1978)

Flourishing of allergen
Nigeria, guinea savannah *Dermatophagoides,* house dust mite, provoking bronchial *Asthma.*
(Warrell et al., 1975); (Cookson & Makoni, 1975).

Nutritional deficiencies
Folic acid –
Tanzania – few fresh vegetables (Foster, 1968)
Gambia – (Bates et al., 1994)
Micronutrients – Gambia; vitamins A, C, riboflavin and folic acid (Bates et al., 1994)

Dry season
Easy transmission of micro-organisms
Bacterial
Anthrax Gambia (Heyworth et al., 1975)
Pneumococci Malawi, cold dry season (Gordon et al., 2001) including pneumococcal meningitis (Gordon et al., 2000),
Nigeria, guinea savannah colder dry season (Tugwell et al., 1976)
Meningococci Nigeria, guinea savannah, warmer dry season (Greenwood, 1999)

Viral
Measles

Lack of water/trauma
Pyoderma in farmers (end of dry season) (Belcher et al., 1977)
Snake bite in farmers (end of dry season/early rains) (Warrell & Arnett, 1976)

the Sudan prevents reproduction of snails of the *Biomphalaria* spp., and in the same way the high temperature of the coastal lowlands limits the distribution of *S. mansoni* infection in these areas. The reproductive activity of the snails, optimal around 25 °C, is also limited by cold, so that in Egypt during the winter, and in the cold season elsewhere, there are fewer snails to act as intermediate hosts so that the incidence of new infections falls.

During the rainy season in East Africa the breeding of snails decreases and there are fewer young snails; after the rains, however, the population of snails rises briskly and transmission increases.

The snail host discharges most cercariae at an optimal temperature of around 24 °C, and it is also at this temperature that the cercariae are most infective to man. At higher temperatures, and below 12 °C, they die. Transmission to humans is therefore more likely in warm weather than when it is very hot or cold.

Bacteria and viruses

Airborne infections

Meningococcal meningitis

The meningitis belt is the savannah country just south of the Sahara where the disease is endemic and large outbreaks occur every year towards the end of the dry season. When the rains begin, the number of cases drops abruptly, indicating that transmission of *N. meningitides* has stopped. The behaviour of this infection cannot be explained solely by overcrowding of people inside huts during the dry season (although this may be a factor in localized outbreaks in army barracks and other institutions) and is explained much better by the need of the organism for an ideal temperature and humidity.

Measles

Measles is epidemic during the dry season, particularly during the colder months: people move more at this season and children at hospital outpatients' departments are at particular risk.

Water-borne infections

Where pit latrines are close to wells, or night-soil contaminates drinking water, infections that spread from faeces are transmitted easily; for example, typhoid, poliomyelitis, hepatitis A and cholera. In many parts of Africa, the incidence of such water-borne diseases increases during the rains, but in other parts it increases at the end of the dry season because the few remaining sources of water are easily contaminated.

Direct contact through skin

Louse-borne relapsing fever

This is still endemic in the highlands of Ethiopia, where it is transmitted by the human body louse, *Pediculus humanus.* Although sporadic cases occur throughout the year, the peak of infection is during the rainy season, particularly July and August. The reason for this is not known, but it has been suggested that people crowd together during the rains and so are liable to crush infected lice on their bodies. This can be only part of the reason, because crowding is also intense during the cold nights of December and January. However, it is probable that the organism survives better when crushed on wet skin.

Endemic syphilis and tropical ulcer

Among the Peuls of Senegal and the Tuareg of Niger, the skin lesions of endemic syphilis become more numerous and florid in the rainy season, only to die down in the dry season. *Borrelia vincenti* is an important organism in tropical ulcer, which can also flare up during the rains.

Yaws

Yaws is no longer the scourge that it was in the hot and wet parts of Africa, for example, the south of Ghana: the lesions of those infected are worse during the rainy season.

People

Infections and contact with vectors or organisms

Although diseases may be limited by the direct effect of temperature and rainfall on organisms or vectors, contact between individuals and the vector or organism is also often governed by climate and the seasons, as mentioned earlier.

Other seasonal influences on health and disease

Just as anyone may be at risk of infections, which reach their peak during the rains, whether the farmer from infection in a wound, the newly weaned infant and the pregnant mother from malaria, or anyone from other infections which reach their peak during the dry season or the rains, the farmer is inevitably seasonally vulnerable to injury, from thorn or hoe, during the rains when work is heaviest; he is therefore caught in a vicious cycle. Some of the seasonal hazards to farmers and their families in the west African guinea savannah are shown in Fig. 2.28. This Figure is an example so that you can construct a similar diagram for your area, as a guide for clinical care and prevention in the community. If a detailed agricultural calendar is available also, it would be possible to study the relationship between health and disease and activity for both men and women (Fig. 2 29).

Births and deaths

In those areas where birth rate is highest during the rains, pregnant mothers and their babies are particularly vulnerable. In some places, deaths are more common during the rains. If a target group, for example, recently weaned children, is identified as vulnerable to a disease prevalent during a specific season, then special attention should be given to such a group when it is at high risk.

Health services

During the rains, health services can become less efficient, particularly as travel and supplies are more precarious.

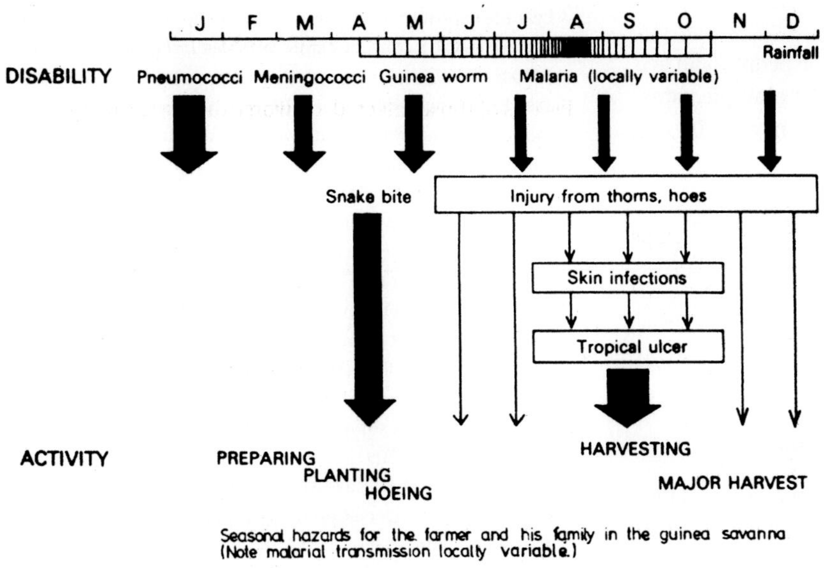

Fig. 2.28. Seasonal hazards and diseases in the guinea savannah of west Africa.

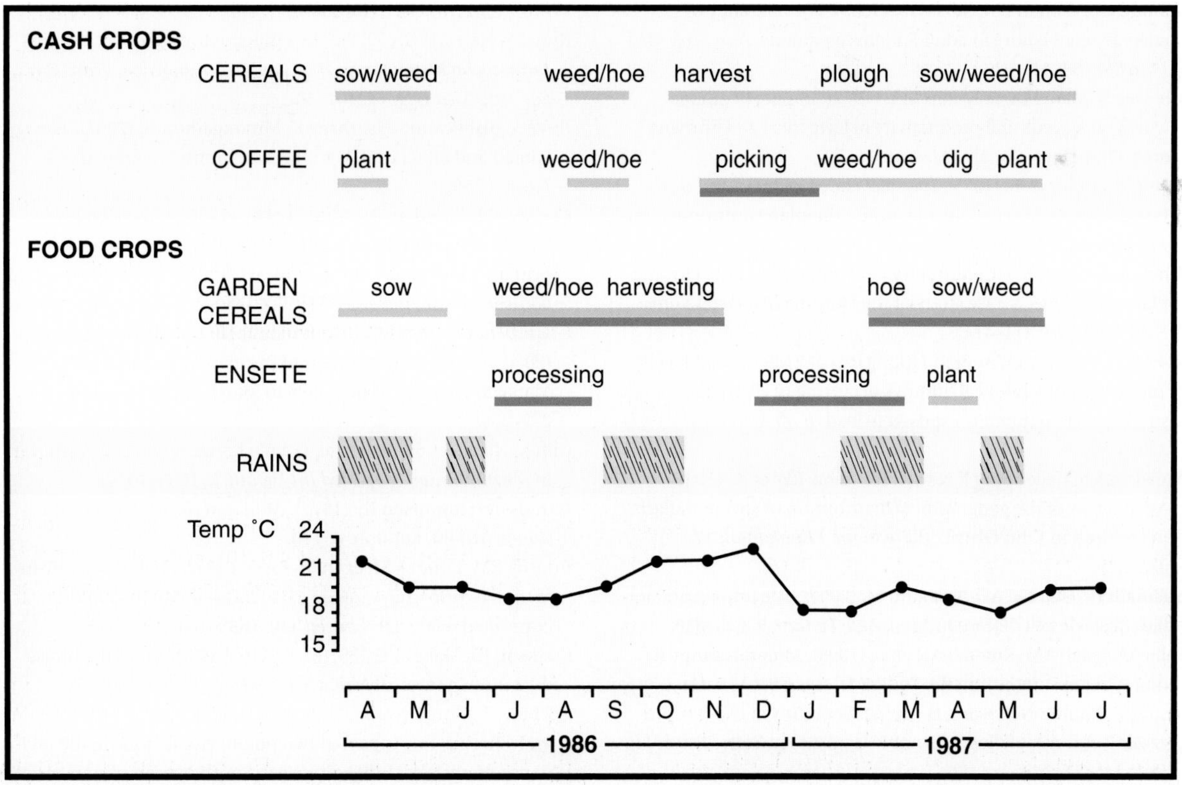

Fig. 2.29. An agricultural calendar to show the activities of men and women in a coffee growing area of southern Ethiopia. (Adapted from Ferro-Luzzi et al., 1990.) Men, blue bars; women, red bars.

Access to health care

If a home is far from a health facility, the people who live there are even further disadvantaged, for example, rains may cut paths so that they are unable to move an ill person.

- Provide an adequate supply of drugs during the rains for anyone from a remote place so that they do not lack what they need when travel becomes impossible because the roads and paths are cut or too muddy.

Travel, leisure, seasonal disease and accident

When farming stops in the dry season, people travel more and so can carry communicable diseases along the major highways. Road accidents are also more common in the hottest time of year when drivers become sleepy in the heat.

References

Abboud OL, Osman EM, Musa AR. (1989). The aetiology of chronic renal failure in adult Sudanese patients. *Ann Trop Med Parasitol*; **83**: 411–414.

Adewale B, Mafe MA, Sulyman MA. (1977). Impact of guinea worm on agricultural productivity in Owo local government area, Ondo State. *W. Afr J Med*; **16**: 75–79.

Alemu T, Lindtjorn B. (1995). Physical activity, illness and nutritional status among adults in a rural Ethiopian community. *Int J Epidemiol*; **24**: 977–983.

Amuyunzu M. (1997). Community perception regarding chronic filarial swellings: a case study of the Duruma of coastal Kenya. *E Afr Med J*; **74**: 411–414.

Ankrah NA, Kamiya Y, Appiah-Opong R et al. (1996). Lead levels and related biochemical findings occurring in Ghanaian subjects occupationally exposed to lead. *E Afr Med J*; **73**: 375–379.

Armstrong Schellenberg J, Newell JN, Snow RW et al. (1998). An analysis of the geographical distribution of severe malaria in children in Kilifi District, Kenya. *Int. J Epidemiol*; **27**: 323–329.

Assimadi JK, Gbadoe AD, Nyadanu M. (2000). The impact on families of sickle cell disease in Togo. *Arch Pediatr*; **7**: 615–620.

Balla AA, Salah AM, Khattab AH et al. (1998). Mineral composition of renal stones from the Sudan. *Urol Int*; **61**: 154–156.

Banea M, Poulter N, Rosling H. (1992). Shortcuts in cassava processing and risk of dietary cyanide exposure in Zaire. *Food Nutr Bull*; **14**: 137–143.

Banea-Mayambu J-P, Tilleskar T, Nahimana G et al. (1997). Geographical and seasonal association between linamarin and cyanide exposure from cassava and the upper motor neurone disease konzo in former Zaire. *Trop Med Intl Hlth*; **2**: 1143–1151.

Barrell RAE, Rowland MGM. (1979). The relationship between rainfall and well water pollution in a West African (Gambian) village. *J Hyg.,Camb*; **83**: 143–150.

Bates CJ, Prentice AM, Paul AA. (1994). Seasonal variations in vitamins A, C, riboflavin and folate intakes and status of pregnant and lactating women in a rural Gambian community: some possible implications. *Eur J Clin Nutr*; **48**: 660–668.

Belcher DW, Wurapa FK, Ward WB et al. (1975). Guinea worm in southern Ghana: its epidemiology and impact on agricultural productivity. *Am J Trop Med Hyg*; **24**: 243–249.

Belcher DW, Afoakwa SN, Osei-Tutu E et al. (1977). Endemic pyoderma in Ghana: a survey in rural villages. *Trans Roy Soc Trop Med Hyg*; **71**: 204–209.

Belew M, Kebede D, Kassaye M et al. (2000). The magnitude of khat use and its association with health, nutrition and socio-economic status. *Ethiop Med J*; **38**: 11–26.

Billington, WR (1968). The problem of the epileptic patient in Uganda. *E Afr Med J*; **45**: 563–569.

Binka FN, Adongo P. (1997). Acceptability and use of insecticide impregnated bednets in Northern Ghana. *Trop Med Intl Hlth*; **2**: 499–507.

Branca F, Pastore G, Demissie T et al. (1993). The nutritional impact of seasonality in children and adults of rural Ethiopia. *Eur J Clin Nutr*; **47**: 840–850.

Bray RS, Harris WG. (1977). The epidemiology of infection with *Entamoeba histolytica* in the Gambia, West Africa. *Trans Roy Soc Trop Med Hyg*; **71**: 401–407.

Buvé A, Bishikwabo-Nsarhaza K, Mutangadura G. (2002). The spread and effect of HIV-1 infection in sub-Saharan Africa. *Lancet*; **359**: 2011–2017.

Ceesay SM, Prentice AM, Cole TJ et al. (1997). Effects on birth-weight and perinatal mortality of food supplementation in a primary healthcare setting in rural Gambia: 5 year prospective controlled trial. *Br Med J*; **315**: 786–790.

Champetier de Ribes G, Rakotanjonabelo LA, Migliani R et al. (2000). One year assessment of the cholera epidemic in Madagascar, from March 1999 to March 2000. *Santé*; **10**: 277–286.

Cliff J., Nicala D, Sante F et al. (1997). Konzo associated with war in Mozambique. *Trop Med Int Health*; **2**: 1068–1074.

Cloudsley-Thompson JL. (1977). *Man and the Biology of Arid Zones*. Arnold, London. p. 118.

Conroy RM, Elmore-Meegan M, Joyce T et al. (1996). Solar disinfection of drinking water and diarrhoea in Maasai children: a controlled field trial. *Lancet*; **348**: 1695–1697.

Cookson JB, Makoni G. (1975). Seasonal asthma and the house dust mite in tropical Africa. *Clin Allergy*; **5**: 375–380.

Corbett EL, Churchyard GJ, Clayton TC et al. (2000). HIV infection and silicosis: the impact of two potent risk factors on the incidence of mycobacterial disease in South African miners. *AIDS*; **14**: 2759–2768.

Costrini AM, Pitt HA, Gustafson AB et al. (1979). Cardiovascular and metabolic manifestations of heatstroke and severe heat exhaustion. *Am J Med*; **66**: 296–302.

Dabis F, Ekpini ER. (2002). HIV1/AIDS and maternal and child health in Africa. *Lancet*; **359**: 2097–2104.

Davidson NMcD, Parry EHO. (1978). Peri-partum cardiac failure. *Quart J Med*; **47**: 431–461.

Demeke T, Kidane Y, Wuhib E. (1979). Ergotism: a report of an epidemic 1977/78. *Ethiop Med J*; **17**: 107–113.

Dieng MT, Ndiaye B, Ndiaye AM. (1998). Scabies complicated by acute glomerulonephritis in children: 114 cases observed in two years in a paediatric service in Daka. *Dakar Med*; **43**: 201–204.

Dumont A, de Bernis L, Bouvier-Colle M-H et al. (2001). Caesarean section rate maternal indication in sub-Saharan Africa: a systematic review. *Lancet*; **358**: 1328–1333.

Elebute EA. (1969). Evaporative fluid loss in adult Nigerian males. *Br J Surg*; **56**; 213–216.

Esterhuizen T, Hnidzo E, Rees D. (2001a). Occurrence and causes of occupational asthma in South Africa – results from SORDSA – a occupational asthma registry, 1997–1999. *S Afr Med J*; **91**: 509–513.

Esterhuizen T, Hnizdo E, Rees D et al. (2001b). Occupational respiratory diseases in South Africa – results from SORDSA, 1997–1999. *S Afr Med J*; **91**: 502–508.

Ferro-Luzzi A. (1990). Seasonal energy stress in marginally nourished rural women: interpretation and integrated conclusions of a multicentre study in three developing countries. *Eur J Clin Nutr*; **44**: 41–46.

Ferro-Luzzi A, Scaccini C, Tafesse S et al. (1990). Seasonal energy deficiency in Ethiopian rural women. *Eur J Clin Nutr*; **44**, 7–18.

Fevre EM, Coleman PG, Odiit M et al. (2001). The origins of a new *Trypanosoma brucei rhodesiense* sleeping sickness outbreak in eastern Uganda. *Lancet*; **358**: 625–628.

Ford, L, Abdullahi A, Anjorin FI et al. (1998). The outcome of peripartum cardiac failutre in Zaria, Nigeria. *QJ Med*; **91**: 93–103.

Foster RM. (1968). The seasonal incidence of megaloblastic anaemia at Mombasa. *E Afr Med J*; 45: 673–676.

Garnham PCC. (1945). Malaria epidemics at exceptionally high altitudes in Kenya. *Br Med J*; **ii**: 45–47.

Ferro-Luzzi A, Branca F, Pastore G. (1994). Body mass index defines the risk of seasonal energy stress in the Third World. *Europ. J. Clin. Nutr*; **48**: S165–S178.

Gernaat HB, Dechering WH, Voorhoeve HW. (1998). Clinical epidemiology of paediatric disease at Nchelenge, north-east Zambia. *Ann Trop Paediatr*; **18**: 129–138.

Getahun H, TekleHaimanot R. (1998). Psychosocial assessment of lathyrism patients in rural Estie district of South Gondar, northern Ethiopia. *Ethiop Med J*; **36**: 9–18.

Getahun H, Lambein F, Vanhoorne M, et al. (2002). Pattern and associated factors of the neurolathyrism epidemic in Ethiopia. *Trop Med Intl Hlth*; **7**: 118–124.

Ghebreyesus TA, Haile M, Witten KH et al. (1999). Incidence of malaria among children living near dams in Northern Ethiopia: community based incidence survey. *Br Med J*; **319**: 663–666.

Gill EL. (1991). *Seasonality and Agriculture in the Developing World*, Cambridge: Cambridge University Press, p. 99.

Gordon SB, Walsh AL, Chaponda M et al. (2000). Bacterial meningitis in Malawian adults: pneumococcal disease is common, severe and seasonal. *Clin Infect Dis*; **31**: 53–57.

Gordon MA, Walsh AL, Chapionda M et al. (2001). Bacteraemia and mortality among medical admissions in Malawi – predominance of non-typhi salmonellae and *Streptococcus pneumoniae*. *J Infect*; **42**: 44–49.

Greenwood BM. (1999). Meningococcal meningitis in Africa. *Trans Roy Soc Trop Med Hyg*; **93**: 341–353.

Gyapong M, Gyapong J, Weiss M et al. (2000). The burden of hydrocele on men in Northern Ghana. *Acta Trop*; **77**: 287–294.

Heyworth B, Ropp, ME, Voos UG et al. (1975). Anthrax in the Gambia. *Br Med J*; **3**: 79–82.

Howlett WP, Brubaker G, Mlingi N & Rosling H. (1992). A geographical cluster of Konzo in Tanzania. *J Trop Geog Neurol*; 2: 102–108.

Kale OO. (1977). The clinico-epidemiological profile of guinea-worm in the Ibadan district of Nigeria. *Am J Trop Med Hyg*; **26**: 208–214.

Khogali M, Weiner JS. (1980). Heatstroke: report on 18 cases. *Lancet*; **ii**; 276–278.

Kigutha HN, van Staveren WA, Wijnhoven TM et al. Maternal nutritional status may be stressed by seasonal fluctuations in food availability: evidence from rural women in Kenya. *Int J Food Sci Nutr*; **46**: 247–255.

Knight R, Merrett TG. (1981). Hookworm infection in rural Gambia: seasonal changes, morbidity and total IgE levels. *Ann Trop Med Parasitol*; **75**: 299–314.

Koram KA, Bennett S, Adiamah JH et al. (1995). Socio-economic risk factors for malaria in a peri-urban area of Gambia. *Trans Roy Soc Trop Med Hyg*; **89**: 146–150.

Kristensen JK. (1991). Scabies and pyoderma in Lilongwe, Malawi. Prevalence and seasonal fluctuation. *Int J Derm*; **30**: 699–702.

Latham MC. (1965). *Human Nutrition in Tropical Africa*, p. 249. Rome: FAO.

Lawoyin TO, Ogunbodede NA, Olumide EA et al. (1999). Outbreak of cholera in Ibadan, Nigeria. *Eur J Epidemiol*; **15**: 367–370.

Lawrence M, Coward WA, Lawrence F et al. (1987). Fat gain during pregnancy in rural African women: the effect of season and dietary status. *Am J Clin Nutr*; **45**: 1442–1450.

London L, Nell V, Thompson ML et al. (1998). Health status among farm workers in the Western Cape – collateral evidence from a study of occupational hazards. *S Afr Med J*; **88**: 1096–1101.

Lynch M, West SK, Munoz B et al. (1994). Testing a participatory strategy to change hygiene behaviour: face washing in central Tanzania. *Trans Roy Soc Trop Med Hyg*; **88**: 513–517.

Mhalu FS, Mntenga WM, Mtango FD. (1987). Seasonality of cholera in Tanzania: possible role of rainfall in disease transmission. *E Afr Med J*; **64**: 378–387.

Molyneux L, Gramiccia G. (1980). *The Garki Project*, pp. 231–490. WHO: Geneva.

Mukiibi JM. (1989). Megaloblastic anaemia in Zimbabwe, 1.Seasonal variation. *Cent Afr J Med*; **35**: 310–313.

Murdoch ME, Asuzu MC, Hagan M et al. (2002). Onchocerciasis: the clinical and epidemiological burden of skin disease in Africa. *Ann Trop Med Parasitol*; **96**: 283–296.

Murray J, Kielkowski D, Reid P. (1996). Occupational disease trends in Black South African Gold Miners. *Am J Respir Crit Care Med*; **153**: 706–710.

Needham DM, Foster SD, Tomlinson G et al. (2001). Socio-economic, gender and health services factors affecting diagnostic delay for tuberculosis patients in urban Zambia. *Trop Med Int Hlth*; **6**: 256–259.

Okonofua F. (2001). Optimising caesarean-section rates in West Africa. *Lancet*; **358**: 1289.

Oladepo O, Brieger WR, Otusanya S et al. (1997). Farm land size and onchocerciasis status of peasant farmers in south-western Nigeria. *Trop Med Int Hlth*; **2**: 334–340.

Parry, EHO, Davidson NMcD, Ladipo GOA et al. (1977). Seasonal variation of cardiac failure in northern Nigeria. *Lancet*; **1**: 1023–1025.

Pastore G, Branca F, Demissie T et al. (1993). Seasonal energy stress in an Ethiopian rural community: an analysis of the impact at the household level. *Eur J Clin Nutr*; **47**: 851–862.

Peters EJ, Esin RA, Immananagha KK et al. (1999). Lung function of some Nigerian men and women chronically exposed to fish drying using burning firewood. *Centr Afr J Med*; **45**: 119–123.

Platt BS. (1975). *Tables of Representative Foods Commonly Used in Tropical Countries*. London: HMSO.

Porter MJ. (1980). Seasonal change and its effect on the prevalence of infectious skin disease in a Gambian village. *Trans Roy Soc Trop Med Hyg*; **74**: 162–168.

Price EW. (1990). *Podoconiosis. Nonfilarial Elephantiasis*. Oxford: Oxford University Press.

Revill WDL. & Barker DJP. (1972). Seasonal distribution of mycobacterial skin ulcers. *Br J Prev Soc Med*; **26**: 23–27.

Sadikali F & Owor R. (1974). Hypothermia in the tropics. *Trop Geog Med*; **26**: 265–270.

Samuelsen H. (2001). Infusions of health: the popularity of vaccinations among Bissa in Burkina Faso. *Anthrop in Med*; **8**; 163–175.

Saungweme T, Khumalo H, Mvundura E et al. (1999). Iron and alcohol content of traditional beers in rural Zimbabwe. *Cent Afr J Med*; **45**: 136–140.

Scott D. (1969). An epidemiological note on guinea-worm infection in North-West Ashanti. *Ann Trop Med Parasit*; **50**: 32–43.

Scott JAG, Hall AJ, Muyodi C et al. (2000). Aetiology, outcome and risk factors for mortality among adults with acute pneumonia in Kenya. *Lancet*; **355**: 1225–1230.

Schellenberg JRMA, Abdulla S, Nathan R et al. (2001). Effect of large-scale marketing of insecticide-treated nets on child survival in rural Tanzania. *Lancet*; 357: 1241–1247.

Schultink JW, Klaver W, van Wijk H et al. (1990). Body weight changes and basal metabolic rates of rural Beninese women during seasons with different energy intakes. *Eur. J. Clin. Nutrit*; **44**: 31–40.

Schultink JW, van Raaij JMA, Hautvast JGAJ. (1993). Season weight loss and metabolic adaptation in rural Beninese women: the relationship with body mass index. *Br J Nutr*; **70**: 689–700.

Shkolnik A, Taylor RC, Finch V et al. (1980). Why do Bedouins wear hot robes in hot deserts? *Nature, Lond*; **283**: 373–375.

Tayeh A, Cairncross S. (1996). The impact of dracunculiasis on the nutritional status of children in South Kordofan, Sudan. *Ann Trop Paediatr*; **16**: 221–226.

Taylor RB, Shakoor O, Behrens RH et al. (2001). Pharmacopoeal quality of drugs supplied by Nigerian pharmacies. *Lancet*; **357**: 1933–1936.

Tewodros W, Muhe L, Daniel E et al. (1992). A one-year study of streptococcal infections and their complications among Ethiopian children. *Epidemiol Infect*; **109**: 211–225.

Theander TG. (1998). Unstable malaria in Sudan: the influence of the dry season. Malaria in areas of unstable and seasonal transmission. Lessons from Daraweesh. *Trans Roy Soc Trop Med Hyg*; **92**: 589–592.

Thomson IG (1956). The pathogenesis of tropical ulcer amongst the Hausas of Northern Nigeria. *Trans Roy Soc Trop Med Hyg*; **50**: 485–495.

Thomson MC, Elnaiem DA, Ashford DA et al. (1999). Towards a kala azar risk map for Sudan: mapping the potential distribition of *Phlebotomus orientalis* using digital data of environmental variables. *Trop Med Intl Hlth*; 4: 105–113.

Tugwell P, Greenwood BM, Warrell DA. (1976). Pneumococcal meningitis: a clinical and laboratory study. *Quart J Med*; **45**: 583–601.

Tumwine JK, Dungare PS, Tswana SA et al. (1989). Tropical ulcers in a remote area in Zimbabwe. *Centr Afr J Med*; **35**: 413–416.

Tylleskart T, Banea M, Bikangi N et al. (1991). Epidemiological evidence from Zaire for a dietary etiology of konzo, an upper motor neuron disease. *Bull Wld Hlth Org*; **69**: 581–589.

Venn AJ, Yemaneberhan H, Bekele Z et al. (2001). Increased risk of allergy associated with the use of kerosene fuel in the home. *Am J Respir Crit Care Med*; **164**: 1660–1664.

Von Schirnding YE, Fuggle RF, Bradshaw D. (1991). Factors associated with elevated blood lead levels in inner city Cape Town children. *S Afr Med J*; **79**: 454–456.

Warrell DA & Arnett C (1976). The importance of bites by the saw-scaled or carpet viper (*Echis carinatus*). Epidemiological studies in Nigeria and a review of the world literature. *Acta Tropica*; **33**: 307–341.

Warrell DA, Fawcett IW, Harrison BDW et al. (1975a). Bronchial asthma in the Nigerian Savanna region. *Quart J Med*; **44**: 325–347.

Warrell DA, Harrison BDW, Fawcett IW et al. (1975). Silicosis among grindstone cutters in the north of Nigeria. *Thorax*; **30**: 389–398.

Widler P, Mathys K, Brenneisen R et al. (1994). Pharmacodynamics and pharmacokinetics of Khat: controlled study. *Clin Pharmacol Ther*; **55**: 556–562.

Wiener JS, Khogali M. (1980). A physiological body cooling unit for the treatment of heatstroke. *Lancet*; **I**: 507–509.

Wolff CG, Schroeder DG, Young MW. (2001). Effect of improved housing on illness in children under 5 years old in Northern Malawi: cross sectional study. *Br Med J*; **322**: 1209–1212.

Workneh W, Fletcher M, Olwit G. (1993). Onchocerciasis in field workers at Baya Farm, Teppi Coffee Plantation Project, south-western Ethiopia: prevalence and impact on productivity. *Acta Trop*; **54**: 89–97.

Food and nutrition

3

Nutritional determinants of health – general principles

Nutrition is amongst the most powerful of the environmental factors influencing health and disease. As Africa passes through the demographic transitions of increasing wealth and urbanization the patterns of diet-related diseases are changing. Non-communicable diseases are overtaking infectious diseases as the leading causes of death and the role of nutrition has become even more crucial.

Recommended nutrient intakes

Nutritional requirements vary from individual to individual, and throughout the different stages of life. In the past these requirements have frequently been summarized in complex tables listing recommended daily allowances (RDAs) for each nutrient (more recently updated to 'dietary reference values' – DRVs). Such tables can still be found, but it is becoming more common to move from nutrient-based recommendations towards food-based dietary guidelines (FAO, 2000). These are often more appropriate in the clinical setting and are more readily adapted to public health messages, since people eat foods not nutrients. However, nutrient-based DRVs still form the basis of designing therapeutic diets, and vitamin and mineral supplementation protocols.

Food-based dietary guidelines vary from country to country but all contain the same basic principles of optimum nutrition. These stress the need for a balanced and varied diet of wholesome foods with only moderate intakes of fat (especially saturated fats), highly refined sugars, salt and alcohol. Most populations are encouraged to raise their intakes of fresh fruits, vegetables and whole-grain foods, and to moderate their intake of dairy products and red meat. In poor communities, and especially in young children, some of this advice, e.g. the low fat target, may need to be reversed in order to ensure an adequate energy and protein density in the diet. Graphical representations of food pyramids (such as in Fig. 3.1) are used frequently to explain the concept of a balanced diet to the general public.

Malnutrition modulates other diseases

Malnutrition and infection frequently create a vicious cycle in which each contributes to the other. This downward cycle can be difficult to break especially in the chronically malnourished child and in patients with 'wasting' diseases such as HIV, TB and cancers. Malnutrition affects the immune response (see Chapter 6) and other aspects of natural resistance to infection. At the same time, cytokine responses triggered by infections cause anorexia and tissue catabolism. Malnutrition in the host may also increase the pathogenicity of certain infections by allowing the propagation of mutated organisms which evade T-cell surveillance. There is evidence that this may be especially so in the case of deficiencies in anti-oxidant nutrients (see page 73) (Fig. 3.2).

Malnutrition is rarely a direct cause of death, but it is a major contributory cause (Rice et al., 2000, Tomkins, 2000). An analysis of hospital patients in The Gambia showed a progressive increase in case-fatality statistics with worsening nutritional status (Table 3.1) (Man et al., 1998). This relationship existed across most disease categories. An audit of case-fatality rates for severe malnutrition since the 1960s showed great divergence in different African hospitals ranging from 20–50 per cent (see Chapter 9) (Schofield & Ashworth, 1996).

In the high-pressure environment of the acute hospital adequate nutritional assessment is rare and aggressive nutritional therapy is given even more rarely. Several

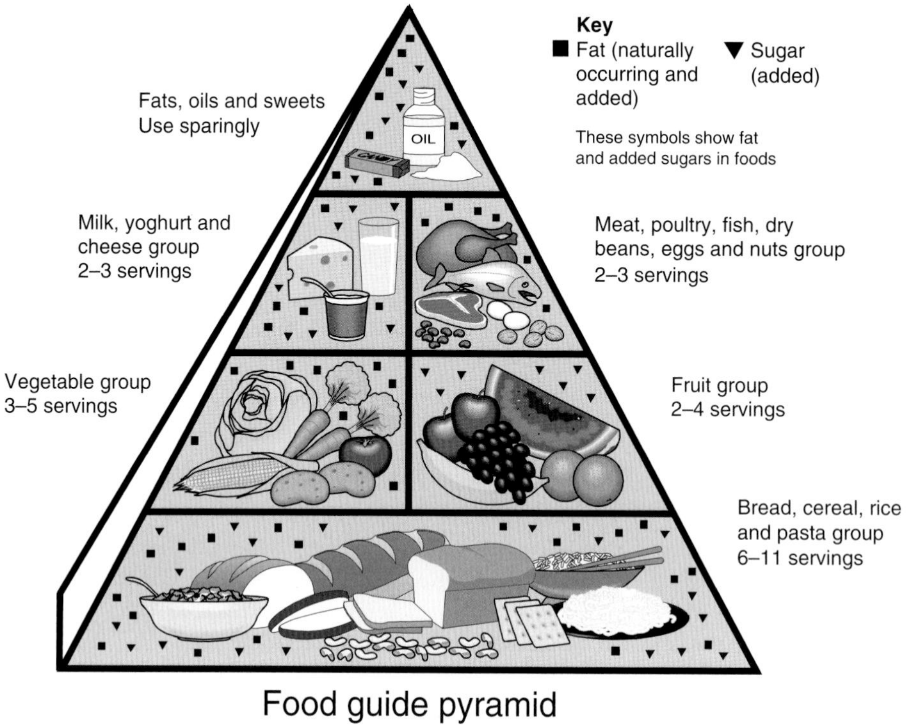

Fig. 3.1. Example of a food pyramid used to indicate the balance of good nutrition.

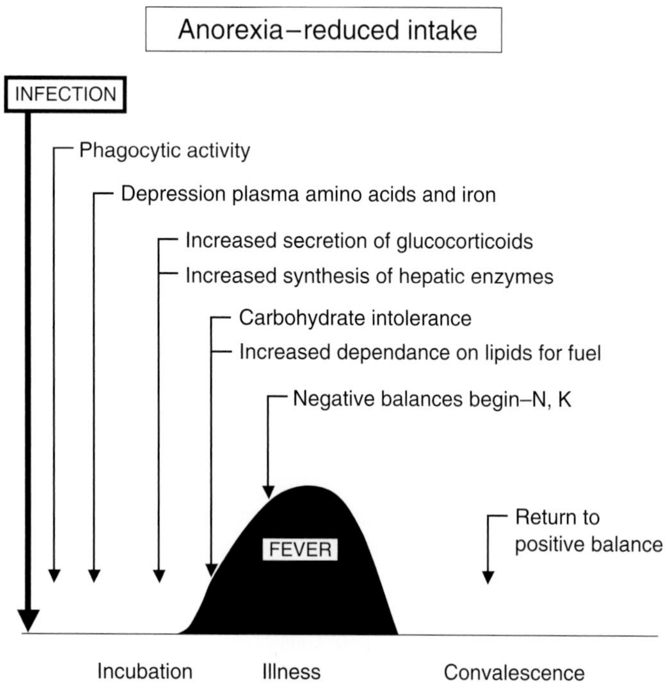

Fig. 3.2. Some metabolic consequences of a febrile infectious illness. (From Beisel, 1977.)

studies suggest that its importance has been undervalued. For example, mortality among elderly Swedish patients was halved virtually in a group randomly assigned to extra nutritional supplementation. Studies among African patients with chronic debilitating infections, especially TB, are required urgently.

At the other extreme of malnutrition – namely overnutrition – obesity is a major contributor to Type 2 diabetes and hypertension (see Chapter 69). The African Diaspora Study revealed that the degree of overweight of the different populations studied was by far the strongest determinant of diabetes and hypertension rates (see Fig 3.3 for diabetes) (Cooper et al., 1997). The emerging epidemic of obesity in urban areas will increase greatly the burden of diabetes in Africa (King et al., 1998).

Malnutrition and immunity

The efficiency of many aspects of immunity depends on adequate nutrition, but the exact details of the effects of malnutrition on immunity remain surprisingly controversial (Beisel, 1982). At the severe end of the spectrum there is no doubt that immunity is greatly compromised. Barrier defences are breached due to breakdown of epithelia. Cell-mediated immunity (which is very energy consuming) is especially depressed. Lymph glands and the thymus are atrophic in the severely malnourished child. There is little secretion of IgA, complement components are low and phagocytic activity is reduced (Golden 1995). Such changes almost certainly contribute to the increased mortality in malnourished children and adult patients with AIDS, TB and cancer.

At less extreme levels of malnutrition, the evidence is complicated by the fact that malnutrition and disease frequently co-exist, making it difficult to separate the immunosuppressive effects of each (Beisel, 1995; Morgan, 1997). Paradoxically, children with persistent gastroenteropathy tend to exhibit an inappropriately active inflammatory response. Likewise, it can be argued that certain marginal nutrient deficiencies (e.g. of iron, zinc or n-3 PUFAs) might be more harmful to certain pathogens than they are to the host. This remains an active area of research.

Essential nutrients

Energy

Energy (though not strictly a nutrient) lies at the heart of nutrition, since a person's energy needs drive hunger and hence their basic food needs. The need for energy therefore drives the consumption of all the other nutrients. Energy is also the only dietary component for which intake needs to be finely balanced with expenditure (the tissue utilization rate) in order to maintain a healthy physiological state, i.e. a constant body weight.

A dietary energy deficit must be met from body stores. In the short term (the meal-to-meal interval) energy is drawn from muscle and liver glycogen and from short-term fat stores. In the medium term adipose tissue buffers any dietary shortages and, in the longer term, muscle protein is also utilized (see below). Sustained energy deficits lead inevitably to wasting. This may arise from simple shortages of food as in famines or serious poverty, from incorrect child feeding practices, or from the anorexia of infections and illness. Children tend to be particularly vulnerable and, although the proportion of malnourished children has been falling in recent decades, the absolute number has been rising (Table 3.2) (de Onis et al., 2000). Classifications of childhood malnutrition are listed in Tables 3.11 and 3.12.

In adults the classification of 'chronic energy deficiency' (CED) is made according to the body mass index (BMI). This is calculated as weight in kilograms divided by the square of height in metres, i.e. kg/m^2, and gives a fairly robust measure of fatness across people of different heights. The accepted cut-off for defining adult CED is a BMI $<18.5\ kg/m^2$: below this people have a reduced work capacity and an increased likelihood of illness (see Fig. 3.4) (Shetty & James, 1994).

Table 3.1. Influence of nutritional status on case-fatality rates in two West African hospitals

Weight-for-age (Z-score)	Proportion of admissions (%)	Case-fatality rate (%)
Better than −2	54	7.2
−2 to −3	24	9.3
−3 to −4	13	15.6
Worse than −4	9	22.7

Source: Results from 13 579 children <5 years of age (from Man et al., 1998).

Table 3.2. Percentage and absolute number of underweight children under 5 years of age in Africa

Year	Percentage underweight	Total number underweight (millions)
1975	30.4	22.9
1990	27.3	31.6
1995	27.0	34.8

Source: WHO (1995).

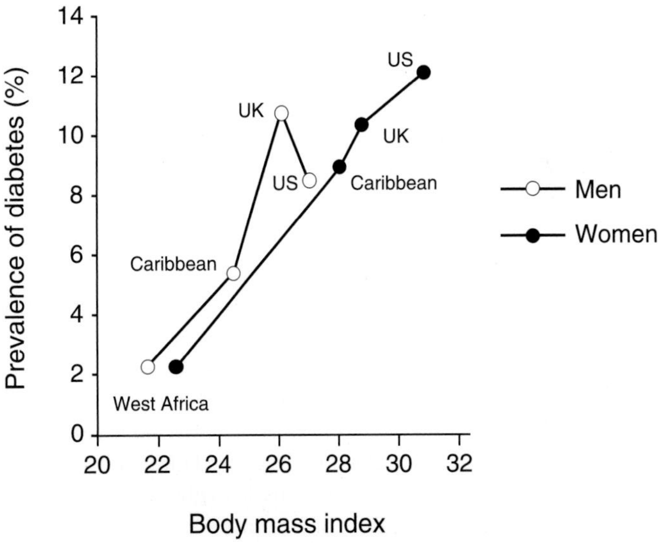

Fig. 3.3. Obesity strongly predicts Type-2 diabetes and hypertension rates. (From Cooper et al., 1997.)

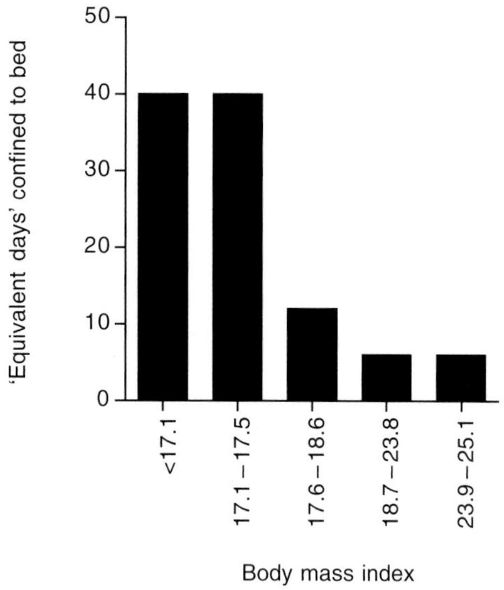

Fig. 3.4. Body mass index and 'equivalent days' illness among Rwandese women. (From Shetty & James, 1994.)

Table 3.3. WHO classification of obesity according to body mass index

Body mass index (kg/m^2)	Classification
<18.5	Underweight
18.5 – 25.0	Normal
25.1 – 30.0	Overweight
>30.0	**Obese**
30.0 – 34.9	Grade I obese
35.0 – 39.9	Grade II obese
>40.0	Grade III obese

Source: International Obesity Task Force (www.iotf.org).

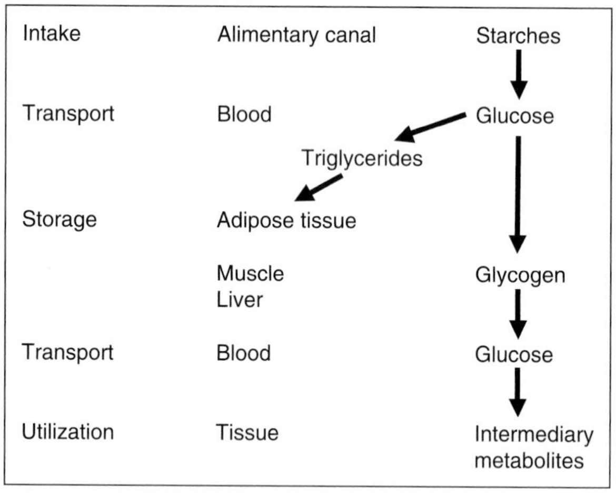

Fig. 3.5. Utilization of carbohydrates. (Adapted with permission from Davidson et al., 1972.)

At the opposite end of the spectrum, the temptations of energy-dense and highly palatable foods, and of a sedentary lifestyle, frequently undermine nature's regulatory systems controlling appetite and energy balance. The result is a progressive accumulation of body fat leading to obesity. The WHO classification system for obesity is shown in Table 3.3 (WHO, 1998).

Carbohydrates

Most of the energy in all diets is provided by carbohydrates, which yield 17.6 joules per gram on combustion: in poor areas of Africa the proportion of energy derived from carbohydrates is 70–80 per cent; in richer areas it may drop to 40–50 per cent due to a greater consumption of fats and oils. The carbohydrate in food is digested by amylase, sucrase, maltase and lactase and is absorbed from the small intestine as monosaccharides. Indigestible cellulose passes on to provide bulk to the stool. Glucose transported in the blood is either used directly by the tissues or stored in liver or muscle as glycogen. It is now known that the amount of fat converted from carbohydrate is extremely low.

Normally, the brain uses glucose for its energy, consuming about 60 per cent of the total circulating glucose supply. However, in prolonged starvation, it is able to use ketones, particularly β-hydroxybutyric acid, which are derived from fats. During light or moderate exercise, glucose or glycogen is oxidized aerobically in muscle to generate energy, which is utilized in the form of high energy phosphate bonds contained in creatine phosphate and adenosine triphosphate (ATP). In severe exercise, when an oxygen debt is incurred, glucose is oxidized anaerobically to lactic acid which later, when oxygen is available, is synthesized to glycogen in the liver (Fig. 3.5).

Insulin increases the rate of uptake of glucose by cells – especially those of muscle and adipose tissue. Cortisol and growth hormone have the opposite effect. The clinically important disturbances of carbohydrate utilization and metabolism are summarized in Table 3.4.

Fats

Fats are a concentrated source of energy yielding 39 joules per gram on complete combustion. Fats occur chiefly in the form of triglycerides. In general, those derived from plant sources are unsaturated, i.e. contain double bonds, and those from animals are saturated. Long-chain polyunsaturated fatty acids (PUFAs) are also essential for health. and are discussed on page 62.

Table 3.4. Clinically significant disturbances in carbohydrate metabolism

Malabsorption	Congenital lactase deficiency
	Acquired lactase deficiency
	Infections of gut
	Persistent gastroenteropathy
	Kwashiorkor
Disturbed metabolism – hypoglycaemia	**Inadequate stores**
	Marasmus
	Kwashiorkor
	Liver damage
	Severe hepatitis
	Severe septicaemia
	Toxins
	Alcohol
	Some herbal drinks
	Drugs
	Insulin
	Chlorpropamide
	Cerebral malaria
Disturbed metabolism – hyperglycaemia	**Hormonal**
	Diabetes (insulin resistance)
	Excess corticosteroids

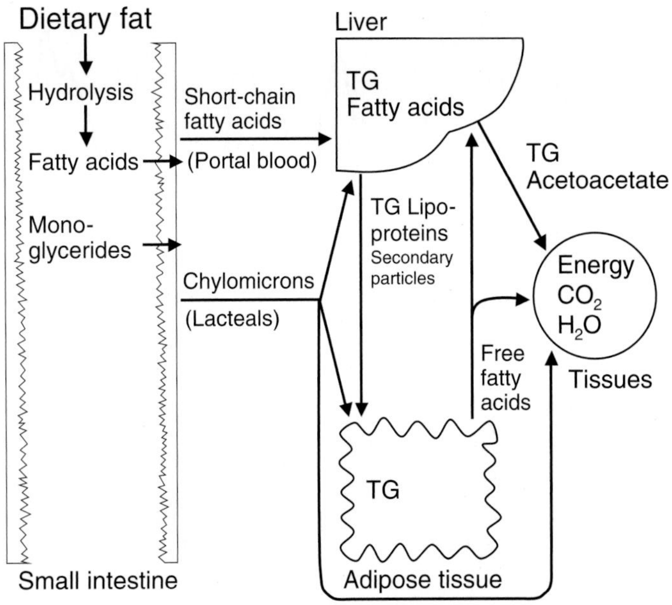

Fig. 3.6. Metabolism of fats. TG = trigycerides. (Adapted with permission from Davidson et al., 1972.)

Dietary fats are emulsified and partially hydrolysed in the small intestine. With the aid of bile salts they are absorbed by the mucosa in the form of micelles rich in monoglycerides. Short-chain fatty acids are transported to the liver in the portal blood. Long-chain fatty acids are synthesized to triglycerides, coated with protein, cholesterol, and phospholipid, and transported as chylomicrons in the lacteals, mainly to the liver and adipose tissue (Fig. 3.6).

In the liver the triglycerides from the chylomicrons are broken down to fatty acids. New triglycerides are resynthesized using, in part, fatty acids derived from adipose tissue which have been transported to the liver, bound to plasma albumin in the blood. These triglycerides leave the liver as very low density lipoproteins (VLDL). The lipoproteins consist of varying amounts of triglyceride, cholesterol, and phospholipid. Sedentary people, whose food is rich in animal fats or who eat much carbohydrate, tend to have high cholesterol levels in the form of the more damaging low-density lipoproteins (LDL) and low concentrations of the cardio-protective high-density lipoproteins (HDL).

When energy balance is negative, fat deposits are depleted by the action of noradrenaline and growth hormone, which stimulate hormone sensitive lipase in the adipocytes. Free fatty acids (FFA) and triglycerides are oxidized in the liver to acetoacetic acid, which is then used for energy by the other tissues. FFA are also used directly by skeletal or heart muscle. In times of plenty, triglycerides are stored in adipose tissue, a process requiring insulin. In poor societies (for instance, those with seasonal food shortages – see Fig. 3.7) adipose tissue acts as an essential buffer against starvation. However, in modern societies obesity has now become a major health problem because the excess adipose tissue (especially when stored in the abdominal cavity and in the intramuscular space) causes profound metabolic disturbances characterized as the 'cardiovascular metabolic syndrome'. This is a cluster of conditions including insulin resistance, secondary hyperinsulinaemia, hypertriglyceridaemia and hypertension (Pi-Sunyer, 1993).

The clinically important disturbances of fat utilization and metabolism are summarized in Table 3.5.

Proteins

Proteins are an essential food providing the amino acids used to synthesize enzymes, hormones, plasma proteins and milk, and to build the tissue cells which are constantly being renewed. During starvation, amino acids are used also to maintain blood glucose levels through gluconeogenesis, a process under the influence of adrenocortical hormones (Fig. 3.8). The use of protein in this way, although acting as an effective short-term adaptation, in the longer term leads to a decrease in muscle mass and damage to vital organs – as in the case of marasmus, cancer cachexia and the wasting of AIDS.

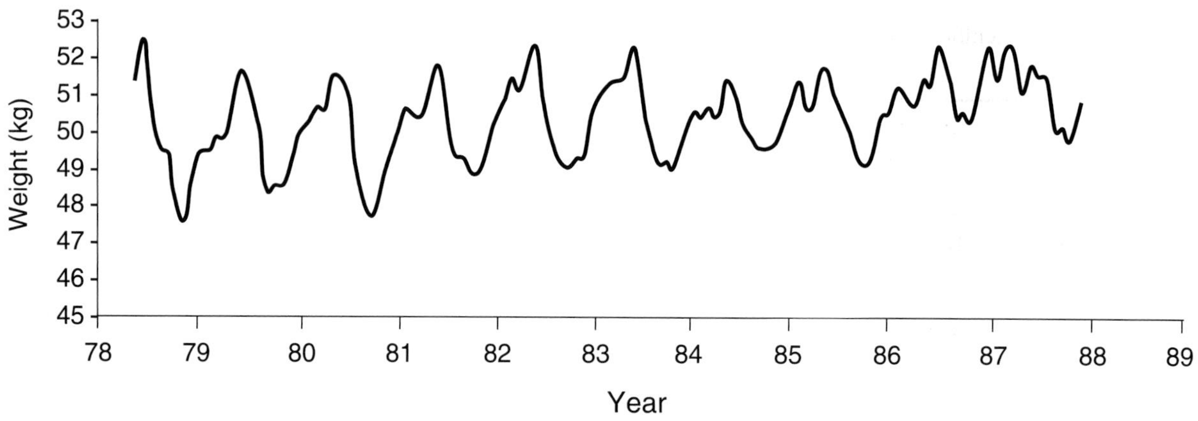

Fig. 3.7. Body weight changes in Gambian women caused by annual 'hungry' and 'harvest' seasons. (From Cole, 1993.)

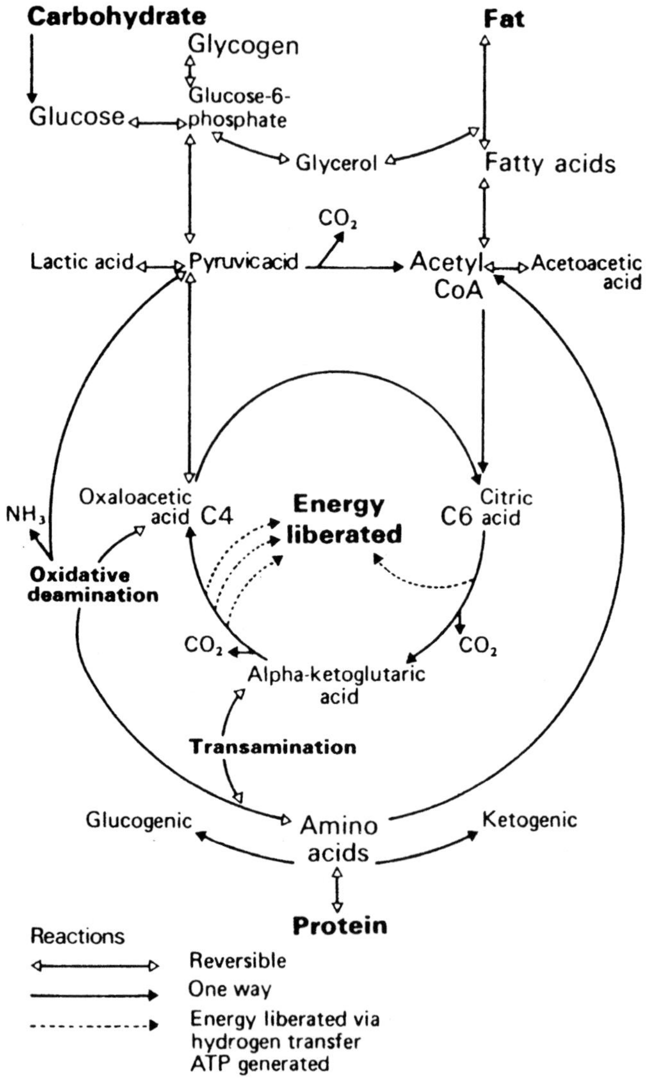

Fig. 3.8. Intermediary metabolism.

Dietary proteins are hydrolysed to polypeptides and amino acids and then absorbed from the small intestine to be circulated via the portal system. The turnover of proteins is reflected in the plasma amino acid pattern and the urinary excretion of nitrogen. If protein intake is reduced, urinary nitrogen excretion falls. After the first few days of starvation, the body adjusts to this state by using a larger proportion of available nitrogen for protein synthesis and by excreting a smaller amount. The liver cells have a limited ability to convert one amino acid to another; those that cannot be made must be found in food and so are termed essential amino acids.

The quality of dietary proteins differs and is measured by their ability to promote the growth of animals. Animal protein, which has a similar amino acid composition to human tissue, is high-quality, or first-class, protein. The most easily digestible form is milk, which thus has a high net protein utilization index (NPU = biological value, i.e. quality × digestibility). Plant proteins vary in digestibility and quality: some, such as zein, which is found in certain varieties of maize, lack essential amino acids. However, mixtures of plant proteins may supplement each other and thus provide high quality protein. The minimum protein concentration of diets compatible with good health and growth is around 5–6 per cent energy. Infants, malnourished children and lactating women require about 6–8 per cent protein in the diet. Table 3.6 lists the utilizable protein contents of various staple foods commonly eaten in Africa. Many of these have almost adequate protein content even if consumed with very little additional protein from animal sources, pulses or nuts. Therefore, primary protein deficiency usually only occurs in areas of very monotonous diets based on matoke (plantain) or cassava.

The clinically important disturbances of protein utilization and metabolism are summarized in Table 3.7.

Table 3.5. Clinically significant disturbances in fat metabolism

Excess	**Obesity**
	Hypertriglyceridaemia
	Insulin resistance (hyperinsulinaemia)
	Hypertension
Inadequate stores	**Dietary**
	Starvation
	Marasmus
	Malabsorption
	Infections of the gut
	Giardia
	Strongyloides
	Others secondary to HIV
	Bile salt deficiency
	Obstructive jaundice
	Gall bladder disease
	Bacterial overgrowth
	Pancreatic damage
	Pancreatitis
	Kwashiorkor
	Congenital
	Lipodystrophy (rare)
Disturbed metabolism	**Fatty liver**
	Kwashiorkor
	Alcoholism

Table 3.6. Utilizable protein expressed as a percentage of the total energy in African staples

Staple	Protein (expressed as % energy)
Grains	%
Maize	4.7
Rice	4.9
Millet	5.3
Wheat	5.9
Roots/fruits	
Cassava	0.9
Plantain	1.6
Yam	4.6

Table 3.7. Disturbances of protein utilization and metabolism

Inadequate stores	Starvation
	Marasmus
	Kwashiorkor
Malabsorption	Pancreatic disease
	Kwashiorkor
Increased catabolism	Infections
	Tumours
Inadequate synthesis	Cirrhosis of liver
	Diabetes
Increased loss	Nephrotic syndrome
	Severe infections of the gut
	Measles
	Amoebiasis
	Bacillary dysentery
	Burns and exudates

Minerals

Minerals in the body have many functions: bone contains the greatest amounts, but all body tissues and fluids contain minerals, which have specialist functions in coenzymes, hormones, and vitamins. In practice, most minerals are available in adequate amounts from a balanced diet. However, many diets in rural Africa are very low in meats, fish, eggs and dairy products. As a consequence they are low in iron (and to a lesser extent zinc) and very low in calcium (see below). The minerals iodide, fluoride and selenium enter the diet through uptake into plants and in the water supply. Intake levels are highly dependent on local soil and rock conditions. Deficiencies in these minerals therefore affect many people in deficient areas and few people elsewhere (Table 3.8). They can be combated by a number of interventions ranging from fortification of essential foodstuffs (e.g. iodization of salt) or the water supply (fluoridation) to supplemented oil drops or injection. Iron and iodine are considered the most damaging causes of micronutrient deficiencies world-wide (along with vitamin A) and are the subject of massive global efforts to eliminate 'hidden hunger' (Micronutrient Initiative, 2002). Much progress has been made especially with iodine and vitamin A.

In certain diseases such as kwashiorkor and chronic diarrhoea a deficiency of potassium and magnesium occurs, and in cardiac and renal disease the regulation of sodium intake and excretion is often compromised.

Vitamins

Minute amounts of these organic substances are vital for life but, with the exception of vitamin D, they are not synthesized by the body and so must be obtained from the diet. They do not enter into the tissue structure and are not degraded for energy, but play a part in metabolic reactions as regulators, e.g. vitamin D regulates calcium absorption, intermediary reactants, e.g. tetrahydrofolate – derived from folic acid acts as a methyl group carrier, or

Table 3.8. Variable prevalence of goitre and urinary iodine levels in different regions of two African countries

	Goitre prevalence	
Shoa region, Ethiopia	**Men**	**Women**
Chebon-Gurage	25	39
Merhabete	39	60
Selale	12	21
Kembatana-Hadya	27	51
Tegultna-Bulga	16	28
Yifatna-Timuga	28	42
Menzena-Gishe	36	52
	Median urinary iodine levels (μg/dl)	
Gambia		
Banjul/Kanifing	7.4	
Western Division	3.6	
North Bank Division	4.8	
Lower River Division	2.8	
Central River Division	6.9	
Upper River Division	3.2	

Sources: Wolde-Gebriel et al. (1992). *Micronutrient deficiencies in Ethiopia and their inter-relationships,* University of Wageningen; Gambian National Nutrition Agency (2001). *Consultancy Report on Iodine Deficiency Disorders Survey in The Gambia.*

cofactors of enzyme systems, e.g. riboflavin is required by all flavoproteins. The vitamins are divided into two groups: the fat-soluble – vitamins A, D, E, and K; and the water-soluble – vitamins C and those of the B complex (Table 3.9).

Vitamin and mineral deficiencies tend to occur together in people on poor monotonous diets, in emergencies, or when food intake is suppressed through illness. Certain other general predictions can be made about the likelihood of encountering vitamin deficiencies in clinical practice in Africa. Mild vitamin A deficiency is common across Africa but severe deficiency with clinical eye signs is less common. Moderate riboflavin deficiency is almost universal amongst populations consuming little dairy produce. Mild to moderate deficiencies of other B vitamins occur, but severe deficiencies are rare and usually attributable to special circumstances (e.g. famine or prison rations). Folate deficiency is rare where fresh green leaves are consumed. Vitamin C deficiency tends to be highly seasonal in many areas and is rare when fruits and vegetables are abundant. Vitamin D deficiency is rare except amongst infants and young children kept indoors. For further details (see p. 68).

Table 3.9. Vitamins essential to life and their dietary sources

Vitamin	
Fat-soluble	
Vitamin A	Liver, fish-liver oils, egg yolk, milk and dairy products, green leafy vegetables (especially kale, amaranth, sweet potato, cowpea and cassava leaves), yellow- and orange-coloured fruits and vegetables (carrots, pumpkin, mango, papaya, oranges), orange-coloured sweet potato, palm oil
Vitamin D	Cod-liver oil, oily fish, liver, egg yolk
Vitamin E	Vegetable oils (such as maize, soybean and sunflower oils), nuts, soybeans, cereals, egg yolk
Vitamin K	Green leafy vegetables, vegetable oils, egg yolk, beef, mutton, poultry
Water-soluble	
Thiamine (vitamin B_1)	Millets, sorghum, wheat, maize, dried beans, rice, liver, kidney, beet, nuts
Riboflavin (vitamin B_2)	Green leafy vegetables, liver, kidney, milk, cheese, eggs, whole grains
Niacin (nicotinic acid)	Lean meat, poultry, fish, groundnuts, dried beans, wheat, yam, potato
Pantothenic acid	Kidney, fish, egg yolk, most vegetables, most cereals
Pyridoxine (vitamin B_6)	Meat, poultry, fish, egg yolk, whole grains, banana, potato, dried beans, lentils, chickpeas
Biotin	Groundnuts, dried beans, egg yolk, mushrooms, banana, grapefruit, watermelon
Folic acid	Green leafy vegetables (losses from cooking can be high), fresh fruits (especially orange juice), dried beans, peas, nuts, egg yolk, mushrooms, banana, liver
Vitamin B_{12}	Liver, kidney, chicken, beef, fish, eggs, milk, cheese
Vitamin C	Citrus fruits, guava, baobab, mango, papaya, green leafy vegetables, green chili, potato, green peppers, tomatoes

A life-cycle approach to optimal nutrition

It is useful for the physician and dietician to consider the various phases of life at which people have special nutritional needs. This life-cycle approach is taken below. From the moment of conception these phases are linked and each affects the next stage of development in a continuous loop of cause and consequence.

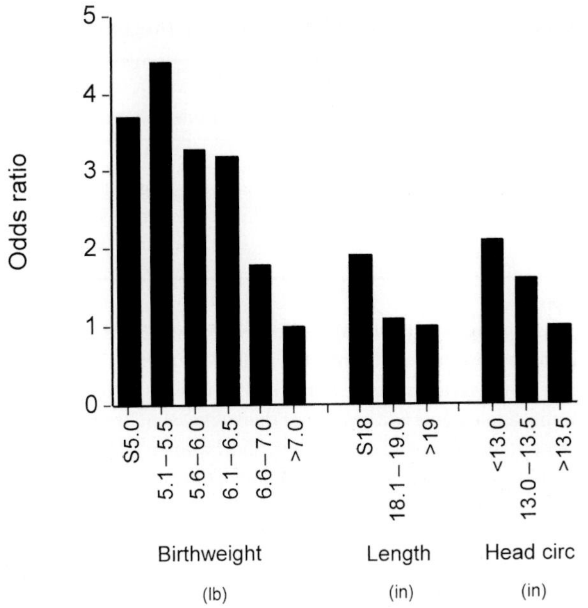

Fig. 3.9. Fetal growth and coronary heart disease in South India. Odds ratios show the risk of heart disease in adults over 45 years in Mysore, India. (Drawn from Stein et al., 1996.)

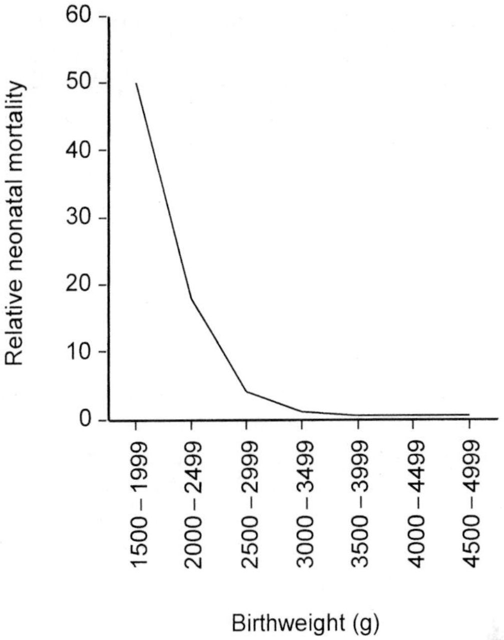

Fig. 3.10. Relationship between birth weight and neonatal mortality. Data are aggregated across the world. Absolute levels of neonatal mortality vary greatly but the proportional effect of low birthweight is very similar. (Drawn from Ashworth & Feachem, 1985.)

Recent discoveries about the 'fetal and infant origins of diseases' have underscored this point by showing that even a short period of undernutrition in utero (leading to low birthweight) can have a major impact on a person's chronic disease risk up to 80 years later (Barker, 1998). Most data in support of this theory comes from European studies but emerging Indian data (Fig. 3.9) supports the concept (Yajnik, 2001). It is proposed that intra-uterine growth retardation causes metabolism to adapt to expect a frugal diet (the so-called 'thrifty phenotype'). This adaptation causes people to become doubly prone to chronic diseases if they migrate towards a better nutritional setting such as is now very common in Africa with rural-to-urban drift.

Importantly, a woman's own birthweight predicts the size of the babies she herself produces, therefore creating an inter-generational cycle of malnutrition, which takes several generations to overcome fully. It is because of these long-term consequences that the nutrition of the pregnant and nursing mother requires special attention.

Fetal growth and the nutritional needs of pregnant women (see also Chapter 87 on Pregnancy)

Nutrition of the fetus is vital to its immediate survival as well as to the lifelong consequences described above.

Low birthweight is strongly predictive of neonatal and even post-neonatal mortality in all populations (Ashworth & Feachem, 1985). The left-hand side of the birthweight mortality curve shown in Fig. 3.10 is extremely steep. A consequence of this is that any interventions (e.g. malaria and anaemia control, dietary supplementation) that can raise the mean birthweight of a population by even as little as 100 g, can have a major impact on neonatal mortality. It should also be noted from Fig. 3.10 that there is a negligible rise in neonatal mortality (e.g. from obstructed labour) until babies are very large. This evidence can be used to combat the 'eating down' syndrome prevalent in some areas of Africa.

The fetus used to be considered a 'perfect parasite' that could extract whatever nutrition it required from the mother without harming her, and was protected by the mother from any external influences. This is a misleading view. Fetal growth is influenced by many factors including infections, smoking, altitude, placental function and nutrition (see Fig. 3.11) (Kramer, 1987).

Nutritional effects on fetal growth

Nutritional effects on fetal growth are both short and long term. In the long term a woman's adult body size is a strong predictor of the size of her babies since the uterine environment constrains growth in small mothers. This is the major reason that many south Asian countries have low-birthweight rates (defined by WHO as babies <2500 g) approaching 50 per cent. In most rural African populations mothers are taller and heavier than in Asia and rates of low birthweight rarely exceed 25 per cent. In affluent urban areas low-birthweight rates are generally lower.

In the short term a mother's energy balance also affects fetal growth. This is most easily judged by her rate of weight gain in pregnancy. Optimal rates of weight gain in affluent populations are recommended to be about 12.5 kg over a full pregnancy (~1.5 kg per month). In America, the Institute of Medicine recommends different optimal rates of weight gain according to women's nutritional status at conception (see Table 3.10) (IOM 1992). According to these, the optimal fetal outcome is achieved when thin women gain more that 12.5 kg and when fat women gain less. No such data are available for Africa but there is no reason to believe that these recommendations should not hold. In practice, however, most rural women gain less than 10 kg and it is often unrealistic to expect greatly enhanced values. In overweight urban women pregnancy represents a risk period for further weight gain, and such women should be encouraged not to gain more than 1 kg per month. Gains greater than this may precipitate gestational diabetes and pregnancy-induced hypertension in addition to contributing to their obesity.

Table 3.10. Recommended weight gain in pregnancy

Pre-pregnancy weight-for-height (kg/m^2)	Recommended total gain (kg)
Low (<19.8)	12.5 – 18.0
Normal (19.8 to 26.0)	11.5 – 16.0
High (>26.0 to 29.0)	7.0 – 11.5
Obese (>29.0)	≤7.0

Notes:
These recommendations where derived for the US but are considered widely applicable. They refer to singleton pregnancies. The range for women carrying twins is 16 to 20 kg. Young adolescents (<2 years after menarche) should strive for gains at the upper end of the range. Short women (<157 cm) should strive for gains at the lower end of the range.
Source: From Institute of Medicine. (1992).

Nutritional needs of pregnancy

According to WHO/FAO calculations a woman only needs to increase her normal energy intake by 10 per cent during pregnancy. This is because the human fetus grows exceptionally slowly compared to other mammals (an evolutionary adaptation that allows the complex brain time to

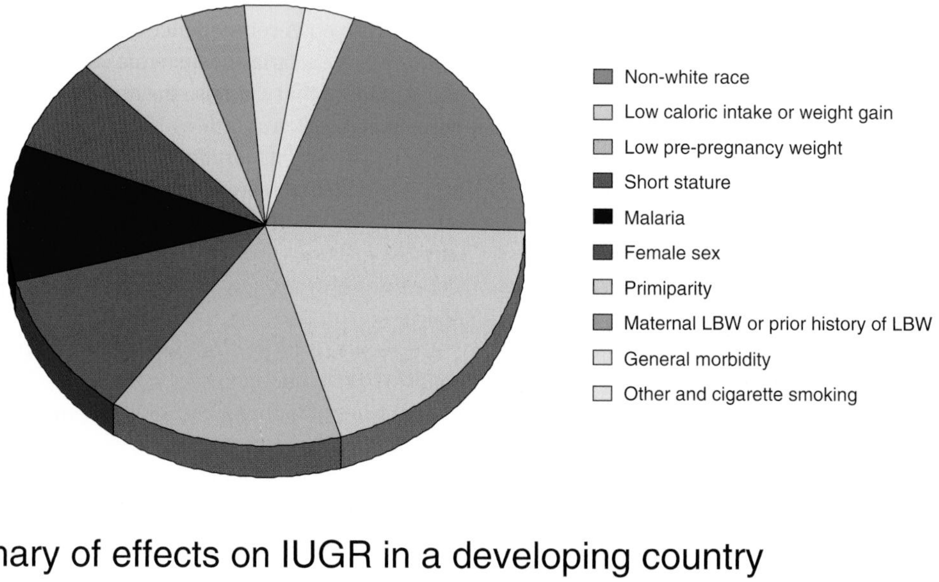

Fig. 3.11. Determinants of low birthweight in developing countries. (From Kramer, 1987.)

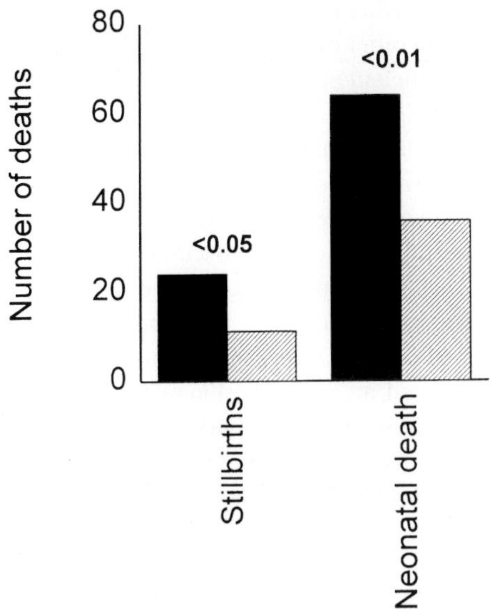

Fig. 3.12. Effect of maternal dietary supplementation on stillbirths and perinatal mortality. Solid bars = unsupplemented, hatched bars = supplemented. (From Ceesay et al., 1997.)

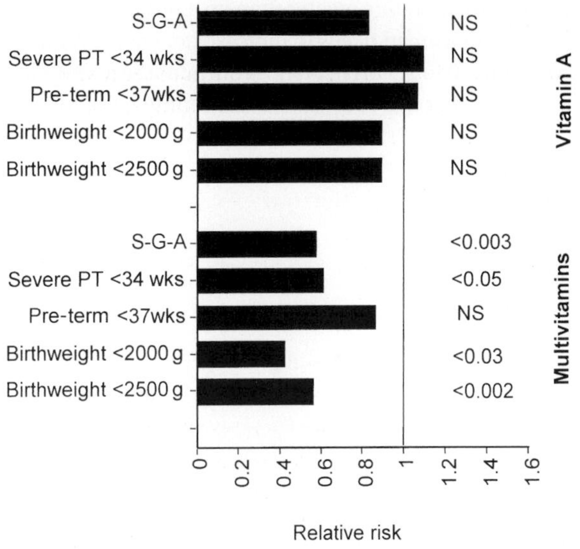

Fig. 3.13. Effect of vitamin A and multivitamin supplementation on low birthweight and prematurity (SGA = small for gestational age: PT = preterm). (From Fawzi et al., 1998.)

develop). Detailed studies with metabolic chambers in The Gambia have shown that under-nourished women have remarkable mechanisms for saving energy in order to support a relatively normal pregnancy when food is short (Poppitt et al., 1993). They also lay down less fat. The existence of these energy-sparing mechanisms helps to explain the remarkable success of human reproduction in poor societies, but should not be used as an excuse to condone poor diets in pregnant women.

The additional protein, vitamin and mineral requirements in pregnancy are also surprisingly small and can usually be considered to be met so long as a woman is gaining weight adequately and eating a well-balanced diet. Exceptions to this general rule occur in the case of women who are simultaneously pregnant and lactating, and in adolescent pregnancies when the mother's own body tissues have not yet fully matured.

Dietary supplements in pregnancy

Community-wide dietary supplementation of poor rural women has been shown to enhance birthweight significantly in Gambian women, especially during the annual hungry season (Fig. 3.12) (Ceesay et al., 1997). The balanced protein–energy supplement consisted of groundnut-based biscuits and was distributed to women in the second and third trimesters by their traditional village birth attendants. The supplement also significantly reduced the number of stillbirths and perinatal mortality, demonstrating that such interventions could be effective if they can be delivered within a health system (Kramer, 2000).

In HIV-positive women in Kenya a micronutrient supplementation trial (without extra energy and protein) also caused a significant reduction in the number of small-for-gestational-age (SGA) babies (see Fig. 3.13) (Fawzi et al., 1998). World-wide there are several trials being undertaken to test whether multiple micronutrient supplementation would have wider benefits in other groups of women.

The intention of such community-based intervention programmes should be to prevent fetal growth retardation rather than to augment fetal growth that is already adequate. To be effective they need to be targeted carefully at populations where there is a genuine problem with low birthweight and with evidence of inadequate pregnancy weight gains in the mothers. Under these circumstances the theoretical concern about inducing cephalopelvic disproportion (CPD) can be discounted. Figure 3.10 confirms that babies have to be extremely large before CPD becomes an issue.

Lactation

The nutritional requirements of an infant are greater than those of a fetus. The stresses on a lactating mother are therefore greater than on a pregnant mother. A lactating woman needs to increase her energy intake by about 2.0 to 2.5 MJ per day – equivalent to about 20–25 per cent of her usual intake. Assuming that this is

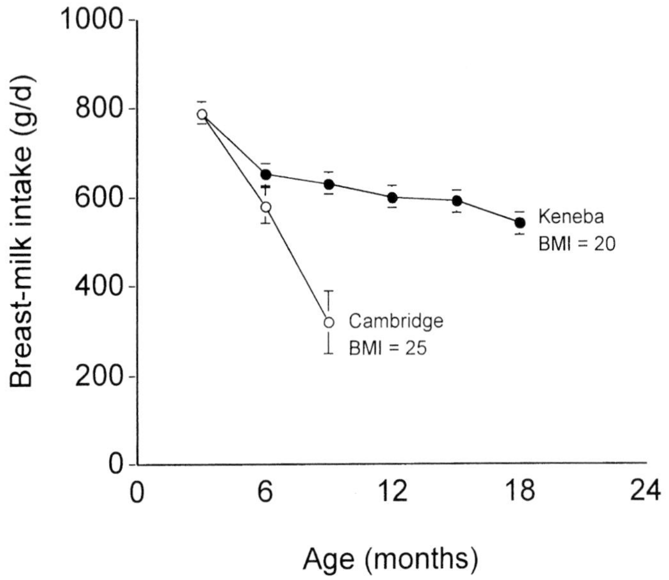

Fig. 3.14. Breast-milk intakes in Keneba, The Gambia vs Cambridge, UK. Note that the much thinner mothers from Gambia produce an equal or better amount of milk. (From Prentice et al., 1994.)

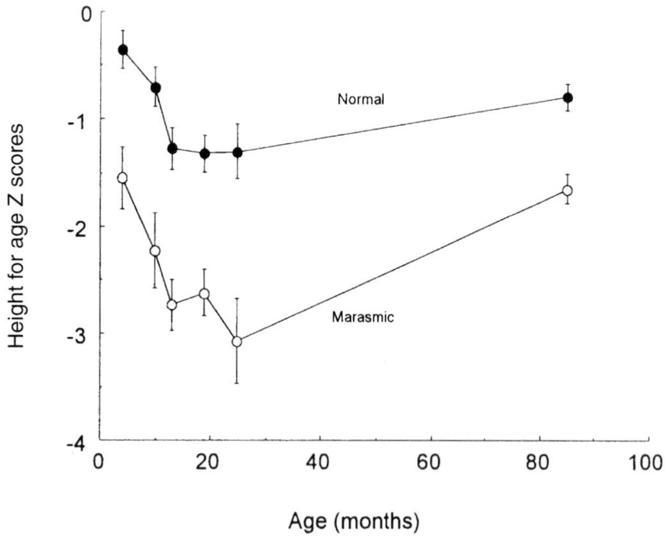

Fig. 3.15. Typical nutritional status of rural African children. The upper line shows normal children in Keneba, The Gambia. The lower line shows a group who were marasmic in the second year of life. Note that this group started with lower birthweights. (Unpublished data from M. Darboe, MRC Keneba.)

met from a balanced diet then she will likely meet her additional needs of other nutrients (except where the diet is generally deficient even in the non-reproductive state).

Comparative studies in many different communities across the world have shown that lactation is a highly robust process and continues to function well even in thin and chronically under-nourished women (Fig. 3.14) (Prentice et al., 1994). As with pregnancy (see above) this should not be used as an excuse not to attend to the special nutritional needs of lactating women – both groups are considered 'at risk' in nutritional terms. Maternal deficiencies in water-soluble vitamins are directly reflected as low concentrations in breast-milk. The same is true for several minerals, especially calcium. Fat soluble vitamins tend to be better buffered and may be quite well maintained in milk. The protein, fat and carbohydrate composition of human milk tends to remain remarkably constant even in poorly nourished women.

Before it was understood that lactational performance is so robust several dietary supplementation studies were undertaken in an attempt to augment milk production. In one trial in The Gambia there was no effect on milk output, and prolactin levels declined in the mothers (Prentice et al., 1980; Lunn et al., 1984). This would be predicted to shorten the inter-birth interval by reducing the period of lactational amenhorreoa. Energy supplementation of lactating women is therefore not generally recommended except in extreme situations.

Infant nutrition

Growth

Affluent children in urban Africa generally grow well. Their nutritional requirements and associated clinical conditions are broadly similar to those of western children and are covered in detail in other paediatric textbooks (but see also the special needs of children with haemoglobinopathies discussed in Chapter 78). This section focuses on the nutrition of children from poor backgrounds where food supplies are insecure, diet is of low quality and infections are frequent.

Even in such settings, breast-fed children grow extremely well over the first 3–4 months of life. On average, their growth curves cross the standard centile charts as they catch up their size deficit from birth (see Fig. 3.15) (Whitehead & Paul, 1984). With the introduction of weaning foods growth starts to falter – frequently in a serious manner. By 1 year of age average weight-for-age for many communities is only 75 per cent of the WHO norm (equivalent to −2 Z-scores – see Box below for definition). Growth does not recover until adolescence, when an extended period of development often allows them to reach a reasonable adult stature. Rural children in Africa are stunted frequently as well as wasted. This makes them look better nourished than they really are and emphasizes the need for keeping good records of age, weight and height. These should be regularly plotted on the child's 'Road to Health' chart as an important part of clinical monitoring (see p. 167, Fig. 9.11). Wasting reflects acute malnutrition and stunting reflects a longer-term deficit. Changes in weight are therefore the best short-term guide to nutritional adequacy and acute weight loss should be investigated urgently.

Stunting (or 'nutritional dwarfism' in extreme cases) is almost universal in poor populations in Africa. Without an immediate visual comparison against a normal child, or reference to a growth curve, it usually goes unnoticed because stunting compensates for wasting and gives the child a relatively normal appearance. Stunting is strongly associated with developmental deficits in both the individual and the community as a whole.

The excellent growth of very young infants arises because breast-milk is an ideal food available in adequate amounts and because young infants suffer few infections. The introduction of weaning foods (generally at an unnecessarily early age) usually triggers weight faltering due to the weaning foods having very low nutrient density and often being contaminated with enteric pathogens.

Methods of assessing growth failure and malnutrition

Against reference growth curves for weight and height
The most common way to assess adequacy of growth is to compare children against standard reference curves from well-nourished healthy populations (for example using WHO or NCHS curves). This is the basis of Road to Health Charts employed in most African countries. A child's weight is simply expressed as a percentage of the expected weight at the same age to derive % weight-for-age (% WFA). The same principle can be used for height to derive % height-for-age (% HFA). Because a child's age is sometimes unknown, curves are also published for weight-for-height so that % weight-for-height can be estimated (% WFH).

Centile curves
The same reference growth curves are sometimes expressed in terms of centiles. The 50% centile (or percentile) is the line up the centre of the distribution of the healthy population (where 50% of children would be above and 50% below the line). The 75% centile represents large children (only 25% would be above this in a normal population) and the 25% centile represents small children.

Z-Scores
One 'Z-score' is defined as 1 standard deviation (SD) for a normal population. These are expressed relative to the mean. Thus a child of average WFH is classified as 0 Z-score. A child whose weight is 1 SD lower than the mean is –1 Z-score and so on. The same calculation can be applied to HFA and WFH. Z-score is sometimes contracted to simply 'Z'.

Other anthropometric measures
Numerous other anthropometric measures can be used. The most common of these are mid-upper arm circumference (MUAC), head circumference (HC) and skinfold thicknesses (frequently triceps and supra-scapular). Mid-upper arm circumference remains relatively constant from 1 to 5 years so has been applied as a simple and easily performed screening tool with the following cut-offs:

MUAC	*Classification*
>14 cm	Normal
12.5–14 cm	Mild/moderate malnutrition
<12.5 cm	Severe malnutrition

Causes of growth failure

Growth failure in later infancy appears to be caused as much by infections as by primary nutrient shortages. A fairly typical growth chart from an actual child is shown in Fig. 3.16. It comes from a highly seasonal setting in the sub-Sahel where each rainy season brings an increase in infectious diseases. The child in question was born small, but showed excellent catch-up growth in the first few months. The introduction of weaning foods coincided with the start of the wet season and caused numerous clinically recorded illnesses (and no doubt many sub-clinical ones). The child failed to gain any weight for the following 6 months. In the subsequent dry season he recovered somewhat and once again showed a degree of catch-up growth, but at the next wet season his growth again stalled for 6 months. Such extreme growth faltering would be grounds for emergency investigations in a western tertiary hospital setting. Although resources limit such responses in many areas of Africa, growth faltering should still be seen as a serious clinical issue.

A persistent 'tropical' gastroenteropathy characterized by villous atrophy and an increased permeability of the gut is extremely common throughout Africa. Studies in rural Gambia using a dual-sugar permeability test show that all children are affected to some degree (Lunn, 2000). The gut damage affects the efficiency of nutrient absorption (particularly of lactose since the lactase enzyme is normally concentrated at the villous tip) and in extreme cases can lead to loss of plasma proteins – a 'protein

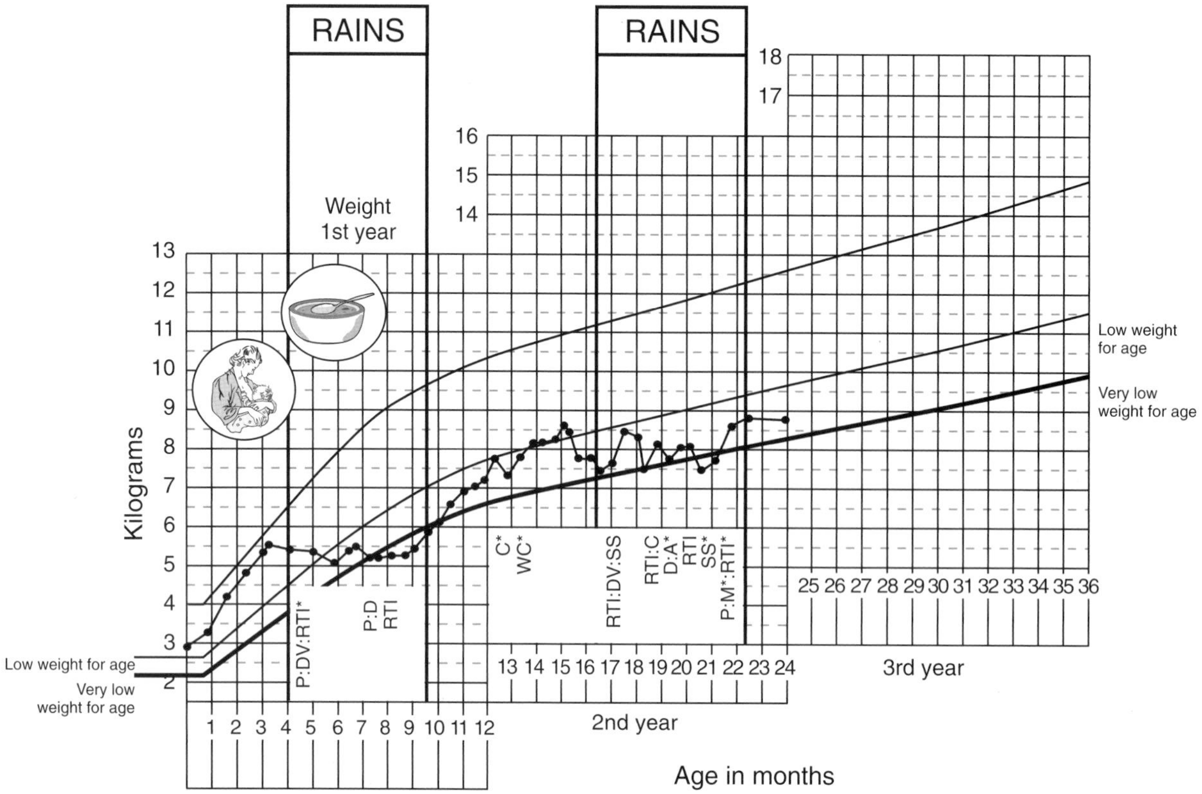

Fig. 3.16. Typical growth chart from a rural child in a seasonal environment. Note that the combination of poor diet, increased infections and deteriorating maternal care in the busy farming season cause growth to virtually cease for many months. Catch-up growth generally occurs in the harvest season but is inadequate.

losing enteropathy' which is common during measles infection. The degree of gut damage seems to strongly predict growth failure. The initial causes of the enteropathy are still not well understood and nor are the factors that perpetuate it. Paradoxically, the histological picture shows an over-active inflammatory response even in severely malnourished children who might be expected to be immunosuppressed.

Severe forms of protein-energy malnutrition

Protein-energy malnutrition (PEM) has a wide spectrum of manifestations (Golden, 1995). The most severe forms present as the clinical syndromes kwashiorkor and marasmus (see below), but there is often a spectrum between these extremes. Marasmus can be thought of as the normal 'adapted' state where prolonged underfeeding forces the child to consume its own fat and protein stores to maintain the function of its vital organs. Kwashiorkor is a 'disadapted' state in which an imbalance in protein supply limits the hepatic production of albumin and other plasma proteins thus causing oedema and multiple other metabolic abnormalities. Because it arises from a poor dietary intake PEM is frequently associated with deficiencies of minerals and vitamins. The causes of poor intake can cover a wide range including: famine, family poverty, poor maternal knowledge, neglect, loss of appetite due to infection, malabsorption (increasingly associated with HIV), handicap in the child, e.g. cleft palate, cerebral palsy, and others.

Severe malnutrition is a common cause of hospital admission in developing countries. Malnutrition is also present, but often unrecognized, in many children admitted to hospital with a wide range of illnesses. It is associated with a markedly increased case-fatality rate (see Table 3.1) which applies across almost all illness categories (Man et al., 1998).

The Gomez classification of malnutrition (Table 3.11) tends to be used in public health screening and emergency situations, and the Wellcome classification (Table 3.12) in clinical settings (WHO Working Group, 1986; Waterlow, 1992).

Table 3.11. Gomez classification

Weight-for-age (% of reference)	Classification
90–110	Normal
75–89	Grade I – mild malnutrition
60–74	Grade II – moderate malnutrition
Less than 60	Grade III – severe malnutrition

Table 3.12. Wellcome classification of clinical types of malnutrition

Weight-for-age (% of NCHS median)	No oedema	With oedema
60–80	Undernutrition	Kwashiorkor
Less than 60	Marasmus	Marasmic kwashiorkor

Marasmus

Marasmus frequently occurs in the first year of life. The patient is very thin with severe muscle wasting (particularly from the shoulders and buttocks) and virtually no subcutaneous fat. Thin, atrophic skin lies in redundant folds. The pinched face makes the child look much older.

Kwashiorkor

Kwashiorkor typically occurs in the second year of life. The child has fine, friable and discoloured (orange) hair and develops skin lesions (flaky paint appearance in severe cases), peripheral oedema and hepatomegaly. The child is apathetic when alone but fractious when picked up or examined. Kwashiorkor is an acute illness, often precipitated by infections such as measles, in which the history of swelling, loss of appetite and mood change is of a few days only.

Guidelines for the treatment of the severely malnourished child are given in Chapter 9.

The importance of breast-feeding

Constituents of breast milk

Breast-feeding is crucially important to the health and survival of infants in Africa (Huffman et al. 2001). This statement holds true even in spite of current concerns about the optimal advice to give to HIV-positive mothers (see below). Breast-feeding is the most important contraceptive agent world-wide and assists maintaining adequate birth-spacing. Breast milk has evolved to match optimally the nutritional and physiological needs of the young infant. It contains numerous specialist nutritional constituents such as lactose (with a high galactose content for neural growth) and long-chain PUFAs (also essential for neural development). Breast-milk also contains numerous signalling molecules (such as insulin-like growth factors, TGF-β, leptin, interleukins, etc.) which appear to stimulate intestinal development and immune function in the infant. It also contains a host of immuno-protective factors designed to guard against infection in both the mammary gland and the infant (Table 3.13) (Hanson et al., 2001). The biological function of many of these is not yet fully understood, but it seems safe to assume that most are there for a purpose. It may be that one of their roles is to protect against diseases

Table 3.13. Immuno-protective factors in breast milk

	Protective against		
	Bacteria	Viruses	Comments
Humoral factors			
Secretory IgA	++	++	Binds to bacteria/viruses and inhibits adherence to gut mucosa
Specific IgG	++	–	Maternal antibodies confer immunity to the infant. Also effective against *Giardia*.
'Bifidus factor'	++	–	Carbohydrate that promotes lactobacilli which in turn produce acid and suppress other bacteria
Lactoferrin	+	–	Bacteriostatic effect by binding of free iron essential to many pathogens
Lysozyme	+	–	Breaks down outer capsule of gram negative bacteria
Milk lipids	+	+	Active against staphylococci and enveloped viruses
Oligosaccharides	+	–	Mimic bacterial cell walls thus blocking specific adhesion sites in the gut
Other unidentified macromolecules	+	+	Active against herpes and rotavirus
Cellular factors			
Polymorphs and macrophages	+	+	Phagocytic against bacteria and *Candida*
B-lymphocytes and plasma cells	+	+	Synthesize antibodies locally. Specific mechanisms allow cells to 'home' to mammary lymphoid tissue from other maternal sites (especially the mother's gut)

Table 3.14. Mortality rates in breast-fed and non-breast-fed babies

	Relative risk of death		
Type of milk	Diarrhoea	Respiratory infections	Other infections
Breast only	1.0	1.0	1.0
Breast + formula	4.5	2.1	0.1
Breast + cows	3.4	1.2	1.4
Formula only	16.3	3.9	2.3
Cows only	11.6	3.3	2.6

Source: From Victora et al. (1987).

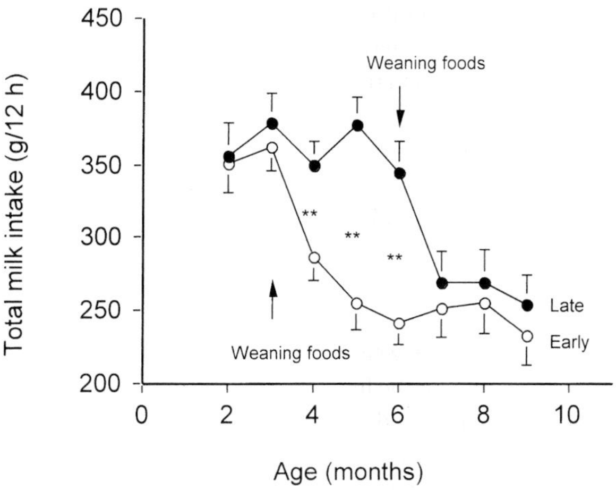

Fig. 3.17. Early introduction of weaning foods reduces milk output. (Infants were randomly assigned to receive an institutional supplement at 3 or 6 months. (Unpublished data from R. Downes and A.M. Prentice.)

in later life by entraining metabolic processes during this crucial early phase of development. This view is increasingly supported by recent research showing that breast-fed babies have less allergy, obesity and diabetes in later life. They are also more intelligent on average.

Breast feeding, infections and HIV

Numerous studies have shown that breast-fed babies are less likely to die from infectious diseases than bottle-fed babies (see, for example, Table 3.14) (Victora et al., 1987). For some disease categories the risk is lowered by as much as five-fold or more. This does not hold true for the babies of HIV-positive mothers in whom there is a moderate increase in the likelihood of vertical transmission of HIV (Coutsoudis et al., 1999). This creates a terrible dilemma for mothers and their health workers alike. There remains significant controversy over the difficult issue of what is the best advice to give to HIV-positive mothers, and the decision must be taken in the light of family circumstances such as the ability to afford alternative infant foods. In formulating such advice it should be remembered that, even in communities with exceptionally high HIV rates, the overall protective effects of breast-feeding in the community as a whole are likely to outweigh the extra risk associated with vertical HIV transmission. The WHO guidelines current at the time of writing are summarized in the Box (WHO, 2000a).

WHO Recommendations for breast-feeding by HIV-infected mothers

- When replacement feeding is acceptable, feasible, affordable, sustainable and safe, avoidance of all breast-feeding by HIV-infected mothers is recommended.
- Otherwise, exclusive breast-feeding is recommended during the first months of life.
- To minimize HIV transmission risk, breast-feeding should be discontinued as soon as feasible, taking into account local circumstances, the individual woman's situation and the risks of replacement feeding (including infections other than HIV and malnutrition).
- When HIV-infected mothers choose not to breast-feed from birth or stop breast-feeding later, they should be provided with specific guidance and support for at least the first 2 years of the child's life to ensure adequate replacement feeding. Programmes should strive to improve conditions that will make replacement feeding safer for HIV-infected mothers and families.

WHO Consultation on Mother-to-Child Transmission of HIV – October 2000

Optimal duration of exclusive breast-feeding

WHO has recommended that all mothers should breast-feed exclusively for at least 6 months (WHO, 2001). This recommendation has been somewhat controversial due to concerns that some mothers may not be able to produce sufficient milk to match their infant's needs for this long. In practice, the amount of milk that a mother produces is very strongly determined by the demand from the child. This affects the frequency, duration and intensity of sucking which, in turn, have a feedback effect to stimulate milk synthesis. Therefore the withholding of alternative foods and fluids does help to stimulate an adequate milk flow and mothers should be given the confidence that this is so (Fig. 3.17). True lactational failure (as opposed to perceived failure due to maternal anxiety) is extremely rare especially in Africa where traditional cultures promote good breast-feeding practices. A tendency for these valuable practices to be undermined by 'modernization' should be combated by the introduction of baby-friendly initiatives in hospitals and clinics.

- Be vigilant against possible infringements of the WHO Code on Marketing Breast-Milk Substitutes (WHO, 1981)
- Take every opportunity to promote breast-feeding.

Weaning foods

Traditional forms of weaning foods vary widely across Africa according to the foodstuffs available. Specific recommendations and formulations will therefore differ from region to region. However, certain basic guiding principles can be offered (see also Chapter 11 on Treatment of Malnutrition).

Energy and nutrient density

The energy and nutrient density of weaning foods is a crucial issue (Walker, 1990; Brown, 1997). Many women in Africa have the mistaken belief that weaning foods should be very thin gruels which approximate the consistency of milk. Sometimes even rice water is offered. Energy densities of these foods are often low and their consumption displaces breast-milk thus leading to malnutrition. The effects of varying the energy density of weaning foods on total energy intake are shown in Fig. 3.18 (Brown et al., 1995). When given free access to foods of different energy densities, infants ingest a greater total nutrient load when the nutrient density is high, in spite of consuming a smaller actual volume. Energy density and the palatability of foods can be raised by the addition of small amounts of sugar and oil, though care must be taken not to dilute out other nutrients including protein. The palatability and energy density of weaning foods becomes especially critical when infants are ill and lose appetite. Under these circumstances they will be unable to eat sufficient bulk to meet their nutrient needs.

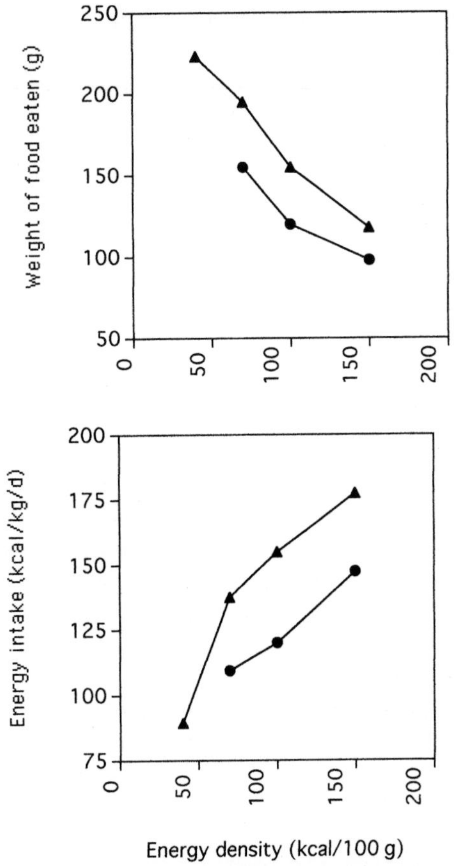

Fig. 3.18. The effect of energy density of weaning foods on total energy intake in infants. Note that although the infants reduce their total volume of intake at higher energy densities, they still obtain a higher overall intake. Circles represent three different energy densities fed three times daily. Triangles indicate four different energy densities fed five times daily. (From Brown et al., 1995.)

Bacterial contamination

The second major problem with any early weaning foods is bacterial contamination (Rowland et al., 1978). Weaning foods are often prepared with unclean water and in unhygienic containers. This problem is confounded by mothers not bringing them fully to the boil for fear of thickening cereal-based gruels. Pathogens can easily survive and then find a warm and nutrient-rich medium in which to multiply if the mothers leave the weaning foods to be fed by nursemaids or grandmothers over the remainder of the day. Tests of weaning foods prepared in this manner have revealed very high levels of bacterial contamination (Barrell & Rowland, 1979). The use of fermented cereals can overcome some of these problems since the amylase produced by fermentation partially hydrolyses starch and reduces glutination. The acid produced by fermentation also inhibits bacterial growth.

As infants reach about 9 months, homogenized adult foods can, and should, be introduced into the diet with increasing frequency. The introduction of eggs, dairy produce, fish and meat should be encouraged whenever affordable.

Childhood and adolescence

Children in Africa generally consume a similar diet to the adults in the family. Due to a higher basal metabolic

Table 3.15. Person first served food in two Anambra State communities in Nigeria

	Opi		Odageri-edda		Total	
Person	Number	%	Number	%	Number	%
Father	132	87	49	98	181	**90**
Mother and children	15	10	1	2	16	**8**
Oldest children	5	3	0	0	5	**2**
Total	152	100	50	100	202	**100**

Source: Okeke & Nnanyelugo, 1989.

rate, their energy requirements are proportionately higher than adults. This is also true for other nutrients. Health workers should ensure that they are given an appropriate share of the family bowl, but this is often not the case (Table 3.15) (Okeke & Nnanyelugo, 1987). During the adolescent growth spurt, nutrient requirements rise, especially for energy, protein and calcium. Post-menarchal girls will have a raised iron requirement due to menstrual losses and it is important that they are not iron deficient as they enter their first pregnancy.

Specific nutrients and consequences of deficiency

Protein

In the 1970s a misconception arose that the most important and widespread nutritional deficiency in children in Africa was that of protein (McClaren, 1975). This is still reflected in the belief of many medical staff that protein is somehow more important than calories for sick children. In fact, there is much evidence to show that energy deficits are more general both in the community and the hospital setting. In a survey of the amounts of protein and energy given to malnourished children in a West African hospital only 15 per cent received inadequate amounts of protein whereas 55 per cent received too little energy (Whittle 1984). Primary protein deficiency in children can occur in areas where the staple food is cassava or plantain (see Table 3.6), or where mothers feed inappropriate foods like sugar water. In these circumstances it is one of the major precipitating factors in kwashiorkor. However, in other areas children's protein needs are likely to be met if their energy needs are met and if they have a relatively varied diet.

A sufficient supply of carbohydrate (not generally a problem to achieve in Africa) spares protein from being used as a substrate for glucose. A varied diet, including proteins from various plant and animal sources, helps to ensure that amino acid imbalances in any one protein source are offset by other proteins thus increasing the net protein utilization (NPU) of the mixture. Once again, the watchwords in human nutrition are variety and balance.

Children recovering from malnutrition have special needs, both in the immediate and the longer-term rehabilitation phases. These are covered in Chapter 9.

Essential fatty acids

Certain long-chain polyunsaturated fatty acids (PUFAs) act as precursors for prostaglandins, leukotrienes and other signaling molecules with potent biological effects. Human metabolism is incapable of inserting all of the double-bonds and is dependant on dietary sources of α-linolenic (so-called n3 or $\omega3$ series) and linoleic (n6 or $\omega6$ series) acids. The requirements for these essential fatty acids (EFAs) are small, and gross EFA deficiency has only been reported in patients after bowel resection. However, a good intake of long-chain PUFAs (especially the n3 variety from fish, which tend to be anti-inflammatory) is beneficial to health, and the balance between n6 and n3 may affect numerous metabolic processes (FAO, 1994).

Breast-milk is a critical source of long-chain PUFAs, and thus probably exerts a major influence on brain development (Uauy & De-Andraca 1995). In many communities the intakes of these essential fatty acids plummet after weaning (Prentice & Paul, 2000). The full consequences of this are not yet known, but it may have multiple long-term effects on community development if it impairs cognitive development.

Minerals

Calcium, phosphorus, magnesium and sulphur are important constituents of bone and hence necessary for optimal physical development.

Calcium

Absorption

Calcium absorption is aided by vitamin D and regulated by parathyroid hormone in response to the body's need. There is considerable scope for changes in the efficiency of calcium absorption since up to 80 per cent of dietary calcium is usually excreted into the faeces.

Dietary intake
Most non-dairy consuming peoples in Africa have very low calcium intakes compared to Europe and America, and compared to international recommended intakes (Abelow et al., 1992; Prentice, 2000). The calcium content of breast milk may also be low in rural African mothers, though it still remains a much better source than most weaning foods and its calcium is highly available. Paradoxically, these low calcium intakes probably do not result in high rates of osteoporotic fractures in the elderly (though accurate figures are not easily found). This may be because of differences in the physical geometry of African hip bones and because lifelong high levels of physical activity help to maintain bone strength. It is predicted that the westernization of African diets and activity patterns will precipitate an epidemic of osteoporotic fractures as currently seen elsewhere in the world.

Deficiency
In children, calcium deficiency may contribute to stunting. In certain, relatively rare cases it may also cause a calcium-deficiency rickets. There is some suggestion that this is becoming more frequent with the increased consumption of polished imported rice, and as improved energy supplies allow growth to outstrip the calcium availability.

Sources
The main sources of calcium are milk of all types and other dairy produce, small fish containing bones that can be eaten, beans, peas and nuts, millet, and dark green leaves (especially baobab and moringa).

Copper

Copper is required by a number of metalloprotein enzymes involved in mitochondrial oxidation, in the synthesis of collagen and blood vessels, and neurotransmitters. Deficiency is most often seen in premature babies or in older babies fed inappropriately on unmodified cow's milk, and in children with protracted diarrhoea. Children recovering from malnutrition may also be copper deficient and supplementation has been found to improve growth and reduce infection rates (Castillo-Duran et al., 1983).

Shellfish, legumes, wholegrain cereals, nuts and liver are good dietary sources of copper. Excess zinc and iron block copper absorption and can induce copper deficiency. This is one reason to urge caution over excessive prescription of mineral supplements (Table 3.16).

Table 3.16. Desirable nutrient intakes for a child in the acute and intermediate recovery phases of malnutrition (see also Chapter 9)

Nutrient	Desirable intake (per kg body weight)
Water	120–140 ml
Energy	420 kJ (100 kcal)
Protein	1–2 g
Electrolytes	
Sodium	<23 mg
Potassium	>160 mg
Magnesium	>10 mg
Phosphorus	60 mg
Calcium	80 mg
Trace elements	
Zinc	2.0 mg
Copper	0.3 mg
Selenium	4.7 μg
Iodine	12 μg
Water-soluble vitamins	
Thiamin	70 μg
Riboflavin	200 μg
Niacin	1000 μg
Pyridoxine	70 μg
Cobalamin	100 ng
Folic acid	100 μg
Ascorbic acid	10 mg
Pantothenic acid	300 μg
Biotin	10 μg
Fat-soluble vitamins	
Retinol	150 μg
Calciferol	3 μg
Tocopherol	2.2 mg
Vitamin K	4 μg
Lipids	
Total lipid	25–55% energy
N-6 fatty acids	4.5% energy
N-3 fatty acids	0.5% energy

Source: From Golden, 1995.

Iron

Functions
Iron lies at the centre of the oxygen-carrying haem pigment in haemoglobin and myogloblin. It is also an essential co-factor for dozens of proteins as a result of its useful redox properties. Although highly necessary for health, iron is also a potential danger because it can induce oxidant damage to tissues. Thus numerous systems have evolved for handling and transporting iron. These require proteins such as ferritin, transferrin,

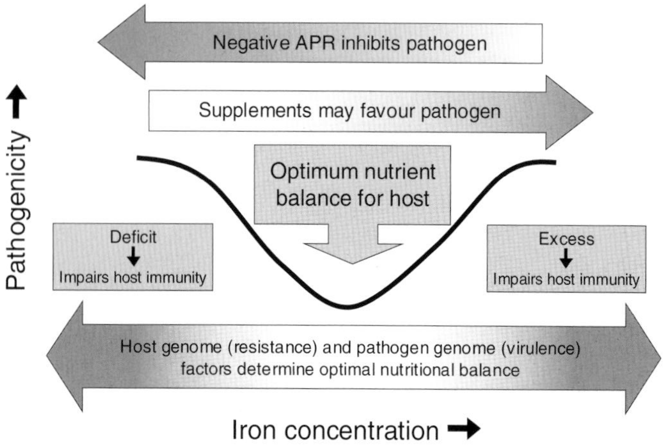

Fig. 3.19. Possible effects of iron on host–pathogen interactions – a delicate balance. (From Doherty et al., 2002.)

Table 3.17. Regional variability in prevalence of iron-deficiency anaemia within a single country

Division	Total n	Hb < 11 g/dl	%	Hb < 7 g/dl	%
Banjul	48	31	65	3	6
KMC	124	74	60	4	3
WD	81	66	81	7	9
LRD	24	22	92	4	17
CRD	95	77	81	19	20
NBD	49	32	65	6	12
URD	94	87	93	33	35
Total	515	389	76	76	15

Notes:
Banjul and KMC divisions represent the richer coastal belt with greatest access to healthcare. URD is the most remote area.
Source: NaNA/MRC/PHPNP, 2000.

lactoferrin, haptoglobin and others which must be in good order if optimal health is to be maintained. Iron is also essential to almost all pathogenic organisms and lies at the centre of a battlefield between the host and the pathogen. The host attempts to starve invading organisms of iron (and zinc) through the acute phase response which increases the levels of iron-binding proteins and drains iron from the circulation. In response most organisms have evolved special transport proteins designed to obtain iron when little is available. There remains much to be discovered about the role of iron in infectious diseases, and it may be preferable to avoid both iron deficiency and iron excess (see Fig. 3.19) (Doherty et al., 2002).

Sources and absorption
Iron occurs in two forms in the diet: haem iron and non-haem iron. Haem iron occurs in the blood and flesh of animals. It is relatively well absorbed. Non-haem iron occurs in plants (especially green leaves), eggs and milk. In general, it is very poorly absorbed (only 5–15 per cent). Absorption can be enhanced by vitamin C when it is consumed (in the form of fruits) in the same meal. Breast-milk iron is well absorbed because it is bound to lactoferrin for which the infant's gut has special receptors and transport mechanisms.

Requirements and deficiency
Iron requirements are high during growth and in any persistent iron-losing condition (for instance heavy menstrual bleeding, heavy hook worm load). The prevalence of iron deficiency in regions is usually inferred from the levels of haemoglobin on the assumption that most anaemia is primarily caused by iron deficiency. By this criterion most of West, Central and North Africa have deficiency rates exceeding 50 per cent. Deficiency levels are lower in East Africa (40–50 per cent) and even lower in Southern Africa (20–40 per cent) (WHO & FAO websites). Even within countries there can be large regional gradients in the degree of deficiency as shown in Table 3.17 (NaNA/MRC/PHPNP, 2000). Reproductive women and young children are most at risk of iron deficiency.

Iron deficiency anaemias are discussed in Chapter 78. Note that in certain diseases iron-deficiency anaemia can occur in spite of high bone marrow iron stores (the so-called 'anaemia of chronic disease'). This is caused by a cytokine blockade of erythropoiesis rather than by iron deficiency *per se.*

Iodine

Iodine deficiency (see p. 1096) has been a major scourge in many populations including some in Africa. Iodine is required for the formation of thyroid hormones and its deficiency leads to hypothyroidism. The body attempts to compensate for iodine deficiency through hypertrophy of the thyroid gland, and this leads to goitre (an enlarged, sometimes massively enlarged, thyroid gland detectable by visual inspection or palpation). The prevalence of goitre gives a good measure of iodine deficiency, but is a rather extreme manifestation. Assessment of urinary levels of iodine (p. 52) are therefore now the method preferred by the International Council for Combating Iodine Deficiency Disorders (see ICCIDD website). Sub-clinical iodine deficiency may have damaging effects on health before the appearance of goitres (Fig. 3.20).

Iodine deficiency, through its effect on the thyroid, retards many aspects of metabolism and is therefore

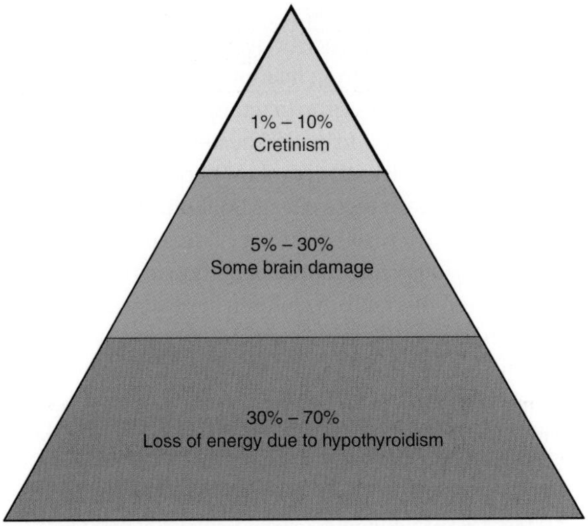

Fig. 3.20. Community-wide effects of iodine deficiency. (From WHO/UNICEF/ICCIDD, 1993.)

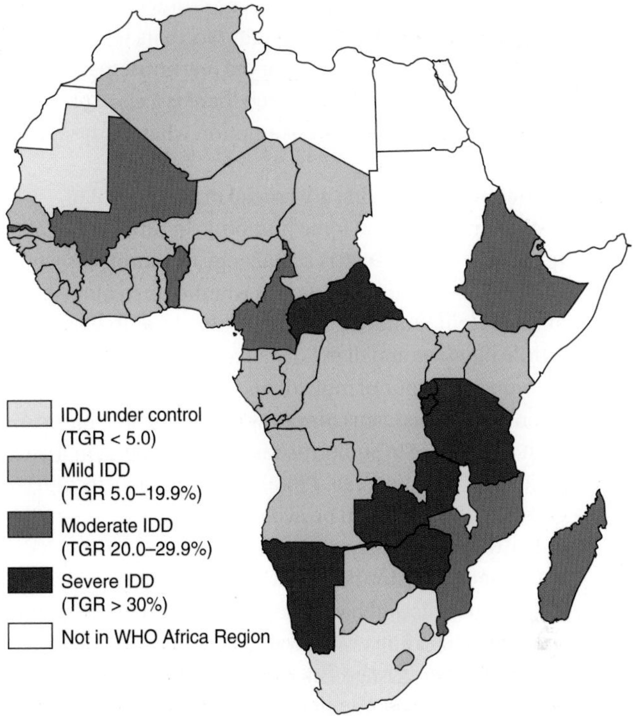

Fig. 3.21. Distribution of iodine deficiency disorders across Africa. (From WHO/UNICEF/ICCIDD, 1993.)

widely debilitating. Iodine deficiency in pregnant women can lead to cretinism in their infants, a condition of mental retardation and stunted growth.

Endemic goitre is determined geographically (see Table 3.8 and Fig. 3.21) since it occurs where the soil is deficient in iodine. In areas of marginal iodine availability a full deficiency can be precipitated by the consumption of goitrogenic agents in food. The classic example of this is the residual cyanide found in poorly cooked cassava roots or leaves.

Magnesium

Magnesium is widely distributed in the soft tissues and bone (which contains about 70 per cent of the total body content) and is involved in a large number of metabolic processes. The plasma magnesium level is remarkably constant and is maintained so by the kidneys; a fall in magnesium intake is rapidly followed by a reduction in urinary output.

Hypomagnesaemia is relatively uncommon but may arise secondary to bowel resection or persistent gastroenteropathy/diarrhoea and PEM. Hence administration of magnesium is recommended in treatment of the severely malnourished child (see Chapter 11).

Potassium

Potassium is also required for the maintenance of cell homeostasis. There are many abnormalities in potassium balance but almost none of these are of a primary nutritional origin since it occurs widely in vegetable foods. Attention to potassium levels is also crucial to the therapy of the severely malnourished child (see Chapter 11).

Selenium

Selenium is important in several enzymes especially glutathione peroxidase which has an important anti-oxidant role in cells (see below). In animal studies selenium deficiency has been shown to increase the virulence of certain viruses including influenza (Beck, 1999). This affects both the immediate host and any animals to which the infection is transferred.

Selenium deficiency is not a problem where the soil has an adequate concentration though over-intensive farming can deplete soils of selenium if it is not replaced in fertilizers. There is little information on the extent of selenium deficiency in Africa.

Sodium

The natural availability of sodium and chloride (as common salt) in different regions has influenced the migration of animals and the trading patterns of people in Africa since the dawn of history. In coastal areas salt is generally available in abundance, but in some inland areas it may become a highly valued commodity. The exchange of gold for salt was a major source of trade in West Africa where salt was literally worth its weight in gold in Timbuctu. Salt is one of the few nutrients, along with energy and water, for which there is a clear physiological drive to increase consumption when body stores are low.

Sodium and chloride are crucial in the control of osmotic pressure and ionic pumping. In Africa the maintenance of salt balance is a challenge in conditions when sodium loss occurs abundantly, whether in health – high ambient temperatures, heavy work loads, or in disease – febrile illnesses and diarrhoea. It is thought that genetic selection in favour of individuals who had effective salt retention mechanisms may now be responsible for the high prevalence of sodium-sensitive hypertension in Africans (Forrester et al., 1998). Thus both deficits and excesses of salt need to be avoided.

The discovery of oral rehydration solutions (ORS) which aid an appropriate sodium absorption has saved millions of lives and had a major impact on reducing the severity of diarrhoea worldwide (Victora et al., 2000). Severely malnourished children have a compromised renal ability to handle salt so must not be given the normal WHO ORS solution. Instead, they should receive a solution with less sodium and more potassium (see Chapter 20 for detailed guidance).

Zinc

Sources

Zinc occurs in high concentration in animal products and especially in some seafoods. In Africa the main source of zinc is from cereals. As most zinc resides in the outer layers of grains their final content is dependent on the level of refinement. As with calcium, zinc absorption is impaired by phytates in foods. Protein seems to act as an anti-phytate and aids zinc absorption.

Functions

Zinc plays a role in cell replication and growth and has a stabilizing function in organic compounds including cell membranes. The total body content of around 2–3 grams of zinc is mostly in muscle (~60%) and bone (~30%). Plasma zinc represents only 0.1 per cent of the total body pool. Levels of zinc in the body are carefully maintained through changes in absorption and excretion in response to deficiency. Severe deficiency is rare. This homeostatic control is so effective that no studies have yet shown a correlation between intakes and plasma indices of zinc status. Excess intakes of zinc may impair the absorption of some other metals (especially copper) since they appear to share the same intestinal uptake transporters.

Deficiency and replacement

Many adverse consequences of mild zinc deficiency have been claimed, especially in relation to growth retardation (including intrauterine growth retardation IUGR), cell-mediated immunity and wound healing. However, numerous trials have failed to show persuasive evidence in favour of some of these effects (Mahomed, 2000; Wilkinson & Hawke, 1998). Strong evidence does support a role for low-dose zinc supplementation in reducing diarrhoea and mortality in children in several areas of the developing world (Black & Sazawal, 2001), but at least one trial of high-dose zinc supplementation in severely malnourished children with chronic diarrhoea showed clear adverse effects (Doherty et al., 1998). As with iron, care should be taken over the administration of zinc in the early recovery phase although withholding of zinc is not part of the IMCI guidelines.

Other trace elements

Molybdenum acts as a cofactor for three enzymes involved in sulphur and purine/pyrimidine metabolism. Chromium potentiates the action of insulin. Deficiencies of these elements are rare. Some other elements may be essential but it is difficult to establish this, and deficiency syndromes have not been described.

Fat-soluble vitamins

Vitamin A (retinol)

Sources

Foods contain vitamin A in several forms. Pre-formed vitamin A (retinol) occurs in animal products especially liver which has very high concentrations (Table 3.9). Carotenoids, which can be converted into vitamin A in the intestinal lumen, occur in yellow and red fruits and vegetables and in leaves. The concentration in foods is often expressed as retinol equivalents (RE) where 1 RE = 1 μg of retinol or 6 μg of beta-carotene.

Functions

Vitamin A is involved in cell differentiation and its deficiency syndromes tend to concentrate in rapidly dividing epithelial cells (the surface of the mouth, gut and respiratory tract), in immune cells, and in periods of reproduction and growth. It is involved in vision both in the retina (where an early clinical sign of deficiency is night blindness) and in maintaining the integrity of the conjunctiva and the cornea.

Deficiency syndromes

Severe vitamin A deficiency leads to Bitot's spots, xerophthalmia and keratomalacia and is a common cause of

Table 3.18. Regional differences in prevalence of vitamin A deficiency in 1–5-year-olds in The Gambia

Division	Total n	Plasma retinol <0.7 μ(mol/l)	%	Plasma retinol <0.35 μ(mol/l)	%
Banjul	20	12	60	0	0
KMC	94	51	54	7	7
WD	55	26	47	0	0
LRD	22	15	68	4	18
CRD	82	63	77	8	10
NBD	42	30	71	2	5
URD	90	62	69	16	18
Total	405	259	64	37	9

Source: NaNA/MRC/PHPNP, 2000.

blindness in Asia (Sommer, 1995). Tissue depletion of vitamin A can occur during persistent illness because the acute phase response suppresses the circulating concentration of retinol binding protein.

Severe vitamin A deficiency is rare in Africa (except as a secondary consequence of measles), but marginal-to-moderate deficiency is common (Fig. 3.22). As with many micronutrient deficiencies it tends to be most common in poor rural areas and can show wide differences in prevalence across countries (Table 3.18).

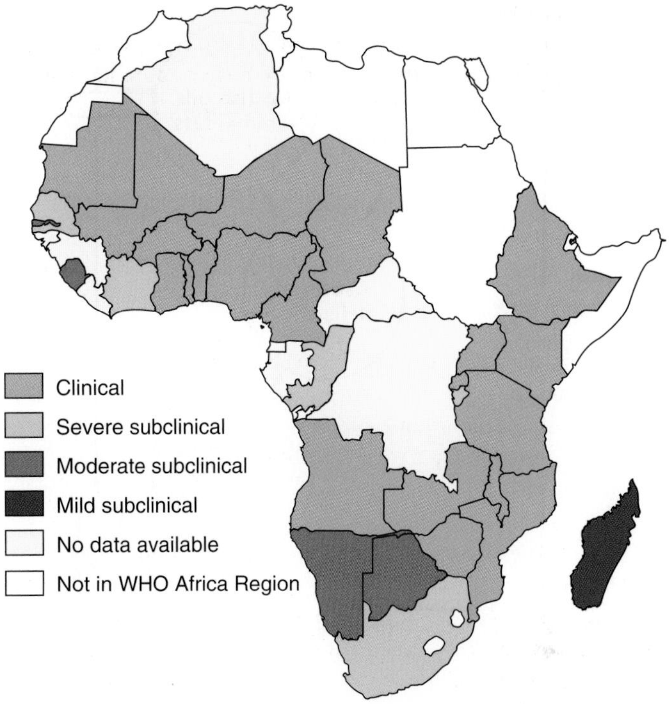

Fig. 3.22. Distribution of vitamin A deficiency across Africa. (From WHO/UNICEF, 1995.)

Significance for health of the community

Many studies have now shown that community-wide administration of vitamin A to children reduces overall mortality (on average by about 25%) (Fawzi et al., 1993; IVACG, 1997). Consequently, WHO and UNICEF have adopted vitamin A as one of the key nutrients in the world-wide push to eliminate micronutrient deficiencies and most African countries now have a policy of nation-wide supplementation of women and children. Since the liver stores vitamin A effectively, its administration does not have to be very frequent and many countries manage its distribution through their national immunization days. At the time of writing, there is a likelihood that the WHO recommended dosing schedules will be increased. Refer to the latest guidelines available for your region.

Vitamin D (calciferols)

Sources

As it is a fat-soluble vitamin the best dietary sources are animal products, especially the fatty parts and liver. Many imported margarines available in Africa are fortified with vitamin D and are labelled accordingly.

Vitamin D occurs in the diet in the form of cholecalciferol or ergocalficerol. These are converted to the biologically most active form (1,25–dihydroxyvitamin D3) through a number of steps in the skin, liver and kidney. The initial step in the skin requires ultraviolet light and this accounts for the fact that vitamin D deficiency occurs through an interaction of low dietary sources and lack of exposure to sunlight.

Functions

Vitamin D stimulates intestinal calcium absorption.

Physiology

The metabolism of the vitamin is shown in Fig. 3.23.

Vitamin D stimulates the active transport of calcium by the upper small intestine, initiates the mineralization of osteoid in bone, raises the serum phosphate and (in cases of dietary deficiency) mobilizes calcium from bone. Vitamin D receptors occur on other cells and may play other roles in relation to, for instance, cell-mediated immunity.

In vitamin D deficiency there is inadequate calcification of osteoid tissue, malabsorption of calcium, and deficient reabsorption of phosphate by the kidney. At the same time more parathormone than usual is secreted to maintain a normal plasma calcium level. This causes increased resorption and thinning of bone because

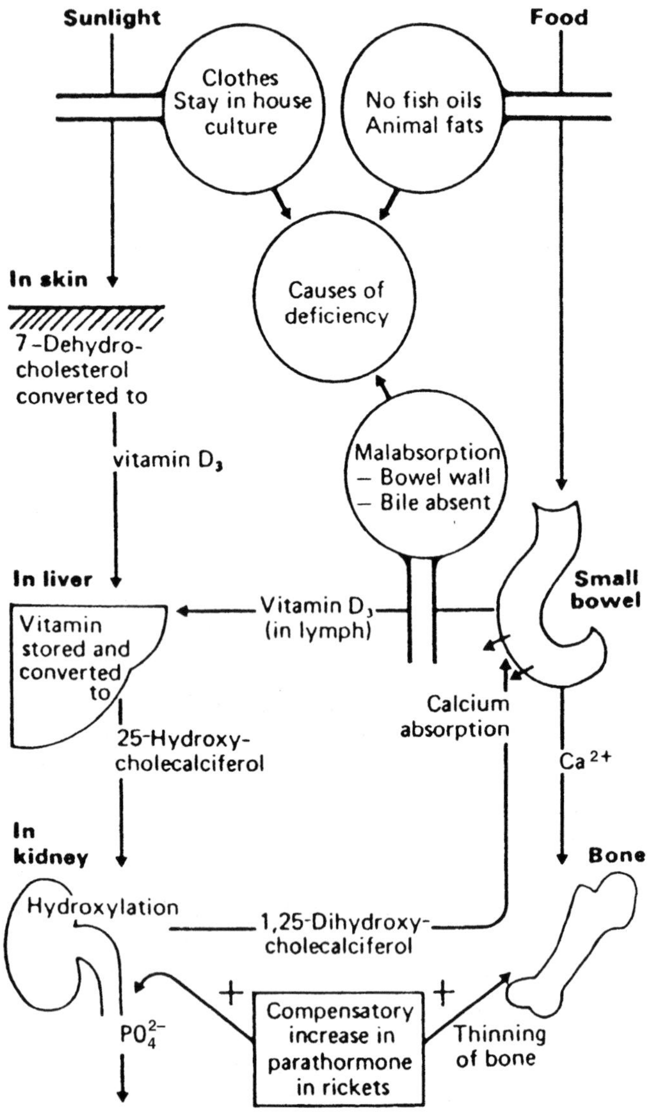

Fig. 3.23. Metabolism of vitamin D.

parathormone stimulates osteoclastic activity, and a lowering of the plasma phosphate due to increased renal loss of phosphate. The raised plasma alkaline phosphatase is an index of amount of bone resorption. In children, there is abnormal growth of cartilage which fails to calcify so that a wide, irregular, soft zone of non-calcified cartilage and osteoid tissue is formed and causes the characteristic deformities at the metaphysis.

Epidemiology

Rickets is common where for cultural and social reasons children are not exposed to sufficient sunlight. Diets, especially of the weanling, are extremely deficient in animal fats and oils, which may not be properly absorbed due to repeated gastrointestinal infections.

In North Africa, rickets is rife because mothers stay at home during daylight and those who venture out conceal themselves and their young children beneath cotton wraps (Lawson et al 1987). Thus the children, especially those in the crowded dark streets of the cities, receive little sun and are unable to synthesize sufficient vitamin D for their requirements. In addition, the high phytate content of the wheat diets may bind calcium in the gut and so limit its absorption. Cultural reasons are also important in Ethiopia, where mothers keep their children at home and risk factors include family size, birth order and crowding (Lulseged, 1990), while in South Africa, infants who are left at home by mothers who go out to work, are at risk. By contrast, in the forest zone of Nigeria, dietary calcium deficiency is largely responsible for rickets (Oginni et al., 1996).

Lack of sun and a poor diet lead to rickets. In most other parts of Africa, especially the rural savannah, children are nearly always in the sun and rickets is rare. Sporadic cases are usually due to vitamin D resistance, a hereditary disorder, or chronic renal disease.

In adults vitamin D deficiency is uncommon except in those with malabsorption, liver disease, or chronic renal disease. However, deficiency may be more common in the old and disabled who stay indoors and take an inadequate diet. Young women who stay indoors during pregnancy are at risk, and signs of vitamin D deficiency may appear during late pregnancy or after delivery. Their breast milk contains little of the vitamin.

Clinical features

The disease is commonest in infants and young children.

Bones. The epiphyses of the long bones are swollen at the wrists and ankles, the costochondral junctions are enlarged (rachitic rosary), the chest is flattened and the sternum appears to project forward. In infants a soft skull (craniotabes) is an early sign and frontal bossing is also seen. When the child begins to sit or walk, kyphosis and lordosis develop and the pelvis becomes narrowed, so that obstructed labour may follow in adult life. The long bones bend, which causes bow legs and knock-knees (Fig. 3.24(*a*)(*b*).

Muscles. Weak and flabby muscles make the child slow to sit and walk. Tetany, carpopedal and laryngeal spasm, and convulsions may occur if the serum calcium is very low.

Pneumonia. Children with rickets have significantly more pneumonia than controls, both due to defective immune function and to the distorted chest, which reduces lung volumes and predisposes to collapse and underventilation (Muhe et al., 1997). Cor pulmonale complicates severe cases (Woldemariam & Sterky, 1973).

Diagnosis

Biochemistry. The fasting serum calcium is normal or low, the serum phosphate low, and the alkaline phosphatase raised. Urinary phosphate, and hydroxyproline excretion, which is an index of collagen turnover in the bone, are increased.

Radiology. The distal ends of radius and ulna are widened, cupped, and frayed: the costochondral junctions are widened and the bones are less dense than usual (osteopenia).

Bone biopsy (iliac crest). This shows inadequate mineralization and an excessive volume of osteoid tissue.

Treatment and prognosis

Straightforward rickets or osteomalacia, due to vitamin D deficiency, will respond to sunlight or ultraviolet light, but this alone is not enough.

Calciferol. A single massive dose of vitamin D2 150 000 i.u. (3750 mg), by mouth or intramuscular injection, is the best and simplest treatment for severe cases although 3000 i.u. (75 mg) calciferol by mouth or cod liver oil (75 i.u./ml or 1.8 mg/ml) may be given daily for 1 month. If healing is inadequate with these doses the patient either has malabsorption or vitamin D resistant rickets.

Tetany. Give calcium gluconate (5–10 ml of a 10 per cent solution) intravenously, or calcium chloride 1 g 6 hourly in milk orally.

Calcium supplements. Healing is accelerated if milk or calcium lactate tablets 5 g three times a day can be given.

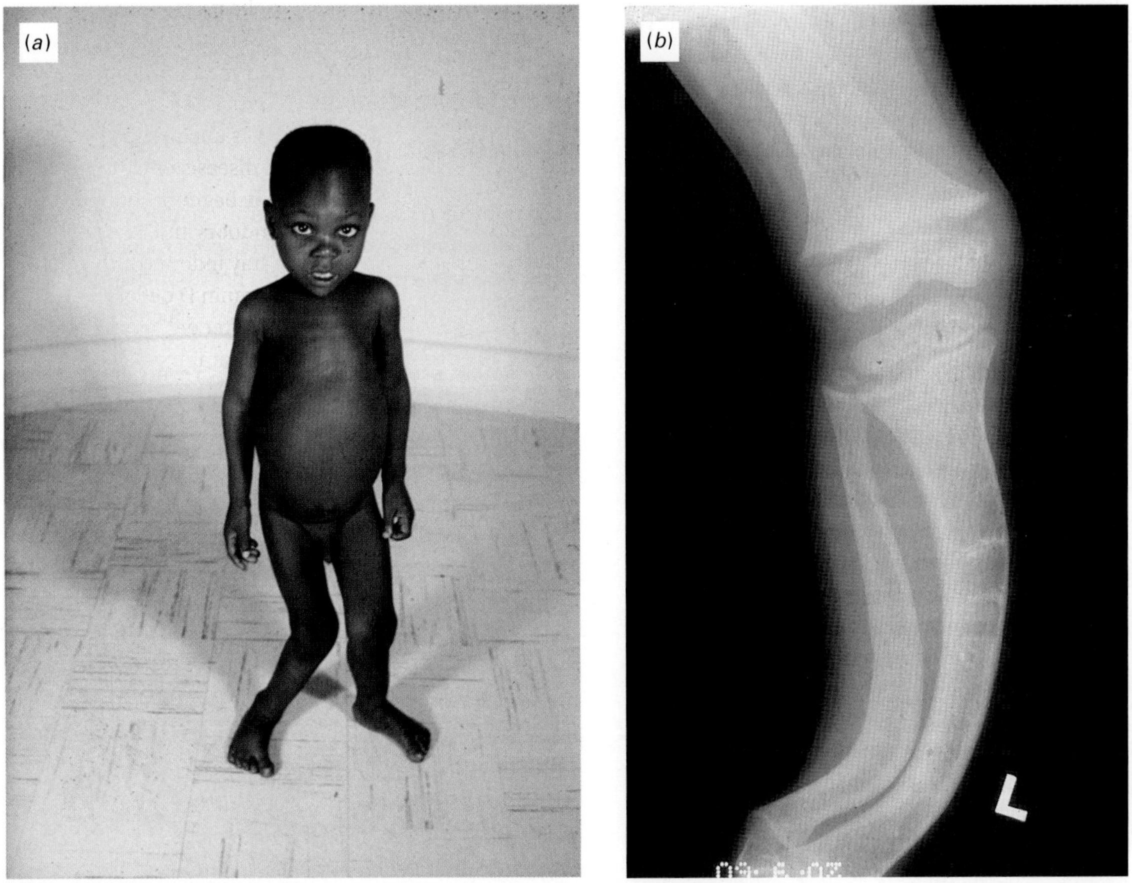

Fig. 3.24. Rickets.
(*a*) Nutritional rickets in a child from the rain forest region of Nigeria: this child had been kept out of the sun for cultural reasons. (Reproduced by courtesy of the Wellcome Trust and Professor R. G. Hendrickse.)
(*b*) Radiograph of the leg of a child with severe rickets. Note the gross curvature of the tibia and fibula.

Evidence of healing. After 6 weeks' vitamin D treatment, the biochemical changes are reversed, but bones heal more slowly and may never become normal.

Prevention

A vigorous health education programme, which involves the community, is the best method for educating the mothers, who should be told emphatically that their children need sunlight and animal foods, such as eggs, which are rich in vitamin D. If economic or religious practices make such teaching impractical in areas where rickets is prevalent, give fish oil to children at risk, premature babies, infants and treated patients.

Vitamin E (tocopherols)

Sources

Vitamin E occurs in vegetable-derived fats and oils and is frequently added as an anti-oxidant to prevent rancidity. It also occurs in whole-grain seeds and nuts and in animal fats.

Functions

Vitamin E plays an important role within cell membranes by protecting polyunsaturated fatty acids from oxidant damage (peroxidation). It does this in partnership with selenium and glutathione peroxidase. Vitamin E deficiency in animals causes a number of syndromes associated with damage to cell membranes probably resulting from an absence of these protective effects. It was discovered originally as an anti-sterility factor and in animals reduces fetal deaths. The absolute requirements in humans are not yet known, but a number of studies have suggested that it protects against coronary disease and some of the damaging effects of smoking.

Deficiency

Frank deficiency is only observed in premature babies or in adults with fat malabsorption.

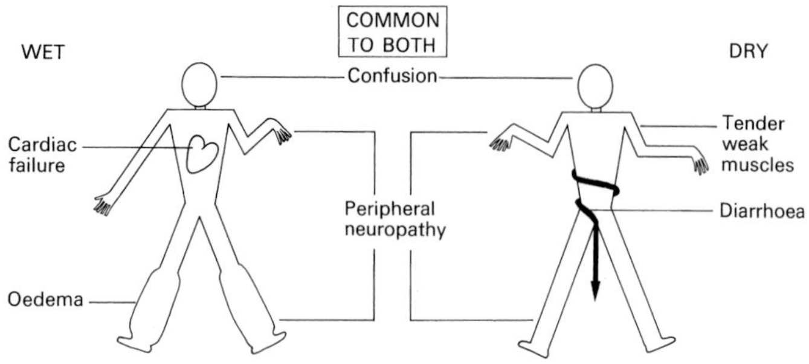

Fig. 3.25. The clinical features of wet and dry beri-beri. By courtesy of the Wellcome Trust.

Vitamin K

Sources

Vitamin K occurs abundantly in dark green vegetables and leaves as well as in some margarines and oils (particularly those based on soya beans). Its activity deteriorates with storage especially when exposed to light. There is virtually no data on vitamin K levels in African populations.

Functions

Vitamin K catalyses the conversion of certain proteins so that they become able to bind calcium ions. It is this property which gives them their biological actions in blood-clotting and bone formation. In the neonate deficiency of vitamin K is associated with haemorrhagic disease of the newborn. It is still not clear whether this arises from poor maternal diet, inadequate placental transfer or intestinal malabsorption. A possible role for vitamin K in influencing heart disease and osteoporosis remains controversial.

Water-soluble vitamins

Thiamin (vitamin B_1)

Sources and problem in Africa

The main dietary sources of thiamin in Africa are unrefined cereals grains and plant seeds (nuts and legumes). Organ meats are also a good source. In Africa deficiency is relatively rare, but it has been described chiefly in casual migrant labourers and alcoholics. It may occur as part of a general malnutrition syndrome associated with the anorexia of illness, e.g. in AIDS patients, alcoholism, poverty among migrant labourers particularly those who also drink a maize based beer. Outbreaks have been observed in poorly fed prisoners and in emergencies (WHO, 1999a). Deficiency used to be common in Asia due to consumption of diets based predominantly on polished rice.

Functions

Thiamin forms a cofactor for many reactions in carbohydrate metabolism and the requirements for the vitamin are therefore related to carbohydrate intake.

Beri-beri

Severe thiamin deficiency leads to beri-beri. The patient first has a peripheral neuropathy with sensory and motor symptoms in the legs, and then arms. Untreated, the disease progresses to wet or dry beri-beri (Fig. 3.25):

- Wet beri-beri. The patient has oedema, and a dilated cardiomyopathy with high output cardiac failure.
- Dry (shoshin) beri-beri. The patient is wasted, acidotic and often has chronic diarrhoea.

In both forms there may be a confusional state.

Treatment

1. Bed rest is essential if there is cardiac failure.
2. Intramuscular thiamine (WHO, 1999a): 10 mg daily for 1 week produces a dramatic response and diuresis. Dry beri-beri responds more slowly.

Riboflavin (vitamin B_2)

Sources

The main sources of riboflavin are dairy products, meat, fish and eggs.

Function

Riboflavin serves as a cofactor for many flavo-enzymes involved in oxidation–reduction reactions and in cellular respiration. Biochemical tests show that marginal deficiency is almost universal in non-dairy consuming rural populations in Africa, but clinical symptoms are less common.

Deficiency

Cracks in the skin at the corners of the mouth(angular stomatitis), cracked lips (cheilosis), and an intense glossitis – the tongue may become purplish in colour and oedematous – are characteristic. The patient may also have cracking and peeling of the skin of the scrotum and of the vulva. Some of these signs may be related to other associated deficiencies (Fig. 3.26).

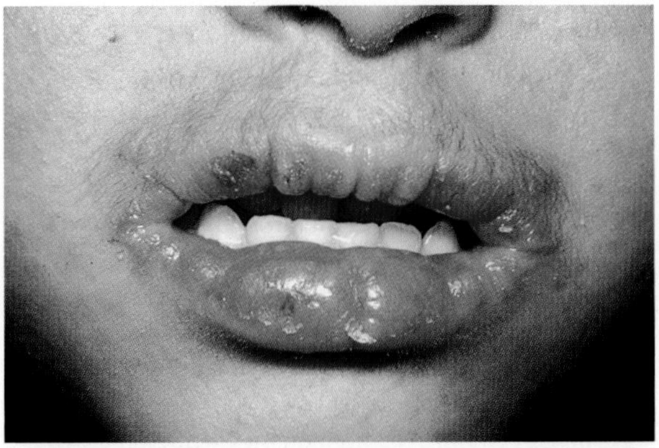

Fig. 3.26. Multiple micronutrient deficiencies, including riboflavin deficiency: angular stomatitis and cheilosis in a 4-year-old child from Bangladesh). By courtesy of the Wellcome Trust.

The full consequences of subclinical deficiency are not known but, as with many micronutrients, it is likely that deficiencies of one nutrient may exacerbate those of another. Several studies indicate that riboflavin deficiency may exacerbate iron-deficiency anaemia by blocking iron transport to the liver.

Treatment

A good mixed diet with yeast tablets is usually curative.

Niacin (nicotinic acid)

Severe deficiency causes pellagra.

Functions

Niacin is the collective term for nicotinic acid and its derivatives, niacinamide and nicotinamide. The latter is incorporated in NAD and NADP and functions in many reactions involved in glycolysis, fatty acid metabolism, respiration and detoxification.

Sources

The best dietary sources of niacin are eggs and dairy products and meat. Maize is deficient in tryptophan, an amino acid that spares niacin (WHO, 2000b).

Epidemiology

Pellagra is endemic in the maize-eating people of central and southern Africa, particularly among poor urban migrants, who subsist on maize and drink a lot of alcohol, or pathetically poor neglected older rural people. Inevitably, prisoners are vulnerable to this as to any dietary deficiency. Significant outbreaks have been reported among Mozambican refugees in Malawi, when groundnuts were no longer issued with their emergency rations of food (Malfait et al., 1993), and among refugees from civil war in Angola (Baquet et al., 2000).

Deficiency

The '3 Ds' – dermatitis, diarrhoea and dementia – are its hallmarks.

- Dermatitis. This is photosensitive, with hyperpigmentation and roughening of the skin, on forearms and around the neck ('Casal's Collar') (Fig. 3.27).
- Diarrhoea, with a smooth red and painful tongue. Oesophagitis can complicate severe pellagra.
- Dementia. This may be acute and can be precipitated by an acute infection, such as typhoid, when the patient presents with confusion, hallucinations and may be thought to have delirium tremens.

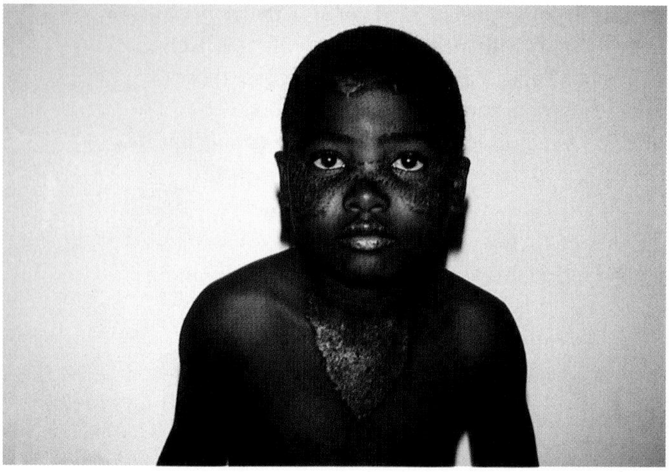

Fig. 3.27. Niacin deficiency: the photosensitive dermatosis in this child has the pattern described as Casal's necklace. By courtesy of the Wellcome Trust.

Treatment

Pellagra responds dramatically to nicotinamide, 50 mg three times a day by mouth. Chlorpromazine, 25–50 mg, is effective for the confusion.

Folic acid (folate)

Deficiency in what was discovered later to be folic acid was demonstrated first as a macrocytic anaemia prevalent among poor pregnant textile workers in Bombay. Folic acid is required, among other things, for DNA synthesis so deficiency is first clinically expressed in tissues with high rates of cell turnover. Megaloblastic anaemia, diagnosable from the appearance of hypersegmented nuclei in circulating neutrophils, is the most common detectable sign.

Folate deficiency can occur through inadequate intakes (especially in elderly people consuming monotonous diets), decreased absorption (e.g. through tropical gastroenteropathy), increased requirements (in pregnancy and lactation), drug interactions (e.g. anti-folate antimalarials) and alcoholism.

Pre-conceptional folate supplementation has been demonstrated conclusively to decrease the risk of neural-tube defects in European populations (MRC, 1991). A deficiency in folic acid (and/or vitamin B_6 and/or vitamin B_{12}) causes an increase in homocysteine levels, which is a risk factor for coronary heart disease.

As folic acid occurs in green leaves, nuts and grains, deficiency may be less likely in African populations than in many more wealthy societies. Nonetheless, many countries support combined iron and folate supplementation (FeFol) of pregnant women in an attempt to counter pregnancy-related anaemia.

Vitamin B_6 (pyridoxine)

Functions

Vitamin B_6 supplies the vital coenzyme pyridoxal phosphate (PLP), which plays a role in numerous reactions related to protein metabolism and the formation of several neurotransmitters. It also participates in glycogen metabolism and sphingolipid synthesis, and hence the formation of the nervous system.

Sources

Animal products are the best sources of vitamin B_6, but in Africa groundnuts, other nuts, and unpolished grains are good sources.

Clinical features

Those most vulnerable are the slow inactivators of isoniazid, which binds to PLP, as does penicillamine (certain natural moulds and fungi, which act as phosphorylation inhibitors, reduce the conversion of pyridoxine to PLP); those with chronic malabsorption; and alcoholics.

- Peripheral neuropathy, with sensory symptoms in feet and hands, is the dominant problem. As with other B vitamins, there may be glossitis, cheilosis and angular stomatitis.
- A sideroblastic anaemia may also occur.
- Subclinical deficiency can contribute to the build-up of homocysteine, which is associated with increased risk of CHD and premature ageing. Thus, like many vitamins, the nutritional target should not merely be to avoid clinical deficiency but rather to promote optimal intakes.

Vitamin B_{12} (cobalamin)

Pernicious anaemia is the classic clinical syndrome of vitamin B_{12} deficiency. It arises from a failure of methionine synthesis and ultimately of DNA synthesis. Folic acid is involved in the same reaction which accounts for the similarity in the megaloblastic anaemia with both deficiencies. Vitamin B_{12} deficiency also may cause megaloblastosis in enterocytes resulting in glossitis and diarrhoea. The vitamin also is involved in the degradation of fatty acids, and through this route deficiency can lead to subacute combined degeneration of the cord and a peripheral neuropathy. One study has shown marked improvement in neuropsychiatric symptoms on treatment with vitamin B_{12} (Bottiglieri, 1996).

All dietary vitamin B_{12} originates from microbial synthesis and subsequent incorporation into animal products. Strict vegetarians are prone to deficiency unless they take supplements. Bacterial contamination of foods and utensils is thought to help in maintaining reasonable dietary intakes in the poorest populations. The absorption of vitamin B_{12} is complex and requires an 'intrinsic factor'. Gastric atrophy can reduce absorption and several compounds interfere with uptake (e.g. colchicines, neomycin, aspirin and ethanol).

Biotin and pantothenic acid

Biotin and pantothenic acid are not covered here since deficiencies are virtually unknown except in cases of bizarre dietary practices or starvation.

Vitamin C (ascorbic acid)

Vitamin C is classically known for its protection against scurvy – hence its name 'ascorbic acid'.

Sources

Vitamin C is abundant in some vegetables and fruits – from wild baobab to mangoes and oranges, which have very high concentrations. Many populations therefore show marked swings in vitamin C status ranging from very good to very poor according to the fruit season (Fig. 3.28).

Epidemiology

Scurvy is uncommon in Africa and, while it has been described in labourers in southern Africa, in southern Sudanese migrants to Khartoum and inevitably in prisoners, it is a constant threat among refugees. The prevalence of clinical scurvy was between 13.6 and 44 per cent in refugees in camps in Somalia and Sudan, particularly among the old and women of child-bearing age (Desenclos et al., 1989). Scurvy may also be seen in patients with severe malabsorption and in alcoholics (WHO, 1999b). Scurvy takes about 6 months to develop on a grossly vitamin C deficient diet.

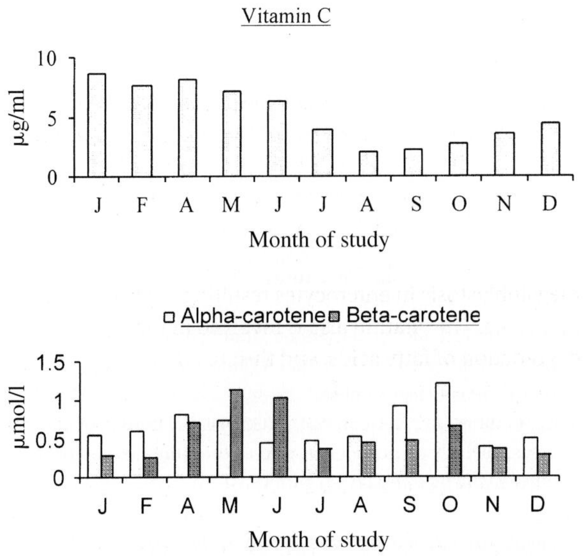

Fig. 3.28. Seasonal swings in vitamin C and carotenoid status in a Gambian subsistence farming community. (From SE Moore, MRC Keneba by kind permission.)

Functions

Ascorbic acid promotes the formation of protein cross-links in collagen. It also influences many other metabolic processes (such as carnitine and noradrenaline synthesis) but its quantitative role remains rather poorly understood. It is a strong reducing agent and hence can act as an anti-oxidant (see below). There is little evidence to support the often-quoted claim that very high intakes of vitamin C can protect against viral infections!

Clinical features

Marginal vitamin C deficiency has been suggested to cause bleeding gums and retarded wound healing, which are the typical signs of scurvy, but formal trials have found it difficult to prove this. Early signs in the skin are perifollicular haemorrhages: later, larger bruises in the skin and subperiosteal haemorrhages may cause an infant scream when moved. Leukocyte ascorbic acid is the best test to prove deficiency. In infants, radiographs of the knee show atrophic bones: a white line, due to calcified cartilage, is seen at the mataphysis and around the epiphysis.

Treatment

Ascorbic acid tablets 250 mg for adults and 50 mg for children, four times a day are curative. Fresh fruit is best as a means of prevention.

Anti-oxidants

The body creates a number of free radicals or 'reactive oxygen species' (ROS). Some of these are an inevitable, and undesirable, by-product of oxidative metabolism. Others are made intentionally in order to kill bacteria by an oxidant burst in phagocytes. If left uncontrolled, the oxidant stress resulting from many of these reactions causes tissue damage. Free radicals therefore need to be quenched by anti-oxidants. Some of these quenching reactions involve enzymic processes such as superoxide dismutase (which requires iron and zinc) and glutathione peroxidase (which requires vitamin E, selenium and reduced glutathione). Other nutrients can act directly as natural anti-oxidants (e.g. vitamin C and to a lesser extent the carotenoids). Nutritional status is critical in maintaining an appropriate oxidant balance, and hence may affect ageing processes by inhibiting tissue degradation.

References

Abelow BJ, Holford TR, Insogna KL. (1992). Cross-cultural association between dietary animal protein and hip fracture: a hypothesis. *Calcif Tissue Int*; **50**: 14–18.

Ashworth A, Feachem RG. (1985). Interventions for the control of diarrhoeal diseases among young children: prevention of low birth weight. *Bull Wld Hlth Org*; **63**: 165–184.

Baquet S, Wuillaume F, Van Egmond K et al. (2000). Pellagra outbreak in Kuito, Angola. Lancet, **355**: 1829–1830.

Barker DJP. (1998). *Mothers, Babies and Health in Later Life*. London: Churchill Livingstone.

Barrell RA, Rowland MG. (1979). Infant foods as a potential source of diarrhoeal illness in rural West Africa. *Trans Roy Soc Trop Med Hyg*; **73**: 85–90.

Beck MA. (1999). Selenium and host defence towards viruses. *Proc Nutr Soc*; **58**: 707–711.

Beisel, WR. (1977). Magnitude of the post-nutritional responses to infection. *Am J Clin Nutr*; **30**: 1236–1247.

Beisel WR. (1982). Single nutrients and immunity. *Am J Clin Nutr*; **35**: 417–469.

Beisel WR. (1995). Herman Award Lecture. Infection induced malnutrition – from cholera to cytokines. *Am J Clin Nutr*; **62**: 813–819.

Black RE, Sazawal S. (2001). Zinc and childhood infectious disease morbidity and mortality. *Br J Nutr*; **85**: S125–S129.

Bottiglieri T. (1996). Folate, vitamin B12, and neuropsychiatric disorders. *Nutr Rev*; **54**: 382–390.

Brown KH. (1997). Complementary feeding in developing countries: factors affecting energy intake. *Proc Nutr Soc*; **56**: 139–148.

Brown KH, Sanchez-Grinan M, Perez F, Peerson JM, Ganoza L, Stern JS. (1995). Effects of dietary energy density and feeding frequency on total energy intakes of recovering malnourished children. *Am J Clin Nutr*; **62**: 13–18.

Castillo-Duran C, Fishberg M, Valenzuela A et al. (1983). Controlled trial of copper supplementation during the recovery from marasmus. *Am J Clin Nutr*; **37**: 898–903.

Ceesay SM, Prentice AM, Cole TJ et al. (1997). Effects on birthweight and perinatal mortality of food supplementation in a primary healthcare setting in rural Gambia: 5 year prospective controlled trial. *Br Med J*; **315**: 786–790.

Cole TJ. (1993). *Seasonal effects on physical growth and development*. In *Seasonality and Human Ecology*, ed. SJ Ulijaszek, SS Strickland, pp. 89–106. Cambridge: Cambridge University Press.

Cooper RS, Rotime CN, Kaufman JS et al. (1997). Prevalence of NIDDM among populations of the African diaspora. *Diabetes Care*; **20**: 343–348.

Coutsoudis A, Pillay K, Spooner E, Kuhn L, Coovadia HM. (1999). Influence of infant-feeding patterns on early mother-to-child transmission of HIV-1 in Durban, South Africa: a prospective cohort study. South African Vitamin A Study Group. *Lancet*; **354**: 471–476.

Davidson SNMcD. (1972). *Human Nutrition and Dietetics*, 5th edn, p. 40. Edinburgh: Churchill Livingstone.

de Onis M, Frongillo EA, Blossner M. (2000). Is malnutrition declining? An analysis of changes in levels of child malnutrition since 1980. *Bull Wld Hlth Org*; **78**: 1222–1233.

Desenclos JC, Berry AM, Padt R et al. (1989). Epidemiological patterns of scurvy among Ethiopian refugees. *Bull Wld Hlth Org*; **67**: 309–316.

Doherty CP, Sarkar MA, Shakur MS, Ling SC, Elton RA, Cutting WA. (1998). Zinc and rehabilitation from severe protein-energy malnutrition: higher-dose regimens are associated with increased mortality. *Am J Clin Nutr*; **68**: 742–748.

Doherty CP, Weaver LT, Prentice AM. (2002). Micronutrient supplementation and infection: a double-edged sword? *J Paed Gastroenterol Nutr*; **34**: 346–352.

FAO (1994). Fats and oils in human nutrition: Report of a Joint Expert Consultation. FAO Food and Nutrition Paper No 57. Rome: Food and Agriculture Organization.

FAO (2000). *Agriculture, food and nutrition for Africa – A resource book for teachers of agriculture*. Rome: Food and Agriculture Organization. (available as pdf file at: http: //www.fao.org).

Fawzi WW, Chalmers TC, Herrera MG, Mosteller F. (1993). Vitamin A supplementation and child mortality: a meta-analysis. *J Am Med Assoc*; **269**: 898–903.

Fawzi WW, Msamanga GI, Spiegelman D et al. (1998). Randomised trial of effects of vitamin supplements on pregnancy outcomes and T cell counts in HIV-1–infected women in Tanzania. *Lancet*; *351*: 1477–1482.

Forrester T, Cooper RS, Weatherall D. (1998). Emergence of Western diseases in the tropical world: the experience with chronic cardiovascular diseases. *Br Med Bull*; **54**: 463–473.

Golden MHN. (1995). Severe malnutrition. In: *Oxford Textbook of Medicine*, ed DJ Weatherall, JGG Ledingham, DA Warrell. Oxford: Oxford University Press, pp 1278–1296.

Hanson L, Silfverdal SA, Stromback et al. (2001). The immunological role of breast feeding. *Pediatr Allergy Immunol*; **12**: 15–19.

Huffman SL, Zehner ER, Victora C. (2001). Can improvements in breast-feeding practices reduce neonatal mortality in developing countries? *Midwifery*; **17**: 80–92.

Institute of Medicine. (1992). *Nutrition during Pregnancy and Lactation – An Implementation Guide*. Washington, DC: National Academy Press.

IOM (1992) *Nutrition during Pregnancy and Lactation: An Implementation Guide*. Institute of Medicine. Washington: National Academy Press.

IVACG. (1997). Policy statement on vitamin A status and child mortality. International Vitamin A Consultative Group (see IVACG website listed above).

King H, Aubert RE, Herman WH. (1998). Global burden of diabetes, 1995–2025: prevalence, numerical estimates and projections. *Diabetes Care*; **21**: 1414–1431.

Kramer MS. (1987). Determinants of low birth weight: methodological assessment and meta-analysis. *Bull Wld Hlth Org*; **65**: 663–737.

Kramer MS. (2000). Balanced protein/energy supplementation in pregnancy. *Cochrane Database Syst Rev*; CD000032.

Lulseged S. (1990). Severe rickets in a children's hospital in Addis Ababa. *Ethiop Med J*; **28**: 175–181.

Lunn PG, Austin S, Prentice AM, Whitehead RG. (1984). The effect of improved nutrition on plasma prolactin concentrations and post-partum infertility in lactating Gambian women. *Am J Clin Nutr*; **39**: 227–235.

Lunn PG. (2000). The impact of infection and nutrition on gut function and growth in childhood. *Proc Nutr Soc*; **59**: 147–154.

McClaren DS. (1975). The great protein fiasco. *Lancet*; **ii**: 93–96.

Mahomed K. (2000). Zinc supplementation in pregnancy. *Cochrane Database Syst Rev*; CD000230.

Malfait P, Moren A, Dillon JC et al. (1993). An outbreak of pellagra related to changes in dietary niacin among Mozambican refugees in Malawi. *Int J Epidemiol*; **22**: 504–511.

Man WD, Weber M, Palmer A et al. (1998). Nutritional status of children admitted to hospital with different diseases, and its relationship to outcome in The Gambia, West Africa. *Trop Med Intl Health*; **3**: 678–686.

Morgan G. (1997). What, if any, is the effect of malnutrition on immunological competence? *Lancet*; **349**: 1693–1695.

MRC. (1991). Prevention of neural tube defects: results of the Medical Research Council Vitamin Study. MRC Vitamin Study Research Group. *Lancet*; **338**: 131–137.

Muhe L, Lulseged S, Mason KE et al. (1997). Case control study of nutritional rickets in the risk of developing pneumonia in Ethiopian children *Lancet*; **349**: 1801–1804.

NaNA/MRC/PHPNP. (2000). *Nationwide Survey on the Prevalence of Vitamin A and Iron Deficiency in Women and Children*. Report of the National Nutrition Agency, The Gambia.

Oginni LM, Worsfold M, Oyelami OA et al. (1996). Etiology of rickets in Nigerian children. *J Pediatr*; **128**: 692–694.

Okeke EC, Nnanyelugo DO. (1987). Intra-familial distribution of food and nutrients in a rural Nigerian population. *Ecol Food Nutr*; 23: 109–123.

Pi-Sunyer FX. (1993). Medical hazards of obesity. *Ann Intern Med*; **119**: 655–660.

Poppitt SD, Prentice AM, Jequier E, Schutz Y, Whitehead RG. (1993). Evidence of energy sparing in Gambian women during pregnancy: a longitudinal study using whole-body calorimetry. *Am J Clin Nutr*; **57**: 353–364.

Prentice AM, Whitehead RG, Roberts SB et al. (1980). Dietary supplementation of Gambian nursing mothers and lactational performance. *Lancet*; **ii**: 886–888.

Prentice AM, Goldberg GR, Prentice A. (1994). Body mass index and lactation performance. *Eur J Clin Nutr*; **48**: S78–S89.

Prentice A. (2000). Calcium in pregnancy and lactation. *Ann Rev Nutr*; **20**: 249–272.

Prentice AM, Paul AA. (2000). Fat and energy needs of children in developing countries. *Am J Clin Nutr*; **72**: 1253S-1265S.

Rice AL, Sacco L, Hyder A, Black RE. (2000). Malnutrition as an underlying cause of childhood deaths associated with infectious diseases in developing countries. *Bull Wld Hlth Org*; **78**: 1207–1221.

Rowland MG, Barrell RA, Whitehead RG. (1978). Bacterial contamination in traditional Gambian weaning foods. *Lancet*; **i**: 136–138.

Schofield C, Ashworth A. (1996). Why have mortality rates for severe malnutrition remained so high? *Bull Wld Hlth Org*; **74**: 223–229.

Shetty PS, James WPT. (1994). Body mass index – a measure of chronic energy deficiency in adults. FAO Food and Nutrition Paper No 56. Rome: FAO.

Sommer A. (1995). *Vitamin A deficiency and its consequences: a field guide to their detection and control*, 3rd edn. Geneva: World Health Organization.

Stein CE, Fall CHD, Kumaran K, Osmond C, Cox V, Barker DJP. (1996). Fetal growth and coronary heart disease in South India. *Lancet*, **348**: 1269–1273.

Tomkins A. (2000). Malnutrition, morbidity and mortality in children and their mothers. *Proc Nutr Soc*; **59**: 135–146.

Uauy R, De-Andraca I. (1995). Human milk and breast feeding for optimal mental development. *J Nutr*; **125**: 2278S-2280S.

UN ACC/SCN. (1992). *Second report on the world nutrition situation*. Vol 1. Global and regional results. Geneva, Switzerland.

Victora CG, Smith PG, Vaughan JP et al. (1987). Evidence for protection by breast-feeding against infant deaths from infectious diseases in Brazil. *Lancet*; **ii**: 319–322.

Victora CG, Bryce J, Fontaine O, Monasch R. (2000). Reducing deaths from diarrhoea through oral rehydration therapy. *Bull Wld Hlth Org*; **78**: 1246–1255.

Walker AF. (1990). The contribution of weaning foods to protein-energy malnutrition. *Nutr Res Revs*, **3**: 25–47.

Waterlow JC. (1992). *Protein-energy malnutrition*. London: Edward Arnold.

Whitehead RG, Coward WA, Lunn PG, Rutishauser I. (1977). A comparison of the pathogenesis of protein-energy malnutrition in Uganda and The Gambia. *Trans Roy Soc Trop Med Hyg*; **71**: 189–195.

Whitehead RG, Paul AA. (1984). Growth charts and the assessment of infant feeding practices in the western world and in developing countries. *Early Hum Dev*; **9**: 187–207.

Whittle HC. (1984). Food, agriculture and disease. In *Principles of Medicine in Africa*, ed. EHO Parry. 2nd edn, pp. 46–103. Oxford/Nairobi: Oxford University Press.

WHO. (1981). International Code of Marketing of Breast-milk Substitutes. Geneva: World Health Organization (available online as pdf file at: http: //www.who.int/nut/documents/code_english.PDF)

WHO Working Group. (1986). Use and interpretation of anthropometric indicators of nutritional status. *Bull Wld Hlth Org*; **64**: 924–941.

WHO. (1995). Bridging the Gaps. Report of the Director-General. Geneva: World Health Organization.

WHO. (1997). Vitamin A supplements: a guide to their use in the treatment and prevention of vitamin A deficiency and xerophthalmia. 2nd edn. Geneva: World Health Organization.

WHO. (1998). Obesity: preventing and managing the global

epidemic. WHO Technical Report Series No. 894. Geneva: World Health Organization.

WHO. (1999a). Thiamine deficiency and its prevention and control in major emergencies, World Health Organization, Geneva (available on-line as pdf file at http: //www.who.int/nut/documents/thiamine_in_emergencies_en g.pdf

WHO. (1999b). Scurvy and its prevention and control in major emergencies, World Health Organization, Geneva (available on-line as pdf file at http: //www.who.int/nut/documents/scurvy_in_emergencies_ eng.pdf)

WHO. (2000a). New data on the prevention of mother-to-child transmission of HIV and their policy implications conclusions and recommendations. *WHO Technical consultation on behalf of the UNFPA/UNICEF/WHO/UNAIDS Inter-Agency Task Team on Mother-to-Child Transmission of HIV. Geneva, 11–13 October 2000* (see http: //www.who.int/child-adolescent-health/New_ Publications/CHILD_HEALTH/MTCT_ Consultation.htm)

WHO. (2000b). Pellagra and its prevention and control in major emergencies, World Health Organization, Geneva (available on-line as pdf file at http: //www.who.int/nut/documents/pellagra_prevention_control.pdf)

WHO. (2001). Recommendations on exclusive breastfeeding. http: //www.who.int/child-adolescent-health/NUTRITION/infant_exclusive.htm

WHO/UNICEF/ICCIDD. (1993). *Global prevalence of iodine deficiency disorders.* MDIS (Micronutrient Deficiency Information System) Working Paper No 1. Geneva, Switzerland.

WHO/UNICEF. (1995). *Global prevalence of vitamin A deficiency.* MDIS (Micronutrient Deficiency Information System) Working Paper No 2. Geneva, Switzerland.

Wilkinson EA, Hawke CI. (1998). Does oral zinc aid the healing of chronic leg ulcers? A systematic literature review. *Arch Dermatol*; **134**: 1556–1560.

Woldemariam T, Sterky G. (1973). Severe rickets in infancy and childhood in Ethiopia. *J Pediatr*; **82**: 876–878.

Yajnik CS. (2001). The insulin resistance epidemic in India: fetal origins, later lifestyle, or both? *Nutr Rev*; **59**: 1–9.

Further Reading

Agriculture, Food and Nutrition for Africa – A Resource Book for Teachers of Agriculture (2000). Rome: FAO. (available as pdf file at: http: //www.fao.org)

Nutrition and Health in Developing Countries (2001). ed. R Semba. Humana: Humana Press.

Nutrition Today Matters Tomorrow: A Report from the March of Dimes Task Force on Nutrition and Optimal Human Development (2002) March of Dimes, White Plains, NY (available free from the March of Dimes Fulfilment Center, outside the US, call 570–820–8104).

Bowman BA & Russell RM, eds. (2001). *Present Knowledge in Nutrition.* Washington: ILSI Press.

Garrow JS, James WPT, eds. (1999). *Human Nutrition and Dietetics.* 10th edn. London: Churchill Livingstone.

World Health Organization. (1999). *Management of Severe Malnutrition. A Manual for Physicians and Other Senior Health Workers.* Geneva.

World Health Organization. (2000). *The Management of Nutrition in Major Emergencies.* Geneva.

Useful websites

Food and Agricultural Organization (FAO). http: //www.unicef.org
International Vitamin A Consultative Group (IVACG). http:// ivacg.ilsi.org/
International Council for the Control of Iodine Deficiency Disorders (ICCIDD). http: //www.people.virginia.edu/~jtd/ iccidd/
International Obesity TaskForce (IOTF) http: //www.iotf.org
Micronutrient Initiative (MI). http: //www.micronutrient.org/
United Nations International Children's Emergency Fund (UNICEF). http: //www.unicef.org
World Health Organization (WHO). http: //www.who.int/nut/
For iron: http: //www.who.int/nut/ida.htm
For iodine: http: //www.who.int/nut/idd.htm
For vitamin A: http: //www.who.int/nut/vad.htm

Refugees and disasters

4

Introduction

This chapter concentrates on the general principles of management of large groups of refugees or displaced people. It has been included because health workers need to understand and manage 'disasters' better.

In Africa, the impact of disasters is particularly severe because so many people are poor and have few reserves to cushion them against crises. In addition, the ability of some African countries to cope with disasters is impaired by poor infrastructure; especially primary and public health care systems.

The aim of this chapter is to encourage a carefully thought-out public health approach to tackling disasters. Both natural and conflict-based events will be discussed. These are often inter-linked, especially in Africa.

Disasters are usually of rapid onset and hence disorganized. Often, many organizations (governments, national and international NGOs) respond to the crisis, each pursuing different approaches creating a need for good co-ordination. The influence of external military peace-keeping forces and the media has also increased since the 1990s, bringing further complications.

This chapter does not include detailed descriptions of disease patterns and clinical case management. These are covered in other sections of the book. However, it is important to be aware that infectious disease is an important component in disasters and that it may not be possible to offer optimal clinical care.

There is a considerable literature available on health care in disasters, with handbooks produced by organizations such as the WHO, MSF, UNHCR and the Red Cross, as well as publications in the general medical literature and in specialist journals (such as *Disasters*). In a short chapter, we can only summarize the main points.

Lessons from previous disasters

Toole (1998) provided an resumé of the main lessons learnt from previous disasters and drew several valuable conclusions, which should be borne in mind when preparing an emergency response.

Summary of principles outlined by Toole (1998)

- Effective refugee health care must be based on accurate information and focus on disease prevention and health promotion
- Highly effective outcomes may be achieved through active involvement of host government staff, utilization of local refugee skills, and the insistence on accountability by relief agencies
- The major causes of mortality in refugee populations in developing countries may be prevented through the prompt use of well-proven, low-cost public health interventions.
- Refugees and internally displaced persons require the same quantity and range of nutrients required by all human beings
- Bold political measures and military support for humanitarian aid operations will only be effective if their application is predictable and consistent, interventions are based on real public health needs, and field personnel are adequately trained to deliver relevant services
- In public health, primary prevention aims to remove the risk of individuals being exposed to potentially harmful agents. Secondary and tertiary prevention measures reduce the harm caused by the agent and the risk of mortality or disability, respectively. When war-related injuries have been the major public health problem in a civilian population, the international community has failed to achieve the goals of primary prevention.

These may seem very obvious statements, but it is sad to reflect how misguided much emergency aid has been over the last few decades. There is no longer any need for inappropriate interventions.

Accountability of agencies

Agencies undertaking disaster response are increasingly held accountable to both donors and beneficiaries. Guidelines on best practice have been laid down in documents such as the *Code of Conduct for the International Red Cross and Red Crescent Movement and Non Governmental Organisations in Disaster Relief.*

The Sphere project (2000),*Humanitarian charter and minimum standards in disaster response,* has set agreed targets and principles for organizations, for example in the provision of water, vaccination priorities, sanitation and nutrition. This was developed with input from accumulated expertise throughout the humanitarian world.

Disasters

Disasters may have a rapid onset and a short duration of the acute phase, e.g. an earthquake, or may be long drawn-out chronic problems (famines, civil wars). In some instances, for example following an earthquake, the response required may be reasonably straightforward.

The types of emergencies often seen in Africa are a combination of human and natural disasters. These require a wide-ranging response. For example, the eruption of Mt. Nyragongo in Goma in eastern DRC in January 2002 compounded serious problems caused by 40 years of underdevelopment capped by the civil war that had affected the area for several years. The term 'complex emergencies' was coined to define these situations following the Rwandan crisis in 1994. Such emergencies are defined as 'relatively acute situations affecting large civilian populations, usually involving a combination of war or civil strife, food shortages and population displacement, resulting in excessive mortality' (Burkholder & Toole, 1995).

Wars

Between 1990 and 2000 at least 30 wars occurred each year throughout the world. Conflicts in Europe, the former Soviet Union and Asia received extensive publicity, but most of these were of short duration. Africa has the most conflicts of any continent but the media rarely reports them. Many of these are unlikely to be resolved in the near future. Some have lasted for over 20 years.

Causes

Unfortunately, resource-rich regions with unstable politics are particularly vulnerable. Disputes over international borders, partly a colonial legacy, continue to prevent stability, security and development. Disputes over resources (water, oil, mineral reserves etc) are likely to generate conflicts in the future.

Effects

The impact of war does not end with a peace accord; the effects on the infrastructure, economy, education and standard of living can be long lasting. The causes may remain unresolved, the psychological and socio-economic effects can last for years and re-establishment of agriculture and re-colonization of war affected areas can be seriously hindered by the physical legacy of conflict, e.g. landmines, unexploded ordnance, etc.

Natural disasters

Most of those affected by disasters world-wide (*c.* 80 per cent) are affected by natural or technological disasters. Nearly 200 million people were affected by this type of disaster during each year of the 1990s, and at least 80 000 people died in such disasters during 1999 (World Disasters Report, 2001).

The proportion (although not the numbers) affected by natural disasters is less in Africa than elsewhere, due to the numbers of conflicts, but the situation in Africa has been complicated because environmental changes have caused increased vulnerability in certain regions. For example, the size of the Sahara Desert has increased, regions to the south becoming drier, and this has affected adjacent regions seriously. The predicted 31 per cent reduction in flow in the River Niger will have a great impact in the sub-Saharan region (P. Walker 1998, personal communication to the IFRC). Changes in sea level due to global warming will affect the level of the Nile and may cause local flooding. The floods in Mozambique in 2001 placed immense pressure on the local infrastructure.

This type of disaster will continue and worsen as shortages of land lead to increased building on flood plains. The impact of such events should be measured not only in lives lost and people displaced but also the damage to social development, agriculture and infrastructure.

Refugees and IDPs

People who have had to flee their homes in the face of disaster are divided into two broad groups, those who have crossed internationally recognized borders in search of sanctuary (refugees) and those who have moved within the borders of their country of residence (internally displaced persons – IDPs). These two groups often have

Table 4.1. Estimated number of people of concern to UNHCR (January 2000)

Region	Refugees	Asylum seekers	Returned refugees	IDPs
Africa	3523250	61110	933890	1732290
Asia	4781750	24750	617620	1884740
Europe	2608380	473060	952060	3252300

similar needs but meeting those needs may pose very different problems.

Scale of the problem

Very large numbers of people fall within these two categories (Tables 4.1 and 4.2).

Legal status of refugees

A precise definition of a refugee was made in 1951 by the Convention Relating to the Status of Refugees.

Definition of a Refugee (Convention Relating to the Status of Refugees 1951)
'Any person who, owing to a well founded fear of being persecuted for reasons of race, religion, nationality, membership in a particular social group or political opinion, is outside the country of his nationality and is unable or, owing to such fear, is unwilling to avail himself of the protection of that country; or who, not having a nationality and being outside the country of his former habitual residence as the result of such events, is unable or, owing to such fear, is unwilling to return to it'.

The Convention also stressed the principle of non-refoulement (refugees cannot be forcibly returned to countries from which they have fled). This Convention is the heart of the international refugee protection system but is rather dated, e.g. its concentration on individuals persecuted for political reasons, reflecting its origins in the immediate post Second World War era. It has now been expanded to include those affected by other types of disaster and the mandate of the UN High Commission for Refugees (UNHCR), the body responsible for the care of refugees, has been enlarged to include those fleeing generalized danger rather than just individual persecution.

Predicament of IDPs

Refugees therefore have, at least in theory, considerable international legal protection. Nations that have ratified the convention have well-defined duties to care for refugees and to allow the UNHCR and other international bodies access to them. IDPs are in a very different legal position. They are still within the boundaries of their country of residence and the ability of the international community to help them may be limited especially if they come from groups politically unacceptable to their national government. The poorly planned repatriation of refugees, especially to countries where war continues, can simply mean that they become IDPs (as occurred in Afghanistan and in West Africa).

Table 4.2. The counties of origin and asylum of the six largest refugee groups in Africa in 1999 (UNHCR)

Country of origin	Main countries of asylum	Number of refugees
Burundi	Tanzania, DR Congo	525700
Sierra Leone	Guinea, Liberia, Gambia	487200
Sudan	Uganda, Ethiopia, DR Congo, Kenya, CA Republic, Chad	467700
Somalia	Ethiopia, Kenya, Yemen, Djibouti	451600
Angola	Zambia, DR Congo, Congo	350000
Eritrea	Sudan	345000

Vulnerability of residents

Other groups that may require aid, as much as those who have moved, are those who have remained at home but who are no longer supported by the original infrastructure or those who accept the burden of IDPs/refugees (e.g. host families).

Meeting their needs

Refugees

Meeting the needs of refugees who are on the move is difficult and it is often hard to predict where refugee movements may occur. However, once they have reached a place of relative safety, they are frequently housed in refugee camps and in this environment their numbers and their needs become relatively easier to define and meet (Toole & Waldeman, 1990).

IDPs

By contrast, enumeration, determination of health needs and provision of health services for IDPs can be extremely difficult, even if access is permitted. Many move into urban areas or remote areas of forest or bush. Their situation is, in some ways, analogous to that of refugees before they have reached a camp.

Appropriate interventions

Aid programmes should be designed to meet needs within the cultural and geopolitical constraints in the area.

It is important not to make things worse.

- The provision of aid to refugees or IDPs without considering the needs of the community that has taken them in may generate resentment and worsen their long-term position.
- Improper provision and use of aid may fuel conflicts if it is seen as a desirable resource.
- Poorly designed interventions can undermine longer-term development of the health sector as well as fail to deliver relief effectively.

A generic or standard initial response

Disaster management has been improved by analysis of past disasters. Each emergency is different and the effects on health differ according to the type of disaster and the population affected, but emergencies have enough in common for agencies to prepare generic responses allowing them to operate reasonably effectively from the beginning while they adjust what they do. Some of the many appropriate handbooks are listed in the references.

Information sources

Improved data collection and the development of prediction and planning tools have aided planning emergency responses. For example, information on the sub-Saharan meningitis epidemics is valuable in identifying the warning signs so that rapid action can be taken in the early stages of an epidemic. One example of these systems is the HINAP (Health Intelligence Network for Advanced Contingency Planning) system launched in 1999. This is intended for use by agencies involved in major public health emergencies with population movements. Other data resources, which are being developed, include *Healthmap*; a geographical information system designed to provide public health resources and information on diseases in the context of the local infrastructure. Reuters have produced a website to provide global news, communication and logistic reviews for the international disaster community (Alertnet).

Once a disaster has occurred, the response of any agency must be based on reliable data collected in the field and assessment of the needs of the affected people that are as accurate as possible.

Overview of medical aspects in disaster context

Changes in disease patterns

Although this chapter is aimed at the problems of refugees and IDPs associated with conflict and/or natural disasters; the impact of massive changes in disease patterns in Africa cannot be ignored, with the resurgence of previously controlled diseases and the emergence of new ones.

The most important is HIV/AIDS. It has been estimated that the number of people who will die from AIDS in the first decade of the twenty-first century will rival the number that died in all the wars in all the decades of the twentieth century (Al Gore, Jan 2000 at the UN Security Council, quoted in the World Disaster Report, 2001). The concomitant rise of TB as a co-infection is well documented and has been a major cause of the world-wide increase in TB cases.

In West Africa the conflicts in Sierra Leone and Liberia have resulted in increases in the numbers of cases of Lassa fever.

Mortality and morbidity

In most wars, more people die from illness than from trauma, and warfare is often accompanied by increases in frequency of disease. In the wars in Angola and Mozambique during the 1980s, for each person killed in combat, 14 died due to other causes. In times of war, excess mortality occurs in all age groups, but death rates are often particularly high in children under 14 years old. Orphaned and separated children and pregnant women are especially vulnerable.

Measured mortality

Deaths from disease can be overwhelming in massive disasters. In the Rwandan crisis of 1994, when between 500000 and 800 000 Hutus crossed into DRC in less than 1 week, it is estimated that 50 000 people died of infectious disease (much of it cholera) within the first month. This is a crude mortality rate of 20 to 35 per 10 000 per day. A significant excess mortality is defined as greater than 1 death per 10 000 per day. The rate inside Rwanda during the genocide was 10 per 10 000 per day

Breakdown in control of disease

Breakdowns in disease control measures such as vector control and water purification lead to upsurges in infections. The war in Bosnia saw large increases in the incidence of diarrhoeal disease, hepatitis A, lice and scabies and there have been vast increases in the incidence of malaria and typhoid following the civil war in Tajikistan.

When considering the diseases likely to affect a displaced population, the area of origin of the people and the route they have taken to their place of refuge must be taken into account. They may have been exposed to unfamiliar infections en route or at their place of refuge, diseases to which they have little natural resistance. Equally, they may bring with them diseases not normally found in their new location, presenting a risk to their host population.

Major causes of mortality and morbidity

Five conditions, acute respiratory infection, diarrhoeal diseases, measles, malaria and malnutrition consistently account for 60–95 per cent of all deaths of refugees and IDPs (Toole et al., 1992). Other potential causes of epidemics, e.g. meningitis, typhus or plague are less common. Some are regional, e.g. typhus in Burundi, and an awareness of past disease patterns in an area, can help planning for particular disease hazards.

Details of the clinical management of these conditions are described elsewhere in this book. We emphasize here aspects of the control of infections that are particularly important among refugees and where control may be affected by the special circumstances. The key elements of control are listed in the next box.

ARI

Attack and case-fatality rates due to acute respiratory infection are particularly high in malnourished children, especially in overcrowded conditions. Effective control is essential when dealing with refugees and IDPs.

Diarrhoea

Disasters provide the ideal setting for outbreaks of diarrhoeal disease, which can be devastating. In 1994, one million Rwandan refugees in Goma were exposed to cholera and dysentery: more than 50 000 died in the first month of the outbreak. If outbreaks occur they must be managed properly (Fig. 4.1).

Any agency operating in a disaster where outbreaks of diarrhoea can be expected must:

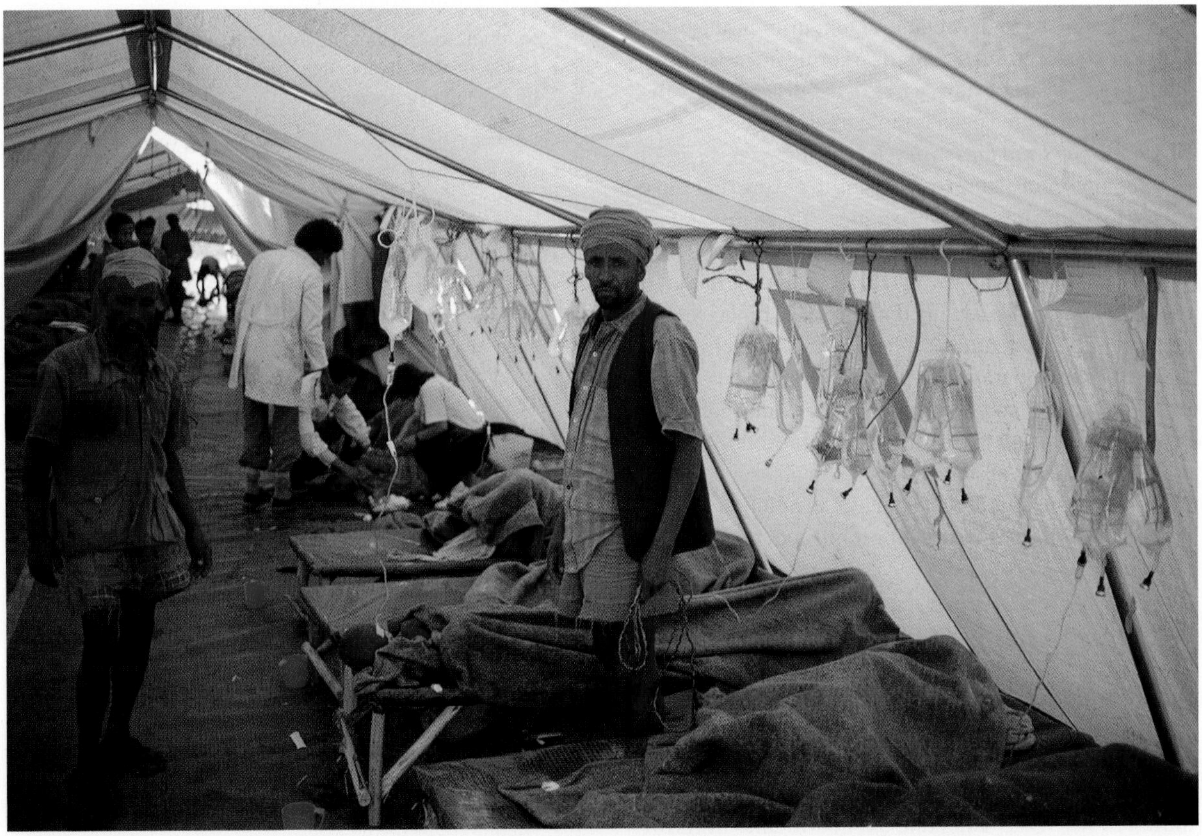

Fig. 4.1. Cholera outbreak in Korem, Ethiopia, 1985. Simple methods of rehydration are being used: a practicable approach.

- set up emergency preparedness programmes;
- train staff properly;
- stockpile appropriate equipment for rehydration points;
- where possible, improve hygiene measures and undertake hygiene education.

Measles

Measles was a major cause of refugee deaths in the 1980s and children under 5 years old are especially vulnerable. For example, there was a 32 per cent case-fatality rate among children with measles in the Wad Kowli camp in the Sudan, in 1985 (Toole & Waldman, 1990). This disease is less of a problem in disasters than it was due, at least in part, to aid agencies undertaking measles immunization as the first health priority when dealing with refugees or IDPs. Measles can precipitate acute kwashiorkor in children with borderline malnourishment and can exacerbate vitamin A deficiency leading to blindness. The risk that children will develop severe measles or die of the disease is greatly increased if they are clinically or subclinically deficient in vitamin A.

Malaria

Population movements often lead to non-immune individuals being exposed to malaria or bring infected individuals into areas previously free of the disease. As with diarrhoea, the prime need is rapid treatment especially where *Plasmodium falciparum* is endemic as this can kill very rapidly. Information campaigns to ensure that those with fever come forward for treatment are an integral part of control programmes.

Malaria control, whether in refugee camps or in the open situations where many IDPs live, is complex and poor control and treatment measures can result in outbreaks. Control operations will depend on the level of information and technical skill available. Anti-malarial drugs are important in treatment and prevention but may not be available to all and public health measures are likely to be much more cost effective. In addition, resistance to anti-malarial drugs is becoming an increasing problem.

Nutrition

Malnutrition remains a serious problem for refugees and IDPs. There is a strong relationship between malnutrition and mortality. Food shortages due to breakdowns in storage and distribution systems are exacerbated when large areas of land are unproductive through land mines, or when the deliberate use of atrocities or terror prevents people settling in an area long enough to produce food, e.g. in Sierra Leone. In a disaster, everyone must receive an adequate general food ration (the World Food Programme suggests at least 1900 kcal/head/day for survival but WHO recommends 2100 kcal/head/day). When malnutrition rates are high, supplementary and therapeutic feeding programmes aimed at vulnerable groups, e.g. the under 5s and pregnant women, are effective in decreasing morbidity and mortality, but are expensive.

The food aid provided for refugees is usually designed to treat or prevent protein energy malnutrition (PEM). Population-based PEM levels are based on sampling those between 6 and 59 months of age. The prevalence of serious PEM depends on the situation and advice should be obtained from a nutritionist. The importance of micronutrients has been recognized more recently (Toole, 1992).

Key measures for disease prevention and control

Health promotion programmes play a central role in prevention and control of all infectious diseases and other health problems in these situations.

ARI
- Better shelter and nutrition
- Less overcrowding
- Immunization against measles and pertussis
- Follow treatment guidelines on management of LRI (may be difficult in emergencies).

Diarrhoea
- Safe food and water
- Proper disposal of waste and dead bodies
- Vermin control
- Oral rehydration salts (ORS)
- Large numbers of rehydration points provided with ORS, disposable cups (or facilities to sterilize reusable mugs), large supplies of safe water, intravenous fluids, giving sets, cover (tents), beds, etc.
- Training of health workers in the management of acute diarrhoeal diseases

Measles
- Vaccination
- Vitamin A supplements

Malaria
- Control mosquito breeding sites
- Residual insecticide spraying
- Treated bed nets
- Anti-malarial drugs

Nutrition
- Therapeutic and supplementary feeding programmes
- Micronutrients
- Vitamin supplements

Scurvy, pellagra, thiamine, iron and iodine deficiencies have all caused problems in different disasters. Most refugees' rations contain less than the recommended daily allowance of 2500 i.u. of vitamin A and the distribution of this vitamin to children is one of the most effective interventions to reduce mortality in refugee populations.

Planning a suitable response

Needs assessment

When disaster strikes, there is a conflict between the desire to start an aid programme immediately, even if this is done without adequate information, and delaying the response to allow time for a proper needs assessment. Do not assume that a useful response can be mounted without preliminary investigation. The initial assessment is the foundation for the whole programme and must contain relevant, accurate, timely, representative and easily analysed information. The agency may wish to follow the ATPAR process (assess – think – plan – act – review), or an equivalent tool. Information is required on the needs of the population (both refugee/IDP and local) of the resources available to meet those needs, and of the capacity of the local population, the host government and of the agency itself to respond. The assessment process must include consultation with those to whom aid is being supplied to ensure that their real needs are met (see the Box).

Needs assessment

- Determine the needs of those affected
- Decide on the order of priority to meet these needs
- Determine resources available in the affected country (i.e. capacity assessment)
- Assess the security and other risks affecting the response
- Decide on the objectives of the agency's response (e.g. mortality reduction, vaccination coverage)
- Draw up plans for the response
- Implement the response
- Monitor progress towards achievement of the predetermined objectives
- Modify the programme in the light of changes in the situation and of new information provided by ongoing assessment

An inadequate assessment can lead to an ineffective response. A balance must be struck between gathering enough information to mount an effective programme, and wasting time gathering unnecessary data. Make a clear distinction between what you need to know and what you would like to know. Each situation will be different and the assessment will reflect this but there will always be a certain core of information that is required making it possible to produce needs assessment protocols. The information requirements are centred on the basic principles of who, what, when, where, why and how.

Monitoring the response

A persistent problem for aid agencies has been producing consistent and repeatable needs assessments that can be used for initial determination of need and as tools to monitor programme progress. Most needs assessments are descriptive, but there is a move towards the use of statistical methods such as the cluster analysis methods developed for the Expanded Programme on Immunization (Henderson & Sundaresen, 1982; Bennett et al., 1991; Drysdale et al., 2000) and of small area statistics to produce objective and repeatable surveys.

Needs assessment is a dynamic concept and continues as the programme progresses:

- Repeat assessments as part of the evaluation process to check the effectiveness of the response.
- Make new assessments at any time if the situation changes or a new crisis point, e.g. a new refugee camp, is established or discovered.

Public health priorities

Initial priorities

Although understanding the priorities of a particular emergency will require a needs assessment, people have certain key needs that must be met in any response to a disaster.

Key needs

- Safe water
- Food, utensils and cooking fuel
- Shelter and blankets
- Sanitation (disposal of refuse, faeces, bodies; vector control)
- Curative health care for acute respiratory infections, diarrhoea and malaria
- Measles vaccination
- Vitamin A distribution to those under 14
- Establishment of simple surveillance system for epidemic disease and nutrition

The relative importance of each of these will vary. Water, food and shelter are of high priority. When temperatures are low, shelters and blankets are the highest priority. Insulation reduces food requirements; an additional

100 kcal/person/day is needed for every 5 °C temperature drop below 20 °C.

The need for the establishment of curative care services must not be overlooked. Many of the displaced will be in urgent need of such services.

Water

Sufficient water must be supplied. It is better to provide large amounts of reasonably clean water than small volumes of pure water. Health education is of supreme importance. Beneficiary participation, an important tool in implementing such measures, is often under-utilized.

Supplies

The stockpiling of appropriate logistic and medical supplies is a priority at the start of an emergency. Analysis of data about types of illness in an area can facilitate prediction of possible problems and allow pre-positioning of appropriate supplies and identification of suitable personnel to ensure rapid responses to developing problems.

Health care

Meeting health needs requires:

- establishment of basic clinics with treatment protocols and limited drug prescribing (oral)
- community outreach
- epidemic management with specific protocols
- decisions on management of surgical/obstetric emergencies
- agreement on referral if possible or appropriate. (Determine availability of referral facilities during than initial assessment.)

Basic health education material should be available from the beginning but as leaders emerge in a camp and medical services become established with increased participation by the camp's inhabitants, outreach and community health education programmes should be developed. Treatment protocols can be modified to suit local conditions. Work can begin to tackle less acute but potentially serious problems such as TB and STIs.

Those who are planning programmes must be aware that logistic and security issues can make needs assessment and epidemiological and microbiological outbreak investigation very difficult.

Logistic considerations

Infrastructure – large actions are needed quickly

In complex disasters it can be difficult for the inexperienced to think in public health terms. However, a camp holding 100 000 people has the same population as a large town (Fig. 4.2). A town usually has an established infrastructure of water, sanitation, housing and shops, but these have to be established for a camp and this has to be done quickly. Good links with local authorities must be established rapidly, however difficult this may be in the circumstances.

Certain organizations (e.g. Oxfam, MSF) have considerable expertise in the provision of water and sanitation systems. Co-operation between agencies with each providing help in its main field of expertise and complementing the work of others is increasingly seen as the most productive way to provide aid in emergencies.

Co-ordination

This is one of the most important aspects of a successful intervention, as there may be as many as 100 different organizations on the ground. In general, the UN agencies (WHO, UNHCR) are best placed to co-ordinate the response.

The media

The press often creates additional strain on resources and personnel. But good relationships with the press are important in order to mobilize public opinion in donor countries and hence ensure financial support (Pelly, 1996). An effective co-ordinating agency can help the situation by providing good press briefings and by removing pressure from individual NGOs (Perrin, 1996).

Constraints

Disasters frequently occur in difficult areas and inevitably there are many constraints to effective intervention.

Constraints

- Security
- Limited access
- Logistics and infrastructure (e.g. roads, distance, water, electricity)
- Communication between host government and outside organizations
- Co-ordination of agencies working in the region and the emergency
- Competition between agencies
- Media pressure to intervene often without appropriate planning

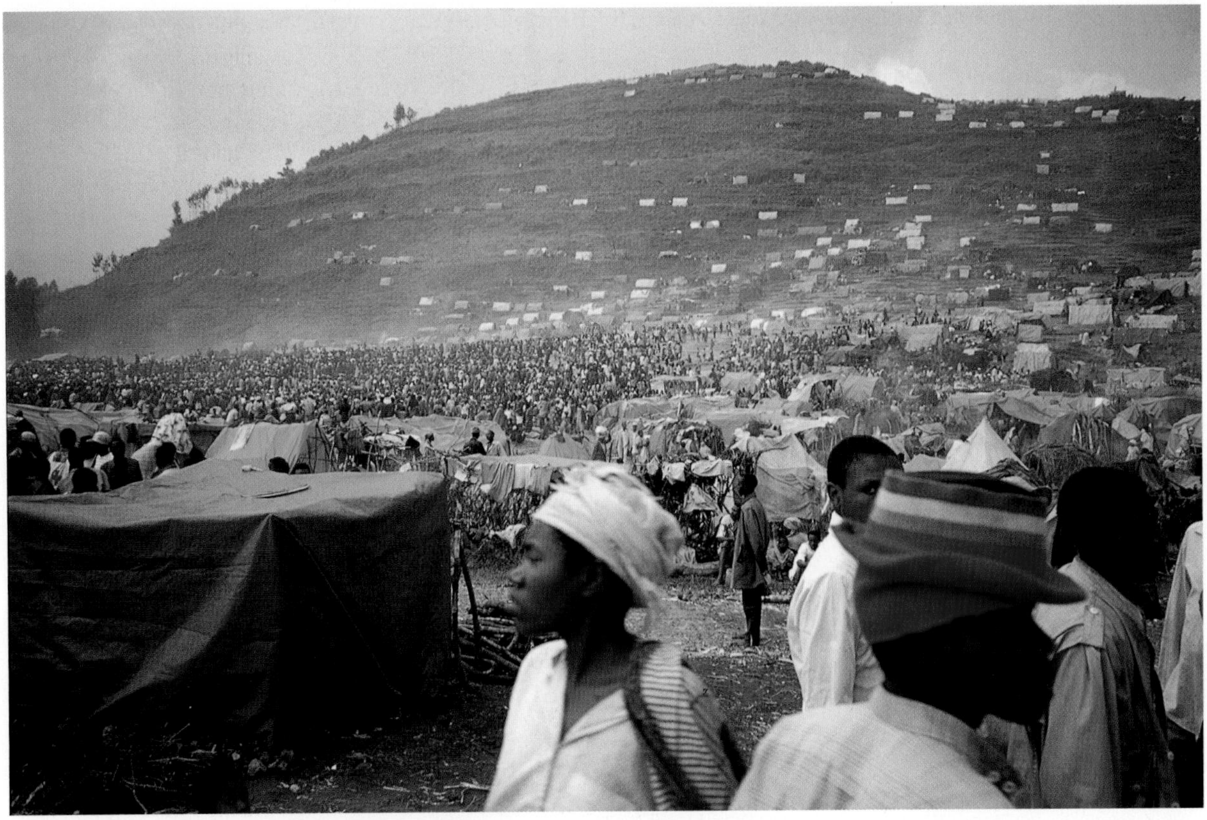

Fig. 4.2. Kibumba Camp, Goma (now Democratic Republic of Congo), 1994.

Conclusions

In any crisis, simple guidelines from one of the many publications on the subject are invaluable in ensuring priorities are tackled appropriately. The pressures on the humanitarian agencies have increased with the major crises since the 1990s and this trend will probably continue. Governments in the region will need assistance, both from the major players and from the NGO community. The potential for effective collaboration is there, but an agreed knowledge of the priorities and best practice is vital for responses to be effective. Unfortunately, disaster preparedness is difficult in countries with poor economies and decaying infrastructure. The responsibility for this has become global.

References

Banatvala N, Laurence B, Healing TD. (1999). Paediatric care in disaster and refugee situations. *Rec Adv Paediat*; **17**; 211–227.

Bennett S, Woods T, Liyange WM, Smith DL. (1991). A simplified general method for cluster sample surveys of health in developing countries. *Wld Hlth Statist Quart*; **44**: 98–106.

Burkholder B, Toole MJ. (1995). Evolution of complex disasters *Lancet*, **346**: 1012–1015.

Drysdale S, Howarth J, Powell, Healing TD. (2000). The use of cluster sampling to determine aid needs in Grozny, Chechnya in 1995. *Disasters*; **24**: 217–227.

Henderson RH, Sundaresen T. (1982). Cluster sampling to assess immunisation coverage: a review of experience with a simplified sampling method. *Bull Wld Hlth Org*; **60**: 253–260.

Howarth JP, Healing TD, Banatvala N. (1987). Health care in disaster and refugee settings. *Lancet*; **348**: 14–17.

International Federation of the Red Cross and Red Crescent (IFRC) Societies (2001). World Disasters Report.

Médecins sans Frontières. (1997). *Refugee Health – An Approach to Emergency Situations.* London: Macmillan.

Noji EK. (ed) (1997). *The Public Health Consequences of Disasters.* Oxford: Oxford University Press.

Perrin P. (1996). *War and Public Health.* Geneva: International Committee of the Red Cross.

Sphere project. (2000). *Humanitarian Charter and Minimum Standards in Disaster Response.* Oxford: Oxfam Publishing.

Pelly MDE. (1996). Humanitarian aid and the media. *Bull Trop Med Intl Hlth*; **4**: 1–2.

Toole MJ. (1992). Micronutrient deficiencies in refugees. *Lancet*; 339: 1214–1216.

Toole MJ. (1998). (Address) Protecting the health of conflict-affected populations: lessons learned, 1976–1998. Presented at the Conference on Humanitarian Aid Challenges in the New Millenium. New York.

Toole MJ, Waldeman RJ. (1990). Prevention of excess mortality in refugees and displaced populations in developing countries. *JAMA*; **263**: 3296–3302.

Toole MJ, Malikki RM. (1992). Famine affected, refugee and displaced populations: recommendations for public health issues. *MMWR*; 41: RR13.

Further reading

Bres P. (1986). *Public Health Action in Emergencies Caused by Epidemics.* Geneva: World Health Organization.

Chin JA. (2000). *Control of Communicable Diseases Manual.* 17th edn. Washington: American Public Health Association.

Davis J, Lambert R. (1995). *Engineering in Emergencies. A Practical Guide for Relief Workers.* IT Publications

Eddleston M, Pierini S. (1999). *Oxford Handbook of Tropical Medicine.* Oxford: Oxford University Press.

Levy BS, Sidel VW. (eds.). (1997). *War and Public Health.* Oxford: Oxford University Press.

Lumley JSP, Ryan JM, Baxter PJ, Kirby N. (eds). (1996). *Handbook of the Medical Care of Catastrophes,* London: Royal Society of Medicine Press.

Useful websites

WHO	www.who.int/
Roll back malaria	www.rbm.who.int
Hinap	www.who.int/disasters/
Healthmap	www.who.int/emc/healthmap
UNICEF	www.unicef.org
FAO	www.fao.org
UNAIDS	www.unaids.org
UNHCR	www.unhcr.ch
IFRC	www.ifrc.org
ICRC	www.icrc.org
Disasters	www.webguide.webmagic.com/disasters.com
Reuters Alertnet	www.alertnet.org

5

Managing a health service

Foundations of health service management

The structure of health services in Africa

Levels of care

Peripheral health units, such as health centres, dispensaries or community health posts, are the first point of contact between patients and the formal public health care system in most rural African districts. People also seek help from more or less well-trained private medical providers, pharmacies and formal or informal drug retailers; and they still use traditional providers, especially in rural areas. These are popular for psychosocial problems, HIV-related disease and other problems, where orthodox medicine does not meet all people's needs. Generally, there are more health care options in cities, towns and settlements along the main roads. Together, these providers represent the primary level of medical care, and we have to consider the performance and quality of all of them when we want to improve health services in the district.

The structure of the health care system, especially in Anglophone African countries, is organized around the district hospital, which is responsible for the health of the district population. The district hospital provides secondary level medical care; whilst regional (provincial) and national hospitals serve as tertiary care institutions. The underlying assumption is that a referral chain exists: a patient is only referred to be seen at the next higher level if the one below it cannot manage the medical problem. In reality, most district and even tertiary hospitals have very busy outpatient departments that act as primary care units for the local community. As countries increasingly become urbanized, urban polyclinics function like district hospitals and are meant to act as an intermediate tier between smaller urban clinics and tertiary and specialist hospitals.

Primary medical care vs. primary health care

The primary level of medical care (also called primary medical care or simply primary care) is often confused with primary health care. Primary medical care refers to the first contact between patients and the health system. It focuses on individuals and is mainly concerned with delivering curative services to those who seek them. Primary health care is a broader concept. It

- focuses on the entire community – not just on those who visit health facilities
- is concerned with disease prevention, health promotion and curative care.

District health system

The district health management team (DHMT) forms the backbone of health services in the district. Led by the district medical officer (DMO) or district manager its task is:

- to plan, manage and monitor public health and community service delivery at lower levels.
- to react swiftly in the case of outbreaks or other public health emergencies, if necessary by calling in help from outside.
- to monitor the care offered by private, commercial and non-commercial health care providers in the district.

The team comprises specialists from a number of key areas, which may differ from country to country but often includes senior staff responsible for nursing care, the expanded programme on immunization (EPI), mother and child care, tuberculosis control, primary health care, AIDS control and drug supply.

Large municipalities and urban areas may also be divided into zones, with zonal teams responsible for the health of defined geographical areas and their populations. These zonal teams are equivalent to the DHMT in a rural district.

Co-ordinating hospital and district health services

In some countries, the DMO is at the same time a senior medical officer or even the medical officer in charge of the district hospital, thus combining the job of a public health service manager with clinical and even hospital management duties. Ideally, such multiple responsibilities should be avoided, because they present an enormous workload, but this may not always be feasible. Where the DMO is a hospital clinician, it is essential that he or she is genuinely interested, and ideally has training in public health management; otherwise, community health services may suffer at the expense of hospital priorities. But, as coordinated disease control for many of the major disease priorities – malaria, HIV/AIDS and tuberculosis – becomes more and more important, there are definite advantages in including senior hospital staff on the DHMT. This provides an integrated approach to curative, outreach and preventive care. Such staff, for example, can include the hospital manager, matron, pharmacy and the senior laboratory staff member.

In many African countries, hospitals that are run by religious organizations are charged with official government functions. They act as designated district hospitals, where they carry responsibility for coordinating community health services in their area, working within a nationally defined policy framework and answerable to higher levels of the ministry of health.

Peripheral health units

The health centre (HC)

The HC has been defined as a unit which provides a family with a basic or 'essential' package of curative and preventive health services, other than those which can only be provided by a hospital such as major surgery or specialist care (King, 1966). They are run by clinically trained medical assistants or experienced nurses and often provide inpatient as well as outpatient care. They usually have trained midwives, and provide basic emergency obstetrical care, other than major interventions such as caesarean sections. They can provide a comprehensive package of preventive and curative services that makes a substantial contribution to the health of the population, and relieve some of the primary care burden from the district hospital.

Each health centre is responsible for the health of the population in a specified area within the district, sometimes called a sub-district. Ideally, the entire country is covered by a network of rural health centres and urban clinics, with rapid and convenient access for anyone who requires these services. The reality in most developing countries, especially in rural areas and those which are difficult to reach, is that health centres need to be complemented by smaller peripheral units and outreach activities. These ensure that at least a minimum set of preventive and curative services are within easy reach of every community.

Smaller peripheral units – dispensaries or community health posts

A dispensary may be staffed by a trained medical aide, community health nurse and/or nurse-midwife. They are trained to cope with common and more easily managed health problems, and to recognize and refer more serious or complicated conditions to the next higher level. In practice, when the condition is urgent (such as an obstetric emergency) or health centres have limited capacity, cases are referred directly to the district hospital.

Community health workers

The type of training and mechanisms for paying health workers in the most peripheral units vary between different African countries. The policy in some cases is only to have ministry of health-salaried workers at the periphery. Following the Alma Ata conference, there was a big drive in many countries to train community health workers (CHWs). The training of CHWs is comparatively short, typically comprising a few weeks to a few months, organized either *en-bloc* or in intervals, and is often conducted with the support of the district hospital and the DHMT. A key feature is that CHWs are usually not government employees and either work as volunteers or are reimbursed by the local community. On occasion, the local traditional midwife or even the local traditional healer may be trained as a CHW. Trained traditional birth attendants (TBAs) are an important source of care for pregnant women, especially in rural areas.

During the late 1980s and the 1990s ministries of health in many countries moved away from the CHW model because often the strategy had not met the expectations. Unfortunately, when these decisions were taken, the importance of CHWs as potential agents of change in the community and their role in community development was often overlooked, because in many cases this strategy did not meet people's and policy makers' expectations. At least in part, the disappointment occurred because the model had not been fully implemented: for example, CHWs often had not been selected carefully and not been supported regularly and supervised from higher levels of the health system.

Primary health care: the principles

Alma Ata revisited: The philosophy and the principles of PHC

The philosophy of Primary Health Care (PHC) has evolved from decades of experience in developing countries. Many countries, when they emerged from colonial rule, invested in a hospital-based model that offered mainly curative care, but found that they could only afford to build and resource hospitals in the major cities and some towns, so that their population, especially those in rural areas, were largely deprived of medical and preventive care. PHC was an answer to the realization that this effort had failed, and that the very limited available resources needed to be spent more fairly and wisely. Countries also realized that many of the determinants of health could only be tackled by going beyond the health sector, working with other sectors and communities, in addressing urgent social and developmental needs.

A new concept was formulated in 1978 during a conference organized by the World Health Organization (WHO) and attended by over 60 countries, held at Alma Ata (now called Almaty), the capital of Kasahkstan.

The conference defined Primary Health Care as:

> essential health care made accessible to individuals and families in the community, by means acceptable to them, through their full participation, and at a cost that the community and country can afford.
>
> (Alma Ata Declaration 1978, cited in Tarimo and Webster, 1994)

Four principles were agreed, which embody the PHC concept. While representing an ideal, they are still accepted as a yardstick for the planning of health programmes in Africa and are used to evaluate their success:

(a) *Universal accessibility and coverage on the basis of need*, acknowledging equity as a value, and thus the need to make essential services available to all. This principle recognized that 70 per cent or more of health care resources were spent on urban hospitals that were accessible to only 30 per cent or less of the population.

(b) *Community and individual involvement and self-reliance*, accepting the need for and the advantages of decentralized decision making and local responsibility and initiative. This principle is based on the belief that communities know many of the causes of their health problems; and that they have essential insights into possible solutions, and can mobilize their own resources to help implement solutions. It recognizes that technical and financial support from higher levels will still usually be required.

(c) *Intersectoral action for health*, recognizing that the health of a population depends on its overall development. This principle comes from an understanding of the underlying determinants of health, especially income and education; but also recognizes that the health care system must work with other sectors to achieve health goals. This requires tackling the immediate determinants of health, working with those sectors that are responsible for providing clean water, sanitation, nutrition, and other services.

(d) *Appropriate technology and cost-effectiveness*, based on available human and material resources. This principle recognizes that even very limited resources can make a big difference to people's health, if they are spent on affordable interventions and on activities that provide best value for money.

PHC: activities and components

Under the guidance of WHO, eight major priorities or interventions were identified to translate the philosophy of PHC into practice (Tarimo and Webster, 1994):

- access to clean water and appropriate sanitation
- provision of sufficient food and balanced nutrition
- immunization against six major diseases
- mother and child health (MCH) care, including family planning techniques to achieve child spacing
- prevention and control of locally endemic diseases
- treatment for common diseases and injuries
- health education about prevention and control of important diseases
- the provision of essential drugs

Comprehensive vs. selective PHC

Comprehensive PHC approach

The concept of PHC implies that all of the components of a basic or essential package of care are made available to communities, with their active involvement and with technical support and resources provided by staff from the health and other sectors. This 'bottom-up' approach can improve not only the health status but also the social capacity of communities. However, the comprehensive PHC approach takes time to deliver results and may sometimes fail, especially where there is lack of commitment and resources from government.

Selective PHC approach

During the 1980s, more targeted (selective) strategies for delivering the primary health care components were recommended by some international agencies. This 'top-down' approach focused on delivering a small range of cost-effective health services, rather than on a broad sector-wide approach to improving health. Such selective PHC activities use vertical management and support structures, with less involvement and development of communities. Typical examples were the Universal Child Immunization initiative of UNICEF in the 1980s, and more recently the polio eradication initiative.

Selective PHC may be more effective than the comprehensive approach in the short term and has achieved some major successes, but is usually more costly and less sustainable. The debate about these different approaches (see Rifkin & Wall, 1986) continues without a conclusion!

District health service managers in Africa usually favour the comprehensive approach, as they have to deal with everyday realities, but will complement it with a selective strategy if emergencies require a rapid and efficient response.

Some diseases, such as onchocerciasis, are best tackled through vertically organized mass campaigns. Other problems, such as malaria or obstetrical emergencies, require the whole health system to be functioning well. Finding the right 'fit' depends on the context, the specific health problem, and the time-span of commitment (Cairncross et al., 1997). Many international policy makers, especially those working within specific international disease control programmes, favour selective approaches that provide quicker results.

The challenges

Health and disease in the community: the ears of the hippopotamus

Disease patterns: hospital vs. community

Managing a health service for a defined population requires addressing the important health needs of the population. But what are the priorities? When working out of hospitals and health centres, our perception of what is important is often moulded by the patterns of morbidity that we are confronted with. However, disease seen in hospital may not be representative of disease in the community. Less obvious health problems, such as HIV in the early stages of the epidemic, which often does not present to the hospital or health centre, may well be bigger threats to the health of the population. Disease encountered in hospitals has rightly been compared with the ears of the submerged hippopotamus: these are clearly visible, but reflect little of the size of the animal that is hidden below the surface.

For example, a hospital may see only a small part of the major burden of morbidity associated with non-communicable diseases such as diabetes, hypertension, asthma or epilepsy (Chapters 70–74), particularly if there is no treatment, or communities think there is no effective treatment for them. Hospitals may see the late complications of chronic disease, but many people with these conditions never reach the hospital. The same applies to chronic anaemia in children, which can result from the combined effects of repeated attacks of malaria and hookworm infection. Patients with anaemia may only present to hospital if their anaemia aggravates another disease, or when it is so severe that it precipitates cardiac failure. However, chronic anaemia is extremely common in many parts of Africa. It can reduce the productivity of rural people, put pregnant women at risk and affect the physical and mental development of their children. Yet such patients may never reach the health services.

Many factors influence whether people make use of the health services and particularly whether they attend a hospital. These include:

- disease severity
- distance to hospital
- lack of money during the growing season
- community beliefs about the best sources of care for particular diseases
- affordability of services
- the opportunity costs associated with the loss of working time when seeking care.

Routine health service data

Many health care priorities can only be detected if we take a closer look at the communities, particularly those that are not in the direct neighbourhood of hospitals. Routine information systems are often weak, so that health service managers get little useful information from health centres and lower levels about the health problems in the community. Still, this is an important first source of information. The DMO and DHMT should use this as a starting point, visiting these facilities and taking steps to improve the quality of information reported. This is just one important activity for strengthening the performance of peripheral health facilities (see below).

Rapid community-based surveys

In areas where useful health-service and population-based health data are lacking, health service managers are strongly encouraged to fill this gap by performing community based surveys. Such surveys do not require sophisticated scientific procedures: for example, most chronic medical problems can be detected through simple medical techniques, such as a brief focused medical history, a physical examination including measurement of

BP, and simple blood, urine and stool examinations. Lower level health workers and even school graduates can be trained to administer simple screening questionnaires.

Random sampling
It is not necessary to screen or survey the entire population to get a good idea of what the rest of the hippopotamus looks like: a random sample of a few hundred individuals or families will usually be enough. Randomization, which means that everybody in the community has an equal chance of being enrolled into the sample to be surveyed, is essential. Simple survey techniques are available (e.g. Bennett et al., 1991). The survey can be combined with assessing the performance of key public health interventions such as the local vaccination programme (Turner et al., 1996). The survey itself provides an opportunity to strengthen the capacity of the local community by actively involving them: a number of extremely useful approaches and techniques are available (Annett & Rifkin, 1995; Chambers, 1994).

The role and importance of peripheral health services

Community-based health data will often confirm that there is an unmet need for basic curative and preventive health services, especially in the less accessible parts of a district. Ensuring that high quality services are available, especially to those who most need them (who are too often those who have least access to them), is one of the biggest challenges for health service managers. Poverty is an important barrier to good services, and this also affects city dwellers as Africa becomes increasingly urbanized.

Components
Essential services, which should be within convenient reach and affordable to the population, include:

- antenatal care
- child vaccination
- treatment of common childhood illnesses
- screening and treatment of patients with acute and chronic diseases, both infectious, e.g. tuberculosis, and non-infectious (Chapter 69).

Whilst the provision of preventive care is essential, peripheral services need to be able to manage routine ailments so that they remain credible to the population. Health centres are the best settings to provide this basic package.

Services as peripheral sensors
Health services also serve as the peripheral sensor of the DHMT to detect unexpected changes of disease patterns in the community before a problem gets out of control. Thus they form an important part of the surveillance system so that local epidemic outbreaks, and important shifts in morbidity, such as the emergence of malaria in areas which were hitherto free of it, can be detected. But surveillance can only succeed if health workers understand the difference between public health and individual patient care, and the significance of careful reporting according to standardized procedures. Health service managers will need to pay attention to these aspects through training of peripheral health workers, regular support and supervision, and prompt data analysis and feedback of information to the periphery.

The influence of the seasons on disease burden and the quality of health services

The effects of seasons on health and disease have been discussed in Chapter 2. The essential lesson for the DHMT is:

Be prepared! Health care managers can take some actions to prevent and reduce seasonal problems.

- Deliver a larger stock of drugs to peripheral units before they become less accessible.
- Assess which communities can be expected to experience serious food supply shortages.
- Collaborate with local government officials so that it is possible to take preventive action.
- Maintain regular supervision, however difficult it is: this will boost staff morale and the performance of peripheral health units.
- Reserve a budget for transport and fuel.
- Maintain transport and fuel for outreach services, which are essential for ensuring rural communities receive a basic standard of care.

The reality of district health services today: frustrations and hopes

Public health care services in Africa: the victims of economics and structural adjustment

In many countries and particularly in rural areas, the public sector is still the main provider of health care in Africa. However, for decades the public sector in most African countries has been in a deep economic crisis, with little prospect of improvement in the foreseeable future. Globally imposed structural adjustment policies in the 1980s and 1990s forced countries to divert resources from the health and other social sectors. As a result, there was little routine maintenance of buildings and equipment and essential consumables are often in short supply. Despite the introduction of essential drug programmes and centralized procurement of drugs, countries have not been able to ensure a reliable provision of the most needed medicines. Whilst some of these problems can be overcome through careful planning and rational prescription strategies (see p. 108) on management and financing of drug supply), low absolute levels of funds and low per capita spending on health are major obstacles.

Public sector health workers: underpaid and undersupported, but still on duty

The scanty pay and the need to make money for survival, and the lack of supervision and in-service training, sap the morale of health workers and seriously affect health services. But in spite of all these difficulties, most workers are still on duty during morning hours, most communities value their services, and many health workers still maintain motivation and enthusiasm for their work.

To combat these problems, the DHMT has to ensure:

- in-service training
- supervision
- visits to all health workers in remote clinics.

Primary health care: successes and failures

More than two decades have passed since PHC was launched in Alma Ata. Has primary health care proved to be a successful strategy in the arsenal of health service managers in Africa?

Some major successes have undoubtedly been achieved. There has been a general political commitment to the principle of 'health for all'. The incidence of diseases that are preventable through childhood immunization decreased dramatically in most countries (WHO, 2001). Infant and under-five mortality decreased and life expectancy increased (although these gains are now threatened due to the advent of HIV infection and AIDS)(WHO, 2001).

But failures have occurred and problems remain that have a direct bearing on the work of health service managers today (Visschedijk, 1997), as can be seen by reviewing the list of principles described on p. 89:

Universal accessibility and coverage on the basis of need

A much higher proportion of the world's population now has access to at least some kind of effective health care than had access up to the late 1970s. But achievements have been patchy, depending on the geographic location and on the type of service: while coverage by immunization services has increased, women have continued problems in getting emergency obstetrical care.

- *Poor people*, in particular, face new barriers to services since user fees and cost-recovery programmes were introduced as part of health sector reforms in the late 1980s and early 1990s in many African countries. These were an attempt to increase sustainability and decrease public sector spending in countries that receive inadequate external support.
- *Women* still face social and economic, cultural and traditional barriers to receiving basic or better health care in some countries.

A chronic lack of resources

The biggest obstacle to success continues to be the underfunding of PHC, with many countries spending less than 5% of GDP on health care.

Community involvement and self-reliance

The interpretation of this principle has varied. While community participation has been encouraged in many PHC systems, this has often focused on eliciting community support for programmes designed at higher levels, while the community has been little involved in making decisions. The reason for this relative lack of success in many areas lies mostly in the resistance to devolving resources and funds to the periphery. Even in highly decentralized health systems, most funding decisions are taken by national programme managers so that district managers, not to mention the communities they serve, have limited power.

Intersectoral action for health

Political support for this has been substantial but, in practice, this principle has met many difficulties. Frequent failures by the health services to work with other sectors, particular at higher levels, have been compounded by poor co-ordination between individual health programmes within the health sector. Structures to promote intersectoral collaboration at different levels of PHC, as well as the detailed functions and roles of the different sectors, have been inadequately defined, or not at all.

Appropriate technology and cost-effectiveness

Many interventions which are appropriate and address the priority needs of the population have been successfully implemented, e.g. oral rehydration therapy and the expanded programme of immunization, but some have had limited success, e.g. control of acute respiratory infections, and the provision of essential drugs. There are serious doubts, or a lack of adequate data and research, about the effectiveness of major components of PHC programmes, such as growth monitoring, antenatal care, and health education.

Health sector reforms

Traditionally, international agencies and bilateral donors have funded health care programmes, aimed at the rehabilitation of health services and the delivery of selective primary health care projects. These have tended to address the most urgent health problems and diseases, such as HIV/AIDS, malaria and tuberculosis. During the late 1980s and 1990s, health sector reforms were introduced in most African countries, building on Alma Ata and the later Bamako initiative, which provided a model for adapting PHC in the light of global economic recession (Hanson and McPake, 1993). Health sector reforms involved organizational and financing reforms.

The most important feature of the reform, from the district health manager's perspective, was the drive to decentralize the planning and organization of community health services to districts, so that some funds are now disbursed from the national level to DHMTs to spend on local priorities. This supports the 'comprehensive' PHC approach, because district health teams can thus involve communities in planning and organizing health services to tackle their own health care needs.

The situation of health service managers in the face of structural and economic problems

Public sector health service managers cannot change the underlying structural and economic problems, but if they plan carefully and use their meagre resources well, they can still make some things better, and, perhaps most importantly, they can keep up the motivation of their health workers.

The challenges:

- to organize refresher seminars at local level
- to ensure regular support supervision
- to make careful contingency plans to facilitate the work of their colleagues within the DHMT.

NGOs and international agencies

Health services that are run by religious bodies, for example, mission hospitals and the primary health care projects they have established within their catchment areas, have generally been better funded than public sector services, although their resources are dwindling in many places. Where non-governmental organizations (NGOs) or international agencies provide resources for specific interventions, their services must be coordinated with the DHMT's work.

The challenges:

- to co-ordinate the work of the NGOs with the DHMT
- to integrate national services with local services
- to use the additional resources to strengthen rather than undermine local services.

Managing a health system: practical aspects

Health management teams

In recent years, hierarchical structures and processes in health service management have been increasingly replaced by the concept of team management, in which power and responsibility are delegated to individuals to carry out different functions, working as self-reliant members of a group of managers. While general guidance and ultimate decision making may still be the responsibility of the most senior person, the team concept allows more flexibility to respond to unforeseen organizational difficulties and can generate a higher level of motivation and enthusiasm among the staff.

Composition of the team

The team comprises specialists for different local priorities and components of the health system. Examples include coordinators for public health or primary health care, clinical services, MCH, tuberculosis and leprosy control, AIDS and STD control, a pharmacist and a statistician or information officer.

Functions of the team

Health management teams plan, manage, monitor and supervise, so as to provide and ensure the quality of the health services within their area of responsibility. Ideally, the DHMT should also monitor and ensure the quality of commercial and non-commercial private providers in their areas.

Support supervision

Many of these tasks require frequent supervision of peripheral health services. Supervision is a supportive and creative activity rather than a strategy to maintain discipline. To emphasize this aspect, the term 'supervision' is increasingly being replaced by 'support supervision'.

Regular effective supervision is the backbone of any health care programme. It is an opportunity to motivate health workers through:

- in-service training
- information feedback
- attention to administrative and sometimes personal staff problems.

A portrait of the supervisor

The best supervisors of peripheral services are those who have themselves worked in these settings, have both managerial and teaching skills, and have substantial working experience in the specific area of work that they are to supervise. In addition to professional competence, physical fitness is often required, as visits to peripheral health units may involve travelling long distances in the heat or rain and over bad roads.

Regular planned visits

It is good practice to keep strictly to a regular supervisory schedule. While surprise visits may be revealing under certain circumstances, much more is gained if health workers know that the supervisor will come on a specific day and will be available for several hours, or most of the day. They can plan their work accordingly, avoid a clash with other major official or personal activities, arrange for problem patients to attend on that day, have all required documents available, and much else. Weaknesses in the organization of the Health Centre (HC) or District Hospital (DH) that would be detected through surprise visits usually become apparent during scheduled visits, if these are carefully planned and thoroughly performed.

A list of activities

The effectiveness of the visit is greatly enhanced if a carefully designed standard supervision checklist is used. Such a list enables both health workers and supervisors systematically to review different aspects of the work. Tailor the list to local needs and include sections related to:

- staff availability and duty rosters
- functioning of equipment such as refrigerators or clinical tools
- availability of consumables such as drugs and laboratory supplies
- assessment of the type of patients seen and of the pattern of disease
- help with problem patients
- identification of health workers' knowledge, skills and training needs.

An example of such a supervision checklist (which has been widely used in AMREF's STD/HIV control programme in NW-Tanzania) is shown in Fig. 5.1.

The community and the visit

The principle is to keep regular cordial contact with the community so that the effectiveness and credibility of the health service can be increased. Therefore,

- visit the authorities of the local community.
- where a community health or development committee has been established (see section on community-based health services, below), involve its members in supervision: get its help to identify problems and their solutions, especially in intersectoral issues such as water, sanitation and environmental health.

Dealing with weaknesses

Where major problems or weaknesses are detected,

- use the problems as an opportunity to retrain the staff and provide technical or organizational advice. This can take time and requires patience.
- try, if problems persist, instead of a reproachful attitude, to detect whether any deep-seated managerial or structural causes lie at the core of the problem.
- discuss this in the health management team, and seek a constructive solution.

Data collection and reporting, feedback: the health information system

Patients' records

When patients first present to health services, they are registered and the name, sex, reasons for presenting, diagnoses and treatments given are recorded. These data will be amended with follow-up information when patients return for review or with a new complaint. Keep records systematically and carefully.

The purpose of records

(i) They contain information on individual patients for subsequent care and treatment.
(ii) They can be used to monitor the consumption of drugs and other supplies.
(iii) They help in the preparation of monthly reports.
(iv) They build up a health information and surveillance system for the country.
(v) Health services are also usually obliged to keep person-specific clinical records for legal reasons.

The range of records

Other records that are often kept at peripheral health units include drug consumption books, vaccination record books and registers, antenatal clinic and MCH records, and tuberculosis and other programme-specific registers.

Unnecessary reports

Health workers are often expected to submit separate monthly report forms for the main services delivered. Many of these various registers, records and reports may not be essential. A critical review of the workload at

This list is being used in the STD/HIV Intervention Programme Mwanza Region, Tanzania

Standard supervision checklist **Part 1**

Personnel, equipment, performance

Health unit: ____________________ Date: _______ Quarter: ________

Supervisor: ____________________

1. Personnel: health workers

Name: Function: present and working Y / N

Name: Function: present and working Y / N

Name: Function: present and working Y / N

2. Equipment

Item	available and in order?	Item	available and in order?
Examination bed	Y / N	Torch	Y / N
Bed sheet	Y / N	Waiting bench	Y / N
Screen	Y / N	Desk	Y / N
Speculum	Y / N	2 chairs	Y / N
Plastic container	Y / N	Register book	Y / N
Water container	Y / N	Treatment flow charts	Y / N
Plastic mug	Y / N	Training manual	Y / N

Repairs or replacement needed: ____________________

3. Supervision checklist

1. Staff availability: any present or anticipated problem ?		Y / N
2. Register book: is the information complete and consistent ? Which problems ?		Y / N
3. Have algorithms been followed ? What type of problem did you observe ?		Y / N
4. Any difficult cases seen jointly with the HWs today? Record details.		Y / N
5. Feed-back and training: Which topics did you discuss today with the HWs ?		

Training needs identified: ____________________

Other action required: ____________________

Standard supervision checklist **Part 2**

Calculation of consumables surplus and deficit / consumables supplied / new stock

Health unit: **Month/year:**

	1 old stock	2 count stock	3 real consump	4 should-be consump	5 =(4 - 3) surplus: + deficit: -	6 reasons/ remarks	7 supplied today	8 new stock
TMS forte 960 mg								
Docycycline 100 mg								
Metronidazole 200 mg								
Erythromycin 500 mg								
Benza-Penicill 2.4 MU								
Cipro-floxacin 500 mg								
Gentian violet 1% 0.5 l								
Syringes 10 ml								
Needles for injections								
Cotton wool								
Antiseptic solution								
Batteries								
Register book								
Pens								

Date: ________ Supplied (name): ____________ Signature: ____________

Received (name): ____________ Signature: ____________

Fig. 5.1. Standard supervision checklist.

health units that are under your supervision may reveal that health workers spend far too many hours filling in record books and report forms, although much of these data does not get used.

This time could be spent much more effectively on health education of the community, delivering outreach services, or other useful activities. Sometimes, health workers have concocted data for inclusion in reports to higher levels, often unaware of the importance of reliable data. The resulting fake data are included in summary statistics, unless detected by supervisors who take the trouble to compare the data with patients' registers and other facility records.

Feedback from reports

Monthly report forms are sent to district, provincial and national offices, where they are sometimes filed without the data being used. Even if data are processed and analysed, health workers often do not receive any feedback, which is essential for their motivation and would help them to see the need for accurate recording and reporting. For example, feedback on how local vaccination coverage compares to other similar areas can stimulate health workers' efforts to maintain or improve it.

Standardized essential data

While some documentation and reporting are definitely required, this should be restricted to the minimum necessary, for example: registers of a limited set of priority preventive services such as immunization and family planning uptake; and the recording of essential data on patients. Reports to higher levels should be requested only for data that will be analysed and used; and the reasons for collecting these data should be explained and feedback routinely be given to health workers in peripheral units, with supervisors and health workers jointly discussing and interpreting the data.

For statistics to be valid, routine data must be collected on a standardized form, to reduce inter-observer variation. Such standardization is difficult to achieve, and requires a major effort in training, supervision and monitoring. Data that are compiled at central level may be much more reliable and the system more easily sustainable if they are not based on reports from all health units in the country, but on a smaller number of representative facilities, also known as surveillance sites.

Outreach services

There is evidence that the utilization of services drops steeply beyond a radius of a few kilometres around a health unit. Most people who seek preventive or curative care come from the surrounding community, some from adjacent communities, and very few from distant places. The reason is not that people do not sufficiently value health, but that the costs in travelling long distances, including waiting time and transport, are just too high. This dilemma can partly be solved through outreach services, where a team of health workers from a fixed facility such as a district hospital or health centre regularly (often monthly) visit and provide services to communities in under-served areas.

Outreach services may include some or all of the following activities:

- EPI vaccination
- antenatal screening
- screening and treatment of children under 5 years of age
- health education
- special screening activities, such as detection of early leprosy and treatment of common conditions such as eye diseases, depending on local conditions
- long-term management of chronic diseases.

The direct costs of such services, mainly vehicle depreciation, maintenance and cost of fuel, may be substantial; the opportunity costs, through the absence of health workers from their routine duties, may also be high.

While one would ideally wish to make services easily accessible to every community in a district, health service managers need to monitor the cost-effectiveness of such services and decide if this is the best use of scarce resources. The more the outreach services are used, the higher the cost-effectiveness. Their use can be enhanced by:

- preparing outreach visits in collaboration with community authorities
- informing the public well in advance that the outreach team is to be expected
- keeping to agreed time tables
- making sure that the services delivered are of high quality.

This includes not only technical quality but also ensuring a friendly and caring attitude of health workers. While this should be a feature of all health care delivery, preventive services in particular will be under-used if people fear being upbraided by health workers.

Community-based health services (CHCs, CHWs, health posts, TBAs)

The potential benefits of well-functioning PHC programmes for the prevention and control of diseases, and for community development, are huge. Furthermore, in much of rural Africa ministries of health cannot afford to build and maintain health centres and staff them with salaried health workers, and the PHC model provides an option to bring health care to otherwise under-served populations. PHC thus addresses a double need. (See the first section of this chapter for the role of CHWs within the structure of health services in Africa, and the second section regarding the principles of PHC.) Organizing and facilitating effective PHC programmes is one of the most important and rewarding tasks of health service managers. This section provides practical information on how this can be done.

Community needs

The preconditions for starting a PHC programme are for the community to:

- recognize that it has health problems
- want to do something about them
- be ready to invest time and resources to tackle the problems. The health management team can assist and guide the community in analysing its problems and identifying ways to solve them. However, the desire and drive for action must come from the people. If a community does not place a high priority on its health problems, a PHC programme will neither be effective nor sustainable, and should not be started.

Community health committees (CHCs)

In many PHC programmes, the formation of CHCs is routinely encouraged. The CHC takes overall responsibility for health care in the community and for the support of its community health workers. Such committees may have anything from a few to 20 active members. They should include both influential individuals in the community, for example, school teachers, and also those who are most affected by and feel most concerned about local health problems.

It is essential, therefore, that women should be involved, to ensure that both children's and women's health problems are addressed. However, some societies do not automatically allow women to take part in making decisions.The health management team or PHC Co-ordinator has to guide the community in selecting a balance of members that is both acceptable and addresses the needs of the whole community, especially those who are most vulnerable and have the greatest need of health services.

Training courses and seminars

CHC members should be offered short seminars and training courses to improve their skills in analysing obstacles to good health, to develop solutions and to implement the programme. Such courses should be quite short and should be conducted within or close to the community. Bringing together CHCs from a number of communities for initial and refresher training can be more efficient, and is a good way of promoting community empowerment and mutual learning between communities.

Community health workers (CHWs)

CHWs are the technical frontline workers who help their community to implement its PHC programme, in close collaboration with the local CHC and the District PHC Co-ordinator. They are potentially important sources of care, in settings where there are no salaried government health workers, and a point of contact for the DHMT. CHWs are usually residents of the community in which they work. They are trained for their task, but usually continue to perform their original occupation.

The tasks of the CHW

There is no firm job description, but the following activities will usually form part of the duties:

(i) To work with the CHC to identify the main health hazards of the community, such as polluted water sources, mosquito breeding sites, other environmental hazards, harmful weaning practices, and unhygienic practices that promote gastrointestinal infections;
(ii) to discuss and help organize solutions to these hazards;
(iii) to support the PHC Co-ordinator and other outreach workers in organizing vaccination days or MCH/ANC clinics;
(iv) to treat common uncomplicated diseases using simple syndromic treatment guidelines;
(v) to identify patients at high risk or with potentially serious health problems and refer them promptly to higher levels of care;
(vi) to support patients who are enrolled in a chronic disease care programme by providing treatment according to prescribed schedules for conditions such as tuberculosis, asthma, epilepsy or high blood pressure, and to monitor whether they attend and take the prescribed medicines.

Selection criteria for CHWs

It is crucial that the community identifies the right individuals to be trained as CHWs. The DHMT and its PHC co-ordinator should help the community to establish a list of selection criteria: CHWs should be:

- well respected,
- highly motivated and hard working,
- able to cope with the intellectual challenge of their task, and
- mature, and ideally have families themselves, as CHWs are expected to discuss health matters with family heads and other senior people in the community
- literate (although there are successful PHC programmes with illiterate CHWs, making use of guidelines and records based on pictorial symbols)
- willing to continue living in their community for the foreseeable future. One reason for the failure of CHW programmes has been the selection of individuals who saw the position as a stepping stone towards a career, in either the public or private sector.

The number of CHWs to be selected and trained will depend on the size of the community, the geographical environment and the nature of the health problems encountered. As a rule-of-thumb, it may be useful to have at least one female and one male health worker per 3000 population.

Training of CHWs

Different training schemes have been tested for CHWs in Africa, lasting from one week to one year. Experience shows that a series of short training courses, conducted in small groups of no more than 15 trainees, are more effective than longer courses, or those with many participants. The training should aim at developing skills rather than acquiring detailed medical knowledge. While some basic knowledge of the causes and main features of common diseases is certainly required, for example how to interrupt the transmission of the locally most important communicable diseases, much of the training time should be used to gain skills in health education and promotion using role play.

The use of drugs by CHWs

Whether or not CHWs should be permitted to use antibiotics for patients with acute infections has been debated for many years. The decision should depend on:

(i) the remoteness of the community

(ii) the skills and experience of the individual worker In our personal experience, CHWs are usually well capable of making correct use of such medicines, provided they are carefully trained, equipped with simple clear guidelines and receive regular support supervision during which cases should be reviewed. In addition, the growing reality in rural Africa is that antibiotics can be easily purchased over the counter, even from small village shops and from market vendors. Therefore, CHWs will lose respect in the community if they do not know when and how such medicines should be correctly used.

Interaction of CHWs, the DHMT and other providers

CHWs require regular support and supervision. This is the task of the DHMT through its PHC Co-ordinator. Support visits should be performed frequently, initially at monthly intervals, and should start immediately after completion of the training. The visits provide an opportunity for further on-the-job training. CHWs and the Coordinator should meet with the CHC, should jointly inspect and discuss problems in the community, and jointly review problem patients.

Record keeping by CHWs

Encourage CHWs to keep records, both on their health promotional activities and on patients treated or referred. However, these records must be very simple and easy to keep, and should include only an essential minimum of information. More detailed information, if required, can be collected by the PHC Co-ordinator during support supervisory visits.

Referrals from CHWs

Make sure that patients referred by CHWs to health centres or hospitals are treated with priority, as this strengthens the position of the CHW, and encourages patients to make use of the PHC programme. Give feedback to the CHWs wherever possible.

Remuneration of CHWs

In the initial phase of a new PHC programme, CHWs often agree to fulfil their new tasks voluntarily, because the training and social recognition they receive are themselves strong incentives, but, sadly, their initial enthusiasm wanes after some months, and CHWs discover that the additional burden is greater than they had expected. The DHMT should urge the community from the beginning to establish a reliable mechanism by which CHWs will be given at least some payment for their work. Otherwise, the PHC programme in that community is likely to collapse.

Direct payment of CHWs by the government or from the budget of an NGO has been introduced in some countries, but this is not sustainable – especially where ministries have difficulty paying their salaried workers – and it also contradicts the principle of self-reliance. An option frequently tried is that the community agrees to provide remuneration in the form of working time, e.g. by clearing the CHWs' farms before the planting season, or through payment in kind, e.g. gifts of farm produce. Experience shows, however, that this system rarely functions effectively as promises will not be honoured by some community members, and this discourages others.

A workable solution is that the CHC collects a small contribution from all community members at the time when cash is more readily available, and pays this money to the CHWs in regular monthly instalments, as a lump sum or according to performance. Other successful models include charging a small fee that is paid by patients when they present for consultation, or putting a small profit margin on drugs sold. The disadvantage of this last approach is that it may lead to an overemphasis on the curative care component of the PHC programme.

Community health posts

For many communities the construction or the establishment of a community health post is perceived as a symbol of their PHC programme. While it certainly demonstrates some commitment by the community, a post is not a prerequisite for a successful programme, and it may even have disadvantages: very often such posts become mere clinics, over-emphasizing the curative medical component of the programme. If a post is newly built, it should have enough space for group health education or for activities such as vaccination days that are organized by CHWs, in collaboration with visiting outreach teams from hospitals or health centres.

Traditional birth attendants (TBAs)

Many PHC programmes provide training courses for TBAs to ensure safe and hygienic deliveries. TBAs are expected:

- to recognize and refer mothers at high risk who require skilled obstetric care
- to prevent tetanus neonatorum through promoting hygienic delivery practices
- to know and apply simple measures to control post-partum haemorrhage

Programmes equip them with sterile gloves, razor blades and threads to cut and ligate the umbilical cord. Such programmes should not be applied blindly: in many societies, it is the neighbour or a friend rather than a 'professional TBA' who provides assistance during delivery, and it is neither possible nor useful to invite all women in the community for training.

Furthermore, although TBA training seems a rational strategy in communities that lack easy access to trained midwives, evidence that such programmes have been able to reduce maternal or neonatal mortality is still uncertain. The most effective way to prevent tetanus of the newborn is still through tetanus toxoid vaccination of pregnant women and those of child-bearing age. Although their benefits to pregnant women are uncertain, TBA training projects provide an opportunity to promote other aspects of PHC, such as general health education, promotion of child vaccination and improvement of weaning practices.

Planning, implementation and evaluation of a programme or service

The planning cycle

Far too often managers plan and start implementing projects based on untested assumptions and perceptions rather than on hard data, and soon run into unforeseen difficulties. Quite often, difficulties resulting from insufficient planning are only discovered when a lot of resources and efforts have been spent, and when it is almost impossible to put things right.

One of the most useful frameworks that can facilitate sound planning and implementation is the planning cycle (Green, 1999). This framework is helpful both for planning new programmes and for making corrections to existing ones. It illustrates planning as a process with a number of logical steps (Fig. 5.2), and is sufficiently flexible to allow adjustment of plans to local needs and constraints. While the proposed sequence of steps may

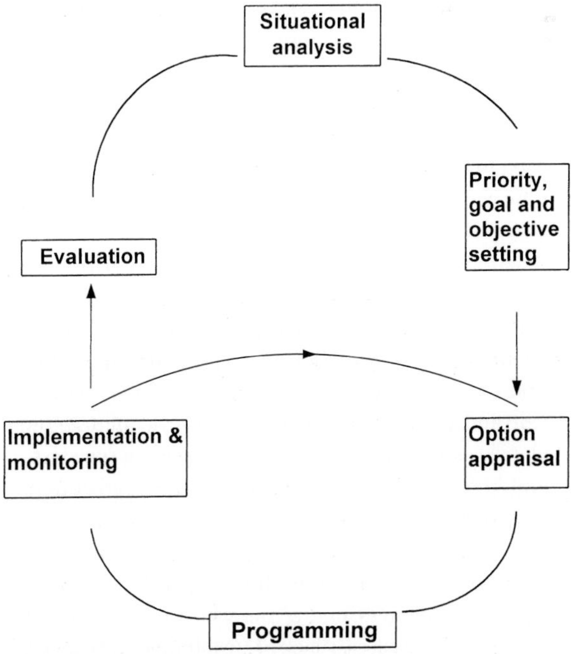

Fig. 5.2. The planning cycle.

not always be so clear-cut in practice, it is a useful way of organizing one's planning.

The key steps of the cycle are:

- Situational analysis: assessment of the present situation through the analysis of existing data, a stakeholder analysis and a series of rapid surveys. This leads to the identification of relevant health related problems, the factors that determine these problems, and those factors that may be of importance for the design of health interventions. Depending on the nature of the programme, the data needed may include population characteristics, local disease patterns, health seeking behaviour, services provided, information on influential individuals and organizations, or a combination of all of these.
- Priority-setting: identification of the most important and urgent problems, based on the results of the situational analysis. These will be translated into a set of objectives for the programme.
- Option appraisal: assessment of the different approaches that are available to achieve the above objectives, with selection of the most feasible and cost-effective approach or combination of approaches. Programming: formulation of a detailed plan identifying the resources needed (staff, equipment, consumables, budget and time) and listing the activities necessary to achieve the objectives.
- Implementation and monitoring: putting the plan into action, with continuous follow-up to observe whether the programme is 'on track' or whether immediate corrective measures are required.
- Evaluation: intermittent investigation of the achievements of the programme , usually conducted through surveys among the target population. Evaluation can be used to make a new set of plans, so that a regular planning cycle is developed: activity – evaluation – plan – new activity.

To illustrate this, we will use the example of a district programme designed to improve care for people with non-communicable diseases (see Chapter 75).

- A situational analysis showed that certain important non-communicable diseases such as asthma, hypertension and epilepsy were much more prevalent than previously assumed, as evidenced from patient registers and from a community based survey, and that patients with such diseases were not receiving adequate care. The problem was so severe that addressing it became a major priority for the authorities.
- A lack of awareness among many health professionals about these diseases, a lack of sustainable strategies to control them, the insufficient skills of health workers, and the non-availability of drugs were identified as the most important causes contributing to the problem. The need to overcome each of these contributing factors defined the specific objectives.
- Three different options to address the problem were suggested:
  - (i) screening of the entire population to identify those with non-communicable diseases and establishing specialist care centres in all communities;
  - (ii) training of peripheral workers so that they could detect and refer patients with non-communicable diseases; initial treatment of such patients in existing centres; and setting-up of a comprehensive follow-up service involving both skilled physicians and peripheral workers;
  - (iii) establishing regular specialist outreach services in the larger communities.

  Option 2 was chosen as likely to be the most cost-effective and sustainable strategy for controlling non-communicable diseases.
- Programming: the health management team calculated the required number of staff, drugs and vehicles, prepared a budget and designed detailed rosters for training, supplies and supervision.
- The programme was implemented according to these plans. The performance of health workers, availability and uptake of drugs in the periphery, and the health status of patients were monitored continuously. Information on difficulties encountered at this stage were immediately used to make corrections to the programme.
- After a year, a thorough evaluation was done, and the data were compiled and used to reformulate plans for the new service.

Stakeholder analysis

Some steps of the cycle deserve a closer look. A thoroughly performed situational analysis should also provide important information on individuals and institutions that are stakeholders in the planned programme. Stakeholders are those who can be expected to gain or to lose as a result of the programme. Programme recipients, that is the community, are often termed 'primary stakeholders'. 'Secondary stakeholders' are, for example, the staff who manage a disease control programme and those who provide support from higher levels.

A stakeholder analysis can help show that some individuals, for example traditional healers, may lose power or benefits because of the programme (see Varvasovszky & Brugha, 2000, for guidance on how to conduct a stakeholder analysis). Stakeholders who are potential threats are not always obvious; however, they may be influential and could jeopardize the programme's success. The process through which this happens may not be obvious and the programme implementers suddenly become confronted with obstacles, the origin of which they may not understand. It is therefore of paramount importance to identify such stakeholders during the situational analysis, to understand their agenda and, if they pose a genuine threat, to plan the programme in such a way that their concerns are either accommodated or neutralized.

Example
In a programme to control HIV infection and other STDs among bar girls and hotel attendants in a large African city, a drop-in centre was established where women were offered health education, condoms and syndromic STD case management. Women were invited to come for regular check-ups and were encouraged to work together to enforce '100 per cent condom use'. Initially, bar and guesthouse owners were fiercely opposed to the programme, thinking that customers would stay away from their establishments, out of fears that participating women had AIDS and because customers would be unhappy about being urged to use condoms. The problem was overcome when bar and guesthouse owners were invited to a series of short seminars in which the rationale of the programme was discussed and fears dispersed.

When the programme was started, it met clandestine opposition from medical practitioners in the area, who formerly were the main STD treatment providers. One of these practitioners was well connected to higher authorities in the municipality, and the programme was suddenly threatened by administrative complaints, which took time to resolve. This problem could have possibly been avoided if the important local STD treatment providers had been identified (situation analysis) and had been invited to participate or benefit from the programme in some way (a possible outcome of a stakeholder analysis), for example through providing them with training on effective STD treatment strategies.

How to overcome obstacles during the implementation phase

Activity plans

Activities of different programmes and team members may rely on and compete for a limited pool of vehicles, support staff, equipment and funds. This will require careful coordination of activities and efficient sharing of scarce resources.

It is extremely helpful to base one's work on detailed activity plans that have been discussed and agreed upon by the team. This principle applies particularly to the work of the DHMT, but also to all other teams of health care providers, be it the hospital management, the staff of a peripheral unit, a PHC programme or a village health committee. Plans should be drawn up well in advance, especially where they involve co-ordinated outreach visits and the need to communicate with distant communities. Planning in quarterly intervals, with monthly fine-tuning, has proved a useful strategy. The Gantt chart is an effective tool to plan and co-ordinate activities. This chart helps to visualize important details and to detect possible bottlenecks in implementation. It also facilitates more detailed planning, necessary for the preparation of an operational budget.

An example of a Gantt chart for the work of a DHMT is given below (Fig. 5.3).

Avoiding planning mistakes

Health service managers will meet frequent difficulties that hamper their plans: for example, funds or supplies may not arrive in time, a vehicle may break down, or the rains may set in early.

Problems
An analysis of such problems in implementation shows that most can be classified in one of two categories, each of which requires different practical remedies in order to avoid the problem in future.

Genuine planning mistakes
Perhaps supply orders were not placed in time; important background information, for example on social or political events in a community, was disregarded or not collected when outreach activities were initially planned; the resources required were underestimated; or, finally, collaborating sectors just did not communicate with each other. The remedy consists of timelier, more detailed and more accurate planning of activities.

Unforeseeable events
Such events often hamper the implementation of activities: a key team member may fall ill, the district commissioner may requisition a vehicle that was allocated to an outreach activity, funds and supplies may have failed to arrive although requests were submitted on time.

Planning in uncertainty is a particular problem in unstable settings, for example where there has been recent conflict and/or movements of refugees into one's district.

(Monthly activity and transport coordination plan for the District Health Management Team)

September		Week 1	Week 2	Weeke 3	
Date	01 02 03	04 05 06 07 08 09 10	11 12 13 14 15 16 17	18 19 20 21 22 23 24	25 26 27 28 29 30
DMO				xx xx xx Provincial DMO meeting Komba	xx xx xx Support SV at Bungam Hosp.
DNO		xx xx xx Support SV at District Hospital	xx xx xx xx Support SV 4 health centres in Bungam Div.		xx xx xx Support SV at Bungam Hosp.
DTLC		xx xx xx FU visit 6 villages Gamba Division		xx xx xx FU visit 6 villages Urkar Division	xx xx xx xx Annual prov. T+L control progr. meeting
D MCH C		xx xx xx Vacc. + ANC Bekondo	xx xx xx xx Support SV 4 health centres in Bungam Div.		xx xx xx Vacc. + ANC in Great Gunga
DSCC			xx xx xx xx Support SV 4 health centres in Bungam Div.	xx Collect supplies from Komba, SV of cotton factory STD services	xx xx xx Support SV at Bungam Hosp.
DACC		xx xx xx Teach at 3 primary schools in Gamba Division	xx xx xx xx Community campaign in Bungam Div.	xx xx Teach staff at Bungam hospital	xx xx xx Comm. Campaign in Great Gunga
D PHC C		xx xx xx Vacc. + ANC Bekondo	xx xx xx xx SV PHC posts in Gamba Division		xx xx xx Vacc. + ANC in Great Gunga
Vehicle 1		xx xx xx -- -- -- Bekondo Quarterly maintenanc e	xx xx xx xx Emergency backup for Bungam and Gamba	xx xx xx Emergency back-up for Urkar, 19/9 + 21/9 to Bungam with DACC	xx xx xx Great Gunga Community
Vehicle 2		xx xx xx xx xx Emergency back-up for Bekondo and Gamba	xx xx xx xx With DNO, DMCHC, + DSCC in Bungam	xx xx xx -- -- With DMO to Quarterly Provinc. Meetg maintenance	x x 26/9 am + 28/9 pm to Bungam (DMO + DNO + DSCC)
Motorcycle		x x x With DTLC + DACC Gamba Division	xx xx xx xx -- -- With D PHC Gamba Monthly mainten.	xx xx xx With DTLC Urkar division	xx xx xx xx With DTLC to Komba
Remarks				!! 19/9 only: arrange for pickup with Komba Cotton Ltd	

DMO District Medical Officer, DNO District Nursing Officer, DTLC District Tbc and Leprosy Control Coordinator, D MCH C District MCH Coordinator, DSCC District STD Control Coordinator, DACC District AIDS Control Coordinator, D PHC C District PHC Coordinator;

xx = officer out of office, vehicle out of station;

-- = vehicle out of service

Fig. 5.3. Example of a Gantt chart.

While there may not be a remedy for every situation, many problems can be overcome with the help of flexible contingency planning, based on the assumption that such things are likely to happen. For example, one may have a mutual and reciprocal agreement with other sectors or even other districts to provide emergency backup transport, where possible. Such arrangements could even be made with private institutions, which may in turn benefit from an extension of health educational services to their workers. A buffer stock of drugs or vaccines can be built up over time in anticipation of unforeseen shortages. All this requires creative flexibility by the DHMT, but overcoming unexpected obstacles can actually be fun and satisfying.

Evaluation of health services

The last step in the planning cycle is the evaluation of health programmes and services. The evaluation will feed into a new round of planning, and is therefore an important managerial tool. The terms 'monitoring' and 'evaluation' are sometimes confused. Monitoring is a continuous effort conducted during the implementation of a service or project. It is often performed as part of routine supervision, and used to keep the service 'on track', just as a driver constantly checks the position of the car on the road and takes immediate corrective action if needed. Evaluation is a more systematic tool, conducted at less frequent intervals. It will often comprise surveys and therefore will require the allocation of additional resources, including funds, staff and sometimes equipment.

Evaluation levels and techniques

In order to document and analyse the achievements of a health service, it is helpful to distinguish between four different levels: evaluation of inputs, outputs, outcomes and impact.

Inputs are the resources that were actually used, such as staff, vehicles, drugs, training or supervision.

Outputs refer to the quantity and/or quality of activities conducted, such as services provided.

Outcomes relate to the programme objectives, for example the proportion of the target population that actually received the service (note that outcome measures capture also the acceptance of the programme by the target population).

Impact is concerned with the improvement that the service achieved in the health status of the population.

Each of these levels requires its own set of evaluation techniques.

Example – vaccination services

An evaluation of inputs would report the number of vaccination days held according to plan, the number of refrigerators provided and of vaccines delivered to peripheral health units. This evaluation step would involve the inspection of documents available at base.

An evaluation of outputs would report the number of vaccination sessions and the quality of services delivered, including the actual technical performance of health workers who vaccinate children. This evaluation step could start with a record review, would include a systematic check of the cold chain, but would also require an observation of actual vaccination sessions.

An evaluation of outcomes would measure the vaccination coverage that has been achieved in the population, and would require a household survey such as the community-based random cluster survey described by Henderson and Sundaresan (1982) and Turner et al. (1996). More recently, an assessment of this important variable has been included in the national demographic and health (DHS) surveys that are conducted in many countries. However such services, whilst collecting representative data, may not provide information on a particular district or area, and health service managers may find the classical EPI cluster survey still useful for their area.

An evaluation of impact would attempt to measure the incidence of vaccine preventable diseases in the catchment area of the health services, through disease surveillance. One could also conduct large-scale sero-epidemiological surveys to measure the immune status of the target population. Unfortunately, such surveys are usually prohibitively expensive.

Techniques to evaluate the quality of health services

The quality of service delivery is what health service managers should be most concerned with. Various techniques have been developed to investigate this important criterion of output.

Evaluating patients' register books for adherence to standard treatment guidelines

Curative services are often facilitated through the use of standardized treatment guidelines. Health workers should keep *brief standardized records* on all patients: date, name, sex, diagnosis, treatment given, follow-up information. If they are well maintained, it is possible to evaluate the quality of health services by checking these records. They will reveal whether the services are used, and whether diagnosis and treatment guidelines have been followed. They can also help to check drug turnover and provide pointers to when drugs may be going astray. It is possible to calculate the proportion of health units or health workers that treat a specified percentage (e.g. 80 per cent) of patients correctly according to available guidelines. The procedures involved are simple, if good quality records are maintained, they can be used in routine supervisory and monitoring visits, as well as in systematic surveys to evaluate health services.

Evaluation of training

Training is often evaluated through pre- and post-training tests. However, strictly speaking, such tests are an evaluation at the input level and should mainly be used to guide the design and content of training courses. The sustained benefits of training cannot be evaluated under classroom conditions. Instead, health workers should be asked to demonstrate knowledge and skills during routine supervisory visits, or special surveys some time after they are back in the field. The evaluator needs a standardized checklist and recording form to ensure that the results can be reproduced and quantified. The technique can be combined with direct observation of the interaction between patient and health worker (see below).

Direct observation

The evaluator sits in and observes the health worker's interactions with patients for an adequate period of time (at least several hours). Observations are recorded using a checklist of issues and skills that the health worker should have mastered and be able to demonstrate. An example of this technique is the measurement of the WHO preventive indicators PI, PI 6 and PI 7 for STD services, developed for the evaluation of AIDS control programmes (WHO, 1994):

$$\text{PI 6} = \frac{\text{No. of patients assessed and treated according to (national) standards}}{\text{No. of patients presenting with specific diseases (STDs)}}$$

$$\text{PI 7} = \frac{\text{No. of individuals receiving appropriate advice on condom use and partner notification}}{\text{No. of individuals seeking STD care}}$$

Similar indicators can be constructed for other health service delivery components. The advantage of this technique is that the evaluator can assess the behaviour of the health worker, including the quality of communication and other skills, and not just knowledge. One disadvantage is that during the evaluation health workers may act differently from their normal practice. However, experience shows that this does not pose a real problem, as most workers return to their routine behaviour, once they get used to the presence of the observer. It is important, therefore, that the observation period is long enough and that the observer does not interrupt.

Exit interviews of patients

This technique has often been recommended, but is difficult to do and rarely done. It requires diplomatic skills and good preparation to avoid ill feelings and embarrassment on the side of the staff member who is to be evaluated.

Surrogate client visits

A surrogate client is a staff member of the evaluation team who pretends to be a patient, presents with certain symptoms, and after the visit records all actions taken by the health worker. The purpose of this is to detect discrepancies between what health workers report about their practices and what they are actually doing. For example, in an STD control programme in East Africa, all health workers had been carefully trained to examine all patients, to promote condom use and to give health education, and all reported that they were actually always doing this. However, an evaluation revealed that only 75 per cent of the patients were examined, 60 per cent received health education and 30 per cent were offered condoms (Grosskurth et al., 2000).

Surrogate clients are best placed to identify such weaknesses in the performance of health services. A standard checklist should be used for this purpose. The surrogate client needs debriefing by the investigator soon after the clinic visit. The surrogate client should not be from the same community, needs to be well prepared and trained, and able to act out the role.

Ethical questions about this technique have been raised. The use of safeguards (surrogate clients need to be trained in how to avoid receiving harmful treatments), and informing health workers well in advance that such techniques may be used, help to address concerns of ethics and acceptability. It also helps to equip surrogate clients with a document that certifies their official mission in case they unexpectedly find themselves detected and accused by the service provider. Surrogate client visits can provide most useful information. They are easy to perform in urban settings, but are much more difficult in rural communities.

Follow-up visits to patients

A related evaluation technique involves follow-up visits to patients who were treated within a recent defined period before the evaluation. Such patients are interviewed by the evaluator(s) about the outcome of their care and how their health is in general. On this occasion, questions can be asked about examinations done at the health facility, treatment received, health education given, health workers' attitudes and the level of the patient's satisfaction. This evaluation of health workers' performance can be 'camouflaged' by including the specific questions about quality in a variety of questions about general health. Consent from health workers, community leaders and the individual former patients should be obtained. Experience shows that this is usually not difficult (Grosskurth et al., 2000).

Focus group discussions with community members

Similarly, during meetings held in the community, questions can be asked which refer to people's perceptions of the attitude and the work performance of the local health services. This should preferably be embedded in a topic regarding general health perceptions of the population. The evaluator acts as discussion facilitator for the group. A second person from the evaluation team should be present as an observer. Depending on the culture and setting, these sessions may be tape-recorded, or written notes are made after the end of the meeting.

Evaluation of outcomes or impacts?
Should health intervention programmes in developing countries be generally evaluated at the outcome rather than at the impact level (see Van Norren et al., 1989; Schrettenbrunner & Harpham, 1993)? Unfortunately, for many health interventions, it is difficult to establish effectiveness at the impact level, because such evaluations often require costly large-scale intervention studies (to ensure the required sample size), because the staff and expertise required to do impact evaluations may not be available and because impact often depends on additional influences, which are outside of the control of the services and cannot easily be measured. Some donor agencies (and many implementing agencies) have not realized these constraints, and 'impact evaluations' are inappropriately requested in the design stage of programmes.

Many commentators believe that it will be sufficient if, for the evaluation outcome, parameters are used that are known to be closely associated with the desired impact. For example, the following parameters have been suggested for the evaluation of comprehensive primary health care services that aim to improve the health status of children, expressed as percentage of the target population reached (Van Norren et al., 1989):

- indicators covering conditions at child-birth: percentage of mothers using child spacing, percentage of mothers with immunization during pregnancy, morbidity of mother during pregnancy (e.g. prevalence of STDs), percentage of mothers having a skilled attendant during childbirth
- indicators covering susceptibility to infection/malnutrition: duration of breast-feeding, immunization coverage (of children), percentage of children receiving Vitamin A supplements
- indicators covering nutrition: duration of breast-feeding, percentage of mothers using appropriate food during weaning
- indicators covering exposure to infection: percentage of households with appropriate water storage, nutritional hygiene, and sanitation practices.

References

Annett H, Rifkin S. (1995). Guidelines for rapid participatory appraisals to assess community health needs. WHO/SDS/DHS/95.8; WHO.

Bennet S, Woods T, Liyanage WM et al. (1991). A simplified general method for cluster-sample surveys of health in developing countries. *Wld Hlth Statist Quart*, **44**: 98–106.

Cairncross S, Peries H, Cutts F et al. (1997). Vertical health programmes *Lancet*, **349**: s20–s22.

Chambers C (ed). (1998). Why seasons matter. In *Challenging the Professions – Frontiers for Rural Development.* London: Intermediate Technology Publications.

Chambers R. (1994). The origins and practice of participatory rural appraisal. *Wld Dev Rep*, **22**: 953–969.

Green A. (1999). *Health Planning in Developing Countries*, 2nd edn. Oxford: Oxford University Press.

Grosskurth H, Mwijarubi E, Todd J. et al. (2000). Operational performance of an STD control programme in Mwanza Region, Tanzania. *Sex Transm Inf*, **76**: 426–436.

Henderson RH, Sundaresan T. (1982). Cluster sampling to assess immunisation coverage: a review of experience with a simplified sampling method. *Bull WHO*, **60**: 253–260.

Hanson K, McPake B. (1993). The Bamako Initiative: where is it going? *Hlth Pol Plan*, **13**: 107–120.

Rifkin S, Wall G. (1986). Why health improves: defining the issues concerning 'comprehensive primary health care' and 'selective primary health care'. *Soc Sci Med*, **23**: 559–566.

Schrettenbrunner A, Harpham T. (1993). A different approach to evaluating PHC projects in developing countries: how acceptable is it to aid agencies? *Hlth Pol Plan*, **8**: 128–135.

Tarimo E, Webster E. (1994). Primary health care – concepts and challenges in a changing world: Alma-Ata revisited. Geneva: WHO.

Turner AG, Magnani RJ, Shuaib M et al. (1996). A not quite as quick but much cleaner alternative to the expanded Programme on Immunisation (EPI) cluster survey design. *Int J. Epidemiol*, **25**: 198–203.

Van Norren B, Boerma JT, Sempebwa EK et al. (1989). Simplifying the evaluation of primary health care programmes. *Soc Sci Med*, **28**: 1091–1097.

Varvasovszky Z, Brugha R. (2000). How to do a stakeholder analysis. *Hlth Pol Plan*, **15**: 338–345.

Visschedijk J. (1997). A fresh look at health for all. *Med Trop*, **35**: 1–18.

WHO (1994). WHO/GPA/TCO/SEF/94.1: Global Programme on AIDS: Protocol for the assessment of STD case management through health facility surveys. Geneva: WHO.

WHO (2001). MacroEconomics and health: investing in health for economic development. *Report of the Commission on MacroEconomics and Health.* Geneva: WHO. Geneva. http://www3.who.int/whosis/cmh

MANAGEMENT AND FINANCING OF DRUG SUPPLY

What can be done at district or provincial level to improve drug supply and use? The simple answer is – much, even when the central supply is not functioning optimally. This section will review steps to be taken at individual health facilities to improve

- procurement and ordering
- storage
- dispensing
- prescription.

Medical officers can, and should, take the lead in organizing the process of selecting and ordering drugs, and in ensuring that drugs are rationally prescribed and dispensed by medical and paramedical personnel. Remember that the public sector may not be the only source of drugs and that the private and non-profit sectors may also be able to supply needed drugs. A book entitled *Managing Drug Supply* has been published to help drug supply managers in developing countries (Quick et al., 1997).

Selection of drugs

Which drugs?

The first step is to review which drugs are genuinely needed and in what quantities. The basis for this is often standard treatment guidelines or agreed protocols for the most common illnesses, so that fewer different drugs are bought, and in larger quantities. Treatment guidelines can also help to reconcile differing prescribing traditions, when physicians and health workers who have been trained in different countries are working together.

The VEN analysis

The next step is to designate which drugs are Vital, which are Essential, and which are Non-essential. The first drugs selected are the vital, next the essential; last of all, non-essential drugs can then be ordered, if there are any funds! This avoids the problem of 'specialty' drugs which are sometimes ordered by a specialist doctor — which may be expensive and not used for many, or even any, patients. Such drugs commonly expire unused on the shelves, which is a costly waste of money.

The ABC analysis

In the ABC analysis, which is another useful guide, drugs are ranked by previous expenditure over a specific period, usually a year: for example, chloroquine accounted for 10 per cent of the funds expended, aspirin 9.5 per cent of expenditure, etc. ABC analysis of existing purchases may reveal that much money is being spent on non-essential items, or on drugs which could be replaced by less expensive alternatives; for example, paracetamol could be replaced by aspirin in many cases.

Quantity

When the selection of drugs is accomplished, the next step is to decide how much to order.

- Base the quantity on:
  - (i) past consumption
  - (ii) the treatment guidelines
  - (iii) the morbidity patterns.
- Concentrate on larger quantities of fewer drugs and dosage forms: this simplifies the process of ordering and reduces the chances of stock-outs. Order tablets or capsules rather than syrups or injections: this saves a great deal of money.
- Maintain an appropriate level of stock to prevent stock-outs: this depends on:
  - (i) how long it will take to replenish supplies
  - (ii) how rapidly the supplies are being consumed
  - (iii) the VEN category of the drug.

If the hospital runs out of stock, it may be forced to buy smaller quantities on the local market, which is often the most expensive source of all.

Procurement and ordering

Generic durgs are almost always at least one-tenth as expensive than brand name drugs, and, if bought in bulk, the price savings can be up to100 times! This of course means that a given budget can buy significantly more drugs when bulk, generic drugs are purchased.

Reference list for prices

International prices are available on line from *Management Sciences for Health.* This is a US-based consulting organization, which produces an *International Drug Price Reference Guide* that can be used to compare prices.[1] Local prices must, of course, include transportation and freight, and local taxes where applicable (see Box).

If you detect that your hospital or organization is paying 50 per cent more than the international price, significant improvements are probably possible.

> **Procurement and ordering of drugs**
> The most important single action: Procure generic drugs in bulk.

[1] http: //erc.msh.org/dmpguide/index.cfm?search_cat=yes&display=yes&module=dmp

Bulk organizations

Organizations that do bulk procurement but then sell smaller quantities, usually to non-profit organizations including hospitals in Africa, can help smaller purchasers to obtain the advantages of competitive tendering – such organizations include IDA, the International Dispensary Association based in the Netherlands, the MEDS or JMS organizations in East Africa or ECHO, a UK-based charity. UNICEF in Copenhagen is also able to supply to government-supported institutions.[2]

Storage

The FEFO rule

In order to avoid drugs expiring while in stock, rotate the stock, and thus follow the FEFO rule – 'First Expiry, First Out'.

- Use older stock first.

but this requires more work by medical store or hospital pharmacy managers to keep putting the fresh stock at the back of the shelf.

Security

Drugs are a source of cash: they are portable, easily concealed in clothing, have a high value on the outside and are easily disposed of. Therefore,

- control access to the storehouse
- select trustworthy persons to control access to the store.

Conditions of storage

Proper storage conditions, including minimizing exposure to heat, light and humidity, are important for some drugs – but most drugs have proven remarkably resistant to poor conditions. Notable exceptions are tetracycline products, which become toxic when exposed to heat, and oxytocin and ergometrine, which lose their potency when exposed to light and heat, and thus should be stored in the refrigerator. Most vaccines also have to be stored in the refrigerator; for insulin (see p. 749). Proper FEFO stock rotation will ensure that exposure to harsh conditions is minimized and the potency is preserved as much as possible. Ensure good air circulation and prevent contact of stored drugs with water.

Monitor levels of stock

- Establish a system to supervise and monitor stock levels regularly.
- Place new orders so that the drugs arrive before the old stock runs out – usually a minimum of 3 months' stock will need to be kept on hand, but in remote areas the stock needed might be as much as a year.
- Keep a reasonable stock level so that you can avoid having to order drugs in emergency, or to use more expensive substitutes.
- Maintain a stock control system. This may be very simple and consist only of stock cards or may be more sophisticated with a ledger (stock book) or even a computer.

A method to check the system

- Select five items randomly in the store, and compare the stock card recorded balances with the actual physical count on the shelf. If all five are exactly correct, you can be very sure that the remaining stock has been correctly recorded as well.
- Take a bottle or box from the back of the shelf, when you are doing the physical count, and compare the expiry date with the same product from the front of the shelf, to check that FEFO is being followed. Such routine checks, enable you to detect losses early and to prevent further loss. WHO has published a simple manual which describes a stock management system for health centres (WHO, 1998).

Donated drugs

Management of donated drugs is a major problem in some areas, particularly where there has been an emergency which has precipitated an influx of drug donations. The best strategy is to accept only invited donations of drugs which the facility has specifically asked for and is expecting. But this is not always possible, so a strategy for rapidly selecting the donated drugs which are useful, and discarding and disposing properly of those which are not, is needed.

Discard

As a rough guide, discard any drug which:

- is neither vital nor essential
- is not labelled clearly with its generic name
- is expired
- is in a package which contains only a few days' dosage
- is not on the national essential drugs list or on the facility's formulary. Reassure your pharmacists that they should feel no guilt about disposing of these useless drugs.

Disposal

These drugs:

- take up space
- require tracking like other drugs
- waste the time of of the pharmacist.

[2] http: //www.ida.nl/engels/ida.html, http: //www.echohealth.org.uk/intro.html, and http: //www.supply.unicef.dk/index.html

- may cause harm to a patient if accidentally dispensed
- must be disposed of safely: they are potential toxic waste, and should be treated as such
- must be disposed of so that they cannot be retrieved and sold or otherwise used.

WHO has produced two useful manuals to deal with donations and disposal of unwanted pharmaceuticals (WHO, 1999 a, b).

Prescription

This book deals with the treatment of major diseases in Africa and thus implicitly with prescription.

Multiple drugs

Few of the recommended treatments involve more than one or two drugs – yet actual practice is often to prescribe multiple drugs, even for uncomplicated cases. If an average of under two drugs per treatment is used:

- important savings will be made
- better care will be given: fewer drugs will reduce the possibility of drug interactions
- the patients themselves, and not the physician, will take part in the selection of the drugs which are actually taken, especially where there is a prescription fee
- patients are less likely to make mistakes, and will probably take them correctly.

Traditions of prescribing

Some prescribing traditions may involve up to seven or eight drugs per prescription – such overuse of drugs will rapidly consume stocks and does not add to the quality of care (although patients may believe that more drugs are better, in part because it allows them to stockpile drugs at home). Clearly, prescribing fewer and absolutely necessary drugs largely increases adherence. The use of injections instead of equally effective oral preparations is also common. This has risks associated with the injections themselves and the cost of these injections is far greater than for the equivalent oral preparations.

If all the prescribers at a hospital or clinic can agree upon, and adhere to, standard treatment guidelines, which can be used as the basis for procurement and storage, the problem of overprescription and stock-outs may gradually be eliminated. Uncertainties about dosages, particularly with pediatric dosages, can also be reduced by the use of standard guidelines by age or weight. Doctors often cite their mistrust or delay of laboratory results as a reason to 'cover' the patient for a variety of conditions – dealing with laboratory efficiency or accuracy issues may be a worthwhile way to improve prescription practices which would also yield great benefits in terms of quality of care. Regularly reviewing a sample of prescriptions or case records and comparing treatments given to the standard treatment guidelines is likely to have a dramatic effect in improving treatment practices. Ten recommendations have been made for improving medication use in developing countries (Laing et al., 2001).

Dispense

The last step in the chain of drug supply is the delivery to the patient. Dispensing is often a neglected step but it is in some ways the most important, and the place where all the efforts expended to get the drugs to the patients may come to nought. Dispensing is often done by untrained staff who know little about the drugs they are dispensing, and are unable to communicate effectively with the patient. Patients need explanations about the drugs they are getting, and how to use them.

- Explain to patients that many pills are white – and not all white pills are the same!
- Increase the use of dispensing materials – paper or plastic bags – if it helps patients to adhere to treatment.
- Explain in simple words what the drug is meant to do and which frequent possible side effects might occur.

The key process in adequate dispensing is to ensure that patients understand why and how to take their medicines. Success or failure can be easily checked by conducting 'exit' interviews with a few patients. Brief training courses for dispensers substantially improve the quality of dispensing.

Fees and revolving drug funds

To ask patients to pay part, or all, of the cost of their drugs has become very popular in the past few years. Such 'user fees' can:

- hold down costs
- improve drug use
- replenish the funds for drugs in the system. Revenue from these fees has been used to replenish drug stocks, and sometimes to buy improvements for patients, such as benches or shading, provide incentives for staff, such as tea and sugar, or even to pay salaries of community health workers.

However, it is important to set realistic objectives for such cost recovery, and to agree in advance on how the money will be used, how it will be stored, accounted for, etc. Rarely have more than 15 per cent of overall costs of care been recovered from patient fees in low-income countries.

In some countries, the government has reduced its allocation to health facilities by the amount recovered, leaving the health facility no better off, and placing a heavier burden on local populations rather than sharing it more equitably throughout the nation.

Effects of user fees

Almost inevitably, attendance at health facilities declines when a user fee is introduced. In urban areas, attendance usually returns after some time to the level before fees were introduced. However, few studies have documented whether the patients who 'return' are the same ones who used the facility before. Have the former, possibly poorer, patients been replaced by better-off patients who are able to afford the fee and who are attracted to the quality improvements such fees usually bring?

Level of user fees

Setting the level of fee is an important issue, and it is essential to plan for 'losses' such as expired or damaged products. The book *Managing Drug Supply* describes the 'cycle of terrors' by which revolving drug funds become decapitalized and eventually fail – these include:

(a) port fees and losses
(b) underestimate of the amount of drugs needed for the 'pipeline'
(c) expiry
(d) theft
(e) losses during transport
(f) deterioration of stored drugs
(g) high operating costs
(h) prices being set too low
(i) excessive granting of both official and unofficial 'exemptions' from fees
(j) unanticipated price increases
(k) lack of foreign exchange
(l) funds being tied up in the banking system
(m) late receipt of money from government.

(Quick et al., 1997)

User fees and the poor

It is also important to consider the role of any existing 'under the table' payments and how a new fee will affect that system – will the fees replace the old payments, or be in addition to them? How will staff, when faced with a possible loss of income, react to the introduction of fees?

What will be the result in terms of overall level of expenditure for patients, and how many will be excluded from obtaining care by these new fees? Where facilities serve subsistence farmers and marginal urban dwellers, it is essential to remember that their cash earnings are extremely limited and are often seasonal and must be used for a variety of expenditures. User fees or prescription fees may be only part of the funds they have to spend in order to get health care. Drugs purchased on the local market may be significantly more expensive than imported drugs. This may pose a burden for lowest income groups who are already incurring other costs for care, such as lost wages, transport, or other fees.

Another issue to consider prior to introducing such a fee is that it will recover local currency, but this may not easily be converted into foreign exchange to buy imported drugs. In deciding on a prescription fee, the effects on the behaviour of patients and providers needs to be taken into account. A flat prescription fee will encourage patients to ask for more drugs; a fee per drug may encourage prescribers to overprescribe, especially if they keep a part of the revenue thus generated.

User fees and communicable diseases

It is especially inadvisable and risky in public health terms to charge for treatment of transmissible diseases such as TB, STDs, malaria – if people who cannot pay are not treated,treatment will be incomplete and/or delayed, and ultimately more people will develop the disease, or resistance to cheaper drugs will be found. The introduction of a cost recovery policy involving a substantial charge for TB treatment in China is thought to have resulted in 1–1.5 million additional TB cases (World Bank, 1993). Charging for STD treatment in Nairobi as the HIV epidemic was accelerating is thought to have increased HIV transmission through people remaining untreated for the STDs (Moses et al., 1992).

Conclusions

- Drug management demands committed work from pharmacists or pharmacy technicians, actively working with clinical staff.
- Clinical staff have to decide how to select and classify drugs by the VEN category and how to use drugs rationally. Insisting on the use of generic drugs, following treatment guidelines and promoting oral rather than liquid or injectable products will all extend the meagre drug budget dramatically. Investing a little time each week on checking stock levels and expiry dates, assessing patients' understanding of their dispensed drugs, reviewing clinical records or prescriptions can have a dramatic effect on drug availability and the quality of care provided by the health facility.

References

Laing RO, Hogerzeil HV, Ross-Degnan D. (2001). Ten recommendations to improve use of medicines in developing countries. *Hlth Pol Plan*, **16**: 13–20.

Moses S, Manji F, Bradley JE et al. (1992). Impact of user fees on attendance at a referral centre for sexually transmitted diseases in Kenya. *Lancet*, **340**: 463–466.

Quick JD, Rankin JR, Laing RO et al. (eds) (1997). *Managing Drug Supply. Management Sciences for Health in Collaboration with the World Health Organization*, West Hartford, CT. Kumarian Press. (May be available from WHO/EDM on request.)

WHO and BASICS. (1998). *Drug Supply Management Training Handbook*. WHO/CHD/98.4d, Geneva: WHO.

WHO. (1999a). *Guidelines for Drug Donations Revised 1999*, 2nd edn. WHO/EDM/PAR/99.4. Geneva: WHO.

WHO. (1999b). *Guidelines for Safe Disposal of Unwanted Pharmaceuticals in and after Emergencies*. WHO/EDM/PAR/99.2, Geneva: WHO (Free on request.)

World Bank. (1993). *World Development Report 1993: Investing in Health*. New York: Oxford University Press.

Part II
Infection

Infection: general principles

6 The immune response to infection

Introduction

Infectious diseases are by far the most important agents of disease in Africa today. Millions of children suffer and die from malaria, respiratory infections and diarrhoeal disease each year. Tuberculosis is the commonest cause of death in adults. In 2001, 24 million people in Africa were estimated to be infected with the Human Immunodeficiency Virus (HIV) (Weiss, 2001). The majority of people are infected with intestinal helminths or schistosomiasis at some time in their lives.

The immune system is the mechanism whereby the human body protects itself against infectious pathogens (Parkin & Cohen, 2001). It has two main components. The first is the non-specific immune system, which acts independently of any previous exposure to a pathogen, and includes the skin and body secretions. The second is the specific immune system, which responds to individual pathogens and has a memory process, so that the response becomes more effective with repeated exposures. When the immune response is most effective, the pathogen is eliminated with little or no damage to the human host and the host retains a memory response, which prevents future episodes of disease. The immune system is usually extremely beneficial. However, some components of the immune response cause adverse effects, which we see as disease. These include fever, inflammation and tissue destruction. Occasionally, abnormal immune responses cause disease directly. This is the case in diseases such as rheumatoid arthritis and asthma.

The immune system is generally very effective, protecting us from the millions of viruses, bacteria, protozoa, fungi and worms in the environment to which we are exposed every day. However, there are a number of general factors which influence the effectiveness of the immune response. These include the dose and virulence of the pathogen and genetic variation, age, nutrition and hormonal factors in the host.

Some pathogens, especially the parasitic helminths, have developed mechanisms to evade the immune response and can live in the human host for years. Recent studies indicate that their effect on the immune system may also have an important influence on responses to other infections. Other pathogens, such as HIV, directly invade and progressively destroy the cells of the immune system, leaving the host vulnerable to a wide spectrum of other infections. The tragic consequences of the HIV epidemic reveal the importance of effective immunity to human health and survival.

New developments in molecular biology offer ever-increasing opportunities for us to explore and understand the interactions between host and pathogen. These developments include the successful sequencing of genomes of several pathogens, and of the human host (International Human Genome Sequencing Consortium, 2001). New techniques, such as flow cytometry, allow us to study the activity of cells in detail, even at the level of the single cell. The study of immunology contributes to the development of improved treatments and vaccines, and immunological methods have been used to develop many important diagnostic tools.

Non-specific or innate immune mechanisms (Table 6.1)

The non-specific immune defence mechanisms, such as skin, secretions, opsonins and phagocytes, function independently of any previous contact with a pathogen. They are important first lines of defence against infection and are often breached in the very young or in the severely

Table 6.1. Non-specific or innate immune mechanisms

Surface defences	Tissue defences
Skin	*Soluble*
Lysozymes	Lysozymes
Gastric acid	Opsonins and natural antibodies
Normal microflora	Interferon
	Complement
	Chemokines
	Cytokines
	Cellular
	Polymorphonuclear neutrophils
	Macrophages
	Interdigitating dendritic cells
	Natural killer cells

malnourished. The non-specific response also has a key role in initiating the specific response which follows it. The non-specific or innate immune responses lack immunological memory; thus they remain unchanged however often a pathogen is encountered (Delves & Roitt, 2000).

The non-specific surface defences

Skin

Bactericidal and fungicidal compounds containing fatty acids are produced by the sebaceous glands of the skin. The skin may be thin, and these secretions are defective in the malnourished. Skin infections are much more common in the wet, humid times of year. Bacteria and fungi are able to multiply easily at these times, possibly because bactericidal secretions are diluted by sweat.

Lysozyme

This powerful enzyme is found in conjunctival, nasal and gastrointestinal secretions and can lyse some bacteria.

Gastric acid

Normal gastric secretions have a low pH which destroys many bacteria. The acid secretion of the vagina is thought to have a similar effect. Gastric acid secretion may be low in the malnourished, in patients treated for peptic ulcers with drugs that reduce gastric acid such as cimetidine, ranitidine, or omeprazole, and in people who smoke cannabis. Such individuals are at higher risk of gastrointestinal infections such as cholera. The malnourished are also susceptible to bacterial colonization of the ileum.

Normal flora

The normal gut bacterial flora protects against invasion of the gut by other pathogenic organisms. The mechanism of this phenomenon is not fully understood but may involve competition for food substances or the production of bacterial toxins. Breast milk influences the bacterial flora of the gut by lowering the pH and favouring growth of lactobacilli: pathogenic organisms do not grow well in this environment. Antibiotics can disturb normal flora so favouring the growth of pathogens such as *Clostridium difficile*, which causes colitis and diarrhoea.

The non-specific tissue defences

An organism which succeeds in penetrating the surface barriers of the host is susceptible to attack by a combination of humoral and cellular defences.

Lysozyme

This enzyme is also present in internal fluids and in polymorphs. It lyses bacteria, especially gram-positive cocci.

Opsonins and natural antibodies

These are substances present in serum that can coat bacteria and make them more susceptible to phagocytosis. A special example is C-reactive protein. This is a protein found in normal serum, and is one of a group of proteins called 'acute phase proteins', which increase in concentration rapidly during the inflammatory response. C-reactive protein is so called because it reacts with C-protein on the surface of pneumococci and makes them susceptible to phagocytosis.

Most so-called natural antibodies are probably cross-reacting antibodies, formed as a result of infection with a harmless gut or throat organism. Thus, infection with a non-pathogenic strain of *Escherichia coli* can induce the formation of protective antibodies against *Haemophilus influenzae* type B (Schneerson & Robins, 1975). Immunization by natural infection with non-pathogenic meningococci, or with the harmless commensal *Neisseria lactamica*, can induce the formation of cross-reacting antibodies, which protect against virulent strains of meningococci (Gold et al., 1978).

Cytokines and chemokines

The outcome of stimulation of cells in the immune system is highly dependent on cytokine production. Cytokines are small protein molecules, which act as messengers in the immune system. They are produced in response to stimulation through both the non-specific or innate immune system and the specific immune system. They can act on cells nearby, or on the cells that produce

Table 6.2. Some cytokines: their sources and effects

Cytokine	Immune system source	Principal effects
Interleukin-1	Macrophages and other cell types	• Lymphocyte activation • Macrophage activation • Increase in adhesion molecules for leukocytes on the endothelium and activation of neutrophils • Synthesis of acute phase proteins • Fever
Interleukin-2	Activated Th1 cells	• T cell proliferation • Activation of T cells • Chemotaxis and activation of macrophages
Interleukin-4	Activated Th2 cells	• B cell proliferation • Isotype selection for IgE and IgG_1
Interleukin-5	Activated Th2 cells	• B cell proliferation and differentiation • Isotype selection for Ig A • Eosinophil proliferation
Interleukin-6	T-cells B-cells	• Induces acute phase proteins • B-cell differentiation • Fever
Interleukin-8	Macrophages	• Chemotaxis • Superoxide and granule release
Interleukin-10	Macrophages Activated Th2 cells Regulatory/suppressor 'Th3' cells	• Inhibition of cytokine synthesis
Interleukin-12	Macrophages	• Promotion of Th1 cytokine responses
Interferon-γ	Activated Th1 cells	• Macrophage activation • Promotion of antigen presentation • Macrophage cytokine synthesis
Tumour necrosis factor-α	Macrophages Mast cells Lymphocytes	• Activation of macrophages and polymorphs • Increased cell adhesion • Induces acute phase proteins • Angiogenesis • Fever • Weight loss
Tissue growth factor-β	Various cells	• Suppression of antigen presentation
Colony stimulating factors	Various cells	• Growth and activation of phagocytic cells

them, by binding to specific receptors on the cell membrane and setting off a series of signals within the cell. Through these signals they can control expression of genes and hence the activities of the cell. More than 100 cytokines have been identified. They include interleukins, interferons, tumour necrosis factors, colony-stimulating factors, growth factors and chemokines. A selection of cytokines that are important in the immune system are described in Table 6.2, and some chemokines in Table 6.3. Some cytokines promote inflammation, others suppress or modulate inflammatory responses. The overall outcome of each immune stimulus is influenced by the spectrum of cytokines that are produced.

Interferons

This family of cytokines is particularly important in protecting cells from viral infection. Interferon gamma (IFN-γ) is involved in the non-specific response to infection. Interferons are produced by virally infected cells, and induce resistance to viral infection in neighbouring cells, thus reducing the spread of viral infection from cell to cell. IFN-γ is produced by T-cells in response to anti-

Table 6.3. Molecules which are chemotactic to leukocytes

	Molecule	Function
Products of micro-organisms	*Bacterial peptides* (f.MLP, the initial peptide of prokaryotic proteins)	Attract • polymorphs • eosinophils • macrophages
Damaged tissue	*Products of the clotting system* (fibrin peptide B, thrombin)	
Products of immune activation	*Complement components* (C_5a) *Chemokines* (products of cells in the immune system which increase the mobility of other cells), e.g. • interleukin-8 • MIP-1α • MIP-1β • RANTES	Activate and attract selected leukocytes according to the expression of receptor molecules on their surfaces.

Notes:
f.MLP: this tripeptide (formylated methionine–leucine–phenylalanine) is typical of prokaryotic proteins which are intiated with a formylated methionine amino acid residue. Eukaryotic proteins are initiated with an unformylated methionine. Receptors for f.MLP on polymorphs and macrophages thus allow them to be attracted specifically to sites of bacterial invasion.
MIP: macrophage inhibitory protein.
RANTES: a chemokine, whose name stands for 'regulated-upon-activation, normal T expressed and secreted'.

genic stimulation in the specific immune response, and has many other activities.

Complement

Complement was first recognized as a component of normal serum that aided the opsonization and lysis of bacteria. Complement, in fact, is not a single substance but a group of at least 20 proteins, which activate one another in turn in a similar manner to the coagulation pathway. This cascade system contains feedback loops which mean that, once activated, the signal is rapidly amplified.

Complement can be activated in three ways: by the classical pathway, the alternative pathway, or the mannan-binding lectin pathway (Fig. 6.1). The 'alternative pathway' is part of the non-specific immune response. It can be activated by endotoxins, such as those in gram-negative organisms. Similarly, the mannan-binding lectin pathway is activated by mannose-containing proteins and

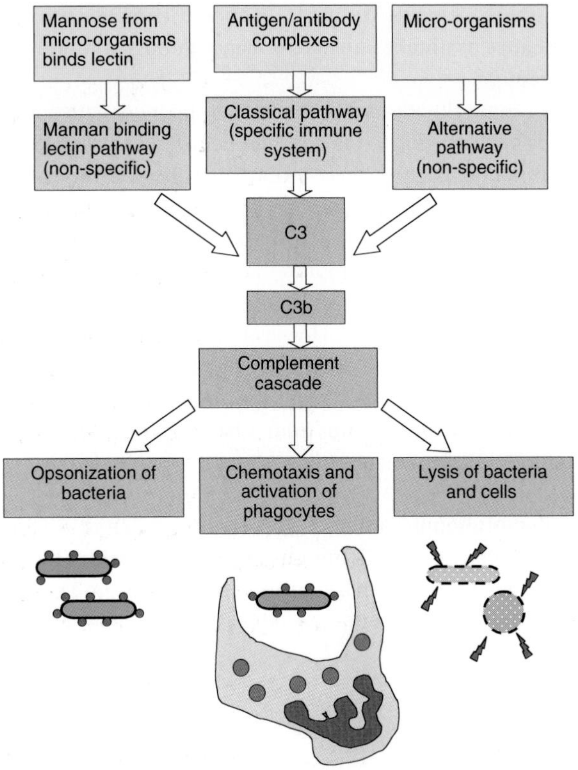

Fig. 6.1. Complement pathways and the results of their activation. (Adapted from Roitt et al., 1998.)

carbohydrates from micro-organisms including yeasts, bacteria and viruses. The 'classical pathway' is started by the binding of the first component of complement (C_1) to an antigen–antibody complex and is part of the specific immune response. All three pathways converge to convert C_3 to C_3b and other active breakdown products. The active breakdown products of complement have three main functions, (a) opsonization, (b) chemotaxis and activation of phagocytic cells, and (c) direct lysis of bacteria and cells. For example, C_3b may opsonize the surface of a bacterium, foreign cell or antigen–antibody complex. This aids their phagocytosis by neutrophils or macrophages which have a receptor for C_3b. Biologically active substances are released at various points in the pathway which increase vascular permeability and attract polymorphs, thus helping to produce acute inflammation. Other activated complement components can cause lysis of bacteria and cells directly, and may help destroy organisms such as *Eschericia coli.*

Some pathogenic organisms have evolved mechanisms to resist complement, for example by developing a capsule that does not activate the alternate pathway. Others even use complement to enhance their pathogenesis. For example, Dengue virus uses C_3-antibody complexes to enhance its uptake into macrophages through antibody receptors.

In some situations the effect of complement activation may be damaging to the host (see below). For example, complement activation contributes to the syndrome of endotoxic shock. Complement activation can also lead to localized tissue damage in diseases where antigen–antibody (immune) complexes are formed.

Low levels of C_3 and total haemolytic complement are found in many diseases. However, measurement is of most clinical value in differentiating post-streptococcal immune-complex acute nephritis (in which complement components are used up) from other renal diseases in which complement levels are normal.

Polymorphonulcear leukocytes (neutrophils)

These phagocytic cells are a most important part of the non-specific defences against microbial invasion. The cells are attracted to the site of invasion, for example a cut, boil, or insect bite, by chemotactic factors (Table 6.3), which are released by damaged tissue, activated complement, and bacteria themselves. Activated polymorphs express molecules on their surface which allow them to stick to vascular endothelia, migrate through the vessel walls, and enter the connective tissue where they first engulf and kill the organisms, and then die (Fig. 6.2). Phagocytosis of most pathogenic organisms, especially those with capsules, is achieved with the aid of serum factors such as complement and antibody, for the cells have surface receptors for both C_3b and the Fc portion of immunoglobulin IgG (see below). Once the microbe is inside the polymorph, the granules, containing powerful enzymes, discharge and kill the organism. The enzymes can kill directly, or through production of toxic chemicals including reactive oxygen intermediates such as superoxide anions ($^{\bullet}O_2^-$) or hydrogen peroxide (H_2O_2).

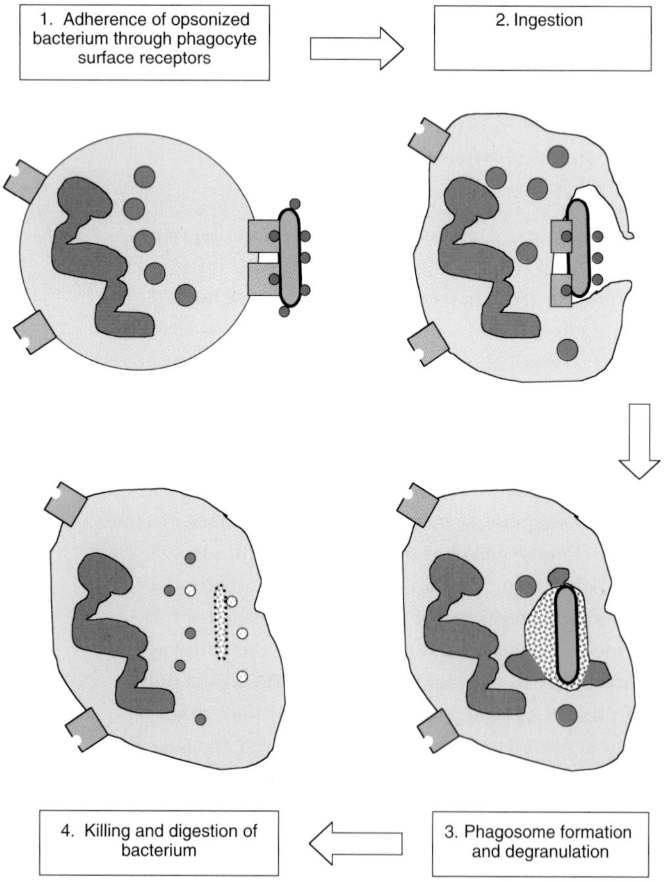

Fig. 6.2. Phagocytosis and killing of a bacterium by a polymorphonuclear leukocyte.

In African practice a variety of secondary polymorph defects are seen: polymorphs from severely malnourished children are unable to kill bacteria efficiently, bactericidal function is impaired in severe septiciaemia, chemotaxis is impaired in measles. Patients with HIV infection often have multiple or recurrent abscesses, or severe pyogenic infections such as pyomyositis. This may be because the specific antibody response is reduced in HIV infection (see below). Hence the coating of bacteria with antibody, and complement activation, required for efficient phagocytosis by polymorphs, is impaired.

The importance of polymorph killing is shown in children with genetic polymorph defects such as chronic granulomatous disease and Chediak–Higashi syndrome, whose polymorphs are able to ingest but not kill bacteria. These children suffer from severe and chronic infections.

Macrophages and interdigitating dendritic cells

Mononuclear macrophages are derived from bone marrow stem cells and migrate to strategic sites throughout the body. These macrophages were previously referred to as the reticulo-endothelial system. They function to remove particulate matter such as bacteria, immune complexes, and denatured proteins from blood and tissues, by phagocytosis or endocytosis. Alveolar macrophages in the lungs contribute to the first line of defence against inhaled pathogens; Kupffer cells in the liver process material entering through the digestive system; splenic and lymph node macrophages process material circulating through the lymphatic system and the blood, and circulating monocytes can migrate to new sites of infection and develop into mature, active phagocytic cells.

Macrophages, unlike polymorphonuclear neutrophils, are long-lived phagocytic cells. However, they engulf and kill organisms by mechanisms very similar to those used by polymorphs. Like polymorphs, they have surface receptors for immunoglobulins and complement and, in addition, they have receptors for carbohydrate molecules found on the surface of bacteria, allowing non-specific recognition, attachment and ingestion. Following ingestion, the phagosome fuses with lysosomes. Like the granules of polymorphs, the lysosomes contain enyzmes which promote killing of ingested bacteria directly, or through production of toxic chemicals such as oxygen radicals and nitric oxide. The pH of the phagosome becomes acidic. Activated macrophages release cytokines which promote inflammation and regulate lymphocyte responses, and enzymes, which can contribute to tissue damage and fibrosis. Besides these non-specific functions, macrophages have a vital role in the induction of the specific immune response, for these cells process and present the antigens of micro-organisms to lymphocytes, and their cytokines influence the lymphocyte response (see below).

Interdigitating dendritic cells are found in tissues such as the skin and lymphoid tissue. They have a similar role to macrophages, bridging the innate and specific immune response. Non-specific receptors allow them to recognize and take up foreign material by endocytosis, and they are susceptible to entry by many viruses. They process and present antigen to lymphocytes, and may be more important than macrophages in initiating the specific response to an antigen when it is encountered for the first time.

However, infection of macrophages and interdigitating dendritic cells by viruses, such as polio, dengue, influenza A and HIV can reduce their ability to process antigens normally. This may be one reason why cell-mediated immunity is impaired during these viral infections. Other organisms have developed mechanisms that allow them to live within macrophages without being killed. These include bacteria, such as *Mycobacterium tuberculosis, Mycobacterium leprae* and salmonella; protozoa such as *Leishmania*; and fungi such as *Histoplasma*. For example, *Mycobacterium tuberculosis* can survive in the macrophage phagosome through mechanisms which prevent fusion of the phagosome with lysosomes, and which prevent the phagosome pH from becoming acidic (Fig. 6.3).

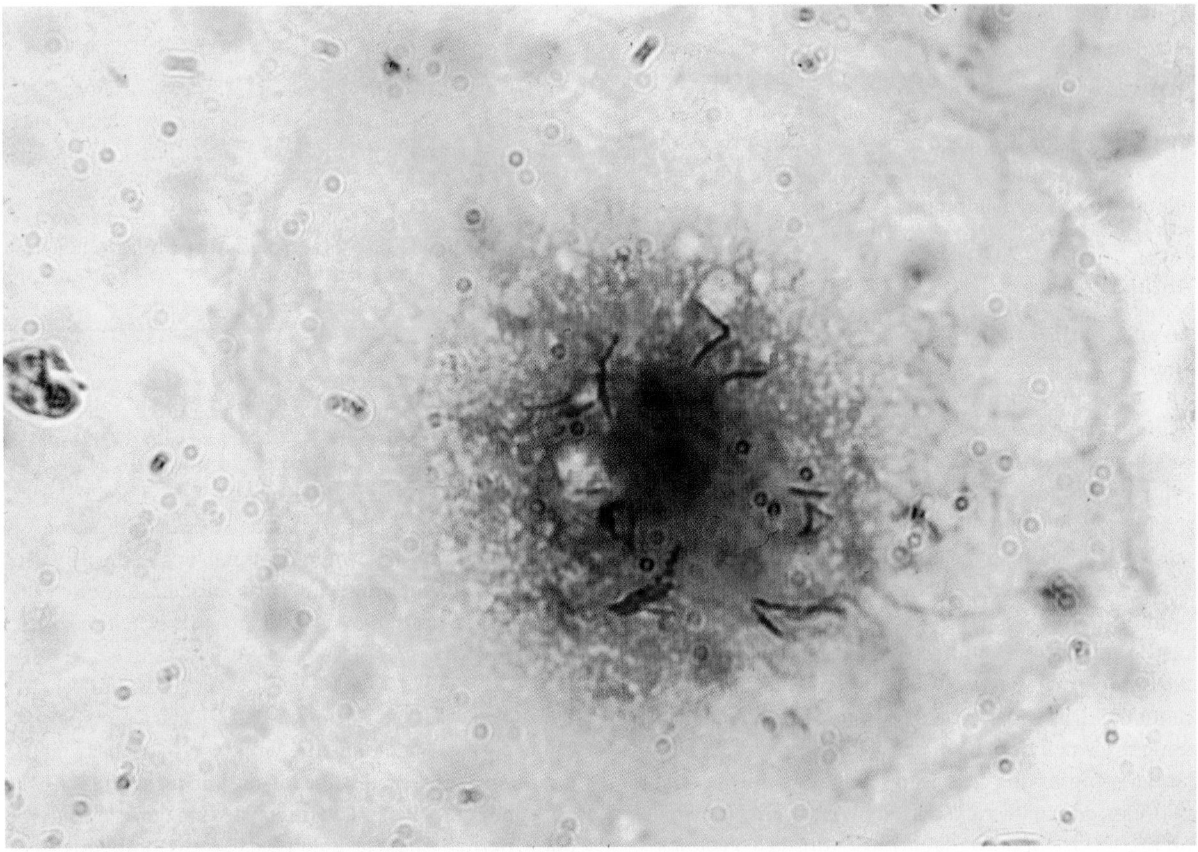

Fig. 6.3. *Mycobacterium tuberculosis* multiplying within a human monocyte-derived macrophage in culture.

Natural killer cells

Natural killer cells also have a role in both innate and specific immune responses. They are especially important early in some viral and bacterial infections. They are activated by IFN-γ, released from cells infected by viruses, and by cytokines such as interleukin-12 released from macrophages as part of the non-specific response. They can produce IFN-γ, which further activates macrophages, and they can recognize and kill abnormal cells, including both infected cells and tumour cells. In the specific immune response, they interact with antibody in antibody-mediated cytotoxic immune responses (see below).

Specific immune mechanisms

Although the non-specific defence mechanisms are of great importance in protection against infection, they are not sufficient in themselves. This is demonstrated in children lacking B- or T-lymphocyte systems, which are responsible for specific immunity, or those with diseases affecting lymphocytes such as the Acquired Immunodeficiency Syndrome (AIDS). Untreated, these people usually die of overwhelming infection. The lymphocyte system, the ways in which these cells confer specific immunity to man, and how they work to augment the non–specific defence mechanism are now described. This specific immune response is sometimes called the adaptive or cognate immune response.

Antigen

An antigen (immunogen) is a molecule that can be specifically recognized by receptors on lymphocytes. This recognition leads to the B-cells producing antibodies, and to the T-cells producing the required cytokines, or killing virus infected cells. Antibody molecules do not bind to the whole of an infectious agent, but to one of the many molecules (antigens) on the micro-organism's surface. Therefore, there are many different antibodies for a given pathogen, each binding to a different antigen on the pathogen's surface. Each antibody binds to a restricted part of the antigen called an epitope. A particular antigen can have several different epitopes. On the other hand, as will be discussed later, T-cells recognize antigens which have been processed or degraded by 'antigen-presenting cells' into small fragments or peptides, which become bound to presenting molecules on the surface of the antigen-presenting cell. Proteins and carbohydrates, especially polymers, are good antigens; nucleic acids and lipids are not. Thus some components of micro-organisms can act as strong antigens whereas others are weak antigens or non-antigenic.

Table 6.4. Characteristics of lymphocytes

	T	B
Characteristic		
Processed by	Thymus	Bursa (in birds) Peyer's patches in animals
Lifespan	Months–years	Days–weeks
Localization		
Lymph node	Deep cortical Perifollicular	Subcapsular Medullary germinal centres
Spleen	Periarteriolar	Peripheral white pulp, Red pulp
Peyer's Patch	Perifollicular	Central follicle
Blood	60–70% of lymphocytes	5–15% of lymphocytes
*Markers**	Form rosettes with sheep red cells; CD2, CD3, CD4 or CD8	Possess immunoglobulin on their surface; CD19, CD20, CD22
Function	Cytotoxic T-cell, cell mediated immunity: key cell in viral immunity	Antibody production
	Helper T-cell: necessary for many antibody responses by B-cells	T-dependent: possess receptor C3b, require T-cell help for antibody production
	Delayed hypersensitivity: T-cells attract and activate other cells, e.g. macrophages	T-independent: makes mainly IgM antibody in direct response to antigen

Notes:
* Lymphocytes express a number of markers on their surfaces termed CD (cluster designation); some are specific; others are found on more than one type of cell (From Roitt et al., 1998).

Lymphocytes

There are two major types of lymphocytes, T-cells and B-cells, which are responsible for specific recognition of antigens (Table 6.4). All lymphocytes are derived from the bone marrow stem cells. However, T-cells, or thymus-dependent lymphocytes, have been processed by the

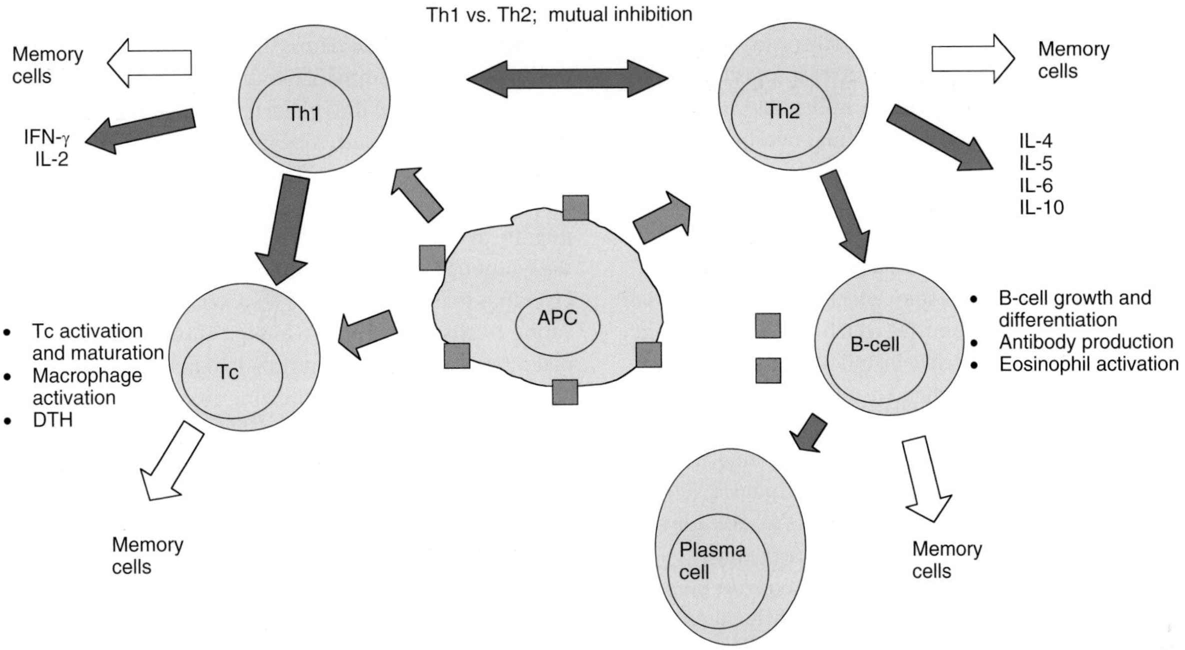

Fig. 6.4. Interactions of cells involved in the specific immune response. The antigen presenting cell (APC) varies according to the responding cells. B-cells can respond to intact antigen and are helped by CD4+ Th cells, which respond to processed antigen presented in association with MHC class II molecules. The presenting cells can be monocyte/ macrophages, dendritic cells or B cells. Th2 helper cells particularly promote selected antibody types, such as IgG1 and IgE, as well as eosinophilia. This type of response is common against helminths and in hypersensitivity against allergens. CD8+ Tc cytotoxic cells respond to processed antigen presented in association with MHC class I molecules which occur on practically all cell types. Their activation can be helped by Th1 cells which also promote macrophage activation. These responses are useful against intracellular pathogens and also cause the responses characteristic of delayed type hypersensitivity. Th1 and Th2 cells each produce cytokines that inhibit the other.

thymus. There are two major subsets of T-cells which are responsible for immunity. The first subset, which helps or induces immune responses through cytokine production (Th), has a CD4 marker. The second subset, which carries a CD8 marker, is predominantly cytotoxic (Tc). A further division of Th cells has also been recognised, defined by the cytokines they produce, which, in turn, defines their function. Th1 cells help in cytotoxic T-cell and macrophage activation. They are probably most important in protection against intracellular pathogens and contribute to delayed type hypersensitivity reactions (see below). Th2 cells help in antibody production and contribute to responses to helminth infections and hypersensitivity reactions to allergens in asthma and hayfever (Fig. 6.4).

B-cells or bursa-dependent cells have been processed during development by the Bursa of Fabricius (in birds) and by the equivalent of this organ (possibly Peyer's patches) in animals. These are responsible for producing antibody, either with help from T-helper cells (T-dependent), or without help (T-independent).

Lymphocytes have the following features.

(a) **Receptors which permit each cell to respond to an individual antigen thus conferring specificity on the cell.** The antigen receptors of B- and T-cells are probably derived from a common ancestor and both belong to the immunoglobulin superfamily of proteins. B-cell antigen receptors are immunoglobulins with two identical heavy chains and two identical light chains. Circulating antibodies (page 124, and Fig. 6.6) have the same structure as the B-cell antigen receptors except that they lack the segments that anchor the receptor antibody in the membrane and cross into the cytoplasm. All classes of immunoglobulins can act as receptors on B-cells.

The T-cell antigen receptor (TCR) comprises an α chain and a β chain, folded into a structure that resembles the antigen binding region of antibodies. A second TCR with γ and δ chains also exists on 5–10% of T-cells. These γ T-cells are especially associated with epithelial tissues. Like immunoglobulins, the TCR chains have external variable and constant chains, as well as segments that anchor the receptor in the membrane and cross into the cytoplasm.

The genes of the lymphocyte receptors allow us to generate a remarkably large number (10^{15}) of antibody variable regions and a similar number of T-cell-receptor variable regions. This diversity enables the immune system to respond to encounters with a huge variety of antigens.

(b) **Clonal proliferation or expansion (triggered by antigen) and long lifespan which provide the basis of memory.** The lymphocytes which respond to specific antigens are numerically insufficient to deal with an infection. However, when an antigen is encountered, mechanisms are activated which allow multiplication of B- or T-lymphocytes which recognize that antigen. This is called clonal proliferation or expansion. For B-cells, the recognition of antigen leads to multiplication of a clone of identical cells which become plasma cells, secreting the same antibody, or persist for many years as memory cells. Similarly, when T-cells encounter an antigen, they proliferate to produce the desired helper and cytotoxic T-cells, or to persist as memory cells. Clonal proliferation provides a highly efficient way to produce an effective response without the necessity to possess large numbers of each specific lymphocyte before exposure to infection.

(c) **Recirculation back into the bloodstream, which ensures that specific memory following a local response is distributed throughout the body.** For example, lymphocytes sensitized by a gut microbe migrate to the mammary gland and produce antibody to the microbe which is secreted in the milk.

The specific immune response takes place in response to antigens in the lymph nodes, spleen, or Peyer's patches and involves the co-operation of a number of cells leading to antibody production and/or cell mediated responses and retention of immunological memory. This is summarized in Fig. 6.4.

Antigen presentation to T-cells

Although antigens activate lymphocytes, very few antigens appear to bind directly to antigen-reactive T-cells. Instead they are usually presented on the surface of other cells known as antigen-presenting cells (APC), some of these being dendritic cells, macrophages and B-cells.

Dendritic cells as antigen-presenting cells

These are now regarded as the most important antigen-presenting cells, important initiators of the immune response. They are widely distributed in the body. B- and T-lymphocytes are mediators of immunity, but their function is under the control of dendritic cells. Dendritic cells in lymph nodes and the spleen trap antigens circulating in the lymph and blood, concentrate these on their surfaces and present them to the resident lymphocytes. They also trap antigens outside the lymphoid tissues and migrate to the lymphoid tissues, carrying the antigens to the lymphocytes. In the lymphoid organs they secret cytokines to initiate immune responses. As well as activating T-cells in response to foreign antigens they also make T-cells tolerant to antigens that belong to the body (self-antigens) thereby minimizing autoimmune reactions (Banchereau & Steinman, 1998). In HIV-1 infection dendritic cells decrease in number contributing to the immune deficiency (Jones et al., 2001).

Macrophages as antigen-presenting cells

When blood monocytes migrate through the blood vessel walls into the various organs, they become macrophages. It has been mentioned above that these bone marrow-derived cells can remove particulate antigens by phagocytosis. In the specific immune responses, they have another important role of ingesting and processing antigens and presenting them to the T-cells. Some antigens, notably those polysaccharides that interact directly with B-lymphocytes, do not need to be processed by macrophages or dendritic cells.

B-cells as antigen-presenting cells

During antibody responses, activated B-cells can also act as APC. They present antigen to T-helper cells that in turn make cytokines that stimulate the B-cells to further differentiate and make more antibodies.

Mechanisms of antigen processing and presentation

Presentation to a T-cell involves the enzymatic degradation of the antigen into small peptides. There are two pathways for processing antigen. The first involves proteins from outside the cell (exogenous antigens) that are taken up by the APC by phagocytosis or endocytosis and degraded within the lysosomal compartment into small peptides. In this process the peptides bind with large molecules called class II MHC (major histocompatibility complex) molecules. These molecules are then transported to the cell surface to display the peptide to nearby T-cells. The second pathway involves peptides that are synthesized within the cell cytoplasm (endogenous antigens) and these peptides associate with MHC class I mol-

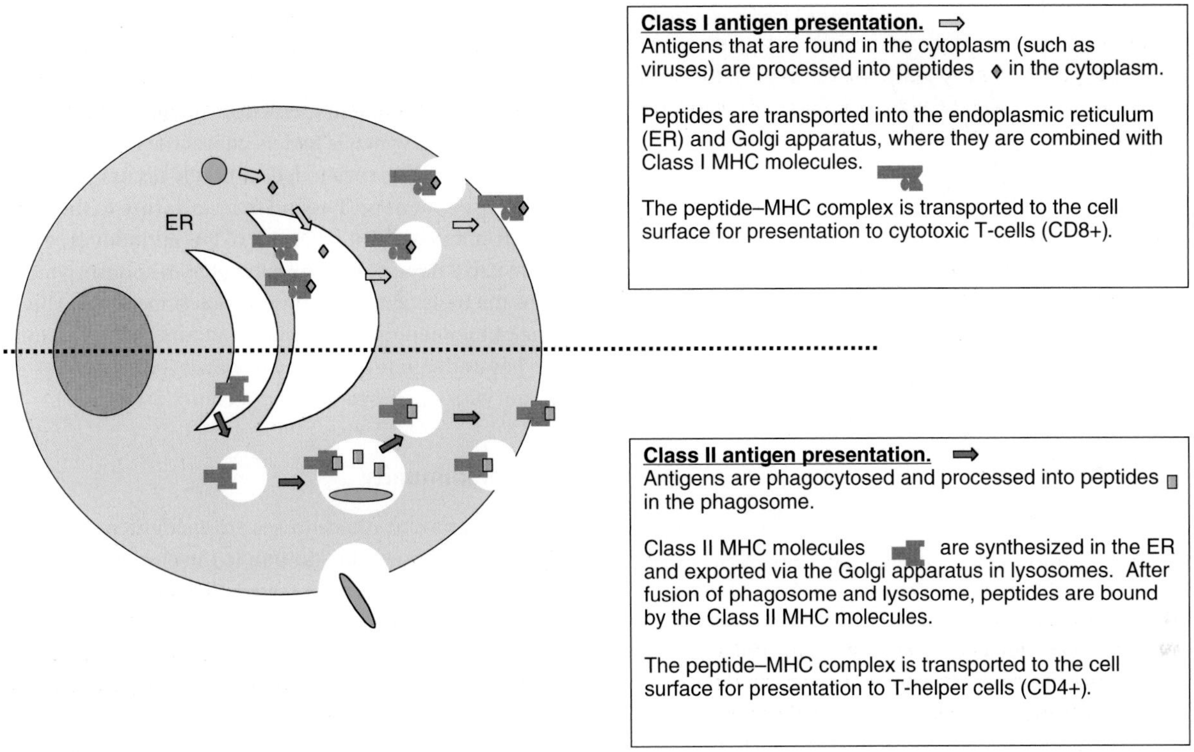

ER
Class I antigen presentation.
Antigens that are found in the cytoplasm (such as viruses) are processed into peptides in the cytoplasm.
Peptides are transported into the endoplasmic reticulum (ER) and Golgi apparatus, where they are combined with Class I MHC molecules.
The peptide–MHC complex is transported to the cell surface for presentation to cytotoxic T-cells (CD8+).
Class II antigen presentation.
Antigens are phagocytosed and processed into peptides in the phagosome.
Class II MHC molecules are synthesized in the ER and exported via the Golgi apparatus in lysosomes. After fusion of phagosome and lysosome, peptides are bound by the Class II MHC molecules.
The peptide–MHC complex is transported to the cell surface for presentation to T-helper cells (CD4+).

Fig. 6.5. Pathways of antigen presentation.

ecules. This is the important pathway for organisms such as viruses that infect and multiply in the cytoplasm of the cell (Fig. 6.5).

The two pathways are concerned with the activation of different types of T-cells. The MHC class II endocytic pathways is concerned with CD4+ T-cells such as T-helper cells. The MHC class I pathway is concerned with CD8+, cytotoxic T-cells.

Co-operation of cells involved in the specific immune response

It is important to note that, with the exception of a few antibody responses, nearly all immune responses depend upon T-cells. (Fig. 6.4). In general, antigens are presented by an appropriate cell (APC) to T-cells and their activation and responses are amplified or restrained by the various types of T-helper cells.

B-cells recognize a native, or unprocessed antigen, but receive help from T-cells which have also recognized the processed peptides of this same antigen. This interaction of T- and B-cells drives B cell division and differentiation. The T- and B-cell may recognize distinct parts of the antigen.

For many infections such as measles and HIV, both humoral and cellular immunity are involved in containing and limiting the virus. Therefore, the interaction of antigen, APC, MHC molecules, accessory molecules and cytokines are important in inducing an effective immune response.

Memory cells

The capacity to mount a secondary response is based on immunological memory. The basis of memory lies in the clonal proliferation or expansion of populations of antigen-specific lymphocytes during primary response, that is, following the fist exposure to antigen. This response increases the frequency of resting B and T cells capable of responding to the same antigen in future.

Antibodies

These is a special class of plasma proteins, known as immunoglobulins, which have a similar basic structure (Fig. 6.6). This structure consists of two heavy and two light chains, each of which is made up of amino-acid residues linked by disulphide bonds assembled in a Y

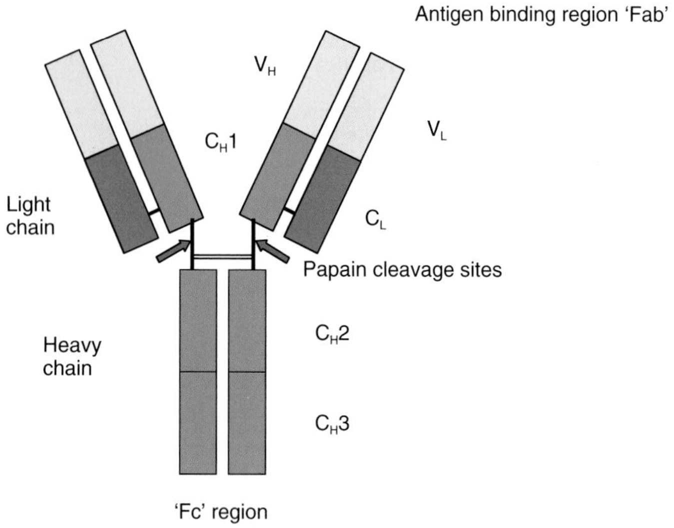

Fig. 6.6. The structure of an antibody. Antibody molecules are made up of two identical heavy polypeptide chains (shown in blue) and two identical light chains (shown in pink). They are joined together by disulphide bonds (shown in black). Each heavy chain has three "constant" domains (C_H1, C_H2, C_H3). These are regions which vary relatively little between antibody molecules of the same class. Each light chain has one constant region (C_L). Each heavy and light chain also has one 'variable' domain (V_H, V_L). These regions include the antigen binding sites, and their high degree of variability acounts for the large number of antigens which can be recognized. The enzyme papain can cleave antibodies at the sites shown, producing two 'Fab' fragments which can bind antigen, and one 'Fc' fragment, the structure of which determines the antibody's characteristics for binding surface receptors on effector cells and fixing complement.

shape. Digestion of the molecule with papain gives two Fab fragments and an Fc fragment. The Fab fragments bind antigen, and the Fc fragment can attach itself to receptors on polymorphs, macrophages, and certain lymphocytes. All immunoglobulins have light chains of one or two types known as kappa (κ) or lambda (λ). However the immunoglobulins differ markedly in the structure of their heavy chains, differentiating them into five classes with differing properties (Table 6.5). Each immunoglobulin class contains many different immunoglobulin molecules each capable of reacting with only one antigen. This specificity is determined by the amino-acid sequence of the variable region lying at the free ends of the light and heavy chains. These regions combine with the antigen by chemical binding. The strength of this binding, or affinity, is important in protecting against infection, as is the ratio of antibody to antigen. Too little antibody may not neutralize a pathogen such as a virus.

Primary and secondary antibody responses

Free antibody cannot be found in the circulation until about a week after the first exposure to antigen. This initial antibody, which is IgM, is part of the primary response; later a change to IgG antibody occurs. This class switching depends on T-cells. On re-exposure to the same antigen, a marked and rapid rise of IgG antibody is seen within 2 to 3 days. This is the secondary response, which forms the basis of most immunization procedures. The same phenomenon occurs when an immune person (one who has undergone a primary response) comes in contact with a pathogen for the second time.

Mucosal immunity

Many bacteria and some viruses are encountered at the mucous membranes. In addition to the non-specific immune mechanisms discussed earlier, antibodies of the IgA type are found at the mucosal surfaces. These can bind to micro-organisms and prevent their adherence to the cells of the mucous membrane thereby stopping the infection. IgA gives protection in tears, saliva, bronchial secretions and in the gut. This immune system is sometimes called the secretory immune mechanism.

T-cell independent antibody production

Antibody response to most antigens depends on both T-cells and B-cells recognizing the antigen in a linked fashion. This is called T-dependent response. However, there are a few antigens that can activate B-cells without T-cell help, these are called T-independent antigens. The major characteristic of T-independent antigens is the structure. They are large polymeric molecules with repeating antigenic determinants. Many are resistant to degradation and are of microbial origin, for example bacterial carbohydrates, and proteins such as endotoxin and flagellin. The way the B-cells are activated is thought to be due to these large molecules cross-linking the B-cells, receptors and triggering responses. Some polysaccharide vaccines, such as the polysaccharide meningococcal and pneumococcal vaccines, work in a T-cell independent fashion.

Antibody and infection

The ways that antibody can protect against infection are shown in Fig. 6.7. The importance of antibody is shown in patients with congenital or acquired defects of antibody production. Children who congenitally are unable to produce immunoglobulins suffer repeated infection by pyogenic cocci. Children with severe malnutrition have a deficiency of secretory antibody: this may explain why they have frequent gut and lung infections. Certain individuals do not respond to hepatitis B vaccines: they are in great danger of being infected. Children with AIDS, malaria or measles have a poor antibody response to other sorts of antigen, which makes them susceptible to secondary infection.

T-cells and infection

We shall now look at some of the effector mechanisms of the T-cells.

CD4 T-helper cells

The activation of these cells is controlled by the presence of the antigen in association with MHC class II and costimulatory molecules on the surface of APC. Naïve CD4 T-cells respond to presented antigen by differentiating into two main subtypes, Th1 or Th2 (Fig. 6.4). Th1 cells produce IL-2 and IFN-γ and these lead to the activation and differentiation of the cytotoxic T-cells and activation of macrophages. The activation of macrophages causes an increase in the respiratory burst and the production of toxic nitrogen and oxygen metabolites in addition to the fusion between phagosomes and lysosomes. All these together help to kill organisms such as mycobacteria that reside in the macrophages. IFN-γ also suppresses the effect of IL-4 on B-cells. On the other hand, Th2 cells produce IL-4, IL-5 and IL-10. IL-4 and IL-10 lead to the activation and differentiation of B-cells, while IL-5 promotes proliferation of eosinophils. IL-4 and IL-10 also suppress Th1 responses, so Th1 and Th2 responses are mutually inhibitory. The bias of the immune response to Th1 or Th2 is influenced by a number of factors. Some antigens, such as mycobacteria, tend to elicit a polarized Th1 response, while others, such as helminths and allergens, elicit a polarized Th2 response. However, many T-cells in humans have cytokine profiles intermediate between the above and are known as Th0 cells.

Cytotoxic T-cells

Cell-mediated cytotoxicity is an essential defence against intracellular pathogens, including viruses, some bacteria and parasites. Cytotoxic T-cells are mostly CD8 T-cells that recognize specific antigens presented by MHC class I. However, there are a few CD4 cytotoxic T-cells that recognize antigens presented by class II molecules. Measles infection is one example where, cytotoxic CD4 T-cells are generated which recognize and kill MHC class II positive cells infected with virus. Cytotoxic cells kill by directing their granules towards the target cells. The granules of Tc cells contain molecules called perforins which can punch holes in the outer membranes of the target. They also contain granzymes which are a cocktail of toxic proteases and esterases. Some Tc cells, including CD4 Tc, can also use a molecule called 'FAS Ligand', which they possess, to cluster FAS molecules on the target cell leading to activation of genes for 'programmed cell death', also known as 'apoptosis' (see below) (Fig. 6.8).

The most important role of Tc cells is in virus infection. Virtually all cells in the body express MHC class I, making it possible to identify and eliminate virus-infected cells.

Table 6.5. Properties of immunoglobulins

Class	Molecular weight and structure	Serum concentration	Properties
IgA	170 000 monomer or dimer	150 mg%	The major immunoglobulin in secretions and bile where the dimer is linked to the secretory piece. Important in mucosal immunity
IgG	160 000 monomer	1200 mg% raised in Africans	Found widely in body tissues. Good all-purpose antibody which fixes complement. Actively secreted across placenta to protect new born
IgM	900 000 pentamer	100 mg% raised in Africans	Rapid production in primary response. Fixes complement and good agglutinating properties
IgD	184 000 monomer	3 mg%	No known specific function
IgE	188 000 monomer	0.03 mg% raised in Africans	Involved in immediate hypersensitivity reactions. Binds to mast cells and leads to histamine release on contact with antigen. Binding of IgE triggers degranulation of eosinophils

Apoptosis

Apoptosis is an important defence mechanism against viruses which has received much attention in the last 10 years. This programmed cell death involves the

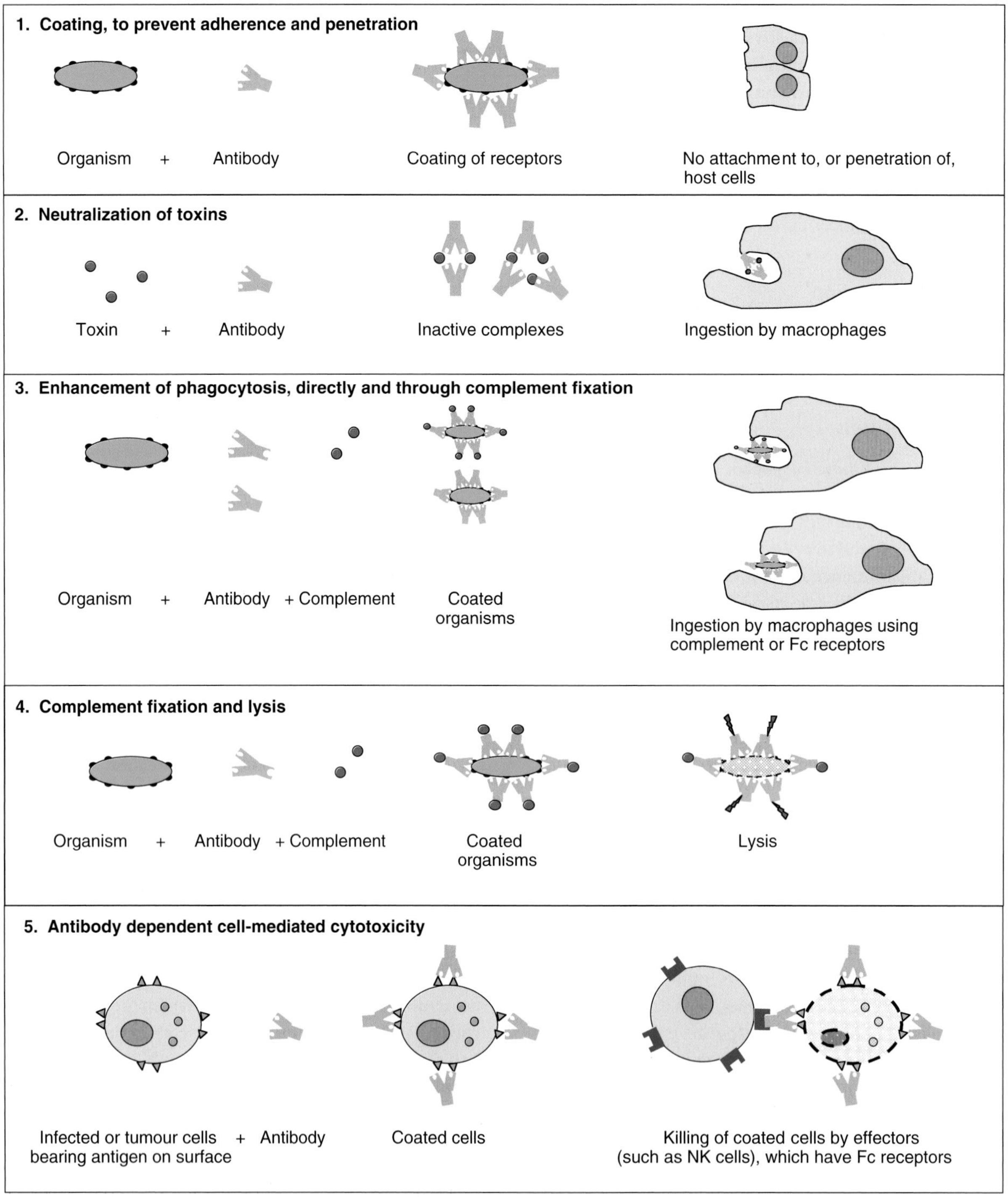

Fig. 6.7. Ways in which antibodies can protect against infection.

activation of several 'suicide' genes which orchestrate first the fragmentation of DNA, followed by the systematic disruption of organelles, and finally the packaging of the digested cellular contents into non-inflammatory membrane-bound packages that are consumed by phagocytes. This is triggered by some cytotoxic T cells as discussed above. For further reading, see Janeway and Travers (1996).

There are some diseases where apoptosis is thought to play a major role in pathogenesis. For example, some HIV gene products lead to activation of the apoptosis pathways. The proportion of CD4 T-cells in the later stages of apoptosis is about two-fold higher in HIV-1 infected individuals than in uninfected people. This may be one way in which CD4 T-cells are lost in HIV infection.

Antibody-dependent cell mediated cytotoxicity

Natural Killer (NK) cells can kill infected cells without use of MHC molecules. They have receptors to recognize target cells. For example, they can use Fc receptors to kill targets that are coated by antibodies. They attach to these targets using their Fc receptors. This is called antibody-dependent-cell mediated cytotoxicity (ADCC). NK cells require IL-2 from Th1 for stimulation and proliferation. ADCC is an example of an effector mechanism that can be triggered by either the innate or the specific (adaptive) mode of recognition.

Mast cells, basophils and eosinophils

These cell types are related to neutrophils but have a role as effector cells in the specific immune response, especially in anti-helminth immunity and in the hypersensitivity reactions of asthma and hay fever. They all contain granules, which are released when triggered through cell membrane receptors. Mast cells are found in quite large numbers in mucosal tissues, while basophils circulate in the blood. IgE is passively absorbed on their surface. When this binds the specific antigen, be it parasite or allergen, the cells degranulate causing local inflammation and chemotaxis of inflammatory cells, especially eosinophils. Eosinophils, on the other hand, depend on IgG or IgE antibodies coating the parasite. Binding leads to degranulation and the granule contents lead to extracellular damage or killing of the target parasite. This is another form of the antibody-dependent cell-mediated cytotoxicity (ADCC), described above.

The role of specific cell-mediated immune reactions in protecting against infection is summarized in Fig. 6.8.

Evasion of the immune response

We have described the immune mechanisms that help man to combat infection. Why is man infected in spite of these defences? Part of the answer is that some organisms, whether bacterium, virus or worm, have also evolved mechanisms by which they can evade the immune response. Some are especially successful in that they can survive and replicate for prolonged periods, while causing little harm to the host. Others, particularly protozoa and helminths, are eventually eliminated, but subsequent infection with the same parasite may occur repeatedly.

Different pathogens have different ways of evading the immune responses depending on how they are normally cleared from the body. We shall now look at some immune evasion mechanisms of bacteria, viruses and parasites

Bacteria

Phagocytosis is one of the main protective mechanisms against bacteria. The presence of antibodies and complement greatly increase the rate of clearance of bacteria. Some bacteria are killed directly by complement-dependent lysis, the activation of the lytic process being initiated by antibody binding to the surface of the bacteria. Antibodies also sometimes directly neutralize bacteria or toxins they produce.

Bacteria that have capsules or adhere poorly to phagocytic cells can resist being killed. This is seen with meningococci. Others, like staphylococci, evade the immune clearance by producing endotoxins that damage neutrophils and prevent their chemotaxis to sites of infection. Meningococci can produce free antigens from their capsules, which neutralize circulating antibodies thus allowing the organism to escape. Blocking antibodies can combine with an antigenic site on the surface of a microbe without damaging it and thus protect it from damage by lethal antibodies. This mechanism may play a role in disseminated gonococcal and meningococcal infections.

Some bacteria resist complement-mediated attack by directing deposition of complement away from cell membrane to sites where it cannot be effective. This is done by some gram-negative bacteria.

Others, like *Listeria monocytogenes*, release enzymes that lyse phagosome membranes thereby moving into the cytoplasm and escaping the phagosome-induced killing. *Mycobacterium tuberculosis* and *M. leprae* can survive in macrophages by preventing their lysosomes from functioning properly.

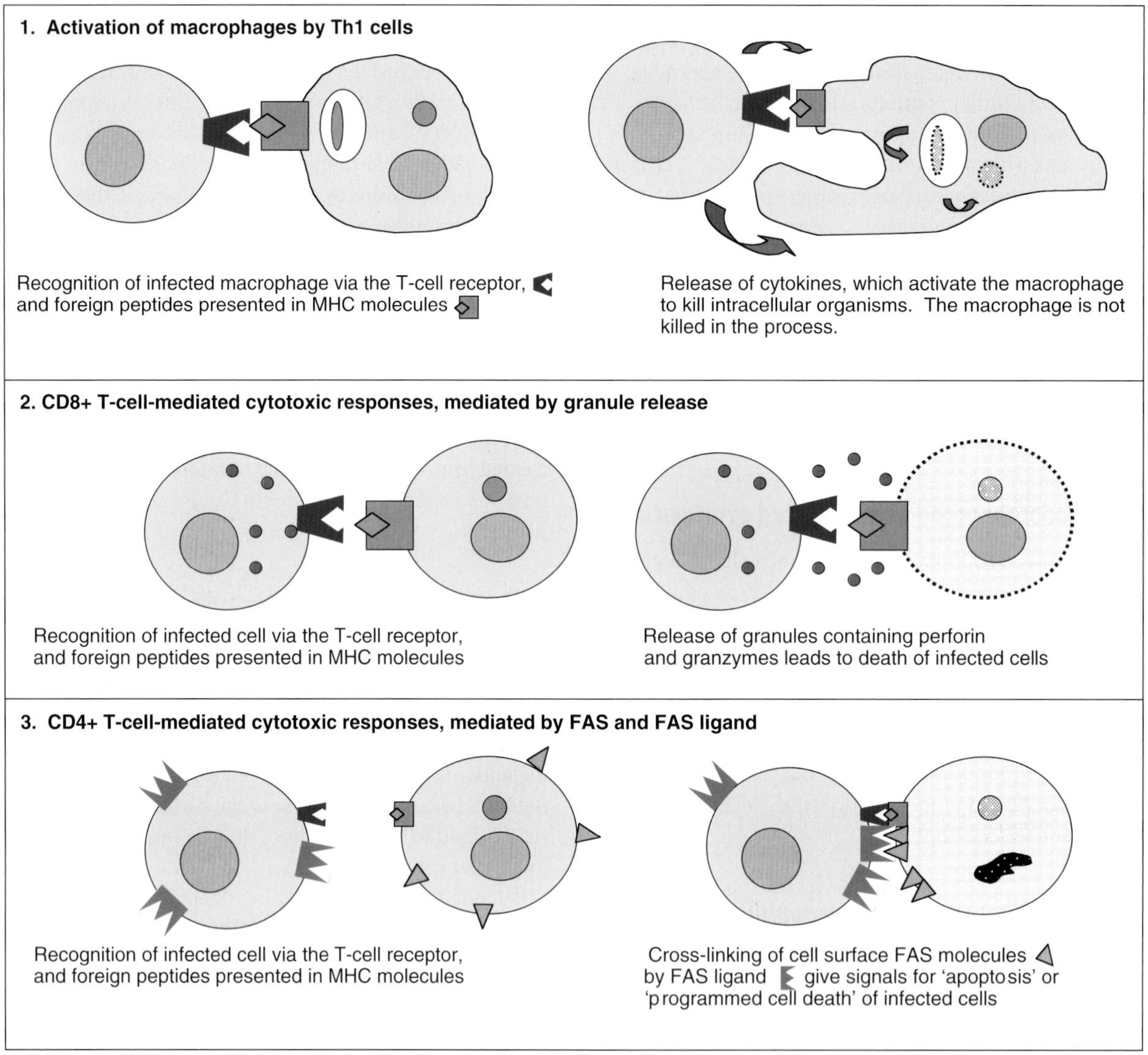

1. Activation of macrophages by Th1 cells
Recognition of infected macrophage via the T-cell receptor, and foreign peptides presented in MHC molecules
Release of cytokines, which activate the macrophage to kill intracellular organisms. The macrophage is not killed in the process.
2. CD8+ T-cell-mediated cytotoxic responses, mediated by granule release
Recognition of infected cell via the T-cell receptor, and foreign peptides presented in MHC molecules
Release of granules containing perforin and granzymes leads to death of infected cells
3. CD4+ T-cell-mediated cytotoxic responses, mediated by FAS and FAS ligand
Recognition of infected cell via the T-cell receptor, and foreign peptides presented in MHC molecules
Cross-linking of cell surface FAS molecules by FAS ligand give signals for 'apoptosis' or 'programmed cell death' of infected cells

Fig. 6.8. Ways in which T-cells can protect against infection.

Viruses

Viruses also have a number of mechanisms to evade the immune response. These include antigenic variation which involves mutations of regions that are normally recognized by antibodies and T-cells. This is seen in influenza virus and HIV. Other viruses such as adenovirus and CMV encode proteins that are able to inhibit the transportation of MHC class I molecule to the cell membrane, hence avoiding being recognized by cytotoxic T-cells. Epstein–Barr virus and adenoviruses produce substances that inhibit the activation of interferon. Many viruses have evolved mechanisms to counteract the effect of apoptosis. For example, adenoviruses encode Bcl-2, a negative regulator of apoptosis.

Parasites

Parasites have many different mechanisms to evade the immune system. Intracellular parasites can avoid destruction by oxgyen metabolites and lysosomal enzymes by penetrating the macrophages through methods other than phagocytosis. This is done by *Toxoplasma gondii. Trypanosma cruzi* can escape from the phagosome into the macrophage cytoplasm. On the other hand, *Leishmania* produces enzymes that protect against the action of the oxgyen radicals. *Leishmania* resist destruction by complement by directing its lytic activity to the surface coat which can be shed off, while the trypomastigotes of *Trypanosomiasis cruzi* have glycoproteins which down-regulate complement reactions.

Like viruses, parasites such as the African trypanasome and various malarial parasites change their surface antigen, thereby evading the antibody responses. The tapeworm *Echinococcus* lives in a hydatid cyst, usually in the liver, out of reach of immune recognition. *Entamoeba histolytica* also forms protective cysts. Others, like the schistosome, incorporate MHC molecules, complement components and immunoglobulin fragments into their own surface coating, making themselves antigenically like the host (disguised) and therefore invisible to the immune system. Some parasites release large amounts of their own antigens into circulation which block potentially damaging lymphocytes and antibodies from reacting against the parasites themselves. Some parasites, such as schistosomes, elicit production of immunosuppressive cytokines such as IL-10, and hence cause immune suppression by interference with macrophage function, and dampening specific immune responses to their own and other antigens. In addition, helminths secrete molecules that can degrade antibodies, interfere with complement activity, inhibit polymorph chemotaxis and inhibit the killing mechanisms of activated phagocytes (Maizels et al., 1993).

Malaria-infected erythrocytes also adhere to dendritic cells, inhibiting the maturation of dendritic cells and subsequently reducing their capacity to stimulate T-cells (Urban et al., 1999).

The consequence of this wide array of evasive mechanisms is that parasite infections tend to be long and chronic as the battle between parasite and immune response goes on.

Clinical features of the immune response to infection

The immune response is generally highly beneficial in protecting us against infection. However, many of the clinical manifestations of infectious diseases are a 'side effect' of the immune response. Often it is difficult to determine how much tissue damage is produced directly by the causative organism and how much is due to the host's immune response because the harmful effects of the host's immune response occur at the same time as the protective effects. Manifestations of disease that are mediated by immunological mechanisms include hypersensitivity reactions, fever, shock, tissue destruction and lymphadenopathy.

Hypersensitivity reactions

Some of the harmful effects of the immune response have traditionally been called 'hypersensitivity reactions', reflecting the idea of an over-active response. Examples of clinical disease that result from hypersensitive immune responses are listed in Table 6.6.

Fever

Body temperature is controlled by the hypothalamus. During infection, release of cytokines from macrophages, especially IL-1, IL-6 and TNF-γ, leads to synthesis of prostaglandins which act on the hypothalamus, leading to fever. In non-infectious diseases similar processes can also lead to fever as a result of tissue damage, or immune activation. Examples include the tissue damage of myocardial infarction, or the fever observed in lymphoma, or autoimmune connective tissue diseases. Antipyretic drugs, such as aspirin, inhibit this pathway by blocking prostaglandin synthesis. However, it has been noted that fever can develop exceedingly quickly following infection, and before measurable increases in cytokines can be detected in the blood. It is now thought that this may be mediated by a neurological pathway. This new hypothesis proposes that synthesis of small amounts of cytokines by liver macrophages (Kuppfer cells) leads to rapid stimulation of sensory fibres of the vagus nerve in the liver. This signal is transmitted by the vagus nerve to the hypothalamus, leading to a rapid rise in body temperature (Blatteis & Sehic, 1998).

Endotoxic shock

Massive release of cytokines in response to infection can lead to shock. This is best known as a complication of septicaemia caused by gram-negative bacteria. The lipopolysaccharide (endotoxin) from the gram-negative bacterial cell wall is a potent stimulant of the release of cytokines such as IL-1 and TNF-γ from circulating white cells. Released in large quantities, these cytokines cause fever, increased expression of adhesion molecules on endothelial cells and increased permeability of blood vessels. Thus platelets and fibrin adhere to the blood vessel walls forming small thrombi throughout the circulation (disseminated intravascular coagulation) and fluid leaks out into the tissues causing a fall in blood pressure and circulatory collapse. In addition, intense activation of

Table 6.6. Harmful effects of the immune response to infection

Allergic reaction	Mechanism	Clinical examples
TYPE 1 Immediate hypersensitivity	IgE antibody, bound to basophils and mast cells, initiates histamine release on contact with antigen. Eosinophils modulate the reaction	Asthma produced by pollens, nematode larvae. Urticaria produced by schistosome cercariae. Anaphylactic shock to injected horse serum (e.g. anti-tetanus)
TYPE II Antibody mediated cytotoxicity	Antibodies bind to an antigen derived from an infective agent but situated on a host cell and cause death of the cell by lysis or phagocytosis	Anaemia in some infections, like malaria or *Mycoplasma* pneumonia
TYPE III Immune complex formation	Formation of antigen/antibody complexes. This may occur: (a) Within the circulation (serum sickness type), with complexes depositing in kidneys, skin, and synovium (b) Within the tissues where there is persistent antigen (Arthus type). Immune complex deposition leads to inflammation by activation of complement, attraction of polymorphs, phagocytosis, enzyme release, and vascular damage	(a) Nephrotic syndrome in *P. malariae* infection. Post-streptococcal nephritis. Arthritis in serum hepatitis and rubella. Endocarditis in Streptococcal and Staphoccocal infection (b) Erythema nodosum leprosum, menigococcal arthritis
TYPE IV Delayed hypersensitivity	Cell-mediated immune response to an organism may result in the development of killer cells capable of destroying host cells carrying the organism	Tuberculoid leprosy, ulceration in cutaneous leishmaniasis, cavitation in tuberculosis

the complement cascade leads to massive release of toxic products from granulocytes, and contributes to increased vascular permeability and tissue damage.

Septicaemia caused by gram-positive bacteria, such as *Staphylococcus aureus*, is sometimes also associated with shock. This may be the result of release of cytokines in response to stimulation of large numbers of T-cells by 'superantigens' which can activate certain T-cell subsets by a mechanism which bypasses normal antigen processing and presentation.

Tissue destruction and fibrosis

Death of bacteria and polymorphonuclear phagocytes at the site of infection with bacteria such as *Staphylococcus aureus* leads to abscess formation. In the specific immune system, the cell-mediated response to pathogens such as *Leishmania* or *Mycobacterium tuberculosis* is associated with progressive destruction of tissue and healing with scarring. Similarly, in tuberculoid leprosy nerve damage is not caused directly by bacilli, but by an extreme immune response which severely damages the nerves in whose sheaths the bacilli are harboured. These are examples of type IV hypersensitivity reactions (Table 6.6).

Lymphadenopathy

During the immune response to a local or systemic pathogen the local or systemic lymph nodes, and the spleen, may become enlarged as responding lymphocytes multiply in these organs.

Factors that influence the immune system

A number of general factors can affect the immune system.

Genetic factors

Genetic factors can influence resistance to infection in several ways (Hill, 1998). Specific hereditary defects in molecules which mediate immune responses increase susceptibility to disease. For example, those with deficiency in the complement system (Alper et al., 1972) or with agammaglobulinaemia (Bruton, 1952) suffer from severe bacterial infections. Those with abnormal receptors for gamma interferon or IL-12 suffer from severe infections with intracellular pathogens such as mycobacteria and salmonella (Newport et al.,1996; Altare et al., 1998).

Genetic variation in 'HLA-type' has subtle effects on the immune response. The name 'HLA' (human leukocyte antigen) was given to these molecules before their function was known. The HLA molecules are the Class I and Class II MHC antigen-presenting molecules which bind peptides from foreign proteins and present them on the surface of macrophages and other antigen-presenting cells, as described above. The genes for MHC molecules have many alleles, and consequently the proteins which they encode vary between individuals in the same population. Since these molecules are involved in the process of antigen-presentation, genetic variation determines which components of an invading pathogen will be presented on the cell's surface, recognized, and hence elicit an immune response. In West Africa, individuals with HLA-B53 are resistant to severe malaria. In these individuals, the HLA-B53 molecule specifically binds a key peptide from the liver stage of the malaria parasite. It is likely that this allows the immune system to recognize and destroy parasitized liver cells particularly efficiently, and hence limit multiplication of the malaria parasites (Hill et al., 1992).

Age

Immune responses change with age. The immune response develops in utero, and factors affecting the mother during pregnancy, such as viral or helminth infections, can influence the neonatal immune response (Malhotra et al., 1999). Then, during infancy, breast milk provides both non-specific protective effects (through a range of antimicrobial agents such as lysozyme, and the influence of pH described above) and specific protective effects (through the presence of maternal antibodies).

Infants themselves differ in their response to some infections, compared with older children and adults. Although they have mature T- and B-cells, there is a significant Th2 bias, which decreases with time. Thus many viral infections, such infection with hepatitis A and B, cytomegalovirus and Epstein–Barr virus, have a less severe clinical presentation in children, and are more likely to go unnoticed, perhaps because Th1-mediated pathological effects of the response to infection are less severe. On the other hand, these subclinical infections may also be associated with persistence of the viral infection. This is especially important for hepatitis B where young children tend to have a prolonged carrier state (Edmunds et al., 1993).

Infants also have a poor response to carbohydrate antigens. This probably accounts for the low efficacy of polysaccharide vaccines in infancy. In addition, the response to bacterial infections, especially to bacteria with polysaccharide capsules, is poor, leading to more severe disease.

The hormonal changes of adolescence may also influence the immune response. This age group appears to be particularly susceptible to tuberculosis, whereas children above 5 years old and mature adults are relatively resistant. Finally, the immune system deteriorates in old age so that infections are less efficiently checked and thus more severe.

Hormonal factors

In addition to the hormonal changes of puberty, three other important hormonal factors should be noted.

(a) Pregnancy is associated with suppression of immune responses with increased risk of several infections, including pneumococcal meningitis and severe malaria.
(b) Uncontrolled diabetes mellitus increases susceptibility to many infections, especially pyogenic infections and tuberculosis.
(c) Large doses of corticosteroids (such as prednisolone) increase susceptibility to many infections. In particular, quiescent infections with *Mycobacterium tuberculosis*, herpes zoster or *Strongyloides stercoralis* may become active.

The causes and effects of immune deficiency

The principal causes of immune deficiency in Africa are malnutrition and infection. Many pathogens cause an element of immunosuppression. Often this is an adaptation that allows them to survive and replicate in the host, as described above. On the other hand, the Human Immunodeficiency Virus (HIV) selectively infects the cells of the immune system, with consequent depletion and immune deficiency.

Malnutrition

Malnutrition has been described as the most common cause of immunodeficiency world-wide (Chandra, 1997).

Protein-energy malnutrition is associated with impaired non-specific defences (thinning of the skin, damage to mucosal surfaces, reduced production of lysozyme; impairment of phagocyte function and reduced levels of complement components) and impaired specific responses (reduction in cell-mediated immune responses, cytokine production and secretory IgA production). Children who are malnourished show atrophy of the thymus and of lymphoid tissue in the spleen and lymph nodes, lymphocyte counts are reduced and the CD4/CD8 T-cell ratio declines. These children are highly susceptible to a wide range of infections, especially tuberculosis, pneumonia, diarrhoea and measles (Chapters 17, 18, 19, 20, 56). Mineral and vitamin deficiencies also have important effects. Vitamin A deficiency weakens epithelial surfaces and allows increased binding of bacteria. Other minerals and vitamins are required by key enzymes in the immune system, and for lymphocyte proliferation.

Perhaps surprisingly, obesity and excess intake of food is also associated with reduced immune responses.

Infections

A number of viral infections are known to suppress the immune response to other pathogens for a period after infection. Measles is of particular note. A general suppression of the cell-mediated response leads to increased susceptibility to infections such as tuberculosis and pneumonia. Many febrile illnesses are associated with a degree of systemic immune suppression, exhibited by the activation of herpes simplex virus, as so-called 'fever blisters'. Chronic diseases such as tuberculosis are associated with reduced lymphocyte counts, and tuberculosis patients may suffer from infections such as oral thrush even in the absence of HIV infection.

Helminths

As described above, helminths have many mechanisms of evading the host immune response. This allows them to persist in the host for long periods, causing relatively little tissue damage. Some of these effects may also alter the response to other pathogens. People with helminths can have reduced specific cytokine responses to other pathogens, or reduced responses to immunization. By inducing a Th2 profile of immune response, or the production of immunosuppressive cytokines such as IL-10 and tissue growth factor (TGF)-γ, helminths may suppress the Th1 response required for protective immunity to other pathogens (Bentwich et al., 1999). The importance of these effects for the response to immunizations and for susceptibility to other infectious diseases still needs to be determined.

HIV infection

HIV interacts very closely with immunological mechanisms and is adapted to use the normal molecules and functions of the immune system to promote its own replication. The principal cells infected by HIV are CD4+ T-cells and macrophages. This is because the viral surface protein gp (glycoprotein) 120 specifically adheres to the CD4 molecule (the normal function of which is to assist in the T-cell response). Following adhesion to the CD4 molecule the viral glycoprotein unfolds, allowing recognition of one of a group of additional molecules on the cell surface. Virologists call these additional molecules 'coreceptors' and, in combination with CD4, they allow fusion of the virus with the cell membrane and entry of the virus into the cell.

Once the virus has entered the cell the RNA is 'reverse transcribed' and a DNA copy is integrated into the host cell genome. This DNA 'provirus' may persist in a latent form in these cells until activated to initiate viral replication. When cells are activated in response to a stimulus, such as another infection, cellular factors which normally activate host genes also activate replication of the integrated virus. Thus viral replication is increased during episodes of opportunistic infection, such as tuberculosis or *Pneumocystis carinii* pneumonia, when many lymphocytes are activated (Goletti et al., 1996).

Immune deficiency develops following HIV infection as infected CD4+ T-cells are progressively destroyed. How the cells are killed is not entirely known and there may be more than one mechanism. The virus itself may cause some cells to die, while other infected cells may be recognized and killed by the immune system (Weiss, 1993). The result is a progressive reduction in the number of CD4+ T-cells and hence in immunity to other pathogens. Marked impairment of cell-mediated immunity, in which CD4+ T-cells contribute cytokine production and macrophage activation, leads to a high degree of susceptibility to intracellular pathogens such as *Mycobacterium tuberculosis*, salmonella and *Leishmania*, to fungal infections such as *Candida* and to viral infections such as herpes zoster. Failure of CD4+ T-cell help in antibody production leads to susceptibility to extracellular bacteria such as *Streptococcus pneumoniae*. Increased malaria parasitaemia and clinical episodes have also been reported with increasing HIV immunosuppression (Whitworth et al., 2000; French et al., 2001).

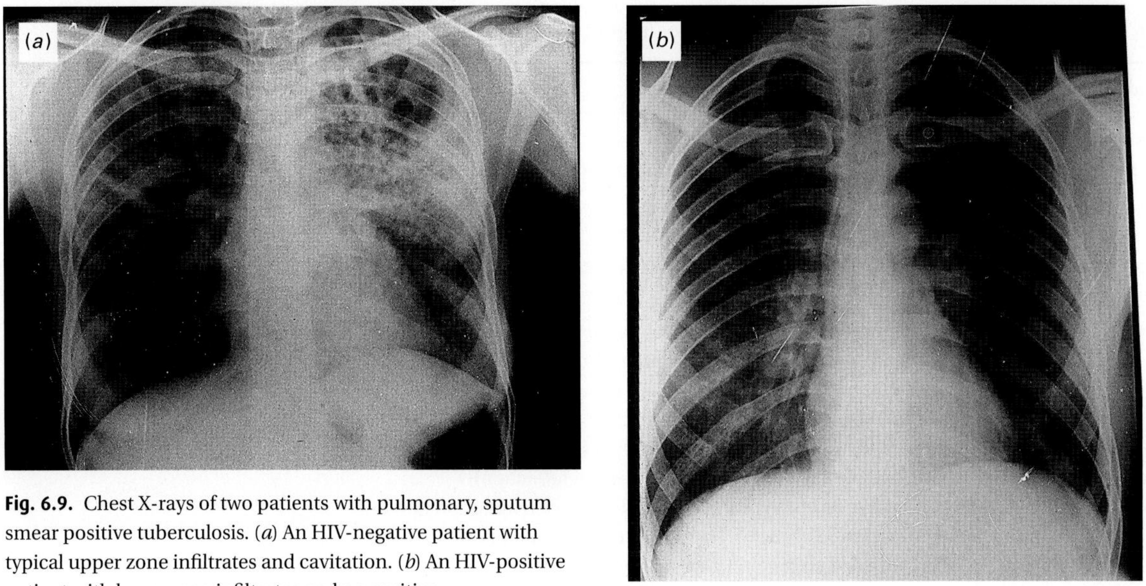

Fig. 6.9. Chest X-rays of two patients with pulmonary, sputum smear positive tuberculosis. (*a*) An HIV-negative patient with typical upper zone infiltrates and cavitation. (*b*) An HIV-positive patient with lower zone infiltrates and no cavities.

As well as causing increased susceptibility to disease, immune suppression by HIV can lead to a change in the clinical presentation of disease, especially where the clinical findings are strongly affected by the immune response. This is strikingly demonstrated in tuberculosis. HIV-negative adults with tuberculosis most commonly present with pulmonary disease confined to the upper part of the lung and with cavitation and fibrosis caused by immunologically mediated tissue destruction (Fig. 6.9(*a*)). Large numbers of tubercle bacilli accumulate in the cavities and are excreted in the sputum, hence the diagnosis can be confirmed by the sputum smear. As HIV disease progresses tubercle bacilli disseminate and can multiply readily in other tissues. Granuloma formation fails and tissue destruction is less prominent. Pulmonary tuberculosis may present with non-specific infiltrates in middle or lower lobes, without cavitation (Fig. 6.9(*b*)), and the sputum smear is more often negative, making the diagnosis very difficult to confirm (Elliott et al., 1990).

Use of immunological tests in the diagnosis of infection

Immunological tests have gained importance in the diagnosis of many bacterial and viral infections. Recent advances have made antibody tests more sensitive and specific. Though we still try to isolate bacterial and parasitic organisms, this is not always possible. Virus isolation is specialized and expensive. Failure to isolate organisms may also occur because of prior use of antibiotics or low levels of infection; organisms may lie latent in an inaccessible site or techniques may be insensitive or difficult to perform.

It is a challenge to transform advances in immunology into diagnostic procedures that will be useful in the practice of medicine. For infectious diseases tests are designed to detect specific antibodies or specific antigens. Table 6.7 shows some of the immunological tests used in the diagnosis of infections.

Detection of antibodies

The detection of antibodies usually indicates that a patient has been exposed to infection with that organism at some time but does not necessarily indicate active infection. However, if the antibody is predominantly IgM (indicating that a primary immune response is occurring), active infection is much more probable. This technique has been successfully used in detecting rubella infection in new-born children. If the antibody titre rises over 2–3 weeks, it is surer confirmation of recent infection.

IgG antibody detection can be misleading in children below the age of 12 months, as this may be due to maternal antibodies transferred across the placenta rather than actual infection.

Table 6.7. Some immunological tests in the diagnosis of infection

Method	Principle	Examples
Detection of antigen and antibody		
1. Precipitation	Antigen and antibody react in agar to give precipitation line or in tubes	Many viral and bacterial diseases. Invasive amoebiasis, Slow, insensitive, but cheap
2. Countercurrent immuno-electrophoresis	Precipitation in agar aided by electric current	Hepatitis B, *Meningococcus, Pneumococcus, Haemophilus influenzae*
3. Agglutination	Antibody may cause visible agglutination of an organism (direct agglutination). This method of antibody detection can be extended by binding antigen to red cells and using these as a marker system (heamagglutination). For those antibodies that do not agglutinate red cells effectively, a second antibody is used to help agglutinate (indirect heamagglutination). Agglutination of antigen-coated red blood cells can be inhibited by homologous antigen (Haemagglutination Inhibition)	Widal test (typhoid) direct agglutination. Haemagglutination is widely used in virology and experimental parasitology
	Latex-coated antibody agglutinates in presence of antigen	Useful for detection of antigen in CSF
4. Radioimmunoassays (RIA)	These techniques use radioactive isotopes to detect antigen or antibody	Hepatitis B, many other viral and bacterial antigens. Very sensitive but use limited due to safety of radioisotopes
5. Enzyme-linked immunosorbentassay (ELISA)	This uses labelled reagents to detect for antibody or antigen. Antibody or antigen is initially coated on solid phase. Then another specific antibody or antigen labelled with enzyme which reacts with substrate to give colour is added	Most widely used for many bacterial and viral infections. Very sensitive and specific
6. Immunoblotting (Western blot)	Can detect different antibodies bound to different antigens of varying molecular weight electrophoretically transferred to a nitrocellulose membrane. The bound antibody is detected by colour using labelled enzyme conjugate and substrate. The principle is similar to that of ELISA	Many viral diseases such as AIDS virus
7. Complement fixation	Reaction of antibody with antigen leads to fixation of complement, which is then not available to lyse sensitized red cells subsequently added to the system	Wassermann reaction (syphilis). Used in virology
8. Fluorescent microscopy	Tissue sections with antigens can be mounted on slides and detected directly by fluoresceinated antibody which gives bright fluorescence on light stimulation (direct immunofluorescence). Antibody binding to antigen can also be demonstrated by the use of anti-immunoglobulin antiserum labelled with fluorescein (indirect immunofluorescence) (Fig. 6.3)	Malaria, syphilis, leishmaniasis, rabies, some viruses, e.g. HIV and HHV8
9. Fluorescence-activated cell sorter (FACS)	Fluorochrome-labelled antibodies bind to cell surface markers (e.g. CD4 or CD8 on lymphocyes). When cells come into contact with the laser light beam the fluorescent light provides information for the instrument to count the cells	Measures levels of CD4 and CD8 T-cells in HIV infection.
10. Biological assay	The presence of antibody is detected by its effects in a biological system	Virus neutralization. TPI (syphilis)
Skin tests		
1. Immediate hypersensitivity	Weal and flare produced within a few minutes. Depends on the presence of bound IgE antibody	Casoni test (hydatid). Identification of allergens in hay fever, asthma
2. Delayed hypersensitivity	Induration produced at 48 hours. Depends on the presence of a cell-mediated immune reaction	Mantoux test (tuberculosis). Lepromin test (leprosy). Leishmanin test (leishmaniasis). Used also in fungal infections, e.g. candidiasis, histoplasmosis

Skin tests

Immediate hypersensitivity reactions (depending on the presence of IgE antibodies) and delayed hypersensitivity reactions have both been used successfully as diagnostic skin tests. Shared or cross-reacting antigens between different organisms may make diagnosis difficult. Thus, the Mantoux test may not only be positive in tuberculosis but also during infection with *Mycobacterium ulcerans* or following immunization with BCG (Bacille Calmette-Guerin). Just as a single raised antibody level indicates no more than infection with that organism at some time, and not necessarily the presence of active disease, so too does a positive skin test. Individuals exposed to tuberculosis may have a positive Mantoux test for the rest of their lives, but may never develop active disease.

Immunization and vaccines

The incidence of infectious diseases has been greatly reduced in the industrialized countries, chiefly on account of clean water, sewerage systems and better housing. Nevertheless, vaccines have further lowered the incidence of infections. Smallpox has been totally eradicated and there are now campaigns to eradicate polio. Other diseases like measles and hepatitis, which are restricted to man and involve no animal reservoir, could also be eradicated. Childhood mortality has been greatly reduced in Africa as a result of immunization.

The ideal vaccine or immunizing agent

(a) The vaccine should promote effective resistance to the disease, although it may not necessarily prevent infection. Meningococcal vaccine stops meningitis but in many people has no influence on passage of the organism in the throat. For a vaccine to be effective it should induce the right type of immune resistance: cell-mediated immunity is necessary against typhoid, tuberculosis, or leprosy; antibody is necessary for yellow fever or poliomyelitis. The antibody must be the right type directed against the right antigen. The killed measles vaccine was not successful because antibody was directed against the wrong viral antigen. The immune response should be in the right place. Secretory antibodies will protect epithelial surfaces. This is appropriate for infections like influenza or cholera, but not for rabies in which the virus enters the body through a bite or wound.

(b) The vaccine should be highly purified so that it consists of one or only a few antigens. Genetic engineering and immunochemistry are enabling important advances in this field.

(c) The vaccine should be safe with minimal side effects. No vaccine is perfectly safe or effective. Close monitoring and timely assessment of suspected vaccine adverse events are critical to prevent loss of confidence and decreased vaccine coverage. However, side effects should be weighed against the worst scenario of disease. Vaccines, like other pharmaceutical products, undergo extensive safety and efficacy evaluations in the laboratory, in animals and in phased human trials before licensing.

(d) The vaccine should be stable and remain potent during storage and shipping. Now vaccine vial monitors (VVM) have been developed which enable failures in the cold chain to be highlighted in a simple way. These are labels that change colour if the vaccine has been exposed to excessive temperature over time and if it is likely to have been damaged. The VVM clearly indicates to health workers whether a vaccine can be used and thus ensures the quality of the cold chain at a minimal cost. Agencies purchasing vaccines should request manufacturers to supply all vaccines with VVMs. VVMs are now available for most vaccines.

(e) The vaccine should be cheap, particularly if it is to be used on a large scale.

Two basic approaches to immunization

An individual can be made artificially immune to an infectious agent by one of two ways. First, an antibody made in another animal or human may be injected (passive immunization): second, an antigen, which may be part of a killed or live organism, is injected so that the host then raises an immune response to protect against that organism (active immunization or vaccination). Each of these two methods has advantages and disadvantages.

Passive immunization

Examples are given in Table 6.8. Details will be found in chapters on each infection.

Advantages. Protection is offered rapidly, which is important if the individual has already been exposed to an infectious agent or its toxins. Thus human gammaglobulins, which contain antibodies to hepatitis A virus, protect against this virus, immediately they are injected and can be beneficial if given before, or for up to 1 week

Table 6.8. Infections for which passive immunization is useful

Infection	Source of anti-sera	Comment
Botulism	Horse	Disease is rare. Sera not generally available
Diphtheria	Horse	Give with toxoid and antibiotics
Hepatitis A	Human	Useful for travellers to tropics
Hepatitis B	Human	Must have high titres of antibody. Use after needleprick with infective blood
Measles	Human	Give as soon as possible. Used for children with immune defects
Rabies	Horse	Give with vaccine
Rubella	Human	Give to pregnant women as soon as possible after exposure
Tetanus	Horse or human	Human anti-sera preferable but more expensive and not widely available

Notes:
Passive immunization can be life-saving if toxin is already circulating, as in tetanus or diphtheria. If the anti-sera are from a human source, they must be screened for blood-borne infections such as HIV and hepatitis.

after exposure to the virus. A live vaccine takes longer to induce immunity and is of little use for protection after exposure. Passive immunization may modify the severity of an infection even if it is not fully protective.

(a) Disadvantages
Use of human antisera has dangers of transmitting infections like HIV and hepatitis. Antisera are expensive, they need to be kept cool and they have a limited life. Protection is short lived, up to 6 months depending on dose, and repeated doses carry danger of sensitization to a foreign protein. This may take the form of an immediate hypersensitivity reaction (Table 6.6) or if large amounts of serum have been given, as for treatment of snake bite, serum-sickness.

Passive immunization with maternal antibody
IgG antibody from the mother crosses the placenta, so it is possible to protect the infant by vaccinating the mother during pregnancy. This approach has proved successful in preventing neonatal tetanus.

Table 6.9. Killed whole-organism vaccines

Cholera
Hepatitis A
Pertussis
Polio
Rabies
Typhoid
Influenza

Active immunization
Vaccines used for active immunization can be divided into: (i) killed whole-organism vaccines (ii) live vaccines (natural and attenuated) (iii) subunit vaccines, and (iv) engineered vaccines.

Active immunization with killed organisms (Table 6.9)
Initially killed vaccines were crude preparations of whole organisms injected into animals and sometimes human beings in the hope of stimulating protective immunity. This hit-or-miss approach has its dangers of unwanted allergic reactions. However, some of these killed vaccines have been very effective, such as the rabies and polio (Salk) vaccines. Others are of moderate efficacy, such as the typhoid, cholera and influenza vaccines.

Other killed vaccines have not worked well. Killed measles vaccine raised antibody to measles haemagglutinin but not the fusion glycoprotein, which is another surface antigen of measles virus. The result was incomplete protection against measles and occasional allergic reactions when vaccinated individuals were later infected with wild measles virus. The killed respiratory syncytial virus vaccine causes severe allergic reactions in the lungs of some children when they encounter the wild virus.

Advantages
(a) Killed vaccines are often more stable, easier to store, and have longer period of potency than live vaccines. They are not necessarily cheaper.
(b) Killed vaccines can usually be combined, a good example being diphtheria, pertussis, and tetanus vaccine.
(c) Killed vaccines do not produce an infection in the host so there is no chance of mutant organisms causing disease in the individual who is vaccinated. By contrast, a few cases of poliomyelitis have been caused by mutant strains of the live, oral polio virus.
(d) Maternal antibody, present in infants up to 6–9 months of age, has little effect on killed vaccines.

Table 6.10. Subunit vaccines

Diphtheria toxoid
H. influenza B
Hepatitis B surface antigen
Meningococcal group A and C polysaccharide
Pneumococcal polysaccharide
Plague (*Yersinia pestis*)
Tetanus toxoid
Vibrio cholerae toxoid

Table 6.11. Live vaccines

BCG
Measles
Mumps
Polio
Rubella
Typhoid
Yellow fever

Disadvantages

(a) Repeated doses of killed vaccines must be given if an adequate immune response is to be raised. This is also necessary to confer long-lasting immunity unless the child is continually re-exposed to the pathogen, in which case subclinical infection may boost immunity. Repeated doses increase the cost and difficulties of delivering the vaccine; this is a particular problem in remote rural areas.

(b) Many killed vaccines need to be given with adjuvant, which is a material that increases the immune response to a given antigen without being antigenically related to it. Lack of a suitable adjuvant for use in man has hindered the development of a variety of vaccines.

(c) If inactivation has been incomplete, the vaccine can lead to infection. On one occasion incomplete inactivation of virulent poliomyelitis virus by formaldehyde caused paralytic poliomyelitis in many children.

Active immunization with subunit vaccines (Table 6.10)

These are vaccines made from parts of a micro-organism or from its toxins.

Some of the most successful bacterial vaccines we have today (tetanus and diptheria) are made from inactivated exotoxins. This works when the disease is caused by the toxin rather than by the organism itself. For organisms that can be controlled by antibody responses, surface antigens constitute a safe and effective vaccine. There are many bacterial vaccines made from inactivated capsular polysaccharides.

These vaccines have some of the same disadvantages as killed vaccines. Subunit polysaccharide vaccines also have the problems associated with T-cell independent antibody responses, with relatively poor function in young children and poor induction of memory. To avoid these problems, the strategy now is to couple them to protein carriers, making conjugate vaccines. Conjugate vaccines, such as the *Haemophilus influenzae* vaccine, and the new conjugate pneumococcal vaccine, elicit T-cell help and T-cell dependent antibody responses.

Active immunization with live vaccines (Table 6.11)

The pathogenicity of micro-organisms can be reduced by growth in artificial media, cell cultures or even in chicken eggs. This method has been used to develop non-pathogenic strains for use as vaccines. Thus one measles vaccine was developed by passage 24 times in human kidney cells, 28 times in human amnion cells, 6 times in a chick embryo and 85 times in chick fibroblasts. The repeated passage of the virus in artificial media selects mutants that are best suited to grow in these media. Such mutants are usually less pathogenic when returned to the original host but, if attenuated too far, many may not replicate sufficiently to induce a good immune response.

With advancement in DNA technology, it is possible to deliberately induce mutations in selected genes known to contribute to virulence. This 'site directed mutation' may be used in development of future vaccines.

Advantages

Live vaccines give longer protection than killed vaccines. Yellow fever and measles vaccine protect for many years and are remarkably effective. One dose of the vaccine is usually sufficient. An exception is oral poliovirus and perhaps other live viruses required to stimulate mucosal immunity.

Disadvantages

(a) Live vaccines are often unstable. Some such as measles and polio vaccines need to be stored at −20 °C and transported either frozen or at 4 °C. They may be inactivated by chemicals such as methanol, which are used to sterilize syringes or the skin.

(b) Live vaccines may not work in the presence of circulating antibodies. Thus measles vaccine has to be given around 9 months of age when maternal antibodies have gone (Siegris, 2000).

(c) Live vaccines may mutate in the host to a more virulent form. Type 1 polio vaccine contains 57 mutations and has never reverted to wild type, while for type 2 and 3, with only 2 mutations, frequent reversion has occurred leading to paralytic polio. Some countries have therefore now reverted to the killed polio vaccine.
(d) Live vaccines may cause disease if the host is immunodeficient, as in leukaemia and AIDS. Measles vaccine, and other live attenuated vaccines are contraindicated in people who are severely immunosuppressed. The World Health Organization recommend that live vaccines such as Bacillus Calmette–Guerin (BCG) should not be given to infants with clinical AIDS, although they should be given to asymptomatic babies, since HIV status cannot be established easily in the first few weeks of life.
(e) Live virus vaccines occasionally interfere with each other so that the immune response is not so great if they are given together. The Sabin oral poliomyelitis vaccine contains three strains, which may interfere with each other when multiplying in the intestine. Naturally acquired enteroviruses may also interfere with polio virus. For these reasons three doses of the vaccine are given.

Genetically engineered vaccines

In the past two decades a revolution in vaccine design has taken place, through recombinant DNA technology. This has allowed scientists to generate four new types of vaccines: recombinant proteins, synthetic peptides, live recombinant organisms (where selected genes from the pathogen are inserted into a vector, such as a non-pathogenic virus) and DNA vaccines. Most of these types of vaccines are still in development and to date the only recombinant vaccine licensed is the hepatitis B surface antigen vaccine.

Advantages of this approach

(a) Safety. Recombinant proteins and peptides are safe since they are neither infectious nor pathogenic. The safety of live recombinant vaccines depends on the vector used. Some vectors are very safe to use. DNA vaccines are very new and safety data is being accumulated, but so far, in small studies, they have been safe.
(b) Unlimited supply. After successful 'cloning', vast amounts of the desired genes or proteins can be produced.
(c) Vaccines can be designed to express the antigens of interest and omit those that are not important or can cause disease. More than one sequence can be included, for example, both B- and T-cell epitopes, to optimize the immune responses.

Failure of vaccination programmes

Many vaccination programmes have not been very successful for a number of reasons.

Lack of political will

Changing politicians and governments may shift their health priorities from preventive to curative medicine, or to other issues such as military expenditure, giving no priority to health issues. Large expensive teaching hospitals in cities are politically attractive and popular whereas vaccination schemes, especially in rural areas, are given lower priority. A successful vaccination scheme needs long-term implementation and planning so that recurrent costs for personnel, vehicles and equipment are met.

Costs of vaccine

Vaccines are expensive. A simple infant immunization scheme, excluding delivery, costs about $4.00 per child. This may be beyond the budget of poorer countries of Africa. In the past, vaccines have been paid for by donors such as UNICEF in many cases, but Governments are now encouraged to contribute partially or fully to the purchase of vaccines, under the Vaccine Independence Initiative.

Failure of the cold chain

Vaccines usually need to be kept refrigerated throughout their journey from factory to patient. However, electricity may fail or be unavailable and health authorities may not budget for standby power to run refrigerators: the cold chain therefore fails and the vaccine deteriorates. Gas or solar-powered refrigerators are useful where electricity is not available.

Administration of vaccine to the wrong person, e.g. to those already immune

This is mainly due to low community awareness and poor mobilization and education strategies.

Poor immune response in vaccinated subjects

Malnutrition is often blamed for the failure of vaccination campaigns, but all evidence suggests that mild malnutrition has little or no effect on the immune response to vaccines. Acute malaria can suppress the response to immunization but it is doubtful whether subclinical malaria has any practical significance on the immune response to vaccines. It has been postulated that exposure to helminth infections in the mother, while the child is in utero, or in the individual at the time of vaccination, may be an important cause of impaired responses to vaccines.

Staff motivation

Many countries in Africa cannot maintain staff due to poor motivation. Poor pay of staff is one of the biggest problems.

Poor records

Some health authorities do not keep careful records so it is not clear who has been vaccinated with what, and when this was done. Tally sheets and immunization cards are often available but are not always used.

Herd immunity

In some communities, there could be decreased chance of exposure of susceptible persons to a pathogen due to herd immunity. This may be due to high immunization coverage in the community that can interrupt the chain of transmission even to the unvaccinated. This could also happen in a community if the majority of people have been affected by the disease in the past, and recovered with lasting immunity.

The future

The World Health Organization and other interested parties have proposed an immunization policy for 2001–2005 on the African Continent. This includes improving the current 'Expanded Programme on Immunisation' through better management, delivery of quality services and increased coverage; polio eradication and continued surveillance for polio through 'Acute Flaccid Paralysis' surveillance; measles control and elimination; maternal and neonatal tetanus elimination. The policy also includes control initiatives for other diseases such as yellow fever and meningitis. Introduction of new vaccines, such as Hepatitis B and *Haemophilus influenzae* type b vaccines, is also proposed.

Some countries like Gambia have already introduced *Haemophilus influenzae* type b (Hib) conjugate vaccine (Adegbola et al., 1999), and this has led to a drastic reduction in the annual incidence of *Haemophilus influenzae* meningitis. The country also introduced Hepatitis B vaccine into the immunization programme from 1986 (Hall et al., 1989). Presently, many African countries do not have the resources to do the same. However, the Global Alliance of Vaccines and Immunization (GAVI) is supporting several countries in Africa: Hepatitis B vaccine in combination with DPT (tetravalent DPT-HepB), and pentavalent DPT-HepB-Hib will be introduced into several countries under this initiative.

Great efforts are being made to develop vaccines against parasites, notably malaria, trypanosomiasis, schistosomiasis and against HIV virus. When these become available, costs should be negotiated so that these vaccines are affordable.

The question of safety now dominates vaccination campaigns in the developed countries. Whole cell pertussis vaccine has been shown to cause some neurological reactions. This has led to some developed countries shifting to the use of subunit and acellular pertussis vaccines. However, the debate should weigh benefit vs. damage.

Vaccination campaigns may be even more effective if combined with other public health interventions in developing countries such as distribution of vitamin A, nutritional monitoring, distribution of oral rehydration salts, health education and case management of acute infection. Vaccination efforts should be a package with delivery of other preventive services.

References

Adegbola RA, Usen SO, Weber M et al. (1999). *Haemophilus influenzae* type b meningitis in The Gambia after introduction of a conjugate vaccine. *Lancet*, **354**: 1091–1092.

Alper CA, Colten HR, Rosen FS, Rabson AR, Macnab GM, Gear JS. (1972). Homozygous deficiency of C3 in a patient with repeated infections. *Lancet*, **ii**: 1179–81.

Altare F, Durandy A, Lammas D et al. (1998). Impairment of mycobacterial immunity in human interleukin-12 receptor deficiency. *Science*, **280**: 1432–1438.

Banchereau J, Steinman RM. (1998). Dendritic cells and the control of immunity. *Nature*, **392**: 245–252.

Bentwich Z, Kalinkovich A, Weisman Z, Borkow G, Beyers N, Beyers AD. (1999). Can eradication of helminth infections change the face of AIDS and tuberculosis? *Immunol Today*, **11**: 485–487.

Blatteis CM, Sehic E. (1998). Cytokines and fever. *Ann NY Acad Sci*, **840**: 608–618.

Bruton OC. (1952). Agammaglobulinaemia. *Pediatrics*, **9**: 722–728.

Chandra RK (1997). Nutrition and the immune system: an introduction. *Am J Clin Nutrit*, **66**: 460–463.

Delves PJ, Roitt IM. (2000). The immune system. *N Eng J Med*, **343**: 37–49.

Edmunds WJ, from Medley GF, Nokes DJ, Hall AJ, Whittle HC. (1993). The influence of age on the development of the Hepatitis B carrier state. *Proc Roy Soc, Lond*, **253**: 197–201.

Elliott AM, Luo N, Tembo G et al. (1990). The impact of Human Immunodeficiency Virus on tuberculosis in Zambia: a cross-sectional study. *Br Med J*, **301**: 412–415.

French N, Nakiyingi J, Lugada E, Watera C, Whitworth JA, Gilks CF. (2001). Increasing rates of malarial fever with deteriorating immune status in HIV-1 infected Ugandan adults. *AIDS*, **15**: 899–906.

Gold R, Goldschneider I, Lepow ML, Draper TF, Randolph M. (1978). Carriage of *Neisseria meningitidis* and *Neisseria lacamica* in infants and children. *J Infect Dis*, **137**: 112–121.

Goletti D, Weissman D, Jackson RW et al. (1996). Effect of *Mycobacterium tuberculosis* on HIV replication: role of immune activation. *J Immunol*, **157**: 1271–1278.

Hall AJ, Inskip HM, Loik F et al. (1989). Hepatitis B vaccination in the Expanded Programme on Immunisation: The Gambia experience. *Lancet*, **i**: 1057–1060.

Hill AV, Elvin J, Willis AC et al. (1992). Molecular analysis of the association of HLA-B53 and resistance to severe malaria. *Nature*, **360**: 434–439.

Hill AV. (1998). The immunogenetics of human infectious diseases. *Ann Rev Immunol*, **16**: 593–617.

International Human Genome Sequencing Consortium (2001). Initial sequencing and analysis of the human genome. *Nature*, **409**: 860–921.

Janeway C, Travers P. (1996). *Immunobiology; The Immune System in Health and Disease* 2nd edn. London: Current Biology Ltd.

Jones GJ, Watera C, Petterson S et al. (2001). Comparative loss and maturation of peripheral blood dendritic cell subpopulations in African and non-African HIV-1 infected patients. *AIDS*, **15**: 1657–1663.

Maizels RM, Selkirk ME, Smith DF, Anderson RM. (1993). Immunological modulation and evasion by helminth parasites in human populations. *Nature*, **365**: 797–805.

Malhotra I, Mungai P, Wamachi A et al. (1999). Helminth- and Bacillus–Calmette–Guerin-induced immunity in children sensitized in utero to filariasis and schistosomiasis. *J Immunol*, **162**: 6843–6848.

Nalin DR, Levine MM, Rhead J et al. (1978). Cannabis, hypochlorhydria and cholera. *Lancet*, **ii**: 859–862.

Newport MJ, Huxley CM, Huston S. et al. (1996). A mutation in the interferon-γ-receptor gene and susceptibility to mycobacterial infection. *N Eng J Med*, **335**: 1941–1949.

Parkin J, Cohen B. (2001). An overview of the immune system. *Lancet*, **357**: 1777–1789.

Roitt I, Brostoff J, Male D. (1998). *Immunology*, 5th edn. London: Mosby.

Schneerson R, Robbins JB. (1975). Induction of serum *Haemophilus influenzae* type B capsular antibodies in adult volunteers fed cross-reacting *Eschericia coli* O75: K100: H5. *N Engl J Med*, **292**: 1093–1096.

Siegrist CA. (2000). Vaccination in the neonatal period and early infancy. *Int Rev Immunol*, **19**: 195–219.

Staines N, Brostoff J, James K. (1999). *Introducing Immunology*. 2nd edn. London: Mosby.

Urban BC, Ferguson DJP, Pain A. et al. (1999). *Plasmodium falciparum*-infected erythrocytes modulate the maturation of dendritic cells. *Nature*, **400**: 73–77.

Weiss RA. (1993). How does HIV cause AIDS? *Science*, **260**: 1273–1279.

Weiss R. (2001). AIDS: unbeatable 20 years on. *Lancet*, **357**: 2073–2074.

Whitworth J, Morgan D, Quigley M et al. (2000). Effect of HIV-1 and increasing immunosuppression on malaria parasitaemia and clinical episodes in adults in rural Uganda: a cohort study. *Lancet*, **356**: 1051–1056.

7

The diagnosis and treatment of infection

Most infections encountered in Africa can be treated with cheap and widely available drugs if an adequate diagnosis is made early enough. The outlook for patients correctly diagnosed with infections such as tuberculosis, typhoid or meningitis is better in even the most basic clinic in Africa at the start of this century than it would have been in the best-equipped hospital in the world at the start of the last century. To be effective, however, the powerful anti-infective agents we have need to be properly used, and this depends on adequate diagnosis. This chapter aims to explore some of the general principles of diagnosis and management of infectious diseases in Africa. These will be expanded on in the chapters on specific diseases.

General principles of diagnosis

Levels of diagnosis

In clinical practice an adequate diagnosis is one which allows the patient to be managed well. How detailed this diagnosis needs to be depends on several factors, including the severity of the illness, the possible causes, and local diagnostic facilities. To illustrate this, let us take three infections which all present with fever and headache: malaria, bacterial meningitis and influenza.

For malaria it is important that the underlying organism is known, as only specific antimalarial treatment will be effective. Knowing the species of malaria will also be useful, as non-falciparum malaria is treated with different drugs from falciparum malaria. This holds true however basic local diagnostic services are.

For bacterial meningitis the exact diagnosis is less critical. It is essential that the clinician has diagnosed it as meningitis, and is happy that it is bacterial rather than tuberculous or cryptococcal meningitis, which need different treatment. Most cases can then be managed using broad-spectrum antibiotics to cover all likely organisms. Where good microbiology services exist, a more specific diagnosis will help to pick up the rare organisms that are not covered by conventional empirical antibiotics; but where these services do not exist most patients can be treated effectively without knowing the underlying organism.

In a patient with influenza, apart from supportive treatment, what the clinician gives will make little difference to the clinical outcome. It is therefore irrelevant what exact diagnosis the clinician makes. It is preferable that s/he has made a sufficient assessment to decide the patient needs no specific treatment, avoiding the risk of side effects from unnecessary drugs.

The first decision clinicians must make, therefore, is how far they need to go in narrowing down a diagnosis. This has to be guided by what facilities are available, and by whether it is likely to change patient management. There is a hierarchy of levels of diagnosis.

Level one: triage. This can be done in the most basic medical facility.

Level two: syndromic diagnosis. This requires a good clinician, but needs no facilities.

Level three: aetiological diagnosis. This often requires laboratory or other diagnostic services

These levels blur into one another, but are useful as a way of ordering thinking.

Triage

Triage is an essential skill in outpatients and emergency departments in Africa. The term triage is now used generally to include rapid assessment of the patient on presentation, and deciding on the basis of that assessment how

urgent their problem is. In the case of infectious diseases the main triage questions are:
(a) is this going to get better on its own?
(b) if not, how urgently does it need to be investigated and treated?

It is often possible, on the basis of a very rapid assessment, to be able to reassure a patient that s/he is likely to recover quickly without treatment. The ability to divide patients into those who have potentially serious disease and those who are not seriously ill is important in all branches of medicine. Even the best clinicians sometimes get it wrong, and it is usually important to tell patients to come back if they get worse, or do not get better. A mild case of fever or watery diarrhoea is unlikely to be anything serious if seen on day 2; if it is still going on after 3 weeks it is much more likely to represent serious pathology.

Syndromic diagnosis

In the cases where further diagnosis is needed the next stage is to narrow the diagnosis down. An accurate history is the key, with examination guided by what the patient (or patient's carer) says. The importance of history cannot be over-emphasized: what are the symptoms, how long have they been there, coming on how fast, and in what order. History and examination will enable the clinician to narrow the diagnosis down to a syndrome: a presentation typical of a small group of diseases that cannot be reliably differentiated by history and examination alone. A decision then needs to be made on how far to go in narrowing the diagnosis further still (see Box).

> A 30-year-old presents with gradual onset headache, and subsequently fever, coming on over 3 weeks. During that time he took 4 doses of amoxycillin bought in the market. On examination he has moderate neck stiffness, a fever and oral candida.

The clinician can reasonably make a diagnosis of the syndrome 'chronic meningitis' with weak evidence of immunosuppression. The differential diagnosis includes TB meningitis, cryptococcal meningitis and partially treated bacterial meningitis, all of which are serious diseases that require very different treatment. This is not an appropriate syndrome for syndromic treatment, and requires further investigation. It would be quite wrong for the clinician to decide it is one or another on clinical grounds alone. No clinician, however good, can reliably differentiate them every time, and trying to do so risks making potentially fatal errors (see Box).

> A 5-year-old child presents with acute onset watery diarrhoea for 2 days. There is no fever or blood in the stool, and examination reveals the child to have moderate dehydration.

There is a wide range of possible infectious agents, viral, bacterial and parasitic, which can cause this as well as some non-infectious causes. The initial management is the same for every case: rehydration, preferably with oral rehydration solution. In most cases this general syndromic management is all that is needed, because in most cases acute viral or bacterial infection will be the cause and these will be self-limiting. Identifying the infectious agent will not affect management. It is therefore usually a waste of time and money. In a few cases, however, making an aetiological diagnosis (finding the microbiological cause) becomes important. One situation is where an infectious diarrhoea persists: this may suggest a cause, such as a parasitic infection, which requires specific treatment. Another would be where an agent of public health importance such as cholera might be the cause. In these cases knowing the cause will make a difference to patient management.

Often, making an accurate syndromic diagnosis is enough to guide treatment, and no further narrowing of the diagnosis is necessary. Where it is not, the careful clinical assessment will have limited the diagnosis down to one of a small number, and a relatively small number of well-directed tests will be all that is needed. This process of narrowing down the clinical diagnosis to a 'syndrome' is therefore essential in every case of moderate or severe infection, however good the diagnostic facilities.

Aetiological diagnosis

Sometimes it is very helpful to make a diagnosis of the actual infecting organism, the *aetiological* diagnosis. This is usually where it requires specific treatment. Making a firm aetiological diagnosis is sometimes possible without investigations. Occasionally history alone is sufficient; for example a patient from south-eastern Nigeria with repeated transient sub-cutaneous swellings, who notices a worm crossing the eye, almost certainly has loa loa. Examination may also be so typical of a specific infection that an aetiological diagnosis can be made with near certainty. This is especially true of some skin infections such as tuberculoid leprosy, Kaposi's sarcoma or cutaneous leishmaniasis.

Often, however, there is an element of doubt about the diagnosis; history and examination may be suggestive, but firm aetiological diagnosis is not possible. To make a firm diagnosis in these cases requires investigations, usually microbiological or parasitological. In many centres in Africa (especially rural health centres) these will not be available. Even where they are, a clinician may have to act before laboratory results are available. In both cases the clinician has to act on a grey area between the clear syndromic diagnosis which can always be treated as a syndrome (for example, penile ulcer), and a clear aetiological diagnosis (such as tuberculous meningitis). This is the working clinical diagnosis, and can be made in all patients, irrespective of diagnostic facilities.

Pre-existing probability and the working clinical diagnosis

By a combination of history and examination good clinicians will narrow a diagnosis down to a few possibilities, but these may have very different treatments. If so, the clinician can either treat every possibility or will have to make a working clinical diagnosis and treat without a firm diagnosis at this stage. This is never ideal, but is realistic. The most important factor in deciding which way to go is the pre-existing probability of a particular disease in that particular patient. Many factors will be important in deciding this, including the patient's age, occupation, location and how common a disease is overall. In much of Africa the likelihood that a patient has underlying HIV infection is the most important single factor in deciding what diagnosis is most likely.

A few examples (see Boxes) serve to illustrate this.

> Consider a patient presenting very unwell with fever and headache.
>
> If this was a 25-year-old man resident in coastal Tanzania, malaria, despite being a common disease, would be an unlikely cause. He is likely to be semi-immune to malaria, so unlikely to become very unwell with it. If, however, he had come from the highlands (where malaria is much less common and immunity lower), or had lived in Europe for several years, malaria would be the most likely cause. In a young child, or a pregnant woman with the same presentation, malaria would also be the most likely diagnosis. Malaria would not even be considered in a young man living and presenting the same way in central South Africa, unless he had recently travelled, because malaria is not transmitted there.
>
> A young man in Malawi with headache, fever and neck stiffness who has oral candida and shingles scars is likely to have one of the HIV-related meningitides such as cryptococcal or pneumococcal meningitis. The same presentation in Niger without signs of HIV-related disease is more likely to be meningococcal meningitis, especially if it occurs during a meningococcal meningitis epidemic.

> In a 30-year-old rural worker living in Zaire with a chronic cough, haemoptysis and weight loss, tuberculosis is by far the most likely diagnosis. The same symptoms in an elderly, wealthy Egyptian, who is a heavy smoker, are more likely to represent lung cancer.
>
> This does not exhaust the possible diagnoses by any means: for example, the lung fluke *Paragonimus westermani* can also present with haemoptysis and chronic cough in Africa, but is so rare that, except in a small number of very localized areas of west Africa, it can reasonably be ignored.

A good working clinical diagnosis, based on the patient's pre-existing probability and local patterns of disease, will be right in the majority of cases, but not invariably. It remains important to make firm aetiological diagnoses in many cases, where facilities exist.

Uses and abuses of diagnostic tests

Central hospitals often have more laboratory and diagnostic facilities than district hospitals and health centres. This does not always lead to better diagnosis. It seems obvious that tests clarify diagnosis and make medicine more scientific, and that the more tests a patient has, the more accurate the diagnosis will be. It is, however, untrue. Unnecessary tests are, at best, a waste of laboratory time and money and inconvenient to the patient. At worst, they are actively misleading, or even harmful. Before requesting tests, clinicians need to be certain in their own minds exactly why they are doing so. They also need to know how to interpret the results. This is not as obvious as it sounds.

> A clinician in central Africa requests a malaria film and Widal test on every adult with a fever. If the malaria film shows a few parasites, he treats as malaria; if the Widal test is 'positive', he treats as typhoid, and if both are positive he treats as 'typhoid and malaria'.
>
> In many cases, however, despite the test being positive the diagnosis (and therefore treatment) will be wrong. The Widal test has a high false-positive rate, and many adults in central Africa carry malaria parasites at low level without being symptomatic. Most patients treated as 'malaria and typhoid' based on these tests will have neither disease.

This is an example where, far from aiding the diagnosis, tests actually make it more inaccurate.

Before requesting a test in an infectious disease, we must be able to say 'yes' to three questions.

(a) *Will the test significantly improve the diagnosis?* A full blood count will, for example, only be really helpful in diagnosing a very small number of infectious conditions (visceral leishmaniasis for example). The same can be said for most 'routine' tests such as electrolytes and liver function tests. Generally, they are of limited help at best. Many tests are requested without any very clear advantage in diagnosis.

(b) *If so, will it actually alter patient management?* If, irrespective of what the test shows, you are going to do the same thing, it should probably not be requested. A patient presenting very unwell with acute purulent sputum, a fever, and clear lobar consolidation clinically is going to be treated with antibiotics for severe pneumonia. A negative sputum culture and microscopy is not going to make you decide not to give the antibiotics, so the test is irrelevant, even though it may 'confirm' the diagnosis.

(c) *Is the use of laboratory time and money justified?* Clinicians often underestimate how long even the simplest test takes to do. If laboratories are flooded with irrelevant work, or tests which do not really make that much difference, they will not have the time (or the reagents) to do the tests well where it is actually going to make a significant difference to a patient.

Tests, properly applied, have revolutionized aetiological diagnosis, in infectious disease. Provided clinicians are asking clear, appropriate questions after proper clinical diagnosis, they improve management of the critically ill patient with certain infectious diseases. They are not, however, a substitute for good clinical diagnosis, but an addition to it.

Accuracy of tests and probability of disease

The key factor in interpreting a test is the pre-existing probability that a patient has the condition for which the test is done. If you do a test for a disease in a patient who has a low chance of having it, and it comes back positive, there is a very high likelihood that the result is wrong. This is not because the test is bad, or because the laboratory has made a mistake (although mistakes can be made in the best laboratories). Tests, like people, are fallible. Even good tests have a false-positive rate, and the less likely it is that the patient has the disease, the more likely this becomes.

Figures 7.1 and 7.2 demonstrate this. We have taken a test with a 95 per cent sensitivity (it will pick up 95% of all

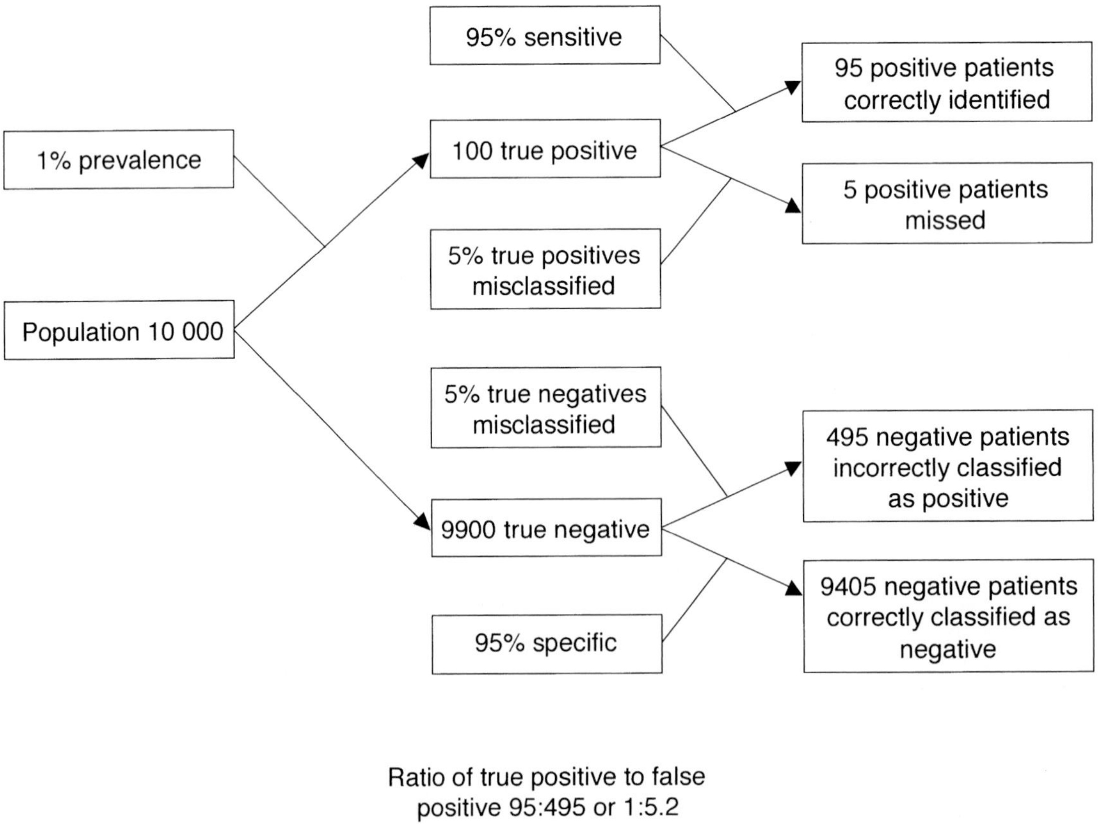

Fig. 7.1. Accuracy of a 95% sensitive and 95% specific test in a population where prevalence of disease is 1%.

cases) and 95 per cent specificity (95% of people without the disease test negative). This is better than many tests in clinical practice. We apply this test to 10 000 people from a population with a true prevalence of 1% (Fig. 7.1) and to a population of 10 000 people where the prevalence is 30 per cent (Fig. 7.2). In this example using the same test the ratio of true positives to false positives is around 1: 5 in the low-prevalence population and 8: 1 in the high-prevalence population. When the pre-test probability is low, the test will be very inaccurate; where it is high, it will be accurate. This applies to individuals as well as to populations. If you do a test on an individual who has very little chance of having a disease and it turns out positive, it is likely to be a false-positive result. In clinical practice this reinforces the fact that specific tests should usually only be requested when there is a reasonably high chance that a patient has the disease. Requesting tests without clear thought is not just wasteful, it is bad medicine and potentially dangerous.

General principles of treatment

An exact aetiological diagnosis is not always necessary to treat a patient well, but a good clinical diagnosis has to be made to guide further investigation or treatment. The most basic decision a clinician has to make once s/he has made an adequate diagnosis is whether any treatment is necessary at all. Many infectious diseases are self-limiting, and drugs make little or no difference to the outcome. All drugs have side effects ranging from trivial rashes to life-threatening gastric bleeding or anaphylactic shock. They also all have a cost to the patient or clinic. Many patients are treated unnecessarily, and whilst patient pressure may sometimes make this unavoidable, it is never good medical practice.

The clinician then has to decide whether to treat syndromically, or whether an exact aetiological diagnosis should be made. This has been discussed earlier. Some conditions can be managed syndromically, some need more accurate aetiological diagnosis. It is worth stressing that a syndromic treatment is not necessarily a less good

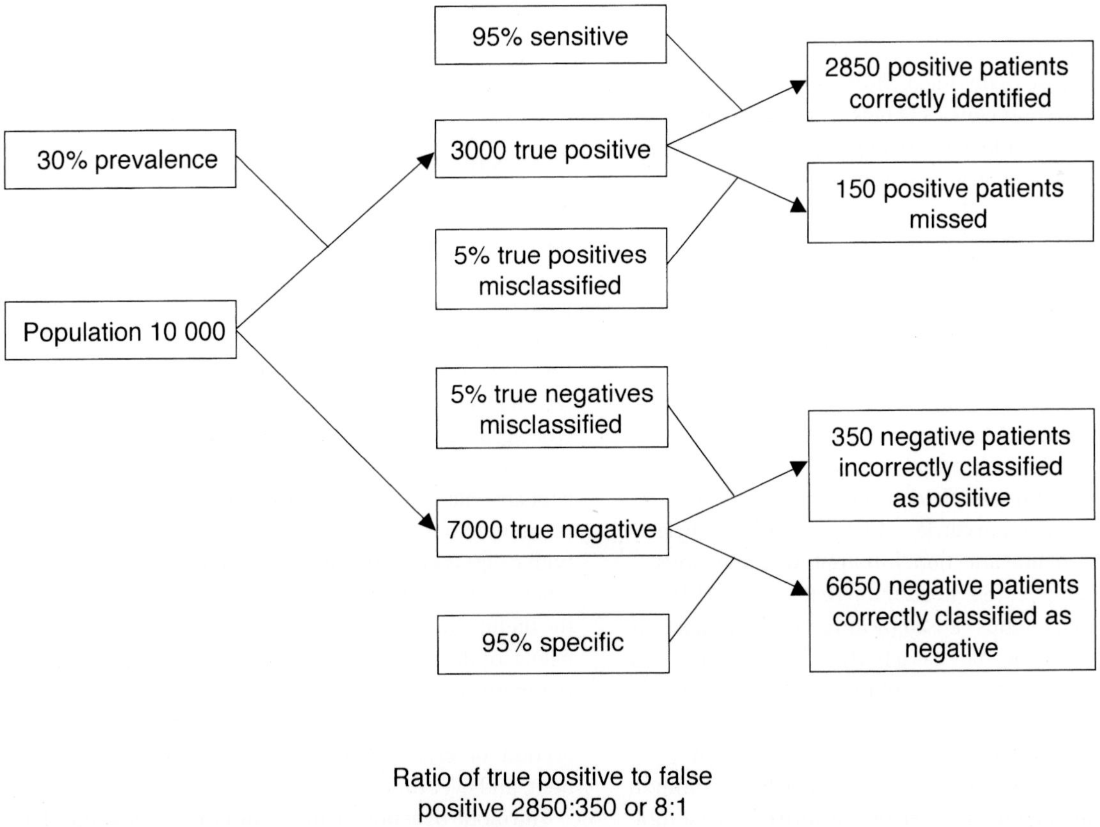

Fig. 7.2. Accuracy of a 95% sensitive and 95% specific test in a population where prevalence of disease is 30%.

treatment- used appropriately it can often be ideal management.

> A patient presents with a penile ulcer and probable HIV. Exact aetiological diagnosis is difficult clinically. Even with full laboratory services, exact diagnosis is not easy. For example, a positive VDRL does not prove the ulcer is due to primary syphilis; neither does a negative one rule it out. Patients may fail to return for their test results. Since penile ulcers significantly increase the risk of HIV transmission, it is far better to give immediate syndromic treatment, covering all the likely aetiologies, to all patients when they present, than to attempt aetiological diagnosis, which may be wrong and will delay treatment.

What treatment, for how long, and by what route

Most infectious diseases are treated with anti-microbial dugs, but the place of surgery should not be overlooked and in some situations it is the most important part of management. Large collections of pus have to be drained in almost all cases. Without doing this, no amount of drug treatment will have any long-term effect. Dead tissue may have to be removed.

The perfect drug is safe, effective, cheap and easy to take. No drug is perfect, but antibiotics for bacterial infections come close to this ideal. Most antibiotics are highly effective with short courses of between 3 days and 2 weeks. Which antibiotic to use depends on the probable infective agent and on local patterns of antibiotic resistance. This is discussed in the chapters on specific diseases, which follow.

In severe infections it is usually best to start with high doses of intravenous or intramuscular drugs, but once adequate steady-state levels have been reached (within 24 hours in most cases) oral drugs are usually equally effective if the patient can tolerate them. Most antibiotics in general use, such as amoxycillin and co-trimoxazole, are well absorbed orally. Oral antibiotics are generally both cheaper and safer than intravenous antibiotics. Intravenous injection carries a higher risk of anaphylaxis, and the risk of line infection. Intramuscular injections also carry a higher risk. In addition to the risk of HIV transmission, tetanus caused by intramuscular injections with non-sterile needles has a particularly high mortality. The exceptions where oral antibiotics will not be adequate are when the infection is in a 'privileged' site where getting adequate antibiotics to the site of infection requires very high levels in the blood. The most common examples are meningitis (CSF penetrance of most antibiotics is poor), endocarditis, cellulitis, osteomyelitis and abscesses that cannot be drained surgically.

Anti-parasitic drugs are covered under the individual disease chapters, but in general the side-effect profile is less good for many of these drugs, ranging from itching or nausea with some anti-malarials to a 5% mortality associated with the arsenical treatment of CNS trypanosomiasis attributable to the drug itself.

Broad-spectrum antibiotics kill a very wide range of organisms, so blind treatment is often effective even if the diagnosis is wrong. For example, a patient treated with chloramphenicol for presumed typhoid usually gets better even if the actual diagnosis was meningococcal septicaemia. The same is not true for parasitic disease: if you treat for malaria and the patient has acute trypanosomiasis, the patient will not be cured. It is therefore more important to make a firm diagnosis before anti-parasitic treatment is started. The decision about which route to use for anti-parasitic disease is simplified by the fact that there is either no parenteral formulation or no oral formulation for most anti-parasitic drugs: once the drug is chosen, the route of administration follows automatically.

Effective anti-fungal drugs are currently either expensive (e.g. fluconazole), or toxic (amphotericin), or both. Blind treatment without proper diagnosis is therefore generally only indicated when all else has failed. Treatment of presumed cryptococcal meningitis without trying to make an aetiological diagnosis is, for example, almost never justified.

Classes of antibiotic

Anti-parasitic and anti-tuberculosis drugs are covered in the chapters on the diseases they treat. This section is a brief refresher on antibiotics and broadly what they are good for and what they are not. Resistance patterns for many common pathogens in Africa are changing fast, however, and antibiotic use should always be guided by recent local information. For example, at the time of writing, in Malawi around 5 per cent of *Streptococcus pneumoniae* isolates are penicillin resistant, and 5 per cent are chloramphenicol resistant, but few isolates are resistant to both. In South Africa, however, resistance to both drugs is currently more common, with dual resistance the norm. This is likely to spread northward during the lifetime of this book. The patterns of activity quoted below for the most commonly used antibiotics in Africa therefore, only give an overview of what antibiotic classes might reasonably be expected to cover: they do not take account of resistance patterns, which vary over the continent, and over time.

The mode of action of antibiotics varies. What they have in common is that they affect bacterial, but not human, cells. Penicillins and cephalosporins act by disrupting the bacterial cell wall. Chloramphenicol, tetracyclines, erythromycin, gentamicin and the other aminoglycosides all act by inhibiting bacterial protein synthesis. The quinolones (such as ciprofloxacin), rifampicin, metronidazole and nitrofurantoin act by inhibiting nucleic acid synthesis. Sulphonamides act on the folate pathway.

Whilst this section concentrates on the anti-bacterial activity of antibiotics, it is worth remembering that many of them also have important anti-parasitic activity, especially against malaria (tetracyclines, co-trimoxazole, macrolides) and other protozoa (metronidazole).

The penicillins

The penicillins (e.g. penicillin G, amoxycillin, ampicillin) are cheap, safe and widely available. They have excellent activity against most streptococci except for a few of the faecal streptococci, and against *Neisseria meningitidis.* They are therefore first-line treatment in chest infections (likely to be due to *S. pneumoniae*) and meningitis in adults (*S. pneumoniae* and *N. meningitidis*). Penicillin and amoxycillin have little activity against *Staph. aureus,* the cause of many wound infections, cellulitis and some joint infections, but flucloxacillin does. Penicillins are seldom useful in the treatment of any gram-negative gut organisms found after surgery or in urinary tract infections (although some enterococci are sensitive). They also do not cover *H. influenzae,* a common cause of childhood meningitis.

The cephalosporins

The cephalosporins are a much more varied group, and it is worth being aware of the differences because they are often included in drug donation programmes. The earlier ('first-generation') cephalosporins are relatively cheap, and have much the same spectrum of activity as penicillins, with some limited additional activity against a few gram-negative organisms including *E. coli.* They have no activity against *N. meningitidis.* The common members of this class are cephalexin, cefadroxyl and cefazolin. The 'second-generation' oral cephalosporins (cefaclor, cefprozil) have a slightly better range of activity against gram-negatives. The 'third-generation' cephalosporins (and some earlier injectable ones) have excellent activity against most gram-negative organisms, and good activity against most gram-positives. Common members of this group are cefuroxime, cefotaxime, ceftazidime and ceftriaxone.

The aminoglycosides

The aminoglycosides (in practice, gentamicin) are excellent against most gram-negative organisms, but not against *N. meningitidis.* They are effective against staphylococci, but not very effective against streptococci on their own, although if used with a penicillin they may enhance the killing activity synergistically. This is only of clinical importance in treating endocarditis. Gentamicin is therefore a good drug to use in severe gram-negative sepsis following gut or urinary tract infection, but in prolonged use or at high doses it is toxic both to the auditory nerve and kidney.

Chloramphenicol

Chloramphenicol is an excellent drug against most common bacteria of medical importance, both gram-positive and gram-negative, and is well absorbed. There is a theoretical risk of aplastic anaemia, but in practice this is very rare. It is particularly useful in childhood meningitis because it has activity against *S. pneumoniae, N. meningitidis* and *H. influenzae.*

Trimethoprim/sulfamethoxazole

Trimethoprim/sulfamethoxazole ('Septrin', Co-trimoxazole, 'Bactrim') also has a wide spectrum of activity against both gram-positive and gram-negative bacteria. There is now quite widespread resistance among some gram-negative bacteria, however, and growing resistance in *S. pneumoniae,* so its usefulness in critical bacterial illness is gradually waning. In less severe infection it remains an important drug for practice in Africa.

Tetracyclines

Tetracyclines have a much more selective range of useful activity, although they have weak activity against many organisms. They are seldom appropriate in severe gram-negative or gram-positive sepsis, although they have some activity against streptococci. They are particularly useful for a few specific indications, including atypical pneumonias, infections (such as non-specific urethritis and trachoma) caused by chlamydia, and brucellosis. Unlike most other antibiotics, out-of-date tetracyclines are not simply ineffective, but actively toxic, and should not be used.

Macrolides

Macrolides (erythromycin, azithromycin, clarithromycin) are ineffective against gut organisms, but have useful activity against most others, including both gram-positive and gram-negative organisms which affect the chest. In clinical practice they are important in treating atypical pneumonias, and can be used as a substitute for penicillins in most situations in the patient who is genuinely penicillin allergic.

Metronidazole

Metronidazole has excellent activity against anaerobic organisms, and virtually none against any aerobic organisms.

Table 7.1. Some suggested empirical treatment of common bacterial infections

	First choice	Alternative	Second line alternative
Pneumonia	Amoxycillin	Erythromycin	
Severe pneumonia	Amoxycillin/ampicillin/benzylpenicillin and erythromycin	Amoxycillin and tetracycline	Cefuroxime and erythromycin
Severe pneumonia where PCP is possible	High-dose co-trimoxazole		
Ear infection	Amoxycillin	Tetracycline	
Meningitis (in adult)	Benzylpenicillin	Chloramphenicol	
Complicated urinary tract infection	Co-trimoxazole	Gentamicin	Cefuroxime *or* ciprofloxacin
Bacterial dysentery	Co-trimoxazole		Ciprofloxacin
Abdominal sepsis	Ampicillin + gentamicin and metronidazole		Cefuroxime and metronidazole
Endocarditis	Penicillin and gentamicin		

Quinolones

Quinolones such as ciprofloxacin and norfloxacin are good antibiotics, but often expensive. They are active against most bacteria, but are best reserved for severe gram-negative bacterial infection likely to be resistant to other drugs. Oral quinolones are generally as effective as intravenous third-generation cephalosporins in this context.

In Table 7.1 we outline a reasonable starting point for empirical treatment of selected significant infections. This will need to be modified by local patterns of resistance and availability of drugs. Where reliable microbiology services exist, this will allow treatment to be modified when resistance is a problem. Bacterial infections that require specific treatment, such as brucellosis or typhoid, are covered in the chapters on individual diseases.

One drug or several

In general, one drug should be used to treat a disease unless there is a clear reason why two or more will be better. Increasing the number of drugs increases the cost and risk of side effects whilst reducing compliance. Some drugs are less good as a combination than alone, for example, mixing bacteristatic drugs (such as erythromycin or tetracycline) with bactericidal drugs (such as amoxycillin) may reduce the effectiveness of both. There are, however, a number of specific situations where a combination of drugs is preferable.

(a) The two drugs act synergistically, and each one enhances the activity of the other in severe infection. An example for bacteria would be gentamicin and penicillin in treating streptococcal endocarditis. Co-trimoxazole (Septrin) or sulphadoxine/pyrimethamine (S/P, Fansidar) are examples of combinations which are put into the same pill because of this synergistic effect. This is not common, however, and most infections can be killed just as effectively with one drug as with two.

(b) The patient is being treated syndromically, and there are several possible infections that could cause the syndrome, which do not all respond to a single antibiotic. An example might be penile ulcer or urethritis.

(c) Local resistance patterns make it difficult to be sure a single antibiotic will be effective in severe infection. In Malawi 5 per cent of *S. pneumoniae* is penicillin resistant and 5 per cent chloramphenicol resistant, but none is resistant to both. It may be necessary to give both drugs to a case of pneumococcal meningitis, where the severity of the disease means we cannot risk giving ineffective treatment.

(d) To prevent drug resistance emerging during treatment. This is the most common situation where more than one antibiotic is not only justified, but necessary. The classic example of this is tuberculosis combination treatment, and more recently antiretroviral treatment. In these diseases, if a single drug is used, resistance will emerge, with potentially disastrous results for the patient and others they infect with drug-resistant strains. Each drug 'protects' the others in the combination. There are moves to introduce combinations of drugs to treat malaria, so as to slow the emergence of drug resistance in Africa.

Supportive treatment

This chapter has concentrated on the process of making a diagnosis and instituting appropriate anti-microbial treatment. This is essential, but is only part of the management of patients with severe infections. General supportive measures, which need to be adjusted throughout a critical illness, are at least as important if a patient is to survive. It is quite common in busy wards with over-worked nurses and over-stretched clinicians for patients with entirely treatable conditions to die because of inadequate supportive treatment, despite an accurate diagnosis and appropriate initial treatment. Since supportive treatments are generally cheap and universally available, this is wholly unnecessary. Most supportive measures appropriate in Africa are obvious, and almost all clinicians will get them right if they think about them. The error is usually not to give them sufficient priority during a busy day.

Adequate fluid replacement

In acute diarrhoeal illness, from childhood diarrhoea to adult cholera, dehydration is virtually the only cause of death. Dehydration can also occur exceptionally fast in other infections in Africa; patients who are not drinking, who have fever and peripheral vasodilatation in a hot climate, are at very high risk of pre-renal failure and other complications. If patients can drink, oral fluids are ideal, and relatives can safely be encouraged to push fluids. If not, intravenous fluids may be needed. Generally, 3 litres fluid intake a day is an absolute minimum in a febrile illness, and in hot climates more may be needed. There are very few conditions where it is possible to over-hydrate patients unless they are elderly. A history of left ventricular failure (or congestive cardiac failure) or nephrotic syndrome are reasons to be cautious, but even in these patients there is generally a greater risk of under-hydrating than over-hydrating during an acute infection.

Maintaining adequate oxygenation

Specific infectious diseases present particular problems. Examples are tetanus (acute upper-airway obstruction), tuberculous pleural effusion (reduced lung volume), polio (reduced respiratory effort) or pneumocystis pneumonia (reduced gas exchange). The management of these specific problems is covered in later chapters; the key here is anticipating they will happen and forward planning rather than reacting to a crisis. Any patient with a chest infection, or with impaired consciousness, is also at risk of reduced oxygenation, and numerically these patients are more common. The level of intervention necessary to improve oxygenation is often quite small. The simplest, available in all hospitals, is clearing secretions. In chest infections encouraging deep breathing to open up the airways is important to help clear sputum, with chest physiotherapy if it is available. Nursing unconscious patients on their side reduces the risk of acute obstruction. Where oxygen is available, this will often be useful. The role of artificial ventilation in Africa is as a last resort. It is very tempting to ventilate all severely ill patients, but there are considerable risks associated with artificial ventilation, ranging from pneumothorax to nosocomial infection to power-cuts. In most severe infections ventilation is likely to do more harm than good, except when reduced respiratory effort or gas exchange is the main clinical problem.

Most of the other aspects of good supportive treatment are fairly obvious. They include preventing pressure sores and maintaining nutrition.

Public health implications of the infected patient

In a hospital context it is important to protect patients and their carers from acquiring infections in hospital that they did not have when they came in. This is very difficult in many African countries, but still important. For example, in countries where both TB and HIV are relatively common, TB suspects may be investigated in open wards surrounded by HIV-positive patients with unrelated problems who do not have TB. The patients with TB are usually segregated once open TB is confirmed, but by then treatment has started and their infectiousness rapidly declines: it is the pre-diagnosis stage which is most dangerous. The best way to reduce hospital-acquired infection is to get patients out of hospital as soon as it is safe, and to do as much investigation as an outpatient as possible. Patients with diarrhoea also need to be nursed separately with barrier methods (gloves) or at least vigorous handwashing between patients. The special case of cholera will be dealt with in Chapter 48.

The clinician also has a wider responsibility to spot diseases with a clear public health implication. These are either diseases where the patient may transmit a serious disease to others (plague, Lassa fever), or where the fact that one patient has a disease may indicate an outbreak which needs vigorous public health measures (cholera, yellow fever or Legionella are examples). An abnormally high cluster of cases of a disease that would normally only occur in ones or twos may be the first hint that an outbreak is occurring (meningococcal disease, for example). Countries vary in how their notification process works, and in some cases theory and practice are different, but with important diseases such as yellow fever or meningococcal meningitis outbreaks all countries will have emergency plans, and it is essential to inform public health officials early.

8 The control and prevention of infection

Epidemiology or endemiology?

Many infections have the ability to spread from one person to another. This is not true of all – tetanus spores are in the soil all around us and it is these that cause infection when they come into contact with open wounds; tetanus does not spread from person to person. However, it is the way in which infections spread from person to person that has led to the special attention they receive in public health control. Epidemics of diseases are usually due to infections (illicit drugs and toxic chemicals are other important causes). The study of health and disease in populations, epidemiology, derives its name from epidemic. Epidemic infections such as meningococcal meningitis and cholera are a cause of great alarm and require well coordinated, usually government led, responses. This is discussed later in terms of outbreak control. Yet the major burden of infection in the community is not from these epidemic diseases but from the endemic (meaning present all the time) conditions such as pneumonia, diarrhoea and skin infections. It might have been better to have called the science of public health endemiology!

Infection and disease

An important point about infectious diseases is the separation of infection and disease. New organisms continuously infect us. The colony of bacteria that lives on the surface of our skin and on the lining of our gut is constantly changing. Every minor break in our skin or mucosa allows bacteria around us to invade the tissues. Viruses in the air and water probe at our defences to try to gain a foothold. Yet most days we are well. So there are two steps to an infectious disease – the exposure to the infectious agent (virus, bacteria, fungus) and then the development of disease as a result of that infection. When we consider what it is that leads to infectious diseases we will consider both steps. In both there are three major determinants: the infectious agent – that is the 'bug'; the route by which it reached you, the human; and what state you are in – your susceptibility.

Types of agent

The type of infectious agent is an important aspect of the relationship between infection and disease. For example, bacteria and fungi can grow without invading a cell and therefore can 'colonize' the surfaces of our bodies. Thus superficial infections with bacteria and fungi are common. They represent a local invasion by a locally resident organism when the chance arises – maybe a cut or poor diet reducing immunity. Viruses in contrast must enter and destroy cells to survive. Thus virus infection always leads to some damage, but it may not be sufficient for us to call it disease.

Different bacteria and viruses vary in their ability to cause infection. Some bacteria can digest local tissue, some damage immune defences (see Chapter 6). Viruses have tricks for evading immune attack by making their proteins look like human ones so the immune system does not recognize them as foreign. Others may hide in parts of the body the immune system cannot reach. Varicella zoster virus (chickenpox) retreats after infection to the inside of nerve cells. When immunity to it falls for some reason, it can re-appear and cause the disease herpes zoster (or shingles), which is a rash like chickenpox but only affecting the distribution of one or a few nerves. We all live with chickenpox virus, and many other viruses, inside us.

Even within what appears to be a single type of organism – *Strep. pneumoniae*, for example – there are many subtypes. Some of these spread very rapidly from person to person, whilst others are hardly infectious at all.

The ability of different organisms to cause disease varies. Measles virus causes the disease we call measles in around 99 per cent of those infected. Hepatitis B virus causes recognizable disease amongst around a third of adults it infects. Hepatitis G virus, which infects around 50 per cent of Ghanaians, does not seem to cause any disease at all. Serotype 1 of *Strep. pneumoniae* is virtually never found in people's noses but is a frequent and important cause of pneumonia. It is assumed that it produces disease in virtually everybody infected. Other serotypes rarely cause disease but are frequent residents of the nose.

Host characteristics

Infection has been one of the great driving forces of evolutionary adaptation. Human genetics have been determined to a large part by the infections that have afflicted mankind. The development of molecular biology has led to great interest in these genetic determinants of susceptibility to infection, to disease and to severity of disease.

However, in Africa the major determinant of host susceptibility remains 'environmental'. By this is meant everything that is not genetic. The integrity of our skin and mucosal surfaces is determined to a large extent by our behaviour (fishing, digging in the fields), by our diet (e.g. vitamin A) and by our access to effective health care (e.g. stitches and dressings for wounds).

The immune system is the major barrier to infectious organisms (see Chapter 6). Many infections produce long-term memory such that when we meet the same 'bug' again we recognize it, have immune cells that know it ready and waiting, and we contain the infection before any harm is done. Prior experience of the infectious agent is important in determining the outcome of infection. This may be in the form of natural infection, or as a result of immunization with all or part of the organism concerned. A special case is the young baby in whom the mother's experience of an infection is important, since maternal antibodies cross the placenta and persist in the baby for the first months of life.

The immune system undergoes marked changes during life. It takes up to the first 10 years of life to fully reach maturity. From then until 40 years of age it is affected by diet and in women by reproduction. After the age of 40 it declines. Infectious disease is particularly a phenomenon of young and old age. Yet surprisingly some infections do not lead to disease at a young age. The very immaturity of the immune system protects against disease. These are infections where immune attack on the infected cell is the cause of the disease. Hepatitis B virus infection does not cause clinical disease in those aged under five years. However, the risk of the virus persisting if a child is infected is very high at around 20–30 per cent. This reflects a balance. Although the immune response to the infection is the main cause of the destruction of liver cells – and hence hepatitis – it is also the mechanism for clearing the virus from the body. Age then is an important host characteristic; not only in determining exposure to infectious agents, but also in determining the infection/disease ratio, the severity of the disease and, for some viruses, whether or not the infection persists.

Transmission

We have already distinguished between infections that have the environment as a source – such as tetanus – and those that have another person as a source. Here we are concerned with the route that the infection takes. This may be important in determining whether the infection leads to disease or not but is also critical in how we attempt to protect ourselves and others against infection.

Direct transmission occurs between two people at close range. It may involve actual physical contact – as in the case of sexually transmitted infections and those spread by kissing, biting and touching. It may be through droplets passing directly from one person to the mucosa of the eyes, nose or mouth of another. This usually only occurs over a distance of up to 1 metre. Indirect transmission occurs where some intermediary object or organism plays a role. For example, faecal bacteria may be spread on clothes to cause diarrhoea (see Box).

Routes of transmission of infectious agents

Route	*Examples*
Respiratory	Measles, influenza viruses
Faecal-oral	Poliomyelitis virus, *Vibrio cholerae*, salmonellae, shigellae, other enteric organisms (note this includes direct and indirect routes through food and water)
Cutaneous	*Bacillus anthracis, Staphylococcus aureus*
Sexual	HIV, *Neisseria gonorrhoea, Treponema pallidum*
Blood-borne	Hepatitis B virus, HIV, hepatitis C virus
Vector borne	*Plasmodium falciparum*, guinea worm
Transplacental	*Toxoplasma gondii, T. pallidum*

Each route of transmission has its own epidemiological pattern. This is important in interpreting surveillance data and when dealing with a disease of unknown cause. The pattern may suggest a particular route of transmission.

Respiratory infections are very efficient at spreading to a large number of people. Each cough or sneeze may reach 10 or 20 people. This leads to epidemics that rise very steeply in numbers and also disappear quickly as everybody becomes immune. The annual influenza epidemic is of this kind, as are epidemics of measles and respiratory syncytial virus. Interestingly rotavirus diarrhoea epidemics also show this pattern, and it is believed that rotavirus can be transmitted both by the respiratory and the faecal–oral route. Respiratory transmission may be associated with overcrowded situations – epidemics of measles are frequently related to school attendance or the opening of the trade season in West Africa. No particular part of society is selected by the infections however.

The faecal–oral route is usually much less efficient. The commonest route is through the contamination of hands by faecal material and the transfer of this to the mouth either by licking or sucking the hands or by handling food. So, any one person rarely infects more than one or two others – and usually only those in close contact. Hand washing is highly effective at interrupting this mode of transmission. For these reasons, diarrhoeal disease tends to be associated with poverty – where access to clean water and soap is limited. Occasionally, food or water may be contaminated and lead to larger outbreaks of disease. Cholera typically does this through contamination of foodstuffs. Here the classical method of control is by cleanliness in food handling and sanitation of water supplies. It is clear that diarrhoeal disease may be spread by multiple routes – hand to mouth, contaminated food, contaminated water and even respiratory. The identification the most important in different communities may be a useful, if difficult, step in choosing how best to control diarrhoeal disease.

Cutaneous transmission is rare through unbroken skin. However ectoparasites (ones that live on the outside) such as head lice or scabies are relatively easily transmitted. Most of these infections occur in children and are associated with close physical contact and overcrowding.

Sexually transmitted infections are typically infections that persist over long periods of time. This is an important adaptation of the organism to this means of transmission since in general people change sexual partners relatively infrequently and for transmission to occur the organism needs to stay around for a long time. The pattern of infection here is sporadic but in some populations with seasonal variation related to seasonal sexual activity. Certain population groups are typically affected – young unmarried people, sex workers, long distance lorry drivers. These drivers have been particularly important in the spread of HIV infection in East Africa (Gysels et al., 2001).

Blood-borne infections are typically represented by hepatitis B, hepatitis C and HIV. Blood transfusion was an important means of transmission prior to the introduction of screening of donated blood. However they all have other routes of transmission. Sexual transmission is the major route for HIV and also a route for hepatitis B. Hepatitis C is particularly transmitted by contaminated needles and the evidence is now strong that mass injection treatment of schistosomiasis in Egypt played the key role in spreading hepatitis in that country (Habib et al., 2001). Egypt has the highest proportion of the adult population infected with the virus of anywhere in the world – around 20 per cent. Transmission of this group of infections is a particular concern in the health setting but can largely be prevented by careful attention to the use of sterile needles and sterile injection practice. In Africa, where people particularly believe that injections are the most effective treatments, minimizing the numbers of injections given is an important, though difficult, means of infection control. Injection-related infections are rarely, if ever, epidemic over a short time-scale: they occur over years rather than days. The people particularly at risk are those most likely to have injections – the young, the old and the sick.

Vector-borne infections are particularly important in Africa. Malaria is the most important vector-borne disease and illustrates the way in which the pattern of infection reflects exposure to the vector. Where domestic mosquitoes are the main vector, we see a pattern of infection affecting children and adults of both sexes. Where the vectors are largely in the forest or fields, then those who work most in the fields are primarily affected – usually adults and sometimes more males than females. This association with the vector is also seen with schistosomiasis – here the snail vector lives in water and water contact is necessary for transmission. Infection is then particularly seen in children who play in water and rural women who spend long hours in pools washing clothes.

Finally, there are the relatively small number of infections that can cross the placenta. These are important because they may cause damage to the growing fetus. With the exception of syphilis, they are relatively rare in most of Africa as most women are exposed to them as children and therefore cannot get them when they are pregnant. However, in wealthier urban communities they may begin to appear. Toxoplasmosis and rubella are two important infections that cross the placenta and may result in fetal damage.

Infection dynamics

Incubation period

The source of an infection is almost invariably a relatively small number of 'bugs'. These then have to multiply and spread within the body before they lead to disease. This interval between exposure to the infection and developing disease is known as the 'incubation period'. For all infections it has the same shape as shown in Fig. 8.1 but the actual period varies from infection to infection. Thus for typhoid fever it varies from 7–21 days, for measles from 7–18 days with a median of 10 and for rabies it is usually 2–8 weeks but may be as short as 5 days or longer than a year. As we will see later, this is important information when investigating an outbreak.

The incubation period represents time to first symptom but this does not necessarily coincide with the beginning of the time that the person is infectious to others. This is often shorter than the incubation period and is known as the latent period. This means that, by the time somebody has symptoms of the disease, they may already have infected others – an important point in terms of disease control.

Epidemic patterns

Epidemics can have different patterns over time. These may be valuable in suggesting what kind of organism is causing them, and in predicting what may happen in the next week or two.

If the infection all comes from one source over a short period of time, then the pattern of the epidemic is essentially the distribution of the incubation periods. This is the kind of epidemic one sees after a group of people eat a contaminated meal – for example, cholera in West Africa has been associated with food eaten at funeral gatherings and has the pattern shown in Fig. 8.2 (St. Louis et al, 1990).

Where there is transmission from one generation of cases to the next, then the waves of a propagated epidemic are seen (Fig. 8.3). One might think that the time interval from one wave of the epidemic to the next is the incubation period – but it is not. Because people may be infectious before they get disease, and what you are observing are diseased people, the interval is different

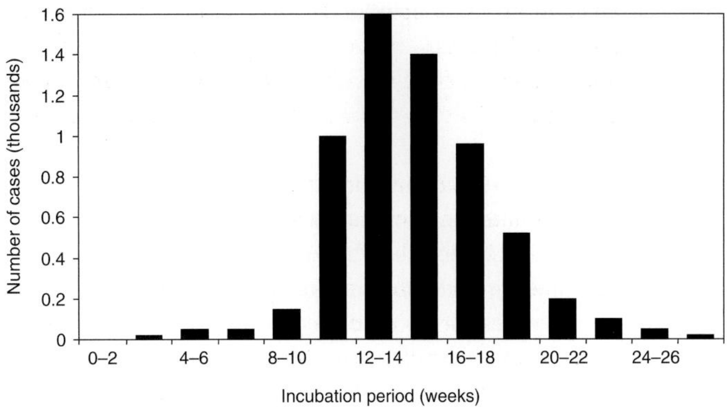

Fig. 8.1. Incubation period distribution of hepatitis B.

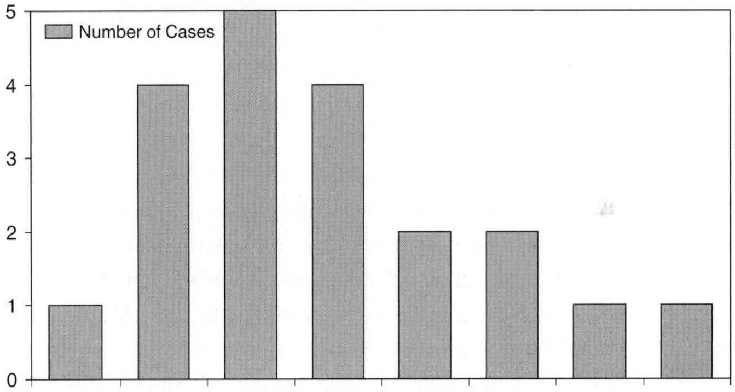

Fig. 8.2. Epidemic curve for a point source outbreak.

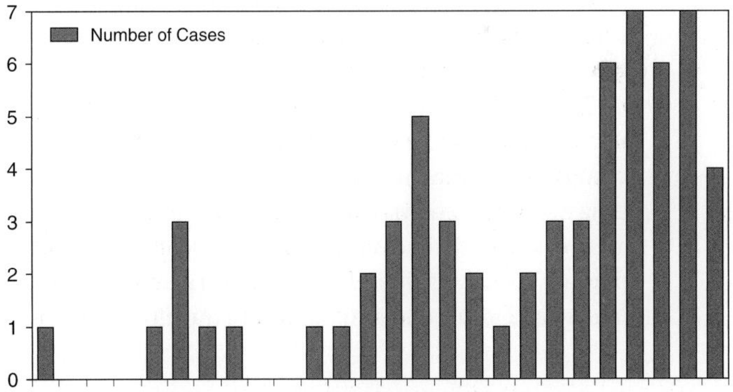

Fig. 8.3. Epidemic curve for a propagated outbreak.

both from the incubation period and the latent period – it is known as the serial interval.

Often the serial interval is too short to see this pattern – the waves all run into one another.

As well as these epidemic patterns, infection may follow two other patterns in communities. When a disease occurs every now and then as one or two isolated cases, it is known as sporadic. If it is present all the time but shows no great variation up or down it is known as endemic infection/disease.

Surveillance

If these patterns of infection are to be recognized in a community, there has to be accurate recording of infectious diseases. Surveillance is the routine collection of data and its analysis in order to generate public health action. All communities are involved in some kind of surveillance.

The key to surveillance is a standardized definition of the disease that you are studying. This will depend on the level at which surveillance is being conducted. A village health worker might record all children who have had more than three liquid stools in the last 24 hours as a definition of diarrhoea – most probably simply on a tally sheet. In contrast, a hospital might record rotavirus diarrhoea as a similar clinical condition with a positive screening test on faecal examination. Definitions are produced by organizations such as the World Health Organization. These are useful because they can be used to compare disease rates between countries. However, it may be necessary to develop your own definition, depending on the diagnostic facilities in your setting.

The second key issue in surveillance is estimating the population at risk. How many people live in the geographical area that the health facility serves? The most recent census is usually the best source of information on this but can be up to 10 years out of date.

It is often necessary to adjust the census data:

- for migration, where large parts of the population may have moved – particularly to cities, and
- for growth, since many African countries have high population growth due to high birth rates.

Data need to be analysed and interpreted. This is best done at as local a level as possible, so that the people who collect the data see the results immediately, and people who understand local conditions can make the interpretation.

Outbreak investigation

This will almost always involve the public health authorities. The first question to ask is whether this needs investigating at all. Although outbreaks can be interesting to investigate, they also consume much time. One needs to be sure that there is truly an outbreak and that it is likely to be sufficiently serious to make an investigation worthwhile.

Once that decision has been made, a team needs to be put together to do the field investigation. You will need people with expertise in the following areas on the team:

- nursing
- environmental health
- clinical diagnosis
- epidemiology
- statistics
- interviewing
- local politics
- microbiology.

Of course, members of the team may have more than one of these skills. The team then needs to carry out the following steps of investigation. They are shown as a list, but in reality they will be carried out almost simultaneously – one cannot wait before treating cases, or instituting simple control measures such as hand washing for a diarrhoeal disease.

- What is the diagnosis?
- Confirm that there is an epidemic.
- Identify affected people and get basic information on age, sex, occupation.
- Search for additional cases.
- Define the population at risk and collect basic information on them (to allow calculation of rates).
- Examine the data and form a theory of how the epidemic started and spread.
- Manage the epidemic.
  Treat cases.
  Prevent further spread through control measures.
  Write a report.
  Set up/strengthen continuing surveillance.
- If possible, carry out an experiment to test your theory of source and spread.

Diagnosis

The diagnosis may be very obvious – measles is so characteristic that serological confirmation is hardly necessary in epidemics. But often it will require laboratory tests to be certain. For example meningitis will require cerebrospinal fluid examination. It is best if this can be done in the field, as transportation to a laboratory and return of the results may take a long time. This has implications for equipment – you may need to take a power supply to the field if the village has none. Microscopes, stains and simple laboratory equipment will be needed. Confirmation of the diagnosis may take a few days; but if you have seen the characteristic vibrios on dark ground illumination of a faecal sample in the field, you can confidently treat an outbreak as cholera without definitive confirmation.

Where there have been deaths from the disease, it may be necessary to conduct some form of examination of the body. This does not have to be a complete post-mortem. For example, if yellow fever is suspected, a needle biopsy of the liver will be sufficient, or in the case of cholera, a rectal swab. In this way the trauma to the bereaved family and community can be minimized.

An experienced clinician is clearly a great asset to the investigating team. This is particularly important when the diagnosis is less obvious, or if there is a possibility that it is a haemorrhagic fever.

Is it an epidemic?

You need to be sure that this is an epidemic. There are various definitions of an epidemic. At one extreme, a single case of a disease that is eradicated or targeted for eradication may represent an epidemic – a case of smallpox for example.

An epidemic can be defined as a situation where two people have a disease or infection linked through a common exposure in person time or place. More usually, though, epidemic refers to the situation where there is a higher incidence of disease than is usually expected for that place at that time. This means that you have to know how much of the disease was there before.

There may be records at a local health centre that you can look at, or a village health worker who has some kind of tally sheet. But often you will be dependent on the knowledge and experience of people in the village and of local health workers. This is important, as sometimes a new health worker may start diagnosing a disease that has been there all along, or the health centre gets a new test for a disease that could not be diagnosed before. In these situations it is not a real epidemic and does not deserve special investigation.

It is important to plot out – on graph paper or using a portable computer – the time distribution of the epidemic where possible, including data about disease in the community from before the start of this outbreak. This confirms the fact that it is an epidemic and the shape of the curve – as discussed above – may suggest what kind of source and what kind of transmission is occurring. From this plot it may be possible to identify primary cases and secondary cases – people infected by the primary cases. Examining these links – who caught it from whom and where it is likely to have happened – can be especially important in detecting the way the infection is spreading. For example, you may find that the secondary cases in a cholera outbreak all get their water from the same home water jar – clearly suggesting that this is contaminated and the source of the secondary cases.

Who got the disease?

So that you can make these kinds of links, you need to make a list of all the people who have the disease – sometimes called a line listing. For each of them you will need to record some basic information – sex, age, where they live, what work they do, if they have travelled recently, if they have had any visitors, and so on. It will be particularly important to find out exactly when they had the first symptom of the disease – possibly down to the hour of the day. This allows you to plot the graph above, and by relating this to the incubation period of the disease concerned you can see if all the cases could have come from one source. If the disease is vaccine preventable, you will also need to find out their vaccination history.

All this information needs to be collected on specially designed forms. These are often best prepared using the software EPI-INFO, which can then be used to enter the data into the computer, to analyse it and to generate the graphs. Thus the team needs to have a printer and supply of paper as well as a portable computer with them, though it may be feasible to do all this at the nearest health office.

Do you have all the cases?

Special efforts may be needed to find everybody who had the disease. Often, it is the most severe cases that you get to hear about – particularly those who ended up at the health centre or hospital. It will be necessary to visit the village or area where cases lived, to find out if there are more, milder cases. It may even be necessary to do a house to house survey. People who died from the disease, particularly early in the epidemic, may be missed because the diagnosis was not made. The team need to particularly ask about these. Finding out exactly what happened in the epidemic will be much more difficult if some cases are not detected and listed.

Who might have got the disease?

You now have as good a list of cases as you can get. This tells you about the age, sex, occupation, place of residence of the cases. To understand this, you now need to find out about these factors in the people who did not get the disease but who might have done – the population at risk.

Whatever statistics or census information is available should be used but with care – it is often inaccurate and/or out of date. If a house-to-house survey for cases is done, this is an opportunity to collect information on everybody in the household. Survey data of this kind is very valuable but can only be done on relatively small populations. If the epidemic is from a single source, then determining the population at risk can be straightforward. For example, cholera epidemics in West Africa have followed funeral feasts – in this situation only those people attending the feast are at risk. In this setting one would then find out what foods were available at the funeral, and who ate what. Differences between those who got disease and those who did not should indicate which food or drink was contaminated.

As well as questioning the population at risk, it may be necessary to perform laboratory tests. People may carry an infection and infect others without being ill themselves. An outbreak of typhoid amongst children being fed food supplements at a NGO (non-government organization) centre was found to be due to one of the workers being a typhoid carrier.

For some epidemics you may want to extend the investigation to the local animal population as well. Yellow fever has an important reservoir in monkeys. If it is a vector borne disease then the local vectors may need to be studied.

Constructing the story

Once all of the evidence has been gathered, it is important to consider all of the factors that have led to the epidemic. Where did the agent come from? This might have been an introduction by a traveller or a returning villager. Why did it spread? The age distribution of those affected may indicate whether this was because people were not immune (younger people usually) or because of particular circumstances of contact – for example amongst all members of a women's community group. The specific elements that must all be addressed are:

- the agent of disease
- the reservoir or source
- how did it leave the source?
- how was it transmitted to the next host?
- how did it enter the next host?
- what was the susceptibility of the next host?

Management of the epidemic

The person managing the investigation team must ensure s/he has enough people to investigate the outbreak properly. It may be necessary to take educated local people and rapidly train them in simple techniques if the epidemic is serious and large – for example a meningococcal epidemic. For some diseases – such as cholera – it may be necessary for the team to take equipment and drugs with them since these will not be available at the local health centre. In severe situations a field hospital may have to be set up – in places such as the market-place – to give emergency treatment.

Once the immediately sick are dealt with, attention needs to turn to preventing more cases. If the source of the infection has been identified, it can be isolated and sterilized. For example, a contaminated well can be closed and treated with lime. Person-to-person spread from people who are not yet cases also needs attention. In faecal–orally transmitted infections attention to hand washing and provision of soap is important. Respiratory spread infections may necessitate isolation of individuals and restrictions on gatherings of people, even school closures.

For some infections the use of antibiotics in contacts of cases can reduce secondary attack rates. Vaccination remains the best means of preventing infectious diseases. Where it is available, vaccinate the susceptible population immediately.

Continued surveillance

Once the epidemic is controlled, consider setting up systems for detecting outbreaks sooner. This applies not only to the setting of this outbreak, but also at the regional or even national level. Whilst this is mainly the responsibility of health workers, there is no reason why others in the community, such as school teachers and senior figures, should not play a part in reporting new outbreaks promptly.

Experimental verification

Finally, it may be possible to carry out experiments in the laboratory to see if the story of the epidemic you reconstructed is true. For example, if you find that certain foods are protective in a cholera epidemic, you can test to see if they inhibit the growth of the organism in a laboratory.

Control

The control of infectious diseases in the community depends either on general measures related to the particular route of transmission concerned (see below), or to specific methods for that agent. The specific measures are vaccines that are tailored to that organism.

Transmission route	Control measures
Faecal–oral	Hand washing, clean food preparation, clean water supply
Respiratory	Reduced household and institutional crowding
Sexual	Barrier contraceptives and safe sex
Blood-borne	Minimize injections and transfusions, safe sterile injections
Vector-borne	Insecticide treated bednets, residual spraying

Vaccines rely on the principle that exposure to an antigen (a molecule that stimulates the immune system) results in memory (discussed in detail in Chapter 6). This memory provides the ability to fend off subsequent attacks from infectious agents that have a recognized antigen on their surface. Individual vaccines are discussed in the relevant disease section. The use of vaccines as a means to intervene in the community and control infection is discussed here.

The World Health Organization introduced the Expanded Programme on Immunization in the late 1970s following the success of vaccination in eradicating smallpox. The aim was to vaccinate children as early in life as possible. This was to ensure that as many as possible had immunological memory before they met the infectious agent. Currently, countries deliver several or all of the following vaccines: BCG (Bacille Calmette–Guerin) for TB and leprosy; oral poliomyelitis vaccine (OPV); diphtheria, pertussis (whooping cough) and tetanus as a triple vaccine (DPT); measles; yellow fever; haemophilus influenzae type b (Hib); hepatitis B (HBV). Pneumococcal and meningococcal vaccines will be introduced soon.

Typical vaccine schedule		
As soon after birth as possible	BCG	OPV
6 weeks	DPT	OPV
10 weeks	DPT	OPV
14 weeks	DPT	OPV
9 months	measles	yellow fever

The emphasis has been very much on childhood diseases. This was because of the very high infant and child mortality rates resulting from these acute infectious diseases. The success of the programme can be seen in the reduction of whooping cough and measles as causes of death. Much of this success has been due to the training and delivery system that the EPI has put in place throughout Africa. All vaccines require some kind of protection against heat that destroys their effectiveness. So a good EPI system has to have a cold chain from the airport or factory to a storeroom and then out to health centres and hospitals. Each of these places needs a reliable, maintained fridge/freezer. Vaccinators need a regular supply of sterile needles and syringes to deliver the vaccine safely, and of course the vaccines themselves. The health workers need regular training and support to do the best job. All of this needs to be monitored to identify and correct problems. This is all the work of the EPI. It is the most effective public health intervention in Africa.

References

Gysels M, Pool R, Bwanika K (2001). Truck drivers, middlemen and commercial sex workers: AIDS and the mediation of sex in south west Uganda. *AIDS Care*; **13**: 373–385.

Habib M, Mohamed MK, Abdel Aziz F et al. (2001). Hepatitis C virus infection in a community in the Nile Delta: risk factors for seropositivity. *Hepatology*; **33**: 248–253.

St Louis ME, Porter JD, Helal A et al (1990). Epidemic cholera in West Africa: the role of food handling and high-risk foods. *Am J Epidemiol*; **131**: 719–728.

9

The integrated management of childhood illness (IMCI)

Background

Although the mortality rate of children less than 5 years old has decreased by almost a third since the 1970s, the reduction has not been evenly distributed throughout the world. According to the *1999 World Health Report*, children in low-to-middle-income countries are ten times more likely to die before 5 years of age than children living in the industrialized world. In 1998, more than 50 countries still had childhood mortality rates over 100 per 1000 live births, and 12 over 200.

In Africa, the majority of these deaths are due to acute respiratory infections (mostly pneumonia), malaria, diarrhoea, measles, or malnutrition, and often to a combination of these conditions (Fig. 9.1). In addition, neonatal problems constitute a major share of these deaths.

Many sick children present with symptoms and signs related to more than one of these conditions. This overlap means that a single diagnosis may also be complicated by the need to combine therapy for several conditions. Therefore, during the mid-1990s, the World Health Organization (WHO) developed the Integrated Management of Childhood Illness (IMCI). Although the major reason for its development resulted from curative care needs, the strategy also addresses aspects of nutrition, immunization, and other elements of disease prevention and health promotion. It focuses on first-level health facilities in low-income countries with health workers with limited training. Diagnosis relies on history and clinical signs to determine management within the context of limited resources.

The IMCI strategy consists of three main components:

- Improvements in the case-management skills of health staff
- Improvements in the functioning of the overall health system
- Improvements in family and community health care practices.

The IMCI case management guidelines for first-level health facilities

The IMCI guidelines are based on the following principles: all sick children under 5 years are examined for general danger signs that indicate the need for immediate referral or admission to hospital. They are then assessed for major symptoms which include: cough or difficult breathing, diarrhoea, fever, ear infections. In addition, all sick children are routinely assessed for nutritional and immunization status, and other potential problems. Only a limited number of clinical signs are used, selected on the basis of their sensitivity and specificity to detect disease. A combination of individual signs leads to a child's classification within one or more syndrome groups rather than a diagnosis. This classification indicates the level of severity and the appropriate initial management. These classifications are colour coded: 'pink' suggests hospital referral or admission, 'yellow' indicates initiation of outpatient treatment, and 'green' indicates symptomatic treatment. The IMCI guidelines address most, but not all, of the major reasons why a sick child is brought to a clinic. The guidelines do not describe the management of trauma or other acute emergencies due to accidents or injuries, skin or musculoskeletal conditions, and a number of chronic and less common conditions. IMCI management procedures use a limited number of essential drugs and encourage active participation of the family in the treatment of children. An essential component of IMCI is counselling of carers about feeding, fluids and when to return for review.

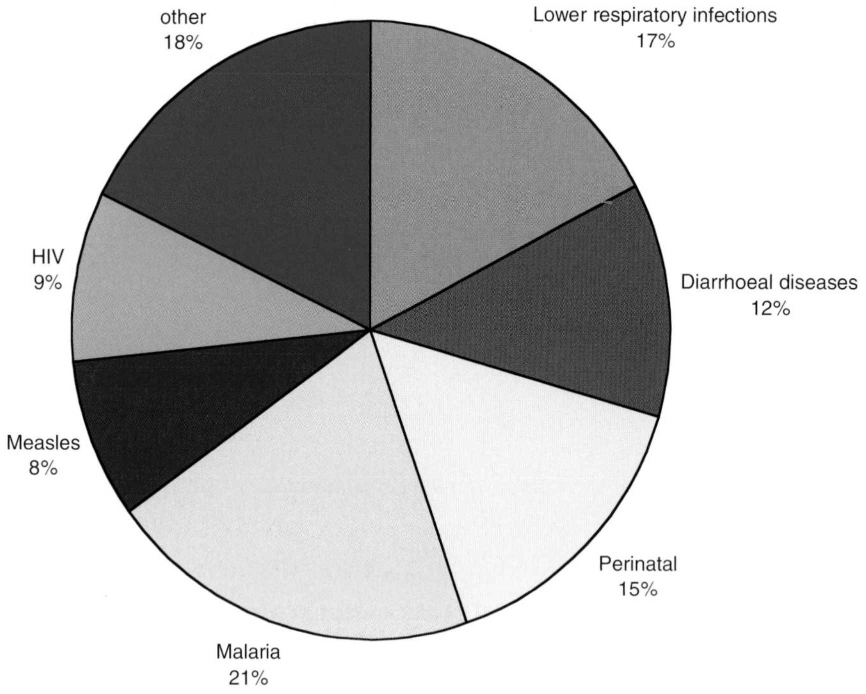

Fig. 9.1. Distribution of the childhood deaths <5 years of age in sub-Saharan Africa (WHO, 2000).

The IMCI case management process

The case management of a sick child brought to a first-level health facility includes a number of important elements (see Fig. 9.2).

At the first-level health facility

During the initial visit at the outpatient facility, the process consists of: the assessment of the child's condition; the classification and identification of treatment; decision regarding referral, treatment or counselling of the child's carer; and follow-up care.

Some clinical signs and symptoms have different reliability and diagnostic value in different age groups, therefore the IMCI guidelines use two age categories:

- Children age 2 months up to 5 years;
- Young infants age 1 week up to 2 months.

At the referral care facility

When the child reaches a referral care facility, typically a small or district hospital, children are prioritized using emergency triage assessment and treatment (ETAT). This is followed by diagnosis, treatment and monitoring of patient progress by more experienced staff than those available at a first-level health facility.

Appropriate home management

For children who are sent home from the first-level facility, care consists of teaching mothers or other carers how to give oral drugs and treat local infections at home, and counselling mothers or other carers about feeding, fluids, and when to return to the health facility.

Adapting the guidelines to a particular country

The underlying principles of the IMCI guidelines are constant. However, in each country the IMCI clinical guidelines need to be adapted to:

- cover the most serious childhood illnesses seen at first-level health facilities;
- be consistent with national treatment guidelines;
- recommend home care that is appropriate and attainable.

Adaptation of the IMCI guidelines is co-ordinated by a national health regulating body (usually the Ministry of

Health) and incorporates decisions made by national health experts. Therefore, some of the details described below may differ from the practice used in a particular country. The principles used for management of sick children, however, are applicable everywhere.

The IMCI guidelines for children aged 2 months to 5 years presenting to an outpatient facility

After the health worker has asked the carer why s/he has brought the child, s/he checks the child for the presence of *general danger signs*. These are:

- a history of convulsions;
- being lethargic or unconscious;
- the inability to drink or breast-feed;
- vomiting everything.

These signs indicate that the child is severely ill. They might be combined with other disease specific signs, such as cough, fever or diarrhoea. Their presence leads to referral of the child (unless they are associated with severe dehydration, and successful rehydration leads to the resolution of the danger sign).

Cough or difficult breathing

In the context of the IMCI clinical algorithm, the entry criterion for the assessment of children for pneumonia is a complaint of 'cough or difficulty in breathing'. The IMCI algorithm uses three clinical signs to assess a sick child with cough or difficult breathing:

- elevated respiratory rate;
- lower chest wall indrawing;
- stridor.

As the respiratory rate decreases with age, the following cut-offs for fast breathing (tachypnoea) are used: 2 months up to 12 months: 50 breaths per minute or more, and 12 months up to 5 years: 40 breaths per minute or more. Based on these findings, the children are classified, as described in Fig. 9.3, into three categories:

Severe pneumonia or very severe disease

This includes children with any general danger sign (inability to feed, vomiting everything, a history of convulsions, or being lethargic or unconscious), lower chest wall indrawing, or stridor at rest. Referral is required for intravenous antibiotics. Before referral, children receive one dose of an antibiotic, e.g. cotrimoxazole or amoxicillin. If an oral antibiotic is not tolerated, give

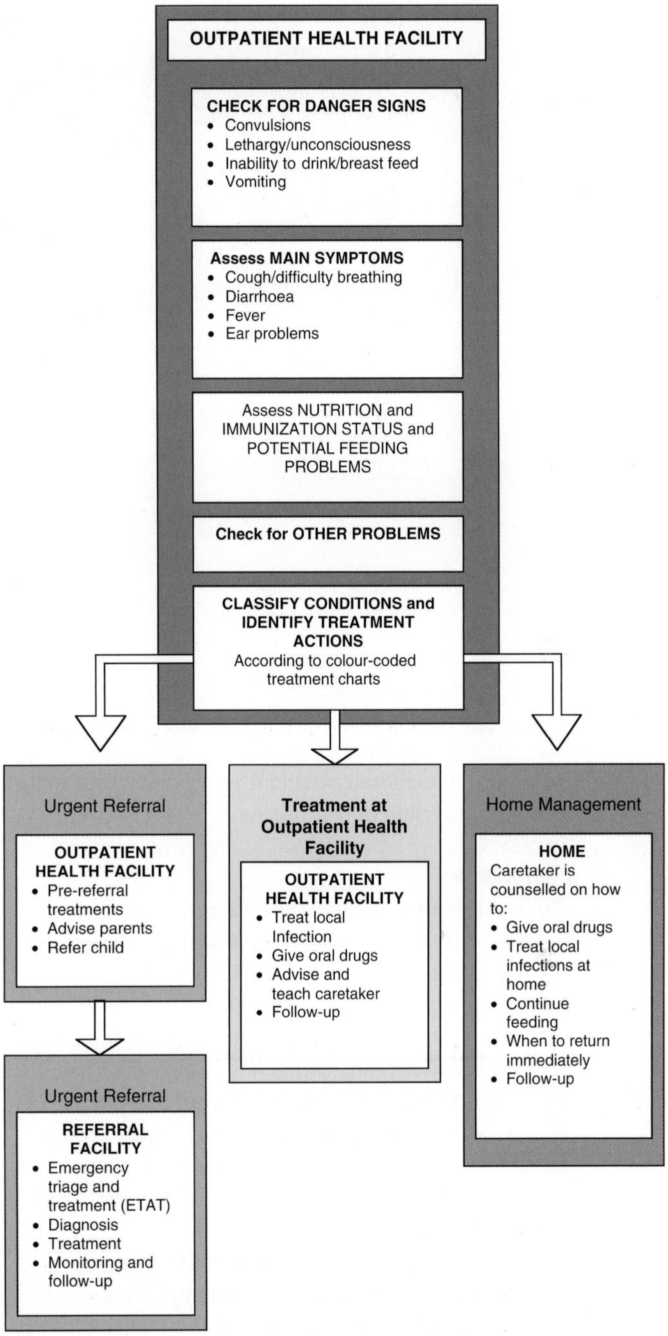

Fig. 9.2. Overview of the process of patient management according to the IMCI process.

SIGNS	CLASSIFY AS	IDENTIFY TREATMENT (Urgent pre-referral treatments are in bold print.)
• Any general danger sign or • Chest indrawing or • Stridor in calm child.	SEVERE PNEUMONIA OR VERY SEVERE DISEASE	➤ **Give first dose of an appropriate antibiotic.** ➤ **Refer URGENTLY to hospital.**
• Fast breathing	PNEUMONIA	➤ **Give an appropriate oral antibiotic for 5 days.** ➤ Soothe the throat and relieve the cough with a safe remedy. ➤ Advise mother when to return immediately. ➤ Follow-up in 2 days.
No signs of pneumonia or very severe disease.	NO PNEUMONIA: COUGH OR COLD	➤ If coughing more than 30 days, refer for assessment. ➤ Soothe the throat and relieve the cough with a safe remedy. ➤ Advise mother when to return immediately. ➤ Follow-up in 5 days if not improving.

Fig. 9.3. IMCI classification for cough or difficult breathing.

intramuscular chloramphenicol, or an alternative such as benzylpenicillin or ceftriaxone.

Pneumonia

This classification includes all children with tachypnoea. Treatment consists of a 5-day course of oral cotrimoxazole or amoxicillin. Both antibiotics are relatively inexpensive, widely available, and on the essential drug list of most countries. Cotrimoxazole is cheaper and is used twice daily, so that it is more likely to be taken. However, an increasing proportion of isolates of *Strep. pneumoniae* are resistant to it in some parts of Africa.

Coughs or colds

These do not require antibiotics. A child with a non-severe respiratory infection normally improves in 1 or 2 weeks. Symptomatic treatment such as cough linctus can be prescribed. However, a child with chronic cough (more than 30 days) needs to be further assessed to exclude tuberculosis, asthma, whooping cough, or other less common respiratory conditions, and will therefore be referred.

Adaptations of the IMCI algorithm which include the presence of wheeze are available for countries where asthma has emerged as major public health problem; but this is not (yet) the case in sub-Saharan Africa.

Diarrhoea

The assessment of diarrhoea in children is directed at three disease entities: the detection of dehydration, the diagnosis of dysentery, and the management of persistent diarrhoea.

The entry question is 'Does the child have diarrhoea?'. If the carer says 'yes', the health worker follows the flow in Fig. 9.4.

Based on the findings, the degree of dehydration is classified into three degrees of severity: no dehydration, some dehydration, and severe dehydration (Fig. 9.5). The principles of rehydration are summarized in three treatment plans, which are described in Chapter 20.

In addition to the classification of dehydration, a child who has bloody diarrhoea is managed for dysentery. If the diarrhoea has lasted longer than 14 days, a diagnosis of persistent diarrhoea is made. The principles of management of both conditions are described in Chapter 20.

Fever

Malaria is the main potentially life-threatening cause of fever in Africa. If the child has a generalized skin rash, together with fever, measles is the main condition to consider. Accordingly, these two diseases are prominent in the IMCI algorithm for fever. If the caretaker answers

Does the child have diarrhoea?

IF YES, ASK:	*LOOK, LISTEN, FEEL:*	
• For how long? • Is there blood in the stool	• Look at the child's general condition. Is the child: Lethargic or unconscious? Restless or irritable? • Look for sunken eyes. • Offer the child fluid. Is the child: Not able to drink or drinking poorly? Drinking eagerly, thirsty? • Pinch the skin of the abdomen. Does it go back: Very slowly (longer than 2 seconds)? Slowly?	***Classify DIARRHOEA***

Fig. 9.4. The IMCI assessment of a child who has diarrhoea.

SIGNS	CLASSIFY AS	IDENTIFY TREATMENT (Urgent pre-referral treatments are in bold print.)
Two of the following signs: • Lethargic or unconscious • Sunken eyes • Not able to drink or drinking poorly • Skin pinch goes back very slowly	**SEVERE DEHYDRATION**	➤ If child has no other severe classification: - Give fluid for severe dehydration (Plan C). OR ***If child also has another severe classification:*** ***- Refer URGENTLY to hospital with mother giving frequent sips of ORS on the way. Advise the mother to continue breast-feeding*** ➤ ***If child is 2 years or older and there is cholera in your area, give antibiotic for cholera .***
Two of the following signs: • Restless, irritable • Sunken eyes • Drinks eagerly, thirsty • Skin pinch goes back slowly	**SOME DEHYDRATION**	➤ Give fluid and food for some dehydration (Plan B). ➤ ***If child also has a severe classification:*** ***- Refer URGENTLY to hospital with mother giving frequent sips of ORS on the way. Advise the mother to continue breast-feeding*** ➤ Advise mother when to return immediately. ➤ Follow-up in 5 days if not improving.
Not enough signs to classify as some or severe dehydration.	**NO DEHYDRATION**	➤ Give fluid and food to treat diarrhoea at home (Plan A). ➤ Advise mother when to return immediately. ➤ Follow-up in 5 days if not improving.

Fig. 9.5. The classification of the severity of dehydration in a child with diarrhoea.

Does the child have fever?
(by history or feels hot or temperature 37.5 °C[a] or above)

IF YES:
Decide the Malaria Risk: high or low

THEN ASK:

- For how long?
- If more than 7 days, has fever been present every day?
- Has the child had measles within the last 3 months?

LOOK AND FEEL:

- Look or feel for stiff neck.
- Look for runny nose.

Look for signs of MEASLES

- Generalized rash and
- One of these: cough, runny nose, or red eyes.

If the child has measles now or within the last 3 months:

- Look for mouth ulcers.
  Are they deep and extensive?
- Look for pus draining from the eye.
- Look for clouding of the cornea.

Fig. 9.6. The IMCI assessment of a child who has fever. Based on axillary temperature.

that the child has fever, the health worker follows the outline in Fig. 9.6.

Malaria or meningitis

The further management decisions depend on the findings, and the malaria risk. If the malaria risk is high, every child with fever receives an anti-malarial. If the malaria risk is low, children with obvious other causes of fever, such as measles or an upper respiratory infection, are not immediately treated for malaria. Figure 9.7 gives the management guidelines for children with fever in a high malaria risk setting. Children who might have meningitis are identified in this category by having any of the danger signs or a stiff neck. As cerebral malaria and meningitis cannot be differentiated at first-level health facilities, pre-referral treatment covers both possibilities with an anti-malarial and an antibiotic to be given to the child prior to referral.

Measles

Children who have fever and a generalized rash are checked further for suggestive signs. The presence of cough, a runny nose or red eyes are considered diagnostic for measles. They are further checked for possible complications of measles, as indicated in Fig. 9.6, and classified as shown in Fig. 9.8.

Ear infections

Although ear infections rarely cause death, they are the main cause of hearing loss in low-income countries. This may result in learning problems. The clinical assessment assumes that otoscopy is not available and is therefore based on the following simple clinical signs:

(a) *Tender swelling behind the ear.* The most serious complication of an ear infection is mastoiditis, which manifests with tender swelling behind one of the child's ears.
(b) *Ear pain.* This is usually present in the early stages of acute otitis, and often causes the child to become irritable and rub the ear frequently.
(c) *Discharge of pus from the ear* may be seen later in the course of disease,. These findings are used for classification as shown in Fig. 9.9.

Malnutrition and anaemia

This part of the algorithm focuses on two contributors to child mortality which are rarely listed as direct causes, but nevertheless are estimated to contribute to over half of all childhood deaths. These are malnutrition and anaemia. Infection, particularly frequent or persistent diarrhoea, pneumonia, measles, and malaria, impair nutritional status. In addition, poor feeding practices such as inadequate breastfeeding, too little food, and poor food choice all contribute to malnutrition and anaemia. All children, irrespective of their complaints, are assessed for both malnutrition and anaemia, as shown in Fig. 9.10.

SIGNS	CLASSIFY AS	IDENTIFY TREATMENT (Urgent pre-referral treatments are in bold print.)
• Any general danger sign • Stiff neck	VERY SEVERE FEBRILE DISEASE	➤ ***Give quinine for severe malaria (fist dose).*** ➤ ***Give first dose of an appropriate antibiotic.*** ➤ ***Treat the child to prevent low blood sugar.*** ➤ ***Give one dose of paracetamol in clinic for high fever (38.5 °C or above).*** ➤ ***Refer URGENTLY to hospital.***
• Fever (by history or feels hot or temperature 37.5 °C[a] or above)	MALARIA	➤ ***If NO cough with fast breathing, treat with oral antimalarial.*** ➤ ***Give one dose of paracetamol in clinic for high fever (38.5 °C or above).*** ➤ Advise mother when to return immediately. ➤ Follow-up in 2 days if fever persists. ➤ If fever is present every day for more than 7 days, REFER for assessment.

[a] These temperatures are based on axillary temperature.

Fig. 9.7. Management of a child with fever in high malaria risk setting.

SIGNS	CLASSIFY AS	IDENTIFY TREATMENT (Urgent pre-referral treatments are in bold print.)
• Any general danger sign or • Clouding of cornea or • Deep or extensive mouth ulcers.	SEVERE COMPLICATED MEASLES[b]	➤ ***Give vitamin A.*** ➤ ***Give first dose of an appropriate antibiotic.*** ➤ ***If clouding of the cornea or pus draining from the eye, apply tetracycline eye ointment.*** ➤ ***Refer URGENTLY to hospital.***
• Pus draining from the eye or • Mouth ulcers	MEASLES WITH EYE OR MOUTH COMPLICATIONS[b]	➤ ***Give vitamin A.*** ➤ ***If pus draining from the eye, treat eye infection with tetracycline eye ointment.*** ➤ If mouth ulcers, treat with gentian violet. ➤ Follow-up in 2 days.
• Measles now or within the last 3 months.	MEASLES	➤ **Give vitamin A.**

[b] Other important complications of measles – pneumonia, stridor, diarrhoea, ear infection, and malnutrition – are classified in other tables.

Fig. 9.8. The classification of the severity of measles (if measles now or within the last 3 months).

For calculating the child's weight for age, use the local Road to Health cards. Figure 9.11 shows an example of such a card.

The classification of malnutrition or anaemia is shown in Fig. 9.12.

Checking immunization status

Illness episodes are not a contraindication to immunization and vaccine efficacy is not reduced in sick children. There are four contraindications to the immunization of sick children:

SIGNS	CLASSIFY AS	IDENTIFY TREATMENT (Urgent pre-referral treatments are in bold print.)
• Tender swelling behind the ear.	**MASTOIDITIS**	➤ ***Give first dose of an appropriate antibiotic.*** ➤ ***Give first dose of paracetamol for pain.*** ➤ ***Refer URGENTLY to hospital.***
• Pus is seen draining from the ear and discharge is reported for less than 14 days, or • Ear pain.	**ACUTE EAR INFECTION**	➤ ***Give an oral antibiotic for 5 days.*** ➤ Give paracetamol for pain. ➤ Dry the ear by wicking. ➤ Follow-up in 5 days.
• Pus is seen draining from the ear and discharge is reported for 14 days or more.	**CHRONIC EAR INFECTION**	➤ Dry the ear by wicking. ➤ Follow-up in 5 days.
• No ear pain and No pus seen draining from the ear.	**NO EAR INFECTION**	No additional treatment.

Fig. 9.9. Classification for ear problems.

THEN CHECK FOR MALNUTRITION AND ANAEMIA

LOOK AND FEEL:

- Look for visible severe wasting.
- Look for palmar pallor. Is it:
  Severe palmar pallor?
  Some palmar pallor?
- Look for oedema of both feet.
- Determine weight for age.

Classify NUTRITIONAL STATUS

Fig. 9.10. Assessment of the child for nutritional status or anaemia.

- Do not immunize children who are being referred urgently to hospital. There is no medical contraindication: but if the child dies, the vaccine may be incorrectly blamed for the death.
- Do not give BCG or yellow fever vaccines to a child with symptomatic HIV infection/AIDS, but do give the other vaccines. Give all immunizations, including BCG and yellow fever vaccines, to a child with asymptomatic HIV infection.
- Do not give DPT-2 or -3 to a child who has had convulsions or shock within 3 days of the most recent dose. Do not give DPT to a child with recurrent convulsions or an active neurological disease of the central nervous system.
- A child with diarrhoea who is due to receive OPV should be given a dose of OPV. However, this dose should *not* be counted in the schedule. Mark the fact that it coincided with diarrhoea on the child's immunization record, so that the health worker will know this and give the child an extra dose.

Table 9.1 shows the generic WHO immunization recommendations, which might have been adapted by countries to include other vaccines such as against hepatitis B, yellow fever, and *Haemophilus influenzae* type b.

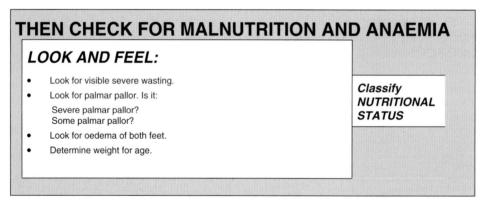

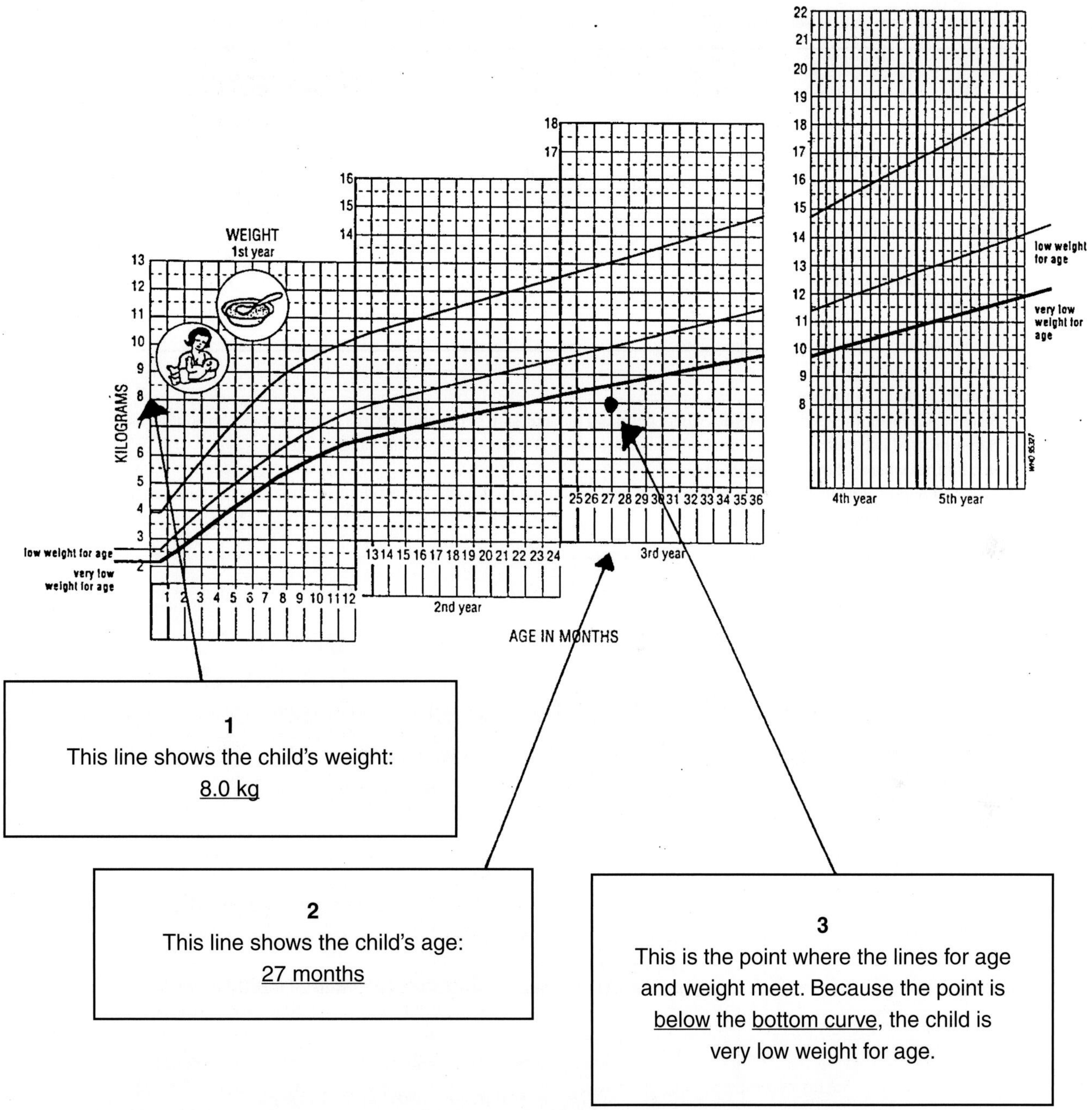

Fig. 9.11. Weight for age ('Road to Health') chart with the example of a child who is 2 years 3 months old and weighs 8 kg.

Neonatal period and early infancy

Mortality is highest in the neonatal period and in early infancy. During this period, young infants are less able to mount a response to infection, and clinical signs are often non-specific. Therefore, a separate chart deals with infants between 1 week and 2 months of life (Chapter 10). The IMCI guidelines were not targeted to include sick newborns less than 1 week old. In the first week of life, illnesses in newborns are often due to perinatal factors, or have conditions that require specific interventions. Common conditions include birth asphyxia, sepsis from premature ruptured membranes or other intrauterine infections, birth trauma, respiratory distress syndrome, or jaundice. For these perinatal problems, separate guidelines called the 'Integrated Management of Pregnancy

Table 9.1. Immunization schedule for infants recommended by the Expanded Programme on Immunization

Vaccine	Age: Birth	6 weeks	10 weeks	14 weeks	9 months
BCG	✗				
Oral polio	✗[a]	✗	✗	✗	
DTP		✗	✗	✗	
Hepatitis B Scheme A[b]	✗	✗		✗	
Scheme B[b]		✗	✗	✗	
Haemophilus influenzae type b		✗	✗	✗	
Yellow fever					✗[c]
Measles					✗[d]

Notes:

[a] In polio-endemic countries.

[b] Scheme A is recommended in countries where perinatal transmission of hepatitis B virus is frequent (e.g. in South-East Asia). Scheme B may be used in countries where perinatal transmission is less frequent (e.g. in sub-Saharan Africa.

[c] In countries where yellow fever poses a risk.

[d] A second opportunity to receive a dose of measles vaccine should be provided for all children. This may be done either as part of the routine or in a campaign.

SIGNS	CLASSIFY AS	IDENTIFY TREATMENT (Urgent pre-referral treatments are in bold print.)
• Visible severe wasting or • Severe palmar pallor or • Oedema of both feet.	SEVERE MALNUTRITION OR SEVERE ANAEMIA	➤ ***Give Vitamin A.*** ➤ ***Refer URGENTLY to hospital.***
• Some palmar pallor or • Very low weight for age.	ANAEMIA OR VERY LOW WEIGHT	➤ Assess the child's feeding and counsel the mother on feeding according to the FOOD box on the *COUNSEL THE MOTHER chart.* - If feeding problem, follow-up in 5 days. ➤ If pallor: - Give iron. - ***Give oral antimalarial if high malaria risk.*** - Give mebendazole if child is 2 years or older and has not had a dose in the previous 6 months. ➤ Advise mother when to return immediately. ➤ If pallor, follow-up in 14 days. If very low weight for age, follow-up in 30 days.
• Not very low weight for age and no other signs or malnutrition.	NO ANAEMIA AND NOT VERY LOW WEIGHT	➤ If child is less than 2 years old, assess the child's feeding and counsel the mother on feeding according to the FOOD box on the *COUNSEL THE MOTHER* chart. - If feeding problem, follow-up in 5 days. ➤ Advise mother when to return immediately.

Fig. 9.12. Classification of malnutrition or anaemia.

and Childbirth (IMPAC)' have been developed, which are adapted to country needs similarly to the IMCI process described above.

For a sick neonate or young infant brought to a health worker, a list of questions and examinations are included in the IMCI algorithm. They reflect the often subtle signs and non-specific response a neonate might show in response to infection. If any of these signs are present, a bacterial infection is assumed to be present, which would require referral for inpatient treatment. Only two signs of focal infection, skin pustules and a red umbilicus, are treated at the health facility. Figure 9.13 shows the details. The management of diarrhoea is similar to that in older children.

Feeding problems or low weight in young infants

Adequate feeding is essential for growth and development. Poor feeding during infancy can have lifelong effects. It is therefore important to assess a young infant's feeding and weight so that feeding can be improved if necessary. The best way to feed a young infant <6 months is to breastfeed exclusively. Exclusive breastfeeding means that the infant takes only breast milk, and no additional food, water or other fluids. (Medicines and vitamins are exceptions.) To determine whether there are any feeding problems, all young infants brought to the health facility are assessed, classified and treated according to the guidelines in Figs. 9.14 and 9.15.

Finally, young infants are checked for their immunization status and assessed for other problems, as is done for older children.

Counselling mothers

The success of outpatient management depends on the mother or carer's understanding of the illness and treatment, and their ability to continue this at home. The child's mother or carer needs to recognize when the child is not improving, or deteriorating.

Counselling a mother or carer includes the following.

SIGNS	CLASSIFY AS	IDENTIFY TREATMENT (Urgent pre-referral treatments are in bold print.)
• Convulsions or • Fast breathing (60 breaths per minute or more) or • Severe chest indrawing or • Nasal flaring or • Grunting or • Bulging fontanelle or • Pus draining from ear or • Umbilical redness extending to the skin or • Fever (37.5 °C[c] or above or feels hot) or low body temperature (less than 35.5 °C[c] or feels cold) • Many or severe skin pustules or • Lethargic or unconscious or • Less than normal movement.	**POSSIBLE SERIOUS BACTERIAL INFECTION**	➤ ***Give first dose of intramuscular antibiotics.*** ➤ ***Treat to prevent low blood sugar.*** ➤ ***Advise mother how to keep the infant warm on the way to hospital.*** ➤ ***Refer URGENTLY to hospital***
• Red umbilicus or draining pus or • Skin pustules.	**LOCAL BACTERIAL INFECTION**	➤ ***Give an appropriate oral antibiotic.*** ➤ Teach the mother to treat local infections at home. ➤ Advise mother to give home care for the young infant. ➤ Follow-up in 2 days.

[c] These thresholds are based on axillary temperature. The thresholds for rectal temperature are approximately 0.5 °C higher.

Fig. 9.13. Classification table for possible bacterial infection in young infants.

THEN CHECK FOR FEEDING PROBLEM OR LOW WEIGHT

ASK:

- Is there any difficulty feeding?
- Is the infant breastfed? If yes, How many times in 24 hours?
- Does the infant usually receive any other foods or drinks? If yes, how often?
- What do you use to feed the infant?

LOOK, LISTEN, FEEL:

- Determine weight for age.

IF AN INFANT: **Has any difficulty feeding,**
Is breastfeeding less than 8 times in 24 hours,
Is taking any other foods or drinks, or
Is low weight for age,

AND

Has no indications to refer urgently to hospital:

ASSESS BREAST-FEEDING:

- Has the infant breast-fed in the previous hour?

If the infant has not fed in the previous hour, ask the mother to put her infant to the breast. Observe the breastfeed for 4 minutes.

(If the infant was fed during the last hour, ask the mother if she can wait and tell you when the infant is willing to feed again.)

- Is the infant able to attach?

no attachment at all not well attached good attachment

TO CHECK ATTACHMENT, LOOK FOR:
- Chin touching breast
- Mouth wide open
- Lower lip turned outward
- More areola visible above then below the mouth

(All these signs should be present if the attachment is good.)

- Is the infant suckling effectively (that is, slow deep sucks, sometimes pausing)?

no suckling at all not suckling effectively suckling effectively

Clear a blocked nose if it interferes with breastfeeding.

- Look for ulcers or white patches in the mouth (thrush).

Fig. 9.14. Checking a young infant for feeding problems or low weight.

Advising on feeding and fluid intake

Children may become anorexic and drink less when they are sick. However, fluid intake should be increased and appropriate food offered frequently to prevent growth faltering.

Counselling to solve feeding problems

Breastfeeding, improved weaning practices with appropriate energy and nutrient rich foods, and offering nutritious snacks to children 2 years or older, can prevent growth faltering. The frequency of feeding is age dependent. Encourage exclusive breast-feeding for the first 4 months, and if possible, up to 6 months. Bottle-feeding should be avoided at any age. For mothers of breastfeeding infants, correct positioning and attachment is important.

Advising on when to return

Every mother or carer needs advice about when to be reviewed or when to return immediately to the health facility.

The process of referral

All infants and children with a severe classification (pink) are referred to hospital after the necessary pre-

SIGNS	CLASSIFY AS	IDENTIFY TREATMENT (Urgent pre-referral treatments are in bold print.)
• Not able to feed or • No attachment at all or • Not suckling at all.	NOT ABLE TO FEED – POSSIBLE SERIOUS BACTERIAL INFECTION	➤ ***Give first dose of intramuscular antibiotics.*** ➤ ***Treat to prevent low blood sugar.*** ➤ ***Advise the mother how to keep the young infant warm on the way to hospital.*** ➤ ***Refer URGENTLY to hospital.***
• Not well attached to breast or • Not suckling effectively or • Less than 8 breast-feeds in 24 hours or • Receives other foods or drinks or • Low weight for age or • Thrush (ulcers or white patches in mouth).	FEEDING PROBLEM OR LOW WEIGHT	➤ Advise the mother to breast-feed as often and for as long as the infant wants, day and night. • If not well attached or not suckling effectively, teach correct positioning and attachment. • If breastfeeding less than 8 times in 24 hours, advise to increase frequency of feeding. ➤ If receiving other foods or drinks, counsel mother about breast-feeding more, reducing other foods or drinks, and using a cup. • If not breast-feeding at all: – Refer for breast-feeding counselling and possible relactation. – Advise about correctly prepared breast milk substitutes and using a cup. ➤ If thrush, teach the mother to treat thrush at home. ➤ Advise mother to give home care for the young infant. ➤ Follow-up any feeding problem or thrush in 2 days. Follow-up low weight for age in 14 days.
• Not low weight for age and no other signs of inadequate feeding.	NO FEEDING PROBLEM	➤ Advise mother to give home care for the young infant. ➤ Praise the mother for feeding the infant well.

Fig. 9.15. Classification table for feeding problem or low weight.

referral treatment is administered. Successful referral of severely ill children to the hospital depends on effective communication with the carer. If referral is not accepted, the child may be managed by repeated clinic or home visits. If the carer accepts referral, s/he should be given advice regarding management during transfer.

Depending on the child's classification, the following pre-referral treatment is given at the health facility:

- appropriate antibiotic;
- quinine (for severe malaria);
- vitamin A;
- breast milk or sugar water to prevent hypoglycaemia;
- oral anti-malarial;
- paracetamol for high fever (38.5 °C or above) or pain;
- tetracycline eye ointment (if corneal clouding or conjunctivitis);
- ORS solution so that the mother can give frequent sips on the way to the hospital.

The first four treatments above are urgent because they can prevent progression of bacterial meningitis or cerebral malaria, corneal rupture due to lack of vitamin A, or brain damage from hypoglycaemia. The other listed treatments can prevent clinical deterioration.

For young infants in the first 2 months of life, urgent pre-referral treatment includes a first dose of intramuscular or oral antibiotic in the case of a possible severe bacterial infection, advice on preventing hypothermia,

Table 9.2. Possible diagnoses of children referred to hospital with four main symptoms included in the ICMI algorithm

Main symptoms and possible diagnoses			
Unconsciousness, lethargy or convulsions	Cough or difficult breathing	Diarrhoea	Fever
• Meningitis	• Pneumonia	• Acute watery diarrhoea	• Malaria
• Cerebral malaria (only in children exposed to *P. falciparum* transmission, often seasonal)	• Malaria	• Cholera	• Septicaemia
• Febrile convulsions (not likely to be cause of unconsciousness)	• Severe anaemia	• Dysentery	• Typhoid
• Hypoglycaemia (always seek the cause)	• Cardiac failure	• Persistent diarrhoea	• Urinary tract infection
• Head injury	• Congenital heart disease	• Diarrhoea with severe malnutrition	• HIV infection
• Poisoning	• Tuberculosis	• Intussusception	• Meningitis
• Shock (can cause lethargy or unconsciousness, but is unlikely to cause convulsions)	• Pertussis		• Otitis media
• Acute glomerulonephritis with encephalopathy	• Foreign body		• Osteomyelitis
• Diabetic ketoacidosis	• Empyema		• Septic arthritis
• Encephalitis	• Pneumothorax		• Skin and soft tissue infection
	• Pneumocystis pneumonia		• Pneumonia
	• Asthma		• Viral infections
			• Throat abscess
			• Sinusitis
			• Measles
			• Meningococcal infection
			• Relapsing fever
			• Typhus
			• Dengue haemorrhagic fever

prevention of hypoglycaemia with breast milk or sugar water, and frequent sips of ORS solution on the way to the hospital in the case of dehydration

Management at the level of the small hospital

Severely ill children referred to hospital should be reassessed using the expertise and diagnostic capabilities of the hospital setting. Triage is the first step in assessing children referred to a hospital (**see** Paediatric Emergencies, Chapter 97). Children with emergency signs such as airway obstruction, severe respiratory distress, central cyanosis, signs of shock, coma, convulsions, or signs of severe dehydration require immediate treatment. Those with priority signs should be assessed and treated without delay: visible severe wasting, oedema of both feet, severe palmar pallor, any sick young infant (less than two months), lethargy, continual irritability and restlessness, major burns, any respiratory distress, or urgent referral note from another health facility. Non-urgent cases have neither emergency nor priority signs and are treated in their turn.

Table 9.2 gives the main differential diagnoses of children referred with severe IMCI classifications.

Further reading

WHO Division of Diarrhoeal and Acute Respiratory Disease Control. (1995). Integrated management of the sick child. *Bull WHO*; **73**: 735–740.

Tulloch J. (1999). Integrated approach to child health in developing countries. *Lancet*; **354**(2): SII16–SII20.

Weber MW, Mulholland EK, Jaffar S, Troedsson H, Gove S, Greenwood BM. (1997). Evaluation of an algorithm for the integrated management of childhood illness in an area with seasonal malaria in the Gambia. *Bull WHO*; **75**(1): 25–32.

World Health Organization. (2000). *Management of the Child with a Serious Infection or Severe Malnutrition. Guidelines for Care at the First-Referral Level in Developing Countries.* Geneva (WHO/FCH/CAH/00.1).

Website of the WHO Department of Child and Adolescent Health and Development, which contains all documents and the above charts as files that can be accessed and downloaded: URL: http://www.who.int/child-adolescent-health/

Neonatal care

10

Introduction

In all countries, a high proportion of infant deaths occur in the first days and weeks of life. In developing countries as a whole, around one-third of the 10 million infant deaths occur before 28 completed days of life. In Africa, the neonatal mortality rate can be as high as 50 per thousand live births. Most of these deaths are avoidable with simple interventions in the antenatal, perinatal and immediately post-natal periods. The purpose of this chapter is to describe the preventive and therapeutic interventions which can be carried out in the neonatal period with the basic skills, drugs and equipment that are usually available at primary care level and at first referral level.

Four sequential and equally important aspects of care can be identified in neonatal care:

- safe delivery
- essential neonatal care for all newborns
- assessment and management of the most frequent and serious problems of newborn babies
- advice for the mother.

Essential steps to good neonatal care prior to delivery

Good prenatal and delivery care play a vital role in ensuring that newborn babies are healthy. It is particularly important to ensure that at risk deliveries are detected and take place in the safest available place. The place of birth may well be at home, provided that a safe and clean delivery can be ensured by a skilled professional and that there are no major risk factors or complications. But in many instances, and particularly in the poorest areas, as many as one-third of mothers are at risk and as many as 15–20 per cent of babies are low birth weight (Bique Osman et al., 2001). Many mothers and babies will need additional care and support due to a variety of medical and social problems.

As a health professional responsible for maternity care make every effort to:

- promote good practices, coordination of care and timely identification of at risk cases.
- work with the community to disseminate information on good practices and on the timely identification of risk signs and symptoms during pregnancy and labour.
- coordinate messages relating to the care of the woman and the newborn during pregnancy, delivery and the post-partum period with health providers, women's groups and other community groups
- establish links with traditional birth attendants and traditional healers who are working in the area. You should recognize their role in the community, seek their collaboration in disseminating information on good perinatal practices, and hold discussions with them to identify safe and unsafe community practices.

Discuss the requirements for essential care for normal deliveries, and if possible reach a consensus with all parties involved. Discuss criteria for identifying at risk women who may need to be transferred before delivery, or who may need additional support from the community. Discuss ways to ensure, perhaps through informal networks, that transport will be available when necessary, and prepare an action plan to respond to emergencies. These aspects need to be planned in advance, as in an emergency transport may not be available, or time may be insufficient given the condition of the mother. Identify a clean place for delivery, and ensure that essential drugs, supplies and equipment are available (Table 10.1).

Table 10.1. Essential steps to good neonatal care prior to delivery

– Community information and networking to coordinate pregnancy delivery and post-partum care
– Identification and recognition of at risk cases
– Organization of timely transport when necessary
– Procurement of essential equipment, drugs and supplies.

Table 10.2. Essential equipment for delivery

– a clean surface for the mother to deliver on to
– a warm room
– clean warm towels and a blanket for drying, covering and wrapping the baby
– a sterile kit to cut and tie the cord
– water and soap for clean hands

Table 10.3. Newborn Resuscitation

1. Clamp and cut the cord if necessary.
2. Place the baby on a dry clean and warm surface (use radiant heater or lamp).
3. Position head so that it is in the neutral position (with the neck neither flexed nor extended).
4. Suction mouth and nose (introduce not more than 5 cm from lips and 3 cm from nostrils and suck while withdrawing).
5. If still not breathing, start ventilating (a newborn face mask should be used and sealed to cover mouth and nose): squeeze first two or three times and observe rise of chest. If not rising, reposition head, check mask seal and squeeze bag with whole hand.
6. When chest is rising, ventilate at 40/min.
7. Stop when newborn starts crying or breathing and observe for 1 minute.
8. If breathing less than 30/min or there is severe chest indrawing, continue ventilating and give oxygen if available.
9. If no breathing or gasping at all after 20 min of ventilation, stop ventilating.
10. If breathing more than 30/min and no severe chest indrawing, stop ventilating, put the baby skin to skin to mother's chest and check breathing and temperature every 15 minutes.

Essential care for all newborn babies at birth

Many serious problems can be prevented through simple interventions carried out at birth in all babies, either at home or at the health facility, by trained birth attendants with the simple skills and basic equipment shown in Table 10.2.

Remember that newborn babies can feel, see and hear and must be handled gently. Treat mothers with respect. Explain procedures to the mother in clear language. If other members of the family are present, explain what you are doing to them too.

There are four essential steps to the care of a newborn baby at birth:

- assessment of breathing and resuscitation if necessary
- management of the cord
- thermal protection of the baby
- support for breast-feeding.

Assessment of breathing and resuscitation

In a normal delivery with clear amniotic fluid there is no need to clean the mouth and throat of the baby by suction or wiping. It is better not to interfere unless there is a good reason to do so. As soon as the baby is born, while drying the baby, check that it is breathing normally. If the baby is crying or breathing regularly (chest rising regularly between 40 and 60 times per minute) there is no need to intervene. If the baby is not breathing, is gasping or breathing irregularly within 1 minute of birth, start resuscitation procedures immediately (Table 10.3) (WHO, 1999).

Thermal protection of the baby

The skin temperature of a newborn baby falls within seconds of birth. This is normal and helps the baby to start breathing. However, if cooling continues, the body temperature will drop below 36.5 °C and hypothermia may occur. To prevent hypothermia, the concept of the 'warm chain', i.e. a set of interlinked procedures, has been introduced (WHO, 1993). They include: a warm (ideally above 25 °C) and draught-free room; immediate drying of the newborn baby; wrapping the baby in a warm clean towel and giving it to the mother quickly after birth, possibly placed on the mother's abdomen; putting the baby on the mother's breast; putting a warm cap on the baby's head unless the ambient temperature is particularly warm (above 25 °C).

At birth, remove only blood or meconium from the baby's skin, with a warm clean cloth. Do not remove vernix or bathe the baby until at least 6 hours of age, to allow for thermal stabilization. If transport is necessary, ensure skin-to-skin contact with the mother or adequate wrapping and protection.

Table 10.4. The necessary steps to help the mother initiate breast-feeding soon after birth

- Avoid giving the mother any medicines during labour which make the baby sleepy after birth.
- After birth, let the baby rest on the mother's chest in skin-to-skin contact.
- Tell mother to help the baby to her breast when the baby seems to be ready.
- Check that position and attachment are correct at the first feed.
- Help the baby have the first feed if the mother feels too tired.
- Keep the mother and baby in close contact as much as possible during the first days.
- Delay routine birth procedures such as weighing until after the first feed.

Management of the cord

Birth attendants should keep their hands clean, wash them often and, if possible, use sterile gloves during delivery. There is no need to clamp and cut the cord in a rush, except when resuscitation is needed. The baby can be dried and given to the mother first, and the cord cut when it stops pulsing (Bergstrom et al., 1994). It does not matter what instrument is used to cut the cord as long as it is sterile. Any sterile tie, such as string boiled for 20 minutes, will work, as long as it is tied very tight and checked in the first hours after birth to make sure there is no bleeding. Infections can enter the cord after birth. The cord should be kept clean and dry. Bandages are not helpful. Cutting the cord and handling the placenta may be bound by tradition in different cultures. It is important that health personnel are aware of these traditions and of the mother's own requests, and that they try to fulfil these as far as possible if they are safe for the mother and the baby. Advise mothers and their families not to apply any other substances such as ash or cow dung. Expose the cord to the air and leave it to dry. If it gets dirty with the baby's urine or faeces, it is sufficient to wash it with clean water. If the cord starts producing pus or has a foul smell, this is a danger sign, which should be appropriately assessed and treated (see below).

Support to breast-feeding

Exclusive and prolonged breast-feeding is very important for the baby's survival and wellbeing in the first year of life (WHO Collaborative Study Team, 2000; WHO, 1998). Counselling on the importance of exclusive breast-feeding should ideally start during pregnancy. Birth is a crucial time for initiation and support of breast-feeding. If put in skin-to-skin contact with their mothers, most newborn babies will start looking for the breast and nipple within 15–30 minutes from birth after a normal delivery. Health workers should help mothers to start breast-feeding (see Table 10.4). See Table 10.5 for recommendations for mothers suspected to be HIV positive.

Breast-feeding should start as soon after birth as possible. Putting a limit on the length and frequency of feeds is not helpful. Bottles and teats should not be used, and other fluids should not be given. Inform mothers about the benefits of breast-feeding, encourage them to sleep in the same room as the baby and support them in case of problems. Teach them correct positioning and attachment (see Figs. 10.1–10.3), especially if first time or adolescent mothers.

Artificial teats or pacifiers should not be used.

Mothers who are not breast-feeding because they are too sick or the baby is ill or too small to suckle should be given special support and advice (see below, management of feeding problems)

Recommendations for known or strongly suspected HIV-positive mothers are shown in Table 10.5.

Other preventive measures

Protection against eye infection must be given routinely to all babies (Bergstrom et al., 1994; WHO, 1997). Wipe the eyes with a clean cloth (wipe each eye with a separate cloth or use a different corner of the cloth) soon after

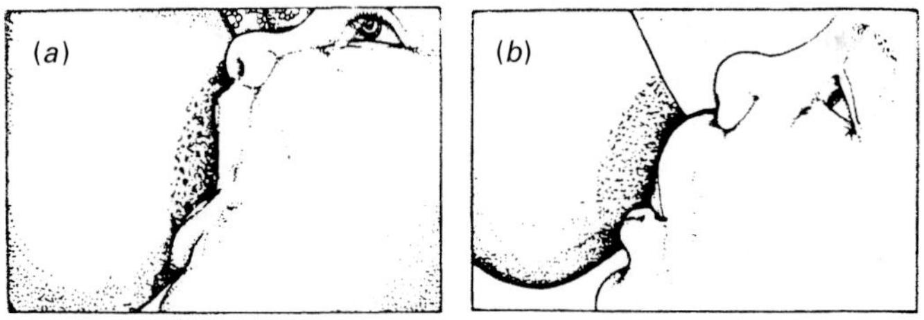

Fig. 10.1. (*a*) Good and (*b*) poor attachment of infant to the mother's breast.

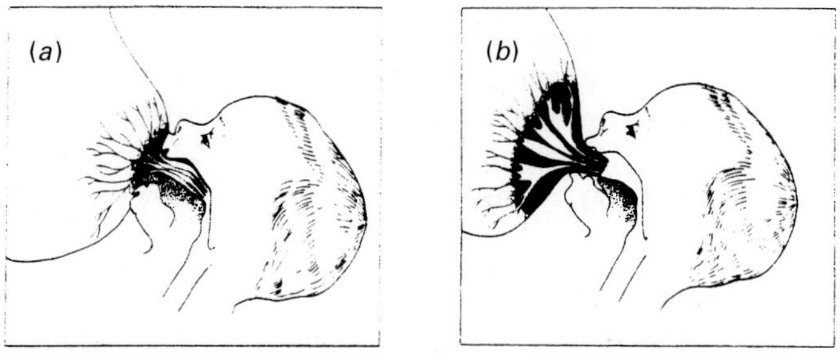

Fig.10.2. (*a*) Good and (*b*) poor attachment – cross-sectional view of the breast and baby.

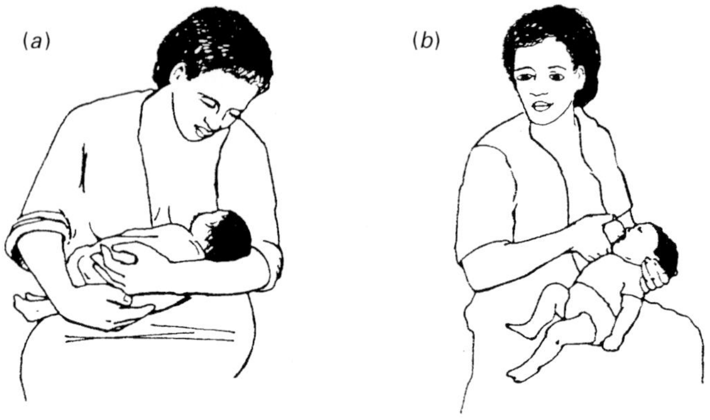

Fig. 10.3. (*a*) Good and (*b*) poor positioning of infant for breast-feeding.

birth. An anti-microbial should then be applied to both eyes, according to national guidelines. The following have been shown to be effective in preventing gonococcal ophthalmia neonatorum (a common and potentially blinding condition):

- 1 per cent silver nitrate solution
- 1 per cent tetracycline ointment
- 2.5 per cent solution of povidone–iodine

Where there is a high risk of TB, a BCG vaccination should be given by intradermal injection soon after birth. The mother should be advised to get the baby immunized according to the local schedule.

Assessment and management of common newborn problems

After birth, all babies should be thoroughly examined: in the first hour of life if a health professional attended the birth, or within 12 hours after birth if the baby is seen for the first time after a home delivery. Babies born at a health facility should be examined at birth and again before discharge. The examination should include an assessment of maternal risk factors and of the newborn baby's danger signs. Chart 1 and the following notes provide a guide to assessment, classification, treatment and advice to mothers (Bergstrom et al., 1994; WHO, 1997; Klaus & Fanaroff, 1995; Sinclair & Bracken, 1998).

Assessing mother's risk factors and baby's danger signs

Mother HIV-positive

Ask the mother and check all available records. Consider also probable HIV infection if high prevalence area and mother shows signs of disease.

Table 10.5. Recommendations for feeding babies from HIV positive mothers

– When replacement feeding is acceptable, feasible, affordable, sustainable and safe, avoidance of all breast-feeding by HIV-infected mothers is recommended.
– Otherwise, exclusive breast-feeding is recommended during the first months of life.
– To minimize HIV transmission risk, breast-feeding should be discontinued as soon as feasible, taking into account local circumstances, the individual woman's situation and the risks of replacement feeding (including infections other than HIV, and malnutrition).
– When HIV-infected mothers choose not to breast-feed from birth or stop breast-feeding later, they should be provided with specific guidance and support for at least the first 2 years of the child's life to ensure adequate replacement feeding.

Source: From: WHO Technical Consultation, 2000.

Maternal TB treatment

Baby at risk if treatment started less than two months before delivery

Signs of infection in the mother

Membranes ruptured more than 18 hours before birth; mother being treated with antibiotics; fever above 38 °C; amniotic fluid stained.

Low birth weight

The traditional definition include babies weighing less than 2500 g. Most babies with a weight above 2000 g at birth will not show any problems if essential care is provided at the time of birth.

Malformations

A standard textbook should be referred to for the management of major malformations. Cleft lip and palate is a rather frequent problem that poses specific feeding problems, due to the difficulty of sucking when the defect is wide. Provide special support for breast-feeding and consider alternative feeding methods.

Breathing

Any among the following: grunting, very fast breathing (>80/min); slow breathing (<30/min); severe chest indrawing; cyanosis.

Temperature

Moderate hypothermia is between 35 °C and 35.9 °C. Severe hypothermia is below 35 °C. Severe hypothermia is a danger sign for possible serious illness.

Chart 1. Assessment classification and treatment of the newborn baby soon after birth

Assess for maternal factors and danger signs	Classify	Treat and advise
Maternal Factors		
Known HIV +	Risk HIV	Counsel on feeding Arrange for follow-up
Syphilis test +	Risk Congenital Syphilis	Give benzathine penicillin[a]
TB treatment	Risk TB	Give isoniazid[a]; BCG when treatment completed; follow-up
Fever or other signs of possible infection	Risk bacterial infections	Give ampicillin + gentamicin[a]
Mother very ill or transferred	Not able to breast-feed	Arrange for alternative feeding
Danger signs		
VLBW (<1500 g)	Risk respiratory distress: risk severe infection	Keep warm; provide care for LBW; consider referral;
LBW (<2500 g)	Risk hypothermia\hypoglycaemia	Provide care for LBW
Malformations	Risk feeding difficulties, mother's concern; specific problems	Consider referral; counsel mother; provide specific care
Breathing difficulty	Possible serious illness	Give oxygen; rewarm; give ampicillin + gentamicin[a]
Temperature <36 °C	Hypothermia	Rewarm; check temperature
Floppy	Possible severe illness	Give oxygen; ampicillin + gentamicin[a]
Stiff/convulsing	Possible severe illness	Give oxygen; give ampicillin + gentamicin[a]; treat convulsions[b]
Not able to feed	Possible serious illness; breast-feeding problems; possible thrush	Check breast-feeding and advise; treat thrush; treat infection
Severe jaundice	Possible severe illness	Give ampicillin + gentamicin[a]; encourage breast-feeding
Umbilicus bleeding	Umbilical bleeding	Stop bleeding; re-tie cord
Umbilicus redness or purulent	Serious umbilical infection	Give antibiotic[a]
Eyes swollen or purulent	Eye infection	Give antibiotic[a]
Swelling of head; asymmetrical arm movements	Birth injury	Advise mother and family;
Ulcers and white patches in mouth	Thrush	Treat with nystatin or gentian violet Advise mother

Notes:

[a] see section on antibiotic therapy below for details.

[b] give phenobarbitone 15–20 mg per kg i.m. or preferably rectal diazepam 1 mg per kg

Floppy

Hypotonia may be due to asphyxia, sepsis or severe hypothermia.

Stiff/convulsing

Usually due to severe asphyxia or CNS infection; newborn babies may show fine tremors at the extremities which should not be confused with convulsions. Neonatal tetanus is not symptomatic before 3 to 10 days after birth.

Jaundice

Should be considered severe when both palms and soles are yellow and in all preterm infants. Mild jaundice after the second day of life in a full-term and otherwise normal baby is not a danger sign, unless it persists after 10 days.

Inflamed umbilicus

Is a danger sign for possible severe infection if extending to peri-umbilical skin.

Birth injury

If an arm is not moving, handle gently, do not pull the arm. In most cases it will recover in 1–2 weeks. Head swelling will also disappear in 1–2 weeks.

Case management

Further diagnostic work-up for newborns with signs of severe infection

Usually signs of infections in the first 7 days of life are quite non-specific, and since the risk of sepsis is very high, newborns should be treated for sepsis when danger signs or maternal risk factors for severe infections are present. If meningitis is suspected, a lumbar puncture (LP) and cerebrospinal fluid (CSF) examination may be performed, provided that the procedure can be safely carried out. Standard treatment for severe infection should be started without delay.

Antibiotic therapy

Ampicillin (if not available, give i.m. benzylpenicillin 50 000 units per kg twice a day) and gentamicin should be administered i.m. for 10 days in babies classified as at risk of severe infection. Asymptomatic babies classified as at risk of severe infection (for example for maternal signs of infection) should be treated for 5 days. A first dose of ampicillin and gentamicin should also be given to babies at risk for infection who need to be referred. Intramuscular antibiotics should be injected in the thigh. A new syringe and needle should be used for each antibiotic. Due to the immature metabolism and slower renal clearance, the dosage of antibiotics must be appropriate to the baby's gestational age and weight (see Table 10.6 for dosages of ampicillin and gentamicin).

If the mother is seropositive for syphilis, benzathine penicillin should be given to baby i.m. in a single dose (50 000 units per kg).

Suspected gonococcal eye infection should be treated with ceftriaxone 50 mg per kg once; kanamicin (25 mg per kg once up to a maximum of 75 mg) is an alternative, albeit less safe and effective.

Thrush (*Candida albicans* infection)should be treated with nystatin (100 000 units/ml suspension), 1–2 ml dropped in mouth, four times a day for 7 days. If not available, apply 0.25 per cent gentian violet solution with clean cloth four times a day.

Isoniazid prophylaxis (5 mg/kg) should be given orally once a day for 6 months to infants of mothers with sputum positive TB. BCG should be delayed until treatment is completed. Mothers should be told that breast-feeding is safe and advised to return to follow-up every 2 weeks to assess the baby's weight gain.

Table 10.6. Recommended dosages of ampicillin and gentamicin according to body weight in the first week of life

Weight	Ampicillin IM Dose: 50 mg per kg every 12 hours. Add 2.5 ml sterile water to 500 mg vial = 200 mg/ml	Gentamicin IM Dose: 5 mg per kg every 24 hours (4 mg in preterm babies) 20 mg per 2 ml vial = 10 mg/ml
1.0–1.4 kg	0.35 ml	0.5 ml
1.5–1.9 kg	0.5 ml	0.7 ml
2.0–2.4 kg	0.6 ml	0.9 ml
2.5–2.9 kg	0.75 ml	1.35 ml
3.0–3.4 kg	0.85 ml	1.6 ml
3.5–3.9 kg	1 ml	1.85 ml
4.0–4.4 kg	1.1 ml	2.1 ml

Feeding

Breast-feeding should be assessed at any time the baby is examined to ensure a good technique and to identify and manage any feeding difficulties (see chart 2).

Alternative feeding methods must be considered when the baby is not able to suckle or when the mother cannot breast feed or when breast-feeding is not advisable (mother HIV +). Expressed breast milk should be used for small preterm babies and babies who are too sick to suckle. In this case cup feeding is recommended. Cup feeding is a very effective technique (Gupta et al, 1999). It can be handled successfully provided that the correct technique is used (Table 10.7).

Assessment of cup feeding is also made by baby's weight. Weight loss should be less than 10 per cent in the first week of life: the baby should gain at least 150 g/week in the following weeks.

Mothers should be taught to express their milk by themselves and to feed the baby by cup. Expressed milk should be used immediately to feed the baby. If not, it should be stored in a cool clean and safe place. Breast milk can be also expressed directly into the baby's mouth. This technique resembles cup feeding in that the baby is allowed to smell and lick the nipple and attempt to suck, then some breast milk is expressed into the baby's mouth: it must be repeated more frequently (every 1–2 hours).

Babies of 30–32 or fewer weeks of gestational age may need to be fed by nasogastric tube. Expressed breast milk should be used if possible. The mother may let the baby suck on her finger while being tube fed: this may stimulate the baby's digestive tract and the suckling reflex. If

Chart 2. Assessment classification and management of feeding difficulties at birth

Assess breast-feeding and mother's breasts	Classify	Treat and advise
Exclusive breast-feeding on demand Good suckling Healthy breasts	Feeding well	Encourage mother to continue Advise to seek help if any difficulty
Not able to feed at all	Serious baby's problem (sepsis, VLBW, malformation, others)	Examine the baby Manage accordingly
Not suckling effectively Not well attached to breast Feeding <8 times per day Receiving other fluids	Feeding difficulties	Assess next feed and examine the baby Advise the mother on exclusive breast-feeding; feeding on demand, correct position and attachment Reassess in 1–2 days
Both breasts swollen and patchy red; no fever or less than 38 °C	Breast engorgement	Improve attachment and increase frequency
Nipple soreness with or without fissures	Sore nipples, fissures	Improve positioning and attachment
Part of breast painful swollen and red Fever < 38 °C Feels ill	Mastitis	Improve attachment Follow up in 24 hours: if no improvement, fever continues: cloxacillin for 10 days

Table 10.7. Cup feeding

- Hold the baby in a semi-upright position on the lap.
- Hold the cup to the baby's lips and tip it so that milk just reaches the baby's lips
- Do not pour milk into the baby's mouth. The baby will become alert and start sucking the milk
- Stop feeding when the baby will not show any interest in taking more
- Give 80 ml/kg on day 1 and increase by 10–20 ml until 150 ml/kg per day
- Give the suggested amount every 2–3 hours in divided doses
- If the baby dose not take the calculated amount during the 24 hours, feed more often

the mother does not express enough milk or cannot breast-feed at all, consider giving donated heat-treated breast milk or home-made or commercial formula.

Mothers who are not breast-feeding at all (baby died, mother chose replacement feeding or advised to do so) may be uncomfortable for a while. Avoid any stimulation of the breast and advise the mother to express just enough milk to relieve discomfort and to seek advice if the breasts become painful, swollen or red or if fever appears.

Oxygen and respiratory support

If the baby shows moderate respiratory distress with spontaneous breathing, oxygen and air under normal pressure can be used. In this situation the oxygen administration technique to the newborn does not differ from that used to older infants (see Chapter 16). Concentrations of up to 40 per cent oxygen can be achieved through a nasal catheter. A flow of 0.5–1 litres/min will be sufficient.

If the child deteriorates, the air-oxygen must be delivered under continuous positive pressure (CPAP). This method requires that compressed air is available. In CPAP the humidified warm gas–air mixture is pressure controlled by a water-lock, and connected to a nasal catheter by a T-piece with a variable leakage. A CPAP of 2–6 cm H_2O is normally used. In wards with limited resources CPAP is an extremely cost-effective method and when used at an early stage most infants with respiratory problems will be successfully treated. Details on CPAP can be obtained from standard neonatal textbooks.

Rewarming

Prompt and effective rewarming is very important as hypothermia can be a contributing factor for generalized infection (sepsis) and asphyxia, and diminish the baby's response to infections. Incubators are traditionally used for this purpose but rewarming can be achieved even more safely and effectively through skin-to-skin contact (Christensson et al., 1998; Ludington et al., 2000). The baby's clothing should be removed and the baby should be placed skin-to-skin on the mother's chest dressed in a pre-warmed shirt open at the front. The baby should wear a hat, socks and a nappy. The mother should be covered with her clothes plus an additional, possibly pre-warmed, blanket. The baby should be kept in this position until the temperature is in the normal range. The temperature of the room should be at least 25 °C.

Care of low birth weight neonates

The major problems that a small baby may encounter are feeding problems and hypothermia. Hypoglycaemia is also frequent, as a consequence of inadequate feeding and hypothermia. It can be prevented by ensuring adequate thermal protection and feeding. Small preterm babies may have suckling difficulties and therefore may need alternative feeding for some time.

Kangaroo mother care (KMC) is an effective strategy for providing comprehensive care for small babies when resources are scarce (Charpak et al., 1997). KMC is defined as early prolonged and continuous skin-to-skin contact between the mother and the baby, both in hospital and after discharge, with exclusive breast-feeding (see Fig. 10.3) (Cattaneo et al., 1998a).

In first-level facilities in countries with very limited resources, KMC will be beneficial for babies weighing 1800 g or more with no respiratory problems (Cattaneo et al., 1999b). In those weighing 1200 to 1799 g mortality and morbidity can also be reduced, though it should be recognized that for babies of gestational age <32 weeks, respiratory support such as CPAP is often required. This is usually available only in secondary or tertiary care, so referral may be indicated, provided that more skilled staff and respiratory equipment are available at the referral level. When referral is not possible, these LBW babies will have to be cared for at the first-level facility, but many of them will die. Since with KMC death will occur at the mother's breast, the acceptability of such an event should be assessed in any given context before establishing a policy.

All KMC infants should be monitored or frequently reassessed for breathing, feeding and temperature. Adequate services for mothers, careful evaluation before discharge and follow-up should be ensured (Cattaneo, et al., 1998a, b).

Small babies should be kept in a warm room. Breathing and temperature should be assessed frequently (every 4 hours or more frequently if abnormal values are present). Weight should also be checked every 24 hours as well as feeding. They should not be discharged until they are feeding regularly and gaining weight for three consecutive days, and the mother is confident in caring for the baby. If a LBW baby is discharged before starting to regain weight, return for follow-up within 2–3 days must be advised.

Breathing difficulties are frequent in small babies. Differential diagnosis includes a variety of conditions, the most common being self-limiting tachypnoea of the newborn, hyaline membrane disease (respiratory distress syndrome) and bacterial pneumonia. Preterm infants younger than 33 weeks of gestational age are at high risk of developing respiratory distress syndrome, which gradually develops over the first 2–3 days of life. Severe RDS requires assisted ventilation, moderate RDS can be managed by CPAP. Respiratory difficulties and irregular breathing, including episodes of apnoea, are common in sepsis, and should be considered as danger signs for possible severe infection

Referral

Referral is a difficult choice, the benefits of which must be weighed against the cost and risk of transport. The severity of the problem, the chances that it will be managed successfully at the referral hospital, and the risks of transport for the well-being of the baby and the mother (including the serious consequences of separation when mother and baby cannot be transferred together) must all be carefully evaluated. Appropriate explanation and advice should be given to the mother and her family. Transport should be arranged so that it is safe. Thermal protection of the baby should be ensured, through skin-to-skin contact if transport incubators are not available. Feeding should be ensured if transport implies a long journey. First treatment with antibiotics should be started before transport if a serious infection is a possible diagnosis.

Advice to mothers at discharge

Babies delivered at a health facility should not be discharged before 12 hours. For home births, the notion of conceptual discharge has been introduced to emphasize the need for support and observation during the first hours, and to recommend that mothers receive the necessary advice before the birth attendant has left her home. Advice should include the general care of the baby, feeding, follow-up visits when necessary, well-child visits and immunization, as well as indications on when to seek help.

General care of the child at home

The baby should sleep on his/her back, and should be kept away from smoke or people smoking. The baby, especially if small, should be kept away from sick children and adults. A bed net should be used night and day when the baby sleeps.

Feeding

Mothers should be encouraged to continue exclusive breast feeding on demand and to seek advice in case of any problems. Other fluids or use of pacifiers should be discouraged. Babies should be weighed monthly if of normal birth weight and breast feeding well.

Follow-up

Follow-up visits are recommended within 1–2 days in case of problems, such as local infection or feeding difficulties that did not require hospital care. Babies of HIV-positive and RPR-positive mothers, or those receiving TB treatment should return for follow-up within 2 weeks.

Well-child and immunization visits

A routine well-child visit should be arranged at home or at the health facility at 7 days of age. First OPV-O can be administered at 1 week of age and HB-1 vaccines if authorized by the local immunization programme. Otherwise, immunizations start at 6 weeks of age.

Danger signs

The mother should be advised to seek help in case of difficult feeding, difficult breathing, fever, diarrhoea or abnormal behaviour.

Case management during the first weeks of life

Newborn babies are in general at higher risk of severe infections during the first weeks of life. LBW babies will be at even higher risk and may remain at risk for a longer time. Danger signs in newborn babies and young infants should therefore be carefully evaluated and assessed. Newborn babies up to 1 month of age should always receive priority in triage systems. Guidelines for assessment and treatment of infants one week to 2 months of age have been developed within the IMCI strategy (see page 161).

References

Bergstrom S, Hojer B, Liljestrand J, Tunell R. (1994) *Perinatal Health Care with Limited Resources.* London: Macmillan Press Ltd.

Bique Osman N, Challis K, Cotiro M, Nordhal G, Bergstrom S. (2001). Perinatal outcome in an obstetric cohort of Mozambican women. *J Trop Ped*, **47**: 30–38.

Cattaneo A, Davanzo R, Bergman N, Charpak N. (1998a). Kangaroo mother care in low-income countries. *J Trop Ped* **44**: 279–282.

Cattaneo A, Davanzo R, Uxa F, Tamburlini G. (1998b). Recommendations for the implementaton of Kangaroo mother care for low birth weight infants. *Acta Paediatr* **87**: 440–445.

Charpak N, Ruiz-Pelaez JG, Figueroa Z, Charpak Y. (1997). Kangaroo mother versus traditional care for newborn infants less than 2000 grams: a randomised controlled trial. *Pediatrics*, **100**: 682–688.

Christensson K, Bhat G, Amadi BC, Eriksson B, Hojer B. (1998). Randomised study of skin to skin versus incubator care for rewarming low-risk hypothermic neonates. *Lancet* **352**: 1115.

Gupta A, Khanna K, Chattree S. (1999). Cup feeding: an alternative to bottle feeding in a neonatal intensive care unit. *J Trop Ped*, **45**: 108–110.

Klaus MH, Fanaroff AA. (1995). *Care of the High Risk Neonate.* Philadelphia: WB Saunders Company.

Ludington SM, Nguyen N, Swinth JV, Satysur RD. (2000). Kangaroo care compared to incubators in maintaining body warmth in preterm infants. *Biol Res Nurs*, **2**: 60–73.

Sinclair JC, Bracken MB. (1998). *Effective Care of the Newborn Infant.* Oxford: Oxford University Press.

WHO (1993). *Thermal Control of the Newborn: A Practical Guide.* Geneva: WHO, Maternal Health and Safe Motherhood Division.

WHO (1997). *Essential Newborn Care and Breastfeeding.* Copenhagen: WHO Regional Office for Europe.

WHO (1998). Evidence for the Ten Steps to Successful Breastfeeding. Geneva: WHO-CHD.

WHO (1999). *Newborn Resuscitation.* Geneva: WHO Maternal Health and Safe Motherhood Division.

WHO (2000). Collaborative Study Team on the Role of Breastfeeding on the Prevention of Infant Mortality. Effect of breastfeeding on infant and child mortality due to infectious diseases in less developed countries: a pooled analysis. *Lancet*, **355:** 451–55.

WHO Technical Consultation on Behalf of the UNFPA/UNICEF/WHO/UNAIDS Inter-Agency Task Team on Mother-to-Child Transmission of HIV (2000). *New Data on the Prevention of Mother-to-Child Transmission of HIV and their Policy Implications: Conclusions and Recommendations.* Geneva: WHO.

11 Severe malnutrition

The problem in Africa

Malnutrition is a serious and widespread problem in sub-Saharan Africa. It contributes to an estimated 54 per cent of deaths in children aged 0–4 years in developing countries (WHO, 1999a). Many of these deaths are because common childhood infections are more severe and longer lasting in malnourished children and are more likely to be fatal compared with the same illnesses in well-nourished children. Infections also undermine nutritional status and young children can quickly enter a cycle of repeated infections and ever-worsening malnutrition (Fig. 11.1). Breaking this cycle is important in preventing malnutrition-related deaths.

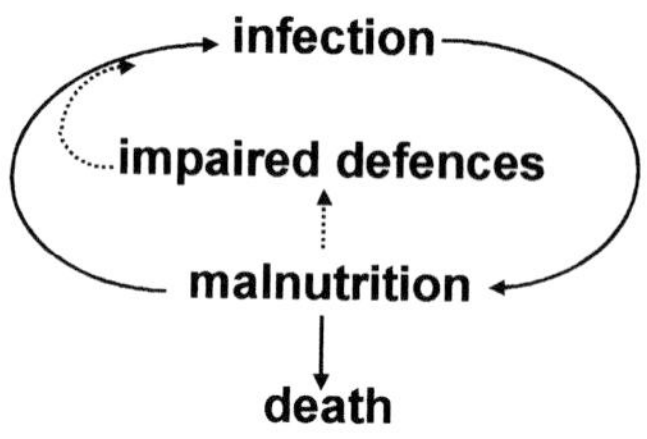

Fig. 11.1. Infection – malnutrition – infection cycle.

Other consequences of malnutrition

Malnutrition contributes to delayed mental development and behaviour problems, leading to poor school performance and poor employment prospects (Grantham-McGregor, 2002). This 'poverty trap' adversely affects families and their communities, and ultimately national economies.

Causes and prevention of malnutrition

Malnutrition can occur at any age but is most common between 6 and 30 months. In famine, all ages are affected. There are many causes of malnutrition but poverty is an underlying factor. Figure 11.2 shows that the causes extend from the family level to the national and international level. Political, economic, and agricultural policies that prevent the equitable distribution of resources often deny poor families their right to adequate food and health. Health professionals must strive to promote human rights and influence decision making at all levels, and be advocates for equity and justice.

Control of childhood infections (particularly diarrhoea, pneumonia, measles, malaria, and HIV/AIDS) and promotion of good feeding practices are important in preventing malnutrition.

The problem of mismanagement of severe malnutrition

Incorrect management is very common and thousands of children die unnecessarily each year. Dangerous practices that we have observed are use of diuretics to treat oedema, indiscriminate use of i.v. rehydration fluids, failure to prescribe broad-spectrum antibiotics, failure to provide potassium and vitamin A, and failure to meet nutritional needs (Puoane et al., 2001). By recording the number of hospital admissions with a diagnosis of severe malnutrition, and the number of these who die, we are discovering mortality rates (case fatality) as high as 40–50 per cent. Inadequate training of doctors in medical schools, lack of awareness of treatment guidelines, and limited hospital resources are common reasons for the high death rates (Schofield & Ashworth, 1996).

With correct treatment and attentiveness, case fatality rates can be reduced to <10%, even where HIV/AIDS is prevalent (Chopra & Wilkinson, 1995). To help improve treatment and reduce mortality, WHO has published treatment guidelines (WHO, 2000) and a manual (WHO, 1999b). We will summarize treatment later in this chapter.

Definition of severe malnutrition

Severe malnutrition is the presence of:

- severe wasting

and/or

- oedema of both feet.

Severe wasting is extreme thinness (<70 per cent of the median weight-for-height of the NCHS reference population or <3 standard deviations).

The term 'protein-energy malnutrition' is now avoided as this oversimplifies the aetiology. Other terms used are *marasmus* (severe wasting), *marasmic-kwashiorkor* (severe wasting + oedema) and *kwashiorkor* (oedema). A widely-used indicator for hospital admission is low weight-for-age. This can lead to stunted (short) children being admitted, which is inappropriate. Using only this indicator to decide whether to admit a child is therefore not recommended.

Clinical features

Severe wasting is most visible where loss of fat and skeletal muscle is greatest, i.e. on the thighs, buttocks and upper arms, and over the ribs and scapulae. The eyes may be sunken due to loss of retro-orbital fat. Tears may be absent and mouth dry as a result of atrophy of the lacrymal and salivary glands. Weakened abdominal muscles and gas from bacteria invading the upper gut (small bowel overgrowth) can lead to a distended abdomen. Wasted children are often anxious and irritable, and cry easily.

In *oedematous malnutrition*, the oedema is most likely to appear first in the feet, and then the lower legs. It can quickly develop into generalized (severe) oedema, affecting the arms and face as well as the legs. Skin changes often occur over the swollen limbs and include abnormally dark, crackled, peeling patches ('flaky paint' dermatosis) with pale skin underneath that is easily

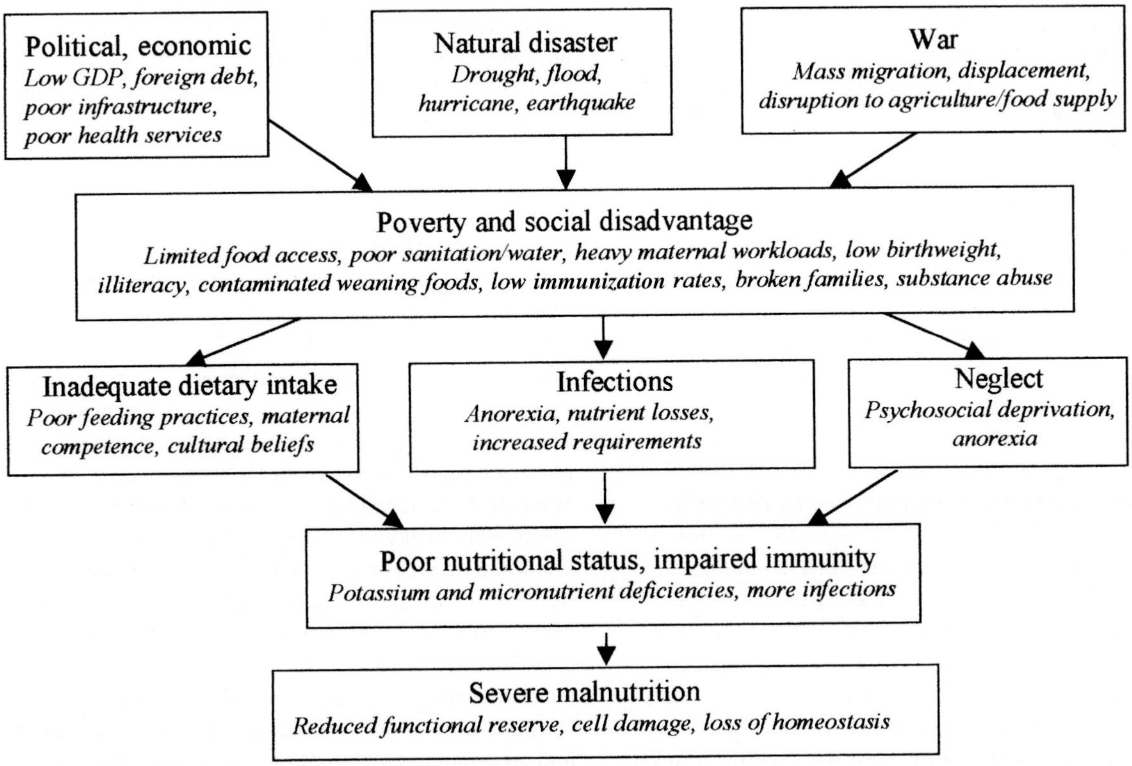

Fig. 11.2. Aetiology of severe malnutrition.

damaged and infected. Hair becomes sparse and easily pulled out. It may turn pale or reddish and lose its curl. The liver may be enlarged with fat. Children with oedema are miserable, apathetic and often refuse to eat.

Oedema can be mistaken for 'fatness'. To diagnose oedema, grasp the child's foot with your thumb on top. Press gently for 10 seconds. The child has oedema if a pit (dent) remains in the foot when you lift your thumb. In the presence of oedema, muscle wasting can be best seen over the upper arms and shoulders. Oedema is usually lost in the first few days of treatment.

Pathophysiology

When a child's intake is too little to cover basic needs, physiological and metabolic changes begin to take place in an orderly progression to conserve energy and support life for as long as possible. This process is called reductive adaptation.

In this process, fat stores are mobilized to provide energy. Eventually muscle, skin and gastrointestinal proteins are also mobilized.

Energy is conserved by cutting down expenditure. This includes:

- reducing physical activity and growth
- reducing basal metabolism by:
  - slowing the rate of protein turnover
  - reducing the functional reserve of organs and the gut
  - slowing the Na^+/K^+ pumps in cell membranes, and reducing their number
- reducing inflammatory and immune responses.

Consequences of reductive adaptation

These changes in body composition, metabolism and cell function have important consequences.

- Heat production is less, making the child more vulnerable to hypothermia.
- The liver makes glucose less easily and produces less albumin, transferrin and other transport proteins. A dysfunctioning liver is less able to excrete toxins like aflatoxin and cannot cope with excess dietary protein.
- The kidneys are less able to excrete excess fluid and sodium. Excess fluid easily builds up in the circulation.
- The heart is smaller and weaker than usual and has a reduced output. Excess fluid in the circulation readily leads to death from heart failure.
- Sodium builds up inside cells due to slower and fewer Na^+/K^+ pumps, leading to excess body sodium, fluid retention and oedema.
- Potassium leaks out of cells and is lost in the urine contributing to electrolyte imbalance, anorexia, fluid retention and heart failure.
- Loss of muscle protein leads to accompanying loss of potassium, magnesium, zinc and copper.
- The gut produces less gastric acid and enzymes. Motility is reduced. Bacteria often colonize the stomach and small bowel, damaging the mucosa and deconjugating bile salts. Damaged, flattened villi are common. Digestion and absorption are impaired.
- Immune function is impaired, particularly cell-mediated immunity. There may be no fever or raised pulse or respiration rates, no redness or swelling, or raised white cell count in infection.
- Red cell mass is reduced, liberating iron. Conversion of liberated iron to ferritin uses scarce glucose and amino acids.

Severe malnutrition is a multi-deficiency state. Coexisting deficiencies of vitamin A, zinc, selenium and other anti-oxidant nutrients limit the body's natural ability to mop up *free radicals*. These damage cell membranes. Oedema and changes in skin and hair are outward signs of cell damage. Giving iron supplements whilst transferrin levels are low can create unbound 'free' iron, which promotes free radical generation. Free iron also makes some infections worse. Giving iron in the initial phase of treatment increases mortality (Smith et al., 1989).

'Best practice' takes these physiological and metabolic changes into account. Failure to do so can kill the patient.

Treatment of severe malnutrition

Many severely malnourished children are admitted to hospital with a primary diagnosis of gastroenteritis, pneumonia, etc. A common and often fatal mistake is to try to tackle the illness first and then the malnutrition afterwards. This ignores the profound metabolic and physiological changes that exist in severe malnutrition. The correct approach is to regard such children as having severe malnutrition with a coexisting infection, and follow the treatment guidelines for severe malnutrition. Routine treatment of severe malnutrition involves ten steps in two phases: an initial stabilization phase to treat acute medical conditions and restore homeostasis, and a longer rehabilitation phase to replace lost tissues (catch-up growth). Treatment procedures are similar for wasted and oedematous children. The approximate timescale is shown in the Box below.

Ten steps in the care of severely malnourished children (approximate timescale)

	Stabilization		Rehabilitation
	Day 1–2	Day 2–7	Week 2–6
1. Prevent/treat hypoglycaemia	→		
2. Prevent/treat hypothermia	→		
3. Treat/prevent dehydration	→		
4. Correct imbalance of electrolytes	———	———	——→
5. Treat infections	———	——→	
6. Correct deficiencies of micronutrients	— no iron —	— with iron —	——→
7. Start cautious feeding	———	——→	
8. Rebuild wasted tissues (catch-up growth)			——→
9. Provide loving care and play	———	———	——→
10. Prepare for follow-up			——→

Severely malnourished children die in hospital from four main causes:

- hypoglycaemia
- hypothermia
- cardiac failure (from overhydration and potassium deficiency)
- missed infection.

Centres with low mortality take steps to prevent these deaths. Centres with high mortality have practices that contribute to these deaths (see the Box below).

Prevent/treat hypoglycaemia

Why are severely malnourished children at increased risk of hypoglycaemia?

- They have a limited glucose supply:
  - gluconeogenesis is impaired
  - they have less glycogen in reserve because their muscles have wasted.
- they have an **increased demand** for glucose to:
  - fight multiple infections
  - convert liberated red cell iron into ferritin.

Treatment practices that delay feeding, e.g. long queuing times for admission, or lead to long gaps between feeds, e.g. no night feeds, contribute to hypoglycaemia.

Hypoglycaemia and hypothermia usually occur together and are associated with infection. Consider them as the 'deadly triad'.

Actions to prevent hypoglycaemia

- Give severely malnourished children priority as soon as they arrive at the hospital and send them quickly to the ward. Do not send to X-ray. This can be done later.
- Give 50 ml of 10 per cent glucose or sucrose solution (1 rounded teaspoon of sugar in 3½ tablespoons water) immediately (orally or by nasogastric tube) or give starter formula (see below). Choose whichever is quickest.
- Feed straightaway (or start rehydration if needed).
- Feed every 2 or 3 hours, day and night. Frequent feeding prevents hypoglycaemia and hypothermia.
- Start antibiotics immediately (see the last Box on p. 187).

To treat hypoglycaemia (blood glucose <3 mmol/l), proceed as above if the child is conscious and feed every 2 hours day and night. If the child is unconscious, treat with 10 per cent sterile glucose i.v. (5 ml/kg). If unavailable, give 10 per cent glucose or sucrose by nasogastric tube.

Prevent/treat hypothermia (see the Box below)

Why are severely malnourished children at increased risk of hypothermia?

- they have increased heat loss:
  - they have lost their fat insulation
  - they have a relatively large surface for their (reduced) weight.
- they have reduced heat production:
  - they are less physically active
  - their basal metabolism is lower than usual
  - fuel (glucose) is diverted to fight infection and convert free iron to ferritin.

Draughty, cold wards add to the risk of hypothermia. Children become chilled if left in wet clothes or if they are not dried carefully after bathing.

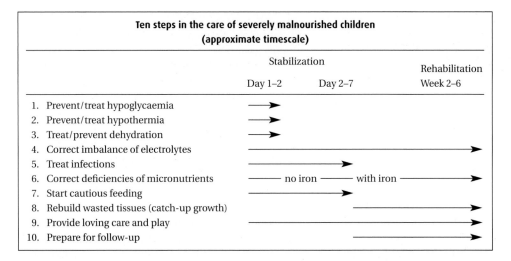

Actions to prevent hypothermia

- Feed immediately (or start rehydration if needed).
- Feed every 2 or 3 hours, day and night. Frequent feeding prevents hypoglycaemia and hypothermia.
- Keep child warm and covered, and away from draughts.
- Keep dry.
- Start antibiotics immediately.

To treat hypothermia (rectal <35.5 °C, axillary <35.0 °C):

- Feed immediately and give antibiotics (including gram-negative cover)
- Rewarm:
  – put the child on the mother's bare chest (kangaroo method) skin-to-skin, and cover them.
  – *or* clothe the child, including head, and cover with a warmed blanket. Place a heater or lamp nearby. Do not use hot water bottles except to warm the blanket.
- Monitor rectal temperature 2-hourly until it rises above 36.5 °C (take every half-hour if a heater is used).

Treat/prevent dehydration (see the Box below)

Why is dehydration often overdiagnosed in severely malnourished children?

- The common signs of dehydration (slow skin pinch, sunken eyes, no tears, dry mouth) are similar to the signs of malnutrition itself.

Why do malnourished children die during rehydration?

- Because signs of malnutrition are confused with signs of dehydration and too much fluid is given. Excess fluid in the circulation causes heart failure.
- Because i.v. fluids are given without good cause and increase the risk of overhydration.
- Children are not monitored carefully during rehydration, so fluid overload is missed.

Severely malnourished children often have diarrhoea. Because it is difficult to diagnose dehydration in a severely malnourished child, all children with watery diarrhoea should be assumed to have some dehydration.

Actions to treat dehydration

- Give low sodium rehydration solution for malnutrition (ReSoMal): see Box p. 187.
- give 5 ml/kg every 30 min for the first 2 hours. Then give 5–10 ml/kg/h for the next 4–10 hours. The exact amount and duration depends on how much the child wants, and the volume and frequency of stools and vomit.
- Monitor pulse and respiration rates every 30 min for the first 2 h and then hourly for signs of overhydration (pulse increases by ≥25 beats/min and respirations by ≥5 breaths/min).
- Do not give severely malnourished children i.v. fluids except in shock.

Treating a child in shock

Common reasons for malnourished children to go into shock are severe dehydration and sepsis. Often, both are present. It is not possible by examining the child to differentiate them. The only way is to see how the child responds to i.v. fluid. Children with dehydration respond to i.v. fluid. Those with septic shock do not and they quickly get fluid overload.

The usual emergency signs of shock (cold hands, capillary refill time >3 seconds, weak fast pulse) may be present in severely malnourished children even if there is no shock, so only give i.v. fluids if the child also has lethargy or is unconscious.

If lethargic or unconscious, keep child warm and give:

- oxygen
- i.v. glucose (5 ml/kg of 10 per cent glucose solution)
- i.v. fluids (see below)
- i.v. antibiotics (see the last Box on p. 187).

The best i.v. fluids for severely malnourished children are Ringer's lactate with 5 per cent glucose (dextrose) *or* 0.45 per cent (half-normal) saline with 5 per cent glucose, or half-strength Darrow's with 5 per cent glucose.

To start treatment

- Give i.v. fluid 15 ml/kg over 1 hour. Use a paediatric giving set.
- record pulse and respiration rates at the start and then every 5–10 minutes to check for fluid overload.

After 1 hour

If there are signs of improvement (pulse and respiration rates are slower):

- Repeat i.v. fluid 15 ml/kg over one more hour. (Do not rehydrate i.v. for >2 hours)
- Then change to oral or nasogastric rehydration with ReSoMal 10 ml/kg/h for up to 10 hours
- After 4 hours, if rehydration is still continuing, replace ReSoMal with starter formula and again whenever a feed is due.

If there is no improvement after the first 15 ml/kg i.v. assume the child has septic shock:

- Give maintenance fluids (4 ml/kg/h) while waiting for blood.
- Transfuse fresh whole blood 10 ml/kg *slowly* over 3 hours; give furosemide first (1 mg/kg i.v.). Use packed cells if the child is in cardiac failure. If blood is not available, use plasma.

- *If the child gets worse* (pulse increases by ≥25 beats/min and respiration by ≥5 breaths/min) stop i.v. fluids (see the Box below).

Recipe for ReSoMal
(Modified ORS solution for severe malnutrition)

Ingredient	Amount
Water	2 litres
WHO-ORS	One 1 litre packet
Sugar	50 g
Electrolyte/mineral solution (see next Box)	40 ml

Correct electrolyte imbalance

Do not be guided by serum electrolyte levels. All severely malnourished children have excess body sodium and deficiencies of potassium and magnesium. Oedema is partly due to these imbalances. Never give diuretics to treat oedema as this makes potassium deficiency worse.

Actions to correct electrolyte imbalance

Give daily:
- extra potassium (4 mmol/kg)
- extra magnesium (0.6 mmol/kg).

The extra potassium and magnesium can be prepared in liquid form (see the Box below) and added to feeds and ReSoMal during preparation. If this is not possible, give priority to finding another source of potassium: for example:
- make a 10 per cent KCl solution (100 g in 1 litre of water) and add 22.5 ml to each 1litre of feed and 45 ml to 2 litres of ReSoMal
- or give crushed slow K, half a tablet/kg/day.

Restrict sodium:
- Use low sodium rehydration fluid (ReSoMal)
- Prepare food without salt.

Recipe for concentrated electrolyte/mineral solution

Ingredient	Amount (g)	mmol/20ml
Potassium chloride	224	24
Tripotassium citrate	81	2
Magnesium chloride	76	3
Zinc acetate	8.2	300 μmol
Copper sulphate	1.4	45 μmol
Water: make up to	2500 ml	

Add 20 ml per litre of feed. Add 40 ml to 2 litres of ReSoMal

Treat infection

In severe malnutrition, the usual signs of infection are often absent. *Therefore, give broad spectrum antibiotics immediately to all children routinely* (Box below).

Doctors are often unaware that the normal signs of infection may be absent in severely malnourished children. Consequently, hidden infections go untreated and mortality is high. Case-fatality rates increased from 18 per cent to 38 per cent when doctors unfamiliar with treatment guidelines replaced 'trained' doctors in a rural South African hospital. The main differences in treatment between the two teams were provision of gram-negative cover to children who were very ill and provision of potassium.

Choice of antibiotics
- For a child **with no complications**, give:
  co-trimoxazole 5 ml (240 mg) orally twice daily for 5 days (2.5 ml if <4 kg).
- For a child who **has complications** (shock, hypoglycaemia, hypothermia, respiratory or urinary tract infections, or skin lesions) or is **lethargic** or **looks sickly**, give:
  gentamicin 7.5 mg/kg i.v./i.m. once daily for 7 days
  plus
  ampicillin 50 mg/kg i.v./i.m. every 6 hours for 2 days then oral amoxicillin 15 mg/kg every 8 hours for 5 days or, if amoxicillin is unavailable, give oral ampicillin 50mg/kg every 6 hours for 5 days.
  plus
  oral metronidazole 7.5mg/kg every 8 hours for 7 days.

Malnourished children are very vulnerable to cross-infection because their immune function is impaired (Chevalier et al., 1998). Good ward hygiene and hand-washing by doctors, nurses, mothers and other family members is therefore very important.

- Avoid overcrowding and sharing of cots.
- Give measles vaccine if the child is >6 months and unimmunized, or is <9 months and immunized (see Table 11.1).

- If the child fails to improve within 48 hours, add chloramphenicol 25 mg/kg i.v./i.m. every 6 hours for 5 days.
- If poor appetite continues after 5–7 days of antibiotic treatment, complete a 10–day course. If poor appetite persists, fully reassess the child.

(These drugs can be modified according to local availability and local patterns of pathogen resistance, but gram-negative cover is essential for children who have complications or who look sickly. Additional antibiotics may be needed for specific infections such as dysentery and severe pneumonia.)

Correct micronutrient deficiencies

All severely malnourished children have vitamin and mineral deficiencies, which must be corrected.

Actions to correct deficiencies

- Give a large single dose of Vitamin A on Day 1 to boost immune function and prevent blindness:

<6 months:	50 000 i.u.
6–12 months:	100 000 i.u.
>12 months:	200 000 i.u.

If there is any sign of xerophthalmia, repeat the dose on Days 2 and 14.

Give daily:

- multivitamin supplement;
- folic acid1mg/day (5 mg on Day 1);
- zinc 2 mg/kg/day;
- copper 0.3 mg/kg/day.

Zinc and copper can be combined with the potassium and magnesium to make a stock solution which can be added to feeds during preparation (see the Box at the top of p. 187).

Delay giving iron until the child has a good appetite and is in the rehabilitation phase. Then give ferrous sulphate, 3 mg Fe/kg/day.

Start cautious feeding

In the stabilization phase, the amount and type of food given is important. Too much protein stresses the liver, too much lactose stresses the gut, and too much fluid stresses the kidneys and heart. In this phase, feeds should provide just enough energy and protein to cover basic needs.

Actions

Give:

- small frequent feeds of a milk-based starter formula with low osmolarity and low lactose (see the Box below);
- 100 kcal/kg/day;
- 1–1.5 g protein/kg/day;
- 130 ml/kg/day of liquid (or 100 ml/kg/day if the child has severe oedema).

If the child is breast-fed, encourage continued breast-feeding (give starter formula first).

Starter formula is also called F-75. It contains 75 kcal and 0.9 g protein/100 ml.

Achieve catch-up growth

Readiness to enter the rehabilitation phase and start catch-up growth is signalled by a return of appetite, usually about 1 week after admission. A controlled transition over 3 days is recommended to prevent a child suddenly consuming huge amounts, which may over-stimulate sodium pump activity and cause rapid efflux of sodium from cells and heart failure (Patrick, 1977).

After the transition, give unlimited amounts of catch-up formula, which is also called F-100 and contains100 kcal and 2.9 g protein/100 ml. Modified porridges or modified family foods can be used if they have similar energy and protein concentrations.

To make the transition

- For 2 days replace the starter F-75 with an equal amount of catch-up F-100.
- Then increase each successive feed by 10 ml until some feed remains uneaten. At this point the child should eat about 200 ml/kg/day of the catch-up formula.

After the transition

- give frequent feeds of F-100 (unlimited amounts)
- 150–220 kcal/kg/day
- 4–6 g protein/kg/day

If the child is breast-fed, encourage continued breast-feeding. Breast milk does not have sufficient energy and protein to support catch-up growth, so give F-100 first at each feed.

Rates of weight gain are considered poor if <5 g/kg/day, moderate if between 5 and 10 g/kg per day and good if >10 g/kg/day.

Recipes for milk-based starter and catch-up formulas

For ***full-cream milk powder*** *use*

Ingredient	Starter	Catch-up
Full-cream milk	35 g	110 g
Sugar	100 g	50 g
Vegetable oil	20 g	30 g
Electrolyte/mineral solution	20 ml	20 ml

Make up to 1000 ml with cooled, boiled water.

For ***dried skimmed milk*** *use:*

Ingredient	Starter	Catch-up
Dried skimmed milk	25 g	80 g
Sugar	100 g	50 g
Vegetable oil	30 g	60 g
Electrolyte/mineral solution	20 ml	20 ml

Make up to 1000 ml with cooled, boiled water.

For ***fresh cows' milk*** *use:*

Ingredient	Starter	Catch-up
Milk	300 ml	880 ml
Sugar	100 g	75 g
Vegetable oil	20 ml	20 ml
Electrolyte/mineral solution	20 ml	20 ml

Make up to 1000 ml with cooled, boiled water.

To make: Place the ingredients in a 1–litre electric blender. Add water *up to* the 1 litre mark and blend. (*Do not add* 1 litre of water as this makes it too dilute.) If a blender is not available, mix the oil and sugar thoroughly, mix in the milk and electrolyte/mineral solution and make up to 1 litre. Whisk thoroughly to prevent the oil from separating out.

Provide loving care and sensory stimulation

Severe malnutrition delays a child's mental and behavioural development. Starting from admission, provide:

- tender, loving interactions
- a cheerful stimulating environment
- maternal involvement (as much as possible: comforting, feeding, bathing, play)
- structured play therapy led by staff
- physical activity as soon as the child is well enough.

Prepare for follow-up

With correct care and feeding, severely malnourished children will achieve a normal weight for their height in 4–6 weeks. Recovery of immunity takes longer. Relapse and death are likely if children are discharged early.

Table 11.1. WHO immunization recommendations

Age	Vaccine
Birth	BCG, oral polio vaccine (OPV-0)
6 week	DPT-1, OPV-1
10 weeks	DPT-2, OPV-2
14 weeks	DPT-3, OPV-3
9 months	measles[a]

Notes:

[a] In exceptional situations, where measles morbidity and mortality before 9 months of age represent more than 15 per cent of cases and deaths, given an extra dose of measles vaccine at 6 months of age. The scheduled dose should also be given as soon as possible after 9 months of age. The extra measles dose is also recommended for groups at high risk of measles death, such as infants in refugee camps, infants admitted to hospitals, HIV-positive infants, and infants affected by disasters and during outbreaks of measles.

Discharge children only if:

- Child has completed antibiotic treatment.
- Child has no oedema.
- Child is eating very well.
- Child shows good weight gain.
- Child has had 2 weeks of potassium and vitamin supplements (or can continue at home).
- Follow-up has been arranged with neighbourhood clinics.
- Parents/carers know what to feed, how much and how often, using foods that will support continued catch-up growth and are affordable and culturally acceptable.
- Parents/carers know how to keep their child healthy at home.
- Parents/carers know how to provide play and stimulation to promote development.
- Parents/carers know to take their child for follow-up at 1, 2 and 4 weeks, then monthly, and for booster immunizations and 6-monthly vitamin A.

Changing treatment practices – unresolved problems

Many factors can limit effective treatment including shortage of staff and essential supplies due to inadequate health budgets, inefficient health management systems, and lack of accountability and supervision. We have found, however, that staff are motivated to take action to improve treatment when they are actively involved in assessing case-fatality rates and quality of care (Puoane et al., 2001). Even in poorly resourced rural African hospitals, case-fatality rates have been halved with in-service training and introduction of treatment guidelines. Sustaining improved care can be difficult and is hampered by rotation and loss of trained staff. Adoption of the WHO guidelines as hospital policy or issuing 'standing orders' can help resolve this problem to some extent, but if mismanagement is to be reversed, doctors and nurses must be taught best practice during their training and those already qualified given in-service training. Lives can be saved when treatment guidelines are followed (Ahmed et al., 1999; Schofield & Ashworth, 1997) and the dramatic and rapid transformations of severely malnourished children can be one of the great satisfactions of professional life.

References

Ahmed T, Ali M, Ullah MM et al. (1999). Mortality in severely malnourished children with diarrhoea and use of a standardised management protocol. *Lancet*, **353**: 1919–1922.

Chevalier P, Sevilla R, Sejas E et al. (1998). Immune recovery of malnourished children takes longer that nutritional recovery: implications for treatment and discharge. *J Trop Pediatr*, **44**: 304–307.

Chopra M, Wilkinson D. (1995). Treatment of malnutrition. *Lancet*, **345**: 788–789.

Grantham-McGregor S. (2002). Linear growth retardation and cognition. *Lancet*, **359**: 542.

Patrick J (1977). Death during recovery from severe malnutrition and its possible relationship to sodium pump activity in leucocytes. *Br Med J*, **1**: 1051–1054.

Puoane T, Sanders D, Chopra M et al., (2001). Evaluating the clinical management of severely malnourished children – a study of two rural district hospitals. *S Afr Med J*, **91**: 137–141.

Schofield C, Ashworth A. (1996). Why have mortality rates for severe malnutrition remained so high? *Bull Wld Health Org*, **74**: 223–229.

Schofield C, Ashworth A. (1997). Severe malnutrition in children: high case-fatality rates can be reduced. *Africa Health*, **19**: 17–18.

Smith IF, Taiwo O, Golden MHN. (1989). Plant protein rehabilitation diets and iron supplementation of the protein-energy malnourished child. *Eur J Clin Nutr*, **43**: 763–768.

World Health Organization (1999a). *Management of Childhood Illness in Developing Countries: Rationale for an Integrated Strategy.* WHO/CHS/CAH/98.1A. Geneva: World Health Organization.

World Health Organization (1999b). *Management of Severe Malnutrition: A Manual for Physicians and Other Senior Health Workers.* Geneva: World Health Organization.

World Health Organization (2000). *Management of the Child with a Serious Infection or Severe Malnutrition. Guidelines for Care at First-referral Level in Developing Countries.* WHO/FCH/CAH /00.1. Geneva: World Health Organization.

Further key references

Waterlow J C. (1992). *Protein Energy Malnutrition.* London: Edward Arnold.

Golden MHN. (1996). Severe malnutrition. In *Oxford Textbook of Medicine*, ed DJ Weatherall, JGG Ledingham, DA Warrell, 3rd edn. Oxford: Oxford University Press.

Internet resources

Wellcome Tropical Medicine Resource. (2000). *Topics in International Health: Nutrition.* London: The Wellcome Trust.

World Health Organization (1999). *Management of Severe Malnutrition: A Manual for Physicians and Other Senior Health Workers.* This manual can be downloaded in English, French and Spanish from the WHO website: http: //www.who.int/nut/ Manageme.pdf.

Training courses

WHO Training course on the management of severe malnutrition (2002). From WHO Regional Offices or from Dr Sultana Khanum, WHO, Geneva. Khanums@who.ch

Ashworth A, Puoane T, Sanders D, Schofield C. (2001). Improving the management of severe malnutrition: a training guide. From Ann.Hill@lshtm.ac.uk, or from tpuoane@uwc.ac.za.

12 The febrile patient

Fever is one of the most common reasons for seeking medical care. The patient may complain of fever, or of symptoms resulting from fever or from the systemic effects of infection, such as headache or general body pain.

The presence of fever is confirmed, usually by placing a thermometer under the tongue, in the axilla or in the rectum for one minute. Axillary temperature is some 0.5 °C lower, and rectal temperature 0.5 °C higher than the normal oral temperature of around 37 °C. In healthy people the temperature is up to 0.5 °C lower at 6 am than at 6 pm, and a similar variation is observed in many febrile patients. It is therefore important to measure the temperature of febrile patients at least twice daily.

Control of body temperature

Body temperature is controlled by the hypothalamus. The release of pyrogenic cytokines from macrophages and mononuclear cells, especially interleukin-1 (IL-1) and tumour necrosis factor (TNFα), acts on the hypothalamic regulatory centre to increase the set point for body temperature. Different infectious agents induce fever in different ways. Bacterial components which stimulate release of inflammatory cytokines include lipopolysaccharide of gram-negative organisms, peptidoglycan of gram-positive organisms, and lipoarabinomannan from mycobacteria. In addition, some bacteria (e.g. *Strep. pyogenes*) secrete soluble toxins that stimulate their release. Inflammatory cytokines may also be released in response to other stimuli, e.g. drugs, cancers, or other inflammatory disorders such as vasculitis.

Causes of fever

Most febrile patients in Africa have an **infection,** but it is important to consider other causes of fever when the infection cannot be diagnosed or there is no response to anti-microbial treatment.

Malignant diseases, particularly lymphomas and leukaemias, but also deep-seated cancers such as hepatocellular or renal carcinomas, can present as unexplained persistent fever.

Autoimmune diseases such as systemic lupus erythematosus (SLE), which are rare in Africa but more common in people of African descent living in western countries, should also be considered in cases of prolonged fever.

Occasionally, fever can result from a *failure of temperature control*, due to damage to the hypothalamus, for example by cerebrovascular disease or trauma; or to excessive heat production or limited heat loss, as in heat stroke.

Immediate assessment of the febrile patient (triage)

Medical emergencies are relatively uncommon, but they do occur, particularly, in an African context, meningococcal septicaemia, meningitis and severe malaria. Therefore, first assess the patient rapidly to see if immediate life-saving interventions are needed.

- Is s/he unconscious or convulsing?
- Is the airway patent?
- Is there evidence of hypovolaemic shock?
- Are there petechiae or other signs suggesting meningococcal septicaemia, which requires immediate antibiotic treatment?
- Is the patient bleeding? If so, could this be yellow fever

or another haemorrhagic fever such as Ebola or Lassa, requiring immediate precautions to avoid infection of hospital staff?

Does the patient need treatment?

In patients who are less unwell, consider whether the patient is likely to be suffering from an acute self-limiting illness, or whether s/he needs specific anti-microbial treatment. The vast majority of febrile illnesses are self-limiting, presumably due to viral infections, and do not require specific treatment.

The identification of those febrile patients who need further investigation and/or treatment is one of the most important tasks facing clinicians working in Africa. No amount of textbook learning will equip you for this task, which can only be learned through clinical experience, but a methodical approach to taking a history and performing a clinical examination is an essential starting point.

One of the many pleasures of practising medicine in Africa is that, in very many cases, the diagnosis is obvious on clinical grounds alone. Cellulitis, other skin sepsis and acute respiratory infection make up a large proportion of febrile cases, and can be confidently diagnosed and treated without any other investigations.

History and examination

After the immediate rapid assessment, take a more detailed history and perform a complete physical examination.

While doing this, ask yourself why this patient, from this place, should be presenting to this hospital at this time with this illness. The patient's age, occupation and place of residence will provide clues that will help you to answer these questions. For example, a severe febrile illness in an adult who has lived all his life in a malaria endemic area will probably not be caused by malaria; but in an immigrant from a non-malarious region, it might be. Cattle herders are at increased risk of brucellosis, rice farmers may be at increased risk of leptospirosis, gold miners in southern Africa have a very high incidence of tuberculosis, and truck drivers or bar workers may be at increased risk of HIV-related diseases.

The history of the present illness usually provides important clues to the diagnosis.

For example,

- A febrile illness that has lasted more than a week is probably not due to a self-limiting viral infection.
- Symptoms associated with the fever may help to localize the site of disease, e.g. cough, diarrhoea or pain in a bone, muscle or joint.
- The way in which the illness began may help to identify the underlying cause. A sudden onset of cough, chest pain and fever suggests pneumococcal pneumonia; the same symptoms with a gradual onset over a few weeks are more likely to be due to tuberculosis.

Knowledge of the local pattern of disease will help you to reach a diagnosis.

For example,

- Many infectious diseases (e.g. malaria, meningococcal meningitis, rotavirus and respiratory syncitial virus infection) are more common at certain seasons
- Some infectious diseases occur in epidemics (Chapter 8). During an epidemic of meningococcal meningitis, many febrile patients are likely to have this disease
- In communities where schistosomiasis is endemic, there is an increased risk of invasive salmonella infections
- Malaria transmission varies greatly in different parts of Africa. Increasing numbers of Africans in urban areas may not develop immunity to the disease.

Taking a history

The answers to the following questions will help you make a diagnosis:

General

- Age
- Occupation
- Address
- How long has s/he lived there?
- If an immigrant, where from?

The present illness

How did it begin? Did it come on suddenly, or gradually over several weeks? What other symptoms did the patient notice in addition to fever?

- A rash?
- A cough – if so, was it productive, was there haemoptysis?
- Diarrhoea – if so, was it bloody?
- Pain passing urine?
- Localized pain: for example in a muscle, suggesting pyomyositis, in a bone, suggesting osteomyelitis, or in the flanks, suggesting pyelonephritis or psoas abscess?

Previous treatment

- Has the patient been treated for this illness?
- If so, where and with what?
- Are any medical records available?
- Is the patient allergic to any medication?

Past medical history

A history of vaccination or previous significant illness may be very useful.

- Has the patient been immunized against measles and meningococcal infection?
- Has s/he had any serious illnesses or operations in the past?
- Does s/he have an underlying condition such as diabetes or sickle cell disease?
- Is s/he taking any medication?

Examination

In many cases you will have a good idea of the probable diagnosis after taking the history. Nevertheless, it is essential to perform a thorough examination in all febrile patients. The patient must be undressed and examined in a good light.

While examining the patient, consider whether s/he is likely to be HIV-positive. HIV-positive patients are at increased risk of serious bacterial infections, e.g. those due to *S. pneumoniae* or salmonella species, and you will need to consider a wider spectrum of possible infections in these patients.

In regions with a high HIV prevalence, which unfortunately include most of sub-Saharan Africa, the social history may not be helpful in identifying individuals at risk. Look particularly for a scar due to herpes zoster (shingles) and for other skin manifestations of HIV, such as papular prurigo, seborrhoeic dermatitis, Kaposi's sarcoma (KS) or severe psoriasis. Stevens–Johnson syndrome is a strong predictor of HIV infection. Look in the mouth for KS and thrush, and at the tongue for oral hairy leukoplakia. Look for generalized lymphadenopathy, especially epitrochlear, and for evidence of weight loss.

Generalized signs

What is the patient's nutritional state? A wasted patient is likely to be suffering from a chronic disease such as tuberculosis or HIV-related illness. A patient who is malnourished for social reasons, e.g. because s/he is a refugee, is at increased risk of serious infection.

Is the patient dehydrated? Dehydration is common in febrile patients in hot climates, due to increased fluid loss, often accompanied by decreased intake, and may be exacerbated if there is diarrhoea or vomiting. Measure the patient's pulse rate and blood pressure, and assess peripheral perfusion. Examine the mucous membranes; and assess skin turgor.

What is the patient's mental state? Is s/he agitated, confused, drowsy or unconscious? If so, consider infections which involve the central nervous system, such as cerebral malaria, meningitis, typhoid, trypanosomiasis or a viral encephalitis; but bear in mind that confusion can be seen in any serious infection, especially in children and the elderly.

Is the patient jaundiced? Jaundice in Africa is unlikely to be due to hepatitis A or B, which are usually asymptomatic infections of childhood. It is commonly seen in severe malaria and other conditions causing haemolysis or hepatitis, such as sickle cell disease, relapsing fever and leptospirosis. It is a well-recognized manifestation of pneumococcal pneumonia and other severe bacterial infections such as typhoid. When seen in a bleeding patient, it suggests yellow fever or another viral haemorrhagic fever.

Is there a rash? Always examine the skin carefully, in a good light, after undressing the patient. There are many conditions which cause a fever and a generalized rash (see Box, p. 192). As rashes may be hard to see in dark-skinned patients, you should also examine the mucous membranes of the mouth and conjunctiva, where characteristic lesions, such as the petechiae of meningococcal disease or relapsing fever, the Koplik's spots of early measles, or the vesicles of chickenpox, are easier to see. Macular rashes, such as those due to early measles, rubella or typhoid are particularly difficult to see in dark-skinned patients. The rash of tick typhus and trypanosomiasis can also be hard to see, but there may be a localized skin lesion at the site of inoculation: the chancre of East African trypanosomiasis or the eschar of tick typhus, which is often found where the clothes are tightest. The rash of secondary syphilis, which usually affects the palms and soles, is more obvious, and may be accompanied by other characteristic lesions such as condylomata lata. The petechial or haemorrhagic rash of meningococcal septicaemia or viral haemorrhagic fever may be quite obvious.

The pattern of fever

In many older textbooks, much is made of the pattern of fever associated with different infections. Classically, the fever of falciparum and vivax malaria is tertian, that is to say it recurs every third day, or has a 48-hour cycle; the fever of brucellosis recurs at irregular intervals, giving rise to a temperature chart that resembles waves in the ocean, an undulant fever; the fever of typhoid is continuously high, and accompanied by a relative bradycardia. These findings, although 'classical', are not necessarily typical. At best, the pattern of fever can suggest a possible cause.

Rashes in febrile patients

Organism	Syndrome	Comment
Measles	Measles	Maculopapular, later desquamation
Varicella-zoster	Chickenpox	Vesicular, generalized Lesions also in mouth
Varicella-zoster	Shingles	Neurological distribution Associated pain Suggests HIV infection,esp. when affects >1 dermatome
Primary HIV infection	Mononucleosis-like illness	Maculopapular rash, often with generalized lymphadenopathy and splenomegaly
Viral haemorrhagic fevers	See Chapter 58	Purpura, ecchymoses
Neisseria meningitidis	See Chapter 39	Petechial/purpuric
Strep. pyogenes	See Chapter 37	Cellulitis, erysipelas
Staph. aureus	See Chapter 38	Pyogenic lesions
Leptospira species	See Chapter 52	Petechiae, haemorrhages
Borrelia species	Relapsing fever 45	Petechiae, haemorrhages
Rickettsia species	See Chapter 44	Maculopapular. Eschar in some syndromes
Treponema pallidum	Secondary syphilis	Maculopapular, usually affects palms and soles
Trypanosoma brucei rhodesiense	East Africa sleeping sickness	Maculopapular. Chancre at site of inoculation

Localized signs

Look in particular for the following signs:
- skin sepsis, such as cellulitis or abscess
- tenderness of bone or muscle, suggesting osteomyelitis or pyomyositis
- neck stiffness or a positive Kernig's sign, suggesting meningitis
- chest signs (rapid breathing, bronchial breathing or crepitations), suggesting pneumonia
- a heart murmur, suggesting bacterial endocarditis.
- tender frontal or maxillary sinuses: sinusitis is often overlooked as a cause of fever.
- an abscess in the gluteal muscles (resulting from a non-sterile injection).

A conscious patient will usually be able to tell you where the pain is.

Examine the abdomen carefully.
- Is it tender? Generalized or localized abdominal tenderness is a common finding in typhoid.
- Is the liver or spleen enlarged? A tender enlarged liver suggests an amoebic abscess, hepatitis or a hepatocellular carcinoma. A palpable spleen in an acutely febrile African patient suggests malaria or typhoid, although there are many other causes of splenomegaly (Chapter 81).
- Do not forget to do a rectal or pelvic examination when indicated. For example, a pelvic examination is essential if you suspect pelvic inflammatory disease or septic abortion.

Investigations

After taking the history and examining the patient, you will have a good idea of the probable diagnosis in most febrile patients. Laboratory tests can be useful in confirming the diagnosis, but are no substitute for good clinical practice. Moreover, the results of laboratory investigations can be misleading; for example, the presence of a few trophozoites of *Plasmodium falciparum* in the blood film of a febrile adult does not necessarily mean that his illness is due to malaria (Chapter 15).

Microscopy

A microscope and reagents to perform a gram stain, Giemsa or Field stain, and a Ziehl–Neilsen (ZN) stain can be of great value in the management of febrile patients.

Stain thick and thin blood films by the Giemsa or Field method, and examine them for malaria parasites. Trypanosomiasis and relapsing fever can also be diagnosed in this way.

Request sputum microscopy in patients with a productive cough. The presence of large numbers of gram-positive cocci in a sputum sample suggests pneumococcal pneumonia in a febrile patient with a cough. The presence of acid fast bacilli (AFB) in a

ZN-stained sample is diagnostic of pulmonary tuberculosis.

Gram stain of pus from abscesses or osteomyelitis can be useful in identifying the causative organism. The presence of pus cells in the urine of a febrile patient suggests a urinary tract infection.

Microscopy of cerebrospinal fluid (CSF) is essential for the diagnosis of meningitis. More than 5 white blood cells per mm^3 is diagnostic. A cell count and differential is helpful in distinguishing acute bacterial meningitis from viral or tuberculous disease, and it may be possible to identify the causative organism on a gram-stained deposit from a centrifuged sample. It is sometimes possible to identify AFBs in the deposit from patients with tuberculous meningitis, and an Indian ink stain is useful in diagnosing cryptococcal meningitis, though many patients with cryptococcal meningitis will not have identifiable fungi in the CSF.

Full blood count and differential can be helpful in reaching a diagnosis. Findings suggestive of particular infections are shown in the Box.

Finding	Suggests
Neutrophilia	Bacterial infection, amoebic abscess
Thrombocytopenia	Malaria, viral infection (e.g. dengue, HIV), DIC
Neutropenia	Brucellosis, typhoid
Lymphopenia	Advanced HIV disease
Pancytopenia	Visceral leishmaniasis, other causes of hypersplenism
Sickle cells, nucleated rbcs	Sickle cell disease

Serology

Since HIV-positive patients are at increased risk of serious infection, and a wider variety of infections must be considered in them, it is useful to know the HIV status of febrile patients. However, patients should not be tested for HIV without their consent, and it is important that both pre- and post-test counselling should be provided. Almost all the serological tests available for HIV diagnosis are highly sensitive and specific, but because of the serious implications of a positive test, results should not normally be given until a positive test has been confirmed, using a different assay.

Serological tests can be useful in the diagnosis of other infections in febrile patients. For example, amoebic serology in patients with a suspected amoebic abscess, or serology for brucellosis, or the Widal test for typhoid. However, the interpretation of these tests can be difficult in populations where the infections are endemic, or in individuals who have been immunised against typhoid, and a single test is insufficient to confirm the diagnosis, which requires a four-fold increase in titre in paired acute and convalescent samples.

Microbiological cultures

Where facilities allow, send appropriate samples of blood, urine, CSF, pus, stool or sputum to the laboratory for culture. The isolation of pathogenic bacteria from normally sterile body fluids, such as blood or CSF, is diagnostic, provided contamination can be ruled out. The significance of organisms isolated from sputum or faeces is less clear, since pathogenic organisms such as *Strep. pneumoniae* or salmonella species can be present at these sites in healthy carriers.

Imaging

A chest X-ray is helpful in the diagnosis of pulmonary tuberculosis in particular; other pulmonary infections, such as pneumonia or empyema, can often be diagnosed clinically. Ultrasound can be extremely useful in the identification of collections of pus in the abdomen, e.g. abscesses in the liver or subphrenic space, and in the diagnosis of pelvic inflammatory disease.

Needle aspirate or biopsy

In cases where the diagnosis remains unclear, consider more invasive diagnostic methods, such as a fine needle aspirate or biopsy. A fine needle aspirate of an enlarged lymph node, or of the bone marrow, can be stained for acid fast bacilli for the diagnosis of tuberculosis, which is high in the differential diagnosis of unexplained fever in African patients. If facilities are available, the sensitivity can be increased by setting up mycobacterial cultures. Trypanosomiasis can also be diagnosed by lymph node aspiration.

The presence of lymphocytes in pleural or peritoneal fluid suggests tuberculosis. Where there is access to histopathology, pleural or peritoneal biopsy can be helpful in patients with pleural or peritoneal effusions. Biopsies of liver and bone marrow can be helpful in diagnosing tuberculosis, lymphoma or disseminated malignancy.

Management of the febrile patient

After taking the history and completing the physical examination, make a working diagnosis. This will guide your choice of investigations, and your initial management of the patient.

Most febrile patients have self-limiting viral illnesses that do not need specific treatment.

In these cases, aim to relieve symptoms, usually with aspirin or paracetamol, and ask the patient to return if his condition does not improve.

In more seriously ill patients, specific treatment may need to be started before the results of investigations are available. In many cases you will have made a clinical diagnosis, eg. of pneumonia, or cellulitis, which will guide your choice of anti-microbial treatment. In other cases the diagnosis will not be certain, and you may need to start empirical treatment, based on your 'best guess' as to the most likely diagnosis. Except in exceptional cases (e.g., suspected meningococcal disease), this can wait until appropriate samples have been taken for microbiological investigation.

In much of Africa, there is a high probability that a persistent fever without localizing signs, in which malaria and pneumonia have been ruled out, is due to typhoid or tuberculosis. A trial of a broad spectrum antibiotic effective against local strains of *Salmonella typhi*, such as chloramphenicol or a quinolone, should be given initially.

Correct dehydration. In mildly or moderately dehydrated patients who are not vomiting and are conscious, oral rehydration is appropriate; this can be by nasogastric tube in patients who are unwilling to drink. A febrile adult in a warm climate requires at least 3 litres of fluid per 24 hours. In more severely dehydrated patients, or those who are unconscious or vomiting, set up an intravenous infusion, and correct any fluid deficit over 2 hours with Ringer's lactate solution or normal saline.

Assessment of dehydration (see Box) (see also Chapter 20)

Moderate dehydration (5% of body fluid)
Any two of the following:
- moderately reduced skin turgor
- increased thirst
- restlessness/ irritability (in children)
- sunken eyes

Severe dehydration (10% + of body fluid)
Any two of the following:
- greatly reduced skin turgor
- sunken eyes
- reduced conscious level
- inability to drink
- poor peripheral perfusion
- hypotension

Follow-up

Ask outpatients to return at any time if their symptoms get worse. Depending on the working diagnosis, routine follow-up appointments may or may not be appropriate.

Febrile patients admitted to hospital should be carefully monitored by medical and nursing staff. Keep the nursing staff fully informed about the patient, as this will improve the quality of the data they collect, for example, on temperature and pulse (which should be measured 6-hourly whenever possible), and fluid balance. Re-examine the patient daily to assess whether or not s/he is improving, and to identify new symptoms or signs that may develop.

The time taken for the temperature to subside after starting appropriate treatment depends on the diagnosis. It is generally rapid (2–3 days) in uncomplicated respiratory or urinary tract infections, but may take longer in typhoid (5–7 days) or tuberculosis (up to 1 month). A persistent fever is likely in patients with collections of pus that have not been drained.

Persistent fever

In patients whose general condition is not improving, or whose fever persists for more than 1 week after anti-microbial treatment is started, consider the following possibilities.

(a) The original diagnosis was wrong.
(b) The organism responsible is resistant to the antimicrobial you have prescribed.
(c) The patient has more than one cause for his/her fever. Many African patients with malaria, for example, have a coexisting serious bacterial infection (Berkley et al., 1999; Prada et al., 1993; Mabey et al., 1987).
(d) The patient has not taken the treatment prescribed.

Patients with fever of uncertain cause should be kept under continuous review, and should be questioned and re-examined daily for new symptoms and signs, since the cause of the fever will often become clear with time.

Because tuberculosis is such a common, and curable, cause of fever in Africa, consider a trial of anti-tuberculous therapy in patients with persistent fever of uncertain origin who do not respond to broad spectrum antibiotics. Patients who fail to improve after a trial of broad spectrum antibiotics and 1 month of anti-tuberculous treatment probably have another cause for their fever, e.g. malignant or autoimmune disease, and should be investigated further for these conditions if facilities are available.

References

Berkley J, Mwarumba S, Bramham K, Lowe B, Marsh K. (1999). Bacteraemia complicating severe malaria in children. *Trans Roy. Soc Trop Med Hyg* **93**: 283–286.

Mabey DC, Brown A, Greenwood BM. (1987). *Plasmodium falciparum* malaria and *Salmonellla* infections in Gambian children. *J Infect Dis* **155**: 1319–1321.

Prada J, Alabi SA, Bienzle U. (1993). Bacterial strains isolated from blood cultures of Nigerian children with cerebral malaria. *Lancet* **342**: 1114.

Major common infections

13 HIV/AIDS

In 1982, physicians in South West Uganda noticed a new disease with prominent symptoms of weight loss and diarrhoea, known locally as slim disease, and in 1983 patients with opportunistic infections and Kaposi's sarcoma were identified in hospitals in Rwanda and Zaïre. These observations were made shortly after reports of clusters of unusual diseases associated with profound immunosuppression among homosexual men in the United States. These reports were the first to draw public attention to the acquired immunodeficiency syndrome (AIDS), initially as an unusual new disease, and now undoubtedly the greatest challenge to global public health in recent years.

The problem in Africa

The global burden of HIV disease falls most heavily in sub-Saharan Africa. The Joint United Nations Programme on HIV/AIDS (UNAIDS) estimates that, of the 42 million people estimated to be living with HIV/AIDS at the end of 2002, 95 per cent were in developing countries, and about two-thirds in sub-Saharan Africa (Fig. 13.1). In some African countries up to one-third of adults aged 15–49 are infected. HIV disease is the most common diagnosis among adults hospitalized in medical wards in many urban centres, and is the major cause of death among young adults. The impact on society of a disease causing severe illness and death primarily among young adults is far-reaching. For example, the incidence of tuberculosis among staff at a district hospital in South Africa increased five-fold from 1991–2 to 1993–6 (Wilkinson & Gilks, 1998) and mortality rates among Zambian nurses increased ten-fold comparing 1980–5 with 1989–91 (Buvé et al., 1994). HIV-related morbidity and mortality among teachers is affecting education: it is estimated that Swaziland will need to train twice as many teachers as previously in order to maintain the same level of service (UNAIDS, 2000). The rapid increase in the numbers of children orphaned by AIDS is also a major cause for concern.

HIV disease is caused by two distinct viruses, HIV-1 and HIV-2. The distribution of these two infections in African countries is illustrated in Fig. 13.2. Unlike HIV-1, HIV-2 has remained confined to a relatively limited geographical area in West Africa, Portugal and countries with historical links to Portugal; this limited spread most probably results from much lower transmissibility. The prevalence of HIV-2 is declining, and HIV-1 infection is 'taking over' in areas where HIV-2 has been prevalent.

The course of the epidemic has varied in different countries. This is illustrated in Fig. 13.3, showing the changes in the prevalence of HIV infection among pregnant women in selected African cities; Kampala, Uganda; Abidjan, Côte d'Ivoire; Yaoundé, Cameroon; and Francistown, Botswana. In the 1980s, countries most severely affected were those of eastern and central Africa, such as Uganda. In Southern Africa, the epidemic started later, in the early 1990s, but has subsequently spread very rapidly and this region now has the highest general population prevalence of HIV infection world-wide.

Transmission of HIV infection

HIV infection may be transmitted from person to person by sexual intercourse (heterosexual or homosexual), from mother to child, by the transfusion of HIV-infected blood or blood products, or via contaminated needles, either by injecting drug use where needles or equipment are shared or by re-use of unsterilized medical equipment.

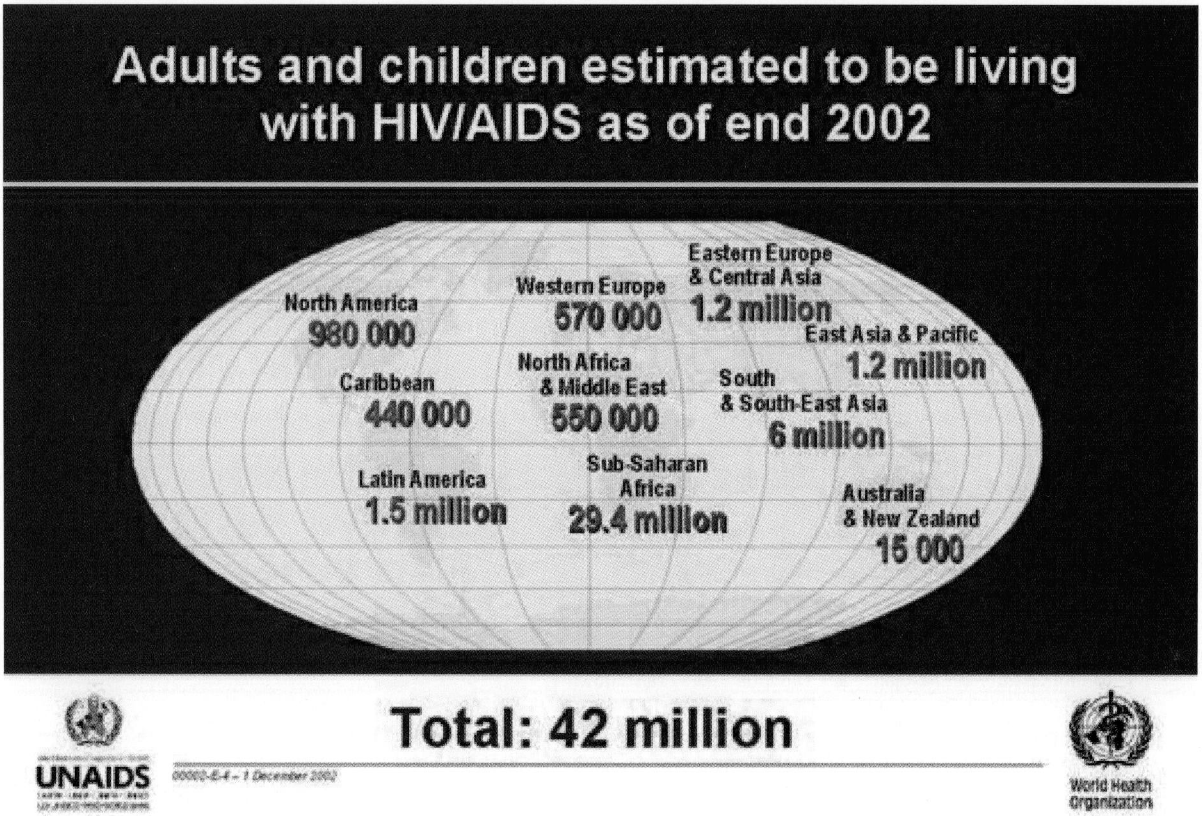

Fig. 13.1. Global distribution of individuals living with HIV/AIDS at the end of 2002.

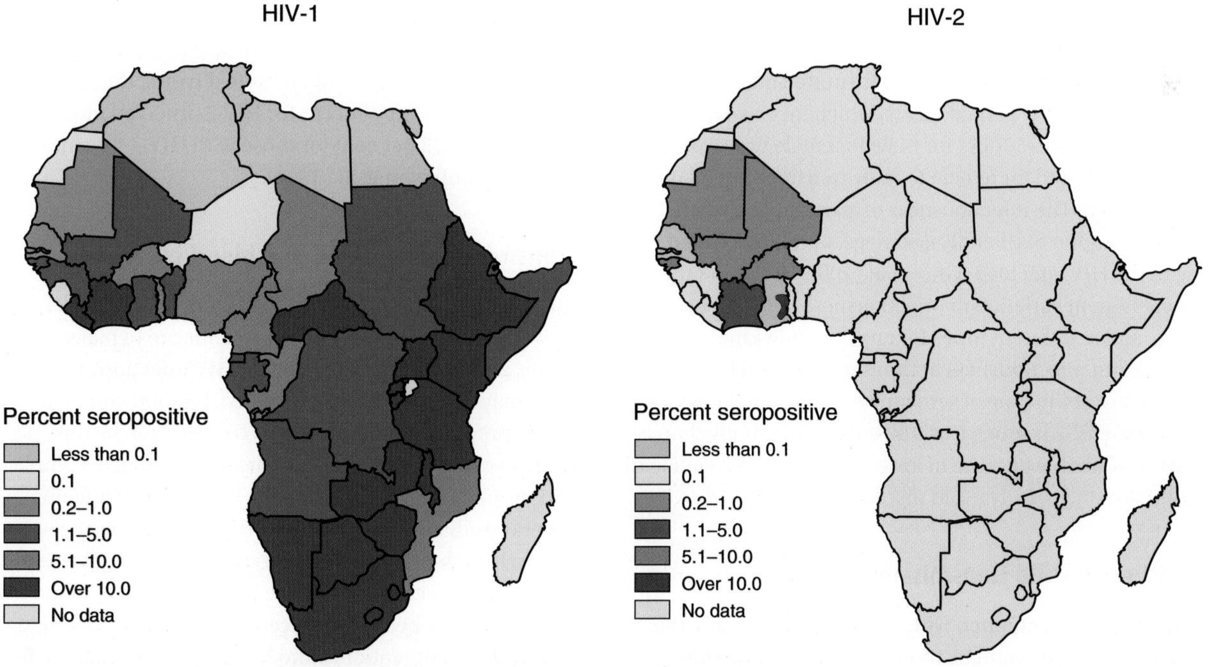

Fig. 13.2. Prevalence of HIV-1 and HIV-2 infections among low-risk urban populations. *Source:* HIV/AIDS surveillance database of the US Bureau of the Census (June, 2001).

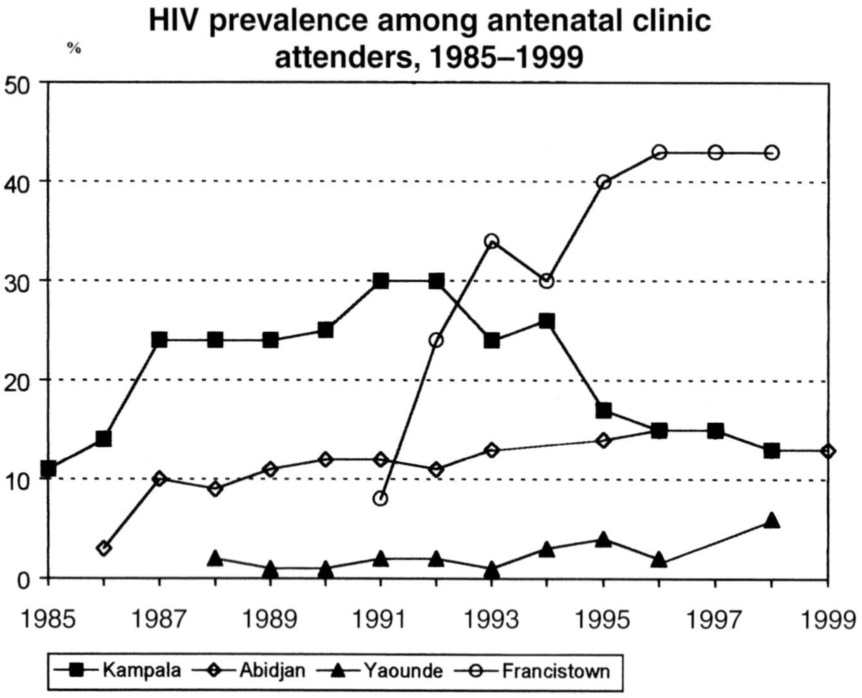

Fig. 13.3. Changes in HIV prevalence among pregnant women in selected African cities, 1985 to 1999. *Source:* HIV/AIDS surveillance database of the US Bureau of the Census (June, 2000).

Sexual transmission

Heterosexual intercourse is responsible for the great majority of HIV infections world-wide, particularly in sub-Saharan Africa. Transmission of HIV is enhanced by the presence of other sexually transmitted infections (STI), particularly genital ulcers, which increase the risk of transmission 10–50-fold for male to female transmission, and 50–300-fold for female to male transmission (Hayes et al., 1995). The infectiousness of an individual also depends upon his/her disease stage, and is correlated with the HIV viral load (Gray et al., 2001). It follows that there is great variation in infectiousness between individuals, and at different times for any one individual, with maximum infectiousness at times of high viral load, which are at the time of seroconversion and in late-stage disease. HIV-2 is much less transmissible sexually than is HIV-1, probably because of lower levels of HIV-2 viral load until the stage of advanced disease.

Mother-to-child transmission

The majority of children with HIV infection acquire the virus from their mothers, though some transmission occurs through blood transfusion, piercing with contaminated instruments, or through sexual abuse of children.

The overall risk of mother-to-child transmission for HIV-1 is reported at between 20 and 42 per cent; this subject is discussed in detail later in this chapter. The risk of mother-to-child transmission of HIV-2 is much lower than that of HIV-1; in Abidjan, Côte d'Ivoire, the risk of transmission was 1 per cent for HIV-2–infected mothers compared to 25 per cent for those with HIV-1 infection (Adjorlolo-Johnson et al., 1994).

Transmission via blood and blood products

Although transmission of HIV by blood products is largely preventable where appropriate systems are in place, estimates are that up to 10 per cent of HIV infections worldwide may be transfusion-associated. Women and children are disproportionately at risk of HIV infection by this route because of the impact of the haemorrhagic complications of childbirth, and malaria as a cause of anaemia. Several studies in sub-Saharan Africa have shown a surprisingly high risk from blood transfusion, as high as 2 per cent overall, in countries where HIV screening of blood had apparently been introduced, the persistent risk being largely due to operational and logistical difficulties such as shortages of supplies and poor laboratory and clerical practices (Moore et al., 2001).

Transmission via contaminated needles

In parts of western and southern Europe, the former Soviet Union, and Asia, injecting drug use is the major mode of HIV transmission. In other parts of the world, including in some countries of sub-Saharan Africa, injecting drug use is rare at present but is emerging or threatening to emerge as a problem of public health significance. In settings as diverse as Bangkok and Edinburgh, the increase in rates of HIV infection among drug injectors escalated more rapidly than in any other population. Injecting drug users act as an important bridge population for sexual and mother-to-child transmission of HIV.

Transmission of HIV may also occur if medical equipment is reused without sterilization, or via needle-stick injuries to health care workers. The risk of HIV transmission following a single percutaneous needlestick injury is estimated at 0.3 per cent; the risk is increased by deep intramuscular injury, visible blood on the needle, needle used to enter a blood vessel and a source patient with end-stage disease. There are few data on the frequency of transmission by this mode in African countries; where studies have been done, health care workers usually have a similar HIV prevalence to individuals from the same community, suggesting that nosocomial transmission is relatively less important than other routes. None the less, facilities and procedures for safe handling of potentially infected sharps are required in order to minimize any excess risk to health care staff.

Regional differences in dynamics of the HIV epidemic

As Fig. 13.3 illustrates, there have been marked regional differences in the dynamics of the HIV epidemic in terms of the speed of increase in HIV prevalence among the general population and the plateau level of prevalence reached. There are many possible explanations for these differences, including differences in sexual behaviour, in the prevalence of sexually transmitted diseases, and in the effect of control measures. These differences were investigated in a study in four African cities, two with a high prevalence of HIV infection (Kisumu, Kenya and Ndola, Zambia, adult HIV prevalence 25.9 per cent and 28.4 per cent, respectively) and two with relatively low HIV prevalence (Cotonou, Benin and Yaoundé, Cameroon, HIV prevalence 3.4 per cent and 5.9 per cent, respectively) (Buvé et al., 2001). The factors most strongly associated with HIV infection were infection with herpes simplex virus type 2 (HSV-2) and lack of male circumcision. Perhaps surprisingly, sexual behaviour patterns did not appear to explain differences in HIV prevalence. The conclusion was that differences in the efficiency of transmission of HIV, due to circumcision and the presence of STIs, outweighed the effect of differences in sexual behaviour. Strategies to prevent HSV-2 infection are now being investigated, and a randomized controlled trial to investigate the protective effect of male circumcision has been proposed.

The organisms

HIV disease and AIDS are caused by two distinct viruses, HIV-1 and HIV-2, which both belong to the lentivirus subfamily of retroviruses. Retroviruses are single-stranded RNA viruses which are unique in having an enzyme, reverse transcriptase, which makes a DNA copy of the viral RNA genome. The DNA copy is then inserted into the host genome.

Structure of HIV

The structure of the virus is illustrated in Fig. 13.4. The virus consists of two copies of the RNA genome and two copies of the enzyme reverse transcriptase contained in the viral core, surrounded by a viral envelope composed of lipids. The viral envelope contains glycoproteins gp120 and gp41 (gp = glycoprotein; the number indicates the approximate molecular weight in kilodaltons); these are encoded by the *env* gene. Most diagnostic tests for HIV detect antibodies to these viral envelope glycoproteins. The *gag* gene encodes the viral core proteins p24, p7 and p6, along with the matrix protein p17. p24 antigen is detectable in blood when it is present in higher concentrations than anti-p24 antibodies, typically in very early and in late-stage HIV infection. p24 antigen has also been used in diagnostic testing at these stages of disease.

HIV replication

The replication cycle of HIV is illustrated in Fig. 13.5. HIV most often uses the CD4 receptor to attach to cells, though other receptors are also involved. Once in the cell, viral RNA is transcribed to double-stranded DNA by reverse transcriptase. Proviral DNA enters the cell nucleus and is integrated into the host genome, promoted by the enzyme integrase. RNA is then transcribed from the integrated proviral DNA, which provides new RNA for the formation of new virions, and also messenger RNA to make viral proteins. The enzyme protease is required to split the

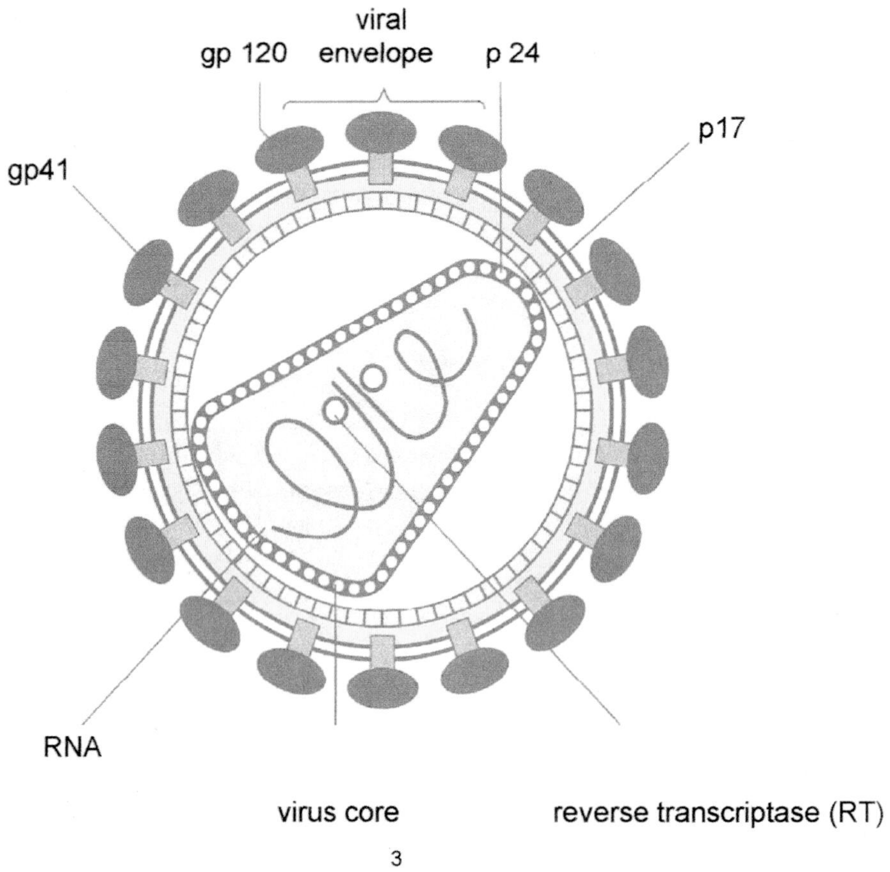

Fig. 13.4. Structure of HIV. (Courtesy of Dr Wolfgang Preiser.)

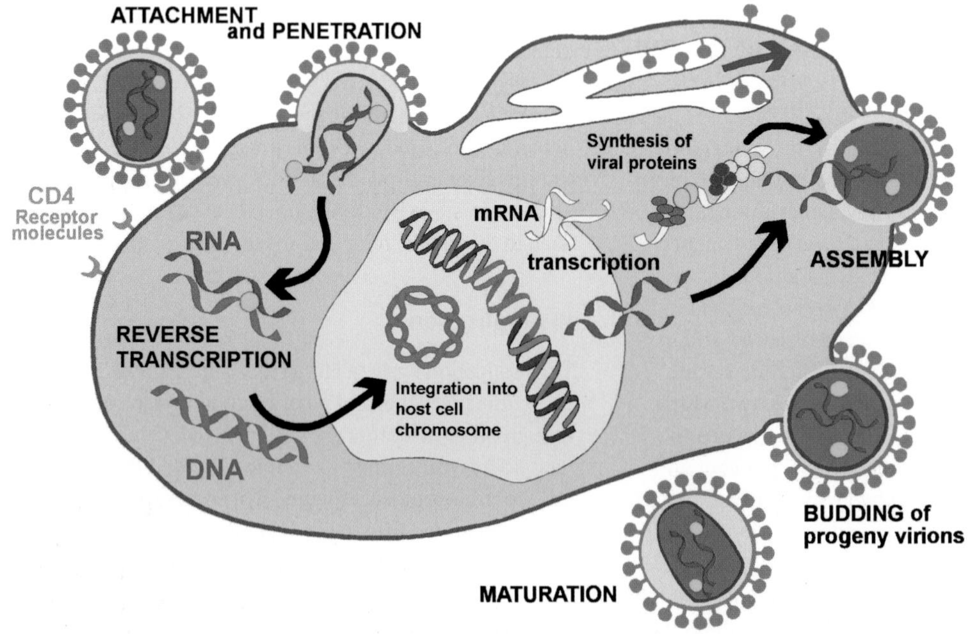

Fig. 13.5. HIV replication cycle. (Courtesy of Dr Lydia Stannard.)

structural viral proteins into appropriate sections to make new virions. The enzymes reverse transcriptase, integrase and protease which are involved in the replication of HIV are important as targets for drugs which inhibit HIV replication – antiretroviral drugs (often abbreviated to ARV, or ART, meaning antiretroviral therapy).

HIV is highly genetically diverse, both within each HIV-infected individual, and within populations. When reverse transcriptase transcribes viral RNA to proviral DNA, transcription errors are frequent. This results in a high rate of production of viral mutants. In addition, there are two strands of viral RNA within each viral particle, and during reverse transcription, there may be genetic recombination between the two strands. Recombinant viruses may thus develop if an individual is infected with more than one subtype of HIV (see below).

Origins of HIV

It is generally accepted that HIV was introduced into human populations from non-human primates. HIV-1 is genetically very similar to simian immunodeficiency virus (SIV) in chimpanzees (SIV_{cpz}) and HIV-2 to SIV in sooty mangabeys (SIV_{sm}). It is most likely that the viruses crossed from primate to man via the hunting and preparation of primate meat, or from primate bites. The earliest human plasma sample providing evidence of HIV-1 infection dates from 1959, from Kinshasa, Democratic Republic of Congo. Analysis of the genetic differences between subtypes of HIV-1 suggests that the virus has probably been present in humans since the early part of the twentieth century. The virus has spread more rapidly during the last 20 years, probably assisted by more rapid means of transportation, the displacement of populations, and changing patterns of sexual behaviour. The three major groups of HIV-1 (M, N and O) have genetic differences which imply that the virus has crossed into human populations on at least three separate occasions (Hahn et al., 2000).

Over the years since HIV was first identified, there has been continuing controversy concerning whether HIV really is the cause of AIDS. Dissenters suggested that the syndromes comprising AIDS were due to recreational or antiretroviral drugs. The evidence supporting HIV as the cause of AIDS is now overwhelming: some of the most compelling data include the greatly increased rates of mortality among HIV-infected compared with uninfected people in rural Uganda in the early 1990s when use of either recreational or antiretroviral drugs was virtually unknown, and the development of AIDS in the children of HIV-infected mothers, who were similarly not exposed to these drugs. Although scientific ideas usually benefit from challenge, further debate over this issue creates confusion among populations badly hit by the epidemic, where strong political leadership and clear messages concerning prevention are desperately needed in order to combat the epidemic.

Subtypes of HIV-1 and HIV-2

On the basis of analysis of the viral genome, HIV-1 can be divided into three distinct strains, known as group M (main or major), N (new) and O (outlier). Group M is the most common group world-wide; groups N and O are much less common, and have remained largely limited to Cameroon and Gabon. Group M is further subdivided into 11 subtypes (or clades), known as subtypes A–K. The geographical distribution of these subtypes is illustrated in Fig. 13.6. Subtype B is predominant in the USA, Europe and Australia: subtype A predominates in West Africa, subtypes A and D in East Africa and subtype C in Southern Africa. Some subtypes, such as subtype E in Thailand, show evidence of having emerged as a result of recombination (as described above). Six subtypes of HIV-2, A-F, are recognized.

This variation in subtype by geographical region may be particularly relevant to vaccine development, because a vaccine giving effective protection against one subtype of HIV-1 might not necessarily be effective against others. It has been suggested that different subtypes of HIV-1 may vary in terms of transmissibility and pathogenesis, but there is little good evidence to support these hypotheses (Hu et al., 1999).

Pathogenesis

HIV causes disease in humans primarily by causing destruction of cells of the immune system, thus making the HIV-infected individual increasingly susceptible to other pathogens as the course of HIV disease progresses. CD4+ lymphocytes are the main target cell infected by HIV, and loss of CD4+ cells is a key feature of HIV-related immunosuppression (see Chapter 6). There are a number of mechanisms by which CD4+ cells are lost, including direct destruction of infected cells, and induction of apoptosis (programmed cell death). It was initially thought that HIV was relatively inactive during the asymptomatic period between seroconversion and the onset of symptomatic disease. However, it is now understood that active viral replication continues throughout the asymptomatic period, which leads to virus- and immune-mediated destruction of CD4 lymphocytes.

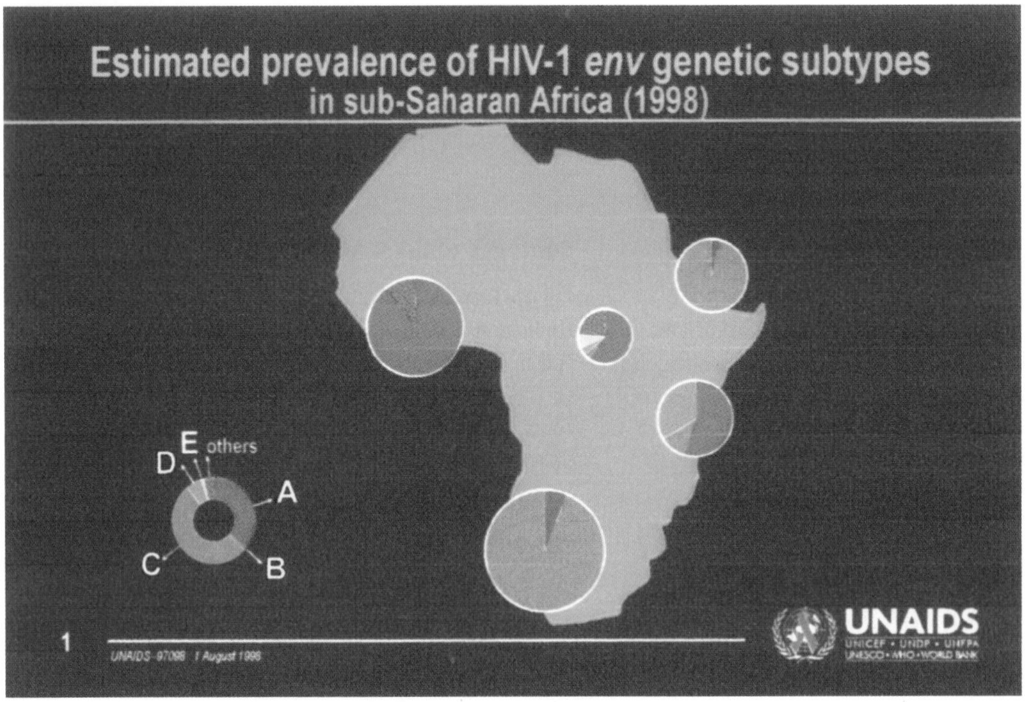

Fig. 13.6. Distribution of HIV-1 subtypes in Africa.

Initially the immune system is able to replenish the CD4 cells, but eventually its regenerative capacity becomes exhausted, leading to the fall in CD4 cell counts typical of advanced HIV-related immunosuppression (Ho et al., 1995).

In addition to destruction of cells of the immune system, HIV can have a direct pathogenic effect on other organ systems, particularly the central nervous system and the gastrointestinal tract.

Diagnosis of HIV infection

Tests for antibodies to HIV-1 and HIV-2

The tests most commonly used to detect HIV infection are tests for antibodies to HIV, most often enzyme immunoassays (EIA). EIAs are relatively easy to use, and a wide range of HIV EIAs with very high sensitivity and specificity are commercially available at around US$1–2 per test.

The Western blot is a way of testing for a range of antibodies to HIV. Western blots use HIV antigens separated by electrophoresis on prepared gels. Antibodies from a patient's serum bind to these antigens, and (when appropriately labelled, for example with a substrate which undergoes colour change when it binds to the antibodies) appear as bands on the gel, which are compared to positive and negative controls. Western blots are generally regarded as the 'gold standard' for HIV antibody testing, but are much more expensive and labour intensive than EIAs, and more difficult to interpret. Now that a range of highly accurate EIAs are available, Western blots are not normally necessary for routine diagnostic purposes.

Different strategies for HIV antibody testing are appropriate for different situations (such as screening blood for transfusion, anonymous surveillance and diagnostic testing of an individual), and recommendations on testing algorithms have been made by UNAIDS and WHO (UNAIDS/WHO, 2001). Only diagnosis of HIV infection in an individual requesting a test will be considered further here. Because the performance of any laboratory test depends upon the prevalence of disease in the population (the higher the prevalence, the greater the probability that a person with a positive test result is genuinely HIV infected), three strategies are recommended to maximize sensitivity and specificity while minimizing cost:

Strategy I is appropriate for diagnostic testing in populations where the prevalence of HIV infection is greater than 30 per cent among persons with clinical signs or symptoms suggesting HIV infection. This requires a single EIA test, with the result of the test accepted as indicative of the HIV status of the individual.

Strategy II is appropriate for diagnostic testing in populations where:

- among persons with clinical evidence suggesting HIV infection, the prevalence of HIV infection is less than 30 per cent; or
- among asymptomatic persons, the prevalence of HIV infection is greater than 10%.

This requires two EIA tests. The two tests should use different antigens: the first ('screening') test should have maximum sensitivity, and the second should have maximum specificity. If the first test is negative, the result is considered negative. If the first test is positive, the second ('confirmatory') test is performed. If the second test is also positive, the result is considered positive. If the second test is negative, the result is considered negative.

Strategy III is recommended for diagnostic testing in populations where the prevalence of HIV infection among asymptomatic individuals is less than 10 per cent.

This requires three EIA tests, and is similar to strategy II, but differs in the procedure if the first EIA is positive and the second negative. In this case, a third EIA (again based on a different antigen) should be performed. If the third EIA is positive, the result is considered positive, but if the third EIA is negative, a negative result is recorded.

For all strategies, when a person is newly diagnosed as HIV-infected, a second blood sample should be tested in order to minimize the risk of an incorrect result due to clerical or administrative error.

Interpretation of HIV test results

HIV antibodies may be undetectable in very early infection (the so-called 'window period') and a negative HIV antibody test result may therefore be misleading in an individual who has been at risk of HIV infection shortly before having the test. If there is doubt, repeat testing should be recommended after a suitable interval: the great majority of individuals will have detectable HIV antibody by 3 months after infection.

So-called 'indeterminate' or 'discordant' HIV test results, where different EIA tests give discrepant results, may occur in very early HIV infection (when only the most sensitive EIAs may be positive), and if this is possible, repeat testing after 2 weeks is recommended. Indeterminate results may also be seen in individuals with advanced HIV disease because of a decrease in antibody levels. In this situation, where the clinical suspicion of HIV is very high, it is not normally necessary to repeat the test.

Recommendations on the selection of appropriate tests are available from UNAIDS and WHO (2001), available at http: //www.unaids.org/publications/documents/epidemiology/surveillance/JC602–HIVSurvGuidel-E.pdf (accessed 11.2.02). There is increasing availability of HIV 'rapid tests' in which all the necessary equipment is provided with the kit, and so laboratory facilities are not required. Results are usually available in under 45 minutes. These tests can be used in geographically remote areas, and for hard-to-reach populations, and are increasingly used for on-site testing, for example at HIV voluntary counselling and testing centres, and antenatal clinics. At US$1–3 per test, the cost is slightly higher than for EIAs. Since rapid tests are often used at multiple sites rather than at a few centralized laboratories, staff training and quality assurance are particularly important. Tests which detect HIV antibodies in saliva or urine are also available, and may be useful in some circumstances, though they are generally less reliable than tests using blood.

Tests for the virus

A number of techniques can be used to detect HIV itself rather than the antibody response to it. The most commonly used of these are:

Detection of p24 antigen

p24 is the viral core protein, which is detectable in plasma when present in greater quantities than antibodies to it, typically in very early infection and in advanced immunosuppression. Commercial ELISA tests are available for p24 detection, but most are limited by low sensitivity. The use of a modified p24 assay as a cheaper and simpler substitute for viral genome detection is currently being investigated.

Detection of the viral genome

A number of tests are available which use the polymerase chain reaction (PCR) to amplify the viral genome. These assays detect either RNA from virus free in the blood, or proviral DNA from circulating mononuclear cells. These assays can be qualitative, i.e. they detect presence or absence of the virus, or quantitative, i.e. they give an estimate of the amount of virus present in the blood. Quantitative PCR tests for HIV RNA or DNA are commonly referred to as 'viral load' tests. These PCR assays are currently very expensive and not widely available in developing countries. These assays may differ in their performance for different viral subtypes, and are not currently commercially available for HIV-2.

Tests which detect HIV itself are particularly useful in:

- diagnosis of very early HIV infection, before HIV antibodies are detectable. p24 detection was previously used for this purpose, but has now been superseded by qualitative PCR

- diagnosis of HIV infection in infants
- assessment of prognosis. As discussed later, the quantity of virus detectable in the blood is closely associated with the risk of disease progression, and viral load testing is now routinely used for this purpose, where available
- monitoring therapy. Viral load testing is also used to monitor the effectiveness of antiretroviral treatment and in making decisions on when to change therapy.

Clinical diagnosis of HIV infection

The clinical diagnosis of HIV infection is difficult because most of the characteristic symptoms and signs of HIV infection are neither sensitive nor specific. A particular problem is that the clinical presentation of advanced HIV disease can be indistinguishable from tuberculosis in an HIV-negative individual. In populations with a high prevalence of HIV infection, herpes zoster and other findings such as prurigo (a generalized itchy maculopapular rash) have a high positive predictive value for HIV infection in adults. This means that if these clinical findings are present, the individual has a high probability of being HIV-infected; however, they are found in a relatively small percentage of HIV-infected individuals, and so their absence does not indicate absence of HIV infection. In all cases, wherever possible, individuals thought to have HIV infection should undergo HIV testing so that appropriate counselling and care can be given.

Counselling before and after testing for HIV infection

Counselling is an interpersonal communication through which a person is helped to assess his/her current situation, explore his/her feelings and come up with a constructive plan of action. Counselling provides an opportunity for health workers to discuss with clients the nature of HIV disease, its implications for health and their choices for the future. A health worker should thus know the facts about HIV, develop counselling skills and incorporate them into his or her daily practice.

Objectives of counselling

Effective counselling aims to:

(a) provide adequate and accurate information on HIV infection (including transmission, prevention, diagnosis and treatment).

(b) help the client deal with feelings commonly associated with HIV infection (e.g. grief, loneliness, anxiety, anger, guilt, hopelessness).

(c) help the client mobilize support from his family, community, religious community, health workers and friends.

(d) help the client adopt appropriate behaviour to reduce the risk of transmission of infection, and to prevent suicide, violence towards others, premature withdrawal from responsibilities, etc.

(e) help the client to deal with death, and make decisions related to his own death.

(f) intervene constructively in crisis situations (e.g. financial problems, loss of spouse, child or job, rejection by friends).

Types of counselling

Pre-test counselling

This is counselling offered before an HIV antibody test. Key issues to be addressed are summarized in the Box. All people taking an HIV test must understand the meaning of a negative and a positive test result: a positive test does not mean an immediate death sentence, nor does a negative test mean being 'immune' to HIV. Effective pre-test counselling also involves helping the client anticipate and cope with emotions that may be the consequence of a positive or negative test.

Key issues to be addressed in HIV pre-test counselling

1. What is HIV?
2. How is HIV transmitted?
3. How to prevent transmission (safer sex, safer injecting if relevant)
4. What is the meaning of a positive and negative HIV test result, and understanding of the 'window' period
5. Difference between HIV and AIDS; a positive HIV test does not indicate AIDS
6. Advantages of knowing status: what care is available if test is positive
7. Disadvantages of knowing status (e.g. possible stigma; exclusion from life insurance, health insurance etc. if relevant.)
8. How would the individual cope with a positive test result: who would they tell? (identify individuals who are isolated or at risk of self-harm who may need additional support; also partner notification issues)
9. Confidentiality of test result (explain local procedures, e.g. in many centres test results are only disclosed to a third party with the client's written permission)
10. How will test result be given (when, by whom)

Post-test counselling

This is counselling after the test result has been given. Receiving a positive result can be an emotionally traumatic experience. A counsellor offers his/her experience and time to help the client cope with his/her feelings and arranges appropriate follow-up. A negative test result provides an important opportunity to reinforce the importance of safe behaviour to preserve negative status.

Pre- and post-diagnosis counselling

This is done before and after a diagnosis of HIV disease is made on clinical grounds alone. This happens when a health worker has no access to HIV testing facilities, but would like to initiate appropriate care for a patient with features suggesting underlying HIV infection. The principle issues to be discussed are similar to those listed for pre-test counselling.

Prevention counselling

This is where information and appropriate skills are passed on to an individual or a group of people to empower them to avoid becoming HIV infected by minimizing high risk behaviour.

Supportive counselling

This is carried out to support those affected and infected by HIV. It helps the patient, the family and friends cope better with the infection.

On-going counselling

Counselling is a continuous process, and further counselling may be needed to deal with issues and problems that arise as the client and their family cope with the disease.

Effective counselling

Anyone who has basic counselling skills and adequate knowledge of HIV infection can be an effective counsellor, for example a health worker, religious leader, community worker or teacher.

Effective counselling requires the following attitudes:

- *Non-judgemental approach:* the counsellor accepts the client and his/her problems without being judgmental or moralistic. A counsellor should not condemn a client's behaviour.
- *Confidentiality:* a counsellor must not reveal anything that a client has shared with him/her to anyone else without the client's permission.
- *Empathy:* a counsellor should try to imagine what it is like to be in a similar situation to the client.
- *Caring:* the counsellor should show that s/he cares about the client by:
  - being approachable, easy to talk to, interested in the client, prepared to take time to talk
  - being reliable – if s/he says will do something, s/he honours that promise.

Good counselling skills

An effective counsellor must be a good communicator; the following are key skills:

- *Active listening* encourages the client to tell his story. A skilled counsellor spends more time listening than talking and thereby learns what the client already knows about AIDS and HIV infection, and his problems, feelings and behaviour.
- *Non-verbal communication*: using appropriate body language and eye contact.
- *Effective use of questions*: using open-ended questions which encourage the client to be open about his/her attitudes, feelings and behaviour.
- *Checking key points* to ensure that client and counsellor understand each other
- *Reinforcing positive attitudes, feelings and behaviour*: identifying existing strengths in the client, and reinforcing them so the client can build his/her own strategies.
- *Providing information*: this must be correct, clear and consistent. A counsellor should be honest if he/she does not know the answer to a question.

An effective counsellor helps the client to tell his/her story, to consider his/her options and to make an informed plan for the future.

Clinical HIV disease in adults

Natural history

The natural history of HIV disease can be divided into a number of stages:

- acute HIV infection
- asymptomatic infection
- early symptomatic disease
- advanced disease.

Figure 13.7 shows how cellular immunity and the concentration of virus detectable in the blood change over time. The function of the cellular immune system is best measured using the CD4+ lymphocyte count when this is available: unfortunately this is rare in low income settings. The total lymphocyte count can be used as a surrogate marker for the CD4 count: it is less satisfactory

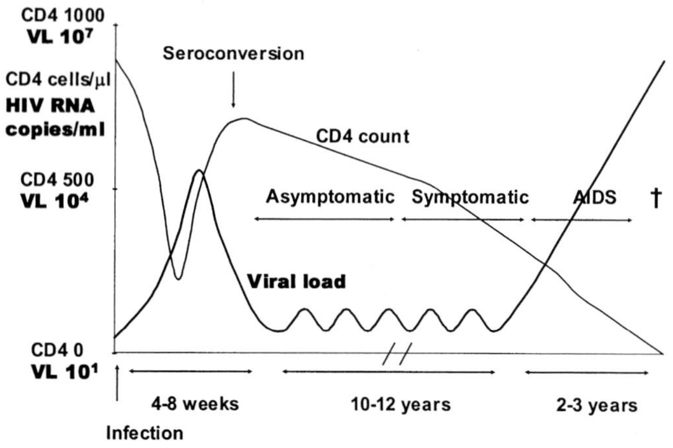

Fig. 13.7. Changes in CD4 lymphocyte count and HIV viral load during the course of HIV disease. (Courtesy of Dr Wolfgang Preiser.)

because it also includes CD8 cells, which are often elevated in HIV-infected patients. However there is some evidence that total lymphocyte count also has prognostic significance.

Acute HIV infection

Shortly after infection with HIV, there may be a symptomatic illness (referred to as acute HIV infection, primary HIV infection or seroconversion illness). This is usually mild and non-specific. The best-known syndrome is a glandular fever-like illness with fever and generalized lymphadenopathy, but a wide range of manifestations are described (Box) including diarrhoea, skin rash and lymphocytic meningitis. Few individuals seek medical attention at the time of seroconversion.

Clinical manifestations of acute HIV infection

- glandular-fever like illness: fever, sore throat, generalized lymphadenopathy
- skin rash
- weight loss
- nausea, diarrhoea, abdominal pain, vomiting
- oral and/or genital ulceration
- headache, photophobia, maningism, peripheral neuropathy, facial palsy

At the time of seroconversion, the HIV viral load rises to a peak (see Fig. 13.7). Since infectiousness is directly related to viral load, individuals are highly infectious at this time. At the same time, the CD4 count may drop transiently, and occasionally falls to very low levels such that conditions typical of more advanced HIV disease, such as oral candidiasis, may be seen. This will normally resolve as the CD4 count returns to its previous level.

Asymptomatic infection

Following seroconversion, HIV-infected individuals remain apparently well and asymptomatic for a variable period of time. This asymptomatic period lasts on average 10 years in industrialized countries, with great variation between individuals. The viral load declines from high levels at the time of seroconversion to a relatively stable level after three to four months, the so-called 'set point', which represents an equilibrium between viral replication and the attempts of the host's immune system to control replication. The set point varies greatly between individuals, and is closely associated with the rate of subsequent disease progression. There is a progressive decline in immune function during the asymptomatic period: the CD4 count falls by an average of $50–75 \times 10^6$/l per year (see Fig. 13.7).

Early symptomatic disease

Early symptoms may include skin and mucous membrane disorders such as reactivation of varicella-zoster virus, fungal skin and nail infections and prurigo (a generalized itchy maculopapular eruption which eventually heals, often leaving pigmented macules). There may also be constitutional symptoms such as unexplained fever and weight loss. Tuberculosis can occur at any stage of HIV disease and should always be considered in individuals with fever, weight loss or persistent cough. Bacterial pneumonia, Kaposi's sarcoma and non-Hodgkin's lymphoma may also occur relatively early as well as at the stage of advanced disease. Oral candida, although generally considered an early manifestation, may be an indicator of more advanced disease (Malamba et al., 1999).

Early symptoms of HIV disease are often non-specific. In regions where diseases such as malaria, tuberculosis and pneumococcal disease are frequent in adults irrespective of HIV status, symptoms of these diseases, such as fever and weight loss, may give the impression of rapid progression of HIV disease. In industrialized countries, symptomatic HIV disease is unusual until the CD4 count falls below about 500×10^6/l. In Uganda, the median CD4 count at the development of symptomatic disease defining WHO stages 2 and 3 (described later) were 516 and 428×10^6/l, respectively (Morgan, 1998). Some of the most important causes of morbidity and mortality in developing countries, particularly tuberculosis and pneumococcal disease, can occur at any stage of disease, but the risk increases with increasing immunosuppression.

Advanced disease

In industrialized countries, diseases due to organisms of relatively low pathogenicity (so-called 'opportunistic' infections), such as *Pneumocystis carinii* pneumonia (PCP), cerebral toxoplasmosis, cryptococcal disease and cryptosporidiosis, are unusual until the CD4 count falls below 200×10^6/l. The limited data on CD4 counts from African countries suggest that the majority of individuals with advanced disease similarly have CD4 counts below 200×10^6/l. HIV-infected individuals dying in African countries have median CD4 counts around 50×10^6/l, whereas in industrialized countries death was rare with CD4 counts above 10×10^6/l before the advent of highly active antiretroviral therapy (HAART). This reflects poor survival at the stage of advanced disease, most probably because of lack of access to diagnosis and treatment of severe infections occurring in advanced disease.

The most common diseases occurring at the stage of advanced disease vary by geographical region: those common in African countries are described in the section on spectrum of disease.

The diseases characteristic of HIV-related immunosuppression occur at different points in the progress of the disease. Figure 13.8 shows data from African studies documenting the mean or median CD4 count at the time of diagnosis of selected HIV-related diseases. It follows that the median survival following an HIV-related disease depends upon which disease it is: survival after a diagnosis of tuberculosis is much better than that after a diagnosis of oesophageal candidiasis.

Determinants of disease progression

Host factors: intrinsic

Older age at the time of seroconversion is the factor most consistently associated with rapid progression from infection to advanced disease, and from the onset of advanced disease to death. Large cohort studies from industrialized countries suggest that gender and mode of HIV transmission do not have a major influence on the rate of disease progression.

After allowing for demographic factors such as age, there is wide variation in the rate of disease progression between individuals. Although the CD4 molecule is the main receptor that HIV uses to enter CD4 cells, other receptors are also involved, in particular chemokine receptors such as CCR5. Some individuals in Caucasian populations who appear to have a high degree of (but not absolute) resistance to HIV infection have been found to be homozygous for a deletion in the gene which codes for

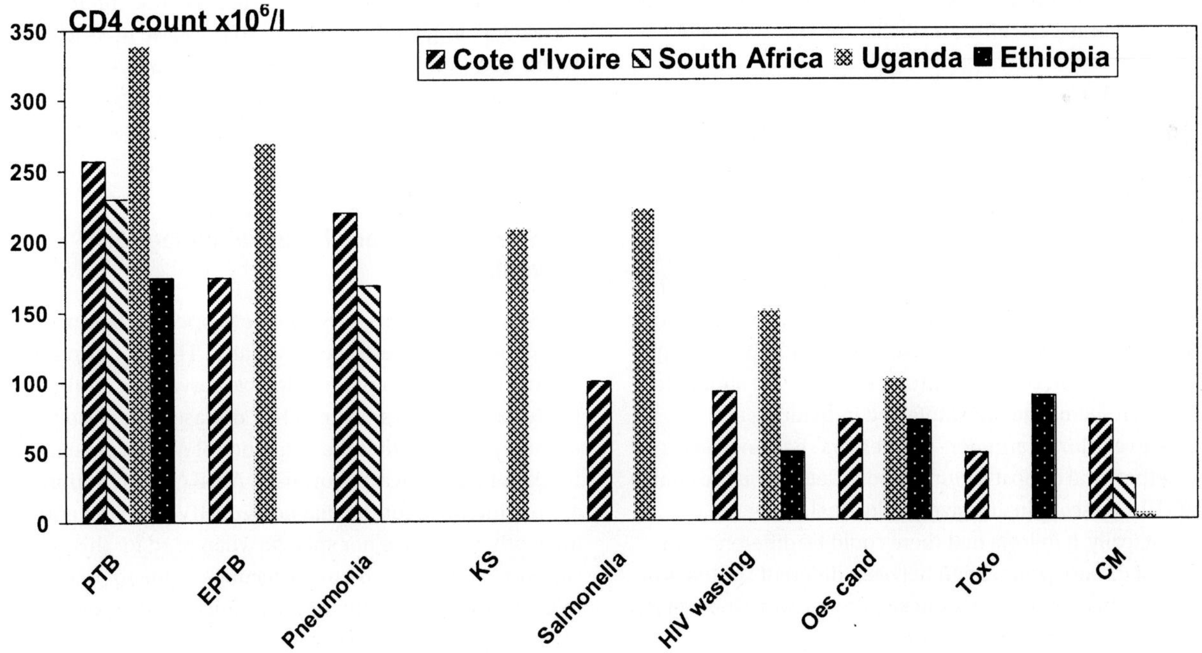

Fig. 13.8. CD4 counts at the time of diagnosis of selected HIV-related diseases in African countries. Key: PTB = pulmonary TB; EPTB = extra-pulmonary TB; KS = Kaposi's sarcoma; salmonella = non-typhoid salmonella septicaemia; oes cand = oesophageal candidiasis; toxo = cerebral toxoplasmosis; CM = cryptococcal meningitis. (Sources: Ackah et al., 1995; Martin et al., 1995; Schwander et al., 1995; Kassa et al., 1999; Morgan et al., 2000; Corbett et al., 2002; Grant, 1998.)

CCR5, resulting in CCR5 not being expressed on the cell surface. Heterozygotes for this deletion appear to have slower disease progression. This gene deletion is rare, and not found in non-Caucasian populations, and hence cannot account for all individual variation in the rate of HIV disease progression. However, this illustrates a genetic determinant of differences in the natural history of HIV infection, and other similar mechanisms may also play a role. Further evidence for genetic determinants of disease progression is provided by associations between certain HLA types and fast or slow disease progression.

Host factors: extrinsic

Many infections have been found to cause a temporary increase in plasma viral load among HIV-infected individuals; this is particularly marked for tuberculosis. It has been suggested that the high incidence of infectious diseases, particularly tuberculosis, among HIV-infected people in developing countries may accelerate the progression of HIV disease by increasing viral replication. This hypothesis is plausible, but there are few data to either support or refute it. If it is true, then prevention of intercurrent infectious diseases, such as tuberculosis, should prolong survival. However, data from trials of tuberculosis preventive therapy suggest that it confers little if any survival benefit, and so it seems that if intercurrent infectious diseases do accelerate the progression of HIV disease, the effect is small.

Virus factors

Individuals infected with HIV-2 progress to advanced immunosuppression much more slowly than those infected with HIV-1 (Marlink et al., 1994). Mortality among HIV-2-infected individuals in Guinea Bissau is about twice that of HIV-negative individuals (Poulson, et al., 1997), whereas HIV-1-infected people have a risk of death about ten times higher than HIV-negative individuals in the same community (Nunn et al., 1997). Although HIV-2 infection can cause progressive disease similar to HIV-1, it seems that most infected individuals are effectively 'long-term non-progressors'. It is unclear whether viral or host factors or both determine the course of HIV-2 disease in any given individual.

Logically, it follows that there could be differences in rate of disease progression between different subtypes of HIV-1. This is not an easy question to answer, since there are few places where different subtypes are found in otherwise similar populations. On the basis of current evidence, however, it does not appear that virus subtype plays a major role in determining the rate of disease progression (Hu et al., 1999).

Environmental factors

It has been widely believed that the progression of HIV disease is much more rapid in developing countries than in industrialized countries. In order to make accurate comparisons, studies comparing the time from seroconversion to the onset of severe disease and death in different settings are required. Because seroconversion may be asymptomatic, or have very non-specific symptoms, HIV-infected individuals are rarely identified at this stage, and therefore cohorts of individuals with well-documented dates of seroconversion are unusual. The assumption of rapid progression has been based largely on a study among female sex workers in Nairobi, where the median interval between seroconversion and AIDS was estimated at 4.4 years (Anzala et al., 1995), compared to 10 years for HIV-infected men in the United States in the 1980s (Rutherford et al., 1990). However, sex workers may not be representative of HIV-infected individuals in developing countries. A more recent study of a population-based cohort of HIV-infected adults in rural Uganda with well-defined dates of seroconversion has found a median interval from seroconversion to AIDS of nearly 10 years, similar to that seen in industrialized countries in the early years of the HIV pandemic (Morgan et al., 2002). Although this estimate is based on a single study, this is a more representative population than the sex workers mentioned earlier, and suggests there is little difference in the rate of progression to severe HIV disease in Africa compared with Europe and the US. This is not true of survival with advanced disease, which is substantially shorter in developing countries, largely as a result of lack of access to care.

AIDS case definitions for epidemiological surveillance

AIDS case definitions were first developed in the early 1980s, before HIV tests were available. They are primarily intended for use in epidemiological surveillance – that is, to identify cases of advanced HIV disease with reasonable accuracy, in order that the incidence of AIDS can be monitored for public health purposes. AIDS case definitions are not intended for the diagnosis of HIV infection and are neither sensitive nor specific when used for this purpose. They are also not an accurate guide to prognosis in an individual patient: for this, clinical staging systems are required (described later).

In industrialized countries, the AIDS case definition most widely used is that published by the US Centers for Disease Control and Prevention (CDC); the most recent version dates from 1993 (Centers for Disease Control and

Prevention, 1992) (Box). The CDC definition is impractical for use in low-income countries because definitive diagnosis of many conditions included requires access to laboratory investigations which are often not available. WHO therefore developed a case definition for AIDS which depends on clinical features alone (WHO, 1986) (Box). This is often referred to as the Bangui case definition and can be used when no laboratory facilities are available. However, it is not ideal, and in particular distinguishes poorly between advanced HIV disease and HIV-negative TB. In order to improve specificity, the Expanded WHO Case Definition for AIDS Surveillance was developed (WHO, 1994) (Box); this requires serological testing for HIV. If serological testing for HIV is available, the expanded case definition should be used for surveillance; in the absence of serological testing facilities, the Bangui case definition should be used.

Principal conditions included in the 1993 CDC surveillance case definition for AIDS among adolescents and adults

- oesophageal, tracheal, bronchial or pulmonary candidiasis
- invasive cervical cancer
- extrapulmonary cryptococcosis
- intestinal cryptosporidiosis for >1 month
- cytomegalovirus disease (other than liver, spleen or lymph nodes)
- cytomegalovirus retinitis with loss of vision
- HIV encephalopathy
- herpes simplex with ulcers for >1 month; or bronchitis, pneumonitis or oesophagitis
- extrapulmonary histoplasmosis
- intestinal isosporiasis for >1 month
- Kaposi's sarcoma
- lymphoma, Burkitt's, immunoblastic, or primary cerebral
- *Mycobacterium tuberculosis*, pulmonary or extrapulmonary
- non-tuberculous mycobacterial infection, disseminated or extrapulmonary
- *Pneumocystis carinii* pneumonia
- recurrent pneumonia
- progressive multifocal leukoencephalopathy
- recurrent salmonella septicaemia
- cerebral toxoplasmosis
- HIV wasting syndrome

Staging systems for HIV disease

Clinicians need to be able to predict prognosis in HIV-infected individuals, in order to counsel patients and to advise on provision of appropriate preventive therapies against opportunistic infections, and, where available, ART.

The CD4 count and viral load give the best guide to the risk of disease progression. CD4 count and viral load are correlated, but also give independent information on the risk of progression. A frequently used analogy is that of a train speeding towards a cliff, where the train represents the HIV-infected individual, and the edge of the

WHO case definition for AIDS surveillance

For the purpose of AIDS surveillance, an adult or adolescent (>12 years of age) is considered to have AIDS if at least two of the following major signs are present in combination with at least one of the minor signs listed below, and if these signs are not known to be due to a condition unrelated to HIV infection.

- *Major signs*
  - weight loss ≥10% of body weight
  - chronic diarrhoea for more than 1 month
  - prolonged fever for more than 1 month (intermittent or constant)
- *Minor signs*
  - persistent cough for more than 1 month[a]
  - generalized pruritic dermatitis
  - history of herpes zoster
  - oropharyngeal candidiasis
  - chronic progressive or disseminated herpes simplex infection
  - generalized lymphadenopathy

The presence of either generalized Kaposi's sarcoma or cryptococcal meningitis is sufficient for the diagnosis of AIDS for surveillance purposes.

[a]For patients with tuberculosis, persistent cough for more than 1 month should not be considered as a minor sign.

Expanded WHO case definition for AIDS surveillance

For the purposes of AIDS surveillance an adult or adolescent (>12 years of age) is considered to have AIDS if a test for HIV antibody gives a positive result, and one or more of the following conditions are present:

- ≥10% body weight loss or cachexia, with diarrhoea or fever, or both, intermittent or constant, for at least 1 month, not known to be due to a condition unrelated to HIV infection
- Cryptococcal meningitis
- Pulmonary or extrapulmonary tuberculosis
- Kaposi's sarcoma
- Neurological impairment that is sufficient to prevent independent daily activities, not known to be due to a condition unrelated to HIV infection (for example, trauma or cerebrovascular accident)
- Candidiasis of the oesophagus (which may be presumptive diagnosis based on the presence of oral candidiasis accompanied by dysphagia)
- Clinically diagnosed life-threatening or recurrent episodes of pneumonia, with or without aetiological confirmation
- Invasive cervical cancer

Table 13.1. Percentage risk of progression to AIDS in 3 years according to HIV-1 concentration and CD4 count

CD4	Viral load (copies/ml, equivalent RT-PCR values)				
(× 10⁶/l)	<1500	1501–7000	7001–20000	20001–55000	>55000
>750	0	2	3	10	33
501–750	3	2	8	16	33
351–500	–	2	8	16	43
201–350	–	–	8	40	64
<200	–	–	–	40	86

Source: US Department of Health and Human Services and the Henry J. Kaiser Family Foundation. Guidelines for the use of antiretroviral agents in HIV-infected adults and adolescents. Washington, DC: US Department of Health and Human Services; August 2001.

Proposed WHO staging system for HIV infection and disease

Clinical staging
Patients with HIV infection who are aged ≥13 years are clinically staged on the basis of the presence of the clinical condition, or performance score, belonging to the highest level.

Clinical stage 1: asymptomatic or persistent generalized lymphadenopathy; performance scale 1 (asymptomatic, normal activity).
Clinical stage 2: weight loss <10% body weight; minor mucocutaneous manifestations, varicella zoster within the last 5 years, recurrent upper respiratory tract infections (bacterial sinusitis); performance status 2 (symptomatic but normal activity)
Clinical stage 3: weight loss >10% body weight, unexplained chronic diarrhoea >1 month, unexplained chronic fever >1 month, oral candidiasis, oral hairy leukoplakia, pulmonary tuberculosis within the past year, severe bacterial infections; performance scale 3 (bed-ridden <50% of day during the last month)
Clinical stage 4: most other CDC AIDS-defining diseases (but not pulmonary tuberculosis); performance scale 4 (bed-ridden >50% of day during the last month)

Clinical/laboratory classification

	Laboratory axis		Clinical axis			
			1	2	3	4
	Lymphocytes or (×10⁶/1)	CD4 (×10⁶/1)	Asymptomatic	Early	Intermediate	Late
A	>2000	>500	1A	2A	3A	4A
B	1000–2000	200–500	1B	2B	3B	4B
C	<1000	<200	1C	2C	3C	4C

cliff represents profound immunosuppression. The CD4 count is represented by the distance between the train and the cliff, analogous to the remaining reserve in immune function before the individual becomes profoundly immunosuppressed. The viral load is represented by the speed of the train, analogous to the activity of viral replication. Data from large cohort studies of homosexual men in the United States (prior to widespread use of ART) have been used to calculate the risk of progression to AIDS based on CD4 and viral load, illustrated in Table 13.1. It is not yet clear whether these estimates are also valid for African populations.

Currently CD4 count and viral load measurements are only available in major centres in African countries. However, a clinical staging system developed by WHO for use in HIV-infected people (WHO, 1990), has been found to be useful in predicting outcome in studies in Uganda (Malamba et al., 1999; French et al., 1999). This system, shown in the Box, in its simplest form is based on clinical manifestations only and can therefore be used in any setting, even if laboratory tests are not available. For example, in a rural population in Uganda, median survival from the first time an individual was seen in each of the four WHO stages was stage 1: greater than 7.2 years; stage 2: 5.4 years; stage 3; 2.8 years; stage 4: 0.8 years (Malamba et al., 1999). If laboratory facilities are available, the prognostic value of the system can be improved by incorporating either the CD4 count, if available, or the total lymphocyte count.

Spectrum of HIV disease in African countries

There are important differences in the spectrum of HIV-related disease in different geographical regions; many of the most common manifestations of advanced immunosuppression in industrialized countries are relatively rare in African countries. There may also be some variation by region within Africa, although there are limited comparable data. Such data are important to develop guidelines for empirical treatment of common syndromes in HIV-infected people, particularly because in many settings the facilities required to make firm aetiological diagnoses are lacking, and hence a syndromic approach to management is required.

Regional variation in the spectrum of HIV disease

The spectrum of HIV-related disease in African countries is illustrated in Table 13.2. Some caution is needed in comparing data from the cited studies because the methods (e.g. selection of the study population, diseases included, methods of diagnosis) were not the same. A common

Table 13.2. Major causes of HIV-related disease in South Africa, Côte d'Ivoire, Kenya, and Ethiopia

Population	South Africa (Corbett et al., 2002) HIV+ hospitalized patients[a]	Côte d'Ivoire (Grant & De Cock, 1998) HIV+ hospitalized patients[b]	South Africa (Wood et al., 1996) HIV+ clinic attenders[c]				Kenya (Gilks et al., 1990a,b, 1992) HIV+ medical admissions	Ethiopia (Kassa et al., 1999) Hospitalized patients with suspected AIDS[d]
			Total	White	Black	Mixed race		
No. of HIV+ patients	599	349	342				95	79
Tuberculosis	21%	28%	30%[c]	12%[c]	51%[c]	29%[c]	18%	51%
Bacteraemia	–	18%	–				26%	–
HIV wasting	0.2%	11%	11%	13%	5%	15%	–	34%
Meningitis	0	10%	–				–	–
Isosporiasis	–	7%	–				–	–
Bacterial pneumonia	17%	6%	–				16%[e]	13%[f]
Cerebral toxoplasmosis	0	6%	3%	1%	2%	4%	–	6%
Bacterial enteritis	5%	5%	–				–	–
Non-specific diarrhoea	–	5%	–				15%	–
Oesophageal candidiasis	0.2%	3%	17%	18%	13%	20%	–	10%
Cryptococcosis	6%	2%	9%	7%	3%	7%	1%	–
Cytomegalovirus	0	0	9%	13%	2%	0	–	–
Kaposi's sarcoma	0	1%	18%	22%	14%	14%	2%	–
Pneumocystis pneumonia	1%	0	22%	34%	8%	18%	–	1%
HIV encephalopathy	0.2%	0	14%	23%	2%	11%	–	8%
Chronic herpes simplex	–	0	13%	15%	10%	10%	–	3%

Notes:

– = Data not available. Patients could have more than one diagnosis. Not all diagnoses are shown, so columns do not total 100%.

[a] Included 599 admissions of HIV-infected individuals in a mining workforce; some individuals had multiple admissions.

[b] Included patients admitted to infectious diseases and respiratory wards.

[c] Reported only World Health Organization (WHO) stage 4–defining conditions. Percentages by ethnic group estimated from graph. TB refers to extrapulmonary disease only.

[d] Patients admitted to referral hospital with clinical suspicion of AIDS or advanced HIV disease: only WHO stage 3– and 4–defining conditions reported.

[e] 'Acute cough and fever'; 46% of this subgroup had pneumcocci isolated from blood culture.

[f] 'Severe/recurrent bacterial infections'.

finding in these studies is the predominance of tuberculosis, but in other respects there are regional differences. The pattern of disease in South Africa is more similar to that seen in the US and Europe, with PCP being relatively frequent, particularly among white South Africans. In other regions, PCP is unusual in adults, and bacterial infections, particularly due to pneumococcal disease and non-typhoid salmonellosis, are more important.

Tuberculosis

Tuberculosis is clearly the most important cause of HIV-related morbidity and mortality in African countries. The clinical features of tuberculosis are described in Chapter 17; the differential diagnosis is discussed later in this chapter. In developing countries, in the absence of other interventions, tuberculosis has a poor outcome in HIV-infected people with a case-fatality usually higher than 20 per cent in the 12 months after diagnosis; most deaths are due to other opportunistic infections rather than tuberculosis itself. Case-fatality is higher among those with more advanced immunosuppression at diagnosis.

Bacteraemia

Bacterial diseases are a major cause of morbidity and mortality among HIV-infected individuals. Bacteraemia is common among HIV-infected patients admitted to hospital, but may not be diagnosed unless blood cultures are performed, and a high index of suspicion is needed. The main organisms isolated are illustrated in Table 13.3; the most common isolates are pneumococci and non-typhoid salmonellae. If blood cultures for mycobacteria are performed, mycobacteraemia is also relatively common in patients with advanced HIV disease. In contrast to industrialized countries, *Mycobacterium tuberculosis* is much more common than *Mycobacterium avium-intracellulare.*

Pneumococcal disease may occur relatively early in the course of HIV disease as well as at later stages and manifests predominantly as acute lobar pneumonia but also sinusitis, otitis media and bacteraemia with no obvious focus (Gilks et al., 1996). Disease due to non-typhoid salmonellae may present as fever, with or without gastrointestinal symptoms, or as diarrhoea; respiratory symptoms may also be present. With both diseases, recurrences are common in HIV-infected individuals.

Diarrhoeal disease

Diarrhoea is a common manifestation of advanced HIV disease; it is often persistent, and symptoms may fluctuate spontaneously. In about 50 per cent of patients, no cause is found. The organisms most commonly identified include protozoa such as *Cryptosporidium parvum, Isospora belli* and microsporidia; *Giardia lamblia* and *Entamoeba histolytica* are much less common (see Chapter 35). Bacterial pathogens, particularly non-typhoid salmonellae, but also *Shigella* spp., *Campylobacter* spp. and *Escherichia coli,* are common although often not identified because of lack of facilities for stool culture. The contribution of viral causes of diarrhoea is unclear; cytomegalovirus may cause enteritis or colitis in advanced HIV disease.

The HIV wasting syndrome, i.e. weight loss of at least 10 per cent, plus fever or diarrhoea or both persisting for at least a month, is a relatively common diagnosis. At autopsy, the most common diagnosis among HIV-infected patients with severe wasting was disseminated tuberculosis, and a high index of suspicion for tuberculosis is required since this may be a difficult diagnosis to confirm, especially where laboratory facilities are limited.

Neurological disease

Two common neurological syndromes are meningitis and cerebral space-occupying lesions. Common causes of meningitis include tuberculosis and cryptococcal disease, in addition to bacterial causes such as *Streptococcus pneumoniae* and *Neisseria meningitidis.* The importance of viral meningitis is unclear. The most common cause of a cerebral space-occupying lesion is toxoplasmosis, followed by primary lymphoma. Cerebral tuberculomata were relatively uncommon in an autopsy study in Abidjan, Côte d'Ivoire, but are said to be common in South Africa, though data documenting the aetiology of space-occupying lesions in Southern Africa are lacking.

A diverse range of neurological syndromes is recognized in HIV-infected individuals: lymphocytic meningitis, Guillain–Barré syndrome and facial nerve palsies may be a manifestation of seroconversion, and Guillain–Barré syndrome may also be an early manifestation of HIV disease. Painful peripheral neuropathy is common: this may be due to HIV disease alone, but may also be a consequence of isoniazid treatment for tuberculosis.

Dermatological disease

Common skin disorders in HIV-infected adults include prurigo, herpes simplex and herpes zoster, bacterial and fungal skin infections, psoriasis and Kaposi's sarcoma. Oral manifestations include candidiasis, herpes simplex and Kaposi's sarcoma. Hair changes (thinning and loss of curly architecture) are also common.

Neoplastic disease

Kaposi's sarcoma is probably the most common HIV-associated neoplasm, believed to be caused by human

Table 13.3. Cause of bacteraemia among human immunodeficiency virus (HIV)-infected patients admitted to hospitals in five African countries

	Côte d'Ivoire (Grant & de Cock, 1998; Grant et al., 1997) Acute medical admissions[a]	Tanzania (Archibald et al., 1998) Febrile medical admissions	Uganda (Ssali et al., 1998) Febrile medical admissions	Côte d'Ivoire (Vugia et al., 1993) Infectious diseases admissions	Malawi (Archibald et al., 2000) Febrile medical admissions	Rwanda (Taelman et al., 2000) Acute medical admissions	Kenya (Gilks et al., 1990b) Acute medical admissions
No. HIV-infected patients	349	282	227	202	173	163	95
No. (%) with bloodstream infections, excluding mycobacteria[b]	63 (18%)	118 (42%)	61 (27%)	39 (19%)	38 (22%)	52 (32%)	26 (27%)
Organisms identified (% of total with bloodstream infection, excluding mycobacteria)							
Non-typhoid salmonella	56%	23 (36%)	13 (41%)	16 (41%)	12 (32%)[c]	10 (19%)	10 (38%)
Streptococcus pneumoniae	17%	6 (9%)	11 (34%)	3 (8%)	21 (12%)	12 (23%)	7 (27%)
Escherichia coli	17%	7 (11%)	2 (6%)	4 (10%)	–	–	2 (8%)
Cryptococcus neoformans	0%	10 (16%)	0	5 (13%)	5 (3%)	13 (25%)	1 (4%)
Other	11%	18 (28%)	6 (19%)	12 (31%)	7 (4%)	17 (33%)	6 (23%)
No. (%) with mycobacteraemia	–	57 (20%)	30 (13%)	10 (5%)	24 (14%)	1 (0.5%)	–

Notes:

– = data not available.

[a] Infectious diseases and respiratory wards combined; a weighted average was used to allow for unequal sampling; therefore, absolute numbers are not given.

[b] Clinically important organisms. Since cultures for mycobacteria were not done in all studies, to facilitate comparison, mycobacterial isolates have been excluded from this analysis, but fungi are included. Some individuals had more than one organism; thus, totals may exceed 100%.

[c] all salmonella sp.

herpes virus-8 (HHV-8). Kaposi's sarcoma is particularly common in Eastern Africa: its incidence increased tenfold in Uganda between the 1960s and 1990s, as HIV prevalence increased. Non-Hodgkin's lymphoma (NHL) doubled in incidence in Uganda over the same period. The incidence of NHL increases with duration of HIV infection; in developing countries, shorter survival of individuals with advanced HIV disease may limit the number of cases observed. Squamous cell carcinoma of the conjunctiva is strongly associated with HIV infection and its incidence has increased markedly in some countries with high HIV prevalence.

Gynaecological disease

Amenorrhoea is common amongst HIV-infected women, as is vaginal candidiasis, which may be recurrent. Pelvic inflammatory disease is more severe among HIV-infected than uninfected women. HIV-infected women are more likely to have detectable cervical human papillomavirus infection, and to have cervical squamous intraepithelial neoplasia. The association between invasive carcinoma of the cervix and HIV infection is much less strong in Africa than has been reported in industrialized countries, perhaps because HIV-infected women die of other HIV-related diseases before invasive carcinoma develops.

Degree of immunosuppression at which HIV-related diseases occur

Most HIV-infected adults admitted to hospital in Africa have advanced disease with CD4 counts in the range indicating advanced immunosuppression. Reported mean or median CD4 counts were 87, 83, 83 and 55×10^6/l, in Abidjan, Côte d'Ivoire; Addis Ababa, Ethiopia; Dakar, Senegal; and Nairobi, Kenya, respectively (Kassa et al., 1999; Grant et al., 1997; Ndour et al., 2000; Rana et al., 2000). It has been suggested that the lack of PCP among adults in African countries is because they die before reaching the stage of advanced immunosuppression at which PCP becomes frequent. This hypothesis is not supported by these CD4 data, which show that adults are admitted to hospital with CD4 counts at which PCP would be expected to be common, especially in a population where preventive therapy is not widely used. The reason for the relative rarity of PCP in African adults, contrasting with its frequency in HIV-infected children, remains unclear. Reported median CD4 counts at the time of diagnosis of selected HIV-related diseases are illustrated in Fig. 13.8.

Some conditions which are relatively common as complications of advanced immunosuppression in industrialized countries, such as disease due to cytomegalovirus (CMV) and non-tuberculous mycobacteria, are unusual in African countries. This is probably because survival with advanced immunosuppression is short where there is limited access to health care.

Interaction of HIV with endemic tropical diseases

Recent evidence suggests that clinical malaria and malarial parasitaemia are more common in HIV-infected people, and become more frequent with increasing immunosuppression (Whitworth et al., 2000; French et al., 2001). However, severe malaria is not a frequent manifestation of advanced HIV disease in malaria endemic regions. Malarial parasitaemia is more frequent and more severe in pregnant women who are HIV infected, and placental malaria is also more common. Children who become anaemic as a consequence of malaria may have an increased risk of HIV infection as a result of the transfusion of inadequately screened blood.

Visceral leishmaniasis behaves as an opportunistic infection in advanced HIV disease, often causing disseminated disease. Strains of *Leishmania infantum* which typically cause cutaneous disease in the immunocompetent may cause visceral disease in the immunosuppressed. Reports of increased incidence of leishmaniasis in HIV-infected people come mostly from southern Europe but cases are also reported from countries in the north and east of Africa (Chapter 32). Maintenance therapy is required to prevent relapse after successful treatment.

Some tropical diseases do not appear to be altered by HIV infection, although data are limited: these include leprosy, amoebiasis, strongyloidiasis and trypanosomiasis.

HIV-infected individuals with schistosomiasis excrete fewer eggs than HIV-negative persons, but it is unclear whether the severity of disease differs, and response to treatment appears to be unaffected.

Spectrum of disease in HIV-1 and HIV-2 disease

The spectrum of advanced HIV-2 disease among adults is very similar to that due to HIV-1. At autopsy, disseminated CMV disease, HIV encephalitis and cholangitis were all more common in individuals with HIV-2 than in those with HIV-1 infection, perhaps because of longer survival of HIV-2 infected individuals (Lucas et al., 1993). Individuals infected with both HIV-1 and HIV-2 have disease clinically indistinguishable from those with HIV-1 only.

Management of HIV-related disease in African countries

Respiratory syndromes

Common causes of respiratory symptoms in HIV-infected adults include:

- pulmonary tuberculosis
- bacterial pneumonia due to *S. pneumoniae*, etc.
- fungal pneumonia:
  - *Pneumocystis carinii*
  - cryptococcal
- pulmonary Kaposi's sarcoma.

Pulmonary tuberculosis Typically, patients give a history of symptoms for at least 3 weeks with cough which may be productive of sputum, and there may be haemoptysis. They usually describe fever with or without drenching night sweats and often have significant weight loss. The key investigation is sputum microscopy for acid-fast bacilli. If sputum microscopy is negative, chest radiography should be performed: typically in TB this shows upper lobe infiltrates with or without cavitation. However, it is important to note that the clinical presentation of tuberculosis may be altered in HIV infection, particularly in advanced immunosuppression, with atypical appearances on the chest radiograph (less cavitation and upper lobe predominance, more hilar lymphadenopathy and diffuse parenchymal abnormalities), and a greater frequency of extrapulmonary and disseminated disease. The appearances of pulmonary nocardiosis may be very similar to pulmonary tuberculosis and this is an important differential diagnosis in some areas, though much less common.

Bacterial pneumonia Patients usually give a short history of cough with or without purulent sputum and fever; they may also describe pleuritic chest pain. Chest examination may reveal signs of consolidation. Sputum microscopy may show bacterial pathogens but is negative for acid-fast bacilli. The chest radiograph shows lobar or segmental consolidation which may be less clearly defined than in HIV-uninfected individuals; there may also be a pleural effusion.

PCP Patients typically have a subacute history with non-productive cough and fever; increasing exertional breathlessness is often prominent. There may be no chest signs except tachypnoea, and the chest radiograph classically shows bilateral symmetrical perihilar infiltrates, referred to as 'bat's wing' shadows because of their shape, but these changes may be subtle and the chest radiograph may appear normal. Pleural effusions are not typical of PCP. The diagnosis is confirmed by identification of the organism on cytological examination of induced sputum or bronchial washings: sputum microscopy is a very insensitive test for *P. carinii.*

Pulmonary Kaposi's sarcoma Patients usually presents with cough and increasing breathlessness: patients usually have cutaneous and/or oral KS lesions. The chest radiograph typically shows bilateral basal coarse reticulonodular shadows: there may also be pleural or pericardial effusions, which are usually blood stained.

Distinguishing between these different conditions can be difficult, especially in individuals with more advanced immunosuppression in whom the presentation of disease may be 'atypical'. If there is cavitation on the chest radiograph then TB is most likely, but do not forget nocardiosis (Chapter 76). Haemoptysis also suggests TB. Lobar consolidation may be due to bacterial pneumonia or TB, but is unlikely to be due to PCP. If there is clear clinical evidence to support a specific diagnosis, then the appropriate treatment should be started. If the diagnosis is unclear, it is logical to treat first with antibiotics to cover common bacterial infections. Patients who fail to respond, or who improve temporarily and then worsen, should be reassessed, and treated for TB if this is a possible diagnosis, or PCP if this appears more likely, although PCP is far less common than TB among adults in Africa. Remember that HIV-infected individuals may have more than one disease. In particular, individuals with pulmonary TB may present with symptoms suggesting bacterial pneumonia, and may improve temporarily on antibiotics: always consider TB in those whose symptoms or chest radiograph abnormalities do not resolve.

The treatment of common HIV-related conditions is outlined in Table 13.4.

Pleural effusion

Common causes of pleural effusion in HIV-infected individuals include TB, bacterial infection and malignancy, especially Kaposi's sarcoma. In *TB* the pleural fluid will normally be clear and on microscopy, white cells will be predominantly lymphocytes. Pleural biopsy has a much higher yield than pleural fluid for culturing *M. tuberculosis,* and typical features of TB (caseating granulomata, with or without acid fast bacilli) may be seen on histological examination. Sputum specimens should also be examined for acid-fast bacilli in the usual way. In *bacterial infection,* the pleural fluid may be purulent, and on microscopy white cells will be predominantly neutrophils; if there is an empyema, drainage is indicated in addition to appropriate antibiotics. In *Kaposi's sarcoma,* the pleural fluid is typically blood stained and usually reaccumulates rapidly after drainage (see also Chapters 18 and 19).

Table 13.4. Treatment of common HIV-related opportunistic infections

Disease	Initial treatment	Prevention of relapse[a]	Comments
Tuberculosis	According to national guidelines (see TB Chapter 17)	Not currently recommended: may be useful if high risk of reinfection and advanced disease	
Bacterial pneumonia	Amoxycillin 500 mg t.d.s. or erythromycin 1g b.d. for 10–14 days	Co-trimoxazole may prevent recurrent pneumonia: indicated in advanced disease	Chapter 18, pneumonia
Non-typhoid salmonella bacteraemia	Ciprofloxacin 500 mg b.d. for 10 days OR chloramphenicol 500 mg q.d.s. for 14 days	Co-trimoxazole 960 mg daily may be useful, depending on sensitivity	Chapter 49, salmonella
Pneumocystis carinii pneumonia	Co-trimoxazole 120 mg/kg/day i.v. or p.o. for 2 days, then reducing to 90 mg/kg/day for 19 days, in two or more divided doses OR clindamycin 600 mg q.d.s. i.v. or p.o. AND primaquine 15 mg o.d. p.o. for 21 days OR pentamidine 4 mg/kg/day i.v. for 21 days AND steroids in moderate and severe disease	Co-trimoxazole 960 mg daily	Nausea and vomiting very common at treatment dose of cotrimoxazole. Avoid cotrimoxazole and primaquine in G6PD deficiency
Oral candidiasis	Nystatin suspension or 1–2 tablets dissolved in the mouth 3–5 times daily OR clotrimazole oral troches 10 mg 5 times daily OR ketoconazole 200 mg sucked or chewed with food o.d. for 3–5 days OR fluconazole 50–200 mg o.d. for 2–3 weeks if unresponsive to other treatment		
Oesophageal candidiasis	Ketoconazole 200 mg o.d. for 5–10 days OR fluconazole 100–200 mg o.d. for 5–10 days	if recurrent, ketoconazole 200 mg o.d. OR fluconazole 100–200 mg o.d.	
Cryptosporidiosis	Symptomatic management		
Isosporiasis	Co-trimoxazole 960 mg q.d.s. for 10 days	Co-trimoxazole 960 mg 3 times weekly	
Microsporidiosis	Albendazole 400 mg b.d. for 28 days	If relapse occurs after treatment, albendazole 400 mg o.d.	
Cryptococcal meningitis	Amphotericin B 0.7 mg/kg i.v. daily for 2 weeks, then fluconazole 400 mg daily for 10 weeks OR Fluconazole 400–800 mg daily for 10 weeks	Fluconazole 200 mg daily for life	Amphotericin highly nephrotoxic: monitor renal function
Cerebral toxoplasmosis	Sulphadiazine 2 g t.d.s (oral or i.v.) AND pyrimethamine 75 mg stat, then 50 mg daily AND folinic acid 15 mg daily, all for 4–6 weeks OR Clindamycin 600 mg q.d.s. (oral or i.v.) AND pyrimethamine as above AND folinic acid as above	Sulphadiazine 1 g t.d.s. AND pyrimethamine 25 mg o.d., AND folinic acid 15 mg daily all for life OR Clindamycin 450 mg t.d.s. AND pyrimethamine as above AND folinic acid as above	Risk of bone marrow depression with pyrimethamine (may need to reduce dose or use alternative drug regime), and of renal stones or crystalluria with sulphadiazine.

Note:
[a] Secondary prophylaxis for most opportunist infections can be stopped if ART sustains the CD4 count above 200×10^6/l.

Gastrointestinal syndromes

Candidiasis

Oral candidiasis is common. The characteristic appearances are of creamy-white plaques in the oral cavity which can be scraped off, leaving a bleeding surface. In atrophic (erythematous) candidiasis the lesions are red rather than white. Possible treatments are listed in Table 13.4: topical gentian violet may be a useful adjunct in the treatment of superficial fungal infections such as angular cheilitis, small red fissures at the angle of the mouth. Oesophageal candidiasis is also a relatively common feature of advanced HIV disease; definitive diagnosis is by endoscopy, but it may be diagnosed presumptively in patients with retrosternal pain on swallowing and oral candidiasis. Less common causes of pain on swallowing include ulcers due to herpes simplex or cytomegalovirus.

Diarrhoea

The principal causes of HIV-related diarrhoea were listed earlier. The spectrum of severity varies from occasional loose stools to severe diarrhoea with ten or more stools daily leading to dehydration. In diarrhoea without blood, the most common identified causes are protozoal diseases, particularly cryptosporidiosis, which causes profuse watery diarrhoea with abdominal pain, vomiting and weight loss but no fever (see Chapter 35). Bacteria such as salmonella spp. may also cause watery diarrhoea. Diarrhoea with blood is more likely to be due to bacteria, such as *Shigella* spp., but may also be caused by amoebic colitis, cytomegalovirus or visceral Kaposi's sarcoma.

Investigation of diarrhoea

The presence of white and red blood cells on stool microscopy suggests colitis. *Cryptosporidium parvum* can be identified microscopically using a modified Ziehl-Neelsen stain, but cysts are excreted intermittently and identification may be difficult. Identification of microsporidia requires special techniques (see Chapter 35). Stool culture for bacterial pathogens is useful if available.

Treatment

Give fluid replacement as necessary, orally or intravenously as appropriate (see Chapter 20). If a specific cause of diarrhoea is found, give appropriate antimicrobial agents. If no specific cause is identified and a bacterial cause seems likely (diarrhoea with fever, and/or bloody stools) the following may be useful:

- ciprofloxacin (500 mg b.d. for 5 days), effective against most enteric bacteria
- cotrimoxazole (960 mg b.d. for 7 days), effective against some enteric bacteria, depending on local resistance patterns. Also effective against *I. belli*, although a higher dose is recommended when used specifically to treat isosporiasis (see Table 13.4).
- chloramphenicol (e.g. 50 mg/kg/day in 4 divided doses for 14 days) is effective against most salmonella spp.

Diarrhoea due to non-typhoid salmonellae commonly recurs after treatment, even when the organism is sensitive to the agent used; recurrence may be less common after treatment with a fluoroquinolone because higher intracellular antibiotic concentrations are achieved. Recurrences may respond to a further course of the agent which was effective initially, but may be multiple. Maintenance treatment may be effective in preventing recurrences.

If bacterial causes seem less likely (watery diarrhoea without fever) then the following may be useful:

- albendazole (400–800 mg twice daily for 2 weeks), effective against microsporidia and strongyloides; a longer course is recommended specifically for microsporidiosis (see Table 13.4)
- cotrimoxazole for *I. belli*, as above
- metronidazole (400 mg or 750 mg three times daily for 7 days), effective against giardiasis and amoebic colitis, respectively.

There is no treatment of proven value for cryptosporidiosis, which is managed symptomatically with fluid replacement and anti-diarrhoeal agents. The following may be useful for symptomatic treatment of persistent diarrhoea:

- Adsorbent agents, e.g. kaolin
- Antimotility drugs such as
  - loperamide 4–8 mg daily in 2 divided doses (up to 16 mg daily may be used)
  - Lomotil 4 tablets initially, then up to 2 tablets every 6 hours
  - codeine phosphate 30–60 mg 3–4 times daily; this may also relieve abdominal pain.

Combinations of agents may be required, e.g. loperamide and codeine. Anti-diarrhoeal agents should not be used in patients with bloody diarrhoea because of the risk of toxic megacolon.

Calorie intake should be maintained as far as possible.

Other gastrointestinal symptoms

Nausea and vomiting suggest an underlying cause, such as gastrointestinal infection or severe dehydration, and improve when this is treated. If no underlying cause can be identified, symptomatic treatment with metoclopramide or chlorpromazine may be helpful. Hiccup can be a troublesome symptom in advanced HIV disease. There

Table 13.5. CSF findings in HIV-infected patients with meningitis

	Indian ink stain for cryptococci	Cryptococcal antigen	White cells ($\times 10^6$/l)	Gram stain	Bacterial culture	Protein (g/l)	Glucose
Normal	negative	negative	<5	negative	negative	<0.45	60–80% of blood glucose
Cryptococcal	positive in 70%	positive in 90%	normal or high, >50% lymphocytes	negative or yeasts	may yield cryptococci	normal or high	normal or low
Tuberculous	negative	negative	high, >50% lymphocytes except very early	negative	negative	1–2, may be very high	very low
Bacterial	negative	negative	high, >50% neutrophils	positive in 60–90%	positive in 70–85%	1–5	low

may be no obvious cause, but chlorpromazine (25 mg 2–3 times daily) may be helpful. Perianal pain can have a number of causes including perianal abscess, which would require incision and drainage; recurrent or persistent perianal ulcers are most likely to be due to herpes simplex and may be treated with aciclovir.

Neurological and psychiatric syndromes

Meningitis

The most important causes of meningitis in HIV-infected patients are bacterial pathogens (*S. pneumoniae* or *N. meningitidis*), tuberculosis and *Cryptococcus neoformans*. Bacterial meningitis presents with features similar to those seen in HIV-negative individuals:

- acute onset of fever
- headache
- vomiting
- neck stiffness.

Tuberculous meningitis is typically less acute in onset, and in HIV infection does not always cause neck stiffness; about 50 per cent of patients will have concomitant pulmonary TB, which may help make the diagnosis. Cryptococcal meningitis usually causes headache, but meningism may be absent; some patients present late, with convulsions, confusion or in coma. Mortality is high even when treatment is available. Cryptococcal meningitis is rare until the stage of advanced disease (CD4 $< 200 \times 10^6$/l) whereas bacterial and tuberculous meningitis can occur in early as well as advanced HIV disease.

Investigation of meningitis

This is discussed in Chapter 20.

When examining the CSF of HIV-infected patients, in addition to counting white cells and doing a Gram stain, always perform an Indian ink stain for cryptococci. This is positive in about 70 per cent of patients with cryptococcal meningitis. If possible, request a cryptococcal antigen test, which has a higher sensitivity (around 90 per cent). A positive result on either of these tests is diagnostic of cryptococcal meningitis. The white cell count may be raised, typically with predominant lymphocytes, the CSF protein may be raised and the glucose low, but CSF findings in cryptococcal meningitis may be normal (see Table 13.5).

Treatment of meningitis

HIV-infected patients with bacterial and tuberculous meningitis are treated in the same way as HIV-negative patients (see Chapter 20).

Cryptococcal meningitis can be treated with amphotericin B or fluconazole (see Table 13.4). The response to amphotericin B is faster, and it is therefore recommended for patients with poor prognostic factors (abnormal mental state, CSF Indian ink stain positive, CSF cryptococcal antigen titre greater than 1: 1024, CSF white cell count $>0.02 \times 10^9$/l, CSF culture positive, disseminated disease). Lifelong secondary prophylaxis (usually with fluconazole) is important, otherwise relapse is likely.

Focal neurological signs

Cerebral toxoplasmosis is the most likely cause of a cerebral mass lesion in an HIV-infected person in most African countries. Cerebral lymphoma is also possible, but less likely, and very difficult to treat effectively. Consider the possibility of a cerebral tuberculoma since this is treatable. Any of these lesions may present with sudden onset of a focal neurological deficit similar to a stroke, or focal or generalized convulsions, but the onset may be more insidious with fever, headache and abnormal behaviour with few if any focal signs.

Investigation of a patient with focal neurological signs
Cerebral imaging is useful to confirm the presence of a mass lesion if this can be done; typically, toxoplasmosis appears as multiple enhancing lesions with surrounding oedema, particularly at the interface between grey and white matter or in the basal ganglia, and lymphoma is a single periventricular lesion. However, even with cerebral imaging it can be very difficult to distinguish between toxoplasmosis and lymphoma. Serology for toxoplasma antibodies is not helpful since a positive result does not confirm the diagnosis, nor does a negative result exclude it.

Treatment of focal neurological signs
Since the most likely treatable cause of a mass lesion is cerebral toxoplasmosis, the most appropriate empirical approach is to treat for toxoplasmosis. Clinical improvement on treatment for toxoplasmosis alone is supportive of the diagnosis; a response should be seen in 10–14 days. If there is significant mass effect it may be necessary to give high dose steroids to reduce oedema, but since most of the likely causes of a mass lesion will improve temporarily with high dose steroids, the specificity of the trial of toxoplasma treatment is lost. Hence steroids should be avoided unless essential. Anticonvulsants may be required to control fitting, and physiotherapy may be helpful. Consider the possibility of a tuberculoma, and look for other evidence of tuberculosis, e.g. by chest radiograph, lymph node aspirate. If there is a good response to treatment for toxoplasmosis, give maintenance therapy, otherwise the risk of relapse is high. If treatment for toxoplasmosis is unsuccessful and further diagnostic tests are not available, a trial of anti-tuberculous treatment with steroids may be justified.

Dementia

HIV-related dementia is a common complication of advanced disease. It is a progressive dementia. Features include cognitive dysfunction with forgetfulness, loss of concentration, mental slowing and impaired performance of complex mental activities; and behavioural symptoms such as apathy, reduced spontaneity and emotional responses, social withdrawal, depression, irritability or emotional lability.

Investigation
Advanced dementia may be obvious clinically, but in early disease, accounts of close relatives and associates are important, plus a detailed mental state and neurological examination; dementia should be distinguished from acute confusion (for example due to hypoxia, severe sepsis or drug side effects). The diagnosis is one of exclusion of other treatable causes, ideally by cerebral imaging and CSF examination. The CT brain scan may appear normal in early disease, though later ventricular enlargement and widening of cerebral sulci are seen.

Management
There is no specific treatment; dementia due to HIV may improve with antiretroviral therapy (ART) if this is available. Management should be symptomatic, including cautious sedation for those who are agitated and aggressive.

Peripheral neuropathy

Distal sensory peripheral neuropathy is common, especially in advanced disease. The most common causes are HIV itself and drugs, either conventional (especially isoniazid) or traditional herbal remedies, and may be exacerbated by poor nutrition. The usual presentation is a painful neuropathy of the feet causing burning, numbness or pins and needles; there may be contact hypersensitivity. There is usually no muscle weakness; pain and temperature sensation may be diminished and ankle jerks may be diminished or lost.

Investigation
Exclude treatable causes of neuropathy, for example diabetes, vitamin B12 deficiency, syphilis and excess alcohol, and review diet and medication. Vitamin supplements may be useful, especially in patients taking isoniazid, e.g. pyridoxine 100 mg daily for 4–6 weeks, if effective continued at 50 mg daily for the duration of isoniazid therapy. If no reversible cause is found, give simple analgesia. Drugs such as amitryptiline may also be helpful.

Psychiatric disorders

Common psychiatric disorders include depression, which manifests as loss of energy or fatigue, difficulty with concentration, insomnia or early morning waking. This is treated in the conventional way with counselling or antidepressant medication. Some HIV-infected patients become excessively anxious over issues such as their own health, their drugs, family or job. Some may be able to control their anxieties but others may become panicky, obsessive or compulsive, in which case they should be referred to an experienced counsellor or physician or psychiatrist. Individuals with psychotic symptoms should be referred to a psychiatrist.

Fever

Fever is a very common symptom in HIV-infected patients (see pp. 192–3). Often there are other symptoms which suggest a specific focus (e.g. respiratory or gastrointestinal symptoms). However, in some cases there may be no obvious focus of infection, in which case important diagnoses to consider include:

- *tuberculosis.* Since tuberculosis and HIV infection are closely associated in African countries, TB should always be considered in HIV-infected patients with fever, especially if the history is long and there is marked weight loss. Pulmonary TB may present with atypical appearances or minimal abnormalities on the chest radiograph; extrapulmonary and disseminated disease also need to be considered.
- *bacteraemia.* As described earlier, bacteraemia, particularly due to non-typhoid salmonellae, is common among HIV-infected individuals admitted to hospital in African countries, but may not be identified, and a high index of suspicion is needed. The most effective treatment for bacteraemia due to non-typhoid Salmonella spp. is with ciprofloxacin or a third generation cephalosporin. If these are not available, chloramphenicol is the best alternative (see Table 13.4). There is a high risk of recurrence and maintenance treatment is recommended.
- *PCP.* Although PCP is much less common than TB or bacterial infections in adults in Africa, bear it in mind as a cause of fever and breathlessness, usually with subacute onset.
- *other sites of infection.* Check for evidence of sinusitis, meningitis, perianal infection, cholecystitis.
- *common pathogens.* HIV-infected people are susceptible to the same organisms that cause disease in the HIV-uninfected population: fever may be due to malaria or a respiratory tract infection.
- *uncommon pathogens.* In individuals with advanced HIV disease, consider organisms which normally have low pathogenic potential. Cytomegalovirus and non-tuberculous mycobacteria were common causes of fever without obvious focus in industrialized countries before the widespread use of antiretroviral therapy. They are less common in low-income countries, probably because survival with advanced disease is shorter.

Skin disorders

Generalized pruriginous dermatitis (prurigo)

This common disorder starts with small itchy papules, usually containing clear fluid which discharges after scratching. The open lesions heal, leaving hyper- or hypopigmented macules or papules. The lesions are most often found on the face and limbs, less often on the trunk, and usually occur in crops, with lesions at different stages of evolution. There may be secondary bacterial infection. Treatment is difficult: antihistamines (e.g. promethazine, chlorpheniramine, astemizole and chlorpromazine) may be helpful, as may betamethasone skin ointment. Treat secondary bacterial infection with antibiotics (e.g. flucloxacillin); abscesses require incision and drainage.

Seborrhoeic dermatitis is a common early manifestation of HIV infection; it may be due to overgrowth of the fungus *Pityrosporum ovale.* It should be distinguished from psoriasis. Treatment includes removal of crusts with 2–3 per cent salicylic acid, ketoconazole topically or systemically (400 mg daily for 14 days) and topical steroids (1 per cent hydrocortisone or betamethasone).

Psoriasis may be unusually aggressive in HIV-infected individuals. It must be distinguished from fungal skin infection. Treatment includes 2–3 per cent salicylic acid for the removal of scale and 10 per cent crude coal tar for individual lesions.

Fungal skin infections tend to be more aggressive and less responsive to treatment in HIV-infected individuals. *Tinea* infections (*Tinea pedis, Tinea capitis, Tinea corporis, Tinea versicolor*) can all be treated with topical anti-fungal creams (miconazole, ketoconazole, clotrimazole) or an oral anti-fungal agent: ketoconazole 400 mg o.d. for 3 weeks is preferable to griseofulvin 500 mg o.d. for 3 weeks.

In moist areas of skin (perineum, axillae, below the breasts, glans penis, interdigital clefts), candidiasis is the most common fungal skin infection. This can be treated with an anti-fungal cream or gentian violet 1 per cent. Systemic anti-fungals (e.g. ketoconazole 400 mg o.d. for 7 days) may be required if topical treatment fails.

Viral skin infections may also be more widespread and difficult to treat in HIV-infected patients. Warts can be treated in with topical podophylline. Herpes zoster is a common early manifestation of HIV disease: aciclovir (800 mg 5 times daily for 7 days) may be useful, especially if the patient presents within 24 hours of the onset of symptoms or if the disease affects the ophthalmic division of the trigeminal nerve. Adequate analgesia is important to reduce the risk of post-herpetic neuralgia. *Molluscum contagiosum* in adults suggests HIV infection: treatment is by enucleation or mechanical expression of the core with a spatula. This may however lead to secondary bacterial infection or scarring, and so asymptomatic lesions may be best left alone.

Drug eruptions may be unusually severe in HIV disease, particularly with sulphonamides. Thiacetazone, previously used as part of anti-tuberculous regimes, can cause life-threatening reactions.

Sensitivity to sunlight is common in HIV disease as is blue–black nail discoloration.

Neoplastic disease

HIV-related cancers become more common with increasing immunosuppression, and are likely to increase in incidence as care of HIV-infected people improves, resulting in better survival.

The commonest cancer in HIV-infected people in Africa is Kaposi's sarcoma (KS), a malignant tumour of the endothelial cells of the lymphatics or blood vessels. In the AIDS clinic in Mulago Hospital, Makerere University, Kampala, Uganda, about 7 per cent of the patients present with KS; 50 per cent are female. HIV-associated Kaposi's sarcoma is also known as 'epidemic' KS, distinguishing it from 'endemic' KS, which was seen in Central Africa in adults (mostly in men) and children before the HIV epidemic. Although the skin lesions look the same, HIV-associated KS runs an aggressive course and is often disseminated, affecting the skin but also lymph nodes, the lungs and the gastrointestinal tract.

HIV-associated KS usually presents with painless, non-itchy skin lesions on the limbs, trunk, face, hard palate or penis which can be macular, papular or nodular. There may be enlarged lymph nodes as a result of lymphatic involvement, and lymphatic obstruction may cause lymphoedema and consequent localized swelling of one or more limbs, the genitals or the face. Pulmonary KS may cause progressive breathlessness, and/or persistent cough with frothy or blood-stained sputum. The chest radiograph typically shows coarse reticulonodular shadowing bilaterally in the lower zones. There may also be blood-stained pleural and/or pericardial effusions, and mediastinal lymphadenopathy. Gastrointestinal KS may present with abdominal pain, gastrointestinal bleeding and occasionally intestinal obstruction. Cerebral KS is described as a cause of a cerebral mass lesion, but is rare.

KS can be diagnosed clinically by experienced clinicians, and can be confirmed by histology of a skin lesion if necessary. Biopsy of oral lesions may be complicated by excessive bleeding, and should be done by an oral surgeon.

KS is usually not itself life-threatening, and treatment carries risks, so management must balance the risks and benefits for the individual patient. Early KS may be asymptomatic, in which case treatment is not indicated. Indications for treatment of KS include:

- extensive skin lesions which are disfiguring, painful or ulcerating
- bulky lesions of the mouth or tongue which interfere with nutrition
- eye lesions interfering with vision
- pulmonary KS causing severe dyspnoea
- lymphatic obstruction causing severe oedema.

KS may improve with ART alone, and this would be appropriate if available. Treatment is otherwise with radiotherapy, which is appropriate for limited skin or palatal lesions, and can also be used for pulmonary KS, or chemotherapy, which is preferred for extensive or visceral disease.

Gynaecological disease

Gynaecological disease becomes more frequent as HIV disease progresses. Some common manifestations include:

Menstrual abnormalities including amenorrhoea and intermenstrual bleeding. Amenorrhoea is common in advanced disease; menses may return if infections are treated and the woman gains weight.

Vaginal candidiasis: this may be recurrent, or persistent in advanced disease. Treatment with topical clotrimazole 1 per cent or nystatin pessaries o.d. or b.d. may be effective. Persistent disease may require systemic anti-fungal agents such as fluconazole or ketoconazole (see Chapter 14).

Genital herpes simplex: recurrent ulceration is common. In advanced disease, lesions may become persistent, extensive and extremely painful. Treatment is with aciclovir 200–400 mg five times daily for at least five days: treatment for 3 weeks or more may be needed.

Pelvic inflammatory disease (PID): women should be counselled to report early symptoms suggestive of PID (fever, pelvic or abdominal pain) so that the diagnosis can be made promptly and appropriate antibiotics given (see Chapter 14). Huge pelvic abscesses may develop in immunosuppressed women following pelvic infection or surgical procedures: these require drainage and appropriate antibiotics to cover aerobic and anaerobic pathogens.

Palliative and home care

In spite of recent advances in the treatment of HIV infection, there is currently no cure, and thus for the vast majority of HIV-infected patients, the final outcome will be death. In HIV disease it may be harder to predict when death is imminent than for other chronic diseases: opportunistic infections may be life-threatening, but the patient may still recover if appropriate treatment is given. Nevertheless, experienced health care workers can identify the point at which further attempts to sustain life are futile. At this point, the main aim of treatment is to provide palliative care; that is, to make the life which remains as comfortable and as meaningful as possible for the patient and his/her family.

Principles of palliative and home care

Palliative care responds to physical, psychological, social, spiritual and cultural needs. It may extend, if necessary, to support of bereaved relatives.

Principles of palliative care include:

- Symptom relief
- Psychosocial and spiritual support
- Teamwork and partnership
- Appropriate ethical considerations
- Sustaining hope with realistic goals.

Consider palliative and home care when advanced HIV disease is diagnosed; it becomes more important as life-prolonging interventions become less appropriate.

Effective home care

Start by assessing the home environment, identifying the family's strengths in terms of human and financial resources, available facilities and support within the home and community. Identify possible sources of stress and conflicts of interest. For example, children within the home may have to leave school in order to provide care or may have to share the limited resources between buying drugs and paying school fees.

Appropriate education for family members who are providing home care is very important. They should be able to recognize changes in their patient and know how and where to get help. They should be taught simple palliative procedures that make the patient more comfortable, such as regular turning to avoid bedsores. Family carers should be able to recognize symptoms and signs of common conditions like oral thrush, dehydration etc. and deal with them appropriately.

Palliative and home care teams should work in partnership. The team should include nurses and medical officers to manage symptoms, counsellors to provide emotional, psychosocial and spiritual care for the patient and his/her carers, and community members to provide additional support.

Prevention of HIV-related disease in African countries

Many of the major diseases affecting HIV-infected adults in African countries are potentially preventable using drugs which are affordable and widely available.

Prevention of tuberculosis

Randomized controlled trials have shown that a 6-month course of isoniazid (isoniazid preventive therapy, IPT) reduces the risk of active TB among HIV-infected individuals with no previous history of TB, and this is recommended by WHO/UNAIDS (1998). The benefit of IPT has only been proven among individuals with a positive tuberculin skin test, but skin testing is often logistically difficult, and therefore IPT is recommended for all HIV-infected individuals if the prevalence of latent TB infection is high (greater than 30 per cent) or if the risk of new TB infection is high, for example among health care workers, household contacts of TB patients, miners or prisoners. It is important that active TB is excluded before starting IPT, because if isoniazid monotherapy were given to individuals with active disease, this would promote the development of resistance.

The recommended regimen is isoniazid 5 mg/kg daily up to a maximum of 300 mg daily for six months: patients should be seen monthly for monitoring of toxicity, adherence and signs of active TB, and only given one month's supply of medication at a time. Routine monitoring of liver function tests is not recommended, although patients should be educated to report immediately any symptoms suggestive of hepatitis, and to discontinue isoniazid should these occur (Table 13.6).

The idea of TB preventive therapy dates from the pre-HIV era, when active TB disease in adults was considered to arise largely due to reactivation of latent infection, and newly acquired infection was thought to be relatively unimportant as a cause of active disease. This may still be true in countries with a low prevalence of TB. However, molecular techniques used to 'fingerprint' TB isolates now suggest that recent infection makes an important contribution to active disease in HIV-infected people in populations where the prevalence of active disease and therefore the risk of new infection are high (as in most African countries) (Sonnenberg et al., 2001). This, along with increasing evidence that the protective effect of 6 months of IPT diminishes over time, suggests that the optimal duration of IPT may be longer than 6 months, perhaps lifelong. In addition, secondary TB preventive therapy (that is, treatment to prevent a further episode in individuals who have previously completed treatment for TB) may be a useful intervention in populations where the risk of new TB infection is high; this is likely to be most useful in individuals with advanced disease where the risk of new infection progressing rapidly to disease is highest. Currently there is relatively little firm evidence to support these suggestions, but guidelines concerning the duration of IPT, whether secondary IPT should be given and to whom may be revised as new evidence emerges.

Prevention of bacterial infections, toxoplasmosis and other infections

Cotrimoxazole is recommended as primary preventive therapy for HIV-infected adults with CD4 counts below

Table 13.6. Recommendations for preventive interventions for HIV-infected people in African countries

Disease targeted	Drug	Duration	Indication	Contraindications
Tuberculosis	Isoniazid 5mg/kg daily (max 300mg)	6 months[a]	TST positive[b]	Active TB, chronic hepatitis, peripheral neuropathy
Bacterial infections, cerebral toxoplasmosis	Cotrimoxazole 960mg daily	lifelong	advanced HIV disease	hypersensitivity to cotrimoxazole
Pneumococcal disease	Pneumococcal polysaccharide vaccine		Not recommended	

Notes:

[a] Current WHO recommendation is for 6 months; lifelong treatment may be more effective, but currently there is no direct evidence of superiority over 6 months.

[b] TB preventive therapy may be given without performing a tuberculin skin test if the prevalence of latent TB infection and/or the risk of new infection is high.

200×10^6/l in industrialized countries, primarily in order to prevent PCP. Since PCP is relatively unusual among adults in Africa, the value of cotrimoxazole was unclear. However, two randomized controlled trials from Abidjan, Côte d'Ivoire, demonstrated a major reduction in morbidity and mortality attributed to cotrimoxazole among HIV-infected adults with TB (Wiktor et al., 1999) and among health care attenders in WHO stages 2 and 3 (Anglaret et al., 1999). This intervention is recommended by WHO and UNAIDS. It is likely that the maximum benefit from cotrimoxazole is seen in individuals at highest risk of severe HIV-related infections, such as those with CD4 counts below 200×10^6/l and those with active tuberculosis. Where CD4 counts are not available, maximum benefit is likely in individuals in WHO stage 3 and 4 (Badri et al., 2001).

There are some concerns that cotrimoxazole may not be effective as preventive therapy in all African countries, particularly those in East Africa where the prevalence of resistance to cotrimoxazole among key bacterial pathogens (non-typhoid salmonellae and pneumococci) is higher than in Côte d'Ivoire. Further randomized trials of cotrimoxazole preventive therapy are under way in Zambia to investigate this issue. There are concerns that widespread use of prophylactic cotrimoxazole will accelerate the development of cotrimoxazole resistance among common bacterial pathogens, and also the development of resistance to anti-malarial drugs whose action is based on anti-folate drugs, particularly sulphadoxine-pyrimethamine.

Prevention of pneumococcal disease

In US guidelines, pneumococcal polysaccharide vaccine (PPV) is recommended for prevention of pneumococcal disease among HIV-infected adults with CD4 $> 200 \times 10^6$/l, and to be 'considered' for those with CD4 $< 200 \times 10^6$/l (USPHS/ISDA, 2001), although the evidence for the efficacy of this vaccine in HIV-infected persons is relatively weak. A randomized controlled trial of PPV among HIV-infected adults in Uganda found that the vaccine did not prevent pneumococcal disease or death, and there was a small excess of pneumonia in the group receiving vaccine compared with placebo (French et al., 2000). The population studied had relatively advanced HIV disease (majority in WHO stage 2 or 3, median CD4 count just over 200×10^6/l) and therefore PPV cannot be recommended in such individuals. The effect of PPV among HIV-infected individuals in African countries at an early stage of disease is not clear.

Prevention of fungal disease

Cryptococcal disease is a major cause of morbidity and mortality in many African countries, perhaps more so in Southern and Eastern than in West Africa. Until recently, the drugs required for treatment of cryptococcal disease have been prohibitively expensive, and so it has been unrealistic to consider the use of these drugs to prevent fungal disease. Fluconazole has been shown to reduce the incidence of fungal disease among HIV-infected adults in industrialised countries, but is not recommended for routine use because of the low incidence of severe fungal disease, and because of concerns about toxicity, drug interactions, the development of resistance and cost. However, as access to imidazole drugs (such as fluconazole) increases, prevention of fungal disease may become achievable, and trials of fluconazole as primary prophylaxis against fungal disease in African countries are planned.

Table 13.7. Recommendations for starting ART in different countries, 2001

	South Africa	United Kingdom	United States
Symptomatic	treat	treat	treat
Asymptomatic			
CD4 < 200	treat	treat	treat
CD4 200–349	treat if high VL	consider, based on CD4 decline and patient's wishes	generally treat
CD4 > 350	treat if high VL	defer	consider if high VL

Note:
VL = HIV viral load.

Antiretroviral drugs

Antiretroviral drugs (ART) are agents which inhibit the replication of HIV. Early ART regimes, using one or two antiretroviral drugs, had a limited effect on the course of HIV disease, probably because of the development of drug-resistant virus. However, the introduction of the protease inhibitor class of ART, and the use of a combination of three or more agents (highly active antiretroviral therapy, HAART), has transformed HIV infection from an almost inevitably fatal condition to a chronic, manageable disease in settings where ART is available. ART is not, however, a cure for HIV infection.

ART has been extremely expensive, and beyond the reach of the vast majority of HIV-infected individuals in developing countries. However, prices are falling fast, and there is mounting pressure to expand access to antiretroviral therapy. The cost of ART is not the only obstacle to implementation in low-income settings: the laboratory tests (CD4 count and HIV viral load) used to monitor therapy are not widely available in developing countries, and the public health infrastructure is also inadequate to assure effective delivery in many places. This section summarizes the principles of ART use. Recommendations for antiretroviral use change rapidly, and readers are advised to consult national and international guidelines to get the most up-to-date advice (US Dept Health, 2001; WHO, 2000; BHIVA; South Africans Clinicians Society, 2000). Physicians unfamiliar with ART use should seek advice from experienced colleagues before starting or changing ART regimes.

The aim of antiretroviral therapy is to reduce disease and prolong survival among HIV-infected people. In order to achieve this, treatment should ideally be started before there is irreversible damage to the immune system, and before the onset of life-threatening opportunistic infections. However, increasing experience of long-term ART use demonstrates that these drugs remain far from ideal. The potential benefit of starting ART must be balanced against the risk of side effects, difficulties with long-term adherence, especially to complex regimes, and the risk of development of resistant virus, especially if adherence is poor. Guidelines for when to start ART change frequently and vary from country to country (Table 13.7). With increasing awareness of long-term side effects, the current trend is towards a more conservative approach, deferring ART until the onset of symptomatic disease or when the risk of progression to advanced disease is high.

Currently, three main classes of antiretroviral drugs are available (Table 13.8). Reverse transcriptase inhibitors (NRTI and NNRTI) inhibit the transcription of viral RNA to proviral DNA by reverse transcriptase, whereas protease inhibitors (PI) inhibit the splitting of the structural viral proteins into appropriate sections to make new virions by viral protease (see Fig. 13.5).

A combination of at least three different antiretroviral agents should be used for the treatment of chronic HIV disease. Monotherapy gives incomplete viral suppression and is only suitable for short-term use, such as the prevention of mother-to-child transmission. Dual therapy is inferior to triple therapy, and is much more likely to lead to the development of resistant virus. Some ART combinations are contraindicated because of the additive risk of side effects or antagonism between the agents: ART guidelines should be consulted for further details.

Popular first-line regimens in developing countries include two NRTI and an NNRTI, e.g. AZT, 3TC and nevirapine, or three NRTI, e.g. AZT, 3TC and abacavir. Two NRTI and a protease inhibitor, e.g. AZT, 3TC, indinavir, are also used as first-line regimes, although protease inhibitors are currently much more expensive than NRTI and NNRTI.

New classes of antiretroviral are in development, including fusion inhibitors, which bind to the viral envelope glycoprotein gp41 and prevent it fusing with the host cell membrane, and integrase inhibitors, which prevent proviral DNA being inserted into the host genome.

One of the limitations of ART is the frequency of side effects. The principal side effects are listed in Table 13.8; minor intolerance is very common, and usually settles within the first few weeks, but more serious side effects are not infrequent, and patients and physicians need to be aware of the possible risks. Another complication is the frequency of drug interactions with ART, particularly protease inhibitors; in developing countries the most important of these is between ART and rifampicin. NNRTI and PI are metabolized by cytochrome p450, which is

Table 13.8. Antiretroviral drugs

Class	Drug	Side effects	Comments
Nucleoside reverse transcriptase inhibitors (NRTI)			
	zidovudine (AZT)	nausea, headache, muscle pain, bone marrow suppression	
	didanosine (ddI)	nausea, diarrhoea, peripheral neuropathy, pancreatitis	best taken 1 hour before food
	zalcitabine (ddC)	stomatitis, peripheral neuropathy	
	lamivudine (3TC)		usually well tolerated
	stavudine (d4T)	peripheral neuropathy	
	abacavir (ABC)	nausea, vomiting, hypersensitivity	hypersensitivity can present non-specifically; rechallenge may be fatal
Non-nucleoside reverse transcriptase inhibitors (NNRTI)			
	nevirapine	rash, hepatitis	caution in liver disease
	efavirenz	rash, neuropsychiatric disturbance	potentially teratogenic, unsuitable for pregnant women
	delavirdine	rash, headache	caution in liver disease
Protease inhibitors (PI)			
	ritonavir	nausea, diarrhoea, hyperglycaemia, lipodystrophy	better tolerated if taken with food. Capsules require refrigeration
	indinavir	nausea, skin/nail problems, renal stones, lipodystrophy	taken on an empty stomach; high fluid intake to avoid renal stones
	saquinavir	nausea, diarrhoea, hyperglycaemia, lipodystrophy	best taken with fatty meal
	nelfinavir	diarrhoea, nausea, hyperglycaemia, lipodystrophy	best taken with food
	amprenavir	nausea, vomiting, diarrhoea, mood disorder, hypersensitivity	fatty food reduces absorption

induced by rifampicin. Rifampicin accelerates the metabolism of these drugs, resulting in lower plasma ART levels, and hence increasing the likelihood of treatment failure and viral resistance. The combination of rifampicin with either NNRTIs or PIs may be contra-indicated or may need dose adjustment.

For individuals whose HIV infection is diagnosed as a result of an episode of tuberculosis, it may help to remember that antiretroviral therapy is not an emergency, whereas treatment of tuberculosis often is. Many physicians would recommend treatment of tuberculosis first, and then reconsider the need for ART when the individual has at least completed the induction phase, if not the full course of anti-tuberculous treatment. If ART must be combined with anti-tuberculous therapy, rifabutin may be substituted for rifampicin, but this may be difficult to obtain if it is not part of the standard national anti-tuberculous regime, and rifabutin is not compatible with all protease inhibitors: detailed guidelines on ART use should be consulted.

If antiretroviral therapy is to be implemented on a wide scale in countries with a high prevalence of HIV infection, it is most likely to be successful if the model of effective TB control is followed. This would require political commitment, the use of standardized ART regimens using quality-controlled products, a secure drug supply and monitoring and evaluation. Maximizing adherence to treatment is another key issue: there is ample evidence that adherence to ART is a key determinant of a successful response to treatment, and that at least 95 per cent adherence is needed to ensure maximum effectiveness. Some people think that ART implementation should follow the TB model by using directly observed therapy as the standard method of delivery, but it is not clear whether direct observation of ART will be effective in promoting adherence and effectiveness of therapy, and if effective, whether it will be feasible to continue this in the long term. Studies to address this issue are planned.

A further challenge is the need for monitoring ART. CD4 counts and viral load assays are performed regularly for HIV-infected patients in industrialized countries to help decide when to start ART, and, once on therapy, to monitor its effectiveness. Such assays are expensive and

Table 13.9. Estimated timing and risk of mother-to-child HIV-1 transmission

	No breast-feeding %		Breast-feeding 6 m %		Breast-feeding 18–24 m %	
Timing	Relative proportion	Absolute rate	Relative proportion	Absolute rate	Relative proportion	Absolute rate
Intrauterine	25 to 35	5 to 10	20 to 25	5 to 10	20 to 25	5 to 10
Peripartum	65 to 75	10 to 20	40 to 55	10 to 20	35 to 50	10 to 20
Early (<2m) breast-feeding	–	–	20 to 25	5 to 10	20 to 25	5 to 10
Late (>2m) breast-feeding	–	–	5 to 10	1 to 5	20 to 25	5 to 10
Total transmission	–	15 to 30	–	25 to 35	–	30 to 45

Source: De Cock et al. (2000).

currently only available in a few centres in Africa. It is not clear whether clinical monitoring of disease stage could be used as an acceptable substitute to decide when to start ART, and to monitor its effectiveness. Trials are planned to investigate this, and also to evaluate alternative methods of estimating CD4 counts and surrogate measures of viral load.

HIV disease in children

Acquisition of HIV infection in infants and children

Transmission from mother to infant occurs through three distinct mechanisms and at different times. During pregnancy 5–10 per cent of exposed infants will become infected. Without antiretroviral treatment an additional 10–20 per cent of infants will be infected during labour and delivery through exposure to cervico-vaginal secretions and maternal blood (see Table 13.9). Breast milk contains both free and cell-associated virus and causes transmission in an additional 5–15 per cent of exposed infants. The mother's viral load and clinical status are the major factors that influence the rate of transmission; a pregnant woman with AIDS, or one who acquires the infection during pregnancy or lactation is more likely to transmit than an asymptomatic HIV-infected mother.

Natural history and spectrum of disease

Infants and children with HIV infection have widely varying clinical courses. During the first year of life 15–25 per cent of infected infants develop severe immunodeficiency associated with serious infections or encephalopathy. These infants have a rapidly progressive clinical course, with failure to thrive and development of AIDS in the first 6–12 months. Other infants experience more frequent infections, malnutrition, and develop AIDS in the second or third year of life. In African natural history studies, approximately one-third of children follow a clinical progression that is longer, similar to adults, with mild or moderate HIV-related symptoms, and may survive into mid-childhood or adolescence. Infection acquired during pregnancy or in the peripartum period, a higher dose of virus, and concurrent disease exposure such as TB may contribute to a more rapid clinical progression, though data to support this are limited.

Clinical presentation of HIV infection in children

Infants and children with HIV infection present with illnesses that are also common in uninfected African children: frequent acute infections, pruritic skin rashes and eczema, oral candidiasis (thrush), fever, and malnutrition or failure to thrive. Chronic diarrhoea or cough, developmental delay or loss of milestones, and persistent conditions, including generalized lymphadenopathy, hepatosplenomegaly, and parotitis, are more common in HIV-infected children. Over 50 per cent of children with symptomatic HIV infection are malnourished, but wasting and stunting are also common in uninfected children. Malnutrition or serious acute infections (bacterial pneumonia, sepsis or meningitis) raise suspicion of HIV infection in young children, especially if HIV infection is confirmed in the mother.

Case definitions for paediatric AIDS

Clinical case definitions for paediatric AIDS were developed to assist the identification of children with AIDS for surveillance purposes, where laboratory facilities were limited. The WHO clinical case definition of AIDS in children requires two of three major signs and two of six

Table 13.10. Mortality in children born to HIV-infected and uninfected mothers

Country of study	IMR in infants of HIV-uninfected mothers	IMR in HIV exposed (HIV-infected mother, HIV-negative child)	IMR in HIV-infected infants	3 year mortality in infants of HIV-uninfected mothers	3 year mortality in exposed (HIV-infected mother, HIV-negative child)	3 year mortality in HIV-infected infants
Malawi[63]	145	235				
Uganda	34	163	336	47	287	663
Zaire[64]	36	262	261	67	365	494

Notes:
IMR (Infant Mortality Rate) = deaths per 1000 live births in first year of life.
3 year mortality = deaths per 1000 live births in first three years of life.

minor signs (Box). It cannot be used for diagnosis of HIV/AIDS in Africa because many children who meet the case definition in Africa do not have HIV infection, but rather malnutrition, fever, or diarrhoea caused by other diseases.

World Health Organization clinical case definition of AIDS in children

Major signs:
Weight loss or failure to thrive
Chronic diarrhoea (>1 month)
Prolonged fever (>1 month)

Minor signs:
Generalized lymphadenopathy (lymph nodes measuring at least 0.5 cm and present in two or more sites with bilateral lymphadenopathy counting as one site)
Oropharyngeal candidiasis
Repeated common infections (otitis, pharyngitis, etc.)
Persistent cough (>1 month)
Generalized dermatitis
Confirmed maternal infection

Paediatric AIDS is suspected in an infant or child presenting with at least two major signs associated with at least two minor signs in the absence of known causes of immunosuppression.

Diagnosis of HIV infection in infants and children

Laboratory diagnosis of HIV infection in children over 18 months follows the same procedures as for adults, but poses special problems in infants and children under 18 months of age. HIV antibodies passively transferred across the placenta cause infants of HIV-infected mothers to test antibody positive whether or not they are infected with HIV. If the infant is uninfected, the amount of antibody diminishes to an undetectable level between 9 and 18 months. Repeated negative HIV EIA tests after 9 months of age confirm that an infant is uninfected, but between 9 and 18 months of age, a positive EIA for HIV does not confirm infection. Definitive diagnosis of HIV infection in infants under 18 months of age requires special tests that directly detect HIV, as described earlier. These are costly, and not widely available.

Mortality in HIV-infected children

HIV-infected mothers have higher rates of stillbirth, spontaneous abortion and neonatal deaths. Maternal mortality is also higher, particularly in breast-feeding mothers (Nduati et al., 2000), and a mother's death is often associated with death of her child, especially in those who are HIV-infected. Infants of HIV-infected mothers have a high mortality in Africa (Table 13.10). Difficulties in early diagnosis limit the accuracy of infant mortality data in HIV-infected children in Africa; diagnosis of HIV infection is uncertain in those who die in the neonatal period or are lost to follow-up. The median survival of HIV-infected children in a closely followed cohort in Uganda was 21 months, while infant mortality was 335 per thousand live births. Similar results have been seen in Kenya, DRC Kinshasa, Malawi, and Rwanda. By 3 years of age, 50–66 per cent of HIV-1 infected infants in African studies have died.

Clinical management of children with HIV infection

Clinical management of acute illnesses in HIV-infected children follows the same principles and protocols as in uninfected children. Acute respiratory infection (ARI), fever and malaria, and acute diarrhoeal diseases are the most common presenting illnesses in infants and children under 5 years age, regardless of HIV status. Children with HIV infection are more likely, however, to present with multiple symptoms and more severe illness, and more likely to be malnourished or anaemic.

The integrated management of childhood illness (IMCI) has been developed by UNICEF and WHO as a care algorithm that assesses, classifies, and treats common syndromes, identifies underlying nutritional problems and anaemia, and provides sound counselling and follow-up plans (WHO, 1997). Each country adapts the management algorithms to their own conditions and treatment policies; these adaptations may include specific guidelines for recognizing and referring those suspected of symptomatic HIV infection, and for inpatient management of sick children.

Growth and malnutrition

Growth failure is frequent and associated with early mortality in HIV-infected children in Africa, where background rates of acute and chronic malnutrition are also high. In Burkina Faso 13.8 per cent of HIV-infected children were marasmic, though kwashiorkor was not seen more frequently than in uninfected children (Prazuck et al., 1993). HIV-infected children admitted for malnutrition had twice as long a hospital stay in Dakar and three times the mortality rate (45 per cent vs. 15 per cent) in Abidjan. In Uganda, HIV-infected children with weight-for-age 1.5 standard deviations below the mean (z-score –1.5) had a five-fold increase in risk of death in the second year of life (Berhane et al., 1997).

Recommendations for weaning at 6 months in infants exposed to HIV present an additional nutritional challenge to those who are already infected, as well as those born to HIV-infected mothers who are not infected. Pay close attention to early signs of faltering growth and develop locally appropriate, available and affordable weaning foods and breast milk substitutes. The risk of micronutrient deficiencies is also increased. Vitamin A is of particular importance and supplementation has been shown to reduce morbidity in HIV-infected children (Coutsoudis et al., 1995; Semba et al., 1999).

Bacterial infections and acute respiratory illness

Pneumonia and bacteraemia are more common and more likely to be fatal in HIV-infected children. *Salmonella typhimurium, S. pneumoniae, Haemophilus influenzae* and *Staphylococcus aureus* were the most common organisms isolated in studies in Kenya, Rwanda, Malawi, and Zimbabwe (Gilks et al., 1991; Lepage et al., 1989; Nathoo et al., 1996). Start appropriate antibiotics early in HIV-infected infants and children.

Tuberculosis

The exponential rise in tuberculosis in Africa in the last decade has been largely due to HIV infection. Children are the group with the largest increase in tuberculosis incidence in Malawi (Kiwanuka et al., 2001). In Africa the overall relative risk of active tuberculosis in children with HIV is 5– to 10–fold higher than in uninfected children (Harries, 1997; Sassan-Morokro et al., 1994). Children with HIV infection are likely to be exposed through a family member with dual HIV infection and tuberculosis, and are more susceptible to primary progressive tuberculosis.

Other respiratory diseases

PCP is an AIDS-defining illness for children that most frequently presents in the 3 to 6-month age group. The prevalence of *P. carinii* varies in different parts of Africa. Among HIV-infected children under 2 years, 8 per cent of those admitted with pneumonia in Malawi (Kamiya et al., 1996) and 31 per cent of those who died in hospital in Abidjan had PCP (Lucas et al., 1996). Treatment is high-dose cotrimoxazole for at least 3 weeks; steroid therapy should also be considered in severe disease (for example, dexamethasone 150 micrograms/kg q.d.s. for the first 5 days).

Lymphoid interstitial pneumonitis commonly presents in the second year of life in HIV-infected children, and may be more frequent in Africa. Lymphadenopathy, parotid gland enlargement, tachypnoea, wheezing and, eventually, finger clubbing are prominent features. Bronchodilators for wheezing and steroids may be useful.

Diarrhoeal diseases and HIV

Acute, recurrent and persistent diarrhoea (>14 days) are all more common in children with HIV infection (see Chapters 20 and 35). In a study in Zambia, acute diarrhoea caused by rotavirus was more severe in HIV-infected children (Oshitani et al., 1994). In a prospective study in Zaire, persistent diarrhoea was more common and had a higher mortality rate (10/11 vs. 1/19) in HIV-infected children (Thea et al., 1993). Stool pathogens are generally similar to those in uninfected children with the exception of a Tanzanian study noting *Blastocystis hominis* only in the HIV-infected (Cigielski et al., 1993).

Childhood cancers

The incidence of Kaposi's sarcoma (KS) in children in Uganda increased 40-fold between the 1960s and 1990s.

In 1989–1993, 78 per cent children with KS were HIV-infected, with a median onset at 33 months of age (Ziegler & Katongole-Mbidde, 1996). KS is nearly twice as common in males. Most children present with mucous membrane involvement, and have oro-facial or genital lesions. Increases in KS and non-Hodgkin lymphomas have been seen in Zambia and Côte d'Ivoire, though shortened survival of HIV-infected children in Africa may limit the occurrence of childhood cancers.

Neurological disease and encephalopathy

More than 50 per cent of children with HIV infection have neurological abnormalities, including delayed motor development, loss of milestones, seizures or encephalopathy, according to cohort studies in African countries. Encephalopathy may result in lack of growth or actual decline in head circumference, and in Uganda was the leading AIDS-defining illness.

Immunization of HIV-infected and exposed infants

Children born to HIV-infected mothers should be immunized following the standard protocols recommended by the WHO Expanded Programme on Immunization (EPI). Though there are concerns about giving live vaccines (measles, oral polio, and Bacillus Calmette–Guerin (BCG)) to persons with symptomatic HIV disease, the immunization schedule should be complete before HIV infection is confirmed and usually before AIDS develops; the benefits of immunization outweigh risks at this stage. BCG vaccination may result in persistent bacteraemia, and should be withheld from older children with confirmed, symptomatic HIV disease.

Breast-feeding by HIV-infected mothers

One of the great dilemmas of paediatric care in the era of AIDS regards feeding practice. The nutritional, immunological, psychological, and economic benefits of breast-feeding are well known. Child survival is significantly better in breast-fed infants, especially in the first 6 months of life in locations where there is a significant risk of death from infectious diseases and malnutrition. Yet breast-feeding contributes substantially to mother-to-child HIV transmission.

Balancing the risk of HIV transmission and the risk of death from malnutrition and diarrhoeal disease requires careful assessment of water supply, sanitation, availability of economic resources and fuel to obtain and prepare safe breast milk substitutes. Replacement feeding must be acceptable, feasible, affordable, sustainable and safe. Where replacement feeding cannot meet these criteria, 6 months of exclusive breast-feeding followed by rapid weaning to other foods and milk may be the most practical recommendation.

Antiretroviral therapy

Just as HAART has had an impact on the mortality and progression of disease in adults with HIV infection in developed countries, so children with HIV infection can benefit from these therapies. High cost, side effects and complicated regimens have put ART out of reach for all but an elite few in Africa. However, with reduced drug prices and simpler, standardized regimes, HAART may become available to some HIV-infected children in urban areas of Africa in the coming years.

Public health measures for prevention and control of HIV/AIDS

The response to HIV/AIDS must be comprehensive in nature, encompassing prevention of new infections, treatment of established disease, and mitigation of impact on the individual and society. The essentials of a comprehensive HIV/AIDS prevention programme are shown in the Box. A first requirement is the involvement and commitment of government to prevent HIV/AIDS and limit its impact, requiring leadership at the highest levels and the creation of technical and organizational infrastructure to address the epidemic. Although the health sector is critical in an organized response, the essential elements for prevention and mitigation of impact extend beyond health to all sectors. Because of the

Essentials of a national HIV/AIDS control programme

- Government commitment; formation and staffing of a national HIV/AIDS control programme
- Surveillance for HIV/AIDS
- General population awareness and education
- Lifeskills education for youth
- Support for voluntary counselling and testing
- Prevention of sexual transmission
- Blood safety
- Prevention of mother-to-child transmission
- Prevention services for injecting drug users
- Services for HIV/AIDS care
- Strengthening of tuberculosis control
- Services for HIV/AIDS orphans

chronic nature of HIV infection, and its association with sex and drug use, HIV/AIDS is frequently stigmatizing and HIV-infected persons may face discrimination. Society's response to HIV/AIDS must balance the rights of infected persons with the public health imperatives to prevent HIV transmission and thus limit social impact.

Surveillance

Surveillance is the routine, systematic collection of data concerning disease frequency and distribution, the analysis of those data, and their dissemination to all relevant parties.

Three broad types of activities support surveillance: case reporting, prevalence and incidence studies, and other, special studies. Surveillance data provide the essential information on descriptive epidemiology (the characterization of disease in time, place, and person) which is the basis for targeting prevention and treatment programmes. Surveillance data also provide important information concerning the impact of prevention and treatment.

When AIDS was first described in the United States in 1981, its infectious nature and cause were unknown. The case definition for AIDS that was introduced served to support a typical epidemiological investigation of an outbreak, the essential first steps of which were to verify that an epidemic was occurring and to describe it in time, place, and person (how have cases occurred over time; where were they; who was affected?). This led to the establishment of surveillance programs which have been instrumental in describing the impact of the epidemic in the industrialized world, the groups affected, trends over time, and the effects of prevention and treatment programs.

Once HIV had become established as the cause of AIDS, a test had become available, and the long natural history of HIV infection was understood, a logical approach to surveillance would have been to switch to the public health reporting of cases of HIV infection, instead of, or in addition to, reporting AIDS cases. This proved controversial because of concerns about privacy and other factors, and is only now being more widely introduced in the industrialized world.

In addition to HIV and AIDS case surveillance, many countries have conducted serological surveys to monitor the prevalence of HIV infection in specific groups such as pregnant women, injecting drug users attending treatment facilities, patients attending sexually transmitted disease clinics, and others. These studies have mostly been done in an unlinked, anonymous fashion, meaning testing has been conducted on specimens collected for other purposes (e.g. testing for syphilis) which have been stripped of their identifiers, thus ensuring bias is avoided from selective testing. Unlike HIV and AIDS case reporting, such surveys are not population-based, and it is uncertain how representative the denominator is in relation to the general population.

In the developing world, AIDS case reporting is widely practiced, but rather ineffectively. The substantial underreporting that occurs largely invalidates the data as an indicator of the burden of disease, but the descriptive characteristics of reported cases have been useful to know what sectors of the population are most heavily affected. Problems also exist with the Expanded WHO case definition for AIDS that is used in developing countries (Box p. 213), which lacks sensitivity, i.e. does not recognize all cases of advanced HIV disease. It must be emphasized that the AIDS case definition was introduced as a tool for surveillance, not as a clinical definition for patient care.

The most useful surveillance approach in developing countries has been screening of pregnant women who undergo syphilis testing routinely, and whose blood can subsequently (once anonymised) be tested for HIV. Extensive data have been generated from many different countries, and such data have served as the basis for making estimates of numbers of infected persons. Antenatal HIV prevalence also gives insight into the likely burden of paediatric HIV disease. Figure 13.3 shows trends in HIV prevalence in antenatal women in a number of different African countries. A current area of interest is to link such surveillance data to behavioural data collected in special surveys; such an approach has allowed more confident interpretation of Ugandan data showing a decline in HIV prevalence in recent years as indicating success in preventive interventions.

General population awareness, and lifeskills education for youth

To prevent HIV infection in the general population, as well as promoting rational and appropriate attitudes to HIV infection and persons living with HIV, it is important to assure a good level of knowledge about HIV, and the ways in which it is transmitted, in the general population.

In established epidemics such as those in sub-Saharan Africa, the highest rates of HIV incidence are in young people. To be effective, HIV education must be started before children become sexually active, and continued through adolescence.

The challenges are formidable. Some influential people believe that provision of HIV prevention and reproductive health education serve to promote sexual activity, and are therefore inappropriate. In many cultures communication between youth and their elders is limited, making provision of prevention messages and services difficult. Youth may be exploited, including sexually, in poor communities, where access to schooling is limited, and provision of information and prevention services may be challenging. A particularly difficult group to reach is out-of-school youth.

Voluntary counselling and testing

Voluntary counselling and testing (VCT) for HIV should be part of any comprehensive HIV prevention programme. Ideally, VCT should be linked to services for family planning, treatment of other sexually transmitted infections, screening, management, or prophylaxis against tuberculosis, and HIV/AIDS care services.

Different models for VCT have been used, such as the provision of this service within health care structures, at specially designated sites ('stand alone'), and with different levels of training for counsellors. Although the term 'VCT' is used in the context of other forms of testing (clinical care, sexually transmitted disease clinics, prevention of mother-to-child transmission), VCT as a prevention activity has its own special requirements and attributes and is largely aimed at people who are well.

VCT can be conducted anonymously (clients do not give names) or confidentially. Increased emphasis is being placed on pre-marital VCT, allowing couples to know their HIV status before starting a family. The efficiency of VCT has greatly improved with the advent of rapid tests which can be done on-site in the presence of the client. This ensures all clients receive their results and makes clerical and logistic mistakes less likely.

Prevention of sexual transmission of HIV

Essential elements of the prevention of sexual transmission of HIV are reduction in numbers of sex partners, promotion of condom use, and treatment and prevention of sexually transmitted infections. Groups that are especially at risk are those with frequent partner change, such as commercial sex workers and their clients, persons living away from their families, and those with high rates of sexually transmitted infections. Early in an epidemic, concentrating prevention efforts on epidemiological "core groups" (those who contribute disproportionately to the spread of a sexually transmitted agents, such as commercial sex workers) is especially effective in curtailing epidemic spread. VCT services can enable individuals to select HIV-negative partners: couples may choose to undertake VCT together.

A randomized, community-based trial in Tanzania showed that provision of effective drugs for STI and training health care providers to treat symptomatic STI resulted in a 40 per cent reduction in HIV incidence (Grosskurth et al., 1995). A trial in rural Uganda of mass therapy for STI did not show any reduction in HIV incidence (Wawer et al., 1999). The results of these two studies are not necessarily in conflict. Relevant issues include the stage of the HIV epidemic (once an epidemic is generalized and severe, STI may be proportionately less important in maintaining it); the local epidemiology of STI, especially genital ulcer disease; and the relative importance of viral STI, especially those associated with ulceration such as herpes (see Chapter 14). Despite the debate about the overall contribution of STI control to HIV/AIDS prevention, there is widespread agreement that STI prevention and control form an important part of any HIV/AIDS prevention programme.

Blood safety

Although blood transfusion contributes relatively little to the overall HIV/AIDS epidemic, prevention of transfusion-transmitted HIV is a priority for ethical reasons and because an unsafe blood supply threatens the credibility of any health service. Screening blood for transfusion for HIV and rejecting positive donors is only one element of an overall strategy to providing a safe blood supply (see the Box). Other essential elements are the recruitment and retention of voluntary donors at low risk for HIV; decreasing the use of blood transfusion as far as possible, and improving the appropriate use of blood; developing and instituting transfusion guidelines and supervisory structures; developing blood banking where this is safe and feasible; monitoring and evaluating transfusion use and safety; and introducing interventions to reduce anaemia, especially among women and children. An overriding problem is the low priority that is given by decision makers to addressing this preventable mode of HIV transmission.

Essentials of a blood safety programme
- National blood transfusion policies and guidelines
- Elimination of unnecessary transfusions
- Recruitment and retention of safe blood donors
- Screening of blood for HIV and other pathogens
- Local blood transfusion committees

An important step is the elimination of commercial blood donation and 'replacement' donors, persons related to or acquainted with individual patients who are recruited to donate on behalf of a patient needing blood. Such donors have been shown to be more likely to be HIV-infected than voluntary donors.

Prevention of mother-to-child transmission

Required components of a mother-to-child transmission prevention programme commonly used treatment regimens are shown in the Boxes below. The nevirapine based regimen is the simplest to use. Although conceptually simple, prevention of mother-to-child transmission in developing countries faces great logistic barriers. Antenatal care should include screening and treatment for anaemia and syphilis, and prevention of malaria, but in reality is weak in many settings. Ensuring universal counselling is challenging, and many women decline HIV testing or do not return for results. Women must be given and remember to take drugs at the beginning of labour, and drugs must be given to the infant after birth (in the case of the nevirapine regimen). Providing safe obstetric practices means at a minimum avoiding unnecessary invasive procedures which can increase the risk of HIV transmission.

Essentials of programmes to prevent mother-to-child transmission of HIV

High-quality antenatal care
HIV counselling and testing
Safe obstetric practices
Short course antiretroviral therapy
Safe infant feeding
Maternal HIV/AIDS care

Commonly used short-course antiretroviral regimes for prevention of mother-to-child transmission of HIV

- Zidovudine 300 mg twice daily from 36 weeks gestation, and 300 mg every 3 hours during labour.
- Nevirapine 200 mg single dose at onset of labour, and single dose of nevirapine 2 mg/kg to the infant in first 72 hours

Competing requirements operate when considering advice about infant feeding, in that breast-feeding is most nutritious and avoids the infectious complications associated with formula feeding, yet prolonged breast-feeding almost doubles the risk of HIV transmission. The advice to practice exclusive breast-feeding, which may be associated with a lower risk of HIV transmission than mixed feeding, is difficult to adhere to, and early weaning is both difficult and challenging from the perspective of assuring adequate nutrition for the infant.

Finally, assuring appropriate care for the mother's own health is difficult. Most mothers would not meet clinical or CD4+ lymphocyte criteria for starting antiretroviral therapy, even if they were available, though a minority would. Linkage with medical services is required. Opportunities exist for prophylaxis of opportunistic infection, and especially exclusion of active tuberculosis and provision of preventive therapy. Infants born to HIV-infected mothers should receive standard vaccinations and infant care, with the exception that children with clinically evident immune deficiency should not receive BCG. Since BCG is given at birth, this means in practice that infants born to HIV-infected mothers are treated like all other infants.

Prevention services for injection drug users

Prevention programmes for injecting drug users must focus not only on drug injecting but also on sexual behaviors, both in the context of individual relations as well as for commercial sex which is frequently engaged in to support drug habits. No one intervention exists that will solve the problem of injecting drug use and its many complications. A first requirement is political will to address the issue; some countries are reluctant to admit they have drug-using populations. A balance is required between public health interventions aiming to limit drug use and its complications, and law enforcement aiming to curb the importation, distribution, and sale of illicit drugs. Public health measures considered efficacious include educational and drug treatment programmes to reduce dependency and use, needle and syringe exchange allowing drug users to exchange used injection equipment for sterile materials, and over the counter sterile syringe and needle sales by pharmacists.

Tuberculosis services, HIV/AIDS care, and services for orphans

Since tuberculosis is the most frequent opportunistic infection in persons with HIV in the developing world, tuberculosis prevention and care constitute important components of HIV/AIDS mitigation. Increased coordination is required between HIV/AIDS and tuberculosis control programmes, and in some developing countries these are being merged. The basic strategy for tuberculosis control is referred to as DOTS (directly observed therapy, short course), whose essential components are government commitment; passive diagnosis based on smear microscopy; direct observation of therapy, at least in the rifampicin-containing part of treatment; a secure supply of drugs; and a standardized reporting system. Although special initiatives need to be explored in the face of escalating tuberculosis rates, such as increased use of preventive therapy, DOTS should remain the backbone of tuberculosis control. HIV counselling and testing services are needed for patients with tuberculosis. Antiretroviral therapy for persons with HIV may play a role in preventing tuberculosis, as it does for other opportunistic infections, although many persons with tuberculosis would not meet the criteria for starting therapy.

HIV/AIDS care is discussed earlier. Care is an essential part of society's response to the epidemic and prevention and care are inseparable. Whether and how to deliver antiretroviral therapy in a resource-poor setting are evolving questions, though it is likely that much more use will be made of antiretroviral drugs in developing countries in the future.

The problem of orphanhood may be the most devastating and long-lasting impact of the HIV/AIDS epidemic. Children who have lost one or both parents face physical, emotional, and economic challenges, and orphans from AIDS have swelled the numbers of underprivileged, homeless, and street children in Africa. A particularly negative consequence for orphans is the premature curtailment of schooling because of inability to pay school fees. Until now the burden of orphans has largely fallen on individuals and families who have had to take in orphaned children of relatives or friends who have died. To date, an organized or innovative response on the part of society has been lacking.

Unresolved issues and prospects for the future

One of the most challenging policy issues today concerns the use of antiretroviral drugs in resource-poor settings. Antiretroviral therapy has changed the face of AIDS in the industrialized world but has been inaccessible to the vast majority of HIV-infected persons in developing countries. Three broad arguments shape the discussion:

- investment in antiretroviral drugs is inappropriate in settings where basic public health measures such as clean water and sanitation cannot be assured
- essential infrastructure for safe use of these drugs, including the appropriate laboratory monitoring, precludes widespread increase in access
- it may be possible to introduce HAART using standardized regimens and approaches, with attention to adherence and minimal monitoring.

Whatever the specific outcome, it is inevitable that antiretroviral drug use will increase in resource-poor settings.

A further balance to seek is that between searching for new approaches and applying what we already know. Our understanding of HIV/AIDS is deep and we have effective interventions, yet the impact of prevention programmes on the epidemic has been limited. The single most important biomedical research objective today is the search for an HIV/AIDS vaccine. A vaccine yielding sterilizing immunity, i.e. which prevents establishment of infection, would be ideal, but one which does not prevent infection but keeps viral load under control may be more likely. This approach would prevent disease and, since viral load is the main determinant of transmission, may reduce transmission. However, even if a vaccine became available, other preventive measures and provision of care to persons already infected would still have to be assured.

Final discussion points for the future concern our attitudes and commitment to HIV/AIDS prevention and control. In heavily affected countries with generalized epidemics, greater emphasis will be required on public health and infrastructure strengthening. Greatly increased resources will be necessary if we are to alter the course of the HIV/AIDS pandemic, undoubtedly the greatest public health challenge ever faced in Africa.

Acknowledgements

Wolfgang Preiser for Figs. 13.4 and 13.7.

Selected reading

Mann J, Tarantola D, eds. (1996). *AIDS in the World – II.* New York: Oxford University Press.

Laga M, ed. (1997). *AIDS in Africa.* 2nd edn. London: Rapid Science Publishers.

Sande MA, Volberding PA. (1999). *The Medical Management of AIDS.* 6th edn. Philadelphia: WB Saunders.

De Cock KM, Fowler MG, Mercier E et al. (2000). Prevention of mother-to-child transmission of HIV-1 in resource-poor countries: translating research into policy and practice. *JAMA*; **283**: 1175–1182.

Grant AD, Kaplan JE, De Cock KM. (2001). Preventing opportunistic infections among HIV-infected adults in African countries. *Am J Trop Med*; **65**: 810–821.

Kaplan JE, Hu DJ, Holmes KK, Jaffe HW, Masur H, De Cock KM. (1996). Preventing opportunistic infections in human immunodeficiency virus-infected persons: implications for the developing world. *Am J Trop Med Hyg*; **55**: 1–11.

Grant AD, De Cock KM. (1998). The growing challenge of HIV/AIDS in developing countries. *Br Med Bull*; **54**: 369–381.

Grant AD, Djomand G, De Cock KM. (1997). Natural history and spectrum of disease in adults with HIV/AIDS in Africa. *AIDS*; **11**: S43–S54.

Gilks CF, Katabira E, De Cock KM. (1997). The challenge of providing effective care for HIV/AIDS in Africa. *AIDS*; **11**(suppl B): S99–S106.

Grant AD, De Cock KM. (2001). HIV infection and AIDS in the developing world. In *ABC of AIDS*, London: BMJ Publishing.

Paediatric HIV

Pizzo PA, Wilfert CM. (1999). *Pediatric AIDS: The Challenge of HIV Infection in Infants, Children and Adolescents*, 3rd edn. New York: Williams and Wilkins.

Preble EA, Piwoz EG. (2001). Prevention of mother-to-child transmission of HIV in Africa: practical guidance for programs. Support for Analysis and Research in Africa (SARA) Project, Academy for Educational Development.

WHO. (1997). Integrated management of childhood illness: a WHO/UNICEF initiative. *Bull WHO*; **75** Suppl 1.

WHO. (1993). WHO guidelines for management of HIV infection in children. Geneva: WHO.

References

Ackah AN, Coulibaly D, Digbeu H *et al.* (1995). Response to treatment, mortality, and CD4 lymphocyte counts in HIV-infected persons with tuberculosis in Abidjan, Côte d'Ivoire. *Lancet*; **345**: 607–610.

Adjorlolo-Johnson G, De Cock KM, Ekpini E *et al.* (1994). Prospective comparison of mother-to-child transmission of HIV-1 and HIV-2 in Abidjan, Ivory Coast. *J Am Med Assoc*; **272**: 462–466.

Anglaret X, Chêne G, Attia A *et al.* (1999). Early chemoprophylaxis with trimethoprim-sulphamethoxazole for HIV-1–infected adults in Abidjan, Côte d'Ivoire: a randomised trial. *Lancet*; **353**: 1463–1468.

Anzala OA, Nagelkerke NJD, Bwayo JJ *et al.* (1995). Rapid progression to disease in African sex workers with human immunodeficiency virus type 1 infection. *J Infect Dis*; **171**: 686–689.

Archibald LK, den Dulk MO, Pallangyo KJ, Reller LB. (1998). Fatal *Mycobacterium tuberculosis* bloodstream infections in febrile hospitalized adults in Dar es Salaam, Tanzania. *Clin Infect Dis*; **26**: 290–296.

Archibald LK, McDonald LC, Nwanyanwu O *et al.* (2000). A hospital-based prevalence survey of bloodstream infections in febrile patients in Malawi: implications for diagnosis and therapy. *J Infect Dis*; **181**: 1414–1420.

Badri M, Ehrlich R, Wood R, Maartens G. (2001). Initiating co-trimoxazole prophylaxis in HIV-infected patients in Africa: an evaluation of the provisional WHO/UNAIDS recommendations. *AIDS*; **15**: 1143–1148.

Berhane R, Bagenda D, Marum L, Aceng E, Ndugwa C, Olness K. (1997). Growth failure as a prognostic indicator of mortality in pediatric HIV infection. *Pediatrics*; **100**: 126.

BHIVA Writing Committee. British HIV Association (BHIVA) guidelines for the treatment of HIV-infected adults with antiretroviral therapy. Available at: www.aidsmap.com/about/bhiva/guidelines.pdf

Bloland PB, Wirima JJ, Steketee RW, Chilima B, Hightower A, Breman JG. (1995). Maternal HIV infection and infant mortality in Malawi: evidence for increased mortality due to placental malaria infection. *AIDS*; **9**: 721–726.

Buvé A, Foster SD, Mbwili C, Mungo E, Tollenare N, Zeko M. (1994). Mortality among female nurses in the face of the AIDS epidemic: a pilot study in Zambia. *AIDS*; **8**: 396.

Buvé A, Caraël M, Hayes RJ *et al.* (2001). Multicentre study on factors determining differences in rate of spread of HIV in sub-Saharan Africa: methods and prevalence of HIV infection. *AIDS*; **15**: S5–S14.

Cegielski JP, Msengi AE, Dukes CS *et al.* (1993). Intestinal parasites and HIV infection in Tanzanian children with chronic diarrhea. *AIDS*; **7**: 213–221.

Centers for Disease Control and Prevention. (1992). 1993 revised classification system for HIV infection and expanded surveillance case definition for AIDS among adolescents and adults. *MMWR*; **41**(RR17): 1–19.

Corbett EL, Churchyard GJ, Charalambous S *et al.* (2002). Morbidity and mortality in South African gold miners: the impact of untreated HIV disease. *Clin Infect Dis*; **34**: 1251–1258.

Coutsoudis A, Bobat RA, Coovadia HM, Kuhn L, Tsai WY, Stein ZA. (1995). The effects of vitamin A supplementation on the morbidity of children born to HIV infected women. *Am J Pub Hlth*; **85**: 1076–1081.

De Cock KM, Fowler MG, Mercier E. (2000). Prevention of mother-to-child-transmission in resource-poor countries: translating research into policy and practice. *J Am Med Assoc*; **283**: 1175–1182.

French N, Mujugira A, Nakiyingi J, Mulder D, Janoff EN, Gilks CF. (1999). Immunologic and clinical stages in HIV-1–infected Ugandan adults are comparable and provide no evidence of rapid progression but poor survival with advanced disease. *J Acquir Immune Defic Syndr*; **22**: 509–516.

French N, Nakiyingi J, Carpenter LM *et al.* (2000). 23–valent pneumococcal polysaccharide vaccine in HIV-1–infected Ugandan adults: double-blind, randomised and placebo controlled trial. *Lancet*; **355**: 2106–2111.

French N, Nakiyingi J, Lugada E, Watera C, Whitworth JAG, Gilks CF. (2001). Increasing rates of malarial fever with deteriorating immune status in HIV-1–infected Ugandan adults. *AIDS*; **15**: 899–906.

Gilks CF, Brindle RJ, Otieno LS *et al.* (1990a). Extrapulmonary and disseminated tuberculosis in HIV-1–seropositive patients presenting to the acute medical services in Nairobi. *AIDS*; **4**: 981–985.

Gilks CF, Brindle RJ, Otieno LS *et al.* (1990b). Life-threatening bacteraemia in HIV-1 seropositive adults admitted to hospital in Nairobi, Kenya. *Lancet*; **336**: 545–549.

Gilks CF, Ojoo SA, Brindle RJ. (1991). Non-opportunistic bacterial infections in HIV-seropositive adults in Nairobi, Kenya. *AIDS*; **5**: S113–S116.

Gilks CF, Otieno LS, Brindle RJ *et al.* (1992). The presentation and

outcome of HIV-related disease in Nairobi. *Quart J Med*; **82**: 25–32.
Gilks CF, Ojoo SA, Ojoo JC *et al.* (1996). Invasive pneumococcal disease in a cohort of predominantly HIV-1 infected female sex-workers in Nairobi, Kenya. *Lancet*; **347**: 718–723.
Grant AD (1998). Spectrum and natural history of HIV disease in Abidjan, Côte d'Ivoire. PhD thesis. University of London.
Grant AD, De Cock KM. (1998). The growing challenge of HIV/AIDS in developing countries. *Br Med Bull*; **54**: 369–381.
Grant AD, Djomand G, Smets P *et al.* (1997). Profound immunosuppression across the spectrum of opportunistic disease among hospitalised HIV-infected adults in Abidjan, Côte d'Ivoire. *AIDS*; **11**: 1357–1364.
Gray RH, Wawer MJ, Brookmeyer R *et al.* (2001). Probability of HIV-1 transmission per coital act in monogamous, heterosexual, HIV-1–discordant couples in Rakai, Uganda. *Lancet*; **357**: 1149–1153.
Grosskurth H, Mosha F, Todd J *et al.* (1995). Impact of improved treatment of sexually transmitted diseases on HIV infection in rural Tanzania: randomised controlled trial. *Lancet*; **346**: 530–536.
Hahn BH, Shaw GM, De Cock KM, Sharp PM. (2000). AIDS as a zoonosis: scientific and health implications. *Science*; **287**: 607–614.
Harries AD. (1997). Tuberculosis in Africa: Clinical presentation and management. *Pharmacolog Ther*; **73**: 1–50.
Hayes RJ, Schulz KF, Plummer FA. (1995). The cofactor effect of genital ulcers on the per-exposure risk of HIV transmission in sub-Saharan Africa. *J Trop Med Hyg*; **98**: 1–8.
Ho DD, Neumann AU, Perelson AS, Chen W, Leonard JM, Markowitz M. (1995). Rapid turnover of plasma virions and CD4 lymphocytes in HIV-1 infection. *Nature*; **373**: 123–126.
Hu DJ, Buvé A, Baggs J, Van der Groen G, Dondero T. (1999). What role does HIV-1 subtype play in transmission and pathogenesis? An epidemiological perspective. *AIDS*; **13**: 873–881.
Kamiya Y, Mtitimila E, Broadhead R, Brabin B, Hart CA. (1996). *Pneumocystis carinii* pneumonia in Africa. *Lancet*; **347**: 1114–1115.
Kassa E, Rinke de Wit TF, Hailu E *et al.* (1999). Evaluation of the World Health Organization staging system for HIV infection and disease in Ethiopia: association between clinical stages and laboratory markers. *AIDS*; **13**: 381–389.
Kiwanuka J, Graham SM, Coulter JBS *et al.* (2001). Diagnosis of pulmonary tuberculosis in children in an HIV endemic area, Malawi. *Ann Trop Paediatr*; **21**: 5–14.
Lepage P, Van de Perre P, Dabis F *et al.* (1989). Evaluation and simplification of the World Health Organization clinical case definition for paediatric AIDS. *AIDS*; **3**: 221–225.
Lucas SB, Hounnou A, Peacock C *et al.* (1993). The mortality and pathology of HIV infection in a West African city. *AIDS*; **7**: 1569–1579.
Lucas SB, Peacock CS, Hounnou A *et al.* (1996). Disease in children infected with HIV in Abidjan, Côte d'Ivoire. *Br Med J*; **312**: 335–338.
Malamba SS, Morgan D, Clayton T, Mayanja B, Okongo M, Whitworth J. (1999). The prognostic value of the World Health Organization staging system for HIV infection and disease in rural Uganda. *AIDS*; **13**: 2555–2562.
Marlink R, Kanki P, Thior I *et al.* (1994). Reduced rate of disease development after HIV-2 infection as compared to HIV-1. *Science*; **265**: 1587–1590.
Martin DJ, Sim JGM, Sole GJ *et al.* (1995). CD4+ lymphocyte count in African patients co-infected with HIV and tuberculosis. *J Acquired Immune Defic Syndr Hum Retrovirol*; **8**: 386–391.
Moore A, Herrera G, Nyamongo J *et al.* (2001). Estimated risk of HIV transmission by blood transfusion in Kenya. *Lancet*; **358**: 657–660.
Morgan D, Ross A, Mayanja B, Malamba S, Whitworth J. (1998). Early manifestations (pre-AIDS) of HIV-1 infection in Uganda. *AIDS*; **12**: 591–596.
Morgan D, Malamba SS, Orem J, Mayanja B, Okongo M, Whitworth JAG. (2000). Survival by AIDS defining condition in rural Uganda. *Sex Transm Infect*; **76**: 193–197.
Morgan D, Mahe C, Mayanja B, Okongo MJ, Lubega R, Whitworth JAG. (2002). HIV-1 infection in rural Africa: is there a difference in median time to AIDS and survival compared with that in industrialized countries? *AIDS*; **16**: 597–603.
Nathoo KJ, Chigonde S, Nhembe M, Ali MH, Mason PR. (1996). Community-acquired bacteremia in human immunodeficiency virus-infected children in Harare, Zimbabwe. *Pediatr Infect Dis J*; **15**: 1092–1097.
Ndour M, Sow PS, Coll-Seck AM *et al.* (2000). AIDS caused by HIV1 and HIV2 infection: are there clinical differences? Results of AIDS surveillance 1986–97 at Fann Hospital in Dakar, Senegal. *Trop Med Int Hlth*; **5**: 687–691.
Nduati R, John G, Mbori-Ngacha D *et al.* (2000). Effect of breastfeeding and formula feeding on transmission of HIV-1. *J Am Med Assoc*; **283**: 1167–1174.
Nunn AJ, Mulder DW, Kamali A, Ruberantwari A, Kengeya-Kayondo J-F, Whitworth J. (1997). Mortality associated with HIV-1 infection over five years in a rural Ugandan population: cohort study. *Br Med J*; **315**: 767–771.
Oshitani H, Kasolo FC, Mpabalwani M *et al.* (1994). Association of rotavirus and human immunodeficiency virus infection in children hospitalized with acute diarrhea, Lusaka, Zambia. *J Infect Dis*; **169**: 897–900.
Poulsen A-G, Aaby P, Larsen O *et al.* (1997). 9–year HIV-2–associated mortality in an urban community in Bissau, west Africa. *Lancet*; **349**: 911–914.
Prazuck T, Tall F, Nacro B *et al.* (1993). HIV infection and severe malnutrition: a clinical and epidemiological study in Burkina Faso. *AIDS*; **7**: 103–108.
Rana FS, Hawken MP, Mwachari C *et al.* (2000). Autopsy study of HIV-1–positive and HIV-1–negative adult medical patients in Nairobi, Kenya. *J Acquir Immune Defic Syndr*; **24**: 23–29.
Rutherford GW, Lifson AR, Hessol NA *et al.* (1990). Course of HIV-1 infection in a cohort of homosexual and bisexual men: an 11 year follow up study. *Br Med J*; **301**: 1183–1188.
Ryder RW, Nsuami M, Nsa W *et al.* (1994). Mortality in HIV-1-seropositive women, their spouses and their newly born

children during 36 months of follow-up in Kinshasa, Zaïre. *AIDS*; **8**: 667–672.

Sassan-Morokro M, De Cock KM, Ackah A *et al.* (1994). Tuberculosis and HIV infection in children in Abidjan, Côte d'Ivoire. *Trans Roy Soc Trop Med Hyg*; **88**: 178–181.

Schwander S, Rüsch-Gerdes S, Mateega A *et al.* (1995). A pilot study of antituberculosis combinations comparing rifabutin with rifampicin in the treatment of HIV-1 associated tuberculosis. *Tuber Lung Dis*; **76**: 210–218.

Semba RD, Kumwemba N, Hoover DR *et al.* (1999). Human immunodeficiency virus load in breast milk, mastitis, and mother to child transmission of human immunodeficiency virus type 1. *J Infect Dis*; **180**: 93–98.

Sonnenberg P, Murray J, Glynn JR, Shearer S, Kambashi B, Godfrey-Faussett P. (2001). HIV-1 and recurrence, relapse and reinfection of tuberculosis after cure: a cohort study in South African mineworkers. *Lancet*; **358**: 1687–1693.

Southern African HIV clinicians society. (2000). Guidelines for antiretroviral therapy in adults. *S Af J HIV Med*; **1**: 22–27.

Ssali FN, Kamya MR, Wabwire-Mangen F *et al.* (1998). A prospective study of community-acquired bloodstream infections among febrile adults admitted to Mulago Hospital in Kampala, Uganda. *J Acquir Immune Defic Syndr Hum Retrovirol*; **19**: 484–489.

Taelman H, Bogaerts J, Batungwanayo J *et al.* (1990). Community-acquired bacteremia, fungemia and parasitemia in febrile adults infected with HIV in central Africa. *V International Conference on AIDS in Africa.* Kinshasa, October 1990 [abstract F.O.D.1].

Thea D, St.Louis M, Atido U *et al.* (1993). A prospective study of diarrhoea and HIV-1 infection among 429 Zairian infants. *N Engl J Med*; **329**: 1696–1702.

UNAIDS. (2000). *Report on the global HIV/AIDS epidemic.* Geneva: UNAIDS; 6.

UNAIDS/WHO. (2001). Guidelines for using HIV testing technologies in surveillance: selection, evaluation and implementation, pp. 1–38. Geneva: World Health Organization.

US Department of Health and Human Services and the Henry J.Kaiser Family Foundation. Guidelines for the use of antiretroviral agents in HIV-infected adults and adolescents. Available at: www.hivatis.org/guidelines/adult/Aug13_01/pdf/AAAug135.pdf

USPHS/ISDA prevention of opportunistic infections working group. 2001 USPHS/IDSA guidelines for the prevention of opportunistic infections in persons infected with human immunodeficiency virus. Available at: hivatis.org/trtgdlns.html#opportunistic

Vugia DJ, Kiehlbauch JA, Yeboue K *et al.* (1993). Pathogens and predictors of fatal septicemia associated with human immunodeficiency virus infection in Ivory Coast, West Africa. *J Infect Dis*; **168**: 564–570.

Wawer MJ, Sewankambo NK, Serwadda D *et al.* (1999). Control of sexually transmitted diseases for AIDS prevention in Uganda: a randomised community trial. *Lancet*; **353**: 525–535.

Whitworth J, Morgan D, Quigley M *et al.* (2000). Effect of HIV-1 and increasing immunosuppression on malaria parasitaemia and clinical episodes in adults in rural Uganda: a cohort study. *Lancet*; **356**: 1051–1056.

Wiktor SZ, Sassan-Morokro M, Grant AD *et al.* (1999). Efficacy of trimethoprim-sulphamethoxazole prophylaxis to decrease morbidity and mortality in HIV-1–infected patients with tuberculosis in Abidjan, Côte d'Ivoire: a randomised controlled trial. *Lancet*; **353**: 1469–1475.

Wilkinson D, Gilks CF. (1998). Increasing frequency of tuberculosis among staff in a South African district hospital: impact of the HIV epidemic on the supply side of health care. *Trans Roy Soc Trop Med Hyg*; **92**: 500–502.

Wood R, O'Keefe EA, Maartens G. (1996). The changing pattern of transmission and clinical presentation of HIV infection in the Western Cape region of South Africa (1984–1995). *S Afr J Epidemiol Infect*; **11**: 96–98.

World Health Organization. (1986). Acquired immunodeficiency syndrome (AIDS): WHO/CDC case definition for AIDS. *Wkly Epidemiol Rec*; **61**: 69–73.

World Health Organization. (1990). Acquired immunodeficiency syndrome (AIDS): interim proposal for a WHO staging system for HIV infection and disease. *Wkly Epidemiol Rec*; **65**: 221–224.

World Health Organization. (1994). WHO case definitions for AIDS surveillance in adults and adolescents. *Wkly Epidemiol Rec*; **69**: 273–280.

World Health Organization. (1997). Integrated management of childhood illness: a WHO/UNICEF initiative. *Bull World Health Organ*; **75**(Suppl 1).

World Health Organization Global Tuberculosis Programme, UNAIDS. (1998). Policy statement on preventive therapy against tuberculosis in people living with HIV. Geneva: WHO. WHO/TB/98.255

World Health Organization. (2000). Safe and effective use of antiretroviral treatments in adults. Geneva: WHO. WHO/HSI/2000.04

Ziegler JL, Katongole-Mbidde E. (1996). Kaposi's sarcoma in childhood: an analysis of 100 cases from Uganda and relationship to HIV infection. *Int J Cancer*; **65**: 200–203.

14

Sexually transmitted infections

Sexually transmitted infections (STIs)[1] are caused by over 30 pathogens, including bacteria, viruses, protozoa, fungi and ecto-parasites (Table 14.1). The most important bacterial STI pathogens are *Neisseria gonorrhoeae, Chlamydia trachomatis, Haemophilus ducreyi* (which causes chancroid) and *Treponema pallidum*) (which causes syphilis). The most important viral infections are HIV, herpes simplex virus type-2, Hepatitis B virus and human papillomavirus (HPV). The most common protozoal agent is *Trichomonas vaginalis.* Infestations with *Sarcoptes scabiei* (scabies) or *Phthirus pubis* (pubic lice) can also be acquired through sexual contact.

Reproductive tract infections (RTIs) have been defined to include STIs, endogenous and iatrogenic infections. Endogenous infections are caused by an overgrowth of organisms that can be present in the genital tract of healthy women (bacterial vaginosis or vulvovaginal candidiasis). Iatrogenic infections are associated with improperly performed medical procedures, such as unsafe abortions, poor delivery practices, pelvic examinations and intro-uterine contraceptive device (IUCD) insertions.

The problem in Africa

Sexually transmitted infections (STIs) impose an enormous burden of morbidity and mortality in Africa, both directly through their impact on reproductive and child health, and indirectly through their role in facilitating the sexual transmission of HIV infection. The greatest impact is among women and infants (Table 14.2). The World Bank has estimated that STIs, excluding HIV, are the second commonest cause of healthy life years lost by women in the 15–44 age group in Africa, responsible for some 17 per cent of the total burden of disease (World Bank, 1993). STIs are also responsible for the two commonest cancers in Africa (cervical and hepatocellular carcinoma).

STIs are among the most common reasons for seeking medical care in many parts of Africa, yet systematic surveillance is almost non-existent. Most epidemiological data have been obtained from prevalence studies, and from sentinel surveillance sites in a few countries. Prevalence surveys suffer from the disparity of population groups surveyed, which have included university students, antenatal clinic attenders, STI clinic attenders and sex workers. Until the 1990s there was little data from rural communities, but large community-based studies conducted in Tanzania and Uganda in recent years have provided a wealth of data on STI incidence and prevalence (Grosskurth et al., 1996; Mayaud et al., 1997; Wawer et al., 1999). Some reasons for the high prevalence of STIs in Africa are shown in the Box below.

Factors underlying the high prevalence of STIs in Africa

- Demographic factors (a large young population which is sexually active)
- Urban migration with accompanying socio-cultural changes
- Migration and displacement (labour, wars, natural catastrophes)
- Increase in levels of prostitution through economic hardship
- Multiple and concurrent sexual partnerships
- Lack of access to effective and affordable STI services
- High prevalence of antimicrobial resistance in some pathogens.

[1] The term 'sexually transmitted infections' (STI) is used throughout this chapter to describe sexually transmitted infections and the diseases, complications and sequelae which result from them. For example, a sexually transmitted infection, *Neisseria gonorrhoeae*, results in a disease, gonorrhoea, manifested by cervicitis, which may lead to a complication, salpingitis. Permanently impaired fertility would be a sequela. This terminology also highlights that infections may exist and be transmissible (thus of public health importance) without causing major clinical manifestations or disease in the host.

Table 14.1. Main STI pathogens and the diseases they cause

Pathogen	Associated disease or syndrome
Bacteria	
Neisseria gonorrhoeae	GONORRHOEA • *Men*: urethritis, epididymitis, orchitis, urethral stricture, infertility, prostatitis (?) • *Women*: cervicitis, bartholinitis, endometritis, salpingitis, pelvic inflammatory disease (PID) and sequelae (infertility), chorio-amnionitis, premature rupture of membranes (PROM), preterm birth and low birthweight, perihepatitis • *Both sexes*: proctitis, pharyngitis, disseminated gonococcal infection (DGI) • *New born*: conjunctivitis, corneal scarring and blindness
Chlamydia trachomatis (strains D-K)	CHLAMYDIAL INFECTION • *Men*: urethritis, epididymitis, orchitis, urethral stricture, infertility • *Women*: cervicitis, bartholinitis, endometritis, salpingitis, PID, infertility, chorio-amnionitis, PROM, preterm birth and low birthweight, perihepatitis (Fitz–Hugh–Curtis syndrome) • *Both sexes*: proctitis, pharyngitis, Reiter's syndrome • *New born*: conjunctivitis, pneumonia
Chlamydia trachomatis (strains L1–L3)	LYMPHOGRANULOMA VENEREUM • ulcer, inguinal bubo, proctitis
Treponema pallidum	SYPHILIS • *Both sexes*: primary (ulcer), secondary (rash and condylomata lata), latent and tertiary (neurological, bone, cardiovascular and other tissue damage) stages of syphilis • *Women*: pregnancy wastage (abortion, stillbirth), premature delivery • *Newborn*: stillbirth, congenital syphilis
Haemophilus ducreyi	CHANCROID • ulcer, inguinal bubo
Calymmatobacterium (reclassified as genus *Klebsiella) granulomatis*	DONOVANOSIS (GRANULOMA INGUINALE) • ulcer, inguinal bubo
Mycoplasma genitalium	*Women*: bacterial vaginosis, PID? *Men*: non-gonococcal urethritis
Ureaplasma urealyticum	*Women*: bacterial vaginosis, PID? *Men:* non-gonococcal urethritis?
Viruses	
Herpes simplex virus type 1 (HSV-1) and type 2 (HSV-2) (also labelled Human Herpesvirus HHV-1 and HHV-2)	Genital and orolabial herpes, aseptic meningitis *Newborn*: neonatal herpes (often fatal)
Cytomegalovirus (HHV-5)	Mononucleosis, congenital CMV infection, CMV disease in immuno-suppressed
Kaposi-sarcoma associated herpes virus (KSHV or HHV-8)	Kaposi's sarcoma

Hepatitis A virus	Acute hepatitis
Hepatitis B virus	Acute and chronic hepatitis, liver cirrhosis, hepatocellular carcinoma
Human papillomavirus (HPV)	Condylomata acuminata (low-risk oncogenic strains HPV-6 and -11) Squamous intraepithelial lesions (SIL) and carcinoma of the cervix, vagina, vulva, anus, penis (high-risk oncogenic strains HPV-16, -18, -35 and related strains) *Neonates*: Laryngeal papilloma
Molluscum contagiosum virus	Genital *Molluscum contagiosum*
Human T-cell lymphotropic virus (HTLV) types I and II	Tropical spastic paraparesis, human T-cell leukaemia or lymphoma
Human immunodeficiency virus (HIV) types -1 and -2, and subtype 0	HIV disease, AIDS
Protozoa	
Trichomonas vaginalis	TRICHOMONIASIS *Women*: vaginitis, preterm birth and low birth weight (?) *Men*: non-gonococcal urethritis
Fungi	
Candida albicans	CANDIDIASIS *Women*: vulvo-vaginitis *Men*: balanitis
Parasites	
Phtirus pubis	Pubic lice infestation
Sarcoptes scabiei	Scabies

Sources: Goeman et al. (1991); Holmes et al., eds. (1999).

Table 14.2. Complications and sequelae of STIs

In adults	In children
• Pelvic inflammatory disease (PID) • Ectopic pregnancy • Spontaneous abortions • Post-partum infections (endometritis) • Infertility (male and female) • Neoplasia (cervical, vaginal, anal, penile, liver, Kaposi sarcoma, leukemia) • AIDS	• Stillbirth • Prematurity and low birth weight • Congenital syphilis • Conjunctivitis and blindness • Pneumonia • Otitis media • Neonatal systemic infections • Meningitis • Laryngeal papillomatosis

Epidemiology

Certain broad generalizations can be made about the epidemiology of STIs. Clearly, they are diseases of the sexually active, although mother-to-child transmission also occurs. None of the sexually transmitted agents described in this chapter has an epidemiologically significant non-human reservoir. They are more common among young adults, among single people of both sexes, and among those who travel. Although no sexually active individual is immune, certain groups can be identified whose behaviour places them at higher risk than others. Such groups include commercial sex workers and their clients, bar workers, the military, truck drivers and sailors, and have been called core groups.

The World Health Organization (WHO) estimates that approximately 340 million new cases of the four main curable STIs (gonorrhoea, chlamydial infection, syphilis, and trichomoniasis) occur every year, 85 per cent of them in developing countries (WHO, 2001a) (Table 14.3). There are substantial geographical variations. Sub-Saharan Africa has the highest prevalence and incidence, with an estimated annual incidence of curable STIs of about 250 per 1000 people of reproductive age (15–49 years).

Table 14.3. Global incidence estimates of curable STIs (excluding chancroid), among adults 15–49 years, 1999

Infection/disease	New cases annually
Gonorrhoea	62 million
Chlamydial infection	92 million
Syphilis	12 million
Trichomoniasis	174 million
Total	**340 million**

Source: WHO (2001b).

STIs in women

STI prevalence among African women has been studied in 'high-risk' and 'low risk' populations. 'High-risk' populations are groups of women frequently exposed to STI pathogens by the nature of their occupation (e.g. sex workers), their environment (e.g. women living in mining communities), or their sexual behaviour (STI clinic attenders). 'Low-risk' populations, typically antenatal clinic or family planning clinic attenders, are supposed to represent the normal sexually active female population. These women generally do not come primarily into contact with health services for the single purpose of STI treatment.

Summarizing 11 studies conducted recently in Africa, median prevalences of gonorrhoea and chlamydial infection in 'low-risk' populations were 2.3 per cent (range 1.6–9 per cent) and 7 per cent (range 4–19 per cent), respectively (Mayaud, 2001). The highest rates were recorded in countries from the Southern and Eastern parts of the continent. Gabon, which lies in the so-called 'infertility belt' of Africa, combined low rates of gonorrhoea (1.9 per cent) with high rates of chlamydial infection (9.9 per cent). In the same populations, the median prevalence of active syphilis was 4.4 per cent, though prevalences ranged from 1 per cent to 29 per cent (Table 14.4).

As expected, the prevalence of most STIs (gonorrhoea, syphilis, *T. vaginalis)* was highest among the high-risk groups. However, the prevalence of *C. trachomatis* was not markedly different between STD clinic attenders and 'low-risk' populations. More than 50 per cent of gonococcal and chlamydial infections were asymptomatic, which has important implications for the control of these infections. Median prevalences obtained in recent studies are comparable to earlier estimates in high-risk and low-risk African populations (Wasserheit & Holmes, 1992; Gerbase et al., 1998), confirming the high prevalence of STIs in women in Africa.

STIs in men

More than 50 per cent of men attending African clinics complaining of urethral discharge have gonorrhoea; 5–15 per cent have chlamydial infections (Mabey, 1994), and dual infections are common. Non-specific urethritis (NSU), after exclusion of gonococcal and chlamydial infection, accounts for about a quarter to a third of cases. In settings where it has been investigated, *T. vaginalis* is found in 2–20 per cent of cases. There is always a

Table 14.4. Prevalence of STIs among women in sub-Saharan Africa in the 1980s and in the 1990s

	High-risk populations				Low-risk populations				Low risk WHO estimates 1995
	1980s		1990s		1980s		1990s		
STI	Median (%)	Range (%)	Median (%)	Range (%)	Median (%)	Range (%)	Median (%)	Range (%)	Mean (%)
Chlamydia	14	2–25	8	2–13	8	1–29	7	4–18	7.1
Gonorrhoea	24	7–66	16	6–31	6	0.3–40	2.3	1.6–9	2.8
Trichomoniasis	17	4–20	28	11–46	12	3–50	18	10–27	14.1
Syphilis	15	4–32	8	2–29	8	0.01–33	4.4	1–29	3.9
Candidiasis	NS	NS	33	28–38	NS	NS	27	7.5–39	NS
Bacterial vaginosis	NS	NS	NS	NS	NS	NS	22	15–35	NS

Note: NS = not studied.
Sources: Reproduced from: Mayaud (2001) with permission. 1980s: Wasserheit & Holmes (1992). 1990s: Mayaud (2001). WHO, 1995: Gerbase et al., (1998).

relatively high proportion of men in whom no diagnosis of STI can be made, partly because of the frequent use of prior self-treatment.

Community-based studies have reported similar rates of *N. gonorrhoeae* and/or *C. trachomatis* among men and women (around 2–4 per cent for each pathogen). The majority (>70 per cent) of these infections are asymptomatic (Grosskurth et al., 1996; Wawer et al., 1999). *T. vaginalis* has recently been shown to be one of the most prevalent urethral pathogens in men in large population-based studies (Jackson et al., 1997; Watson-Jones et al., 2000).

STI–HIV interactions

Earlier reports of an association between the 'classical' STIs and HIV infection have now been supplemented by virological studies showing that STIs increase levels of HIV in genital fluids, and that treatment of those STIs decreases HIV genital excretion (Fleming & Wasserheit, 1999). Moreover, a randomized community intervention trial has demonstrated that provision of STI services in general primary health care clinics in Tanzania led to a 40 per cent decrease in the number of new HIV infections (Grosskurth et al., 1995).

HIV and STIs may interact with each other in the following ways (Fig. 14.1):

- HIV, by causing immunosuppression, can modify the natural history (duration), clinical presentation (severity), and response to treatment of certain STIs, notably other viral infections such as genital herpes simplex virus infection or human papillomavirus;

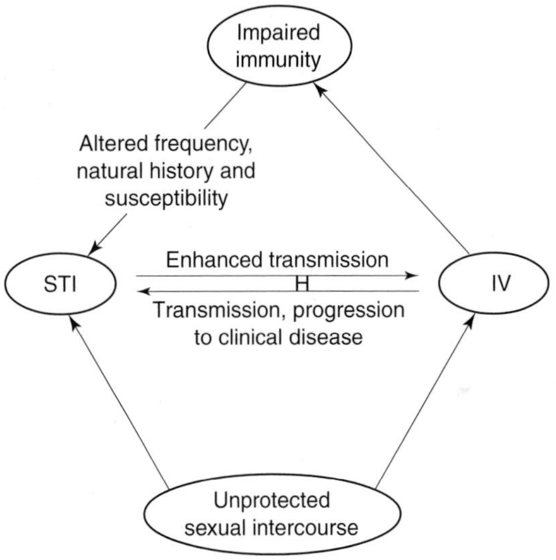

Fig. 14.1. Relationships between HIV and other STIs (Mayaud & McCormick, 2001).

- STIs, by causing ulceration or inflammation of the genital tract, may enhance the transmission of HIV by increasing the infectiousness of HIV-positive individuals and/or the susceptibility of HIV-negative persons. Many STI increase HIV viral load in the genital tract and/or activate target cells for HIV.

The high prevalence of STI has contributed to the disproportionately high HIV incidence and prevalence in Africa. Conversely, HIV may have contributed to some extent to STI increases, especially of viral agents such as herpes simplex virus (genital herpes) or human papilloma viruses (condylomata acuminata or genital warts).

Control of STI

STI control programmes have three objectives:

- to interrupt the transmission of STIs
- to prevent the development of diseases, complications and sequelae; and
- to reduce the transmission of HIV infection.

Health education and condom promotion can modify behaviour, and hence reduce the incidence of STIs. Improved access to care and improved case management can prevent complications, and also reduce transmission, by shortening the duration of infection.

Primary prevention of STI

Behavioural interventions

Primary prevention aims to modify sexual behaviour towards 'safer sex' through information, education and communication (IEC), or peer-assisted education programmes. It is particularly important in adolescents, as they have high rates of STI and are more likely to change their behaviour.

Barrier methods

When used properly and consistently, condoms are one of the most effective methods of protection against STI. They can be made readily available on a large scale through free distribution or social marketing. In Thailand, the 100 per cent Condom Programme, which has been promoting 100 per cent use of condoms in commercial sex establishments, overcame many cultural and logistical barriers. The programme has been linked to a decrease in reported STI rates and HIV prevalence among military recruits.

STIs disproportionately affect women, and in particular adolescent women are at increased risk, due to ignorance of appropriate preventative measures, and unplanned or forced sexual intercourse where it may be difficult or impractical to negotiate safer sex. Female controlled methods of protection are badly needed. These could include:

- female condoms
- vaginal microbicide compounds.

Unfortunately, both types of methods have proven rather disappointing or of limited use. The female condom has important advantages such as efficacy, safety and in some areas increasing acceptance by women. However disadvantages include high cost, lack of visual and auditory appeal, difficulty of use, pre-planning of intercourse and mixed reactions among male partners. Vaginal microbicides have been under development since the early 1990s. A detergent based chemical (nonoxynol 9, or N-9) with virucidal and bacterial activity raised initial hopes, but eventually proved disappointing for HIV prevention (Mauck et al., 2001). There is also concern that repeated use of these compounds can disrupt the vaginal epithelium and actually make users more susceptible to infection. A number of new compounds are currently under development.

Vaccines

Hepatitis B is the only STI for which an effective vaccine is currently available. Unfortunately lasting immunity to most STIs is not conferred by natural infection, suggesting that it may prove difficult to develop effective vaccines, although intensive research continues for viral STIs in particular.

STI case management

One of the cornerstones of STI control is accessible, affordable and effective STI case management for patients presenting with symptomatic infections.

History-taking, examination and counselling in the STI clinic

It is not possible to provide a good clinical service for STIs without gaining the confidence of the patient. This requires privacy and the avoidance of a moralistic attitude.

It is usually possible to take a history and examine a patient with an STI in 10 minutes. When taking a history, collect the following information in addition to name, occupation, address and date of birth.

1. The nature and duration of the symptoms.
2. The nature of any treatment already taken for this condition.
3. A sexual history, which should include marital status and the nature and frequency of recent sexual contacts with regular or casual partners. This information is essential in order to attempt contact tracing and/or partner notification.
4. Past medical history.
5. In female patients, take a menstrual and obstetric history.

Always counsel patients about ways to reduce the risk of STIs and their complications:

Table 14.5. Role of the laboratory in STI case management

	Peripheral/PHC level	Intermediate/district level	National/reference level
Clinical activities			
Diagnosis	• (Optional – Simple tests for vaginal infections: pH, wet mount microscopy)	• Microscopic diagnosis of vaginal infections • Gram stain for diagnosis of gonorrhoea in men • Optional: *N. gonorrhoeae* culture	• Culture: *N gonorrhoeae* • Chlamydia EIA • Optional – PCR or LCR for Chlamydia
Case finding	• RPR/VDRL	• RPR/VDRL • Confirmatory tests for syphilis (TPHA)	• RPR/VDRL • Confirmatory tests for syphilis (TPHA)
Public health activities			
Contribution to STD guidelines	• Clinical efficacy of algorithms (in selected sentinel sites)	• Participating in aetiological/algorithm validation studies	• Conducting/coordinating aetiological studies • Evaluation of algorithms
Epidemiological and microbiological monitoring	• Syphilis rates in ANC	• District/regional level syphilis statistics • Quality control of peripheral syphilis testing • Antimicrobial susceptibility of *N gonorrhoeae* (disk diffusion)	• National level syphilis statistics • Quality control of syphilis testing • Monitoring antimicrobial susceptibility of *N gonorrhoeae* and *H ducreyi* (MIC or E-test) • Guiding choice of drugs to be included in essential drug list • Training, supervision, quality control schemes

Notes:
RPR: rapid plasma reagin, VDRL: venereal disease reference laboratory, TPHA: *Trepanoma pallidum* haemagglutination assay, EIA: enzyme immuno-assay, PCR: polymerase chain reaction, LCR: ligase chain reaction.

- Use condoms, including in marital relationships during the course of treatment
- Complete the full course of treatment
- Refer sexual contacts for treatment.

The examination should be carried out in private with good light. After examining the mouth and palms, ask the patient to undress so that you are able to examine him/her from the umbilicus to the knees. Examine the skin of the abdomen, groins and perineum in particular for evidence of scabies and pediculosis, and palpate the inguinal glands.

In males inspect the penis, after retraction of the foreskin in uncircumcized patients. If a urethral discharge is not apparent, look for evidence of urethritis by milking the urethra forward and examining the meatus for discharge. Palpate the scrotum for evidence of epididymitis.

Examine female patients lying down. Palpate the lower abdomen for evidence of PID (masses and/or tenderness) and, after inspection of the vulva, pass a vaginal speculum. Examine the cervix and slowly withdraw the speculum while examining the walls of the vagina. Perform a bimanual examination to identify pelvic masses and/or tenderness. The presence of pain on moving the cervix (cervical motion tenderness) suggests the presence of PID. In both sexes, inspect the perianal skin and, if receptive anal intercourse is suspected, examine the rectum with a proctoscope.

The laboratory investigations requested will depend on the facilities available. See Table 14.5 for the role of the laboratory in the control of STIs at different levels of health care. In general, lab tests should be selected on the principle that a patient with one STI is also at increased risk of other STIs; that is, they should not be limited to tests designed to identify the cause of the present symptoms. All patients with an STI should be screened for syphilis. Whether they should also be screened for HIV depends on the availability of counselling and treatment for those found to be positive.

Table 14.6. Important Syndromes associated with STIs

Urethral discharge in men (suspected urethritis), caused by
- *Neisseria gonorrhoeae*
- *Chlamydia trachomatis*
- *Trichomonas vaginalis* and/or
- Other organisms, eg *Mycoplasma genitalium*

Testicular pain and swelling (suspected epididymo-orchitis), caused by
- *Neisseria gonorrhoeae*
- *Chlamydia trachomatis*
- Other organisms

Abnormal vaginal discharge, caused by
- organisms causing vaginal infection, such as
  - *Trichomonas vaginalis,*
  - *Candida albicans* or
  - bacterial vaginosis
- organisms causing cervical infection, such as
  - *Neisseria gonorrhoeae*
  - *Chlamydia trachomatis*

Lower abdominal pain in women (suspicion of pelvic inflammatory disease – PID) caused by
- *Neisseria gonorrhoeae*
- *Chlamydia trachomatis*
- anaerobic bacteria

Genital ulcers – caused by
- *Haemophilus ducreyi* (chancroid)
- *Treponema pallidum* (syphilis)
- Herpes simplex virus (HSV) type-2
- *Klebsiella* (formerly *Calymmato bacterium*) *granulomatis* (Donovanosis or granuloma inguinale)
- *Chlamydia trachomatis* (L1–L3 strains) (lymphogranuloma venereum (LGV))

Inguinal bubo caused by
- *Haemophilus ducreyi* (chancroid)
- *Chlamydia trachomatis* (L1–L3 strains) (LGV)

Neonatal conjunctivitis (ophthalmia neonatorum), caused by
- *N. gonorrhoeae*
- *C. trachomatis*

STI syndromes and the syndromic approach to STI case management

STI (and RTI) manifest themselves as clinical entities called 'syndromes' (associations of symptoms and physical signs), which are readily recognizable by patients and clinicians. Each syndrome can be caused by a variety of STI pathogens, and mixed infections are common. The main syndromes and their aetiological agents are summarized in Table 14.6.

Where laboratory diagnosis is not feasible, the World Health Organization (WHO) has recommended a syndromic approach to patient management. In syndromic management patients with a syndrome, for example urethral discharge, are treated for all the likely and important causes of that syndrome (in this case gonorrhoea and chlamydial infection) (WHO 2001b). Figures 14.2–14.7 show flowcharts recommended by WHO for the management of common STI syndromes.

Even when laboratory diagnosis is available, syndromic management has the advantage that treatment can be given at the patient's first visit, rather than relying on the patient to return for his/her results. Effective syndromic treatment depends on knowledge of local disease patterns and antimicrobial susceptibilities; a laboratory is required to monitor these, preferably in each country or province (Mayaud & Mabey, 2000). Syndromic patient management of men with urethral discharge, and of men and women with genital ulcers, works well. Syndromic management of women presenting with the syndrome of vaginal discharge, however, is not as satisfactory as many women with this syndrome do not have an STI as the primary causes of the discharge (Dallabetta et al., 1998). The advantages and disadvantages of syndromic management are shown in Table 14.7.

Treatment of sexual partners

Partner notification, or contact tracing, is the process of contacting sexual partners of index STI cases in order to offer them STI screening and/or treatment. This strategy aims to avoid complications and sequelae in partners who may have asymptomatic infections, to avoid onward transmission of the infection, and to prevent reinfection of the index case. It is often done by providing a partner notification card to the index STI patient. Treatment is given irrespective of symptoms and should be similar to that received by the index patient.

Screening/case-finding for STIs

Since many STIs are asymptomatic, case finding may be a useful complementary strategy for individuals coming into contact with health care services for reasons other than STI. For example, STI screening can be offered to women attending family planning or antenatal clinics, to young people attending adolescent health clinics, or to men in occupational health clinics.

Table 14.7. Advantages and disadvantages of syndromic management of STIs

Advantages	Disadvantages
• Problem-orientated (responds to patient's symptoms) • Highly sensitive and does not miss mixed infections • Treatment given at first visit • Provides opportunity and time for education and counselling • Avoids expensive laboratory tests • Avoids unnecessary return visit for laboratory results • Curtails referral to specialist centres • Can be implemented at PHC level	• Overdiagnosis and overtreatment with the following consequences: – Increased drug costs – Possible side effects of multiple drugs – Changes in vaginal flora – Potential for increased drug resistance – Domestic violence • Requires (re)training of staff • Possible resistance to its introduction from medical establishment

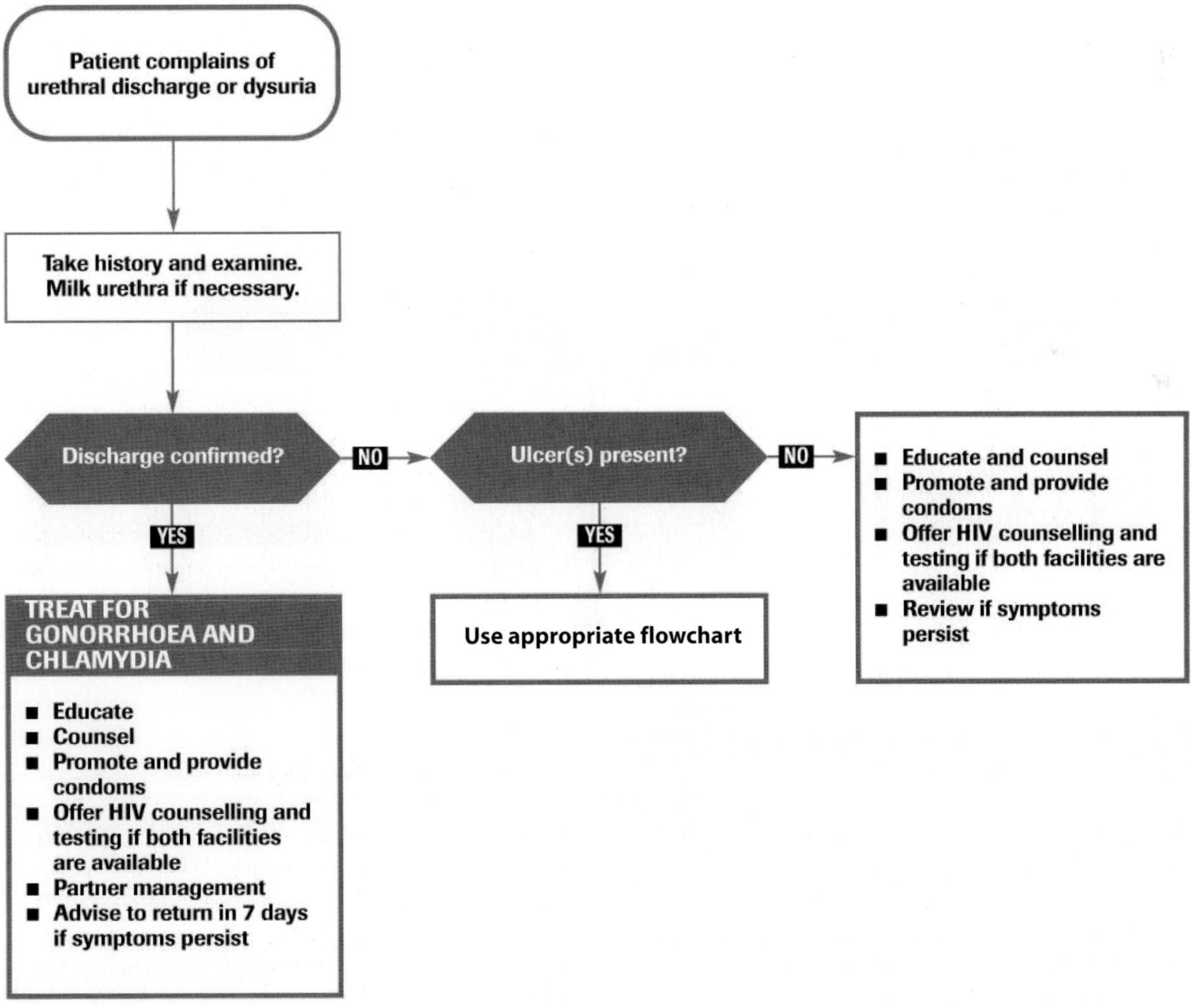

Fig. 14.2. Flowchart for urethral discharge syndrome (WHO, 2001).

Basic examination

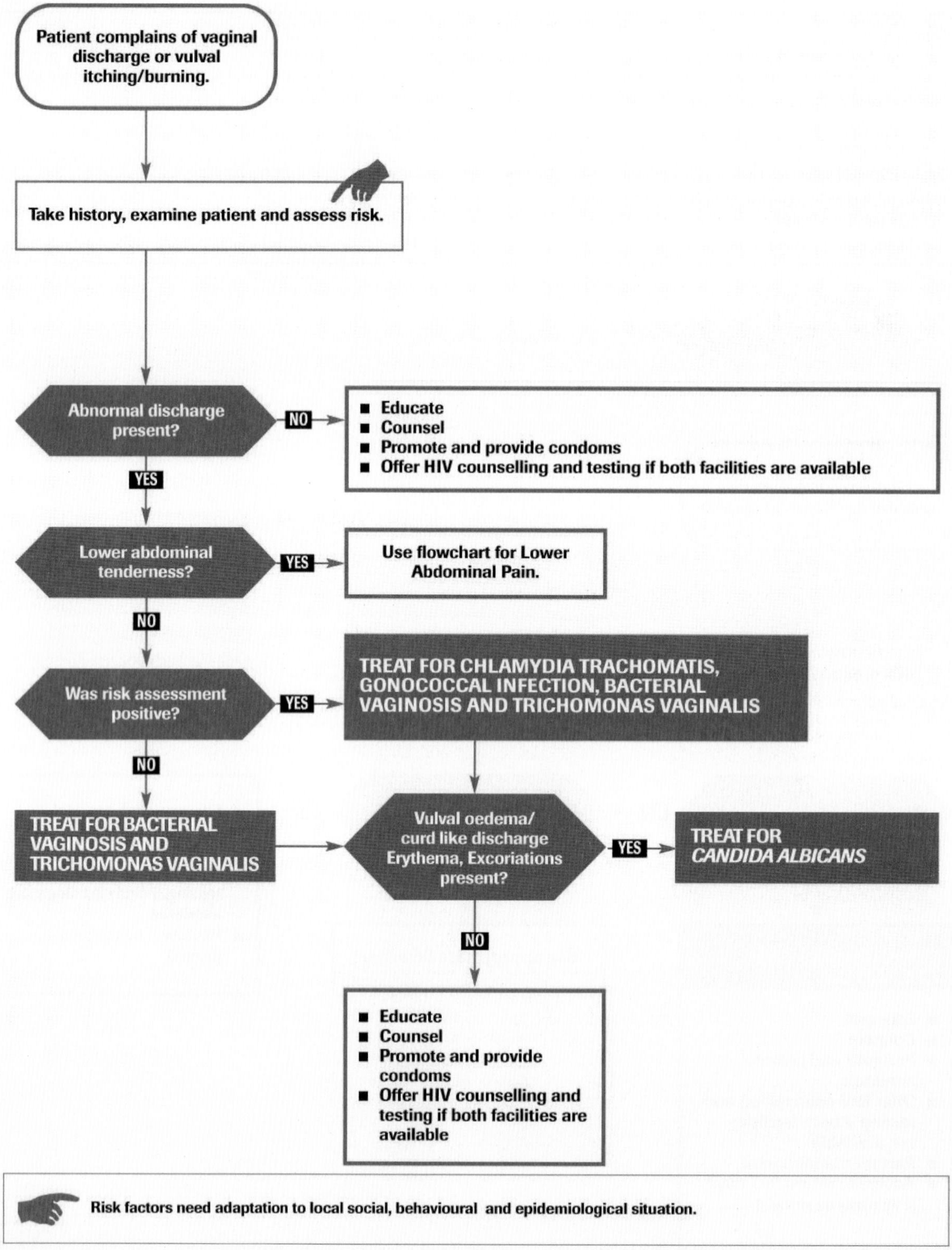

Fig. 14.3.1. Flowchart for vaginal discharge syndrome in the absence of speculum and microscope (WHO, 2001).

If speculum is available

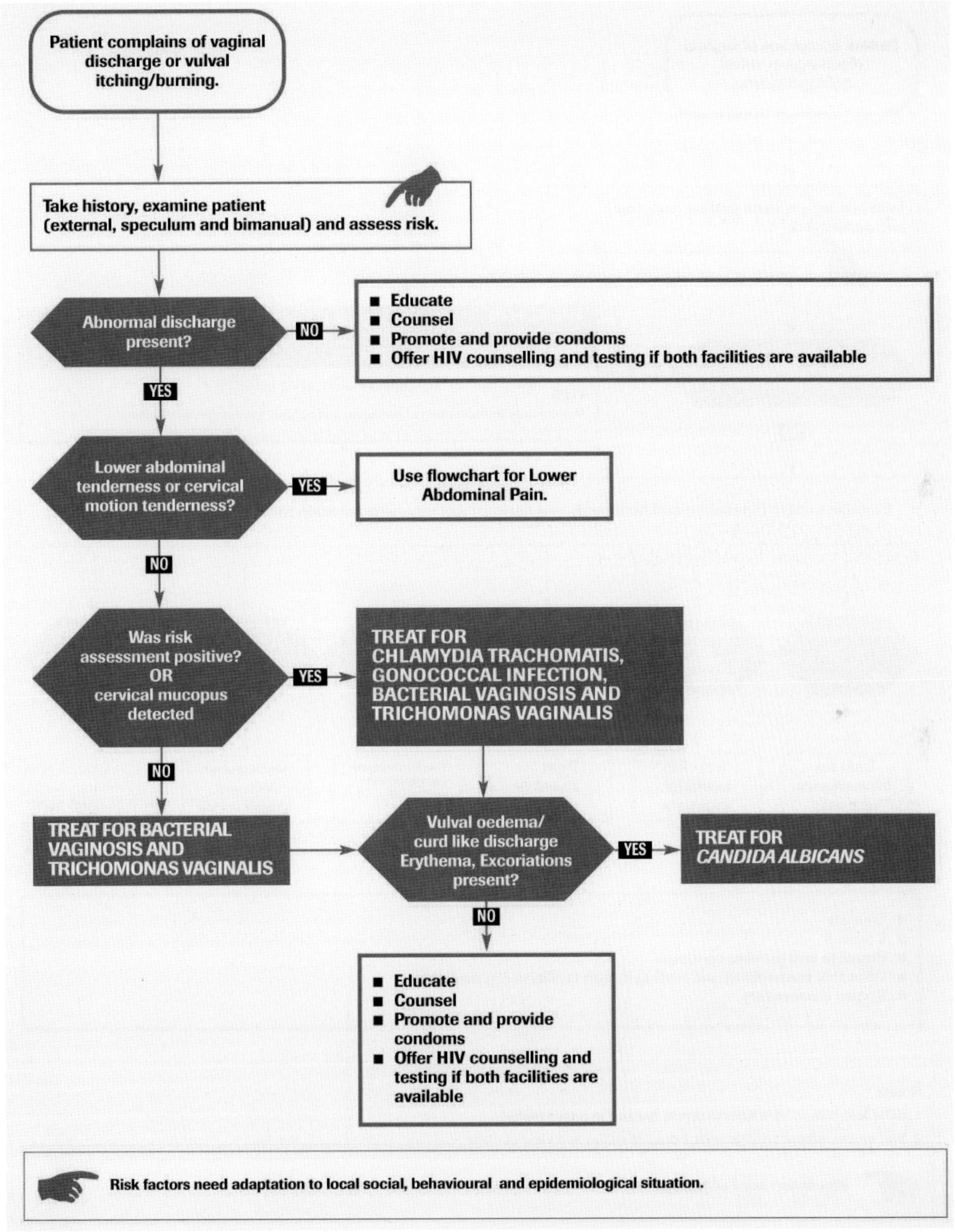

Fig. 14.3.2. With speculum.

If speculum and microscope are available

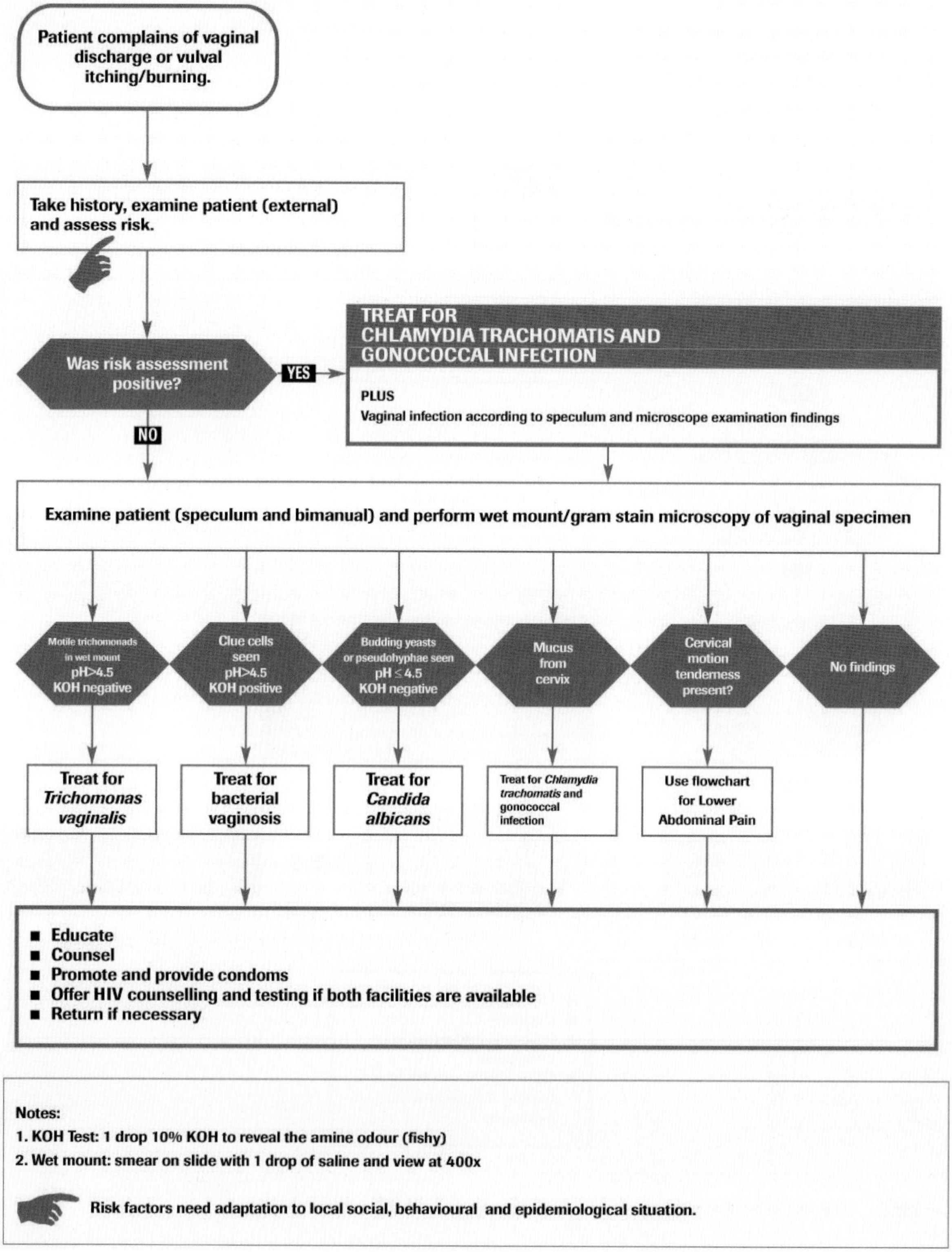

Fig. 14.3.3. With speculum and microscope.

Serological testing of pregnant women for syphilis is one of the most cost-effective health interventions and can help reduce congenital syphilis (Hira et al., 1990). However, it is often poorly implemented (Temmerman et al., 1993). There is an urgent need for simple and cheap diagnostic tests to identify asymptomatic men and women with gonococcal or chlamydial infections.

Improving access to services

A substantial proportion of people with symptomatic STI treat themselves or seek treatment in the informal or private sector; from traditional healers, unqualified practitioners, street drug vendors, pharmacists or private practitioners. Many patients only attend formal public health services after alternative treatments have failed (see Box below).

Reasons for seeking care in private sector
- More confidential
- Less judgemental
- More convenient
- Less stigma.

Although many patients are prepared to pay for treatment, high cost may deter patients from seeking care in the public sector. The introduction of user-fees led to a sharp drop in attendance at a large STI clinic in Nairobi. Lifting of the fees a few months later resulted in increased attendances (Moses et al., 1993).

Public services should aim to offer confidential non-judgemental STI services, and seek ways to harness the collaboration of private providers.

Community and targeted treatment approaches

Special services should be provided for groups at higher risk of, or more vulnerable to, STIs. Outreach programmes for such groups have been introduced in several African countries (Vuylsteke et al., 2001), often led by individuals with easier access to those communities such as fellow workers/members ('peers'), or influential leaders ('gate keepers' such as pimps, 'madams' union leaders). Broad health care services with a particular emphasis on reproductive health, STI care and HIV/AIDS prevention and care can be provided through static or mobile clinics. STI care should be easily available at convenient times (see Box below).

Reasons why STI control programmes often fail
- Low priority for policy makers and planners in allocating resources, because STI are perceived to result from discreditable behaviour
- Failure to recognize the magnitude of the problem in the population
- Failure to associate the diseases with serious complications and sequelae
- Control efforts concentrated on symptomatic patients (usually men) and failing to identify asymptomatic individuals (commonly women) until complications develop
- Service delivery through specialized STI health care facilities which provide inadequate coverage and tend to confer stigma
- Treatment strategies focused on unrealistic requirements for definitive diagnosis rather than on practical decision making
- Ineffective low cost antibiotics continuing to be used for reasons of economy
- Little emphasis on educational and other efforts to prevent infection occurring in the first place, especially among adolescents in and out of school
- Absence of authoritative guidance on a rational, practical and well-defined package of activities for prevention and care programmes.

Pathogens causing genital discharge

Gonorrhoea

The organism

Neisseria gonorrhoeae (described by Albert Neisser in 1879), also known as the gonococcus, is a small gram-negative, non-motile, aerobic, or facultatively anaerobic coccus. Usually, these organisms are found arranged in pairs with their adjacent surfaces flattened, giving a kidney-shaped appearance, hence the term diplococci. The organisms are delicate and fastidious with specific nutritional and environmental requirements. They are typically intracellular, especially adept at colonizing the epithelial surfaces of the male and female uro-genital tract, conjunctiva, pharynx and rectum. Outside the body they are easily killed by drying and by disinfectants such as soap.

Epidemiology

Due to the poor viability of *N. gonorrhoeae* away from the mucosal surfaces of the host, the infection is typically acquired by sexual intercourse with an infected sexual partner. The risk of contracting infection after a single sexual exposure to gonorrhoea is about 20 per cent for males, and probably higher for females. Even in young

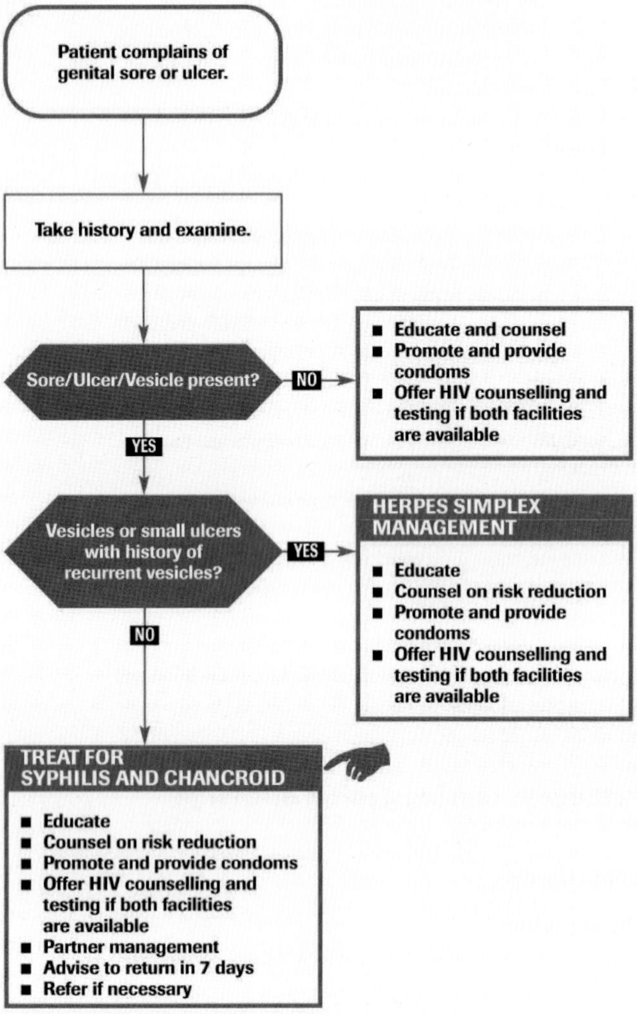

Fig. 14.4. Flowchart for genital ulcer syndrome (WHO, 2001).

children and prepubertal girls sexual transmission is the most frequent cause of infection. However, fomites such as shared towels, may cause transmission of infection to the girl child. Rectal infection is possible in women due to the anatomical proximity of the anus to the vaginal introitus. In men rectal infection is due to anal intercourse.

Pathogenesis

The gonococcus has an affinity for columnar and transitional epithelium found at most of the body's orifices, such as the urethra, rectum, conjunctiva and endocervix.

The surface components of the gonococcus are largely responsible for the interaction of the organisms with the host cells. Surface components include pili (protein spikes that attach the bacteria to the mucosa) assembled from pilin protein, opa outer membrane proteins and lipo-oligosaccharide (LOS).

Pili confer virulence by enabling adherence sufficient to withstand hydrodynamic forces within the urethra, and by inhibiting phagocytosis. The pilus antigens and the LOS are capable of antigenic variation sufficient to permit repeated reinfection of the same host within a short period. For this reason there is no development of any significant protective immunity during infection with the organism, although IgA, IgM and IgE antibodies to *N. gonorrhoeae* are found at infected mucosal surfaces, which can inhibit adherence, and facilitate phagocytosis by opsonization. Gonococci evade the immune response by producing an IgA protease, an enzyme which inactivates IgA, and also by intracellular growth. A neutrophil response, leading to a purulent discharge at the site of infection, is usually seen.

Clinical features

In men

Most men develop symptoms within 2 to 5 days of infection; the incubation ranges from 1 to 10 days. Common symptoms and signs are:

- urethral discharge (often profuse and purulent, but may be scanty or mucoid)
- dysuria
- frequency of micturition.

Less common symptoms and signs include:

- meatal itching
- meatal reddening
- oedema
- acute proctitis (mucopurulent anal discharge, diarrhoea, rectal bleeding or anal pruritus). However, the majority of patients with ano-rectal gonorrhoea have no symptoms.

Complications of gonorrhoea in men

Early:

- inflammation of the parafrenal glands
- inflammation of the para-urethral glands, on either side of the urethral meatus
- inflammation of the bulbo-urethral glands
- epididymitis (see box)
- disseminated gonococcal infection.

Late:

- urethral stricture.

Disseminated gonococcal infection presents as an acute arthritis, tenosynovitis or dermatitis. Its incidence in Africa is not known. Although generally benign, the rare complications of endocarditis, myocarditis and pericarditis are serious (see Box).

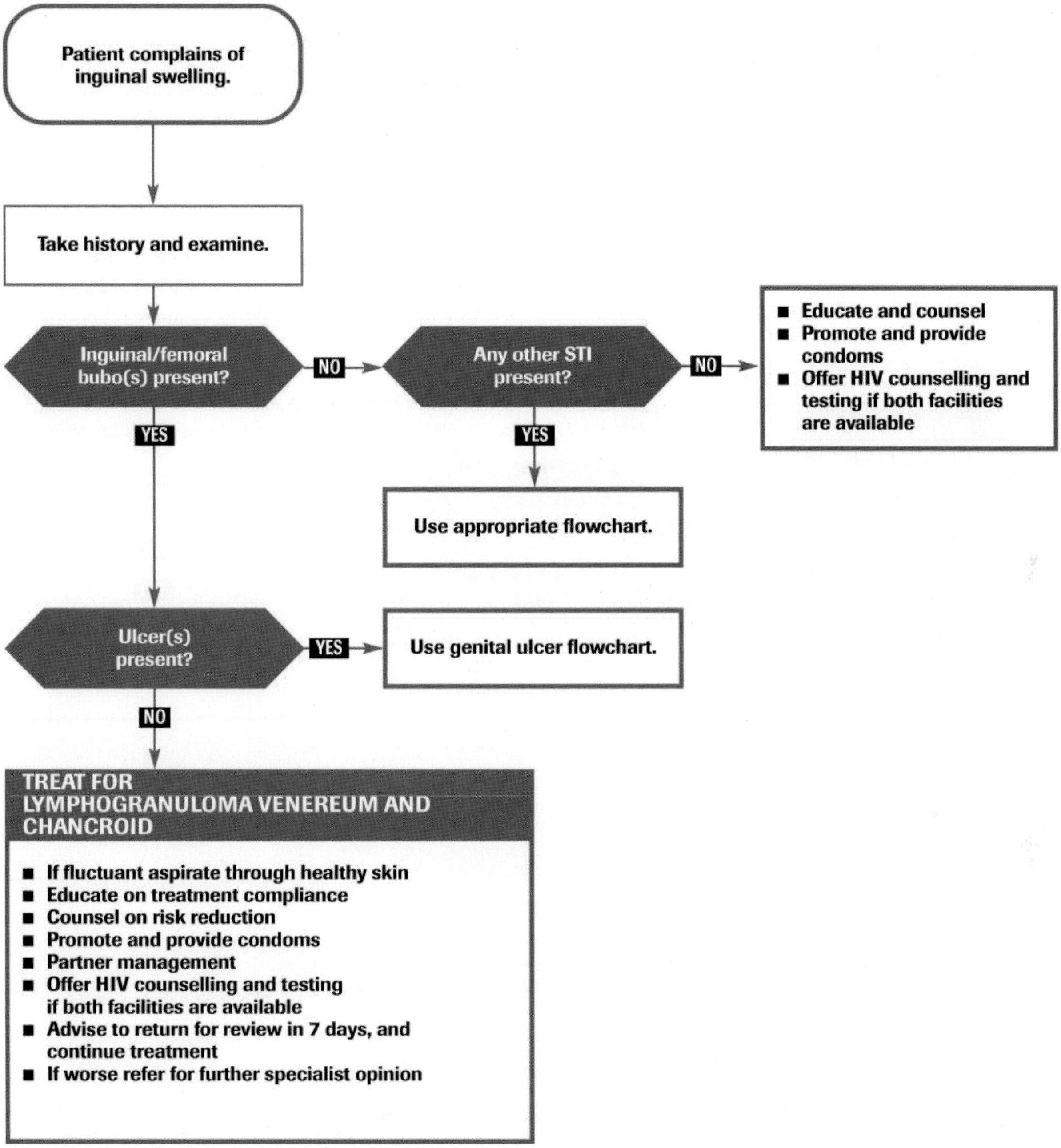

Fig. 14.5. Flowchart for bubo syndrome (WHO, 2001).

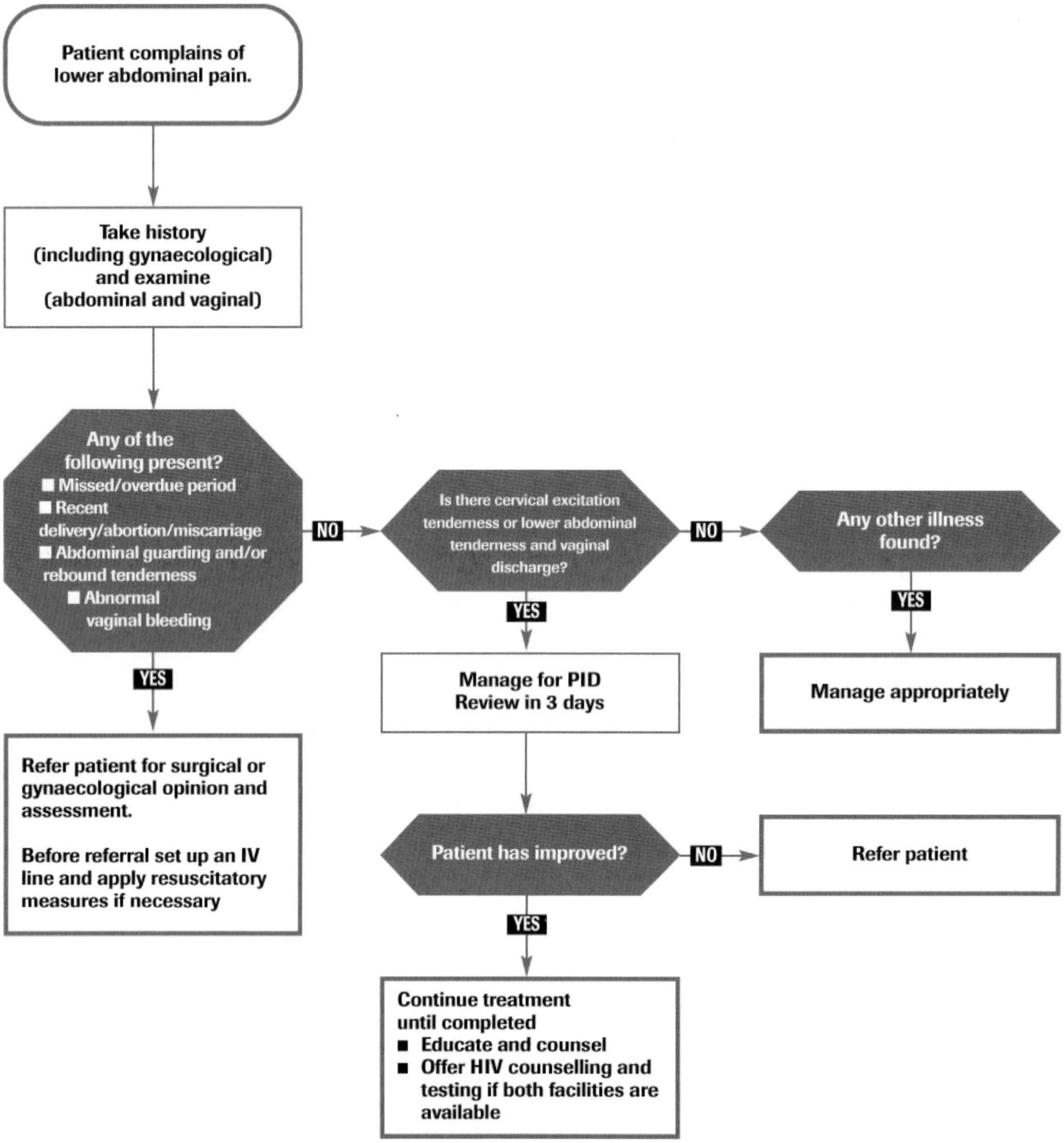

Fig. 14.6. Flowchart for low abdominal pain (PID) syndrome (WHO, 2001).

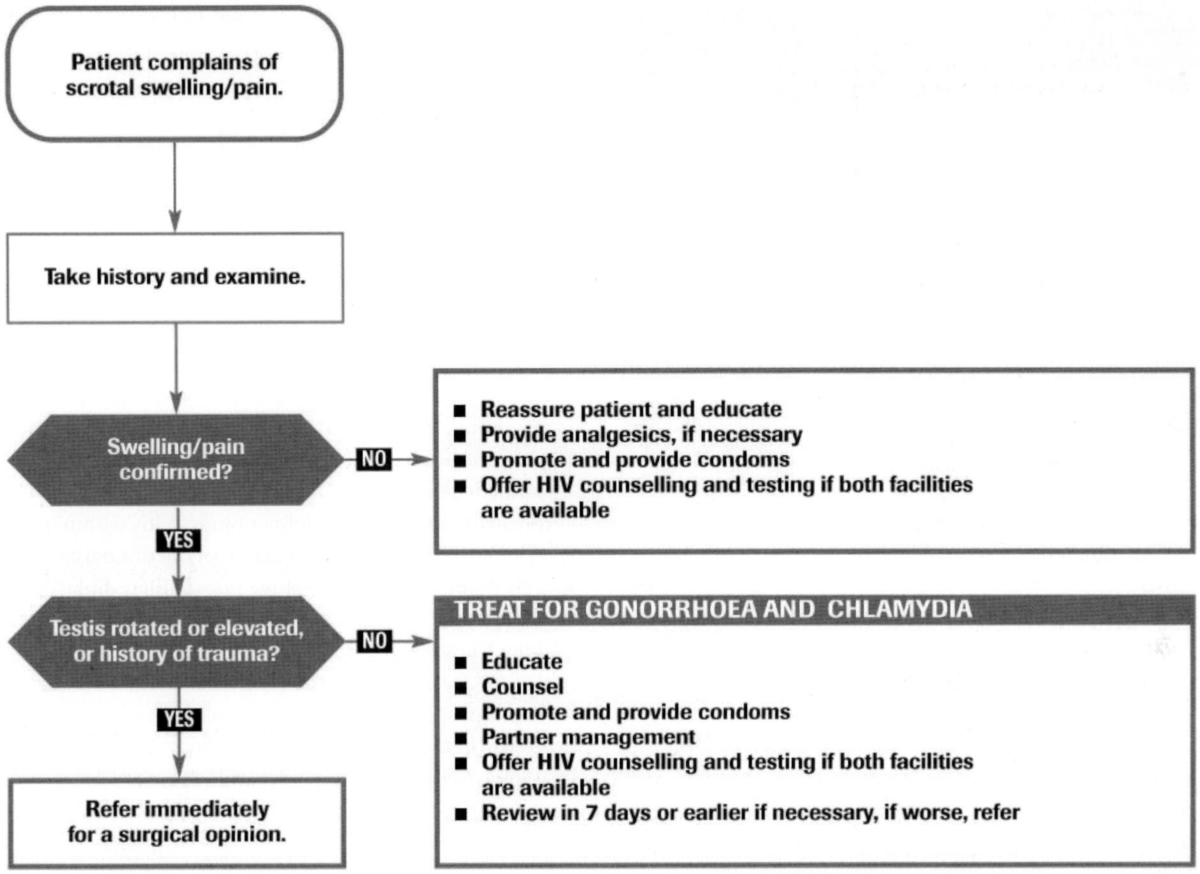

Fig. 14.7. Flowchart for painful swollen scrotum syndrome (WHO, 2001).

Epididymitis

The epididymis, situated on the posterior border of the testis, can become infected with STI, causing an acute epididymitis. In men under the age of 35 years *N. gonorrhoeae* and *C. trachomatis* are the common causes; in older men, coliforms are more commonly implicated, as a complication of urinary tract infection.

The patient complains of a painful swelling in the scrotum.

Examination reveals an enlarged and tender epididymis, usually unilateral:

The differential diagnosis includes:

- testicular torsion, which requires urgent surgical referral
- hydrocoele (usually painless and chronic)
- tuberculous epididymitis (usually bilateral, non tender and firm)
- mumps orchitis. Ask for a recent history of mumps
- testicular carcinoma (hard irregular mass involving testis).

See Fig. 14.7 for syndromic management of painful swollen scrotum.

Urethral stricture has been common in many parts of Africa (Osegbe & Amaku, 1981; Bewes, 1973). In Zaria, Nigeria, infection caused stricture in about 66 per cent of 556 urethral strictures treated, and gonococcal infection was reported to be the commonest cause (Ahmed & Kalayi, 1998).

In women

Most women (up to 80 per cent) with gonorrhoea have no symptoms. Early symptoms of uncomplicated gonococcal infection include:

- increased vaginal discharge
- dysuria.

In pre-pubescent girls gonococcal infection may present as a vulvovaginitis; but after puberty the acid environment of the vagina does not allow replication of *N. gonorrhoeae*, which infects primarily the endocervix.

Complications in women

Early:

- pelvic inflammatory disease (PID)
- perihepatitis
- Bartholin's abscess

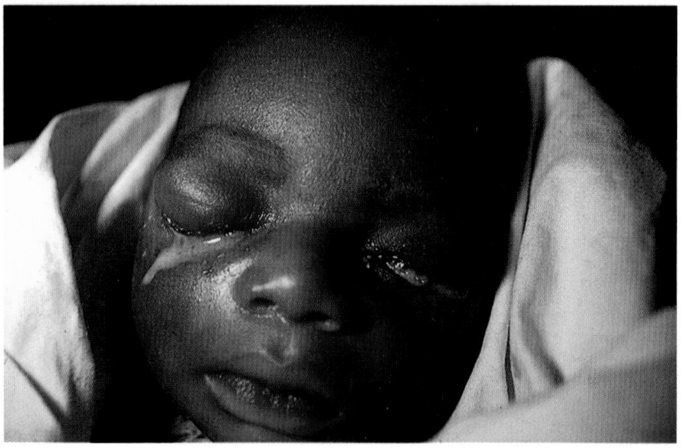

Fig. 14.8. Ophthalmia neonatorum.

- adverse pregnancy outcome
- disseminated gonococcal infection.

Late:
- ectopic pregnancy
- tubal infertility.

Pelvic inflammatory disease (PID) is the most common, and most important complication of gonorrhoea in women. It is caused by spread of the infection to the upper genital tract, which is facilitated by manipulation of the cervix, e.g. during childbirth, termination of pregnancy or insertion of an intrauterine contraceptive device (IUCD). PID may affect the endometrium or fallopian tubes, and may lead to peritonitis. Patients present with a variety of symptoms, including fever, nausea and vomiting, lower abdominal pain, vaginal discharge, dysmenorrhoea, irregular menstrual bleeding and pain on intercourse. A few patients may be asymptomatic. The cardinal findings on examination are lower abdominal and cervical motion tenderness.

See Fig. 14.6 for a flowchart for the management of lower abdominal pain in women.

A perihepatitis (Fitz–Hugh–Curtis syndrome) may complicate PID. It causes pain in the right upper quadrant of the abdomen, which may mimic that due to gall bladder disease, hepatitis or hepatocellular carcinoma.

Gonorrhoea in pregnancy has been associated with low birthweight, premature rupture of membranes, chorioamnionitis and post-partum upper genital tract infection (Elliot et al., 1990; Plummer et al., 1987).

Untreated gonorrhoea may lead to chronic PID, ectopic pregnancy (the risk of which is increased tenfold after a single episode of salpingitis), or infertility. In a study from Central Africa, fallopian tube occlusion was present in 83 per cent of infertile women (Collet et al., 1988). Acute salpingitis has been estimated to produce sterility in 17% of patients, the risk rising with multiple episodes or more severe inflammation.

Ocular gonococcal infections

Ocular gonococcal infection in adults is presumed to follow autoinoculation, e.g. with a contaminated finger. It presents as an acute purulent conjunctivitis which may progress rapidly to corneal perforation.

Neonatal conjunctivitis (ophthalmia neonatorum), defined as conjunctival inflammation in the newborn occurring within 28 days of birth, is commonly due to gonococcal or chlamydial infection acquired from the maternal genital tract at the time of delivery. The risk of transmission from an infected mother is between 30 and 50 per cent (Laga et al., 1989).

Gonococcal ophthalmia neonatorum presents as a severe acute bilateral purulent conjunctivitis within one week of birth (Fig. 14.8). Gram stain of the discharge reveals numerous gram-negative intracellular diplococci. Give both systemic and topical treatment to the neonate (Table 14.8), and treat the mother and her sexual partner(s) for both gonorrhoea and chlamydial infection.

Ocular prophylaxis with either 1 per cent silver nitrate drops or 1 per cent tetracycline ointment, administered by midwives or traditional birth attendants to all infants at delivery, prevents gonococcal ophthalmia neonatorum (Laga et al., 1988).

Diagnosis

The laboratory diagnosis of gonorrhoea depends on identification of *N. gonorrhoeae* at infected sites, through microscopic examination of stained smears or by culture. In experienced hands a gram stain demonstrating gram-negative intracellular diplococci in urethral smears (Fig. 14.9) has a sensitivity and specificity of more than 95 per ent in males and neonates, but both sensitivity and specificity are considerably lower in females, where culture is the method of choice.

Isolation of *N. gonorrhoeae* on antibiotic-containing selective culture media (e.g. modified Thayer–Martin medium) is the gold standard diagnostic test. *N. gonorrhoeae* is a delicate organism, highly susceptible to drying; ensure that swabs are inoculated immediately on to culture medium, or placed in Stuarts transport medium and sent to the lab without delay.

The sites to be swabbed depend on the history and examination findings. In males with urethritis, insert the swab in the urethra for 5 seconds and rotate it. In women wipe the ectocervix clean, insert the swab into the cervical os and rotate it for 10 seconds. Take rectal swabs through a proctoscope.

Table 14.8. Recommended treatment regimens for STI

Disease	Drug	Route	Dose	Duration	Notes
Gonorrhoea					
Uncomplicated genital or pharyngeal infection	*Recommended regimens*				
	Ciprofloxacin	Oral	500 mg	STAT	
	Cefixime	Oral	400 mg	STAT	
	Ceftriaxone	IM	250 mg	STAT	
	Azithromycin	Oral	2 g	STAT	
	Alternative regimens				
	Spectinomycin	IM	2 g	STAT	
	Kanamycin	IM	2 g	STAT	
	Pregnancy/lactation				
	Avoid ciprofloxacin				
Disseminated gonococcal infection (DGI)	*Recommended regimens*				
	Ceftriaxone	IV or IM	1 g every day	24–48H	
	Spectinomycin	IM	2 g twice a day	24–48H	
	Followed by:				
	Cefixime	Oral	400 mg twice a day	5–6 days	
	Ciprofloxacin	Oral	500 mg twice a day	5–6 days	
Ophthalmia neonatorum	*Recommended regimens*				
	Ceftriaxone	IV or IM	25–50 mg/kg	STAT	Max 125 mg
	Alternative regimens				
	Kanamycin	IM	25 mg/kg	STAT	Max 75 mg
	Spectinomycin	IM	25 mg/kg	STAT	Max 75 mg
	Tetracycline or Erythromycin eye ointment and saline irrigation	Topical			
Chlamydia					
Uncomplicated genital or pharyngeal infection	*Recommended regimens*				
	Doxycycline	Oral	100 mg twice daily	7 days	
	Tetracycline hydrochloride	Oral	500 mg four times daily	7 days	
	Azithromycin	Oral	1 g	STAT	
	Alternative regimens				
	Erythromycin (base or ethylsuccinate)	Oral	500 mg four times daily 500 mg twice daily	7 days 14 days	Compliance and side effects
	Pregnancy/lactation				
	Avoid doxycycline, tetracycline, and erythromycin estolate. Use erythromycin base or ethylsuccinate				
Ophthalmia neonatorum	*Recommended regimens*				
	Erythromycin syrup	Oral	50 mg/kg in 4 doses	10–14 days	
Trichomoniasis	*Recommended*				
	Metronidazole	Oral	2 g	STAT	Avoid alcohol
	Alternative				
	Metronidazole	Oral	400–500 mg twice daily	7 days	
	Pregnancy/lactation				
	Metronidazole is safe after first trimester				

Table 14.8 (*cont.*)

Disease	Drug	Route	Dose	Duration	Notes
Bacterial vaginosis	*Recommended*				
	Metronidazole	Oral	400–500 mg twice daily	5–7 days	Caution with alcohol
	Alternative regimens				
	Metronidazole	Oral	2 g oral. Avoid alcohol	STAT	
Candidiasis	*Recommended regimens*				
	Clotrimazole pessaries/ vaginal tablets	Intra-vaginal	500 mg	STAT	
	Miconazole pessaries/ovules	Intra-vaginal	200 mg at night	3 nights	
	Nystatin pessaries 100 000 u	Intra-vaginal	1 pessary at night	7–14 nights	
	Alternative regimens				
	Fluconazole	Oral	150 mg	STAT	Repeat weekly for 6 months if frequent recurrences
	Pregnancy/lactation				
	Oral therapy contraindicated				
Pelvic inflammatory disease (PID)	*Recommended regimens* (treat for gonorrhoea, Chlamydia and TV/BV/ anaerobic infections)				Intra-uterine contraceptive device (IUCD) removal recommended
	Inpatient regimen				
	Gentamicin	IV/IM	1.5 mg/kg three times daily	Until improved +2 days	
	+Clindamycin	IV	900 mg three times daily	Until improved +2 days	
	Followed by:				
	Doxycycline	Oral	100 mg twice daily	14 days	
	+Metronidazole	Oral	400–500 mg twice daily	7 days	Avoid alcohol
	Alternative regimens				
	Ciprofloxacin	Oral	500 mg twice daily	Until improved +2 days	
	OR				
	Ceftriaxone	IM	250 mg once daily	Until improved +2 days	
	Followed by:				
	+Doxycycline	Oral	100 mg twice daily	14 days	
	+Metronidazole	Oral	500 mg twice daily	7 days	
	Outpatient regimen				
	Ciprofloxacin	Oral	500 mg	STAT	
	+Doxycycline	Oral	100 mg twice daily	14 days	
	+Metronidazole	Oral	400 mg twice daily	7–14 days	
Epididymo-orchitis (acute scrotal swelling syndrome)	*Recommended regimens* – if gonorrhoea and/or Chlamydia or NGU suspected:				
	Ciprofloxacin	Oral	500 mg	STAT	
	OR				
	Ceftriaxone	IM	250 mg	STAT	
	AND				

Table 14.8 (*cont.*)

Disease	Drug	Route	Dose	Duration	Notes
	Doxycycline AND Bed rest, scrotal elevation and analgesics/non-steroidal anti-inflammatory drugs as required	Oral	100 mg twice daily	14 days	
Syphilis					
Early syphilis (ie. primary, secondary, or early latent <2 years duration)	*Recommended regimens*				
	Benzathine penicillin	IM	2.4 million units (1.2 MU in each buttock)	STAT	(Lidocaine solution can be added to solvent to reduce pain)
	Procaine penicillin	IM	600 000 units daily	10–14 days	
	Benzyl penicillin	IM	1 million units daily	10–14 days	
	Alternative regimens (if penicillin allergy or parenteral treatment refused)				
	Doxycycline	Oral	100 mg twice daily 200 mg once a day	 14 days	
	Tetracycline hydrochloride	Oral	500 mg four times daily	14 days	
	Erythromycin	Oral	500 mg four times daily	14 days	
	Ceftriaxone	IM	250 mg daily	10 days	
	Azithromycin	Oral	1 or 2 g 500 mg once daily	STAT 10 days	Trials are under way
Late latent syphilis (i.e. serological >2 year duration) or tertiary syphilis	*Recommended regimens*				
	Benzathine penicillin	IM	2.4 million units (1.2 in each buttock)	Once weekly for 3 weeks	
Neurosyphilis	Procaine penicillin	IM	600 000 units daily	21 days	
	Benzyl penicillin	IM	1 million units daily	21 days	
	Alternative regimens (if penicillin allergy or parenteral treatment refused)				
	Doxycycline, tetracycline, erythromycin	Oral	same doses as above	28 days	Some authors recommend doubling doses of doxycycline
Management of reactions	(i) *Jarisch–Herxheimer reaction*				
	Prednisolone + antipyretics	Oral	10–20 mg three times daily	3 days	
	(ii) *Anaphylactic shock*				
	Adrenaline/epinephrine (1:1000)	IM	0.5 ml	STAT	
	Followed by:				
	Antihistamine (e.g. chlorpheniramine) +hydrocortisone	IM/IV	10 mg	STAT	
Congenital syphilis	*Recommended regimens*				
	Benzyl penicillin	IM	150 000 U/kg daily (in 6 doses 4-hourly)	10–14 days	

Table 14.8 (*cont.*)

Disease	Drug	Route	Dose	Duration	Notes
	Procaine penicillin	IM	50 000 U/kg daily	10–14 days	
	Alternative regimens				
	Benzathine penicillin	IM	50 000 U/kg	STAT	If CSF is normal
Chancroid	*Recommended regimens*				
	Ciprofloxacin	Oral	500 mg	STAT	
	Ciprofloxacin	Oral	500 mg twice daily	3 days	if HIV+ patient
	Azithromycin	Oral	1 g	STAT	
	Ceftriaxone	IM	250 mg	STAT	
	Alternative regimens				
	Co-trimoxazole (trimethoprim/ sulphamethoxazole – TMP-SMX)	Oral	80 mg/400 mg × 5 tablets twice daily	1 day	Only where reliable susceptibility data on TMP-SMX is available
	Spectinomycin	IM	2 g	STAT	
	Erythromycin (base)	Oral	500 mg three–four times daily	7 days	
	Pregnancy/lactation				
	Use ceftriaxone or erythromycin regimens				
Lymphogranuloma venereum (LGV)	*Recommended regimens*				
	Doxycycline	Oral	100 mg twice daily	14–21 days	
	Tetracycline	Oral	500 mg four times daily	14–21 days	
	Alternative regimens				
	Erythromycin	Oral	500 mg four times daily	14–21 days	
	Azithromycin	Oral	1 g daily	14–21 days	
	Pregnancy/lactation				
	Use erythromycin				
Donovanosis	*Recommended regimens*				
	Azithromycin	Oral	1 g weekly	4 weeks	Treatment to be provided until complete resolution or slightly beyond
			500 mg daily	1 week	
	Doxycycline	Oral	100 mg twice daily	7–21 days	
	Tetracycline hydrochloride	Oral	250 mg four times daily	7–21 days	
	Alternative regimens				
	Erythromycin base/stearate	Oral	500 mg four times daily	14 days	
	Cotrimoxazole (TMP-SMX)	Oral	80 mg/400 mg × 2 tablets twice daily	14 days	
	Gentamicin	IM/IV	1 mg/kg every 8 H		To be added if improvement not seen with above regimens
Genital herpes					
Primary or recurrent episode	*Recommended regimens*				
	Acyclovir (ACV)	Oral	400 mg three times daily	5–10 days	The longer regimen is preferred if primary case suspected
		Oral	200 mg five times daily	5–10 days	
	Alternative regimens				
	Valaciclovir	Oral	500 mg–1 g twice daily	5–10 days	As above

Table 14.8 (*cont.*)

Disease	Drug	Route	Dose	Duration	Notes
Severe episode (immunosuppressed or possible ACV resistance)	*Recommended regimens*				
	Acyclovir	Oral or IV	400–800 mg 5 times daily	Until complete healing	
	Valaciclovir	Oral	1 mg twice daily		
Suppressive therapy (if >6 recurrences per year)	*Recommended regimens*				
	Acyclovir	Oral	400 mg twice daily	Max 1 year	Re-assess after 1 year
		Oral	200 mg four times daily		
	Alternative regimens				
	Valaciclovir	Oral	250 mg twice daily	1 year?	In HIV-infected persons
Pregnant women	*Women with first or recurrent lesions of genital herpes*		500 mg twice daily		
	ACV is preferred for treatment of episodes as required				Continuous treatment in last 4 weeks of pregnancy may prevent neonatal herpes
	Genital lesions at onset of labour				
	Consider Caesarean section				
Anogenital warts	*Recommended regimens*				
	Trichloracetic acid (TCA) 80–90%	Topical	Once weekly at clinic	Until cure	Cytotoxic – protect surrounding skin with petroleum jelly, zinc oxide or plaster
	Podophyllin 15–25%	Topical	Once or twice weekly, wash 4h later	Until cure	Protect as above. Oncogenic and teratogenic effects
	Podophyllotoxin 0.5% solution or 0.15% cream	Topical	Twice daily (self) application for 3 days	Repeat for 4 weeks	Use with protective cream
	Imiquimod 5% cream	Topical	Three times weekly – wash after 6–10h	Repeat for up to 16 weeks	
	Alternative regimens				
	Excision, cryotherapy, loop excision, electrosurgery, laser treatment	Physical ablation			
	Special considerations				
	Pregnancy/lactation				
	• Avoid podophyllin, podophyllotoxin, imiquimod during pregnancy				
Scabies	*Recommended regimens*				
	Permethrin 5% cream (2.5% formulation for children)	Topical	One application	Wash after 12h	Safe during pregnancy and breastfeeding
	Lindane (gamma-benzene HCL) 1% cream/lotion	Topical			Possible toxicity for children <2 yrs
	Benzylbenzoate 25% solution (10% formulation for children)	Topical			
	Special considerations				
	• Treatment can be repeated at one week				

Table 14.8 (*cont.*)

Disease	Drug	Route	Dose	Duration	Notes
	• Disinfection of bedding and clothing through laundering and use of pyrethrins				
	Ivermectin	Oral	200 μg/kg	STAT	For crusted (Norwegian) or disseminated infestation (AIDS)
Lice	*Recommended regimens*				
	Malathion 0.5% lotion	Topical	Wash out after 12 h		
	Permethrin 1% hair lotion	Topical	Wash out after 10 minutes		
	Phenotrin 0.2%	Topical			

Management (see Box)

> **Principles underlying choice of STI drugs**
> Ideally, treatment for STIs should be:
> - single dose, and supervised
> - oral
> - free from side effects
> - at least 95 per cent effective.
>
> *N. gonorrhoeae* and *H. ducreyi* are resistant to many antibiotics. Their susceptibility varies in different regions and over time, and should be monitored regularly.

See Table 14.8 for recommended treatment regimens. Most gonococcal isolates in Africa are now resistant to penicillins, tetracyclines, and other older antimicrobial agents, which can therefore no longer be recommended for the treatment of gonorrhoea (Fig. 14.10) (Ison et al., 1998; Mayaud et al., 2002). It is important to monitor local in vitro susceptibility, as well as the clinical efficacy of recommended regimens.

Chlamydial infections

The organism

Chlamydia trachomatis is a non-motile, gram-negative obligate intracellular bacterium, with an unusual life cycle. The metabolically inert infectious elementary body (EB) has a rigid cell wall and is adapted for extracellular survival. It infects preferentially columnar epithelial cells, by which it is actively taken up. After entering the host cell it differentiates over a number of hours to the metabolically active reticulate body, which divides by binary fission until an intracellular inclusion is formed, which may contain several thousand organisms. The life cycle is completed when reticulate bodies condense to form elementary bodies, which are released from the inclusion after lysis of the host cell.

A number of serotypes of *C. trachomatis* have been identified. Serotypes A–C cause ocular infection in trachoma endemic areas, whereas serotypes D–K cause genital tract infections worldwide. Serotypes L1, L2 and L3 are more invasive, and cause lymphogranuloma venereum (LGV).

Pathogenesis

The pathological hallmarks of *C. trachomatis* infection are: (i) the subepithelial lymphoid follicle; and (ii) fibrosis and scarring. The host immune system is believed to play an important part in the pathogenesis of chlamydial infections, and a chlamydial heat shock protein of 57 kDa, which has been shown to elicit a delayed hypersensitivity reaction in previously infected animals, may also be a determinant of immunopathology in humans (Peeling et al., 1997).

Clinical features and complications

The clinical spectrum of disease due to chlamydial infection is similar to that seen in gonococcal infection. Genital tract infection with *C. trachomatis* is asymptomatic in 50–80 per cent of men and women. When symptoms are present, in general, those due to *C. trachomatis* are less severe than those due to *N. gonorrhoeae*. However, chlamydial infection is more likely to cause serious sequelae, particularly in women.

Men present with urethral discharge and/or dysuria. Epididymitis is the most important complication.

Women may complain of vaginal discharge or dysuria. A muco-purulent discharge at the cervical os on speculum examination is suggestive of chlamydial or gonococcal cervicitis. Ascending infection of the female genital tract may

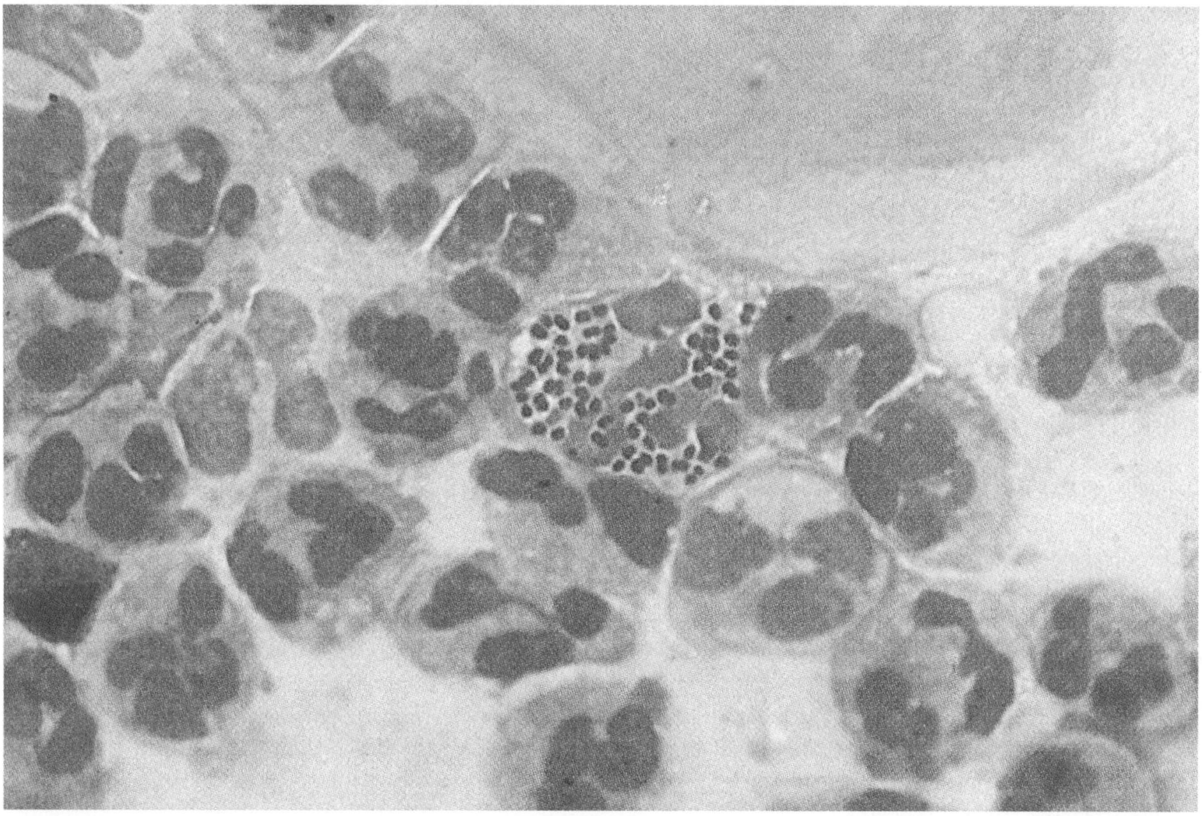

Fig. 14.9. Gram stain of urethral smear showing gram-negative intracellular diplococci.

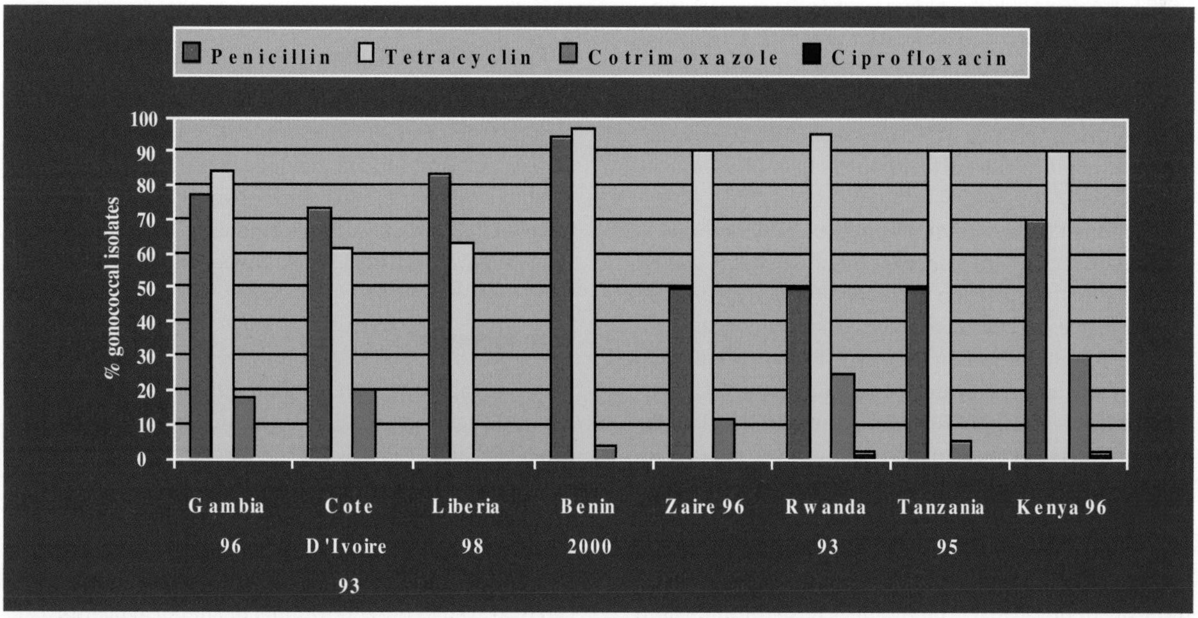

Fig. 14.10. Antimicrobial resistance of *N gonorrhoeae* to commonly used antibiotics in Africa.

lead to PID. Often women present only when the sequelae of irreversible damage to the fallopian tubes (infertility, ectopic pregnancy) become apparent. Infection may track to the right upper quadrant, giving rise to a perihepatitis with characteristic adhesions between the liver capsule and peritoneum (the Curtis–FitzHugh syndrome).

Neonatal chlamydial infections

Some 30 per cent of infants born to infected mothers become infected. In the majority of cases the only consequence of this is a self-limiting conjunctivitis presenting within the first 2 weeks of life, but occasionally chlamydial ophthalmia is more severe. A small proportion of infected infants develop chlamydial pneumonitis, presenting usually between the ages of 6 weeks and 3 months with a paroxysmal cough and tachypnoea in the absence of fever. Rales may be heard on clinical examination, and a chest radiograph often reveals extensive bilateral pulmonary infiltrates with hyperinflation (Beem & Saxon, 1977).

Diagnosis

Few laboratories in Africa are able to diagnose chlamydial infection. Syndromic management of urethral and vaginal discharge, and of lower abdominal pain in women, covers chlamydial infection, but fails to identify the majority of infected people, who have no symptoms. A simple, rapid, dipstick-type test to diagnose chlamydial infection is badly needed, and may soon be available.

Microscopy is of little value except in chlamydial ophthalmia neonatorum, in which characteristic intracellular inclusions may be seen in conjunctival epithelial cells stained by Giemsa's method. *C. trachomatis* can be identified in smears stained with fluorescein-labelled monoclonal antibodies, but only with the help of a fluorescence microscope.

Isolation of *C. trachomatis* is rarely possible, since it requires tissue culture. Enzyme immunoassays (EIAs) are available for the detection of chlamydial antigen, but they are expensive, and detect at most 70 per cent of cases. Nucleic acid amplification tests (NAAT) and such amplification tests such as polymerase chain reaction (PCR) or ligase chain reaction (LCR) are now the gold standard for the diagnosis of genital chlamydial infection, but they are expensive, and require expensive equipment as well as careful laboratory practice. These tests are more sensitive than antigen detection tests (Black, 1997), and a speculum examination is not required, since they give good results with first-catch urine samples or self-administered vaginal swabs.

Serology is of no value in the diagnosis of uncomplicated chlamydial infection, except for lymphogranuloma venereum (LGV, see below).

Management

See Table 14.8 for recommended regimens. Doxycycline (and other tetracyclines) are contraindicated in pregnant women, in whom erythromycin or amoxycillin are preferred. Erythromycin estolate is contraindicated during pregnancy because of drug-related hepato-toxicity; only erythromycin base or erythromycin ethylsuccinate should be used.

Bacterial vaginosis

The organisms

Bacterial vaginosis (BV) is a syndrome in which a malodorous vaginal discharge is associated with an alteration in the vaginal bacterial flora, from a pattern in which *Lactobacillus* species are predominant, to a mixed flora pattern in which *Gardnerella vaginalis*, genital mycoplasmas and a variety of anaerobes (e.g. *Prevotella* spp., *Mobiluncus* spp.) are more numerous. Women with BV have an increase in vaginal fluid pH, increased quantities of amines and other products of bacterial metabolism and a characteristic vaginal discharge (Hillier & Holmes, 1999).

The problem in Africa

The reported prevalence of BV has varied from 10 per cent to 40 per cent in clinical studies conducted in Senegal, Central African Republic, Burkina Faso, and Tanzania (Mayaud, 2001), and between 38 per cent and 51 per cent in population-based studies in The Gambia and Uganda (Walraven et al., 2001; Sewankambo et al., 1999).

Pathogenesis

Bacterial vaginosis is an imbalance in the vaginal ecosystem rather than a sexually transmitted infection, and it can be found in sexually inexperienced women. However, onset of the condition has been associated with a change of sexual partner and with vaginal douching.

The underlying causes of BV are not well understood. Hygiene practices (menstrual or sexual) have been implicated, as well as other hormonal or chemical factors which may trigger alterations in the vaginal flora. BV seems to recur more frequently in women following their menstruation, or after sexual intercourse (possibly as a result of sperm-associated chemical factors).

As the term 'vaginosis' (rather than 'vaginitis') implies, no inflammatory response accompanies the syndrome, although increased levels of pro-inflammatory cytokines may be found in genital secretions of women with BV.

Clinical features and complications

Typically, women complain of a malodorous (fishy) discharge, which is homogeneous and white/grey, and adherent to the vaginal walls. BV has been associated with complications of pregnancy including preterm labour, premature rupture of membranes, premature delivery of low birthweight infants and histologic chorioamnionitis, and with PID following the insertion of intrauterine contraceptive devices or termination of pregnancy (Hillier & Holmes, 1999). An increased prevalence of HIV infection was found in women with BV in Uganda and Malawi suggesting that it may be a risk factor for HIV acquisition (Sewankambo et al., 1997; Taha et al., 1998).

Diagnosis

BV is diagnosed using one of two methods. The clinical diagnosis according to the *Amsel's method* requires the presence of three of the following four criteria (Hillier & Holmes, 1999):

- vaginal pH >4.5
- characteristic homogeneous greyish and adherent vaginal discharge
- release of a strong fishy odour on adding potassium hydroxide (10% KOH) solution to a sample of vaginal fluid ('Whiff' test)
- presence of 'clue cells' (epithelial cells to which many bacteria are attached) on wet preparation microscopy.

Increasingly, BV is diagnosed using a gram-stained smear of a vaginal swab, according to *Nugent's method*, which relies on a quantitative scoring system for three bacterial morphotypes (*Lactobacilli; Gardnerella* and *Bacteroides* spp.; and curved, gram-variable rods, taken as evidence of *Mobiluncus* spp.) (Nugent et al., 1991). The sum of the three individual scores gives a final score between 0 and 10, which classifies the flora pattern as normal, intermediate or bacterial vaginosis.

Several studies have found a good correlation between the two methods (Hillier & Holmes, 1999). However, both require microscopy and some clinical expertise, which may not be available in many primary health care settings in developing countries.

Management

Give oral metronidazole 2 g single dose or 400 mg twice daily for 7 days. Topical preparations of metronidazole (0.75 per cent gel and vaginal tablets) and clindamycin 2 per cent cream can also be used (Table 14.8).

Relapses

BV follows a relapsing remittent course in some women who may require repeated or prolonged treatment.

Male partners

Treatment of male partners does not reduce the rate of recurrence of BV.

Trichomoniasis

The organism

Trichomoniasis is caused by the protozoal parasite *Trichomonas vaginalis*. *T. vaginalis* has a characteristic appearance with a body slightly larger than a pus cell, from which four motile flagella project anteriorly, while one extends backwards, to which an undulating membrane is attached. In a wet preparation, it can be recognized easily by the lashing movements of its flagella.

The problem in Africa

T. vaginalis is the most common curable STI world-wide, with an estimated 170 million cases occuring annually (Gerbase et al., 1998). It is a frequent cause of vaginal discharge in Africa. It is found in 10–30 per cent of antenatal clinic attenders, and in a high proportion of asymptomatic women in community-based studies in Africa (Wawer et al., 1999; Walraven et al., 2001). *T. vaginalis* has been isolated from 1–15 per cent of cases of non-gonococcal urethritis in men. Recent community-based studies in East Africa have found prevalences of around 10 per cent among truck drivers in Mombasa (Jackson et al., 1997) and rural men in Tanzania (Watson-Jones et al., 2000).

Transmission and pathogenesis

T. vaginalis is usually transmitted by sexual contact, but can survive on inanimate objects providing moist conditions (lavatory seats, towels), and non-sexual transmission may sometimes occur (Adu-Sarkodie, 1995).

Following attachment to the vaginal mucosa, *T. vaginalis* multiplies and deprives the protective vaginal lactobacilli of glycogen, resulting in their disappearance, a corresponding elevation of the pH (>4.5), and an increase in the anaerobic flora. An inflammatory response with polymorphonuclear leukocytes (PMN) is seen. *T. vaginalis* can colonize the vulva, vagina, and para-urethral glands (Bartholin's and Skene's ducts), but does not usually colonize the upper genital tract. The infection does not confer immunity and repeated infections are common.

Clinical features and complications

Infected women may have no symptoms (10–50 per cent), but usually complain of at least one of the following:

- vaginal discharge
- vulval itching
- dysuria
- dyspareunia
- post-coital or intermenstrual bleeding.

On examination, up to 75 per cent of infected women have a vaginal discharge, which may be typically abundant, greenish-yellow and frothy. There may be tender labial oedema and erythema, and occasionally small abscesses of Bartholin's or Skene's glands. The cervix, like the vagina, is reddened and bleeds easily on contact, and may have a 'strawberry' appearance (punctate cervicitis).

In men, the infection is commonly asymptomatic (around 50 per cent). The commonest presentation is with urethral discharge and/or dysuria, indistinguishable from that caused by other organisms, although it tends to be thin and watery. Occasionally small erosions are seen on the glans penis, which may be associated with a subpreputial discharge.

Diagnosis

Microscopy of a drop of discharge mixed with saline shows increased numbers of polymorphonuclear leukocytes, and motile flagellated parasites, which are slightly larger. They are best seen under phase contrast. Compared with culture, direct microscopy is less than 80 per cent sensitive, so that culture (using Diamond's medium or the InPouch® system) should also be performed when available. The organisms are more difficult to demonstrate in male patients; culture of a centrifuged first catch urine specimen may be the most sensitive method.

Management

See Table 14.8. Metronidazole tablets should be taken after meals to avoid gastric side effects and alcohol should be avoided for 48 hours after treatment is completed. Other side effects of metronidazole include metallic taste, dizziness, headache and nausea.

Cure rates are usually high (>95 per cent) but metronidazole resistance can occur. Treatment failures may need a higher dose (400 mg orally three times daily for 7 days), plus metronidazole pessaries 1 g intravaginally each night for 7 days.

There is increasing evidence that *T. vaginalis* infection can cause adverse pregnancy outcomes (preterm delivery and low birthweight) (Cotch et al., 1997). Trichomoniasis should therefore be treated in pregnancy, and metronidazole is safe, although it should probably be avoided in the first trimester.

Candidiasis

The organism

Vulvovaginal candidiasis (VVC), or 'thrush' is a common fungal infection. It affects most females at least once during their lifetime, and 40–50 per cent suffer from it more than once. *Candida albicans* causes more than 80 per cent of cases; the remainder are caused by *C. glabrata (Torulopsis glabrata), C. parapsilosis* and *C. tropicalis.*

Transmission and pathogenesis

Candida species inhabit the mouth and genitalia without causing symptoms, and can be isolated from the genital tract in 20–50 per cent of asymptomatic women.

Colonization is by adherence to epithelial cells. All *C. albicans* strains adhere well to exfoliated vaginal and buccal epithelial cells, but there seems to be variation from one person to another in vaginal epithelial cell receptivity. No epithelial cell receptor has yet been described for *Candida* spp.

The vaginal milieu determines whether *Candida* spp. becomes a commensal or a pathogen. Factors predisposing to symptomatic infection include:

- pregnancy
- diabetes mellitus
- use of broad-spectrum antibiotics
- treatment for trichomoniasis
- immunosuppression (in HIV infection or malignancy).

Symptomatic disease is associated with an increase in the number of yeasts in the vagina. In general, blastospores are associated with asymptomatic colonization and germinating forms are found in symptomatic individuals.

Tight, poorly ventilated nylon underclothing, by increasing perineal moisture, may predispose to symptomatic disease in warm climates.

Clinical features

In women the commonest presenting symptom of VVC is vulval itching, with or without a vaginal discharge. If there is a discharge it is typically white, with curd-like plaques adhering to the vaginal wall, and does not smell. There may be erythema and/or oedema of the vulva and vaginal walls.

Men with genital Candida infection often have no symptoms. They may experience a transient erythema and itching of the glans penis after acquisition from an infected partner, or present with an acute or chronic inflammation of the glans penis (balanitis). The typical case is mild with erythema and symptoms of burning.

Diagnosis

Microscopic examination of a wet preparation of the vaginal discharge, or a smear from the glans penis, reveals budding yeasts or mycelia, which are more easily seen after addition of 10 per cent potassium hydroxide. Culture is the most sensitive method for the detection of *Candida*, but a positive culture can be obtained even from asymptomatic individuals.

Management

See Table 14.8.

Vulvovaginal candidiasis during pregnancy

Only topical azoles should be used in pregnancy.

Recurrences

Advise patients not to take antibiotics or antiseptic/antibiotic vaginal preparations. Exclude other underlying factors, such as uncontrolled diabetes mellitus, immunosuppression, and corticosteroid use.

Vulvovaginal candidiasis and HIV infection

Candidiasis is an important correlate of HIV disease. It is often quite severe and frequently relapses. Prolonged treatment is generally required, and chronic suppressive therapy is frequently given.

Balanitis

Clotrimazole cream twice daily for 7 days or single dose fluconazole 150 mg.

Pathogens causing genital ulceration

Syphilis

Syphilis, a young shepherd boy who succumbed to an apparently new disease which had swept across Europe a few years earlier, was the eponymous hero of a Latin poem written in 1530 by the Italian G. Fracastorio.

The problem in Africa

Syphilis is highly prevalent among antenatal clinic attenders and in the general population in many African countries (**Table** 14.4). The relative rarity of late syphilis in parts of Africa where early syphilis is common suggests that the disease has become more common in recent years, perhaps reflecting loss of herd immunity following the mass treatment campaigns against endemic treponemal disease in the 1950s and 1960s.

The organism

Syphilis is caused by *T. pallidum (*first described by Schaudin in 1905), one of a small group of treponemas (of the order Spirochaetales) pathogenic to man. It cannot be distinguished in the laboratory from the agents responsible for yaws and pinta (*T. pallidum* subsp. *pertenue* and *T. carateum*, respectively). It is a spiral organism 6–15 mm in length and 0.15 mm in width, visible by light microscopy only under conditions of dark-field illumination, and cannot be grown on artificial media. In tissue culture and in animal models it divides slowly, with a replication time of approximately 30 hours. It is highly susceptible to drying.

Transmission by sexual contact requires exposure to moist mucosal or cutaneous lesions; experiments in the rabbit suggest that an inoculum of some 50 organisms is sufficient to initiate infection.

Pathogenesis

T. pallidum has not been shown to produce either exotoxins or endotoxins. Following experimental infection in the rabbit, *T. pallidum* begins to replicate once it has passed through the epithelium. An initial polymorphonuclear leukocyte response at the lesion is soon replaced by an infiltrate of T- and B-lymphocytes. The primary chancre also contains mucoid material, mainly hyaluronic acid and chondroitin sulphate, which may modulate the host immune response. Both circulating *T. pallidum* specific T-cells and specific antibody can be found in the majority of

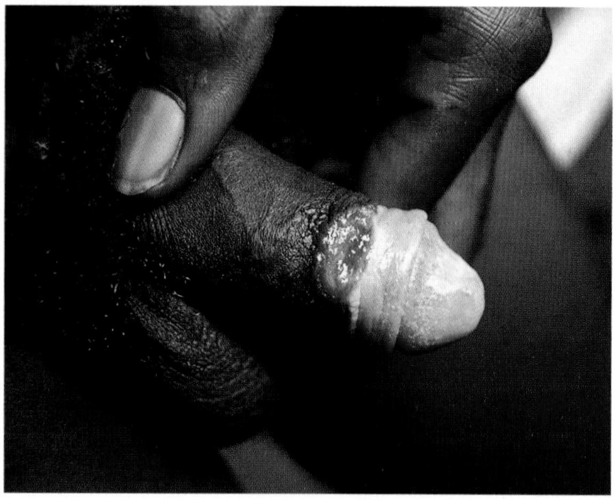

Fig. 14.11. Syphilitic primary chancre (D. Mabey).

cases of primary syphilis. At the same time as these are first noted, the number of organisms in the lesion decreases and the ulcer begins to heal, suggesting that the immune system is controlling the infection.

The appearance of secondary lesions some weeks later, due to the dissemination of organisms and circulating immune complexes, indicates that this is not the case, although the mechanism by which such a slow growing organism evades the host immune response is not clear. Much of the pathology of secondary syphilis may be immune complex mediated. High levels of antitreponemal antibody are present in the circulation, but cell-mediated immune responses are depressed.

Eventually cell-mediated immune responses to *T. pallidum* are restored as the lesions are brought under control, leading to the latent stage. Follow-up studies in the pre-penicillin era showed that relapse of infectious secondary lesions occurred in up to 25 per cent of cases. The organism can survive in the body for many years thereafter, causing tertiary lesions characterized by the presence of a small number of organisms and a lymphocytic host response giving rise to an endarteritis.

Clinical features

After an incubation period of 10–70 days (median 21 days), a *primary chancre* (Fig. 14.11) develops at the site of inoculation. The chancre is typically painless, indurated, with a clean base and a raised edge, and does not bleed on contact. There is usually only a single lesion; in the male it is most commonly on the glans, the foreskin, the coronal sulcus or the shaft of the penis, and in the female on the cervix or vulva. The primary chancre is often accompanied by inguinal lymphadenopathy; the glands are characteristically hard (the 'bullet bubo' of Hutchinson) and painless.

The primary chancre generally resolves spontaneously over several weeks. Between 3 and 6 weeks after its first appearance the features of *secondary syphilis* appear, which commonly include:

- rash
- condylomata lata
- oral ulceration
- generalized lymphadenopathy.

And more rarely include:

- fever
- hepatitis
- glomerulonephritis
- uveitis
- meningitis.

The rash of secondary syphilis may take many forms: papular, macular, pustular or annular. It often desquamates, but in moist areas of the body (e.g. perineum, axilla) soft raised condylomata lata may be seen (Fig. 14.12). It generally affects the palms (Fig. 14.13) and soles, and does not itch. The mucous membranes may be involved, with mucous patches or oral ulceration sometimes in the form of the characteristic 'snail track' ulcer.

The lesions of secondary syphilis generally resolve after several weeks, although relapses commonly occurred in the pre-antibiotic era. In the absence of adequate treatment the patient then enters the latent stage of the disease, and is liable to develop tertiary syphilis at some time in the future, perhaps after many years.

The lesions of tertiary syphilis fall into three categories: the gumma, cardiovascular disease and central nervous system disease. The most common manifestation is the gumma, a painless 'punched out' ulcer with little or no inflammatory reaction, usually affecting the skin, but occasionally involving bones or viscera. Cardiovascular lesions include aortitis, aortic valve disease or coronary ostial occlusion, and neurological manifestations include tabes dorsalis and general paresis. It is surprising that tertiary syphilis, and in particular neurosyphilis, appears rather uncommon in Africa in spite of the high incidence of early syphilis.

Congenital syphilis

Early congenital syphilis

Pregnant women with untreated early or latent syphilis are liable to give birth to congenitally infected infants. The risk is highest among those with primary or secondary syphilis during pregnancy, and diminishes as the duration of latent syphilis increases. Studies conducted in

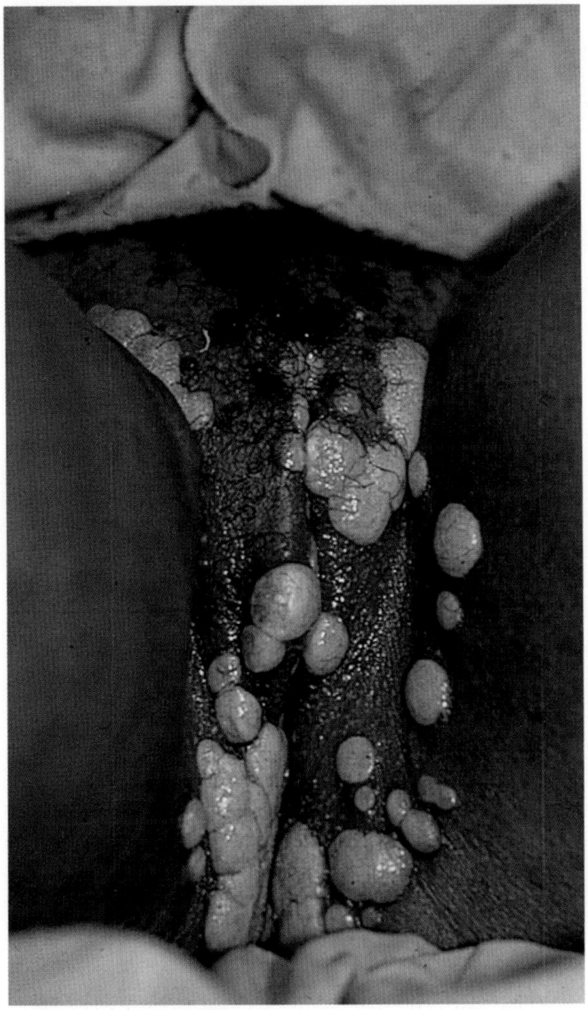

Fig. 14.12. Condylomata lata of secondary syphilis (J. Richens).

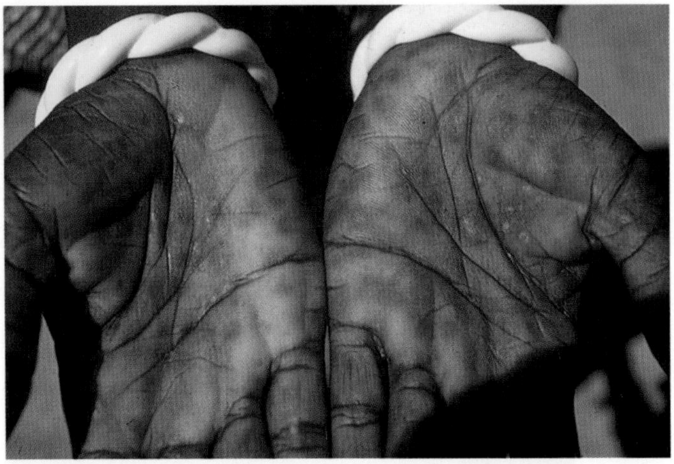

Fig. 14.13. Typical palmar rash of secondary syphilis (D. Mabey).

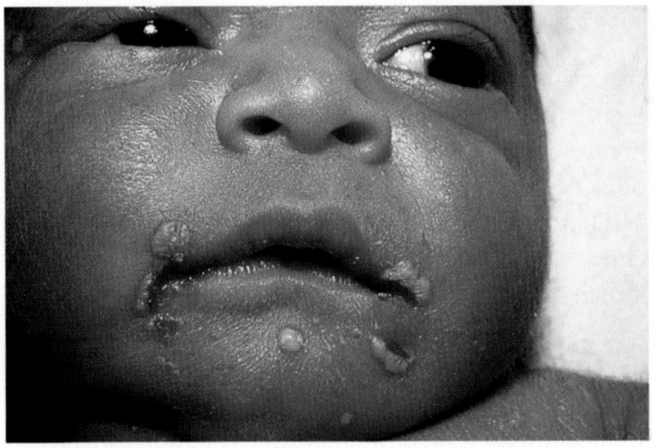

Fig. 14.14. Bullous rash of congenital syphilis in a neonate (J. Richens).

the preantibiotic era found that untreated early syphilis in the mother led to stillbirth in 25 per cent of cases, neonatal death in some 15 per cent of cases and a syphilitic infant in about 40 per cent of cases. Corresponding figures for untreated late syphilis were 12, 9 and 2 per cent. Congenital syphilis was the most common reason for admission to hospital in infants aged less than 3 months in Lusaka, Zambia in the pre-AIDS era (Hira et al., 1982). A recent study in Tanzania found that 50 per cent of stillbirths were caused by syphilis (Watson-Jones et al., 2002).

Signs of congenital syphilis in the neonate include a bullous rash (Fig. 14.14), anaemia, jaundice and hepatosplenomegaly. The infant is often small for dates and may have feeding difficulties. The prognosis is poor in infants with signs of congenital syphilis at birth. More commonly, the syphilitic infant appears normal at birth, and presents in the first 3 months of life with: failure to thrive; a rash which resembles that of secondary syphilis, with desquamation usually involving the palms (Fig. 14.15) and soles; persistent nasal discharge (sometimes bloodstained); and anaemia or hepatosplenomegaly. Periostitis of the long bones, with or without metaphyseal abnormalities, is radiologically evident in more than 90 per cent of cases, and may present clinically as pseudoparalysis of one or more limbs. The prognosis is very much better in those presenting in the post-neonatal period.

Late congenital syphilis

Late congenital syphilis in the child or adolescent corresponds to tertiary syphilis in the adult, although the cardiovascular system is seldom involved. Manifestations include bony and dental abnormalities (skull bossing, Hutchinson's teeth) and inflammatory lesions of the

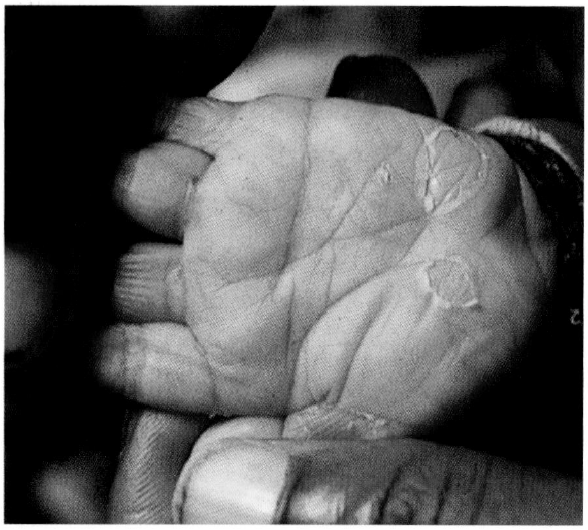

Fig. 14.15. Palmar rash in an infant aged 3 months with congenital syphilis (D. Mabey).

cornea (interstitial keratitis) and joints (Clutton's joints). Eighth nerve deafness is commonly seen, and symptomatic neurosyphilis may occur, corresponding to tabes dorsalis or general paresis in the adult. In view of the high incidence of early congenital syphilis in many African cities, late manifestations of the disease are surprisingly rare in Africa.

Diagnosis

Clinically it may not be possible to distinguish a syphilitic primary chancre from other causes of genital ulceration. In most parts of Africa chancroid is the most important differential diagnosis, but in areas where donovanosis is prevalent this should also be considered. The primary chancre should also be distinguished from LGV, herpes and nonvenereal causes of genital ulceration. Syndromic management of genital ulcer disease should always include treatment for syphilis (Fig. 14.4).

Secondary syphilis may resemble a variety of other skin conditions, but rashes which do not itch and affect the palms and soles are syphilitic until proved otherwise. Early congenital syphilis in the neonatal period may be confused with perinatally acquired herpes simplex on account of the bullous rash, or with other intrauterine infections causing hepatosplenomegaly, anaemia and jaundice (e.g. cytomegalovirus, toxoplasmosis, rubella).

Dark-field microscopy

T. pallidum may be demonstrated by dark-field microscopy in fluid from ulcerated or moist lesions of early syphilis, or in bulla fluid from lesions of early congenital syphilis. It can be distinguished from other spirochaetes which may be present under the foreskin by its characteristic shape and motility. Dark-field microscopy is likely to be negative in patients who have applied antiseptics to the lesion or taken antibiotics.

Serological diagnosis

Two categories of test are available for the serological diagnosis of syphilis: non-specific or reagin tests (e.g. Venereal Disease Research Laboratory (VDRL), rapid plasma reagin (RPR)) and treponemal tests (*T. pallidum* haemagglutination (TPHA), *T. pallidum* particle agglutination (TPPA), fluorescent treponemal antibody (FTA)).

The reagin tests are useful for monitoring the response to treatment because they exhibit a falling titre after successful therapy, but they may give false-positive reactions in subjects with other chronic infections. The treponemal tests generally remain positive for life, and cannot therefore distinguish between a current and a past infection. They are more specific than the reagin tests but cannot distinguish between sexually acquired and endemic treponemal infections. The RPR and TPHA tests are simple to perform and do not require sophisticated laboratory equipment. In the neonate it is necessary to demonstrate IgM antibodies by the FTA test in order to distinguish between true infection and passively acquired maternal antibody; however, in an infant with signs of congenital syphilis, a positive maternal reagin test is sufficient grounds for treatment.

Management

See Table 14.8. *T. pallidum* remains fully sensitive to penicillin. Because it is a slowly dividing organism it is necessary to ensure adequate circulating penicillin levels for at least 10 days. Standard treatment regimens appear equally effective in HIV positive patients. Give epidemiological treatment to sexual contacts. In cases of congenital syphilis, investigate and treat the mother and her sexual partner(s) appropriately. If possible, follow up infants after 6 months to ensure that the RPR or VDRL test has reverted to negative.

Prevention

Congenital syphilis can be prevented by serological screening of pregnant women at antenatal clinics. Experience in Lusaka, Zambia, has shown that in a developing country setting this is only successful if serological tests are performed in the clinic and treatment given immediately (Temmerman et al., 1993).

Chancroid

Chancroid, or soft chancre, was first differentiated clinically from syphilis, or hard chancre, in France in the 1850s. In 1889, Ducrey showed that inoculation of purulent ulcer material from a chancroidal ulcer caused lesions in the skin of the forearm, and identified the causative organism which bears his name, *Haemophilus ducreyi*.

The problem in Africa

Chancroid is an important cause of genital ulceration in Africa. Before the HIV epidemic it accounted for more than 60 per cent of ulcers seen in clinics; but in recent years an increasing proportion of ulcers has been due to herpes simplex virus type-2, with a corresponding decrease in the proportion due to *H. ducreyi* (O'Farrell, 1999) (Fig. 14.16). Co-infections of chancroid with *Treponema pallidum* or herpes simplex virus (HSV) are frequent, and occur in more 10 per cent of ulcer patients in some centres.

More than any other STI, chancroid is a disease of core groups, especially commercial sex workers and their clients. There is no reservoir of asymptomatic infections in the general population, and transmission from asymptomatic individuals is rare. The incidence of chancroid appears to be falling in some African cities where condom use has increased among sex workers and their clients and where coverage of appropriate STi case management has increased.

The organism

H. ducreyi is a small facultatively anaerobic gram-negative bacillus which requires haemin (X factor), reduces nitrate to nitrite and forms typical streptobacillary chains on gram stain. It is a fastidious organism which will only grow on enriched media and grows best at 30–33 °C in an atmosphere of 5 per cent carbon dioxide.

Pathogenesis

Histopathologically, chancroidal ulcers contain three distinct zones: a superficial zone consisting of necrotic tissue, fibrin and numerous bacteria; an intermediate zone showing oedema and new vessel formation; and a deep zone containing a dense infiltrate of neutrophils and plasma cells with fibroblastic proliferation.

The application of *H. ducreyi* to the human forearm does not produce a lesion unless the skin is traumatized. Certain strains are avirulent in the human and in a rabbit model, but lack of virulence in the rabbit does not necessarily imply a strain is avirulent in the human. There is some evidence that virulent strains are relatively resistant to phagocytosis by human polymorphonuclear leukocytes and to complement-mediated killing by normal

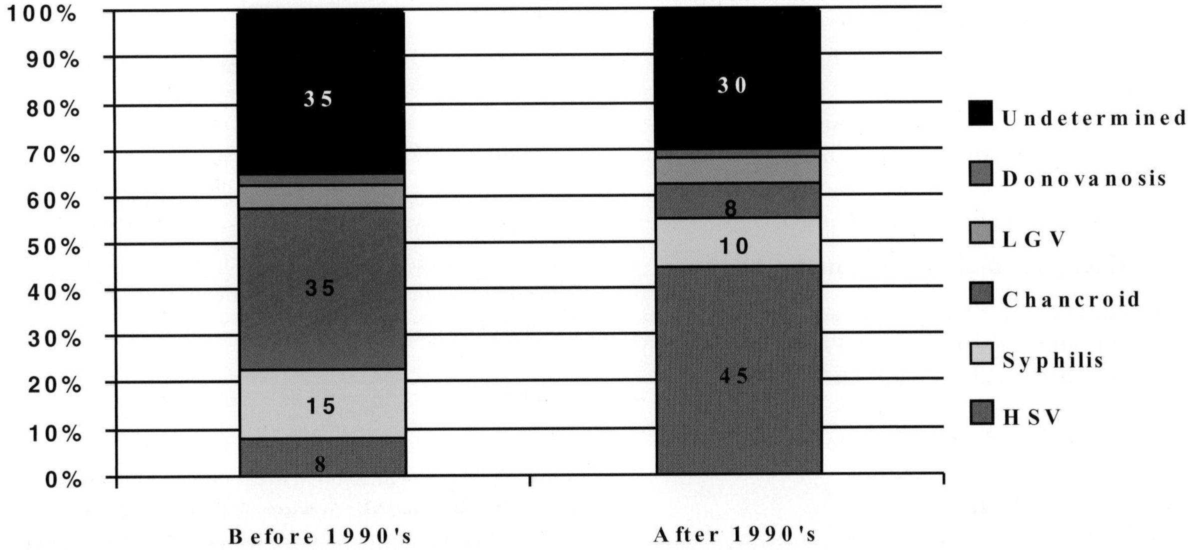

Fig. 14.16. 'Typical' distribution of agents causing genital ulcer disease (GUD) in Africa before and after the 1990s.

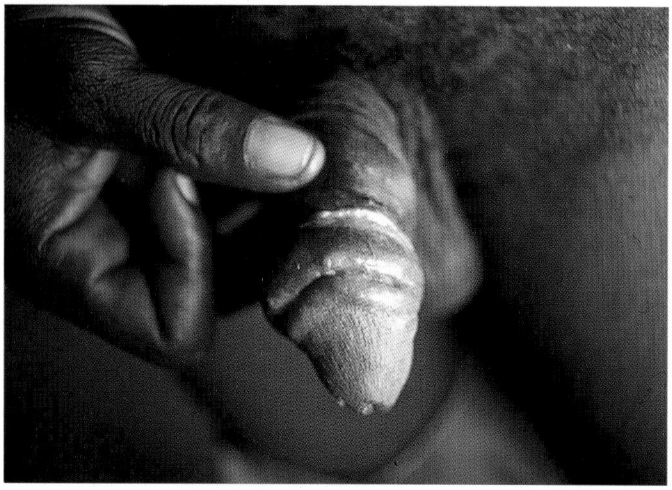

Fig. 14.17. Ulcer due to chancroid (D. Mabey).

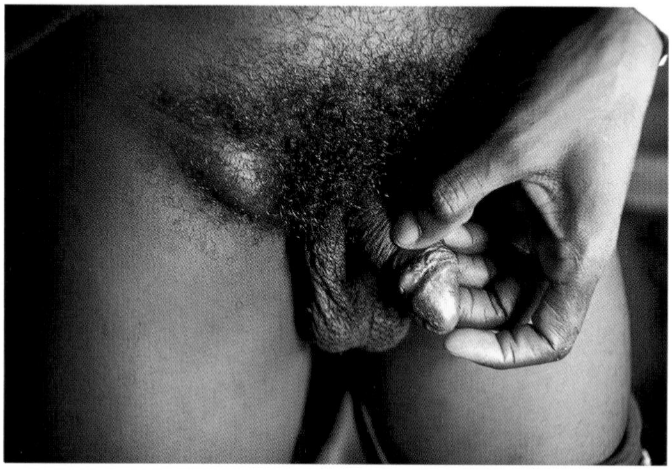

Fig. 14.18. Chancroidal ulcer with bubo (D. Mabey).

human and rabbit serum. The suppurating lymphadenopathy of chancroid is notable for the large number of neutrophils and small number of bacilli present.

Clinical features and complications

The incubation period ranges between 3 and 10 days. In contrast to other STIs, most cases of *H. ducreyi* infection are symptomatic. Symptoms include:

Ulceration at the site of primary inoculation

The ulcer is classically described as:

- single or (often) multiple
- not indurated ('soft sore')
- with a necrotic base and purulent exudate
- bordered by ragged undermined edges
- bleeding easily on contact
- painful.

In males, most ulcers are found on the prepuce near the frenulum or in the coronal sulcus (Fig. 14.17). In females, most are at the entrance of the vagina, particularly the fourchette. Several lesions may merge to form gigantic ulcers.

Inguinal lympahdenopathy

Painful inguinal adenitis is also a characteristic feature of chancroid and is present in about 50 per cent of cases (Fig. 14.18). The adenitis is unilateral in most patients. Buboes form and can become fluctuant and rupture, releasing thick pus, resulting sometimes in extensive ulceration. See box for the differential diagnosis of inguinal adenopathy.

Differential diagnosis of inguinal lymphadenopathy

With genital ulcer or history of recent ulcer	
• Chancroid	(usually painful, may be fluctuant)
• Syphilis	(usually painless)
• Herpes simplex	
• Lymphogranuloma venereum	(no ulcer in 50% or more)
With no genital ulcer or history of ulcer	
HIV infection	(look for generalized lymphadenopathy)
Pyogenic infection of foot or leg	(examine interdigital clefts if nothing obvious)
Tuberculosis	(usually painless)
Lymphoma	(look for generalized lymphadenopathy)
Carcinoma	(hard glands; examine anus and rectum)
Plague	(severe systemic illness)

Complications

Ulcers may cause extensive tissue destruction, particularly on the glans penis (so-called 'phagedenic' ulcers, Fig. 14.19). There can be mild constitutional symptoms but *H. ducreyi* does not cause systemic infection or spread to distant sites.

Diagnosis

Clinical diagnosis is unreliable, with an accuracy ranging from 33–80 per cent, even in areas of high prevalence and good clinical expertise. Syndromic management of genital ulcers in Africa should always include treatment for chancroid.

Gram stain of smears obtained from ulcers lacks both sensitivity and specificity. The laboratory diagnosis of chancroid depends on the isolation of *H. ducreyi* from the ulcer, which is difficult, as it is a fastidious and slow growing organism.

Take swabs for isolation from the ulcer base or its undermined edge, and plate them directly on appropriate enriched blood-containing media made selective with vancomycin. For optimal rates of isolation, inoculate media made up from both gonococcal agar and Mueller–Hinton agar base. Incubate plates for at least 72 hours in an atmosphere of 5 per cent carbon dioxide at 33 °C. *H. ducreyi* is identified by its typical colonial morphology (colonies are difficult to break up and can be moved intact across the surface of the agar), gram stain and inability to ferment sugars.

Management

See Table 14.8. Chancroidal ulcers should be kept clean and dry, with regular washing in soapy water. The mainstay of antimicrobial treatment has for a number of years been co-trimoxazole or erythromycin in standard dosage given by mouth for 7 days. However, an increasing proportion of strains worldwide are now resistant to sulphonamides, and many trimethoprim-resistant strains have been isolated in Thailand and Kenya.

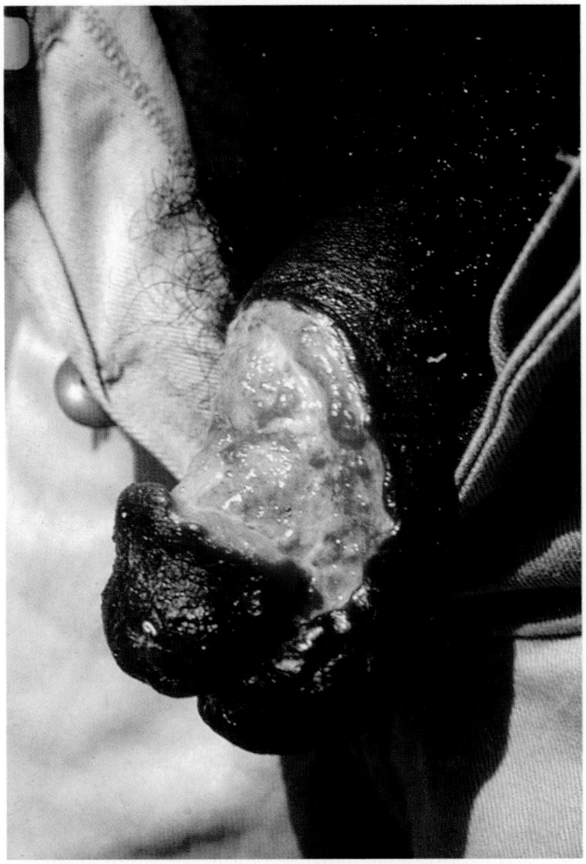

Fig. 14.19. Phagedenic ulcer (D. Mabey).

If treatment is successful, ulcers improve symptomatically within 3 days and substantial re-epithelization occurs within 7 days after onset of therapy. The time required for complete healing is related to the size of the ulcer (and perhaps HIV status); large ulcers may take more than 2 weeks to heal.

Management of fluctuant buboes

The classic strategy has been to needle-aspirate fluctuant buboes from adjacent healthy skin. The procedure is simpler and safer than incision, which is prone to complications (sinus formations). A randomized study conducted during an outbreak of chancroid in the US (Ernst et al., 1995) has shown that careful incision and drainage was also an effective and safe method for treating fluctuant buboes and avoided frequent needle re-aspirations. This procedure should always be performed under effective antibiotic cover.

LGV

Lymphogranuloma venereum (LGV) has in the past also been known as lymphogranuloma inguinale, lymphopathia venereum, tropical or climatic bubo and Durand–Nicolas–Favre disease.

Epidemiology

The epidemiology of LGV is not well defined, as there is no widely available test that is both sensitive and specific, but it is largely confined to the tropics. In most places it accounts for only a small proportion of patients with STIs. It is seen more often in men than women, though the late anorectal complications are more prevalent in women.

Aetiology

LGV is caused by the invasive L1, L2 and L3 strains of *C. trachomatis.*

Pathology

The characteristic pathological features are a thrombolymphangitis and perilymphangitis with proliferation of the endothelial cells of the lymphatics. In the lymph nodes prominent migration of neutrophils leads to characteristic stellate abscess formation.

Clinical features

The disease is important chiefly as a cause of bubo. Up to 50 per cent of cases of confirmed LGV presenting with buboes may not recall having had a genital ulcer (Viravan et al., 1996).

The primary stage, occurring 3–30 days after exposure, is a small, painless ulcer of the genitalia which may pass unrecognized and resolves spontaneously.

The secondary stage is a painful inguinal lymphadenitis, accompanied by fever and malaise.

The infected nodes (bilateral in a third of cases) coalesce into a matted mass which may project outwards below or above the inguinal ligament to give the classical 'groove sign'. The nodes are liable to rupture, forming multiple sinuses. Untreated, the disease may cause extensive lymphatic damage resulting in elephantiasis of the genitalia. The combination of elephantiasis with skin breakdown sometimes seen in late cases is referred to as 'esthiomène'. An additional characteristic feature in long-standing cases is the development of fenestrations in the labia.

In women and homosexual men the disease may present as an acute proctocolitis which, in a proportion of cases, leads much later to abscess formation, fibrosis, fistula and rectal stricture. Chronic LGV may predispose to vulval or rectal carcinoma.

Diagnosis

The laboratory diagnosis of LGV is difficult, and is not possible in most African hospitals. For this reason, syndromic management of inguinal buboes is recommended (Fig. 14.5), which covers both LGV and chancroid. The most reliable laboratory method is the identification *of C. trachomatis* in fluid aspirated from a bubo. It may be necessary to inject 2–5ml of sterile saline in order to aspirate sufficient fluid. *C. trachomatis* can be identified by direct immunofluorescence, antigen detection EIA, PCR or culture (Viravan et al., 1996). High levels of serum antibody (IgG and IgM) to *C. trachomatis* are found, but serological tests lack specificity due to cross-reaction with non-LGV serotypes, and with the common respiratory tract pathogen *Chlamydia pneumoniae.*

Treatment

See Table 14.8. Benefit in late cases, e.g. with rectal stricture, is slight. Plastic surgical operations may be of benefit in cases with extensive elephantiasis or deformity. Biopsy suspicious areas in healed scars to exclude malignant change. Aspirate buboes through adjacent healthy skin.

Donovanosis

Synonyms: granuloma inguinale, granuloma venereum. It is important not to confuse this disease with *lympho*granuloma venereum (see above) or to confuse Donovan bodies (see below) with Leishman–Donovan bodies (leishmaniasis). The disease was first recognized in India, where Donovan observed the bodies that bear his name in an oral lesion.

The problem in Africa

Donovanosis is endemic in southern Africa (O'Farrell & Hoosen, 1997). The disease is strongly associated with prostitution and low socio-economic status. There is strong evidence that it is sexually transmitted in most patients, although some authors have put forward arguments for a non-sexual mode of transmission. The risk of transmission to partners appears to be lower than for other STis, and perinatal transmission is rare.

The organism

Donovanosis is caused by a poorly characterized, encapsulated, Gram-negative coccobacillus, previously called *Calymmatobacterium granulomatis*, recently re-classified as a *Klebsiella* on the basis of ribosomal RNA sequences. It is an intracellular parasite that can be grown in tissue culture.

Pathology

The disease primarily attacks the skin. Bacteria are carried to inguinal nodes where they occasionally cause a suppurating periadenitis ('pseudobubo'), but more often they escape to produce ulcers in the overlying skin. The key histological features are (i) epithelial hyperplasia, (ii) a dense dermal infiltrate of plasma cells, and (iii) scattered large macrophages containing clusters of Donovan bodies. Donovan bodies stain poorly with haematoxylin and eosin but with Giemsa they typically display a capsule and bipolar densities which give a characteristic closed safety-pin appearance.

Clinical features

The first manifestation, appearing after a 3–40-day incubation period, is usually a small papule which ruptures to form a granulomatous lesion that is characteristically pain

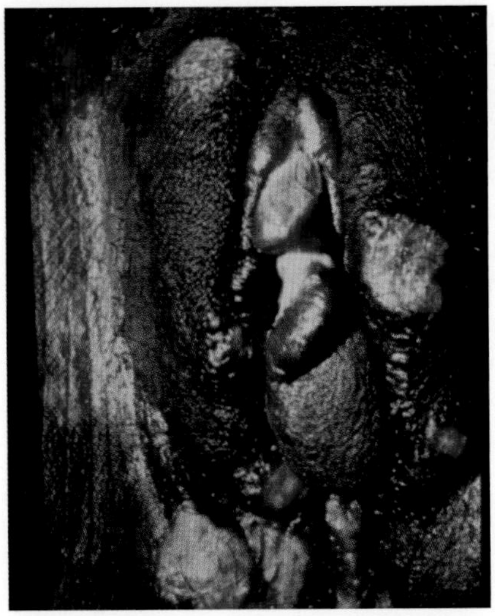

Fig. 14.20. Ulcer due to Donovanosis.

free, 'beefy-red' in colour, bleeds readily on contact and is often elevated above the level of the surrounding skin (Fig. 14.20). The lesion has to be differentiated from other forms of genital ulcer. Most likely to cause confusion are chancroid, condylomata lata, ulcerated warts and squamous carcinoma. Untreated, the ulcers slowly extend, particularly along skin folds towards the groins and anus. Special features are extragenital lesions (mostly neck and mouth), cervical lesions (resemble carcinoma or tuberculous cervicitis), involvement of uterus, tubes and ovaries (hard masses, abscesses, 'frozen pelvis', hydronephrosis) and rare cases of haematogenous dissemination to lung, liver, spleen and bone. Complications include rapid extension of lesions secondarily infected with fusospirochaetal organisms, scarring (in some populations very prominent), elephantiasis, and the development of squamous carcinoma.

Diagnosis

The diagnosis requires the demonstration of intracellular Donovan bodies in either biopsy material (best stained with silver stains or Giemsa) or smears taken from active areas which can be stained by Giemsa or Leishman stains. When collecting specimens, thoroughly clean the lesions of surface debris, detach a small piece of tissue by any suitable means (local anaesthetic is not always necessary) and then, between two glass slides, crush it and spread it for staining.

Treatment

See Table 14.8. Recent studies in Australia have shown that azithromycin is the treatment of choice (Bowden & Savage, 1998). Treatment should be continued until lesions have resolved and, if possible, a little longer to reduce the risk of relapse. Plastic surgical procedures are required in some patients. Treatment of contacts without lesions is not thought necessary.

Herpes simplex virus type 2

Infections with herpes simplex hominis virus type 1 and type 2 (HSV-1 and HSV-2) are amongst the commonest human viral infections. There are two main clinical presentations. HSV-1 is the usual cause of orolabial herpes and HSV-2 of genital herpes, although either viral type can cause either clinical syndrome. HSV-1 is usually horizontally transmitted in childhood and HSV-2 is almost always sexually transmitted, except vertically from mother to baby during delivery.

The problem in Africa

High seroprevalence rates of HSV-2 (40–70 %) and near universal infection by HSV-1 (>90%) have been recorded in population-based studies in Africa (Obasi et al., 1999; Weiss et al., 2001). Prevalence is higher among women and increases sharply around adolescence. HSV-2 seropositive status has been shown to be a marker of high-risk sexual behaviour, correlating with early sexual debut and number of lifetime sexual partners.

HSV-2 is one of the commonest causes of genital ulceration world-wide, but the relative importance of infection appears to vary from place to place. Recent data from Africa indicate that HSV-2 has become an increasingly frequent cause of genitourinary disease (GUD) (O'Farrell, 1999 (see Fig. 14.16)). In countries where co-infection with HIV and HSV-2 is common, HSV-2-associated ulcerations would be expected to increase since HSV-2 reactivation is known to be more frequent and more prolonged in immuno-compromised individuals

Natural history and pathogenesis

Following initial (primary) infection, HSV-2 establishes latency in the sacral dorsal root ganglia. In most HSV-2 infected individuals there is intermittent virus reactivation, with viral shedding occurring on mucosal surfaces. Most recurrences occur in the first year following primary infection, with an average of four to five episodes per year Recurrences are usually shorter and less clinically severe than the primary episode. Asymptomatic viral shedding in the genital tract is common, and most HSV-2 infections are probably transmitted by asymptomatic patients.

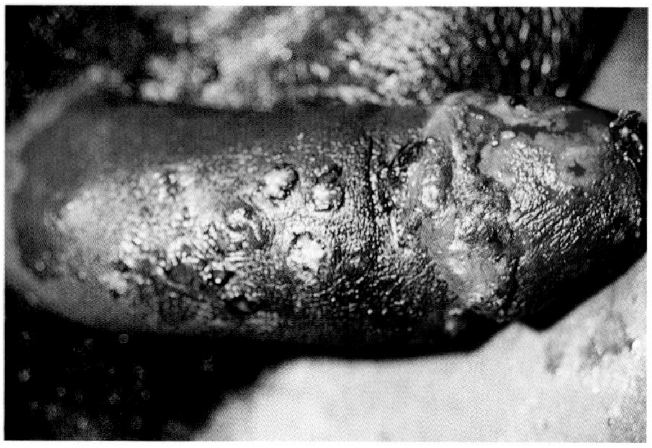

Fig. 14.21. Genital herpes with HIV (P. Mayaud).

The natural history of HSV-2 infection is poorly documented in Africa. Clinical features of HSV-2 infection are less severe in people with prior HSV-1 infection, which is almost universal in African children.

Patients with immunosuppression caused by HIV are more likely to have severe clinical disease and chronic large ulcers. Asymptomatic HSV-2 shedding is also more frequent among women with HIV infection. Conversely, HIV shedding is increased in the presence of HSV shedding. It is likely that HSV and HIV each increases the transmission of the other (Mbopi-Keau et al., 2000).

Clinical features and complications

Primary infection

After an incubation period of 3–5 days, small painful vesicles develop either singly or in clusters surrounded by a zone of erythema (Fig. 14.21). Consitutional symptoms, such as low-grade pyrexia and malaise may accompany this stage. The vesicles soon break into multiple superficial tender ulcers, sometimes accompanied by tender inguinal lymphadenopathy. In the absence of secondary infection, this is followed by crust formation and healing usually occurs within 1–2 weeks.

Lesions may develop anywhere on the external genitalia but rarely occur on the scrotum of men. When the urethra is involved patients may present with symptoms of urethritis (severe dysuria can be caused by the contact of urine with the ulcers). In women, the cervix may be involved either alone or together with the vulva. In both men and women, the rectum, perianal region and pharynx can also be involved.

Recurrent episodes

Lesions follow the same pattern as in primary attack, but with a less severe course. The appearance of vesicles is sometimes preceded by a prodromal phase of pruritus. Consitutional symptoms or lymphadenopathy are rare.

Complications include secondary infections, tender adenitis and urine retention. More serious neurological sequelae such as neuralgia, radiculomyelitis or aseptic meningitis are rare and self-limiting. Frequent recurrent genital herpes episodes may lead to anxiety and depression and put considerable strain upon relationships. In pregnant women recurrences and dissemination are more frequent and premature delivery may complicate primary attacks. Severe and intractable ulceration due to HSV-2 occurs in patients immunosuppressed by HIV.

Diagnosis

Typical herpetic vesicles are recognised clinically (particularly if accompanied with a history of recurrences), but concomitant infections with other ulcerative STI (syphilis, chancroid, LGV or granuloma inguinale) occur frequently and must be excluded by specific tests or managed adequately.

The differential diagnosis includes other vesicular or ulcerative diseases, such as Behçet's syndrome, molluscum contagiosum, erosive balanitis, erythema multiforme and other dermatoses, as well as trauma during sexual intercourse.

The definitive diagnosis rests on viral isolation by culture. Kits for antigen detection are available commercially, and NAAT (nucleic acid amplification tests) have been successfully used to identify HSV-2 in symptomatic and asymptomatic shedders. Serological diagnosis is only of value in a primary attack and in epidemiological studies.

Management

See Table 14.8. No cure is yet available for genital herpes. Patients require explanation, reassurance and advice. Tell them that the disease is likely to recur, and that they will transmit the infection to others if they have sexual intercourse while they have lesions. Advise them to keep the lesions clean and dry. Acyclovir and other antiviral agents have been shown to be beneficial in reducing the severity and duration of the primary attack, in treatment of infected neonates and among adults with immunosuppression or disseminated disease.

Herpes in pregnancy

Transmission from mother to child occurs in 50 per cent of cases with a primary attack at term, but is much lower in patients with recurrences (about 1 per cent). It occasionally occurs as a result of asymptomatic viral shedding by the mother at term. Neonatal herpes carries a 60 per cent mortality which has changed little with the introduction of acyclovir. The presence of active herpetic lesions of the cervix at term is an indication for caesarean section, though this operation does not fully protect against infection developing in the neonate. The use of acyclovir in late pregnancy is being investigated.

Human papilloma viruses (anogenital warts and genital cancers)

The problem in Africa

Infection with human papillomaviruses (HPV) is ubiquitous, and it is one of the most prevalent viral STI. In most populations, prevalence is high in the young sexually active population and declines dramatically after 55 years of age.

There has been only one published truly population-based study of HPV infection among women in Africa to date. Using self-administered vaginal swabs, Serwadda and colleagues (Serwadda et al., 1999), found an overall prevalence of 16 per cent among women in the rural Rakai district of Uganda, being highest among women 15–19 years (25%) with a four-fold decline among women aged 40 and over (7%). Other studies have been conducted in various high-risk groups such as sex workers in Zaire, Abidjan and Kenya, gynaecology outpatients in Abidjan, HIV/infectious disease outpatients in Dakar. Less selected populations have been studied in several African countries (Mayaud et al., 2001), all of which have shown high rates of infection with oncogenic HPV genotypes (between 12 and 34% of women tested). In keeping with these high HPV prevalences, carcinoma of the cervix is the most common cancer among women in the developing world. The incidence and prevalence of anogenital warts are not known in African populations.

The organism

Human papilloma viruses (HPV) are small DNA viruses which can cause a range of diseases from simple skin warts, to genital warts and anogenital cancers. Based on DNA homologies, over 75 different HPV types have been characterized from mucosal (oral and genital) and cutaneous sites. Of the several anogenital HPV types identified, HPV -6 and -11 are typically associated with genital warts with a lower potential for causing neoplasia, whilst genotypes -16, -18, -31, -33, -35 and others are associated with cancers.

Pathogenesis

HPV infects the basal layer of differentiating squamous epithelium and produces a pathognomonic large, clear, perinuclear zone known as koilocytotic atypia. Full assembly of viral particles is confined to the more superficial layers of the epithelium.

Clinical features and complications

Warts caused by HPV vary from the pathognomonic soft, flesh-coloured broad-based or pedunculated lesions characteristic of 'condylomata acuminata' which may become exuberant ('cauliflower-like') and offensive in moist areas, to papular flat warts on drier areas (e.g. shaft of the penis), which resemble those seen on other parts of the body. They can be seen anywhere in the genitalia, including the perianal region, even in those denying anal intercourse. In males, warts are more commonly seen on the fraenum and coronal sulcus. Intraurethral warts may be accompanied by dysuria, discharge and bleeding. In females, the introitus and labia minora are most commonly infected. In pregnancy and in immunosuppressed patients there is a tendency for warts to grow rapidly. Laryngeal papillomas have been reported in infants born to mothers with genital warts at delivery.

Subclinical cervical HPV infections can only be visualized by colposcopy after application of 5 per cent acetic acid or detected in tissue specimens by techniques such as the polymerase chain reaction.

Diagnosis

Condylomata acuminata are diagnosed clinically, but can be confused with condylomata lata of secondary syphilis, molluscum contagiosum and occasionally, verrucose forms of donovanosis.

Cervical cytology using Papanicolaou staining method, where available, is recommended for female patients and female contacts in order to detect progression of lesions to cervical intraepithelial neoplasia (high grade squamous intraepithelial lesions or HSIL).

Management

See Table 14.8. Treatment is generally reserved for macroscopic lesions because subclinical infections show high spontaneous regression rates and also show a strong tendency to relapse with currently available forms of treatment. Care is needed to avoid burning normal skin, which can be protected with glycerine. Podophyllin should be washed off after 4 hours and is contraindicated in pregnant women. Larger warts can be removed with cryotherapy or diathermy.

Persistent cervical lesions and suspicious lesions should be excised surgically. Detection programmes based on cervical cytology screening and colposcopy have been successful in curbing the incidence of cervical cancers in industrialized countries, but are expensive and logistically difficult to run in developing countries.

Ectoparasitic STIs (scabies and pubic lice)

Scabies

The organism

Scabies is caused by the acarus mite *Sarcoptes scabiei*, identified in 1867. Adult scabies mites have an oval non-segmented body structure and 4 pairs of short legs, the front ones with suckers and claws that facilitate entry into the skin. The adult gravid female causes pathology. To lay its eggs during its lifespan of 4–6 weeks, it tunnels into the horny layer of the skin, apparently attracted by specific lipids of human skin, leaving a trail of eggs and faeces, creating the characteristic wavy dark 'burrow'. Eggs hatch within 3–5 days and either tunnel laterally or migrate to enter adjacent hair follicles.

The scabies mite elicits an immune response with IgE antibodies and immediate hypersensitivity reactions that cross-react with dust mites, but it is not clear whether these phenomena help control infestation.

Epidemiology

Infestation occurs during close and prolonged bodily contact, so is often sexually acquired, but can be transmitted by non-sexual contacts in families through sharing of bed linen and clothing, rarely by casual contact.

Clinical features

The most common manifestation of scabies is intense itching, which is worse at night, accompanied by papular eczematous lesions on the sides of the fingers and in the interdigital spaces. The demonstration of burrows is pathognomonic. These can be found on flexor aspects of wrists, ulnar border of the hands and extensor surface of the elbows.

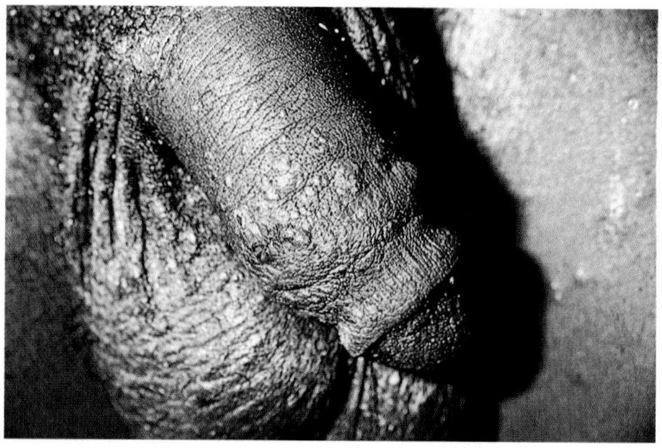

Fig. 14.22. Genital scabies (P. Mayaud).

Genital scabies

When scabies is sexually acquired, lesions occur on the genital organs: in men, on the penis and scrotum (Fig. 14.22); in women, around the umbilicus, on the lower abdomen and buttocks.

Scabies in immunocompromised hosts, including HIV/AIDS

Crusted or Norwegian scabies is a rare, severe form of scabies with florid scaling, itchy lesions. It is more commonly found in patients who are physically or mentally disabled, or immunocompromised. The lesions are highly contagious. The face and scalp, which are rarely involved in immuno-competent patients, may be affected.

Diagnosis

Diagnosis is made on history and clinical examination. Patients present with itchy papular lesions and burrows, sparing the face. Burrows can be made more easily visible by rubbing ink in the area, then wiping it off – the ink remaining visible inside the burrow.

Management

A number of topical acaricidal preparations are available (Table 14.8). In all cases, the preparation must cover the whole body from neck to toe, and help may be necessary to reach the back. Treatment should be applied after washing, and left in place for 12–24 hours (depending on compound used). Treat sexual contacts and those sharing beds simultaneously. Bedding and clothing must be washed in hot water, which effectively kills the mites.

Oral ivermectin (200 μg/kg stat) has been used successfully to treat scabies during epidemics and in HIV patients with diffuse scabies.

Pubic lice or pediculosis pubis

The organism

The crab louse *Phthirus pubis* is the cause of pubic lice. This small wingless insect depends for survival on human blood, and all development stages from egg (or nit) to adult are found on the human host. The pubic louse is about 1–2 mm in length, and can be seen with the naked eye. It is made of three parts (head, thorax and abdomen) with 3 powerful pairs of legs with distal claws giving it the appearance of a 'crab', and enabling it to maintain its hold on hair. It penetrates the skin using its mouth part and producing an anti-coagulant to facilitate blood sucking.

Epidemiology

Phthirus pubis infestation is frequently associated with the presence of other STI; screen patients with pubic lice for such infections. Human lice are transmitted from one person to another primarily by intimate contact, but there are documented cases of transmission by fomites.

Clinical features

The infestation may be asymptomatic, but most frequently causes itching of the pubic area and groins, leading to excoriation, sometimes superinfection, erythema and maculopapular rash. The patient may have noted the presence of lice.

Diagnosis

Careful examination of pubic hair reveals both adult lice and nits clinging to hair. Other hairy parts of the body, with the exception of scalp hair and eyebrows may also be involved. Nits may be differentiated from other foreign material by their cemented oblique attachment to hair whilst foreign material may slide up and down. Crusts or scabs can be removed and observed under the microscope for characteristic morphology and movement.

Management

See Table 14.8. Treatment relies on disinfection of clothing (laundering in hot water or dry cleaning) and application of a pediculocide that can kill both the adult and the egg. The application is to the hairy parts only, and is washed off after 12 hours. Dead lice and nits are removed with a fine-tooth comb. Some authors recommend reapplication 7 days later to kill any surviving nits. Treat sexual partners simultaneously.

Unsolved problems

Operational research to validate treatment algorithms

Before recommending a particular treatment flowchart for STI syndromic management, it is important to have **local** information on the causes of those syndromes, and the antimicrobial susceptibility of *N. gonorrhoeae*. It is particularly important to know the prevalence of *N. gonorrhoeae* and *C. trachomatis* infection in women presenting with vaginal discharge, in order to decide whether to include treatment for these infections in that flowchart.

Rapid, simple, point-of-care diagnostic tests for STIs

These, especially for *N. gonorrhoeae* and *C. trachomatis,* are badly needed, to guide the treatment of symptomatic women, and to enable those without symptoms to be screened, e.g. at antenatal, family planning or occupational health clinics.

Strategies for treating sexual partners

Possible strategies include giving either contact slips or courses of treatment to index cases to pass on to their partners. Few studies in Africa have evaluated either method.

Involving the private sector

There is a need to explore ways of working with private practitioners, pharmacy staff, and traditional healers to improve STI case management in the private sector.

Oral treatment for syphilis

This would simplify the treatment of this condition, and make it easier to eliminate congenital infection. Clinical trials of oral azithromycin are being conducted in some African countries.

References

Adu-Sarkodie Y. (1995). *Trichomonas vaginalis* transmission in a family. *Genitourin Med.*; **71**: 199–200.

Ahmed A, Kalayi GD. (1998). Urethral stricture at Ahmadu Bello University Teaching Hospital, Zaria. *East Afr Med J*; 75: 582–585.

Beem MO, Saxon EM. (1977). Respiratory tract colonisation and a distinctive pneumonia syndrome in infants infected with *Chlamydia trachomatis. N Engl J Med*; **296**: 306–310.

Bewes P C. (1973). Urethral stricture. *Trop Doct*; **3**: 77–81.

Black CM. (1997). Current methods of laboratory diagnosis of *Chlamydia trachomatis* infections. *Clin Microbiol Rev*; **10**: 160–184.

Bowden FJ, Savage J. (1998). Azithromycin for the treatment of donovanosis. *Sex Transm Infect*; **74**: 78–79.

Collet M, Reniers S, Frost E et al. (1988). Infertility in Central Africa: infection is the cause. *Int J Gynaecol Obstet*; **26**: 423–428.

Cotch MF, Pastorek JG, Nugent RP et al. (1997). *Trichomonas vaginalis* associated with low birth weight and preterm delivery. *Sex Transm Dis*; **24**: 361–362.

Dallabetta GA, Gerbase AC, Holmes KK. (1998). Problems, solutions, and challenges in syndromic management of sexually transmitted diseases. *Sex Transm Infect*; **74**: S1–S11.

Elliot B, Brunham R C, Laga M et al. (1990). Maternal gonococcal infection as a preventable risk factor for low birth weight. *J Infect Dis*; **161**: 532–536.

Ernst AA, Marvez-Valls E, Martin DH. (1995). Incision and drainage versus aspiration of fluctuant buboes in the emergency department during an epidemic of chancroid. *Sex Transm Dis*; **22**: 217–220.

Fleming DT, Wasserheit JN. (1999). From epidemiological synergy to public health policy and practice: the contribution of other sexually transmitted diseases to sexual transmission of HIV infection. *Sex Transm Infect*; **75**: 3–17.

Gerbase AC, Rowley JT, Mertens TE. (1998). Global epidemiology of sexually transmitted diseases. *Lancet*; 351**:** SIII2–SIII4.

Grosskurth H, Mosha F, Todd J et al. (1995). Impact of improved treatment of sexually transmitted diseases on HIV infection in rural Tanzania: randomised controlled trial. *Lancet*; **346**: 530–536.

Grosskurth H, Mayaud P, Mosha F et al. (1996). Asymptomatic gonorrhoea and chlamydial infection in rural Tanzanian men. *Brt. Med. J.*; **312**: 277–280.

Hillier SL, Holmes KK. (1999). Bacterial vaginosis. In *Sexually Transmitted Diseases*, 3rd edn, ed. KK Holmes, PF Sparling, PA Mardh et al., pp. 563–586. New York: McGraw-Hill.

Hira SK, Ratnam AV, Sehgal D, Bhat GJ, Chintu C, Lulenga RC. (1982). Congenital syphilis in Lusaka I. Incidence in a general nursery ward. *E Afr Med J*; **59**: 241–246.

Hira SK, Bhat GJ, Chikamata DM et al. (1990). Syphilis intervention in pregnancy: Zambian demonstration project. *Genitourin Med*; **66**: 159–164.

Ison CA, Dillon JR, Tapsall JW. (1998). The epidemiology of global antibiotic resistance among *Neisseria gonorrhoea* and *Haemophilus ducreyi. Lancet* 1998; **381**: SIII8–SIII11.

Jackson DJ, Rakwar JP, Chohan B et al. (1997). Urethral infection in a workplace population of East African men: evaluation of strategies for screening and management. *J Infect Dis*; **175**: 833–838.

Laga M, Meheus A, Piot P. (1989). Epidemiology and control of gonococcal ophthalmia neonatorum. *Bull Wld Hlth Org*; **67**: 471–478.

Laga M, Plummer F A, Piot P et al. (1988). Prophylaxis of gonococcal and chlamydial ophthalmia neonatorum; a comparison of silver nitrate and tetracycline. *N Engl J Med*; **318**: 653–657.

Mabey, DCW. (1994). The diagnosis and treatment of urethritis in developing countries. *Genitourin Med*; **70**: 1–2.

Mauck C, Rosenberg Z, Van Damme L. (2001). Recommendations for the clinical development of topical microbicides: an update. *AIDS*; **15**: 857–868.

Mayaud P. (2001). Infertility in Africa: the role of reproductive tract infections. In: Boerma T, Mgalla Z (Eds), *Women and infertility in Africa: a multi-disciplinary perspective with special reference to Tanzania.* Royal Tropical Institute, KIT Press, Amsterdam, 2001.

Mayaud P, Mabey D. (2000). Cutting edge review. Managing sexually transmitted diseases in the tropics: is a laboratory really needed? *Tropical Doctor*; **30**: 42–47.

Mayaud P, Gill D, Weiss HA et al. (2001). The interrelationship of HIV, cervical human papilloma virus and neoplasia, and other sexually transmitted infections in antenatal clinic attenders in Mwanza, Tanzania. *Sex Transm Infect*; **77**: 248–254.

Mayaud P, Mosha F, Todd J et al. (1997) Improved treatment services significantly reduce the prevalence of sexually transmitted diseases in rural Tanzania: Results of a randomised controlled trial. *AIDS*; **11**: 1873–1880.

Mayaud P, Lloyd-Evans N, West B, Seck K. (2002). GASP-WAR: West African network to tackle gonorrhoea. *Lancet*; **259**: 173.

Mbopi-Keau F-X Grésenguet G, Mayaud P et al. (2000). Interactions between herpes simplex virus type-2 and HIV-1 infection in African women: opportunities for intervention. *J Infect Dis*; **182**: 1090–1096.

Moses S, Manji F, Bradley NE, Nagelkerke NJ, Malisa MA, Plummer FA. (1992). Impact of user fees on attendance at a referral centre for sexually transmitted diseases in Kenya. *Lancet*; **340**: 463–466.

Nugent RP et al. (1991). Reliability of diagnosing bacterial vaginosis is improved by a standardized method of Gram stain interpretation. *J Clin Micro*; 29: 297–301.

Obasi A, Mosha F, Quigley M et al. (1999). Antibody to herpes simplex virus type 2 as a marker of sexual risk behavior in rural Tanzania. *J Infect Dis*; **179**: 16–24.

O'Farrell N, Hoosen AA. (1997). Sexually transmitted diseases in South Africa: epidemic donovanosis in Durban? *Genitourin Med*; **73**: 76.

O'Farrell N. (1999). Increasing prevalence of genital herpes in developing countries: implications for heterosexual HIV transmission and STI control programmes. *Sex Tranm Infect*; **75**: 377–384.

Osegbe DN, Amaku EO. (1981).Gonococcal strictures in young patients. *Urology*; **18**: 37–41.

Peeling RW, Kimani J, Plummer F et al. (1997). Antibody to chlamydial hsp60 predicts an increased risk for chlamydial pelvic inflammatory disease. *J Infect Dis*; **175**: 1153–1158.

Plummer FA, Nagelkerke NJD, Moses S, Ndinya-Achola JO, Bwayo J, Ngugi E. (1991). The importance of core groups in the epidemiology and control of HIV-1 infection. *AIDS*; **5**: S169–S176.

Plummer F A, Laga M, Brunham R D et al. (1987). Postpartum upper genital tract infections in Nairobi, Kenya: epidemiology, etiology, and risk factors. *J Infect Dis*; **156**: 92–98.

Serwadda D, Wawer MJ, Shah KV et al. (1999). Use of a hybrid capture assay of self-collected vaginal swabs in rural Uganda for detection of human papillomavirus. *J Infect Dis*; **180**: 1316–1319.

Sewankambo N, Gray RH, Wawer MJ et al. (1997). HIV-1 infection associated with abnormal vaginal flora morphology and bacterial vaginosis. *Lancet*; **350**: 546–550.

Taha TE, Hoover DR, Dallabetta GA et al. (1998). Bacterial vaginosis and disturbances in vaginal flora: associations with increased acquisition of HIV. *AIDS*; **12**: 1699–1706.

Temmerman M, Mohamedali F, Fransen L. (1993). Syphilis prevention in pregnancy: an opportunity to improve reproductive and child health in Kenya. *Hlth Policy Planning*: **8**: 122–127.

Temmerman M, Hira S, Laga M. (1996). STDs and pregnancy. pp. 169–186. In: Dallabetta G, Laga M, Lamptey P, (eds), *Control of Sexually Transmitted Diseases. A Handbook for the Design and Management of Programs*. AIDSCAP/FHI/USAID.

Viravan C, Dance DAB, Ariyarit C et al. A prospective clinical and bacteriologic study of inguinal buboes in Thai men. *Clin Infect Dis*; **22**: 233–239.

Vuylsteke B, Jana S et al. (2001). Reducing HIV risk in sex workers, their clients and partners. In: Lamptey P, Gayle H, Mane P (eds), *HIV/AIDS Prevention and Care in Resource-Constrained Settings: A Handbook for the Design and Management of Programs*, ed. P Lamptey, H Gayle, P Mane, Chapter 8, pp. 187–210. Washington: FHI Publications.

Walraven G, Scherf C, West B et al. (2001). The burden of reproductive-organ disease in rural women in The Gambia, West Africa. *Lancet*; **357**: 1161–1167.

Wasserheit JN, Holmes KK. (1992). Reproductive tract infections: challenges for international health policy, programs, and research. In: Germain A, Holmes KK, Piot P & Wasserheit JN, eds. *Reproductive Tract Infections: Global Impact and Priorities for Women's Reproductive Health*. For IWHC, Plenum Press, New York 1992: pp. 7–33.

Watson-Jones D, Mugeye K, Mayaud P et al. (2000). High prevalence of trichomoniasis in rural men in Mwanza, Tanzania: Results from a population-based study. *Sex Transm Infect*; **76**: 355–362.

Watson-Jones D, Gumodoka B, Changalucha J et al. (2002). Syphilis in pregnancy in Tanzania II. The effectiveness of antenatal syphilis screening and single dose benzathine penicillin treatment for the prevention of adverse pregnancy outcomes. *J Infect Dis*; **186**: 948–957.

Wawer MJ, Sewankambo NK, Serwadda D, et al. (1999). Control of sexually transmitted diseases for AIDS prevention in Uganda: a randomised community trial. Rakai Project Study Group. *Lancet*; **353**: 525–535.

Weiss HA, Buve A, Robinson NJ et al. (2001). The epidemiology of HSV-2 infection and its association with HIV infection in four urban African populations. *AIDS*; Suppl 4: S97–S108.

World Bank. (1993). *World Development Report 1993: Investing in Health*. New York: Oxford University Press.

World Health Organization (2001a). Guidelines for the management of sexually transmitted infections. Geneva: WHO/HIV_AIDS/2001.01.

WHO (2001b). Global prevalence and incidence of selected curable sexually transmitted infections. Overview and estimates. Geneva: WHO/HIV_AIDS/2001.02.

15 Malaria

Malaria is caused by protozoan parasites of the genus plasmodium. Infection usually results from the bite of female Anopheline mosquitoes, though it can also be transmitted by the transfusion of infected blood. The clinical manifestations range from a self-limiting fever to a severe illness, which may mimic many other infectious diseases. Malaria kills around a million people a year in Africa (Snow et al., 1999), the majority of these are children under 5 years of age and in many areas it accounts for around a quarter of all deaths in this age group. However, malaria also causes significant illness and death in a large number of adults and it therefore needs to be considered in the differential diagnosis of any febrile illness in children or adults.

The organisms

There are around 120 species of plasmodia, causing infections in a wide range of animals including reptiles, birds and mammals. Four species commonly infect humans: *P. falciparum*, *P. malariae*, *P. vivax* and *P. ovale*. All four species are found in the tropics and sub-tropics around the world, though their distribution is variable. *P. vivax* is essentially absent from West Africa because the majority of the population do not carry the Duffy determinant, which the parasite uses as a receptor to enter the host red cell. *Plasmodium malariae* and *P. ovale* are found in most of Africa, but usually cause low density parasitaemia with relatively little serious acute morbidity because they are well adapted to humans (though *Plasmodium malariae* is an important cause of renal disease – see Chapter 83). The key fact is that the vast majority of clinical disease and practically all malaria related deaths in Africa are due to *P. falciparum*. Therefore, except where specifically stated, this chapter concentrates on the epidemiology, clinical features, treatment and prevention of *P. falciparum*.

Life cycle

The life cycle of the malaria parasite is shown in Fig. 15.1.

The parasite in the vector

Female Anopheline mosquitoes become infected when they ingest blood from an infected human. The infective stage of the parasite is known as the *gametocyte*. In the mosquito's stomach the gametocytes undergo a series of changes known as *exflagellation*, followed by a process of sexual division. The dividing parasite forms an *oocyst* attached to the gut wall, before releasing many thousands of *sporozoites* which migrate to the mosquito's salivary glands, from where they are injected when the mosquito next takes a blood meal.

The exoerythrocytic (liver) stage

Sporozoites, which are uninucleate and approximately 11 microns long, circulate in the blood stream for a short time before entering hepatocytes. Here, they replicate rapidly by asexual division before bursting out of the hepatocyte to enter the bloodstream. The length of this hepatic phase varies with species and in *P. falciparum* it is typically about 6 days, by which time the single sporozoite has divided to form a multinucleate schizont with up to 30 000 daughter merozoites packing the hepatocyte. A proportion of the sporozoites of *P. vivax* and *P. ovale* may not develop immediately into hepatic schizonts but enter into a dormant phase, known as the *hypnozoite*, which may go on to form schizonts at intervals many months later. These later infections are known as *relapses*. *P. falciparum* and *P. malariae* do not have a dormant liver stage, though if not adequately treated, the blood stages

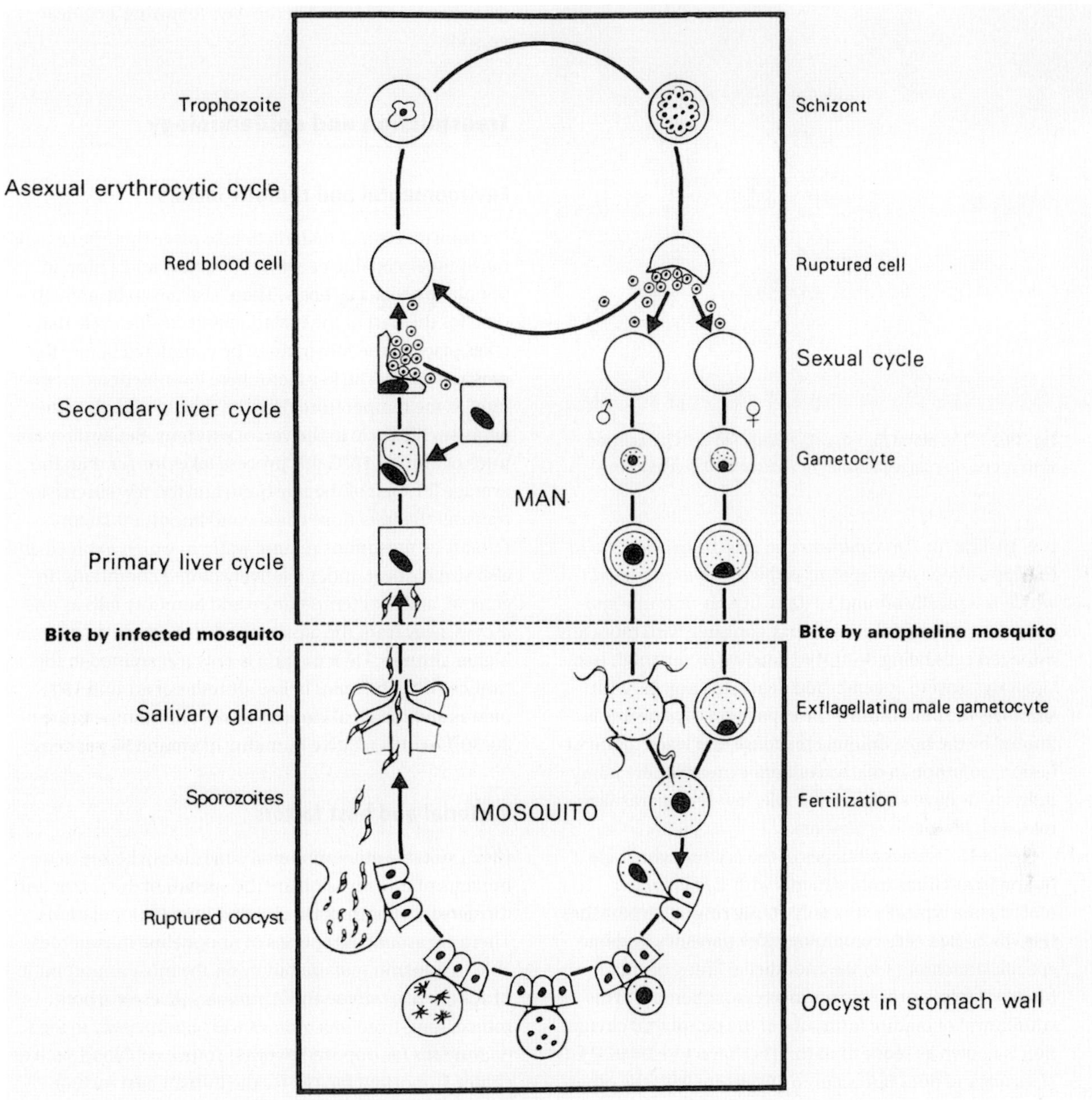

Fig. 15.1. The life cycle of the malaria parasite.

may persist at undetectable levels for long periods. The subsequent reappearance of parasites in the blood stream is known as a *recrudescence.*

The erythrocytic (blood) stage

Merozoites released from the hepatic schizonts have only a short life before being either cleared or entering host red cells. Once inside the red cell, the parasite again undergoes a process of asexual division to form a multinucleate schizont, which then bursts releasing daughter merozoites which attach to and enter new red cells, and so repeat the cycle. The whole red cell cycle takes around 48 hours in *P. falciparum.* These repeated cycles of asexual division lead to rapid exponential growth of the number of infected red cells and it is during this period that the characteristic symptoms of malaria appear. The time from infection to the appearance of parasites detectable on a blood film is known as the *pre-patent period* and

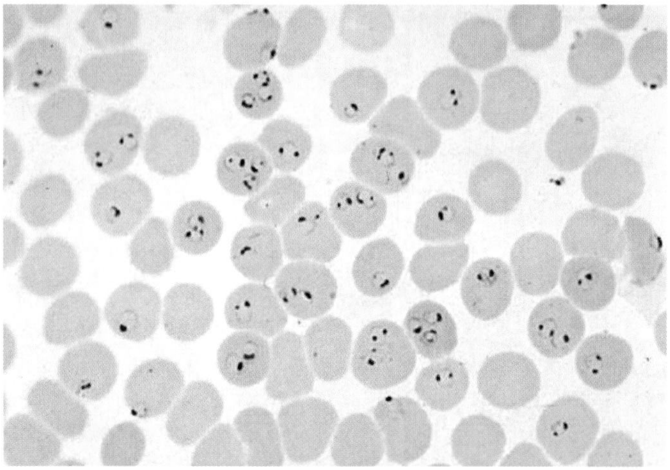

Fig. 15.2. Thin blood film showing many red cells parasitized with young ring stage parasites of *Plasmodium falciparum.*

is 9–10 days for *P. falciparum.* The time from infection to the appearance of symptoms is the *incubation period,* which is typically around 12 days. In non-immune subjects the exponential growth may continue with more and more red cells being destroyed, leading to very high parasitaemias, severe anaemia and death. In subjects with some degree of immunity the expansion of parasites is limited by the host immune response and leads to the situation, common in malaria endemic areas, where many individuals have a relatively stable, low-level parasitaemia, with few or no symptoms.

Figure 15.1 shows all stages of the erythrocytic cycle, but on blood films from patients with *P. falciparum* malaria one typically sees only young ring stage parasites (Fig. 15.2). Red cells containing older parasites undergo specific attachment to the endothelial lining of small blood vessels, a process known as cytoadherence. This withdrawal of mature forms out of the peripheral circulation is known as sequestration. It is characteristic of *P. falciparum* and does not occur to any extent with the other malaria parasites that infect humans. Blockage of small blood vessels by sequestered parasites is believed to be central to many aspects of the pathogenesis of severe malaria.

At some point in the erythrocytic cycle a proportion of the merozoites entering red cells follow a different developmental path and rather than dividing to form yet another schizont, develop instead into the sexual stage of the parasite, forming either a male or female gametocyte. The exact stimuli to form gametocytes are not fully understood, but it is likely that this is a response to various forms of stress as, typically, large numbers of gametocytes are found in the days following a clinical episode.

Transmission and epidemiology

Environmental and climatic factors

For transmission of malaria to take place there have to be mosquitoes capable of acting as vectors and a human population to act as hosts. There also has to be enough time for the part of the malaria parasite's life cycle that takes place in the mosquito to be completed before the mosquito dies. The key factor here is ambient temperature: as the temperature rises the time to complete the parasites life cycle in the vector shortens. Below temperatures of around 18 °C this process takes longer than the average lifespan of the mosquito and too few survive to transmit the infection. The second important factor is rainfall, as mosquitos require water in which to breed and also survive best under relatively humid conditions. In general, ambient temperature and humidity falls as one moves away from the equator and also as one moves to a higher altitude. Thus malaria is only transmitted in the tropics and subtropics below altitudes of around 1600 metres and the ideal circumstances are a temperature of 20–30 °C with a relative humidity of around 60 per cent.

Vectorial and host factors

Given suitable environmental conditions, the key determinants of transmission are the species of the vector and the density of both the vector and human populations. There are around 60 species of Anopheline mosquitoes able to transmit malaria but by far the most important in Africa are *A. gambiae* and *A. funestus.* These are both robust, long-lived mosquitoes with a propensity to feed on humans (as opposed to other sources of blood such as cattle). Important factors for the human host include social and behavioural characteristics, such as the type and density of housing and the use of bed nets, as well as the immune status of the population (see below).

Transmission and endemicity

The complex interactions of climatic, vector and host factors in different parts of Africa leads to a great variation in the amount of transmission, expressed as the average number of infected bites per person per year, or entomological inoculation rate (EIR). This may vary from less than one a year on the edges of the Sahel, to a thousand per year in areas of high rainfall near the equator. This affects both the amount and pattern of clinical malaria seen in a population and a key distinction is that between stable and unstable endemicity. Malaria may be said to be stably endemic when transmission occurs from year to year and leads to a characteristic pattern of immunity whereby older children and adults become immune to the worst effects of the disease. Malaria is said to be *unstable* when there is not reliable year-to-year transmission, for instance where long dry periods followed by rain lead to practically no transmission for long periods and then a sudden epidemic. Under these conditions there is little evidence of acquired immunity to disease and deaths occur in all age groups.

Immunity and age

Repeated exposure to malaria eventually leads to the development of some degree of immunity to the parasite. Immunity to malaria is never complete, in the sense that even adults in highly endemic areas continue to be susceptible to parasitization. They even experience clinical illness, though less frequently than children and illness is rarely more than a short-lived fever. The key point is that, as subjects age, and experience more exposure to malaria, they acquire the ability to limit the consequences of infection, and in particular they are protected from dying from malaria. Under conditions of very high transmission, this may result in the majority of malaria deaths occurring in infants under one year. Under moderate transmission the risk of death is concentrated in children under five years, whereas under conditions of low stable endemicity the ability to limit severe malaria and death may not be established until the early teens. Under all conditions of stable endemicity, asymptomatic parasitization for long periods is part of the normal process of developing immunity. Where the majority of children have a positive blood film at any time, it may be difficult to decide whether any symptoms that do occur are actually caused by the parasites or whether they have another cause (such as a viral infection in a child who just happens to be parasitized).

Risk groups

The subjects most at risk of developing malaria, and particularly severe malaria are those with the least immunity. Thus anyone from a non-endemic area, such as tourists or other travellers, is at high risk at any age. Within areas with stable transmission children under 5 years of age are at particular risk of severe malaria. Pregnancy carries special risks in relation to malaria: women from non-endemic areas or areas of unstable endemicity are prone to develop more severe disease when pregnant. In areas of stable endemicity, where adults have significant degrees of immunity, pregnant women become more susceptible to episodes of parasitization, which may not cause severe symptoms but are associated with the development of both severe anaemia and low birthweight.

Individuals with sickle cell disease are usually considered to be at increased risk of malaria, though the evidence for this is not clear cut. Finally, there is increasing evidence that HIV infection may lead to increased susceptibility to severe disease.

The clinical picture

Uncomplicated malaria

The vast majority of cases of malaria seen in the community or at dispensaries and clinics in Africa are initially mild or uncomplicated. This can be a misleading term because some of these episodes would undoubtedly progress to become severe or life threatening if not treated promptly. In endemic areas the textbook picture of cyclical fevers, rigors and cold sweats is rare. The most common presentation of malaria is as a non-specific febrile illness. A wide range of symptoms may occur, none of which are specific or diagnostic. Headache, backache, general body pains, malaise and vomiting are all common. A mild cough and diarrhoea are both common, especially in children. Many patients and some health workers feel that they can diagnose malaria from the clinical picture. This is a dangerous and mistaken idea and the consequences of being wrong may be serious. The key point is that malaria is a common illness that may mimic many other common illnesses, and therefore the only safe rule is to consider any febrile illness in an endemic area as potentially due to malaria.

Severe malaria

In most African settings severe malaria is predominantly a disease of childhood, though in areas of unstable endemicity all ages may be affected and even in endemic areas a small proportion of patients present with severe disease. The sections below are therefore focused on childhood disease. The principles are essentially the same for adults with severe malaria, though there are some specific differences in presentation and management and these are indicated where relevant.

Table 15.1. Features of severe malaria in children and adults

	Children	Adults
Prostration	+++	+++
Impaired consciousness	+++	++
Respiratory distress	+++	+
Multiple convulsions	+++	+
Circulatory collapse	+	+
Pulmonary oedema (radiological)	+/−	+
Abnormal bleeding	+/−	+
Jaundice	+	+++
Haemoglobinuria	+/−	+
Severe anaemia	+++	+
Renal failure	+/−	++
Hyperparasitaemia	+	++
Hypoglycaemia	++	++

Notes:
See text for definitions +/++ indicates frequency, +/− indicates occurs rarely.

Table 15.2. Practical classification of severe malaria in children (indications for admission to hospital)

[a] Prostrated or any neurological impairment [a] Respiratory distress	High risk, require parenteral and supportive therapy.
Convulsions Haemoglobin <5 g/dl	In absence of prostration or respiratory distress can be managed with oral antimalarials but admit because of risk of deterioration.
Persistent vomiting	Needs parenteral therapy and fluids

Notes:
[a] See text for details.

Definitions of severe malaria

There have been a number of attempts to define and classify severe malaria. Definitions based on the presence of key signs and symptoms, or results from investigations, are useful in identifying specific problems and in allowing standardized comparisons. A definition based on clinical and laboratory features, any one of which should be taken to indicate severe disease, is given in Table 15.1.

In many settings not all desired investigations will be available and in practice the most important decision is whether the patient needs admitting to hospital. Fortunately, a simple set of clinical criteria perform at least as well as the more complex definition above in identifying patients at high risk (World Health Organization, 2000), and a practical classification based on this approach is given in Table 15.2.

The pathogenesis of severe malaria

Malaria is a multi-system disease and not all aspects of its pathogenesis are fully understood. However, there are several key factors which interact to make the difference between a mild self-limiting infection and an acute life-threatening disease.

Exponential parasite growth and red cell destruction

P. falciparum is able to invade red cells of any age, has a relatively short cycle and produces large numbers of merozoites. The result is that the number of parasites in the body can increase with great rapidity, sometimes multiplying by a factor of between 10 and 20 every 48 hours. Even in the absence of any other pathogenic process this would lead to death of the host, as the majority of the body's red cells would be rapidly destroyed. Clearly, the host's ability to control rapid parasite expansion, either by innate mechanisms or acquired immunity, is critical in limiting the ill effects of malaria infection.

It is important to note that it is not only infected red cells that are destroyed as parasites multiply; many uninfected cells are also destroyed, probably by a variety of mechanisms including immune sensitization leading to either haemolysis or mechanical clearance in the spleen. Furthermore, the ability of the bone marrow to respond by producing more red cells is often impaired. The end result of the combination of rapid parasite growth and uninfected red cell destruction is severe anaemia, which leads to a reduction of oxygen carrying capacity. This, in turn, together with obstruction to the microcirculation by sequestered parasites (discussed below) may lead to widespread tissue hypoxia and consequent metabolic acidosis, which is one of the most important prognostic indicators in severe malaria.

Sequestration of infected red cells

A characteristic feature of *P. falciparum* infection is the accumulation of mature parasites in capillaries and post-capillary venules in many tissue of the body, including muscle, brain and kidneys. This process of withdrawal from the peripheral circulation is known as sequestration. When sequestration is heavy the flow of red cells through tissues is likely to be compromised, leading to tissue hypoxia. Sequestration is caused by infected red cells adhering to specific molecules (cytoadherence receptors) expressed on the endothelial cells lining blood vessels. Although several cytoadherence receptors have been identified, two key ones are CD36 and intracellular adhesion molecule 1 (ICAM 1) (for review see Miller et al., 2001). CD36 is distributed widely throughout the body but is largely absent on the endothelium of cerebral vessels, whereas ICAM 1 is present on cerebral vessels. This difference in distribution has led to the idea that cerebral malaria may be caused by parasites with a particularly strong ability to adhere to ICAM1. There is some evidence to support this hypothesis, though in practice it is likely to be more complex (Heddini et al., 2001). Another example of cyto-adherence to specific receptors being associated with a particular clinical picture occurs in placental malaria in pregnant women. Here, parasites with the ability to bind to chondroitin sulphate, which is found on the surface of syncytiotrophoblast, are concentrated in the placenta of infected women (Beeson et al., 2001).

Cytokine activation

Cytokines are chemical mediators, acting either locally or at a distance, released by a range of cells of the immune system, such as macrophages. They include molecules like gamma interferon, tumour necrosis factor (TNF) and a wide range of interleukins. They have multiple effects, such as stimulating further cytokine release from other cells, activating immune responses and causing fever. Many infections lead to different patterns and degrees of cytokine release, and these responses play an important role in protection of the host. However many cytokines in excess also have important negative effects, for instance causing cell damage or death, and the concept has arisen that there may be a critical balance between the protective role of cytokines and their role in damaging the host. In *P. falciparum* infections there are often very high levels of circulating cytokines and for some, including notably TNF, there is a clear relationship between their concentration and the chances of becoming severely ill or dying (Kwiatkowski et al., 1997). The mechanisms of damage are likely to include direct effects on cellular metabolism and stimulation of the release of other toxins. One important aspect may be the role of cytokines in up-regulating receptors mediating the cytoadherence of parasitized red cells (see above) and thus leading to more widespread obstruction to tissue blood flow and consequent hypoxia and metabolic acidosis.

From the above brief discussion it can be seen that there is no single feature of the parasite or host response that can be said to explain the pathogenesis of severe malaria. Rather, it is likely to be the interaction of several processes including the destruction of red blood cells by a combination of rapid parasite expansion and other processes, blocking of the microcirculation leading to tissue hypoxia and a range of effects of cytokine activation. Important consequences are tissue hypoxia and metabolic acidosis in many parts of the body, giving rise to a generalized and multisystem severe illness. In certain circumstances these effects may be focused in particular organs such as the brain, giving rise to characteristic clinical pictures (Marsh et al., 1996).

The clinical features of severe malaria

Although patients with severe malaria may have many different manifestations, the majority of malaria deaths in children occur with one or more of three main clinical syndromes: impaired consciousness, respiratory distress and severe anaemia (Marsh et al., 1995). The relative proportions of the clinical syndromes, and their case-fatality, may vary in different settings and different age groups; however, this classification does none the less provide a fairly robust framework to describe severe malaria in children. The clinical picture of severe malaria in African adults has been less well documented but in most settings impaired consciousness is a major presentation. Renal failure and pulmonary oedema, which are rare as presenting features in children, are important complications in adults in some parts of Africa.

Malaria with impaired consciousness

Definitions

Prostration

Malaria may lead to a range of impairments of neurological function, from lethargy to deep coma. A useful clinical concept to define the milder end of the spectrum is prostration, defined as the inability to sit up in a patient who can normally do so, or inability to feed or drink in a younger child. Prostrated patients are a high-risk group and require urgent and careful assessment and management.

Cerebral malaria

In the past the term *cerebral malaria* has been used loosely to describe patients with any degree of neurological impairment. More recently a rigorous definition based on the presence of deep coma has become widely

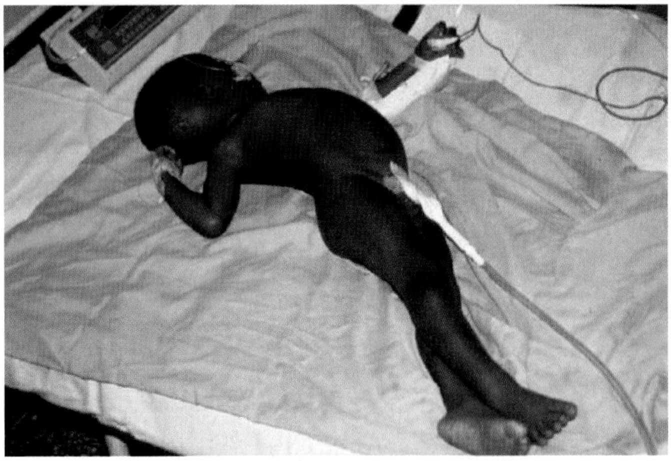

Fig. 15.3. Kenyan child with cerebral malaria showing opisthotonic posturing.

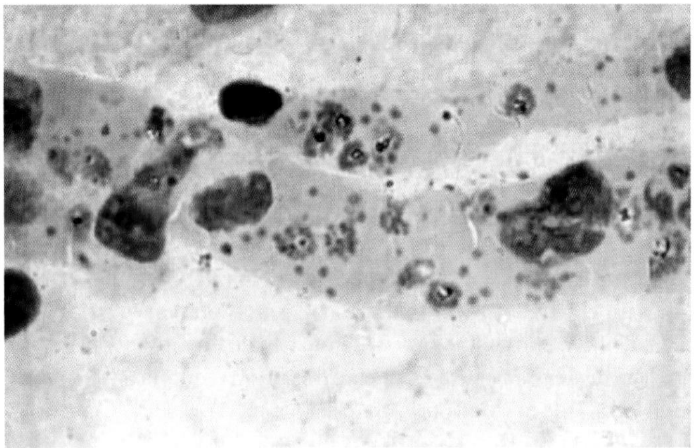

Fig. 15.4. Cerebral microvasculature blocked by sequestered *P. falciparum* parasites in a fatal case of cerebral malaria.

accepted. Cerebral malaria is defined as unrousable coma with the inability to localize a painful stimulus, in the presence of a peripheral parasitaemia and after the exclusion of other causes of coma. In adults this corresponds with a Glasgow coma score of 9 or less. In the section below we will restrict the term cerebral malaria to this more limited definition.

Clinical features of cerebral malaria

Patients presenting in coma typically have had a febrile illness for several days, though exceptionally children present within 24 hours of the first signs of illness. Coma often occurs suddenly following a convulsion, though in some cases the patient may simply become increasingly drowsy and finally unrousable over a period of several hours. On examination the signs are typically of a symmetrical encephalopathy. Muscle tone and reflexes may be either increased or decreased and may fluctuate. In a minority of patients there may be signs of a hemiparesis, which may either resolve rapidly or persist even after the patient has recovered consciousness. Plantar reflexes are often up-going or equivocal. Children in coma typically have their eyes open, which may mislead clinicians more used to examining adult patients. Corneal reflexes are often lost but pupillary reflexes are usually normal, and the development of signs such as asymmetrical pupils or loss of response to light indicate worsening prognosis. Retinal examination may reveal a range of abnormalities including haemorrhages and exudates (Lewallen et al., 1999). Although some degree of raised intracranial pressure is the norm in cerebral malaria, papilloedema is a rare finding. Examination of the cranial nerves is usually normal. A proportion of children exhibit opisthotonic posturing (Fig. 15.3), which may be extreme and lead to the suspicion of meningitis. The cause is not known but recent evidence suggests that in at least some cases this is a form of seizure activity, with implications for therapy (see below). In a small proportion of children (probably around 5 per cent) neurological impairment follows a biphasic course, typically the child recovers consciousness for a period of anything between a few hours and two days, before lapsing back into coma. The pathogenesis of this syndrome is not known and, although the child often makes a full recovery, these children do have a significantly higher risk of permanent sequelae.

Pathogenesis of cerebral malaria

The classical view is that cerebral malaria is a specific syndrome, probably caused by blocking of the cerebral microvasculature by sequestered parasites (Fig. 15.4). However, it has recently become clear that the clinical picture described above can be the result of several different processes, with important implications for treatment. The sections below describe the clinical–pathological syndromes seen in children. It seems likely that cerebral malaria in adults is similarly heterogenous but the relative contribution of different processes is less clear.

Prolonged post-ictal state

Convulsions are common in malaria, and the large majority do not lead to prolonged coma. Usually, such fits are followed by complete recovery of consciousness within half an hour. However, a proportion of children who present in coma have a history of a preceding fit, have no evidence of any other feature of severe disease and regain consciousness between one and eight hours following cessation of the fit. These children have a good prognosis.

Covert status epilepticus

Convulsions are reported at some stage in up to 80 per cent of children in coma with malaria. Recent studies using EEG have shown that, in a proportion of children in coma, there is persistent status epilepticus in the absence of obvious external clinical signs (Crawley et al., 1996). Close examination may reveal minimal signs, such as the occasional twitching of a finger or the corner of the mouth. Some children have intermittent nystagmus, excessive salivation or abnormalities of respiratory pattern, typically shallow irregular breathing. It is extremely important to search carefully for these signs and, in the absence of EEG facilities, to give a careful trial of anti-epileptic therapy, which may lead to surprisingly rapid recovery. In a proportion of children with opisthotonic posturing there is also evidence of electrical seizure activity and, when sustained, these patients should also be given a trial of anti-epileptic therapy. This syndrome has not been described in adults with cerebral malaria, but it is not clear whether this is because it is not a feature or simply that it is difficult to diagnose.

Coma as a response to metabolic stress

Many patients with severe malaria have multiple metabolic disturbances. Hypoglycaemia alone may result in a range of neurological signs, from altered behaviour to profound coma. The commonest and most important metabolic abnormality in severe malaria is a metabolic acidosis (see below). In a proportion of such patients, appropriate management of the acidosis by fluid resuscitation leads to rapid regaining of consciousness, suggesting that in these patients coma is a host response to protect the brain, rather than the expression of a primary neurological problem.

Coma as a primary problem

In addition to the three groups above, one is left with a group of patients who either do not have persistent convulsions or metabolic disturbances, or in whom coma persists after they have been treated. It is assumed that the primary problem in this group is a cerebral insult related to blockage of cerebral blood vessels by sequestered parasites. Survivors typically recover consciousness over a period of between 8 to 72 hours.

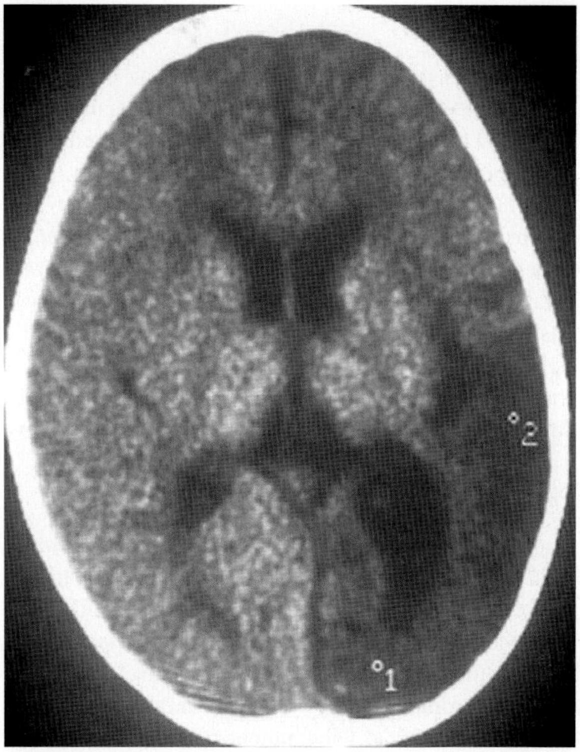

Fig. 15.5. CT scan of the head showing a large occipital infarct in a case of cerebral malaria.

Prognosis of cerebral malaria

The case-fatality of cerebral malaria varies between 10 and 30 per cent (Waller et al., 1995). Around 10 per cent of survivors have obvious neurological sequelae, ranging from relatively mild ataxia to severe global deficits (Brewster et al., 1990) (Fig. 15.5). Around half of these either recover or improve markedly over time. Survivors with cortical blindness typically have a good prognosis, the majority recovering their sight over the following 6 months or so. As well as obvious motor sequelae, more subtle cognitive and behavioural impairment also occurs in around 12 per cent of survivors (Holding et al., 1999). Neurological sequelae are less frequently reported in adults following cerebral malaria.

Respiratory distress

Definition

Respiratory distress is the clinical observation of abnormally deep breathing, intercostal recession or indrawing of the bony structures of the chest wall.

Clinical features

In most cases the episode of malaria will have begun as a febrile illness. In around 20 per cent of patients the only abnormal feature is increasing respiratory effort often developing gradually but occasionally quite rapidly. The other 80 per cent of patients have additional signs of severe disease, either impaired consciousness or severe anaemia or both. In the majority of patients the main respiratory sign is increased depth of breathing and this can easily pass unnoticed unless one specifically examines for it. In the majority of children with respiratory distress there are no abnormalities on auscultation, the oxygen saturation is normal and the lung fields are clear on X-ray.

Pathogenesis

There are a number of possible reasons for a patient with malaria to develop respiratory distress and their relative importance seems to vary between children and adults. In the large majority of children respiratory distress reflects a severe underlying metabolic acidosis, leading to an attempt to compensate by blowing off carbon dioxide (English et al., 1996a). Other potential causes for respiratory distress include congestive cardiac failure or a concomitant pneumonia (English et al., 1996b). Although emphasis has traditionally been put on congestive cardiac failure, in children with malaria, this is probably relatively uncommon (this is discussed below in the section on management of anaemia). In adults, respiratory distress often is a sign of pulmonary oedema and in some cases the patient develops the clinical and radiographic features of adult respiratory distress syndrome (ARDS).

Prognosis

Respiratory distress carries a high mortality. When it occurs as the single major sign or in association with severe anaemia, mortality is around 20 per cent. If the patient also has impaired consciousness, mortality rises to over 30 per cent. In adults ARDS carries a grave prognosis. Children with respiratory distress who survive seem to do so without any specific sequelae, other than those that may be associated with concomitant impaired consciousness.

Severe anaemia

Definition

Severe malarial anaemia is defined in children as a haemoglobin concentration of 5 g/l or less in the presence of asexual parasites on a peripheral blood film. In pregnant women a haemoglobin of 7 g/l or less is usually considered to indicate severe anaemia

Clinical features

The majority of patients with malaria who are severely anaemic present with a simple febrile illness and are noticed to have marked pallor. However, a proportion of such patients present with respiratory distress. At first this may be relatively mild, with the mother reporting that the child has some difficulty breathing. On examination the respiratory rate may be raised and the child may have nasal flaring, a clinical picture that often leads to the diagnosis of a chest infection. A more extreme presentation is the pale child with severe respiratory distress. The patient is tachycardic and tachypnoeic, the depth of breathing is usually markedly increased and there may also be intercostal recession. In such children the presence of a gallop rhythm and a palpable liver often lead to the diagnosis of congestive cardiac failure; however in the large majority of cases the lung fields are clear on auscultation and there is no evidence of pulmonary oedema on the chest X-ray. If blood gases are measured, the patient is usually acidotic, with a negative base excess and a low pCO_2.

Pathogenesis

Some degree of red cell destruction, usually far more than can be accounted for by the loss of only infected cells, accompanies all malaria infections. Destruction of non-infected red cells probably occurs predominantly by removal in the spleen and liver, either because the cells become coated in antibody or complement, or because the cells are damaged by host or parasite products and lose some of their normal deformability. In addition to the loss of infected and uninfected red cells, there is also commonly a degree of dyserythropoeisis, with the bone marrow not producing replacement cells as efficiently as would normally be expected. The clinical presentation is probably more determined by the rapidity of red cell destruction than the absolute haemoglobin concentration. Rapidly developing severe anaemia leads to a reduction in delivery of oxygen to tissues resulting in lethargy, which when severe may lead to the child being prostrated, and to the development of a metabolic acidosis which causes respiratory distress. It is important to recognize that the definition of severe anaemia by haemoglobin concentration is arbitrary; a patient with an acute attack of malaria in which the haemoglobin has fallen quickly from 11 g to 6 g may be extremely ill, while one who has been chronically anaemic may tolerate a haemoglobin of 5 g with remarkably few obvious symptoms. It should also be recognized that it is usually not possible to talk confidently of pure malarial anaemia; patients in malaria endemic environments have multiple reasons to be anaemic, particularly helminth infestation and nutritional deficiency (Newton et al., 1997). The current acute attack of malaria may, in some cases, be the straw that breaks the camel's back.

Prognosis

Patients who are severely anaemic, but who do not have other features of severe disease, usually do well when managed conservatively with oral anti-malarials and haematinics as required. The presence of either impaired consciousness or respiratory distress markedly increases the chance of dying and patients who present with both commonly have a case-fatality rate of 30 per cent or more.

Other manifestations of severe malaria

Convulsions

Convulsions are common with cerebral malaria. However, the large majority of convulsions in children suffering from malaria do not lead to coma. In many cases there is a limited number of relatively brief convulsions, with complete recovery between fits. It has often been argued that these are febrile fits, and are common in malaria because malaria is such a common cause of fever. However, there are persuasive grounds for thinking that this is not the complete story (Waruiru et al., 1996): febrile fits are typically single episodes with no evidence of lateralization. Malaria, by contrast, often gives rise to multiple and complicated fits. Most importantly, the majority of fits with malaria occur at temperatures below 38 °C. Finally, although other species of malaria infecting humans often give rise to higher fever, the incidence of fits is significantly higher in children with *P. falciparum* malaria. Thus falciparum malaria appears to be specifically epileptogenic, though the basis of this remains to be determined.

Hypoglycaemia

Hypoglycaemia is not specific to malaria but is a common finding in severely ill children with a range of diagnoses. In most settings around 15 per cent of children with severe malaria are hypoglycaemic on admission to hospital (English et al., 1998). This may be manifest in a number of ways, from slightly odd behaviour to profound coma. Although hypoglycaemia is normally caused by malaria itself, it can also be a complication of treatment with quinine, which may lead to hyperinsulinaemia. For reasons that are not understood, quinine-induced hyperinsulinaemia seems to be mainly a problem in adults and particularly in pregnant women but rarely occurs in children (Taylor et al., 1988). Hypoglycaemia is associated with an increased risk of death and in survivors is associated with the risk of developing neurological and cognitive sequelae

Circulatory collapse

Circulatory collapse, or shock, occurs when the blood pressure cannot be maintained within normal limits. The patient becomes prostrated and may have impaired consciousness ranging from confusion to deep coma. The patient typically has cool peripheries and prolonged capillary refill time. The reduction in tissue oxygen supply will lead to, or exacerbate already existent metabolic acidosis and this may be manifested by respiratory distress. Established shock is a commoner finding in adults with severe malaria than in children, probably because children maintain their blood pressure well for a while but when circulatory collapse occurs it leads rapidly to death. Circulatory collapse carries a grave prognosis and requires immediate aggressive resuscitation.

Hyperparasitaemia

The importance of high parasite density as a risk factor varies with patient group and transmission conditions and needs to be defined locally. As a rule of thumb, in children in endemic areas a parasitaemia of 20 per cent or more should be considered to indicate severe malaria. In areas of unstable endemicity a parasitaemia of 4 per cent indicates potentially severe disease.

Renal failure

Renal failure may occur in severe malaria in non-immune adults and older children. It typically occurs as part of multi-organ involvement in patients who present prostrated or in coma, or as a late event in patients who are recovering following treatment. Acute tubular necrosis leads usually to oliguria or anuria, though occasionally the patient enters a polyuric phase relatively quickly. In children in endemic areas established renal failure is very unusual, though pre-renal failure reflected in a raised serum creatinine or urea is common, due to hypovolaemia.

Haemoglobinuria

Haemoglobinuria is an occasional finding, commoner in adults than in children. The pathogenesis is unclear. Although G 6PD deficiency may play a role, this is by no means always the case. These patients are not usually in renal failure and the haemoglobinuria usually resolves within a few days.

Hepatic dysfunction

Hepatic dysfunction, reflected in mild disturbances of liver enzymes, is common in malaria. Clinically obvious jaundice is common in adults with severe malaria but relatively rare in children in endemic areas. Deep jaundice or clinically evident liver failure are not features of severe malaria and their presence should prompt the search for an additional or alternative diagnosis.

Bleeding abnormalities

Thrombocytopenia is common in malaria and is not in itself related to the severity of the disease. Mild disturbances of laboratory tests of coagulation are not uncommon. Clinical evidence of a bleeding tendency, including petechiae and oozing at injection sites may occur, particularly in adults with evidence of multi-system involvement. It is rare in children, occurring in less than 1 per cent of severe cases.

Management

The management of malaria in an outpatient setting

The circumstances of busy outpatient clinics often preclude detailed history taking. It is therefore important to concentrate on key information, which may alter management.

- Does the patient really have malaria?

Whenever possible the diagnosis should be confirmed by examination of a thick blood film stained with Giemsa or Fields stain. However, in practice management often has to be initiated without this information. Even when it is available, interpretation is not always straightforward because many subjects in an endemic area have a positive blood film and it may be difficult to know whether this accounts for the symptoms or whether it is simply a coincidental finding. It is therefore essential to think of, and to actively exclude, other possible causes of febrile illness such as otitis media, chest infections or urinary tract infection. One is often left in a position of having to apply clinical judgement and the key point is that in patients who are susceptible to severe malaria (children, pregnant women or non-immune patient of any age) it is best to err on the side of caution and to treat with antimalarials all patients with a febrile illness.

- Has the patient already received treatment?

In most African countries home treatment of febrile illness is extremely common. If the patient has already received an adequate dose of an acceptable first-line drug, a decision will have to be made as to whether to give symptomatic treatment only and keep under review, or whether to use a second-line drug.

- Has the patient travelled?

It is easy to assume that older children or adults in an endemic area are at lower risk but it may be that the patient is a visitor from a non-endemic part of the country. Similarly, in an area of low endemicity it is easy to forget the possibility of malaria but the patient may have travelled to an area of active transmission.

- Does the patient need admitting or referring?

Patients should be assessed for two key signs: prostration and respiratory distress (see Table 15.2). Prostration is the inability to sit up in a patient who is old enough to do so normally, or inability to drink or suck in a younger child. Respiratory distress is any visible impression of increased depth or effort of breathing (intercostal recession or retraction). All such patients should be admitted to hospital for parenteral treatment. Other patients who may be capable of taking oral treatment but who should be admitted because of the risk of clinical deterioration include those with severe anaemia (haemoglobin less than 5 g per litre) and those who have had convulsions in the current illness. Ideally, any patient with a history of convulsions should be admitted and fully investigated, including performance of a lumbar puncture, but in practice many children with a previous history of febrile fits are safely managed as outpatients if they have had a single brief fit and are fully conscious and have no other signs of being severely ill. Febrile fits are uncommon before 6 months of age and after the age of 6 years, and all such patients with even a single fit should be admitted and fully investigated. Patients who have none of the above signs or symptoms but who have persistent vomiting require admission for parenteral therapy.

Treatment of uncomplicated malaria

The management of uncomplicated malaria is, in principle, straightforward, requiring a full course of an effective anti-malarial. For many years in Africa this essentially meant treatment with chloroquine, a safe, effective and easily affordable drug. Unfortunately, chloroquine resistance is now widespread, worst in south and eastern Africa but an increasing problem in all countries. Many countries are in the process of re-evaluating their national policies. Some countries have already changed to sulphadoxine–pyrimethamine (SP) as first-line treatment and others are now recommending that SP be used in combination with chloroquine or amodiaquine. In a rapidly changing situation it is no longer possible to give a single treatment recommendation for all areas and the key point is for clinicians to be aware of local resistance patterns and of the national policy. Drugs commonly used for the treatment of uncomplicated malaria are summarized at the end of this chapter.

In addition to anti-malarials it is usual to give antipyretics for symptomatic relief. Aspirin should be avoided in children, in whom paracetamol is the drug of choice. Opportunity should also be taken to inform the patient, or the patient's parents, on important issues relating to malaria, for instance the desirability of using a bed net, and what to do for future fevers. In the case of children, vaccination and nutritional status should also be checked.

The management of severe malaria

At the point of first contact, one is essentially dealing with the assessment of the severely ill patient. There may be no definite diagnosis and even if a blood film result is available, it may not be clear what role the malaria parasites are playing in the illness. Therefore, the assessment and initial management is essentially that of any severely ill patient.

- Is the airway clear?

The airway may be blocked by secretions, particularly if the patient has been convulsing, or vomitus if the patient is in coma, and this requires immediate clearance and establishment of a clear airway.

- Is the patient breathing normally?

A number of abnormalities of breathing pattern may be noted in children with cerebral malaria (Crawley at al., 1998). The most immediately important is that the child may be hypo-ventilating, often with an irregular rhythm. If a transcutaneous pulse oximeter is available, use it as a guide to the seriousness of the situation and to monitor management. If not available, management must be guided by careful clinical assessment of rate, depth and rhythm. The commonest cause of hypo-ventilation is that the chid is having a convulsion and the abnormal breathing pattern may be the only manifestation of this. Occasionally during a fit the child may develop laryngeal spasm, clinically evident as ineffective and uncoordinated chest movements. If there is any suspicion that the child is hypo-ventilating, try to improve airflow by bag and mask and by the use of oxygen. If the hypoventilation persists, give a rapidly acting anti-convulsant. If diazepam (0.3 mg/kg) is used, it should not be given as a rapid bolus but injected slowly over several minutes while maintaining assisted ventilation with bag and mask.

- Is circulation adequate?

Assess the circulatory state by feeling the temperature of the peripheries and by taking the blood pressure, which should be compared against standard tables of the range for age. Very cool peripheries and delayed capillary bed refill are a sign of severe circulatory compromise and should lead to immediate attempts to restore circulating fluid volume. Give twenty mls per kilogram of resuscitation fluid intravenously as rapidly as possible. The fluid used will depend on availability; most commonly this will be normal saline. If available, colloids are more appropriate for immediate resuscitation. Whole blood is an ideal resuscitation fluid, especially in a setting where the patient is likely to be anaemic, however it is unlikely that this will be immediately available and on no account should resuscitation be delayed whilst waiting for blood to become available. The aim is to restore circulation, judged by improvements in blood pressure and detection of peripheral pulses, thereafter the patient will require careful assessment of further fluid requirements (see below).

- Is the patient hypoglycaemic?

If there is any evidence of disturbed consciousness, check immediately for hypoglycaemia. This is best done by bedside dipsticks. If these are not available, assume that any unconscious patient is potentially hypoglycaemic and give dextrose, preferably 2 ml per kg of 25 per cent dextrose or 5 ml per kg of 10 per cent dextrose. The dextrose should run in over several minutes and not be injected as a rapid bolus, as this may lead to hyperglycaemia and subsequent rebound hypoglycaemia.

- Is the patient convulsing?

Terminate convulsions lasting beyond five minutes with a rapidly acting anti-convulsant such as diazepam given intravenously over five minutes at a dose of 0.3 mg per kg (up to a maximum dose of 10 mg).

Management once immediate emergencies have been dealt with

Perform a complete physical examination, paying particular attention to assessing the level of consciousness, request investigations and consider the differential diagnosis. If facilities are available, request the following investigations:

Blood film

To confirm the diagnosis and assess parasite density.

Full blood count

The most important parameter is the haemoglobin concentration. Other measurements have less immediate relevance to management. A low mean cell volume may indicate the presence of iron deficiency but normal values do not exclude it. The total white cell count or neutrophil count may be normal or raised but in children is not a reliable guide to the presence of additional bacterial infection. The platelet count is commonly reduced, sometimes to less than 10 000 but is rarely associated with clinical manifestations and has no prognostic value.

Measure ***blood glucose***: in any patient with neurological impairment.

Hypoglycaemia is defined as a blood glucose concentration of less than 2.2 mmol/l.

Blood gases

Metabolic acidosis is a common feature of severe malaria and the degree of acidosis is directly correlated with prognosis. A base excess greater than minus 10 is an indication for specific fluid management. Monitoring changes in base excess allows careful adjustment of fluid regimens.

Creatinine

Patients often have a mildly raised creatinine at presentation, due to a degree of dehydration. In adults a creatinine concentration of greater than 265 μmoles/l, which persists despite rehydration, indicates acute renal failure.

Blood cultures

Septicaemia is an important differential diagnosis and a proportion of children with severe malaria are also bacteraemic.

Serum electrolytes

Whilst part of the assessment of any severely ill patient, electrolyte abnormalities requiring specific management are unusual in malaria. A degree of hyponatraemia is common, but usually self-correcting as the patient improves.

Request a *chest X-ray* in any patient with respiratory distress, looking for evidence of concomitant infection or pulmonary oedema.

Lumbar puncture

Examine the CSF in any patient with evidence of neurological dysfunction to exclude meningitis. If there are concerns over the safety of this, for instance in patients with lateralizing signs or very deep coma, it may be necessary to delay until the patient is neurologically stable. If this is done, the patient should be covered with broad-spectrum antibiotics as for the treatment of bacterial meningitis.

Differential diagnosis

Severe malaria may be confused with practically any cause of severe illness in both children and adults. In endemic areas the presence of a positive blood film *per se* does not establish that malaria is the primary problem, though it does indicate that the patient should receive a full course of anti-malarials, whatever other pathology may be present.

The other diagnoses to consider depend on the clinical features but the most important are severe bacterial infections, including septicaemia, pneumonia and meningitis, intoxications and poisonings (for example alcohol or pesticide ingestion), metabolic problems (for example, diabetes, renal failure or hepatic failure) or cerebrovascular accidents.

Anti-malarials

Anti-malarials should be given as soon as possible. Patients who can definitely take and retain oral medication should be treated with the current nationally recommended first-line anti-malarial, unless they have already received this, in which cases they should be given the recommended second-line drug. All other inpatients require parenteral anti-malarials. At the time of writing, quinine remains the parenteral drug of choice throughout Africa. There is evidence that achieving therapeutic levels quickly is important (White, 1996), and where feasible treatment should begin with a loading dose of 20 mg per kg in normal saline run in over 4 hours. Maintenance doses of 10 mg per kg should be given at intervals of either 12 or 8 hours and run in over 2 hours (where there is no reduced parasite sensitivity to quinine 12-hourly maintenance is sufficient. Eight-hourly maintenance should be used where stipulated by local guidelines or where parasite quinine sensitivity status is unknown). Quinine is cardiotoxic and must never be given as a bolus. Absorption characteristics following intramuscular injection are very similar to those achieved by intravenous administration and this route may be used if quinine can not be safely or reliably given intravenously. For intramuscular injection, the quinine solution should be diluted one in five in sterile water; the loading dose should be split between both thighs and subsequent doses given in alternate thighs. Parenteral treatment may be discontinued and the patient put on oral therapy with either quinine or the recommended first line anti-malarial once the patient is eating and drinking. In practice, many patients dislike continuing with quinine and it may be easier to switch to an alternative. However, this decision needs to be made in the light of local knowledge on levels of resistance to the first line oral anti-malarial drug.

The artemesinins (particularly artemether or artesunate) have been shown to be at least as effective as quinine in the management of severe malaria and are an appropriate alternative. Dosages are given at the end of this chapter.

Management of anaemia

Many patients with severe malaria are markedly anaemic. The key decision is whether the patient needs a blood transfusion. Because blood is often in short supply and because there are inherent risks in transfusion, the need for transfusion needs careful weighing. Many children with haemoglobin concentrations between 4 and 6 gm/dl, but without other signs of severe disease, do well with oral anti-malarials and haematinics and the clinical state of the patient is more important than the absolute haemoglobin concentration. Any of the following is a definite indication for transfusion in children with haemoglobin concentrations less than 6 g/dl:

- any evidence of circulatory collapse
- significant respiratory distress (deep breathing or in drawing)
- impaired consciousness
- a haemoglobin concentration of 4 g/dl or less.

In other cases, for example a patient without the above signs, hyperparasitaemia may push one to transfuse if blood is readily available because of the chance that the patient may deteriorate as the haemoglobin continues to fall. The key point is that, if transfusion is withheld in an anaemic patient, it is essential to review the patient at regular intervals and to be prepared to reverse this decision.

It is common practice to give the transfusion very slowly in patients with malaria because of the perception that they may be in cardiac failure. However, in most cases the main problem is a metabolic acidosis, giving rise to an increased respiratory drive. Most of these patients are in high-output cardiac failure, i.e. they can not deliver enough oxygen to the tissues despite maximum cardiac effort, rather than congestive cardiac failure. This presents a management problem, as acidotic patients in high-output failure require rapid transfusion, whereas this may be dangerous in patients in left ventricular failure. It may be extremely difficult to make the distinction; clinical signs such as an enlarged liver or a gallop rhythm are not particularly useful as they are common in children with malaria. The clinical finding of bilateral basal crackles on auscultation is strongly suggestive of left ventricular failure, as is radiographic evidence of marked cardiomegaly or pulmonary congestion.

In the absence of these findings, it is sensible in the majority of patients, who have a degree of respiratory distress but who are not *in extremis*, to give blood at an intermediate speed of 20 ml per kg over 4 hours. In patients who are severely distressed begin the transfusion at a rate of 10 ml per kg to be given over the first 30 minutes, thereafter giving the second 10 ml per kg over 3 hours. The key point is that all such patients should be observed continuously as the transfusion proceeds. In the event of worsening condition, particularly if accompanied by the new appearance of basal crackles, the transfusion should be slowed down to run over 6 hours and, if necessary, a dose of a diuretic (frusemide) given intravenously.

Fluid management

Patients with severe malaria are often relatively dehydrated due to a combination of decreased intake and increased loss (English et al., 1996c). This would argue for patients needing a higher than normal fluid intake. On the other hand, patients in coma may have raised intracranial pressure, giving rise to concern that a high fluid intake may lead to cerebral oedema. In such a situation blanket recommendations are not useful and may be dangerous and it is essential that each patient be carefully assessed. However, patients are likely to fall into the following four categories:

Patients who can be managed with oral fluids

Those patients admitted because of anaemia or repeated convulsions but with none of the other signs of severity can usually be managed with oral fluids as required. Diarrhoea is common in children with malaria. Children with diarrhoea should be encouraged to take oral rehydration fluid.

Patients requiring maintenance with parenteral fluids

Patients unable to take oral fluids but who have no clinical signs of dehydration, circulatory collapse, or deep breathing should be given isotonic maintenance fluids at a rate appropriate for their size (this can be calculated by giving 4 ml per kg for the first 10 kg of body weight, 2 ml per kg for the second 10 kilos and 1 ml per kg for each additional kg. Thus a 10 kilo child would require 40 ml per hour while a 70 kg adult would require 110 ml per hour. In adults normal saline is an appropriate replacement fluid. In children appropriate maintenance fluids include half strength Darrow's solution, half-strength Hartmann's solution or 0.18 per cent saline with 4 per cent dextrose. These may be alternated with normal saline.

Patients who require increased maintenance fluids

The resuscitation of the patient in circulatory collapse is dealt with above, as is the special case of the patient who requires acute blood transfusion. Other patients requiring increased fluids are those with clinical signs of dehydration or of respiratory distress (indicative of underlying metabolic acidosis). The amount of fluid required and time over which it needs to be given has to be based on assessment of the individual – the more severely ill the higher the volume and the more rapidly it should be given initially. As a general guide patients with obvious signs of dehydration or respiratory distress should receive an initial infusion of 20 ml per kg over 30 minutes to an hour and then continue at twice normal maintenance rates. It is essential that the requirements for additional fluids be continually re-assessed. Normal maintenance rates should be given after 24 hours and the patient returned to oral fluids as soon as s/he is able to take them.

Patients who require reduced maintenance fluids

As indicated above, there is a concern that patients in coma may be susceptible to cerebral oedema and these patients should be maintained on 60 per cent of normal maintenance fluids. However, it should be stressed that establishment of normal circulating volume and resolution of acidosis should take precedence, therefore the initial fluid management of patients in coma who have any signs of dehydration or respiratory distress should be as above, only switching to reduced maintenance levels when the patient is in a stable condition.

Management of convulsions

Convulsions are a common feature of malaria in children. In the majority of cases the child recovers consciousness quickly, though this may be followed by further convulsions. Convulsions are also an important feature of cerebral malaria in both children and adults. The principles of management are the same whether they occur as an isolated problem or as part of cerebral malaria. In the acute situation it is important to ensure that the patient is lying in the recovery position and that the airway is not compromised. It is also important to reassure relatives, who usually find the situation very worrying. The majority of convulsions are self-limiting within a few minutes and do not require specific intervention. This is, however, required when the convulsion continues for more than 5 minutes, or when shorter convulsions occur repeatedly with only short intervening periods. In such cases, give a rapidly acing anti-convulsant such as diazepam or paraldehyde. Diazepam is given in a dose of 0.3 mg per kg (up to a maximum of 10 mg in older children and adults) intravenously; it should be injected slowly over 5 minutes. If intravenous access is not possible it can be given intrarectally in a dose of 0.5 mg per kg. Diazepam should not be given by intramuscular injection, as its absorbtion may be unpredictable. If the convulsion is not controlled within five minutes a second dose of diazepam may be given cautiously. Diazepam is a respiratory depressant and the patient's breathing should be closely monitored.

Paraldehyde is an anti-convulsant with less risk of leading to respiratory depression. Unfortunately its use has declined and it is not available in many settings. Where it is available, it is a good alternative to diazepam in either primary management or as an alternative agent in patients whose convulsions are not controlled by diazepam. It should be drawn up in a glass rather than a plastic syringe, is given as an intramuscular injection in a dose of 0.2 ml per kg (max 10 ml) and may safely be repeated. If convulsions are not controlled following the above approach, the patient should be given phenobarbitone 15 mg per kg, either as a slow intravenous injection or as an intramuscular injection. Phenytoin is an alternative; however it is more expensive, slower to act in the acute situation and has to be given by slow infusion in saline (18 mg per kg over 20 minutes).

The use of antibiotics

Pathogenic bacteria are isolated from blood cultures in a significant minority of patients with severe malaria (Prada et al., 1993). There are probably two things going on here: first, at the time of admission it may be impossible to be sure whether a low-level parasitaemia in a severely ill patient is really the cause of the problem, i.e. the primary diagnosis may not be malaria. Second, it does seem that bacteraemia may be a feature of severe malaria in some situations, particularly non-typhoid salmonellae in children. This presents a problem in management. Many hospitals are not able to perform blood cultures and even when this is possible results will not be available in time to affect management over the critical first 48 hours. One alternative is to begin all severely ill patients on broad spectrum antibiotics, but this may not always be possible because of cost. A reasonable compromise is to target antibiotics to those at highest risk, such as patients with respiratory distress or impairment of consciousness, particularly those under 3 years of age.

The comatose patient in whom meningitis remains a possibility presents a special case. Ideally all such patients require immediate lumbar puncture and examination of CSF but in practice this may not be possible due either to lack of resources or because the patient is neurologically unstable and there is a concern over raised intracranial pressure and therefore the risk of coning. The key point is that, if an immediate lumbar puncture cannot be carried out, the patient should be covered with the locally recommended parenteral antibiotic for the treatment of meningitis.

Adults with malaria

Adults born and living all their lives in non-malarious areas have no immunity to malaria and are just as susceptible to severe disease as young children from endemic areas. This may be obvious in the case of a visitor from a non-tropical country but it is important to remember that in some African countries quite large areas, particularly those at high altitude, are not malarious but people born there may travel to other parts, for example for schooling or in search of work. In general, severe malaria and the principles of management in adults are similar to that described above for children. However, there are significant differences. For instance, pulmonary oedema and ARDS are commoner in adults, as is renal failure, while convulsions are considerably less common. Important differences have been noted in the main text above and are summarized in Table 15.1.

Malaria in pregnant women

Malaria presents a special risk for both the pregnant women and her baby. In non-immune women clinical attacks may be especially severe and the woman is particularly prone to pulmonary oedema and to hypoglycaemia (White et al., 1996). There is an increased risk of miscarriage or premature delivery. Women who have grown up in an endemic area, and who have therefore developed a considerable degree of immunity, are at increased risk of parasitization. This appears to be due not so much to a generalized failure of immunity but to the specific targeting of malaria parasites to the placenta. The woman may not be obviously symptomatic at the time of her antenatal visit but may develop severe anaemia, particularly if she also has other risk factors such as poor iron intake or hookworm infestation.

The presence of malaria parasites in the placenta interferes with placental function and may reduce birthweight, which in turn predisposes the baby to increased risk of death from a range of causes. All episodes of malarial parasitization, whether symptomatic or not, should be treated promptly with an effective anti-malarial. In the past, chemoprophylaxis with chloroquine was recommended for all pregnant women, but widespread chloroquine resistance has now rendered this ineffective in most settings. Recent studies have demonstrated that intermittent treatment with a sulphadoxine–pyrimethamine combination, two or three times during the course of the pregnancy, significantly reduces the incidence of severe anaemia and increases mean birthweight. This policy has been adopted in a number of countries. It is likely that the effectiveness of this approach will be compromised as resistance to SP drugs spreads and other drugs for intermittent treatment of pregnant women are urgently needed. The approach taken should be that recommended in the national policy guidelines but the key point is to recognize the importance of malaria in pregnancy in all settings.

The prevention of malaria

Whenever a patient presents with clinical malaria, it represents to some degree a failure of prevention. Malaria can be prevented in two main ways: avoidance of biting by Anopheline mosquitoes and the use of prophylactic drugs. Even when malaria occurs, the progression to life threatening disease can be prevented by early appropriate treatment.

Anti-vector strategies

In the middle of the last century a group of powerful insecticides, such as DDT, were developed which were so effective that they seemed to offer the prospect of actually eradicating malaria by attacking its vector. Whilst this was achieved in many areas at the outer limit of malaria's distribution, such as southern Europe, it quickly became clear that this would not be possible in sub-Saharan Africa where the environment, in terms of temperature and rainfall, allows both maximum growth of mosquito populations and maximum chance that the mosquito will live long enough to transmit malaria. In these circumstances the aim has to be to reduce the chances of being bitten by *Anopheline* mosquitoes to a minimum. This can be achieved by a variety of approaches.

Environmental management

Anopheline mosquitoes can breed in a variety of water sources including both natural collections, such as ponds and ditches, and man made collections such as discarded car tyres and potholes. It is common sense to reduce such breeding sites to a minimum in the vicinity of dwellings and in many countries legal provisions exist to enforce this. For bodies of water too large to be drained, various approaches such as larviciding or the introduction of natural predators for mosquito larvae, such as fish, have been used. Whilst environmental control alone is unlikely to have a major effect on the incidence of malaria in most settings, it may none the less be important as a highly visible way for public health authorities to stress the importance of mosquitoes in transmitting malaria as part of a concerted programme to apply other approaches, such as the use of impregnated bed nets.

House spraying

In many parts of the world residual house spraying has formed the corner-stone of vector reduction activities for many years. It is based on the application of long-acting preparations of insecticides to the walls of houses, so that any mosquitoes resting there will be killed. Whilst undoubtedly effective, its use requires substantial resources in terms of manpower and transport. It is also difficult to apply in rural areas with dispersed housing, which of course includes the majority of high-risk areas. These difficulties have led to a reduction of its use in many areas in favour of approaches such as impregnated bed nets (see below). However it remains an important tool for malaria control in defined situations such as densely populated urban areas and in the control and prevention of outbreaks in areas of unstable transmission.

Impregnated bed nets

Mosquito nets have been used for personal protection in malaria endemic areas around the world for many years. The rationale for their use in Africa is strengthened by the fact that practically all biting by *Anopheline* mosquitoes takes place at night. A properly used net in good condition provides a complete barrier between the person sleeping under it and mosquitoes. Impregnation of mosquito nets with insecticides adds to the physical barrier by repelling or killing any mosquito landing on the net. This is a particular advantage when nets have holes in them, which is almost always the case after a short time. A series of large trials have demonstrated major effects in reducing the number of cases of malaria and in significant reductions in all causes of childhood mortality (Lengeler, 1998). Impregnated bed nets are now one of the main strategies for malaria control in practically all endemic areas. Constraints on their use remain the relatively high cost and the need to re-impregnate the nets at intervals. A number of initiatives such as social marketing or the supply of nets through antenatal clinics to pregnant women are increasing coverage in many countries, and the recent development of nets that do not need re-impregnation should remove some of these barriers.

Personal protection

Anopheline mosquitoes tend to target their biting on peripheral areas such as ankles and wrists. Approaches to reducing biting by wearing clothes that limit exposed areas, such as long trousers and long-sleeved shirts, or the use of repellant sprays or creams are useful adjuncts to measures such as sleeping under impregnated bed nets.

Chemoprophylaxis

A wide range of anti-malarial drugs have been used to prevent malaria, either by killing the malaria parasites in the liver, or by acting on the erythrocytic stages once they emerge from the liver. This approach is limited by considerations such as the safety of long-term exposure to drugs, and cost. Its use is therefore usually limited to relatively short periods of exposure, such as travellers from non-endemic areas visiting malaria endemic areas for periods of weeks or months. Although attention is often focused on tourist travel from Europe and America, it should be remembered that there are many areas of Africa with little or no malaria and, when people travel from these to neighbouring endemic areas, they are also at risk and should consider using prophylaxis. Two groups within endemic areas in whom prophylaxis has been considered important are pregnant women and patients with sickle cell disease.

Malaria infection in pregnancy is associated with a high incidence of severe maternal anaemia and reductions of mean birthweight. As birthweight is the key risk factor for infant mortality, this may lead to a major increase in indirect mortality secondary to malaria. Both of these complications can be markedly reduced by protecting pregnant women with chemoprophylaxis. For many years it was policy in most African countries to recommend the weekly use of chloroquine through out pregnancy. As chloroquine resistance has spread, this has become less effective and in many areas the practice was effectively discontinued, even if not actively withdrawn. Unfortunately, there are few other drugs affordable or safe enough to replace chloroquine. However, recent trials in several countries have shown that an alternative approach of intermittent therapy with SP drugs is effective in markedly reducing the effects of malaria in pregnancy (Shulman et al., 1999) and this approach is being adopted in many countries. Currently, in most areas that have adopted this approach a treatment course is recommended once in the second trimester and once in the third trimester.

Traditionally individuals with sickle cell disease are placed on malaria prophylaxis under the assumption that they are more prone to the severe consequences of malaria. In fact, there is little systematic evidence to support this. However, where chloroquine prophylaxis is effective there is little reason to change this practice, as reducing any risk seems a reasonable approach in individuals who have many other health problems However, as chloroquine fails, the issue of what drug to use becomes problematic. SP is not recommended for prophylaxis, and if used in sickle patients there may be reduced efficacy due to the usual practice of giving folate supplements. Other drugs are too expensive for long-term use for most patients. There is clearly a need for better data in order to weigh the relative risks of malaria vs. the risks and costs of various prophylactics. In its absence the only advice that can be given is to follow any individual country's policy guidelines.

There is no doubt that effective chemoprophylaxis given to non-immune children in endemic areas is effective in reducing morbidity and mortality. However, under most circumstances this is impractical from the point of view of logistics of delivery, cost and chances of inducing resistance. However, recent evidence indicates that intermittent therapy in the first year of life confers marked protection against developing severe anaemia (Schellenberg et al., 2001). At the time of writing there is insufficient evidence in a range of endemic settings to recommend this policy, but a number of large-scale trials are planned by WHO and it may well be that this approach will be incorporated into some countries' malaria control policies over the coming years.

Early appropriate treatment

Even with the most vigorous attempts at prevention, clinical attacks of malaria will remain common as a public health problem. The priority here is to prevent progression to severe life-threatening disease. The key issue is the provision of access to early appropriate treatment. Malarial fevers treated with a full course of effective anti-malarials begun in the first 24 hours have a negligible chance of becoming severe. Unfortunately, this is all too often not achieved due to a combination of reasons including difficulty of access, poor understanding by both patients and health care staff and drug resistance. A key point is that, in most of Africa, first-line treatment of childhood fevers is at home, with drugs bought from small shops or drug sellers. Such treatment is often with the wrong drugs at the wrong doses. Given the scale of the practice, education of parents, patients and drug sellers for more appropriate early treatment represents a major window of opportunity to reduce severe morbidity and mortality (Marsh et al., 1999).

APPENDIX

Notes on commonly used anti-malarial drugs (Table 15.3)

Chloroquine

Although at the time of writing this remains the most commonly used anti-malarial drug in the world, the inexorable spread of resistance severely limits its usefulness. It is rapidly absorbed following oral administration and there is no justification for the common practice of initiating treatment with an intramuscular or sub-cutaneous injection in uncomplicated disease. In therapeutic doses chloroquine is a safe drug, common side effects include nausea, vomiting, headache and pruritus. The latter may be severe and patients who have experienced it may refuse to complete a course. In overdose chloroquine leads to coma, convulsions, hypotension and cardiac dysrhythmias. The cardiac side effects are important if the drug is give parenterally.

Sulphadoxine–pyrimethamine

The combination of these two anti-folate agents in a single preparation has been adopted as first-line treatment in a number of African countries. Generic products generally cost about the same, on a course for course basis, as chloroquine. Both components have long half-lives; whilst this gives the advantage of a single dose treatment it also carries the risk of resistance developing rapidly as patients have sub-therapeutic levels for several weeks, during which time they may be re-infected with malaria, an ideal situation for selecting resistant parasites. Both drugs are well absorbed following oral administration and are well tolerated with few minor side effects. Despite their anti-folate action the combination has been used extensively in pregnancy, though caution should be exercised in the first trimester. The combination should not be given to neonates because of the risk of kernicterus. Patients who are allergic to sulpha drugs may develop a range of skin rashes. The most severe form presents as a Stephens Johnson syndrome and may be fatal. The risk of fatal reactions when used prophylactically was estimated to be in the region of between 1in 11 000 and 1 in 25 000. There are no data on the risk when used for treatment but it may be lower.

Amodiaquine

Amodiaquine is a 4-aminoquinolone. Despite its similarity to chloroquine it has often been reported to remain effective against chloroquine resistant parasites and so there is increased interest in its possible use as a replacement for chloroquine. It has received a bad press due to reports of fatal agranulocytosis and hepatitis when used prophylactically. Many have seen this as a barrier to promoting its use for treatment, though interestingly the reported fatality rate when used for prophylaxis is the same order as that of SP combinations. There have been no reports of serious toxicity when used for treatment and the drug has been used widely in some countries. It seems likely it will be more widely used as chloroquine resistance worsens.

Artemisinin derivatives

This group of drugs was identified as the active components in the traditional Chinese anti-malarial qinghasou, prepared from the plant *Artemesia annua*. They are very fast-acting and effective anti-malarials. These drugs have been used very extensively in South East Asia and there have been no reports of serious toxicity. Three oral formulations, artesunate, artemether and di-hydroartemesinin are available in many African countries. At the moment use is mainly restricted to the private sector; however, the combination of falling prices and great efficacy is likely to lead to increased use. Because they have short half-lives it is essential that full courses are taken; recrudescence is common if the course is shortened but may occur even following a full course. This is a cause for concern both in terms of failed treatments and the possibility of selecting for resistance. Given the potential massive importance of this group of drugs, it is essential that all steps are taken to prevent the development of resistance and most experts feel that they should always be used in combination with other effective anti-malarials. Recently, a fixed dose combination of artemether with lumefantrine has been introduced in many countries and is likely to be used increasingly.

Quinine

Quinine is the drug of choice for the parenteral treatment of severe malaria. Its widespread use as an oral treatment of uncomplicated malaria is therefore not recommended because of the risk of selecting for resistance. However, it must be recognized that quinine is, in fact, widely used for treating both children and adults in some countries. As with the artemesinin derivatives it is important that a full course be completed. Although absorbtion is good, side effects, including tinnitus, high tone deafness, nausea

Table 15.3. Doses of commonly used anti-malarial drugs

	Oral	Parenteral
Chloroquine	10 mg/kg of base day 1 10 mg/kg of base day 2 5 mg/kg of base day 3	3.5 mg/kg base Subcutaneously every 6 hours, until taking orally, they complete to total dose of 25 mg/kg as for oral regime.
Sulphadoxine Pyrimethamine	Sulphadoxine 25 mg/kg Pyrimethamine 1.25 mg/kg as single dose (Max = 1500 mg sulphadoxine 75 mg pyrimethamine	As i.m. injection, doses as for oral.
Amodiaquine	10 mg/kg per day for 3 days	N/A
Artemether	3.2 mg/kg day1 1.6 mg/kg days 2–7	3.2 mg/kg i.m. day 1 1.6 mg/kg for 3 days then complete course orally.
Artesunate	4 mg/kg once daily for 7 days	2.4 mg/kg i.v. on day 1 1.2 mg/kg i.v. for 3 days then complete course orally
Artemether/lumefantrine	Fixed dose combination of 20 mg artemether and 120 mg lumefantrine dose given twice daily for 3 days = <15kg 1 tab, 15 – <25 kg 2 tabs, 25–<35 kg 3 tabs, >35 kg 4 tabs	N/A
Mefloquine	15 mg/kg base day 1, 10 mg/kg base day 2	N/A
Halofantrine	8 mg/kg 6 hrs for 3 doses Repeat the course after 1 week	N/A
Quinine	10 mg/kg salt (max 600 mg) 8 hourly for 7 days	20 mg/kg salt in 10mls/kg isotonic fluid over 4 hours. Thereafter, 10 mg/kg given over 2 hours every 12 hours in children and every 8 hours in adults

and malaise are common and often lead to premature discontinuation of treatment.

Halofantrine

Halofantrine is a phenanthrene–methanol drug effective against multi-drug resistant malaria. It is available in most African countries but its high cost means that it has no role in public health and its use is restricted to private practice; however, within this context it has been widely used. Although well tolerated its absorption is variable, and for this reason the dose is split into three. It is cardiotoxic and produces a dose-dependent delay in atrio-ventricular conduction. There have been a number of sudden deaths reported following treatment which are assumed to be due to arrhythmias; for this reason ideal practice is to perform an ECG before treatment to exclude any pre-existent abnormities, particularly prolonged QT interval. Because of its potential cardiotoxic effect it should not be used in combination with quinine or mefloquine.

Mefloquine

Mefloquine is a quinoline–methanol related to quinine. It is well absorbed and has a long half-life of 2 to 3 weeks. It is a relatively expensive drug but is available increasingly and is used in the private sector. In Africa it is effective against most parasite isolates that are resistant to chloroquine or SP drugs. In most patients it is well tolerated, though many travellers who take it for prophylaxis report mood changes and unpleasant feelings of dissociation. In treatment doses it can lead to neurological side effects including acute psychosis and convulsions. This may occur in as many as 1 per cent of patients and, though transient, may be serious. It should be avoided in patients with a history of neurological disease, including epilepsy.

References

Beeson JG, Reeder JC, Rogerson SJ, Brown, CV. (2001) Parasite adhesion and immune evasion in placental malaria. *Trends Parasitol*; **17**: 331–337.

Brewster DR, Kwiatkowski K, White NJ. (1990). Neurological sequelae of cerebral malaria in children. *Lancet*; **336**: 1039–1043.

Crawley J, Smith S, Kirkham F, Muthinji P, Waruiru C, Marsh K. (1996). Seizures and status epilepticus in childhood cerebral malaria. *Q J Med*; **89**: 591–597.

Crawley J, English M, Waruiru C, Mwangi I, Marsh K. (1998). Abnormal respiratory patterns in childhood cerebral malaria. *Trans Roy Soc Trop Med Hyg*; **92**: 305–308.

English M, Waruiru C, Marsh K. (1996). Transfusion for respiratory distress in life threatening childhood Malaria. *Am J Trop Med Hyg*; **55**: 525–530.

English M, Waruiru C, Amukoye E et al. (1996a). Deep breathing reflects acidosis and is associated with poor prognosis in children with severe malaria and respiratory distress. *Am J Trop Med Hyg*; **55**: 521–524.

English M, Punt J, Mwangi I, McHugh K, Marsh K. (1996b). Clinical overlap between malaria and severe pneumonia in hospitalized African children. *Trans Roy Soc Trop Med Hyg*; **90**: 658–662.

English MC, Waruiru C, Lightowler C, Murphy SA, Kirigha G, Marsh K. (1996c). Hyponatraemia and dehydration in severe malaria. *Arch Dis Childh*; **74**: 201–205.

English M, Wale S, Binns G, Mwangi I, Sauerwein H, Marsh K. (1998). Hypoglycaemia on and after admission in Kenyan children with severe malaria. *Q J Med*; **91**: 191–197.

Heddini A, Pettersson F, Kai O et al. (2001). Fresh isolates from children with severe *Plasmodium falciparum* malaria bind to multiple receptors. *Infec Immun*; **69**: 5849–5856.

Holding PA, Stevenson J, Peshu N, Marsh K. (1999). Cognitive sequelae of severe malaria with impaired consciousness. *Trans Roy Soc Trop Med Hyg*; **93**: 529–534.

Kwiatkowski D, Bate CA, Scragg IG, Udalova I, Knight JC. (1997). The malarial fever response – pathogenesis, polymorphism and prospects for intervention. *Ann Trop Med Parasitol*; **91**: 533–542.

Lengeler C. (1998). Insecticide treated bednets and curtains for malaria control. *Cochrane Rev.* The Cochrane Library, issue no.3 *http://www.update-software.com/cochrane/abstracts/ab000363.htm* (Update Software, Oxford).

Lewallen S, Harding P, Ajewole J et al. (1999). A review of the spectrum of clinical ocular fundus findings in *P. falciparum* malaria in African children with a proposed classification and grading system. *Trans Roy Soc Trop Med Hyg*; **93**: 619–622.

Marsh K, Forster D, Waruiru C et al. (1995). Indicators of life threatening malaria in African children. *N Engl J Med*; **332**: 1399–1404.

Marsh K, English M, Crawley J, Peshu N. (1996). The pathogenesis of severe malaria in African children. *Ann Trop Med Parasitol*; **90**: 395–402.

Marsh VM, Mutemi WM, Muturi J et al. (1999). Changing home treatment of childhood fevers by training shop keepers in rural Kenya. *Trop Med Int Hlth*; **4**: 383–389.

Miller LH, Baruch DI, Marsh K, Doumbo OK. (2001). The pathogenic basis of malaria. *Nature*; **415:** 673–679.

Molyneux ME, Taylor TW, Wirima JJ, Borgstein A. (1989). Clinical features and prognostic indicators in paediatric cerebral malaria: a study of 131 comatose Malawian children. *Q J Med*, **71**: 441–459.

Newton CRJC, Warn PA, Winstanley PA et al. (1997). Severe anaemia in children living in a malaria endemic area of Kenya. *Trop Med Int Hlth*; **2**: 165–178.

Prada J, Alabi SA, Bienzle U. (1993). Bacterial strains isolated from blood cultures of Nigerian children with cerebral malaria. *Lancet*, **342**: 1114.

Schellenberg D, Menendez C, Aponte J et al. (2001). Intermittent treatment for malaria and anaemia control at time of routine vaccinations in Tanzanian infants: a randomised, placebo-controlled trial. *Lancet*; 12: 1471–1477.

Shulman CE, Dorman EK, Cutts F. et al. (1999). Intermittent sulphadoxine–pyrimethamine to prevent severe anaemia secondary to malaria in pregnancy: a randomised placebo-controlled trial. *Lancet*; **353**: 632–636.

Snow RW, Omumbo JA, Lowe B et al. (1997). Relation between severe malaria morbidity in children and level of *Plasmodium falciparum* transmission in Africa. *Lancet*; **349**: 1650–1654.

Snow RW, Craig M, Deichmann V, Marsh K. (1999). Estimating mortality and disability due to malaria among Africa's non-pregnant population. *Bull Wld Hlth Org*; 77: 624–640.

Taylor TE, Molyneux ME, Wirima JJ, Fletcher K, Morris K. (1988). Blood glucose levels in Malawian children before and during the administration of intravenous quinine for severe falciparum malaria. *N Engl J Med*; **319**: 1040–1047.

Waller D, Krishna S, Crawley J et al. (1995). Clinical features and outcome of severe malaria in Gambian children. *Clin Infect Dis*; **21**: 577–587.

Waruiru C, Newton CRJC, Forster D et al. (1996). Epileptic seizures and malaria in Kenyan children. *Trans Roy Soc Trop Med Hyg*; **90**: 152–155.

White N. (1996). The treatment of malaria. *N Eng J Med*; **335**: 800–805.

Meningitis

16

Introduction

Meningitis, a clinical syndrome that results from inflammation of the meninges, can be caused by a wide range of organisms – viruses, bacteria, yeasts or helminths and, rarely, it has a non-infectious cause (Table 16.1). Inflammation of the pia and arachnoid membranes results in the leakage of plasma proteins across the blood–brain barrier and the accumulation of inflammatory cells in the cerebrospinal fluid.

Depending upon its cause, meningitis may present as an acute or as a chronic illness. In tropical Africa, acute bacterial meningitis is the most important form of meningitis. Major causes of chronic meningitis are tuberculosis and cryptococcal infection, conditions whose incidence has increased as a consequence of the HIV epidemic.

Table 16.1. Some of the many organisms that can cause meningitis

Bacteria	Viruses[a]	Yeast	Helminth
Streptococcus pneumoniae	Enterovirus	*Cryptococcus neoformans*[c]	*Angiostrongylus cantonensis*[d]
Haemophilus influenzae	Mumps		
Neisseria meningitidis	Polio virus		
Escherichia coli	Herpes simplex		
Salmonella species	Herpes zoster		
Other gram-negative bacilli	EBV		
Group B streptococci	Arboviruses		
Streptococcus suis[b]			
Listeria monocytogenes			
Staphylococcus aureus			
Leptospira species			
Treponema pallidum			
Mycobacterium tuberculosis[c]			

Notes:

[a] Other viruses cause an encephalitis without meningeal inflammation.

[b] *Streptococcus suis* is an important cause of meningitis in South East Asia.

[c] *Mycobacterium tuberculosis* and *Cryptococcus neoformans* produce a chronic meningitis.

[d] *Angiostrongylus cantonensis* larvae cause meningitis with a predominance of eosinophils in the CSF. This infection occurs predominantly in South East Asia. In Africa, detection of eosinophils in the CSF should suggest a diagnosis of schistosomiasis.

Acute bacterial meningitis

The problem in Africa

Acute bacterial meningitis is a major cause of mortality and morbidity throughout tropical Africa. Surveys of the cause of death in children that have employed the post-mortem questionnaire technique suggest that about 2 per cent of deaths in children under the age of 5 years are due to meningitis. This proportion may be substantially higher in countries of the African 'meningitis' belt (section x.x) during epidemic years. Similarly, acute bacterial meningitis accounts for 2–4 per cent of admissions to the paediatric wards of referral hospitals. Extrapolation of these data suggests that about 200 000 cases of acute bacterial meningitis occur in African children each year and that about 70 000 of these children die.

Epidemiology

Aetiology

A large number of bacteria can occasionally cause acute bacterial meningitis, but throughout tropical Africa, the majority of cases are caused by just three bacteria – *Streptococcus pneumoniae* (the pneumococcus), *Haemophilus influenzae* type b (Hib) and *Neisseria meningitidis* (the meningococcus) (Fig. 16.1) (Cadoz et al., 1981; Campagne et al., 1999; Molyneux et al., 1998; Palmer et al.,

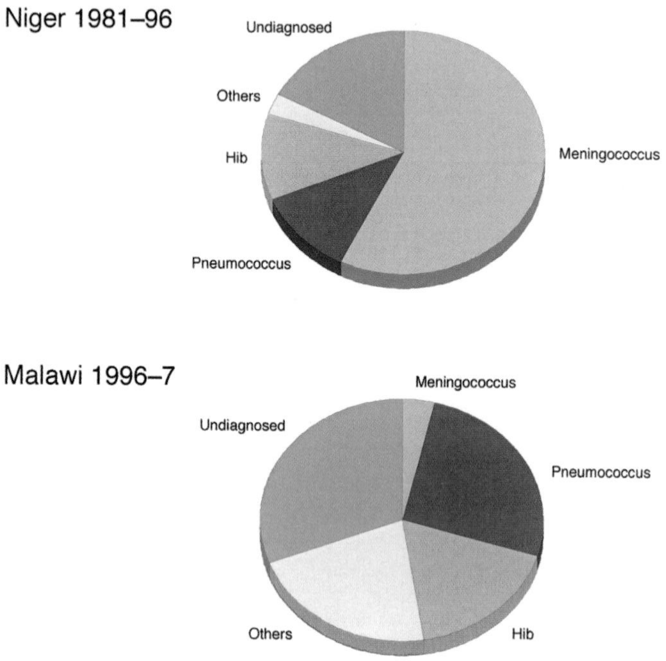

Fig. 16.1. The aetiology of acute bacterial meningitis in Niger, which is in the African meningitis belt, and in Malawi, which is not (Campagne et al., 1999; Molyneux et al., 1998).

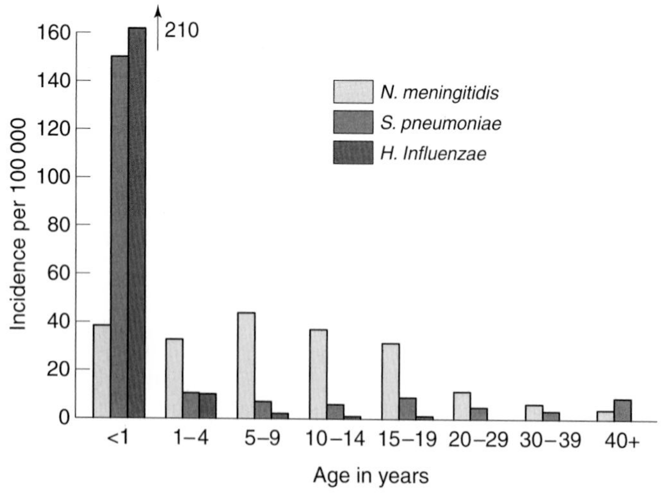

Fig. 16.2. The age incidence of the three major types of acute bacterial meningitis in Niamey, Niger (Campagne et al., 1999).

1999). Non-typhoidal salmonella septicaemia, which may result in meningitis, is seen most frequently in children who are HIV-positive or in those who have recently experienced an episode of severe malarial anaemia. Other gram-negative bacilli cause meningitis in immunocompromised children, such as those with malnutrition, and a wide range of bacteria may cause meningitis in neonates. The group B streptococcus, which is an important cause of neonatal meningitis in the developed world, rarely causes meningitis in tropical Africa for reasons that are not understood.

Geographical distribution

The pneumococcus and Hib are the most important causes of acute bacterial meningitis in children in most parts of Africa. However, in countries of the African 'meningitis belt' (Chapter 40, p. 521), the meningococcus is a major cause, even in years between epidemics (Fig. 16.1).

Age distribution

Each of the three main types of acute bacterial meningitis has a characteristic age distribution (Fig. 16.2). Invasive Hib disease is seen primarily in very young children, with a peak at about 6 months of age (Chapter 40); this peak occurs earlier in Africa than in industrialized countries. The incidence of pneumococcal meningitis is also highest during the first year of life but cases of pneumococcal meningitis occur throughout childhood and into adult life (Chapter 36). In both Africa and in industrialized countries, there is a rise in the incidence of invasive pneumococcal disease, including cases of meningitis, in the elderly. Most studies have shown that the incidence of meningococcal meningitis is highest in the first year of life but cases continue to occur throughout childhood and adult life so that children aged 5–14 years account for the largest proportion of cases, especially during epidemics.

Predisposing factors

The pneumococcus, the meningococcus and Hib are transmitted from person to person by respiratory droplets. In most instances, this results in asymptomatic colonization of the nasopharynx. In developing countries, nasopharyngeal carriage of the bacteria that can cause acute bacterial meningitis is common; nearly all children carry a pneumococcus and the nasopharyngeal carriage rates of Hib and of meningococci may be as high as 10–20 per cent. In a few unfortunate individuals, colonization is followed by invasion of the circulation, widespread dissemination of bacteria and meningitis. What determines whether an exposed subject becomes an asymptomatic nasopharyngeal carrier or develops invasive disease is not fully understood, but some of the risk factors that are thought to be involved are considered in the Box.

Risk factors for acute bacterial meningitis

Only a small proportion of subjects exposed to the pneumococcus, the meningococcus or *H. influenzae* type b develop meningitis, the majority become asymptomatic nasopharyngeal carriers. Factors that predispose to the development of meningitis include the following.

Bacterial factors

- Virulence factors such as type of polysaccharide capsule – some serotypes of pneumococci are more likely to cause invasive disease than others.
- Dose – crowding may favour transmission of a large dose of bacteria.

Environment

- Crowding favours transmission.
- Adverse environmental conditions – dry season in the Sahel and winter in northern countries.

Prior virus infection

- Influenza and RSV may damage the nasopharyngeal or bronchial mucosae predisposing to invasion by bacteria.
- HIV predisposes to pneumococcal, salmonella, and other bacterial infections.

Host factors

- Genetic factors may increase susceptibility to acute bacterial meningitis. Genetic risk factors include sickle cell disease, complement deficiencies and mutations in cytokine genes.
- Impairment of immunity due to malnutrition or other diseases increases susceptibility to infection with relatively non-pathogenic bacteria.

Pathology and pathogenesis

In most instances, meningitis results from colonization of the nasopharynx and subsequent invasion of the circulation. If invasion occurs, it usually does so within a week or two of colonization. Once invasion of the circulation has occurred, bacteria may multiply rapidly, causing the clinical features of septicaemia. However, in most patients, the bacteraemic phase of the illness is contained and illness appears only when bacteria are seeded to a peripheral site, such as the sub-arachnoid space, and multiply. Occasionally, acute bacterial meningitis results from the direct spread of bacteria to the meninges from a nearby focus of infection such as suppurative otitis media and/or mastoiditis. Even more rarely, meningitis follows a penetrative injury of the skull or invasion through the cribriform plate in patients who have a cerebrospinal (CSF) leak from the nose (rhinorrhoea) as a result of a congenital abnormality or trauma.

Examination of the brain of a patient who has died from acute bacterial meningitis shows purulent fluid in the sub-arachnoid space and thickening of the meninges, especially at the base of the brain. Histological examination of the meninges shows the characteristic features of an acute inflammatory reaction with oedema, hyperaemia and infiltration with polymorphonuclear neutrophil leukocytes, which may contain bacteria. There may be signs of damage to large blood vessels with thrombosis of cerebral veins. Widespread damage to small vessels may be found in patients in whom the septicaemic phase of the illness has been prominent.

Studies in experimental animals have shown that the immune response of the host contributes to the inflammatory response seen in acute bacterial meningitis (Quagliarello & Scheld, 1992). Meningococcal and Hib endotoxins and pneumococcal cell wall glycans activate cytokine, complement and coagulation pathways causing acute inflammation and vascular damage. High levels of the cytokines tumour necrosis factor (TNF) and interleukin-6 (IL 6) are found in the CSF of patients with acute bacterial meningitis reflecting these processes.

Immunity to pneumococcal, meningococcal or Hib meningitis depends primarily on bactericidal antibodies. These may be acquired as a result of asymptomatic nasopharyngeal carriage or by infection with a bacterium with cross-reacting antigens; immunity increases with age. Immunity is usually capsular group specific so it is possible for a patient to be infected more than once with a meningococcus or a pneumococcus if each infection is caused by a bacterium of a distinct capsular serogroup.

Clinical features

Symptoms

Most patients with acute bacterial meningitis present with a characteristic two or three day history of fever, headache and a painful, stiff neck. There may be photophobia and/or vomiting. There may be a history of convulsions, especially in young children. However, these characteristic symptoms may not be present in the very young or in the old. In infants, failure to feed may be the only indication of the presence of meningitis and, in the elderly, confusion may be the most prominent symptom.

Physical signs

Patients with meningitis are often dehydrated, drowsy and confused by the time that they reach hospital so that it may be necessary to take a history from a relative.

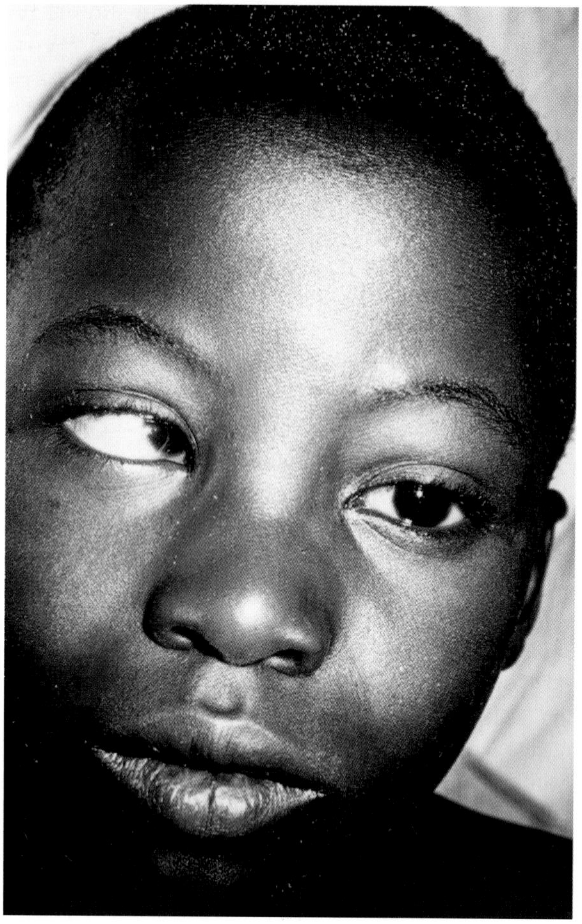

Fig. 16.3. A sixth nerve palsy in a Nigerian patient with acute bacterial meningitis (copyright D. A. Warrell).

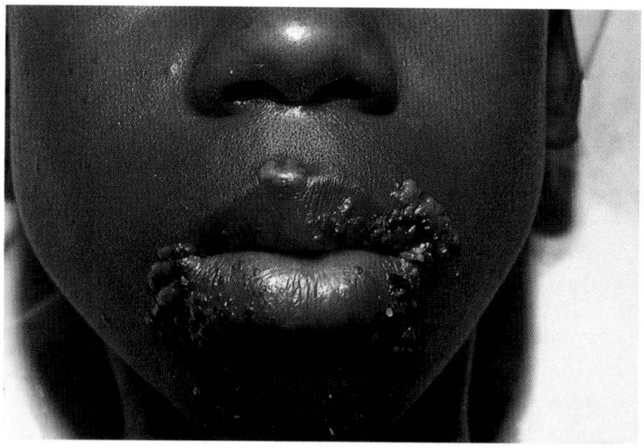

Fig. 16.4. Severe herpes simplex infection complicating acute bacterial meningitis (copyright D. A. Warrell).

Occasionally, patients are already comatose on arrival; this is a bad prognostic sign. Inflammation of the meninges produces characteristic clinical signs. Flexion of the neck is resisted. Flexion of the hips and subsequent straightening of the leg produces pain in the back (Kernig's sign). Bright light is painful and patients with meningitis often lie facing away from the light. Neurological examination may show localizing signs. The most frequent of these is a sixth cranial nerve palsy which may be a consequence of raised intracranial pressure (Fig. 16.3). Less frequently, other cranial nerve palsies, such as a third nerve palsy, are found. Examination of the optic fundi may show distended veins but papilloedema is unusual. In infants, raised intracranial pressure may lead to bulging of the anterior fontanelle. Examination of the limbs may show a motor deficit but this is uncommon. Testing for lack of co-ordination or loss of sensation is usually difficult because of the patient's general condition.

General examination may show signs of septicaemia, such as the presence of petechiae. In dark skinned subjects, these are detected most readily in the conjunctivae and on the soft palate. If the septicaemic component of the illness is prominent, there may be hypotension and other cardiovascular abnormalities. Lesions of herpes simplex infection may be seen on presentation, or may appear during the subsequent few days, and are often severe (Fig. 16.4).

A search should be made for any predisposing cause for the meningitis such as a chronic ear infection or pneumonia. There may be signs, such as severe wasting and/or Candida infection, which suggest underlying HIV infection.

Diagnosis

Clinical diagnosis

Clinical diagnosis of acute bacterial meningitis is not difficult in a patient who presents with a characteristic history, who is confused and who has a stiff neck. However, diagnosis is more difficult in the very young and in the elderly who may not have neck stiffness. Cessation of feeding, perhaps with some fever, may be the only feature of meningitis in an infant and meningitis should be considered as a possible diagnosis in any elderly patient who suddenly becomes confused. Under the Integrated Management for Childhood Illness (IMCI) guidelines, most children with meningitis are found to require hospital admission on the basis of the presence of danger signs (Chapter 9).

Cerebral malaria is an important differential diagnosis in the unconscious patient in areas where infection with *Plasmodium falciparum* is prevalent. Patients with cerebral malaria do not usually have a stiff neck but it may not be possible to differentiate meningitis from cerebral malaria on clinical grounds alone. Patients with a cerebral abscess may have fever and localizing neurological signs but they do not usually have neck stiffness. Meningitis may occasionally be confused with tetanus or rabies but the characteristic spasms seen in these two conditions usually clarify the diagnosis rapidly. Neck stiffness due to spasm of the neck muscles (meningism) may occur in the absence of meningitis. It may accompany an inflammatory lesion in the upper respiratory tract, such as a peritonsillar abscess; it may be due to a torticollis (a painful spasm of the neck muscles of unknown cause which is usually asymmetrical); or it may be caused by drugs such as the phenothiazines. If there is any doubt as to whether a patient has meningitis or meningism, and there are no contraindications, a lumbar puncture should be done.

Clinical examination may give a clue to the cause of a patient's meningitis. The presence of petechiae strongly suggests meningococcal infection but petechiae may occur occasionally in other forms of acute bacterial meningitis. The presence of pneumonia or a chronic ear infection favours a diagnosis of pneumococcal or Hib infection. If a patient is severely malnourished or has signs suggesting immune impairment the possibility of infection with a more unusual bacterium should be considered.

Laboratory diagnosis

Lumbar puncture

Unless there are contraindications to lumbar puncture, examination of the cerebrospinal fluid is essential. Some physicians are very cautious about undertaking lumbar puncture in patients with suspected meningitis because of concerns that this could precipitate coning in patients with raised intracranial pressure. It has also been suggested that lumbar puncture could introduce bacteria into the CSF of a patient who had septicaemia but not meningitis. However, the consequences of missing a diagnosis of acute bacterial meningitis are so serious that a strong case can be made for undertaking lumbar puncture in any patient in whom meningitis is a possible diagnosis unless there are clinical signs of raised intracranial pressure such as papilloedema, abnormalities of respiration or decerebrate spasms. If lumbar puncture is not done for any reason, but acute bacterial meningitis remains in the differential diagnosis, then a broad spectrum antibiotic must be given in addition to any other medication that is prescribed.

Blood

Examination of the blood will usually show a raised white blood cell count with a predominance of polymorphonuclear neutrophil leukocytes. There may be thrombocytopenia. In malaria endemic areas, always examine a blood film for malaria parasites. Absence of malaria parasites makes cerebral malaria very unlikely, unless the patient has already been treated. However, the presence of malaria parasites does not exclude a diagnosis of meningitis as the patient may have both infections. Detection of malaria parasites is not necessarily a reason for not undertaking a lumbar puncture. Blood culture is positive in about 30 per cent of patients with acute bacterial meningitis.

Cerebrospinal fluid

Examination of CSF usually shows a turbid or purulent fluid, thus confirming the diagnosis immediately. However, about 200 cells per μl are required to produce turbidity so that the finding of a clear CSF does not rule out a diagnosis of meningitis and microscopy is required. Chemical examination of the CSF usually shows an increase in CSF protein and a low CSF glucose which is lower than the blood glucose concentration measured at the same time. It has been suggested that a urine 'labstick' can be used to detect a raised CSF protein (Moosa et al., 1995) but simple turbidity methods can be used. A number of other biochemical changes may be found, such as raised CSF levels of lactic acid and lactic dehydrogenase, but these are not usually used as diagnostic tests.

Microscopy of CSF usually shows a raised white cell count with a predominance of polymorphonuclear neutrophil leukocytes. Occasionally, only a few white cells are found and turbidity of the CSF is produced by the presence of enormous numbers of bacteria. This is a bad prognostic sign. Examination of a gram-stained deposit of CSF may show the causative organism either free or in polymorphonuclear neutrophil leukocytes: bean shaped, gram-negative cocci suggest meningococcal meningitis; gram-positive cocci pneumococcal meningitis; and gram-negative cocco-bacilli Hib meningitis. However, diagnosis by gram stain should be confirmed by culture whenever possible and culture may be positive in samples negative on microscopy. Isolation of the causative organism allows determination of its antibiotic sensitivity and, in good laboratories, some of its other characteristics, such as its capsular serogroup, can be determined.

Some patients with acute bacterial meningitis have already received antibiotics before they reach hospital and this may make isolation of the causative organism from the blood or CSF difficult. In these circumstances, tests which depend upon the detection of bacterial products, and not viable bacteria, may be useful. Latex tests which detect bacterial capsular polysaccharide are commercially available and give results comparable to those obtained

Table 16.2. Doses of antibiotics commonly used in the treatment of acute bacterial meningitis

Antibiotic	Adults	Children
Ampicillin	500 mg 6 hourly i.v. or i.m. then orally	50 mg/kg 6 hourly i.v. or i.m. then orally
Ceftriaxone	5 g daily i.v. or i.m.	50 mg/kg 12 hourly i.v. or i.m.
Cefotaxime	2 g 8 hourly i.v. or i.m.	50 mg/kg 6 hourly i.v. or i.m.
Chloramphenicol[a]	500 mg 6 hourly i.v. or i.m. then orally	25 mg/kg 6 hourly i.v. or i.m. then orally
Gentamicin	50 mg 8 hourly i.v. or i.m.	2.5 mg/kg 8 hourly i.v. or i.m.
Penicillin (crystalline)	2–4 mega units 6 hourly i.v. or i.m.	60 mg/kg 6 hourly i.v. or i.m.

Note:

[a] Do not give neonates more than 50 mg/kg/day of chloramphenicol. It should be given parenterally.

with culture within a few minutes but they are relatively expensive. Molecular techniques based on the polymerase chain reaction (PCR) are being used increasingly frequently in industrialized countries to establish the cause of acute bacterial meningitis but these tests are not yet widely available in developing countries.

Management

General

Patients with acute bacterial meningitis are often severely ill and so require the best nursing and medical care that is available. They should be managed in an intensive care unit if this is possible. Hyponatraemia may occur as a result of inappropriate secretion of anti-diuretic hormone and it has been recommended in the past that fluids should be restricted. However, there is no evidence that this improves outcome and dehydration, which is often present, should be treated with intravenous fluids. Headache may be severe and it is an important cause of restlessness and irritability; its control may require powerful analgesics. Convulsing patients need an anticonvulsant such as diazepam. Neonates with meningitis require especially skilled management (p. 178).

Corticosteroids

Whether or not patients with acute bacterial meningitis should be given corticosteroids is controversial. Studies in experimental animals have shown that corticosteroids are beneficial and there is reasonably strong evidence that their administration has reduced the incidence of neurological sequelae in European and American children with Hib meningitis (McIntyre et al., 1997). There is less evidence to support their use in pneumococcal or meningococcal meningitis. A study in Malawian children did not show any benefit (Molyneux et al. 2002). If steroids are given, a high dosage is necessary; for example dexamethasone in a dose of 0.6 mg/kg daily for 2–4 days, and this is expensive. If the cost of treatment is a major concern, it is probably best to give ceftriaxone without steroids to a patient with pneumococcal meningitis or acute bacterial meningitis of unknown cause rather than to give steroids and a less effective antibiotic. It has been suggested that glycerol which, like dexamethasone, reduces intracranial pressure could be used as a cheaper alternative (Kilpi et al., 1995).

Antibiotics

Always give antibiotic therapy to patients with acute bacterial meningitis as soon as possible. It is advisable to give an initial dose of a broad spectrum antibiotic to a patient with suspected meningitis at a peripheral clinic if their journey to a referral hospital is likely to take many hours. The disadvantage of this approach is that it may make it more difficult to isolate the causative organism.

If a patient has not received an antibiotic before reaching hospital, it is reasonable to wait until a lumbar puncture and an initial microscopical examination of the CSF has been done before initiating therapy but not to wait for the results of culture which may take two or three days. If a bacterial diagnosis is established by examination of the CSF (gram stain or antigen test) immediately after initial clinical evaluation, antibiotic therapy can be tailored to the cause of the meningitis. If microscopy is negative or lumbar puncture cannot be done for logistic or financial reasons, antibiotic treatment has to be initiated in the absence of a microbiological diagnosis.

Thus, each facility where cases of acute bacterial meningitis are treated regularly should have a standard treatment protocol for the management of patients with this condition. This should follow regional or national guidelines or, when these are not available, it should be developed locally on the basis of knowledge of the most important bacterial causes of meningitis in the area and their antibiotic sensitivity patterns. Financial constraints may limit the antibiotics that can be recommended and simpler regimens than those recommended for industrialized countries (Quagliarello & Scheld, 1997) may be needed. A possible schema for use in hospitals in Africa is shown in the Box. Doses of the antibiotics commonly used in the treatment of acute bacterial meningitis are shown in Table 16.2.

Treatment of acute bacterial meningitis

Anti-microbial treatment of a case of acute bacterial meningitis should be guided by the results of initial CSF examination provided that this will not delay the start of treatment. Choice of therapy will be guided by local knowledge and the availability of drugs but the following schema is applicable in most parts of Africa for initial treatment.

	Antibiotic		
CSF finding	*First choice*	*Second choice*	*Duration of treatment (days)*
Gram +ve diplococci and/or pneumococcal antigen positive.	Ceftriaxone	Chloramphenicol	10–14
Gram-negative diplococci and/or meningococcal antigen positive.	Penicillin	Chloramphenicol	5
Gram-negative cocco-bacilli and/or Hib antigen positive.	Ceftriaxone	Ampicillin + chloramphenicol	7
No organism or CSF not examined			
Neonates	Cefotaxime	Ampicillin + gentamicin	10–14
Older children	Ceftriaxone	Chloramphenicol	10–14
Adults	Ceftriaxone	Chloramphenicol	10–14

Once the results of CSF culture and antibiotic sensitivity testing of the causative bacterium become available it may be possible to change to a more readily available or cheaper antibiotic. A change of treatment may also be indicated if a patient does not improve after 2–3 days of treatment.

Until recently, penicillin was the recommended treatment for pneumococcal meningitis. However, the emergence and rapid spread of penicillin-resistant pneumococci in many parts of the developing world, including parts of southern and eastern Africa, now makes penicillin a hazardous choice for treatment of this condition. Initial treatment of cases of pneumococcal meningitis should now be with a third generation cephalosporin, such as ceftriaxone. A strong case can be made for using any supplies of a third generation cephalosporin that are available for the treatment of patients with this condition because of its severity. Some pneumococci are now partially resistant to third generation cephalosporins and, in industrialized countries, some physicians recommend that patients with pneumococcal meningitis should also be given vancomycin, but this antibiotic is expensive. Penicillin and chloramphenicol are often given together as the initial treatment of acute bacterial meningitis in developing countries but there is no evidence that this combination is any more effective than chloramphenicol alone and it is substantially more expensive (Shann et al., 1985; Kumar & Verma, 1993).

Outcome

Patients with acute bacterial meningitis treated with an effective antibiotic should begin to improve within two to three days. If the conscious level fails to improve, or new neurological signs appear, it is possible that the bacterium is not responding to the antibiotic that is being given, and that a change in antibiotic therapy is needed. Formation of an extradural effusion or abscess is another cause for deterioration; these may require surgical drainage.

The overall outcome of acute bacterial meningitis is influenced by a number of variables but by far the most important is its cause (Fig 16.5). In Africa, mortality from pneumococcal meningitis is around 50 per cent, mortality from Hib meningitis around 25 per cent and mortality from meningococcal meningitis around 10 per cent. Why mortality from pneumococcal meningitis is so high, even when treatment is started early with an effective antibiotic, is not understood.

Clinical factors that determine the outcome of acute bacterial meningitis regardless of its cause include:

- age
- genetic background
- duration of symptoms before presentation
- conscious level at the time of presentation
- presence of clinical features of septicaemia and
- associated illness.

Unfortunately, many of the survivors of acute bacterial meningitis are left with permanent neurological damage – intellectual impairment, psychological problems, deafness, cortical blindness, cranial nerve palsies or hemiplegia. Obstruction to the flow of CSF may result in hydrocephalus. Neurological sequelae are especially common after pneumococcal meningitis and, in Africa, only a quarter of patients with this infection recover completely (Fig. 16.5). Mortality among patients with severe neurological sequelae is high after their return home.

Prevention

The incidence of acute bacterial meningitis is increased by poverty, so mortality and morbidity from this condition

Table 16.3. Characteristics of polysaccharide and polysaccharide/protein conjugate vaccines

	Polysaccharide	Conjugate
Immunogenicity in very young	Poor	Good
Induction of immunological memory	No	Yes
Predominant class of antibody	IgG2	IgG1
Effects on nasopharyngeal carriage	Little or none	Good
Cost	Cheap	Expensive

should decrease as living conditions in Africa improve. Chemoprophylaxis with penicillin is recommended for young patients with sickle cell disease (p. 940) in order to protect them against invasive pneumococcal disease and chemoprophylaxis is used occasionally in the control of localized outbreaks of meningococcal disease (p. 523). However, vaccination provides the most promising approach to the prevention of this group of infections.

Polysaccharide vaccines

Vaccines based on the capular polysaccharides of the pneumococcus, meningococcus and Hib have been available for several decades. Some of their characteristics are shown in Table 16.3. Pneumococcal polysaccharide vaccines protect immunocompetent adults from invasive pneumococcal disease (Fedson, 1999) but they are less effective in immunocompromised subjects and in preventing pneumonia (Mangtani et al., 2003). A recent study showed that a 23-valent pneumococcal polysaccharide vaccine gave no protection to Ugandan adults with HIV infection and may even have made them more susceptible to pneumococcal infection (French et al., 2000). Meningococcal polysaccharide vaccines are effective in controlling epidemics but they are poorly immunogenic in young children. The same is the case for Hib polysaccharide vaccines which are no longer used.

Polysaccharide/protein conjugate vaccines

Linkage of a polysaccharide to a protein carrier changes its immunological properties so that it becomes immunogenic in young children and able to induce immunological memory. The application of this technique to the development of vaccines against Hib disease has been one of the most successful recent developments in public health. Hib disease has largely disappeared from the many countries in the developed world, and a few countries in the developing world such as The Gambia and Chile, where these vaccines have been introduced into the EPI programme (Steinhoff, 1997). Pneumococcal polysaccharide conjugate vaccines are being developed but this is more difficult as it is necessary to vaccinate against each of the main serotypes of pneumococci causing disease in a given area. Fortunately, a vaccine that contains about ten conjugates will cover about 80 per cent of the pneumococci responsible for invasive pneumococcal disease in most parts of the world. The first trial of a pneumococcal conjugate vaccine, undertaken in California with a seven-valent vaccine, showed that it gave more than 90 per cent protection against invasive pneumococcal disease (Black et al., 2000) and there are expectations that trials of 9 or 11 valent vaccines that are now under way in South Africa, The Gambia and the Philippines will be equally effective. A group C meningococcal polysaccharide conjugate vaccine has been developed and introduced into the

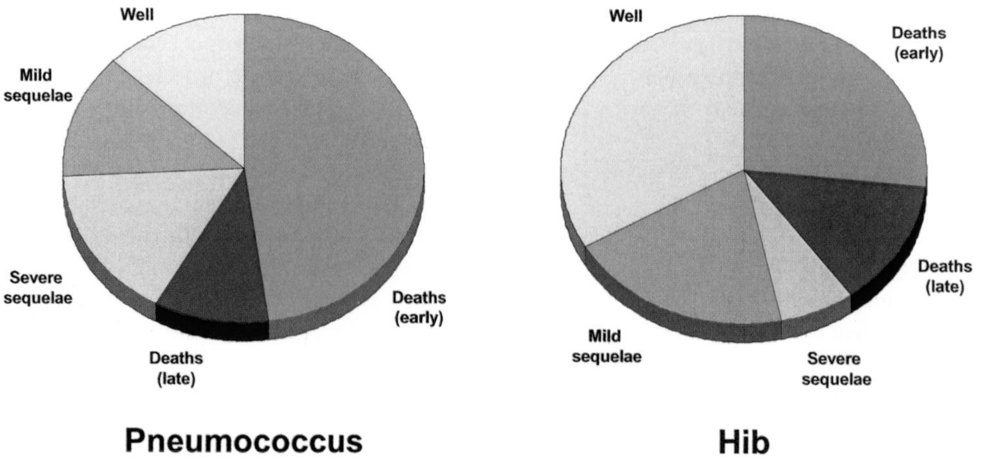

Fig. 16.5. The outcome of acute bacterial meningitis caused by the pneumococcus or Hib in Gambian children.

routine EPI programme in the UK. However, there is presently no commercially available group A meningococcal vaccine, although this is badly needed pp. 524, 528.

Viral meningitis

A large number of viruses can cause meningitis, sometimes in association with inflammation of the brain (meningo-encephalitis). Thus, polio virus can cause meningitis, damage to anterior horn cells or a combination of the two. A transient meningitis may occur during infection with mumps virus and meningitis occurs occasionally in other common viral infections. Some of the most frequent causes of viral meningitis are indicated in Table 16.1. Little information is available about the incidence of acute viral meningitis in Africa. Hospital statistics suggest that it is uncommon, but this may be due in part to the fact that, in Africa, patients with this condition seldom seek hospital treatment.

The clinical features of viral meningitis are indistinguishable initially from those of acute bacterial meningitis; headache may be very severe. Clinical examination usually shows the characteristic features of meningeal inflammation, but the patient is not usually as generally unwell as a patient with acute bacterial meningitis. There may be other systemic features of a viral infection such as a rash.

Diagnosis is made by lumbar puncture. CSF is usually clear or only slightly turbid; laboratory tests usually show a raised CSF protein, a normal glucose and a moderately raised white cell count composed mainly of lymphocytes. A predominance of lymphocytes suggests a diagnosis of viral rather than bacterial meningitis but this is not a definitive finding as a mixed population of polymorphonuclear neutrophil leukocytes and lymphocytes may occasionally be found in the CSF of patients with bacterial meningitis, especially after treatment and in patients with tuberculous meningitis. Viruses can be isolated from the CSF of patients with most forms of viral meningitis and measurement of antibody concentrations in acute and convalescent phase sera may provide a diagnosis. Virological investigations may be important epidemiologically, for example, in determining the cause of an outbreak, but they are not required for the management of an individual patient.

Management of a patient with acute viral meningitis is symptomatic. Headache may be difficult to control and require powerful analgesics. Progressive recovery over a period of a few days is usual.

Chronic meningitis

The two forms of chronic meningitis most likely to be encountered in tropical Africa are tuberculous meningitis and cryptococcal meningitis.

Tuberculous meningitis (see p. 328)

The incidence of tuberculous meningitis varies substantially between different countries in Africa. BCG may be especially effective at preventing tuberculous meningitis so its incidence would be expected to be low in countries with good EPI coverage. Tuberculous meningitis is now seen most frequently in countries where the HIV epidemic has taken hold.

Tuberculous meningitis may occur in patients who are known to have tuberculosis elsewhere or it may be the presenting feature of their illness. The clinical features of tuberculous meningitis are similar to those of acute bacterial meningitis, except that the patient usually has a longer history of illness extending over several weeks. Patients may present with confusion or localizing neurological signs; failure to thrive may be the presenting finding in young children. Examination usually shows signs of meningeal inflammation and there may be localized neurological signs. Occasionally choroidal tubercles are seen in the ocular fundi. Radiological scanning techniques have shown that many patients with tuberculous meningitis also have space-occupying lesions (tuberculomas) in the substance of the brain.

Diagnosis of tuberculous meningitis is confirmed by lumbar puncture. The CSF shows a raised protein, a low sugar (in contrast to viral meningitis) and a raised white cell count comprising both lymphocytes and polymorphonuclear neutrophil leukocytes. Acid-fast bacilli may be found in a CSF deposit but this unusual. However, culture of CSF will usually be positive. Because of the delay in obtaining the results of culture, many attempts have been made to develop chemical, immunological and molecular biological tests to diagnose tuberculous meningitis. These have met with varying degrees of success but no individual test has been adopted uniformly.

Treatment of tuberculous meningitis should follow the standard protocol for treatment of patients with tuberculosis described in Chapter 17. Whether or not patients with tuberculous meningitis should be treated with corticosteroids is controversial. The aim of this practice is to reduce brain oedema, especially at the time that treatment is started. Most physicians now recommend that steroids (dexamethasone 16 mg/day for an adult) should be given from the start of anti-microbial treatment for a period of 4–6 weeks.

Recovery from tuberculous meningitis may be protracted, taking many weeks. Provided that the illness is detected early in its course complete recovery can be anticipated but many patients who present in an advanced state are left with permanent neurological sequelae.

Cryptococcal meningitis

Cryptococcal meningitis, caused by infection with the yeast *Cryptococcus neoformans,* was rarely encountered in Africa until the advent of HIV. It is now commonly seen in the late stages of HIV infection (Chapter 13). Infection of the meninges with *C. neoformans* differs from that seen with most other pathogens in that the yeast invokes little inflammatory response. Thus, the patient may have few of the classical signs of meningitis. Headache is often a predominant feature, probably due to a raised intracranial pressure. Localizing neurological signs may be found. Diagnosis is made by the detection of yeast cells in an Indian ink preparation of a CSF deposit or by an antigen assay. Treatment of cryptococcal meningitis in patients with HIV infection and a low CD4 count is difficult. Treatment is with intravenous amphotericin B or oral fluconazole, but must be lifelong, as it is only able to suppress but not to eradicate the infection. Both drugs are very expensive.

Conclusions

The development of Hib, pneumococcal and meningococcal polysaccharide/protein conjugate vaccines offers, for the first time, a way of drastically reducing the burden of acute bacterial meningitis in Africa. It is essential that these vaccines should reach those who need them most. Unfortunately, conjugate vaccines are inherently costly to produce, so that even when costs are reduced as a result of production on a global scale, it is likely to cost several dollars to protect a child against the three main forms of acute bacterial meningitis.

Where will this money come from? It is possible that some of the richer countries of Africa will be able to raise the necessary resource internally through reorganization of government spending, perhaps with some contribution from individual families. However, at least in the short term, it seems unlikely that the poorest countries of Africa will be able to buy meningitis vaccines at commercial rates and that some form of financial assistance will be needed. This has recently been recognized by the international community which, with substantial support from the Bill and Melinda Gates Foundation and other donors, has established a Children's Vaccine Programme (CVP) and the Global Alliance for Vaccines and Immunization (GAVI). The aims of these new programmes include improving overall levels of vaccine coverage in developing countries and making new vaccines, such as Hib conjugate and hepatitis B vaccines, available to children throughout the world. Thus, a precedent has been set which could, if sustained, provide for the introduction of other new vaccines, such as a pneumococcal conjugate vaccine, raising hopes that the next decade could see the disappearance of the major forms of acute bacterial meningitis from Africa and the rest of the developing world.

References

Black S, Shinefield H, Fireman B et al. and the northern California Kaiser Permanente Vaccine Study Center Group. (2000). Efficacy, safety and immunogenicity of heptavalent pneumococcal conjugate vaccine in children. *Pediat Infect Dis J*; **19**: 187–195.

Cadoz M, Denis F, Diop Mar I. (1981). Etude épidémiologique des cas de méningites purulentes hospitalisés à Dakar pendant la décennie 1970–1979. *Bull Wld Hlth Org*; **59**: 575–584.

Campagne G, Schuchat A, Djibo S, Ousséini A, Cissé L, Chippaux JP. (1999). Epidemiology of bacterial meningitis in Niamey, Niger, 1981–96. *Bull Wld Hlth Org*; **77**: 499–508.

Fedson DS. (1999). The clinical effectiveness of pneumococcal vaccination: a brief review. *Vaccine*; **17**: S85–S90.

French N, Nakiyingi J, Carpenter LM et al. (2000). 23-valent pneumococcal polysaccharide vaccine in HIV-1-infected Uganda adults: double-blind, randomised and placebo controlled trial. *Lancet*; **355**: 2106–2111.

Goetghebuer T, West TE, Wermenbol V et al. (2000). Outcome of meningitis caused by *Streptococcus pneumoniae* and *Haemophilus influenzae* type b in children in The Gambia. *Trop Med Int Hlth*; **5**: 207–213.

Kilpi T, Peltola H, Jauhiainen T, Kallio MJT and the Finnish Study Group. (1995). Oral glycerol and intravenous dexamethasone in preventing neurologic and audiologic sequelae of childhood meningitis. *Ped Infect Dis J*; **14**: 270–278.

Kumar P, Verma IC. (1993). Antibiotic therapy for bacterial meningitis in children in developing countries. *Bull Wld Hlth Org*; **71**: 183–188.

McIntyre PB, Berkey CS, King SM et al. (1997). Dexamethasone as adjunctive therapy in bacterial meningitis. A meta-analysis of randomized clinical trials since 1988. *J Am Med Assoc*; **278**: 925–931.

Mangtani P, Cutts F, Hall AJ, (2003). Efficacy of polysacchasicle pneumococcal vaccines in adults in more developed countries: the state of the evidence. *Lancet Infect Dis*; **3**: 71–78.

Molyneux EM, Walsh AL, Forsyth H et al. (2002). Dexamethasone treatment in childhood bacterial meningitis in Malawi: a randomised controlled trial. *Lancet*, **360**: 211–218.

Molyneux E, Walsh A, Phiri A, Molyneux M. (1998). Acute bacterial meningitis in children admitted to the Queen Elizabeth Central Hospital, Blantyre, Malawi in 1996–97. *Trop Med Int Hlth*; 3: 610–618.

Moosa AA, Quortum HA, Ibrahim MD. (1995). Rapid diagnosis of bacterial meningitis with reagent strips. *Lancet*; **345**: 1290–1291.

Palmer A, Weber M, Bojang K, McKay T, Adegbola R. (1999). Acute bacterial meningitis in The Gambia: a four-year review of paediatric hospital admissions. *J Trop Pediat*; **45**: 51–53.

Quagliarello V, Scheld WM. (1992). Bacterial meningitis: pathogenesis, pathophysiology, and progress. *N Engl J Med*; **327**: 864–872.

Quagliarello VJ, Scheld WM. (1997). Treatment of bacterial meningitis. *N Engl J Med*; **336**: 708–716.

Shann F, Barker J, Poore P. (1985). Chloramphenicol alone versus chloramphenicol plus penicillin for bacterial meningitis in children. *Lancet*; **ii**: 68–84.

Steinhoff MC. (1997). *Haemophilus influenzae* type b infections are preventable everywhere. *Lancet*; **349**: 1186–1187.

17 Tuberculosis

Tuberculosis has become one of the most serious threats to public and individual health in Africa. In 1993, the World Health Organization (WHO) took the unprecedented step of declaring tuberculosis to be a global emergency. The disease is responsible for millions of lives lost each year, and the situation could worsen unless there is effective action to curb its spread. Africa has the highest burden of disease per head of population, with an incidence rate in 1997 estimated at 260 per 100 000 (Dye et al., 1999). The great driving force behind the current tuberculosis epidemic in Africa is the other major epidemic of human immunodeficiency virus (HIV) infection. Not only is HIV responsible for the tremendous increase in case numbers, but it threatens tuberculosis control efforts by further stigmatizing the disease, complicating the diagnosis, reducing the effectiveness of treatment, increasing recurrence rates, and diminishing the already small band of health care staff who are trying to grapple with the problem.

In this chapter we discuss the epidemiology, pathogenesis, clinical features, diagnosis, treatment and prevention of tuberculosis. In all these areas, we emphasize the strong link with HIV. The best chance of detecting the disease, curing the patients and halting transmission lies in having a strong country-wide tuberculosis control programme, and we highlight the important aspects of good programmatic control.

History of tuberculosis in Africa

There is evidence that tuberculosis occurred in Egypt in 3000BC; northern parts of Ethiopia and the Sudan have also had the disease for centuries. Elsewhere in the interior of Africa, tuberculosis may have been an ancient plague, present for centuries, perhaps re-introduced by Arab traders and perhaps further re-introduced by early Europeans (Daniel, 1998). It seems as if the disease was not uniformly distributed across the vast continent, and some areas such as the interior of West Africa, probably had little tuberculosis. Tuberculosis was recognized as an important communicable disease in the early and mid-1900s, but it was with the advent of human immunodeficiency virus infection (HIV) in the 1980s that the dramatic upsurge in case notifications started to occur. Today, sub-Saharan Africa (particularly the southern region of the continent) is gripped by the devastating dual epidemic of HIV and tuberculosis, which threatens to spiral out of control with serious consequences for both immunocompetent and immunocompromised sectors of the population.

Epidemiology of tuberculosis

General aspects of tuberculous infection and tuberculosis disease

Tuberculous infection

About one-third of the world's population is infected with *M.tuberculosis*. Being infected means that a person carries the tubercle bacilli inside the body, but the bacteria are small in numbers and are dormant. These dormant bacilli are kept under control by the body's defences and do not cause disease.

Tuberculosis

Tuberculosis is a state in which one or more organs of the body become diseased as shown by clinical symptoms and signs. This is usually because the tubercle bacilli in the body have started to multiply and become numerous enough to overcome the body's defences.

Sources of infection

The most important source of infection is the patient with pulmonary tuberculosis. Infection occurs by inhaling droplet nuclei (these are infectious particles of respiratory secretions usually less than 5 μm which contain tubercle bacilli). They are spread into the air by coughing, sneezing, talking, spitting and singing, and they can remain suspended in the air for long periods of time. A single cough can produce 3000 infectious droplet nuclei. Direct sunlight kills tubercle bacilli in 5 minutes, but they can survive in the dark for long periods of time. Droplet nuclei are so small that they avoid the defences of the bronchi and penetrate the terminal alveoli of the lungs where multiplication and infection begins.

Risk of infection

The risk of infection is determined by the infectiousness of the source case (i.e. how many tubercle bacilli are being coughed into the air), the closeness of contact and the immune status of the host. Patients with smear-positive sputum (i.e. tubercle bacilli visible under the microscope when appropriate stains are used) are much more infectious than those with smear-negative sputum.

Risk of progression of infection to disease

The risk of progressing to disease is determined by the size of the infecting dose of tubercle bacilli and by the immune status of the host. The likelihood of developing disease is greatest immediately after infection, and declines steadily from that point.

Natural history of pulmonary tuberculosis

Follow-up studies before anti-TB treatment was available showed that the natural history of pulmonary tuberculosis in the absence of HIV infection is that, with **no** anti-tuberculosis treatment, 50 per cent of patients will die within 5 years. Another 25 per cent cure themselves through their own defence mechanisms. The remaining 25 per cent continue chronically ill as smear-positive sources of infection within the community.

Measurements of tuberculous infection and tuberculosis disease

Measurements and estimates of the global burden of tuberculosis are made using defined epidemiological tools. Recent estimates of the global burden of tuberculosis for 1997 were carried out by the World Health Organization (WHO). Estimates for Africa are based on this report (Dye et al., 1999).

Prevalence of tuberculous infection

This is measured by the tuberculin test. In 1997, Africa had a population of approximately 610 million of whom 211 million (35 per cent) were thought to be infected with *M.tuberculosis.*

Annual risk of tuberculous infection

The annual risk of infection (ARI) with *M.tuberculosis* is the probability that an uninfected person will become infected with the bacilli in one year; it reflects the extent of transmission of tubercle bacilli in the community. The ARI is measured by carrying out tuberculin surveys in school children in the general population. In sub-Saharan Africa, the ARI is the highest in the world with estimates of 1.5–2.5 per cent. The ARI has been a useful measurement which has helped in estimating the number of smear-positive pulmonary tuberculosis cases in a community. An ARI of 1 per cent has meant that there will be approximately 50 new smear-positive pulmonary tuberculosis cases per 100 000 per year. However, there are two major problems with use of ARI in Africa. First, BCG vaccination at birth of a large sector of the population means that many children have positive tuberculin skin tests as a result of BCG. Second, the equation between ARI and smear-positive pulmonary tuberculosis cases does not hold true in the presence of HIV infection.

Annual incidence rate of tuberculosis

This is the number of new cases of tuberculosis that occur each year in a defined population. In 1997 there were an estimated 1.6 million new cases of tuberculosis in Africa. Incidence rates are often expressed in terms of the number of new cases of tuberculosis per 100 000: for Africa this was 260 per 100 000 in 1997 (Dye et al., 1999). Because of undetected cases in the community as a result of poor service coverage, the incidence rate cannot be known with certainty, and instead most TB control programmes report an annual case notification rate. In 1997, 500 000 new cases of tuberculosis were notified, giving an estimated case detection rate of 31 per cent.

Prevalence of tuberculosis

This means the number of tuberculosis cases in a community at a given point in time. In 1997 there were an estimated 2.3 million prevalent tuberculosis cases in Africa with a prevalence rate of 380 per 100 000. The prevalence of tuberculosis (i.e. new and old cases together) is not frequently used when describing the tuberculosis health problem.

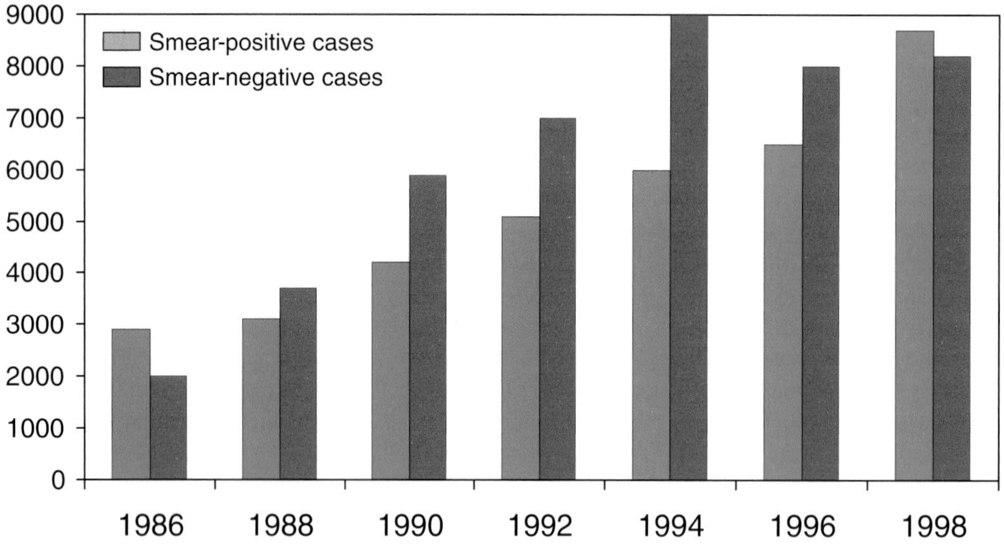

Fig. 17.1. Smear-positive and smear-negative pulmonary tuberculosis notifications in Malawi: 1986–1998.

The association of tuberculosis with HIV infection

HIV infection and AIDS: the size of the problem

According to UNAIDS Reports, at the end of 2000 an estimated 36.1 million people were living with HIV infection or AIDS (acquired immunodeficiency syndrome), of whom 25.3 million (70 per cent) lived in sub-Saharan Africa (UNAIDS, 2000). There are two types of the virus, HIV-1 and HIV-2. HIV-1 is distributed throughout the continent, while HIV-2 is largely confined to West Africa. Both types of virus are associated with an increased risk of tuberculosis.

Dual infection with HIV and the tubercle bacillus

In 1997, nearly 11 million people globally were thought to be co-infected with HIV infection and *M.tuberculosis*, of whom 7 million (68 per cent) were living in Africa (Dye et al., 1999). HIV infection causes a progressive decline in the number of CD4–T-lymphocytes and progressive dysfunction of those lymphocytes which survive. CD4–T-lymphocytes play an important role in the body's defence against tubercle bacilli, and it is therefore not surprising that HIV infection is probably the highest risk factor for reactivation of tuberculosis in those with *M.tuberculosis* infection. HIV-infected persons are also more susceptible to new tuberculous infections, which can progress much more frequently and more quickly to overt disease. In HIV-negative persons infected with *M.tuberculosis* the lifetime risk of developing tuberculosis is 5–10 per cent. In contrast, in HIV-positive persons infected with *M.tuberculosis* the risk is much higher with an annual risk of 5–15 per cent, and a lifetime risk estimated to be 50 per cent or higher.

The HIV and tuberculosis interaction

In 1997, about one-third of all tuberculosis cases in Africa were thought to be HIV-seropositive (Dye et al., 1999). This proportion is unevenly distributed geographically with HIV-seroprevalence rates in tuberculosis cases (adults and children) varying from 15–75 per cent. In some countries such as Malawi, Zambia and Botswana over 70 per cent of tuberculosis cases are HIV-seropositive. From a different perspective, tuberculosis is probably the most important opportunistic disease found among HIV-infected patients in Africa, because it is so common, transmissible to everyone and life-threatening. In autopsy studies as many as 54 per cent of patients with HIV infection or AIDS have been found to have tuberculosis as the cause of death (Raviglione et al., 1997).

Consequences of dual infection with HIV and tuberculosis

Tuberculosis case numbers

Most sub-Saharan African countries with high HIV-seroprevalence rates have experienced a huge upsurge in tuberculosis cases since 1986. For example, the annual notifications in Tanzania rose from 12 000 in 1986 to 49 500 in 1998. Along with this rise has been a disproportionate increase in the number of patients with smear-negative pulmonary tuberculosis (Fig. 17.1). Extra-pulmonary tuberculosis cases have also risen, and in many TB programmes, patients with extrapulmonary tuberculosis represent about 20–25 per cent of all cases. The diagnosis of TB in patients with negative sputum smears and with extrapulmonary tuberculosis depends on clinical and radiographic features combined with other circumstantial evidence and whatever laboratory support is available. It is likely that a proportion do not have TB but rather HIV-related disease. Nevertheless, all registered cases are placed on anti-tuberculosis treatment and therefore consume resources.

Hot spots of TB transmission

Hot spots of TB transmission, fuelled by concurrent HIV infection, may occur in places where people are crowded together such as prisons, refugee camps, boarding schools and health care institutions (Nyangulu et al., 1997).

Increased illness and mortality

HIV-positive TB patients often run a stormy course while on anti-tuberculosis treatment with fevers, chest infections and recurrent diarrhoea. Infections such as oral candidiasis can cause considerable discomfort, and bacteraemia due to *Salmonella typhimurium* and *Streptococcus pneumoniae* is potentially life-threatening. Adverse reactions to anti-tuberculosis drugs are more frequent, leading to interruptions of treatment and occasional fatalities. HIV-positive patients have a much higher death rate during and after anti-tuberculosis treatment compared with HIV-negative patients (Raviglione et al., 1997).

Recurrence of TB after completing treatment

Recurrence rates are increased in HIV-positive patients (Raviglione et al., 1997).

Drug resistance

Several outbreaks of multi-drug resistant TB (MDR-TB) have been reported from industrialized countries amongst patients with HIV. HIV does not itself cause MDR-TB, but it can increase the spread of this dangerous condition by increasing susceptibility to infection and accelerating the progression from infection to disease. MDR-TB rates are currently low in most parts of sub-Saharan Africa (Pablos-Mendez et al., 1998).

Pathogenesis of tuberculosis

The tuberculoid granuloma

At a microscopic level, the classical inflammatory response to infection with *M. tuberculosis* is the granuloma (Fig. 17.3). The granuloma is a collection of activated

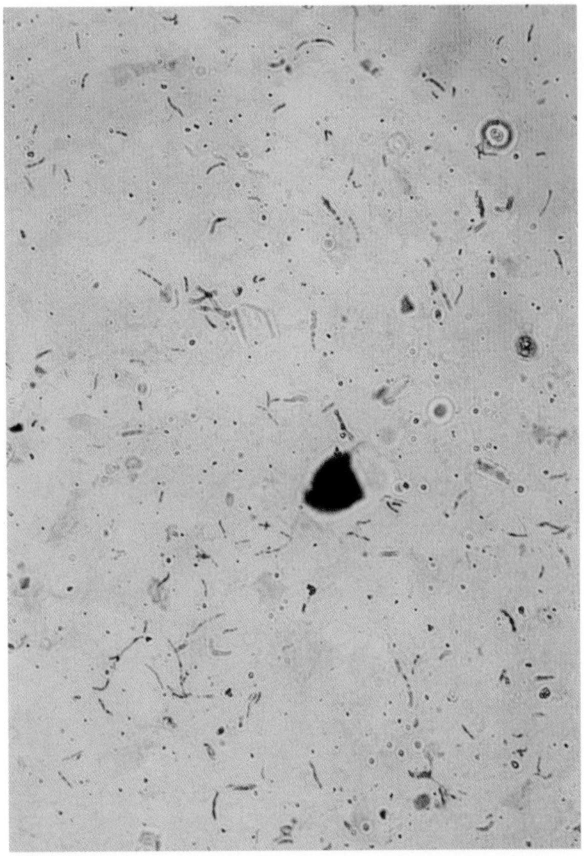

Fig. 17.2. Tubercle bacilli (acid-fast bacilli) in a sputum smear stained by the Ziehl–Neelsen stain as seen under the light microscope.

macrophages, so-called 'epithelioid cells', which surround the tubercle bacilli. Often these macrophages fuse together to form multi-nucleated giant cells. When these giant cells contain nuclei in a peripheral rim within the cell, they are called 'Langhans giant cells' (Fig. 17.3). Epithelioid cells and Langhans giant cells produce and secrete enzymes and free radicals at a higher rate than ordinary macrophages, and hence are more capaple of inhibiting and killing bacteria such as *M.tuberculosis.* Another common type of inflammatory cell in and around granulomas is the lymphocyte. Granulomas in tuberculosis characteristically fuse together. Single or fused granulomas may undergo necrosis in the centre. The resulting firm, pale and yellowish appearance gives rise to the description 'caseous necrosis' or 'cheese-like necrosis'.

The histopathological appearances relate to the host immune status. With strong host immunity, the histological appearances are those of caseating, giant cell and epithelioid cell granulomas with scanty or no tubercle bacilli. As immunity decreases, the histological appearances change

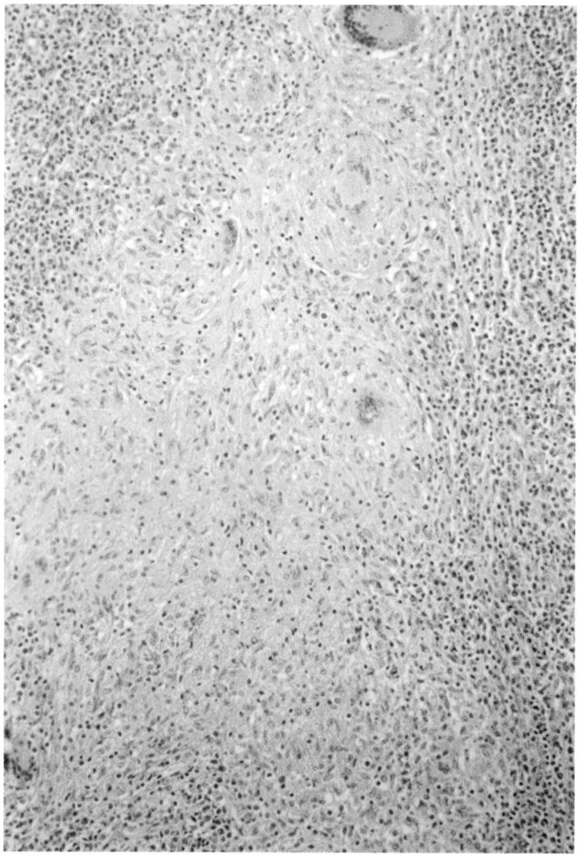

Fig. 17.3. A classical tuberculosis granuloma taken from a lymph node. Note the Langhans giant cell right (top).

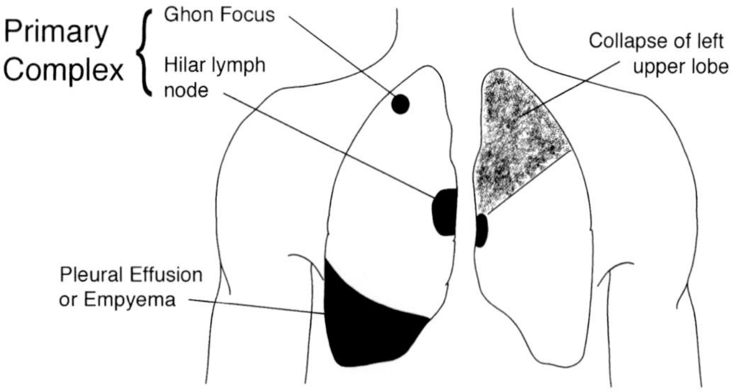

Fig. 17.4. Primary TB and some of the pulmonary complications.

Table 17.1. Outcome of the primary infection

90% of cases	Positive tuberculin test No clinical disease
Pulmonary outcome	Primary complex (Ghon focus plus hilar lymphadenopathy) Complications from primary complex: Advancing pneumonia Bronchial compression → lobar collapse Pleural effusion Pericardial effusion
Disseminated disease	Lymph node enlargement Meningitis Miliary disease
Hypersensitivity reactions	Erythema nodosum, i.e. nodular lesions of the skin usually on the front of the legs Phlyctenular conjunctivitis, i.e. painful irritation of the eye with small conjunctival spots Dactylitis, i.e. swelling of the fingers

to a more granular necrosis with reduced macrophage reaction and abundant tubercle bacilli.

The primary infection of tuberculosis

Primary infection occurs in persons who have not had any previous exposure to tubercle bacilli. The tubercle bacilli, which are inhaled into the lungs, lodge in the alveoli where they multiply. They then spread to the hilar lymph nodes, from where they spread throughout the body via the lymphatic system and blood stream. About 6 weeks after the primary infection, the body develops an immune response to the tubercle bacilli. This is delayed hypersensitivity, which in turn is associated with the development of cellular immunity and evidenced by a positive tuberculin skin test. These two factors together with the concentration of tubercle bacilli in the body determine the outcome of the infection. In the majority of cases, the immune response stops the multiplication of the tubercle bacilli, and the only external evidence of infection is a positive tuberculin test. In a few cases, disease does occur.

The outcome of the primary infection is illustrated in Table 17.1. The clinical manifestations of primary infection are usually seen in children or adults with HIV infection. The sputum is generally smear negative on microscopy and the radiographic findings are those of lung infiltrates, intrathoracic lymphadenopathy and pleural effusion (see Fig 17.4).

Table 17.2. Outcome of post-primary tuberculosis

Pulmonary disease	
Cavitating pulmonary lesions	
Upper lobe infiltrates	
Lung fibrosis	
Progressive pulmonary and endobronchial disease	
Extra-pulmonary disease	
Common	*Uncommon*
Lymphadenopathy	**Male genital tract** epididymitis; orchitis
Pleural effusion/empyema	**Female genital tract** tubo-ovarian; endometrium
Central nervous system meningitis; tuberculomas	**Kidney**
Cardiovascular pericarditis	**Endocrine** adrenal gland
Gastrointestinal ileocaecal; peritoneal	**Skin** miliary skin disease; lupus vulgaris; tuberculids
Bone commonest site is the spine	

Post-primary tuberculosis

After the primary infection resolves, small numbers of tubercle bacilli remain dormant in scarred areas of the body for many years. Post-primary tuberculosis may then occur due to reactivation of the tubercle bacilli acquired from a primary infection. It may also occur as a result of another infection with tubercle bacilli in a person who has already been exposed to the organism. The immune response of the patient results in a pathological lesion which is characteristically localized, often with extensive tissue destruction and cavitation. These cavitating lesions occur most commonly in the lungs (usually the apical and posterior segments of the upper lobes) and contain many actively dividing tubercle bacilli. Patients with these lesions are usually sputum smear-positive for tubercle bacilli, and are the main transmitters of infection in the community. Post-primary disease due to reactivation may also occur in any organ system to which the tubercle bacilli were seeded during primary infection.

The outcome of post-primary tuberculosis is illustrated in Table 17.2. Figures 17.5 and 17.6 show examples of pulmonary and extrapulmonary complications. The clinical manifestations of post-primary infection are usually seen in adults.

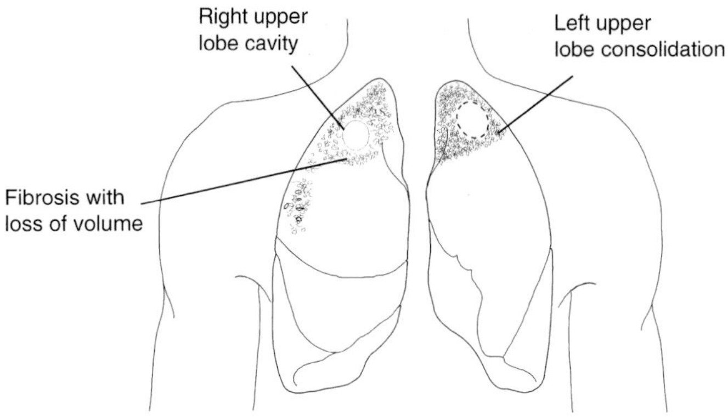

Fig. 17.5. Post-primary TB and some of the pulmonary complications.

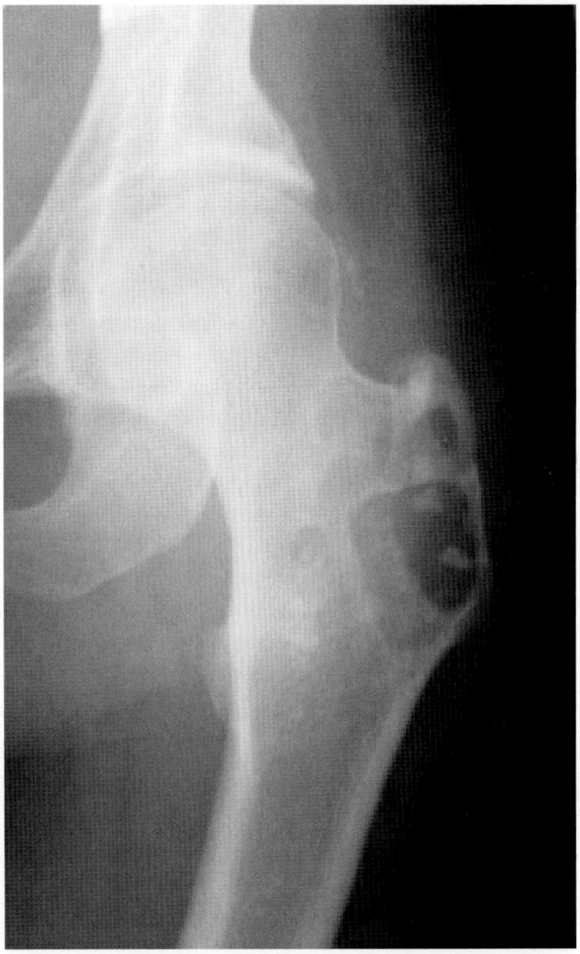

Fig. 17.6. Chronic tuberculosis of the greater trochanter. There is a large cystic lesion which is also expansile within the greater trochanter extending into the shaft of the upper femur. Calcific debris is demonstrated within the lesion but also proximal to it. The appearances are those of an inactive lesion. (By courtesy of the Wellcome Trust and the Institute of Orthopaedics.)

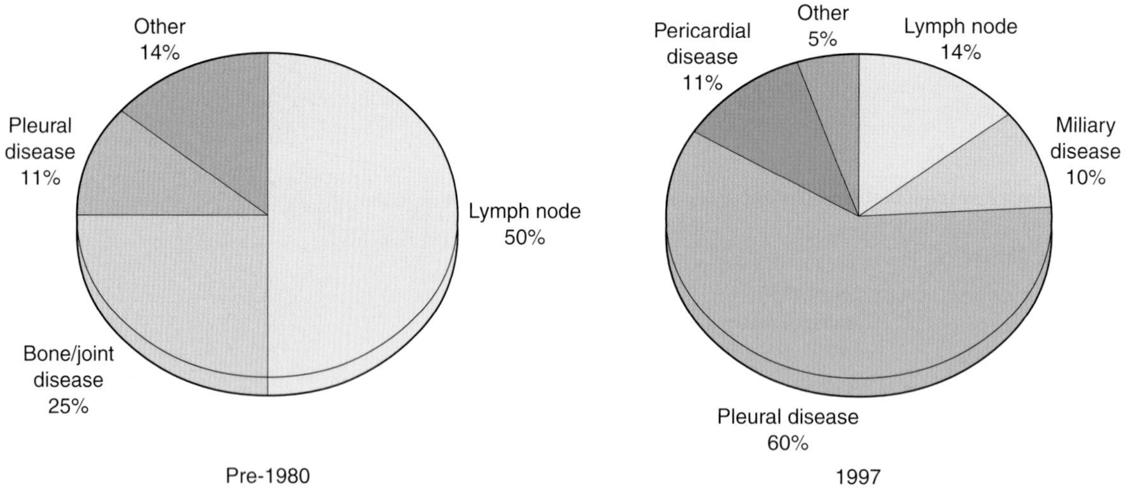

Fig. 17.7. Extrapulmonary tuberculosis in the pre-HIV-era and at the present time. (Data from East Africa, Harries et al., 1997.)

Clinical features and diagnosis

African tuberculosis before the advent of HIV infection

Large surveys carried out in Kenya and Tanzania between 1964 and 1984 provide excellent data on the pattern of tuberculosis prior to the HIV epidemic – see Figures 17.7, 17.8, 17.9, 17.10 (Kenya/British Medical Research Council, 1989). Almost 90 per cent of all patients had pulmonary disease. Amongst adults with pulmonary disease, nearly 80 per cent had sputum smears positive for tubercle bacilli on Ziehl–Neelsen stain and nearly 70 per cent had cavitation on chest radiography. Of those with extra-pulmonary tuberculosis, lymphadenopathy (mainly cervical in distribution), bone/joint disease and pleural effusion were responsible for 85 per cent of the total. Miliary disease, pericardial and peritoneal tuberculosis were uncommon.

African tuberculosis in association with HIV infection.

HIV-infected patients may develop tuberculosis across a wide spectrum of immunodeficiency. The clinical pattern of pulmonary tuberculosis correlates with the patient's immune status (De Cock et al., 1992). If tuberculosis occurs in the early stages of HIV infection, when immunity is only partially compromised, the features are characteristic of post-primary tuberculosis and resemble those seen in the pre-HIV era. As immune deficiency advances, HIV-positive patients present with atypical pul-

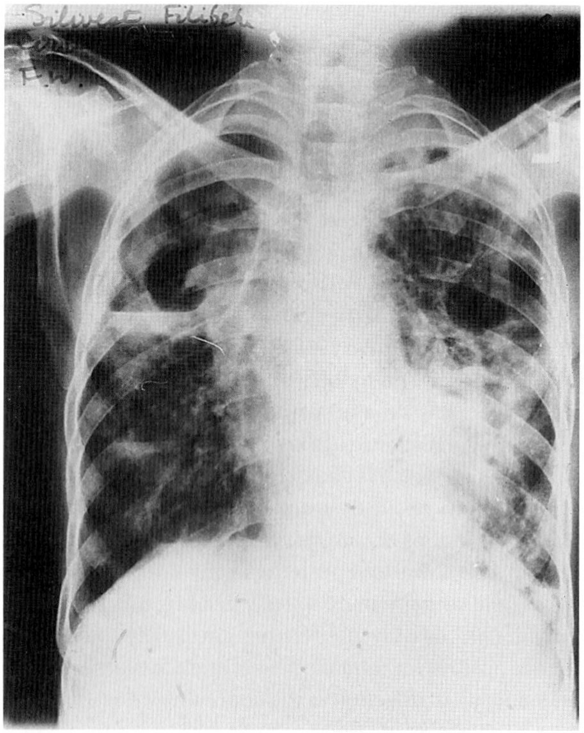

Fig. 17.8. Chest X-ray of smear-positive pulmonary tuberculosis patient.

monary disease resembling primary disease, or with extrapulmonary disease. Studies in sub-Saharan Africa have shown that the ratio of pulmonary to extrapulmonary disease is approximately 70 : 30 in HIV-positive patients. The pattern of HIV-associated extrapulmonary disease is in Fig. 17.7.

Pulmonary tuberculosis

Clinical features

Clinical features which may be found in patients with pulmonary tuberculosis are illustrated by this typical case.

A 35-year-old man presented to the outpatient department at a district hospital with cough productive of sputum for 4 months (see Fig. 17.11). He had visited a traditional healer who had given herbal medicines, and had also taken several different types of antibiotic purchased from a local grocery shop. He was starting to cough up blood, and in the last 2 weeks was experiencing right chest pain and breathlessness on exertion. He had lost weight, had intermittent fever and night sweats and was feeling tired. Physical examination showed that he was wasted, febrile and had some mild finger clubbing. Auscultation of the chest revealed inspiratory crackles throughout the right chest and amphoric bronchial breathing over the right anterior chest. Investigations showed that he had smear-positive pulmonary tuberculosis.

The most important clinical features for suspecting the diagnosis of pulmonary tuberculosis are cough for more than 3 weeks, sputum production, no response to antibiotics and weight loss (see Box).

When to suspect pulmonary tuberculosis
- Cough for 3 weeks or more which has not responded to a full course of antibiotics
- Cough which initially improves and then returns after a course or courses of antibiotics
- Haemoptysis (blood in the sputum)

Cough occurs in a variety of circumstances, notably in acute upper and lower respiratory infections. However, these acute infections often resolve within 3 weeks.

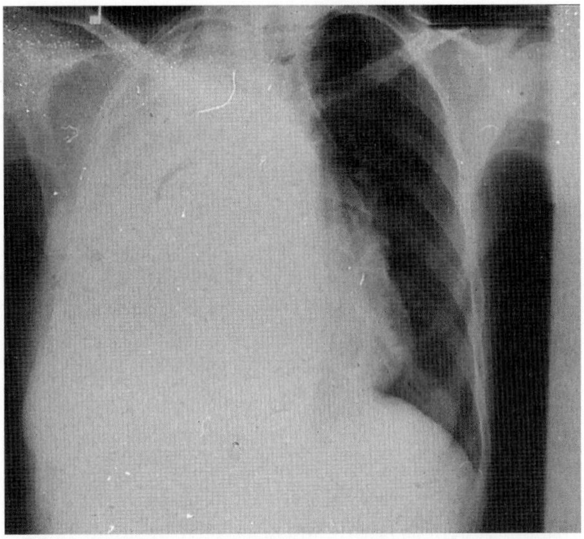

Fig. 17.9. Chest X-ray showing right tuberculous pleural effusion.

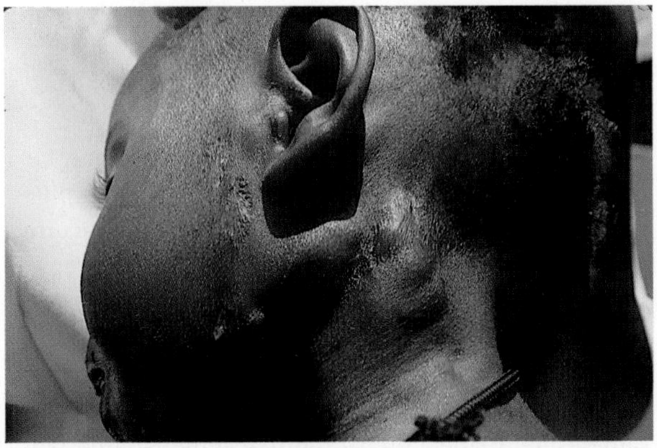

Fig. 17.10. Patient with tuberculous lymphadenopathy.

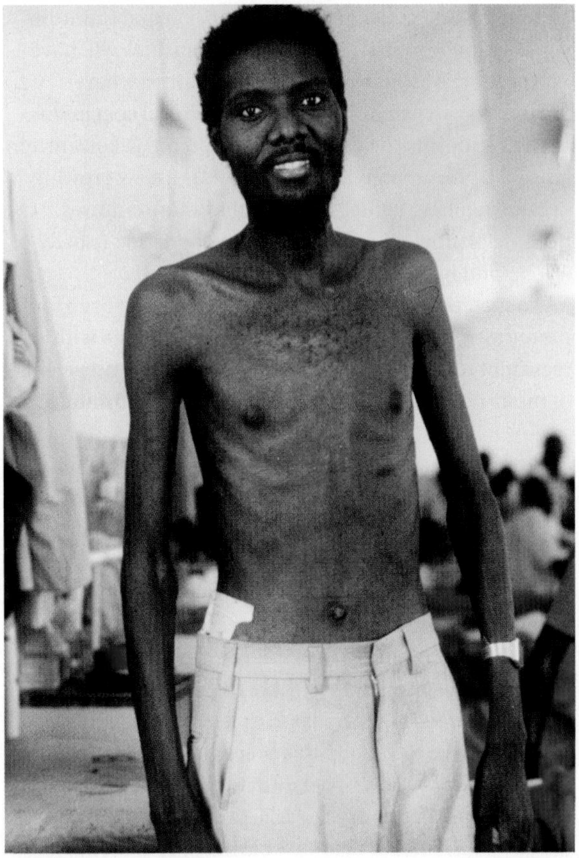

Fig. 17.11. A patient with smear-positive pulmonary tuberculosis.

Therefore, a patient with a cough longer than 3 weeks, especially after a course of antibiotics, must undergo investigations for tuberculosis. Patients with tuberculosis may have co-infection with other bacteria such as *Streptococcus pneumoniae* (Scott et al., 2000). In such patients, the symptom of cough may initially disappear after antibiotics only to return a few weeks later. Patients with recurring cough must also be investigated for tuberculosis.

The physical signs in patients with pulmonary tuberculosis are non-specific, and do not help in deciding whether the patient has tuberculosis or another respiratory disease. Particularly in immunosuppressed patients, there may be no abnormal signs in the chest.

Diagnostic approach in pulmonary tuberculosis.

The diagnosis of pulmonary tuberculosis in most African hospitals is based on simple techniques: sputum smear microscopy and chest radiography. While the tuberculin skin test is useful for measuring the prevalence of tuberculous infection in the community, it is of much less value for individual adult diagnosis because of (i) false-positives from exposure to environmental mycobacteria and (ii) false-negatives from malnutrition and immunosuppression from HIV. Most African countries will have one or more hospital/reference laboratories where *M.tuberculosis* can be cultured from clinical specimens such as sputum. The usual culture medium is Lowenstein Jensen. Unfortunately, *M.tuberculosis* is a slow growing organism taking up to 2 or 3 months before cultures become positive. Culture results are, therefore, usually not helpful in making an individual diagnosis. Mycobacterial culture facilities are more often used for monitoring drug-sensitivity patterns in patients with recurrent tuberculosis and for monitoring the prevalence of multi-drug resistant tuberculosis in the community.

Sputum smear examination

The most cost-effective way to screen pulmonary tuberculosis suspects is for them to first submit three sputum specimens. Two of the specimens can conveniently be collected on consecutive days in the clinic, with the third specimen being an early morning sample produced at home before coming to the clinic on day 2. In well-run laboratories, submission of more than three sputum specimens does not increase the yield of smear-positive cases (Toman, 1997), and this practice is therefore wasteful of resources and scarce laboratory time. Mycobacteria are 'acid-and alcohol-fast' (AAFB), although the term is usually shortened to 'acid-fast bacilli' or AFB. In most laboratories sputum smears are made and stained with the Ziehl–Neelsen stain (see Box and Fig. 17.2).

Ziehl–Neelsen stain for acid-fast bacilli

- Place a small portion of sputum (purulent material if possible) on a glass slide and spread thinly.
- Allow the sputum smear to dry in the air for about 15–30 minutes.
- Fix the smear by passing three times through a flame (Bunsen-burner or spirit lamp).
- Cover the whole surface of the slide with carbol fuschin.
- Heat very gently until vapour rises and leave the warm stain for five minutes.
- Rinse the slide in a gentle stream of running water.
- Cover the slide with 25% sulphuric acid, leave for 3 minutes and rinse (this decolorizes the smear).
- Cover the slide again with 25% sulphuric acid, leave for 1–3 minutes and rinse.
- Counter-stain with methylene blue for 60 seconds, rinse and allow to dry in air.

The organisms observed with the oil immersion objective are slightly bent rods, red in colour and beaded. Another technique for detection of AFB uses a fluorochrome stain with auramine, acid-alcohol decolorization and a methylene blue counterstain. The AFB fluoresce yellow against a dark background, and smears can be scanned under low magnification with a special fluorescent microscope. This provides a more rapid means of screening several sputum smears than Ziehl–Neelsen staining. Most mycobacteria seen under the microscope in Africa are *M.tuberculosis* complex.

Sputum smears are conveniently reported either as positive or negative. If AFBs are present they can be recorded on a scale ranging from scanty when less than 9 are seen in 100 high power fields, to +++ when there are more than 10 in every field. The clinician can then categorize the patient as having smear-positive or smear-negative pulmonary tuberculosis, Table 17.3 (WHO, 1997). In patients with pulmonary tuberculosis, AFB will only be detected on microscopy if there are 10 000 organisms or more per ml of sputum. If there are less than 10 000 organisms per ml of sputum, the sputum smear will usually be negative.

Negative results of sputum smear microscopy may be because (i) the patient has genuine smear-negative pulmonary tuberculosis, (ii) the clinical diagnosis is incorrect and the patient has another condition such as left ventricular failure, asthma, bacterial pneumonia, *Pneumocystis carinii* pneumonia or pulmonary Kaposi's Sarcoma, or (iii) there are false-negative results of smear microscopy due to technical inadequacies (poor sputum sample, faulty smear preparation) or administrative failures (incorrect labelling of specimens).

Chest radiography

The usual indications for a chest X-ray are shown in the Box.

When to request a chest X-ray

In pulmonary TB suspects:
- Cough for 3 or more weeks, no response to antibiotics and negative sputum smears
- Haemoptysis
- Severe breathlessness.

In confirmed smear-positive pulmonary TB patients
- Severe breathlessness to rule out complications
- Frequent haemoptysis.

Pulmonary tuberculosis suspects should proceed to chest radiography after negative sputum smear results have been obtained and providing there has been no response to a course of antibiotics. In general, patients with positive sputum smears do not need a chest X-ray. Exceptions to this rule include

(i) patients with dyspnoea in order to rule out associated complications such as pneumothorax, pleural effusion and pericardial effusion which may be helped by specific therapy,
(ii) patients with frequent haemoptysis to determine the presence or absence of bronchiectasis or aspergilloma,
(iii) patients with only one positive sputum smear for AFB in whom an abnormal chest radiograph is required to fulfil the criteria for diagnosis of smear-positive PTB (see Table 17.3).

The following clinical case illustrates the vital need for a chest X-ray in a breathless patient:

A 24-year old woman diagnosed ten days previously with smear-positive pulmonary tuberculosis suddenly developed dyspnoea while on anti-TB treatment. Examination revealed a resonant percussion note and absent breath sounds over the right chest.

Chest radiography showed a large right-sided tension pneumothorax (see Fig. 17.12). Immediate insertion of a chest drain with underwater seal resulted in prompt relief of symptoms.

No chest radiographic pattern is absolutely diagnostic of tuberculosis. Classical and atypical patterns are shown in Fig. 17.13 and Fig. 17.14. The classical radiographic pattern is more common in HIV-negative patients. The chest radiographic manifestations in HIV-infected patients correlate with the degree of immunosuppression. Patients with relatively well-preserved immune function will show cavitation and upper lobe infiltrates (the classical pattern). Those with severe immunosuppression will show atypical changes. It is well recognized that the chest radiograph can be normal in HIV-positive pulmonary tuberculosis patients, rendering the diagnosis of tuberculosis very difficult if the sputum smears are also negative (Colebunders & Bastian, 2000).

Table 17.3. Classification of patients by sputum smear

Smear-positive	Indeterminate	Smear-negative
At least two smears examined and both positive (i.e. scanty or greater)	Only one smear examined	At least 2 two smears reported 0 (i.e. negative)
	Three smears examined but only one positive	
One smear positive with an abnormal chest X-ray	(In either of these situations, further sputum smears needed or a chest X-ray needed before the patient can be classified)	

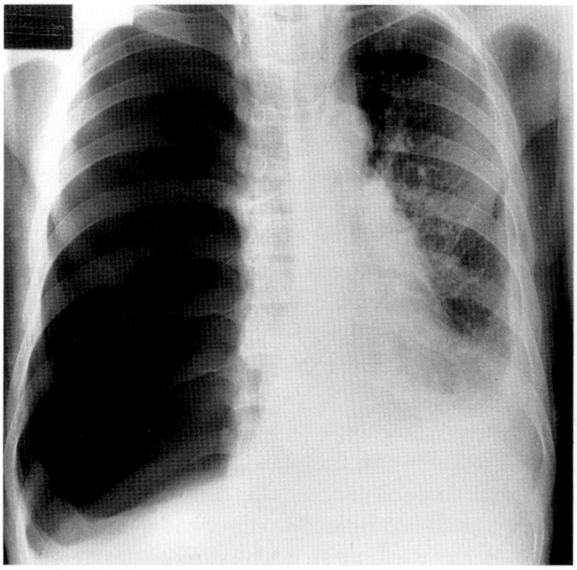

Fig. 17.12. Chest X-ray showing large right pneumothorax in a patient being treated for smear-positive pulmonary TB.

Extra-pulmonary tuberculosis

General features

The common forms of extra-pulmonary tuberculosis are shown in Fig. 17.7. Patients usually present with

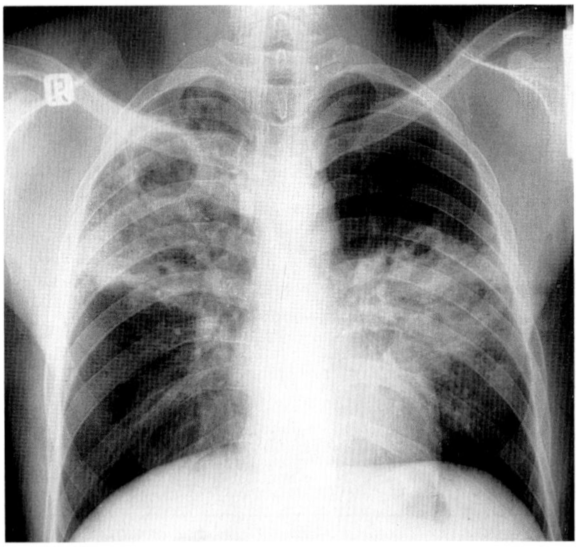

Fig. 17.13. Chest X-ray showing the classical features of post-primary pulmonary TB.

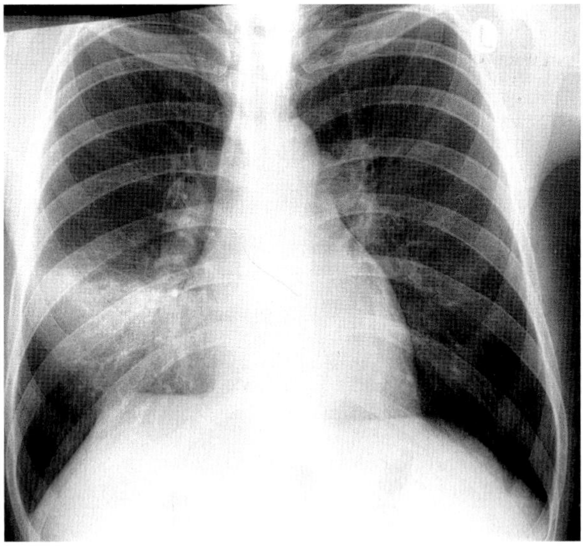

Fig. 17.14. Chest X-ray showing atypical features of pulmonary TB: the patient was sputum smear-negative.

constitutional symptoms and local features related to the site of disease. If patients cough for longer than 3 weeks, sputum smear examination and chest radiography should be carried out as patients may have co-existing pulmonary disease. Definitive diagnosis of extrapulmonary disease depends on available diagnostic tools: such as radiographs, ultrasound scanning, procedures to obtain and analyse fluid samples and procedures for tissue biopsies and histological analysis. This degree of diagnostic sophistication is often unavailable in district hospitals in Africa: in one study in Tanzania only 18 per cent of patients with extra-pulmonary TB had laboratory confirmation of the diagnosis (Richter et al., 1991). If laboratory confirmation cannot be made, a clinical diagnosis of tuberculosis is quite permissible, provided other conditions have been carefully excluded.

Tuberculous lymphadenopathy

Cervical lymph node involvement (scrofula) (Fig. 17.10) is the commonest presentation, regardless of HIV-serostatus. Lymphadenopathy can also be found in the axilla and in the groin. Initially, lymph nodes are firm and discrete, but later they become matted together and fluctuant. The overlying skin may break down with formation of abscesses and chronic discharging sinuses, which heal with scarring. In the immunosuppressed patient the lymphadenitis may be acute and resemble an acute pyogenic bacterial infection.

The important differential diagnoses in a patient presenting with tuberculous lymphadenopathy includes HIV-related persistent generalized lymphadenopathy, lymphoma, Kaposi's sarcoma, carcinoma, chronic lymphatic leukaemia, sarcoidosis, and secondary syphilis. HIV-related persistent generalized lymphadenopathy (PGL) is the most common differential diagnosis. PGL is symmetrical, often involving the posterior cervical chain or the epitrochlear regions, and is non-tender. In high HIV-prevalence areas, many patients with lymphadenopathy will have PGL and it is neither feasible nor cost-effective to investigate all such patients. However, investigation of lymphadenopathy is required if there are features to suggest a disease other than PGL (see Box).

Clinical features of lymphadenopathy that indicate the need for investigation

- Lymph nodes abnormally large (>4 cm in diameter)
- Asymmetrical lymphadenopathy
- Rapid increase in size of lymph nodes
- Painful/tender lymph nodes not associated with local infection
- Adherent or fluctuant lymph nodes
- Fever, weight loss or malaise
- Hilar or mediastinal lymphadenopathy.

In hospitals with no histology or tuberculous culture facilities, a needle aspirate of a suitable lymph node is the best first line investigation. The aspirated material can be

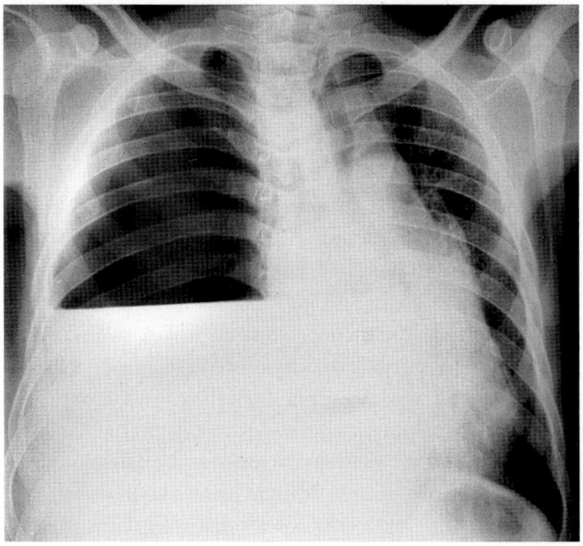

Fig. 17.15. Chest X-ray showing a large tension hydropneumothorax in a patient with confirmed pulmonary TB.

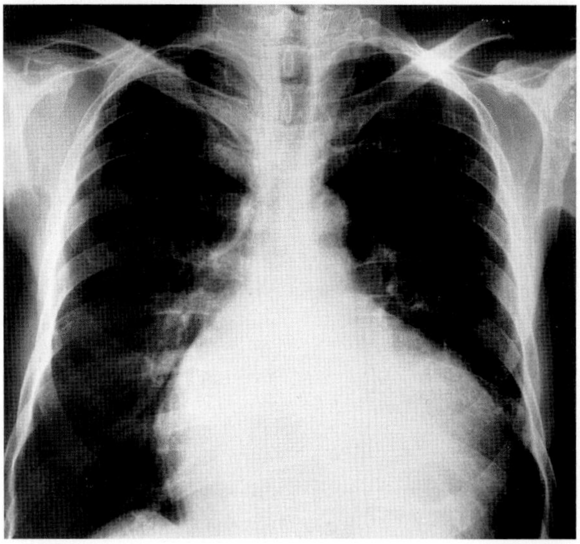

Fig. 17.16. Chest X-ray showing tuberculous pericardial effusion.

examined macroscopically for caseation and also smeared on a slide for AFB examination. If no diagnosis is made after lymph node aspirate, a lymph node can be biopsied, and the cut surface examined for caseation and a smear made from the cut surface for AFB examination. This approach is an effective and cheap way of reaching a diagnosis. Needle aspiration of peripheral TB lymphadenopathy in HIV-positive patients reveals AFB in up to 70 per cent of cases, and macroscopical examination of lymph nodes together with a cut-surface smear/aspiration smear may give a correct diagnosis in almost 80 per cent of cases. In hospitals with access to histopathological services, histological findings in TB lymph nodes from HIV-positive patients depend to some extent on the degree of immunosuppression of the individual: (i) in patients with mild degrees of immunosuppression there may be caseating, giant cell and epithelioid cell granulomas associated with scanty or no visible AFB – this is similar to what is seen in patients who are HIV-seronegative; (ii) in patients with marked immunosuppression there may be necrosis, poor cellular reactivity and numerous bacilli.

Tuberculous serous effusions

Serous effusions occur in the pleural cavity, in the pericardium and in the peritoneum, and they are more common in HIV-infected patients. The aspirate from such lesions is an exudate with a high protein content and white cells consisting predominantly of lymphocytes and monocytes. Ziehl–Neelsen staining of the aspirate is positive in less than 5 per cent of patients. In district hospitals the presence of a serous effusion which clots on standing for 30 minutes, in a patient with a chronic illness is highly suggestive of tuberculosis. Proof of diagnosis in serous effusions would require positive culture from the serous fluid and culture/histology from adjacent tissue (e.g. pleural or peritoneal biopsy), none of which is usually possible in a district hospital.

The development of a pleural effusion is thought to be a result of primary infection (see Fig. 17.9). Sometimes there is a broncho-pleural fistula, which results in a hydro-pneumothorax (see Fig. 17.15). This can be diagnosed clinically by finding a succussion splash, and its importance lies in the fact that drainage with an under-water seal is required for treatment. A pericardial effusion (see Fig. 17.16) is also most likely to be the result of a primary infection, and often develops as a result of rupture of a mediastinal lymph node into the pericardial space. Peritoneal tuberculosis often arises as a result of spread from mesenteric lymph nodes which become matted together, rupture and cause an exudative effusion within the peritoneal cavity. The most appropriate ways of diagnosing each serous effusion is shown in Table 17.4. Because of the need for chest radiography, the diagnosis of these conditions will usually need to be made at a hospital. Use of other investigations such as ultrasound, electrocardiography or pleural biopsy will depend on the diagnostic facilities available. Diagnosis of pericardial effusion can sometimes be difficult, and a high index of suspicion is required in order that the diagnosis is not overlooked

Table 17.4. diagnosis of tuberculous serous effusions

Pleural effusion	
Investigation	*Findings*
Chest X-ray	Unilateral white opacity
Pleural aspiration	Lymphocytic exudate
Pleural biopsy (if available)	Tuberculous granulomas
Pericardial effusion[a]	
Investigation	*Findings*
Chest X-ray	Large globular heart
ECG	Low voltage QRS complexes
Ultrasound	Fluid, often with fibrin strands
Tuberculous Ascites[b]	
Investigation	*Findings*
Chest X-ray	Look for evidence of pulmonary tuberculosis
Ascitic aspiration	Lymphocytic aspirate
Ultrasound	Mesenteric lymph nodes

Notes:

[a] Pericardiocentesis is a potentially dangerous procedure, and is mainly recommended for relief of pericardial tamponade

[b] Blind percutaneous needle biopsy of the peritoneum is not recommended because of low sensitivity and high complication rate. In experienced hands, laparoscopy under local anaesthesia has a high diagnostic success rate.

A 36-year-old man presented with an enlarged liver, ascites and peripheral oedema. A clinical diagnosis of liver cirrhosis was made. On review, there was a tachycardia with 15 mm Hg pulsus paradoxus, an elevated jugular venous pressure of 15 cm, an impalpable apex beat and quiet heart sounds. Chest radiography and ultrasound confirmed the presence of a large pericardial effusion (see Fig. 17.16). The patient responded well to anti-TB treatment with corticosteroids also given for the first 8 weeks.

Tuberculous meningitis (see also p. 313)

Tubercle bacilli usually gain access to the cerebrospinal fluid via small cerebral tuberculomata. Sometimes the disease can occur as part of miliary tuberculosis. Clinically, there is evidence of a chronic meningitis with gradual onset of fever, headache, and altered consciousness. Involvement of the base of the brain may cause cranial nerve palsies. Tuberculomata, vascular occlusion and hydrocephalus may give rise to focal neurology and seizures. The spinal meninges can also be affected causing a spastic or flaccid paraplegia. The diagnosis rests almost entirely on examination of the cerebrospinal fluid (CSF). CSF is obtained by lumbar puncture (always first checking the optic fundi for papilloedma, which if present is a contraindication to LP). CSF opening pressure is elevated. The CSF is usually clear, and the typical findings are a white cell count of 500/mm^3, predominantly lymphocytes, with an elevated protein and reduced glucose. It is not common to find AFB in CSF, although large volumes of CSF (up to 10 ml) may give a higher yield of AFB after centrifugation. In both HIV-positive and HIV-negative patients the CSF parameters may be normal, and on occasions the CSF may be completely normal, leading to difficulties in diagnosis. In high HIV-prevalent areas the other main diagnoses to consider are cryptococcal meningitis and partially treated bacterial meningitis. Indian ink stain (to look for the capsules of *Cryptococcus neoformans*) should always be performed on patients with clinical features suggesting chronic meningitis or lymphocytic meningitis.

Untreated tuberculous meningitis is fatal, and the earlier it is diagnosed and treated then the more likely the patient is to recover without serious permanent damage. Therefore, if the clinical and CSF findings are at all suggestive of the disease and other conditions can be excluded (i.e. lymphocytic meningitis with negative Indian ink stain), treatment should be given. A useful objective response to treatment is a progressive rise in CSF glucose, which can therefore be monitored on a weekly basis when the diagnosis has been in doubt.

Miliary tuberculosis

Miliary tuberculosis occurs when tubercle bacilli are spread through the blood stream. The disease occurs either from a recent primary infection or from reactivation of a tuberculous lesion with erosion of a blood vessel. The disease presents with gradual onset of fever, malaise and weight loss. Physical examination may reveal hepatosplenomegaly, and choroidal tubercles may rarely be found on fundoscopy. Often the presentation is part of a fever of unknown origin and the diagnosis can easily be missed, especially if the clinical presentation is atypical. Autopsy studies on HIV-positive patients with 'wasting disease' in Cote d'Ivoire showed the presence of disseminated tuberculosis in up to 40 per cent of cases, the diagnosis in many cases not having been made ante-mortem (Lucas et al., 1994).

In suspected cases of miliary TB, a chest radiograph should be carried out (see Fig. 17.17). The chest X-ray shows diffuse, evenly distributed, small miliary shadows. However, in the early stages of the disease, the chest X-ray may be normal. Other useful investigations (if available) are: (i) full blood count – which shows a pancytopenia, (ii) liver function tests – which show elevated transaminases and/or alkaline phosphatase, (iii) sputum smears – which may be positive, (iv) liver biopsy – which may show granulomas and (v) bone marrow aspiration – which may show granulomas. The main differential diagnosis of miliary tuberculosis is bacteraemia, especially enteric (typhoid) fever, the AIDS wasting syndrome, disseminated carcinoma, connective tissue diseases, and in endemic regions, trypanosomiasis. Here is an illustrative case.

A 33-year-old man presented with fever, weight loss, right sided abdominal pain and mild jaundice. On examination, there was an enlarged liver with a loud friction rub. A clinical diagnosis of hepatocellular carcinoma was made. A chest radiograph showed classical miliary tuberculosis (see Fig. 17.17). An ultrasound of the liver revealed an inflammatory hepatic capsule with normal liver architecture – there was no evidence of hepatoma. The patient recovered completely on anti-TB treatment.

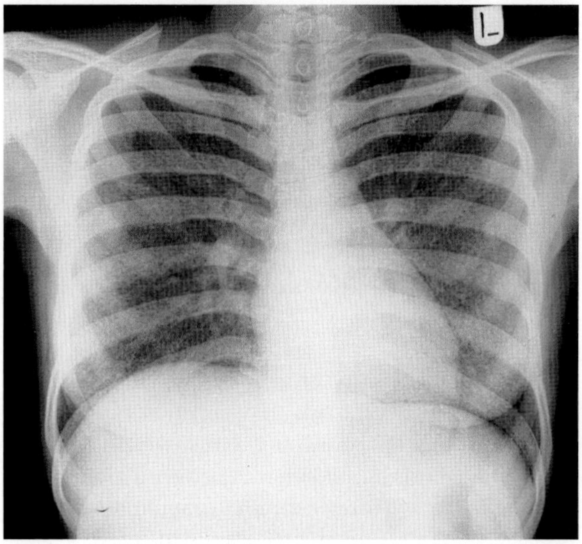

Fig. 17.17. Chest X-ray of miliary tuberculosis.

Tuberculosis of the spine

Tuberculosis starts as an inflammation of the intervertebral disc, which then spreads along the anterior and longitudinal ligaments to involve the adjacent vertebral bodies. Tuberculosis of the spine is important because in the thoracic or cervical region the consequences of missing the diagnosis can lead to irreversible paraplegia. Patients present with back pain, sometimes a gibbus, and paraparesis/paraplegia if there is spinal cord involvement. The diagnosis can usually be made on plain radiography. The classical radiographic appearance is erosion of the anterior edges of the superior and inferior borders of adjacent vertebral bodies with narrowing of the disc space (Figs. 17.18, 17.19, 17.20). The

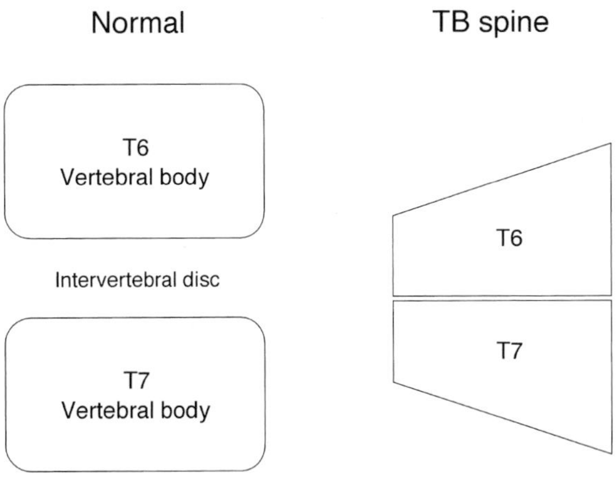

Fig. 17.18. Drawing of lateral spine showing classical features of spinal TB.

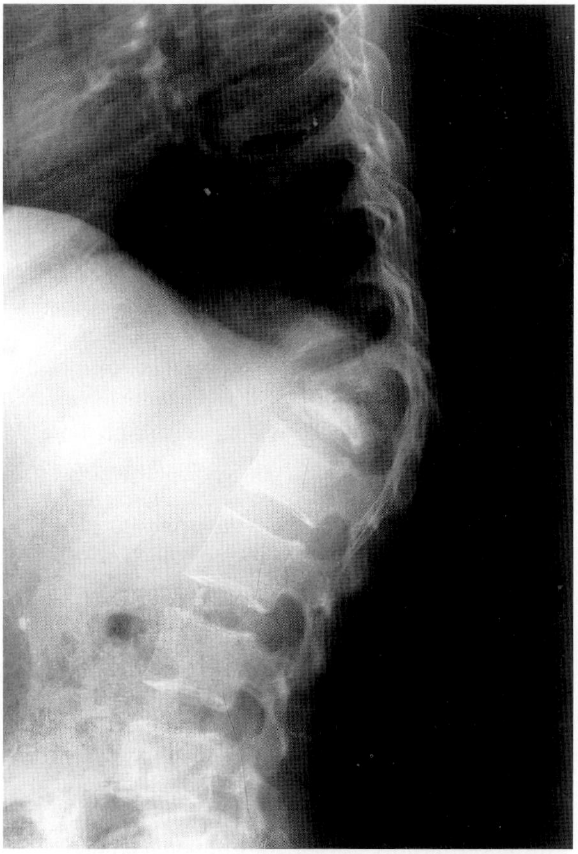

Fig. 17.19. X-ray of the spine – lateral view – showing tuberculosis of the spine.

Table 17.5. Less common forms of extra-pulmonary tuberculosis

Site of disease	Clinical features	Diagnosis
Upper respiratory tract	Hoarseness Pain in ear Pain on swallowing	Usually complication of pulmonary disease
Bone	Chronic osteomyelitis	Tissue biopsy
Peripheral joints	Usually monoarthritis	Plain radiography Synovial biopsy
Renal and urinary tract *M.tuberculosis*	Micturition frequency Dysuria	Sterile pyuria Urine culture
	Haematuria Loin pain/swelling	Intravenous pyelogram
Ileocaecal TB	Chronic diarrhoea Mass Rt iliac fossa	Barium X-ray Colonoscopy
Adrenal gland	Features of hypo-adrenalism (hypotension, low sodium, normal/high potassium, raised blood urea, low blood glucose)	Plain X-ray (calcification) Ultrasound
Female genital tract	Infertility Pelvic inflammatory disease Ectopic pregnancy	Pelvic examination X-ray genital tract Tissue biopsy
Male genital tract	Epididymitis	Often evidence of renal/urine TB

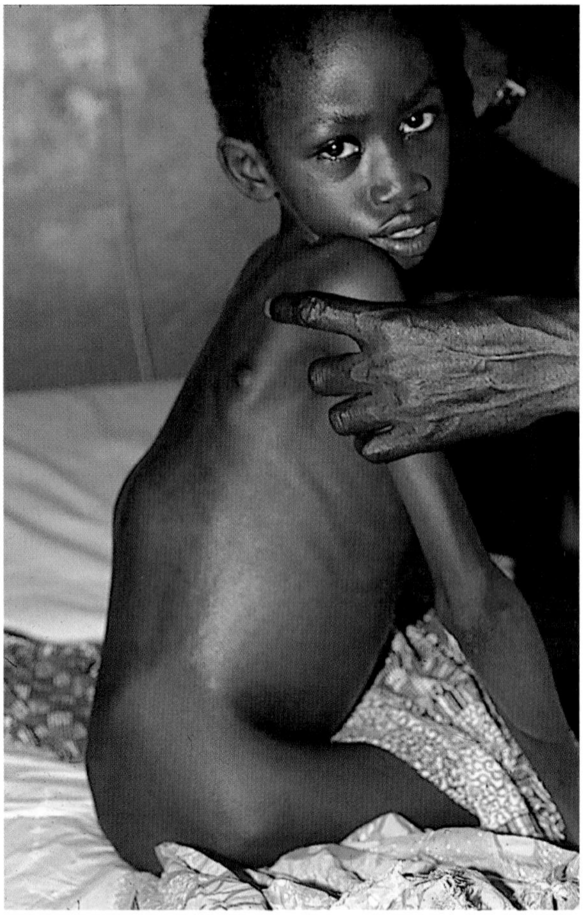

Fig. 17.20. Child with Pott's disease of the lower thoracic spine.

thoracic, lumbar and lumbosacral vertebrae are the sites most commonly involved. The main differential diagnoses are other pyogenic spinal infections and malignancy. Malignant deposits in the spine tend to erode the pedicles and spinal bodies and leave the disc intact. Pyogenic infection tends to be more acute with more severe pain.

Other forms of extrapulmonary tuberculosis

Other forms of extrapulmonary tuberculosis are not common. The clinical features and usual diagnostic tests are shown in Table 17.5.

Tuberculosis in children

General

Children are infected with *M.tuberculosis* as a result of transmission from an adult (often a family member) with smear-positive disease. Most children remain asymptomatic, the only evidence of infection being a positive tuberculin test. The risk of progressing to disease is influenced by the age of the child (the younger the child the higher the risk), HIV infection, nutritional status and other infections such as measles. The diagnosis of tuberculosis in children may be very difficult. Although there is a propensity for extrapulmonary disease, pulmonary tuberculosis is still the most common manifestation in HIV-negative and HIV-positive children. Bacteriological confirmation in children is usually not possible. There are the usual difficulties with extra-pulmonary tuberculosis, and children with pulmonary tuberculosis usually swallow their sputum rather than cough it up. Gastric aspiration and laryngeal swabs are sometimes used to identify swallowed organisms, and these procedures can be useful in the diagnosis of tuberculosis in children.

Diagnosis of pulmonary tuberculosis in children

The diagnosis is based on clinical features, history of contact with a sputum positive case, chest X-ray and

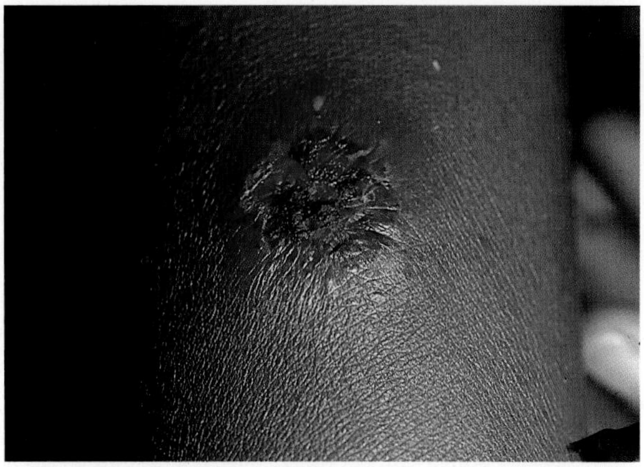

Fig. 17.21. A strongly positive Mantoux test, with ulceration.

tuberculin skin test. Clinical features are non-specific, the most important being weight loss, poor appetite and failure to thrive. Chest X-ray findings are also non-specific, the most common being a broad mediastinum from hilar or mediastinal lymph glands, miliary infiltrations and a pleural effusion. In the presence of other features, a strongly positive tuberculin skin test (Fig. 17.21) is very suggestive of tuberculosis. However, a positive skin test occurs after recent BCG immunization, and a negative test may occur in the presence of TB if there is HIV infection, malnutrition and severe disseminated TB.

Impact of HIV on diagnosis of tuberculosis in children

HIV infection makes the diagnosis of tuberculosis more difficult because several HIV-related respiratory diseases have similar features. Weight loss is a common problem, chest X-ray features are often atypical and interpretation of the tuberculin skin test is even more unreliable than usual. Common conditions which occur in HIV-positive children younger than 5 years and which may be misdiagnosed as tuberculosis, are *Pneumocystis carinii* pneumonia and bacterial pneumonia.

Diagnosis of HIV infection amongst patients with tuberculosis

About 50 per cent of HIV-positive patients with tuberculosis in Africa have no other features to suggest HIV infection except for TB. Voluntary HIV testing with pre- and post-test counselling for TB patients has a number of individual and public health benefits. Knowledge of HIV-serostatus can lead to: (i) improved diagnosis and management of other HIV-related illnesses, (ii) use of co-trimoxazole prophylaxis to prevent opportunistic infections and reduce mortality, (iii) recognition that there is an increased frequency of adverse drug reactions, and therefore the potential for avoiding these reactions, and (iv) the opportunity to counsel patients and relatives about HIV infection, and so adopt measures to prevent further HIV transmission.

Treatment of tuberculosis

Anti-tuberculosis chemotherapy – general aspects

There are five main aims of chemotherapy:

(a) Cure of the patient
(b) Prevention of death from active disease or its late effects
(c) Avoidance of relapse or recurrent disease
(d) Prevention of spread of drug-resistant organisms
(e) Protection of the community from infection.

Essential anti-tuberculosis drugs and their mode of action

Essential drugs

There are six essential drugs. Four are predominantly **bactericidal – isoniazid, rifampicin, pyrazinamide and streptomycin**, and two are predominantly **bacteriostatic – ethambutol and thiacetazone.** The bacterial population consists of (a) metabolically active, continuously growing bacteria which are found within the walls of tuberculous cavities, (b) bacteria inside cells and macrophages, (c) semi-dormant bacteria which undergo spurts of metabolism and (d) dormant bacteria, which die off gradually on their own.

Isoniazid is the most potent bactericidal drug, and kills 90 per cent of the bacillary population during the first few days of chemotherapy. It is most effective against metabolically active, continuously growing bacteria. Rifampicin is another good bactericidal drug. Streptomycin and pyrazinamide are less strongly bactericidal. With the use of these powerful drugs, most smear-positive PTB patients are probably rendered non-infectious after 2 weeks of treatment.

Rifampicin is active against semi-dormant bacilli, and the drug is therefore regarded as a good sterilizing agent. Semi-dormant bacilli undergo spurts of metabolism, but while they are in their semi-dormant state they are capable of surviving the bactericidal action of isoniazid. They are therefore important in causing relapse after treatment. Rifampicin is therefore effective in preventing relapse of disease. Pyrazinamide is another important sterilizing drug which kills bacilli that are well protected in an acid medium inside cells and macrophages.

Thiacetazone, which was such a useful and cheap bacteriostatic drug in Africa in the pre-HIV era, developed a bad reputation amongst the community and health care staff with the advent of HIV infection. This was due to the high frequency of cutaneous skin reactions, which occurred in up to 20 per cent of HIV-positive patients (Nunn et al., 1991). Some of these reactions were severe with skin exfoliation or mucous membrane involvement (Stevens–Johnson syndrome), sometimes resulting in death of the patient. Many tuberculosis control programmes have now removed thiacetazone from their essential drug list, which therefore has five instead of six drugs.

Preventing the emergence of drug resistance

Tubercle bacilli which have not been exposed to antituberculous drugs contain a few drug-resistant mutants. If only one or two drugs are used in patients with high bacillary loads, drug-resistant mutants may replace susceptible bacilli and give rise to drug-resistant disease. Isoniazid and rifampicin are the most effective drugs in preventing the emergence of drug resistance.

Dosage for daily and intermittent treatment

Anti-tuberculosis drugs come as streptomycin for injection, with other drugs formulated as single tablets and combination tablets. Doses of anti-tuberculosis drugs for daily and for intermittent treatment are shown in Table 17.6. All anti-TB regimens are effective when given two or three times a week. It is very important to ensure that the correct doses are given – the doses are usually higher with the intermittent regimens compared with the daily regimens. In order to simplify drug doses, many tuberculosis control programmes use weight bands for calculating doses. In adult patients, these weight bands are:

>55 kg, 40–55 kg, and 25–39 kg. For example, any adult weighing 40–55 kg who is taking rifinah (combination rifampicin 150 mg and isoniazid 100 mg), pyrazinamide (400 mg) and ethambutol (400 mg) on a daily basis would receive 3 tablets of rifinah, 3 tablets of pyrazinamide and 2 tablets of ethambutol (Enarson et al., 1996).

Principles of anti-tuberculosis chemotherapy

As a result of the different populations of bacteria within any individual with tuberculosis, it is important that anti-tuberculosis drugs are always used in combination. If they are administered singly (i.e. monotherapy), then they will not adequately control the bacillary population and this will encourage the emergence of drug resistance (see below). In addition to the important principle of combination chemotherapy, anti-tuberculosis drugs must be given for several months in order to kill off the slow-dividing or semi-dormant bacilli. If regimens shorter than 6 months are used, then a significant proportion of patients will suffer relapse disease arising from semi-dormant bacilli which were not adequately sterilized.

Table 17.6. Dosage of anti-tuberculosis drugs in relation to body weight

Drug	Daily	Three times per week	Twice per week
Isoniazid	5 (4–6)	10 (8–12)	15 (13–17)
Rifampicin	10 (8–12)	10 (8–12)	10 (8–12)
Pyrazinamide	25 (20–30)	35 (30–40)	50 (40–60)
Ethambutol	15 (15–20)	30 (25–35)	45 (40–50
Streptomycin	15 (12–18)	15 (12–18)	15 (12–18)
Thiacetazone	3	Not used	Not used

Notes:
Doses given in mg/kg with the range shown in parenthesis.

Drug resistance

General

Drug-resistant *M. tuberculosis* develops from spontaneous, random mutations of the bacterial chromosome. These mutations are generally unlinked, ie resistance to one drug is not associated with resistance to an unrelated drug. In a bacterial population which has not been exposed to anti-tuberculosis drugs, the highest proportions of drug-resistant mutants that will occur have been estimated to be, for example, 3×10^{-6} for isoniazid, 4×10^{-6} for streptomycin and 3×10^{-8} for rifampicin. The likelihood of spontaneous mutations causing resistance to both isoniazid and rifampicin is the product of these possibilities, or 1 in 10^{15}. It has been estimated that pulmonary cavities contain about 10^7 to 10^9 bacilli. Thus, cavitatory lesions are likely to contain a small number of bacilli resistant to a single drug, but the development of spontaneous dual resistance is highly improbable. This is the cardinal principle underlying modern anti-tuberculosis treatment. By treating tuberculosis with two or more drugs in combination, mutants resistant to a single drug are killed by one of the other drugs in the regimen, and the selection of drug-resistant organisms is prevented.

Definitions of drug resistance

Drug resistance is defined as initial, primary and acquired.

Initial resistance

Resistance observed in newly presenting patients who have or do not report previous treatment with anti-TB drugs.

Primary resistance

Resistance observed in newly presenting patients who have **never** taken anti-TB drugs.

Acquired resistance

Resistance observed in a patient who has a record of having taken anti-TB drugs.

In most countries in Africa, accurate knowledge of previous treatment is difficult to obtain and therefore 'initial resistance' is used to indicate resistance in patients who are not thought to have had any previous treatment. Initial drug resistance is the presence of drug-resistant organisms occurring in a new patient with tuberculosis who was exposed to another patient with drug-resistant tuberculosis. Acquired drug resistance arises during the course of anti-tuberculosis treatment because of bad prescribing practice (i.e. monotherapy with streptomycin), inadequate doses of drugs or non-adherence to the recommended regimen. Acquired resistance is always higher than initial resistance.

Multi-drug resistant tuberculosis (MDR-TB) is defined as resistance to both isoniazid and rifampicin, with or without resistance to other drugs. As with acquired drug resistance, the most powerful predictor of MDR-TB is a history of inadequate treatment for tuberculosis.

Drug resistance in Africa and relationship with HIV infection

Levels of drug resistance vary widely across the continent (Pablos-Mendez et al., 1998). Some countries, such as Ghana and Mali, have high levels of initial drug resistance to isoniazid (30 per cent or more), while others in East and Central Africa have isoniazid resistance levels of about 10 per cent. Some countries such as Malawi have maintained stable isoniazid resistance levels over time, while others such as Sierra Leone have seen an increase in resistance levels reflecting deteriorating TB control programme performance (Harries, 1997). Although HIV infection can fuel the spread of drug resistant tuberculosis because of the increased potential for transmission, HIV does not seem to be associated with drug resistance in Africa.

Rates of MDR-TB are also not associated with HIV infection in Africa, and are generally low. However, a few countries such as Cote d'Ivoire, Sierra Leone and Zimbabwe have MDR-TB incidence rates of >5/100 000 per year (Becerra et al., 2000). This is of concern because of the difficulty of providing effective treatment for this type of patient.

Use of anti-tuberculosis drugs in special situations

Tuberculosis sometimes occurs in special situations, and this can influence the choice of drugs and their dosage.

Pregnancy

There is no evidence that isoniazid, rifampicin, pyrazinamide and ethambutol are teratogenic, and these drugs may be used in pregnancy. However, streptomycin is potentially ototoxic and may cause deafness in babies.

> Streptomycin should not be given in pregnancy, and ethambutol should be substituted.

Renal impairment and renal failure

Drugs such as rifampicin, isoniazid and pyrazinamide are excreted almost entirely by non-renal routes (i.e. by metabolism or biliary excretion), and therefore they can be given in normal dosage to patients with renal failure. Streptomycin is excreted exclusively and ethambutol predominantly by the kidney, and their doses should be reduced and given less frequently in renal failure.

Liver impairment and liver failure

Isoniazid, rifampicin and pyrazinamide are recognized to be hepatotoxic. Patients with active liver disease (i.e. with jaundice or ascites) who develop tuberculosis should not receive pyrazinamide and rifampicin. Although isoniazid is hepatotoxic, it should still be included in the treatment regimen. The safest regimen for this type of problem would be streptomycin, isoniazid and ethambutol for intensive phase of treatment, and isoniazid and ethambutol for maintenance treatment.

Corticosteroids and tuberculosis

Adjunct therapy with corticosteroids, in conjunction with anti-tuberculosis drugs, may be appropriate in particular forms of tuberculosis. Prospective controlled trials carried out in the pre-HIV era have shown that corticosteroids are beneficial in serious forms of tuberculous meningitis, tuberculous pericardial effusion, tuberculous constrictive pericarditis, and large tuberculous pleural effusions (Alzeer & Fitzgerald, 1993). The only published controlled trial in HIV-positive patients also confirmed the benefit of corticosteroids in decreasing mortality in tuberculous pericardial effusion (Hakim et al., 2000).

Response to anti-tuberculosis treatment: effect of HIV

General

If patients are given an appropriate treatment regimen, infectiousness usually disappears within 2 weeks, symptoms improve within 4–8 weeks and the majority of patients who were sputum smear positive become sputum smear negative at 2 months. Although tubercle bacilli may still be coughed up after 2 weeks of treatment, these bacilli are in most instances no longer capable of infecting new contacts. The response of patients to treatment occurs irrespective of HIV-serostatus.

Deaths during anti-tuberculosis treatment

HIV-positive patients experience a high death rate. Between 20 and 30 per cent of HIV-infected smear-positive tuberculosis cases are dead by the end of treatment. Even higher death rates are seen in HIV-infected smear-negative tuberculosis cases, probably because these patients are more immunosuppressed (Harries et al., 1998; Colebunders & Bastian, 2000). Studies in Africa have shown that about one-third of the deaths are due to tuberculosis (from late presentation and severe disease) and about two-thirds are due to HIV-related complications, particularly bacteraemia, diarrhoea, pneumonia and cryptococcal meningitis (Greenberg et al., 1995; Perriens et al., 1995). Death rates appear to be higher in HIV-positive patients treated with standard regimens which do not contain rifampicin, possibly because rifampicin has a broad spectrum antibacterial activity and gives some protection against pyogenic infections (Okwera et al., 1994). Prophylactic cotrimoxazole (960 mg daily), taken during anti-tuberculosis treatment, has been shown to reduce death rates in HIV-positive tuberculosis cases by almost 50 per cent (Wiktor et al., 1999), and in the next few years it may become standard practice to administer adjunctive cotrimoxazole with anti-tuberculosis treatment to tuberculosis cases who are HIV-positive.

Recurrence of TB after completing anti-TB treatment

Recurrence rates in patients who have successfully completed treatment appear to be higher in patients infected with HIV. This is particularly the case in patients treated with regimens which do not contain rifampicin (Hawken et al., 1993). The extent to which recurrent tuberculosis is due to reactivation of disease (as a result of failure to kill off all the semi-dormant bacilli) or the acquisition of a new infection is not known.

Table 17.7. The most common adverse reactions to anti-tuberculosis drugs

Drug	Reactions
Isoniazid	Hepatitis Peripheral neuropathy
Rifampicin	Gastrointestinal reactions Hepatitis Thrombocytopenic purpura Intermittent dosage 'Flu syndrome'
Pyrazinamide	Arthralgia Hepatitis
Streptomycin	Cutaneous hypersensitivity Vestibular and auditory nerve damage including that of the fetus Renal damage
Ethambutol	Optic neuritis
Thiacetazone	Gastrointestinal reactions Cutaneous hypersensitivity reactions

Adverse drug reactions and their management

Side effects of anti-tuberculosis drugs

Side effects of anti-tuberculosis drugs should be looked for and treated if possible. Some of them can be hazardous for the patient's health or may force the patient to stop treatment. All of the anti-tuberculosis drugs potentially have a large number of documented side effects, the most common of which are shown in Table 17.7.

Management of cutaneous hypersensitivity reactions

If the patient complains of itching without a rash or itching with a mild rash, symptomatic treatment with anti-histamines may be tried and the anti-tuberculosis treatment continued. However, the patient must be very carefully watched. If a moderate or severe rash develops, then all treatment should be **stopped**.

If the rash is severe, or if there is evidence of mucosal involvement, hypotension or severe illness, corticosteroid treatment should be instituted. High dose oral prednisolone should be given daily until there is a response. The amount of prednisolone is gradually reduced in the fol-

Table 17.8. Re-introduction of anti-TB drugs after cutaneous reactions

Day	Drug and dose
1	Isoniazid 50 mg
2	Isoniazid 300 mg
3	Combination rifampicin–isoniazid – half a tablet
4	Combination rifampicin–isoniazid – one tablet
5	Combination rifampicin–isoniazid – full dose
6	Day 5 regimen + pyrazinamide – half tablet
7	Day 5 regimen + pyrazinamide – one tablet
8	Day 5 regimen + pyrazinamide – full dose
9	Day 8 regimen + ethambutol – half tablet
10	Day 8 regimen + ethambutol – one tablet
11	Day 8 regimen + ethambutol – full dose
12	Full dose of rifampicin–isoniazid + pyrazinamide + ethambutol

lowing days according to the patient's response. Anti-tuberculosis treatment should be withheld until the reaction has completely subsided.

Once the reaction has subsided, drugs are re-introduced according to the schedule shown in Table 17.8. If the initial cutaneous reaction was severe, smaller initial doses should be given. If the patient is restarted on an adequate anti-tuberculosis treatment regimen (e.g. isoniazid, rifampicin and pyrazinamide), then re-challenging with the implicated drug (e.g. streptomycin) is not advisable.

Management of drug-induced hepatitis

Mild transient symptomless increases in serum liver transaminases occur during the early weeks of treatment. There is no need to interrupt or change treatment unless there is anorexia, malaise, vomiting or clinically evident jaundice with hepatic enlargement. Clinical features of concern include protracted vomiting, mental changes and signs of bleeding – these all suggest acute liver failure. If jaundice or any of the clinical features suggestive of acute liver failure develops, all drugs must be stopped until the jaundice or hepatic symptoms have resolved and the liver function tests have reverted to normal. If liver function tests cannot be measured, then it is advisable to wait an extra two weeks after the jaundice has disappeared before recommencing anti-tuberculosis therapy.

Once the drug-induced hepatitis has resolved, the same drug regimen can be re-introduced either gradually or all at once. However, if there has been a severe hepatitis, it is probably safer to use the standard regimen of streptomycin, isoniazid and ethambutol.

Table 17.9. Symptom-based approach to management of drug reactions

Symptoms	Responsible drug and management
Abdominal pain, nausea	related to rifampicin management: give oral drugs to the patient last thing at night
Burning of the feet	related to isoniazid peripheral neuropathy management: continue isoniazid; give pyridoxine 50 mg – 75 mg daily (wherever possible, pyridoxine 10 mg daily should be given routinely with isoniazid to prevent peripheral neuropathy.)
Joint pains	related to pyrazinamide management: continue pyrazinamide; use aspirin or non-steroidal anti-inflammatory drug.
Red urine	related to rifampicin management: reassure the patient.
Women on rifampicin	rifampicin may reduce the effectiveness of the oral contraceptive pill management: if she is on the 'pill', another form of contraception should be given.

Note: All the above minor side effects not requiring treatment are to be stopped.

Symptom-based approach to management of drug reactions

Clinicians are often faced with patients who are taking anti-tuberculosis treatment and who complain of problems, which may or may not be due to the medication. Tables 17.9 and 17.10 show a symptom-based management approach to adverse drug reactions. An illustrative case history is as follows:

A 50-year-old man developed pain and numbness of the feet 6 weeks after taking anti-tuberculosis treatment which included isoniazid. Anti-tuberculosis treatment was continued, and pyridoxine was added at 75 mg daily. There was partial relief of symptoms after two weeks. Amitryptiline (a tricyclic antidepressant which is useful for managing neuropathic pain) was then also added with almost complete relief of symptoms.

Tuberculosis control in Africa

Framework for tuberculosis control

The overall objective of tuberculosis control is to reduce mortality, morbidity and transmission of the disease.

Table 17.10. Symptom-based approach to management of drug reactions.

Symptoms	Responsible drug and management
Deafness	related to streptomycin management: auroscopy to rule out wax: *stop* streptomycin if no other explanation. Use ethambutol instead
Dizziness	if true vertigo and nystagmus, related to streptomycin management: *stop* streptomycin; if just dizziness with no nystagmus, try dose reduction for one week, but if no better stop streptomycin. Use ethambutol instead
Generalized reactions including shock, purpura	may be due to rifampicin, pyrazinamide and/or streptomycin management: *stop* all medication Use different combination of drugs
Jaundice	related to drug-induced hepatitis. management: *stop* all antituberculosis drugs until jaundice and liver function tests revert to normal
Skin itching	related to all anti-tuberculosis drugs management: s*top* antituberculosis drugs
Visual impairment	related to ethambutol management: visual examination; *stop* ethambutol
Vomiting +/− confusion	suspect drug-induced hepatitis management: urgent liver function tests; if LFTs not available, *stop* antituberculosis drugs and observe.

Note: All the above are major side effects requiring treatment to be stopped.

WHO has set targets for tuberculosis control which are: (i) to cure 85 per cent of the detected new cases of smear-positive pulmonary tuberculosis and (ii) to detect 70 per cent of the existing cases of smear-positive tuberculosis (WHO, 1997). Achieving a high cure rate is the highest priority because TB programmes with high cure rates are often able to attract a majority of existing cases in their catchment area. Giving priority to case finding before achieving high cure rates contributes to the tuberculosis problem by producing chronic cases and multi-drug resistant tuberculosis. The strategy for tuberculosis control is the provision of standardized short course chemotherapy (see below) to all identified smear-positive tuberculosis cases. This should be administered through DOTS (directly observed treatment, short course). The success of the tuberculosis control strategy depends on the implementation of a TB Control Policy package, the five essential elements of which are:

- Government commitment to a TB control programme aiming at nationwide coverage
- Case detection through passive case finding
- Short course chemotherapy to (at the least) all smear positive cases)
- Regular and uninterrupted supply of essential anti-TB drugs
- A monitoring and evaluation system.

Government commitment is most important ensuring that the country's TB control programme is permanent, organized on a country-wide basis (serving rural and urban areas), integrated into the existing health structure, and is accesible, available and convenient for the consumer. Anti-TB drugs should also be available and free to every patient, otherwise there is a strong tendency once patients feel better to default from the lengthy treatment. The TB programme needs a central unit with a permanent team qualified in the management of TB control which co-ordinates, supervises and evaluates the key activities of the National TB programme and which also can link up with TB experts to regularly update knowledge on all relevant aspects of TB. Government also has to assure the continuation of sustained local and/or external funding for all the essential aspects of the programme and support the preparation of a national TB control manual which contains all the necessary information about the structure of the programme and the key operations needed to ensure success.

Standardized case finding and registration

Tuberculosis cases should be diagnosed, classified and categorized in a standard way. Within a country, this allows a uniform approach to tuberculosis control with less room for confusion and mistakes. At an international level, such standardization facilitates uniform data gathering, valid comparisons between countries and a firm template for global tuberculosis control.

Standardized case definitions

Both WHO and the International Union against Tuberculosis and Lung Disease (IUATLD) have issued guidelines for the classification of tuberculosis cases (Enarson et al., 1996; WHO, 1997), and most good TB programmes adhere to these guidelines. Tuberculosis cases are classified and categorized in a standard way, and this information is recorded in a tuberculosis register and on tuberculosis treatment cards (see Table 17.11). One of the most important questions to ask is

Table 17.11. Standardized case definitions of tuberculosis

Classification of tuberculosis patients

Smear-positive patient: a patient with at least two sputum smears positive for acid fast bacilli (AFB) *or* a patient with one sputum smear positive for AFB and radiographic abnormalities consistent with active pulmonary tuberculosis.

Smear-negative patient: a patient with at least two sputum smears negative for AFB and radiographic abnormalities consistent with active tuberculosis. All such patients should have received a course of antibiotics to which there has been no response.

Extrapulmonary tuberculosis: a patient with clinical and/or laboratory evidence consistent with active tuberculosis. This includes patients with pleurisy, pleural effusion and miliary tuberculosis

Categorization of tuberculosis patients

New patient: a patient who has never taken anti-tuberculosis drugs, or who has taken the drugs for less than one month

Relapse patient: a patient who has previously been treated and completed treatment and has now developed active tuberculosis with smear-positive sputum

Failure patient: a newly diagnosed tuberculosis patient who is sputum-smear positive 5 months or more after the start of chemotherapy

Return after default patient: a patient who returns to treatment smear-positive after having left treatment for more than 2 months after the start of treatment. A patient who on return to treatment is found to be smear-negative should not be newly registered but should continue treatment until the completion of the total amount originally prescribed has been completed.

Transfer in patient: a patient who has been started on treatment in another district and been registered in another tuberculosis register and who has been transferred to the district to continue treatment

Other patient: a patient who does not fulfil any of the above categories. Examples are (i) the chronic case who is a patient who remains smear-positive after completing a retreatment regimen under supervision; (ii) recurrent TB case who is a patient who has previously been treated and completed treatment and has now developed active tuberculosis with smear-negative TB or extra-pulmonary TB.

whether the patient has ever been diagnosed and treated for tuberculosis in the past, and if so whether the treatment regimen was completed and when the drugs were stopped.

Registration of tuberculosis cases

All patients diagnosed with tuberculosis should be entered into a TB Register. These registers are kept at all hospitals that diagnose and treat tuberculosis patients, and are completed by tuberculosis officers. For each TB patient, a record is made of the date of diagnosis, the name, age, sex, address, type of tuberculosis and category (i.e. new case, relapse case, transferred in from another district), and the patient is given a unique TB registration number. Only one type of TB is recorded for each patient, and if the patient has a combination of pulmonary and extrapulmonary TB the patient is recorded as having pulmonary TB.

Standardized anti-tuberculosis treatment regimens

General

Patients registered with tuberculosis should also be treated in a standard and effective way. Effective treatment is vital for tuberculosis control because, when applied correctly, it can reduce transmission of infection and decrease the magnitude of tuberculosis in the community. Patients are categorized according to priority for treatment. In general, newly diagnosed cases and those with smear-positive pulmonary tuberculosis and other clinically serious forms of the disease are accorded highest priority (WHO, 1997).

The initial phase and continuation phase of treatment

All treatment regimens have two phases. There is an initial phase designed for the rapid killing of actively growing bacilli and the killing of semi-dormant bacilli. This means a shorter duration of infectiousness with usually rapid smear conversion (80–90 per cent) after 2 to 3 months of treatment. The initial phase involves supervised drug administration and therefore good drug adherence. The initial phase usually involves three or four drugs, depending on the degree of initial drug resistance in the community. If initial resistance rates are high, use of a three drug regimen runs the risk of selecting out drug-resistant mutants especially in patients with high bacillary loads, i.e. with cavitating smear-positive pulmonary tuberculosis. In such situations, a four-drug regimen decreases the risk of developing drug resistance, and reduces failure and relapse rates. If default occurs after the initial intensive phase, relapse is less likely.

The continuation phase eliminates bacilli which are still multiplying and reduces failures and relapses. At the time of starting the continuation phase there are low numbers of bacilli with less chance of selecting drug-resistant mutants, and therefore smaller numbers of drugs (usually two) are needed. Directly observed treatment is the ideal when the patient receives rifampicin in the continuation phase. However, in rural areas this ideal may be difficult to achieve, and close weekly supervision of rifampicin-containing treatment has to suffice. The risk of drug resistance is less during the continuation phase when there are fewer TB bacilli. If the continuation phase does not include rifampicin (e.g. isoniazid and ethambutol), the patient usually receives monthly drug supplies for self-administered treatment.

New cases of tuberculosis

Treatment regimens have an initial phase lasting two months and a continuation phase usually lasting 4–6 months. During the initial phase, consisting usually of four drugs, tubercle bacilli are killed rapidly. Infectious patients become non-infectious within about 2 weeks. Symptoms improve, and many patients become asymptomatic by 4–8 weeks. The majority of patients with sputum smear-positive PTB become smear-negative within 2 months. Pyrazinamide is given during the initial phase, and has its maximum sterilizing effect within this time. No further benefit is obtained from using pyrazinamide for a longer period of time, and the drug is therefore not used in the continuation phase. In the continuation phase, two drugs are usually used and these eliminate the remaining bacilli.

In patients with smear-negative PTB or extrapulmonary TB there is a smaller chance of selecting drug-resistant mutants because these patients harbour fewer bacilli in their lesions. Short course chemotherapy regimens with three drugs during the initial phase, and two drugs in the continuation phase, are of proven efficacy. These are the regimens recommended by the World Health Organization. In patients with smear-negative PTB or extrapulmonary TB, some resource-poor countries in Africa still use a 12-month regimen (streptomycin, isoniazid and ethambutol for one or two months in the initial phase followed by isoniazid and ethambutol for 10 or 11 months in the continuation phase). This regimen is referred to as the 'standard regimen'. It requires a 12-month period of treatment because it does not contain drugs (rifampicin and pyrazinamide) which sterilize the tubercle bacilli. The regimen therefore relies on semi-dormant bacilli becoming metabolically active during the treatment period, and becoming susceptible to the killing effects of isoniazid. However, there are problems with the 'standard regimen'. Under routine conditions, treatment completion rates are low, default rates are high because of the long duration of treatment, there is evidence that death rates in HIV-positive patients are higher because there is no rifampicin to protect against pyogenic infections and there is also evidence that recurrent rates of TB after completing treatment are higher compared with rifampicin-based regimens. For these reasons, 'standard regimens' are not recommended by the World Health Organization.

Re-treatment cases

Previously treated TB patients may have acquired drug resistance, and they are more likely than new patients to harbour and excrete bacilli resistant to at least isoniazid. The re-treatment regimen consists of initially five drugs with at least three drugs in the continuation phase. The patient should receive at least two drugs in the initial phase which are still effective, and this reduces the risk of selecting further resistant bacilli.

Standard codes for TB treatment regimens

There are standard codes for Treatment Regimens. Each anti-TB drug has an abbreviation (see Table 17.12). There are two phases of the regimen, the initial phase and the continuation phase. The number before a phase is the duration of that phase in months. A number in subscript (e.g. $_3$) after a letter is the number of doses of that drug per week. If there is no number in subscript after a letter, then treatment is with that drug on a daily basis. An alternative drug (or drugs) appears as a letter (or letters) in brackets. An example is as follows. 2HRZE/ 6HE is a common regimen. The initial phase is 2 HRZE. The duration of the phase is 2 months. Drug treatment is daily (no subscript number after the letters) with isoniazid (H), rifampicin R, pyrazinamide (Z) and ethambutol (E). The continuation phase is 6 HE. The duration of the phase is 6 months. Drug treatment is daily with isoniazid (H) and ethambutol (E).

Categories for treatment and treatment regimens

There are four different categories for treatment. Table 17.12 shows these four categories and gives examples of the type of regimen recommended by WHO divided into the initial phase and continuation phase of treatment. There are several possible regimens, the selection of which depend on the country's budget, health coverage by primary health care facilities and qualifications of staff at peripheral level.

Patients are categorized according to priority for treatment, especially in resource-poor settings where it is important to get the 'best value for money'. Priorities are based on cure of the patient, prevention of death, prevention of spread of drug-resistant organisms and reduction of transmission to the community. The highest priority is given to patients with smear-positive pulmonary TB and other serious forms of the disease.

Table 17.12. Recommended treatment regimens.

TB treatment category	TB patients	TB treatment initial phase (daily or 3 times per week)	TB treatment continuation phase
I	New cases with smear+ve PTB; New cases with severe EPTB; New cases with severe smear-ve PTB	2EHRZ (SHRZ) 2EHRZ (SHRZ) 2EHRZ (SHRZ)	6HE 4HR $4H_3R_3$
II	Previously treated smear+ve PTB: relapse; treatment failure; treatment after default	2SHRZE/1HRZE 2SHRZE/1HRZE	5 $H_3R_3E_3$ 5 HRE
III	New cases with smear-ve PTB; New cases with less severe forms of EPTB	2HRZ 2HRZ 2HRZ	6HE 4HR $4H_3R_3$
IV	Chronic cases (still smear+ve after supervised re-treatment)		

Notes:

1. Abbreviations are: H = Isoniazid; R = Rifampicin; Z = Pyrazinamide; S = Streptomycin; E = Ethambutol
2. In patients with TB meningitis, miliary TB, spinal TB with neurological involvement, some authorities recommend a 7-month continuation phase with daily isoniazid and rifampicin (7HR).
3. For category IV TB patients, the World Health Organization provides guidelines for the use of second-line drugs.

Category 1

This includes: (i) patients with new smear-positive pulmonary tuberculosis because of their high transmission potential and high risk of death without effective treatment, (ii) new patients with serious forms of extrapulmonary disease such as miliary disease, pericardial disease, meningitis and spinal disease with spinal cord involvement because they have a high risk of death unless treated with effective drug combinations, and (iii) new patients with severe and extensive smear-negative pulmonary tuberculosis because, especially in the HIV era, these patients have a high risk of death.

Category II

This includes patients with previously treated TB who have developed smear-positive PTB. This includes relapses, treatment failures and defaulters. These patients are given multi-drug combination regimens because they are highly infectious and are likely to have drug-resistant organisms, which will be spread to the community unless effectively treated.

Category III

This includes patients with smear-negative pulmonary tuberculosis and less serious forms of extrapulmonary tuberculosis such as pleural effusion and lymphadenopathy. These patients are given a regimen which is less strong than for Category I because they are less infectious than smear-positive cases and there is less risk of death. However, in high HIV-prevalent areas these beliefs are being challenged. HIV-positive smear-negative PTB patients have a higher risk of death compared with HIV-positive smear-positive PTB cases because the former are more immunocompromised. Furthermore, smear-negative patients may also contribute to spread of TB in the community (Behr et al., 1999).

Category IV

These are smear-positive PTB cases who have completed a supervised re-treatment regimen and are still sputum smear positive. They have a high chance of multi-drug resistant TB. They are accorded lowest priority for treatment because cases are few, cure in the case of multi-drug resistant TB is unlikely and the cost of second-line drugs is very high. If chronic cases harbour bacilli which are resistant to at least isoniazid and rifampicin (i.e. multi-drug resistant TB), their management is highly problematic (Iseman, 1993). If resources permit, treatment with second-line drugs can be considered. However, there are problems with second-line drugs because (i) they are generally less effective than first-line agents in drug-susceptible cases, (ii) they are associated with a higher incidence of side effects and (iii) they are considerably more expensive. A regimen recommended by WHO consists of intramuscular kanamycin, ethionamide, pyrazinamide, ofloxacin and ethambutol for 3 months followed by ethionamide, ofloxacin and ethambutol for 18 months (Table 17.12).

Monitoring and recording the results of treatment

General

A proper monitoring and evaluation system, based on meticulous recording and reporting of cases, is essential to assess the effectiveness of the treatment given and the particular TB programme's performance. A unique monitoring, recording and reporting system designed by the International Union against Tuberculosis and Lung Disease (IUATLD) under the guidance of Dr K. Styblo was started in Tanzania in the 1980s, and is used nowadays – with slight variations only – in many national TB control programmes. It represents the WHO recommended recording and reporting system. Monitoring in patients with smear-positive pulmonary tuberculosis is carried out with sputum smear examination at regular, defined intervals during treatment. For other tuberculosis patients, clinical monitoring is the usual guide to treatment response. Routine monitoring of treatment response by chest radiography is believed to be wasteful of resources and unnecessary.

Monitoring of new patients with sputum-positive PTB

Smear-positive pulmonary tuberculosis patients have their sputum tested at 2 months: if the sputum is still positive, the initial phase is continued for another 4 weeks. Sputum is checked again at 4 weeks, but the continuation phase is started regardless of sputum smear results. Patients are monitored during the continuation phase of treatment, and additional sputum smears are examined at month 4 and at the end of therapy in 6-month regimens, and at month 5 and at the end of therapy in 8-month regimens. If the sputum is smear positive at month 5 or at any time after 5 months of treatment, then the patient is classified as a treatment failure and changed to the re-treatment regimen for category II patients.

A 34-year-old man with new smear-positive pulmonary TB started short course chemotherapy with 2SRHZ/6 HE. At the end of two months initial phase his sputum smears were still positive for acid-fast bacilli (AFB). The initial phase was continued for another 4 weeks, at the end of which his two sputum smears showed scanty AFB. He was changed to continuation phase treatment with EH at this time. At five months sputum specimens were examined for AFB and found to be still positive on smear microscopy. He was defined as a treatment failure and started on a re-treatment regimen (2SHRZE/1HRZE/5HRE). He completed the re-treatment regimen, during which his sputum smears became negative for AFB, and he made a full clinical recovery.

Monitoring of patients with recurrent sputum-positive PTB

When the patient has completed the initial phase of treatment and the sputum is smear-negative, the continuation phase is started. If the sputum is still smear-positive at 3 months, the initial phase of treatment is extended for another 4 weeks. If the patient is still smear-positive at the end of the fourth month (16 weeks), all drugs are stopped for 2 days and a sputum specimen is obtained for culture and sensitivity. The continuation phase is then started. Patients complete the continuation phase. If they are still smear positive at the end of treatment, the course is discontinued and the patients are defined as a chronic case (Category IV).

Table 17.13. Standardized definitions of treatment outcome for smear-positive pulmonary tuberculosis

Smear negative (cured)	patient who is smear negative at, or 1 month prior to, the completion of treatment and on at least one previous occasion
Smear not done (treatment completed)	patient who has completed treatment but in whom smear results are not available
Smear positive (failure)	patient who remains or becomes again smear positive at 5 months or more during chemotherapy
Died	patient who dies for any reason during the course of their chemotherapy
Defaulted	patient who has interrupted the treatment for more than 2 consecutive months before the end of course of treatment
Transferred out	patient who has been transferred to another treatment centre and in whom the treatment results are not known.

Recording treatment outcome in patients with tuberculosis

At the end of the treatment course in each individual patient, the treatment outcome is recorded by the district TB officer according to standardized definitions. In smear-positive tuberculosis patients there are six defined treatment outcomes (Table 17.13). In smear-negative and extrapulmonary tuberculosis patients, there are four defined treatment outcomes only because no sputum examination is carried out during treatment.

Reporting case finding and treatment outcome

The reporting system is based mainly on two reports, which are compiled at district level by district TB officers, for each respective district four times a year, i.e.

Table 17.14. Treatment outcome in a cohort of patients with new smear-positive pulmonary TB in Lilongwe District, Malawi

Number	308
Cured	202 (66%)
Completed treatment (sputum smears not done)	20 (7%)
Died	61 (20%)
Defaulted	14 (4%)
Failed	1
Transferred out	10 (3%)

Notes:
Cohort: Patients registered between January and March 1999
Comment: The most effective way to improve cure rates is to reduce the number of patients who complete treatment with no smears examined. The high death rate require several approaches, including reduction of delays in presentation, improved case management, and adjunctive interventions such as cotrimoxazole prophylaxis.

quarterly reports. They are the district quarterly report on case-finding and the district quarterly report on treatment results in smear-positive patients. The basic information is taken from the district TB register, which, being an individual case register, contains all relevant patient information on the cases enrolled for treatment and on outcome of treatment (i.e. smear results at 0, 2, 5 and 8 months in an 8-month short course regimen and defined treatment outcome). District quarterly reports are sent to central level for compilation and analysis.

Case finding reports enable information on trends in disease to be obtained, which are useful for planning staff needs, drug supplies, etc. Reports on results of treatment are called cohort reports, and these are the key management tool used to evaluate the effectiveness of TB control programme delivery (see Table 17.14).

Prevention of tuberculosis

While identification and treatment of infectious cases of tuberculosis is believed to be the most cost-effective way of interrupting the cycle of TB transmission and reducing the burden of TB cases, prevention of tuberculosis is another option to be considered. There are three ways of preventing tuberculosis: (i) BCG vaccination, (ii) isoniazid preventive therapy and (iii) measures to reduce nosocomial transmission (i.e. hospital-based transmission).

BCG vaccination

General

The Bacillus Calmette–Guérin (BCG) vaccine is a live, albeit attenuated, vaccine of several strains of *Mycobacterium bovis*. In most African countries, BCG is given at birth as part of the routine childhood immunization. It is given by intradermal injection, the dose being 0.05 ml in children under 3 months of age and 0.1 ml in others. In routine programmes, BCG is given direct without prior tuberculin skin testing. The injection is administered in the upper arm. After injection there is a weal followed by a papule followed by an ulcer which leads to scarring and healing in about 6–12 weeks. BCG should not be administered at the same time as other live injected vaccines, although it may be given at the same time as oral polio vaccine. BCG can cause local cutaneous side effects and regional lymphadenopathy, but serious or systemic side effects are rare.

Efficacy

There have been a large number of controlled clinical trials, case control studies and household contact studies to derive estimates of efficacy (Fine, 1995). Variable results have been recorded. The consensus is that BCG vaccine protects against tuberculous meningitis and miliary TB in immunocompetent children, but it does not prevent primary infection with *M. tuberculosis*, nor does it prevent an appreciable number of infectious cases of pulmonary tuberculosis. The effect probably lasts about 15 years, and there is no evidence that re-vaccination provides additional protection.

BCG and HIV infection

Although there have been some case reports of local complications and disseminated *M.bovis* infection after BCG in HIV-positive children, population-based studies have found no evidence of adverse effects in HIV-infected children. Whether BCG protects against tuberculosis in HIV-infected children is not known. Conversion to a positive tuberculin test after BCG is less frequent in HIV-positive children, but whether this means a reduction in efficacy is not known. Current WHO recommendations are that BCG should be given to children with asymptomatic HIV infection, but it should not be given to children with clinical AIDS (WHO, 1995).

Isoniazid preventive therapy

Isoniazid may be given as chemoprophylaxis either:
(i) to prevent the establishment of infection, or

(ii) to prevent disease in individuals already infected by diminishing or destroying a relatively small bacterial population. There are two situations where isoniazid chemoprophylaxis could be used in Africa.

Management of childhood contacts of smear-positive tuberculosis cases

In children born to mothers with smear-posiitve tuberculosis, isoniazid prophylaxis should be given for 6 months with BCG administered at the end of this time. Breastfeeding is safe and should be continued. In children aged 5 years and below who have had close contact with a smear-positive adult, isoniazid chemoprophylaxis should be given for 6 months provided there is no evidence of tuberculosis. Children of this age are at high risk of developing active disease if infected, and prevention is considered fully justified. In all children the dose of isoniazid is 5 mg/kg.

Preventive therapy in HIV-positive individuals

There is now good evidence that preventive therapy with isoniazid at a dose of 300 mg daily for 6–12 months reduces the occurrence of tuberculosis in HIV-infected persons, especially if they are co-infected with *M.tuberculosis* (Wilkinson et al., 1998). WHO recommends that isoniazid is indicated for tuberculin-positive, HIV-infected persons who do not have tuberculosis (WHO, 1999). It is therefore important to screen HIV-positive persons for tuberculous infection and for tuberculosis. Isoniazid prophylaxis is contraindicated in individuals with chronic liver disease and should be used with caution in those who consume regular amounts of alcohol. Recent research suggests that after stopping isoniazid, the risk of developing tuberculosis again starts to increase, which supports the belief that many HIV-infected individuals develop tuberculosis as a result of a new infection acquired in the community. If this is the case, life long isoniazid prophylaxis may be necessary.

Feasibility studies in Africa using isoniazid preventive therapy have been disappointing (Aisu et al., 1995), and no country has yet adopted chemoprophylaxis as a strategy for tuberculosis control. However, the intervention could be used safely and selectively in certain situations such as in occupational health services for private businesses and factories, for personnel working in international agencies and missions and amongst high risk groups such as health care workers and prisoners.

HIV-positive patients who complete a course of treatment for tuberculosis are at increased risk of recurrent tuberculosis. Post-treatment isoniazid for 12 months reduces this risk of recurrent tuberculosis (Fitzgerald et al., 2000), and could be considered for secondary preventive therapy.

Protection of health care workers against tuberculosis

Health care workers in the busy wards and outpatient clinics of African hospitals are at high risk of acquiring tuberculosis (Harries et al., 1999). The best way of preventing tuberculosis transmission is to rapidly diagnose and treat patients with smear-positive tuberculosis (Harries et al., 1997). Tuberculosis suspects should ideally be investigated in the outpatient setting. If patients are admitted to hospital for investigation, they should be placed in a sector of the ward which is well ventilated, receives plenty of sunlight and which is separated from patients with other illnesses. Suspects should be taught cough hygiene (i.e. placing a hand in front of the mouth when coughing and turning the head away from the person they are next to). Sputum smear examination should be carried out as rapidly as possible, and once diagnosed tuberculosis patients should be treated in a separate isolation ward. Tuberculosis wards should also be properly ventilated and have plenty of sunlight. Although difficult to apply in practice, health care workers should have the opportunity of being counselled and tested for HIV infection, and HIV-positive individuals should not work with tuberculosis suspects or patients.

The future of tuberculosis control in Africa

The DOTS-TB Control Strategy, if properly implemented, works well. DOTS-TB programmes have better data on case finding, more smear-positive pulmonary tuberculosis cases and better treatment outcomes. However, implementation is not easy, and by the end of 1998 only 21 per cent of smear-positive tuberculosis cases globally were notified through DOTS programmes (WHO, 2000). The DOTS-TB Control Strategy requires strong government commitment, a well-functioning national programme and for resource-poor countries additional support from the donor community. In addition, there are two other major threats to tuberculosis control in Africa, which must be tackled if efforts are to be rewarded with success.

The on-going threat of HIV

Tuberculosis case numbers in high HIV-prevalent countries show no sign of abating, despite well-functioning TB control programmes. Passive case finding in 'hot spots' of TB transmission is associated with delays in diagnosis, and this may not be the best option for case detection. Active case finding may be a better strategy leading to a reduction in the potential period of transmission and a better chance for individual cure. Involving the community in case finding, particularly traditional healers who are often the first port of call for sick patients (Brouwer et al., 1998), is another practical way of reducing diagnostic delays. The increased case burden throws an immense strain on TB control efforts with a need for more staff, more drugs and more resources. Tuberculosis wards are already overcrowded, especially in urban hospitals, and there is a great need for TB programmes to start decentralizing services to health centres and the community (Maher et al., 1999). This is a patient-friendly approach. However, decentralization runs the risk of loss of control and abuse of anti-tuberculosis drugs for conditions other than tuberculosis, with the subsequent development of drug-resistant TB. Multi-drug resistant tuberculosis must not be allowed to develop, for that would be a catastrophe for TB control efforts. The high death rate in tuberculosis patients threatens the credibility of TB programmes amongst patients, the community and health care staff. Ways of reducing death rates have to be found, and will include reducing the time between illness and treatment, improving the diagnosis of smear-negative and extrapulmonary disease, providing better care of patients especially for HIV-related complications, the use of prophylaxis for opportunistic infections (e.g. cotrimoxazole), and assessing how best to use combination antiretroviral therapy. Health care staff need to be protected against the ravages of HIV and nosocomial tuberculosis, and health training institutions must increase their output of trained professionals. The feasibility of using primary and secondary isoniazid preventive therapy must be tested. Strong links must be made with AIDS control programmes, because HIV control is essential for TB control.

Health sector reform

Many countries in Africa, in conjunction with the donor community, are embarking on health sector reform. Health sector reform with its emphasis on district autonomy and the dismantling of vertical programmes, poses a threat to TB control. The health sector reform programme in Zambia lead, within 2 years, to the complete collapse of the country's TB control programme, the most serious effect being the interruption of the supply of anti-tuberculosis drugs in 1998 (Bosman, 2000). Health planners and policy makers need to be aware that chronic diseases like tuberculosis, which needs 6–8 months uninterrupted treatment, need specialist staff at central, provincial, and district level for their effective control. This structure is tampered with at peril.

References

Aisu T, Raviglione M, van Praag E et al. (1995). Preventive therapy for HIV-associated tuberculosis in Uganda: an operational assessment at a voluntary counselling and testing centre. *AIDS*; **9**: 267–273.

Alzeer AH, Fitzgerald JM. (1993). Corticosteroids and tuberculosis: risks and use as adjunct therapy. *Tuberc Lung Dis*; **74**: 6–11.

Becerra MC, Bayona J, Freeman J, Farmer PE, Kim JY. (2000). Redefining MDR-TB transmission 'hot spots'. *Int J Tuberc Lung Dis*; **4**, 387–394.

Behr MA, Warren SA, Salamon H et al. (1999). Transmission of *Mycobacterium tuberculosis* from patients smear-negative for acid-fast bacilli. *Lancet*; **353**: 444–449.

Bosman MCJ. (2000). Health sector reform and tuberculosis control: the case of Zambia. *Int J Tuberc Lung Dis*; **4**: 606 – 614.

Brouwer JA, Boeree MJ, Kager P, Varkevisser CM, Harries AD. (1998). Traditional healers and pulmonary tuberculosis in Malawi. *Int J Tuberc Lung Dis*; **2**: 231–234.

Colebunders R, Bastian I. (2000). A review of the diagnosis and treatment of smear-negative pulmonary tuberculosis. *Int J Tuberc Lung Dis*; **4**: 97–107.

Daniel TM. (1998). The early history of tuberculosis in central East Africa: insights from the clinical records of the first twenty years of Mengo Hospital and review of relevant literature. *Int J Tuberc Lung Dis*, **2**, 784–790.

De Cock KM, Soro B, Coulibaly IM, Lucas SB. (1992). Tuberculosis and HIV infection in sub-Saharan Africa. *J Am Med Assoc*, **268**, 1581–1587.

Dye C, Scheele S, Dolin P, Pathania V, Raviglione MC for the WHO Global Surveillance and Monitoring Project. (1999). Global burden of tuberculosis. estimated incidence, prevalence, and mortality by country. *J Am Med Assoc*, **282**, 677–686.

Enarson DA, Rieder HL, Arnadottir T, Trebucq A. (1996). *Tuberculosis Guide for Low Income Countries*. 4th edn. Paris, France: *International Union against Tuberculosis and Lung Disease*.

Fine PEM. (1995). Variation in protection by BCG: implications of and for heterologous immunity. *Lancet*, **346**, 1339–1345.

Fitzgerald DW, Desvarieux M, Severe P, Joseph P, Johnson Jr WD, Pape JW. (2000). Effect of post-treatment isoniazid on prevention of recurrent tuberculosis in HIV-1-infected individuals: a randomised trial. *Lancet*; **356**: 1470–1474.

Greenberg AE, Lucas S, Tossou O et al. (1995). Autopsy-proven causes of death in HIV-infected patients treated for tuberculosis in Abidjan, Cote d'Ivoire. *AIDS*; **9**: 1251–1254.

Hakim JG, Ternouth I, Mushangi E et al. (2000). Double blind randomised placebo controlled trial of adjunctive prednisolone in the treatment of effusive tuberculous pericarditis. *Heart*; **84**: 183–188.

Harries AD, Nyirenda T, Banerjee A, Boeree MJ, Salaniponi FML.

(1999). Tuberculosis amongst health care workers in Malawi. *Trans Roy Soc Trop Med Hyg*; **93**: 32–35.

Harries AD. (1997). Tuberculosis in Africa: clinical presentation and management. *Pharmacol. Ther*; **73**: 1–50.

Harries AD, Maher D, Nunn P. (1997). Practical and affordable measures for the protection of health care workers from tuberculosis in low-income countries. *Bull World Health Organization*; **75**: 477–489.

Harries AD, Nyangulu DS, Kang'ombe C et al. (1998). Treatment outcome of an unselected cohort of tuberculosis patients in relation to human immunodeficiency virus serostatus in Zomba hospital, Malawi. *Trans Roy Soc Trop Med Hyg*; **92**: 343–347.

Hawken M, Nunn P, Gathua S et al. (1993). Increased recurrence of tuberculosis in HIV-1-infected patients in Kenya. *Lancet*; **342**: 332–337.

Iseman MD. (1993). Treatment of multi-drug resistant tuberculosis. *N Eng J Med*, **329**: 784–791.

Kenya/British Medical Research Council. (1989). Tuberculosis in Kenya 1984: a third national survey and a comparison with earlier surveys in 1964 and 1974. *Tubercle*; **70**: 5–20.

Lucas SB, De Cock KM, Hounnou A et al. (1994). Contribution of tuberculosis to slim disease in Africa. *Br Med J*; **308**: 1531–1533.

Maher D, van Gorkom JLC, Gondrie PCFM, Raviglione M. (1999). Community contribution to tuberculosis care in countries with high tuberculosis prevalence: past, present and future. *Int J Tuberc Lung Dis*; **3**: 762–768.

Nunn P, Kibuga D, Gathua S et al. (1991). Cutaneous hypersensitivity reactions due to thiacetazone in HIV-1 seropositive patients treated for tuberculosis. *Lancet*; **337**: 627–630.

Nyangulu DS, Harries AD, Kang'ombe C et al. (1997). Tuberculosis in a prison population in Malawi. *Lancet*, **350**: 1284–1287.

Okwera A, Whalen C, Byekwaso F et al. (1994). Randomised trial of thiacetazone and rifampicin-containing regimens for pulmonary tuberculosis in HIV-infected Ugandans. *Lancet*; **344**: 1323–1328.

Pablos-Mendez A, Raviglione MC, Laszlo A et al. (1998). Global surveillance for antituberculosis-drug resistance, 1994–1997. *N Engl J Med*; **338**: 1641–1649.

Perriens JH, St.Louis ME, Mukadi YB et al. (1995). Pulmonary tuberculosis in HIV-infected patients in Zaire. A controlled trial of treatment for either 6 or 12 months. *N Engl J Med*; **332**: 779–784.

Raviglione MC, Harries AD, Msiska R, Wilkinson D, Nunn P. (1997). Tuberculosis and HIV: current status in Africa. *AIDS*; **11**: S115–S123.

Richter C, Ndosi B, Mwammy AS, Mbwambo RK. (1991). Extrapulmonary tuberculosis – a simple diagnosis? *Trop Geogr Med*; **43**: 375–378.

Scott JAG, Hall AJ, Muyodi C et al. (2000). Aetiology, outcome, and risk factors for mortality among adults with acute pneumonia in Kenya. *Lancet*; **355**: 1225–1230.

Toman K. (1997). *Tuberculosis. Case Finding and Chemotherapy. Questions and Answers.* Geneva, Switzerland: World Health Organization.

UNAIDS. (2000). Joint United Nations Programme on HIV/AIDS. *AIDS Epidemic Update*: December.

Wiktor SZ, Sassan-Morokro M, Grant AD et al. (1999). Efficacy of trimethoprim-sulphamethoxazole prophylaxis to decrease morbidity and mortality in HIV-1 infected patients with tuberculosis in Abidjan, Cote d'Ivoire: a randomised controlled trial. *Lancet*; **353**: 1469–1475.

Wilkinson D, Squire SB, Garner P. (1998). Effect of preventive treatment for tuberculosis in adults infected with HIV: systematic review of randomised placebo controlled trials. *Br Med J*; **317**: 625–629.

World Health Organization. (1997). *Treatment of Tuberculosis. Guidelines for National Programmes.* Geneva, Switzerland: World Health Organization. WHO/TB/97.220.

World Health Organization. (1999). Preventive therapy against tuberculosis in people living with HIV. *Wkly Epidemiol Rec*; **74**: 385–400.

World Health Organization. (2000a). Global Tuberculosis Control. WHO Report 2000.

World Health Organization. (2000b). Geneva, Switzerland. WHO/CDS/TB/2000.275.

18

Pneumonia in adults

The problem of pneumonia in Africa

For many decades pneumonia ranked second only to malaria as a cause of admission to adult medical wards across Africa (Williams et al., 1986, Harries et al., 1990). However, in the last decade the pattern of hospital admissions has changed, reflecting the dominance of HIV-related problems. Nonetheless, the two commonest reasons for admission among HIV-infected adults are tuberculosis and pneumonia (Grant et al., 1998; Karstaedt, 1992) so pneumonia continues to present a considerable burden to hospital services across the continent.

Pneumonia also affects the sub-group of society that is most economically productive. Although its incidence is higher among those with chronic underlying diseases, the typical patient in Africa is a healthy individual with a short history of illness. Although mortality is higher in the elderly, the majority of pneumonia related deaths in hospital occur among young adults, less than 40 years old; and among survivors, 60 per cent of pneumonia patients have not recovered sufficiently well to return to work 3 weeks after their admission (Scott et al., 2000).

For the clinician, pneumonia is usually straightforward to diagnose and treat. The challenges in management are identifying the severely ill patient, predicting the aetiology of disease, dealing with resistance among respiratory pathogens, and anticipating complications.

Aetiology of acute community acquired pneumonia

Our description of the aetiology of pneumonia is constrained by the insensitivity of gold-standard diagnostic methods, like blood culture, and by the lack of specificity of more accessible diagnostic procedures like sputum culture. Across the globe studies of pneumonia fail to identify an aetiology in-between 10 and 50 per cent of all presenting cases, yet empiric treatment guidelines rely on the assumption that the undiagnosed portion is composed of similar organisms to the diagnosed portion. The spectrum of organisms that can cause pneumonia is illustrated in Fig. 18.1. in which data are taken from a study of Kenyan adults (Scott et al., 2000). Respiratory viruses include Influenza and Parainfluenza viruses, Adenovirus and Respiratory Syncytial Virus. One-third of the patients have no aetiological diagnosis and potential causes of these cases include *Pneumocystis carinii,*

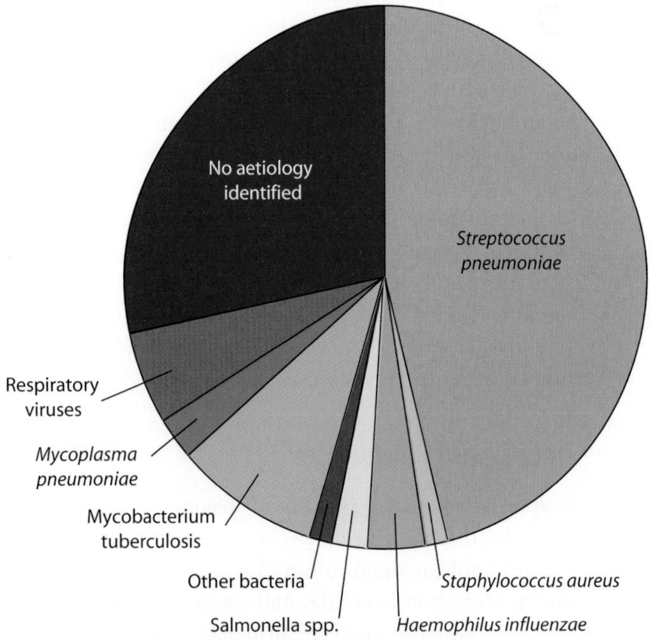

Fig. 18.1. Organisms that can cause pneumonia.

Klebsiella pneumoniae, Escherichia coli, Pseudomonas aeruginosa, anaerobic bacteria, *Chlamydia psittaci, Legionella pneumophila, Coxiella burnetti, Histoplasma capsulatum,* Aspergillus spp., Paragonimus spp. or other migrating parasites. However, even among patients with no defined aetiology, *Streptococcus pneumoniae* is likely to be the commonest causative organism and, where culture and antigen detection methods have been combined in aetiological studies, up to 70 per cent of inpatient pneumonias have been attributable to the pneumococcus (Macfarlane et al., 1979; Scott et al., 2000). This remains the rationale for primary empiric treatment with penicillin.

Bacterial pneumonia

Streptococcus pneumoniae

A gram-positive coccus, commonly found in pairs on microscopy, it colonizes the nasopharynx of healthy individuals, especially young children, and is transmitted by airborne droplet spread and direct contact with infected nasal mucus on hands and fomites. Human immunity is serotype specific, i.e. determined by antibodies to variants of the bacterial polysaccharide capsule of which 90 serologically distinct types have been identified. Among African adults 80 per cent of episodes of pneumonia are caused by only nine serotypes.

Patients with hypogammaglobulinaemia, asplenia, nephrotic syndrome and sickle cell anaemia are at especial risk of pneumococcal pneumonia. Individuals infected with HIV are at increased risk of all bacterial pneumonias, an association that is not unique to *S. pneumoniae.* Pneumococcal pneumonia is typically lobar, multi-lobar or segmental and only rarely causes diffuse bronchopneumonia. An accompanying pleural effusion occurs in 20 per cent of patients, but empyema is rare in patients treated with antibiotics. The pneumococcus does not often lead to cavitation but can produce a destructive pneumonia leading to necrosis of lung parenchyma and fibrotic healing in rare cases.

Haemophilus influenzae

Responsible for 3 to 5 per cent of episodes of pneumonia in adults, this gram-negative coccobacillus is found uncommonly in blood cultures but is found with much greater frequency in studies that employed lung aspirate cultures. It exists in both encapsulated and non-capsulated forms and both are capable of causing pneumonia in adults. As with the pneumococcus, serotyping is based on the serological differentiation of reactions to the capsule; most pathogenic isolates are of serotype b, the non-encapsulated forms are 'non-typable'. The epidemiology and transmission of *H. influenzae* is similar to that of *S. pneumoniae* and the two organisms are occasionally found together in a single case of pneumonia.

Staphylococcus aureus

S. aureus is a gram-positive coccus causing 1–2 per cent of adult pneumonia episodes. The incidence of *S. aureus* pneumonia, and the proportion of cases of pneumonia caused by *S. aureus,* have been shown to rise coincidentally with epidemics of influenza suggesting it has a particular role as a cause of secondary bacterial pneumonia. The bacterium colonizes the nose and the prevalence of colonization is 15–30 per cent in healthy individuals and 50 per cent in hospital workers.

S. aureus also obtains access to the lung by haematogenous spread from existing foci of infection in skin, wounds or via intravenous devices and needles. Staphylococcal pneumonia tends to be severe and cavitation, abscess formation and empyema are all common. Haematogenous infection may lead to multiple lung abscesses.

Gram-negative bacilli

Collectively gram-negative bacilli account for approximately 5 per cent of all episodes of pneumonia. *Klebsiella pneumoniae* is the most frequently isolated. Others include *E. coli,* and bacteria from the genera Pseudomonas, Enterobacter, Serratia, Acinetobacter, Citrobacter and Proteus. *Neisseria meningitidis* is a rare cause of pneumonia; *Yersinia pestis* pneumonia is seen only in very rare outbreaks of plague.

Klebsiella pneumonia is common in alcoholics, diabetics, and inpatients with HIV or neoplastic disease. It has a predilection for the upper lobes and also causes a cavitating pneumonia which may lead to diagnostic confusion with tuberculosis.

Atypical pneumonia

Pneumonias caused by the bacteria *Legionella pneumophila, Mycoplasma pneumoniae, Chlamydia psittaci* and the Rickettsia *Coxiella burnetti* are collectively described as atypical. Despite this label, pneumonia caused by atypical organisms is usually indistinguishable clinically and radiologically from that caused by conventional bacteria. It is difficult to estimate the prevalence of these pathogens in sub-Saharan Africa because diagnosis depends on serological, or on in-vitro culture techniques, which are not routinely available. Several studies have shown that antibodies to atypical organisms are prevalent in African populations, for example, among Somali refugees (Gray et al., 1995). However, the demonstration of a rising antibody titre to any of the atypical antigens during the course of pneumonia is uncommon (Aderaye, 1994b; Rolfe, 1986).

Mycoplasma pneumoniae

In industrialized countries *Mycoplasma pneumoniae* causes pneumonia in older children and young adults with an epidemic cycle of 4–5 years. In studies from Kenya and Ethiopia 3–4 per cent of adult pneumonia patients had serological evidence of Mycoplasma infection. (Aderaye, 1994b; Scott et al., 2000) One study from Zaria, Nigeria, described culture or serological evidence of Mycoplasma in 16 per cent of pneumonia episodes but half of these also had evidence of pneumococcal infection (Macfarlane et al., 1979). The spatial and temporal epidemiology of Mycoplasma infection in African has not been investigated.

Legionella pneumophila

In Europe and North America *Legionella pneumophila* causes outbreaks of severe pneumonia frequently associated with a common source of contaminated aerosolized water (Stout & Yu, 1997). Over 70 per cent of cases are caused by *L. pneumophila* serogroup 1. In three studies of pneumonia, in Nigeria, Zambia and Kenya, not one patient among over 400 demonstrated a four-fold rise in antibody titre against *L. pneumophila* type 1 (Macfarlane et al., 1979; Rolfe, 1986; Scott et al., 2000); in contrast Legionella has been widely observed in South Africa (Working groups of the South African Pulmonology Society and the Antibiotic Study Group of South Africa, 1996). At a clinical level, Legionella more frequently produces severe pneumonia. The pneumonia is more likely to be accompanied by symptoms of headache and diarrhoea, and hyponatraemia occurs in approximately 50 per cent of cases. None of these features, however, is specific for *Legionella pneumophila* pneumonia. During treatment, paradoxical deterioration in the radiographic picture may accompany clinical improvement.

Chlamydia species

Chlamydia psittaci pneumonia is a zoonosis transmitted by birds and the key to making the diagnosis is to obtain a history of bird contact. Cases of psittacosis have been reported, mainly from South Africa, and the birds responsible are parrots, budgerigars, cockatoos and pigeons. In Addis Ababa, 4 per cent of patients with acute pneumonia had a single antibody titre of $\geq 1/320$, though none was shown to produce an antibody response coincident with disease (Aderaye, 1994b).

Chlamydia pneumoniae causes pneumonia with a subacute onset and mild clinical course. In industrialized countries chronic infection with *Chlamydia pneumoniae* has also been associated with the development of ischaemic heart disease though the causality of the association is not clear. A single raised antibody titre to *C. pneumoniae* was found in 4 per cent of pneumonia patients in Yaounde, Cameroon (Koulla-Shiro et al., 1996), but there is no direct evidence of its role in pneumonia on the continent.

Coxiella burnetti

This is the Rickettsial organism that causes Q fever, a systemic illness that may involve pneumonitis. The disease is acquired through contact with goats, sheep, cattle or domestic animals. It is observed uncommonly in hospital practice, but may be encountered in the investigation of an outbreak. In a multi-centre study of pneumonia in the UK, responses to *Coxiella burnetti* infection were found in only 1 per cent of patients (British Thoracic Society Research Committee and the Public Health Laboratory Service, 1987) and in a series of almost 300 Kenyan hospital inpatients with pneumonia not one had serological evidence supporting a diagnosis of Q fever (Scott et al., 2000).

Other aetiologies

Fungal pneumonia

Aspergillus fumigatus is geographically widespread and causes four distinct types of respiratory illness (i) asthma, following sensitization with Aspergillus antigens, (ii) allergic bronchopulmonary aspergillosis, a condition characterized by recurrent episodes of cough, wheeze, and fever with mucus plugging, atelectasis and collapse, eventually leading to proximal bronchiectasis, (iii) aspergilloma, which is a large fungal culture loosely inhabiting an existing lung cavity following for example tuberculosis, (iv) severe invasive Aspergillus pneumonia. Histoplasmosis, blastomycosis, coccidioidomycosis and paracoccidioidomycosis are rare outside the Americas; *Histoplasma capsulatum* causes a benign self-limiting hypersensitivity pneumonitis and a less common chronic fibrotic lung disease; sporadic cases have been reported from East Africa. *Cryptococcus neoformans* pneumonia occurs in HIV-infected adults.

Viral pneumonia

A viral aetiology is described in only 1–5 per cent of cases but this is likely to underestimate the contribution of viruses to pneumonia morbidity and mortality because the diagnosis of viral infections is insensitive. Viruses most frequently associated with pneumonia are influenza A and B, parainfluenza and adenoviruses. Respiratory syncytial virus (RSV) has been shown to be pathogenic, causing pneumonia in adults as well as children (Dowell et al., 1996). Cytomegalovirus (CMV) and herpes simplex virus (HSV) cause pneumonia in immunodeficient patients and primary infections with measles virus or varicella-zoster virus can lead to severe or fatal pneumonia in adults; pregnant women with chickenpox are especially susceptible to varicella-zoster virus pneumonia.

Influenza can either cause a primary viral pneumonia, which evolves directly from the more common flu-like illness associated with the virus, or it may predispose to secondary bacterial pneumonia 5–14 days later. The second illness presents in the same fashion as any bacterial pneumonia, and the organisms most commonly isolated in this situation are *S. pneumoniae* and *S. aureus*. Pathogenic bacteria are frequently isolated from patients with primary viral pneumonia, though the mechanism of the interaction suggested by these observations has not been elucidated.

Mycobacterium tuberculosis

Between 5 and 15 per cent of patients presenting with acute pneumonia in Africa have positive sputum cultures for *M. tuberculosis* or acid fast bacilli on sputum smears (Allen, 1984, Scott et al., 2000). The finding is yet more common among HIV-positive individuals (Scott et al., 2000). *M. tuberculosis* can cause a primary acute pneumonia but it is more commonly isolated in pneumonia alongside other conventional respiratory pathogens. Tuberculosis may be a risk factor for bacterial pneumonia; alternatively, bacterial pneumonia may re-activate latent infection with *M. tuberculosis*, the direction of the association is not known. At a practical level, a sputum smear for acid fast bacilli (AFB) should be considered in patients with acute pneumonia, particularly if there is incomplete resolution on antibiotics.

Aetiology of hospital-acquired (nosocomial) pneumonia

Hospital-acquired pneumonia has been studied little in Africa. Pneumonia developing 3 days or more after admission to hospital is a major problem in industrialized countries, and the largest single cause of infection-related mortality among inpatients. Patient characteristics that increase the likelihood of nosocomial pneumonia are coma, malnutrition, severe metabolic acidosis, alcoholism, burns, pre-existing neurological disease and chronic obstructive pulmonary disease. The elderly are at especial risk. Anaesthesia, sedation or use of corticosteroid drugs are also predisposing factors as are manipulations of the pharynx and larynx, in particular intubation and ventilation. In Africa lack of facilities for hand-washing and sharing a bed with an infected patient are likely to be significant causes of nosocomial disease.

Figure 18.2 shows the aetiology of nosocomial pneumonia in an industrialized setting. The organisms identified are normally resistant to multiple antibiotics. Infection with tuberculosis is an additional risk in African hospitals

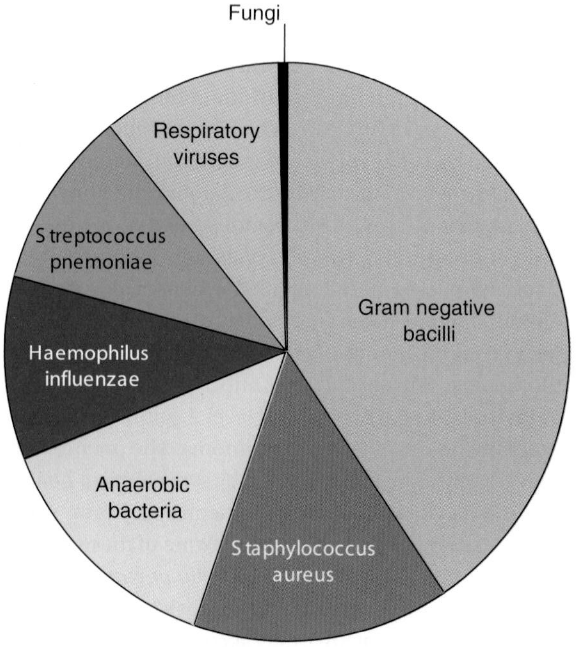

Fig. 18.2. Aetiology in industrialized setting.

that is not included in this list. In a patient who is already severely ill nosocomial pneumonia may not be recognized. Even when it is recognized it is difficult to distinguish from other common complications of hospital in-patients, e.g. pulmonary embolism and adult respiratory distress syndrome (ARDS). The case fatality of nosocomial pneumonia in unventilated patients is approximately 30 per cent. The experience of hospitals in Europe and the USA, coupled with hospital hygiene practice in Africa, suggests that nosocomial pneumonia is a significant, if currently unquantified, cause of inpatient mortality.

Aspiration pneumonia

Aspiration pneumonia is a distinct clinical syndrome caused by aspiration of pharyngeal contents either through depressed conscious level or dysphagia. It is caused by a combination of chemical pneumonitis and aspirated infection with oropharyngeal commensal bacteria that are particularly abundant in the presence of periodontal disease. Culture of sputum typically yields multiple bacteria of the genera Bacteroides, Streptococcus and Fusobacterium. The clinical presentation of aspiration pneumonia varies from a mild pneumonitis to a severe necrotizing pneumonia, lung abscess and empyema. It should be suspected in the presence of any of the specific risk factors listed in the Box below, or when expectorated sputum is foul smelling.

Risk factors for aspiration pneumonia

- Altered conscious level
  - coma
  - seizures
  - sedation
  - alcoholism
- Dysphagia
  - oesophageal malignancy
  - motor neurone disease
  - brain stem stroke
- Periodontal disease

HIV-associated pneumonia

In contrast to industrialized countries, the presentation and aetiology of most respiratory disease among HIV-infected adults in Africa is indistinguishable from that among HIV-uninfected adults. Patients with an acute history most commonly have bacterial pneumonia (Koulla-Shiro et al., 1996; Scott et al., 2000), those with a longer history have tuberculosis (Kamanfu et al., 1993; Daley et al., 1996); the remainder are few in number but it is here that the immunodeficiency influences the likely aetiology.

HIV-positive patients have the same spectrum of bacterial pathogens causing acute pneumonia, principally *S. pneumoniae*, as do HIV-negative patients. However, they are more likely to have bacteraemia, and are more likely to develop recurrent disease. *Salmonella* species, in particular *S. typhimurium* and *S. enteritidis*, have been found in 4–10 per cent of HIV-positive pneumonia patients though they are extremely rare in immunocompetent hosts (Kamanfu et al., 1993; Scott et al., 2000). It is not clear whether these blood-borne isolates are causal in the pneumonia process or merely coincidental bacteraemic infections in acutely sick patients. The short-term outcome of acute bacterial pneumonia among HIV-positive patients is also similar to that in HIV-negative patients (Koulla-Shiro et al., 1996; Scott et al., 2000).

In studies of sub-acute and chronic pneumonia, tuberculosis is the most common diagnosis in both HIV-positive and HIV-negative groups (Kamanfu et al., 1993; Daley et al., 1996). Among the HIV-infected patients 12–17 per cent have neither tuberculosis nor bacterial pneumonia and it is among this sub-population that cases of non-specific interstitial pneumonitis, cryptococcosis, Kaposi's sarcoma and *Pneumocystis carinii* pneumonia (PCP) have been found in bronchoscopic and autopsy studies (Kamanfu et al., 1993; Batungwanayo et al., 1994a; Daley et al., 1996). Other aetiologies associated with pneumonia in immunocompromised patients include herpes simplex virus, cytomegalovirus, *Nocardia* spp., *Aspergillus fumigatus, Strongyloides stercoralis* and *Toxoplasma gondii*, but all of these are rare (Lucas et al., 1994).

The importance of PCP among HIV-infected adults in Africa has been the subject of controversy. PCP was the commonest pulmonary manifestation of HIV/AIDS in industrialized countries, prior to the use of chemoprophylaxis, but in early African studies PCP was found to be uncommon (Elvin et al., 1989; Abouya et al., 1992). Later studies, that excluded patients with acute pneumonia and tuberculosis, found relatively more PCP than early unselective studies. *Pneumocystis carinii* does cause pneumonia in HIV-infected adults in Africa, but its incidence is dwarfed by that of pulmonary tuberculosis. It causes a sub-acute pneumonia with diffuse bilateral pulmonary changes on X-ray and severe hypoxaemia. In an HIV-positive patient with a pneumonia that is unresponsive to antibiotics, in whom smears for *M. tuberculosis* are negative, PCP should be considered a possible diagnosis – but tuberculosis is still more probable (Malin et al., 1995) (see Box overleaf).

Pulmonary complications of HIV in Africa
Pulmonary tuberculosis
Typical bacterial pneumonia
Non-specific interstitial pneumonia
Pneumocystis carinii pneumonia
Kaposi's sarcoma
Unusual bacterial pneumonias (*Nocardia* spp., *Pseudomonas* spp., *Salmonella* spp.)
Fungal pneumonia – *Cryptococcosis, Aspergillus*
Viral pneumonia – CMV, HSV
Non-Hodgkin's lymphoma

Parasites and acute pneumonia

Malaria

Deterioration of an adult patient with malaria, accompanied by new pulmonary shadowing on the chest radiograph, may be due to (a) complicating bacterial pneumonia, (b) pulmonary oedema and fluid overload and (c) ARDS as a direct complication of malaria. Like ARDS due to other causes this complication carries a mortality of over 70 per cent.

Amoebiasis

Amoebic liver abscess (ALA) may be difficult to distinguish from a right lower lobe pneumonia. Elevation of the right hemi-diaphragm, right lower lobe collapse and a right-sided pleural effusion are commonly seen on the chest radiograph. Consider ALA in the differential diagnosis of a right lower lobe pneumonia that has not responded to antibiotics. Lung abscess is a rare complication of amoebiasis, due to rupture of a liver abscess across the diaphragm or to haematogenous spread. Clinically it presents like a bacterial lung abscess.

Ascaris, hookworm and strongyloides

These helminths have a phase of trans-pulmonary migration in their life cycles which precipitates a transient pneumonitis accompanied by eosinophilia. Symptoms, which include fever, dyspnoea, cough and haemoptysis, are related to the size of the migrating worm burden and are usually mild.

Paragonimus

Infection with *Paragonimus africanus* and *Paragonimus uterobilateralis* can be acquired in West Africa by ingesting raw crab or crayfish. They cause a mild respiratory illness with chronic cough and occasional small haemoptyses. The diagnosis is confirmed by finding eggs in sputum or stool. In African cases radiological signs are uncommon and the disease responds well to praziquantel.

Schistosomiasis

In established hepatosplenic schistosomiasis, ova or adult worms can bypass the liver through porto-systemic collaterals and become trapped in lung capillaries where they elicit a granulomatous reaction. If many such granulomata occur the patient develops pulmonary hypertension with dyspnoea and right ventricular hypertrophy. Noted in Far Eastern schistosomiasis, it is uncommon in *S. mansoni* infection and rare with *S. haematobium.*

Echinococcus granulosus

Globally, the highest incidence of hydatid disease is among the Turkana community of Northern Kenya. Infection is acquired from ingesting dog faeces or intestines, and dogs are infected by eating the offal of intermediary hosts, sheep, cattle, camels and possibly dead human remains. Lung cysts are chronic and usually asymptomatic, being discovered incidentally on chest radiographs, but they can cause cough, chest pain, haemoptysis and dyspnoea. Cyst rupture may lead to anaphylactic shock or, if adjacent to a bronchus, the cyst contents (grape skins) may be expectorated.

Tropical pulmonary eosinophilia

Acute hypersensitivity to circulating microfilariae leads to clearance of microfilariae from the circulation but also to an asthma-like illness with cough, wheeze, fever, weight loss and fatigue. Characteristically the eosinophil count is extremely high. Treatment with diethylcarbamazine (DEC) is very effective. Although lymphatic filariases are endemic over a wide geographical area in sub-Saharan Africa, tropical pulmonary eosinophilia is rare; host factors, particularly an association with Indian ethnic origin, appear to make an important contribution to the aetiology of the disease.

Epidemiology of pneumonia

Incidence

Community-based observations on pneumonia are few and the incidence can only be calculated using epidemi-

Table 18.1. Community-based estimates of pneumonia incidence in Africa

Setting	Study	Year	Group	Endpoint	Incidence/ 100 000/year
Migrant workers at the South African Mines	Pneumococcal vaccine miners study	1970–1975	placebo/meningo-coccal vaccine controls	radiographic pneumonia	2600
HIV-positive individuals in Entebbe, Uganda	Pneumococcal vaccine HIV study	1995–1998	placebo treated controls	radiographic pneumonia	3000
Routinely collected data and models for sub-Saharan Africa	Global burden of disease study	2000	adults aged 15–59 years	episodes of LRTI	1000
Routinely collected data and models for sub-Saharan Africa	Global burden of disease study	2000	adults aged ≥60 years	episodes of LRTI	7000
Routinely collected data and models for sub-Saharan Africa	Global burden of disease study	2000	adults aged 15–59 years	deaths from LRTI	6.2–15.4
Routinely collected data and models for sub-Saharan Africa	Global burden of disease study	2000	adults aged ≥60 years	deaths from LRTI	522–553

Source: Austrian et al. (1976), Murray & Lopez (1996), French et al. (2000).

ological models (Table 18.1). The Global Burden of Disease study estimated the annual incidence of non-tuberculous lower respiratory tract infections was 1 episode per 100 adults and 7 episodes per 100 elderly adults (≥60 years) (Murray & Lopez, 1996). Miners and HIV-positive individuals, both constitute high risk groups, and have an incidence of pneumonia 3–5 times as great (Austrian et al., 1976; French et al., 2000). Annual mortality attributable to lower respiratory tract infections is estimated at 1/10 000 for younger adults and 1/200 for older adults (Murray & Lopez, 1996). The absolute number of episodes of lower respiratory tract infection in adults in sub-Saharan Africa is estimated at 4 million per year, with 200 000 deaths.

In America and Britain the risk of pneumonia is higher in those aged 60 years or more (Foy et al., 1973; Macfarlane et al., 1993), and this risk rises progressively with increasing age. Given the demographic structure of African populations, however, the typical pneumonia patient is 15–45 years old. Among inpatient series 54–72 per cent of all patients are male (Allen, 1984; Aderaye, 1994a; El-Amin, 1978; Scott et al., 2000) though it is not known whether this represents a true increased risk of pneumonia in men or a difference in health seeking behaviour between the sexes.

In temperate zones, e.g. in South Africa, mortality from pneumonia is associated with areas of cold climate (Wyndham, 1986) whereas in tropical zones the incidence of pneumonia is associated more strongly with the rains, peaking early in the dry season (Harries et al., 1988; Macfarlane et al., 1979).

There is little data to suggest that the risk of pneumonia varies with occupation, but activities that bring a large number of individuals into close proximity, such as mining and military training, are associated with high risk; new miners on first joining the gold mines of the South Africa Rand in the 1970s were found to have an incidence of putative pneumococcal pneumonia of 9/100 person years of observation (Austrian et al., 1976).

Risk factors

HIV is a strong risk factor for pneumonia, increasing the risk of pneumococcal pneumonia 20-fold (García-Leoni et al., 1992), and that of *H. influenzae* pneumonia approximately 100-fold (Steinhart et al., 1992). Invasive pneumococcal disease (IPD), with blood or lung aspirate cultures positive for *S. pneumoniae,* is even more strongly associated with HIV. Among sex workers in Nairobi IPD was 40 times more common among HIV-positive than among HIV-negative study subjects (Gilks et al., 1996).

In other parts of the world, alcoholism, malignancy, diabetes mellitus, cirrhosis, chronic obstructive pulmonary disease, nephrotic syndrome and chronic renal failure have all been observed more frequently among patients with pneumonia. In the USA cigarette smoking increases the risk of IPD by a factor of 4, and half of all cases observed are attributable to smoking alone (Nuorti et al., 2000).

The incidence of pneumonia in sub-Saharan Africa is so high that it raises the question of genetic susceptibility. For example, African–Americans are at higher risk of IPD than white Americans. It is extremely difficult to define and measure potential environmental confounders of these associations, including childhood exposure to pneumonia pathogens, previous vaccination history, current socioeconomic status and access to health care. A study conducted among US Navy and Marine Corps personnel, who are relatively homogeneous with regard to current environmental confounders, demonstrated a 25 per cent increased risk of pneumonia hospitalization among white servicemen compared to black servicemen, though the pneumonias observed were relatively mild (Gray et al., 1994).

Transmission

Most pathogens causing pneumonia may be found in the upper respiratory tract of healthy individuals or of those experiencing a mild upper respiratory tract infection (URTI). Influenza virus, parainfluenza virus and adenovirus are transmitted from individuals with URTIs to uninfected individuals by droplet spread. Bacteria that colonize the nasopharynx, such as *S. pneumoniae, H. influenzae* and *S. aureus*, can be transmitted from cases of pneumonia but a history of direct contact with a primary case is rarely obtained suggesting that most transmission is mediated by asymptomatic carriers. The prevalence of *S. pneumoniae* colonization in healthy Gambian children <5 years old is 76 per cent, representing a considerable pool of potential infection to the adult population with whom they live (Lloyd-Evans et al., 1996).

Antimicrobial resistance

Bacterial resistance to available antibiotics is now commonplace in Africa, and is rising. For example, intermediate resistance of *S. pneumoniae* to penicillin in Kenya has increased over the last two decades from 10 to 27 per cent (Scott et al., 1998). High level penicillin resistance and resistance to multiple antibiotics including chloramphenicol, tetracycline and cephalosporins has been identified in strains from South Africa.

Causes of emergence of drug-resistant respiratory pathogens	
• antibiotic pressure	over-treatment with antibiotics, especially for viral URTI
• anti-malarial pressure	sulphadiazine-pyremethamine use leading to co-trimoxazole resistance (Feikin et al., 2000)
• importation	spread, by travellers and tourists, of resistant strains that have evolved elsewhere, e.g. Spain (Munoz et al., 1991)

Outside South Africa, resistance of pneumococci to penicillin is almost exclusively at the intermediate level, with an MIC greater than 0.1 μg/ml but less than 2.0 μg/ml. There have been reports of penicillin treatment failure for intermediate resistant isolates among patients with meningitis and pneumonia but it remains unknown whether this is a common cause of treatment failure.

Vaccination

Pneumococcal polysaccharide vaccine has been available for 30 years. It has proven efficacy among gold miners in South Africa, reducing the incidence of pneumonia by 79 per cent (Austrian et al., 1976). In the highlands of Papua New Guinea it reduced pneumonia-associated mortality in otherwise healthy adults by 42 per cent (Riley et al., 1977). However, as adult vaccination has not been seen as a priority for health expenditure, and as the efficacy of the vaccine was much less evident in the USA, enthusiasm for its use has been tempered worldwide. Targeting a high risk group, such as those with HIV infection is an attractive public health policy but a placebo controlled trial of pneumococcal vaccine in Uganda demonstrated no protection from pneumonia associated with vaccinating HIV-positive individuals (French et al., 2000).

Conjugation of capsular polysaccharides to protein carriers has produced pneumococcal vaccines that are highly effective in children and may be shown to be capable of preventing pneumonia in adults; the major limitation of these vaccines is that they protect against only a few serotypes (Hausdorff et al., 2000). In temperate climate countries, influenza vaccine has an established role in protection of the elderly but it has not been evaluated in Africa.

Prognosis and outcome

Inpatient mortality from pneumonia varies from 6–23 per cent in studies across Africa; the variation is most likely to be due to differences in patterns of presentation and admission to hospital in different populations (Table 18.2).

Features of the illness at presentation can be used to identify those most at risk of death. For example, the British Thoracic Society Study of over 500 hospitalized patients showed that the presence of any two of the following factors was associated with a 21-fold increase in morality; (i) admission respiratory rate ≥ 30/min, (ii) admission diastolic BP ≤ 60 mm HG, (iii) urea >7mmol/l during admission (British Thoracic Society Research Committee and the Public Health Laboratory Service, 1987). In Kenya factors that were associated with mortality in hospitalized

Table 18.2. Inpatient mortality of pneumonia

Study	Country	No. of pts	Year	Mortality
Allen	Zambia	502	1981–83	5.6%
Aderaye	Ethiopia	110	1987–89	11%
Sofowora	Nigeria	88	1969–71	23%
Sow	Guinea-Conakry	218	1994–5	6.0%
Scott	Kenya	281	1994–96	10%
Koulla-Shiro	Cameroon	110	1991–92	7.3%

Source: (Allen, 1984, Aderaye, 1994b, Sofowora and Onadeko, 1973, Sow et al., 1996, Scott et al., 2000, Koulla-Shiro et al., 1996)

pneumonia patients were increasing age, tachycardia and, in HIV-positive patients, presence of herpes labialis. Socioeconomic factors such as unemployment or visiting a traditional healer were also predictive of poor outcome, and visiting a pharmacy during the illness was associated with a better outcome (Scott et al., 2000).

It is useful to define a syndrome of 'severe pneumonia' to guide management decisions. The scheme shown in the Box below has not been validated in an African population but, extrapolating from existing global evidence, the presence of any one of the features suggests an increased likelihood of a fatal outcome.

Features of severe pneumonia

Examination

- heart rate ≥120/min
- respiratory rate ≥30/min
- diastolic blood pressure ≤60 mmHg
- systolic blood pressure ≤90 mmHg
- core temperature ≤35.0 °C
- confusion
- hepatomegaly
- pleural effusion

Investigations

- Leukocyte count $<4.0\times10^9$/l
- Leukocyte count $>22.0\times10^9$/l
- Plasma urea >7 mmol/l
- Oxygen saturation <90%
- Multi-lobar disease
- Bacteraemia

Pathophysiology

Host defences

Adaptations to prevent or eliminate infection of the lung are either natural or acquired. Figure 18.3 illustrates the natural anatomical and physiological features that create an environment hostile to pathogen survival. Absence or failure of these components leads to chronic or recurrent infection. For example, the mucociliary escalator is defective in two genetic conditions, Kartagener's syndrome and cystic fibrosis (CF). In Kartagener's syndrome changes in ciliary structure prevent beating of cilia in the respiratory epithelia (and similar changes in sperm tails lead to infertility) and in CF the production of viscid mucous prevents ciliary movement. Both conditions result in bronchiectasis. Cigarette smoking also disrupts ciliary movement making the smoker more susceptible to bronchitis and pneumonia.

Acquired immune defences are pathogen-specific and dependent upon previous exposure. The dominant immunoglobulin sub-type of the upper airways is IgA which is secreted in nasopharyngeal mucous, saliva and respiratory tract fluid. Serum IgG also leaks into these fluids particularly in the alveoli. IgA binding of bacteria prevents attachment and multiplication in the nasopharynx and so reduces colonization. In the lower respiratory tract encapsulated bacteria are opsonized by specific IgG and phagocytozed by polymorphonuclear cells recruited from blood by chemokine-signalling from lymphocytes and alveolar macrophages.

Pathogen virulence factors

Respiratory pathogens are similarly adapted to survive the hostile environment of the respiratory tract. For example, the pneumococci secrete proteases that lyse IgA, the polysaccharide capsule of *Streptococcus pneumoniae* inhibits phagocytosis and pneumolysin released at the death of a pneumococcus has both cytotoxic and complement stimulating properties. Viruses also enhance their own survival and cause disease by interfering directly with the ciliary function of respiratory epithelia.

Pathogenesis of pneumonia

The pathology of lobar pneumococcal pneumonia follows four stages.

1. Congestion: pneumococcal cell wall components (Tuomanen et al., 1995) stimulate the release of a protein rich serous fluid within alveoli, and activate the pro-coagulant cascade leading to local fibrin deposition.

2. Red hepatization: cell wall components also bind to epithelial and endothelial cells causing them to separate from each other disrupting their barrier

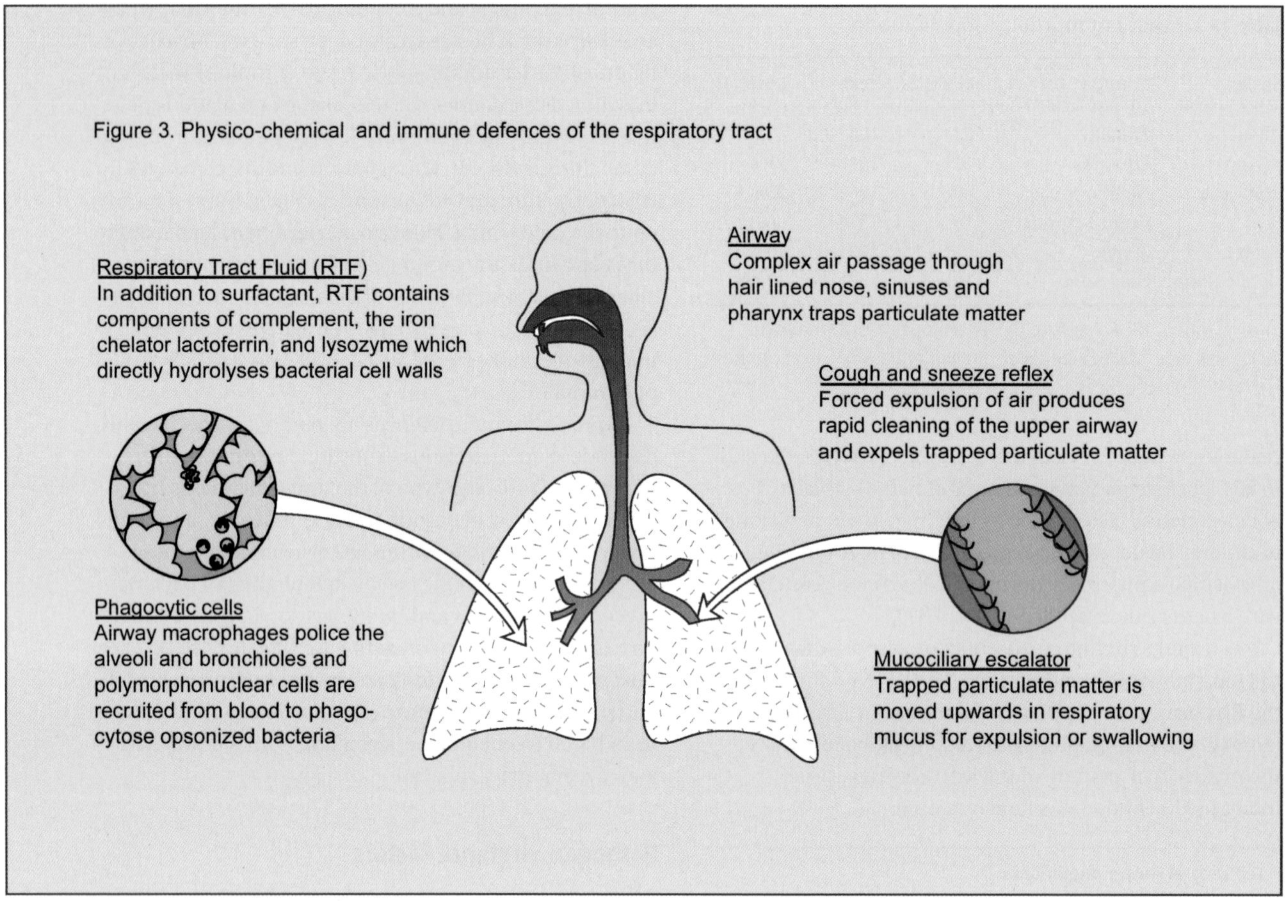

Figure 3. Physico-chemical and immune defences of the respiratory tract
Respiratory Tract Fluid (RTF)
In addition to surfactant, RTF contains components of complement, the iron chelator lactoferrin, and lysozyme which directly hydrolyses bacterial cell walls
Airway
Complex air passage through hair lined nose, sinuses and pharynx traps particulate matter
Cough and sneeze reflex
Forced expulsion of air produces rapid cleaning of the upper airway and expels trapped particulate matter
Phagocytic cells
Airway macrophages police the alveoli and bronchioles and polymorphonuclear cells are recruited from blood to phagocytose opsonized bacteria
Mucociliary escalator
Trapped particulate matter is moved upwards in respiratory mucus for expulsion or swallowing

Fig. 18.3. Host defences.

function and allowing passage of red blood cells to the lesion.

3. Grey hepatization: expression of adhesion molecules or integrins on endothelial cells leads to the recruitment of large numbers of leukocytes and to a gross pathological specimen that appears grey. The complement cascade amplifies the inflammation

4. Resolution: The inflammatory process usually heals without scarring though there may be fibrosis and abscess formation

Pneumonia causes hypoxia by two mechanisms. Firstly consolidation makes the lung stiff and less compliant which, combined with voluntary splinting to reduce pleural pain, leads to lower ventilation. Secondly, fibrin deposition in small pulmonary vessels leads to poor perfusion and shunting, disturbing ventilation–perfusion matching.

Diagnosis and clinical evaluation

There are three components to the clinical evaluation of pneumonia; (i) differentiation of pneumonia from other conditions with a similar presentation; (ii) identification of patients with severe pneumonia and (iii) definition of the aetiology.

History

The typical case has fever, cough, purulent sputum, dyspnoea and pleuritic chest pain. Haemoptysis is less frequently encountered. General symptoms such as myalgia, arthralgia, sweating, anorexia, nausea and headache are also common but of little specific value. A history of recent upper respiratory tract infection is obtained in approximately one-third of patients. The history is neither sensitive nor specific in the diagnosis of pneumonia. Patients who present early in the course of the illness are unlikely to have sputum and the absence of cough should not rule out pneumonia. Conversely cough is a very common symptom in outpatient presentations but only a small percentage of such patients will have pneumonia. The single most important feature of the history is duration of illness; a history of illness greater than two weeks is unusual in viral or bacterial pneumonia and raises the possibility of tuberculosis or HIV-associated pneumonias.

Examination

Chest signs of pneumonia are splinting of the affected hemithorax (to reduce pleural pain) dullness to percussion, increased vocal resonance, bronchial breathing and crepitations. However, intraobserver variation in the evaluation of chest signs is considerable and it is desirable, if possible, to confirm abnormalities with a chest X-ray. Occasionally a patient presenting early in the course of illness lacks radiographic abnormalities despite chest signs on physical examination.

Measurement of the vital signs is more useful. A patient with a pulse rate of <100/min, respiratory rate of <30/min and temperature <37.8 °C is extremely unlikely to have pneumonia. At the same time the vital signs identify those patients with severe pneumonia (see the Box on p. 358). Examine the blood pressure, lying and standing, and evaluate the degree of cyanosis. Measure the oxygen saturation where possible; patients with incipient respiratory failure will exhibit accessory muscle use, sternal retraction, and nasal flaring together with a rapid respiratory rate.

Complete the assessment of pneumonia by looking for oral candidiasis, lymphadenopathy, and weight loss suggestive of HIV. Herpes labialis occurs in 5–30 per cent of patients with pneumonia, particularly pneumococcal. Skin sepsis suggests a staphylococcal aetiology. Poor dentition is a clue to aspiration pneumonia. In patients who have already developed complications, a pleural or pericardial rub may be heard.

Chest radiograph (Fig 18.4)

Look for asymmetrical expansion or a fine or streaky opacity in the distribution of a single lobe. The classical presentation is of a lobar opacity with an air-bronchogram but a pleural effusion or partial lobar collapse may

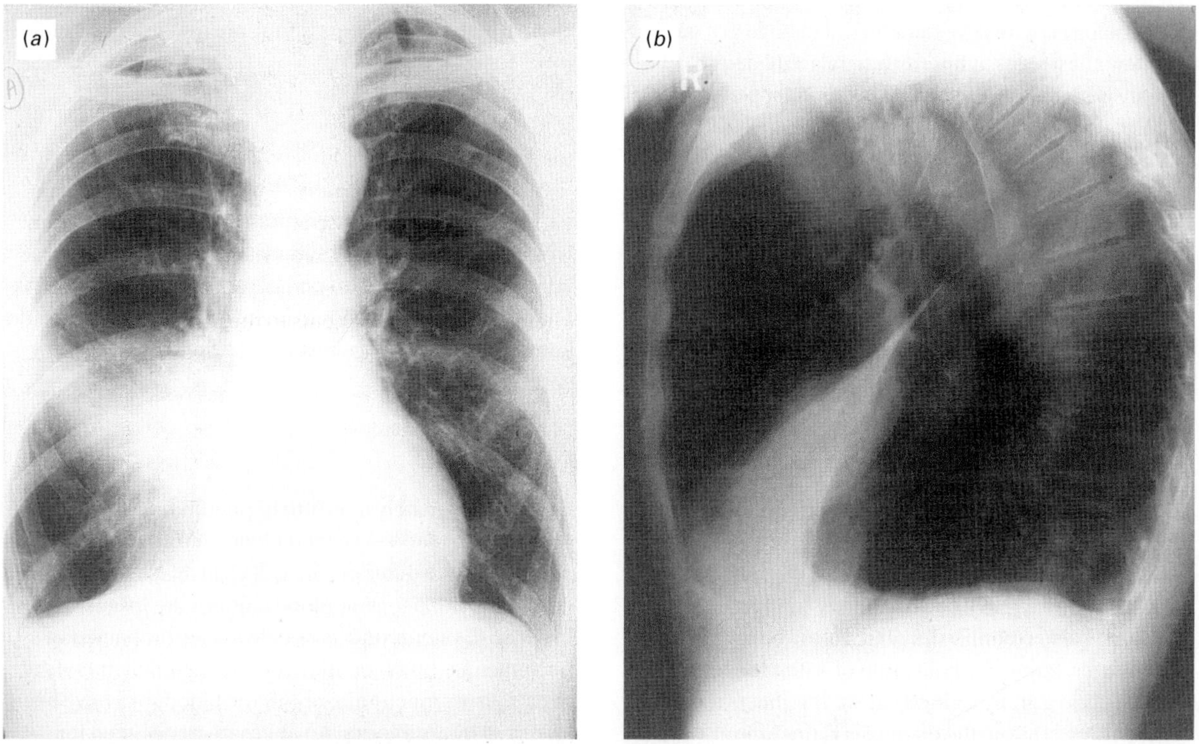

Fig. 18.4. (*a*) PA and (*b*) right lateral radiographs of the chest showing consolidation and partial collapse of the right middle lobe. (Courtesy of Dr Basil Shepstone, Oxford, UK.)

make the diagnosis less clear cut. Complete opacity of the whole of one lung field with little or no deviation of the trachea or the visible heart border suggests a dominance of consolidated lung rather than of pleural fluid. The pattern of lobar involvement can provide supporting evidence of a diagnosis of aspiration pneumonia; in the upright position aspirated liquids pass to the right lower lobe; in the supine position they pass most readily to the apical segment of the lower lobe or the posterior segment of the upper lobe. A peripheral wedge-shaped opacity, with or without a small effusion, may be caused by embolic pulmonary infarction.

Cavitation indicates a destructive pneumonia which can occur with any aetiology but is associated especially with *K. pneumoniae* and *S. aureus*. Upper lobe cavitation or hilar lymphadenopathy suggest underlying tuberculosis. The single most difficult distinction to make is between acute pneumonia superimposed on the scarred lung of old tuberculosis and currently active tuberculosis. Although tuberculosis is extremely common, remember, particularly in the elderly, that hilar lymphadenopathy, partial collapse or pleural effusion can also be caused by underlying malignancy. 'Atypical' pneumonia can present with diffuse, bilateral shadowing but the majority of cases have the same radiological appearance as classical bacterial pneumonias. A feature which does suggest an 'atypical' aetiology is extensive radiological change in a patient with few chest signs. A fine, diffuse bilateral pattern of opacity is seen in PCP as well as pulmonary oedema (Fig. 18.5).

There are two circumstances in which to repeat the radiograph; (i) to confirm that the area of consolidation has extended on therapy, indicating progression of disease and failure of current treatment (ii) to detect complications, lung abscess, pleural effusion and pleural empyema. There is no point in using the radiograph to monitor successful therapy in the acute phase as regression of radiological signs takes up to 12 weeks.

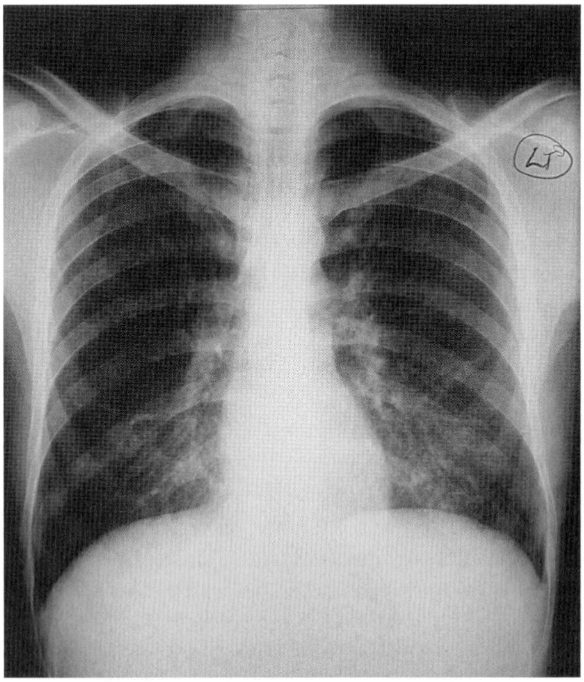

Fig. 18.5. This patient had *Pneumocystis carinii* pneumonia. The chest radiograph shows a fine diffuse bilateral pattern of shadowing characteristic of PCP.

Sputum

Sputum is often not available from patients in the first 48 hours of illness. In hospital the quality of routinely collected specimens is often poor and the specificity of sputum cultures is low because many pneumonia pathogens also colonize the pharynx and contaminate the cultures. Supervise collection of a fresh specimen and examine a gram-stained smear. If it meets the following three criteria, the diagnosis is pneumonia and if the organism cultured is consistent with the gram stained appearance it is likely to be the cause. Unfortunately, these conditions are met in only a minority of specimens.

(i) >25 leukocytes per low power field
(ii) <10 epithelial cells per low power field
(iii) an abundance of a single class of bacteria.

Given that approximately 10 per cent of pneumonia patients have tuberculosis, sputum smear examination with Ziehl–Neelsen (ZN) stain is likely to prove useful at admission. Patients who do not recover following a week of antibiotic therapy should be investigated for tuberculosis with three sputum smears and, where available, sputum culture.

Culture

Only approximately one-fifth of pneumonia cases yield an isolate in blood. A second blood culture taken simultaneously from a different site will yield an isolate in an additional 2–3 per cent. Blood cultures are insensitive because (i) pneumonia is not always accompanied by bacteraemia, (ii) blood may contain insufficient density of organisms for culture, or (iii) the blood may have been sterilized by antibiotics. An alternative specimen for culture is pleural effusion, which is present in a quarter of all patients at presentation and is simple to obtain.

Culture of lung juice from percutaneous lung aspiration leads to an aetiological diagnosis in 50 per cent of cases but may cause pneumothorax and is not recommended as a routine investigation.

Detection of antibodies and antigens

No antibody assay has been developed that can reliably diagnose the cause of pneumonia at presentation. Analysis of acute-convalescent serum pairs using complement fixation tests, micro-agglutination tests and immunofluorescent antibody titres can provide epidemiological information about the relative prevalence of viral pneumonias, *Mycoplasma pneumoniae, Chlamydia psittaci, Chlamydia pneumoniae, Coxiella burnetti* and *Legionella pneumophila.* Detection of type 1 Legionella antigen in urine is a sensitive diagnostic test at admission but the disease is rare in Africa. Pneumococcal capsular antigens can be detected in urine of about half of patients with pneumococcal pneumonia but the assay is cumbersome and labour intensive (Tugwell & Greenwood, 1975; Scott et al., 1999). Cold agglutinins are present in more than half of all patients with *Mycoplasma pneumoniae* but the specificity of the test in Nigerian patients is poor (Macfarlane et al., 1979).

HIV-associated pneumonia

Although cryptococcosis, nocardiosis and Kaposi's sarcoma have all been shown to occur in this context (Kamanfu et al., 1993; Lucas et al., 1994; Batungwanayo et al., 1994a,b) the additional effort required to make these diagnoses routinely, especially the use of bronchoscopy, is not usually justified by the small additional diagnostic yield (Daley et al., 1996). Bronchoscopy, where available, can yield a higher diagnostic return when targeted at patients with chronic symptoms who are ZN smear negative.

Pneumocystis carinii pneumonia is diagnosed by identifying trophozoites on sputum smears stained with methenamine silver or toluidine-blue-O. The sensitivity of sputum microscopy can be improved by inducing sputum with a nebulizer of hypertonic saline.

Diagnostic problems

Acute bronchitis

This is a common cause of productive cough, but pyrexia is usually low-grade and there are no focal signs in the chest. Transmitted sounds from bronchial mucous can be mistaken for coarse respiratory crackles. The infective causes, and treatments, are similar to those for pneumonia.

Malaria/typhoid

A patient who presents *in extremis*, with a short history of fever and tachypnoea, confusion, hypotension, cyanosis, and leukopenia but no focal abnormality of the lung fields is likely to be diagnosed malaria in an area of endemicity, or with typhoid. Remember that in bacterial pneumonia there may be few chest signs during the first 48–72 hours of the illness and this is a typical presentation of early disease.

Acute chest syndrome

Adults with sickle cell disease are prone to episodes of dyspnoea, breathlessness, cough and fever, which are thought to be due to pulmonary infarction. The differentiation from acute bacterial pneumonia, to which sickle cell patients are also susceptible, is difficult and the possibility of infection should always be covered with antibiotics.

Chronic lung disease/tuberculosis

A patient with chronic respiratory symptoms will reduce the length of the history to describe only the current exacerbation. If the patient is emaciated, or has radiological changes suggesting a chronic process, probe directly to elicit an antecedent history.

Treatment and follow-up

Admission to hospital

How can we decide which patients need to be admitted to hospital? Admission to hospital ensures compliance, it allows parenteral antibiotics, resuscitation, nursing and supportive therapy, and a rapid response to both results of investigations and clinical deterioration. Patients who are likely to benefit from admission are those who have severe pneumonia, those likely to deteriorate into severe pneumonia, or those in whom compliance is doubtful. The first Box on p. 358 lists clinical features that may be used to guide this decision.

Table 18.3.

	Outpatient	Inpatient	Severe
First-line	Penicillin V orally	Penicillin G i.m./i.v.	Ampicillin or amoxycillin i.m./i.v. plus gentamicin i.m./i.v. plus cloxacillin i.m./i.v.
Alternative	Ampicillin orally or Amoxycillin orally	Ampicillin i.m./i.v. or Amoxycillin i.m./i.v.	Ampicillin or amoxycillin i.m./i.v. plus chloramphenicol orally/i.v.
Second-line therapy following deterioration	Treat as inpatient	Treat as severe	*Consider addition of:* Erythromycin i.v./orally or anti-tuberculous drugs or high dose co-trimoxazole orally
Duration of therapy	5 days	5–10 days	10–14 days

Indications for admission to hospital

Severe pneumonia (see Box on p. 353)
age >55
pregnancy
poor compliance
poor socioeconomic conditions
underlying medical conditions *(diabetes, chronic lung disease, chronic heart disease, chronic liver disease, chronic renal disease)*
respiratory distress *(nasal flaring, use of accessory muscles, sternal retraction)*
wheeze/hyperexpansion
likelihood of underlying malignancy
cachexia
severe immunosuppression
jaundice
complications on chest X-ray *(cavitation, abscess, collapse, hilar lymphadenopathy)*

Antibiotic therapy

It is not possible to define a single treatment regimen for the whole of Africa. The relative importance of 'atypical' organisms varies, as do both the availability of parenteral antibiotics and local antibiotic susceptibility profiles. The table (Table 18.3) of empiric treatments has not been formally evaluated in any African setting and must be adapted to suit both local circumstances and the unique presentation of the individual patient.

For outpatients with known penicillin allergy, use erythromycin or tetracycline. The inpatient regime assumes that the majority of bacterial pneumonias are caused by *Streptococcus pneumoniae.* In a patient with recent influenza, with evidence of skin sepsis, or with a destructive or cavitating pneumonia, add in cloxacillin i.m./i.v. at the outset; with suspicion of atypical pneumonia add in erythromycin. In aspiration pneumonia, add in metronidazole orally. Treat nosocomial pneumonia as severe pneumonia irrespective of the clinical grading. For severe pneumonia a second generation cephalosporin, e.g. cefuroxime, is preferable to ampicillin though it is rarely available. Give gentamicin in a once daily regimen to reduce the probability of nephrotoxicity and ototoxicity and, ideally, stop the drug after 48 hours. Do not use gentamicin in older patients (e.g. >70 years) or in those with renal impairment.

Dose and duration

Suggested doses are given in the Box below. Bear in mind that intermediate resistant pneumococci comprise 15–30 per cent of all isolates of *S. pneumoniae* and that it is not known whether pneumonia caused by these organisms can be reliably treated by penicillins, nor with what dose. Increase the dose if the patient deteriorates to the severe category. For inpatients, aim to give at least 5 days therapy in total, with at least 2 days of parenteral therapy.

Antibiotic doses in pneumonia treatment

Amoxycillin i.m./i.v. 500–1000 mg 8 hourly
Ampicillin i.m./i.v. 500–1000 mg 6 hourly
Chloramphenicol orally/i.v. 12.5 mg/kg 6 hourly
Cloxacillin i.m./i.v. 500–1000 mg 6 hourly
Erythromycin orally 500–1000 mg 6 hourly
Gentamicin i.m. 7 mg/kg once, repeat once more at 24 hours if renal function is normal
Metronidazole orally 400 mg 8 hourly
Penicillin G i.m./i.v. 600 mg 6 hourly
Penicillin V orally 500 mg 6 hourly
Where ranges are given use higher doses for patients in the severe pneumonia category.

Supportive therapy

Advise bed rest and treat any pleuritic pain vigorously with non-steroidal anti-inflammatory drugs or paracetamol which, together with physiotherapy encourages adequate ventilation and facilitates coughing. Cough is the normal mechanism for clearing infected sputum and should not be suppressed pharmacologically. Treat hypoxia (oxygen saturation <90%) with oxygen if available. Correct hypovolaemia with physiological saline and monitor urine volume. Transfuse patients who have both severe anaemia (e.g. Hb < 6 g/dl) and respiratory distress. Ensure patients have an adequate diet including, if necessary, iron and folate and treat nausea and vomiting with prochlorperazine, especially in those taking erythromycin.

Response to therapy

Worsening tachypnoea or deterioration in oxygen saturation may be due to (a) extension of the area of disease, (b) shunting of the pulmonary circulation, (c) accumulation of pleural fluid, (d) associated bronchospasm, (e) shock, (f) pulmonary embolism or (g) pericarditis/pericardial effusion. Monitor the temperature to evaluate the clearance of infection; the temperature can fall dramatically after 24 hours on treatment or can remain high or fluctuating for 5–7 days even in uncomplicated lobar pneumonia. If you observe persistent or spiking pyrexia beyond 5–7 days consider (i) antibiotic spectrum may be inadequate, (ii) the bacteria may be resistant and (iii) a focal collection may have developed, e.g. empyema or lung abscess.

If an inpatient on beta-lactam antibiotics deteriorates quickly or fails to improve after 5–7 days repeat the aetiological investigations, switch to therapy for severe pneumonia and consider atypical pneumonia. If subsequently there is no improvement, consider empiric treatment for tuberculosis or PCP. Treatment of PCP is co-trimoxazole 1920 mg 6 hourly for a 60 kg adult. In the presence of hypoxaemia prednisolone 40 mg twice daily for 5 days, reduced slowly thereafter, has been shown to improve survival.

Communication

Patients have little notion of the mechanisms of the therapies used on them. Take time to explain both the illness and the therapy to the patient to ensure full compliance. Patients may abscond if they have improved before the end of the treatment course, especially if they are paying accommodation charges, so discuss the treatment plan early with the patient and provide oral therapy at an agreed discharge date. Compliance is not just related to tablets. After one of us failed to explain the working of a chest drain to one patient with *S. aureus* empyema, he removed the drain tube from the underwater seal, put the end in his pocket, and strolled out of the hospital to buy some soap. Fortunately, the pus that filled his pocket was sufficiently tenacious to prevent him developing a pneumothorax. Had he collapsed in the street, it would have been for want of information.

Complications

Lung abscess

Cavitating pneumonia can lead to formation of a lung abscess, detected as a rounded, thick-walled, fluid-filled opacity on the chest radiograph. Primary lung abscess, caused by aspiration, can also come to light after an area of pneumonia surrounding the abscess is successfully treated. If an abscess communicates with the bronchial tree sputum is plentiful and foul smelling; culture reveals a mixed infection of anaerobes. Treat with high-dose benzylpenicillin (e.g. 9.6 g/day) and metronidazole. *Staphylococcus aureus* and gram-negative aerobes require additional treatment if cultured. Postural drainage and chest percussion aids the clearance of pus. Continue the treatment for 4–6 weeks, and approximately 80 per cent of patients will recover; the only options for the remaining patients are bronchoscopic aspiration or surgical resection (Fig. 18.6).

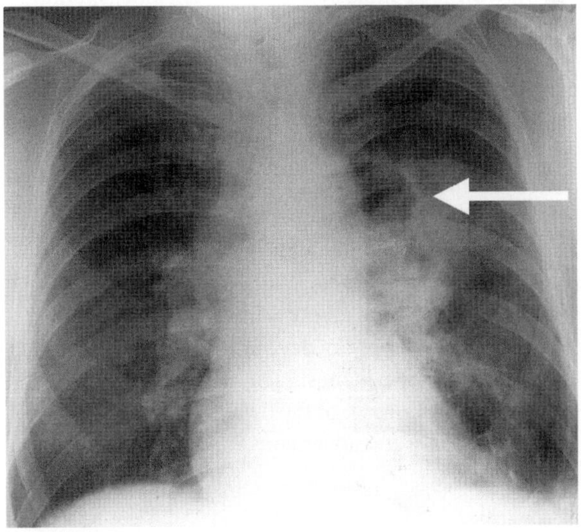

Fig. 18.6. The chest radiograph shows a translucent circle defined by densely opaque margins which are the walls of a lung abscess, associated here with left upper lobe consolidation. (Courtesy of Dr Basil Shepstone, Oxford, UK.)

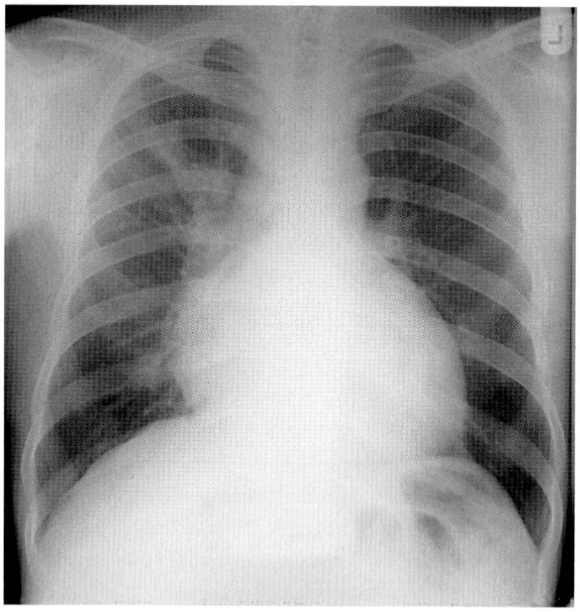

Fig. 18.7. This chest X-ray shows a large globular heart suggestive of pericardial effusion.

Empyema

Infection can spread from the lungs to the pleural space either directly or through rupture of a lung abscess into an inter-lobular septum. The chest radiograph shows a pleural effusion which is often loculated. The diagnosis is made by passing a wide gauge needle into the pleural cavity at the area of the broadest effusion and aspirating pus, often thick and viscid. The microbial aetiology and antimicrobial therapy are similar to that of lung abscess but the most effective part of treatment is pleural drainage. Pass an intercostal tube into the area of the effusion and allow it to drain via an underwater seal. If the pus is viscid and the bore of the drain small, flush the tube with sterile saline. Loculated collections require a series of discrete aspirations without necessarily leaving a drain *in situ.* If the pleural space cannot be drained effectively or if pus is obtained simultaneously from the pleural space and the sputum, implying development of a broncho-pleural fistula, the patient should be referred for surgical pleurodesis and closure of the fistula. Potential causes of treatment failure are tuberculous empyema and pleural malignancy.

Pericarditis

Patients with a severe pneumonia are susceptible to acute bacterial pericarditis by haematogenous spread or direct extension from lung or pleura. The complication is associated, though not exclusively, with *S. pneumoniae* and *S. aureus* pneumonia. The heart sounds are quiet and there may be a pericardial rub. Chest X-ray (Fig. 18.7) shows a large globular heart. Look for the signs of pericardial tamponade, arterial pulsus paradoxus and a grossly elevated JVP; a paradoxical rise in the JVP may be seen on inspiration. If, in addition, there is arterial hypotension the pericardial fluid requires emergency aspiration and later surgical drainage to prevent reaccumulation.

References

Abouya YL, Beaumel A, Lucas S et al. (1992). *Pneumocystis carinii* pneumonia. An uncommon cause of death in African patients with acquired immunodeficiency syndrome. *Am Rev Resp Dis*; **145**: 617–620.

Aderaye G. (1994a). Community acquired pneumonia in adults in Addis Ababa: etiologic agents and the impact of HIV infection. *Tuberc Lung Dis*; **75**: 308–312.

Aderaye G. (1994b). The etiology of community acquired pneumonia in adults in Addis Ababa. *W Afr J Med*; **13**: 142–145.

Allen SC. (1984). Lobar pneumonia in Northern Zambia: clinical study of 502 patients. *Thorax*; **39**: 612–616.

Austrian R, Douglas RM, Schiffman G et al. (1976). Prevention of pneumococcal pneumonia by vaccination. *Trans Assoc Am Phys*; **89**: 184–192.

Batungwanayo J, Taelman H, Lucas S et al. (1994a). Pulmonary disease associated with Human Immunodeficiency virus in Kigali, Rwanda. *Am J Resp Crit Care Med*; **149**: 1591–1596.

Batungwanayo J, Taelman H, Bogaerts J et al. (1994b). Pulmonary cryptococcosis associated with HIV-1 infection in Rwanda: a retrospective study of 37 cases. *AIDS*; **8**: 1271–1276.

British Thoracic Society Research Committee and the Public Health Laboratory Service. (1987). Community-acquired pneumonia in adults in British hospitals in 1982–1983; a survey of aetiology, mortality, prognostic factors and outcome. *Q J Med*; **62**: 195–220.

Daley CL, Mugusi F, Chen LL et al. (1996). Pulmonary complications of HIV infection in Dar es Salaam, Tanzania. Role of bronchoscopy and bronchoalveolar lavage. *Am J Respir Crit Care Med*; **154**: 105–110.

Dowell SF, Anderson LJ, Gary Jr HE et al. (1996). Respiratory Syncytial Virus is an important cause of community-acquired lower respiratory infection among hospitalized adults. *J Infect Dis*; **174**: 456–462.

El-Amin AM. (1978). Bacterial pneumonias in the rural society of Solwezi District of the North-Western Province of Zambia. *Med J Zambia*; **12**: 42–45.

Elvin KM, Lumbwe CM, Luo NP, Bjorkman A, Kallenius G, Linder E. (1989). Pneumocystis carinii is not a major cause of pneumonia in HIV infected patients in Lusaka, Zambia. *Trans Roy Soc Trop Med Hyg*; **83**: 553–555.

Feikin DR, Dowell SF, Nwanyanwu OC et al. (2000). Increased carriage of trimethoprim/sulfamethoxazole-resistant *Streptococcus pneumoniae* in Malawian children after treatment for malaria with sulfadoxine/pyrimethamine. *J Infect Dis*; **181**: 1501–1505.

Foy HM, Cooney MK, McMahan R et al. (1973). Viral and mycoplasmal pneumonia in a prepaid medical group during an 8 year period. *Am J Epidemiol*; **97**: 93.

French N, Nakiyingi J, Carpenter LM et al. (2000). 23-valent pneumococcal polysaccharide vaccine in HIV-1-infected Ugandan adults: double-blind, randomised and placebo controlled trial. *Lancet*; **355**: 2106–2111.

García-Leoni ME, Moreno S, Rodeñó P, Cercenado E, Vicente T, Bouza E. (1992). Pneumococcal pneumonia in adult hospitalized patients infected with the Human Immunodeficiency Virus. *Arch Int Med*; **152**: 1808–1812.

Gilks CF, Ojoo SA, Ojoo JC et al. (1996). Invasive pneumococcal disease in a cohort of predominantly HIV-1 infected female sex-workers in Nairobi, Kenya [see comments]. *Lancet*; **347**: 718–723.

Grant AD, Sidibe K, Domoua K et al. (1998). Spectrum of disease among HIV-infected adults hospitalised in a respiratory medicine unit in Abidjan, Cote d'Ivoire. *Int J Tuberc Lung Dis*; **2**: 926–934.

Gray GC, Mitchell BS, Tueller JE, Cross ER, Amundson DE. (1994). Pneumonia hospitalizations in the US Navy and Marine Corps: rates and risk factors for 6,522 admissions, 1981–1991. *Am J Epidemiol*; **139**: 793–802.

Gray GC, Rodier GR, Matras-Maslin VC et al. (1995). Serologic evidence of respiratory and rickettsial infections among Somali refugees. *Am J Trop Med Hyg*; **52**: 349–353.

Harries AD, Speare R, Wirima JJ. (1988). A profile of respiratory disease in an African medical ward. *J Roy Coll Phys Lond*; **22**: 109–113.

Harries AD, Speare R, Wirima JJ. (1990). Medical admissions to Kamuzu Central Hospital, Lilongwe, Malawi in 1986: comparison with admissions to Queen Elizabeth Central Hospital, Blantyre in 1973. *Trop Geog Med*; **42**: 274–279.

Hausdorff WP, Bryant J, Paradiso PR, Siber GR. (2000). Which pneumococcal serogroups cause the most invasive disease: implications for conjugate vaccine formulation and use, part I. *Clin Infect Dis*; **30**: 100–121.

Kamanfu G, Mlika-Cabanne N, Girard PM et al. (1993). Pulmonary complications of human immunodeficiency virus infection in Bujumbura, Burundi. *Am Rev Respir Dis*; **147**: 658–663.

Karstaedt AS. (1992). AIDS – the Baragwanath experience. Part III. HIV infection in adults at Baragwanath Hospital. *S Afr Med J*; **82**: 95–97.

Koulla-Shiro S, Kuaban C, Belec L. (1996). Acute community-acquired bacterial pneumonia in Human Immunodeficiency Virus (HIV) infected and non-HIV-infected adult patients in Cameroon: aetiology and outcome. *Tuberc Lung Dis*; **77**: 47–51.

Lloyd-Evans N, O'Dempsey TJ, Baldeh I et al. (1996). Nasopharyngeal carriage of pneumococci in Gambian children and in their families. *Pediat Infect Dis J*; **15**: 866–871.

Lucas SB, Hounnou A, Peacock A, Beaumel A, Kadio A, De Cock KM. (1994). Nocardia in HIV-positive patients: an autopsy study in West Africa. *Tuberc Lung Dis*; **75**: 301–307.

Macfarlane JT, Adegboye DS, Warrell MJ. (1979). *Mycoplasma pneumoniae* and aetiology of lobar pneumonia in northern Nigeria. *Thorax*; **34**: 713–719.

Macfarlane JT, Colville A, Guion A, Macfarlane RM, Rose DH. (1993). Prospective study of aetiology and outcome of adult lower-respiratory-tract infections in the community [see comments]. *Lancet*; **341**: 511–514.

Malin A, Gwanzura LKZ, Klein S, Robertson VJ, Musvaire P, Mason PR. (1995). *Pneumocystis carinii* pneumonia in Zimbabwe. *Lancet*; **346**: 1258–1261.

Munoz R, Coffey TJ, Daniels M et al. (1991). Intercontinental spread of a multiresistant clone of serotype 23F *Streptococcus pneumoniae*. *J Infect Dis*; **164**: 302–306.

Murray CJL, Lopez AD. (1996). *Global Health Statistics*. Cambridge: Harvard School of Public Health on behalf of the World Health Organization and the World Bank.

Nuorti JP, Butler JC, Farley MM et al. (2000). Cigarette smoking and invasive pneumococcal disease. Active Bacterial Core Surveillance Team. *N Engl J Med*; **342**: 681–689.

Riley ID, Tarr PI, Andrews M et al. (1977). Immunisation with a polyvalent pneumococcal vaccine. Reduction of adult respiratory mortality in a New Guinea Highlands community. *Lancet*; **1**: 1338–1341.

Rolfe M. (1986). A study of Legionnaire's disease in Zambia. *Ann Trop Med Parasitol*; **80**: 325–328.

Scott JAG, Hall AJ, Hannington A et al. (1998). Serotype distribution and prevalence of resistance to benzylpenicillin in three representative populations of *Streptococcus pneumoniae* isolates from the coast of Kenya. *Clin Infect Dis*; **27**: 1442–1450.

Scott JAG, Hannington A, Marsh K, Hall AJ. (1999). Diagnosis of pneumococcal pneumonia in epidemiological studies: evaluation in Kenyan adults of a serotype-specific urine latex agglutination assay. *Clin Infect Dis*; **28**: 764–769.

Scott JAG, Hall AJ, Muyodi C et al. (2000). Aetiology, outcome, and risk factors for mortality among adults with acute pneumonia in Kenya. *Lancet*; **355**: 1225–1230.

Sofowora EO, Onadeko BO. (1973). Complications and prognostic factors in pneumonia among Nigerians. *Niger Med J*; **3**: 144–145.

Sow O, Frechet M, Diallo AA et al. (1996). Community acquired pneumonia in adults: a study comparing clinical features and outcome in Africa (Republic of Guinea) and Europe (France). *Thorax*; **51**: 385–388.

Steinhart R, Reingold AL, Taylor F et al. (1992). Invasive *Haemophilus influenzae* infection in men with HIV infection. *J Am Med Assoc*; **268**: 3350–3352.

Stout JE, Yu VL. (1997). Legionellosis. *N Engl J Med*; **337**: 682–687.

Tugwell P, Greenwood BM. (1975). Pneumococcal antigen in lobar pneumonia. *J Clin Path*; **28**: 118–123.

Tuomanen EI, Austrian R and Masure HR. (1995). Pathogenesis of pneumococcal infection. *N Engl J Med*; **332**: 1280–1284.
Williams EH, Hayes RJ, Smith PG. (1986). Admissions to a rural hospital in the West Nile District of Uganda over a 27 year period. *J Trop Med Hyg*; **89**: 193–211.
Working groups of the South African Pulmonology Society and the Antibiotic Study Group of South Africa. (1996). Management of community-acquired pneumonia in adults. *S Afr Med J*; **86**: 1152–1163.
Wyndham CH. (1986). Are mortality rates for respiratory diseases in the RSA affected by climate? *S Afr Med J*; **69**: 223–226.

19 Pneumonia and acute respiratory infections in children

Introduction

Minor viral respiratory infections are common in childhood, while pneumonia is the most important cause of serious illness and death in young children globally. It is estimated that pneumonia causes over 2 million deaths in children under 5 years of age each year. In African countries where malaria is an important problem, pneumonia causes a similar number of child deaths (Fig. 19.1). Pneumonia is generally a more common cause of death in those countries that have the highest infant mortality rates. Lack of basic medical care is behind most pneumonia deaths. This remains a problem in many African countries. Untreated, the case-fatality rate is particularly high in the first 6 months of life.

In general wheezing disorders are less common in African countries than in developed parts of the world. Where it has been studied, acute bronchiolitis, usually due to respiratory syncytial virus (RSV), is an important cause of severe respiratory infections in young infants, but asthma remains uncommon, except in the urban areas. Viral laryngotracheobronchitis ('croup') is uncommon in African countries, so an acute presentation with upper airways obstruction should prompt a search for more serious conditions such as abscess, foreign body or diphtheria in an unvaccinated child.

This section focuses on the most important causes of acute cough (pneumonia and the common cold). For details about asthma, see Chapter 71, for bronchiolitis, see Chapter 59 (RSV), and for chronic cough, see Chapter 17 (tuberculosis) (Fig. 19.2).

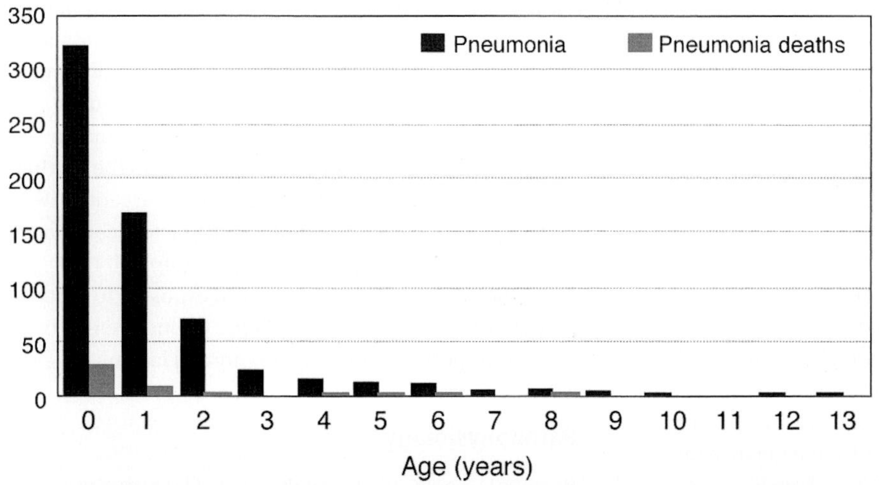

Fig. 19.1. Age distribution of admissions and deaths with ARI to the Royal Victoria Hospital, Banjul during 1995.

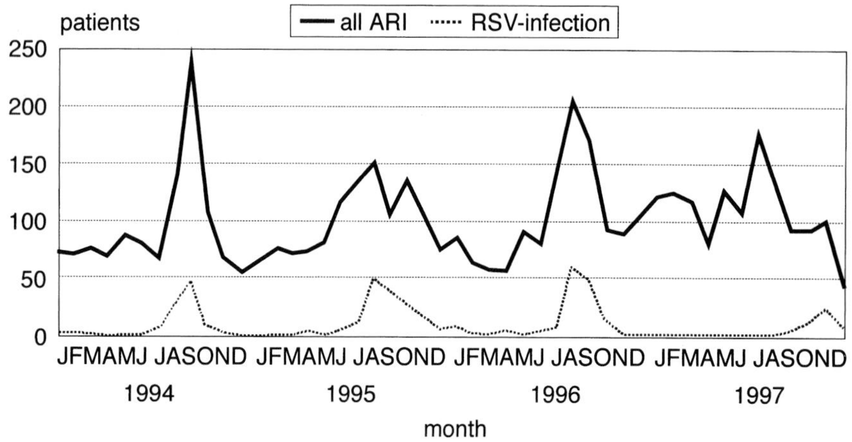

Fig. 19.2. Admissions with acute respiratory infection to three hospitals in the Western region of the Gambia over a period of 4 years, 1994–1997. Note the seasonality of admissions which coincides with the rainy season and in the first 3 years with RSV epidemics.

Pneumonia

Aetiology

Research studies using lung aspiration and blood culture have demonstrated the importance of bacteria in the aetiology of pneumonia in African children. The main causes in children 2 months to 5 years of age are *Streptococcus pneumoniae* (pneumococcus), and *Haemophilus influenzae* (mainly type b but non-serotypable strains have been shown to be important in some Asian studies) (Adegbola et al., 1994).

In addition, some studies have identified a role for *Salmonella* spp. in causing a pneumonia-like illness (O'Dempsey et al., 1994). Pneumonia in neonates and young infants under 2 months of age is associated with a wider range of bacterial agents including *Streptococci* Group A, *Staphylococcus aureus* and gram-negative bacteria such as *E. coli* and *Klebsiella* (WHO Young Infants Study Group, 1999). The most important viral cause of severe lower respiratory tract infection is respiratory syncytial virus (RSV) (Weber et al., 1998).

Prevention and control

Protein conjugate vaccines against *H. influenzae* type b (Hib) have been available for children in developed countries for several years, and have virtually eliminated Hib disease. The vaccine is not available in many African countries because it is still too expensive, but recently vaccine prices have fallen and the Global Alliance for Vaccines and Immunization (GAVI) has made funds available for purchase of Hib vaccines in several poor African countries. Conjugate *S. pneumoniae* vaccines covering 9–11 of the most important pneumococcal serotypes are likely to reduce ARI mortality in developing countries even more effectively than Hib vaccine. A 7-valent pneumococcal conjugate vaccine is now licensed in the USA and other developed countries. Nine and 11-valent vaccines, covering serotypes that are more important in developing countries, are under evaluation in several developing countries including the Gambia. The role of the unconjugated 23-valent polysaccharide *S. pneumoniae* vaccine (an inexpensive vaccine that has been available for 20 years) has not been fully evaluated and it may still have an important role in developing countries.

Some important risk factors have been identified for pneumonia in African children. Malnutrition is a major risk factor, and, in settings where effective treatment is available, a substantial burden of the severe pneumonia is in malnourished children. A number of studies have identified exposure to indoor air pollution, specifically smoke from biomass fuel such as wood or charcoal used for cooking, as a risk factor for childhood pneumonia. In Africa two studies identified being carried on the mother's back while cooking as a risk factor, but these cannot be considered conclusive as confounding factors could have explained the findings (Armstrong & Campbell, 1991). Nevertheless, it is likely that reduced exposure to indoor air pollution will reduce a child's risk of pneumonia, but data to support and quantify this are still lacking.

Pathophysiology

Bacterial pneumonia is usually caused by organisms found in the upper respiratory tract. These organisms

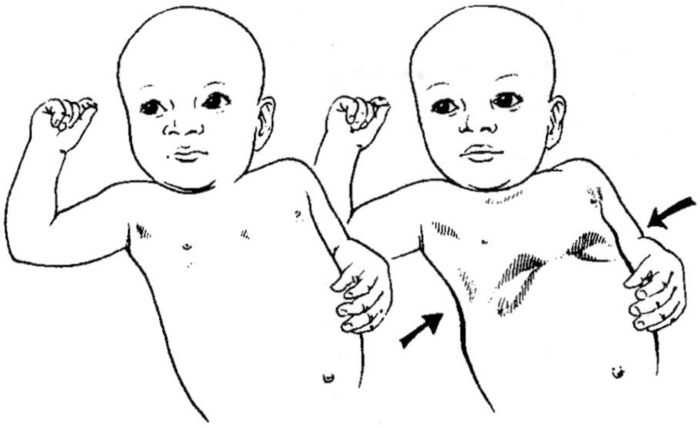

Fig. 19.3. Lower chest wall indrawing, a sign of severe pneumonia indicating the need for treatment with injectable antibiotics according to the IMCI guidelines. During inspiration, the lower, bony part of the chest wall moves in.

could spread to the lung tissue directly via the airways or via the blood stream following an episode of bacteraemia. Inflammatory exudate then fills the alveoli in the affected area of lung inhibiting oxygen transfer and producing the pathological consequences of pneumonia. This may be localized to a single lobe or segment of the lung, or may be widespread and diffuse. A combination of inflammatory fluid in the alveoli and a mismatch between ventilation and perfusion in the lungs can interfere with the transfer of oxygen into the blood and cause hypoxia. The infection and inflammation in the alveoli (pneumonia) and small airways (bronchiolitis) leads to decreased compliance (increased stiffness) of the lungs leading to an increase in the respiratory rate and lower chest wall indrawing. These are the two clinical signs that are most useful for the diagnosis and evaluation of pneumonia at the primary care level.

Clinical presentation

Children with pneumonia typically present with a short history of 2–3 days cough or difficulty breathing. Fever is often present but, in general, it is a poor guide to the presence of pneumonia. In some cultures mothers identify chest pain as an important symptom. The clinical presentation in most cases is with fast breathing and/or lower chest wall indrawing (Fig 19.3).

The IMCI approach to acute respiratory infections (Table 19.1)

In the context of the IMCI clinical algorithm (see Chapter 9), the entry criterion for the assessment of children for

Table 19.1. Differential diagnosis of the child presenting with cough or difficult breathing without wheeze, stridor or chronic cough

Diagnosis	In favour
Pneumonia	• Cough with fast breathing • Lower chest wall indrawing • Fever • Crackles on auscultation • Nasal flaring • Grunting • Head nodding
Malaria	• Fast breathing in febrile child • Blood smear: high parasitaemia • Lives in or travelled to a malarious area • In severe malaria: deep (acidotic) breathing/lower chest wall indrawing • Chest clear on auscultation
Severe anaemia	• Severe palmar pallor • Haemoglobin <6 g/dl
Congenital heart disease or **cardiac failure**	• Cyanosis • Difficulty in feeding or breast-feeding • Gallop rhythm • Raised jugular venous pressure • Basal fine crackles • Apex beat displaced • Enlarged palpable liver • Heart murmur
Tuberculosis	• Chronic cough (more than 30 days) • Poor growth/wasting or weight loss • Positive contact history with tuberculosis patient • Diagnostic chest X-ray such as primary complex or miliary tuberculosis
Pertussis	• Paroxysms of cough followed by whoop, vomiting, cyanosis or apnoea • No fever • No history of DPT immunization
Foreign body	• History of sudden choking • Sudden onset of stridor or respiratory distress • Focal areas of wheeze or reduced breath sounds
Empyema	• Stony dullness to percussion
Pneumothorax	• Sudden onset • Hyper-resonance on percussion on one side of the chest • Shift in mediastinum
Pneumocystis pneumonia	• 2–6-month-old child with central cyanosis • Hyper-expanded chest • Fast breathing • Finger clubbing • Chest X-ray changes, but chest clear on auscultation • Enlarged liver, spleen, lymph nodes • Wasting

Table 19.2. WHO classification of the severity of pneumonia

Sign or symptom	Classification	Treatment
• Central cyanosis • Severe respiratory distress • Not able to drink	**Very severe pneumonia**	– Admit to hospital – Give chloramphenicol – Give oxygen – Manage the airway – Treat high fever if present
• Chest indrawing	**Severe pneumonia**	– Admit to hospital – Give benzylpenicillin – Manage the airway – Treat high fever if present
• Fast breathing ≥60 breaths/minute in a child aged <2 months; ≥50 breaths/ minute in a child aged 2–12 months; ≥40 breaths/ minute in a child aged from 12 months to 5 years. • Definite crackles on auscultation	**Pneumonia**	– Home care – Give appropriate oral antibiotic for 5 days – Soothe the throat and relieve cough with a safe remedy – Advise the mother when to return immediately – Follow up in 2 days
• No signs of pneumonia, or severe or very severe pneumonia	**No pneumonia: cough or cold**	– Home care – Soothe the throat and relieve cough with safe remedy – Advise the mother when to return – Follow up in 5 days if not improving – If coughing for more than 30 days, follow chronic cough instructions in Chapter 77

pneumonia is a complaint of 'cough or difficulty in breathing'. The algorithm uses three clinical signs to assess a sick child with cough or difficulty breathing: ***elevated respiratory rate, lower chest wall indrawing***, and ***stridor***. The child is then classified into three main categories:

- severe pneumonia or very severe disease
- pneumonia or
- cough and cold.

Fast breathing detects a higher proportion of pneumonia cases in young children than auscultatory signs such as reduced air entry, bronchial breathing or coarse crepitations, but where skilled auscultation is available those signs add valuable diagnostic information (Mulholland et al., 1992). Cut-off rates for the diagnosis of fast breathing have been set to balance the need to detect most cases of pneumonia (high sensitivity) against the need not to label too many children with minor respiratory infections as having pneumonia (high specificity or low false positive rate). Since normal respiratory rate falls with age, the cut-off points for respiratory rate vary with age (60 or more for young infants under 2 months; 50 or more in children 2 months to 1 year; 40 or more in children 12 months up to 5 years, Table 19.2). WHO guidelines suggest that children with severe pneumonia (with chest wall indrawing or signs of hypoxia) should be admitted to hospital (WHO programme for the control of acute respiratory infections 1990). Where possible, children with severe pneumonia should have a chest radiograph performed to identify complications or signs of staphylococcal pneumonia (Figs 19.4, 19.5, 19.6; Tables 19.3, 19.4, 19.5).

Hypoxia is best identified by use of a pulse oximeter (which measures reduced oxygen saturation) (Fig. 19.7) but can also be recognized clinically by signs such as central cyanosis, respiratory distress causing inability to drink, severe lower chest wall indrawing; very fast breathing (70 per minute or more), grunting with every breath or head nodding (caused by the use of accessory muscles in an infant) (Usen et al., 1999).

Malnourished children may not exhibit the same clinical signs as well-nourished children (Falade et al., 1995). When managing malnourished children, it is important to have a lower threshold for diagnosis and treatment of pneumonia. The aetiology of pneumonia is likely to be the same as for well-nourished children so the same antibiotics are likely to be effective. However absorption of oral agents may be poor in malnourished children (Adegbola et al., 1994).

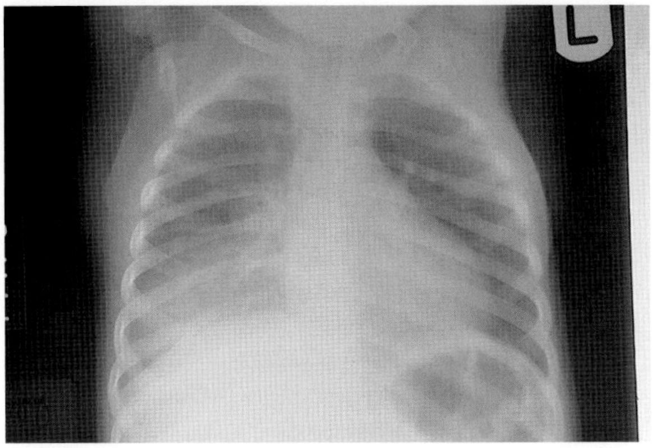

Fig. 19.4. Lobar pneumonia: the chest radiograph shows consolidation of the right middle and lower lobe.

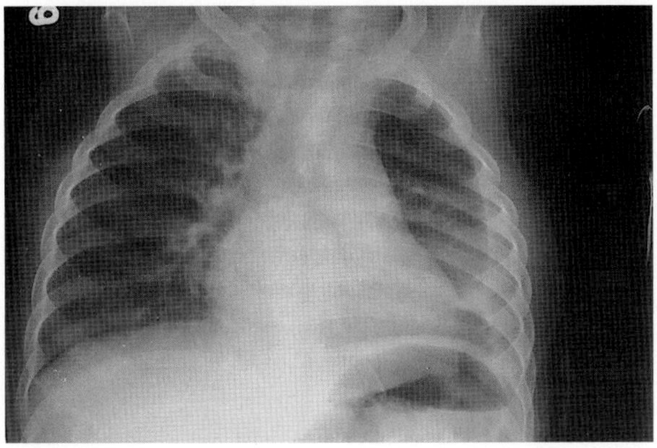

Fig. 19.5. Pleural effusion left side of thorax. The effusion extends along the pleural cleft upwards. On aspiration *Haemophilus influenzae* was grown from the fluid.

Management

Management of pneumonia involves both effective anti-microbial therapy and supportive therapy, particularly oxygen and fluids.

Anti-microbial treatment

Management of pneumonia is usually empirical as the aetiological agent is usually not known. Most cases of pneumonia in children older than 2 months of age can be treated at home with simple, inexpensive oral antibiotics such as co-trimoxazole or amoxicillin. (Campbell et al., 1988). Penicillin V (phenoxymethyl penicillin) does not have good activity against *Haemophilus influenzae* type b, and so is not recommended. Children with severe pneumonia, or malnourished children with pneumonia have a

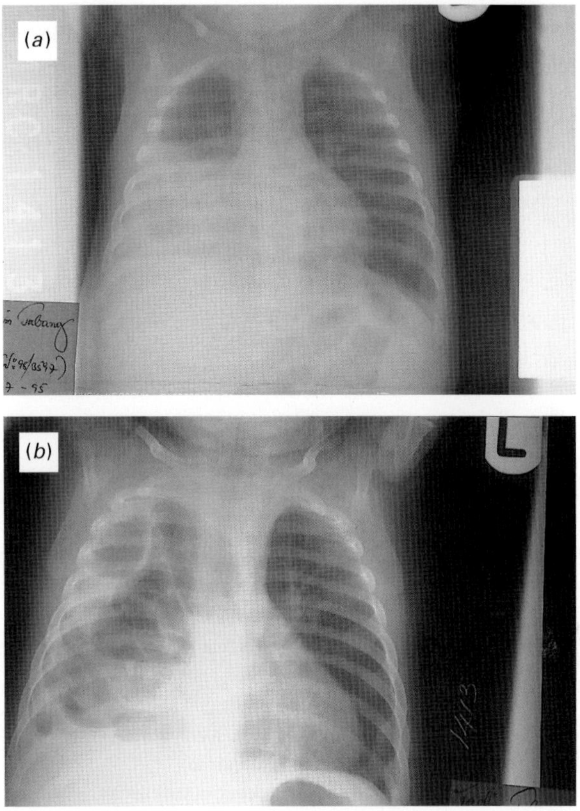

Fig. 19.6. Staphylococcal pneumonia: (*a*) consolidation of the right lower lobe. Lung aspiration was performed and yielded *Staphylococcus aureus*. (*b*) same child 5 days later: multiple pneumatocoeles and some air fluid levels indicating abscesses with connection to the bronchial system can be seen.

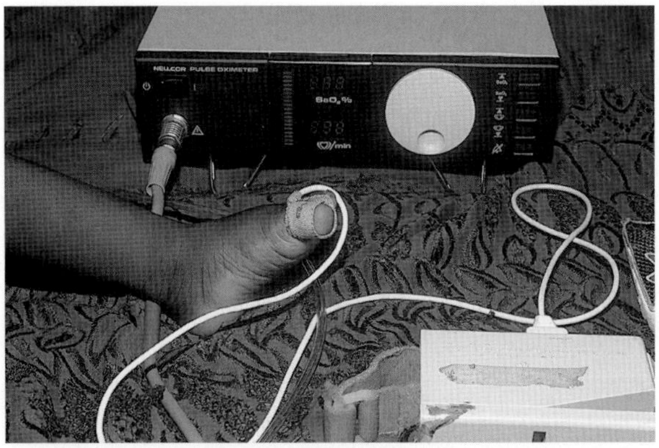

Fig. 19.7. Pulse oximeter. A pulse oximeter determines the proportion of oxygen-saturated haemoglobin in the arterial blood by measuring the absorption of a red light beam, which is transmitted from a probe through the tissue of a finger or a toe. The picture shows a paediatric probe fixed to the toe of an infant, and the machine which displays the saturation and the heart rate. A saturation of <90% is considered to indicate severe hypoxaemia.

Table 19.3. Differential diagnosis of the child presenting with wheeze

Diagnosis	In favour
Asthma	• History of recurrent wheeze, some unrelated to coughs and colds • Hyperinflation of the chest • Prolonged expiration • Reduced air entry (if very severe, airway obstruction) • Good response to bronchodilators
Bronchiolitis	• First episode of wheeze in a child aged <2 years • Wheeze episode at time of seasonal bronchiolitis peak • Hyperinflation of the chest • Prolonged expiration • Reduced air entry (if very severe, airway obstruction) • Poor/no response to bronchodilators
Wheeze associated with cough or cold	• Wheeze always related to coughs and colds • No family or personal history of asthma/eczema/hay fever • Prolonged expiration • Reduced air entry (if very severe, airways obstruction) • Good response to bronchodilators • Tends to be less severe than wheeze associated with asthma
Foreign body	• History of sudden onset of choking or wheezing • Wheeze may be unilateral • Air trapping with hyper-resonance and mediastinal shift • Signs of lung collapse: reduced air entry and impaired percussion note • No response to bronchodilators
Pneumonia	• Cough with fast breathing • Lower chest wall indrawing • Fever • Coarse crackles • Nasal flaring • Grunting

poorer prognosis and so should be admitted to hospital for treatment with parenteral antibiotics. Benzyl penicillin is the first-line treatment as it is effective against the two major bacterial pathogens. Chloramphenicol should be restricted to the few children with very severe pneumonia since this limits the development of drug resistance and its use is sometimes associated with rare but serious adverse effects (Shann et al., 1985). It is active against a wider range of bacterial pathogens including gram-negative organisms. A second-line treatment would be benzyl penicillin or ampicillin plus gentamicin which provide a broader spectrum. In cases not responding to antibiotics a chest radiograph should be taken and antibiotics changed to a regimen that includes effective anti-staphylococcal treatment (see below).

Table 19.4. Differential diagnosis of the child presenting with stridor

Diagnosis	In favour
Viral croup	• Barking cough • Respiratory distress • Hoarse voice • If due to measles, signs of measles (Chapter 56)
Diphtheria	• Bull neck appearance due to enlarged cervical nodes and oedema • Red throat • Grey pharyngeal membrane • Blood-stained nasal discharge • No evidence of vaccination
Foreign body	• Sudden history of choking • Respiratory distress
Congenital anomaly	• Stridor present since birth

Pneumonia in young infants under 2 months of age is associated with a much higher case-fatality rate so all cases should be admitted to hospital for parenteral treatment. In addition, since the range of bacterial agents causing pneumonia is much wider, the first-line treatment is benzyl penicillin and gentamicin (see section on neonatal sepsis).

The classification of severity and the recommended anti-microbial therapy based on the severity is shown in Table 19.2.

Oxygen therapy

Children with hypoxia have a higher mortality and should be given oxygen therapy to bring their arterial oxygen saturation into the normal range. Two methods of oxygen delivery have been recommended by WHO; purpose-built paediatric nasal prongs; and a paediatric feeding tube used as a nasopharyngeal or nasal catheter (WHO, 2000) (Fig. 19.8).

The nasopharyngeal catheter has been associated with acute complications such as acute gastric distension and

Table 19.5. Differential diagnosis of the child presenting with chronic cough

Diagnosis	In favour
Tuberculosis	• Weight loss • Anorexia, night sweats • Enlarged liver and spleen • Chronic or intermittent fever • History of exposure to infectious tuberculosis • Signs of fluid in chest (dull to percussion/reduced breath sounds)
Asthma	• History of recurrent wheeze, some unrelated to coughs and colds • Hyperinflation of the chest • Prolonged expiration • Reduced air entry (in very severe airway obstruction) • Good response to bronchodilators
Foreign body	• Sudden onset of choking • Respiratory distress
Pertussis	• Paroxysms of cough followed by whoop, vomiting, cyanosis or apnoea • Subconjunctival haemorrhages • No history of DPT immunization • Apnoeic episodes in infants
HIV	• Known or suspected maternal or sibling HIV infection • History of blood transfusion • Failure to thrive • Oral thrush • Chronic parotitis • Skin infection with herpes zoster (past or present) • Generalized lymphadenopathy • Chronic fever • Persistent diarrhoea
Bronchiectasis	• History of tuberculosis or aspirated foreign body • Poor weight gain • Purulent sputum, bad breath • Finger clubbing
Lung abscess	• Reduced breath sounds over abscess • Poor weight gain/chronically ill child • Typical chest X-ray appearance

acute upper airways obstruction. Trials have shown that with these delivery methods low oxygen flow (0.5–1 litres per minute) is effective in treating hypoxia and that nasal prongs and the nasal catheter perform as well as the nasopharyngeal catheter without the risk of side effects.

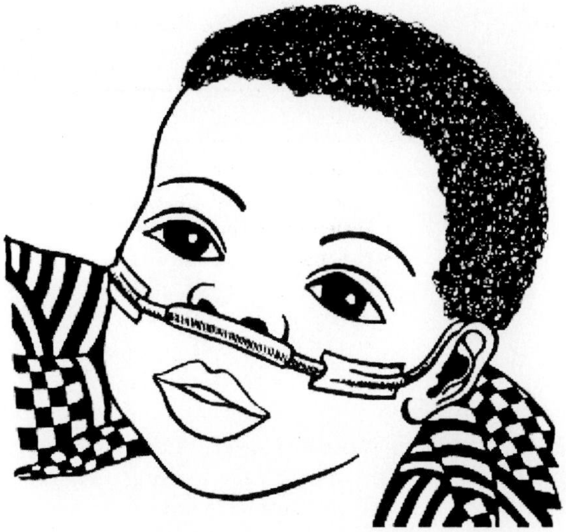

Fig. 19.8. Child with nasal prongs for oxygen delivery.

(Weber et al., 1995) Facemasks are inefficient and not tolerated well by children, while head boxes can be dangerous and require large flows of oxygen. These methods are not recommended. The two main sources of oxygen are cylinders and oxygen concentrators. It is important that all equipment is checked for compatibility and properly maintained, and that staff are instructed in its correct use (Fig. 19.9).

Oxygen therapy should be restricted to children with signs of hypoxia (see above), but, if readily available, oxygen may be given to any child with severe lower chest wall indrawing or a respiratory rate of ≥70/minute.

The management of pneumonia in children with HIV infection follows the same principles. *Streptococcus pneumoniae* is the commonest cause of pneumonia in these children and responds well to the antibiotics described above. However, in countries where the prevalence of HIV infection is very high, infants in the first 6 months of life who present with signs of hypoxia are commonly found to have *Pneumocystis carinii* pneumonia (PCP) and require treatment with high dose cotrimoxazole and prolonged oxygen therapy.

Other supportive therapy

If the child has fever (≥39 °C) which appears to be causing distress, paracetamol may be given. If present, wheeze should be treated with a bronchodilator. Removal by gentle suction of any thick secretions in the throat, which the child cannot clear, will help the child. As with all sick children it is important to pay attention to

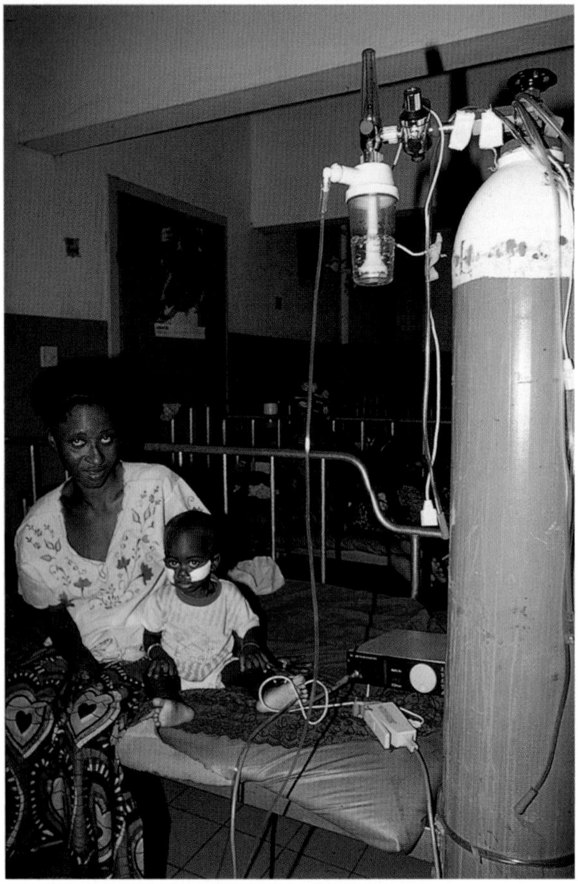

Fig. 19.9. A child with severe pneumonia receives oxygen from an oxygen cylinder. The oxygen passes though a flow meter which makes it possible to adjust the flow, a humidifier, and is delivered to the child by nasal prongs.

fluids and nutrition in children with pneumonia. Frequent breast-feeding, a suitable diet and free oral fluids should be encouraged. If a child is not drinking, a nasogastric tube may be required, but this should be used with great care to avoid airways obstruction. If a nasogastric tube and a nasopharyngeal oxygen catheter are used together they should both be passed through the same nostril.

Monitoring

The child should be checked by nurses at least every 3 hours and by a doctor at least twice a day. In the absence of complications, within two days there should be signs of improvement (breathing not so fast, less indrawing of the lower chest wall, less fever, and improved ability to eat and drink).

Complications

If the child has not improved after two days, or if the child's condition has worsened, look for complications or other diagnoses. If possible, obtain a chest X-ray. The most common complications are given below.

Staphylococcal pneumonia

This is suggested by rapid clinical deterioration despite treatment, by a pneumatocoele or pneumothorax with effusion on chest X-ray (see Fig 19.5 and 19.6), numerous gram-positive cocci in a smear of sputum, or heavy growth of *S. aureus* in cultured sputum or empyema fluid. The presence of septic skin pustules supports the diagnosis. Treat with cloxacillin (50 mg/kg i.m. or i.v. every 6 hours) and gentamicin (7.5 mg/kg i.m. or i.v. once a day). When the child improves, continue cloxacillin orally four times a day for a total course of 3 weeks. Note that cloxacillin can be substituted by another anti-staphylococcal antibiotic such as oxacillin, flucloxacillin, or dicloxacillin.

Empyema

This is suggested by persistent fever, and physical and chest X-ray signs of pleural effusion (see Fig. 19.10). On examination, the chest is dull to percussion and breath sounds are reduced or absent over the affected area. A pleural rub may be heard at an early stage before the effusion is fully developed. A chest X-ray shows fluid on one or both sides of the chest. When empyema is present, fever persists despite antibiotic therapy and the pleural fluid is cloudy or frankly purulent. Where possible, pleural fluid should be analysed for protein and glucose content, cell count and differential count, and examined after gram and Ziehl–Neelsen staining, and bacterial and *Mycobacterium tuberculosis* culture (Fig. 19.10).

Pleural effusions should be drained, unless they are very small. If effusions are present on both sides of the chest, drain both. It may be necessary to repeat drainage 2–3 times if fluid returns. Subsequent management depends on the character of the fluid obtained. Antimicrobial therapy may be with chloramphenicol, but if evidence of staphylococcal infection is present, treatment should be for staphylococcal pneumonia.

Tuberculosis

A child with persistent fever for more than 14 days and signs of pneumonia should be evaluated for tuberculosis. If another cause of the fever cannot be found, a trial of anti-tuberculosis treatment, following national guidelines, may be required (Chapter 17).

Minor acute respiratory infections

These infections ranging from common colds to bronchitis are very common and usually viral in origin. Children present with cough or difficulty breathing that is not associated with signs of pneumonia (see above). Nasal discharge that can vary from clear to purulent is common. Fever may be present. There is no curative treatment. In particular there is no evidence that antibiotics reduce the duration of symptoms, the severity of symptoms or prevent complications such as otitis media or pneumonia from occurring. A purulent nasal discharge does not imply bacterial infection and does not indicate the need for antibiotic treatment. Treatment of high fever may be helpful. The majority of cough and cold remedies are ineffective in young children and some may be harmful or expensive. The treatment of the common cold with antibiotics is an important example of the over-use of antibiotics which drives the development of drug resistance in populations. In the individual child unnecessary use of antibiotics for the common cold may increase the risk of more severe forms of pneumonia (such as staphylococcal pneumonia) or pneumonia with drug resistant bacteria. Complications include otitis media, poor feeding and pneumonia and these should be treated appropriately.

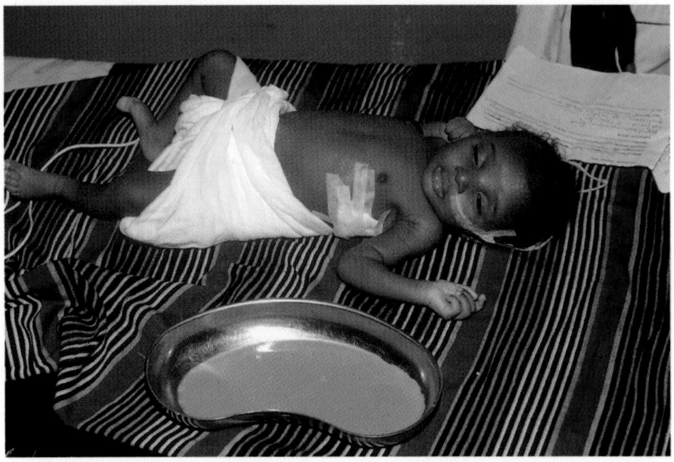

Fig. 19.10. A 1-month-old child with pneumonia and empyema on the left side after aspiration of 70 ml of pus (in kidney dish). The culture of the pus grew *Staphylococcus aureus*. The child receives oxygen by nasopharyngeal catheter.

References

Adegbola RA, Falade AG, Sam BE et al. (1994). The etiology of pneumonia in malnourished and well-nourished Gambian children. *Pediat Infect Dis J*; **13**: 975–982.

Armstrong JR, Campbell H. (1991). Indoor air pollution exposure and lower respiratory infections in young Gambian children. *Int J Epidemiol*; **20**: 424–429.

Campbell H, Byass P, Forgie IM et al. (1988). Trial of co-trimoxazole versus procaine penicillin with ampicillin in treatment of community-acquired pneumonia in young Gambian children. *Lancet*; **ii**: 1182–1184.

Falade AG, Tschappeler H, Greenwood BM, Mulholland EK. (1995). Use of simple clinical signs to predict pneumonia in young Gambian children: the influence of malnutrition. *Bull Wld Hlth Org*; **73**: 299–304.

Mulholland EK, Simoes EA, Costales MO et al. (1992). Standardized diagnosis of pneumonia in developing countries. *Pediat Infect Dis J*; **11**: 77–81.

O'Dempsey TJ, McArdle TF, Lloyd-Evans N et al. (1994). Importance of enteric bacteria as a cause of pneumonia, meningitis and septicemia among children in a rural community in The Gambia, West Africa. *Pediat Infect Dis J*; **13**: 122–128.

Shann F, Barker J, Poore P. (1985). Chloramphenicol alone versus chloramphenicol plus penicillin for severe pneumonia in children. *Lancet*; **ii**: 684–686.

The WHO Young Infants Study Group. (1999). Bacterial etiology of serious infections in young infants in developing countries: results of a multicenter study. *Pediat Infect Dis. J*; **18**: S17–S22.

Usen S, Weber M, Mulholland K et al. (1999). Clinical predictors of hypoxaemia in Gambian children with acute lower respiratory tract infection: prospective cohort study. *Br Med J*; **318**: 86–91.

Weber MW, Palmer A, Oparaugo A, Mulholland EK. (1995). Comparison of nasal prongs and nasopharyngeal catheter for the delivery of oxygen in children with hypoxemia because of a lower respiratory tract infection. *J Pediat*; **127**: 378–383.

Weber MW, Mulholland EK, Greenwood BM. (1998). Respiratory syncytial virus infection in tropical and developing countries. *Trop Med Int Hlth*; **3**: 268–280.

WHO. (2000). Management of the child with a serious infection or severe malnutrition. Geneva: World Health Organization.

WHO programme for the control of acute respiratory infections. (1990). Acute respiratory infections in children: case management in small hospitals in developing countries. WHO/ARI/90.5, Geneva.

20 Diarrhoea

Definitions

Diarrhoea (WHO, 1995) is the passage of loose or watery stools at least three times in 24 hours. In *acute diarrhoea* the illness lasts less than 14 days and the stools do not contain visible blood. *Dysentery* is diarrhoea with visible blood in the stool. *Persistent diarrhoea* is diarrhoea that begins acutely and lasts at least 14 days. These conditions differ with regard to pathogenesis, treatment and risk of death.

The problem in Africa

In Africa, children below age 3 years experience 3–10 episodes of diarrhoea each year and may spend 10–15 per cent of their days with diarrhoea (Bern et al., 1992). World-wide, about 1.5 million children below age 3 years die each year from diarrhoea. Acute diarrhoea causes about 80 per cent of diarrhoea episodes and 50 per cent of deaths. Dysentery causes about 10 per cent of diarrhoea episodes and 15 per cent of deaths whilst persistent diarrhoea causes about 10 per cent of episodes and 35 per cent of deaths.

The incidence of diarrhoea may vary markedly with season; outbreaks of acute diarrhoea due to rotavirus infection, in particular, tend to occur in well-defined epidemics (Fig. 20.1).

Diarrhoea is also common in African adults. Cholera epidemics have occurred in many countries in recent years, and outbreaks of bacillary dysentery, often resistant to multiple antibiotics, have caused many deaths.

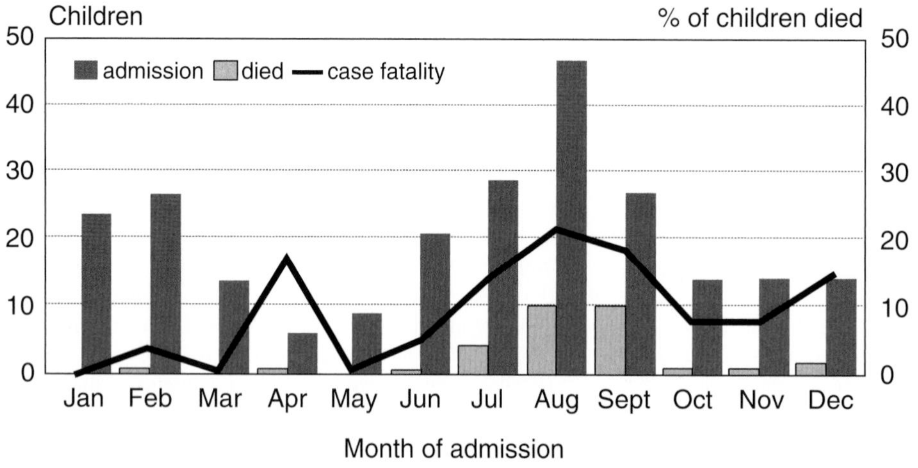

Fig. 20.1. Seasonality of diarrhoeal admissions to the Royal Victoria Hospital, Banjul, The Gambia, 1995. The first peak in January and February is predominantly caused by rotavirus, and has a low case-fatality. The second peak coincides with the rainy season, is associated with malnutrition, and has a higher case-fatality.

Table 20.1. Main organisms causing acute diarrhoea in Africa

Viruses	Rotavirus
Bacteria	Enterotoxigenic *E. coli*
	Enteropathogenic *E. coli*
	Enteroinvasive *E. coli*[a]
	Campylobacter jejuni[a]
	Shigella[a]
	Salmonella
	Vibrio cholerae
Protozoa	*Cryptosporidium*
	Giardia

Notes:
[a] Also causes dysentery.

Control and prevention

There are a number of options to decrease the burden of diarrhoea in Africa, some more feasible than others (Feachem et al., 1983). Promoting exclusive breast-feeding for the first 6 months of life and improved weaning practices are highly effective. Improving water supply and sanitation, and promoting personal and domestic hygiene have a beneficial effect in the prevention of diarrhoea.

Vaccination against measles prevents measles-associated diarrhoea. A vaccine against rotavirus was effective in the prevention of diarrhoea episodes, but was unfortunately associated with an increased incidence of intussusception, which led to its withdrawal.

Control of diarrhoeal disease in hospitals also depends on the provision of safe drinking water, appropriate sanitation and surface water drainage from the ward, and adequate access to water for handwashing by staff and patients. All hospital staff should wash their hands between each patient contact on the ward or in the out-patient clinic, and a sink or bowl with water, soap and a towel is a simple minimum requirement in all clinical areas. Patients admitted with infectious diarrhoea are best isolated in a separate ward or bay whenever possible.

ACUTE DIARRHOEA

Aetiology

Most episodes of acute diarrhoea are caused by intestinal infection; the most common causes are shown in Table 20.1.

Table 20.2. Electrolyte content of stool and several rehydration solutions (average electrolyte content, mmol/l)

	Na^+	K^+	Cl^-	HCO_3^-
Cholera stool	101	27	92	32
Non-cholera stool	56	25	55	14
ORS solution[a]	90	20	80	30
Ringer's lactate	130	4	109	28[b]
Normal saline	154	0	154	0

Notes:
[a] Also contains glucose, 111 mmol/l.
[b] Lactate is converted to HCO_3^-.

Pathophysiology

Several mechanisms contribute to the diarrhoea caused by enteric bacterial infections. These include:

- the ability to produce secretory and other kinds of **exotoxins**
- the ability to **adhere** to and colonize the mucosa using surface adhesins, and to manipulate the mucosal cell morphology
- the ability to **damage** intestinal epithelial cells and cause inflammation.

Escherichia coli has provided a good model for understanding the importance of these mechanisms in producing disease, because different strains of *E. coli* demonstrate different pathogenic mechanisms, which may be coded for in chromosomal, plasmid or bacteriophage DNA.

The term 'exotoxin' is used to describe bacterial toxins, which are proteins, which are released extracellularly, and which cause pathogenic effects in the host. Many of these exotoxins share a common overall structure, with a binding 'B' subunit or domain, and an enzymatic 'A' portion which is responsible for the toxic effect on the host cell. The toxins produced by different bacteria may be closely structurally related. For example, there is considerable homology between cholera toxin and the *E. coli* (ETEC) heat labile toxin, and between the cytotoxins secreted by enterohaemorrhagic *E. coli* (EHEC) and *Shigella dysenteriae* (the Shiga toxin).

Secretory diarrhoea caused, for example, by the heat-labile adenylate cyclase toxin of ETEC or *V. cholerae*, causes secretion of water and electrolytes (sodium, potassium, chloride, and bicarbonate) from the small intestine (Table 20.2). The loss of water and electrolytes causes isotonic dehydration with reduced blood volume, potassium

Table 20.3. Classification of dehydration in children with diarrhoea

Classification	Signs or symptoms	Treatment
Severe dehydration	*Two* or more of the following signs: – lethargy / unconsciousness – sunken eyes – unable to drink or drinks poorly – skin pinch goes back *very* slowly (≥2 seconds)	• Give fluid for severe dehydration (see Treatment Plan C in hospital, Box p. 378)
Some dehydration	*Two* or more of the following signs: – restlessness, irritability – sunken eyes – drinks eagerly, thirsty – skin pinch goes back slowly	• Give fluid and food for some dehydration (see Treatment Plan B, Box p. 377) • Advise mother on home treatment and when to return immediately • Follow up in 5 days if not improving.
No dehydration	Not enough signs to classify as some or severe dehydration	• Give fluid and food to treat diarrhoea at home (see Treatment Plan A, Box p. 377) • Advise mother on when to return immediately • Follow up in 5 days if not improving.

depletion, and base-deficit acidosis. Dysentery, caused by the Shiga-like toxin of EHEC or *S. dysenteriae*, results from damage to the epithelial cells of the large intestine, although it may also be accompanied by increased secretion of fluids and electrolytes.

Clinical features

The IMCI approach to the management of diarrhoea, outlined in Chapter 9, is based on the recognition and treatment of three conditions:

- dehydration
- dysentery
- persistent diarrhoea.

History

The history should establish when the diarrhoea started, and whether it contains blood. It is important also to enquire about vomiting, since if this is frequent, oral rehydration may be difficult. Assess the patient's nutritional state by examination and weighing or, in the case of children, inspection of the 'road to health' card, since failure to thrive, or wasting, suggests chronic diarrhoea with malabsorption, or an underlying illness such as HIV infection or tuberculosis. Enquire about previous treatment; remember that antibiotics frequently cause diarrhoea.

Assessment of dehydration

Rehydration is the mainstay of treatment for acute diarrhoea. The choice of rehydration strategy is guided by a clinical assessment of the severity of dehydration, which is classified into three categories (see Table 20.3).

A fluid deficit equal to 5 per cent of body weight (50 ml/kg) causes few physical signs or symptoms, other than thirst. When losses equal 7–8 per cent of body weight (70–80 ml/kg), thirst increases, infants become restless and irritable, eyes become sunken and skin turgor is diminished. When losses approach 10 per cent of body weight (100 ml/kg) dehydration is severe, blood volume is reduced and hypovolaemic shock develops. Signs and symptoms include lethargy or coma, very poor skin turgor, and inability to drink normally. Death from cardiovascular collapse occurs if the deficit of water and electrolytes is not replaced rapidly.

Assessment of dehydration is based on four signs (Table 20.3):

- conscious level
- skin turgor
- sunken eyes and
- ability to drink.

Standard procedures have been developed to assess skin turgor (see Fig. 20.2). Interpretation of this sign may be complicated by malnutrition (which causes reduced skin turgor), obesity, or oedema (which may mask signs in dehydrated children). Sunken eyes in a dehydrated child are illustrated in Fig. 20.3. In a severely malnourished child the eyes may always look sunken, even if the child is not dehydrated.

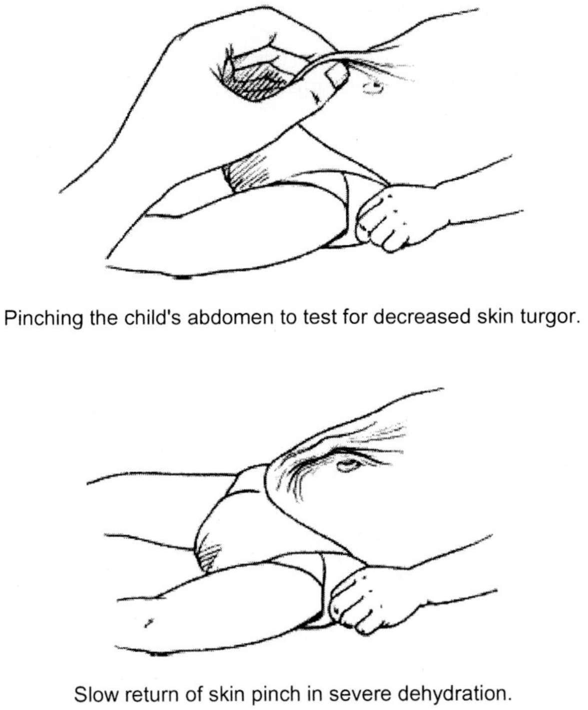

Pinching the child's abdomen to test for decreased skin turgor.
Slow return of skin pinch in severe dehydration.

Fig. 20.2. Pinching the child's abdomen to assess skin turgor. In severe dehydration, skin fold returns very slowly.

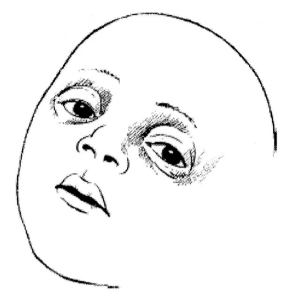

Fig. 20.3. Sunken eyes as a sign of dehydration.

Diagnosis

Investigations are often unnecessary in simple acute diarrhoea, and management should be supportive as outlined below.

Stool microscopy may be useful in distinguishing colitis from secretory enteritis in adults, and in diagnosing parasitic causes of diarrhoea such as giardiasis, cryptosporidiosis and schistosomiasis. A drop of methylene blue is mixed with the stool, and a smear examined at $\times 40$ magnification for leukocytes and red blood cells. A fresh iodine preparation is examined for ova and parasites. The presence of leukocytes in the stool suggests inflammatory or invasive disease of the colon; consider empiric antibiotic treatment in patients in whom they are found. Note that, in amoebic colitis, there may be no leukocytes visible, but motile trophozoites containing ingested red cells confirm the diagnosis.

Stool culture is not routinely recommended as it is expensive, takes several days, and most laboratories are unable to detect many of the important pathogens causing diarrhoea.

In adults, radiology can be helpful if the abdomen is distended, quiet or shows localized tenderness or evidence of generalized peritonism. A plain abdominal X-ray is required to look for evidence of ileus, thickened bowel or toxic dilatation. An erect chest X-ray should be taken when perforation is suspected, to look for free gas under the diaphragm.

Management

Treatment of diarrhoea has three components:
- *rehydration,* to correct dehydration and prevent its recurrence until diarrhoea stops
- *feeding an appropriate diet,* to sustain nutrition
- *anti-microbial treatment* in certain specific situations (e.g. cholera, dysentery).

Rehydration therapy

Rehydration therapy treats dehydration by restoring the deficit of water and electrolytes, and prevents its recurrence by fully replacing any further losses as they occur until the diarrhoea stops (Heymann et al., 1990). Most patients can be treated by oral rehydration; when dehydration is severe rapid intravenous rehydration is needed. In either case, the fluid given must contain sufficient salt and, if possible, potassium and bicarbonate to correct the deficits and replace ongoing losses (Table 20.2 and Box p. 376).

Composition of oral rehydration salts solutions

ADULTS – For the management of dehydration due to acute watery diarrhoea, including cholera, an ORS formulation corresponding to the standard WHO/UNICEF is recommended. This formulation, containing 90 mmol/l of sodium, is best suited to limit the already rare occurrence of hyponatraemia in adult patients.

CHILDREN – Although standard WHO/UNICEF ORS solution has proven safe and effective for children with acute non-cholera diarrhoea,[1] ORS solutions with osmolarity of 215 mmol/l (see individual substance concentrations below) have been shown to be as effective as standard WHO/UNICEF ORS solution and associated with less frequent use of supplemental i.v. therapy.

CHOICE OF ORS SOLUTION – In industrialized countries as well as in developing countries **without cholera**, two different ORS solutions could be used:

- **for children** an ORS solution with the formulation described in paragraph 2, and
- **for adults** the standard WHO/UNICEF ORS formulation described in paragraph 1.

However, in countries where **cholera is present**, it may be more practical to use a single ORS formulation, which in this case should be the standard WHO/UNICEF ORS formulation described in paragraph 1.

	ORS for adults	ORS for children
Glucose	111 mmol/l	75–90 mmol/l
Sodium	90 mmol/l	60–75 mmol/l
Potassium	20 mmol/l	20 mmol/l
Citrate	10 mmol/l	10 mmol/l
Chloride	80 mmol/l	50–65 mmol/l
Sodium: glucose ratio		1: 1 to 1: 1.3

[1] Oral rehydration salts (ORS) solutions with substance concentrations which meet the following criteria can also be used for the treatment and prevention of dehydration due to diarrhoea:

Glucose should not exceed	111 mmol/l
Sodium should be within the range	60–90 mmol/l
Potassium should be	20 mmol/l
Citrate should be	10 mmol/l
Chloride should be within the range	50–80 mmol/l
Sodium: glucose ratio should be within the range	1:1 – 1:3

Solutions with higher sodium and higher osmolarity may be less effective for treating dehydration due to non-cholera diarrhoea in children. On the other hand, solutions with lower sodium and lower osmolarity may be less desirable for treating dehydration in adults.

Severe dehydration

Intravenous fluids should be given in the outpatient clinic according to WHO Treatment Plan C (see Box p. 378).

Intravenous rehydration

When dehydration is *severe*, fluids must be given intravenously to correct shock *rapidly*. Ringer's lactate is the preferred solution because it provides the required salt and bicarbonate. If it is not available, normal saline may be given. Dextrose solution (5 per cent or 10 per cent) is not effective because it contains no salt; it should *not* be given. The objective of initial i.v. therapy is rapidly to restore an effective blood volume. This can be done by infusing 30 ml/kg over one hour for infants, and within 30 minutes for all others. The remaining deficit of 70 ml/kg is replaced more slowly: 5 hours in infants and 2 hours in older children and adults.

If i.v. infusion is not possible, urgent referral to the hospital for i.v. treatment is recommended. When referral takes more than 30 minutes, fluids should be given by nasogastric tube. If the child can drink, ORS should be given orally.

Monitoring

Details of reassessment and adjustment of the speed of rehydration are included in Diarrhoea Treatment Plan C (see Box, p. 378). All children should start to receive some ORS solution (about 5 ml/kg/hour) by cup when they can drink without difficulty (usually within 3–4 hours for infants, or 1–2 hours for older children). This provides additional base and potassium, which may not be adequately supplied by the i.v. fluid.

Some dehydration

These children have a fluid deficit equalling 5–10 per cent of their body weight (Table 20.3). This classification includes both 'mild' and 'moderate' dehydration, which are descriptive terms used in most paediatric textbooks.

Oral rehydration

When dehydration is not severe, or after shock has been corrected, rehydration may be given by mouth. ORS solution is designed efficiently to replace faecal losses. It contains salt, potassium and citrate (which is metabolized to bicarbonate) to replace faecal losses, and glucose (Table 20.2).

ORS solution does not cause stool output to increase or

Diarrhoea treatment plan A: treat diarrhoea at home

Counsel the mother on the three rules of home treatment: give extra fluid, continue feeding, when to return

1. **Give extra fluid** (as much as the child will take)
   - **Tell the mother:**
   - Breast-feed frequently and for longer at each feed.
   - If the child is exclusively breast-fed, give ORS or clean water in addition to breast-milk.
   - If the child is not exclusively breast-fed, give one or more of the following: ORS solution, food-based fluids (such as soup, rice water, and yoghurt drinks), or clean water.

   It is especially important to give ORS at home when:
   - *the child has been treated with Plan B or Plan C during this visit.*
   - *the child cannot return to a clinic if the diarrhoea gets worse.*
2. **Teach the mother how to mix and give ORS. Give the mother 2 packets of ORS to use at home.**
3. **Show the mother how much fluid to give in addition to the usual fluid intake:**

(a) Up to 2 years
50 to 100 ml after each loose stool

(b) 2 years or more
100 to 200 ml after each loose stool

Tell the mother to:
- Give frequent small sips from a cup.
- If the child vomits, wait 10 minutes. Then continue, but more slowly.
- *Continue giving extra fluid until the diarrhoea stops.*

4. **Continue feeding**
5. **When to return**

Diarrhoea Treatment Plan B:

Treat some dehydration with ORS

Give in clinic recommended amount of ORS over 4-hour period

Determine amount of ORS to give during first 4 hours.

	Up to	**4 months up**	**12 months**	**2 years up**
Age[a]	**4 months**	**to 12 months**	**up to 2 years**	**to 5 years**
WEIGHT	<6 kg	6–<10 kg	10–<12 kg	12–19 kg
In ml	200–400	400–700	700–900	900–1400

[a] *Use the child's age only when you do not know the weight. The approximate amount of ORS required (in ml) can also be calculated by multiplying the child's weight (in kg) by 75.*

- If the child wants more ORS than shown, give more.
- For infants under 6 months who are not breast-fed, also give 100–200 ml clean water during this period.

Show the mother how to give ORS solution.
- Give frequent small sips from a cup.
- If the child vomits, wait 10 minutes. Then continue, but more slowly.
- Continue breast-feeding whenever the child wants.

After 4 hours:
- Reassess the child and classify the child for dehydration.
- Select the appropriate plan to continue treatment.
- Begin feeding the child in clinic.

If the mother must leave before completing treatment:
- Show her how to prepare ORS solution at home.
- Show her how much ORS to give to finish 4-hour treatment at home.
- Give her enough ORS packets to complete rehydration. Also give her 2 packets as recommended in Plan A.
- Explain the three rules of home treatment:
  1. **Give extra fluid**
  2. **Continue feeding**
  3. **When to return**

decrease. It is important to make this clear to patients and carers, since failure to do so has been cited as an important reason for non-compliance and under-use of ORS.

It is effective because glucose continues to be absorbed in the small intestine, even during diarrhoea, and this causes the simultaneous absorption of sodium, other electrolytes and water. A solution of salt and water without glucose, however, is not absorbed well and will not treat or prevent dehydration. ORS solution containing 50 g/l of cooked rice powder in place of glucose is also effective because rice is converted to glucose in the small intestine. Thirst is a valuable guide for oral rehydration therapy. Most children, when offered ORS solution, will drink the amount required to maintain adequate hydration and then stop.

For the management of 'some dehydration', WHO has developed the guidelines contained in 'Treatment plan B' (see Box).

No dehydration

Children with diarrhoea but no signs of dehydration usually have a fluid deficit less than 5 per cent of their body weight. They should be given more fluid than usual to prevent dehydration. The mother is asked to return if the child develops blood in the stool, drinks poorly, becomes sicker, or is not better in 3 days.

Unrestricted fluids should be given as soon as diarrhoea begins. ORS may be used at home to prevent dehydration. However, other fluids that are commonly available in the home may be less costly, more convenient, and almost as effective. Most fluids that a child

Diarrhoea Treatment Plan C: Treat severe dehydration quickly

→ FOLLOW THE ARROWS. IF ANSWER IS 'YES', GO ACROSS. IF 'NOT', GO DOWN.

START HERE

Can you give intravenous (I.V.) fluid immediately? — YES →

- Start i.v. fluid immediately. If the child can drink, give ORS by mouth while the drip is set up. Give 100 ml/kg Ringer's lactate solution (or, if not available, normal saline), divided as follows:

Age	First give 30 ml/kg in:	Then give 70 ml/kg in:
Infants (under 12 months)	1 hour*	5 hours
Children (12 months up to 5 years)	30 minutes*	2.5 hours

* *Repeat once if radial pulse is still very weak or not detectable.*

- Reassess the child every 1–2 hours. If hydration status is not improving, give the i.v. drip more rapidly.
- Also give ORS (about 5 ml/kg/hour) as soon as the child can drink: usually after 3–4 hours (infants) or 1–2 hours (children).
- Reassess an infant after 6 hours and a child after 3 hours. Classify dehydration. Then choose the appropriate plan (A, B, or C) to continue treatment.

NO ↓

Is I.V. treatment available nearby (within 30 minutes)? — YES →

- Refer URGENTLY to hospital for i.v. treatment.
- If the child can drink, provide the mother with ORS solution and show her how to give frequent sips during the trip.

NO ↓

Are you trained to use a nasogastric (NG) tube for rehydration? — YES →

NO ↓

Can the child drink? — YES →

- Start rehydration by tube (or mouth) with ORS solution: give 20 ml/kg/hour for 6 hours (total of 120 ml/kg).
- Reassess the child every 1–2 hours:
  - If there is repeated vomiting or increasing abdominal distension, give the fluid more slowly.
  - If hydration status is not improving after 3 hours, send the child for i.v. therapy.
- After 6 hours, reassess the child. Classify dehydration. Then choose the appropriate plan (A, B, or C) to continue treatment.

NO ↓

Refer URGENTLY to hospital for i.v. or NG treatment

NOTE: If possible, observe the child for at least 6 hours after rehydration to be sure the mother can maintain hydration giving the child ORS solution by mouth.

normally takes can also be used for home therapy especially when given with food.

Acceptable home fluids should be the following:

- Safe when given in large volumes

Therefore, avoid very sweet tea, soft drinks, and sweetened fruit drinks as they are hyperosmolar and can cause osmotic diarrhoea, dehydration and hypernatraemia. Other fluids to be avoided are those with purgative actions and stimulants (e.g. coffee, some medicinal teas or infusions).

- Easy to prepare

The recipe should be familiar and its preparation should not require much effort or time. The ingredients and utensils should be readily available and inexpensive.

- Acceptable

The fluid should be one that the mother is willing to give freely to a child with diarrhoea and that the child will readily accept.

- Effective

Fluids that are safe are also effective. Most effective are fluids that contain carbohydrates, protein, and some salt. However, the same result is obtained when fluids are given freely along with weaning foods that contain salt.

The management guidelines are summarized in 'Treatment plan A' (see Box p. 377).

Feeding

The objective of feeding during diarrhoea is to maintain or improve nutrition, prevent weight loss and sustain growth (Brown et al. 1988). This requires continued full-strength feeding. Following rehydration, most children regain their appetite and eat.

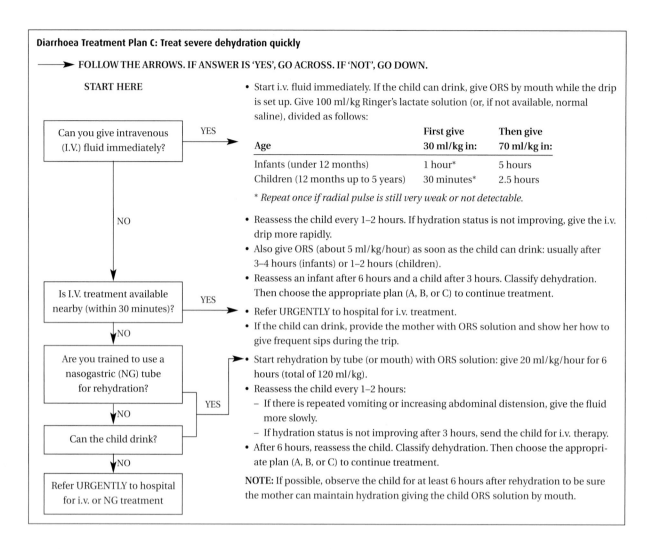

During acute diarrhoea the digestion and absorption of nutrients is only slightly reduced. Overall, 80–90 per cent of nutrients continue to be absorbed. Clinically important malabsorption of lactose is unusual and malabsorption of glucose is rare. A child given a nutritious diet during acute diarrhoea, including the child's usual milk, continues to grow. If food is reduced or withheld, growth will slow or stop, weight is lost and diarrhoea may be prolonged. Feeding during diarrhoea does not increase stool volume; continued breast-feeding actually reduces stool volume.

Use of anti-microbials

Anti-microbials are only useful when the cause of diarrhoea is known and an effective anti-microbial is available. For children with acute watery diarrhoea, the cause cannot be determined when the child is seen and many episodes are due to agents for which anti-microbials are ineffective, such as rotavirus. Routine anti-microbials are not useful for patients with acute watery diarrhoea and they should not be given.

'Anti-diarrhoeal' drugs

Many products are claimed to reduce or stop diarrhoea. These include drugs, such as loperamide, diphenoxylate, tincture of opium, paregoric and codeine. Also included are adsorbents, such as kaolin, attapulgite, smectite and activated charcoal. Many have been studied in well designed clinical trials. None has proven effective and none should be given, either alone or in combination. Some are dangerous. Loperamide has caused fatal intestinal paralysis in infants.

Cholera (see Chapter 48)

Suspect cholera in patients over 2 years old who have acute watery diarrhoea and signs of severe dehydration, if cholera is occurring in the local area. The mainstay of cholera treatment is successful rehydration and prevention of dehydration, as for other causes of watery diarrhoea. In addition, give an oral antibiotic to which strains of *Vibrio cholerae* in the area are known to be sensitive. Possible choices are: tetracycline, doxycycline, cotrimoxazole, erythromycin, and chloramphenicol. If the cause is cholera, diarrhoea will stop within 48–72 hours. Failure to improve suggests that *V. cholerae* is resistant to the anti-microbial given, or that the illness is not due to cholera.

Diarrhoea in children with severe malnutrition

(see Chapter 3)

Dehydration tends to be overdiagnosed and its severity overestimated in severely malnourished children (WHO, 2000). This is because it is difficult to estimate dehydration status accurately in the severely malnourished child using clinical signs alone. Assume that all malnourished children with *watery diarrhoea* may have *some* dehydration. Note that low blood volume can co-exist with oedema.

Treatment

Do *not* use the i.v. route for rehydration in severely malnourished children except in cases of shock (see Chapter 97 'Paediatric emergencies'). Standard WHO–ORS solution for general use has a high sodium and low potassium content, which is not suitable for severely malnourished children. Instead, give special rehydration solution for malnutrition (ReSoMal see Chapter 11 'Severe malnutrition'). Give the *ReSoMal rehydration fluid*, orally or by nasogastric tube, much more slowly than you would when rehydrating a well-nourished child:

- give 5 ml/kg every 30 minutes for the first 2 hours
- then give 5–10 ml/kg per hour for the next 4–10 hours.

The exact amount depends on how much the child wants, volume of stool loss, and whether the child is vomiting. If rehydration is still occurring at 6 hours and 10 hours, give a starter formula (such as 'F75', see Chapter 11 'Severe malnutrition') *instead* of ReSoMal at these times. Use the same volume of starter F-75 as for ReSoMal. Then initiate refeeding with starter formula.

Monitoring

Monitor the progress of rehydration half-hourly for 2 hours, then hourly for the next 6–12 hours. Be alert for signs of overhydration, which is very dangerous in severely malnourished children and may lead to heart failure. Check respiratory rate, pulse rate, urine frequency and the frequency of stool and vomit. During treatment, the child's breathing and pulse rate should decrease and the child should begin to pass urine. Continued fast breathing and a rapid pulse rate during rehydration suggest co-existing infection or overhydration. If you find signs of overhydration (increasing respiratory and pulse rates), stop ReSoMal immediately and reassess after 1 hour.

The return of tears, a moist mouth, less sunken eyes and fontanelle, and improved skin turgor are also signs that rehydration is proceeding, but many severely malnourished children will not show these changes even when fully rehydrated.

DYSENTERY (BLOODY DIARRHOEA)

Bloody diarrhoea in young children is usually a sign of invasive enteric infection that carries a substantial risk of serious morbidity and mortality. Dysentery is especially severe in malnourished, dehydrated, and non-breast-fed infants and children. It is more likely to cause growth faltering and persistent diarrhoea than acute watery diarrhoea. Dysentery occurs with increased frequency and severity in children who have measles, or have had measles recently. Although dysentery is often described as a syndrome of bloody diarrhoea with fever, abdominal cramps, rectal pain and mucoid stools, these features do not always accompany bloody diarrhoea.

Aetiology

Most episodes of dysentery are caused by intestinal infection with Shigella, *Campylobacter jejuni*, or enteroinvasive *E. coli*. *Entamoeba histolytica* is a rare cause in infants and children. The aetiology of dysentery can only be determined by stool culture and microscopic examination.

Prevention and control

The risk factors for dysentery are the same as for acute watery diarrhoea. A vaccine against Shigella and other organisms causing dysentery is currently not available.

Pathophysiology

Bloody diarrhoea results when the intestinal mucosa is damaged by invasive bacteria or protozoa. Important complications of dysentery due to Shigella and enterohaemorrhagic *E. coli* include haemolytic–uraemic syndrome, renal failure and rectal prolapse. Bacteria that cause dysentery may also cause acute non-bloody diarrhoea (Table 20.1). Children with dysentery may also develop dehydration due to excessive loss of water and electrolytes in liquid stool.

Clinical features

Stools contain visible blood; they may be large and watery or frequent and small. The patient often appears listless, irritable and toxic, and refuses to eat. Fever, abdominal pain, and pain or crying when stool is passed are common. A single convulsion may occur in children, even without fever, and sometimes before diarrhoea begins.

Management

Use of anti-microbials

The most common cause of dysentery is Shigella. (Bennish et al., 1990). All children with dysentery should be treated for 5 days with an oral anti-microbial to which local strains of Shigella are known to be sensitive. Examples of antibiotics to which Shigella strains **can be sensitive** (in the absence of resistance) are:

- cotrimoxazole
- ampicillin
- pivmecillinam
- nalidixic acid and
- fluoroquinolones.

Note that metronidazole, streptomycin, tetracyclines, chloramphenicol, sulfonamides, nitrofurans (e.g. nitrofurantoin, furazolidone), aminoglycosides (e.g. gentamicin, kanamycin), first- and second-generation cephalosporins (e.g. cephalexin, cefamandole), and amoxycillin are **not effective** in the treatment of Shigella.

If Shigella is the cause, and an effective oral anti-microbial is given, definite improvement will occur within 48 hours (less fever, less blood in the stool, better appetite, more active) and the child will fully recover within 4–5 days.

Children with severe malnutrition and dysentery, and young infants (<2 months old) with dysentery should be admitted to hospital. Others can be treated at home.

The following groups of children (aged 2 months to 5 years) should be treated at home and asked to return for re-assessment after 2 days:

- those who were initially dehydrated
- those who have had measles during the past 3 months
- infants aged 2–12 months
- any child who is not getting better.

In the follow-up visit in 2 days, look for the following signs of improvement: disappearance of fever, less blood in the stool, passage of fewer stools, improved appetite, and a return to normal activity.

If there is no improvement after 2 days, check for other conditions, stop the first antibiotic, and give the child a second-line antibiotic, which is known to be effective against Shigella in the area. In most countries the second- or third-line anti-microbial for children aged 2 months to 5 years will be either nalidixic acid, pivmecillinam (amidinocillin pivoxil) or ciprofloxacin. If the two antibiotics that are usually effective for Shigella in the area have produced no signs of clinical improvement, check for other conditions. Admit the child if there is another condition requiring hospital treatment. Otherwise treat as an outpatient for possible amoebiasis. Give the child metronidazole (10 mg/kg, 3 times a day) for 5 days.

Hospital treatment

Admit young infants (aged <2 months) who have blood in their stools and severely malnourished children with bloody diarrhoea.

Young infants

Examine the young infant for surgical causes of blood in the stools (for example, intussusception) and refer to a surgeon, if appropriate. Otherwise give the young infant i.m. ceftriaxone (100 mg/kg) once daily for 5 days.

Severely malnourished children

See Malnutrition chapter for the general management of these children. Treat bloody diarrhoea with an antibiotic against Shigella or amoebiasis, as described above. If microscopic examination of fresh faeces in a reliable laboratory is possible, check for trophozoites of *E. histolytica* within red blood cells and treat for amoebiasis, if present.

Other treatment

Rehydration and feeding guidelines follow the same principles as for acute watery diarrhoea (see above). Children with dysentery, however, often remain anorexic and must be encouraged to eat. *Never* give drugs to reduce the frequency of stools ('Anti-diarrhoeal' drugs), as they can increase the severity of the illness.

Nutritional management

Ensuring a good diet is very important as dysentery has a marked adverse effect on nutritional status. However, feeding is often difficult because of lack of appetite. Return of appetite is an important sign of improvement. Breast-feeding should be continued throughout the course of the illness, more frequently than normal, if possible, because the infant may not take the usual amount per feed. Children aged 4–6 months or more should receive their normal foods. Encourage the child to eat and allow the child to select preferred foods.

Complications

Rectal prolapse

Gently push back the rectal prolapse using a surgical glove or a wet cloth. Alternatively, prepare a warm solution of saturated magnesium sulphate and apply compresses with this solution to reduce the prolapse by decreasing the oedema. The prolapse often recurs but usually disappears spontaneously after the diarrhoea stops.

Haemolytic–uraemic syndrome

Where laboratory tests are not possible, suspect haemolytic–uraemic syndrome (HUS) in patients with easy bruising, pallor, altered consciousness, and low or no urine output. Where laboratory support is available, make the diagnosis of HUS on the basis of the blood smear showing fragmented red blood cells, reduced or absent platelets, or both; and an elevated blood urea nitrogen or serum creatinine, indicating renal failure. When a patient develops low urine output and HUS is suspected, stop giving foods or fluids containing potassium, such as ORS solution, and transfer the patient to a facility where haemodialysis or peritoneal dialysis and blood transfusion can be performed.

PERSISTENT DIARRHOEA

Aetiology

Persistent diarrhoea usually begins with intestinal infection (see Table 20.1), but malnutrition and malabsorption, often in combination, cause diarrhoea to be prolonged (Black, 1993). If the stool contains visible blood, *Shigella* is the likely cause.

Prevention and control

Persistent diarrhoea rarely occurs in infants who are exclusively breast-fed.

Pathophysiology

The underlying causes of persistent diarrhoea include protein-calorie malnutrition, concurrent extra-intestinal infection, such as pneumonia, and zinc deficiency, often in combination. The intestinal epithelium may be markedly abnormal, villi are shortened or flat, and crypts are deepened. Disaccharidase enzymes are reduced and disaccharides may not be hydrolysed efficiently; clinically important malabsorption of lactose is common. When the diet contains animal milk, unabsorbed lactose is fermented in the ileum and colon, an osmotic effect causes diarrhoea to worsen, and stools become acidic. Mother's milk, however, is well tolerated. A few children with persistent diarrhoea also malabsorb starch and other complex carbohydrates. Reduced feeding, or continued feeding of an inappropriate diet, usually containing animal milk, causes further weight loss, worsening malnutrition, and eventually death, usually due to severe infection.

Dehydration can occur and is managed as described above for children with acute diarrhoea.

Clinical features

Liquid stools are often passed after eating, sometimes explosively. Occasionally stools contain visible blood. Weight loss is often evident and signs of malnutrition are often present; malnutrition varies in degree and may be severe. In children with marasmus the loss of subcutaneous fat gives the appearance of decreased skin turgor and causes eyes to appear sunken, making these sign useless for detecting dehydration.

Management

Treatment of persistent diarrhoea includes: (i) *rehydration therapy*, to correct dehydration and prevent its recurrence; (ii) *feeding an appropriate diet*, to sustain nutrition and support the recovery of intestinal function, and (iii) *treatment of serious infections* with an appropriate antimicrobial (Anon, 1996).

Rehydration therapy

This follows the principles described for acute watery diarrhoea (see above). If, however, the child is severely malnourished, there is an increased risk that i.v. or oral rehydration would cause heart failure. In such children, rehydration should be done slowly by mouth with the low-sodium solution, ReSoMal, as described above.

Children with severe persistent diarrhoea who also have dehydration should be referred to hospital. Treatment of dehydration should be initiated first. ORS solution is effective for most children with persistent diarrhoea. In a few, however, glucose absorption is impaired and ORS solution is not effective. When given ORS, their stool volume increases markedly, thirst increases, signs of dehydration develop or worsen, and the stool contains a large amount of unabsorbed glucose. These children require i.v. rehydration until ORS solution can be taken without causing the diarrhoea to worsen.

Children with persistent diarrhoea and no signs of dehydration can be managed as outpatients.

Feeding

Careful attention to feeding is *essential* for all children with persistent diarrhoea. Besides giving the child energy and nutrition, feeding helps the gut to recover. In addition to its treatment role, it can have an important preventive value. The normal diet of a child with persistent diarrhoea is often inadequate, so treatment is an important opportunity to teach the mother how to improve her child's nutrition.

Breast-feeding should be continued for as often and as long as the child wants. Other food should be withheld for 4–6 hours – *only* for children with dehydration who are being rehydrated following treatment plans B or C.

Hospital diets

Children treated in hospital require special diets until their diarrhoea lessens and they are gaining weight. The goal is to give a daily intake of *at least* 110 calories/kg.

Infants aged under 6 months

Encourage exclusive breast-feeding. Help mothers who are not breast-feeding exclusively to do so. If the child is not breast-feeding, give a breast milk substitute that is low in lactose, such as yoghurt, or is lactose-free. Use a spoon or cup, do *not* use a feeding bottle. Once the child improves, help the mother to re-establish lactation. If the mother is not breast-feeding because she is HIV-positive, she should receive appropriate counselling about the correct use of breast milk substitutes.

Children aged 6 months or older

Feeding should be restarted as soon as the child can eat. Food should be given six times a day to achieve a total intake of at least 110 calories/kg/day. Many children will eat poorly, however, until any serious infection has been treated for 24–48 hours. Such children may require nasogastric feeding initially.

Given in the table on next page are two diets recommended for children and infants aged >6 months with severe persistent diarrhoea. If the first diet is given for 7 days, some 60–70 per cent of children will improve with this treatment. If there are signs of dietary failure (see

Table 20.4. First diet: a starch-based, reduced milk concentration (low lactose) diet

The diet should contain at least 70 calories/100 g, provide milk or yoghurt as a source of animal protein, but no more than 3.7 g lactose/kg body weight/day, and should provide at least 10 per cent of calories as protein. The following example provides 83 calories/100 g, 3.7g lactose/kg body weight/day and 11 per cent of calories as protein:

• Full-fat dried milk (or whole liquid milk: 85 ml)	11 g
• Rice	15 g
• Vegetable oil	3.5 g
• Cane sugar	3 g
• Water to make	200 ml

Table 20.5. Second diet: a no milk (lactose-free) diet with reduced cereal (starch)

The second diet should contain at least 70 calories/100 g, and provide at least 10 per cent of calories as protein (egg or chicken). The following example provides 75 calories/100 g:

• Whole egg	64 g
• Rice	3 g
• Vegetable oil	4 g
• Glucose	3 g
• Water to make	200 ml

Finely ground, cooked chicken (12 g) can be used in place of egg to give a diet providing 70 calories/100 g.

below) or if the child is not improving after 7 days of treatment, the first diet should be stopped and the second diet given for 7 days.

Successful treatment with either diet is characterized by adequate food intake, weight gain, fewer diarrhoeal stools and absence of fever.

The most important criterion is weight gain. Many children will lose weight for 1–2 days, and then steadily gain weight as the infections get under control and the diarrhoea subsides. There should be at least 3 successive days of increasing weight before one can conclude that weight gain is occurring; for most children the weight on day 7 will be greater than on admission.

Dietary failure is shown by an increase in stool frequency (usually to >10 watery stools a day), often with a return of signs of dehydration (this usually occurs shortly after a new diet is begun), or a failure to establish daily weight gain within 7 days. Of the children who do not improve on this first diet, more than half will improve when given the second diet, in which milk has been totally removed and starch (cereals) partly replaced with glucose or sucrose.

Supplementary multivitamins and minerals

Give all children with persistent diarrhoea daily supplementary multivitamins and minerals for two weeks. These should provide as broad a range of vitamins and minerals as possible, including at least two recommended daily allowances (RDAs) of folate, vitamin A, zinc, magnesium and copper.

Monitoring

Nurses should check the following daily:
- body weight
- temperature
- food taken and
- number of diarrhoea stools.

Give additional fresh fruit and well-cooked vegetables to children who are responding well. After 7 days of treatment with the effective diet, they should resume an appropriate diet for their age, including milk, which provides at least 110 calories/kg/day. Children may then return home, but follow them up regularly to ensure continued weight gain and compliance with feeding advice.

Identify and treat specific infections

Many children with persistent diarrhoea also have other infections, such as pneumonia, urinary infection or skin infection. In such children the persistent diarrhoea will not improve until the concomitant infection is also treated. A child with persistent diarrhoea should be examined carefully for these infections. When an extra-intestinal infection is diagnosed, give an appropriate anti-microbial. If the stool contains visible blood, give an anti-microbial effective for Shigella, as described for children with dysentery. The routine use of anti-microbials for persistent diarrhoea, however, is not effective and is not recommended.

Give treatment for giardiasis (metronidazole: 5 mg/kg, three times a day, for 5 days) if cysts or trophozoites of *Giardia lamblia* are seen in the faeces. In areas where HIV is highly prevalent, suspect HIV if there are other clinical signs or risk factors.

Follow-up

Ask the mother to bring the child back for reassessment after 5 days, or earlier if the diarrhoea worsens or other problems develop. Fully reassess children who have not gained weight or whose diarrhoea has not improved in order to identify any problems, such as dehydration or infection, which need immediate attention or admission to hospital. Those who have gained weight and who have less than three loose stools per day may resume a normal diet for their age.

References

Anon (1996). Evaluation of an algorithm for the treatment of persistent diarrhoea: a multicentre study. International Working Group on Persistent Diarrhoea. *Bull Wld Hlth Org*; **74**: 479–489.

Bennish ML, Salam MA, Haider R, Barza M (1990). Therapy for shigellosis. II. Randomized, double-blind comparison of ciprofloxacin and ampicillin. *J Infect Dis*; **162**: 711–716.

Bern C, Martines J, de Zoysa I, Glass RI (1992). The magnitude of the global problem of diarrhoeal disease: a ten-year update. *Bull Wld Hlth Org*; **70**: 705–714.

Black RE (1993). Persistent diarrhea in children of developing countries. *Pediat Infec Dis J*; **12**, 751–761.

Brown KH, Gastanaduy AS, Saavedra JM et al. (1988). Effect of continued oral feeding on clinical and nutritional outcomes of acute diarrhea in children. *J Pediat*; **112**: 191–200.

Feachem RG, Hogan RC, Merson MH (1983). Diarrhoeal disease control: reviews of potential interventions. *Bull Wld Hlth Org*; **61**: 637–640.

Heymann DL, Mbvundula M, Macheso A, McFarland DA, Hawkins RV (1990). Oral rehydration therapy in Malawi: impact on the severity of disease and on hospital admissions, treatment practices, and recurrent costs. *Bull Wld Hlth Org*; **68**: 193–197.

WHO (1995). *The Treatment of Diarrhoea: A Manual for Physicians and Other Senior Health Workers*. Geneva: World Health Organization.

WHO (2000). *Management of the Child with a Serious Infection or Severe Malnutrition*, 1st edn. Geneva: World Health Organization.

Helminths

21 Intestinal helminths – the burden of disease

Parasitic worms may be the commonest agents of chronic infection in humans

It is estimated that there are more than 3 billion worm infections in the world today (Chan et al., 1994). In many low-income countries it is more common to be infected than not. Indeed, children growing up in an endemic community can expect be infected soon after weaning, and to be infected and constantly re-infected for the rest of their lives.

Infection is most common amongst the poorest and most disadvantaged communities, and is typically most intense in children of school age, and since the risk of morbidity is directly related to intensity of infection these children are also at greatest risk from the morbid effects of disease. Multi-parasite infections are also common, and there is evidence that children harbouring such infections may suffer exacerbated morbidity, making them even more vulnerable. Thus, worm infections pose their most serious threat to the health and development of the poorest children in the poorest countries.

There are approximately 20 major helminth infections of humans that all, to some extent, have public health significance (for review, refer to Warren et al., 1993), but amongst the most common of all human infections are the geohelminthiases. Recent global estimates indicate that more than one-quarter of the world's population are infected with one or more of the most common of these parasites: the roundworm, *Ascaris lumbricoides*; the hookworms, *Necator americanus* and *Ancylostoma duodenale*; and the whipworm, *Trichuris trichiura* (Chan et al., 1994). In addition, more than 200 million people are estimated to harbour schistosome infections (World Bank, 1993).

All worm infections are not equal

The distribution of helminths amongst hosts is over-dispersed: whilst the majority of the hosts harbour few or no worms, a few harbour much larger numbers of parasites (Anderson & Medley, 1985). This fact has clinical consequences for the host, as it is the intensity of infection that is the central determinant of the severity of morbidity (Stephenson, 1987; Cooper & Bundy, 1988). As shown in Fig. 21.1, the age-intensity profile for *Trichuris trichiura* and *Ascaris lumbricoides* is typically convex with maximum intensity at 5–10 years of age. After peak intensity has been attained there is a dramatic decline in intensity to a low level, which then persists throughout adulthood.

A similar profile is apparent for *Schistosoma* infections, but with maximum intensity attained at a slightly later age, usually 10–14 years. A different profile is apparent for hookworm infections, as maximum intensity is usually not attained until 20–25 years (Stephenson, 1987).

It is strikingly apparent that it is the school-age child who is particularly at risk from the clinical manifestations of disease. Indeed, it was estimated that, for girls and boys aged 5–14 years in low-income countries, intestinal worms account for 12 per cent and 11 per cent of the total disease burden of this age group. An estimated 20 per cent of disability adjusted life years (DALY's) lost due to communicable disease among school children are a direct result of intestinal nematodes (World Bank, 1993).

Worm infections constrain child development

Many children in low-income countries underachieve and never realize their full potential. The aetiology of this

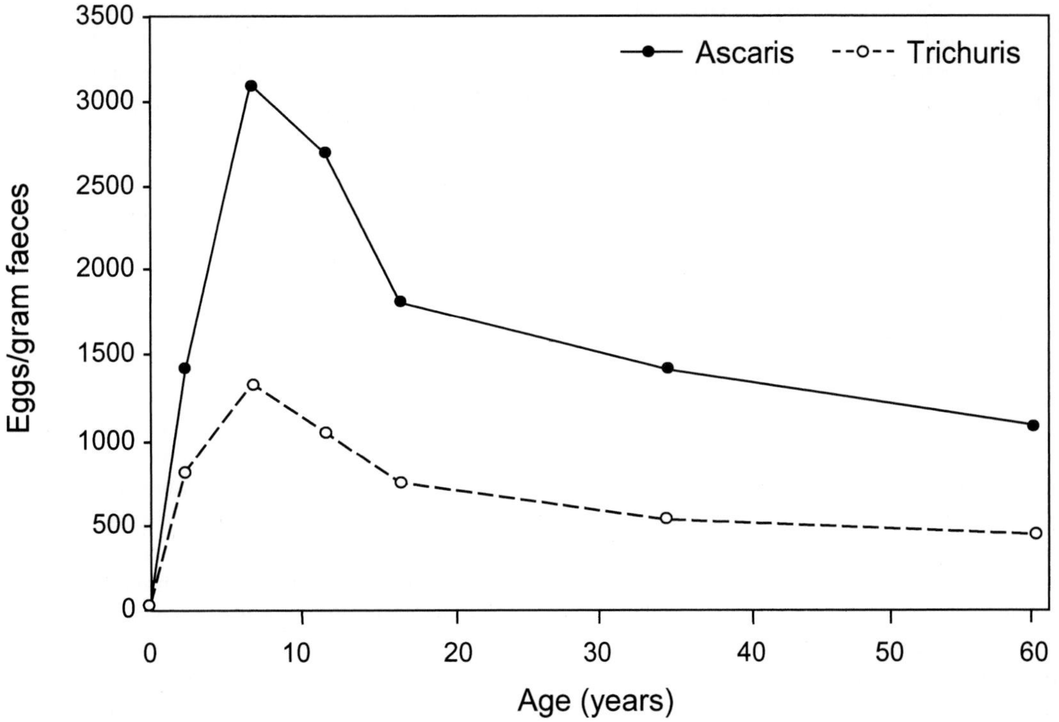

Fig. 21.1. Age intensity profile of *Ascaris lumbricoides* and *Trichuris trichiura.*

underachievement is complex since numerous factors experienced during a child's formative years may have a detrimental effect upon development and functional efficiency. However there has been growing recognition of the specific deleterious effects of helminth infections upon both physical and intellectual development. As children suffer most at an age when they are both growing and learning, the entire developmental process is placed in jeopardy.

By far the most common effect on health is a subtle and insidious constraint on normal physical development, resulting in children failing to achieve their genetic potential for growth and suffering from the clinical consequences of iron deficiency anaemia and other nutritional deficiencies: heavy hookworm burdens have long been recognized as an important cause of iron deficiency anaemia (Roche & Layrisse, 1966); intense whipworm infection in children may result in *Trichuris* Dysentery Syndrome, the classical signs of which include growth retardation and anaemia (Bundy & Cooper, 1989); heavy burdens of both roundworm and whipworm are associated with protein energy malnutrition (PEM) (Stephenson et al., 1993).

Worms may also constrain intellectual development

There is an increasing body of evidence that these infections can have a detrimental effect on cognition and educational achievement in children (Sternberg et al., 1997). The mechanism by which mental processes are affected is uncertain, but evidence suggests that the mechanism is indirect. The most plausible mediators are the common sequelae of infection: iron deficiency anaemia (IDA) and undernutrition (Pollitt et al., 1989; Pollitt, 1999).

IDA in infants and young children is associated with significantly lower scores on psychological tests. Deficits of 0.5–1.5 standard deviation units in scores on infant development scales or IQ tests for children have been found quite consistently across studies and age groups. Moreover, these effects of IDA during infancy are associated with lower developmental test scores at 5 years of age (Cooper & Bundy, 1988). Similar effects have been shown during school age, although the relationship is less clear for children with mild IDA. Treatment studies have consistently found improvements in cognitive function following iron supplementation in middle childhood (Soewendo et al., 1989). IDA also leads to long-term deficits in cognitive functioning (Grantham-McGregor et al., 2000).

Recent studies in Tanzania have shown that schoolchildren infected with worms achieved significantly lower scores in some tests of cognitive ability, and that the degree of deficit was related to the intensity of infection (Sternberg et al., in press). But treatment of these children did not result in an immediate improvement in the ability of the children to do these tests. However, using a battery of different tests, when children were both treated and taught how to do the tests they performed significantly better than children who were taught but not treated (Grigorenko et al., personal communication). These results suggest that children who have lived with infection all their lives, and suffered the constrained development that results from this, will need not only improved health but also a good education to catch up.

A quite different sort of study in Kenya has examined the effects of worm infection on the attendance of children at school (Miguel & Kremer, unpublished observations (http://elsa.berkeley.edu/users/emiguel/miguel worms.pdf)). Schools were randomized to receive health education with or without anthelmintic treatment, and the attendance records of children were followed for 2 years. Within 6 months there was a significant improvement in attendance of children at the treatment schools and this difference was then sustained throughout the 2-year study. Interestingly, the children in the treatment schools did not perform better in academic tests, which probably reflects the fact that they received no remedial education, as discussed above. But an even more interesting observation was that even untreated children in treatment schools showed improved school attendance. This may be a consequence of the general impact of mass treatment on the transmission of infection, such that the untreated children also benefit from the overall reduction in transmission (Bundy et al., 1991).

Thus, these infections may have an insidious and less overt impact upon the developmental process: delays in the development of these abilities may leave a child lacking in the interpersonal and emotional skills vital to making positive life decisions. This is particularly worrying given the current spread of the HIV/AIDS pandemic, and the importance of effective life skills at an early age in avoiding infection.

Even a few worms can have consequences

The effects of infection have tended to be underestimated. One important new factor is that the clinical consequences of infection can manifest themselves at much lower worm burdens than previously thought. Intervention studies have shown that infection with as few as 10 roundworms is associated with deficits in growth and physical fitness in school-age children and moderate whipworm infections can cause growth retardation and anaemia in children. Studies have also demonstrated that even light hookworm infection can lead to anaemia. This is evident not only in the adult population, but also in pre-school and schoolchildren in certain populations (Stolzfus et al., 1998; Beasley et al., 1999).

Children, adolescents and pregnant women are particularly at risk from hookworm morbidity as the physiological demands for iron are high during these periods. Evidence suggests that anaemia during pregnancy may adversely influence intrauterine growth rate, cause prematurity and reduce birth weight. Thus, there may be important maternally programmed consequences for children (Partnership for Child Development, 1997). In addition, it has been suggested that the clinical consequences of hookworm infection occur at a lower threshold in individuals who have a diet low in bioavailable iron (Tatala et al., 1998). Sadly, poor diet is all too common an occurrence in communities in low-income countries where worm infection is most common.

Multiple species infections cause more morbidity

Crompton and Tulley (1987) listed 47 different protozoan and helminth species found in association with *A. lumbricoides* infections, of which 24 were common. The presence of a variety of human parasites that occur in the same environment each with a high prevalence increases the likelihood of significant rates of co-infection. Another study estimated that multiple infections including *P. falciparum*, *P. malariae*, *S. haematobium* and three common nematodes occurred in approximately 60 per cent of a Kenyan population (Ashford et al., 1992).

Howard et al. (2000) found that, in general, associations between geohelminth species were positive, which implies that more multiple species infections are observed than would be expected by chance. Predisposition has been demonstrated for all the major helminth infections, and it has been suggested that perhaps certain individuals may be predisposed to multiple infection.

Behavioural factors could be responsible for multiple species infection. For example, *T. trichiura* and *A. lumbricoides* are both transmitted faeco-orally, thus behavioural factors that lead to exposure and infection with one parasite may also lead to exposure to and infection with the other parasite (Booth & Bundy, 1995). It has been noted that *A. lumbricoides* and *T. trichiura* infections can cluster within households (Forrester et al., 1990). Whether this is caused by genetic factors, behavioural factors or a combination of the two has not been conclusively determined. Analyses do suggest that even if there is a genetic basis for predisposition, its effects tend to be overwhelmed by other household-specific effects (Chan et al., 1994). However, it is now clear that genetic factors do partly regulate susceptibility to *S. mansoni* infection (Marquet et al., 1996).

Individuals harbouring multiple species infections have higher than expected levels of each infection individually, and thus will be at a higher risk of morbidity (Booth et al., 1998). Needham et al. (1998) demonstrated that high intensity *A. lumbricoides* infections were significantly more likely to occur with high intensity *T. trichiura* infections than would be expected by chance; children with multiple species infections have higher egg counts of each species than children with single species infections (Brooker et al., 2000).

Worm infection can be cost-effectively treated in the community

Health can be viewed in terms of the life cycle starting with intrauterine development, moving through birth, infancy, childhood, the school years, adolescence, adulthood and aging. Thus human development and the benefits of health interventions are cumulative in effect – the health status at a given age is at least partially dependent on interventions in an earlier age group. Prioritizing interventions at several points during the life cycle is necessary for sustained, high-impact improvements in health outcomes.

The major difficulty in low-income countries, where capacity and infrastructure are often lacking, is how to reach people in need. Success in reaching pregnant mothers and infants (under the age of five) has been attained through mother and child programmes and community-based IMCI (integrated management of childhood illness) and ECD (early child development) initiatives. Children above the age of five can be most easily reached through school based health and nutrition programmes, exploiting the existing educational infrastructure. By continuing interventions through the childhood years, the success of ECD and other early interventions can be built upon and strengthened.

Ensuring that children are healthy and able to learn is now recognized as an essential component of an effective education system. This is especially relevant to efforts to achieve 'Education For All' in the most deprived areas, as now more of the poorest and most disadvantaged children, many of whom are girls, have access to school. It is these children, who are often the least healthy and most malnourished, who have the most to gain educationally from improved health.

Good health and nutrition are not only essential inputs but also important outcomes of basic education of good quality. On the one hand, children must be healthy and well nourished in order to fully participate in education and gain its maximum benefits. Thus, programmes which improve health and nutrition can enhance the learning and educational outcomes of school children. On the other hand, quality education, including education about health, can lead to better health and nutrition outcomes for children and, especially through the education of girls, for the next generation of children as well.

Positive experiences by WHO, UNICEF, UNESCO and the World Bank suggest that there is a basic framework that could form the basis for an effective school health and nutrition programme upon which to build. This *FRESH* partnership seeks to Focus Resources on Effective School Health. The framework includes four basic interventions: school-based health policies, provision of safe water and adequate sanitation; skills-based health education; and school-based health and nutrition services.

The cost-effectiveness of mass deworming as the school-based services part of an effective school health and nutrition programme can be maximized by combining control of both schistosome and geohelminth infections, using two drugs: praziquantel and a benzimidazole derivative, such as albendazole. Key to the design of such a strategy is the quantification of the pattern of multiple infections, as this approach will only be cost-effective when these infections are endemic in the same communities (Bundy & de Silva, 1998).

Methods to identify communities warranting a combined control approach will enhance the efficacy of this approach. Geographical information systems (GIS) are being used to develop predictive maps of infection prevalence rates (Brooker et al., 2000). A rapid assessment tool has been developed that can be used to identify target communities/schools warranting treatment of *Schistosoma haematobium* infections (Lengeler et al., 1992). This is a questionnaire-based approach using self-reporting of blood in urine as a reliable indicator of infection.

Conclusion

The combination of impact on physical growth and education gives helminth infection an importance to child development that far outweighs the apparent clinical consequences of infection. A single, oral treatment is sufficient to significantly reduce worm burdens in all but the most intensely infected populations. Mass delivery of anthelmintics is one of the most cost-effective, simple and safe school-based health services that can be delivered by trained teachers. Evaluation of large-scale demonstration school health programmes has shown that school-based health services can have an impact on a broad range of health and education outcomes (Partnership for Child Development, 1998).

References

Anderson R, Medley G. (1985). Community control of helminth infections of man by mass and selective chemotherapy. *Parasitology*: **90**: 629–660.

Ashford RW, Craig PS, Oppenheimer SJ. (1992). Polyparasitism on the Kenyan coast. 1. Prevalence, and association between parasitic infections. *Ann Trop Med Parasitol*: **86**: 671–679.

Beasley N, Tomkins A, Hall A et al. (1999). The impact of population level deworming on haemoglobin levels in Tanga, Tanzania. *Trop Med Int Hlth*: **4**: 744–750.

Booth M, Bundy DAP. (1995). Estimating the numbers of multiple-species geohelminth infections in human communities. *Parasitology*: **111**: 645–653.

Booth M, Bundy DAP, Albonico M, Chiwaya H, Alawi K, Savioli L. (1998). Associations among multiple geohelminth infections in schoolchildren from Pemba Island. *Parasitology*, **116**: 85–93.

Brooker S, Miguel E, Moulin S. (2000). Epidemiology of single and multiple species of helminth infections among schoolchildren in Busia District, Kenya. *E Afr Med J*; **77**: 157–161.

Bundy DAP, Cooper ES. (1989). *Trichuris* and trichuriasis in humans. *Adv Parasitol*; **28**: 107–173.

Bundy DAP, Chandiwana S, Homeida MM, Yoon S, Mott KE. (1991). The epidemiological implications of a multiple species approach to the control of human helminth infections. *Trans Roy Soc Trop Med Hyg*; **85**: 274–276.

Bundy DAP, de Silva NR. (1998). Can we deworm this wormy world? *Br Med Bull*; **54**: 421–432.

Chan L, Bundy DAP, Kan KP. (1994). Aggregation and predisposition to *Ascaris lumbricoides* and *Trichuris trichiura* at the familial level. *Trans Roy Soc Trop Med Hyg*; **88**: 46–48.

Chan MS, Medley GF, Jamison D, Bundy, DAP. (1994). The evaluation of potential global morbidity due to intestinal nematode infections. *Parasitology*, **109**: 373–387.

Cooper ES, Bundy DAP. (1988). *Trichuris* is not trivial. *Parasitol Today*, **4**: 301–306.

Crompton DWT, Tulley JJ. (1987). How much ascariasis is there in Africa? *Parasitol Today*, **3**: 123–127.

Forrester JE, Scott ME, Bundy DAP, Golden MH. (1990). Predisposition of individuals and families in Mexico to heavy infection with *Ascaris lumbricoides* and *Trichuris trichiura*. *Trans Roy Soc Trop Med Hyg*; **84**: 272–276.

Grantham-McGregor SM, Walker SP, Chang S. (2000). Nutritional deficiencies and later behavioural development. *Proc Nutrit Soc*; **59**: 1–8.

Grigorenko E, Sternberg R, Ngorosho D, Jukes M, Bundy D. (2002). Effects of antiparasitic treatment on dynamically assessed cognitive skills (submitted).

Howard SC, Donnelly C, Chan MS. (2000). Methods for estimation of associations between multiple species parasite infections. *Parasitology* (in press).

Lengeler C, Sala-Diakanda D, Tanner M. (1992). Using questionnaires through an existing administrative system: a new approach to health interview surveys. *Int J Epidemiol*; **20**: 796–807.

Marquet S, Abel L, Hillaire D et al. (1996). Genetic localisation of a locus controlling the intensity of infection by *Schistosoma mansoni* on chromosome 5q31–q33. *Nat Genet*; **14**: 181–184.

Miguel E, Kremer M. (2002). Worms: education and health externalities in Kenya. *Econometrica* (submitted).

Needham CS, Kim H, Cong L. (1998). Epidemiology of soil-transmitted nematodes in Ha Nam province, Viet Nam. *Trop Med Int Hlth*; **3**: 904–912.

Partnership for Child Development (1997). Better health, nutrition and education for the school-age child. *Trans Roy Soc Trop Med Hyg*; **91**: 1–2.

Partnership for Child Development (1998). The health and nutritional status of schoolchildren in Africa: evidence from school-based programmes in Ghana and Tanzania. *Trans Roy Soc Trop Med Hyg*; **92**: 254–261.

Pollitt E. (1999). Early iron deficiency anemia and later mental retardation. *Am J Clin Nutrit*; **69**: 4–5.

Pollitt E, Hathirat P, Kotchabhakdi N et al. (1989). Iron deficiency and educational achievement in Thailand. *Am J Clin Nutrit*; **50**: 687–697.

Roche M, Layrisse M. (1966). Hookworm anaemia. *Am J Trop Med Hyg*; **15**: 1029–1102.

Soewondo S, Husaini M, Pollitt E. (1989). Effects of iron deficiency on attention and learning processes in preschool children: Bandung, Indonesia. *Am J Clin Nutrit*; **50**: 667–674.

Stephenson LS. (1987). *Impact of Helminth Infections on Human Nutrition: Schistosomes and Soil Transmitted Helminths*. London: Taylor & Francis.

Stephenson LS, Latham M, Adams EJ. Kinoti SN, Pertet A. (1993). Physical fitness, growth and appetite of Kenyan schoolboys with hookworm, *Trichuris trichiura* and *Ascaris lumbricoides* infections are improved four months after a single dose of albendazole. *J Nutrit*; **123**: 1036–1046.

Sternberg RJ, Powell C, McGrane P. (1997). Effects of a parasitic infection on cognitive functioning. *J Exp Psychol*; **3**: 67–76.

Sternberg R, Grigorenko E, Ngorosho D et al. (2002). Assessing intellectual potential in rural Tanzanian school children. *Intelligence*; **30**: 141–162.

Stolzfus RJ, Albonico M, Chwaya HM, Tielsch JM, Schulze KJ, Savioli L. (1998). Effects of the Zanzibar school-based deworming programme on iron status of children. *Am J Clin Nutrit*; **68**: 179–186.

Tatala S, Svanberg U, Mduma B, (1998). Low dietary iron is a major cause of anaemia: a nutrition survey in the Lindi District of Tanzania. *Am J Clin Nutrit*; **68**: 171–178.

Warren KS, Bundy DAP, Anderson RM. (1993). Helminth infection. In: *Disease Control Priorities in Developing Countries*, ed. DT Jamison et al. Oxford: Oxford University Press.

World Bank (1993). *World Development Report: Investing in Health*. Oxford: Oxford University Press.

22 Intestinal helminths: epidemiology and clinical features

STRONGYLOIDIASIS

The problem in Africa

Strongyloides stercoralis is not an obligatory parasite but a soil worm that is also an opportunistic pathogen in several species of mammal, including humans and also dogs. The factors leading to its acquisition are contact with soil contaminated by faeces, intimate contact with other infected people, e.g. in a household, and modification of the host's immune defences. Two known contributors to the last factor are undernutrition and infection with the retrovirus HTLV1. Reproduction of filariform larvae within the host tissues is further enhanced by extreme immunodeficiency as with cancer, corticosteroid treatment, AIDS, etc. Therefore strongyloidiasis is widespread in Africa and a threat to life under extreme conditions (Genta, 1989).

The parasite

This is a small nematode, just visible to the naked eye. The female is far more prevalent than the male and exists in two juvenile forms, rhabditiform (rod-like, relatively thick) and filariform (thread-like, almost microscopically fine). In soil, the rhabditiform juveniles complete a life cycle involving moults to adulthood, sexual reproduction, female egg production and larval moulting which can produce either further rhabditiform larvae or a filariform parasitic stage. The latter can penetrate skin and enter a parasitic life cycle in the host via the lung's alveoli, the bronchi, swallowing and finally invading the upper small intestinal mucosa. Here adults (all female) produce eggs parthogenetically. The larvae may develop into further filariform juveniles capable of repeating the cycle entirely within the host. The abundance of this form is clearly controlled by immune responses, although it often escapes sufficiently to maintain a lifetime, low level infection. Some eggs and rhabditiform larvae are passed in the faeces to renew the free-living cycle and some filariform larvae invade the skin close to the anus to renew the parasitic cycle (Fig. 22.1).

Epidemiology and prevention

The prevalence of *Strongyloides* infection varies widely among human communities, mostly in warm and moist environments. Crowding and poor sanitation are predictive of higher prevalences. The role of dogs in human transmission is not clear. Good faecal disposal is probably the most effective community preventive measure, although the wearing of shoes may contribute some protection. The parasite is probably often acquired in childhood and carried for life, but symptoms may appear only in adult life during intercurrent disease.

Clinical features

Skin

The classic eruption is called larva currens. Itchy wheals on the buttocks become elongated and serpiginous, moving at several centimetres an hour. In chronic strongyloidiasis stationary urticarial lesions in crops may also appear on the trunk and last a day or so at a time.

Lungs

As with other species of migrating larvae, cough and wheeze may occur. This is accompanied by eosinophilia

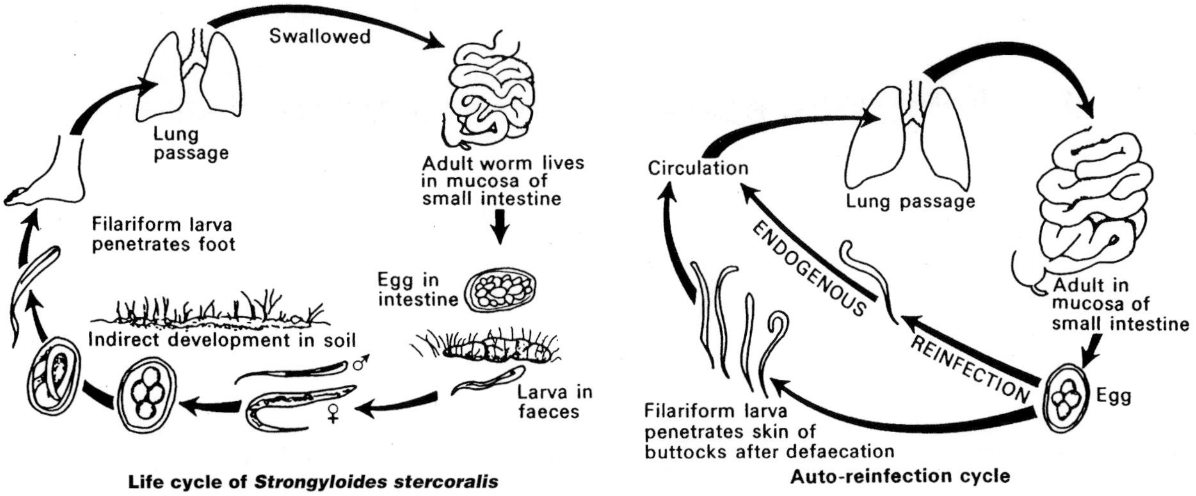

Fig. 22.1. The life cycle of *Strongyloides stercoralis* and the auto re-infection cycle. (Derived from Eshuis & Manschot, 1978.)

and hilar enlargement and pulmonary shadows may be seen on X-ray (Loeffler syndrome).

Gut

There are non-specific symptoms that have not been rigorously associated with the infection, but frank malabsorption and protein-losing enteropathy have been described. On biopsy it is often striking how little inflammation surrounds the adult female worms in the duodenum and jejunum and how intact the villous architecture remains. Rigidity of the duodenum has often been noted by radiologists and the appearance suggests oedema of the upper small intestinal mucosa.

Disseminated strongyloidiasis

This is a possibility to include in the differential diagnosis of any severely ill patient in whom diarrhoea has been a symptom. It is associated with predisposing conditions such as treatment with steroids, malignancy, immunosuppression or cachexia. Fever, shock, jaundice, disseminated intravascular coagulation and coma may occur. Biopsy or necropsy often shows enormous numbers of filariform larvae in every tissue. Secondary gram-negative sepsis is a frequent complication.

Diagnosis

Examination of stool is not a sensitive test. Microscopy after formol-ether concentration may detect rhabditiform larvae or occasionally filariform larvae or eggs, but sensitivity is improved either by Harada–Mori culture (on filter paper) or charcoal culture. Baermann's technique using the larval tropism to light to collect larvae in a Petri dish improves the yield further. An alternative to stool examination is to use the Enterotest capsule in which a sticky thread encased in a digestible gelatine capsule is swallowed and allowed to pass through the pylorus, pulling it back up from the externally fixed upper end after some hours. The adherent mucus is then examined under a microscope: *Giardia* trophozoites are found by the same technique. Where available, serology is far more sensitive, although less specific since (i) the infection may be past, (ii) there may be a cross-reaction with hookworm, filaria or other nematode antigens (Capello & Hotez, 1998).

Treatment

Ivermectin is the drug of choice. A single dose of 200 μg/kg is effective. In disseminated strongyloidiasis it may be needed for 7 days. Thiabendazole 25 mg/kg/day (divided into three doses) may also be used for a similar period, but is less effective in disseminated strongyloidiasis because of relatively poor absorption. It is also more toxic (Marti et al., 1996; Datry et al., 1996; Zaha et al., 2000).

ASCARIS LUMBRICOIDES (Fig. 22.2)

The problem in Africa

ROUNDWORM

This infection is prevalent, affecting up to 90 per cent or more, in both tropical and temperate climates, wherever

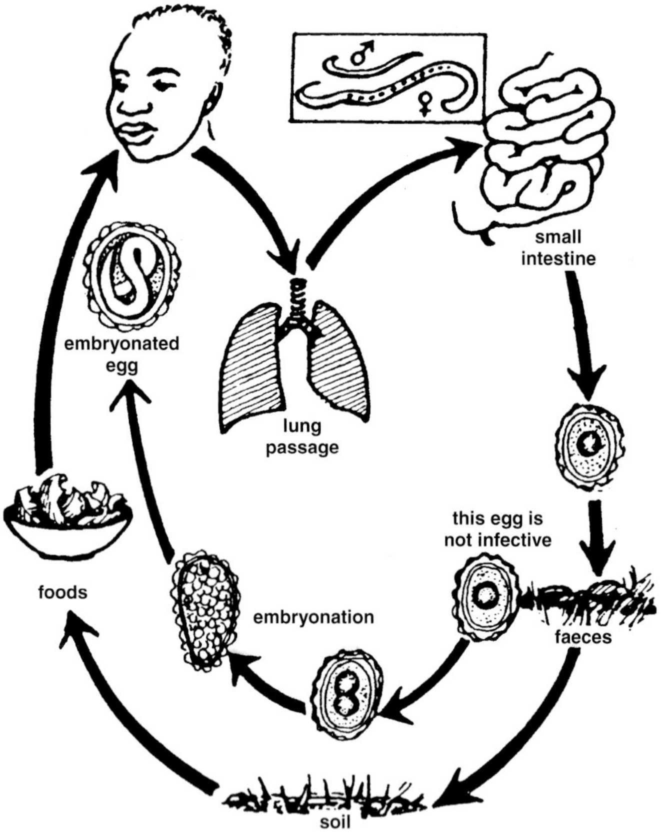

Fig. 22.2. Life cycle of *Ascaris lumbricoides*. (Derived from Eshuis & Manschot, 1978.)

human faeces contaminate soil. People of all ages carry the infection, but young children have higher worm loads and are correspondingly more vulnerable to morbidity.

The parasite

The adult nematode is smooth, muscular, non-segmented and 20–35 cm long. The adults maintain their position in the small intestine by muscular action bracing against peristalsis. They can live for several years and the females produce as many as 200 000 eggs per day. These eggs are not directly infective when passed as they need to embryonate (develop the larva within) while lying in the soil. This means that soil without visible faecal contamination, many months later, may be infective if it is ingested. This occurs either on unwashed food or directly by children who eat soil (pica; geophagia). When swallowed the embryonated eggs release the larvae in the stomach. These invade the small intestinal mucosa, pass to the liver through the portal vein and then through systemic veins to the right heart and pulmonary arteries. From the alveoli they pass in bronchial mucus to be swallowed again, maturing by moulting on this journey. Back in the small intestine, they mature to adulthood. The complete cycle, egg to egg, takes two months.

Epidemiology and infection

All over the developing or non-industrialized world, this is an important parasite, particularly among children, and it is also important in paediatric surgical practice. The parasite will continue to be endemic until faeces are disposed of without contaminating surface soil. This applies to both rural and urban areas. Prevention goes hand in hand with community development (Feachem et al., 1983).

Clinical features

Given the enormous prevalence of the infection and the variation of worm burden that should allow the observation of a gradient of morbidity, perhaps the most remarkable feature is that there is so little agreement about the harmful consequences of harbouring these big worms. Because they inhabit the lumen of the bowel and do not invade tissue except in the larval phase, the host pays a price in accidents rather than in inflammation.

Abdominal pain and discomfort

These symptoms are common both in infected and uninfected children and adults and it is impossible to assess the contribution of worms.

Mechanical effects

A large burden of worms can cause an obstruction requiring emergency surgery, particularly in the small intestine of children, or they may be found at the apex of an intussusception or be the cause of volvulus. If worms migrate into the common bile duct and occlude it, obstructive jaundice, recurrent cholangitis or acute pancreatitis and peritonitis can follow. Ectopic migration of the worms to the larynx, trachea, bronchi, eyes, ENT system, etc., can cause obstructive effects or even fatalities. Migration is promoted by fever, explaining the common vomiting of worms, worms in the nose, etc., of febrile children (Beckingham et al., 1998).

Allergic effects in the lung

As the larvae migrate through the lungs, coughing, wheezing, eosinophilia and sometimes shadows on chest radiography can occur. This is well described in previously uninfected individuals who have entered an endemic zone, but the size of these effects is difficult to assess in local populations. Where soil is contaminated by *A. lumbricoides* eggs, it is also likely to be contaminated by *Toxocara* and other zoonotic nematode eggs and larvae, which may provoke stronger allergic reactions, and so it is impossible to assess the burden of *Ascaris* larva morbidity.

Nutritional effects

Experience from animal husbandry, e.g. the close similarity between *A. suis* infection in the pig and *A. lumbricoides* in man, makes it highly likely that there is an overall negative contribution of roundworm infection to human nutrition and growth. This has not been easy to show in the intricate ecologies of human communities. The most established effect is of exacerbation of Vitamin A deficiency, which will itself have secondary effects on infection, especially mucosal infection, in turn leading to further malnutrition.

Diagnosis and intensity of infection

Eggs of *Ascaris* in the stool confirm the infection. These are easily recognized on microscopy. The counting of eggs per unit weight of faeces is a useful method both in the individual and the community for measuring the intensity of infection, although the correlation with the adult worm burden is only approximate. There are specific laboratory techniques, e.g. the Kato-Katz method which is cheap, quick and easy.

Treatment and prevention

Mebendazole and albendazole are the drugs of choice, equivalent in their efficacy. The dose of mebendazole is 100 mg twice daily for three days or, especially in mass treatment, 500 mg once. Albendazole can be given 200 mg twice daily for three days or 400 mg once (Bennett & Guyatt, 2000).

HOOKWORM INFECTION

The problem in Africa

Hookworm infection is more localized than *Ascaris* and *Trichuris* infections, with some communities heavily infected and others, quite close by, spared. Wet, loamy soil in areas of heavy rainfall promotes the survival and infectivity of the larvae. The adult parasites are long-lived so that an individual's infection can be maintained for many years without re-exposure. If the iron balance is negative, this can mean that an infection acquired in childhood finally leads to severe anaemia in adulthood. Much emphasis has been put on the effects of this on adult workers' productivity, but the infection in childhood also leads to protein-losing enteropathy, growth retardation and delay in physical and possibly mental development. The morbidity is thus directly related to worm burden through gut mucosal inflammatory damage, and to duration of infection through negative nutritional balance, especially for iron (Brooker et al., 1999).

The parasite

The two species that cause disease in man are *Ancylostoma duodenale* and *Necator americanus. Necator* is the more prevalent overall although both species occur in similar environments, except in North Africa where *A. duodenale* predominates completely. The essential, medically relevant, difference between them is that *A. duodenale* causes more morbidity at a smaller worm load. There are morphological differences in the cutting plates that attach the adult mouth to the intestinal mucosa, but otherwise the juvenile forms and the life cycles are very similar.

The adult worms release eggs into the intestinal lumen, which, outside the host, can hatch within 24 to 48 hours. The eggs are relatively thin walled and require warm, moist, shaded conditions for embryonation. The released rhabditiform L1 larvae requires 2–3 days before it moults to the L2 stage and the second moult occurs after a further 5 days, producing the ensheathed (filariform) infective third stage larva. The L3 are non-feeding active stages which move to the periphery of the faecal mass or into the soil, where they can remain active and infective for up to three weeks, depending on the climatic conditions. Hookworms require a moist environment to survive and develop as free-living organisms. Once a host is contacted, the filariform larvae leave their sheaths behind. Hookworm larvae are sensitive to changes in temperature and on contact with a warm-blooded host penetrate the skin rapidly. They enter the capillaries and venous circulation from where they are carried to the alveoli of the lungs, where they undergo the next moult to the L4 stage. After a period of development in the lungs they migrate up the trachea and are swallowed and pass down the oesophagus, through the stomach and into the small intestine. Here they undergo the final moult to produce the young adult stages. The adult hookworms, about 1 cm long, attach to the mucosa of the small intestine with their powerful stoma, abrading the mucosa until they puncture the blood capillaries and can suck the host blood. Heavy hookworm infections can account for as much as 200 ml of blood loss per day.

Humans become infected usually by walking barefoot in contaminated soil. Soil contamination can be extremely heavy, particularly in those communities that use human faeces, known as nightsoil, as fertilizer. Skin penetration is not the only route of infection: *A. duodenale* can also be acquired by ingestion of larvae, for example with unwashed vegetables. Another feature of *A. duodenale* is its ability, using larval hypobiosis within the host, to time maturation and egg production to correspond with the end of the dry season and the maximum chance for survival of the eggs and rhabditiform larvae (Hotez, 1989) (Fig. 22.3).

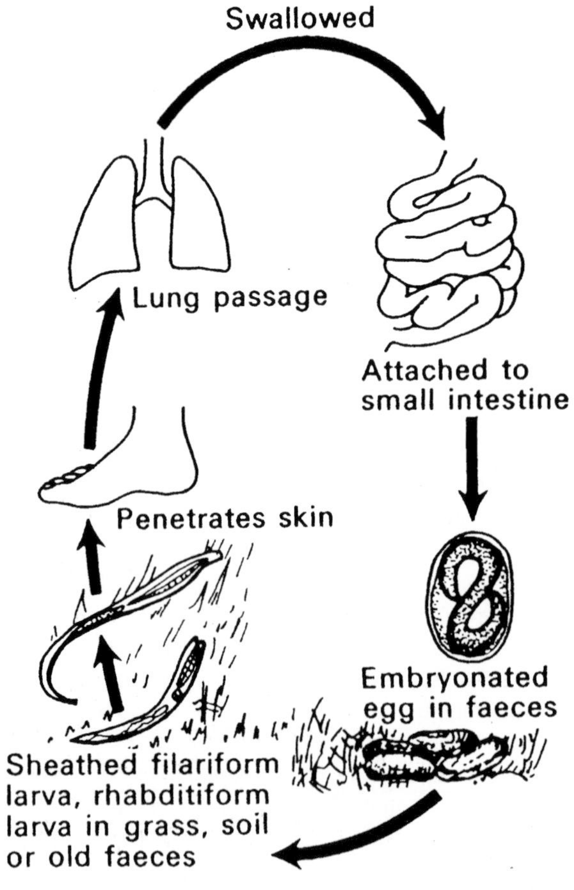

Fig. 22.3. Life cycle of hookworm. (Derived from Eshuis & Manschot, 1978.)

Control

Mass chemotherapy has been relatively effective in hookworm control, at least as compared with *Ascaris*, perhaps because the infective stages do not live so long in the soil. If the water table allows the digging of pit latrines this is also highly effective. Wearing shoes is a traditional recommendation, but the economic advance necessary to allow this would also usually accompany changes in sanitary behaviour and agricultural practice in the same village. Education, especially delivered to school children and accompanied by deworming, appears to be a cost-effective health intervention (Jinabhai et al., 2001).

Clinical features

Ground itch–larval invasion

Larval invasion of the skin is associated with a local dermatitis called ground itch. This is urticarial and there may be a papulovesicular eruption. Where there is intense itching and a serpiginous inflamed area that moves a few centimetres each day, the larva is likely to be that of a zoonotic species such as *Ancylostoma brasiliensis*, a dog hookworm, which will not be able to complete its life cycle in the human host. This will respond to thiabendazole in a steroid ointment, but is eventually self-limiting as the zoonotic invader dies. Ground itch is more transient and is not a common complaint among local children. The phase of larval invasion of the lungs causes cough.

Anaemia – chronic phase

The adult worm phase of infection is chronic.

Children

Oedema, hypoalbuminaemia and growth failure, possibly with diarrhoea and finger-clubbing, are important manifestations but they are not necessarily specific to hookworm infection and may also occur with amoebic dysentery or with intense trichuriasis (see below).

Anaemia is cumulative and is hypochromic and microcytic.

Other nutritional defects such as zinc deficiency, folate deficiency and Vitamin A deficiency are likely to be found in children in a community where children suffer from hookworm infection; it may not be possible to establish specific causality.

Adults

Anaemia affects adult males who have the least access to health services and who may progressively lose physical fitness without recognizing that they are ill. Heart failure is a late manifestation.

Women may be recognized as anaemic in pregnancy, possibly resulting in diagnosis of their helminth infection, although the anaemia itself is also a significant contributor to morbidity and mortality in pregnancy.

Diagnosis

The eggs are seen on stool microscopy. The Kato-Katz method is sensitive and allows quantification of eggs per gram of stool, provided the slide is examined within a few hours as hookworm eggs are fragile. Formol-ether concentration is worth using in light infections, but these may be of little clinical significance anyway. Differentiation between *Necator* and *Ancylostoma* infections is not possible.

Treatment

Mebendazole and albendazole are effective. As with ascariasis, the dose of mebendazole is 100 mg twice daily for 3 days or, especially in mass treatment, 500 mg once. Albendazole can be given 200 mg twice daily for three days or 400 mg once.

ENTEROBIASIS (PINWORM)

The parasite

Enterobius vermicularis is a nematode. The worms are small, white and thread-like. They are often called threadworms, although that name has sometimes also been given to *Strongyloides*. The female is about 10 mm long and larger than the male. They live on intestinal content in the large bowel. The female emerges from the anus, usually at night, and sheds eggs coated in sticky material around the anus. They embryonate rapidly. Perianal itching leads to scratching so that the infective eggs may now lead to a new cycle of auto-infection or to cross infection to other children in family or school. They also survive in dust if it is not too dry (Fig. 22.4).

Epidemiology

This is a cosmopolitan human parasite of little health importance. Infection is not associated with socio-economic deprivation: it can occur in any family or school.

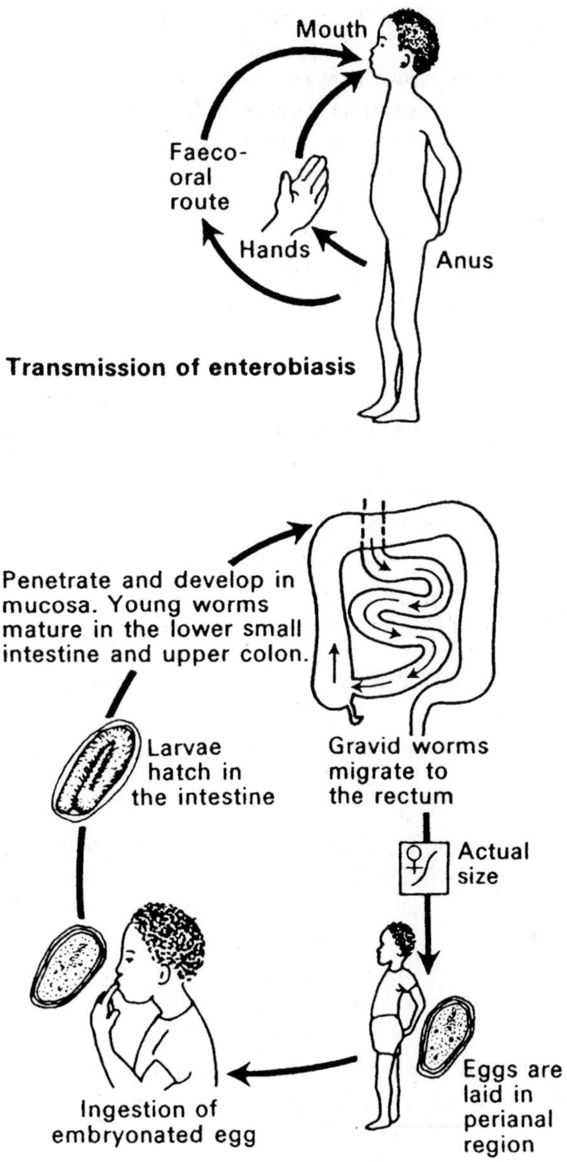

Fig. 22.4. Life cycle of *Enterobius vermicularis*. (Derived from Eshuis & Manschot, 1978.)

Clinical features

Itching around the anus at night can lead to loss of sleep. The other problem is that forward migration of the female worms in female children can lead to inflammation of the vulva and introitus with subsequent discharge and secondary bacteriosis.

Diagnosis

The eggs are seldom seen in stool, so no conclusions on prevalence should be drawn from routine laboratory records. The eggs can be found if sticky tape is placed over the anus at night and peeled off on to a glass slide in the morning. This technique sometimes catches *Strongyloides* rhabditiform larvae also. The effort is usually unnecessary: treatment can be given on the history alone.

Treatment

The parasite is sensitive to mebendazole and albendazole and single doses will kill the adults. However, it is advisable to treat all the children in the household and to repeat the treatment several times as embryonated eggs on the host or on siblings may escape.

TRICHURIS TRICHIURA (WHIPWORM)

The parasite

The adult is shaped like a whip, with the handle representing the wider posterior section containing the reproductive organs and the intestine, while the long, fine anterior part, called the stichosome, contains the long pharynx. The whole is about 4 cm long. The male's posterior end is curled into a flat spiral, making it easy to distinguish: the sex ratio is close to unity. The stichosomes lie within the colonic mucosa in superficial tunnels while the posterior ends are free in the lumen where both copulation and egg release can occur.

Life cycle

Eggs, passed in the faeces, contain a zygote and are not infectious until embryonation, which takes place in the soil over 2 to 4 weeks. The egg now contains the L1 larva. Following human ingestion, the larva is released in the stomach, and passes into the intestine. It penetrates the epithelium in the mucosal crypts of the caecum. The larva develops by moulting, and the adult develops from the L4 stage, by now having migrated with the epithelial cells up the sides of the crypts. Each female produces up to 20 000 eggs per day; the life expectancy of a worm within the host has been estimated at 1–3 years, which would imply that some adults live far longer.

Epidemiology and control

The conditions that favour soil contamination with *Trichuris* eggs, their survival and ingestion are similar to those for *Ascaris*, and the two intestinal parasites have similar human distributions and prevalences. Co-infections of a single host are also common, although intense and pure infections with one parasite are also commonly found. In some communities nearly 100 per cent of stools contain the eggs. More intense infections occur in children and worm burdens of several thousand involve the terminal ileum, the whole colon and the rectum, whereas the more common light burdens of only a few worms are confined to the caecum. The gradient of intensity of infection corresponds predictably with a gradient of morbidity (*cf. Ascaris*): once more than 100 worms are present, involving colonic mucosa beyond the caecum, effects on a child's growth are apparent.

Control in the community, similar to that for *Ascaris* and hookworm, involves the disposal of faeces without contaminating surface soil. Repeated chemotherapy using mebendazole or albendazole, targeted towards children, will reduce transmission, although rebound is inevitable if other conditions are not improved (Phiri et al., 2000).

Clinical features

This nematode was mistakenly regarded as harmless for many years, despite sporadic reports in the literature describing a clinical syndrome of chronic dysentery with rectal prolapse, accompanied by anaemia. Four things led to the underestimation of *Trichuris trichiura* as a pathogen:

- low-intensity infections, which are by far the most common, are asymptomatic
- *Trichuris* is seldom found as the only pathogen but is commonly just one of multiple health and environmental threats to a child
- the onset of significant symptoms is often too slow to be noticed by the family
- it produces a transient, although prolonged, disease of the developing child, while seldom causing disability to adults.

Intense infections are associated with:

- geophagia
- frequent mucoid stools often with frank blood
- rectal prolapse
- extreme hypochromic, microcytic anaemia, comparable to that in hookworm infection

- stunting of growth and delayed development, that is also similar
- clubbing of the fingers. The latter feature was first described in South Africa, where trichuriasis is a common clinical problem (Bundy & Cooper, 1989).

Diagnosis

Eggs of *Trichuris* in the stool, which are robust, confirm the infection. As with *Ascaris*, these are easily recognized on microscopy and the Kato–Katz method for the counting of eggs per unit weight of faeces is an equally useful method. Because intense whipworm infection causes a clinical colitis, double contrast barium enemas or colonoscopies are sometimes performed as part of the investigation. The carpeting of the mucosa with the worms is then seen. Anoscopy can be done in the clinic, using an otoscope for a young child: if worms are seen in the rectal mucosa then the infection is intense and treatment will be curative.

Treatment

Trichuris is more resistant to chemotherapy than *Ascaris* and hookworm, although mebendazole and albendazole are highly and equally effective. However, single dose treatment is unlikely to clear the infection. The dose of mebendazole is 100 mg twice daily for 3 days and albendazole 200 mg twice daily for 3 days. For symptomatic infections in children whose environment remains unchanged, re-treatment every 3 months is advised.

Tapeworm infection (Taeniasis)

These are flat, segmented worms: cestodes. They are quite different from the roundworms, nematodes. The species in Africa in which man is the definitive host are members of the order Cyclophyllidea, of the genera *Taenia* and *Hymenolepis*, although *Diphyllobothrium latum*, native to the Eurasian land mass, is one member of a different order, Pseudophyllidea, which can be introduced to Africa with migration.

The adult worms seldom cause serious disease, but the larval cysts in tissue are responsible for serious morbidity (human cysticercosis from *Taenia solium*) and economic loss (animal cysticercosis from *Taenia saginata* and *Taenia solium*). Although the intestinal adult worms are relatively harmless parasites, the motile segments (proglottids) are passed in stool and have psychological, social, cultural and mythological impact as a visible manifestation of infection and personal invasion.

Tapeworms in which man is not the definitive host, mainly *Echinococcus granulosus* responsible for hydatid disease in man, are considered elsewhere (Chapter 23).

Taenia saginata

The problem in Africa is largely in the cattle-raising regions of East and Central Africa, but individual cases will be found throughout the continent as this is a truly cosmopolitan infection.

Parasite

Since the human is the only definitive host, intermediate hosts such as cattle can only become infected by eating grass contaminated by human faeces. The eggs hatch in the ruminant's intestine and emerging larvae (oncospheres) penetrate the intestinal mucosa and end up via the lymphatics and the circulation in muscles. There the scolex of a future tapeworm develops within the bladder of the complete cysticercus. If this is then eaten as a component of undercooked meat, the scolex will attach itself to the luminal surface of its new host's small intestine by its four suckers. New segments, proglottides, will develop distally until the entire worm (strobila) attains a length up to 12 metres. The most distal proglottids are the most mature, containing a branched uterus full of eggs. These become detached so that the human passes six or so such segments every day. The period of maturation is about three months, during which the proglottids will not appear in the stool. After passage through the anus the uteri expel the eggs which can remain viable in the grass for many months, and the cycle can be completed by further ingestion by a ruminant (Fig. 22.5).

Epidemiology and control

The opportunity for parasite multiplication is confined to the proglottids within the definitive (human) host. The highest human prevalence is attained in nomadic communities where people live with and for their herds of cattle. The cattle themselves are not all infected: this is likely to be through immunological control of the larvae since epidemic cysticercosis is observed in naïve cattle freshly infected by a single human source. Treatment of human hosts is an important control measure as this interrupts the cycle. Meat inspection is important and

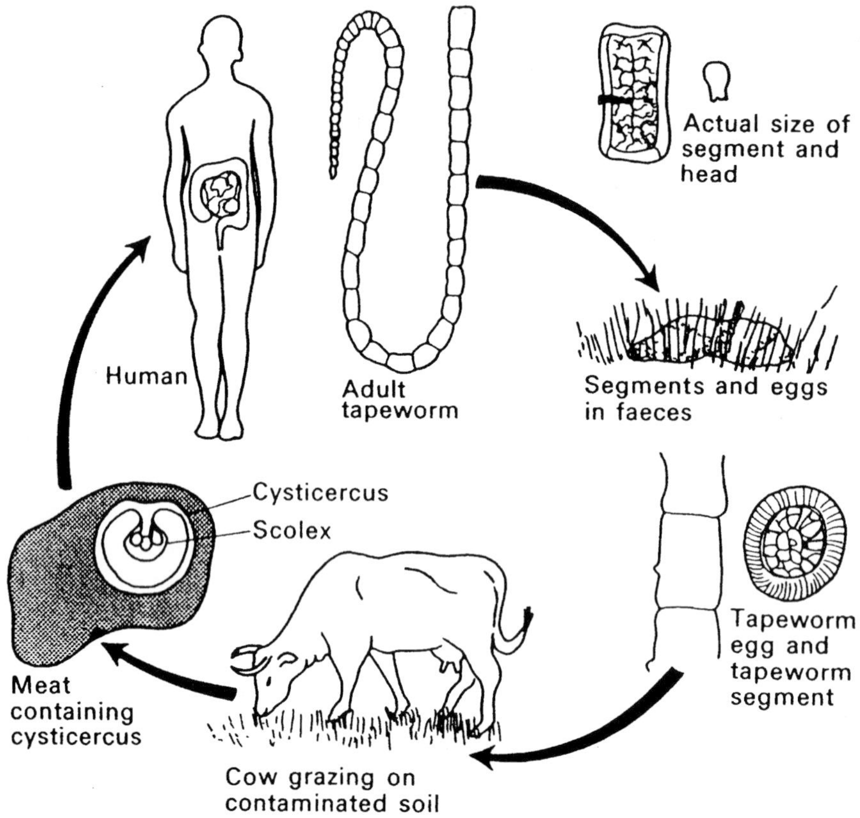

Fig. 22.5. Life cycle of *Taenia saginata*. (Derived from Eshuis & Manschot, 1978.)

infected meat should be condemned, but this is not so effective in control of the parasite life cycle. Sanitation would be effective but is difficult to introduce to nomadic herders. Thorough cooking of the inside of meat is difficult when barbecuing on charcoal is the chosen method, but boiling will sterilize it.

Clinical features

It is difficult to separate mythology from reality in the symptoms: weight loss, colic, irritability and insomnia are mentioned and seem plausible, appetite gain less so. The proglottids can be felt moving at the anus and seen in the stool: this may upset the patient.

Treatment

Praziquantel is the drug of choice. A single dose of 10 to 20 mg/kg is effective. Niclosamide is an alternative. The adult dose is 2 g, reduced to 1 g for children 11–34 kg and 1.5 g for children over 34 kg (Schantz, 1996).

Taenia solium

Cysticercosis in man is the most important consequence of this infection, in which man can act as an aberrant intermediate host as well as the definitive host. Neurocysticercosis is the most common specific cause of epilepsy in the world. Cysticercosis is common in central and southern Africa, and is described in Chapter 23.

Hymenolepis nana

This is both the smallest and the most common tapeworm of man. It grows only to a length of 4 cm with a width of 1 mm. However, the parasite burden in the human ileum can number thousands. There is no requirement for an intermediate host, although insects can provide the cysticercoid phase and rodents are alternative definitive hosts: infection is by person-to-person spread with faecally contaminated hands or food. Internal auto-infection occurs. It is most common in dry climates, suggesting that it may be one of the diseases associated with poor water supply in the 'water-washed' rather than 'water-borne' categories. High prevalence has been noted in Egypt and Zimbabwe.

Clinical features

Most infections are asymptomatic, although allergic manifestations such as phlyctenular conjunctivitis have been described (cf. primary tuberculosis). The situation is somewhat analogous to strongyloidiasis, although the organisms are totally unrelated: it is an opportunistic pathogen with the capacity for auto-infection, with extremely ill-defined symptoms in light infections but uncontrolled internal reproduction in immunodeficient states.

Diagnosis

This is entirely by microscopy of stool. The eggs are fragile and fresh stool should be examined, repeatedly if possible.

Treatment

Both praziquantel and niclosamide are effective. However, the total dosage is higher than for taeniasis: praziquantel is given in a single dose of 25 mg/kg and niclosamide is given as for taeniasis, but following the initial dose by half the initial dose daily for the 6 following days (Wittner & Tanowitz, 1999).

References

Beckingham IJ, Cullis SN, Krige JE et al. (1998). Management of hepatobiliary and pancreatic Ascaris infestation in adults after failed medical treatment. *Br J Surg*; **85**: 907–910.

Bennett A, Guyatt H. (2000). Reducing intestinal nematode infection: efficacy of albendazole and mebendazole. *Parasitol Today*; **16**: 71–74.

Brooker S, Peshu N, Warn PA et al. (1999). The epidemiology of hookworm infection and its contribution to anaemia among pre-school children on the Kenyan coast. *Trans Roy Soc Trop Med Hyg*; **93**: 240–246.

Bundy AP, Cooper ES. (1989). Human *Trichuris* and trichuriasis. *Adv Parasitol*; **28**: 107–173.

Cappello M, Hotez P. (1998). Strongyloides and Capillaria. In Topley & Wilson's *Microbiology and Microbial Infections*, Vol.5, *Parasitology*, ed FEG Cox, JP Kreier, D Wakelin, 9th edn, pp. 583–590. Arnold.

Datry A, Hilmarsdottir I, Mayorga-Sagastume R et al. (1996). Treatment of Strongyloides stercoralis infection with ivermectin compared with albendazole: results of an open study of 60 cases. *Trans Roy Soc Trop Med Hyg*; **88**: 344–345.

Feachem RG, Guy MW, Harrison S et al. (1983). Excreta disposal facilities and intestinal parasitism in urban Africa: preliminary studies in Botswana, Ghana and Zambia. *Trans Roy Soc Trop Med Hyg*; **77**: 515–521.

Genta RM. (1989). Global prevalence of strongyloidiasis: critical review with epidemiologic insights into the prevention of disseminated disease. *Rev Infect Dis*; **11**: 755–767.

Hotez PJ. (1989). Hookworm disease in children. *Pediatr Infect Dis J*; **85**: 16–20.

Jinabhai CC, Taylor M. Coutsoudis A et al. (2001). Epidemiology of helminth infections: implications for parasite control programmes, a South African perspective. *Public Health Nutr*; **4**: 1211–1219.

Marti H, Haji HJ, Savioli L et al. (1996). A comparative trial of a single-dose ivermectin versus three days of albendazole for treatment of Strongyloides stercoralis and other soil- transmitted helminth infections in children. *Am J Trop Med Hyg*; **55**: 477–481.

Phiri K, Whitty CJ, Graham SM et al. (2000). Urban/rural differences in prevalence and risk factors for intestinal helminth infection in southern Malawi *Ann Trop Med Parasitol*; **94**: 381–387.

Schantz PM. (1996). Tapeworms (cestodiasis). *Gastroenterol Clin North Am*; **25**: 637–653.

Wittner M, Tanowitz HB. (1999). Other cestode infections. In *Tropical Infectious Diseases: Principles, Pathogens, and Practice*; pp. 1026–1030. Philadelphia: Churchill-Livingstone.

Zaha OA, Hirata T, Kinjo F et al. (2000). A. Strongyloidiasis – progress in diagnosis and treatment. *Intern Med*; **39**: 695–700.

23 Cysticercosis

The problem in Africa

Cysticercosis is an important cause of epilepsy and other acute and chronic neurological problems in some parts of Africa (Table 23.1). The diagnosis may not be obvious from the clinical presentation, and without sophisticated imaging, the extent to which cysticercosis is at the root of local neurological disease may be substantially underestimated. A soundly based knowledge of the local prevalence of the disease, best obtained by a serological survey, is an invaluable guide to understanding neurological disease in Africa.

The organism

Cysticercosis is caused by the larval, or metacestode, form of the pork tapeworm, *Taenia solium*. Humans are the only host for the adult tapeworm, which lives in the small intestine. Apart from a small head (scolex) equipped with suckers and hooks for attachment to the intestinal mucosa, the bulk of the tapeworm, divided into numerous segments, has the sole function of generating eggs, which it does with great efficiency.

An adult worm is typically about 2 m long, has several hundred segments, and is estimated to generate some hundreds of millions of eggs each year for 5 to 10 years. Eggs are passed in the faeces directly, or within intact motile segments that have separated from the end of the worm. Tapeworm segments that are noticed by a patient emerging from the anus by their own motility, unrelated to defaecation, are much more likely to belong to *Taenia saginata*, the beef tapeworm, which does not cause human cysticercosis.

Cysticercosis is acquired by ingesting *T. solium* eggs. Only pigs and humans are susceptible. Eggs hatch in the duodenum to an invasive larval stage known as an oncosphere. These migrate through the tissues until they further develop into the characteristic static metacestode stage; the cysticercus. Cysticerci are small (around 0.5 cm) bladders made up of a translucent sack containing clear fluid and a central white protoscolex. When dissected out they resemble a miniature raw egg. They are found most commonly in muscle and brain but may occur in many tissues. The life cycle is maintained by humans ingesting live cysticerci in pork meat which then develop into new tapeworms in the gut.

Human cysticercosis is therefore acquired by the faeco-oral route from tapeworm carriers. *T. solium* tapeworm carriers themselves may acquire cysticercosis through autoinfection and sometimes have very heavy infection (Garcia & Del Brutto, 1999). Members of their household are also at increased risk.

Epidemiology

The prevalence of cysticercosis is determined by pig-rearing practices and by the quality of human hygiene and sanitation. The parasite is much more prevalent in pigs that live in close association with humans. The common rural African practice of keeping pigs within a village where they can be conveniently fed on household waste, and may be allowed to scavenge, promotes the possibility of their ingesting material contaminated by human faeces. Cysticerci are easily visible in heavily infected pork meat ('measly pork'), but their significance is often not understood. Sanitation is of central importance in reducing transmission from human faeces to both pigs and people.

In regions where pigs are not eaten by any section of the community, as in the Islamic countries of North

Table 23.1. Examples of some reported prevalences of cysticercosis in Africa

Country	Setting	Method	Population	Prevalence (%)	Reference
South Africa	Rural Hospital	CT Scan	Patients with epilepsy	28	(van As & Joubert, 1991)
Mozambique	City Hospital	Serology	Blood donors and mixed hospital attenders	12	(Vilhena et al., 1999)
Togo	Community	Serology (and clinical)	1. Rural population 2. Patients with epilepsy	2.3 29	(Dumas et al., 1990)
Madagascar		Serology	Patients with epilepsy	22	(Andriantsimahavandy et al., 1997)
Burundi	Community	Serology	Patients with epilepsy	5	(Newell et al., 1997)

Africa, cysticercosis is a rarity. In mixed communities, those who do not eat pork may be infected by tapeworm eggs from those who do. Prevalences in Sub Saharan Africa vary widely and in many regions have not been well investigated. The disease appears to be most common in Southern Africa. Examples of some reported prevalences are in Table 23.1.

Prevention and control

Cysticerci are killed by thorough cooking, but may survive inadequate cooking and can survive for up to four weeks in refrigerated meat. The parasite has been controlled in formerly high prevalence areas, such as Central Europe, by the systematic inspection of pork meat at abattoirs. This, combined with public health improvements in the sanitary disposal of human faeces, interrupts the life cycle at two points and effectively eliminates the parasite.

In rural Africa, where the resources for these changes may not be present, control traditionally depends on providing education about safe pig rearing practices and the significance of measly pork, together with whatever can be achieved towards improved sanitation. A newer strategy is to reduce tapeworm carriage by mass population treatment with antihelminthics (Allan et al., 1997). Although, depending on resources and the local prevalence of the disease, this strategy may be difficult to justify for the control of cysticercosis alone, it could be an important additional benefit from mass treatment programmes for the control of schistosomiasis with praziquantel.

Clinical features

The important clinical consequences of cysticercosis are caused by cysts in the central nervous system, or less commonly the eye. Cysts in the brain occur as small (up to 2 cm) space occupying lesions, sometimes with moderate surrounding inflammation (Fig 23.1). They are usually multiple. They may occur at any intracranial site. Neurocysticercosis is a common incidental post mortem finding in endemic areas, implying that most affected individuals have no symptoms.

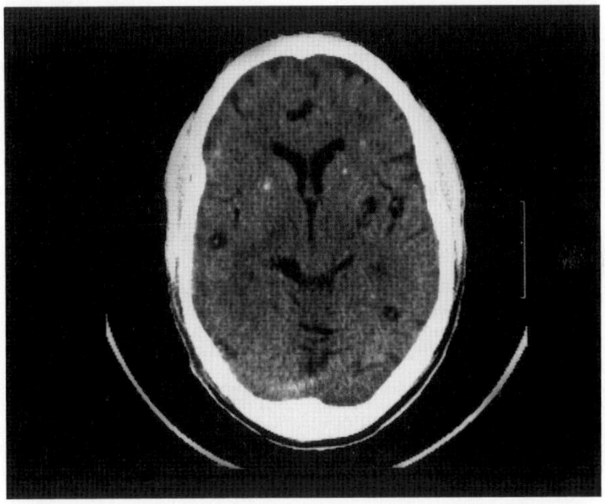

Fig. 23.1. CT brain scan of a Zimbabwean man presenting with new onset epilepsy. There are old calcified cysts appearing as small white densities as well as viable cysts, appearing as dark round lucencies, some with a visible central dense protoscolex.

Epilepsy is the most frequent clinical presentation. It occurs in approximately 80% of symptomatic cases and may be generalized or focal (White, 1997). Headache occurs in around a third of cases. A variety of focal neurological deficits can occur, depending on the location of the parasite, including paraparesis from cysts in or around the spinal cord. Cysts in the ventricular system or basal cystern may cause obstructive hydrocephalus. When there are many actively inflamed cysts, most typically in children, the presentation may resemble a

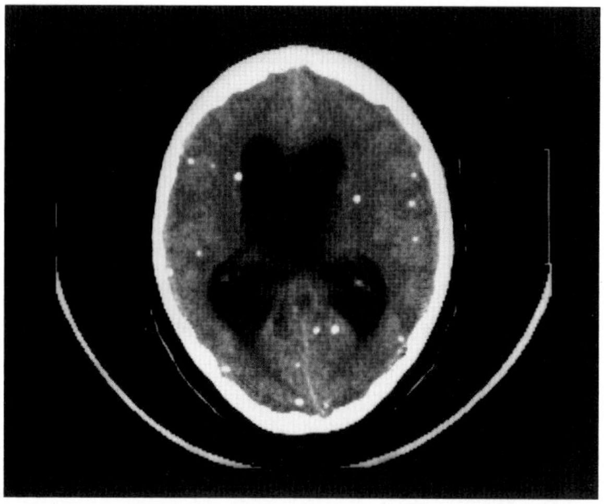

Fig. 23.2. The catastrophic sequelae of severe cysticercosis: This is a CT brain scan of a young Zimbabwean woman who was investigated for dementia and cortical blindness of several years duration. She has numerous old clacified cysticerci as well as gross hydrocephalus. There are no longer any viable cysts and anticysticercal treatment will have no effect.

sub-acute encephalitis, with confusion, and often raised intracranial pressure. The most severely affected patients may sustain severe irreversible damage with hydrocephalus and dementia (Joubert, 1990) (Fig 23.2).

Diagnosis

Cysticercosis may be difficult to distinguish from a wide variety of other focal neurological diseases such as tumours, tuberculomas and vascular accidents as well as idiopathic epilepsy. There may be evidence of cysticerci in other tissues. Sub-cutaneous cysticerci are easily palpable, soft, non-tender swellings that can be confirmed on biopsy. Cysticerci in muscle appear radiologically as spindle shaped calcifications about 0.5 cm long. They may be a chance finding on a chest X-ray in the muscles of neck and shoulder girdle. Unfortunately these clues are seldom present. Plain X-ray of the skull for calcified cysts has too low a yield to be easily justified. In post-mortem studies, more than 75 per cent of cysticerci have some contact with the meninges. In about half of cases there is some abnormality of the CSF; a mild pleocytosis or raised protein, but these changes are not specific.

A large variety of serological tests for cysticercosis have been described. They are not completely sensitive and may cross react with other related cestode infections but are a valuable aid to diagnosis if they are available. Recently, whole blood dried on filter paper has been shown to give satisfactory results when eluted for an ELISA (Peralta et al., 2001). This may make the technique more easily applicable to field conditions. The diagnosis is most directly made by modern imaging techniques, which show cysticerci in the brain as small lucent defects with the protoscolex sometimes visible as a central density. Cysts that show contrast enhancement are probably degenerating and may have disappeared on repeat scanning after a few months (Mitchell & Crawford, 1988). Dead, calcified cysts are also commonly seen.

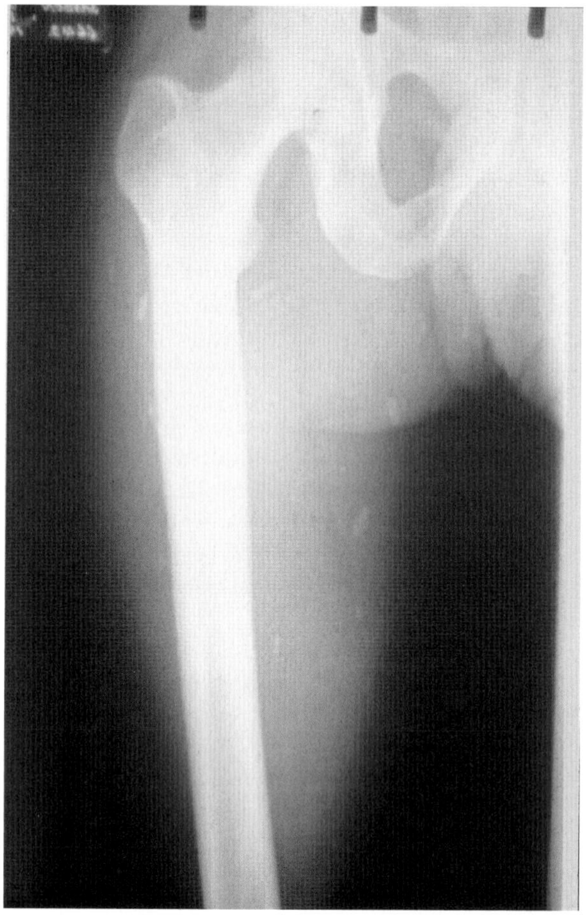

Fig. 23.3. Radiograph to show calcified cysticerci in muscles of thigh and buttock.

In the absence of these diagnostic tools, the management of neurological disease needs to be informed by an awareness of cysticercosis and some idea of its prevalence in the local community, which can be greatly underestimated if only clinical impressions are relied upon. A serological survey or a post mortem series can provide invaluable information.

Management

Epilepsy should be controlled in the normal way.

Raised intracranial pressure may respond to corticosteroids, which must be given as early as possible in the childhood encephalitic manifestation of the disease if permanent neurological damage is to be minimized. If raised intracranial pressure is secondary to obstructive hydrocephalus, only surgical shunting procedures are likely to be of benefit. Even if their intracranial pressure is not raised, children are more likely to have inflamed cysts than adults and may have some symptomatic benefit from corticosteroids, but in the absence of a definite diagnosis this is unwise, as tuberculosis and other infections remain possible.

The role of **anti-helminthics** is controversial (Salinas & Prasad, 2000). The effective drugs are praziquantel and albendazole. The number and size of cysts seen on imaging can be reduced with treatment, but the extent to which this improves epilepsy and other symptoms is more variable. Cysts may in any case disappear spontaneously, especially in children (50–80% in 1 year; Singhi et al., 2000). Early studies have used intense and prolonged treatment, commonly praziquantel 50 mg/kg/day for 15 days (Sotelo et al., 1984) or albendazole 15 mg/kg/day for 28 days. Shorter courses, that are more achievable in resource-poor countries, may be nearly as effective. Albendazole is now more often given for 8 days. Three doses of praziquantel, 25 mg/kg, given 2-hourly on a single day have been reported as effective (Corona et al., 1996). All these treatments, by disrupting cysts, may provoke inflammation and a temporary exacerbation of symptoms, which may occasionally be dangerous. Steroids are commonly given with anticysticercal therapy in an attempt to prevent these complications but significant problems may still occur. Praziquantel is metabolized by cytochrome P450 and blood levels may be reduced if other drugs that induce this enzyme system are also given; for example many anti-convulsants, rifampicin and steroids (Sotelo & Jung, 1998). Given the expense and modest benefits of specific anti-cysticercal treatment, it may not be regarded as a priority in many African health care settings.

References

Allan JC, Velasquez-Tohom M, Fletes C et al. (1997). Mass chemotherapy for intestinal Taenia solium infection: effect on prevalence in humans and pigs. *Trans Roy Soc Trop Med Hyg*; **91**: 595–598.

Andriantsimahavandy A, Lesbordes JL, Rasoaharimalala B et al. (1997). Neurocysticercosis: a major aetiological factor of late-onset epilepsy in madagascar. *Trop Med Int Hlth*; **2**: 741–746.

Corona T, Lugo R, Medina R, Sotelo J. (1996). Single-day praziquantel therapy for neurocysticercosis. *N Eng J Med*; **334**: 125.

Dumas M, Grunitzky K, Belo M et al. (1990). [Cysticercosis and neurocysticercosis: epidemiological survey in North Togo]. [French]. *Bull Soc Path Exotique*; **83**: 263–274.

Garcia HH, Del Brutto OH. (1999). Heavy nonencephalitic cerebral cysticercosis in tapeworm carriers. The Cysticercosis Working Group in Peru. *Neurology*; **53**: 1582–1584.

Joubert, J. (1990). Cysticercal meningitis – a pernicious form of neurocysticercosis which responds poorly to praziquantel. *S Afr Med J*; **77**: 528–530.

Mitchell WG, Crawford TO. (1988). Intraparenchymal cerebral cysticercosis in children: diagnosis and treatment. [Review] [24 refs]. *Pediatrics*; **82**: 76–82.

Newell E, Vyungimana F, Geerts S, Van Kerckhoven I, Tsang VC, Engels D. (1997). Prevalence of cysticercosis in epileptics and members of their families in Burundi. *Trans Roy Soc Trop Med Hyg*; **91**: 389–391.

Peralta RH, Macedo HW, Vaz AJ, Machao LR, Peralta JM. (2001). Detection of anti-cysticercus antibodies by ELISA using whole blood collected on filter paper. *Trans Roy Soc Trop Med Hyg*; **95**: 35–36.

Salinas R, Prasad K. (2000). Drugs for treating neurocysticercosis (tapeworm infection of the brain). [Review] [4 refs]. *Cochrane Database Syst Rev* [computer file] CD000215.

Singhi P, Ray M, Singhi S, Khandelwal N. (2000). Clinical spectrum of 500 children with neurocysticercosis and response to albendazole therapy. *J Child Nuerol*; **15**: 207–213.

Sotelo J, Escobedo F, Rodriguez-Carbajal J, Torres B, Rubio-Donnadieu F. (1984). Therapy of parenchymal brain cysticercosis with praziquantel. *N Engl J Med*; **310**: 1001–1007.

Sotelo J, Jung H. (1998). Pharmacokinetic optimisation of the treatment of neurocysticercosis. [Review] [75 refs]. *Clin Pharmacokinet*; **34**: 503–515.

van As AD, Joubert J. (1991). Neurocysticercosis in 578 black epileptic patients. *S Afr Med J*; **80**:327–328.

Vilhena M, Santos M, Torgal J (1989). Seroprevalence of human cysticercosis in Maputo, Mozambique. *Am J Trop Med Hyg*; **61**: 59–62.

White AC (1997). Neurocysticercosis: a major cause of neurological disease worldwide. *Clin Infect Dis*; **24**: 101–115.

24 Hydatid disease

The problem in Africa

Hydatid disease of animals and man is prevalent in many parts of Africa, where man, sheep and dogs live in close contact (Fig. 24.1). The parasite causes human morbidity and mortality, and also contributes indirectly to human disease by its effects on domestic animals. One of the highest incidence rates of hydatid disease anywhere in the world exists among the Turkana pastoralists of northwest Kenya. In this tribe of 200 000 there are approximately 200–300 new cases of hydatid disease each year. High rates are also seen in Islamic Africa (MacPherson et al.,1989).

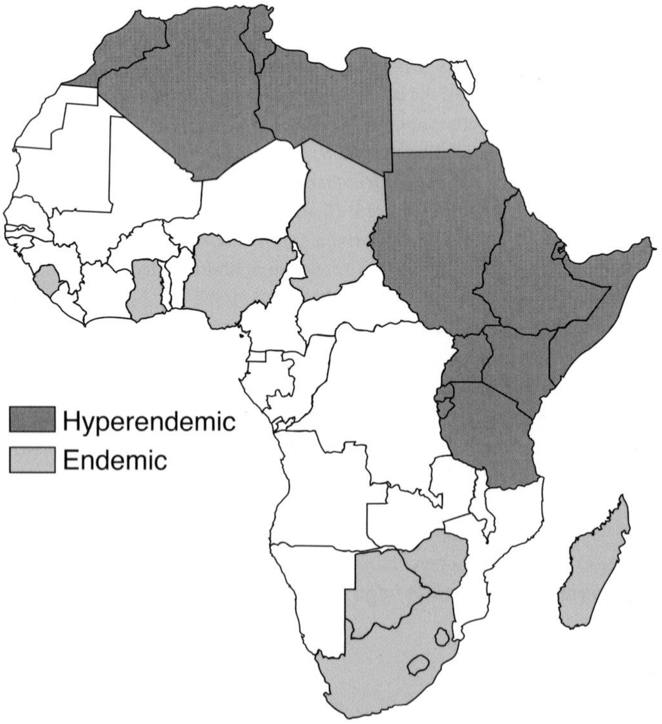

Fig. 24.1. The distribution of hydatid disease in Africa

Organism and vector

The adult stage of *Echinococcus granulosus,* a tapeworm about 3–6 mm long, is found in enormous numbers, deeply embedded in the gut mucosa of the definitive host, a carnivore such as the domestic dog or jackal. Proglottids containing thousands of ova are discharged in the dog's faeces and are eaten by grazing animals such as camels, cattle, sheep, goats, pigs, and horses which become the intermediate hosts. Humans may become infected by hand-to-mouth transfer of ova picked up by stroking a dog, or by drinking water or eating food contaminated by dog faeces (Fig. 24.2).

In all these intermediate hosts the ova hatch in the duodenum, larvae penetrate the gut wall and travel via the portal vein to the liver where most are retained. A few may end up in the lungs, bone, and other tissues. The larvae develop into cysts with an outer laminated layer and an inner germinal layer which produces protoscolices, or from which daughter cysts and brood capsules – full of protoscolices – arise. Protoscolices are the embryonic invaginated tapeworm heads.

The cysts grow slowly over many years and may reach a diameter of 20 cm or more in soft tissues. The cycle is completed when, after the death of the intermediate host, a carnivore ruptures the cysts and ingests the protoscolices which become attached to the gut mucosa and develop into adult worms (Fig. 24.2).

Many cysts die young for there is a contest between parasite and host: later, they may be seen as round calcified opacities on a radiograph. When a live cyst is

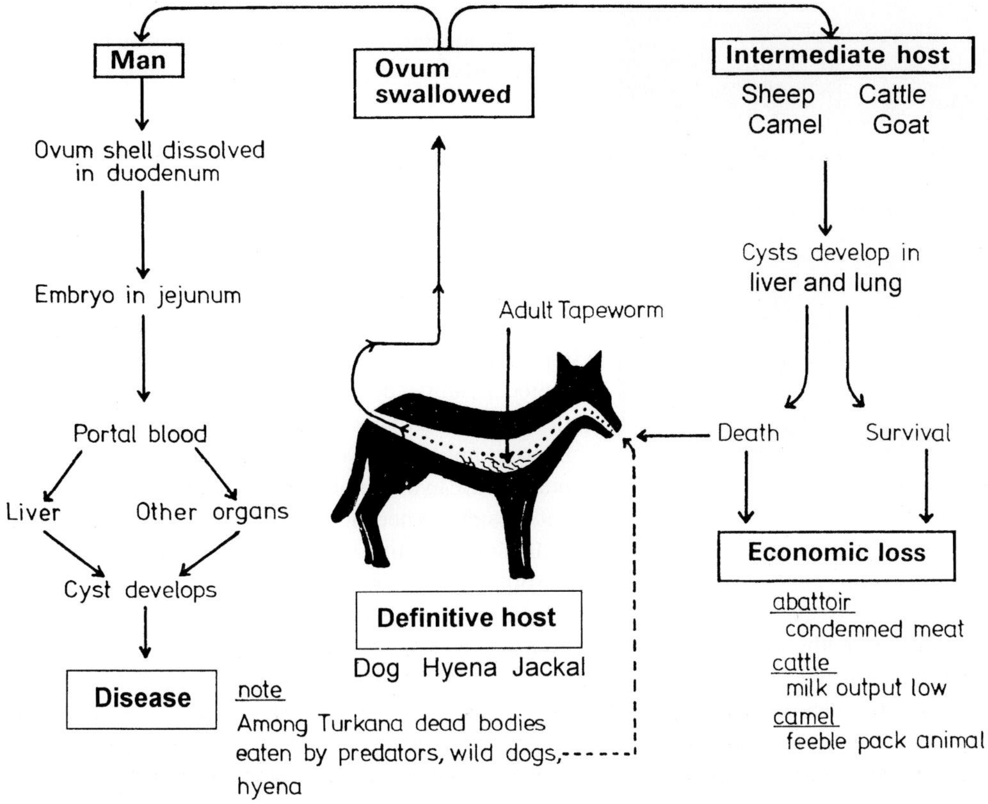

Fig. 24.2. The life cycle of *Echinococcus granulosus*

opened it may be found to be filled with small daughter cysts (Fig. 24.3) or a suspension of hydatid sand consisting of separated brood capsules and liberated protoscolices. Some cysts are sterile and contain only clear water.

Scolices may be cultured in vitro in diphasic medium containing bile. This method has revealed differences between parasites from different animal species such as horses and sheep. The strain differences may explain some of the epidemiological variations in hydatid disease in different parts of the world.

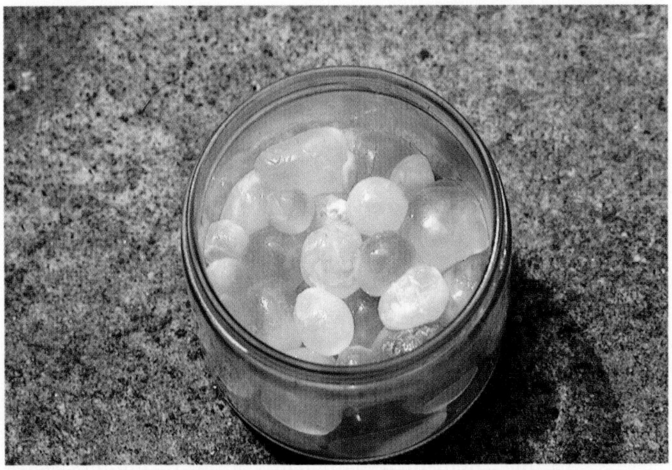

Fig. 24.3. Daughter cysts.

Epidemiology

The animal host and its ecology

Dogs are the main source of human infection, getting infected themselves by eating the viscera of sheep. Goats, camels, cattle and wild herbivores are usually less important reservoirs of infection.

The Turkana people are nomadic over an area of some 24 000 square miles in north-west Kenya and south-eastern Sudan (French et al., 1982). They herd sheep, and goats, cattle, camels, and donkeys. About 6 per cent of the Turkana population have hydatid cysts demonstrable by ultrasound scanning, and about 40–70 per cent of the dogs are infected. The high incidence of hydatid disease is explained by the intimate relationship between humans and their dogs (Watson-Jones & Macpherson,

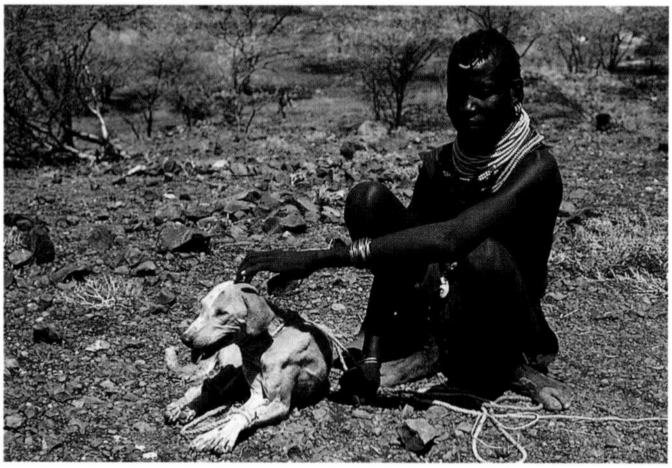

Fig. 24.4. A Turkana herdsman with his dog.

1998) (Fig. 24.4). Dogs are infected by eating raw infected sheep or human remains. The young children are closely attended by dogs which guard and clean them (an alternative to washing encouraged by mothers in this very arid area). This close contact between dog and child ensures that most of the children will be infected with hydatids by the time they are a few years old. Water drawn from wells dug in river beds in times of drought may be heavily contaminated with infected dog faeces (Macpherson,1993).

The Turkana leave their dead to be scavenged by hyenas and other carnivores, so producing a wild animal reservoir of the parasite (Fuller & Fulller, 1981). Other pastoral nomadic people in Africa, such as the Dassanetch of south-western Ethiopia show a comparable prevalence of hydatid infection. In Islamic Africa, viscera of sheep are thrown to dogs after ritual slaughter for religious feasts. In Libya and Morocco, for example, about 40 per cent of dogs are infected, but the lower prevalence in humans of about 2 per cent reflects a less intimate human contact with dogs than in Turkana (Pandey et al.,1988, Shambesh et al., 1999).

People at risk

Farmers, herdsmen (particularly of sheep), hunters, skinners, tanners, and those exposed to dogs are the most likely to develop hydatid disease.

Economic burden

The types of economic loss resulting from hydatid disease are indicated in Fig. 24.2, while the size of the problem is indicated by the prevalence of the disease in different kinds of domestic animals. In Botswana in 1956, 77 per cent of slaughtered animals were condemned because of hydatidosis.

Prevention

Animal host

Dogs must not be fed uncooked offal and the refuse from slaughtered animals should be burnt or heated at temperatures above 55 °C. Stray dogs should be eliminated. Essential domestic dogs should be isolated and treated twice a year with a taenifuge such as arecoline hydrobromide, followed by a taenicide such as bunanidine hydrochloride or praziquantel. Some encouraging experimental work has suggested the possibility of protecting dogs by vaccination. At present, the only reliable way to diagnose hydatid disease in dogs is to examine stools for adult worms after purgation.

Man

People must be educated to avoid close contact with dogs and their faeces. This is easier in Islamic communities, which regard dogs as unclean.

Although impracticable in many developing countries, these preventive measures have reduced the prevalence of hydatidosis in countries such as Iceland, New Zealand and Tasmania. The development of reliable serological tests for hydatid disease in animals could provide a basis for international shipping restrictions, which would limit the geographical spread of the disease.

Clinical features

Many hydatid cysts cause no symptoms and are discovered by accident, for example, when liver calcification is seen on an abdominal radiograph. Two types of symptoms can result from hydatidosis: anaphylactoid reactions resulting from rupture of the cyst and release of hydatid antigens into the circulation; and mechanical effects of the enlarging cysts.

Liver cysts

Fifty to 70 per cent of all cysts occur in the liver, especially the right lobe. Abdominal distension is the commonest presentation amongst the Turkana. Abdominal, pleuritic or shoulder tip pain may indicate leakage from a hydatid cyst, and may be accompanied by fever and eosinophilia. Cysts may rupture into the biliary tree causing colic, or into the peritoneal cavity and thus present as an acute abdomen with severe pain and shock. Cysts in the porta hepatis or bile ducts may cause obstructive jaundice. Very large cysts may occasionally be palpable: they impart a peculiar type of thrill.

Lung cysts

Between 12 and 30 per cent of hydatid cysts are found in the lungs. Cysts were seen in routine chest radiographs of 0.3 per cent of Libyan Arab nomads. Respiratory symptoms may include breathlessness, cough, haemoptysis, pleuritic pain and fever (Jerray et al., 1992).

Other sites

In decreasing order of frequency, omentum, mesentery and retroperitoneal tissues, mediastinum, muscle, bone (0.8–9.1 per cent) (Fig. 24.5), and rarely brain, are affected. Cysts in the posterior mediastinum are particularly difficult to diagnose and may erode vertebral bodies. Cysts in vertebral bodies cause collapse and paraplegia: cysts in long bones cause pathological fractures and the spread of the infection into surrounding muscle and fascial planes. Multiple cysts occur in 22–41 per cent of cases.

Systemic effects

Fever and generalized pruritus are systemic symptoms often associated with hydatid disease. Rupture of cysts, particularly into serosal cavities, may cause acute and sometimes fatal anaphylactoid reactions.

Diagnosis (Babba et al., 1994)

Operation specimens

These must be examined to see whether viable parasites remain or whether the cyst is 'burnt out'.

Imaging

Scanning with ultrasound, with a fixed or portable machine, is the most convenient method of diagnosing abdominal cysts. About 15 per cent of cysts, however,

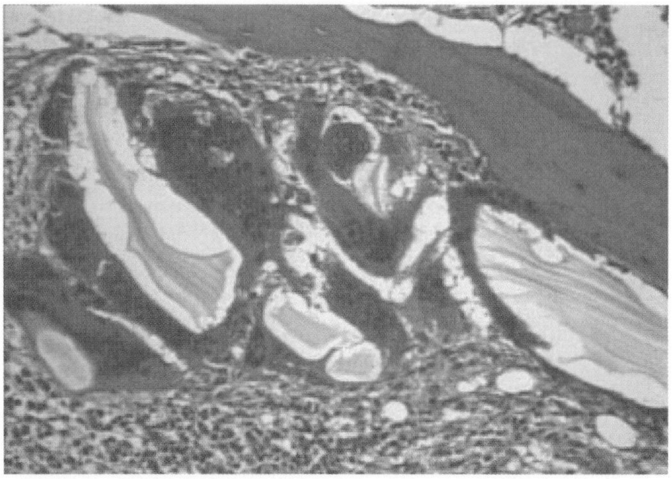

Fig. 24.5. Hydatid cyst in bone – often evident as a pathological fracture. (Courtesy of the Wellcome Trust.)

which were thought to be hydatids will turn out to have another cause – for example, simple cysts, arteriovenous aneurysms, tumours or abscesses, unless serology is also performed. Sometimes computerized tomography or arteriography is needed. Plain abdominal radiographs show only calcified cysts. Cysts in the lung or the pleural cavity are well seen on chest radiographs.

Serology

Enzyme-linked immunosorbent assay (ELISA) and indirect agglutination tests are useful for diagnosis as they are over 90 per cent sensitive, although they are less sensitive in Turkana. Titres do not fall appreciably after successful treatment, so they are not as useful for follow up as the much less sensitive immuno-precipitation and complement fixation tests.

Treatment (Fenton-Lee & Morris, 1996,1997)

In older patients, asymptomatic liver cysts less than 5 cm in diameter do not need to be treated especially if they are calcified.

Surgery

Excision of cysts is indicated if they are accessible and are causing mechanical complications. The complications of rupture at operation are:

(i) dissemination of scolices into the wound or body cavities giving rise to multiple new cysts.

(ii) anaphylaxis. Once the cyst is exposed, it should be carefully packed off with towels soaked with a scolicide solution such as 5–10 per cent formalin, 1 per cent aqueous iodine, 0.5 per cent silver nitrate, or hypertonic (2.7 per cent) saline. Cyst fluid is then aspirated and replaced with scolicide and left for 2–5 minutes in an attempt to kill the parasite. The cyst is then aspirated completely and excised. Adrenaline, antihistamines, and corticosteroids must be available to deal with anaphylactoid reactions.

(iii) Small unilocular cysts, less than 5 cm in diameter, may be aspirated and injected with 70 per cent alcohol. Despite the risk of anaphylaxis, this method is as successful as open surgery (Khuroo et al., 1997).

Chemotherapy

Praziquantel quickly kills protoscolices in a cyst or after spillage, but does not damage the germinal membrane. Albendazole penetrates cysts slowly and gradually damages the germinal membrane. Its action against protoscolices is enhanced by praziquantel. Albendazole is most effective against mesenteric and hepatic cysts and least effective against bone cysts. Treatment with albendazole 400 mg twice daily for an adult, for 4 to 12 weeks preoperatively, damages the germinal membrane, reduces the tension in the cyst and makes surgery safer. The addition of praziquantel 25 mg/kg daily for 2 weeks kills all protoscolices and reduces the risk of postoperative recurrence. Long-term chemotherapy has proved successful in the treatment of inoperable abdominal hydatid disease. Albendazole may cause temporary elevation of liver enzymes, which should be monitored, but rarely liver damage. Both drugs are expensive (Wen et al., 1994).

Unsolved problems

In any endemic focus of hydatid disease, the microepidemiology and dynamics need to be understood in order to plan sensible control measures. Very few foci have been carefully studied. The economic impact of hydatid disease and the cost-effectiveness of control measures are poorly known. The sensitivity and specificity of imaging techniques are still too low, and a single serological test for diagnosis and follow-up after treatment would be useful. Controlled trials of chemotherapy are needed in endemic areas to establish its usefulness in different types of hydatid disease.

References

Babba H, Messedi A, Masmoudi S et al. (1994). Diagnosis of human hydatidosis: comparison between imagery and six serologic techniques, *Am J Trop Med Hyg*; **50**: 64–68.

Fenton-Lee D, Morris DL. (1996). The management of hydatid disease of the liver: Part 1 [see comments]. *Trop Doct*; **26**: 173–176.

Fenton-Lee D, Morris DL. (1997). The management of hydatid disease of the liver: Part 2, *Trop Doct*; **27**: 87–88.

French CM, Nelson GS, Wood M. (1982). Hydatid disease in the Turkana District of Kenya I. The background to the problem with hypotheses to account for the remarkably high prevalence of the disease in man, *Ann Tro Med Parasitol*; **76**: 425–437.

Fuller GK, Fuller DC. (1981). Hydatid disease in Ethiopia: clinical survey with some immunodiagnostic test results, *Am J Trop Med Hyg*; **30**: 645–652

Jerray M, Benzarti M, Garrouche A, Klabi N, Hayouni A. (1992). Hydatid disease of the lungs. Study of 386 cases, *Am Rev Respir Dis*; **146**: 185–189.

Khuroo MS, Wani NA, Javid G et al. (1997). Percutaneous drainage compared with surgery for hepatic hydatid cysts, *N Engl J Med*; **337**: 881–887.

Macpherson CN. (1983). An active intermediate host role for man in the life cycle of Echinococcus granulosus in Turkana, Kenya, *Am J Trop Med Hyg*; **32**: 397–404.

Macpherson CN, Spoerry A, Zeyhle E, Romig T, Gorfe M. (1989). 'Pastoralists and hydatid disease: an ultrasound scanning prevalence survey in east Africa, *Trans Roy Soc Trop Med Hyg*; **83**: 243–247.

Pandey VS, Ouhelli H, Moumen A. (1988). Epidemiology of hydatidosis/echinococcosis in Ouarzazate, the pre- Saharian region of Morocco, *Ann Trop Med Parasitol*; **82**: 461–470.

Shambesh MA, Craig PS, Macpherson CN, Rogan MT, Gusbi AM, Echtuish EF. (1999). An extensive ultrasound and serologic study to investigate the prevalence of human cystic echinococcosis in northern Libya, *Am J Trop Med Hyg*; **60**: 462–468.

Watson-Jones DL, Macpherson CN. (1988). Hydatid disease in the Turkana district of Kenya. VI. Man: dog contact and its role in the transmission and control of hydatidosis amongst the Turkana, *Ann Trop Med Parasitol*; **82**: 343–356.

Wen H, Zou P-F, Yang W-G et al. (1994). Albendazole chemotherapy for human cystic and alveolar echinococcosis in northwestern China, *Trans Roy Soc Trop Med Hyg*; **88**: 340–343.

25

Schistosomiasis

Schistosomiasis is the generic name given to diseases caused by parasitic blood flukes of the genus *Schistosoma*. An older name, still widely used in Africa, is bilharzia. Of the three major species that commonly infect humans, two occur predominantly in Africa:

- *S. mansoni*, a cause of intestinal schistosomiasis, which is also found in Brazil and the Caribbean, and
- *S. haematobium*, the cause of urinary schistosomiasis, which is also found in the Middle East.

The third major species, *S. japonicum*, causes another form of intestinal schistosomiasis but is found only in the Far East, especially China and the Philippines. A minor species, *S. intercalatum*, causes infection but insignificant disease in small areas of Central Africa.

Schistosomiasis is typically a chronic infection. Adult worms slowly accumulate from early childhood over a period of 10 to 20 years, and the deposition of eggs in the tissues leads to fibrosis in the intestines and liver (*S. mansoni*) or the urinary tract (*S. haematobium*). Mild or moderate symptoms occur in most infected children: severe disease develops in later life in only a minority (usually $<10\%$) of individuals. For detailed reviews of different aspects, the reader is referred to books edited by Jordan et al. (1993) and Mahmoud (2000).

The problem in Africa

The impact of high profile conditions such as malaria and HIV-associated disease often leads to the importance of schistosomiasis being underestimated at both local and national levels. Although exact figures are hard to obtain, it is estimated that, out of 600 million people at risk of schistosome infection world-wide, 200 million are infected, of whom three-quarters live in Africa, and 20 million suffer from severe sequelae (Savioli et al., 1997).

Although temporary success in controlling disease has sometimes been achieved, both infection and disease are probably increasing in the continent as a whole. This is the result of increased absolute numbers of people living in rural and peri-urban areas in which transmission occurs, together with the development of irrigation schemes or other water engineering programmes that encourage the spread of the snail intermediate host. Striking examples of this have been seen in large scale programmes, such as:

- the upsurge in *S. mansoni* infection that occurred in the Nile Delta following the completion of the Aswan High Dam in 1968
- the spread of *S. mansoni* infection following the expansion of the Gezira and Managil irrigation schemes in the Sudan during the 1970s, and
- more recently, the epidemic outbreak of *Schistosomiasis mansoni* that occurred in the Senegal River basin, especially around the sugar plantations of Richard Toll, following the construction of the Diama Dam across the Senegal River in 1986 (Talla et al., 1990).

Other examples include the spread of *S. haematobium* infection around the artificial lakes Kossou, Volta, Kainji and Kariba in Côte d'Ivoire, Ghana, Nigeria and Zimbabwe respectively. However, small scale irrigation or water development schemes can be equally important. As marginal agricultural land becomes more intensively used, and access to water more of a constraining factor, such water as is available becomes more widely used for household or farming activities and more liable to contamination with schistosome eggs by the increased human population.

The distribution within Africa of *S. mansoni*, *S. intercalatum* and *S. haematobium* is shown schematically in Figs 25.1 and 25.2 (modified from Doumenge et al., 1987). Both of the major species are patchily distributed

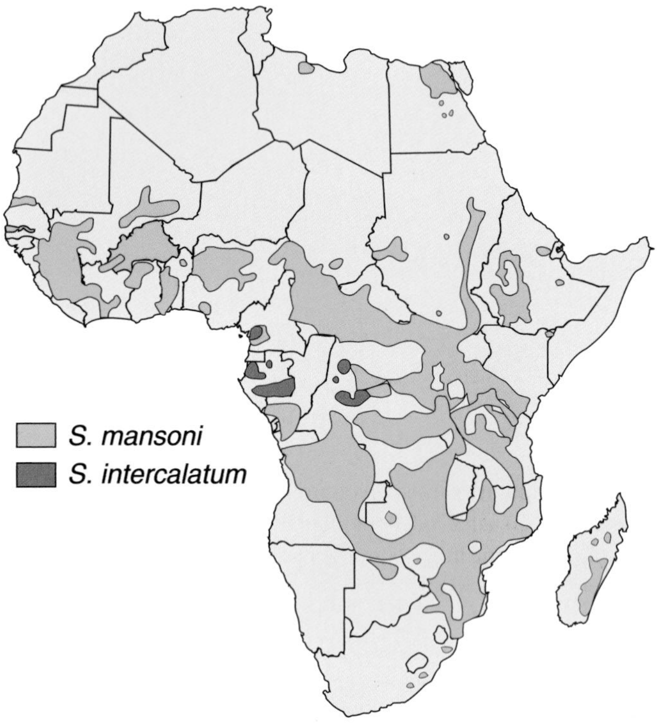

Fig. 25.1. The distribution in Africa of *Schistosoma mansoni* and *S. intercalatum*. (Redrawn from Doumenge et al., 1987.)

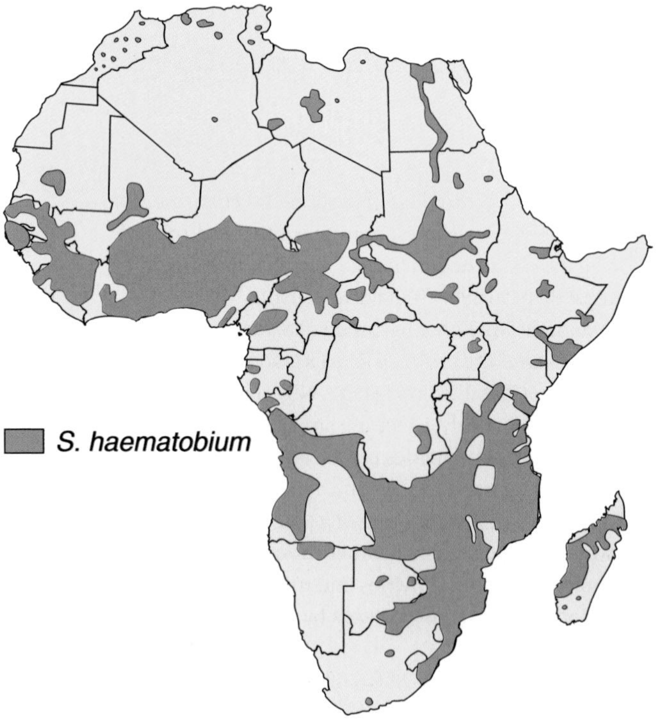

Fig. 25.2. The distribution in Africa of *Schistosoma haematobium*. (Redrawn from Doumenge et al., 1987.)

throughout the continent. *S. haematobium* is more frequent than *S. mansoni* north of the Sahara and along the Nile Valley in Upper Egypt, while *S. mansoni* predominates in the Nile Delta in Lower Egypt. *Schistosomiasis mansoni* is more important in East than in West Africa, with major foci in the Democratic Republic of Congo (DRC), Kenya, Uganda and Burundi, while *Schistosomiasis haematobia* tends to predominate in West Africa, especially in Côte d'Ivoire, Ghana, Togo, Benin and Nigeria. In South Africa, *S. haematobium* is more common than *S. mansoni* in the north and east of the country, while both species are found in Zimbabwe, Malawi and Zambia. In Madagascar, there is a striking dichotomy between the species, with *S. haematobium* being found in the drier, western part of the island, *S. mansoni* in the wetter, eastern part.

Within each affected country, the distribution is usually strongly focal, according to the presence of suitable snail intermediate hosts. The species can overlap, and mixed infections can occur, but less commonly than might be expected. In Kenya, for example, *S. mansoni* is absent from the coastal areas where *S. haematobium* is highly prevalent, but is common in Machakos, Makueni and Kitui Districts where *S. haematobium* is rare. Mixed infections occur in the Taveta region, and also near Lake Victoria, where *S. mansoni* is found mainly around the lake shore, *S. haematobium* further inland.

The parasite and its hosts

The schistosome life cycle is shown in diagrammatic form in Fig. 25.3. The parasite alternates between two hosts:

- the definitive human host, in whom pairing of adult worms and sexual replication occurs, and
- an intermediate snail host, in which asexual replication occurs.

The snail intermediate host

The intermediate hosts are aquatic snails of certain restricted genera, *Biomphalaria* for *S. mansoni* and *Bulinus* for *S. haematobium*. It is the distribution of the snails that determines the distribution of schistosomiasis in any given area or country. They typically live in rivers, streams, dams or pools, but can inhabit virtually any body of open water where there is appropriate vegetation, including large natural or artificial lakes. In Lake Albert in Uganda, for example, transmission occurs both close to the shore, where *Biomphalaria sudanica* lives on reeds close to the surface, and at some distance into the lake,

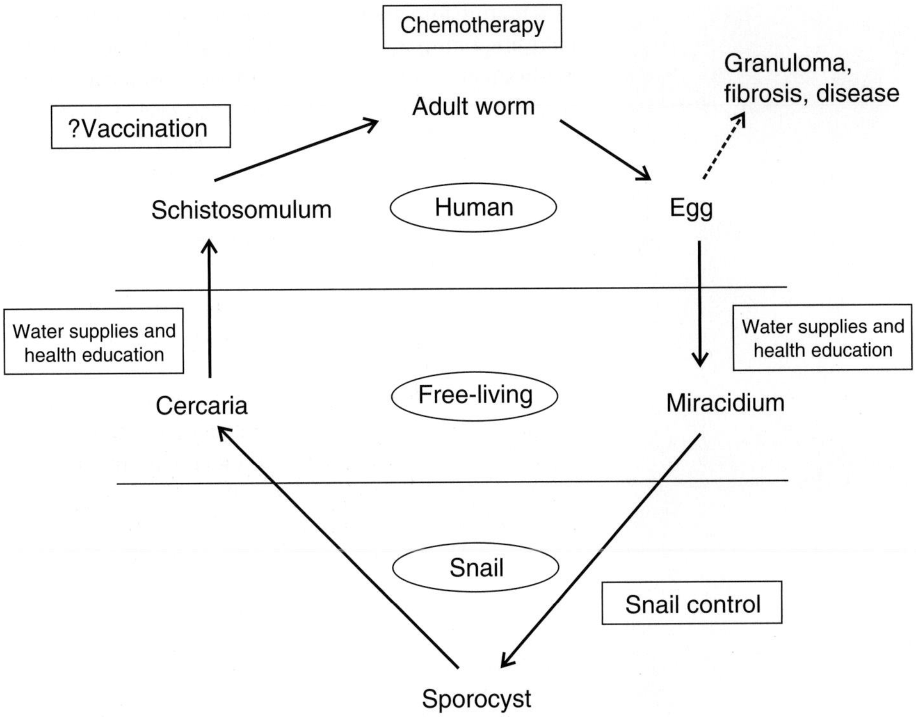

Fig. 25.3. Diagrammatic representation of the schistosome life cycle, showing points of possible intervention.

where *Biomphalaria stanleyi* can live on vegetation at depths of several metres.

Release of infective cercariae

The phase of asexual replication in the snail is characterized by the development of primary and secondary sporocysts in the hepatopancreas and by the subsequent release into the surrounding water of the infective larvae or cercariae (Fig. 25.4). Snails start to release cercariae between 4 and 6 weeks after infection, depending on the water temperature, and can then live for a further 1 or 2 months, each snail shedding up to 1000 cercariae daily. The cercariae are actively motile organisms, about 200 μm long, with characteristic forked tails that propel the organisms with a whip-like motion upwards towards light through the water. They have a water impermeable outer coat or glycocalyx and are unable to absorb nutrients, instead surviving on glycogen reserves. Under experimental conditions they can live for up to 24 hours before their glycogen reserves are depleted, but under natural conditions they die within 6 to 12 hours. Cercariae are shed from snails during the day, as the water temperature rises and, more importantly, the light increases. Thus, peak cercarial densities are found during the middle of the day, and this is the time when water containing infected snails is most infectious (Prentice & Ouma, 1984).

Human infection and maturation of the adult worm

People can come into contact with water containing cercariae for a wide range of reasons, including washing themselves or their clothes and collecting water for drinking or cooking or for irrigation. Among children, playing or swimming in water is an important activity (Fig. 25.5), while some adults, such as fishermen or canal cleaners, may be occupationally exposed at high levels. Cercariae are chemotactically attracted to human skin and, upon contact, they penetrate directly through the skin, losing their tails and their water-resistant outer coats and transforming into young schistosomes or schistosomula. Penetration takes about 1 minute from contact and is assisted by surface tension if, for example, a limb is removed from the water and allowed to dry naturally.

Schistosomula stay in the skin for 2 days before migrating via the bloodstream, first to the lungs and then to the liver, where they arrive about 10 days after infection. Here

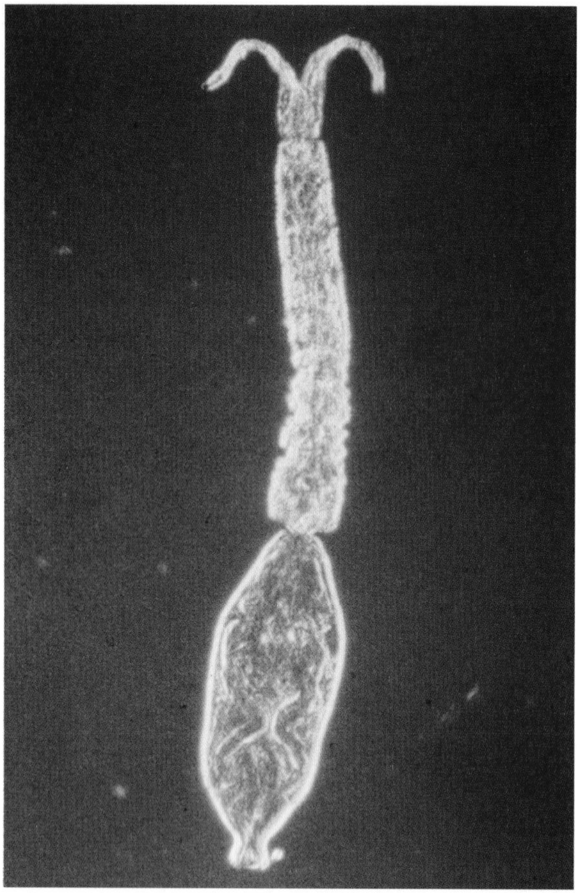

Fig. 25.4. Cercaria of *Schistosoma mansoni*. Note the forked tail, which propels the cercaria vertically through the water.

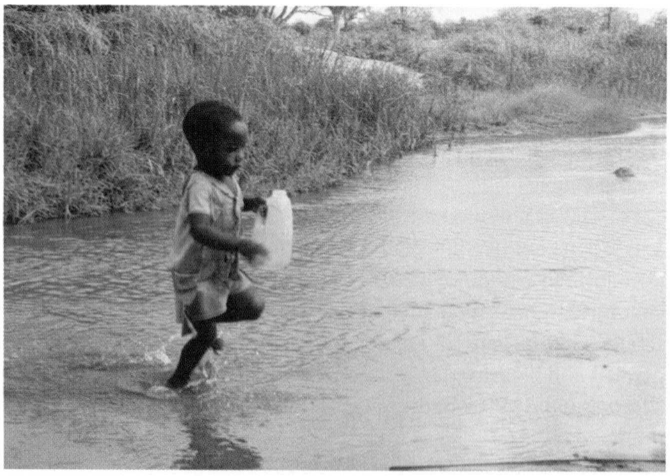

Fig. 25.5. Children are exposed to infection by playing in contaminated water.

they mature into male or female adult worms and form pairs, migrating against the flow of hepatic portal blood to the small venules draining the large intestine in the case of *S. mansoni* or the bladder in the case of *S. haematobium*. The adult male, about 1 cm long and with a flattened body, enfolds the longer and thinner female in its gynaecophoric canal or 'schist'. Once established, adult worms have a mean lifespan of 3 years (*S. haematobium*) to 7 years (*S. mansoni*).

Role of other mammalian hosts

Although the role of other mammals in the transmission of *S. japonicum* is important and well documented, there are insufficient data to be certain that other mammals play a major role in the transmission of either *S. mansoni* or *S. haematobium*. However, it should be noted that various primate and non-primate species have been found to be naturally infected with either of the two species.

Deposition of eggs and infection of snails

The female of the paired adult worms lays eggs at a rate of 300 to 3000 per day, depending on the species. Egg laying starts about 6 (*S. mansoni*) to 10 (*S. haematobium*) weeks after infection, and each egg contains a larval form, the miracidium, surrounded by a hard shell with a characteristic spine, lateral in the case of *S. mansoni* (Fig. 25.6), terminal in the case of *S. haematobium*. These eggs can do one of two things. First, they can lodge in the tissues, where they elicit the development of a cell-mediated granulomatous reaction which, with its subsequent fibrosis, is responsible for the chronic clinical manifestations of disease. Alternatively, the eggs can pass out through the intestinal wall or bladder, being subsequently voided in the faeces or urine. Upon contact with water, the eggs then hatch, releasing the free-living miracidia, which swim actively until they encounter an appropriate snail host. They then penetrate the snail and begin the cycle of asexual replication with the formation of primary and secondary sporocysts and release of cercariae that completes the life cycle.

Epidemiological aspects of transmission and disease

Disease depends on intensity of infection

It is important to remember that, like other helminths, adult schistosomes do not replicate within their defini-

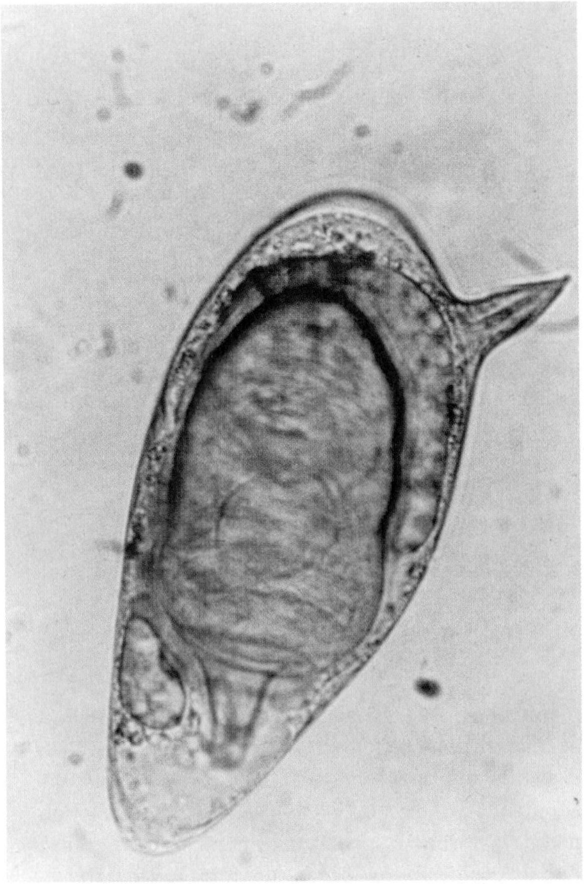

Fig. 25.6. Egg of *Schistosoma mansoni*. Note the distinctive lateral spine, and the larval miracidium within the hard shell.

tive (human) hosts. Each cercaria has the opportunity to become a single worm, either male or female, and infection is cumulatively acquired over a period of years. Each paired female worm then has the capacity to deposit several hundred eggs per day throughout its lifetime of several years. Since most of the clinical manifestations of disease are attributable to the retention of eggs in the tissues, with subsequent fibrosis, it follows that schistosomiasis is a 'dose-dependent' disease. That is, the severity of disease is related not just to the presence or absence of infection, but rather to its intensity and duration. Intensity can be measured indirectly by counting the eggs in a sample of urine or faeces, as an estimate of the adult worm burden, and a relationship between intensity and disease has now been demonstrated in many studies.

A second important feature is that the distribution of adult worms in a host population is statistically overdispersed, showing a high degree of aggregation. Even in a community in which the overall prevalence of infection is high, most individuals have only light infections that cause little morbidity, while only a small proportion have very heavy infections that may lead to severe disease. The reasons for such aggregation are unclear but potentially diverse, and may include:

- a genetic predisposition to heavy or light infections
- a heterogeneity in the acquisition of protective immunity, or
- a heterogeneity, which may be either behavioural or geographical, in exposure to infection. In this context, transmission is often very focal even within a small geographical area, reflecting the heterogeneous distribution of infected snails. Such foci can vary markedly from year to year, as local changes in climate and habitat affect snail populations.

Age distribution of infection

Although in some localities high intensities of infection may persist into adult life (Ongom & Bradley, 1972), the shape of the distribution of infection by age is more usually convex (Fig. 25.7). This holds true both for prevalence of infection (that is, the proportion of individuals in each age group who have detectable infection) and also more markedly for intensity of infection (that is, the mean worm burden for each age group, estimated indirectly as egg output in the faeces or urine). A typical picture is that young children begin to acquire infection from the age of 3 or 4 years, when they start to have regular contact with infected water. Both prevalence and intensity then rise sharply, reaching a peak during the second decade of life. Thereafter, both prevalence and, more markedly, intensity decrease with increasing age. This decline is attributable to:

- a progressive spontaneous death of adult worms from early infections acquired during childhood
- reduced exposure to contaminated water in older children and adults, and
- an age-related development of an acquired immunity to infection.

The relative contribution of reduced exposure and the development of immunity is difficult to resolve, since both are dependent upon age. A useful way of investigating this problem has been to measure intensities of reinfection 1 or 2 years after treatment of cohorts of individuals of different ages, at the same time measuring the levels of exposure of those individuals to contaminated water (Butterworth et al., 1988). As a broad generalization, children have more frequent, prolonged and extensive contact with water than adults through swimming, bathing and

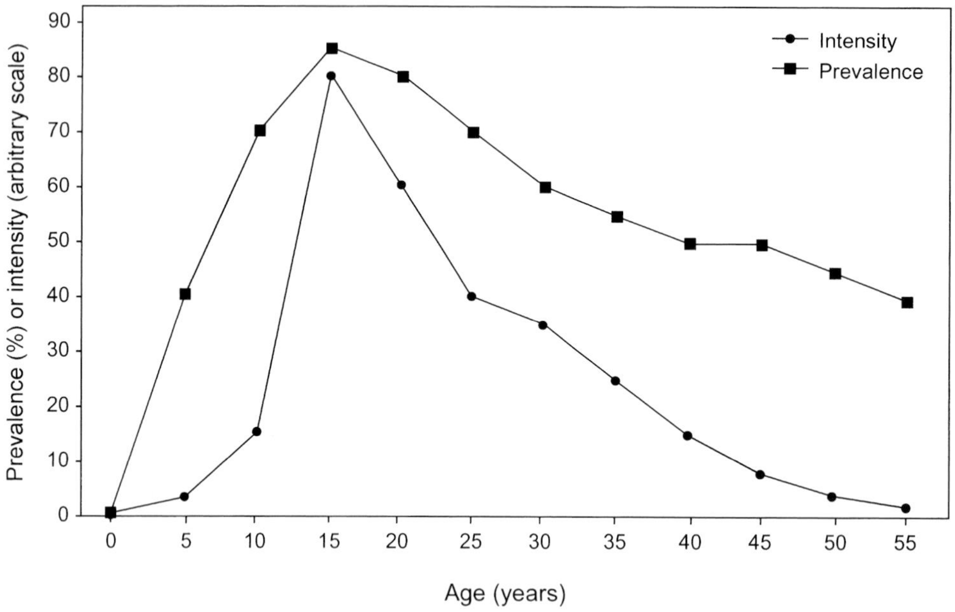

Fig. 25.7. Hypothetical distribution by age of prevalence and intensity of *Schistosoma mansoni* infection.

playing. However, water contact patterns vary markedly between different communities, and some communities show very high levels of occupational exposure among adults. If exposure were the sole determinant of infection, it would be expected that a similar heterogeneity would be seen in patterns of infection. This is not the case. In many studies in different parts of Africa and in Brazil, re-infection has shown a strikingly constant relationship with age, with a peak of re-infection at 10 to 12 years and very much lower levels among older children and adults (Fig. 25.8). A particularly good example has come from studies in fishing villages on Lake Albert, which have shown the typical pattern of re-infection in spite of very high levels of demonstrable exposure among adult fishermen (Kabatereine et al., 1999). This argues strongly for the development at, or shortly after, puberty, of an immunity to re-infection.

Age distribution of disease

A consequence of the relative lack of heavy infection among adults is that, in communities living in endemic areas, schistosomiasis is perceived as a disease of children of primary school age. The late sequelae of infection that result from fibrosis of granulomas that develop in response to eggs deposited in childhood may affect and may kill older children and adults, but these are rare events in comparison with the extensive, although mild, morbidity that is seen in the younger age groups. A typical picture in an area of high transmission is that a majority of children are infected and have detectable but mild signs or symptoms. In most of these children there is a spontaneous reduction in clinical morbidity as they grow older, even without specific treatment: but, in a minority, disease progresses to a severe and irreversible state.

A second consequence of the high intensities of infection among young children is that it is this age group that contributes most to contamination of the environment with excreted eggs, and hence to continued transmission. In the case of *S. haematobium*, contamination occurs when urine is voided directly into water, especially during bathing. In the case of *S. mansoni*, defaecation directly into water is less common. Instead, faeces may be deposited, for example, among bushes on the banks of streams. Eggs survive in drying faeces only for a few days, depending on temperature. They may be flushed by rain into ponds or streams, but this occurs largely during rainy seasons, when snail numbers may be low. Instead, during the dry season, faeces containing eggs may reach water in various ways: for example, by washing of soiled clothes, by washing the anal region after defaecation on dry land, on cattle hooves or bird claws, or even by dogs that drink water after eating faeces (J.H. Ouma, unpublished observations). None of these methods is very efficient, but the reproductive capacity of the organism is sufficiently great that transmission is maintained even if only a small proportion of eggs hatch and go on to infect snails.

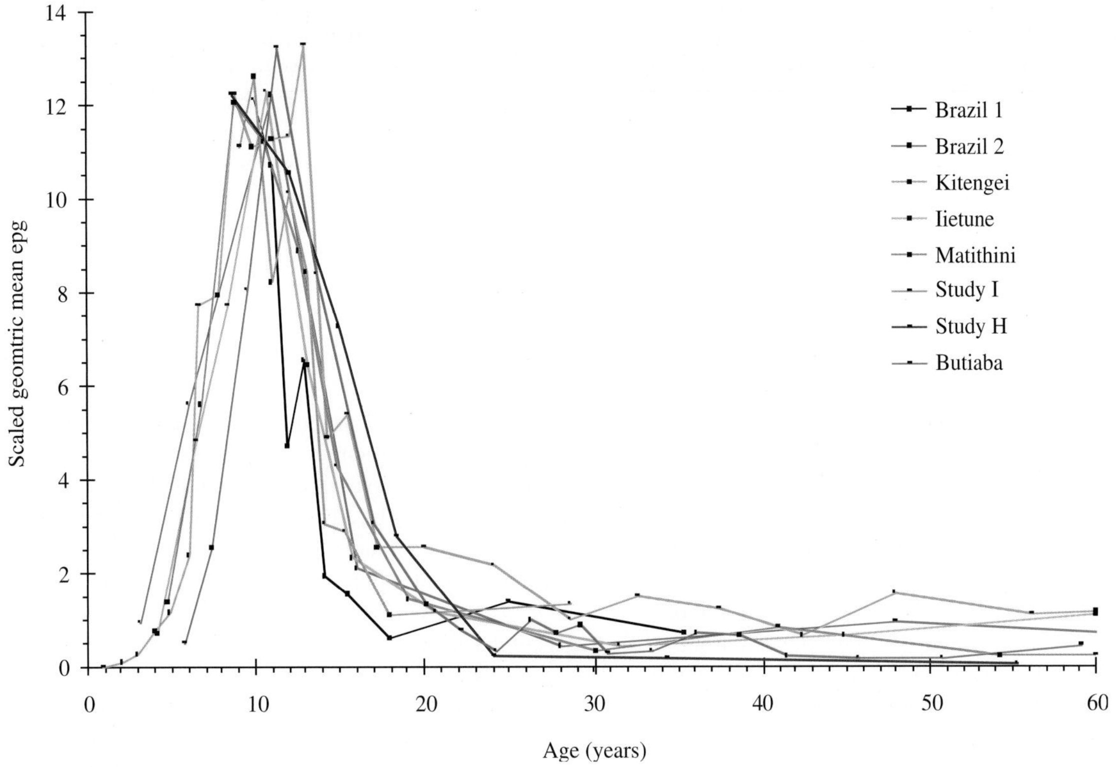

Fig. 25.8. Distribution by age of intensities of reinfection with *Schistosoma mansoni* after treatment: summary of published data from eight communities in Kenya and Brazil. (By kind permission of Dr A.J.C. Fulford, 2000.)

Control of disease in communities

During recent years, emphasis has shifted away from attempts to prevent transmission altogether, which is both impracticable and unsustainable. The aim now is to prevent severe disease, by reducing transmission to levels that are sufficiently low that they do not cause high intensities of infection (WHO, 1993). Even an incomplete control of transmission can have a useful impact in terms of reduction of disease (Fig. 25.9).

Theoretical approaches to control

In theory, control might be achieved by intervening in the schistosome life cycle at one or more of a number of vulnerable points (Fig. 25.3):

- Treatment of the human host with drugs that kill the adult worms and hence prevent the excretion of eggs into the environment. This approach has the added advantage that it has an immediate impact on morbidity (separate from its effect on transmission) by preventing the further deposition of eggs in the tissues.

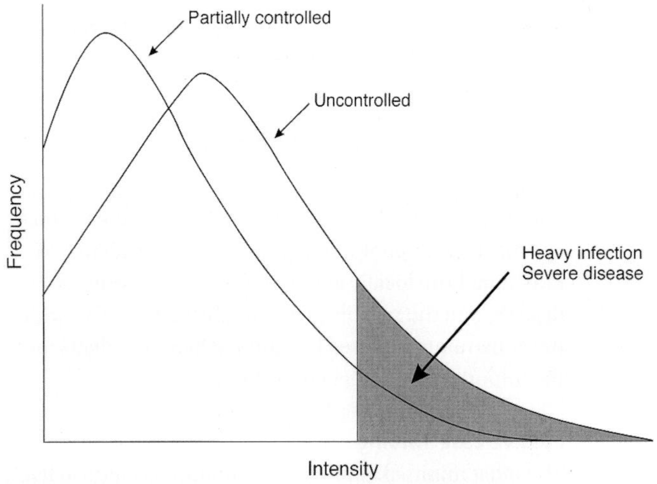

Fig. 25.9. Hypothetical diagrams of the frequency distribution in a population of intensity of infection to show the effect on morbidity of partial control.

- Reduction of excretion of eggs into the water, through improved sanitation and health education. These non-specific measures can also affect other water-borne diseases.
- Reduction in numbers of the snail intermediate host. This can be achieved by the application of molluscicides to water containing snails, on either a small or a large scale; by biological methods, through the introduction of competitors or predators; or by environmental modification to destroy snail habitats.
- Reduction of human contact with contaminated water, through improved water supplies and health education, measures that again can affect other water-borne diseases.
- Vaccination, to prevent the development of the adult worm in the human host.

No vaccine yet exists, although considerable progress has been made in recent years towards understanding the mechanisms of immunity and the antigens against which such immunity may be directed, that might be suitable for use in a vaccine (see below). Each of the other methods has been used, alone or in combination, and sometimes with considerable success. In particular, *S. japonicum* has been eliminated from Japan, and its distribution markedly restricted in China, through the use of environmental methods to control snail populations.

At present, however, the mainstay of control is drug treatment (chemotherapy), usually in combination with other methods. Safe and effective drugs for the treatment of schistosomiasis have now been available for over 20 years. One in particular, praziquantel, which is effective against all three major species of schistosome, is active in a single dose and has only mild side effects, making it ideal for use at the community level.

Ways of delivering chemotherapy

Various approaches to the administration of chemotherapy are possible. There are no hard and fast rules: which approach is adopted will depend on the prevalence of infection, both locally and nationally, the severity of disease, and the priority given to schistosomiasis within the constraints imposed by national health budgets and the importance of other conditions.

Passive case-finding

The most minimal approach: no attempt is made actively to find infected individuals in a community. Instead, patients present spontaneously with signs or symptoms compatible with infection, a diagnosis is made, and treatment is offered. It has been argued that this is an acceptable approach to the problem of schistosomiasis in resource-poor settings where the prevalence of disease is very low. The problem with it is that, when patients present with advanced disease attributable to fibrosis, such as portal hypertension or severe renal dysfunction, it is too late for drug treatment of the infection to have an effect on the progress of disease.

Mass chemotherapy

At the other extreme, the most extensive approach, in which entire communities are treated without previous individual diagnosis. This approach was adopted in an early national control programme in Brazil, in communities in which stool surveys in an index group of schoolchildren showed prevalence to be greater than 20 per cent (Machado, 1982). The advantage is that diagnostic costs are low, being confined to the preliminary survey of a sample of school children. The disadvantages are that drug costs are high, and that it may not be considered acceptable to give drugs to people who are not known to be infected. Maximum impact on morbidity, infection and transmission can be expected, but only if the compliance of the population is good.

Targeted chemotherapy

An intermediate approach, in which quantitative egg counts are carried out on stool or urine samples from entire communities, and treatment is offered to those individuals with heavy infections, on the basis that they are the ones who may go on to develop severe disease. The advantage of this approach is that drug costs are low, since only a small proportion of a population is heavily infected. The disadvantages are that costs of diagnosis are high, since quantitative stool counts are required. In addition, it might be considered unacceptable to leave untreated a person known to bear a light infection, since factors other than intensity may contribute to the development of disease. The targeted chemotherapy approach has little effect on transmission (Ouma et al., 1985), and the approach is currently not widely used.

Selective chemotherapy

Another intermediate approach in which stool or urine samples are collected from each individual in the community, and treatment is offered to those who are infected, irrespective of the intensity of infection. Costs of diagnosis are again high, but may be reduced by using simple, indirect indicators of infection, such as reagent strips for haematuria in the case of *S. haematobium*. Drug costs are low, although not as low as when targeted chemotherapy is used. The approach depends on high levels of compliance in providing stool or urine samples, as well as attending for treatment. The impact on transmission may be less than when mass chemotherapy is used, since the diagnostic tests are insufficiently sensitive to detect all infected individuals. Some infected individuals will therefore remain untreated and will maintain transmission (De Vlas & Gryseels, 1992).

Selective chemotherapy of school children

Finally, another intermediate approach, and the one most currently favoured. In this approach, stool or urine samples are collected on one or more occasions from all children attending primary school, usually in the age range 6 to 16 years, and treatment is given to those detected to be infected. The approach has many advantages. Children usually include the most heavily infected members of the community, who would later go on to develop severe and irreversible disease: they suffer from morbidity that is reversible by treatment: they contribute most to transmission, by indiscriminate defaecation or urination in or around the waterbodies: and they are easily and cheaply accessible for both diagnosis and treatment within the framework of the primary school system. The cost of drugs is low, since they are given on the basis of body weight. The approach, which has proved effective in reducing morbidity, infection and transmission (Butterworth et al., 1991), is dependent on a primary school system sufficiently strong that a high proportion of school age children do indeed attend school. The method can be combined with passive case-finding and treatment among the remaining, adult members of the community and among pre-school children or those who do not attend school.

Whichever method of administering chemotherapy is chosen, the problem remains of surveillance and retreatment. Chemotherapy never eliminates transmission completely: therefore, after a single round of drug treatment, infection will sooner or later recur. Re-infection is particularly important in children less than 15 years old, who have not yet developed immunity. Whatever the starting method adopted, surveillance in subsequent years should be directed at such children, with retreatment as necessary. The frequency of surveillance will depend on the intensity of transmission at the start of the control programme and on the efficacy of the programme, but will typically be required at intervals ranging from 1 year in heavily infected to 3 or 4 years in lightly infected foci.

Ancillary control measures

These include snail control, health education, improved sanitation and provision of water supplies.

Snail control

Before the advent of safe and effective drugs, the most generally used control measure, and still extremely useful when carried out in combination with other measures. The commonest technique is the application of molluscicides, especially niclosamide (Bayluscide®), either on a large scale (for example, the canals feeding an irrigation scheme) or more focally in small individual streams or pools. The cost of niclosamide is high, and treatment of waterbodies needs to be carried out at frequent and regular intervals by well-trained personnel, in order to prevent the reappearance of snail populations. An alternative approach is environmental modification to remove snail breeding sites, especially in irrigation schemes or other water projects, and including, for example, the construction of lined canals or ditches, prevention of seepage, management of water flow and removal of vegetation. A third approach is the introduction of competitors, such as tiariid snails, or predators, such as the fresh water crayfish: such approaches have worked under experimental conditions, but have not been widely applied.

Health education

A desirable component of any disease-specific control programme. In the case of schistosomiasis, it has received much lip service but little serious attention to development of new and effective teaching methods. In particular when diagnosis and drug treatment is undertaken through the primary schools, much could be done to promote both child-to-child and child-to-adult learning. The aims should be to reduce contamination, by education about the role of inappropriate defaecation and urination in maintaining the life cycle, and to reduce exposure. For example, while it may not be realistic to prevent children from playing or swimming in water, it could be emphasized that the middle of the day is a 'dangerous' time for such activities.

Improved sanitation

In parallel with health education, a non-specific measure that can lead to the reduction not only of schistosomiasis but also of other water-borne diseases. The aim should be to ensure not only that latrines are built, but also that they are used by all members of a family, including children. Again, schools can play a major role, both by providing adequate latrines and by ensuring that they are properly used.

Safe water supplies

A final approach to reduce the extent to which people have contact with infected water for domestic activities. In the authors' experience of several hundreds of meetings with village elders or communities, in which the control of schistosomiasis is discussed, the one question that is invariably asked is: 'Why can you not provide us with safe water?' At a large-scale level, this is usually outside the jurisdiction of health authorities, and liaison is needed at a national level between health and water development ministries. On a smaller scale, however, much can be done, through the encouragement of the use of water tanks, boreholes, wells and low cost water pumps.

In summary, the control of schistosomiasis is not a simple problem that is amenable to a single, prescriptive recipe. A reactive and integrated approach is required, in which a number of methods are applied, which may vary from area to area (WHO, 1993). They may frequently involve some form of repeated school-based treatment campaign, together with passive case-finding among those not covered by the school programme, health education in the schools, attention to sanitation and water supplies, and focal mollusciciding of local water bodies at those times of year when snail populations are most abundant.

Pathogenesis and clinical manifestations

For both *S. mansoni* and *S. haematobium* infection, the disease process is conventionally divided into four stages, although these merge into each other. They are associated with:

- invasion of the skin by cercariae, and the subsequent migration of schistosomula through the lungs to the liver
- maturation of the adult worms, and early egg laying
- established infection, with disease mainly attributable to granulomatous reactions around eggs deposited in the tissues
- late infection, with irreversible lesions caused by extensive fibrosis of egg granulomas.

Stage of invasion: cercarial dermatitis

Penetration of the skin by cercariae, both of species that cause human disease and of avian or other 'non-human' schistosomes, can be associated with a cercarial dermatitis, also called 'swimmer's itch'. In the case of the non-human schistosomes, cercarial dermatitis can occur after primary exposure as well as re-exposure: it may be observed in areas endemic for human schistosomiasis as well as non-endemic areas, and is associated with death of the cercariae in the skin. In the case of human schistosomes, dermatitis follows re-exposure in older, putatively immune individuals. A transient immediate hypersensitivity reaction that occurs within 15 minutes of exposure of the skin to water is followed by a delayed reaction that develops 12 to 24 hours after exposure and may persist for up to 15 days. The characteristics of the pruritic rash are that its distribution corresponds to those parts of the body that were immersed in water. It is a trivial condition that does not usually require treatment, and its main interest lies in the fact that it may help in the description of cercarial exposure. Fishermen on Lake Albert in Uganda, for example, report emphatically that itching of the skin after exposure to water is usually more pronounced in the middle of the day; in sunny rather than cloudy weather; in the dry season, when lake levels are low; and at particular sites that are associated with large numbers of infected snails (A.E. Butterworth, Booth and N.K. Kabatereine, unpublished observations).

Stage of maturation: acute schistosomiasis

This condition is common in adults exposed to heavy infection for the first time, such as visitors or immigrants to an endemic area. It is less common among long-term residents of an endemic area. Originally described in *S. japonicum* infection as 'Katayama fever', it is seen in Africa more often with *S. mansoni* than with *S. haematobium*. It resembles classical serum sickness, and is associated with the development of adult worms during the first 5 weeks after infection, and thereafter with the early stages of egg deposition. The aetiology is somewhat controversial. Although usually associated with early egg laying and the formation of florid granulomas, it can precede maturation of the adult worms, occurring as early as 9 to 13 days after infection. In this case, it may be associated with an immune response to dying worms, and with the formation and systemic deposition of immune complexes.

Acute schistosomiasis is usually a mild, self-limiting condition, but can be severe. Symptoms may include fever, rigors, sweating, headaches, muscular aches, weakness and malaise, together with an unproductive cough, abdominal pain, nausea, vomiting, diarrhoea and loss of weight. Physical signs include pyrexia, usually intermittent with evening peaks, oedema, generalized lymphadenopathy, tender enlargement of the liver, sometimes with jaundice, and slight enlargement of the spleen. Patients may become confused or stuporose, or show visual impairments or papilloedema. There is usually a massive eosinophilia, elevation in total IgE levels and the development of specific anti-schistosome antibodies. Eggs become detectable in the faeces or urine from about 6 weeks after exposure.

Localized central nervous system lesions in acute schistosomiasis can be severe. Lesions are most frequently observed in the spinal cord: a myelopathy results from the inflammatory reaction that accompanies the deposition of eggs in venules in and around the spinal cord. Diagnosis depends on a history of exposure and the detection of eggs: the cerebrospinal fluid usually contains eosinophils, while myelography or computerized tomography can be of value.

Stage of established infection

Once adult worms have formed pairs and egg production has begun, most of the pathogenesis of disease is attributable to the formation of granulomatous reactions around eggs deposited in the tissues. These reactions are mediated by T cells, and are characterized by the presence of lymphocytes, macrophages and eosinophils. There is some controversy as to the exact nature of the T cell reactions involved, but recent studies have indicated that Th1 responses with production of tumour necrosis factor (TNFα) and interferon gamma (IFNγ) are associated with severe morbidity in children infected with *S. mansoni*, while Th2 responses with IL-5 production are associated with mild or absent morbidity (Mwatha et al., 1998). As in lepromatous leprosy, the T cell response is a two-edged sword: as well as contributing to disease, it may simultaneously serve to protect the host against the effects of toxic egg products.

This is the stage that is characteristically seen in children in endemic areas. Before the onset of the fibrosis that characterizes the later stages, it is entirely reversible, both spontaneously and more markedly following removal of the adult worms by specific anti-schistosomal treatment. The clinical manifestations of the granulomatous reactions depend on the anatomical location of the deposited eggs, and therefore vary according to the species of schistosome.

In *S. mansoni* infections, eggs are deposited mainly in the large intestine and the liver. This stage may be asymptomatic, and infection is only revealed by detection of eggs in the faeces following school or community surveys. Alternatively, there may be abdominal pain and diarrhoea, often with blood. The liver may be enlarged, especially the left lobe, and is firm, regular and may be tender. The spleen may also be enlarged, but is usually soft. The organomegaly at this stage regresses readily, either spontaneously or after treatment.

In *S. haematobium* infections, eggs are deposited mainly in the bladder wall and the lower parts of the ureters. Some eggs may also be found in the rectal wall, where they cause no pathology but may aid in diagnosis at rectal biopsy. Eggs are also deposited in the genital tract in both males and females: genital schistosomiasis is discussed below. The main symptoms of infection at this stage are suprapubic pain, frequency, dysuria and haematuria, typically terminal. The presence and severity of haematuria is related to the intensity of infection, and in areas of high transmission haematuria in boys may be so common as to be considered by the local community to be a normal process of maturation, comparable to menstruation in girls. The extent of pathology in the upper urinary tract depends on the exact location of the granulomas. If they are found at or near the ureteric orifice, then there may be evidence of obstruction, with ureteric dilatation that may progress to hydronephrosis. As in *S. mansoni* infections, the lesions of this early stage characteristically resolve, either spontaneously or after anti-schistosomal treatment, leaving no residual damage.

Stage of late infection

The stage of established infection, typical of young children, may progress in one of two different directions.

- In most individuals, the adult worms of early infections die, and the host becomes immune to new infection. The worm burden, and therefore the number of new eggs being deposited in the tissues, declines. At the same time, previously formed granulomas resolve, following the destruction of the eggs within them: and newly formed granulomas are smaller than those that arise during early infection, a process referred to as modulation. The end result is that the net burden of pathology spontaneously diminishes, even without specific treatment to kill the adult worms.
- In some individuals, however, previously formed granulomas do not resolve, but instead progress to fibrosis. Fibrous tissue also forms, for example, around the portal tracts (periportal fibrosis), in a distribution that does not correlate exactly with the distribution of eggs. In these individuals, severe, progressive and irreversible pathology develops.

The reasons why severe pathology only develops in some individuals and not in others are not clear. Apart from intensity and duration of infection, various factors may be involved, including for example:

- host genetic constitution
- parasite strain differences
- host nutritional status
- interactions with other infections, especially malaria and hepatitis.

Evidence for such factors is generally lacking, and is the subject of current research. However, there are some indications that host genetic elements may be involved. It has been recognized for many years, from studies in Brazil and the Sudan, that people of black African origin are less likely to develop severe, progressive fibrotic disease than those of Arab or Caucasian origin. Subsequently, in studies in Egypt, evidence was obtained for an association between the HLA haplotypes A1 and B5 and susceptibility to severe disease, but it is not clear whether this association reflected the fact that these haplotypes were in linkage disequilibrium with other, unidentified loci. More recently, in studies in the Sudan by Dessein and colleagues (1999), segregation analysis has provided evidence for a codominant major gene predisposing to advanced fibrosis as detected by ultrasonography. Linkage analysis has shown that this gene maps to a region of chromosome 6 that is closely linked to the interferon-γ receptor.

In *S. mansoni* infections, the most important late complication is hepatic fibrosis leading to portal hypertension (Fig. 25.10). The fibrosis is typically periportal in distribution, and is described as Symmers' or 'clay pipe stem' fibrosis, so-called because it resembles a clay pipe in cross-section, with a thick white wall and a narrow lumen. There is usually no nodule formation or hepatic parenchymal cell damage, and hepatic function usually remains normal except when there is associated hepatitis B infection or after repeated gastrointestinal bleeding ('decompensated' hepatosplenic disease). The liver is usually enlarged, especially the left lobe, smooth and firm or hard, but may be normal in size or even shrunken. The presinusoidal fibrosis leads to portal hypertension, and the spleen is enlarged due to chronic passive congestion and reticuloendothelial hyperplasia. The enlarged spleen may be massive, and is firm or hard, and there may be peri-umbilical or 'Medusa head' collaterals. There may also be ascites and anaemia, as well as reduced growth, infantilism, amenorrhoea or loss of libido.

The most important consequence of portal hypertension is that in 80 per cent of patients with hepatosplenic disease there is evidence of oesophageal varices detectable by endoscopy. Bleeding from such varices leads to haematemesis, melaena or both. Blood loss is frequently massive, and exsanguination is the usual cause of death, rather than hepatic encephalopathy. Repeated episodes of gastrointestinal bleeding, preceding a massive terminal event, are characteristic.

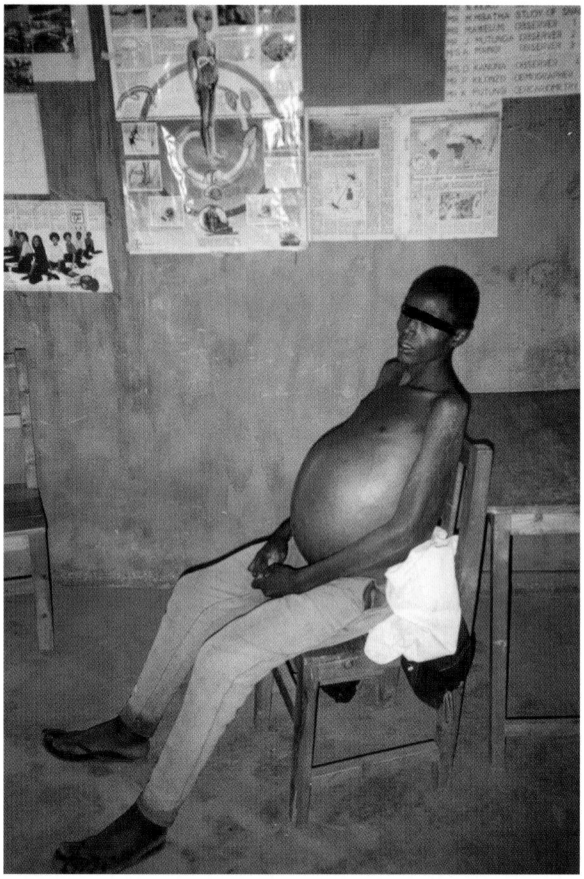

Fig. 25.10. A 19-year-old man from Machakos District, Kenya with massive hepatosplenomegaly and ascites attributable to *Schistosoma mansoni* infection.

Other chronic intestinal manifestations of *Schistosomiasis mansoni* include inflammation, fibrosis and sometimes polyposis in the large intestine. There is chronic intermittent diarrhoea, with or without the passage of blood, and the colon may be tender. Polyposis coli occurs mainly in Egypt, and is associated with anaemia, a protein-losing enteropathy and sometimes ascites.

In *S. haematobium* infections, the common late complication is an irreversible obstructive uropathy that may progress to uraemia. Calculus formation and secondary infections are common. Various changes occur in the bladder, including calcification, ulceration and papilloma formation. At cystoscopy, 'sandy patches', composed of eggs surrounded by dense fibrous tissue with an atrophic mucosal surface, are seen in the bladder walls. As the bladder lesions develop, there may be nocturia, precipitancy, dribbling and severe pain. The ureters are less commonly affected than the bladder, but their involvement is an important cause of morbidity, especially when bilateral, leading to hydronephrosis and loss of renal function. An association, possibly causal, has also been described between *S. haematobium* infection and squamous cell carcinoma of the bladder.

In *S. haematobium* infection, egg deposition, granuloma formation and fibrosis can also occur in the genital tract in both sexes. In males, there may be haematospermia and a sensation of 'lumpy semen' with pain on ejaculation: the sperm contains eggs, together with eosinophils and lymphocytes. In females, lesions of the cervix and vagina are observed. Eggs can be recovered by cervical biopsy when none are found in the urine, especially in women between 20 and 30 years old. There may be dyspareunia, contact bleeding and lower back pain. Genital schistosomiasis in either males or females could theoretically be a risk factor for the transmission of HIV: studies to test this are under way, but with no definite outcome at present.

Other manifestations of schistosomiasis

Apart from the local manifestations of schistosomiasis that are characteristic of each species, there may be others.

In both *S. mansoni* and *S. haematobium* infections, schistosomiasis can compromise growth and development in children. There may be stunting, delayed puberty, disorders of cognitive ability and poor school performance, all of which may be reversed by anti-schistosomal treatment.

Apart from the severe central nervous system lesions, sometimes associated with paraplegia, that are regularly observed in acute schistosomiasis, paraplegia can also rarely occur as a late complication of *S. mansoni* infection in individuals with heavy egg loads, attributable to ectopic egg deposition around the spinal cord, presenting as a slowly developing space occupying lesion, usually in the region of the cauda equina.

Deposition of eggs can also occur in the lungs. This is especially seen as a late complication of hepatosplenic schistosomiasis, in which the opening of porto-systemic collaterals allows the passage of eggs directly via the heart to the lungs. Granulomatous reactions and fibrosis develop in the pulmonary vasculature leading to pulmonary hypertension and cor pulmonale. Symptoms include fatigue, dyspnoea on exertion, cough and sometimes haemoptysis. Patients may progress to congestive cardiac failure, or sudden death may follow cardiovascular collapse.

Renal lesions can occur in *S. mansoni* infection, especially in Egypt, and consist of a chronic glomerulonephritis attributable to the deposition of immune complexes and complement components in the mesangium. The condition develops slowly, up to ten years after the onset of hepatosplenic disease, and presents as proteinuria, the nephrotic syndrome or hypertension.

Rare manifestations include hypopituitarism; chronic dermatitis, due to ectopic eggs; musculoskeletal involvement with polyarthritis in *Schistosomiasis mansoni*; and osteomalacia in *S. haematobium* infections resulting from renal tubular lesions.

Diagnosis and investigations

Diagnosis has two distinct purposes:

- To determine the presence of infection or disease in individual patients, to assist in decisions on individual treatment and management. In this case, *qualitative* evidence of the presence of infection is sufficient, but additional investigations may be necessary to determine the nature and extent of pathology.
- To determine the extent of infection or disease in populations, to assist decisions on the need for and approaches to control. In this case, and especially in epidemiological research studies, *quantitative* estimates of intensity of infection or disease may be needed.

Diagnosis of infection

Diagnosis of infection can be by direct demonstration of parasites or their products, or by indirect methods. The commonest techniques are the examination of faeces for *S. mansoni* and of urine for *S. haematobium.*

For *S. mansoni*, resuspension of faeces and sedimentation of the eggs, followed by microscopy, is a simple and useful qualitative technique. For quantitative studies, the Kato thick smear method is used, based on examination of a known amount of faeces. A stool sample is collected and homogenised by passing through a sieve, and a fixed amount, usually 50 mg, is sampled with a metal template. The sample is squashed on a slide under a cellophane coverslip previously soaked in glycerol and Malachite Green, and allowed to clear for 24 or more hours. The eggs are counted, and results expressed as eggs per gram of faeces. Between-sample variation in egg counts is high, and for detailed studies three to five stools are collected, with duplicate Kato preparations being made from each.

For *S. haematobium*, sedimentation or centrifugation of urine followed by microscopy is a useful qualitative technique. For quantitative studies, urine is collected, preferably at about mid-day, and a sample of 10–20 ml is passed, using a syringe, through a Nucleopore® (polycarbonate) or Nytrel® (polyamide) filter, which is then examined microscopically. Intensities are expressed as eggs per 10 ml of urine. Again, for detailed studies, examination of 3 to 5 urine samples is desirable.

In light infections, eggs can also be detected in rectal biopsies ('rectal snips'), which are crushed between glass slides and examined microscopically. This method is useful not only for *S. mansoni* but also for *S. haematobium*.

Recently, methods have been developed that allow the detection of schistosome antigens (circulating anodic antigen, CAA, or circulating cathodic antigen, CCA) in blood or urine. The assays have high sensitivity and specificity, and are extremely useful in detailed epidemiological studies, although they are not yet commercially available.

Indirect techniques include:

- The detection of antibodies to schistosome antigens. This may be done either by enzyme-linked immunosorbent assays (ELISAs) for antibodies to crude or partially purified egg antigens, or by indirect immunofluorescence tests on sections of adult worms. The tests are sensitive, and can detect changes following treatment, but their specificity is much less good than for the direct tests.
- In *S. haematobium* infections, the detection of protein or blood in the urine, by various dipstick tests, has proved to be a cheap and easy way of screening for infection in epidemiological and control studies, and can be used as a basis for treatment (Lwambo et al., 1997).
- Eosinophiluria is a characteristic of *S. haematobium* infection, and detection of the eosinophil cationic protein ECP has recently been used for the quantitative assessment of eosinophil infiltration in the bladder mucosa and hence of local inflammation.

Investigation of disease: the role of ultrasonography

Once a diagnosis is made, investigation of disease in individuals or populations generally follows conventional methods. However, one technique, ultrasonography, deserves particular mention (Hatz et al., 1992). During recent years, cheap and robust instruments have been developed that make it possible to carry out ultrasonographic examinations under field conditions. This has revolutionized the epidemiological investigation of morbidity, as opposed to infection, both for bladder and urinary tract lesions in *S. haematobium* infection and more recently for assessment of periportal fibrosis and portal hypertension in *S. mansoni* infections. Protocols for standardized investigations have been produced by WHO, and ultrasonography has proved particularly useful for monitoring the decline in morbidity after chemotherapy programmes.

Treatment and management

Treatment of infection

Treatment of schistosomiasis has been revolutionized over the past twenty years by the introduction of a number of drugs that are effective, safe and relatively inexpensive.

Two of the early drugs are still sometimes used:

- Oxamniquine (Vansil®) is used for the treatment of *S. mansoni* infections at a total dose of 30 mg/kg, given with food in two doses over 24 hours, or 60 mg/kg given in four doses over 48 hours. It is generally well tolerated, but can cause dizziness or epileptiform convulsions than can be severe. It is currently used only in South America, where there is now evidence for the emergence of drug-resistant strains of parasite.
- Metrifonate (Bilarcil®) is an inexpensive organophosphorus compound active only against *S. haematobium*. It needs to be given in three doses, each of 10 mg/kg, separated by two weeks. This makes it inconvenient for use in large scale control programmes. In addition, because of its effect on acetylcholinesterase, its use should be avoided in farmers exposed to organophosphorus pesticides.

Instead, treatment now depends mainly on praziquantel (Biltricide®, Distocide®). This is highly active against all three major species of schistosome that infect humans, as well as against other trematode and cestode infections. It is given as a single oral dose of 40 mg/kg, preferably with food. It has not been shown to be teratogenic, but is not recommended for use during pregnancy: treatment should be delayed until after delivery. Side effects are rarely severe, and include abdominal pain and vomiting in about 10 per cent of treated schoolchildren, rarely lasting for more than 24 hours, especially in children with high intensity of infection; urticarial skin reactions or periorbital oedema in about 2 per cent of treated children, especially in teenagers; and non-specific reactions including headache, dizziness, fatigue and fever.

In most areas, complete cure is achieved in up to 85 per cent of treated individuals, while the overall mean reduction in egg counts is 95 per cent or greater. This result is acceptable in population-based chemotherapy campaigns, in which the aim is to reduce the numbers of people with heavy infections that may lead to severe morbidity. If complete cure in an individual patient is required, treatment may be repeated on one or more occasions. Although not clearly proven, some individuals may be refractory to treatment: in these, retreatment may be with 60 mg/kg, given in two doses at an interval of 24 hours. There is no evidence for the emergence of drug resistance: poorer than usual treatment results in the epidemic focus of *S. mansoni* in Senegal may have been due to high starting levels of infection, rapid re-infection in a non-immune population, or a need for synergy between praziquantel and an immune response that was lacking in this newly exposed population.

Praziquantel is not a prophylactic drug, and is not effective against young migrating schistosomula. After initial treatment, a recently infected patient may need re-examination and retreatment after three months.

Management of complications

Acute schistosomiasis is potentially dangerous and difficult to diagnose positively before egg laying starts. Once suspicion has been aroused, it is acceptable to base treatment with praziquantel on clinical indications alone. If symptoms are severe, and especially if there are spinal cord lesions, patients should be hospitalized and given prednisolone, 40 mg for 3 to 5 days, in addition to praziquantel.

The management of the *long-term sequelae* of fibrosis, such as portal hypertension, haematemesis, obstructive uropathy or renal failure is beyond the scope of this section. In general, it is important to note that treatment of children during the early established stage of infection generally leads to a complete resolution of disease, although in areas of high transmission it may take two or three rounds of annual treatment to achieve this. Treatment with praziquantel may also, somewhat surprisingly, lead to a reduction in early fibrosis. However, once fibrosis is advanced, then specific anti-schistosomal treatment has little or no effect on the disease process: advanced fibrosis is anyway seen in older patients, in whom intensities of infection have already fallen to low levels. In such patients, praziquantel may be given to prevent further progression of disease, but the emphasis should be on managing the consequences.

Problems for future study

A number of significant advances have been made in recent years both in understanding the biology of human schistosomiasis and in applying such understanding to control of the disease. These include particularly:

- the introduction of safe and effective anti-schistosomal drugs (oxamniquine and metrifonate, and more recently praziquantel)
- the change in emphasis from control of infection to control of morbidity
- the introduction of ultrasonography as a tool for the large-scale assessment under field conditions of the extent of morbidity in populations, and
- advances in immunoepidemiology that have allowed us to begin to understand both the mechanisms of protective immunity and the events that contribute to severe disease.

In spite of these advances, however, schistosomiasis remains a major and poorly controlled public health problem in many African countries, and much remains to be done, both theoretically and practically. In particular:

- Drug treatment is not a final and definitive solution to the question of control, because of the problems of costs, the need for repeated treatment, and the possible emergence of drug-resistant parasites. A vaccine would be a useful adjunct to control. Progress has been made in experimental animal models, and candidate vaccines are reaching the stage of Phase 1 testing in humans. However, much work remains to be done in understanding the extent, nature and mechanisms of human immunity.
- The mechanisms of disease are beginning to be understood, but little is known about the reasons, other than intensity of infection, for the variation in disease seen between different countries, different communities and different individuals. The recently proven contribution to such variation of human genetic differences needs more work, while very little is known about the possible role of parasite genetic differences, host nutritional status, the role of maternal infection in the development of morbidity in the offspring, or interactions with other conditions such as malaria. Understanding the contribution of such factors might open up new approaches towards reducing the development of morbidity in individuals, which is now the main aim of control.

- As an extension of this point, there is a tendency to think about schistosomiasis in isolation, as if it exists separately from other conditions. In practice, of course, schistosomiasis occurs in conjunction with a multitude of other infections and conditions, and the possible interactions between schistosomiasis and such conditions have been poorly investigated. Such interactions might work in two directions, each of which deserves study. First, other conditions, especially malaria, hepatitis and HIV infection, may affect the severity and outcome of schistosome infection. Secondly, and equally importantly, schistosome infection might affect the outcome of other infections. This is potentially of great importance in the context of HIV, for which schistosomiasis might affect both initial susceptibility to infection and (through systemic changes in overall immune responses) the progress of disease. Evidence is lacking, but this is a major area for future research.

References

Butterworth AE, Fulford AJC, Dunne DW, Ouma JH, Sturrock RF (1988). Longitudinal studies on human schistosomiasis. *Phil Trans Roy Soc Lond, B*; **312**: 495–511.

Butterworth AE, Sturrock RF, Ouma JH et al. (1991). Comparison of different chemotherapy strategies against *Schistosoma mansoni* in Machakos District, Kenya: effects on human infection and morbidity. *Parasitology*; **103**: 339–355.

Dessein AJ, Hillaire D, Elwali NEMA et al. (1999). Severe hepatic fibrosis in *Schistosoma mansoni* infection is controlled by a major locus that is closely linked to the interferon-γ receptor gene. *Am J Hum Genet*; **65**: 709–721.

De Vlas SJ, Gryseels B. (1992). Underestimation of *Schistosoma mansoni* prevalences. *Parasitol Today*, **8**:274–277.

Doumenge JP, Mott KE, Cheung C et al. (1987). *Atlas of the Global Distribution of Schistosomiasis.* Geneva: World Health Organization Talence: Presses Universitaires de Bordeaux. 400 pp.

Fulford AJC, Butterworth AE, Sturrock RF, Ouma JH. (1992). On the use of age-intensity data to detect immunity to parasitic infections, with special reference to *Schistosoma mansoni* in Kenya. *Parasitology*; **105**: 219–227.

Hatz C, Jenkins JM, Tanner M, eds. (1992). Special issue: ultrasound in schistosomiasis. *Acta Trop*; **51**: 1–100.

Jordan P, Webbe G, Sturrock RF, eds. (1993). *Human Schistosomiasis.* Wallingford, UK: CAB International, 465 pp.

Kabatereine NK, Vennervald BJ, Ouma JH et al. (1999). Adult resistance to schistosomiasis mansoni: age-dependence of reinfection remains constant in communities with diverse exposure patterns. *Parasitology*; **118**: 101–105.

Lwambo NS, Savioli S, Kisumku UM, Alawi KS, Bundy DAP. (1997). Control of *Schistosoma haematobium* morbidity on Pemba Island: validity and efficiency of indirect screening tests. *Bull W H Org*; **75**: 247–252.

Machado PA. (1982). The Brazilian programme for schistosomiasis control 1975–1979. *Am J Trop Med Hyg*; **31**: 76–86.

Mahmoud AAF. (Ed). (2000). *Schistosomiasis.* In *Tropical Medicine. Science and Practice*; *Vol 3*. ed. G Pasvol, SL Hoffman. London: Imperial College Press. 550 pp.

Mwatha JK, Kimani G, Kamau T et al. (1998). High levels of TNF, sTNF receptors, sICAM-1 and IFN-g, but low levels of IL-5, are associated with hepatosplenic disease in human *Schistosomiasis mansoni. J Immunol*; **160**: 1992–1999.

Ongom VL, Bradley DJ. (1972). The epidemiology and consequences of *Schistosoma mansoni* infection in West Nile, Uganda. I. Field studies of a community at Panyagoro. *Trans Roy Soc of Trop Med Hyg*; **66**: 835–851.

Ouma JH, Wijers DJB, Siongok TKA. (1985). The effect of repeated targeted mass treatment on the prevalence of *Schistosomiasis mansoni* and the intensity of infection in Machakos, Kenya. *Ann Trop Med Parasitol*; **79**: 431–438.

Prentice MA, Ouma JH. (1984). Field comparison of mouse immersion and cercariometry for assessing the transmission potential of water containing the cercariae of *Schistosoma mansoni. Ann Trop Med Parasitol*; **78**: 169–172.

Savioli L, Renganathan E, Davis A, Behehani K. (1997). Control of schistosomiasis – a global picture. *Parasitol Today*, **13**: 444–448.

Talla I, Kongs A, Verle P, Belot J, Sarr S, Coll AM. (1990) Outbreak of intestinal schistosomiasis in the Senegal River basin. *Ann Soc Belge Med Trop*, **70**: 173–180.

World Health Organization. (1993). The control of schistosomiasis: second report of the WHO Expert Committee. *WHO Technical Report Series 830.* Geneva: WHO.

Paragonimiasis

26

The problem in Africa

Paragonimus spp. parasites only infect humans in Africa when they eat improperly cooked crustaceae (crabs mostly), infected with the metacercariae of the paragonimus parasite. In communities with a tradition for thorough cooking of meat and fish, or where crabmeat is taboo for whatever reason, clinical human disease is very rare.

There is evidence, however, that the parasitic cycle is continuous among the intermediate hosts, non-human definitive and reserve hosts such as wild cats, civet cats, crab-eating mongooses, pigs and dogs, as well as monkeys and lower primates (Nwokolo, 1974). Sudden deterioration in cooking standards due to an emergency, as, for example, during the Nigerian civil war (1967–70), greatly exaggerates the chances of human disease (Nwokolo, 1972a,b). The disease is endemic in parts of West Africa.

The parasite and its life cycle

In Africa, two *Paragonimus* species have been identified in those countries where the disease is endemic: *Paragonimus uterobilateralis*, the dominant parasite in Nigeria, Cameroon, Liberia, Guinea and Gabon (Voelker & Nwokolo, 1973; Sachs & Voelker, 1982) and *Paragonimus africanus* found in Cameroon (Kum & Nchinda,1982). The parasites are identified by the peculiarities of such anatomical features as ovaries, testes, suckers, cuticular spines and eggs.

The adult parasite is a fleshy fluke 6–12mm × 4–6mm × 3.5mm. The eggs of *P. westermani* are the largest (97 × 59μm) (Cabaret et al., 1999), those of *P. africanus* are intermediate in size (91 × 49μm), while *P. uterobilateralis* has the smallest (69 × 42μm): these are operculated.

Table 26.1. The known parasites and intermediate hosts of paragonimiasis

	Asia	Africa
Parasite	*P. westermani* *P. ohirai* *P. miyazakii*	*P. africanus* *P. uterobilateralis*
First intermediate host (snails)	Snails of *Melania* genus	Unknown ? Snails of *Ampullariidae spp.* ? *Potadoma freethii*
Second intermediate host (crabs)	*Eriocheir japonicus* and *Potamon dehaani*	*Sudanonates africanus* (fresh water) *Sudanonautes pelii* *Sudanonautes (Convexonautes) aubryi (Land crabs)*

Life cycle

When the eggs of *Paragonimus* are discharged from the sputum, they hatch within weeks into miracidia which swim around any available stream or brook and ultimately enter a snail (the first intermediate host). Here, they develop into rediae and later cercariae. The cercariae are ultimately released from the snails and seek and enter the muscles of the nearest suitable crab where they develop into metacercariae. Humans, or other definitive or reservoir hosts such as civet cats, become infected when they eat the infected crab. After ingestion, the metacercariae enter the duodenum or jejunum, pierce the peritoneum, the diaphragm and pleura and develop in the lungs.

The intermediate hosts

Unlike schistosomiasis, where there is just one intermediate host, paragonimiasis uses two: a mollusc (or snail) as the first, and a crustacean (crab or crayfish) as the second. Despite an intensive search, the snail (first) intermediate host has not yet been identified in Nigeria. The crustacean (second) intermediate hosts identified in West Africa are crabs of the *Sudanonautes* species, i.e. *Sudanonautes africanus, Sudanonautes aubryii* and *Sudonautes pelii* in Nigeria and *Liberonautes lactidactylus* in Liberia. In some areas of Easter Nigeria, *Sudanonautes aubryii* behaves as a land crab and in the rainy season some infected crabs have been caught in farms up to 1 km from the nearest stream.

Other hosts

As already indicated, the human is probably not an important definitive host in the total cycle of the *paragonimus* parasite in Africa. Other reservoir hosts, including wild carnivorous animals of the cat family, are probably more important than humans.

Epidemiology

In eastern Nigeria, the major ecological centre of paragonimiasis was found between the Cross River and the Imo River and along their tributaries. Infected crabs were found in the streams, and for sale in the market places that served the homes of *Paragonimus* patients. The River Niger area and its tributaries were free of infected crabs and patients. Areas east of the Cross River near the Cameroon border, however, harboured infected patients, suggesting that the well-known Cameroon focus may have been the genesis of a westward advance of the infection.

The finding of the appropriate intermediate hosts in other foci of human infection in West Africa such as Liberia, Guinea, Gabon and Benin, suggests that the ecological conditions favouring the spread of paragonimiasis are probably widespread in tropical Africa (Sachs & Voelcker, 1982).

The prevalence varies in endemic areas from about 5 per cent to over 12 per cent (Arene et al., 1997). In Cross River State in Nigeria (Ibanga & Eyo, 2001), where the prevalence was 8.7 per cent, the 11–15 age group had both the highest intensity and prevalence of infection (m= 18.5, f= 14 per cent).

Control and prevention

Adequate cooking of crabs before eating is the obvious preventive measure and must be part of health education in all endemic areas, but prevention can be difficult. For example, when crabs are caught in traps, young men may bite their heads and legs to prevent their escape, so inevitably the young men can become infected (Ibanga & Eyo, 2001).

Clinical features

The incubation period probably ranges from 3 to 24 months, from the time the crabmeat is eaten to the first episode of haemoptysis.

The host response

In the lungs, (Fig. 26.1) the parasites usually pair up and encyst in caverns in which they provoke a granulomatous tissue response consisting of polymorphs, eosinophils, macrophages and fibroblasts (Voelker & Sachs,1977). Each cavern develops a link with the nearest bronchus through which the eggs ultimately reach the sputum, and so lead to the classical clinical picture.

Evasion by the parasite

The newly excysted metacercariae of the parasite elaborate an excretory secretory product (ESP) which contains cysteine proteases. These attenuate the effector functions of the host's eosinophils, stimulated with IgG, so that they show abnormal degranulation and diminished superoxide production. This allows the parasite to evade the normal immune response of the host (Shin et al., 2001).

Respiratory symptoms

The frequency of blood-stained or coffee-coloured sputum, of cough, dyspnoea and of chest pains is highest in those with a heavy egg load in the sputum. Symptoms thus depend on the parasite load.

Blood stained sputum

The commonest symptom is blood-stained or coffee-coloured sputum. Massive haemoptysis is uncommon.

Clinically the patient looks well except in the presence of complications such as pneumothorax, pleurisy or empyema.

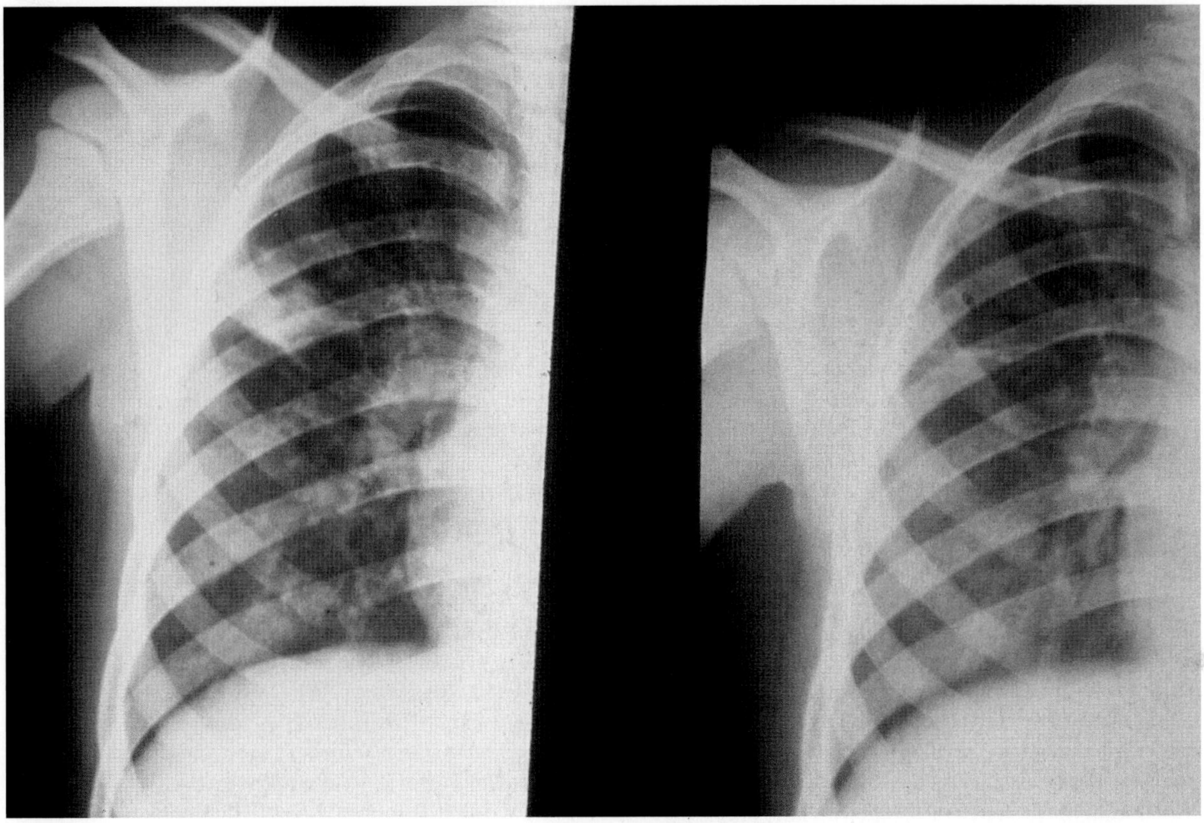

Fig. 26.1. Chest radiographs in a young boy infected with *Paragonimus uterobilateralis*, treated with praziquantel. R. upper zone infiltrate disappears: linear fibrosis only 11 months later. (Courtesy: Wellcome Trust and Bernhard Nocht Institute.)

Extra-pulmonary disease

Rarely, a patient may develop hemiparesis or epileptic fits.

Chest radiograph

Over three-quarters of patients with paragonimiasis show abnormal shadows in the chest radiograph; these are usually of low density and resemble the early shadows of pulmonary tuberculosis. The shadows are well defined in about one third of patients, ill defined in another third, while streaky shadows and bubble type cavitation are seen (Ogakwu & Nwokolo, 1973) in the remainder.

Diagnosis

The diagnosis of paragonimiasis depends on a careful history and microscopic examinations of the sputum and faeces; immunological diagnostic procedures, where available, are useful in epidemiological evaluation.

Sputum

Specimens collected between 06 00 h and 10 00 h have the highest sensitivity. In suspicious cases, where there is no contra-indication, a short brisk exercise improves the prospects for producing an egg-rich sputum, which can be scooped up and examined immediately without staining, under the low power of a microscope.

Paragonimus eggs

These are relatively large and unmistakable – golden brown, ovoid, operculated and 7–10 times the length of the red blood cells that usually surround them. Where eggs are absent, and the diagnosis of paragonimiasis is strongly suspected, the sputum or faeces can be concentrated and examined again. Mix sputum 5 ml with 10 ml NaOH (4%) for 20 min at 37 °C, centrifuge for 3 min at 1200 *g* and examine the sediment with the low-power lens.

CAUTION - TUBERCULOSIS!
Always stain the sputum with Ziehl–Neelsen
Look for acid-fast bacilli:
Tuberculosis and paragonimiasis sometimes co-exist.

Paragonimus skin test

A special antigen derived from extracts of the parasite is used. Patients with paragonimiasis develop an enlarged wheal within 20 minutes. Even after the disease is cured, the test remains positive and so it is valuable in epidemiological surveys. About 50 per cent of Paragonimus patients have blood eosinophilia of more than 1000/μl.

Treatment

Bithionol, the mainstay of the treatment of paragonimiasis for three decades, has been superseded by praziquantel because of its low toxicity and broad spectrum anti-helminthic qualities against not only paragonimiasis, but also schistosomiasis.

For paragonimiasis, a suitable dose is 40 mg per kg body weight daily for 2 days.

Unsolved problems

Land crabs in the life cycle of African paragonimiasis need to be investigated further to define where they are involved in the system. The possibility that rodents, which sometimes share crab holes with land crabs, may act as reserve definitive hosts needs to be studied. Also, the snail intermediate host needs to be identified or the apparent heresy of a single intermediate host re-examined.

References

Arene FOI, Ibanga ES, Asor JE. (1997). Epidemiology of paragonimiasis in Cross River Basin, Nigeria; prevalence and intensity of infection due to *Paragonimus uterobilateralis* in Yakurr local Government Area. *Public Hlth*; **111**: 1–4.

Cabaret J, Bayassade-Dufour C, Tami G et al. (1999). Identification of African Paragonomidae by multivariate analysis of the eggs. *Acta Trop*; **15**: 79–89.

Ibanga ES, Eyo VM. (2001). Pulmonary paragonimiasis in Oban community in Akamkpa Local Government Area, Cress River State, Nigeria: prevalence and intensity of infection. *Trans Roy Soc Trop Med Hyg*; **95**: 159–160.

Kum PN, Nchinda TC. (1982). Pulmonary paragonimiasis in Cameroon. *Trans Roy Soc Trop Med Hyg*; **76**: 768–771.

Nwokolo C. (1972a). Outbreak of paragonimiasis in eastern Nigeria. *Lancet*; **i**: 32–33.

Nwokolo C. (1972b). Endemic paragonimiasis in eastern Nigeria. *Trop Geog Med*; **23**: 128–147.

Nwokolo C. (1974). Endemic paragonimiasis in Africa. *Bull Wld Hlth Org*; **50**: 569–581.

Ogakwu M, Nwokolo C. (1973). Radiological findings in pulmonary paragonimiasis as seen in Nigeria: a review based on 1000 cases. *Br J Radiol*; **46**: 699–705.

Sachs R, Voelker J. (1982). Human paragonimiasis caused by *Paragonimus uterobilateralis* in Liberia and Guinea, West Africa. *Tropenmed Parasitol*; **33**: 15–16.

Shin MH, Kita H, Park HY et al. (2001). Cysteine protease secreted by *Paragonimus westermani* attenuates effector functions of human eosinophils stimulated with immunoglobulin G *Infect Immun*; **69**: 1599–1604.

Voelker J, Nwokolo C. (1973). Human paragonimiasis in eastern Nigeria caused by *Paragonimus uterobilateralis. Tropenmed Parasitol*; **24**: 323–328.

Voelker J, Sachs R. (1977). Monkeys and lower primates as natural and experimental hosts of African lung flukes. *Tropenmed Parasitol*; **28**: 137–144.

Loiasis

27

The problem in Africa

Loiasis is a purely African filarial infection and is endemic in the rainforest belt of West Africa, especially Cameroon and Southern Nigeria, Congo, Gabon and equatorial Sudan (See Fig. 27.1). The prevalence of microfilaraemia may be as high as 33 per cent in some areas (Gardon et al., 1997). *Loa loa*, the responsible helminth, only rarely causes disability or serious ill health. It is, however, responsible for episodes of recurrent subcutaneous swellings, especially in the limbs and face, called Calabar swellings after the Eastern Nigerian town in the heart of the endemic area. As it can cause a significant and sustained eosinophilia, it may well be one of the helminths which, on account of the pathological effects of eosinophils on the heart, can lead to endomyocardial fibrosis.

The parasite and its life cycle

Loa loa is a thread-like, creamy white parasite. The female measures 5–7cm and the smaller male about 3 cm. The microfilariae are diurnal, measure about 250 microns, are sheathed and have nuclei reaching the very end of the tail, which may also be curved (see Fig. 29.3). By contrast, those of *Mansonella perstans,* which is found in many areas where *Loa loa* is prevalent, are not sheathed.

The vector

The vector is a blood-sucking 'mango fly' C*hrysops dimidiata* or *C. silacea* which ordinarily lives in the treetops of the rainforest and is attracted downwards in the daytime towards humans by smoke and human movement. The female C*hrysops* bites and transmits infective larvae of *Loa loa* into the subcutaneous tissues of the host. Here they mature and begin to produce symptoms 3 to 18 months later. Microfilariae produced by the parent worms appear in the blood and, unlike those of *Wuchereria bancrofti,* are found in the blood by day. Warmth in the daytime attracts microfilariae towards the cutaneous blood vessels where they are easily picked up by the tabanid mango flies for ultimate transmission to other victims after a period of development.

Fig. 27.1. Distribution of *Loa loa* in Africa. (Adapted from Muller, 1975.)

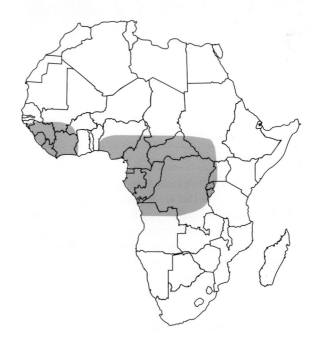

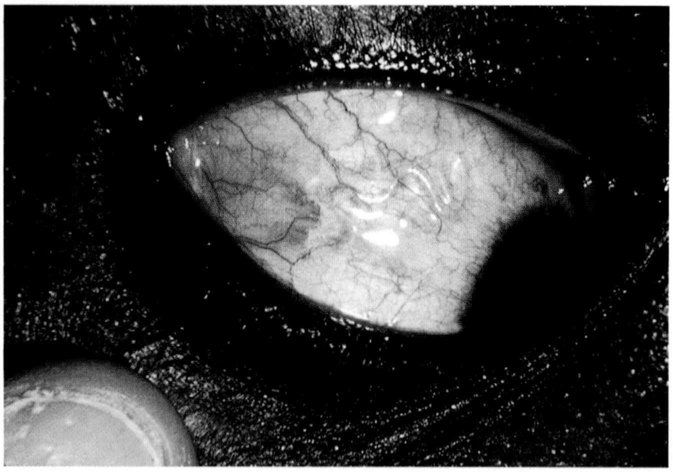

Fig. 27.2. Adult *Loa* crossing the eye.

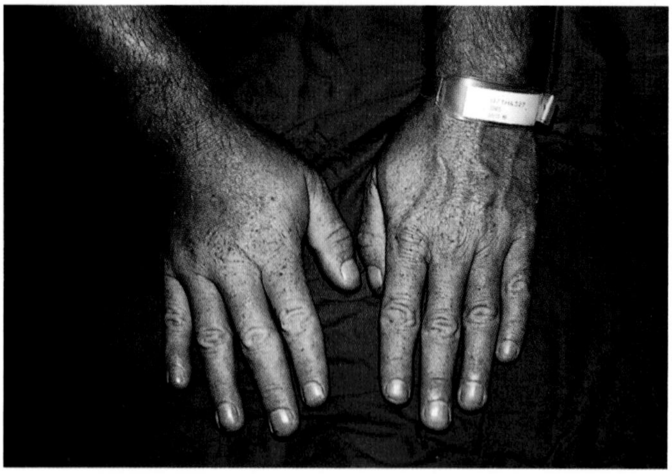

Fig. 27.3. Calabar swelling on dorsum of right hand.

Epidemiology

The principal victims of loiasis infection are the inhabitants, of all ages, of huts in the villages of the African rainforest belts, from the Gulf of Guinea to the Great Lakes. The female tabanid flies lay their eggs in batches in the sandy or muddy beds of the streams in these villages, attaching them to the vegetation or rocks. Within 1 week the eggs hatch and the larvae burrow into the mud or sand, taking up to 1 year to mature into pupae and later adults.

Female tabanid flies are the blood suckers. Their mouth parts, unlike those of the males, are specially designed for this purpose. Adult tabanid flies live in the treetops but the females come down and suck blood from and transfer infective microfilariae to hut dwellers below. When dwelling houses are widely separated from the breeding places of tabanid flies, the incidence of loiasis falls.

Clinical features

Calabar swelling

The major clinical sign of loiasis is the Calabar swelling, which appears in about one-third of those who are microfilaraemic, and about a third of those who report an ocular passage of a worm (Fig. 27.2) (Akue et al., 1996). This is a puffy, diffuse, subcutaneous swelling, usually on the limbs or face. It lasts from a few hours to several days and is often precipitated by vigorous use of affected limbs (Fig. 27.3).

Eye worm

The adult worm can sometimes be seen as it passes across the eye under the conjunctiva, for several minutes or for up to 3 hours. There may also be pruritus, but this is not specific to loiasis. A peripheral blood eosinophilia is common.

Diagnosis

A Calabar swelling in a patient who has lived in, or visited, an endemic area in the rainforest belt is highly suggestive of loiasis, but it is only reported in about one-third of those who are microfilaraemic. Ocular passage of a worm is diagnostic.

Other clinical features

Hydrocoele Adult worms in the scrotum can cause hydrocoele (Negesse et al., 1985)

Laboratory diagnosis

Detection of microfilariae

Prepare a daytime wet (anticoagulated) blood sample and examine directly for microfilariae under the microscope. Sensitivity can be increased by filtering up to 20 ml of anticoagulated blood through a 5 micron Nuclipore filter, and examining the filter under low power.

Serology

Filarial specific IgG, measured by ELISA, is not specific for loa.

Treatment

Diethycarbamazine (DEC), albendazole and ivermectin are all filaricidal drugs which reduce *Loa* microfilaraemia significantly, but only DEC has an effect on the adult worm, which is assumed to cause the clinical effects of the disease. The dose of DEC is 8–10mg per kg per day, in divided doses, for 21 days. DEC can lead to severe reactions in those with onchocerciasis, so should usually be avoided in onchocersiasis endemic areas. A single dose of ivermectin (200 μg/kg) has been shown to reduce microfilaraemia, in patients with loiasis, in Gabon by 87 per cent for up to 10 to12 months (Duong et al., 1997).

Treatment with either DEC or ivermectin can lead to severe encephalopathic reactions 3–4 days after treatment in those with high microfilarial counts in the peripheral blood (Gardon et al., 1997). The risk of this is probably reduced by steroids: prednisolone 20mg daily is recommended, starting 3 days before treatment and continuing for 3 days after the start of treatment.

Prevention and control

Barrier protection

Protective clothing, which is worn to cover all parts of the body during visits to an endemic area, can prevent or minimize the bite of tabanid flies.

Ivermectin in primary and secondary control

Ivermectin, given in a dose of 200 μg/kg, every 3 months to the population of an endemic area, reduces both the prevalence of microfilaraemia and also, therefore, the infectivity of *Chrysops* (Chippaux et al., 1998). The Onchocerciasis Control Programme (OCP) has radically changed the problem of loiasis in some areas where the two infections co-exist, for example in Cameroon, because of the filaricidal effects of the ivermectin. But this strategy is not without risk so that ivermectin cannot be recommended as a means of primary control of loiasis.

References

Akue JP, Hommel M, Devaney E. (1996). Markers of *Loa loa* infection in permanent residents of a loiasis endemic area of Gabon. *Trans Roy Soc Trop Med Hyg*; **90**: 115–118.

Boussinesq M, Gardon J, Gardon-Wendel N, et al. (1998). Three probable cases of *Loa loa* encephalopathy following ivermectin treatment for onchocerciasis. *Am J Trop Med Hyg*; **58**: 461–469.

Chippaux J-P, Bouchite B, Boussinesq M et al. (1998). Impact of repeated large scale ivermectin treatment on the transmission of *Loa loa*. *Trans Roy Soc Trop Med Hyg*; **92**: 454–458.

Duong TH, Kombila M, Ferrer A et al. (1997). Reduced *Loa loa* microfilaria count ten to twelve months after a single dose of ivermectin. *Trans Roy Soc Trop Med Hyg*; **91**: 592–593.

Gardon J, Gardon-Wendel N, Demanga-Ngangue et al. (1997). Serious reactions after mass treatment of onchocerciasis with ivermectin in an area endemic for *Loa loa* infection. *Lancet*; **350**: 18–22.

Muller, R. (1975). *Worms and Disease*, p. 100. Heinemann.

Negusse, Y. Lanoie LO, Neafie RC et al. (1985). Loiasis: 'Calabar' swellings and involvement of deep organs. *Am J Trop Med Hyg*; **34**: 537–546.

28 Onchocerciasis

The problem in Africa

Onchocerciasis, or river blindness, is caused by the filarial worm, *Onchocerca volvulus* and transmitted by blood-sucking Simulium blackflies which breed near fast-flowing rivers. The disease is endemic in 27 countries in sub-Saharan Africa. The first manifestation of infection is usually intense pruritus. Subsequently, a wide variety of acute and chronic skin and eye changes develop. Approximately 270 000 people are blind and 500 000 have significant visual loss directly as a consequence of onchocerciasis and onchocerciasis is the world's fourth most common cause of blindness. There are no comprehensive estimates for the burden of skin disease and severe itching, but such symptoms probably cause suffering in some 6 million people (WHO, 1995a; Okello et al., 1995; Makunde et al., 2000). The socioeconomic consequences are most marked in hyperendemic areas in sub-Saharan Africa.

Organism, life cycle, vector and host

Onchocerciasis is spread by a small black fly of the genus Simulium. Subspecies of this fly have rainforest, sudan and guinea savannah as their natural habitat. All require fast flowing, turbulent water for their larvae to develop, hence infection occurs in communities living near breeding sites and the illness has become known as river blindness.

The disease itself is caused by a filarial worm *Onchocerca volvulus*. After mating, a female Simulium takes a blood meal for the maturation of her eggs. If this meal is taken from an infected host, then she also ingests microfilariae which subsequently mature in her to L3 infective larvae. The cycle is completed when these enter the next human she feeds upon (Fig. 28.1).

Inside the human host, L3 larvae develop into adult worms, which may be found in nodules over bony prominences. These worms produce millions of microfilariae which cause a majority of the symptoms and signs of onchocerciasis.

Epidemiology and sociology

Because the disease is limited to populations who are bitten by the Simulium fly, it occurs in pockets around the fast flowing water breeding sites. In savanna areas of sub-Saharan Africa, up to one in ten people in affected communities may be blind. In the context of the developing world population age distribution, this means one in three or even one in two individuals aged 40 years and above are blind. This has a major effect on communities (Evans, 1995) and life expectancy (Kirkwood et al., 1983; Prost & Vaugelade, 1981).

In Kaduna State, Northern Nigeria we interviewed 97 blind individuals in communities mesoendemic for onchocerciasis. The reported effect on family income and social position was telling, with over two-thirds being definitely financially worse off since becoming blind.

In the same study of blind individuals a majority reported that they had no idea why they were blind. Furthermore, enquiry of local populations in hyperendemic areas in the Hawal Valley, Nigeria about why some of the villages had been abandoned, almost never yielded blindness or onchocerciasis as a reason. In the Onchocerciasis Control Programme (OCP), it has been noted that communities move when the level of blindness exceeds 10 per cent. It is probable that this level of blindness existed in the Hawal Valley villages. The workers in OCP have also reported a similar apparent denial of the true reason for moving by populations in their study areas.

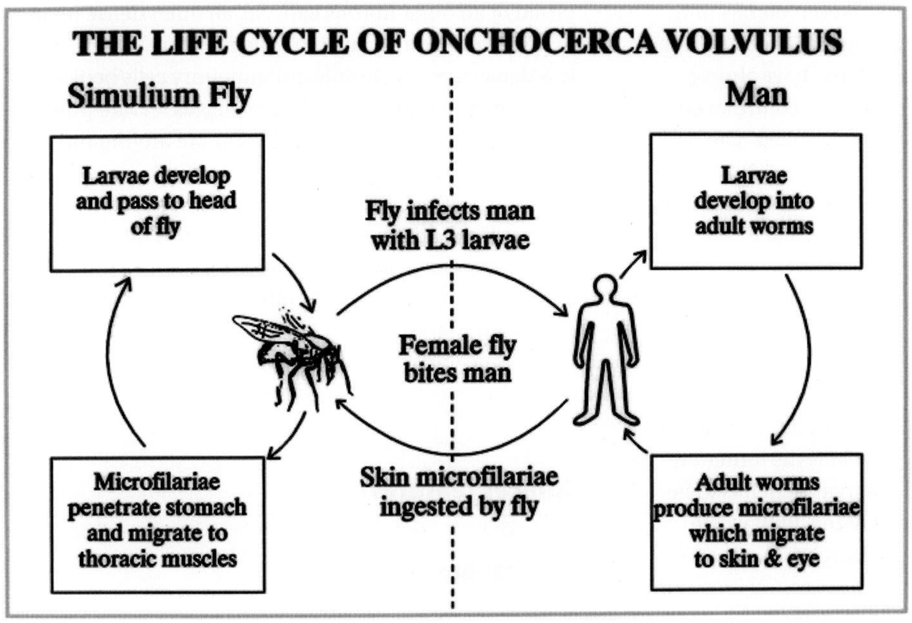
THE LIFE CYCLE OF ONCHOCERCA VOLVULUS
Simulium Fly
Man
Larvae develop and pass to head of fly
Fly infects man with L3 larvae
Larvae develop into adult worms
Female fly bites man
Microfilariae penetrate stomach and migrate to thoracic muscles
Skin microfilariae ingested by fly
Adult worms produce microfilariae which migrate to skin & eye

Fig. 28.1. The life cycle of *Onchocerca volvulus* showing Simulium black fly vector and human host. (By permission from International Centre of Eye Health, London – Teaching Slide Set).

Rainforest areas have lower levels of onchocercal blindness but here skin manifestations are the main complications of disease. It is now appreciated that there are harmful stigmatizing and other psychosocial effects from onchocercal skin disease (OSD) (Ovuga et al., 1995; Brieger et al., 1998a; Vlassoff et al., 2000). For example, in a community in the forest area of Nigeria, adolescent girls considered onchodermatitis to be their most significant health problem because of its severe social consequences. In fact, the Ettehs and local people in other Igbo-speaking areas of Eastern Nigeria describe onchodermatitis as *'Osepuru nwanyi aka na di'* meaning a disease which 'prevents a girl from getting married' (Amazigo, 1993). Futhermore, women with OSD breast-fed their infants for a shorter period than non-infected women because of fatigue from constant itching (Amazigo, 1994). There is also an economic impact of OSD in that farmers with OSD had significantly less farmland under cultivation and had a lower value of personal wealth indicators (e.g. iron sheet roofing, motorcycle) than those without OSD (Oladepo et al., 1997).

Prevention

The most common form of prevention is avoidance of infected areas, and prior to effective control programmes, abandoned villages were often seen in heavily infected regions. Elimination of breeding sites such as bridges or dams which cause turbulent water flow may be helpful and care must always be taken with new projects to ensure that fresh breeding sites are not created. The blackflies bite in the early morning and late evening, but avoidance of the peak biting times by working in the heat of the day is not very practical. Similarly, insect repellents and long clothing are not very expedient.

Control

The Onchocerciasis Control Programme (OCP) 1974–2002

This first major control programme aimed to eliminate the vector blackfly by regular aerial larviciding of rivers in areas with known high rates of onchocercal blindness. The project started with seven member countries in West Africa (Burkina Faso, Niger, Benin, Ivory Coast, Ghana, eastern Mali and Togo), and in 1986 the programme was extended to include parts of Guinea, Guinea Bissau, western Mali, Senegal and Sierre Leone. The OCP now has 11 participating countries, covering an area of 1.23 million sq. km and a combined population of about 30 million people.

The larviciding programme has to be continued throughout the lifespan of the adult worms in the human host (i.e. 10–14 years). The parasite reservoir has now been virtually eliminated in the original 7-country operational area where vector control efforts have almost ceased. Ivermectin is now being used to control recrudescence in areas where larviciding has stopped. The programme is scheduled to come to an end by 2002.

The OCP has been an outstanding success resulting in resettlement and economic development of fertile areas previously deserted.

Global control strategy

In 1987 ivermectin (Mectizan) became widely available for treatment trials of onchocerciasis in humans. It is a safe, effective microfilaricide (i.e. it kills the immature larval stages of filarial worms) but treatment has to be repeated throughout the lifespan of the adult worm (10–14 years). The manufacturer, Merck & Co., Inc., pledged to provide **free** all the drug necessary for as long as necessary to overcome onchocerciasis as a public health problem. It established the Mectizan Donation Programme, which has collaborated with WHO, health ministries and non-governmental organizations in a new global strategy based on yearly administration of single doses of ivermectin to affected populations.

The African Programme for Onchocerciasis Control (APOC) 1995–2007

The objective of this most recent programme, is to establish within 12 years sustainable community-directed ivermectin distribution systems in the 19 countries outside the OCP where onchocerciasis still is a public health problem (Angola, Burundi, Cameroon, Chad, the Cental African Republic (CAR), the Congo, the Democratic Republic of the Congo, Ethiopia, Equatorial-Guinea, Gabon, Kenya, Liberia, Malawi, Mozambique, Nigeria, Rwanda, Uganda, Sudan and Tanzania). In these countries it is estimated that 6.4 million heavily infected people live in areas where the parasite strains cause high rates of blindness and some 6 million heavily infected people live in areas where the parasite strains produce severe pruritus and skin disease.

Pathology and pathogenesis

The adult worms become encapsulated by fibrous tissue and form relatively asymptomatic subcutaneous nodules. They are particularly prevalent around the pelvic girdle and over other bony prominences. The nodules are composed of an outer fibrous capsule, an inner dense inflammatory cell infiltrate surrounding the adult worms, and a less dense layer of chronic inflammatory cells between the outer and inner layers. Macrophages feature prominently in the inflammatory cell infiltrate around the adult worms (Ottesen, 1994).

The microfilariae migrate out of the nodule and concentrate in the dermis of the skin, the eye and lymph nodes where host inflammatory reactions to dead and dying microfilariae result in inflammation and pathology (Murdoch, 1992).

The range of immunological responses in onchocerciasis has been well reviewed (Ottesen, 1994).

Clinical features

Eye changes

Typical

Microfilariae

Using a slit lamp, microfilariae may be seen in the cornea using scatter and/or retro-illumination. Similarly, they may be visualized in the anterior chamber of the eye after adopting a head down posture for over a minute.

Punctate keratitis

White cell infiltrates occur in the anterior third of the corneal stroma around dead microfilariae, particularly at 3 and 9 o'clock positions (Fig. 28.2*a*) (Tonjum & Thylefors, 1978).

Scelerosing keratitis

Sclerosing keratitis comprises a full thickness fibrovascular change in the cornea continuous with the limbus. These corneal changes occur typically at the three and nine positions but can extend to cover the entire cornea (Figs 28.2*b*, *c*).

Uveitis

The typical uveitis of onchocerciasis is flare without cells. Intraocular pressures are lower in infected populations and peripheral anterior synechiae are related to infection (Yang et al., 2001).

Optic atrophy

In the posterior segment, optic atrophy is common and may be the only clinical sign. Optic disc pallor is often secondary to an episode of optic neuritis (Fig. 28.3*a*, *b*).

Onchochorioretinitis

The retinal pigment epithelium is the first of the chorio-retinal layers to be damaged. The most common site for initial loss of this layer is just temporal to the macular area. Loss of the pigment epithlial layer may then extend to involve the entire posterior pole with atrophy and loss of the underlying choroid and death of the overlying retina (Bird et al., 1976). The end-stage fundal appearance is termed a Hisset–Ridley fundus after the authors who gave the first detailed descriptions of it. There is advanced optic atrophy with sheathing of the peripapillary vessels and extensive chorioretinal atrophy of the entire posterior pole leaving only attenuated major retinal vessels, large choroidal vessels and some clumps of pigment covering the sclera (Fig. 28.3*c*, *d* and Fig. 28.4).

Less commonly noted

Microfilariae

These have been reported as being seen in the lens, vitreous and retina.

Uveitis

The pupil may become pear shaped.

Inflammation in the posterior segment

Active chorioretinitis is occasionally observed.

Forest/savannah differences

Typically forest areas have individuals with higher microfilarial loads and less blinding disease. In savannah areas sclerosing keratitis is more common. Posterior segment lesions are seen in both savannah and forest areas (Anderson et al., 1974). Duke introduced the hypothesis of different Onchocerca–Simulium complexes in a series of papers in 1966 (Duke, 1966).

Skin changes

Pruritus

Generalized itching is often the first manifestation of infection.

A classification of the cutaneous changes in onchocerciasis has been developed (Murdoch et al., 1993). This defines the following five main categories of skin disease which may co-exist.

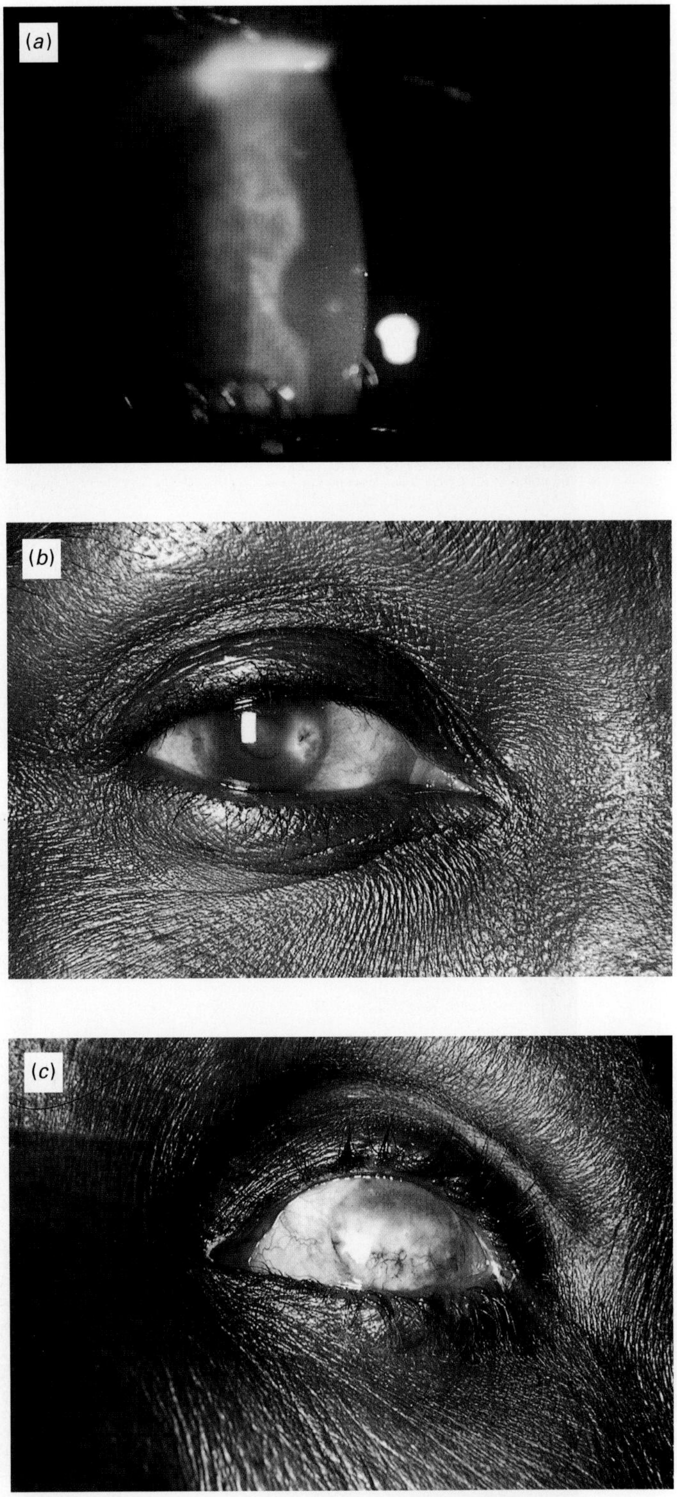

Fig. 28.2. Onchocercal punctate keratitis with dead microfilaria in cornea surrounded by white cell infiltrate (*a*). Sclerosing keratitis at 3 and 9 o'clock positions (*b*), and affecting entire cornea (*c*) (I. Murdoch).

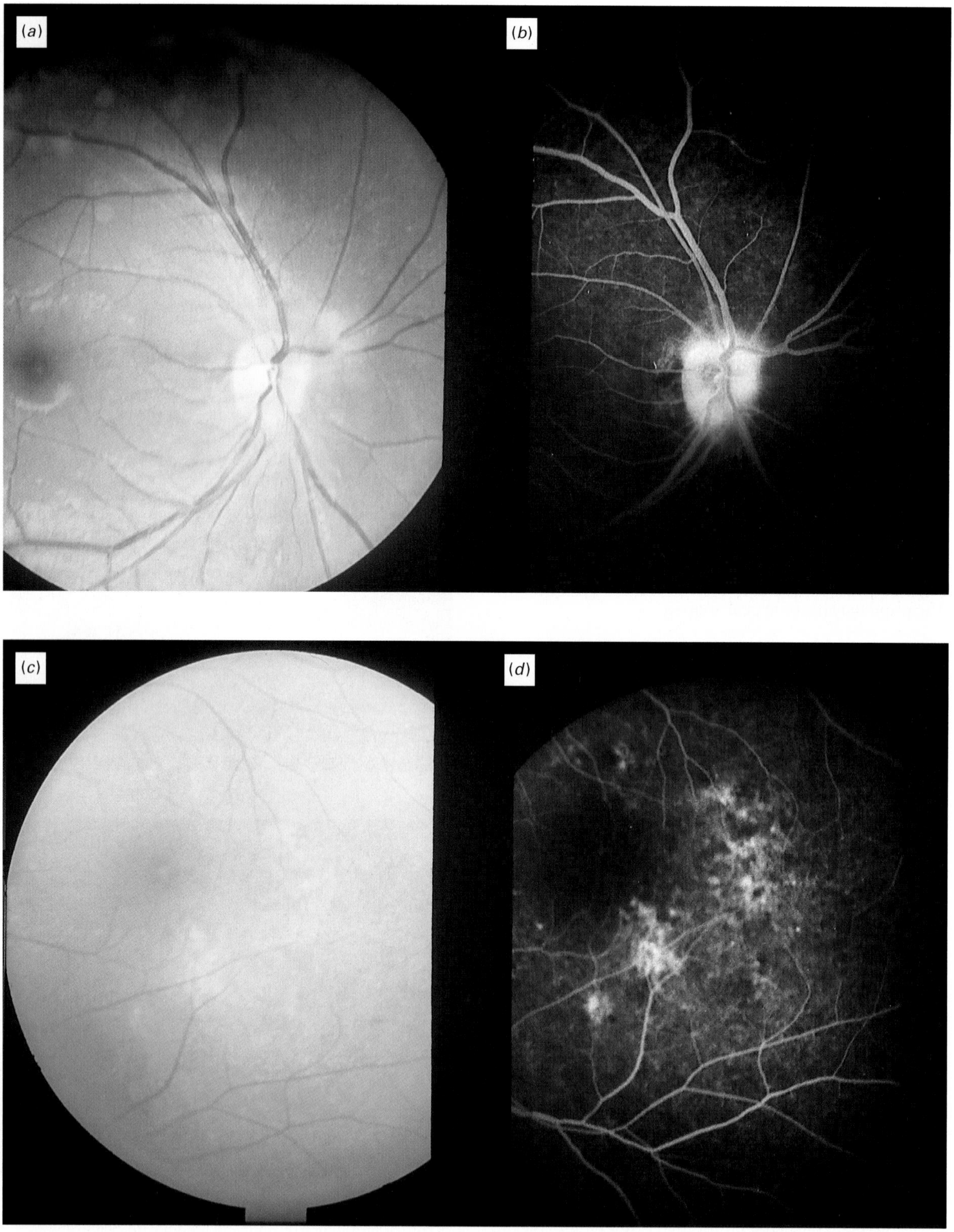

Fig. 28.3. (*a*) Active optic neuritis; (*b*) with leakage of fluorescein on angiography;. (*c*) Retinal pigment epithelial disease; (*d*) with window defects on angiography (I. Murdoch).

Acute papular onchodermatitis

Acute papular onchodermatitis (or APOD) is common in children and young adults and consists of small itchy skin-coloured papules and sometimes small pustules which are usually scattered over the upper trunk and arms (Fig. 28.5).

Chronic papular onchodermatitis

Chronic papular onchodermatitis (or CPOD) is also common in children and adults. The itchy papules are larger and more variable in size than APOD and are often flat-topped (Fig. 28.6). The waist, buttocks and limbs are common affected sites. The papules may heal leaving post-inflammatory hyperpigmentation.

Lichenified onchodermatitis

Lichenified onchodermatitis (or LOD) typically occurs in adolescent and young adult males. Extremely itchy hyperpigmented papules and plaques are characteristically located on a single limb, usually the leg, associated with enlargement of the draining lymph nodes (Fig. 28.7).

Atrophy

Atrophy of the skin is seen around the buttocks, waist and upper thighs in adults (Fig. 28.8). In order to avoid confusion with senile atrophy of the skin, the term onchocercal atrophy is restricted to individuals aged less than 50 years old.

Hanging groin is seen in males and females. Inguinal lymph nodes are thought to enlarge within a sac of atrophic skin on the medial thigh, then as the nodes shrink and become fibrotic, they leave redundant folds of loose skin (Fig. 28.9).

Depigmentation

Depigmentation characteristically occurs on the anterior shins in elderly people (Fig. 28.10). The inguinal regions and external genitalia may also be affected.

Diagnosis

Skin snipping

After cleaning the skin, a small tent of skin is raised with the point of a needle and the apex shaved off with a scalpel.

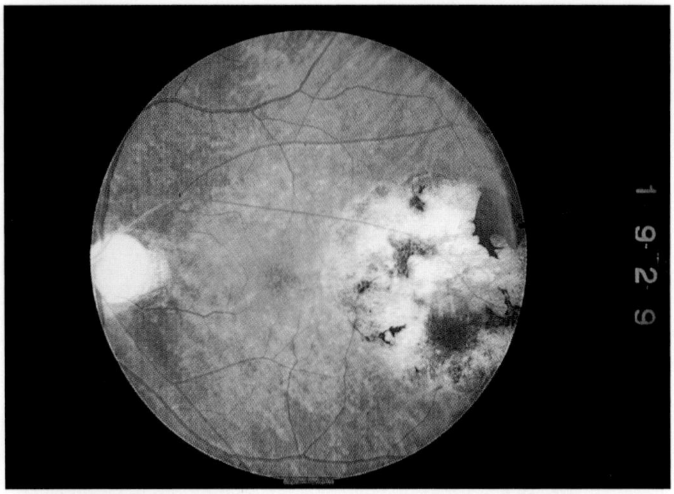

Fig. 28.4. Onchocercal chorioretinitis with optic disc pallor. (From Murdoch et al., 1993.)

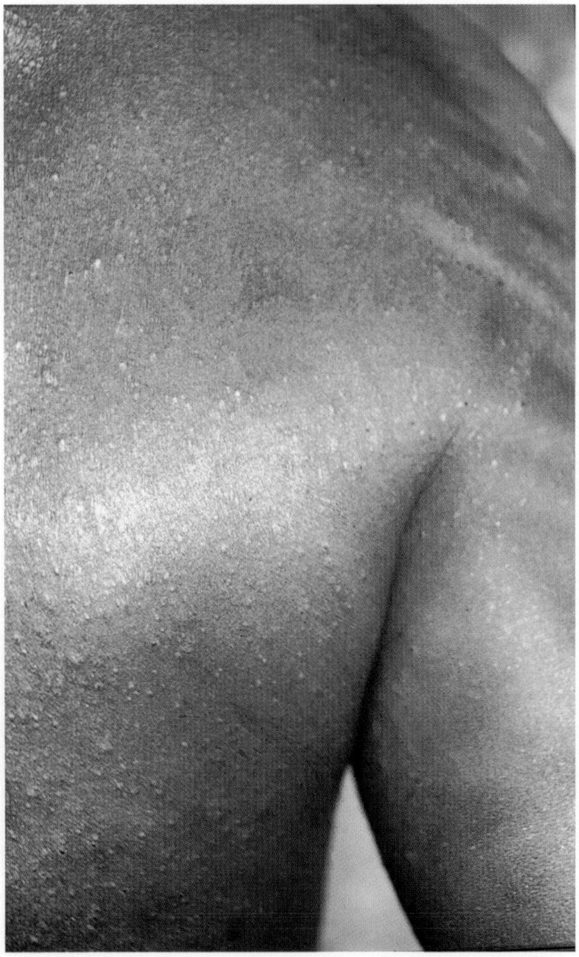

Fig. 28.5. Acute papular onchodermatitis. (From Murdoch et al., 1993.)

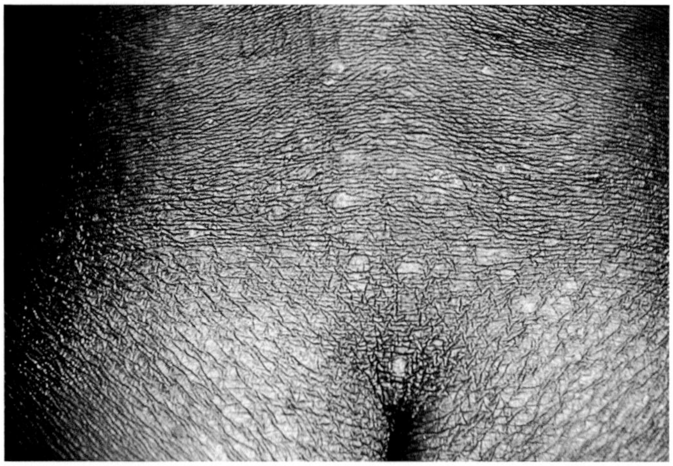

Fig. 28.6. Chronic papular onchodermatitis. (From Murdoch et al., 1993.)

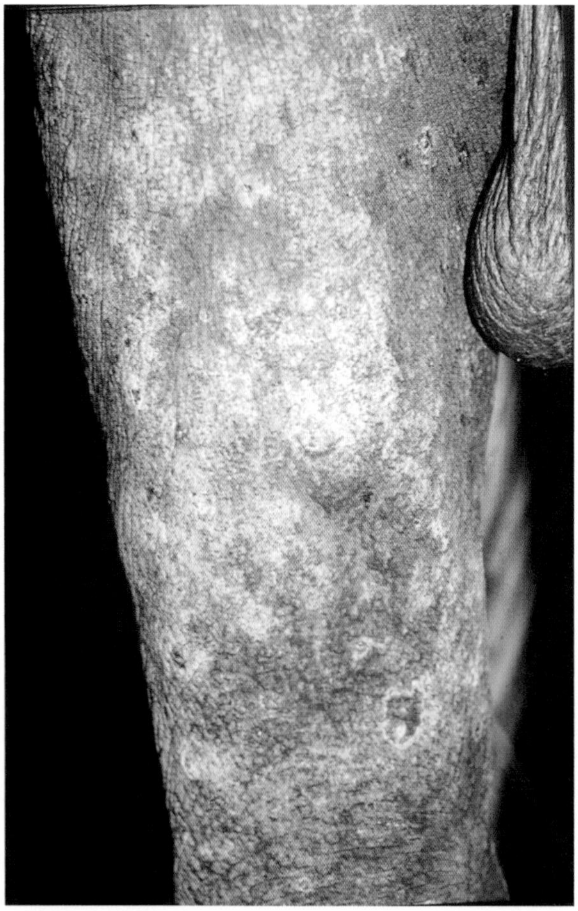

Fig. 28.7. Late confluent stage of lichenified onchodermatitis. (From Murdoch et al., 1993.)

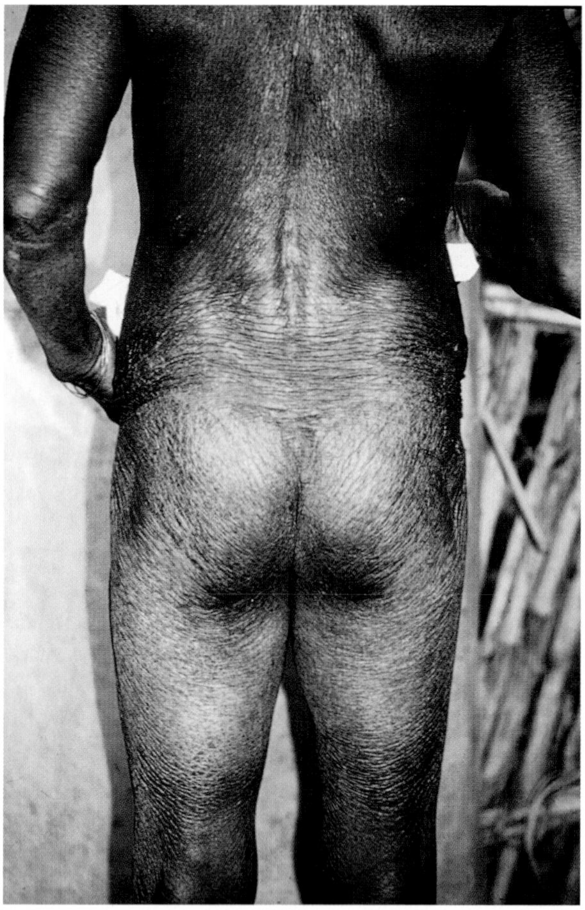

Fig. 28.8. Onchocercal atrophy confined to the buttocks. (From Murdoch et al., 1993.)

A corneoscleral punch is more convenient to use for large-scale surveys. Usually at least 2 snips are taken, one from each iliac crest. For individual diagnosis, the sensitivity is increased by taking additional snips from the scapular region and the calf. The skin-snip is placed in saline in a well of a microtitre plate and after 30 min–24 hours microfilariae may be seen on low power microscopy to have migrated out of the tissue. For research purposes the skin snip may be weighed and the result expressed as the number of microfilariae/mg skin. Skin snips may be negative in pre-patent and early or light infections (WHO, 1987).

Other parasitological forms of diagnosis

Detection of intra-ocular microfilariae using a slit lamp

If the patient is asked to put their head between their knees for at least 1 minute and then examined on a slit

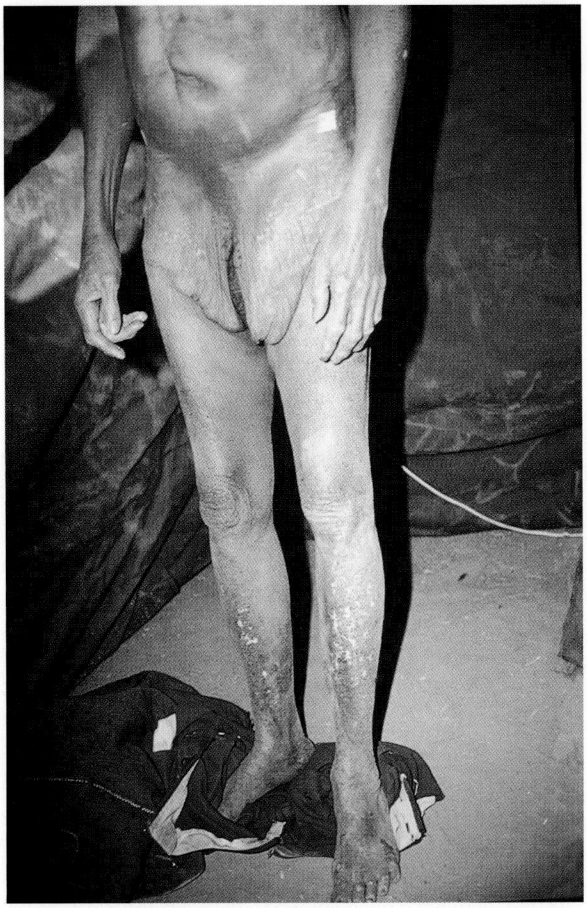

Fig. 28.9. Late hanging groin, with redundant folds of atrophic skin. (From Murdoch et al., 1993.)

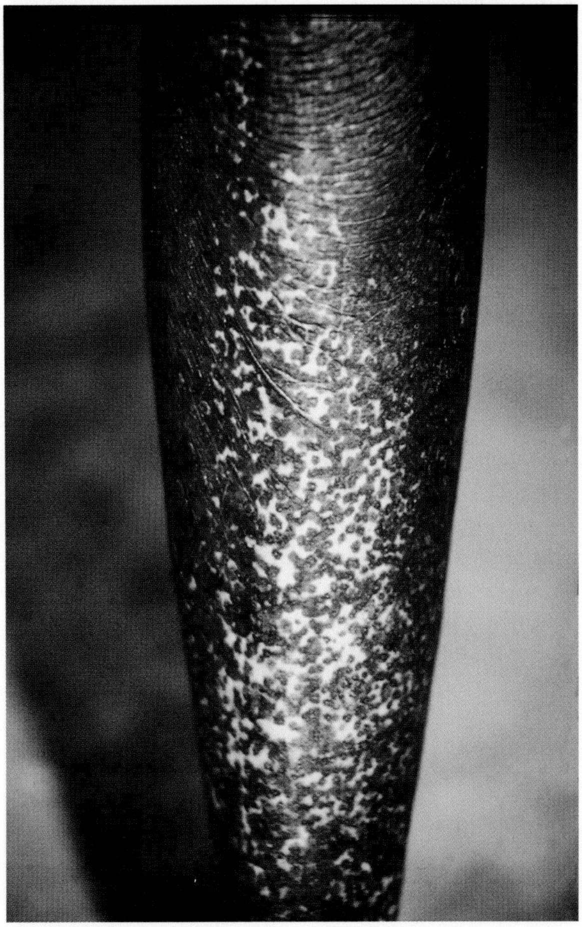

Fig. 28.10. Depigmentation or 'leopard skin'. (From Murdoch et al., 1993.)

lamp, microfilariae may be seen wriggling in the anterior chamber. Live microfilariae in the cornea are more difficult to see as they are transparent. Dead microfilariae in the cornea, however, may be seen as 'fluffy' opacities which are straightened-out microfilariae surrounded by an inflammatory infiltrate. These lesions of punctate keratitis resolve spontaneously.

Demonstration of adult worms by collagenase digestion of excised nodules

Collagenase digestion and dissection of excised nodules will reveal coiled adult worms but this is not a routine procedure (Schulz-Key et al., 1977).

Mazzotti test

If the skin snips are negative but a diagnosis of onchocerciasis is still suspected, a single 50 mg oral dose of diethylcarbamazine may be given and the patient observed carefully over the next 24–48 hours. Infected persons may develop onset or worsening of pruritus about 20–90 min later. An acute papular rash with oedema, fever, cough and musculoskeletal symptoms may also occur. Symptoms and signs reach a peak at about 24 hours and then subside over the next 48–72 hours. The Mazzotti test is contraindicated in heavily infected individuals (who will have positive skin snips) as severe reactions can occur including pulmonary oedema and collapse. The Mazzotti test is also contraindicated in patients with optic nerve disease as it may trigger deterioration in vision (WHO, 1995b).

Full blood count

A peripheral eosinophilia is often present.

Future investigative tools

Serodiagnosis

A specific serological test for onchocerciasis is not routinely available yet but it is anticipated that such a test will become available using a cocktail of recombinant *O. volvulus* antigens (Ramachandran, 1993; Bradley & Unnasch, 1996).

PCR

PCR-based assays are only available as research tools at present, but are more sensitive than skin snips in lightly infected individuals. The PCR-based assay to detect the repetitive DNA sequence known as O–150 (found only in *O. volvulus*), has a sensitivity of 100 per cent and a specificity approaching 100 per cent (Zimmerman et al., 1994). This O–150 PCR assay has also been shown to detect the presence of parasite DNA in superficial skin scrapings (Toé et al., 1998).

Treatment

Ivermectin

As ivermectin has minimal side effects, it has become feasible to conduct mass treatment of endemic communities. The exact mode of action of the drug is unclear. It causes paralysis of microfilariae, possibly as a result of lowered cell membrane resistance produced by increased chloride ion influx. At higher experimental concentrations it interferes with GABA-mediated transmission of nerve impulses. Ivermectin also blocks the release of microfilariae from the uteri of adult female worms but the gradual build-up of microfilariae in the skin is not prevented so ivermectin has to be re-administered every 6–12 months throughout the lifespan of the adult worm. Current control programmes distribute doses of 150 μg/kg of ivermectin annually.

Effects of ivermectin on onchocercal eye disease

After the introduction of ivermectin for onchocerciasis in humans, numerous papers appeared uniformly reporting a remarkable lack of effect on disease involving the anterior segment of the eye. This was in direct comparison to diethylcarbamazine which causes an acute exacerbation of any ocular inflammation around the newly dead microfilariae. Since ivermectin produces a mild inflammatory skin reaction in heavily infected individuals, the anxiety remained that it could precipitate optic neuritis and/or exacerbate posterior segment disease. Happily this was shown not to be the case in a large placebo controlled trial in Northern Nigeria (Abiose et al., 1993).

Effects of ivermectin on onchocercal skin disease

A multicountry placebo-controlled trial has examined the effects of 3-monthly, 6-monthly and annual doses of ivermectin on itching and onchocercal skin disease (Brieger et al., 1998b). From 6 months onwards there was a 40–50 per cent reduction in the prevalence of severe itching after ivermectin therapy compared with placebo. A greater decrease in the prevalence and severity of APOD, CPOD and LOD was also seen in those receiving ivermectin. The difference between ivermectin and placebo was significant for prevalence at 9 months and for severity at 3 months. There was no significant difference among the various ivermectin regimes, so annual treatment for control of onchocerciasis in areas where skin disease predominates seems adequate.

Future therapies

Albendazole

Patients treated with a 10-day course of albendazole (400 mg/day) have been shown to have a significant reduction in microfilarial densities at 12 months (Cline et al., 1992). Albendazole was well tolerated and is believed to interfere with embryogenesis in adult *O. volvulus* worms.

Macrofilaricides

A safe macrofilaricide (i.e. a drug which can kill adult worms) would allow a greater impact to be made in controlling onchocerciasis as a single course of treatment would be curative. Clinical trials of moxidectin are planned to start soon.

Future integration of control programmes for onchocerciasis and lymphatic filariasis

Onchocerciasis and lymphatic filariasis commonly coexist. A new initiative to combat lymphatic filariasis in endemic African communities consists of annual mass administration of single-dose combination therapy with albendazole (donated by SmithKline Beecham) and ivermectin (donated to the lymphatic filariasis programme in sub-Saharan Africa by Merck & Co). This combined drug regimen may be enough to stop transmission of lymphatic filariasis and onchocerciasis simultaneously.

Unsolved problems

The major task for APOC is to maintain and expand annual community-directed ivermectin treatment programmes. Such operational research continues with an overall goal of developing with the affected communities, competent delivery systems that can serve as an example for the delivery of other drugs to control other tropical diseases. The addition of timed larviciding (at the height of the breeding season for *Simulium*) to ivermectin distribution may be beneficial at selected sites. There remains a need for a safe, effective macrofilaricide.

Future immunological research will help to determine the mechanisms of immune evasion employed by the parasite. With respect to the development of a vaccine for onchocerciasis, the differences between protective and pathogenic immune responses need to be clarified.

References

Abiose A, Jones B, Cousens S et al. (1993). A randomized, controlled trial of ivermectin for onchocerciasis: evidence for a reduction in incidence of optic nerve disease. *Lancet;* **341**: 130–134.

Amazigo U. (1993). Onchocerciasis and women's reproductive health: indigenous and biomedical concepts. *Trop Doctor;* **23**: 149–151.

Amazigo UO. (1994). Detrimental effects of onchocerciasis on marriage age and breast-feeding. *Trop Geog Med;* **46**: 322–325.

Anderson J, Fuglsang H, Hamilton PJS, Marshall TF dE C. (1974). Studies on onchocerciasis in the United Cameroon Republic II. Comparison of onchocerciasis in rain-forest and sudan-savanna. *Trans Roy Soc Trop Med Hyg*; **68**: 209–222.

Bird AC, Anderson J, Fuglesang H. (1976). Morphology of posterior segment lesions of the eye in patients with onchocerciasis *Br. J Ophthalmol*; **60**: 2–20.

Bradley JE, Unnasch TR. (1996). Molecular approaches to the diagnosis of onchocerciasis. *Adv Parasitol*; **37**: 57–106.

Brieger WR, Oshiname F-O & Ososanya, OO (1998a). Stigma associated with onchocercal skin disease among those affected near the Ofiki and Oyan Rivers in Western Nigeria. *Soc. Sci Med*; **47**: 841–852.

Brieger WR, Awedoba AK, Eneanya CL et al. (1998b). The effects of ivermectin on onchocercal skin disease and severe itching: results of a multicentre trial. *Trop Med Int Hlth*; **3**: 951–961.

Cline BL, Hernandez JL, Mather FJ et al. (1992). Albendazole in the treatment of onchocerciasis: double-blind clinical trial in Venezuela. *Am J Trop Med Hyg*; **47**: 512–520.

Duke BOL. (1966). Onchocerca–*Simulium* complexes: III – the survival of *Simulium* damnosum after high intakes of microfilariae of incompatible strains of Onchocerca volvulus, and the survival of the parasites in the fly. *Ann Trop Med Parasitol*; **6**: 495–500.

Evans TG. (1995). Socioeconomic consequences of blinding onchocerciasis in west Africa. *Bull Wld Hlth Org;* **73**: 495–506.

Kirkwood B, Smith P, Marshall T, Prost A. (1983). Relationships between mortality, visual acuity and microfilarial load in the area of the Onchocercal Control Programme. *Trans Roy Soc Trop Med Hyg*; **77**: 862–868.

Makunde WH, Salum FM, Massaga JJ, Alilio MS. (2000). Clinical and parasitological aspects of itching caused by onchocerciasis in Morogoro, Tanzania. *Ann Trop Med Parasitol*; **94**: 793–799.

Murdoch ME. (1992). The skin and the immune response in onchocerciasis. *Trop Doctor*; **22**: 44–55.

Murdoch ME, Hay RJ, Mackenzie CD et al. (1993). A clinical classification and grading system of the cutaneous changes in onchocerciasis. *Br J Dermatol*; **129**: 260–269.

Okello DO, Ovuga EB, Ogwal-Okeng JW. (1995). Dermatological problems of onchocerciasis in Nebbi District, Uganda. *E Afr Med J*; **72**: 295–298.

Oladepo O, Brieger WR, Otusanya S, Kale OO, Offiong S, Titiloye M. (1997). Farm land size and onchocerciasis status of peasant farmers in south-western Nigeria. *Trop Med Int Hlth*; **2**: 334–340.

Ottesen EA. (1994). Immune responsiveness and the pathogenesis of human onchocerciasis. *J Infect Dis*; **171**: 659–671.

Ovuga EBL, Okello, DO, Ogwal-Okeng JW, Orwotho N, Opoka RO. (1995). Social and psychological aspects of onchocercal skin disease in Nebbi District, Uganda. *E Afr Med J*; **72**: 449–453.

Prost A, Vaugelade J. (1981). La surmortalite des aveugles en zone de savane oust-africaine. *Bull W Hlth Org*; **59**: 773–776.

Ramachandran CP. (1993). Improved immunodiagnostic tests to monitor onchocerciasis control programmmes – a multicentre effort. *Parasitol Today*; **9**: 76–79.

Schulz-Key H, Albiez EJ, Buttner DW. (1977). Isolation of living adult *Onchocerca volvulus* from nodules. *Tropenmed Parasitol;* **28**: 428–430.

Toé L, Boatin, BA, Adjami A. Back C. Merriweather, A, Unnasch TR. (1998). Detection of *Onchocerca volvulus* infection by O-150 polymerase chain reaction analysis of skin scratches. *J Infect Dis*; **178**: 282–285.

Tonjum AM, Thylefors B. (1978). Aspects of corneal changes in onchocerciasis. *Br J Ophthalmol*; **62**: 458–461.

Vlassoff C, Weiss M, Ovuga EBL, Eneanya C, Nwel PT, Babalola SS. (2000). Gender and the stigma of onchocercal skin disease in Africa. *Soc Sci Med*; **50**: 1353–1368.

World Health Organization. (1987). Expert Committee on Onchocerciasis: Third Report. *WHO Tech Rep Ser*, **752**: 114–121.

World Health Organization. (1995a). The importance of

onchocercal skin disease. Report of a multi-country study by the Pan-African Study Group on Onchocercal Skin Disease. Geneva: *TDR/AFR/RP/95.1.*

World Health Organization. (1995b). Onchocerciasis and its control. Report of a WHO Expert Committee on Onchocerciasis Control. *WHO Tech Rep Ser,* **852**: 57–63.

Yang YF, Murdoch IE, Cousens S, Babalola OE, Abiose A, Jones B. (2001). Intraocular pressure and gonioscopic findings in rural communities mesoendemic and nonendemic for onchocerciasis, Kaduna State, Nigeria. *Eye, in press.*

Zimmermann PA, Guderian RH, Aruajo E et al. (1994). Polymerase chain reaction-based diagnosis of *Onchocerca volvulus* infection: improved detection of patients with onchocerciasis. *J Infect Dis,* **169**: 686–689.

29

Lymphatic filariasis

The problem in Africa

The World Health Organization considers lymphatic filariasis to be the fourth leading cause of permanent disability world-wide, and it will continue to be a major problem in areas of Africa for many years, and probably decades, to come. The outlook for the management and control of lymphatic filariasis in Africa is, however, far better now than when the last edition of this book was published. This is not due to the discovery of new drugs, but to the discovery of new ways of using drugs that were previously known. Coupled to this has been a generous donation programme by two of the drug companies involved, and advances in rapid diagnosis of filariasis. There is now a realistic chance of effective control using a combination of drugs and vector control. In the long term, filariasis is a potential candidate for eradication from Africa, but even if all transmission stopped today, some individuals with filariasis would continue to deteriorate symptomatically over several years.

Organism, lifecycle and vector

In Africa lymphatic filariasis is due almost exclusively to *Wuchereria bancrofti*, although occasionally onchocerciasis can produce similar symptoms. Larvae of *W. bancrofti* are ingested by female mosquitoes during feeding, and undergo further development within the mosquito. They can be transmitted from around 10 days after mosquitoes are infected. Larvae are then injected into humans during mosquito feeding and develop further, eventually migrating to the lymphatic system. It takes from 7 months to a year before adult female worms produce microfilariae. If left untreated, females will continue to produce microfilariae for the rest of their lives, generally around 5 years, although over 10 has been reported. Anopheles, Culex, and Aedes mosquitoes can all act as vectors of *W. bancrofti*.

Epidemiology

Several widely spread vectors are able to transmit *W. bancrofti*, and lymphatic filariasis is therefore widely spread in a broad band across Africa (Fig 29.1). In general, climatic conditions which favour mosquitoes favour the

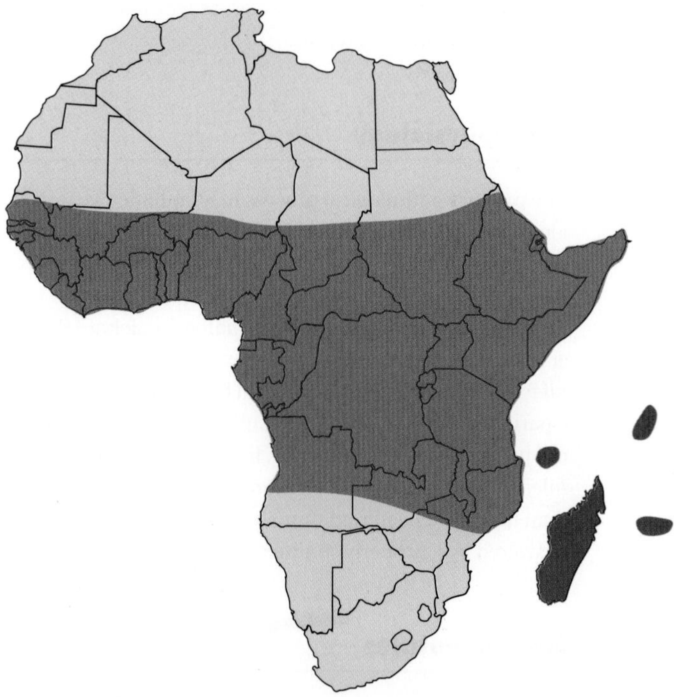

Fig. 29.1. Distribution of filiariasis due to *Wuchereria bancrofti* in Africa.

disease, so it is, for example, less common in highland areas than low-lying humid areas.

Control and prevention

There are two elements to control: vector control and mass treatments with antifilarial drugs. In areas of Africa where there is a high incidence of filarial infections, effective vector control has a significant impact. In many areas *Anopheles* species are the principal vectors, and here malaria control programmes using impregnated bednets and other anti-anopheles measures will help filariasis control. In other areas *Culex* species are the principal vectors, and here specific control measures aimed at peridomestic breeding sites (such as polystyrene balls in latrines) have proved highly effective at reducing transmission (Maxwell et al., 1990).

The new short-course drug regimes based on albendazole, diethylcarbamazine (DEC) and ivermectin, which allow mass treatment, are covered in detail below under treatment. We know from previous campaigns using low-dose DEC in cooking salt that reducing population microfilariae burden leads to a significant reduction in transmission. Because the new regimes are both safe and logistically easy to use in intermittent mass treatment, there is now a real chance that these tools can be used effectively in highly endemic areas, as ivermectin has been against onchocerciasis.

Pathophysiology

The primary pathological process in lymphatic filariasis is local damage to lymphatics, especially at points of drainage, almost certainly as a result of local inflammatory response to adult worms and microfilariae. The exact mechanism of damage remains a matter for debate (Dreyer et al., 2000). Damage may well be exacerbated by local infection; the extent to which local bacterial infection plays a part in irreversible damage is still debated. The point is not just an academic one since, if bacteria play a major role, antibiotics may well be more central to management than they have been traditionally, but this can only be answered by a properly conducted clinical trial.

Clinical features

The initial presentation in a significant infection is usually of repeated fever with painful lymphadenopathy and lymphangitis. This is often associated with transient oedema of the limb or appendage drained by the lymph nodes involved. There may also be redness and tenderness of the skin overlying lymph nodes. If the patient is not re-infected, this will usually die out over time. In people living in endemic areas who are repeatedly infected or in a heavy infection, the oedema of infected limbs and appendages becomes more frequent, and eventually permanent. Over time, oedema is replaced by brawny swelling, and at this point some of the swelling must be considered irreversible. In Africa the legs are most often affected, followed by upper limbs, breasts (in women) and external genitalia (in men) (Fig 29.2).

Where the lymphatics involved do not drain limbs and appendages, other local effects of blocked lymphatics can occur, with probably the most common being chyluria where lymph drains into the bladder. This is diagnosed relatively easily, since the urine has a typical milky appearance; this may cause acute retention. Chyle in the scrotal sac can give rise to massive and rapid scrotal enlargement.

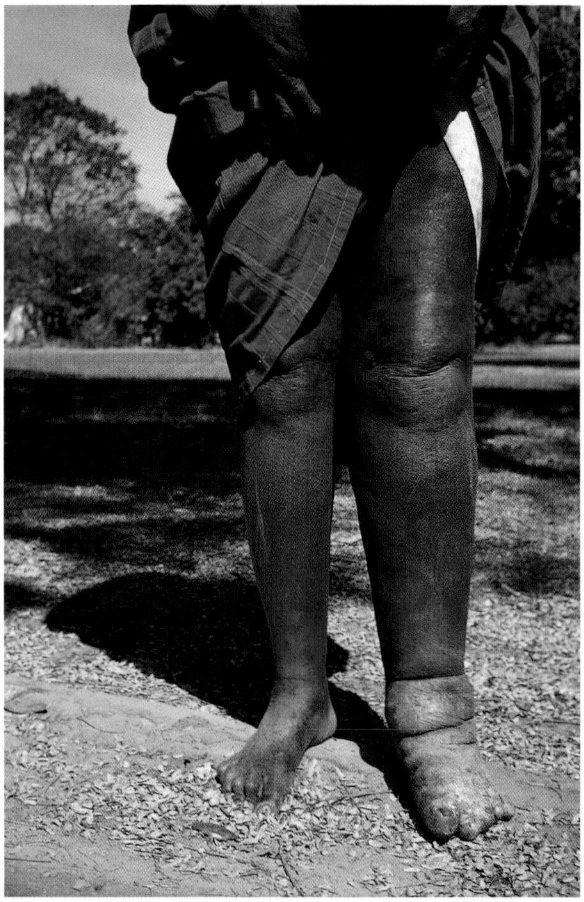

Fig. 29.2. Lymphoedema due to lymphatic filiariasis.

In Africa other presentations of filariasis seem to be rare compared to Asia. The most important of these is tropical pulmonary eosinophilia (TPE). This can cause various chest symptoms, especially wheezing, and is accompanied by a mottled, or miliary appearance of the chest X-ray. Where blood tests are available, eosinophilia is almost invariable, and this helps to differentiate this condition from miliary TB and other chest conditions. Mono-arthritis is a relatively common symptom of acute filariasis. Both this and TPE should disappear rapidly if the filariasis is treated.

The differential diagnosis of limb swelling is very wide. For bilateral pitting oedema of the lower limbs it includes cardiac failure or any of the causes of low albumin (both common throughout Africa and world-wide). In addition, bilateral non-pitting oedema can be caused by damage to the lymphatics caused by prolonged exposure to silica-containing soils by walking barefoot in certain highland areas of Africa. In those without HIV disease the differential diagnosis of unilateral limb swelling includes deep vein thrombosis and cellulitis and metastases to the limb lymphatics (which are rare). In those with HIV disease the most common cause of unilateral limb swelling in Africa is probably Kaposi's sarcoma, usually (but not invariably) associated with skin changes.

Diagnosis

Clinical diagnosis may be so suggestive that laboratory tests are of largely academic interest in late disease, but in early disease (where treatment is most useful) aetiological diagnosis may be important since the differential diagnosis is wide.

The only useful part of routine investigation that is helpful in the diagnosis of lymphatic filariasis is eosinophil count. Where this is raised in the context of someone with typical symptoms, it supports the diagnosis. Specific tests are, however, needed to make a firm aetiological diagnosis in early disease, since eosinophilia is relatively common. The traditional (gold standard) method of diagnosis remains a thick film of blood taken from the patient looking for microfilariae at the right time of day, using either finger prick or whole blood (McMahon et al., 1979a). Except in heavy infections, blood has to be taken at or near the peak biting time of the vector; microfilariae only circulate freely in the blood at around the peak biting time, probably as a way of escaping destruction by the immune system. Since the vectors in Africa are almost exclusively night-biting mosquitoes, microfilariae peak at around midnight. Blood taken more than a few hours either side of this time may well fail to detect light infections. This poses obvious practical problems, especially with outpatients. Yield can be increased by filtering blood with specific filters, but these are unlikely to be available in most hospitals, and it does not overcome the need to take blood at night. An alternative method to increase yield is to give diethylcarbamazine (DEC) at a dose of 6 mg/kg; microfilaria then peak 15 minutes later (McMahon et al., 1979b).

A recent immunological card-based test has proved very sensitive and specific and is not dependent on the time of day. The company producing them (AMRAD ICT) has volunteered to produce them at cost price, and the test is easy to perform. This means that they can be used realistically in lymphatic filarial control programmes, although it is unlikely that they will be available in most routine laboratories in central or district hospitals in Africa.

Both microscopic and immunological diagnosis are good for detecting early active infection when the microfilariae are in the circulation. In later disease, due to the long-term effectiveness of damage to the lymphatic system, there may be no microfilariae or viable adult worms. Deciding whether limb oedema is due to previous filarial infection or due to other causes may therefore end up being a clinical decision based on probability. Negative tests do not rule out the possibility of previous infection. Positive tests are helpful, however, since they suggest active infection that may benefit from anti-filarial treatment.

Treatment and follow-up

Issues surrounding treatment and control now overlap very considerably with treatment of early lymphatic filariasis. It is in the use of anti-filarial drugs where the majority of the new advances have happened. The management of those with chronic limb oedema in late disease remains a difficult area where there have been small advances.

Anti-filarial drugs

The mainstay of anti-filarial treatment for many years has been diethylcarbamazine (DEC). DEC is cheap, generally safe, and effective at reducing microfilariae burdens. It has, however, had drawbacks. For treatment in individual cases a prolonged course has been used traditionally, which can cause logistical problems. In addition, in patients who are co-infected with onchocerciasis, DEC can cause a severe reaction. This means that using it in most parts of West Africa is inappropriate in public health campaigns, and DEC has to be used with great caution in individual patients known to be infected.

Two major advances have made the outlook better than it was a few years ago. The first is the finding that a short course (single-dose or 2 days) with DEC, combined with albendazole, will clear microfilariae from most people for up to year (Ottesen et al., 1999). This will both reduce morbidity in individual cases, and (since the microfilariae are the infective form) will also reduce transmission. The drug combination probably does not kill most adult worms, but they act to kill microfilariae and sterilize the adult females. Since the single-dose course of albendazole and DEC is easy to administer, safe and effective, it provides a very useful tool both for treatment and control in those parts of Africa where onchocerciasis is not a problem. SmithKline Beecham, the manufacturers of albendazole, have generously donated it to microfilaria control programmes, which means that, for the first time, there is a realistic chance of control programmes based on anti-filarial drugs, especially in East Africa.

Ivermectin, which has, for several years, been used as part of the onchocerciasis control programme in West Africa, also has a anti-filarial activity against *W. bancrofti*. Again, a single day's treatment has been shown to be effective in killing microfilariae and sterilizing adult females (Dunyo et al., 2000; Cao et al., 1997). At present, it remains an open question whether adding albendazole increases the efficacy with trials pointing both ways, but at present the evidence is probably in favour of combination treatment. Merck Sharpe & Dohme, the manufacturers of ivermectin, have generously extended their donation programme to include control of lymphatic filariasis in areas of Africa where onchocerciasis makes using DEC impossible.

These two short-course combinations (albendazole and DEC, and ivermectin +/− albendazole) means that, for the first time, we have drugs that can be used in Africa, which require only 1 or 2 days' administration. They can be used for the treatment of patients with early stage disease, and also in mass campaigns to reduce microfilariae.

Treatment of late stage disease

If patients with early lymphatic filariasis due to *W. bancrofti* are treated early, lymphatic damage should be minimal and the long-term effects of lymphatic filariasis may be avoided. In those living with chronic infection, often since childhood, damage will already have occurred to the lymphatic vessels. Since bacterial super-infection may play an important role in making lymphatic damage worse, and eventually irreversible, the balance of opinion is currently to give early treatment with antibiotics (including topical antibiotics) for any infections of the affected limb.

Once a significant disabling oedema has set in, the treatment options are limited, but with careful attention to detail further damage can be limited. The steps that have been demonstrated to have a beneficial effect are:

- elevating the limbs
- washing affected limbs with soap and water
- treating infections
- using topical anti-fungals and antibiotics.

Various drug regimes have been used in an attempt to restore lymphatic flow and reduce swelling. Good evidence that they work is lacking. It is likely that no drugs, apart from antibiotics, are effective for treating intercurrent infections.

Surgical reconstruction of the lymphatics is exceptionally difficult and usually disappointing even in highly specialized units. Surgical de-bulking is occasionally appropriate.

Unsolved problems (Fig 29.3)

The recent advances in diagnosis and anti-filarial treatment mean there is a very real possibility that lymphatic filariasis could become a negligible public health problem in Africa within a generation. It remains to be seen if the theory works in practice. This will need both political will and good operational scientific assessment. The prob-

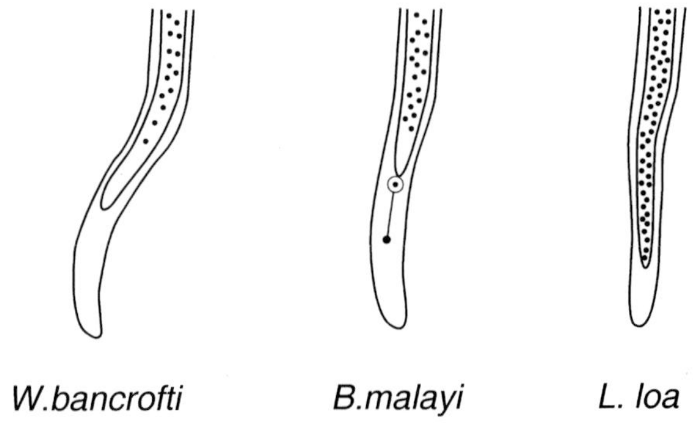

Fig. 29.3. Sketch of *W. bancrofti* and other sheathed microfilariae, *B. malayi* and *L. loa*.

lems of managing those with chronic disease will be with us for many years to come, and further advances to reduce morbidity are clearly needed. It seems likely that multiple small steps are more likely to work than one major breakthrough.

References

Cao WC, Van der Ploeg CP, Plaisier AP, van d SI, Habbema JD. (1997). Ivermectin for the chemotherapy of bancroftian filariasis: a meta-analysis of the effect of single treatment. *Trop Med Int Health*; **2**: 393–403.

Dreyer G, Noroes J, Figueredo-Silva J. (2000). New insights into the natural history and pathology of bancroftian filariasis: implications for clinical management and filariasis control programmes. *Trans Roy Soc Trop Med Hyg*; **94**: 594–596.

Dunyo SK, Nkrumah FK, Simonsen PE. (2000). A randomized double-blind placebo-controlled field trial of ivermectin and albendazole alone and in combination for the treatment of lymphatic filariasis in Ghana. *Trans Roy Soc Trop Med Hyg*; **94**: 205–211.

Maxwell CA, Curtis CF, Haji H, Kisumku S, Thalib AI, Yahya SA. (1990). Control of Bancroftian filariasis by integrating therapy with vector control using polystyrene beads in wet pit latrines. *Trans Roy Soc Trop Med Hyg*; **84**: 709–714.

McMahon JE, Marshall TF, Vaughan JP, Abaru DE. (1979a). Bancroftian filariasis: a comparison of microfilariae counting techniques using counting chamber, standard slide and membrane (nucleopore) filtration. *Ann Trop Med Parasitol*; **73**: 457–464.

McMahon JE, Marshall TF, Vaughan JP, Kolstrup N. (1979b). Tanzania Filariasis Project: a provocative day test with diethylcarbamazine for the detection of microfilariae of nocturnally periodic *Wuchereria bancrofti* in the blood. *Bull Wld Hlth Org*; **57**: 759–765.

Ottesen EA, Ismail MM, Horton J. (1999). The role of albendazole in programmes to eliminate lymphatic filariasis. *Parasitol Today*; **15**: 382–386.

30 Guinea worm

The problem in Africa

This disease has been transformed since the last edition of this book, thanks to the magnificent efforts of the campaign to eradicate guinea worm and the committed support of the Carter Foundation. While it is still a potential threat if methods of control break down, the lives of hundreds of thousands of people have been transformed: what was regarded as an inevitable part of village life is now known to be a wholly unnecessary disablement: people whose families were economically crippled, because the active farming members were physically crippled by painful ulcers on their feet, now enjoy a little more (see Fig. 2.7): and many communities which depended on infected water can now boast a protected and safe supply of water (bore-hole, well, stand-pipe or other protected source). Because the disease is still important it is described below in the hope that, when the next edition of this book is published, it will be a historical memory and no more. Many people were disabled by this infection and suffered much economic loss in parts of West and East Africa.

Eradication

Key components of the campaign
- Protected water supply
- Health education
- Case management
- Vector control

Organism and life cycle

Humans are infected with *Dracunculus medinensis* when they swallow water containing *Cyclops*, a small crustacean. The infective larvae of the worm break out of *Cyclops* within the gastrointestinal tract and pass into the connective tissue, probably via the lymphatics. Male and female worms mature within the connective tissues in about a year. After fertilization, the small male worm dies and is absorbed. The adult female worm, which may be up to a metre long, migrates in the subcutaneous tissues to a part of the body which comes into contact with water, particularly the feet and legs. A toxin is then released and a skin bleb forms which ruptures, producing an ulcer. On contact with water, a loop of uterus prolapses into the ulcer and numerous larvae are released. Having discharged her larvae, the female worm dies.

Defined pattern of transmission

In any village, define the source of infected water and how it is drawn, carried and used. Village people may contract the disease if they drink infected water, or may transmit to *Cyclops* if they are already infected and wash and bathe in the village's water pool. When the source of transmission and any seasonal change is identified, action can follow.

Education of the people

- Community leaders and village health workers have been at the forefront of the campaign. Village health volunteers, motivated by their responsibility and their status and by the fact that they were really doing something of benefit to their own people, have been trained in northern Ghana to monitor the number of cases and thus to establish a system of surveillance (Cairncross et al., 1996).
- Vigorous health education programmes have enrolled many helpers from among the people to explain, for example, what the infection is and to demonstrate how water can be drunk safely, for example, through milli-

pore filters(see Fig. 2.8). These were tested, again in northern Ghana, where polyester cloth filters were found to be both better and cheaper than nylon filters (Olsen et al., 1997).
- Strong measures were adopted too: in one village a man was appointed to guard the pool of water from which people got water and he kept away all those with active infection.
- The method of transmission was explained again and again: repeated teaching has been very important in communities, which regarded the infection as inevitable as the coming of the dry season! People were told what is done when chemical crustacicides are added to their water: the reasons for all preventive and control activities were fully and repeatedly explained

Vector control with chemical crustacicides

These should not be added to water until transmission is defined.

Temephos, 1 p.p.m., is effective for 6 weeks.

Abate (an organophosphorus compound) kills 100 per cent of *Cyclops* at 0.1 p.p.m. and can be modified to have a long residual action. It should be added to give an estimated concentration of 0.5 mg/litre and it should be reapplied after 3 days if normal living *Cyclops* are seen. *Abate* should be applied again 5–7 weeks later to give a concentration of 1 mg/litre if living *Cyclops* are seen.

Example of effect of eradication campaign
Far North Province of Cameroon, Mayo Sava Health District: (Sam-Abbenyi et al., 1999)

	1990	1995
Number of endemic villages	82	6
Number of cases	772	15
Proportion of cases identified within first 24 h	19%	73.5%

Pathology

A local inflammatory reaction with eosinophils and neutrophils occurs where the vesicle forms. Later, secondary pyogenic infection may destroy tissues which subsequently fibrose. The synovium of affected joints may be infiltrated by a variety of different cells. Dead segments of worm may invoke a foreign-body giant-cell reaction.

Clinical features

Guinea worm infections are seen at any age but are not common in unweaned children. Ulcers can occur anywhere but they are most often on the feet, legs and genitalia. Patients may be infected with more than one worm at a time. When the itchy skin bleb appears, the patient may have urticaria, fever, dyspnoea and nausea. The bleb bursts and forms an ulcer, which usually lasts for 2–3 weeks and then, in uncomplicated cases, heals spontaneously. Segments of dead, calcified guinea worms can often be seen on radiographs as small coiled linear shadows in the soft tissues.

Complications

Pyogenic infection

Local
This may occur after unsuccessful attempts to remove the worm, for example, 45 per cent of infected Ghanaian farmers had secondary pyogenic infection.

Systemic
Pyogenic bacteria, particularly *Staphylococcus aureus*, may spread along the worm and cause a septic arthritis, pyomyositis, osteomyelitis or a septicaemia. Joints may become greatly deformed.

Aseptic arthitis
This is most often seen at the knee. It may be due to a discharge of larvae into the joint or perhaps to an immunological reaction to the worm.

Tetanus
The dead tissue of the guinea worm ulcer allows *Clostridium tetani* to become established.

Other sites
Adult worms have been seen in the pleural fluid in patients with a pleural effusion, but eruption of the adult worm is almost invariably on the leg. Paraplegia may follow if worms enter the extradural space.

Diagnosis

Local
An itching painful blister develops and the worm erupts about 4 days later. The thread-like adult worm is obvious. Embryos can be detected if cold water is put on an ulcer and examined under the lower power of a microscope; an ethyl chloride spray also releases them. A coiled calcified

worm is often seen in a radiograph and if it overlies a lung it may be confused with a calcified focus.

Systemic
An eosinophilia is common when worms are emerging.

Immunological
An indirect fluorescent antibody technique can be used; it is specific but a cross-reaction may occur in patients who have onchocerciasis. Antibodies are at their peak when worms emerge and decline over the next 2–9 months until none can be detected.

Treatment

Worm

The best drug has yet to be found, but the following have all been tried: niridazole in a daily dose of 25 mg/kg for 28 days, thiabendazole 100 mg/kg for 1–3 days and metronidazole 25 mg/kg for 10–15 days. Their action is chiefly that of reducing pain and the local inflammatory reaction round the worm, so that it can be removed painlessly and easily. None of these drugs kills the female worms.

The traditional treatment of rolling the worm out on a stick may easily burst the worm and cause a serious local reaction.

Complications of worm

Secondary infection
The worm ulcer must be cleaned and kept clean. Antibiotics, preferably procaine penicillin, can be given daily for 5 days. This dramatically shortens the disability, which can be prolonged (Fig. 2.7).

Tetanus
In areas where tetanus is prevalent, give patients toxoid.

References

Cairncross S, Braide EI, Bugri SZ. (1996). Community participation in the eradication of guinea worm. *Acta Trop*; **61**: 121–136.
Olsen A, Magnussen P, Anemana S. (1997). The acceptability of a polyester drinking-water filter in a dracunculiasis-endemic village in northern region, Ghana. *Bull Wld Hlth Org*; **75**: 449–452.
Sam-Abbenyi A, Dama M, Graham S et al. (1999). Dracunculiasis in Cameroon at the threshold of elimination. *Int J Epidemiol*; **28**: 163–168.

Trichinosis

31

Definition

Trichinosis (trichinellosis) results from the ingestion of under-cooked meat infected with microscopic *Trichinella* species nematode worms. Trichinosis is characterized by fever, diarrhoea, peri-orbital oedema, myositis and eosinophilia.

Epidemiology

Trichinosis has been reported world-wide including most African countries. However, this infection is not common in Africa, probably because meat is an expensive and therefore infrequent food. Trichinosis does not occur in strict vegetarians and pork is often the source of infection, so trichinosis is rare in Muslim communities. *Trichinella spiralis nelsoni* predominates in Africa south of the Sahara and may be transmitted to man by eating under-cooked bush pigs, as well as other animals as diverse as ostrich and crocodile. *Trichinella spiralis* cysts have been identified in a 3200-year-old Egyptian mummy.

Life-cycle and pathology

Enteric phase

Larvae of *Trichinella spiralis* (or other *Trichinella species*) ingested in under-cooked infected meat develop into adult worms (2–4 mm long) that live for a few weeks in the small intestine, causing inflammation.

Migratory/invasive phase

Each female worm releases hundreds of larvae (0.1–1 mm long) that are carried in the blood stream to skeletal muscles where they burrow into muscle fibres. This is associated with a type I hypersensitivity reaction.

Encystment phase

In skeletal muscle the larvae grow, coil, encyst and then remain viable for several years. Eventually, these cysts may calcify.

Control and prevention

Cooking meat until there is no visible pink flesh or fluid (>55 °C) or storage at –15 °C for 3 weeks kills the parasites but salting, smoking and drying are unreliable for sterilizing this infection. Meat inspection allows infected meat to be identified and condemned before ingestion, but this is difficult to implement in resource-poor settings.

Clinical features

Most infections are sub-clinical, caused by <10 larvae per gram of tissue (see Clausen et al., 1996).

Enteric phase

The growth of adult worms over the first week of infection causes inflammation in the small intestine, resulting in diarrhoea, vomiting and abdominal discomfort that may resemble acute food poisoning.

Migratory/invasive phase

More frequently, symptoms result from the invasion of muscles by the new-born larvae and therefore develop 1–3 weeks after infection. Fever, peri-orbital oedema, myositis (with pain, swelling and weakness) are frequent. Headache, cough, shortness of breath, macular or petechial rashes and retinal, sub-conjunctival or sub-ungual splinter haemorrhages, lymphadenopathy, parotid swelling and occasionally splenomegaly may occur. Urinalysis reveals haematuria and proteinuria.

Encystment phase

Malaise and weakness may persist for weeks or months. Death rarely occurs in severe infections (>1000 larvae per gram of tissue) due to enteritis, myocarditis or encephalitis.

Diagnosis

The characteristic clinical features of trichinosis together with marked eosinophilia (from about the 10th day) may allow the diagnosis to be made, especially if undercooked meat has recently been consumed or if there is an outbreak in several people who have eaten the same meat. The ESR is normal but muscle enzymes (creatine phosphokinase and lactic dehydrogenase) are elevated. Larvae may be identified in the peripheral blood by filtration. Antibody tests do not become positive until 3 weeks after infection and then remain positive for many years, as do skin tests. Biopsy of a swollen, tender muscle can be used to confirm the diagnosis by histology or enzymatic digestion of muscle tissue.

Treatment and follow-up

Treatment is directed against both the larvae and the immune reaction they invoke. In the only double-blind randomized placebo-controlled trial of larvicidal therapy, 10 days' treatment was given for trichinosis in Thailand (Watt et al., 2000). Mebendazole (200mg b.d.) proved to be the treatment of choice, improving symptoms compared with fluconazole or placebo. Thiabendazole (25 mg/kg b.d.) was similarly effective but 30 per cent could not tolerate its side effects. Albendazole has also been used and in another trial was marginally more effective than combined thiabendazole + flubendazole; but in mice albendazole is less active than mebendazole. In the rare cases when trichinous meat is known to have been ingested in the previous day then thiabendazole or mebendazole may be administered for 1 week to prevent intestinal and subsequent systemic infection. Once muscle infection has occurred, bed rest and salicylates are often recommended. Corticosteroids may be given to severely ill patients (e.g. Prednisolone 10–20 mg TDS) and this is associated with a good symptomatic response.

References

Clausen MR, Meyer CN, Krantz T et al. (1996). Trichinella infection and clinical disease. *Quart J Med*; **89**: 631–636.

Watt G, Saisorn S, Jongsakul K, Sakolvaree Y, Chaicumpa W. (2000). Blinded, placebo-controlled trial of antiparasitic drugs for trichinosis myositis. *J Infect Dis*; **182**: 371–374.

Protozoa

32 Leishmaniasis

The leishmaniases are a group of diseases that are caused by the protozoan parasite Leishmania, which belongs to the order of Kinetoplastidae. Infection affects the skin and mucosal surfaces or causes disseminated disease or a combination. The geographical distribution, clinical manifestations and prevalence of each form of disease are the result of an intricate interplay between a particular strain of Leishmania, the immunity of the affected individual (the presence of) the reservoir and the sandfly vector (Berman, 1997). Eighty-eight countries are affected with a global annual incidence of $1.5–2 \times 10^6$ cases to $1–1.5 \times 10^6$ cutaneous cases and 500 000 cases of visceral disease (Desjeux, 1996).

The problem in Africa

There are five major clinical syndromes of leishmaniasis, all of which may be found in Africa (Table 32.1); of these, VL and CL are by far the most common. Although scattered cases of VL and CL have been reported from all parts of Africa, the endemic areas are in the northern part (along the Mediterranean coast: Morocco, Algeria, Tunisia, Libya, Egypt) and north east (Sudan, Ethiopia, Kenya, Chad).

Organism and life cycle

Leishmania parasites may appear in two forms: the amastigote (oval shaped, no flagellum; Fig. 32.1) is the form that occurs in the vertebrate host and the promastigote (longitudinally shaped, with a flagellum) form occurs in the sandfly vector (*Phlebotomus* spp.). In the host, parasites are found typically in macrophages, where they divide by binary fission. In diagnostic material (skin smear, bone marrow aspirate) all strains of Leishmania look similar, but the clinical presentation and geographical data will suggest which strain of Leishmania may be present, which is important for management. In routine clinical practice, no further typing is necessary, but epidemiological surveillance demands typing of the parasite by its determining parasite isoenzyme patterns (called zymodemes). In research laboratories monoclonal antibody techniques or PCR can be used directly on the specimens (Evans, 1989).

CUTANEOUS LEISHMANIASIS

CL is caused mainly by *L. major* and *L. tropica*; other leishmania parasites that may cause CL are *L. aethiopica* and *L. infantum*; these parasites also may cause other clinical forms of leishmaniasis (Table 32.1).

L. donovani also may cause skin lesions, but they are the initial manifestations of VL infection in the skin from which the infection may arrest or spread further to fully developed VL; these lesions usually are called leishmaniomas and are not a form of CL.

Epidemiology

CL caused by *L. major* is also referred to as the rural form or zoonotic form of CL (ZCL). The incidence of ZCL is increasing on account of urbanization, settlements in endemic areas, domestication of animals and increase in rodent population. It occurs along the Mediterranean in hot and dry areas; rodents (*Psammomus obesus*) and gerbils (*Meriones* spp.) are the main animal reservoir (Figs. 32.2, 32.3). The vector is *Phlebotomus papatasi.*

Table 32.1. Frequency, principal endemic areas, morbidity, mortality and type of leishmanial parasite involved in various types of leishmaniasis found in Africa

	VL	PKDL	CL	ML	DCL	LR
Frequency	Common	Common	Common	Rare	Rare	Rare
Endemic area	Sudan	Sudan	Sudan	Sudan	Ethiopia	Kenya
	Kenya	Kenya	Kenya		Kenya	
	Ethiopian		Ethiopia			
	Morocco		Morocco			
	Algeria		Algeria			
	Tunisia		Tunisia			
	Libya		Libya			
			Mauritania			
			Senegal			
			Mali			
			Burkina Faso			
			Niger			
			Nigeria			
Morbidity	High	Variable	Mild	High	Moderate	Moderate
Mortality	High	Absent	Absent	Low	Low	Absent
Parasite	*L. donovani*	*L. donovani*	*L. major*	*L. major*	*L. aethiopica*	*L. tropica*
	L. infantum	*L. infantum*	*L. tropica**	*L. donovani*		
	L. tropica		*L. infantum*			
			L. aethiopica			

Notes:
VL, visceral leishmaniasis.
PKDL, post-kala-azar dermal leishmaniasis.
LR, Leishmania recidivans.
ML, mucosal leishmaniasis.
DCL, diffuse cutaneous leishmaniasis.
CL, cutaneous leishmaniasis.

Major epidemics occur, as in Sudan in the 1980s, with a hundred thousand cases; here the reservoir is the rodent *Arvicanthis niloticus*; the vector is as in northern Africa *P. papatasi*, which lives in rodent burrows.

Sub-Saharan Africa, another area of generally low endemicity for *L. major*, CL is seen in Mauritania, Gambia, Senegal, Mali, Burkina Faso, Niger, northern Nigeria, Central African Republic, Cameroon, Ethiopia, and Kenya. The reservoir has not been described fully, but rodent species (*Tatera, Arvicanthis, Mastomys*) have been proved to be reservoirs in some areas. The principal vector is *P. duboscqi*.

An outbreak of ZCL is reported from Ouagadougou (Burkina Faso), which started in 1996. Of 75 patients, 65 had ZCL only and 10 were co-infected with HIV. All had *L. major* of the same zymodeme (MON 74). There was no clinical difference between those co-infected with HIV and those without HIV. Co-infected patients appeared at increased risk of relapse (or new infections), unlike immunocompetent patients, as no immunity was induced (Guiguemdé et al., 2001).

L. tropica

CL caused by *L. tropica* is also known as the anthroponotic form of CL (ACL) with *P. sergenti* and *P. guggisbergi* as vectors. The sandflies live in crevices in houses; ACL is best described from Asia in urban areas hence ACL is also described as the 'urban' type. Main endemic countries in Africa are Morocco, Tunisia and Kenya. The human is the main reservoir. There is another focus in Namibia where the hyrax (*Procavia capensis*) is thought to be a reservoir and the vector is *P. rossi*.

L. aethiopica

CL caused by *L. aethiopica* occurs in the highlands of Ethiopia and Kenya, where *P. longipes* and *P. pedifer* are the vectors and hyraxes the animal reservoir. Some cases of CL caused by *L. aethiopica* may become chronic and proceed to DCL.

L. infantum

CL caused by *L. infantum* has been reported from some countries along the Mediterranean, e.g. Tunisia, as being the cause of CL, but the epidemiology is unclear.

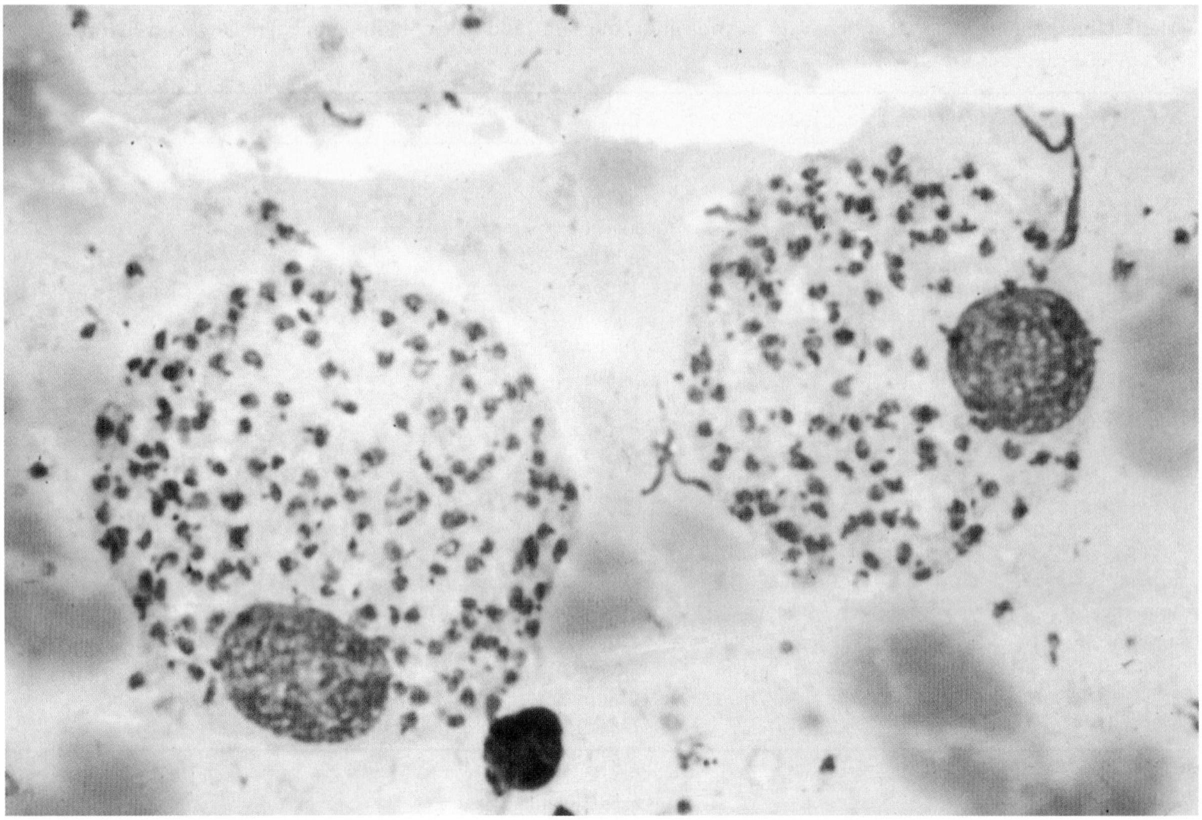

Fig. 32.1. *Leishmania* amastigotes in mononuclear cells in a bone marrow aspirate from a patient with VL (courtesy H. M. Gilles, 1999).

Control and prevention

Individual protection may include:
- the use of impregnated bednets
- the use of repellents
- wearing long sleeves and trousers as sandflies usually bite on exposed areas of the skin.

Other control measures have been implemented rarely; in ZCL these would be directed against rodent reservoirs. Destruction of Rhombomys (a gerbil) colonies in the former USSR proved very effective as it eliminated the reservoir and the resting places for the vector. Vector control by insecticiding has only a temporary effect (Desjeux, 1996).

Leishmanization has been done in Iran and refers to the practice of infecting non-immune individuals with material from active ulcers in order to induce immunity because the vaccinee will develop a single ulcer at a 'convenient' place. In ACL active case-finding is useful in particular in periods of low transmission; peri-domestic insecticiding and improved construction of houses not suitable for breeding of sandflies is recommended (WHO, 1990). No vaccine is yet available.

Pathology

The parasites only spread in the skin, causing characteristic satellite lesions, and to the regional lymphatics, causing metastatic lesions (sporotrichoid spread) and regional lymphadenopathy. Lymphocytes and plasma cells are attracted to developing lesions and the dermis becomes oedematous. The epidermis then breaks down and an ulcer develops, covered by a debris of dead cells and dried exudate. Later, macrophages and amastigotes become less numerous and multinucleated cells appear. Parasites are eliminated by destruction of the macrophages and the developing immune response. The lesion heals with fibrosis leaving a scar (El-Hassan & Zijlstra, 2001).

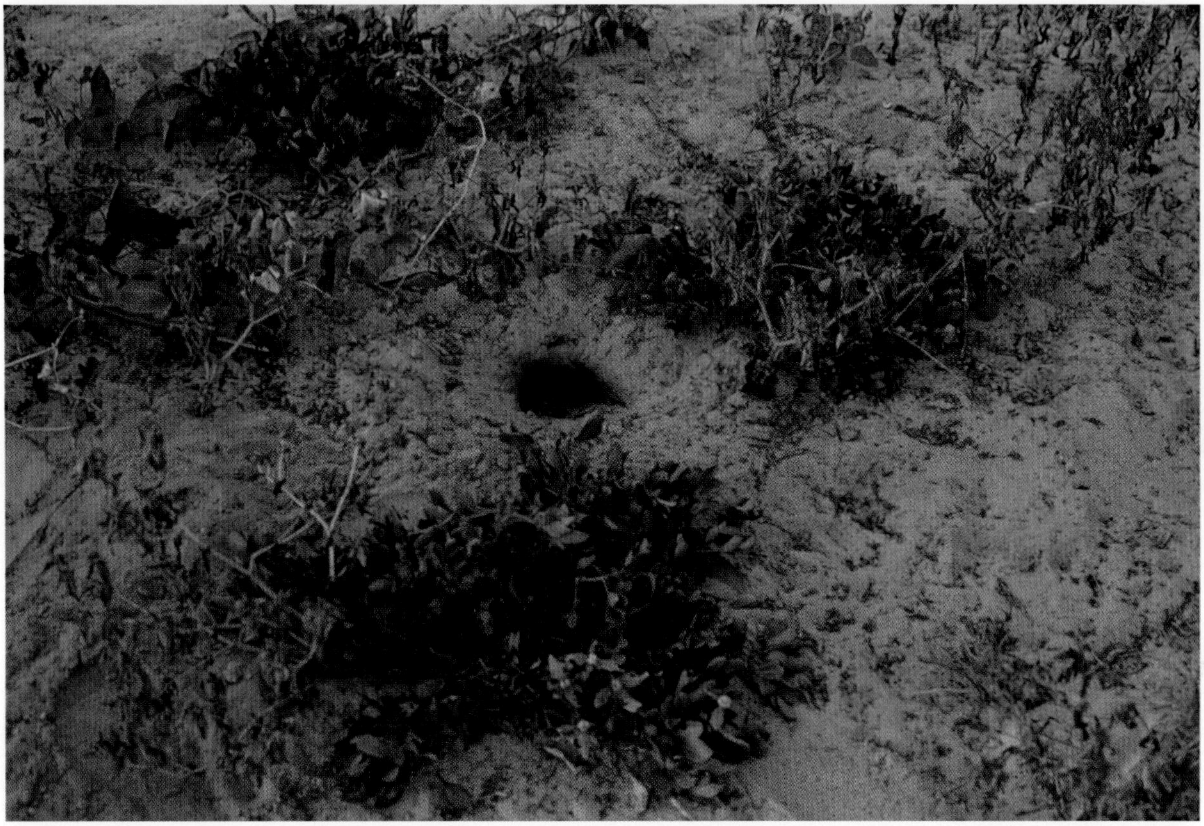

Fig. 32.2. Zoonotic cutaneous leishmaniasis in Morocco: A rodent burrow of *Psammomys obesus.* (courtesy Dr P. Desjeux, WHO, Geneva).

Ulcers and species of parasite

The severity of the ulceration depends on the type of leishmanial parasite, *L. major* being the most immunogenic causing necrosis and more rapid healing, whereas *L. tropica* is less immunogenic and lesions are slower to heal. The immunological reaction induced by *L. aethiopica* is weak; in some patients cell-mediated immunity is persistently suppressed so lesions may become chronic – diffuse cutaneous leishmaniasis (DCL).

Lymph node

Around 10 per cent of patients have enlargement of regional lymph nodes with follicular hyperplasia, germinal centres and expansion of the paracortex. Parasites are scanty or may not be demonstrable. Discrete epitheloid granulomas, with or without Langhan's giant cells are found and, occasionally, the granuloma shows central necrosis resembling tuberculosis, but parasites may be found at the edge of the necrotic focus.

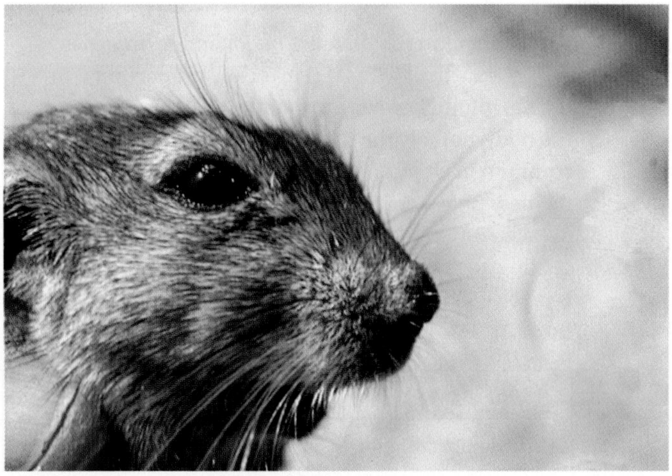

Fig. 32.3. *Psammomys obesus* (courtesy Dr P. Desjeux, WHO, Geneva).

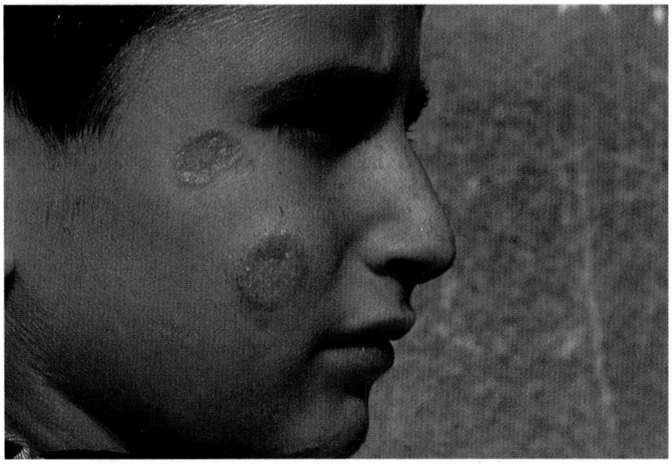

Fig. 32.4. Two active lesions of cutaneous leishmaniasis caused by *L. major* in a Moroccan boy (courtesy Dr P. Desjeux, WHO, Geneva).

Peripheral blood

Mononuclear cells proliferate in response to Leishmania antigen in vitro; a Th1-like reaction (production of interferon-gamma, no interleukin (IL)-4) is found in patients with mild disease but in severe disease a Th2-like pattern (low interferon-gamma with IL-4 production) is seen.

Clinical features

The incubation period for *L. major* and *L. tropica* is 2–4 weeks – it varies as it is inversely proportional to the inoculum. Lesions are mainly on exposed parts of the body, notably the limbs and the face, where they are common in children. The lesions are usually painless unless there is secondary infection: they may itch.

Clinically, one cannot tell with certainty which parasite is involved, but some characteristics may be helpful (see Box).

	L. major	*L. tropica*
Usual number of lesions	multiple[a]	single
Appearance	inflamed, wet (exudative)	less inflamed, dry
Tendency to heal	within months	one year or more

[a] Most patients present with 1–3 lesions, although some patients have tens of lesions up to over 100.

- The lesion starts as a papule that looks like an insect bite. It does not regress, rather the papule persists and gradually increases in size.
- Next, several common types develop – nodular, nodulo-ulcerative and ulcerative.
- The ulcer has a flat base with slightly or moderately rolled-up margins. The base consists of granulation tissue and may be covered by pus if it is secondarily infected.
- The nodulo-ulcerative form looks like a volcano with a broad base in the dermis and subcutaneous tissue (Fig. 32.4). The crater may be covered by a scab.
- Other important features are:
  1. satellite papules; these are small (2–4 mm) papules at the edge of the lesion.
  2. Skin crease orientation.
  3. Clustering, which is common in multiple lesions, because the sandfly bites repeatedly at the same place, each time depositing parasites with the bite.

Enlarged regional lymph nodes, which contain parasites, are found in approximately 10 per cent of cases (see Box).

Special clinical features of *L. major* infection (El-Hassan & Zijlstra, 2001)

1. Diffuse thickening without ulceration (erysipeloid form)
2. Leishmanial cheilitis
3. Chiclero's ulcer; this is an ulcer on the pinna of the ear
4. Mycetoma-like lesions
5. Leishmanial dactylitis
6. Cutaneous leishmaniasis of the nose
7. Sporotrichoid cutaneous leishmaniasis: the infection spreads along the lymphatics as in sporotrichosis.

A special clinical type of *L. tropica* infection is *Leishmania recidivans* or lupoid leishmaniasis. The sore seems to heal but recurs at the edge of the lesion, a process that may continue for many years and may be disfiguring (Fig. 32.5). It resembles cutaneous tuberculosis (*Lupus vulgaris*). Parasites are typically scanty and the leishmanin, skin test (LST) is strongly positive.

L. infantum causes small nodular lesions which may persist for many years.

L. aethiopica causes single lesions that tend to be central on the face and slowly increase in size. Crusts form and ulcers may not occur. In 1: 10000 of cases diffuse cutaneous leishmaniasis (DCL) follows CL caused by *L. aethiopica*. From the original CL lesion, the disease spreads to other parts of the skin, forming large numbers of papules and nodules that may coalesce to form plaques (Fig. 32.6). Ulceration does not occur – a sign of the weak immunogenic reaction elicited by the

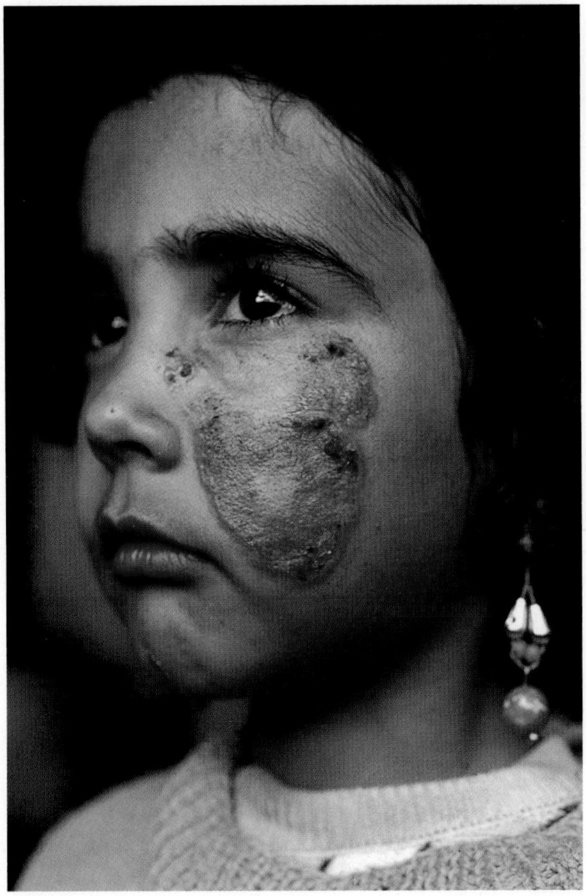

Fig. 32.5. Leishmania recidivans (courtesy Dr P. Desjeux, WHO, Geneva).

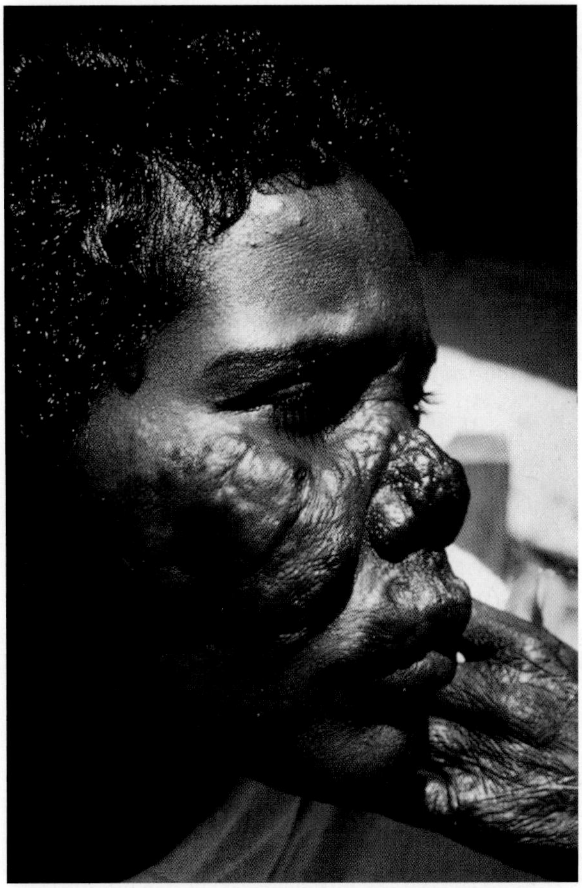

Fig. 32.6. Diffuse cutaneous leishmaniasis caused by *L. aethiopica* (courtesy Dr P. Desjeux, WHO, Geneva).

parasite. This is also demonstrated by the negative LST. In a smear macrophages contain large numbers of parasites and in a biopsy lymphocytes are few (Bryceson, 1970).

Differential diagnosis

The most important differential diagnoses include insect bite, impetigo, furuncle, syphilitic gumma, sporotrichosis, myiasis, mollusca contagiosa, tropical ulcer, anthrax, and basal cell carcinoma (Kubba et al., 1987).

Diagnosis

Clinical

A definite diagnosis is made by demonstration of *Leishmanial* amastigotes in the lesion, but sometimes parasites cannot be found as the yield of various techniques is variable. Clinical features, highly indicative of CL, are:

- persistent lesion in an exposed part of the body
- volcanic nodule
- skin crease orientation
- satellite papules
- subcutaneous extension
- sporotrichoid spread (El-Hassan & Zijlstra, 2001).

Parasitological

Parasites may be demonstrated by slit skin smear with a lancet or dental broach, fine needle aspiration, or surface abrasion with sandpaper. Spread the material on a slide, fix with methanol and stain with Giemsa; the sensitivity is 50–80 per cent. Parasites may also be seen in paraffin sections stained with haematoxylin and eosin in 70 per cent.

Technique of slit skin smear

Take smear from edge of the lesion, not from the necrotic centre
Press the skin firmly between thumb and index finger until it looks pale (to avoid blood)
Make incision in pale skin
Introduce lancet and turn 90°
Scrape along incision, also from deep tissue
Spread material on slide.

Technique of fine needle aspiration

Use 5 or 10 ml syringe and 23-gauge needle
Inject 0.1 ml of saline in edge of lesion
Re-aspirate and push material on a slide

Culture

Schneider's medium is most commonly used but bacterial or fungal contamination is common: this may be overcome by animal inoculation. After culture, parasites may be typed to determine the species and, within the species, the zymodeme by isoenzyme electrophoresis. In clinical practice, culture is rarely done as it requires a well-equipped laboratory.

Molecular biological tools
Leishmanial DNA can be detected by PCR in biopsies in >90 per cent and the species can be identified. For African CL, this is rarely necessary and the technique is not suitable for routine use.

Serological
All tests, ELISA and direct agglutination test (DAT) are of little value.

Leishmanin skin test (LST) (also known as Montenegro test)
After intradermal injection of killed amastigotes, the skin induration is measured after 48–72 hours and a test result of 5 mm or more is considered positive. A positive reaction indicates cell-mediated immunity to *Leishmania*; the test is mainly of value in epidemiological surveys but not in diagnosis of individual cases.

Treatment and follow-up

General

Lesions may be left to heal unless they are cumbersome for the patient. Many patients, however, demand treatment and for multiple lesions or disfiguring lesions it is clearly needed. If the lesions are secondarily infected, use gentian violet or systemic antibiotics to clear the infection after which the lesion may heal.

After healing (spontaneous or after treatment), a thin scar is formed. Multiple lesions heal asynchronously. The patient is usually immune to re-infection, although in 10 per cent re-infection has been reported, but this may run a milder course (Killick-Kendrick et al., 1985). Early treatment may prevent immunity from developing.

Systemic treatments

Pentavalent antimonials

These include sodium stibogluconate (Pentostam, Wellcome, UK): (100 mg antimony per ml) and meglumine antimoniate (Glucantime, Rhone-Poulenc): (85 mg antimony per ml).

For *L. major*, *L. tropica* and *L. infantum*, give 10–20 mg/kg/day for 20 days, which produces good results. No serious toxicity will be met if the dosage is within this range, but be careful in elderly patients and in those with cardiac, hepatic or renal disease (Kubba & Al-Gindan, 1989).

Follow-up at 6 weeks as lesions may regress further. If treatment fails, repeat the course of antimony.

Ketoconazole 600 mg for 30 days has been reported to give good results in Israel in ZCL: hepatotoxicity may occur.

Topical treatment

Intra-lesional antimony

The place of this possibly painful injection directly into the lesion is uncertain, but it may be indicated if there are contraindications to systemic antimonials or in early and solitary lesions (Kubba & Al-Gindan, 1989; El-Hassan & Zijlstra, 2001).

Ointment

A topical preparation of 15 per cent paromomycin (aminosidine) and 12 per cent methylbenzethonium (MBCL) gave better cure rates than placebo in *L. major* infection (77% vs. 27%), respectively (El-On et al., 1992). MBCL may cause severe local inflammation.

Heat

Leishmania parasites are sensitive to heat and do not survive temperatures above 37 °C. A water sack at 40–42 °C applied for several days may cure the lesion.

Cryotherapy

This may be used in single lesions without sub-cutaneous spread; but a bullous reaction may occur and it leaves a depigmented scar which may take 6 months to repigment.

Specific treatment

L. major

Most of the sores are self-healing within 3–5 months: no treatment is necessary. Systemic treatment with antimony is indicated in the patient with multiple lesions (more than five), severe lesions, lesions over the eyelids or nose, sporotrichoid spread or a systemic disease such as diabetes. In other cases where topical treatment is considered antimony may be given into the lesion.

L. tropica, L. infantum

Sores caused by *L. tropica* take longer to heal (10–14 months), and those of *L. infantum* may last for 1–3 years; for these lesions, earlier topical or systemic treatment can be given.

Leishmania recidivans lesions are treated with antimony 20 mg/kg per day for 6 weeks or until cure.

L. aethiopica

These lesions may last 2–5 years and may be best left to heal spontaneously. The response to higher doses of antimony is slow. The dose is 20 mg/kg b.d. for 8 weeks with careful monitoring for toxicity (Bryceson, 1996). In DCL, give aminosidine 15 mg/kg combined with stibogluconate 20 mg/kg; an alternative is pentamidine 3–4 mg salt per kg once weekly, for 4 months or longer with regular skin smear examination to monitor disappearance of parasites (Teklemariam et al., 1994; Bryceson, 1970).

MUCOSAL LEISHMANIASIS

The Sudanese type of ML is a primary infection by *L. major*, or by *L. donovani*, when it may occur as a separate illness or in the course of VL.

ML differs from muco-cutaneous leishmaniasis of South America, which follows a previous episode of CL caused by *L. brasiliensis* in a minority of cases.

Epidemiology

ML is mainly reported from Sudan, where around 100 cases have been described, mainly restricted to adult males belonging to certain tribes from Darfur province. Sporadic cases have been reported from Chad and Ethiopia.

ML has also been reported among patients co-infected with Leishmania and HIV in Spain and France. It may therefore be seen more frequently in endemic areas of Africa as the HIV epidemic spreads.

Prevention

General measures as described under CL apply; early diagnosis is important to prevent irreversible damage.

Pathology

It is unclear how the parasite reaches the nasal or oral mucosa, but hematogenous spread from an unnoticed primary skin lesion seems most likely. There are two types: the fungating or tumour-like form and the dry atrophic form. There is a mixture of lymphocytes, plasma cells and macrophages in the subepithelial tissues. Parasites are seen mainly in the fungating form; parasitized macrophages appear activated in the presence of lymphocytes and scattered granulomas are seen. Parasites appear to be destroyed in activated macrophages, but there is no necrosis as seen in CL, where this is thought to play a major role in elimination of the macrophages. Vascular changes including fibrinoid necrosis, vasculitis and hyalinosis have been described and are thought to be due to deposition of circulating immune complexes (Veress et al., 1986).

In contrast to the lymph nodes in VL, those in ML show granulomas with few parasites.

Clinical features (Fig. 32.7)

These depend on the site of the disease.

- Nasal ML: nasal obstruction, deformity, discharge, bleeding and anosmia are the main complaints.
- Oral and pharyngeal ML: patients complain of a fullness in the mouth with difficulty in mastication and swallowing, and may have bleeding of the gums and toothache. Teeth may become loose and are sometimes shed.
- Laryngeal ML: stridor, hoarseness of voice and cough may occur.

In the fungating form, the mucosa is red, swollen and fissured. When the nose is affected, the whole of the nose is

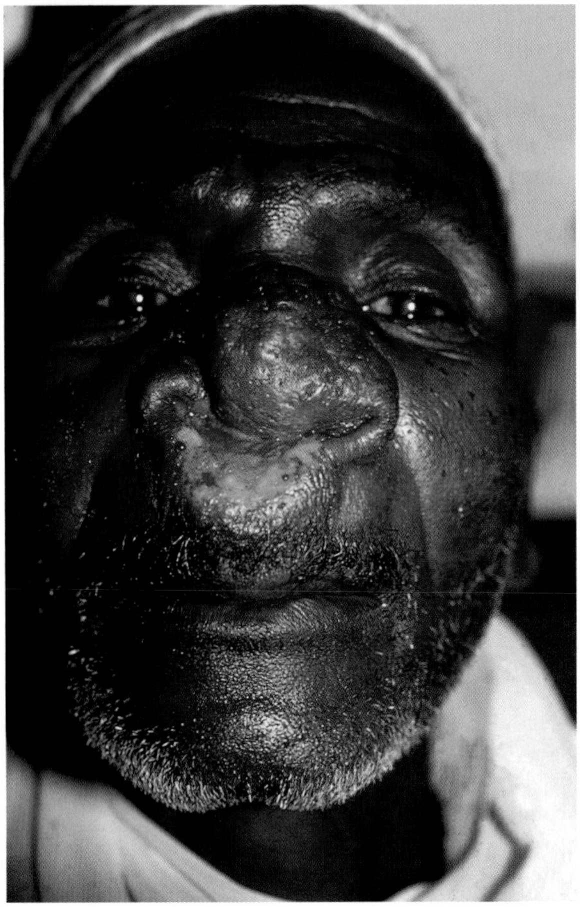

Fig. 32.7. Mucosal leishmaniasis (Sudan) (courtesy Royal Society of Tropical Medicine and Hygiene).

swollen and the skin is oedematous. The cartilaginous but not the bony septum is affected and may be completely destroyed, leading to collapse of the nose.

In the dry atrophic form, the mucosa is only slightly swollen, dry and covered with a scab. Removal of the scab causes bleeding. Perforation of the septum or of the hard palate may occur.

Regional lymph nodes are non-tender, mobile and may contain amastigotes.

In some patients, ML occurs in the course of VL and all classical features of VL may be present. However, VL in these patients runs a milder course and they may show evidence of some form of immunity to Leishmania parasites. When ML follows successful recovery from VL, it should therefore be referred to as post-kala-azar mucosal leishmaniasis.

The differential diagnosis is with paranasal sinus aspergilloma, rhinoscleroma, Wegener's granulomatosis, leprosy, histoplasmosis, rhinosporidioisis and benign and malignant tumours (El-Hassan et al., 1995).

Diagnosis

Parasitological

In the fungating tumour-like form, parasites may be readily demonstrated in a smear from the lesion, but in the diffuse atrophic form they may be scanty. A biopsy may be useful to exclude other conditions. PCR may be useful (El-Hassan et al., 1995) and may be more sensitive than smears.

Serological

Data are scanty, but in the 13 cases reported and tested 12 were positive in either ELISA or DAT (El-Safi & Evans, 1991; El-Hassan et al., 1995).

Leishmanin skin test

The LST is usually positive in particular in those with long-standing disease and extensive tissue damage, e.g. perforated nasal septa. As with serology, a positive LST gives support to the clinical diagnosis.

Treatment

The drug of choice is sodium stibogluconate in a dose of 10 mg/kg for 30 days; other regimens have not been evaluated.

Ketoconazole (400 mg daily for 4–6 weeks) may also be useful (El-Hassan et al., 1995).

VISCERAL LEISHMANIASIS

The problem in Africa

Epidemiology

It is estimated that, world-wide, 500 000 cases of VL occur per year (Desjeux, 1996); the majority being in India and, within Africa, Sudan. Other countries affected by VL are Kenya, Ethiopia and coastal Mediterranean countries.

VL is caused by parasites belonging to the *L. donovani sensu lato* family. These include *L. donovani* species,

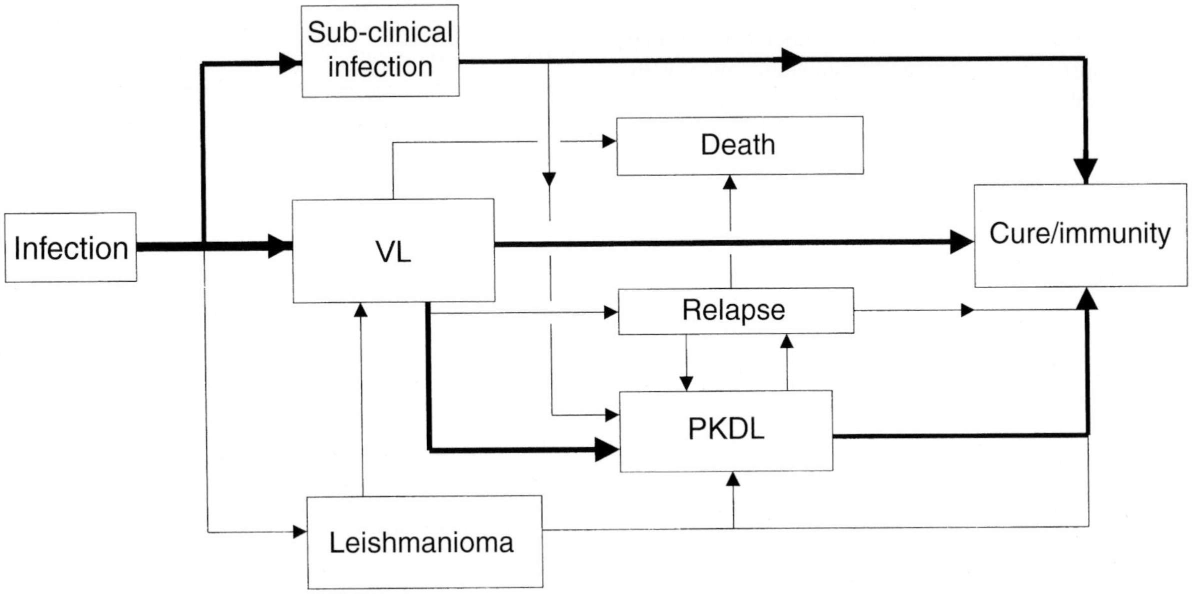

Fig. 32.8. Outcome of *Leishmania donovani* infection in Sudan. The thickness of the lines indicates the importance of that pathway.

which are involved in VL in Sudan and Kenya, as well as *L. infantum*, which is mainly found in areas along the Mediterranean.

In the Sudan, *L. donovani* s.l. is the species involved with *P. orientalis* as the vector. The disease may be zoonotic as rodents, servals and genets have been found infected and intense transmission occurs in relatively sparsely populated areas such as Dinder National Park (eastern Sudan); in other areas anthroponotic transmission is likely (but not proved) in the presence of large numbers of PKDL cases.

In Kenya both *L. donovani* and *L. infantum* have been isolated; in the Kitue focus of *L. donovani*, genets and mongooses have been reported infected; in Baringo district no definite host has been found. *P. martini* seems the most important vector.

In Ethiopia, *L. infantum* and *L. donovani* have been found and *P. orientalis* and *P. martini* have been incriminated as vectors.

P. orientalis has its typical habitat in *Acacia seyal* and *Balanites aegyptiaca* woodland on alluvial clay; *P. martini* is found in lightly wooded areas in the vicinity of termite hills built by *Macrotermes bellicosus*, on laterite clays (Ashford, 1999).

VL in the endemic areas is typically a disease of children; most adults are immune to the infection as shown by a positive leishmanin skin test (LST). They develop immunity by either recovering from a clinical episode of VL or after subclinical infection as may be evidenced by seroconversion followed by LST conversion. The outcome of infection with *Leishmania donovani* in Sudan is shown in Fig. 32.8. Development of VL is twice as common as sub-clinical infection; after VL, either cure or cure after PKDL is the rule; the death rate and relapse rate are around 5 per cent.

In epidemics individuals of all ages may be affected as was the case in the southern Sudan epidemic (western Upper Nile province); also non-immune travellers from non-endemic areas are at risk at any age to contract VL. Similarly, migrants or nomads may introduce the parasite to previously non-endemic areas as in the Sudan epidemic when soldiers, trained along the Ethiopian border, returned home while harbouring the parasite.

In some areas transmission seems stable, but elsewhere there are cycles of activity.

Prevention and control

Personal protection

Few conclusive studies have been done, but impregnated bednets and protective clothing, for example, long sleeves, and repellents are likely to be useful.

Reservoir control

The geographical area often governs the control effort.

(i) Mediterranean VL: current reservoirs, e.g. killing of infected dogs; treatment of dogs is not recommended as relapses are common and repeated treatment with pentavalent antimonials may create resistance.
(ii) Sudan: strategies aiming at the prevention and treatment of patients with PKDL may prove effective as these patients may be a human reservoir.

Sandfly control

Widespread application of insecticides is not useful as, in Africa, sandflies are not peri-domestic. Focal application or destruction of termite hills (the habitat of *P. martini*) has been done in Kenya.

Case detection

Passive case detection and continued surveillance for outbreaks is the minimum required in all areas and a prompt response to new outbreaks is mandatory.

General

(i) Public education in school and villages.
(ii) Making leishmaniasis a notifiable disease.
(iii) Establishment of a central referral centre with extended diagnostic and therapeutic services.

Clinical features

Symptoms (Table 32.2)

Fever is the rule usually without a particular pattern. Weight loss may be severe but may not be obvious in early infections. Life-threatening epistaxis may occur: the pathogenesis is unknown. There is no generalized haemorrhagic diathesis. Cough may result from interstitial leishmanial pneumonia or the common intercurrent infections; diarrhoea may be the result of leishmanial enteritis or another gastrointestinal infections such as amoebic dysentery. The enlarging spleen may cause left upper quadrant pain.

Signs

The spleen is palpable and is often massive (Fig. 32.9); if it is not felt, do not reject the diagnosis of VL. The liver is also enlarged, but less commonly than the spleen. Generalized lymphadenopathy is more common in African VL than in European or Indian VL. Jaundice is rare and may indicate

Table 32.2. Most common symptoms and signs found in Sudanese patients with VL

Symptoms	%
Fever	97–100
Weight loss	70–100
Epistaxis	47–88
Anorexia	70–87
Abdominal pain	41–81
Cough	63–76
Diarrhoea	17–45
Nausea/vomiting	22–27
Signs	
Fever	100
Splenomegaly	96–100
Hepatomegaly	56–100
Enlarged lymph nodes	36–84

Source: From Zijlstra & El-Hassan (2001).

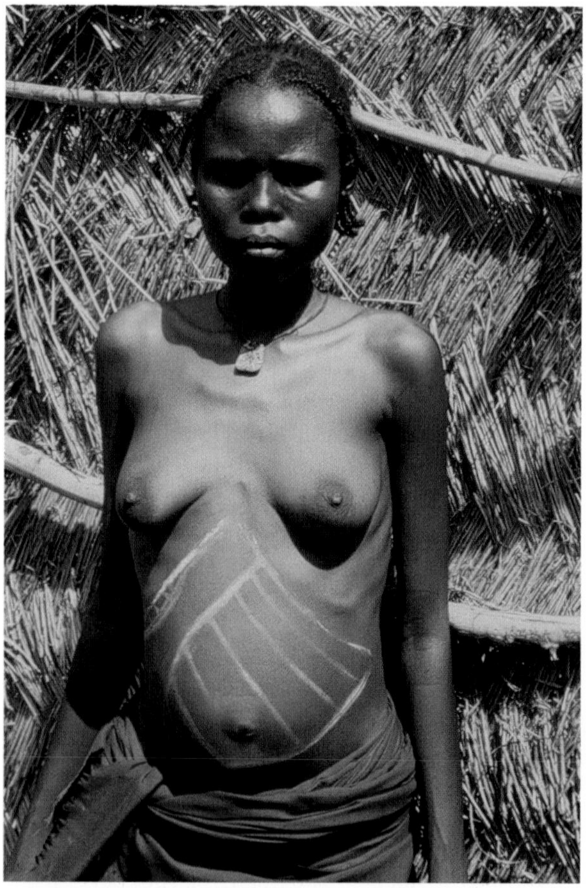

Fig. 32.9. Visceral leishmaniasis (Sudan), showing huge splenomegaly.

advanced disease or other liver pathology. Oedema is also uncommon and may result from anaemia or hypoalbuminaemia. Psychosis and depression are sometimes encountered and disappear after treatment.

CNS

Neurological manifestations in up to 46 per cent of cases. Burning feet are most common; other changes include foot drop, cranial nerve palsies and sensori-neural deafness. These improve after anti-leishmanial treatment.

Although kala-azar in Hindi means the black disease, referring to the hyperpigmentation that is described from India, this is rarely seen in African VL. Other skin changes include the leishmanioma, which is an ulcer at the site of the sandfly bite. These ulcers are flatter and less well circumscribed, without satellite lesions and subcutaneous nodules, in contrast to those in CL. The true incidence of leishmaniomas is unknown as they are easily overlooked. The infection may arrest when a leishmanioma has formed, without further spread, and will leave immunity or it may spread to become overt VL. Progression straight to PKDL without prior VL has also been described. Other skin conditions include tinea versicolor, which may be particularly severe in VL: it has been shown to clear after anti-leishmanial therapy only. Other conditions that reflect decreased immunity are herpes zoster and cancrum oris (noma).

VL in HIV infection

In countries north of the Mediterranean, in particular Spain, hundreds of cases of VL have now occurred in HIV-infected individuals. In Africa, in particular in Kenya and Ethiopia, increasing numbers of patients co-infected with HIV have been reported. Co-infection with HIV and Leishmania may manifest itself as a primary infection or a relapse of a previous episode of visceral or cutaneous leishmaniasis. In addition, Leishmania isolates are found that are not known to cause disease in immunocompetent individuals. The presentation is often atypical and may be masked by other opportunistic infections. Sometimes the diagnosis is made by chance as parasites may be found in uncommon places, e.g. rectal biopsy or bronchoalveolar lavage. Usually CD4 counts are below 200×10^9/l. Serological tests are unreliable and frequently negative in spite of high parasite burden; the leishmanin test is of limited value (Alvar et al., 1997).

Post-kala-azar manifestations

After apparently successful treatment of VL, parasites may persist in certain organs and, with restored immunity, may lead to a spectrum of clinical manifestations. The most frequent is PKDL, in which parasites persist in the skin (see below). All others are rare; post-kala-azar mucosal leishmaniasis is described under ML. Post-kala-azar uveitis, blepharitis and conjunctivitis, when parasites may be demonstrated in smears or biopsies, may have disastrous consequences. Other rare manifestations include laryngitis and colitis.

Laboratory findings

Pancytopenia is the classical finding, with anaemia, leukopenia and thrombocytopenia and hypersplenism. Anaemia may be aggravated by iron or folate deficiency or haemolysis.

The leukopenia is caused by neutropenia and there is relative lymphocytosis. Eosinophils are absent except in concurrent helminthic infection. It is unclear whether significant clotting abnormalities occur.

Albumin levels are low. Globulin levels, both total IgG and anti-parasite IgG, are raised.

Liver enzymes, notably ALT and AST are markedly raised, and to a lesser extent alkaline phosphatase and gamma-glutamyl transferase (GGT), which revert to normal after treatment. Proteinuria may be found.

ECG often shows flat or negative T-wave changes, which may become frequent during treatment with antimony; they are of limited clinical relevance (see Box).

Most important clinical features in VL
- Fever >2 weeks
- Splenomegaly
- Wasting

Most important laboratory findings
- Pancytopenia
- Low albumin
- High gammaglobulin

Pathology

Parasites may be found in all parts of the body, but in particular in the reticuloendothelial system. In the enlarged spleen areas of infarction may be found; microscopically, the white pulp is atrophied and the red pulp is infiltrated with parasite-laden macrophages. The normal architecture of the lymph nodes is destroyed and the lymphocytes are replaced with parasitized macrophages. Unlike in CL, there are no granulomas. The bone marrow is hypercellular with hyperplasia of all cell lines. The pancytopenia is thought to be caused by peripheral destruction of cells rather than decreased production, possibly by auto-antibodies.

Evidence from the animal model, as well as from human studies, shows that in active, progressive VL peripheral blood mononuclear cells show a mainly Th2 type of response as evidenced by IL-10 production, whereas in patients cured of VL Th1 responses are found with production of interferon-gamma and IL-12.

Diagnosis

Principles

- Try to demonstrate the parasite in a smear from a lymph node or bone marrow aspirate; if this is negative,
- A positive serological test combined with the clinical picture and the absence of another obvious diagnosis warrants start of treatment.
- A positive LST (if available) is against current active VL.

Parasitological diagnosis

Demonstration of Leishmania amastigotes is still the most important and simple way of diagnosing VL. Parasites may be found in a lymph node, bone marrow or spleen aspirate.

Lymph node aspiration is easy with minimal discomfort for the patient. Usually inguinal nodes are selected and, even if they do not seem enlarged, it is worth attempting to aspirate (see Box). The sensitivity of lymph node aspiration is around 55 per cent.

Technique of lymph node aspiration

Cleaning the skin:
Fix the node between fingers:
Insert a 20–22 gauge needle into the node:
Rotate the needle gently:
Withdraw it and attach a 2 ml syringe:
Expel the contents onto a slide,
Fix with methanol and stain with Giemsa.
Or attach the needle to the syringe beforehand and, after insertion, suck fluid into the syringe.

Bone marrow aspiration may be done if no parasites can be demonstrated in the lymph node aspirate, but it is much more painful. The sensitivity is higher, 70–90 per cent, than with lymph node aspiration.

Spleen aspiration has a sensitivity of >95 per cent; it carries a minimal risk of bleeding and rupture of the spleen and should preferably be done in hospital by an experienced person (see Box). It is useful to do a prothrombin time, which should not be more than 5 seconds longer than the normal control and the platelet count should not be $<40 \times 10^9$/l (WHO, 1990). Despite these cautions, the procedure has been often done under field conditions in thousands of patients without any laboratory support and apparently without major complications.

Technique of spleen aspiration

- Explain the procedure fully to the patient or, if a child, to the parents. In small children mild sedation may be helpful.
- With the patient lying on his back, draw the outline of the spleen with a marker pen on the skin, and draw a cross where the needle should enter.
- Use a 5 ml syringe with a 21- or 22-gauge needle.
- Puncture the spleen while the patient is breathing normally: in crying children, do the puncture on expiration.
- Clean the skin, introduce the needle in a quick to and fro movement at at an angle of 45°, aiming cranially to avoid the hilar vessels.
- Withdraw the needle and apply suction by withdrawing the plunger slightly.

Or pierce the skin first, then apply negative pressure by pulling the plunger to the 1 ml mark and then enter and exit in a swift motion. Speed and identical angles of the needle entering and coming out are essential. A tiny amount of splenic pulp will be sucked into the needle and pushed out on a slide and processed as described.

Patients often react with disbelief because the procedure is so quick and because it only causes minor discomfort (Zijlstra & El-Hassan, 2001).

The parasite load in spleen aspirates can be monitored before and after courses of treatment and graded as proposed by Chulay and Bryceson (1983):

6+	>100 amastigotes per oil immersion field
5+	10–100 amastigotes per oil immersion field
4+	1–10 amastigotes per oil immersion field
3+	1–10 amastigotes per 10 oil immersion fields
2+	1–10 amastigotes per 100 oil immersion fields
1+	1–10 amastigotes per 1000 oil immersion fields
0	zero amastigotes per 1000 oil immersion fields

Animal inoculation and culture (specialized units)

Materials obtained from aspirates may be cultured, e.g. in Schneider's medium, NNN or RPMI medium. This is potentially more sensitive than smears and, after treatment, may give an indication whether parasites demonstrated in a smear are viable. The parasite may be typed using isoenzyme analysis, a technique that is particularly useful for epidemiological study when cases occur in new areas and in patients with unusual clinical presentation.

If the material is collected from a potentially contaminated area, animal inoculation may be used, e.g. in Syrian hamsters.

Parasites may be demonstrated in all organs and in a blood smear. For example, parasites can be found in 50 per cent of patients co-infected with HIV and in 67 per cent when the buffy coat is cultured (Alvar et al., 1997). PCR is more sensitive than conventional methods so that parasites in a blood film may be detected in more than 90 per cent of patients.

Serological diagnosis

Many tests have been developed, using a variety of antigens and detection methods, chiefly employing whole promastigotes as antigen, but more specific antigens have been identified, which give better tests.

Before a test result is interpreted, one should have some understanding of the natural history of VL. Although most patients will have a positive serological test at diagnosis, some remain negative in particular when diagnosed early. After treatment, positive results may be found for months or years before, if ever, they revert to negative. In sub-clinical infections an individual may convert serologically without developing clinical disease and may continue to show a positive test for a long time. No currently available test reliably distinguishes between active VL, sub-clinical infection and past infection.

Direct agglutination test

This test uses whole promastigotes as antigen and is particularly useful to screen large numbers of cases in the field where it is read by eye. Cross-reactions may occur, for example, with African trypanosomiasis, but better antigen delivery now makes these rare. There is now a freeze-dried antigen, which does not deteriorate outside the refrigerator. The sensitivity and negative predictive value is >90 per cent; specificity (72%) is influenced by persistence of antibodies after previous (sub)clinical infection (Zijlstra & El-Hassan, 2001).

Enzyme-linked immunosorbent assay (ELISA)

There is the standard ELISA, which uses soluble or whole promastigotes and needs an ELISA reader making it less suitable for field use. An adaptation is the DOT–ELISA that can be read visually. The standard ELISA was reported to give a positive result in all patients with VL (El-Safi & Evans, 1989); in CL 60 per cent of patients gave a positive result. A more specific antigen is the gp63 antigen; an ELISA using this antigen could distinguish between past and current infection and gave negative results in CL. Another antigen is recombinant K39 antigen, which gave sensitivity of 93 per cent; as with the DAT, titres remained positive for 24 months after treatment. The rK39 ELISA is adapted to an immunochromatographic strip test; a drop of blood is applied on the strip and 200 microlitres (or 2 drops) of water or saline are added to make the fluid migrate along the strip. When the control line becomes visible, the test can be considered valid; if the test line becomes visible this indicates the presence of anti-rK39 antibodies. In a study in Sudan, the sensitivity was found to be 79 per cent; as with the DAT, positive test results may be found after successful treatment but to a lesser extent than with the DAT. At present, the rK39 strip test costs around US$ 1.00.

Indirect immunofluorescence test (IFAT)

The sensitivity is 100 per cent but an immunofluorescence microscope is needed.

Abandon non-specific serological tests such as the formol geltest and the albumin/globulin ratio as their performance is poor.

Test of cellular immunity

Leishmanin skin test (LST)

The LST is typically negative in active VL; after treatment it becomes positive in 80 per cent after 6 months. A positive LST is thought to correlate well with acquired immunity.

Treatment

Treatment of VL

1. specific anti-leishmanial drugs – expensive, parenteral, prolonged
2. treatment of concurrent infections – such as tuberculosis, malaria
3. adequate nutrition
4. adjuvant treatment of anaemia.

Specific anti-leishmanial treatment

Pentavalent antimonials

Pentavalent (SbV) antimonials, which have been used since the 1940s, remain the drugs of choice: they are effective and safe. While not outrageously expensive, the price of the drug burdens the health budgets of many countries. The cost of treatment for an adult lies around USD 150.

Most countries in Africa use sodium stibogluconate, which contains 100 mg SbV per 100 ml (Pentostam[R] Glaxo Smith Kline). Other countries, mainly French and Spanish speaking, use meglumine antimoniate, which contains 85 mg SbV per ml (Glucantime[R], Rhône–Poulenc). Generic sodium stibogluconate (Albert David Company, Calcutta, India) is equally effective and safe and costs 1/14 of the price of branded stibogluconate (Pentostam[R]). The drug can only be given parenterally; in remote and difficult conditions, when very many patients need to be taken care of daily, it may be necessary to divide the dose between two syringes and to inject both buttocks, as 5 ml is usually considered the maximum amount that can be given in one i.m. injection. If the drug is given repeatedly in the same vein it may cause thrombophlebitis.

The WHO recommends 20 mg/kg for at least 20 days, but the optimum dose should be established in each endemic area. In remote areas where even the most basic health systems do not exist and follow-up cannot be guaranteed, it is probably advisable to over-treat rather than to under-treat, with a total treatment time of 30 days. The injections are given once daily and are usually well tolerated. The full dose is given from the start.

It is perfectly possible to use stibogluconate under desperately difficult field conditions, as was demonstrated during the VL epidemic in southern Sudan in the 1990s.

Side effects

These are mild.

1. Heart – ECG. Flat or inverted T-waves may occur, but are of little clinical importance. A prolonged QT-interval is serious but unlikely to occur at the recommended dosage.
2. Liver and pancreas – enzymes. Both raised liver enzymes and amylase have been reported. In the Sudan hepatic transaminases were found to be raised but returned to normal after treatment, and we found no evidence of liver failure or jaundice, nor clinical features of pancreatitis, in hundreds of patients, and treatment with stibogluconate was rarely if ever interrupted.
3. Other: mild arthralgias are seen, but are easily controlled by analgesics. Idiosyncratic reactions are rare.

Pentamidine

This drug should only be used as a second-line drug, should be given by slow intramuscular injection or slowly i.v. over 2 hours; usually 2–4 mg/kg is given 1–3 times per week. The duration should be determined by clinical response and preferably parasitological cure. Nephrotoxicity and hepatotoxicity may occur and hyperglycaemia may be the result of pancreatitis. Hypoglycaemia may also occur but the mechanism is unknown. It is not suitable for use in the field, but should be reserved for hospital in-patient treatment with careful laboratory monitoring.

Amphotericin B

This drug has excellent activity against Leishmania, but is not used widely because of side effects, which include fever and rigors, renal toxicity with hypokalaemia and metabolic acidosis, and bone marrow depression toxicity. It can only be given in hospital, where toxicity can be monitored. In India, 0.5 mg/kg on alternate days for a total of 14 doses gave cure rates 98–100 per cent without serious side effects.

Liposomal amphotericin

This is the most effective drug but it is so expensive that it is beyond the health budgets of most countries. Liposomal particles containing amphotericin B are eliminated specifically by macrophages, which harbour leishmanial parasites, so that little drug remains in the circulation and toxicity is therefore minimal. A suitable regimen is 3–4 mg/kg given in >5 doses in 10 days with a total dose of 20–30 mg/kg.

Aminosidine (paromomycin; Gabromicina[R], Farmitalia)

This inexpensive aminoglycoside drug may be given either as an alternative for stibogluconate, or in combination with it, as has been advocated in AIDS. The dose is 15 mg/kg per day i.m. or i.v. (infusion over 90 min) for 21 days, although its use as a single drug is not well established.

Other drugs

Allopurinol may be used as a second-line drug in combination with stibogluconate; the dose is 20 mg/kg which is three times higher than is used in treatment of gout. Toxic epidermal necrolysis is a serious side effect. Gamma-interferon may be added to stibogluconate as a second-line drug but is expensive. Ketoconazole and fluconazole have been found of little use.

Miltefosine

Originally developed as an anti-neoplastic agent, it has excellent anti-leishmanial efficacy. It may well be the first effective oral treatment for VL. It is not yet marketed.

Splenectomy

Although effective in some cases that were refractory to treatment, do not consider splenectomy until full drug treatment has been given because of the severe pneumococcal infection and malaria in splenectomized patients.

Response to treatment

There is little resistance to antimonials in Africa: cure should be the rule. In Sudan 98 per cent of 1593 patients responded to first-line treatment. Use clinical signs – fever, spleen size, nutritional state and general well-being – to assess progress. Repeated parasitological investigation is usually not necessary except in those who do not respond. In 80 per cent of patients a positive LST will develop after 6 months, which may be used as a marker for developed immunity in those who are not immunosuppressed.

Failure of treatment

Those who do not respond or who relapse need second-line treatment (see Box). Examine each patient carefully to exclude concurrent disease such as tuberculosis. Repeated spleen aspirates to estimate parasitological load may be useful. It is advisable to refer these cases to a specialist hospital where there is relevant expertise.

Treatment and HIV

In HIV-infected individuals, response to treatment is slower and relapses are more likely. It is advisable to give combination treatment from the start, e.g. stibogluconate and aminosidine, allopurinol or gamma-interferon. When a remission is induced, give maintenance treatment with antimony (once a month), pentamidine (one injection every 3–4 weeks), gamma-interferon (2–3 injections per week) or (liposomal) amphotericin B. Highly active antiretroviral treatment (HAART) in co-infected patients seems to reduce the number of relapses and increase their interval.

First-line treatment

Stibogluconate 20 mg/kg for 30 days
Alternatives:
- Aminosidine 15 mg/kg for 21 days
- Pentamidine 2–4 mg/kg 1–3 times per week
- Amphotericin B 0.5 mg/kg on alternate days for 14 days

Treatment of resistant or relapsing cases (in order of preference)

Second course of stibogluconate for 30–60 days
Stibogluconate plus allopurinol
Stibogluconate plus aminosidine
Stibogluconate plus gamma-interferon
Amphotericin B

Post-kala-azar dermal leishmaniasis (PKDL)

PKDL is a sequel of visceral leishmaniasis that is increasingly recognized in Africa, in particular in Sudan. It causes considerable morbidity as lesions may persist for months and large numbers of cases in an area endemic for VL may act as a human reservoir for parasites.

Pathology

Leishmania parasites can be demonstrated in the skin of patients with VL, but these do not cause disease. After treatment for VL, parasites disappear from lymph node, bone marrow or spleen in most patients, but in PKDL persist in the skin. In 16 per cent of PKDL patients parasites may still be demonstrated in inguinal lymph nodes or bone marrow, suggesting that visceral disease persists (para-kala-azar dermal leishmaniasis). When immunity against Leishmania parasites develops, a rash appears. Figure 32.10 shows the relationship between parasites, immunity and clinical diagnosis.

The changes in the skin resulting from the interaction between parasites and immune response include hyperkeratosis, parakeratosis, acanthosis, follicular plugging and liquefaction in the epidermis and degeneration of the basal layer, sometimes in different combinations. Damage to melanocytes causes hypopigmentation. In the dermis varying degrees of inflammation are seen with scanty parasites. Lymphocytes, macrophages and scattered epitheloid cells may be found. In 20 per cent of cases lesions consisting of mainly discrete granulomas with, or without, Langhans giant cells may be seen. Neuritis of small cutaneous nerves has been described.

In regional lymph nodes there is follicular hyperplasia and enlargement of the paracortex, sometimes with epithelioid granulomas.

The presence of IL-10 in the sweat glands or keratinocytes in VL predicts the development of PKDL: this was also shown in the plasma and peripheral blood mononuclear cells (PBMC). Apparently, IL-10 drives the immune response to a Th2-type of reaction. After treatment for VL there is a shift to a mixed Th1/Th2 type of reaction and the Th1-type cells may play a role in the pathogenesis of PKDL (Gasim et al., 1998; Zijlstra & El-Hassan, 2001).

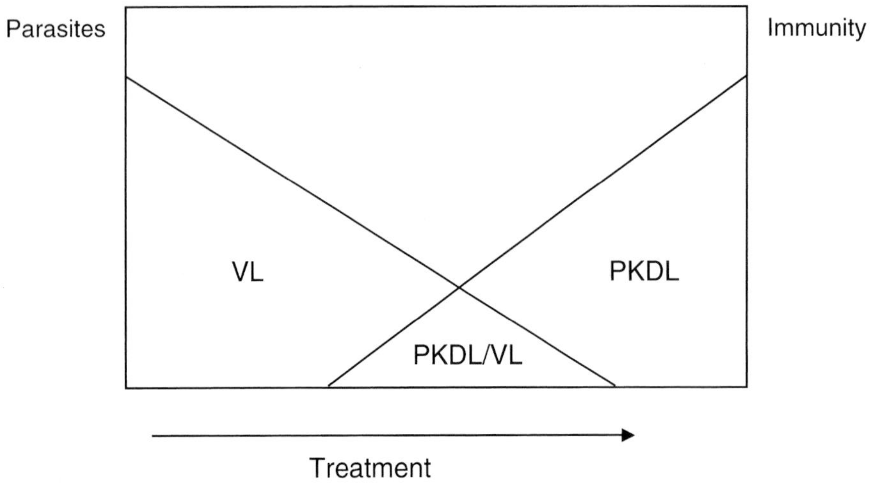

Fig. 32.10. This simplified diagram shows the relationship between decreasing numbers of parasites, developing immunity and resulting clinical presentation in those who develop PKDL after the start of treatment of VL.

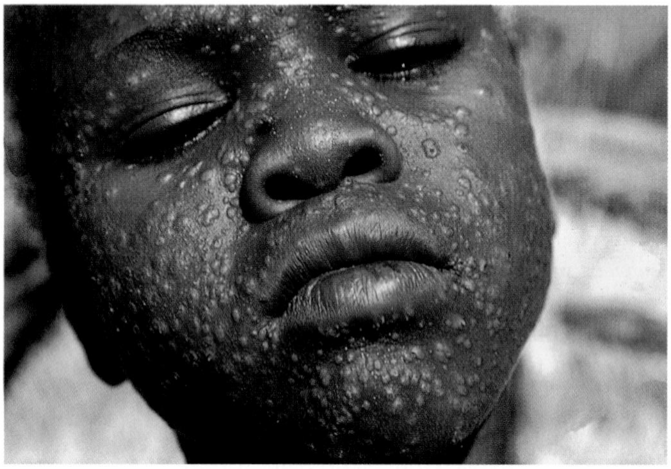

Fig. 32.11. Post-kala-azar dermal leishmaniasis (Sudan): papular and nodular lesions, typically on the face, concentrated in the peri-oral area.

Clinical features

PKDL follows VL in Sudan in 56 per cent of cases, with an interval between 0 and 6 months (mode 3 months). In some cases PKDL occurs during treatment for VL. Typically, PKDL presents as a macular, maculo-papular, papular or nodular rash several weeks or months after the patient has been successfully treated for VL (Fig. 32.11). While the patient no longer shows the systemic signs of VL and is feeling healthy, a rash appears first on the face around the mouth from where it may spread to other parts of the body. There are three grades of severity.

PKDL – Grades of severity

Grade 1

Lesions mainly on the face and head with some scattered lesions on (upper) arms, chest and back.

Grade 2

Lesions involving the head, scalp, forearms, upper legs, upper chest and back, gradually becoming reduced distally. The hands and feet are free.

Grade 3

All parts of the body are affected, including hands and feet.

It is not possible to predict who will, and who will not, develop PKDL. There is some evidence that PKDL occurs in those inadequately treated for VL and in those in whom Leishmanial parasite DNA can be demonstrated by PCR in bone marrow or lymph node aspirates at the end of treatment of VL.

After cure of PKDL either with treatment (see below) or spontaneously, the rash disappears in reverse order with the peri-oral lesions lasting longest. When PKDL relapses, the peri-oral lesions will again be the first to appear.

The lesions are not painful, but may itch. They appear preferentially on pre-existing scars, which become more prominent (Köbner phenomenon). Healing without scarring is the rule, but in severe long-standing cases depressed scars may occur. Others have extensive desquamation of the skin before healing.

Unless there is concurrent VL, patients are otherwise well. Fifty per cent of patients have splenomegaly, but the spleen is much smaller than in VL.

Diagnosis

Clinical

The appearance of the rash, its distribution and its temporal relationship is usually enough to make the diagnosis.

Parasitological

If the diagnosis is uncertain, make a slit skin smear and stain it with Giemsa. A biopsy may show histology which is suggestive of PKDL, but parasites are difficult to find. The sensitivity of both methods is 20–30 per cent. Other methods such as monoclonal antibodies and PCR are more sensitive (>80%). In systemic illness, diagnosis of concurrent VL should be made as already described in the VL section.

Serological

DAT, ELISA or other tests may help to differentiate PKDL from other conditions if clinically indicated. A positive result shows that antibodies formed during VL are persisting. There is no difference in DAT positivity between those with PKDL and those who were cured from VL without PKDL.

Leishmanin skin test

The LST is positive in up to 50 per cent of cases, but the frequency is lower in severe disease than in mild PKDL. This probably reflects the less well-developed immunity in patients with severe PKDL.

Differential diagnosis of PKDL

The most common condition to mimic PKDL is miliaria rubra (prickly heat) but its lesions are usually on the forehead and pressure points and not around the mouth as in PKDL. It occurs typically during hot summer months in infants, almost completely wrapped in cloth, carried on their mother's back.

Differentation from leprosy is more difficult and any form of leprosy may be confused with PKDL. Careful clinical examination is essential – thickening of nerves and madarosis are not features of PKDL: the lesions in PKDL are not anaesthetic. If in doubt, do a slit skin smear to demonstrate acid fast bacilli. Many common and less common conditions may be confused with PKDL.

Treatment

Most PKDL rashes are mild and will heal without treatment within 1–2 months. Reserve treatment for those with severe and persistent lesions; in practice these will be those with grades 2 and 3 PKDL. Give sodium stibogluconate 20 mg/kg for at least 2 months and then assess the patient's condition. In resistant cases, try (liposomal) amphotericin B.

References

Al Gindan Y, Kubba R, El Hassan AM et al. (1989). Dissemination in cutaneous leishmaniasis. III. Lymph node involvement. *Int J Dermatol*; **28**: 248–254.

Alvar J, Canavate C, Gutiérrez-Solar B et al. (1997). Leishmania and human immunodeficiency virus coinfection: the first ten years. *Clin Microbiol Rev*; **10**: 298–319.

Ashford RW. (1999). Visceral leishmaniasis: epidemiology, prevention and control. In *Protozoal Diseases*, ed. HM Gilles. London: Arnold Publishers.

Berman JD. (1997). Human leishmaniasis: clinical, diagnostic, and chemotherapeutic developments in the last 10 years. *Clin Infect Dis*; **24**: 684–703. (excellent and complete review on leishmaniasis).

Bryceson ADM. (1970). Diffuse cutaneous leishmaniasis in Ethiopia II. Treatment. *Trans Roy Soc Trop Med Hyg*; **64**: 369–379.

Bryceson ADM. (1996). Leishmaniasis. In *Oxford Textbook of Medicine*, 3rd edn, Oxford, UK: Oxford University Press.

Chulay JD, Bryceson ADM. (1983). Quantitation of amastigotes of *Leishmania donovani* in smears of splenic aspirates from patients with visceral leishmaniasis. *Am J Trop Med Hyg*; **32**: 475–479.

Desjeux P. (1996). Leishmaniasis: public health aspects and control. *Clin Dermatol*; **14**: 417–423.

El-Hassan AM, Meredith SEO, Yagi HI et al. (1995). Sudanese mucosal leishmaniasis: epidemiology, clinical features, diagnosis, immune responses and treatment. *Trans Roy Soc Trop Med Hyg*; **89**: 647- 652.

Evans D. (1989). (Eds) *Handbook on Isolation Characterization and Cryopreservation of* Leishmania, UNDP/ World Bank/ WHO Special Program for Research and Training in Tropical Diseases (TDR). Geneva: WHO.

El-Hassan AM, Zijlstra EE. (2001). Leishmaniasis in Sudan. 1. Cutaneous leishmaniasis. *Trans Roy Soc Trop Med Hyg*; **95**: S1–S18.

El-On J, Halvey S, Greenwald M. (1992). Topical treatment of Old World cutaneous leishmaniasis caused by *Leishmania major*: a double blind controlled study. *J Am Acad Dermatol*; **27**: 227–231.

El Safi SH, Evans DA. (1989). A comparison of the direct agglutination test and enzyme-linked immunosorbent assay in the sero-diagnosis of leishmaniasis in the Sudan. *Trans Roy Soc Trop Med Hyg*; **83**: 334–337.

El Safi SH, Peters W. (1991). Studies on the leishmaniases in the Sudan. 1. Epidemic of cutaneous leishmaniasis in Khartoum. *Trans Roy Soc Trop Med Hyg*. **85**: 44–47.

Gasim S, Elhassan AM, Khalil EAG et al. (1998). High levels of plasma IL-10 and expression of IL-10 by keratinocytes during visceral leishmaniasis predict subsequent development of post-kala-azar dermal leishmaniasis. *Clin Exp Immunol*; **111**: 64–69.

Guiguemdé R, Sawadogo O, Bories C et al. (2001). *Leishmania major* HIV co-infection. Abstract: Worldleish II, Crete, 20–24 May.

Killick-Kendrick R, Bryceson ADM, Peters W et al. (1985). Zoonotic cutaneous leishmaniasis in Saudi Arabia; lesions healing naturally in man followed by a second infection with the same zymodeme of *Leishmania major*. *Trans Roy Soc Trop Med Hyg*; **79**: 363–365.

Kubba R, Al Gindan Y, El Hassan AM et al. (1987). Clinical diagnosis of cutaneous leishmaniasis (oriental sore). *J Am Acad Dermatol*; **16**: 1183–1189.

Kubba R, Al-Gindan Y. (1989). Leishmaniasis. *Dermatol Clin*; **7**: 331–351.

Teklemariam S, Hiwot AG, Frommel D et al. (1994). Aminosidine and its combination with sodium stibogluconate in the treatment of diffuse cutaneous leishmaniasis caused by *Leishmania aethiopica*. *Trans Roy Soc Trop Med Hyg*; **88**: 334–339.

Veress B, El Hassan AM, Kutty MK et al. (1986). Immunological investigations in chronic cutaneous leishmaniasis in Saudi Arabia. *Trop Geog Med*; **38**: 380–385.

WHO Expert Committee. (1990). Control of leishmaniasis. *WHO Technical report Series No. 793*. Geneva: WHO.

Zijlstra EE, El-Hassan AM. (2001). Leishmaniasis in Sudan. *Trans Roy Soc Trop Med Hyg*; **95**: 27–58.

Resources

Laboratories where typing by isoenzymes can be done include the Laboratoire de Parasitologie, Centre Hôpitalier Universitaire, Montpellier and the London School of Hygiene and Tropical Medicine; strains are referred to, e.g. as *L. major* MON 1 or *L. donovani* LON 46.

African trypanosomiasis

33

Sleeping sickness or human African trypanosomiasis (HAT) is an important health problem in Africa. It is caused by sub-species of the protozoan parasite *Trypanosoma brucei*, which is transmitted to man by tsetse flies. The disease occurs in two clinically and epidemiologically distinct forms, termed West (*gambiense*) and East African (r*hodesiense*) sleeping sickness. An established infection in both forms has invariably a lethal outcome if left untreated. Proper diagnosis and correct patient management are therefore crucial. Treatment, however, is difficult, expensive and hampered by the restricted availability of the essential trypanosomicidal drugs.

The problem of sleeping sickness in Africa

Sleeping sickness is confined to the African continent. Due to the biology of the vector, its distribution is restricted to areas between 14° N and 29° S, the 'tsetse belt' of Africa (Mulligan 1970) (Fig. 33.1).

First reports of the disease go back to the fourteenth century. Caravanners to the Southern Kingdoms and slave traders have recognized the symptoms of a 'sleepy distemper leading to an untimely death'. Its impact on health for the African population had been enormous in the past, and many areas were inaccessible for human settlers and livestock for a long time. During the first decades of the twentieth century, when the parasite, its vector and life cycle were described (Box), sleeping sickness killed hundreds of thousands, possibly millions of people in Central Africa around Lake Victoria and in the Congo basin. The control of sleeping sickness became a focus of colonial activities with the objective of reducing disease burden and economic loss. Offices for planning and implementation of vertical programmes against human and animal trypanosomiasis were established in nearly every country of sub-Saharan Africa (Box).

> 1895: Sir David Bruce (1855–1931) suggests an association between trypanosomes and the 'cattle fly fever', a major problem of livestock in Southern Africa.
>
> 1902: Robert M. Forde and Everett Dutton identify trypanosomes in the blood of a patient during a scientific expedition to the Gambia.
>
> 1903: Sir David Bruce recognizes the tsetse fly as vector of trypanosomes.

> Autonomous structures in the fight against sleeping sickness in colonial times:
>
> - anglophone countries: Sleeping Sickness Bureau
> - francophone countries: Service Général Autonome de la Maladie de Sommeil
> - lusophone countries: Missão de Combate as Tripanosomiases

It took half a century to bring down sleeping sickness. In the 1960s, prevalence was reduced to a few sporadic cases. The impressive success of control programmes suggested that sleeping sickness would imminently disappear as a public health problem. Priorities in health policies were therefore gradually shifted, and funds were decreasing. Surveillance and control activities were diminished and finally put on hold, although sleeping sickness nowhere disappeared completely. The result has been a gradual resurgence, usually unnoticed by the international community. Recent epidemics in the Democratic Republic of Congo, Northern Angola, Sudan, Uganda and increasingly in many other countries, are proof of a major and extremely worrying evolution of events (Smith et al., 1998). There is evidence to believe

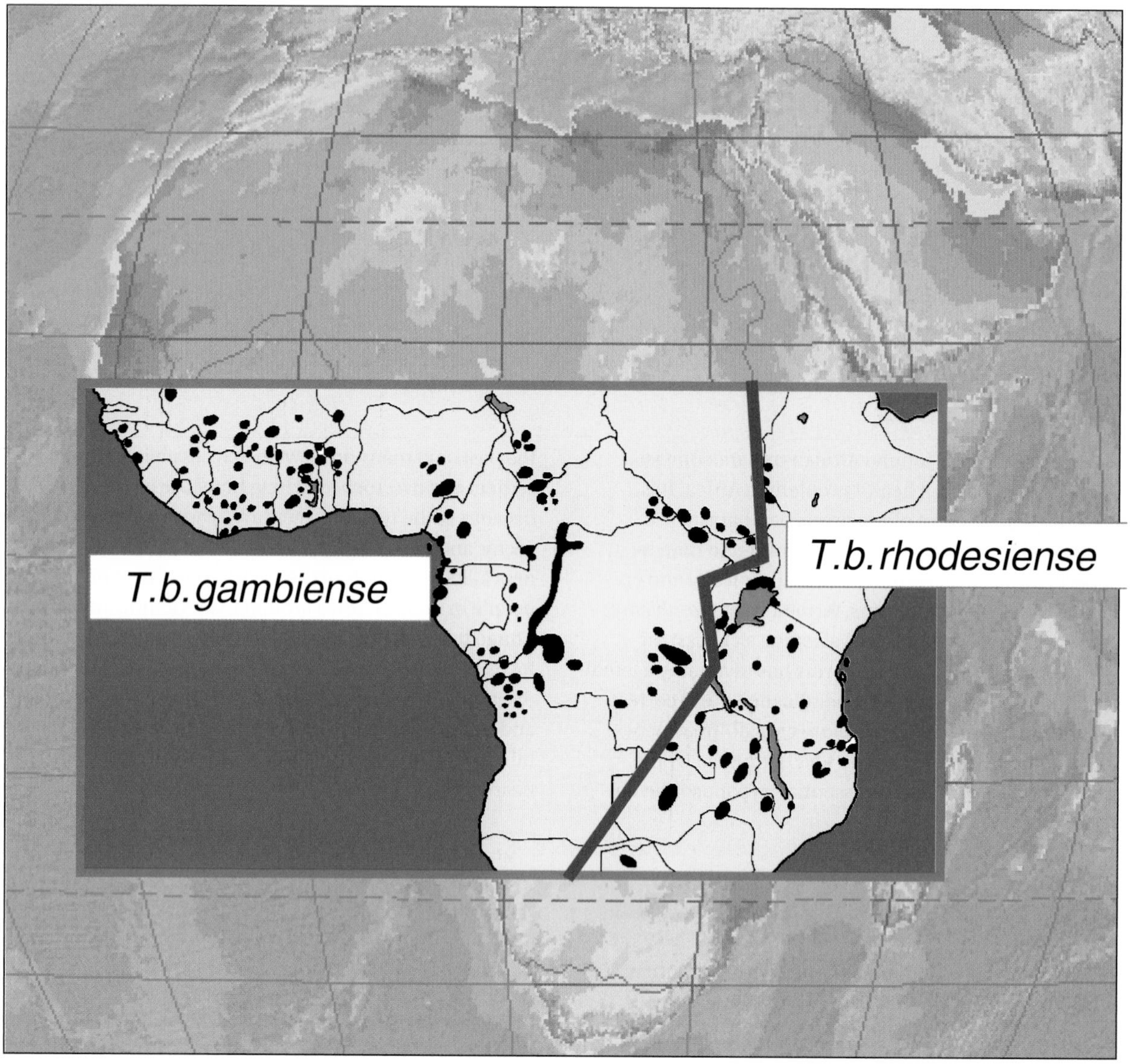

Fig. 33.1. The distribution of sleeping sickness in Africa.

that the achievements in sleeping sickness control during colonial times will be completely reversed in the near future.

Today, some 60 million people in 36 countries are at risk, but less than 4 million are under professional and constant surveillance. 40 000 cases are reported annually to the WHO, nearly all of them *T.b. gambiense* infections. The most affected areas are virtually inaccessible for epidemiological surveys, and the reported numbers have to be multiplied by ten to receive a proper estimate of the magnitude of the problem (World Health Organization, 1998) (Fig. 33.2).

War

The recent resurgence of sleeping sickness in areas ridden by war and civil unrest, the decreasing availability of drugs on the international market and the general loss of interest in issues of health in Africa gives rise to the fear that sleeping sickness might soon be untreatable again. It is already out of control! The fight against sleeping sickness in the field is often left to a few compassionate non-governmental organizations. African health politicians are just beginning to realize the threat and to revive the tradition of a national sleeping sickness bureau, long forgotten since colonial times.

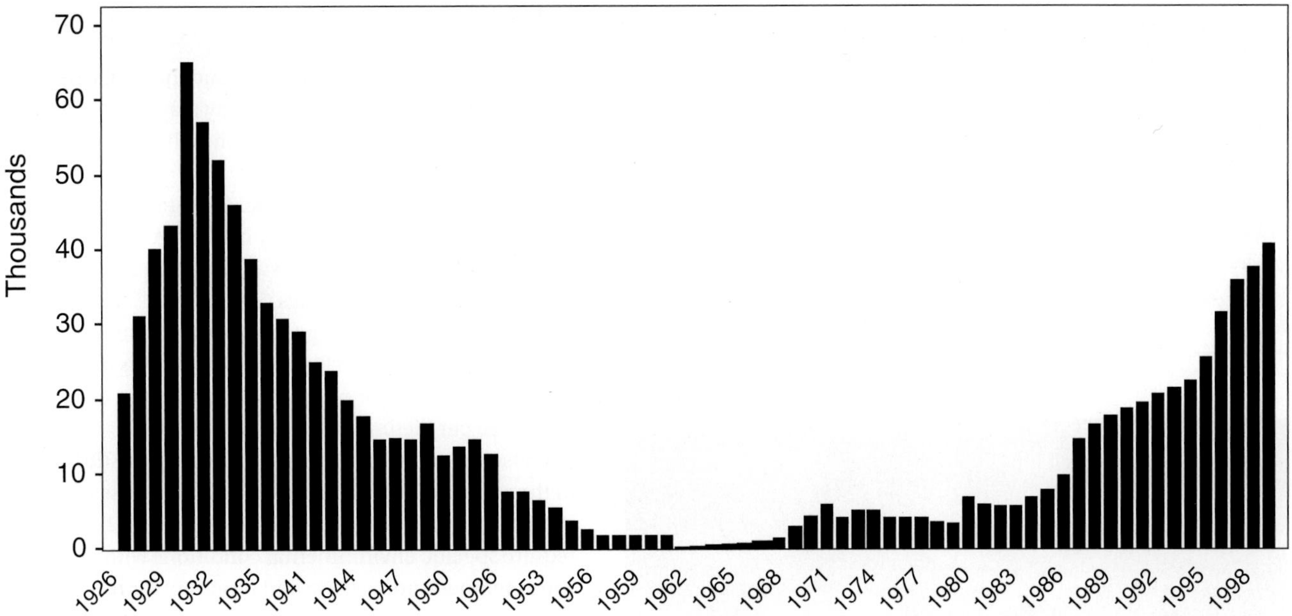

Fig. 33.2. Newly registered cases of sleeping sickness, annually reported to WHO.

So far, activities against sleeping sickness are just getting together on an international level. Under the umbrella of WHO, the 'Programme for Surveillance and Control of African Trypanosomiasis' is set up to co-ordinate field activities, implement international networks, provide training material and foster inter-agency collaboration (Dumas et al., 1999).

The organism

Trypanosoma brucei (phylum Sacromastigophora, order Kinetoplastida) is an extracellular protozoan parasite. Like Leishmania, it possesses a centrally placed nucleus and a kinetoplast, a distinct organelle with extranuclear DNA. The kinetoplast is the insertion site of an undulating membrane, which extends over nearly the whole cell length and continues as a free flagellum (Fig. 33.3).

The three sub-species of *Trypanosoma brucei* are indistinguishable by morphological methods. They differ, however, considerably in the interaction with their mammalian host and the epidemiological pattern of the diseases they cause. Formerly, *T.b. gambiense* and *T.b. rhodesiense* isolates were characterized either by isoenzyme analysis or animal inoculation. Today molecular tools are used for their differentiation (Table 33.1).

Genomic analyses of various isolates taken from the field revealed an extreme and more than expected complexity among the members of the *T. brucei* group:

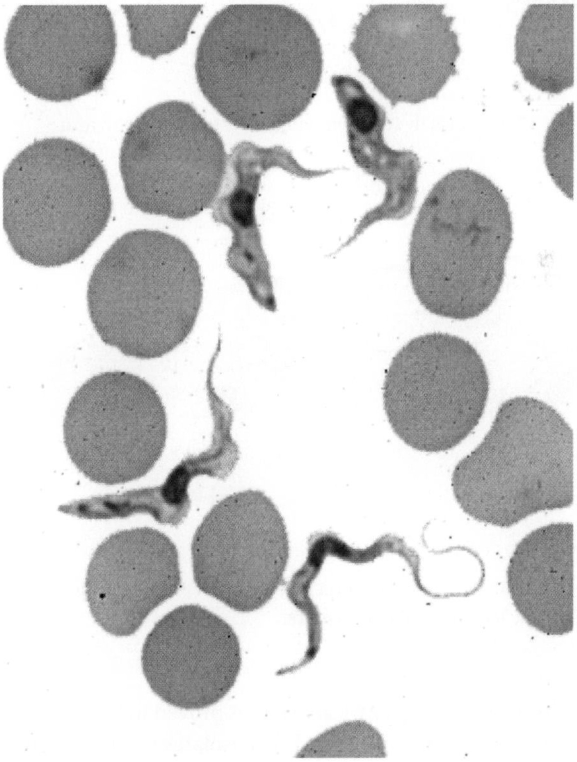

Fig. 33.3. *Trypanosoma brucei* in human blood; thin film, Giemsa stain, oil immersion field ×1000 magnification.

Table 33.1. The three species of African trypanosomiasis

Subspecies	Disease	Major characteristics
Trypanosoma brucei gambiense	West African sleeping sickness	Insidious onset, chronic course, death after months or years
Trypanosoma brucei rhodesiense	East African sleeping sickness	Rapid onset, acute illness, death often within weeks
Trypanosoma brucei brucei	Nagana disease in cattle	Considered apathogenic to humans

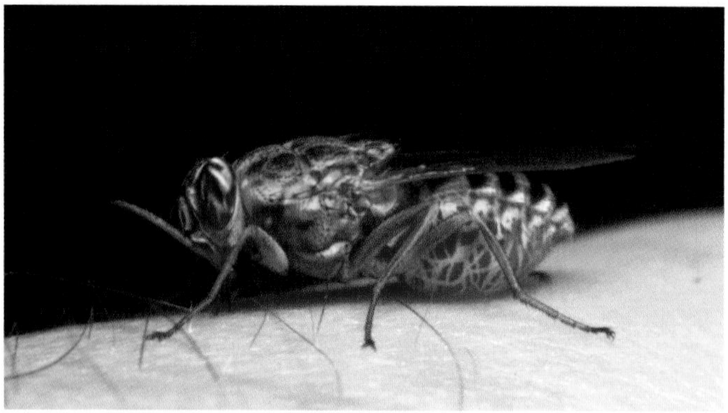

Fig. 33.4. Tsetse fly (*Glossina morsitans*) feeding on an arm.

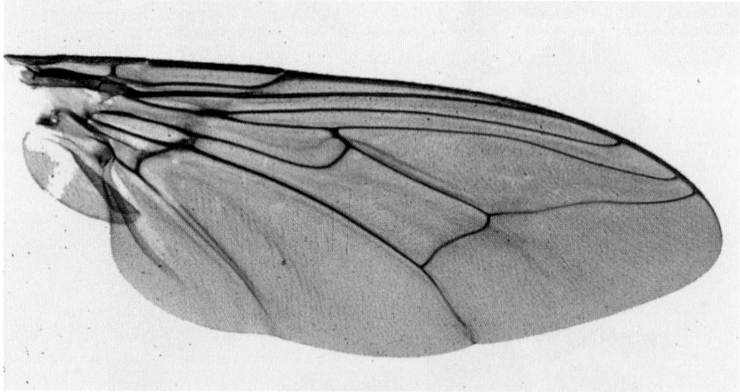

Fig. 33.5. Pattern of venation in the wing of a tsetse fly; note the typical 'hatchet cell' in the centre.

whereas most West African isolates proved to be relatively homogeneous, East African isolates from humans and animals did not follow a regular pattern. There seems to be a complex and very close relationship of what is still called *T.b. rhodesiense* and *T.b. brucei*. There is even evidence of some sexual genetic exchange in the vector.

The vector

Although congenital, blood-borne and mechanical transmission have been reported and may play an occasional role, the main mode of transmission is through the bite of infected tsetse flies (Fig. 33.4).

Tsetse flies (*Glossina* spp., order Diptera) are biologically unique insects, which only occur in Africa. They are easily recognizable by their resting position and by the pattern of veins in their wings (Fig. 33.5).

Tsetse flies are strong, aggressive insects. Both sexes feed on blood. They can live for many months in the wild, but have only a very limited offspring of about eight to ten larvae per lifetime.

Tsetse flies occur in 31 distinct species and sub-species in three groups, of which less than half are possible vectors of human sleeping sickness (Table 33.2). As they require specific environmental conditions with constant warm temperatures, shade and humidity for resting and larviposition, their distribution in Africa is very focal. The distinct biological behaviour, and the ecological preconditions they pose on their preferred habitat, explain many epidemiological features of sleeping sickness. Recently, the mapping and monitoring of possible foci has become possible with the use of satellite imaging techniques.

The life cycle

During the blood meal on an infected mammalian host, the tsetse fly takes up trypanosomes (short-stumpy form) into its mid-gut, where they develop into procyclic forms and multiply. After about 2 weeks, they migrate towards the salivary glands as epimastigotes, where they finally develop into infective metacyclic forms. With the next blood meal, they are then injected into the new vertebrate host as long, slender trypomastigotes. This 'metamorphosis' of the parasite is accompanied by distinct metabolic changes leading to the expression of different protein coats on the cell surface.

Prevention and control of sleeping sickness

Individual protection

Sleeping sickness among tourists and occasional visitors to endemic areas is rare, although occasional clusters of infection might occur. The use of anti-trypanosomal drugs like pentamidine as chemoprophylaxis is historical, and can no longer be recommended: instead, long-sleeved, bright clothing and insecticide repellents are a useful defence against attacking tsetse flies.

Sleeping sickness control

In the past, tremendous efforts have been undertaken to control sleeping sickness as a threat to human lives, live-stock and rural development. Control programmes are based on the five complementary pillars given in Table 33.3.

The most important strategy in the control of sleeping sickness is active case-finding. This requires mobile teams which visit villages in endemic areas regularly. Mostly depending on the results of a brief clinical evaluation and CATT screening (see below), patients – preferably in the early stage of the disease – are identified, treated and thus removed as reservoir for the infection. Prevalence in highly affected communities can be as high as 20 per cent, rarely even 50 per cent. The percentage of patients in late stage trypanosomiasis which are detected during active case-finding is a useful indicator for the success of a control programme (Fig. 33.6).

Glossina is a relatively incompetent vector of trypanosomiasis. Even in the endemic foci, usually less than 1 per

Table 33.2. Tsetse flies

	Palpalis group (subgenus Nemorhina)	Morsitans group (subgenus Glossina)	Fusca group (subgenus Austenia)
Importance	Vectors for *T.b. gambiense*	Vectors for *T.b. rhodesiense* and *T.b. brucei*	Vectors for animal trypanosomiasis
Ecology	Riverine habitat in West and Central Africa: forested lake shores, river banks	Woodland savannah, forest edges in East and Southern Africa	Forest savannah and edges of tropical moist forest in Central Africa
Principal vector species for human disease	*G. palpalis* *G. tachinoides* *G. fuscipes*	*G. morsitans* *G. pallidipes* *G. swynnertoni*	–

Table 33.3. Elements of a sleeping sickness control programme

1. Diagnosis and treatment of patients
2. Active case-finding
3. Vector control
4. Implementation and continuation of a surveillance system
5. Health education and community participation

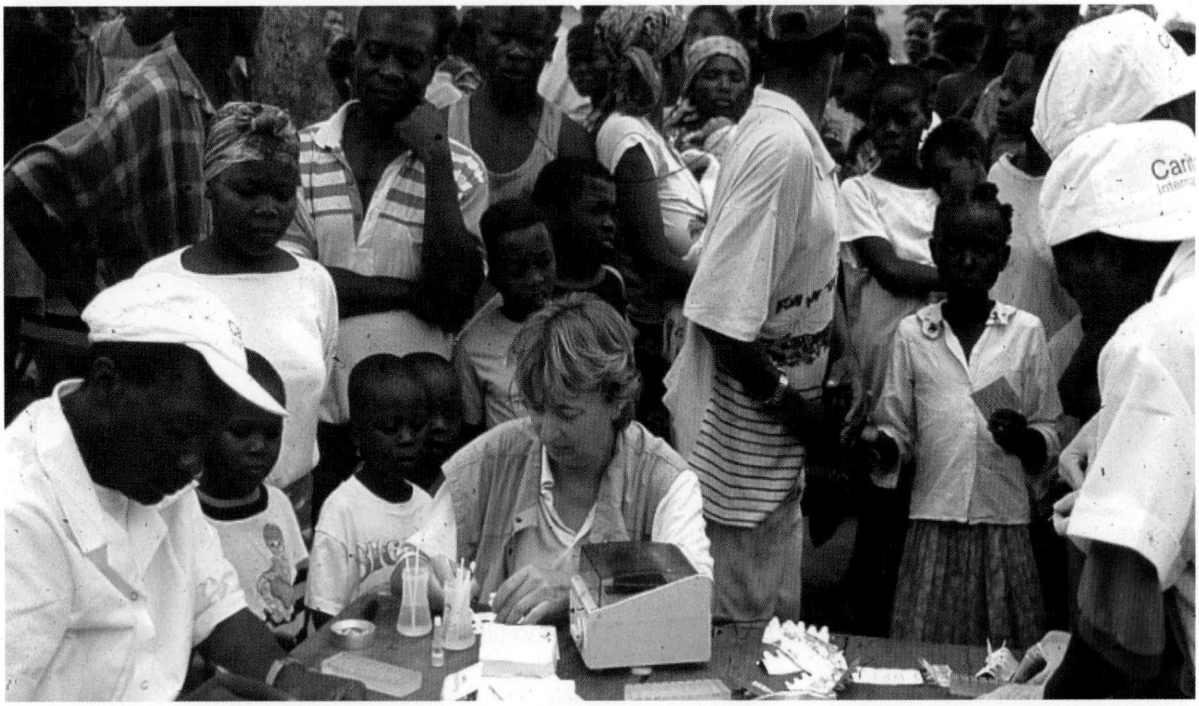

Fig. 33.6. Active case-finding in a village in Northern Angola: the whole village population is examined for clinical signs of trypanosomiasis and screened serologically using the CATT. Villagers with a positive result have to undergo further parasitological investigations.

cent of the flies are infective. The slow generation cycle makes tsetse flies susceptible to various control measures including insecticides. Insecticidal resistance has not yet occurred in the wild.

Tsetse flies are visually attracted to their host. Special traps have been designed, which can be placed at the sites of man–fly contact. They are highly effective especially when impregnated with an insecticide (Fig. 33.7).

The combination of various approaches in trypanosomiasis control can result in a complete break of the transmission cycle. The conditions for a success, however, are the existence of a professional programme, experienced and dedicated personnel, sustainable funding and the political will of the decision makers.

Clinical features

Sleeping sickness is a dreadful disease, causing great suffering to the individual, the family and the affected community. Often, the infection has an insidious onset, but *Trypanosoma brucei*, regardless of its East or West African sub-species, will invariably kill, if the patient is not treated in time. The natural course of sleeping sickness can be divided into different and distinct stages. Their recognition and differentiation is important for the subsequent management of the patient.

The trypanosomal chancre

Tsetse bites can be quite painful, and usually leave a small, self-healing mark. In the case of a trypanosomal infection, the local reaction can be quite pronounced and longer lasting. A small raised papule develops after about 5 days, which increases rapidly in size. It is surrounded by a heavy erythematous tissue reaction with local oedema and regional lymphadenopathy. This chancre heals without treatment after 2 to 4 weeks, leaving a permanent hyperpigmented spot.

In *T.b. rhodesiense* infection, trypanosomal chancres occur in about half of the cases. In *T.b. gambiense*, they are much rarer. Chancres are more inconspicuous on pigmented skin and often remain undetected in populations of endemic areas (Fig. 33.8).

Haemolymphatic stage (HAT Stage I)

After local multiplication at the site of inoculation, the trypanosomes invade the haemolymphatic system, where they can be detected 7 to 10 days after the bite of the infective fly. During this period of systemic spread, trypanosomes are exposed to vigorous defence mechanisms of the host, which they evade by constant antigenic variation. This continuous battle between antigenic switches and humoral defence results in an undulating parasitaemia with parasite numbers frequently decreasing below detection level, especially in Gambiense sleeping sickness. The cyclic release of cytokines during periods of increased cell lysis results in intermittent, non-specific symptoms: fever, chills, rigor, headache and joint pains. Hepatosplenomegaly and generalized lymphadenopathy are common, indicating activation and hyperplasia of the reticulo-endothelial system. All these signs can be easily misdiagnosed as malaria, viral infection or many other conditions and broaden the range of possible differential diagnoses.

A reliable sign, particularly in *T.b. gambiense* infection, is enlargement of lymph nodes in the posterior triangle of the neck ('Winterbottom's sign'). Other typical signs are a fugitive patchy rash, usually only seen on a pale skin, a myxoedematous infiltration of connective tissue ('puffy face syndrome') and an inconspicuous periostitis of the tibia with delayed hyperaesthesia ('Kérandel's sign').

In *T.b. rhodesiense*, this haemolymphatic stage is usually very pronounced with severe, acute symptoms and heavy bouts of recurrent fever, frequently resulting in early death through cardiac involvement (myocarditis). In *T.b. gambiense* infection, the early stage usually has few symptoms. Febrile episodes become less severe as the disease progresses.

Meningoencephalitic stage (HAT Stage II)

Within weeks in *T.b. rhodesiense*, and months in *T.b. gambiense*, cerebral involvement will invariably follow. Trypanosomes cross the blood–brain barrier and start to destroy central nervous tissue. In children sleeping sickness progresses even more rapidly towards this meningoencephalitic stage.

The onset of stage II is insidious. The exact timing of CNS involvement cannot be determined clinically. As the disease progresses, patients complain of increasing headache, and their families may detect a marked change in behaviour and personality. Neurological

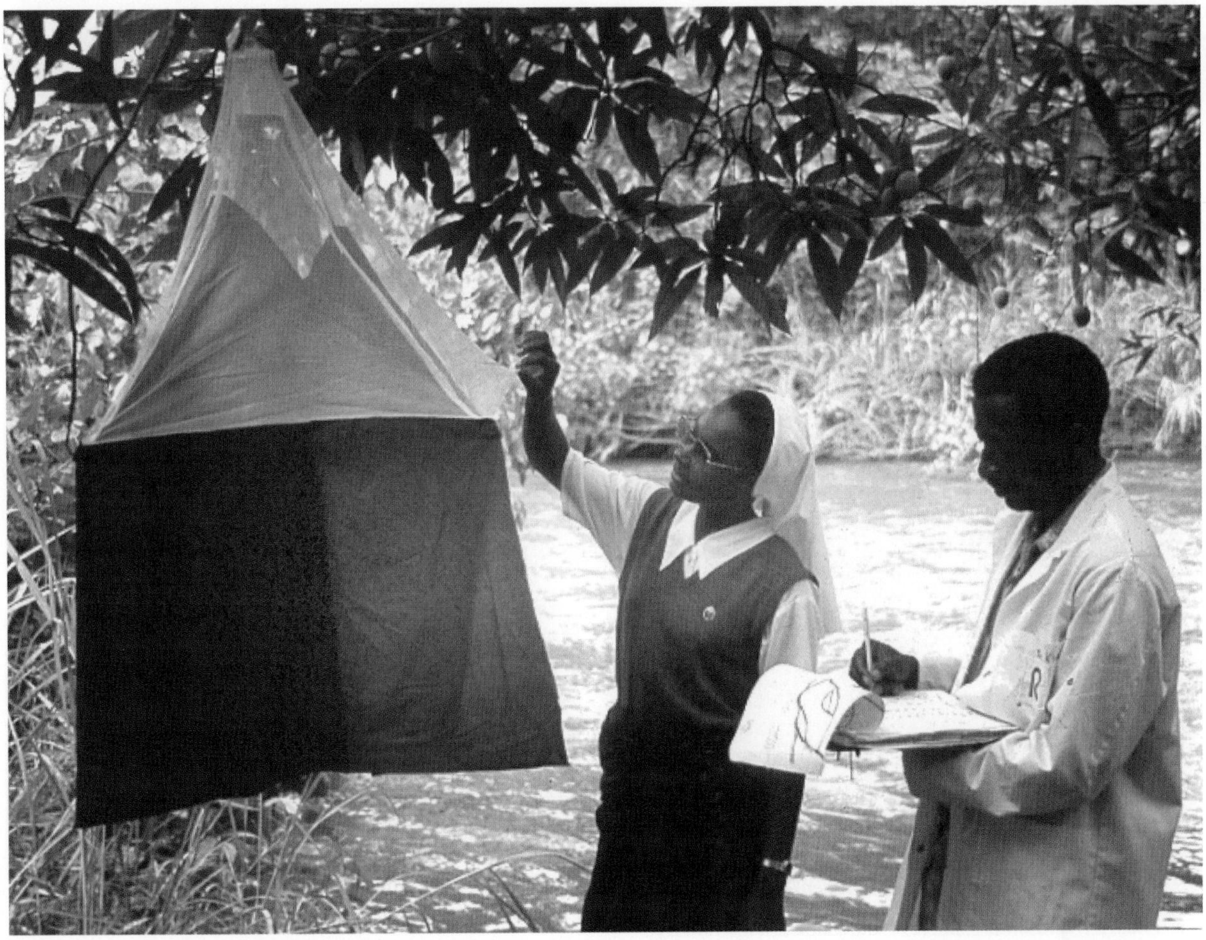

Fig. 33.7. Tsetse trap (Lancien type), placed under a tree along a small river in Northern Angola. Tsetse flies are attracted by the blue cloth and rest on black parts of the trap. They eventually get caught in the mosquito net at the top where they can then be collected in a small container for further counting.

symptoms, which follow gradually, can be focal or generalized, depending on the site of cellular damage in the central nervous system. Convulsions are common, usually indicating a poor prognosis. Periods of confusion and agitation slowly evolve towards a stage of distinct apathy when individuals lose interest in their surroundings and their own situation. Sleep abnormalities result finally in a somnolent and comatose state. Progressive wasting and dehydration follows the inability to eat and drink.

Histologically, perivascular infiltration of inflammatory cells ('cuffing') and glial proliferation can be detected. The picture suggests endarteritis which might be immune-mediated. Pathognomonic for the cerebral involvement of trypanosomiasis is the appearance of the morular cells of Mott in brain tissue and CSF. These are activated plasma cells with characteristic eosinophilic inclusions (Fig. 33.9).

There is no unique clinical sign of late stage sleeping sickness; instead a wide range of possible neurological and psychiatric differential diagnoses opens up. However, the appearance of a patient with apathy and the typical expressionless face must alert health workers in endemic areas immediately and prompt them to investigate for trypanosomes without delay (Fig. 33.10).

Diagnosis

Sleeping sickness cannot be diagnosed with certainty on clinical grounds alone. There is no valid clinical case definition. Trypanosomiasis has to be considered in all

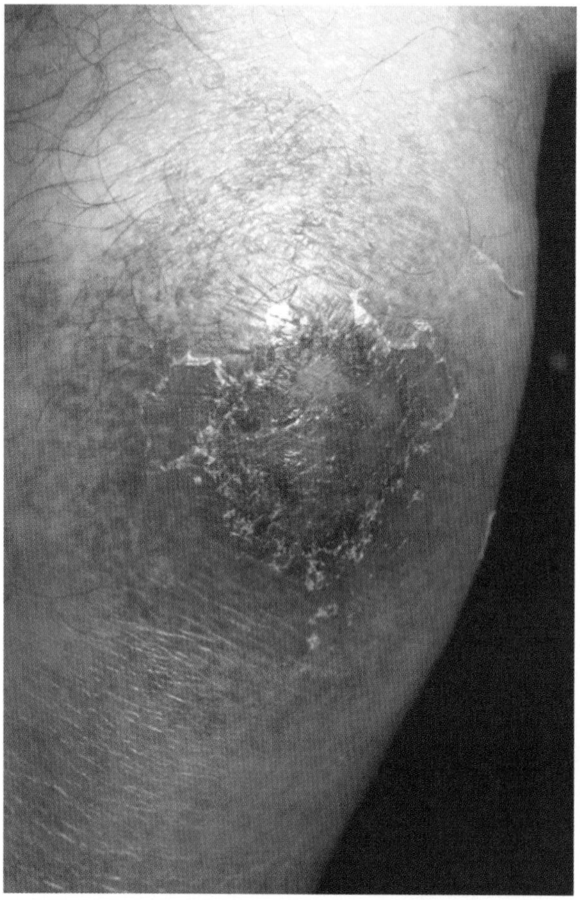

Fig. 33.8. Trypanosomal chancre on the shank of a missionary returning with high fever from the Congo.

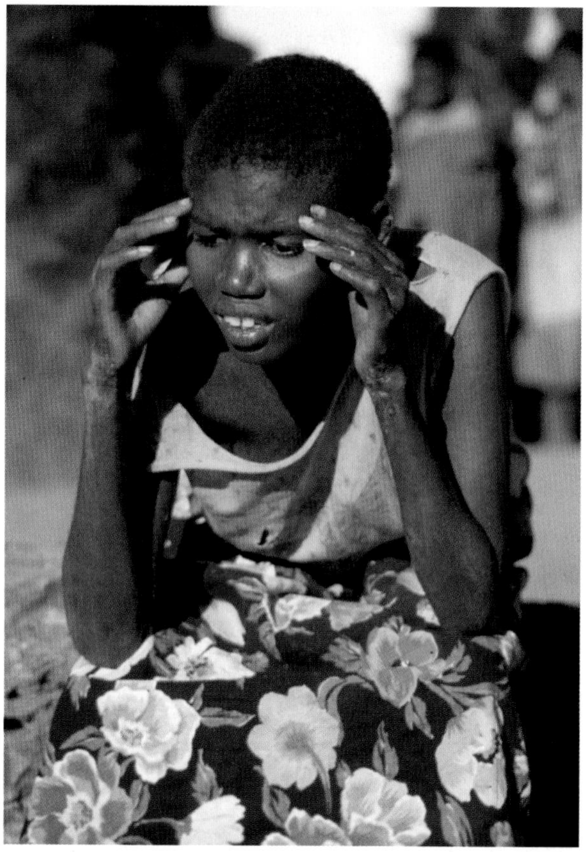

Fig. 33.10. Patient with severe headache, mental confusion and progressive wasting in late stage trypanosomiasis.

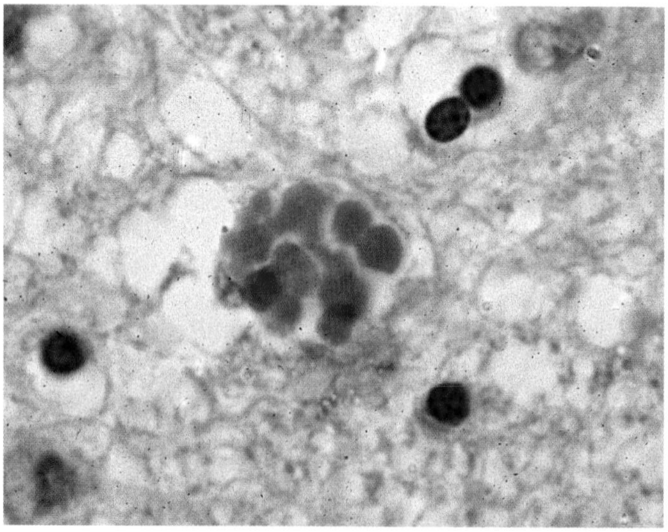

Fig. 33.9. Morula cell of Mott in a histological section, H&E stain, ×1000 magnification.

patients with fever and neurological signs in endemic areas.

Various laboratory abnormalities can occur. Anaemia and thrombocytopenia are caused by a systemic effect of cytokine release, especially TNF-α. Hypergammaglobulinaemia can reach extreme levels as a result of polyclonal activation of immunoglobulins. The IgM serum levels detected in trypanosomiasis are among the highest observed in any infectious disease. In addition, autochthonous production of IgM is commenced in the CSF.

The correct diagnosis of sleeping sickness always requires the detection of the parasite in the aspirate from a chancre, blood, lymph juice or CSF using various parasitological techniques. The methods for diagnosis are essentially the same for *T.b. gambiense* and *T.b. rhodesiense* sleeping sickness.

Table 33.4. Detection limits of various techniques in the parasitological diagnosis of sleeping sickness

Technique	Detection limit no of parasites/ml sample
In vitro isolation	100
Lymph node aspirates	50–100
Thin blood film	33
Wet blood film	25
Thick blood film	17
CTC	16
QBC	16
Inoculation in mice	3–5
Inoculation in immunosuppressed mice	<1
m-AECT	3–4
CSF with double centrifugation	1

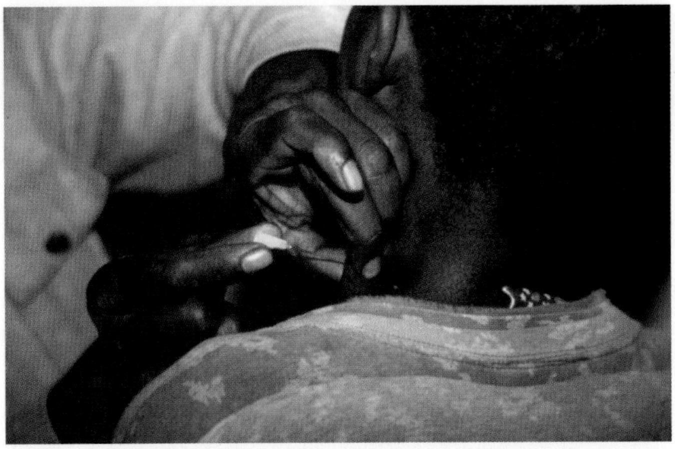

Fig. 33.11. Aspiration of lymph juice from enlarged glands in the posterior triangle of the neck (Winterbottom's sign) for immediate wet preparation.

Lymph node aspiration

The technique of lymph node aspiration is widely used, especially for the diagnosis of *T.b. gambiense* infection. Fluid of enlarged lymph nodes, preferably of the posterior triangle of the neck (Winterbottom's sign), is aspirated and examined immediately at × 400 magnification. Mobile trypanosomes can be detected between the numerous lymphocytes for about 15 minutes until they become immotile and dry out (Box) Fig. 33.11.

> **Lymph node aspiration**
> Enlarged lymph nodes are identified, preferably in the posterior triangle of the neck (Winterbottom's sign). One suitable lymph node is fixed between the fingers of the left hand. After local disinfection a canula (19 G) is directed with the right hand into the node which is then squeezed for several seconds. The canula is withdrawn and its content blown out on a clean glass slide. The drop of clear yellowish lymph juice is covered with a cover slip and immediately examined for motile trypanosomes under a microscope using the ×40 lens.

Wet preparation, thin and thick blood film

During all stages of the disease, trypanosomes appear in the blood where they can be detected in unstained wet or in stained preparations. The yield of detection is highest in the thick blood film, as used for the diagnosis of malaria. Giemsa or Field-staining techniques are appropriate.

In *T.b. gambiense* infection, parasitaemia is usually scanty and undulating, often below detection level. Repeated examinations on subsequent days are sometimes necessary until trypanosomes can finally be documented. In *T.b. rhodesiense* sleeping sickness, parasites are much more numerous in the blood and usually easily detectable (Table 33.4).

Concentration methods

To increase the sensitivity of blood examinations, various concentration assays have been developed. Trypanosomes tend to accumulate just above the buffy coat layer after centrifugation of a blood sample. The best results in the field have been obtained with the m-AECT (mini anion exchange column technique), where trypanosomes are concentrated after passage through a cellulose column, and the QBC® method (quantitative buffy coat), which was originally developed for the diagnosis of malaria.

Serological assays

Serology is a useful tool to detect antibodies against trypanosomiasis. Various test methods have been described and are now commercially available. They are mainly

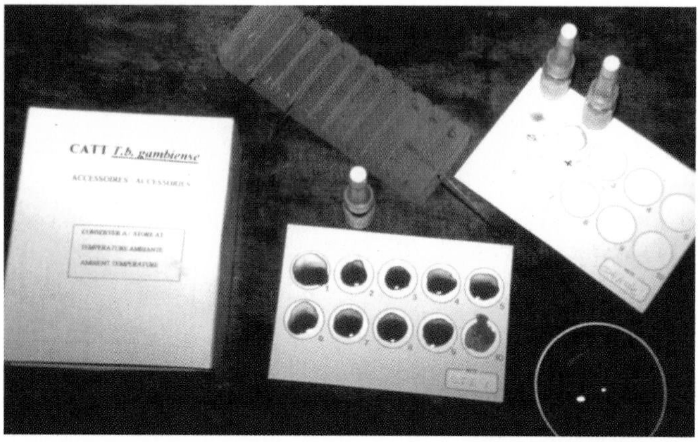

Fig. 33.12. The card agglutination test for trypanosomiasis (CATT), a serological screening tool for West African sleeping sickness.

based on the ELISA technique or immunofluorescence but provide reliable results only in *T.b. gambiense* infection. Their use for diagnosis in an endemic area has to be evaluated locally.

For rapid screening under field conditions, the CATT (card agglutination test for trypanosomiasis) is an excellent tool in areas of *T.b. gambiense* infection. It is easy to perform and delivers results within 5 minutes. A visible agglutination in the CATT suggests the existence of antibodies, but does not necessarily mean florid disease (Fig. 33.12 and Box).

> The CATT can be obtained from:
>
> Department of Parasitology
> Prince Leopold Institute of Tropical Medicine
> Nationalestraat 155
> B-2000 Antwerp, Belgium
> www.itg.be

Diagnosis of Stage II

Stage determination is crucial for the correct management of a patient. This cannot be done following exclusively clinical criteria. Therefore, a lumbar puncture for the examination of about 5 ml of CSF has to be performed in every patient found positive for trypanosomes in blood or lymph aspirate. A lumbar puncture has to be done also in patients with the clinical suspicion of sleeping sickness even if peripheral examinations have been negative (Box).

> Examinations of CSF for determination of late-stage sleeping sickness:
> - Leukocytes
>   pleocytosis, mostly lymphocytes: >5 cells per mm^3
> - Morular cells of Mott
>   activated plasma cells with numerous vacuoles; rare but pathognomonic for cerebral involvement of trypanosomiasis
> - Trypanosomes
>   highest yield with double centrifugation
> - Protein
>   40 mg of protein per 100 ml CSF (dye-binding protein assay) as result of autochthonous production of IgM antibodies in the CSF

Treatment

General considerations

Sleeping sickness can be cured, especially if the diagnosis is made in an early stage of the disease, and if the treatment is administered correctly. In the grim reality of the African situation, however, successful management of patients is facing many constraints.

(a) Sleeping sickness is a disease of rural places, which are often remote and insecure. Patients in the endemic areas have only little access to health care.
(b) The diagnosis and exact staging of trypanosomiasis requires sophisticated methods, which are dangerous in the hands of the unskilled. They are only justified when performed by experienced personnel, who need constant supervision, repetitive training programmes and decent salaries.
(c) The treatment of trypanosomiasis is extremely expensive, and invariably exceeds the locally available resources.
(d) The treatment of trypanosomiasis is dangerous, long-lasting and usually requires admission to hospital. Patients with late stage trypanosomiasis are often severely ill and malnourished. Their management requires considerable medical expertise and good nursing care.
(e) The essential anti-trypanosomal drugs are often unavailable or at the verge of disappearance in spite of an increasing demand. Some of them have even been taken off the market for economic reasons. The range of drugs is diminishing, and new treatments, in spite of promising drug targets, are not in sight (Keiser et al., 2001)

Table 33.5. The choice of drugs in the treatment of sleeping sickness

Gambiense sleeping sickness	*Rhodesiense* sleeping sickness
Stage I	
First-line: Pentamidine	First-line: Suramin
Second-line: Suramin; Melarsoprol	Second-line: Melarsoprol
Stage II	
First-line: Melarsoprol	First-line: Melarsoprol
Second-line: Eflornithine; Melarsoprol + Nifurtimox	Second-line: Melarsoprol + Nifurtimox?

(f) Trypanosomal treatment is not standardized, regimens vary considerably between countries and treatment centres. Only a few properly conducted and sufficiently powered clinical trials are available to evaluate duration, dosage and possible combinations of drugs. A suitable research environment around major trypanosomiasis foci is mostly non-existent.

Treatment of Stage I

The treatment of sleeping sickness varies according to the trypanosome sub-species and the stage of the disease (Table 33.5).

Suramin

In the early twentieth century, the development of suramin, resulting from German research on the trypanosomicidal activity of various dyes (Bayer 205), was a major breakthrough in the field of tropical medicine. African trypanosomiasis, at least in its early stage, became treatable.

After more than 80 years, suramin has still a firm place in the treatment of stage I sleeping sickness, especially in *T.b. rhodesiense* infection. It is injected intravenously after dilution in distilled water.

Adverse effects of suramin are dependent on the nutritional status, concomitant illnesses (especially onchocerciasis) and the general clinical condition of the patient. Although many even life-threatening events have been described, the drug is still one of the safest in trypanosomiasis treatment, and serious adverse effects are rare.

Pentamidine

Since its introduction in 1937, pentamidine became the drug of first choice for early stage *T.b. gambiense* infection where cure rates are reported to be as high as 98 per cent. A low cellular pentamidine uptake in *T.b. rhodesiense* limits its use for East Africa. As for suramin, CSF drug levels are not sufficiently high to guarantee a reliable trypanosomicidal effect in the central nervous system.

Usually, pentamidine is given as deep intramuscular injection, which can safely be given to outpatients. If hospital treatment and reasonable monitoring conditions are available, an intravenous infusion, given in normal saline over two hours, might be used instead.

Adverse effects of pentamidine are related to the route of administration and/or its dose. They are usually reversible.

Treatment of Stage II

Melarsoprol

Up to the first half of the twentieth century, late stage trypanosomiasis had to be considered untreatable. The introduction of the arsenic compound melarsoprol in 1949 became the important turning point. Since then, melarsoprol is the most widely used stage II anti-trypanosomal drug for both *T.b. gambiense* and *T.b. rhodesiense* infection. It has saved many lives, but its reputation is still blurred by the high rate of dangerous adverse effects. In addition, increasing rates of relapses and refractoriness have been reported in some foci of Uganda, Congo and Angola. In spite of these disadvantages and in the absence of an available and affordable alternative, melarsoprol remains the most powerful drug in the fight against sleeping sickness.

Melarsoprol rapidly clears trypanosomes in blood, lymph and CSF. Its toxicity, however, confines its application to the late stages of the disease. Melarsoprol is given as slow intravenous injection; a paravasal deposition of the drug has to be strictly avoided.

Be very careful with i.v. injection
Never inject melarsoprol into the tissues

A wide range of different therapeutic regimens have been used, most of them not supported by prospective clinical trials. Recently acquired knowledge in the pharmacodynamics and effects of the drug have led to a new, less complicated dose regimen, which in the future might make the treatment of stage II trypanosomiasis easier and cheaper (Burriet et al., 2000).

Adverse effects of melarsoprol may be severe and life threatening. The most important is an acute encephalopathy provoked in the first half of the treatment course in 5 to 14 per cent of all treated patients. This complication will be lethal in about half of the cases, depending on their general condition as well as the quality of medical and nursing care. The onset of the reaction is characterized by severe headache, convulsions, the rapid deterioration of neurological symptoms or a deepening of the coma. Characteristically, the eyes of the comatose patient remain open.

The exact cause of this 'treatment-induced' encephalopathy is not known. Most likely, it is an immune-mediated reaction precipitated by the release of parasitic antigen in the first days of treatment. The simultaneous administration of corticosteroids (prednisolone 1 mg/kg body weight, maximum of 40 mg daily) has been shown to reduce this treatment-related mortality, especially in cases with high cell counts in the CSF (Pepin et al., 1989). However, steroids administered in an environment where tuberculosis, amoebiasis or strongyloidiasis are highly prevalent, have dangers of their own!

Melarsoprol has to be considered teratotoxic but the prospect of leaving a trypanosomal infection untreated is too dangerous to withhold the drug from pregnant women.

Eflornithine (DFMO)

Eflornithine was developed as an anti-tumour agent, but with little success. When introduced as an anti-trypanosomal drug, however, it was initially the centre of hope ('resurrection drug') and was believed to be able to replace melarsoprol as first-line treatment in stage II trypanosomiasis. However, *T.b. rhodesiense* isolates show a varying, usually much lower degree of sensitivity. Finally, exorbitant costs (US$ 800 per patient treatment) and limited availability restricted its use only to melarsoprol-refractory cases of *gambiense* sleeping sickness.

The drug can be taken orally, but intravenous administration leads to a much higher bioavailability and success rate. Eflornithine is administered slowly over a period of at least 30 minutes. A continuous 24-hour application is preferable if there are adequate facilities for such treatment.

The range of adverse reactions is considerable and resembles other cytotoxic drugs in cancer treatment. Their occurrence and intensity increase with the duration of application and the severity of the general condition of the patient. Generally, all adverse effects of eflornithine are reversible.

Since 1999, pharmaceutical production of intravenous eflornithine ceased as a result of market considerations in spite of the increasing demand in Africa. Patients with sleeping sickness are no sales target. However, the discovery of the therapeutic effect of eflornithine against facial hair in ladies' cosmetic creams might help to re-stimulate production and thus even have a beneficial 'spin-off effect' on trypanosomiasis. A promising agreement between the pharmaceutical industry and WHO was signed in May 2001.

Nifurtimox

Ten years after its introduction for use against American trypanosomiasis in 1967, nifurtimox was discovered as an effective agent in the treatment of *Gambiense* sleeping sickness. It has a place as second-line treatment in melarsoprol refractory cases or as an element in a combination chemotherapy. So far, experiences with nifurtimox are limited to its use on compassionate grounds for only a few cases. Prospective clinical trials do not exist and are urgently needed.

Nifurtimox is generally not well tolerated, but adverse effects are usually not severe. They are dose-related and rapidly reversible after discontinuation of the drug (Table 33.6).

Combination treatments

Melarsoprol, eflornithine and nifurtimox all interfere at different levels with trypanothione synthesis and activity. There is also experimental evidence that combinations of suramin and stage II drugs might be beneficial. Therefore, by reducing the overall dosage of each individual component, drug combinations could perhaps contribute to reduce the inherent problems of serious side effects, treatment refractoriness and limited drug availability, which are so commonly attributed to pharmaceuticals in the treatment of sleeping sickness.

So far, experiences on the use of drug combinations in trypanosomiasis are mostly confined to single case reports. Properly conducted clinical trials are overdue.

Follow-up of sleeping sickness patients

Patients with sleeping sickness are often severely ill due to malnutrition and concomitant infections. Good medical and nursing care will be decisive for the final outcome.

Depending on the extent of cellular damage, some

Table 33.6. Drugs in the treatment of human African trypanosomiasis

	Dosage regimen	Adverse drug reactions
(a) Stage I drugs		
Pentamidine	4 mg/kg body weight i.m. daily or on alternate days for 7 to 10 injections	• hypotensive reaction with tachycardia, dizziness, even collapse and shock, especially after intravenous application; • inflammatory reactions at the site of injection (sterile abscesses, necroses); • renal, hepatic and pancreatic dysfunction; • neurotoxicity: peripheral polyneuropathy • bone marrow depression.
Suramin	Day 1: Test dose of 4–5 mg/kg body weight Day 3, 10, 17, 24 and 31: 20 mg/kg body weight, maximum dose per injection 1 g	• pyrexia • early hypersensitivity reactions like nausea, circulatory collapse, urticaria; • late hypersensitivity reactions: skin reactions (exfoliative dermatitis), haemolytic anaemia; • renal impairment: albuminuria, cylinduria, haematuria (high tissue concentrations in the kidneys); regular urine checks! • neurotoxicity: peripheral neuropathy; • bone marrow toxicity: agranulocytosis, thrombocytopenia.
(b) Stage II Drugs		
Melarsoprol	Traditionally several dosage regimen were used; example: Day 1: 1.2 mg/kg body weight i.v. Day 2: 2.4 mg/kg body weight i.v. Day 3 + 4: 3.6 mg/kg body weight i.v. repeat course 2–3 times with a 7–10 days interval New regimen: D 1–10: 2.2 mg/kg body weight i.v.	• treatment-induced encephalopathy • pyrexia • neurotoxicity: peripheral motoric or sensorial polyneuropathy • dermatological reactions: pruritus, exfoliative dermatitis • cardiotoxicity • renal and hepatic dysfunction.
Eflornithine	100 mg/kg body weight i.v. every 6 hours for 14 days	• gastrointestinal symptoms like nausea, vomiting and diarrhoea; • bone marrow toxicity: anaemia, leukopenia, thrombocytopenia; • alopecia, usually towards the end of the treatment cycle; • neurological symptoms, convulsions
Nifurtimox	5 mg/kg body weight orally three times daily for 30 days	• abdominal discomfort, nausea, pains and vomiting; • neurological complications: convulsions, impairment of the cerebellar function, polyneuropathy; • skin reactions

neurological symptoms will only be partially reversible. Sequelae have to be distinguished from persisting infections as a result of resistant or incompletely treated trypanosomes. Even re-infections have to be considered in endemic areas as there is no reliable and lasting immunity after infection.

For reasons of individual care and epidemiological surveillance, patients have to be re-examined regularly. In patients with late stage trypanosomiasis, repeated lumbar punctures are necessary in order to assess the efficacy of treatment, preferably 1, 3 and 6 months after the end of treatment.

Trypanosomiasis – the unsolved problem?

There is hardly any other tropical disease, which demonstrates more clearly the dichotomy of our modern age: On one side, trypanosomes are kept in culture and worked on extensively in numerous research laboratories. They are one of the best studied organisms. Their genome is currently sequenced, and many molecular, biochemical and immunological phenomena were discovered for the first time in the trypanosome system as a result of expensive basic research. Novel drug targets have been identified.

On the other hand, diagnostic and especially therapeutic tools are increasingly made unavailable, as the hundreds of thousands of infected people in Africa are non-existent in market terms. Clinical and epidemiological research is grossly under-represented.

The prospect for a future success in the fight against trypanosomiasis looks grim. African countries are increasingly unable to implement effective control programmes, be it due to political instability or financial incapacity. Whether there will be more concern about the reality of sleeping sickness in Africa has to be seen as a question of scientific ethics and international solidarity.

References

Bailey JW, Smith DH. (1992). The use of the acridine orange QBC technique in the diagnosis of African trypanosomiasis. *Trans Roy Soc Trop Med Hyg*; **86**: 630.

Burri C, Nkunku S, Merolle A, Smith T, Blum J, Brun R. (2000). Efficacy of new, concise schedule for melarsoprol in treatment of sleeping sickness caused by *Trypanosoma brucei gambiense*: a randomised trial. *Lancet*; **355**: 1419–1425.

Dumas M, Bouteille B, Buguet A, eds. (1999). *Progress in human African trypanosomiasis, Sleeping Sickness*. France: Springer-Verlag.

Dumas M, Bouteill B. (2000). Treatment of human African trypanosomiasis. *Bull Wld Hlth Org*; **78**: 1474.

Keiser J, Stich A, Burri C. (2001). New drugs for the treatment of human African trypanosomiasis: research and development. *Parasitol Today*; **17**: 42–49.

Laveissière C, Vale GA, Gouteux J-P. (1990). Bait methods for tsetse control. In *Appropriate Technology in Vector Control*, ed. CF Curtis. CRC Press, Inc.

Mulligan HW, ed. (1970). *The African Trypanosomiases*. London: George Allen and Unwin Ltd.

Pepin J, Milord F, Guern C et al. (1989). Trial of prednisolone for prevention of melarsoprol-induced encephalopathy in gambiense sleeping sickness. *Lancet*; **i**: 1246–1250.

Smith DH, Pepin J, Stich A. (1998). Human African trypanosomiasis: an emerging public health crisis. *Br Med Bull*; **54**: 341–355.

World Health Organization. (1998). Control and surveillance of African trypanosomiasis. *WHO Technical Report Series 881*. Geneva: WHO.

Amoebiasis

34

The problem in Africa

Amoebiasis is caused by the protozoan parasite *Entamoeba histolytica* and has a world-wide distribution. It is estimated that 40–50 million cases of amoebic colitis and liver abscess occur annually with 40 000–110 000 deaths (WHO/PAHO/UNESCO report, 1997). The infection occurs all over Africa. Transmission is through the faecal–oral route and therefore the infection can flourish when hygiene is poor. Outbreaks of amoebiasis are frequent during disasters or crises when people are crowded together in refugee camps, after floods and during famine or war.

The organism and its life cycle

Entamoeba histolytica can take two forms: cysts and trophozoites. The cystic form is responsible for transmission from one person to another, but does not have the potential to become invasive and cause disease. Finding cysts in a stool sample therefore only signifies amoebic infection and does not necessarily indicate amoebic disease. The cysts are shed with the faeces and remain viable for 100 hours at 25 °C under moist conditions (Warhurst, 1999) but much longer in water of lower temperature. Infection of the next person occurs by intake of food or water that is contaminated, often by flies. The cysts can survive gastric acidity so that amoebae can cause infection with a low infective dose (<100 organisms) (Warhurst, 1999). Once in the large intestine, the quadrinucleate cysts may release eight trophozoites that are the potentially invasive form which can cause disease. The trophozoites may invade the colonic mucosa causing amoebic colitis or amoeboma; further spread within the portal blood may lead to amoebic liver abscess or abscesses at other sites.

Pathogenic strains vs. non-pathogenic strains of *E. histolytica*

Some strains of *E. histolytica* are pathogenic while others are not. It has now been accepted that there are, in fact, two species: *Entamoeba dispar* which is non-pathogenic and *E. histolytica* which is capable of causing disease. Unfortunately, these two species cannot be distinguished from each other by routine light microscopy, but only by tests normally done in well-equipped laboratories (culture and PCR, antigen detection tests). When haematophageous trophozoites (those that have ingested red blood cells) are seen, the presence of invasive *E. histolytica* strains is proved.

In temperate climates, 90 per cent of all individuals in whom amoebic cysts are demonstrated in stool samples have *E. dispar* and 10 per cent have *E. histolytica*, but only 10 per cent of these (1% of the total) have *E. histolytica* strains that are pathogenic. The prevalence of *E. histolytica* in Africa may be higher (30% or more).

Pathology

Amoebae typically cause flask-shaped ulcers as they undermine the mucosa and penetrate the sub-mucosa. Parts of the mucosa between ulcers remain unaffected but ulcers may coalesce: in severe cases this leads to denuding of the mucosa over large areas. As blood vessels become involved, they may thrombose or bleed which, in severe cases, may lead to necrosis of the bowel wall (toxic megacolon). Amoebae may enter the portal circulation and spread to the liver. Hepatomegaly in patients with amoebiasis is probably the result of accumulation in the portal tracts of leukocytes originating from the gut. It is only when haematophagous trophozoites are seen in a fresh stool sample that the patient's current illness is

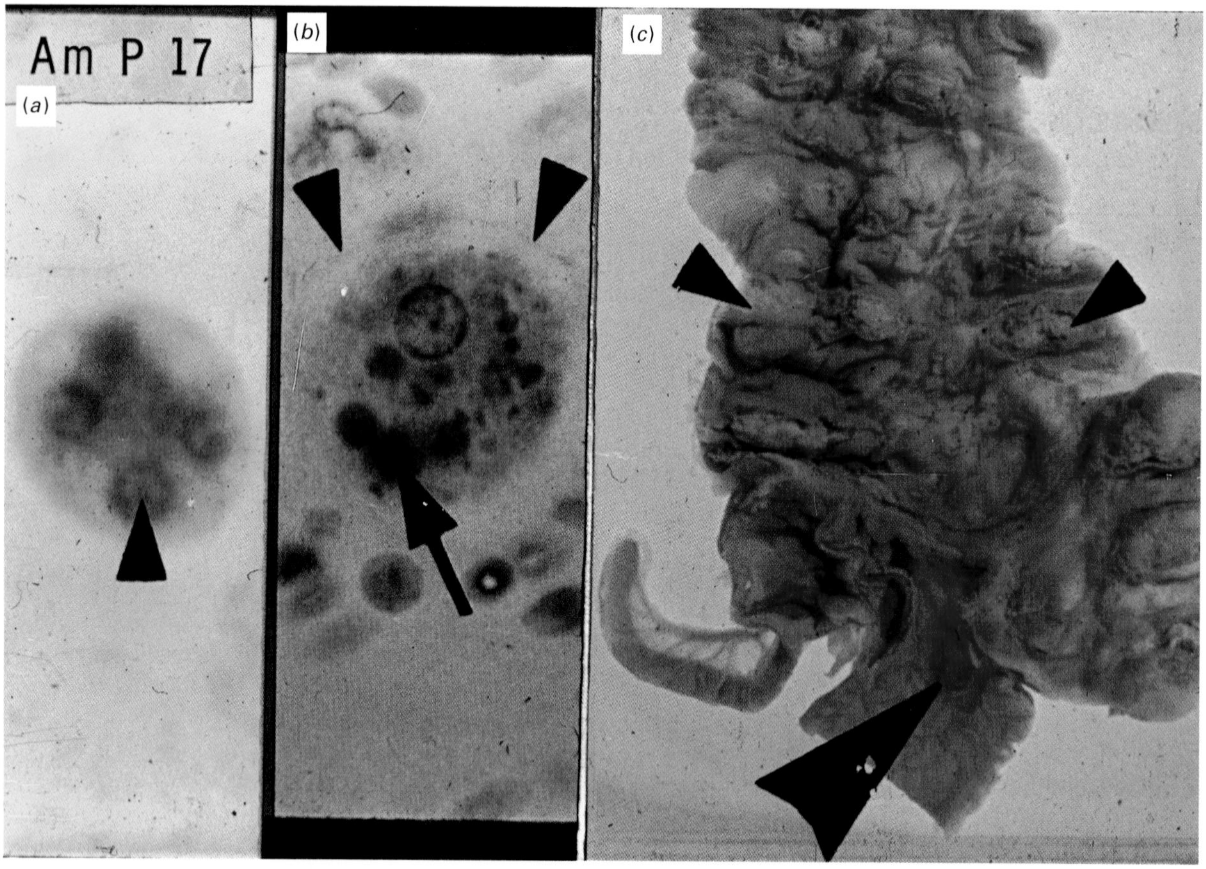

Fig. 34.1. (*a*) Left. The image shows the typical quadrinucleate cysts of *E. histiolytica*. (*b*) Middle: haematophagous trophozoites. The long arrow indicates ingested erythrocytes. Finding these trophozoites is proof of underlying amoebic disease in this patient. (*c*) A pathological specimen of the caecum showing areas of redness and ulcers with sharp edges indicating the undermined base (flask shaped ulcer). (Reproduced by courtesy of TALC, London.)

proved to be caused by *E. histolytica*. If stool samples are not examined immediately, they may give a false negative result. If the quadrinucleate cysts only are found in a stool sample, the diagnosis is amoebic infection, not amoebic disease (Fig 34.1*a*, *b*).

Amoebiasis and immune suppression

Immune suppression associated with pregnancy or induced by treatment with steroids places any patient infected with amoebae at risk of fulminant colitis which may perforate, requiring immediate surgery.

- ALWAYS screen, and if necessary treat, any patient for amoebic infection before starting treatment with steroids for whatever indication.
- In patients with HIV/AIDS there is also an increased risk of severe invasive amoebiasis.

Clinical syndromes of intestinal disease

There are four clinical syndromes of intestinal disease: asymptomatic infection, acute amoebic colitis, toxic megacolon and amoeboma.

Asymptomatic infection

This describes the state in which there is passage of amoebic cysts in the stool, without any clinical symptoms. If such a patient develops diarrhoea from another cause, the number of cysts excreted may increase, but this cannot be taken as proof of current amoebic illness.

Acute amoebic colitis (amoebic dysentery)

Clinical features

This is the classical manifestation of amoebic illness. Although all parts of the large bowel may become involved, the disease typically presents as right-sided colitis affecting the rectosigmoid and caecum (Fig. 34.1*c*).

Colitis develops gradually with loose, semi-formed stools with mucus and visible blood, and colicky abdominal pain usually in the lower abdomen. Patients remain fairly well, but the infection continues intermittently for weeks or months, until they become more ill and start to lose weight.

When the caecum or ascending colon, and rarely the terminal ileum, are involved, patients present with changed bowel habits and flatulence. On examination, the right lower abdomen may be tender. These patients may have some rectal blood loss, but dysentery with blood and mucus is usually absent.

Rarely, the appendix is also affected. This is important to recognize because, if appendicectomy alone is performed, the patient may not be cured and the gut may perforate.

Diagnosis

Clinically, the gradual onset, the absence of high fever, the presence of stools with blood and mucus, and the lack of faecal leukocytes, suggest the diagnosis and warrant the start of treatment.

The diagnosis from bacillary dysentery is shown below (Box).

Demonstrate haematophagous trophozoites in the stool

- Examine a fresh specimen after staining with iron haematoxylin or trichrome stain, or fix by polyvinyl alcohol and stain later.
- Cysts may be demonstrated best in a specimen that is centrifuged and then suspended in formalin ether and stained with iodine.
- Examine at least three separate stool samples, as daily excretion of amoebae may vary.
- Process scrapings from ulcers seen at endoscopy by making a wet mount in saline: look for motile amoebae containing RBC.
- Process the samples immediately.

- Other diagnoses include ileocaecal tuberculosis, schistosomal colitis and *Trichuris* infection and, rarely in Africa, colonic carcinoma and inflammatory bowel disease (Crohn's disease and ulcerative colitis). The distinction is important as steroids can be lethal in amoebic colitis.
- Unusual clinical presentations:
  - (i) Children are often more toxic and tend to have more prominent abdominal pain, which may sometimes mimic an acute abdomen.
  - (ii) When the caecum or ascending colon is involved, stools may be watery with only intermittent blood loss, flatulence, and pain in the right iliac fossa.

Antigen detection

These tests are easy to use and rapid and they differentiate between strains. A variety of tests are based on monoclonal antibodies, ELISA, immunofluorescence or radioimunoassay with good sensitivity.

Serology

Invasive amoebiasis elicits a humoral immune response: antibodies, detected by several tests including indirect haemagglutination and ELISA, are of little use in most endemic areas as a positive test result does not distinguish between current and past infection (Box).

Differences between amoebic and bacillary dysentery

	Amoebic	Bacillary
Fever	none or subfebrile (30%)	prominent
Onset	subacute over weeks, months	days
General condition	adults; fair initially children: ill	ill from the start
Vomiting	no	yes
Tenesmus	uncommon	mild
Dehydration	mild, if any	common
Stool appearance	blood, mucus semi-formed fishy odour	blood, mucus mainly watery odourless
Stool volume	low	high
Faecal leukocytes	rare	common
Natural history	weeks, then remission relapses	3–14 days no relapses

Fulminant colitis

Predisposing factors

Immunosuppression – HIV or the use of steroids, malnutrition, pregnancy or malignancy.

Clinical features

High fever, generalized abdominal pain, frequent bloody stools, sometimes with profuse rectal blood loss. Toxic megacolon may develop with distension of the abdomen or perforation at one or multiple sites.

Diagnosis

Demonstrate trophozoites containing RBC in the stool, leukocytosis in the peripheral blood, and plain X-rays of the abdomen suggesting perforation (paralytic ileus) or toxic megacolon. Barium enema and endoscopy are contraindicated because of risk of perforation.

Management

It is advisable to be as conservative as possible, but total colectomy may be needed in toxic megacolon.

Amoeboma

This is a swelling usually in the caecum or ascending colon caused by thickening of the colon wall with an ulcerating mucosa. It presents as a palpable mass in the right iliac fossa or with evidence of bowel obstruction, or it may be an incidental finding on a barium enema. The pathogenesis is not clear but it may be the result of an unrecognized subacute perforation. It should be differentiated from colonic carcinoma or ileocaecal tuberculosis. Diagnosis is by barium enema or endoscopy; treatment with metronidazole has good results.

Clinical features of extraintestinal disease

Amoebic liver abscess

Abscesses usually occur in the right lobe of the liver and may eventually perforate into the pleural cavity, peritoneal cavity or, if located in the left lobe of the liver, into the pericardial cavity with risk of cardiac tamponade. The clinical features therefore depend on the site and spread of the abscess.

Symptoms

(i) Fever and sweating. Fever is an important symptom (it is not in amoebic dysentery): some patients present because of a PUO.

> If you suspect a liver abscess, ask about a previous attack of bloody diarrhoea, chronic diarrhoea, or abuse of alcohol, which is a risk factor.

(ii) Pain in the right hypochondrium, which may be aggravated by inspiration or which may be referred to the right shoulder.
(iii) Cough. A dry cough may be present if the lung is involved – if there is a pleural effusion, or an empyema, or the lung parenchyma is affected. If the abscess ruptures into a bronchus (broncho-pleural fistula) the patient may cough up a red–brownish fluid.
(iv) Difficult breathing. This may be secondary to pleural effusion and chest pain, or may be due to tamponade if the abscess ruptures into the pericardium, or it may be a feature of severe anaemia.
(v) Weight loss, in chronic cases.

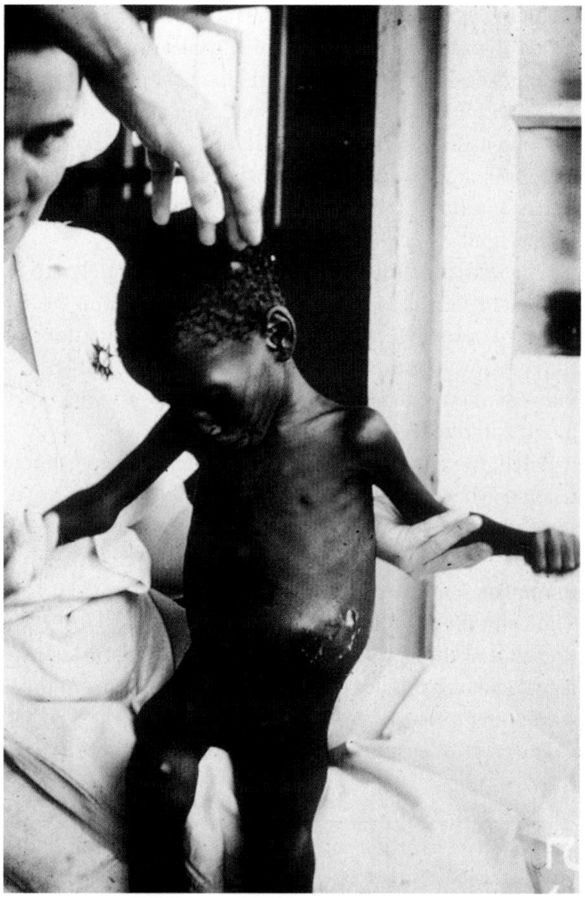

Fig. 34.2. A febrile, ill-looking Sudanese child with an enlarged, tender liver with bulging of the ribcage because of a liver abscess. No diagnostic facilities were available locally and the diagnosis was made clinically. Response to treatment with metronidazole was excellent (Copyright M. Weber).

Signs

(i) Fever.
(ii) Liver: enlarged and tender. Sometimes the tenderness is very localized, with erythema and oedema of the overlying skin. The rib cage may be bulging, with a friction rub over the abscess (Fig. 34.2).

> If the signs are minimal, and you suspect an abscess (and there is no ultrasound), palpate the intercostal spaces over the liver one at a time and press with one finger at intervals of about 2 cm: this may reveal a point of extreme but very localized tenderness. Jaundice is not a feature unless the abscess is very large.

(iii) At the right lung base, dullness and reduced breath-sounds may suggest a pleural effusion.

Diagnosis

Parasitological

Look for amoebae in the last part of an aspirate of the abscess as they are often only present in the peripheral parts of the abscess; in 80 per cent amoebae may be found. Unless there is a pyogenic abscess, no degenerate pus cells are found, but only necrotic liver cells.

Warning: Diagnostic aspiration is no longer recommended as the risk (haemorrhage, bacterial infection, spillage/perforation) outweighs the toxicity of a therapeutic trial of drugs and sensitive serological tests are now available.

Serological

Antibodies against amoebae can be found in virtually all patients with amoebic liver abscess after the first week of illness, by an ELISA, an indirect immunofluorescence test and a latex particle agglutination test. The level of antibody is usually high which is important in endemic areas where many people will have positive antibody tests with low levels of antibody as a result of previous exposure. Recombinant *E. histolytica* antigens are being developed that return to negative after treatment.

Radiological

Ultrasound is excellent to demonstrate abscesses that may be single or multiple and to exclude pericardial effusion (Fig. 34.3). A chest X-ray may be useful to demonstrate a raised right hemidiaphragm and/or a pleural effusion (Fig. 34.4).

Laboratory

Blood: a raised white count (leukocytes $>10^9$/l) with a shift to the left is usual. There is no eosinophilia. In chronic cases there will be normocytic anaemia.

Liver function tests: alkaline phophatase raised, but other liver enzymes are less commonly raised.

Stool: of little value unless there is concurrent dysentery. Many patients with amoebic liver abscess have no detectable amoebae in their stool; in addition, in endemic areas, cysts are common and have no direct relationship with the patient's current illness.

Diagnosis of the abscess and its complications

The possible differential diagnoses in the liver include:

(i) Pyogenic liver abscess, secondary to unrecognized appendicitis, diverticulitis or even a colonic carcinoma.

(ii) Hydatid cyst(s): but the liver is not tender and the patient is not febrile unless the cysts are infected.

The possible diagnoses if the abscess ruptures depend on the site of rupture:

(i) Peritoneum. If the abscess ruptures into the peritoneal cavity, there may be a small and slow leak, or a sudden rupture which may mimic bowel perforation and give classical signs of peritonitis.

(ii) Pericardium. This is a desperate problem. Very commonly fatal, it leads to cardiac tamponade with its typical signs. Prevention is by aspiration, therefore:

> Aspirate a large abscess in the left lobe prophylactically in the course of routine management.

Remote sites

Cerebrum

Patients may present acutely with hemiplegia or altered mental status. A CT scan may show a space-occupying lesion without enhancement after contrast. The condition is rapidly progressive within 2–3 days unless adequate treatment is given with metronidazole, which passes the blood–brain barrier easily, and so has excellent penetration into the CSF. In case of raised intracranial pressure, surgical decompression may be considered.

Genito-urinary

In genito-urinary amoebiasis, there may be sexually acquired penile lesions or anal ulceration; rectovaginal fistulas may develop in the course of amoebic colitis.

Treatment

General principles

There are two classes of amoebicidal drugs:

Tissue amoebicidal drugs kill amoebae in affected tissues; these include metronidazole, tinidazole and emetine.

Luminal amoebicidal drugs eradicate amoebae from the lumen of the gut; examples are diloxanide furoate (Furamide®), paromomycin and clioquinol.

> Always use two drugs when treating invasive amoebae in order to prevent relapse.

For dosages see Table 34.1.

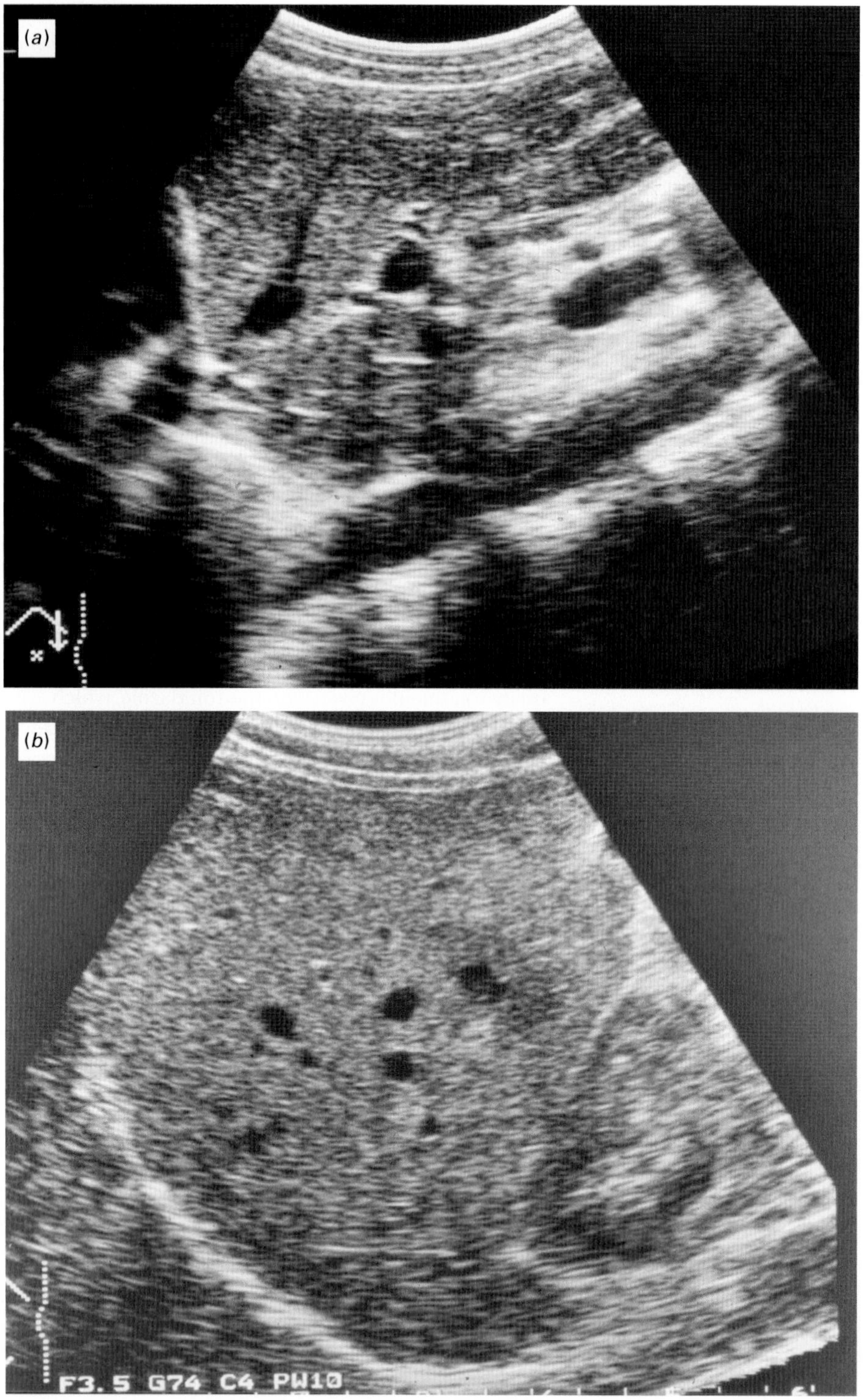

Fig. 34.3. (*a*) An ultrasound of a patient with fever and right upper quadrant pain and weight loss for 3 months; he had a total white count of 12 500/ mm^3 with 80% polymorphs and a raised alkaline phosphatase. An ELISA test for amoebic antibodies was positive: at least four amoebic liver abscesses can be seen.

(*b*) Same patient 3 weeks after treatment with metronidazole; the abscesses have decreased in size; in a follow-up scan 6 weeks after treatment the lesions were no longer detectable (not shown).

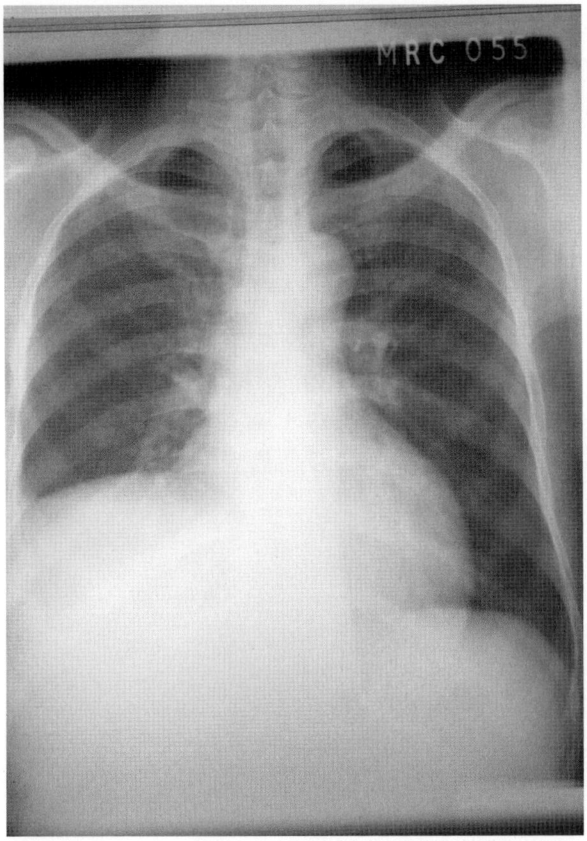

Fig. 34.4. Chest radiograph to show a raised right hemi-diaphragm: this patient had a liver abscess.

Asymptomatic cyst passers

In developing countries in certain areas up to 40 per cent of people may have cysts in their stool without having symptoms; these are not treated as this is costly and re-infection is common. In industrialized countries all patients who are asymptomatic cyst passers routinely receive a luminal agent.

Amoebic dysentery

- Metronidazole (Flagyl®) is the drug of choice; it is widely available and inexpensive. Although it has not been shown to be safe in pregnancy, it should not be withheld in any form of invasive amoebiasis.
- Give intravenous metronidazole to severely ill patients. Tinidazole (Fasigyn®) when available is preferred: it can be given for a shorter period and it has fewer side-effects than metronidazole.
- Emetine can only be given parenterally: it is useful in severe cases when a parenteral drug is needed. The

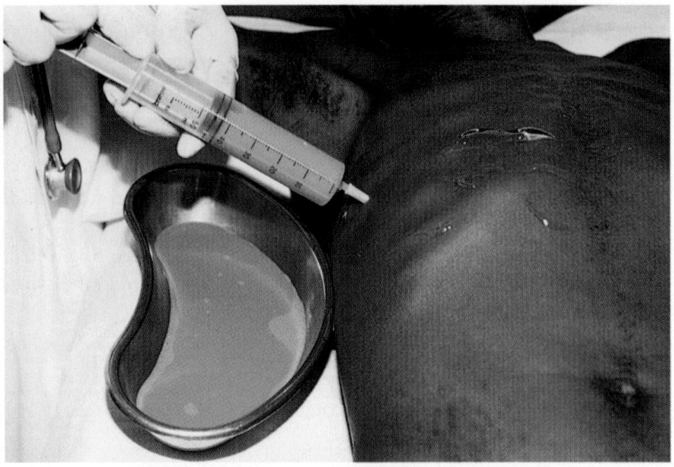

Fig. 34.5. Aspiration of pus from an amoebic liver abscess: the needle was inserted at the point of maximal tenderness. (Copyright M. Weber)

drug has cumulative cardiotoxicity and so ECG monitoring is recommended.

Amoebic liver abscess

Patients can usually be managed by medical treatment alone. Metronidazole or tinidazole will give rapid improvement of the clinical condition.

Indications for drainage of the abscess include:
(i) poor response to medical treatment:
(ii) a large abscess at risk of rupturing:
(iii) a left lobe abscess as this may rupture into the pericardium.

- Drain the abscess percutaneously or surgically. The choice depends on its site and on the skills of the doctor. If there is no ultrasound or imaging, aspirate at the point of maximal tenderness: take great care not to spill the pus outside the abscess (Fig. 34.5).
- Follow patients for 3–6 months after successful treatment. Repeated ultrasound shows that most abscesses disappear completely.
- In about 20 per cent a cavity may persist, which is harmless and should not be aspirated in an otherwise asymptomatic patient.

Free-living amoebae

Naegleria fowleri infection may cause primary amoebic meningoencephalitis in young adults or children after exposure to fresh water. The amoebae are believed to

Table 34.1. Treatment of various amoebic infections in adults and children

Condition	Drug	Adult	Child	Toxicity
Asymptomatic cyst-passers				
Developing countries	none			
Industrialized countries	diloxanide furoate	500 mg p.o. t.d.s × 10 days	7 mg/kg p.o. t.d.s × 10 days	Flatulence; not in pregnancy
	clioquinol	250 mg p.o. t.d.s × 10 days	3–5 mg/kg p.o. t.d.s × 10 days	Not in pregnancy
	di-iodohydroxyquin (iodoquinol)	650 mg p.o. t.d.s × 20 days	10 mg/kg t.d.s × 20 days (max. 2g/day)	Nausea, rashes
	paromomycin	500 mg p.o. t.d.s. × 7 days	10 mg/kg p.o. t.d.s. × 7 days (max. 2 g/day)	Mild diarrhoea safe in pregnancy
Amoebic dysentery	metronidazole[a]	800 mg p.o. t.d.s × 5 days	10–15 mg/kg p.o. t.d.s. × 5 days (max. 2250 mg/day)	Nausea, vomiting, alcohol intolerance
	or			
	tinidazole	2 gram p.o. stat × 3 days	50 mg/kg p.o. once daily × 3 days (max. 2 grams)	
	and			
	diloxanide furoate	see above		
	or clioquinol	see above		
If unresponsive add:	emetine hydrochloride	65 mg i.m. once daily × 10 days	1 mg/kg once daily	Cardiotoxic
	or			
	dihydroemetine	1–1.5 mg/kg i.m. once daily (max. 90 mg/day)	Idem as adult	Less toxic than emetine
	or tetracycline	500 mg t.d.s × 5 days		
Liver abscess	metronidazole[a]	800 mg p.o. t.d.s. × 5 days i.v. 500 mg 6 hourly for 5 days	10–15 mg/kg t.d.s. × 5 days	
	or tinidazole	2 gram p.o. × 3 days		
If very ill nor not responding add	chloroquine	600 mg loading dose, then 150 mg b.d. × 30 days	10 mg/kg daily	Rare

Notes:
[a] If luminal agents are not available, it is advisable to increase the duration of metronidazole treatment to 10 days.

penetrate the CNS through the nose and the olfactory nerve. The incubation period is 2–14 days after which there is a sudden onset of fever, headache, vomiting and signs of meningitis, usually with no focal signs. Most patients have altered mental status. A lumbar puncture will show a typical purulent picture with raised white cells and a shift to the left, raised protein and low glucose; amoebae may be seen. Prognosis is very poor even with treatment for which amphotericin B seems most successful. Accompanying myocarditis has been found at autopsy.

Infection with *Acanthamoeba* may cause granulomatous amoebic encephalitis in immunocompromised individuals; the onset is insidious with focal neurological signs, fever, headache, altered mental status and convulsions. Treatment is with pentamidine or ketoconazole.

Acanthamoeba also causes keratitis often accompanied by anterior uveitis in those who suffer minor corneal trauma or who wear soft contact lenses. Differentation from herpes simplex infection may be difficult. Treatment is with surgical debridement and topical agents such as miconazole, propramidine or neosporin.

References

Petri WA, Singh U. (1999). Diagnosis and management of amebiasis. *Clin Infect Dis*; **29**: 1117–1125.

Warhurst DC. (1999). Amoebiasis. In Protozoal Diseases, ed HM Gilles, pp. 548–559. Oxford: Arnold Publishers.

WHO/PAHO/UNESCO. (1997). Report of a consultation of experts on amoebiasis. *Wkly Epidemiol Rep Wld Hlth Org*; **72**: 97–99.

Intestinal protozoa

35

The problem in Africa

The epidemiology of intestinal infectious disease has changed substantially since the 1980s in Africa and in the rest of the world. With the spread of HIV, parasites previously thought to be of minor importance have assumed a major profile and some previously unrecognized parasites have been found in human hosts. Cryptosporidiosis (infection with *Cryptosporidium parvum*) and isosporiasis (infection with *Isospora belli*) were thought of as unimportant occasional infections with protozoa of minor significance, while human infection with microsporidia was completely unknown before it was recognized in HIV-infected patients. These infections are now understood to pose important public health problems throughout the continent. *Giardia intestinalis* (also called *G. lamblia* or *G. duodenalis*), the first human protozoal parasite to be identified over 200 years ago with the first microscopes, remains an important parasite, especially of children.

These infections, with the exception of giardiasis, have a major impact on people who are immunocompromised because of HIV infection. Cryptosporidiosis is also very important in children as it makes a major contribution to the persistent diarrhoea–malnutrition syndrome (PDM). Table 35.1 presents a summary of studies of infection with intestinal protozoa in AIDS patients from several countries around Africa. Few of the studies included microsporidiosis as this infection is difficult to diagnose.

It appears that cryptosporidiosis and microsporidiosis are equally prevalent all over the continent, but isosporiasis seems to be rare in the Sahel and in the Horn of Africa, while being common in sub-equatorial Africa.

It is also clear from Table 35.1 that these infections are common among AIDS patients, and our own work indicates that multiple infections occur in up to 25 per cent of patients with AIDS-related diarrhoea. We therefore

Table 35.1. Frequency of major protozoa in adults with HIV-related diarrhoea in African studies

				Percentage with protozoan				
Author	Year	Setting	*n*	C	I	M	G	E
Henry et al.	1986	Zaire	46	8	19	–	0	0
Sewankambo et al.	1987	Uganda	23	48	13	–	4	9
Colebunders et al.	1987	Zaire	106	22	7	–	0	3
Colebunders et al.	1988	Zaire	42	31	12	–	5	0
Floch et al.	1989	Burundi	100	15	20	–	1	16[a]
Kadende et al.	1989	Burundi	100	13	16	–		
Lucas et al.	1989	Zambia Uganda	77	–	–	6.5	–	–
Conlon et al.	1990	Zambia	63	32	16	2	2	0
Pichard et al.	1990	Mali	59	38	3	–	1	0
Hunter et al.	1992	Zambia	105	2	8	–	0	0
Mengesha	1994	Ethiopia	63	40	–	–	–	–
Khumalo-Ngwenya	1994	Zambia	27	11	7	–	4	0
Kelly et al.	1996	Zambia	75	25	28	35	1	0

Notes:
C = *Cryptosporidium parvum*, I = *Isospora belli*, M = microsporidia, G = *Giardia intestinalis* and E = *Entamoeba histolytica*. First authors only are shown. The use of '-' implies that a given organism was not looked for or not reported; the use of '0' indicates that none was found.
[a] Includes *Entamoeba coli*.

believe that it makes sense to offer combination anti-infective chemotherapy to our AIDS patients who present with a persistent diarrhoea – malnutrition syndrome. Ultimately, we hope that complex diagnostic tests will not be necessary and should be reserved for research protocols. We have previously demonstrated that anti-protozoal therapy with albendazole has some effect in reducing diarrhoea even when the precise parasitological diagnosis is not known (Kelly et al., 1996). The final protocol for use in our AIDS patients in Lusaka will be decided when current clinical trials are complete, but our current practice is to look for, and treat, isosporiasis with high dose co-trimoxazole (see below) as a first step.

Cryptosporidiosis

The first recorded case of human infection with *C. parvum* was in 1976, but since then it has emerged as one of the most important enteropathogens. It is closely related to *I. belli, Toxoplasma gondii* and *Plasmodium* species, but unlike these organisms it is notoriously difficult to treat.

The organism and its life cycle

Infection is transmitted by the ingestion of oocysts, which are small and spherical (around 5 μm). These excyst in the small intestine and penetrate the host enterocytes. Trophozoites develop inside the cell, undergoing stages of asexual reproduction (forming merozoites and schizonts) and sexual reproduction (forming micro- and macrogametes) to form new oocysts which may excyst further down the gut or may be passed out in faeces to infect someone else. There is still debate as to whether cryptosporidiosis is a zoonosis, i.e. whether it is primarily an infection of animals which occasionally infects man, in temperate or in tropical environments. Substantial evidence has accumulated over the last decade that *C. parvum* exists in at least two major genotypes, as demonstrated by isoenzyme studies and by DNA analysis. Genotype 2 infects a wide range of animal hosts as well as humans, but genotype 1 exclusively infects humans. These genotypes can now be distinguished by molecular techniques. There is little information on transmission of *C. parvum* in Africa, but it seems likely that most cases are acquired either from contaminated drinking water or by direct contact with other people with infection.

Epidemiology

Exposure to *C. parvum* oocysts occurs commonly in childhood in African populations, and as immunity to this organism is strong, cryptosporidiosis is an uncommon cause of diarrhoea in adults with a healthy immune system. *C. parvum* causes diarrhoea in African adults principally when there is a problem with immune function, as in AIDS (see Table 35.1). In Africa, cryptosporidiosis is common in children with or without HIV infection. In population based studies in Lusaka, 17 per cent of diarrhoeal episodes in 222 children were associated with this infection (Nchito et al., 1998). In malnourished children with diarrhoea admitted to the University Teaching Hospital, Lusaka the prevalence was 25 per cent, and only slightly higher in HIV seropositive than in HIV seronegative children (Amadi et al., 2001). Studies in Guinea–Bissau have demonstrated that cryptosporidiosis is associated with malnutrition and with increased mortality (Molbak et al., 1993). For many years it has been known that there is a vicious circle of malnutrition, immune failure and infection. However, with respect to cryptosporidiosis, work in Guinea–Bissau has dissected out the relationship between cryptosporidiosis and malnutrition, and has revealed that episodes of cryptosporidiosis preceded periods of growth failure (Molbak et al, 1997).

Control/prevention

There is no vaccine against *C. parvum*. Cryptosporidiosis will continue to be a major public health problem as long as drinking water is not microbiologically pure. To achieve eradication from the water supplies would require that all sources be free of faecal contamination (from human or animal sources) or efficient filtration as chlorination does not kill the oocysts. Even in industrialized countries with good water purification systems large outbreaks can occur such as a spectacular outbreak in the USA, which affected 400 000 people in 1993. It is a difficult infection to control as the infectious dose is low, with around 100 oocysts being enough to establish infection in adults with no prior immunity.

Clinical features

The commonest manifestation of infection is diarrhoea. This may be indistinguishable from any other acute diarrhoeal illness, but cryptosporidiosis is more likely to become persistent. The severity of illness is variable even in AIDS patients and a minority develop a high volume diarrhoea with fulminating illness and high mortality. There is a relationship between the severity of symptoms and the number of helper T cells, i.e. CD4+ cells in peripheral blood, a marker of the severity of the cellular immune deficiency. As the CD4 count falls as HIV infection progresses, the severity of the illness associated with cryptosporidial infection increases. It is often associated with nutritional problems, as persistent diarrhoea causes severe anorexia and the diarrhoea also leads to malabsorption of micronutrients. Cryptosporidiosis may also cause biliary disease (an infective but not suppurative cholangitis) and this usually presents with right upper quadrant pain with or without jaundice. Few data exist as to the incidence of this complication, but our experience in Lusaka suggests that this is not common.

Diagnosis

Stool microscopy is the standard approach to diagnosis. Thin smears are prepared and stained with a modified Ziehl–Neelsen stain (similar to that used for detection of acid-fast bacteria but without warming the slide). Oocysts stain red on a blue background (Fig. 35.1). The technique is slow and requires skill as the oocysts must be differentiated from yeast and other spores which may cause confusion; important distinguishing features include size and the pattern of staining. Many laboratories will be unable to give this test the time and expertise it requires, and the director of the service will have to decide if this is an appropriate use of resources, given the difficulty providing specific treatment (see below). More rapid diagnosis may be achieved with an auramine stain or with immunofluorescence, but both of these require a fluorescence microscope and the diagnosis should still be confirmed with the ZN stain. Other tests, such as antigen detection tests or PCR are expensive and not yet proven to be of value; in Lusaka we have found these tests to be insensitive.

Treatment

There is no treatment readily available that is effective in cryptosporidiosis, but recent trials from Mali and from Egypt suggest that nitazoxanide may fill that role (Doumbo et al., 1997). This relatively inexpensive drug was superior to placebo in immunocompetent children. The efficacy of treatment in routine clinical practice can be monitored by symptomatic response; there is no need for routinely repeating stool microscopy.

Unsolved problems

The most pressing needs are two-fold. First, to identify a cheap effective therapy. Trials with nitazoxanide in malnourished and/or HIV-infected children and adults are currently under way in Lusaka. Second, to determine the extent to which cryptosporidiosis can be prevented at a population level by developing clean water facilities or better sanitation practices.

Isospora belli

Isospora belli is a coccidian intracellular parasite that has become a major cause of gastrointestinal disease associated with AIDS especially in sub-Saharan Africa (Ackers, 1997). There is little information available on this infection, despite its frequent occurrence in the wake of the HIV epidemic.

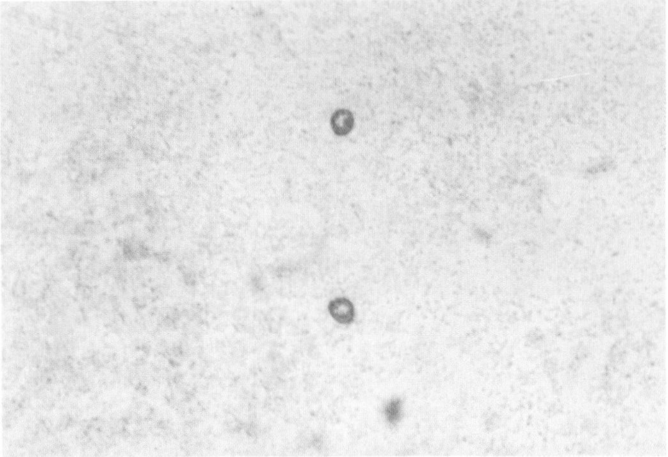

Fig. 35.1. *Cryptosporidium parvum*: thin smear of stool (× 1000). Ziehl–Neelsen stain demonstrates the red oocyst.

Epidemiology

The organism has varying distribution world-wide being prevalent in some parts of Africa. Prevalence in AIDS patients with persistent diarrhoea ranges from 0–28 per cent, with a higher rate of occurrence in West, East and Southern Africa (Table 35.1). Countries in Northern parts of Africa and the Sahel seem to have lower frequency of detection of the parasite. The organism is found mainly in immunocompromised people and HIV has lead to the dramatic increase of *Isospora belli* infection in Africa.

Transmission

Isospora belli is transmitted by ingestion of infective oocysts in contaminated food and water, but the relative importance of different routes of transmission is completely unknown. We have found no evidence of seasonality in the frequency of detection of *I. belli* among patients in Lusaka, in contrast to cryptosporidiosis which is seasonal. Once in the intestine of the host, oocysts excyst and develop through asexual and sexual stages (Lindsay et al., 1997).

Clinical features

I. belli infects both immunocompetent and immunocompromised people. Infection may be asymptomatic

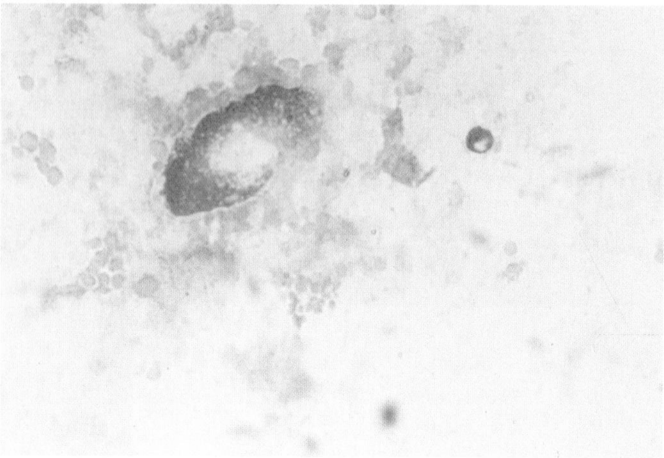

Fig. 35.2. *Isospora belli*: thin smear of strool (× 1000). Ziehl–Neelsen stain. Note the large oocyst of *I. belli*.

in immunocompetent individuals or it may lead to a mild, self-limiting diarrhoea. Persistent non-bloody diarrhoea, indistinguishable from that caused by microsporidia and *Cryptosporidium parvum*, is the major manifestation in immunocompromised individuals. Vomiting, steatorrhoea, headache, fever, malaise, abdominal pain, may also be present. Patients may become dehydrated and weight loss is a common feature. Persistent diarrhoea may occur in immunocompetent persons as well but the features are less marked (Lindsay et al., 1997).

Diagnosis

The organism is identified by light microscopy of wet preparations of faecal samples and/or by staining with the modified Ziehl–Neelsen stain (Fig. 35.2). The oocysts are much larger than *C. parvum* oocysts, around 30 μm long, and may be sporulated, in which case two round sporocysts are seen within the oocyst.

Treatment

The organism responds to a 10-day course of therapy with co-trimoxazole trimethoprim/sulfamethoxazole 960mg four times daily. Longer periods of therapy may be required if the first course is not effective, but these trials suggest that this is uncommon. An 8-week course of pyrimethamine–sulfadiazine also achieves clinical and parasitological response. Secondary prophylaxis (i.e. to prevent relapse) is usually required, suggesting that true eradication is not achieved. The dose required is 960 mg orally three times per week.

Prevention

Improved sanitation and water supply may reduce transmission of the organism, but there is no evidence for this at present, and boiling drinking water may help reduce chances of infection. Infection in immunocompromised individuals is reduced by prophylactic co-trimoxazole (Anglaret et al., 1999). Giving co-trimoxazole prophylaxis to HIV-infected adults has not been adopted as policy by most sub-Saharan African countries. Most of the benefit in the trials reported from Abidjan (Anglaret et al., 1999; Wiktor et al., 1999) was in reduction of bacterial infections, and there is doubt as to the reproducibility of the trial results in countries where bacterial resistance to co-trimoxazole is common, such as Zambia.

Microsporidia

Microsporidia are members of the phylum *Microspora* (Farthing et al., 1996). They are obligate intracellular parasites ubiquitous in nature. They infect both vertebrate and invertebrate organisms and have been described in various animal species such as birds, fish, insects and mammals. There are four species known to be responsible for disease in humans: (i) *Encephalitozoon intestinalis*, (ii) *Enterocytozoon bieneusi*, (iii) *Encephalitozoon hellem* and (iv) *E. cuniculi*. *E. bieneusi* only causes disease of the digestive system, whereas *E. intestinalis* causes both intestinal and disseminated disease.

Epidemiology

Microsporidia have been identified in different parts of the world, including sub-Saharan Africa, in association with AIDS. There is some evidence that these organisms can also cause disease in individuals with immunosuppression not related to HIV such as that following chemotherapy for malignant disease. The prevalence of microsporidia in patients with HIV-related persistent diarrhoea in Africa has been reported as high as 35 per cent (Table 35.1).

Transmission

The sources and routes of transmission are not known. Water and infected animals are possible reservoirs but there is no conclusive evidence to support this. Preliminary evidence suggests a relationship between incidence and rainfall in studies in Lusaka, which might indicate water-borne transmission. One water-borne outbreak has been reported from France.

Clinical features

Diarrhoea is the main clinical feature of intestinal microsporidia infections. The diarrhoea is non-bloody and is indistinguishable from that caused by *Cryptosporidium parvum* or *Isospora belli*. Occasionally, high faecal volumes (1–3 litres) per day can be passed. Vomiting and weight loss are also common features. Other features that may be present are fever and abdominal pain, but in AIDS patients these may also indicate other opportunistic infections. Disseminated disease may occur with *Encephalitozoon intestinalis* and almost any organ can be involved, causing hepatitis, renal failure, encephalitis, and kerato-conjunctivitis. Cutaneous manifestations may very rarely occur as nodular lesions. Sclerosing cholangitis, as in cryptosporidiosis, leads to right upper quadrant abdominal pain, sometimes to jaundice, and is associated with abnormal liver function tests (a raised alkaline phosphatase).

Diagnosis

Microsporidial infection should be suspected in an immunocompromised patient presenting with chronic diarrhoea, but most laboratories in Africa may be unable to spare the time to look for these difficult organisms, and diagnosis is technically demanding. Staining of very thin stool smears is the established method of identification, using one of the modified trichrome stains (Sianongo et al., 2001) or one of the fluorochromes. Examination of several stool samples collected on three consecutive days may be necessary. Gram stain or Giemsa stain can be used to detect microsporidia in tissue biopsies. Three chitin-staining fluorochromes (Calcafluor white, Fungiflor and Fungiqual) are useful in identifying *E. intestinalis* and *E. bieneusi* spores, which fluoresce brightly in stool, intestinal fluids and tissue biopsies. The polymerase chain reaction (PCR) is a newly developed method, which can also be used in the identification of species, but this is currently only a research tool, as is electron microscopy.

Treatment

The usual regimen for treatment of *Encephalitozoon intestinalis* infection is albendazole 400 mg twice daily for 28 days. This drug is also useful for disseminated infection and tissue eradication is achieved. *E. bieneusi* can be suppressed but usually not eradicated (for a review, see Farthing et al., 1996). Patients on antiretroviral therapy usually have a clinical response as their immunity improves.

Unsolved questions

There is a need to define the epidemiology of microsporidiosis more precisely, particularly its occurrence in adults and children without HIV infection, and identify of the sources of infection.

Giardiasis

Infection with *Giardia intestinalis* was first recognized in 1681 by Anthony van Leeuwenhoek in his own stool samples with his own first microscopes. Preceding the discovery of *Entamoeba histolytica* in 1875 and of *Plasmodium* spp. in the 1880s, this was the first protozoal infection of man to be identified. The parasite has a simple life cycle. Trophozoites inhabit a strictly extracellular niche in the proximal small intestine and are never invasive. They are attached to enterocytes but remain in the lumen of the gut, and in the more distal small intestine they encyst to form cysts which are excreted in the faeces to be transmitted to other hosts.

Epidemiology

Giardiasis is very common in children throughout the tropics. Highest prevalence rates have been recorded in studies from Guatemala in which all children in one birth cohort had infection by 3 years of age, or from the Gambia where the prevalence was 45 per cent in children with diarrhoea. However, there seems to be considerable variation in its epidemiology as in Lusaka we have not found giardiasis to be as common as the 20 per cent recorded in neighbouring Zimbabwe.

Many examples of water-borne outbreaks have been recorded, usually related to breakdown of the water filtration system. Chlorination does not kill *Giardia* cysts. As might be expected of an infection that can be transmitted in drinking water, local contamination can lead to high prevalence, and examples of this can be found throughout the world. Travellers to certain areas may be at high risk of giardiasis, and high attack rates have been recorded in travellers to St Petersburg in Russia or to certain North American national parks.

As with *C. parvum*, genetic differences between isolates of *G. intestinalis* suggest that there are two different genotypes with different transmission characteristics.

Transmission

Transmission occurs through ingestion of contaminated drinking water or food or by direct person-to-person contact, presumably carried on unwashed hands touching cooking utensils or drinking vessels. The infectious dose is small, perhaps 100–1000 cysts being sufficient to initiate infection. This probably explains why prevalence can reach high levels in children's day-care centres and in residential institutions.

Clinical features

Giardiasis may be asymptomatic or associated with diarrhoea of varying severity and persistence. The diarrhoea may be steatorrhoea (i.e. laden with fat) and is often persistent, but it is important to remember that there is variation and therefore anyone with persistent diarrhoea should be investigated for giardiasis. The fact that a high proportion of infections may be asymptomatic may explain why some case-control studies may fail to detect an association between giardiasis and diarrhoea.

There is disagreement as to whether giardiasis leads to malnutrition or not. Giardiasis is common in malnourished children, but careful studies in The Gambia found no association between serological evidence of infection and growth faltering (Lunn et al., 1999). In Brazil, cryptosporidiosis was associated with more severe long-term adverse effects on development than giardiasis (Guerrant et al., 1999).

Diagnosis

There are no diagnostic tests that can be used for all cases. Stool microscopy is the most important technique. Cysts can be seen in wet preparations or in smears stained with trichrome stain, with or without concentration. Examination of a single stool sample will be positive in 70 per cent of cases and of three stools in 85 per cent. Trophozoites are seen only in fresh stools passed during heavy infections. Newer techniques include antibody-based tests (Chan et al., 2000) using cartridge membranes and colour change results, but these are expensive. Microscopy of duodenal aspirates may diagnose cases which are negative on stool microscopy, but this is not a readily available procedure. In many instances the diagnosis is not attempted, and a therapeutic trial of metronidazole is often used as an early step in management. However, this is not a specific therapy and cannot be used to infer a diagnosis of giardiasis.

Treatment

Treatment with metronidazole (400 mg t.i.d. for 5 days) or tinidazole (2 g single dose) is usually effective. Albendazole (400 mg b.d. for 3 days) and nitazoxanide (100 mg b.d. for 3 days) are also useful in refractory cases.

Prevention

Strategies for prevention must be seen as part of a coherent programme of prevention of intestinal infectious disease, and will depend on local epidemiology and transmission patterns. One would expect that improved water quality would reduce incidence, but there is little evidence that this is true in practice.

References

Ackers JP (1997). Gut coccidia – *Isospora, Cryptosporidium, Cyclospora* and *Sarcocystis*. *Semin Gastrointest Dis*; **8**: 33–44.

Amadi BC, Kelly P, Mwiya M et al. (2001). Intestinal and systemic infection, HIV and mortality in Zambian children with persistent diarrhoea and malnutrition; *J Ped Gastroenterol Nutr*; **32**: 550–554.

Anglaret X, Chene G, Attia A et al. (1999). Early chemoprophylaxis with trimethoprim-sulphamethoxazole for HIV-1 infected adults in Abidjan, Cote d'Ivoire: a randomised trial. *Lancet*; **353**: 1463–68.

Chan R, Chen J, York MK et al. (2000). Evaluation of a combination rapid immunoassay for detection of *Giardia* and *Cryptosporidium* antigens. *J Clin Microbiol*; **38**: 393–394.

Colebunders R, Francis H, Mann JM et al. (1987). Persistent diarrhea, strongly associated with HIV infection in Kinshasa, Zaire. *Am J Gastroenterol*; **82**: 859–864.

Colebunders R, Lusakumuni K, Nelson AM et al. (1988). Persistent diarrhoea in Zairian AIDS patients: an endoscopic and histological study. *Gut*; **29**: 1687–1691.

Conlon CP, Pinching AJ, Perera CU, Moody A, Luo NP, Lucas SB. (1990). HIV-related enteropathy in Zambia: a clinical, microbiological, and histological study. *Am J Trop Med Hyg*; **42**: 83–88.

Doumbo O, Rossignol JF, Pichard E et al. (1997). Nitazoxanide in the treatment of cryptosporidial diarrhea and other intestinal parasitic infections associated with AIDS in tropical Africa. *Am J Trop Med Hyg*; **56**: 637–639.

Farthing MJG, Cevallos AM, Kelly P. (1996). Intestinal protozoa. In *Manson's Tropical Diseases*, 20th edn, ed. GC Cook. London: Saunders.

Floch PJ, Laroche R, Kadende P, Nkurunziza T, Mpfizi B. (1989). Parasites, etiologic agents of diarrhea in AIDS. Significance of duodenal aspiration fluid test. *Bull Soc Pathol Exot Filiales*; **82**: 316–320.

Guerrant DI, Moore SR, Lima AA et al. (1999). Association of early childhood diarrhoea and cryptosporidiosis with impaired physical fitness and cognitive function 4–7 years later in a poor urban community in northeast Brazil. *Am J Trop Med Hyg*; **61**: 707–713.

Henry MC, De Clercq D, Lokombe B et al. (1986). Parasitological observations of chronic diarrhoea in suspected AIDS adult patients in Kinshasa (Zaire). *Trans Roy Soc Trop Med Hyg*; **80**: 309–310.

Hunter G, Bagshawe AF, Baboo KS, Luke R, Prociv P. (1992). Intestinal parasites in Zambian patients with AIDS. *Trans Roy Soc Trop Med Hyg*; **86**: 543–545.

Kadende P, Nkurunziza T, Floch JJ et al. (1989). Infectious diarrhea in African acquired immunodepression syndrome (AIDS). A propos of 100 patients studied in Bujumbura (Burundi). *Med Trop (Mars)*; **49**: 129–133.

Kelly P, Lungu F, Keane E et al. (1996). Albendazole chemotherapy for treatment of diarrhoea in patients with AIDS in Zambia: a randomised double blind controlled trial. *Br Med J*; **312**: 1187–1191.

Kelly P, Baboo KS, Woolf M, Ngwenya B, Luo N, Farthing MJG. (1996). Prevalence and aetiology of persistent diarrhoea in adults in urban Zambia. *Acta Trop*; **61**: 183–190.

Khumalo-Ngwenya B, Luo NP, Chintu C et al. (1994). Gut parasites in HIV-seropositive Zambian adults with diarrhoea. *E Afr Med J*; **71**: 379–383.

Lindsay DS, Dubey JP, Blagburn BL. (1997). Biology of *Isospora* spp. from humans, non-human primates, and domestic animals. *Clin Microbiol Rev*; **10**:19–34.

Lucas SB, Papadaki L, Conlon CP et al. (1989). Diagnosis of intestinal microsporidiosis in patients with AIDS. *J Clin Pathol*; **42**: 885–887.

Lunn PG, Erinoso HO, Northrop-Clewes CA et al. (1999). *Giardia intestinalis* is unlikely to be a major cause of the poor growth of rural Gambian infants. *J Nutr*; **129**: 872–877.

Mengesha B. (1994). Cryptosporidiosis among medical patients with the acquired immunodeficiency syndrome in Tikur Anbessa Teaching Hospital, Ethiopia. *E Afr Med J*; **71**: 376–378.

Molbak K, Hojlyng N, Gottschau A et al. (1993). Cryptosporidiosis in infancy and childhood mortality in Guinea Bissau, West Africa. *Br Med J*; **307**: 417–420.

Molbak K, Andersen M, Aaby P et al. (1997). *Cryptosporidium* infection in infancy as a cause of malnutrition: a community study from Guinea-Bissau, West Africa. *Am J Clin Nutr*; **65**: 149–152.

Nchito M, Kelly P, Sianongo S et al. (1998). Cryptosporidiosis in urban Zambian children: an analysis of risk factors. *Am J Trop Hyg*; **59**: 435–437.

Pichard E, Doumbo O, Minta D, Traore HA. (1990). Role of cryptosporidiosis in diarrhea among hospitalized adults in Bamako. *Bull Soc Pathol Exot*; **83**: 473–478.

Sewankambo N, Mugerwa RD, Goodgame R et al. (1987). Enteropathic AIDS in Uganda. An endoscopic, histological and microbiological study. *AIDS*; **1**: 9–13.

Sianongo S, McDonald V, Kelly P. (2001). A method for diagnosis of microsporidia adapted for use in developing countries. *Trans Roy Soc Trop Med Hyg*; **95**: 605–607.

Wiktor SZ, Sassan-Morokro M, Grant AD et al. (1999). Efficacy of trimethoprim-sulphamethoxazole prophylaxis to decrease morbidity and mortality in HIV-1 infected patients with tuberculosis in Abidjan, Cote d'Ivoire: a randomised controlled trial. *Lancet*; **353**: 1469–1475.

Bacteria

36 *Streptococcus pneumoniae*

The problem in Africa

Streptococcus pneumoniae (the pneumococcus) causes lobar pneumonia (Chapter 18), meningitis (Chapter 16), otitis media, bacteraemia and acute sinusitis as well as rarer conditions such as peritonitis, endocarditis and myositis in immunocompromised patients. Patients infected with the human immunodeficiency virus (HIV) have more than 20 times increased risk of infection and re-infection compared to matched HIV-negative patients (Gilks et al., 1996). This association with HIV is stronger in those with low CD4 counts. In recent hospital studies, 95 per cent of African inpatients with invasive pneumococcal disease were found to be HIV-positive (Gordon et al., 2001). Pneumococcal infections therefore rank with tuberculosis salmonellae (Archibald et al. 2000) and non-typhoid as the most important infections in HIV-positive patients in Africa – see Table 36.1.

Table 36.1. Blood culture isolates from adult patients admitted to Queen Elizabeth Central Hospital, Blantyre, Malawi 1998–99

Organism	Number of isolates	% of total isolates
Non-typhi salmonellae	164	36.5
Streptococcus pneumoniae	136	30.3
Escherichia coli	43	9.6
Klebsiella spp.	19	4.2
Neisseria meningitidis gp A	16	3.6
Other streptococci	16	3.6
Salmonella typhi	12	2.7
Cryptococcus neoformans	8	1.8
Staphylococcus aureus	6	1.3
Miscellaneous[a]	29	6.5

Notes:

Significant pathogens were grown from 16.1% of 2789 cultures. Culture for *Mycobacterium tuberculosis* was not done.

[a] Includes *Enterobacteria* (11), *Pseudomonas* spp. (7), *Acinetobacter* spp. (6), *Aeromonas* spp. (2), *Haemophilus influenzae* type b (1), *Vibrio cholerae* 01 Ogawa (1), *Salmonella enteritidis* and *S. pneumoniae* (1).

The organism

S. pneumoniae is a gram-positive diplococcus found only in humans. In 1997, it became the first gram-positive organism to have a sequenced genome on-line. (www.tigr.org/tdb/mdb/mdb.html)

Virulence factors – capsule, adherence and pneumolysin

The most important virulence factor is a thick polysaccharide capsule that makes the bacteria resistant to phagocytosis unless opsonized with antibody and complement (Tuomanen et al., 1995). Unlike other streptococci, pneumococci do not have binding pili, but they have other cell wall components that bind avidly to carbohydrates and to specific receptors on the surface of respiratory epithelium. These receptors can be up-regulated by viral infection, increasing the chance of subsequent bacterial invasion. Pneumococci make pneumolysin, a cytotoxic agent released when the bacteria are damaged. Pneumolysin binds to cholesterol and damages host cells, which allows bloodstream invasion.

Phase variation

Most capsular types of *S. pneumoniae* have two types of colony morphology (opaque and transparent phase) on clear agar (Kim & Weiser, 1998). Opaque colonies consist of bacteria with thicker capsules and altered cell wall constituents. This phase shows decreased epithelial binding but increased resistance to phagocytosis compared to bacteria from transparent colonies. Regulation of capsule expression may confer increased capacity to colonize (transparent form) the nasal mucosa before invading (opaque form) the distal respiratory tract.

Epidemiology

Carriage and transmission

Ten to 40% of healthy adults, and a higher percentage of children, carry pneumococci in the nasopharynx. Colonization typically lasts 4 to 6 weeks. Transmission is by droplet infection.

Susceptibility to pneumococcal disease

Pneumococcal disease occurs shortly after colonization with a new type. Disease is most common at the extremes of age and in immunocompromised adults. Table 36.2 shows factors that predispose to pneumococcal disease. In *immunocompetent* adults, *cigarette smoking* is the most important risk factor (Scott et al., 2000; Nuorti et al., 2000)

Control/prevention

Vaccination

There are 90 different types of pneumococcal capsular polysaccharide, and immunity is type specific. A different pattern of local types is found in different parts of the world, but the presently available 23-valent polysaccharide vaccine covers over 80 per cent of the types prevalent in Africa. Unfortunately, it is minimally effective in the young and the elderly, and ineffective in HIV-infected adults (French et al., 2000a, b). Newer protein conjugate vaccines are safe, immunogenic, expensive and under clinical trial (Hausdorff et al., 2000; Jaffar et al., 1999).

Chemoprophylaxis

Cotrimoxazole prophylaxis reduces the incidence of severe bacterial infections in HIV-infected adults (Anglaret et al., 1999; Wiktor et al., 1999), but widespread use of antibiotics in this way may lead to increased antimicrobial resistance (Feikin et al., 2000).

Clinical features

Pneumococcal infections range from asymptomatic carriage, through mild local disease to severe disseminated infections. The clinical presentation is a result of the host-

Table 36.2. Risk factors for pneumococcal disease

Congenital	Acquired
Male sex	**Physiological**
Black race	Infancy and ageing
Primary immune	Cold, fatigue, malnutrition
deficiency (antibody,	Pregnancy
complement,	**Bacteriological**
phagocytes)	Excess exposure (prisons, mines)
Sickle cell disease	**Drugs**
	Cigarette smoking
	Alcohol abuse
	Steroids
	Disease
	Immune deficiency
	HIV infection
	Haematological malignancy
	Prior viral infection
	COPD and asthma
	Liver disease
	Renal failure
	Diabetes mellitus

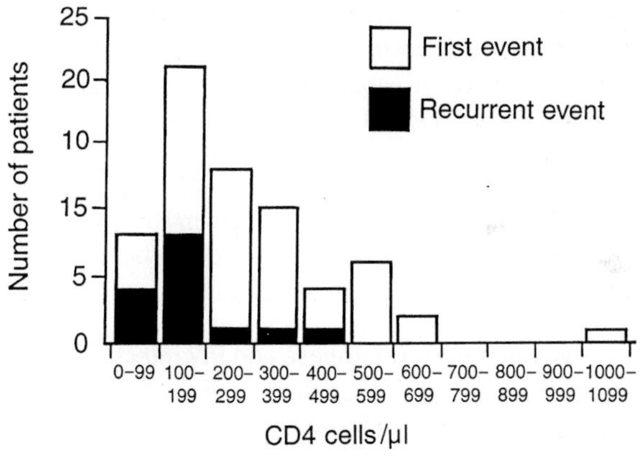

Fig. 36.1. The number of patients presenting with a first episode of pneumococcal disease (light bars) and recurrent episodes of invasive pneumococcal disease (filled bars) according to CD4 count. CD4 counts were not measured during the acute episode. (Figure reproduced from Gilks et al., 1996 with permission).

pathogen balance, which is influenced by host immunity and bacterial virulence (Fig. 36.1).

The host response

Pneumococcal carriage in the nasopharynx is asymptomatic, and small numbers of aspirated bacteria are ingested by alveolar macrophages without acute inflammation. Overwhelming numbers of pneumococci at distal respiratory sites, or in the meninges, result in acute inflam-

Table 36.3. Mortality by clinical presentation for 214 consecutive cases of invasive pneumococcal disease in Queen Elizabeth Central Hospital, Blantyre 1998–99

Diagnosis	Number of cases	Number died	Percentage mortality
Pneumonia	95	25	26
Bacteraemia alone	35	15	43
Meningitis	34	22	65
Meningitis and bacteraemia	28	16	57
Meningitis and pneumonia	19	14	74
Empyema	3	0	0
Total	214	92	43

Notes:
95% of these cases were also HIV-positive (Mas Chaponda, unpub.).

mation (Spellerberg & Tuomanen, 1994). Pneumococcal cell wall constituents cause activation of complement, release of pro-inflammatory cytokines by macrophages and epithelium, recruitment of neutrophils and increased vascular leakiness (see also Chapters 6, 18, 20). This tissue response allows invasion of the bloodstream by pneumococci, where the primary defence mechanisms are specific for antibody, complement and phagocytes, particularly neutrophils. Tissue macrophages in the liver and spleen are important for removal of opsonized bacteria.

Bacteraemia

Pneumococcal bacteraemia is common in HIV-positive adults who present with fever and headache but may have no localizing signs (Gilks et al., 1996).

Invasive pneumococcal disease and HIV infection

In Africa, the majority of patients with invasive pneumococcal disease are also infected with HIV. HIV-infected patients with pneumococcal disease are more likely to have positive blood cultures (French et al., 2000), and have a high mortality (Table 36.3).

Pneumonia

See Chapter 18.

Meningitis

See Chapter 16.

Acute sinusitis

Following an acute viral infection, prolonged nasal discharge, fever and pain made worse by pressure over the sinuses are suggestive (but not diagnostic) of acute sinusitis. These infections are most commonly caused by *S.pneumoniae*, other Streptococci or *Haemophilus influenzae.*

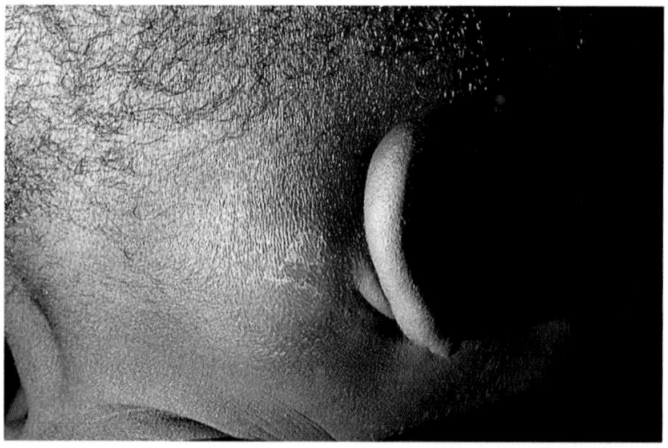

Fig. 36.2. Acute mastoiditis in a child: note swelling behind the ear caused by this pyogenic complication of pneumococcal infection.

Otitis media

This is an important infection in children: the fretful febrile infant, who may put a hand up towards the ear, often has pneumococcal otitis media.

Local complications are:

- acute mastoiditis (Fig. 36.2)
- cerebral abscess
- cerebral venous sinus thrombosis
- chronic suppurative otits media.

Tissue infections

Rarely, pneumococcal infection results in empyema, endocarditis, peritonitis, and even myositis.

Pneumococcal empyema follows partially treated pneumonia or infected pleural effusion. Patients at first get a little better but then may develop pleural pain, shortness of breath and intermittent fever and sweats, with signs of fluid at the lung base. Aspiration of pus (with culture if possible) confirms the diagnosis. Treatment must include drainage until minimal drain output is evident, and antibiotics (see below) for a minimum of 6 weeks. Pneumococcal endocarditis is a rare severe infection causing rapid heart valve damage and septic emboli. It is more common following puerperal infection and in the presence of damaged heart valves.

Pneumococcal peritonitis classically complicates the nephrotic syndrome in children.

Diagnosis

Gram stain and sputum

Gram stain of a sample from a sterile site is useful as the paired pneumococci have a characteristic appearance. Sputum samples must be interpreted with caution, since asymptomatic nasopharyngeal carriage is common, and samples are often inadequate. Sputum samples containing polymorphonuclear cells, few epithelial cells and large numbers of bacteria suggest pneumococcal pneumonia.

Culture

Samples from sterile sites (blood, CSF, pleural fluid, joint aspirate) may grow pneumococci in 24–48 hours even when gram stain has been negative. Isolation in culture confirms the diagnosis and enables antibiotic sensitivity testing.

Antigen tests

Antigen testing of urine and CSF for pneumococcal antigen is still a research tool because of methodological difficulties. Promising new tests are based on the detection of protein antigens, or on the amplification of specific DNA by the polymerase chain reaction (PCR) or related techniques.

Treatment and follow-up

Treatment guidelines

Therapy is usually started empirically, rather than waiting for the results of laboratory tests. Pneumococcal sinusitis should be treated with amoxycillin 500 mg t.d.s. orally for 3 days. Pneumonia is managed according to severity (see Chapters 18, 19). Most community-acquired cases can be treated with amoxycillin 500 mg t.d.s. by mouth for 5 days. The treatment of meningitis is described in Chapter 16.

Resistant organisms

Penicillin resistant pneumococci are still only a limited clinical problem in Africa as most resistance is of intermediate level (Scott et al., 2000; Jones et al., 1998). An increased mortality has been observed in children with meningitis caused by these organisms (Klugman & Madhi, 1999). It is important to note the following.

- Resistant isolates are rarely resistant to high levels of penicillin.
- In most patients from whom a resistant laboratory isolate is grown, a good clinical response can still be obtained by doubling the dose of penicillin used.
- Resistance should not be inferred from a poor clinical response to antibiotics in the first 48 hours of therapy, because it is well known that antibiotics do not alter mortality during this period.

It is inevitable, however, that penicillin resistance will increase in the future. Resistance to other antibiotics is common in penicillin-resistant isolates. Clinicians should therefore remain alert to the possibility of antibiotic resistance in pneumococcal infections, and base empiric therapy on advice gained from the nearest expert microbiology laboratory.

Follow-up and recurrent disease

Immunocompetent adults with pneumococcal disease are not at risk of recurrent infection. Most adult patients with pneumococcal disease in many parts of Africa are now HIV-positive, and pneumococcal disease is a stronger predictor of further bacteraemic episodes. Patients should be warned to seek medical help early.

Unsolved problems

There are two particularly pressing issues in African pneumococcal disease:
- prevention of the disease in vulnerable groups, and
- treatment to reduce the mortality in severe illness, particularly meningitis.

These priorties have not changed since the second edition, but the conjugate vaccine offers some hope.

References

Anglaret X, Chene G, Attia et al. (1999). Early chemoprophylaxis with trimethoprim-sulphamethoxazole for HIV-1-infected adults in Abidjan, Cote d'Ivoire: a randomised trial. Cotrimo-CI Study Group [see comments]. *Lancet*; **353**: 1463–1468.

Archibald LK, McDonald LC, Nwanyanwu O et al. (2000). A hospital-based prevalence survey of bloodstream infections in febrile patients in Malawi: implications for diagnosis and therapy. *J Infect Dis*; **181**: 1414–1420.

Feikin, DR, Dowell SF, Nwanyanwu OC et al. (2000). Increased carriage of trimethoprim/sulfamethoxazole-resistant *Streptococcus pneumoniae* in Malawian children after treatment for malaria with sulfadoxine/pyrimethamine. *J Infect Dis*; **181**: 1501–1505.

French N, Hart CA, Beeching NJ et al. (2000a). Infections in Aids: invasive pneumococcal disease in HIV-infected adults. *J Med Microbiol*; **49**: 947–967.

French N, Nakiyingi J, Carpenter LM et al. (2000b). 23-valent pneumococcal polysaccharide vaccine in HIV-1-infected Ugandan adults: double-blind, randomised and placebo controlled trial. *Lancet*; **355**: 2106–2111.

Gilks CF, Ojoo SA, Ojoo JC et al. (1996). Invasive pneumococcal disease in a cohort of predominantly HIV-1 infected female sex-workers in Nairobi, Kenya [see comments]. *Lancet*; **347**: 718–723.

Gordon MA, Walsh AL, Chaponda M et al. (2001). Bacteraemia

and mortality among adult medical admissions in Malawi – predominance of non-typhi salmonellae and *Streptococcus pneumoniae*. *J Infect*; **42**: 44–49.

Hausdorff WP, Bryant J, Paradiso PR et al. (2000). Which pneumococcal serogroups cause the most invasive disease: implications for conjugate vaccine formulation and use, part I. *Clin Infect Dis*; **30**: 100–121.

Jaffar S, Leach A, Hall AJ et al. (1999). Preparation for a pneumococcal vaccine trial in The Gambia: individual or community randomisation? *Vaccine*; **18**: 633–640.

Jones N, Huebner R, Khoosal M et al. (1998). The impact of HIV on Streptococcus pneumoniae bacteraemia in a South African population. *AIDS*; **12**: 2177–2184.

Kim JO, Weiser JN. (1998). Association of intrastrain phase variation in quantity of capsular polysaccharide and teichoic acid with the virulence of *Streptococcus pneumoniae*. *J Infect Dis*; **177**: 368–377.

Klugman KP, Madhi SA. (1999). Emergence of drug resistance. Impact on bacterial meningitis. *Infect Dis Clin North Am*; **13**: 637–646, vii.

Nuorti JP, Butler JC, Farley MM et al. (2000). Cigarette smoking and invasive pneumococcal disease. *N Engl J Med*; **342**: 681–689.

Scott JA, Hall AJ, Muyodi C et al. (2000). Aetiology, outcome, and risk factors for mortality among adults with acute pneumonia in Kenya. *Lancet*; **355**: 1225–1230.

Spellerberg B, Tuomanen EI. (1994). The pathophysiology of pneumococcal meningitis. *Ann Med*; **26**: 411–418.

Tuomanen EI, Austrian R, Masure HR. (1995). Pathogenesis of pneumococcal infection. *N Engl J Med*; **332**: 1280–1284.

Wiktor SZ, Sassan-Morokro M, Grant AD et al. (1999). Efficacy of trimethoprim-sulphamethoxazole prophylaxis to decrease morbidity and mortality in HIV-1-infected patients with tuberculosis in Abidjan, Cote d'Ivoire: a randomised controlled trial [published erratum appears in *Lancet* 1999 Jun 12; **353**(9169): 2078]. *Lancet*; **353**: 1469–1475.

Streptococcus pyogenes

37

The streptococci are a group of 30 species of bacteria. These are usefully divided according to the appearance of their colonies on blood agar plates.

Colonies with a surrounding green pigmented zone (described as α-haemolysis) are *Streptococcus pneumoniae* (see Chapter 36) or one of the large group of *Streptococcus viridans*, which are common oral and nasopharyngeal flora only occasionally causing severe disease (see endocarditis Chapter 76). Non-haemolytic streptococci are rarely pathogenic.

Streptococcal colonies with a surrounding zone of complete haemolysis (clear appearance) are called β-haemolytic streptococci. These were further classified by Rebecca Lancefield in 1933, using serological techniques, into groups A to H and K to V. Of these, Group A β-haemolytic streptococci (also known as *Streptococcus pyogenes*) are by far the most important in causing human disease, and form the subject of this chapter. Some Group B streptococci may cause puerperal sepsis and neonatal infections (including meningitis) in Africa, and Groups C,D and G organisms may cause upper respiratory infections, urinary infections and endocarditis.

The problem in Africa

S. pyogenes causes pharyngitis and pyoderma. Both conditions can be complicated by deep tissue invasion, suppurative (pus-forming) and non-suppurative complications. The important non-suppurative complication of streptococcal pharyngitis is acute rheumatic fever (ARF, see Chapter 76). The important non-suppurative complications of streptococcal pyoderma are ARF or acute glomerular nephritis (AGN, see Chapter 83) (Kechrid et al., 1997). Valvular damage following more severe episodes of ARF causes an estimated 25–40 per cent of all cardiac disease in Africa with 12.6/1000 schoolchildren in Zambia and 10.2/1000 schoolchildren in Sudan affected (WHO, 1992; Kaplan, 1993). Despite the vast excess of pneumococcal disease in HIV-infected adults and children described in Chapter 36, there has not been a marked increase in other streptococcal infections as a result of the HIV pandemic. The reasons for this are unclear.

The organism

S.pyogenes are ovoid gram-positive cocci which grow in long chains in broth, but can be seen in pairs in clinical samples. They have several features which favour virulence:

- a hyaluronic acid capsule which resists phagocytosis
- M protein – a filamentous (hair-like) macromolecule causing inhibition of complement activation at the bacterial surface
- Haemolysins – streptolysin O (*O*xygen-labile), which is toxic to red and white blood cells, and streptolysin S (produced when growing in *S*erum) which causes most of the haemolysis seen on blood agar.
- Liquefaction agents – DNA-ases (A, B, C and D), hyaluronidase, streptokinase, proteinase, amylase and esterase.

Several of these virulence factors are antigenic, e.g. ASO, DNA-ase B (Mhalu & Matre, 1995) hyaluronidase, streptokinase. *S. pyogenes* may also produce streptococcal pyogenic exotoxin which causes the rash of scarlet fever.

Epidemiology

Asymptomatic oro-pharyngeal carriage and skin colonization with *S. pyogenes* are common in children (8–20%)

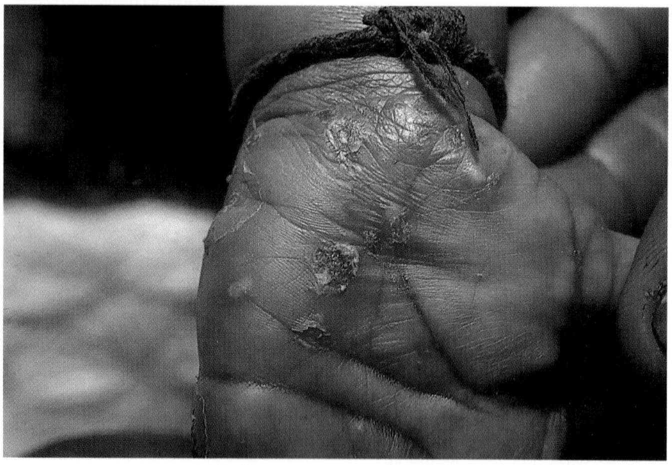

Fig. 37.1. Infected scabies.

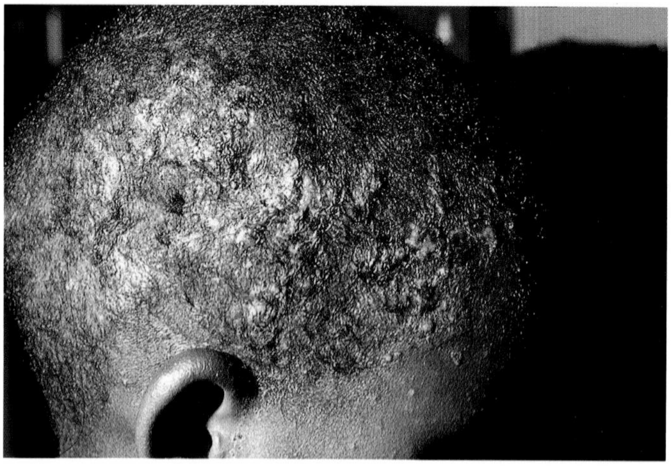

Fig. 37.2. Impetigo scalp: thick crusts.

and adults (5%) (Lawal et al., 1990). Oro-pharyngeal colonization is increased by crowding (as in schools and barracks) and by cold weather. The source of skin infection is uncertain, but spread to the throat takes 10 days. Nasal and oropharyngeal colonization is primarily by droplet infection but food and water-borne outbreaks also occur. Secondary infection of scabies is common, and may become epidemic in crowded unhygienic conditions (Fig 37.1).

Control and prevention

Streptococci are sensitive to penicillin. Prompt treatment prevents local spread and suppurative complications. Unfortunately, one-third of non-suppurative complications follow very mild infections. ARF is only prevented by complete eradication of the streptococcus from the throat. This is achieved with prolonged rather than high dose treatment with penicillin. A single injection of 1.2 megaunits benzathine penicillin G (or a 10-day course of oral penicillin V 250 mg t.d.s.) can be used successfully as late as 9 days after the onset of symptoms. Patients allergic to penicillin are given erythromycin or an oral cephalosporin. There is less evidence that bacterial eradication prevents AGN.

Clinical syndromes

Acute pharyngitis

Most sore throats are caused by viruses (adenovirus, CMV). Streptococcal pharyngitis is most common between 5 and 15 years (Omer et al., 1985) but is also seen in adults. Features suggestive of bacterial pharyngitis are abrupt onset of pain, fever, painful swollen lymph nodes and a greyish exudate with a raised leukocyte count. It is not possible to be certain using clinical or laboratory tests which patients have streptococcal sore throats as 20 per cent of patients will be carriers of *S.pyogenes* regardless of symptoms. These infections are usually self-limiting (3 to 5 days) but prolonged carriage of bacteria is a threat as described above and so penicillin is indicated. If treatment is given in cases with either an exudative tonsillitis or swollen neck glands, this will be 84 per cent sensitive (treated positive cases) and 40 per cent specific (appropriate non-treatment of negative cases)(Steinhoff et al., 1997). Patients treated with 250–500 mg penicillin V orally t.d.s. will feel well after 3 days but will have 50 per cent bacteriological relapse if treatment is stopped then. Treatment should continue for 10 days (34% relapse rate if given for only 6 days).

Streptococcal pyoderma

So-called 'skin strains' of *S. pyogenes* have different M proteins than those causing pharyngitis. Skin infection is associated with hot climate, crowding, scabies (Adjei & Brenya, 1997) and poor hygiene in children under 5 years and with multiple abrasions in adults (e.g. farmers at work- see Chapter 2). Spread of skin infection is by direct contact and environmental contamination. Papules progress to vesicles and then to a crusting impetigo indistinguishable from that caused by *Staphylococcus aureus* (see Chapter 38) (Fig. 37.2). The lesions heal slowly and leave depigmented skin. Treatment is by improved hygiene, difficult unless adequate water is available for washing. Erythromycin 250 mg daily can be given if healing is slow. This antibiotic has the additional benefit that it is more likely to treat disease caused by *S. aureus* in Africa than penicillin.

Invasive streptococcal disease

Erysipelas is marked inflammation of the face following a sore throat. It is seen in infants and adults over the age of 30 and is characterized by a raised swollen edge to the area of erythema, marked peri-orbital oedema and a butterfly distribution on the face. The same raised reaction can be seen as a spreading wound infection. *Cellulitis* is a rapidly spreading infection often complicating burns, characterized by tenderness, swelling and the lack of a distinct edge. Cellulitis and erysipelas are more common in limbs with blocked lymphatics, e.g. following filariasis, and patients often present with features of systemic toxicity. Erysipelas and cellulitis are treated with high dose penicillin (penicillin V 500mg q.d.s. p.o. or benzyl penicillin 2 megaunits 4 hrly i.v.; alternatively use erythromycin in patients allergic to penicillin).

Necrotizing fasciitis

This is extensive rapidly spreading necrosis with gangrene of the skin and underlying tissue. It progresses rapidly from erythema to purplish discolouration with fluid collection and then extensive sloughing of the skin. Treatment is with extensive surgical debridement and high dose penicillin. Failure of adequate debridement is fatal – even optimally treated this condition has a mortality of 20 per cent.

Toxic shock syndrome (TSS)

This is a rare complication of streptococcal skin infections or puerperal sepsis. TSS is found in all ages and has equal incidence in male and females. It differs from staphylococcal toxic shock syndrome (Chapter 38) in that 60 per cent of patients with streptococcal TSS have positive blood cultures. After a 'flu-like prodrome, intense pain, fever, prostration, swelling and erythema are followed by hypotensive collapse and multiorgan failure. The mortality of this syndrome is 30–70 per cent with full intensive care support. It is important to note that the strains causing the syndrome are highly contagious and prophylactic benzathine penicillin should be given to staff and family contacts.

Local and suppurative complications of streptococcal infection

Pharyngitis can be complicated by peritonsillar cellulitis, retropharyngeal abscess, otitis media, sinusitis and suppurative cervical adenitis. Extension of pharyngeal infection can lead to meningitis, brain abscess, venous sinus thrombosis and pneumonia. Haematogenous spread can lead to arthritis, endocarditis and osteomyelitis.

Diagnosis

Identification of the organism

Throat swabs to diagnose streptococcal pharyngitis should be collected by vigorous swabbing of both tonsillar fossae and the posterior pharynx. Success is dependent on the size of the collected inoculum, but the bacteria are resistant to drying and so swabs can be transported dry for 48–72 hours. The organism can be plated on selective blood agar or grown in nutrient broth for 24–48 hours. Skin lesions are best sampled from fluid collections. Resulting isolates are identified by gram stain and serology.

Immunological tests

These are not very helpful. Raised or rising anti-streptolysin O antibodies (ASOT) help to distinguish episodes of pharyngitis with an increased risk of ARF. This test is of limited benefit as the antibody does not rise acutely and is not available in many hospitals. For streptococcal pyoderma, ASOT is weak but anti-DNAase B is strong.

Non-suppurative complications

ARF and AGN are dealt with in Chapters 76 and 83, respectively.

Unsolved problems

- There is still no fast, cheap and accurate method of distinguishing streptococcal pharyngitis from other sore throats.
- There is no vaccine against streptococcal disease, or particularly against the strains causing aggressively invasive disease or severe complications.

References

Adjei O, Brenya RC. (1997). Secondary bacterial infection in Ghanaian patients with scabies. *East Afr Med J*; **74**: 729–731.

Kaplan EL. (1993). T. Duckett Jones Memorial Lecture. Global assessment of rheumatic fever and rheumatic heart disease at the close of the century. Influences and dynamics of populations and pathogens: a failure to realize prevention? [published erratum appears in *Circulation* 1994 Mar; 89(3): A98]. *Circulation*; **88**: 1964–1972.

Kechrid A, Kharrat H, Bousnina S, Kriz P, Kaplan EL. (1997). Acute rheumatic fever in Tunisia. Serotypes of group A streptococci associated with rheumatic fever. *Adv Exp Med Biol*; **418**: 121–123.

Lawal SF, Odugbemi T, Coker AO, Solanke EO. (1990). Persistent occurrence of beta-haemolytic streptococci in a population of Lagos school children. *J Trop Med Hyg*; **93**: 417–418.

Mhalu FS, Matre R. (1995). Antistreptolysin O and antideoxyribonuclease B titres in blood donors and in patients with features of nonsuppurative sequelae of group A streptococcus infection in Tanzania. *East Afr Med J*; **72**: 33–36.

Omer EF, Hadi AE, Sakhi ES. (1985). Bacteriology of sore throats in a Sudanese population. *J Trop Med Hyg*; **88**: 337–341.

Steinhoff MC, Abde KM, Khallaf N et al. (1997). Effectiveness of clinical guidelines for the presumptive treatment of streptococcal pharyngitis in Egyptian children *Lancet*; **350**: 918–921.

WHO. (1992). WHO programme for the prevention of rheumatic fever/rheumatic heart disease in 16 developing countries: report from phase 1 (1986–1990). *Bull Wld Hlth Org*; **70**: 213–218.

38

Staphylococcus aureus

The staphylococci are a group of common skin commensal bacteria that also cause disease when the epidermis is breached. The most important pathogen is *Staphylococcus aureus* which causes skin and deep infections, and toxic shock syndromes. *Staphylococcus epidermidis* is a common skin commensal that also causes disease in association with lines used for venous access and other foreign material inserted into the body.

The problem in Africa

Skin and tissue infections are common in Africa, and pyomyositis is a particular regional problem (Selassie, 1995) that has been exacerbated by the HIV epidemic. An increased HIV seroprevalence was noted in cases of pyomyositis in Uganda in 1996 (Ansalonl et al. 1996). A recent study in Blantyre, Malawi, found that 85 per cent of patients with pyomyositis were HIV-positive, compared to 30 per cent of control patients (M. Callaghan, unpublished observations).

The organism

Staphylococci are hardy gram-positive ovoid bacteria, which grow in clusters on solid media (*staphyle* is the Greek word for bunch of grapes), but can remain viable in dry dust for months. When cultured in liquid media or taken from clinical samples, they do not clump and may stain deceptively poorly with gram stain (and so appear gram-negative). Colony morphology and production of enzymes as well as antibiotic resistance patterns distinguish the different species of staphylococci causing human disease. *S. aureus* has 1–4 mm beige or gold colonies on blood agar and is coagulase-positive, while *S. epidermidis* has white colonies and is the most common of 32 coagulase-negative species.

Virulence factors that are important in staphylococcal invasion and disease include peptidoglycan, protein A, enzymes and toxins. Peptidoglycan (a gram-positive cell wall component) elicits a substantial inflammatory response even in the absence of viable bacteria. Protein A (a soluble extracellular staphylococcal product) binds immunoglobulin F_c fragment and reduces the concentration and effectiveness of local and circulating immunoglobulin. Enzymes produced by staphylococci include catalase (reduces H_2O_2 to H_2O and makes bacteria more resistant to neutrophil attack), coagulase, hyaluronidase, β-lactamase and clumping factor, all of which are associated with virulence. Toxins produced by staphylococci include epidermolytic toxins (Adesiyun et al., 1991) enterotoxins (which cause diarrhoea), toxic shock syndrome toxins, and toxins which cause cell lysis, particularly of red blood cells. The toxic shock staphylococcal toxins (e.g. TSST-1) are the most dangerous and are found in 11 per cent of Nigerian isolates (Adesiyun et al., 1992).

Host risk factors play an important part in susceptibility to pyogenic infection (discussed in Chapter 6). Particular vulnerability to staphylococcal infection is found in patients with diabetes mellitus, HIV infection, or implanted foreign material (intravenous catheters, sutures, ventriculo-peritoneal shunts). Patients with diabetes and HIV infection have increased nasopharyngeal carriage of *Staphylococcus aureus* (Amir et al., 1995), together with increased infections due to altered antibody production and phagocyte function. The presence of a foreign body stimulates invading staphylococci to produce a protective glycocalyx, which reduces polymorphonuclear cell activity, allows bacteria to bind to surface-coated fibronectin and reduces antibiotic sensitivity.

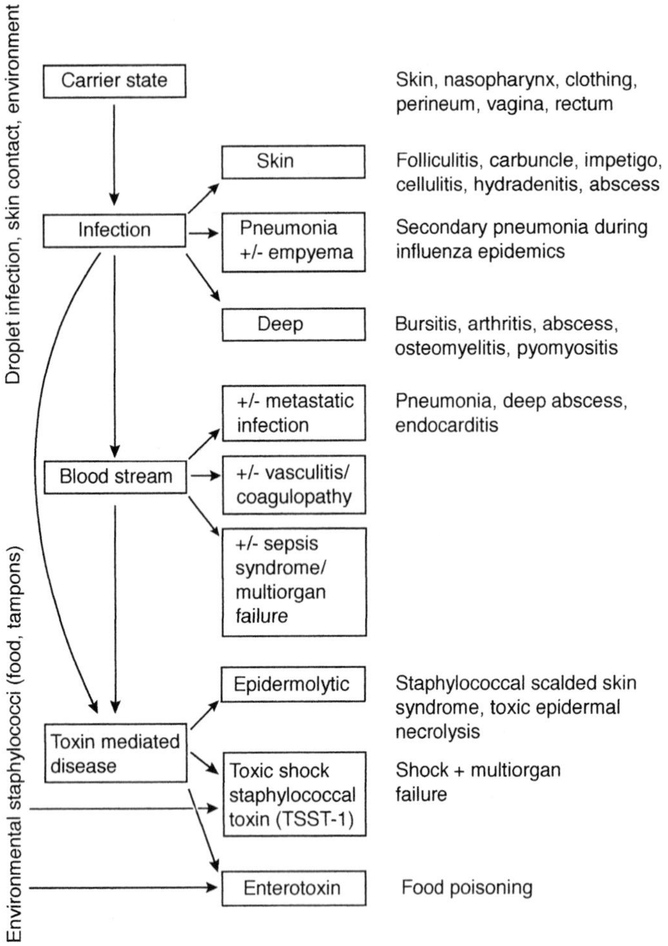

Fig. 38.1. Variety of clinical syndromes caused by staphylococci.

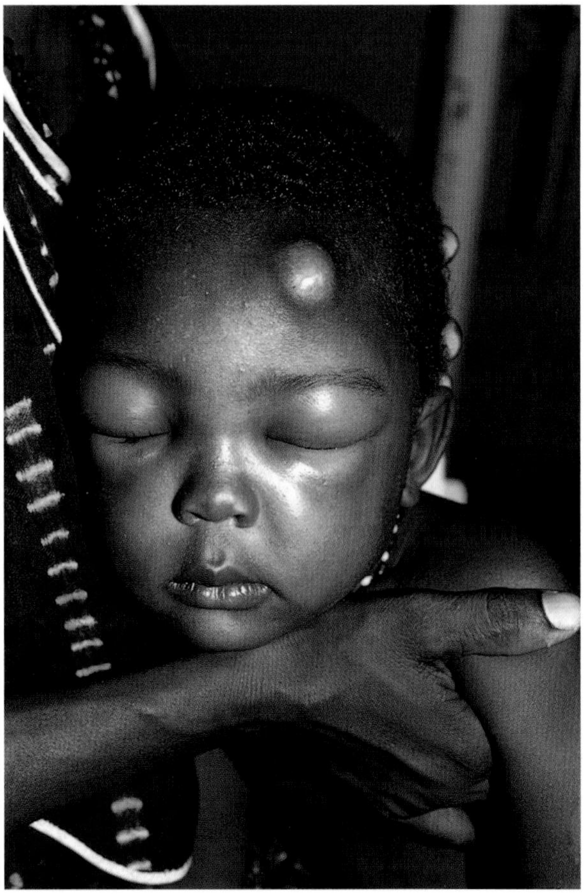

Fig. 38.2. Carbuncle.

Epidemiology

Staphylococci are ubiquitous and colonize the skin, nasopharynx, vagina and perineum in 25–40 per cent of people of all ages. New strains are acquired from other body sites, skin contact, droplet infection and the environment. Carriage is increased in hospital staff, intravenous drug abusers and patients with diabetes mellitus. The carrier state progresses to disease when the epidermis is breached and local, blood stream or metastatic infections result. Toxic syndromes occur when toxin producing strains cause any of these infections.

Control and prevention

Staphylococci are commonly carried by hospital staff and dangerous when infecting hospital patients (Olusanya et al., 1991). Control depends on detailed attention to hygiene and in particular, to hand washing on wards. Disease only occurs when the organism breaches the epithelium. Prevention of disease is therefore achieved by meticulous hygiene in wound management (Kotisso & Aseffa, 1998), the care of intravenous lines and during operative procedures.

Clinical syndromes

Staphylococci cause a variety of clinical syndromes illustrated in Fig. 38.1 and described below.

Skin infections with no rash

S.aureus causes superficial and deep purulent skin infections. Infection can occur in single hair follicles (folliculitis; sycosis barbae), in multiple follicles causing a coalescent abscess (carbuncle; boil, Fig. 38.2), in apocrine sweat glands (hydradinitis suppurativa) and in breasts, particularly in lactating mothers (mastitis). In children, red macules develop to a crusting infection (impetigo, Fig. 38.3). Following minor trauma, burns or infection of a surgical wound, an increase of pain and swelling after 2 days (cellulitis) may be complicated by the formation of a wound abscess, or spread to the lymphatics (lymphangitis) or soft tissues (necrotizing fasciitis). The more extensive skin infections cause fever and symptoms of malaise. Recurrent staphylococcal skin infections may be caused by an underlying defect in host defence, e.g. diabetes mellitus (Archibald et al., 1997), or by the presence of scabies (Adjei & Brenya, 1997).

Skin infections with a rash

In children infected with a toxin-producing strain of *S.aureus*, a severe red rash is followed by extensive skin loss (staphylococcal scalded skin syndrome, Fig. 38.4). This condition is rare in adults in whom toxic epidermal necrolysis is most commonly caused by adverse drug reactions.

Septicaemia and endocarditis

Skin infections may spread to the bloodstream in adults with impaired immunity (e.g. diabetes mellitus, intravenous drug abuse). *S.aureus* septicaemia can be complicated by destructive endocarditis (see Chapter 76)(Hodes, 1993), with multiple septic infarcts in the spleen, brain and kidney. Coagulase-negative staphylococci cause septicaemia by infection of intravenous catheters and implanted foreign bodies including heart valves and joint replacements (Okoro & Ohaegbulam, 1995). Vegetations on the right side of the heart can lead to septic pulmonary infarcts, which rapidly cavitate.

Pneumonia and empyema

Staphylococcal pneumonia occurs with increased frequency during influenza outbreaks (see Chapters 18 and 19) and can also be a complication of septicaemia and measles. This is a severe, rapidly progessive, cavitating pneumonia which fails to respond to standard treatment. Empyema due to staphylococci is frequently complicated by bronchopleural fistula.

Deep tissue infections, osteomyelitis and pyomyositis

Deep tissue infections may occur due to septicaemia but are more usually due to extension from a local skin infection. Osteomyelitis of the long bones is more common in children (Figs 38.5 and 38.6). Vertebral osteomyelitis is seen in adults and has a high risk of neurological complication. Staphylococcal septic arthritis occurs in previously damaged joints and can cause complete joint destruction in days if untreated. Pyomyositis is rare in developed countries but common in Africa (Fig. 38.7). Patients usually present with advanced tissue infection and destruction in large muscles. A history of preceding blunt trauma to the site was reported to be common, but this has not been confirmed in the recent Blantyre series where HIV infection was the most important risk factor (M. Callaghan, unpublished observations).

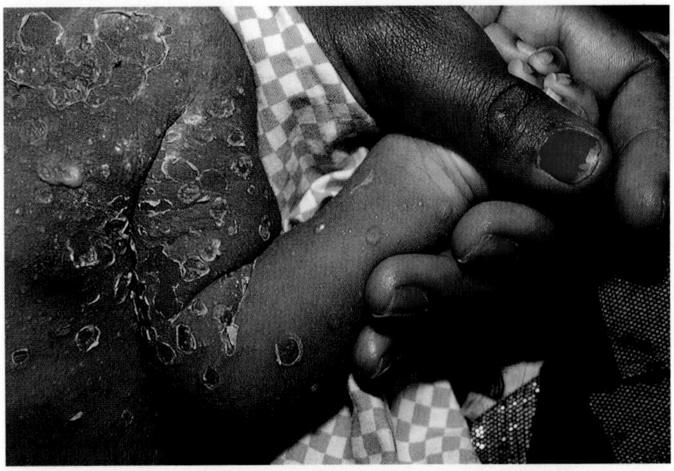

Fig. 38.3. Impetigo.

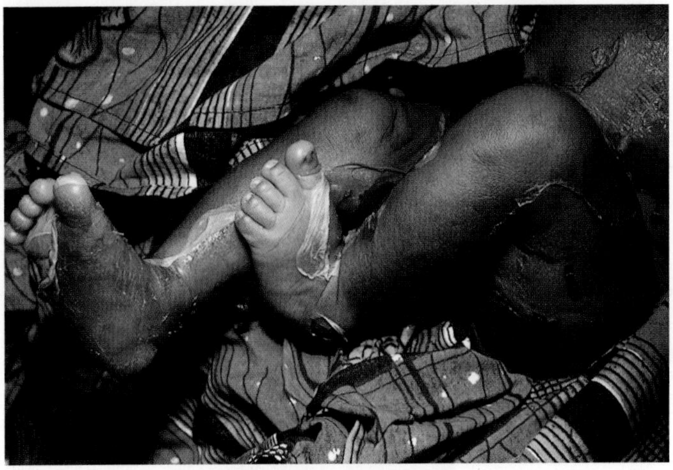

Fig. 38.4. Staphylococcal scalded skin syndrome.

Shock syndromes

Staphylococcal toxins released at the site of skin or deep infections can cause a syndrome of severe hypotension, high fever and rash. Diarrhoea and mucous membrane swelling, cramps (with raised muscle enzymes), confusion and renal failure may accompany this. Multi-organ failure follows. Toxic shock syndromes are associated with the prolonged use of tampons by menstruating women, and with previous antibiotic use and nosocomial infection in other adults.

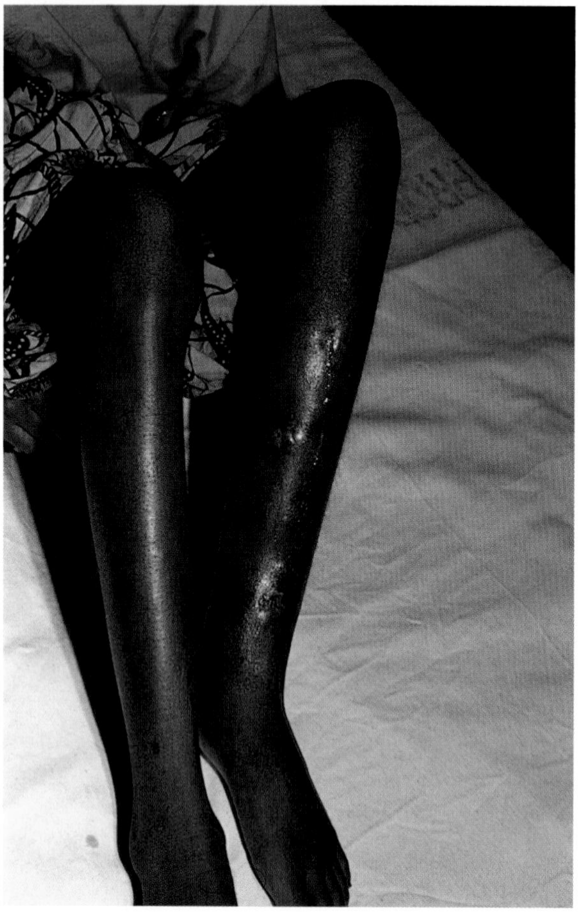

Fig. 38.5. Osteomyelitis: discharging sinuses.

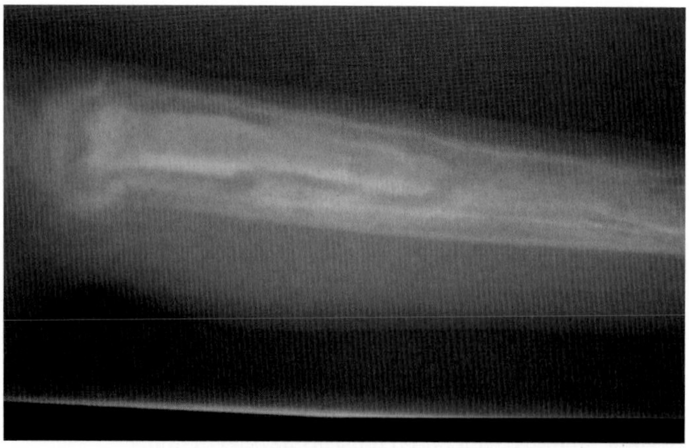

Fig. 38.6. Osteomyelitis: bone changes.

Food poisoning

A milder toxin-related illness due to staphylococcus occurs when toxin-producing strains colonize food handlers. Enterotoxin in milk-based foods is heat stable (Ombui et al., 1992) and produces acute salivation, vomiting and watery diarrhoea 2–6 hours after ingestion of contaminated food. This is not accompanied by rash or fever and is a self-limiting illness diagnosed on the history. Contaminated food sources should be traced.

Diagnosis and treatment

Diagnosis of skin infections is by clinical presentation. Septicaemia is diagnosed by positive blood culture with appropriate clinical signs. Staphylococci in blood culture isolates are more likely to be clinically significant if the isolate is coagulase-positive (*S. aureus*) and a focus of infection can be identified. Patients with toxic syndromes usually have negative blood cultures and the organism must be cultured from the focal site of infection to determine antibiotic sensitivity. This may include searching for pelvic causes of infection, including retained tampons and prostatic abscess (Angwafo et al., 1996).

Identification of the organism

This is by culture of blood, pus, biopsy material, swab or urine according to clinical presentation. *S.saprophyticus* is a coagulase-negative cause of asymptomatic bacteriuria (Gebre-Selassie, 1998).

Penicillin resistance and MRSA

Most staphylococci are resistant to penicillin.
This resistance is due to production of β-lactamases (carried on plasmids, which may also carry erythromycin

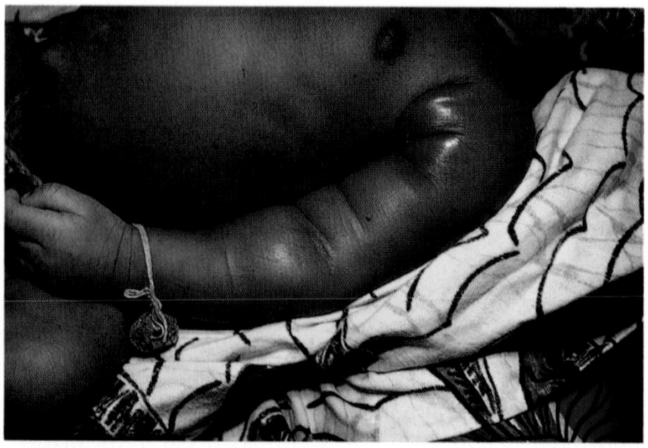

Fig. 38.7. Pyomyositis.

resistance) and mutation of penicillin-binding proteins (chromosome derived resistance). Antibiotic resistance patterns are therefore variable and should be determined wherever possible to guide treatment (Adeleke & Odelola, 1997). Methicillin resistant *S. aureus* (MRSA) are resistant to almost all antibiotics and present a severe risk in vulnerable patients (Hayanga et al., 1997; Musa et al., 1999). Where staphylococcal infections occur in several patients, ward staff should have nasal swabs collected and carriers should be treated with topical neomycin.

Treatment

Treatment of uncomplicated skin infections is by drainage of pus, careful daily washing with antiseptic and dressing. Patients with systemic infections require antibiotic therapy with penicillinase-stable penicillin. This must be started empirically in the ill patient while awaiting sensitivities. For skin infections with systemic symptoms, give cloxacillin or flucloxacillin 500 mg q.d.s. orally for 7 days. For deep tissue infections, osteomyelitis and endocarditis, consider vancomycin 1g b.d. by slow i.v. infusion (100 minutes) or sodium fusidate 500 mg t.d.s. in combination with flucloxacillin. Toxic syndromes are treated supportively once the focus of infection has been found and treated aggressively.

Prognosis

In the pre-antibiotic era, *S.aureus* bacteraemia had a mortality of 80 per cent. The appropriate use of antibiotics has reduced this to 20 per cent. Septic shock has a mortality of 40 per cent (Smith et al., 1991) and the mortality of toxic shock syndrome with multi-organ failure is higher still.

Unsolved problems

Antibiotic resistance is the big problem in staphylococcal infections. Newer effective agents are few in number and very expensive.

Summary points

1. Staphylococcal infections are common and potentially serious.
2. Many infections are preventable.
3. Most staphylococci are penicillin resistant.

References

Adeleke OE, Odelola HA. (1997). Plasmid profiles of multiple drug resistant local strains of *Staphylococcus aureus*. *Afr J Med Sci*; **26**: 119–121.

Adesiyun AA, Lenz W, Schaal KP. (1991). Exfoliative toxin production by Staphylococcus aureus strains isolated from animals and human beings in Nigeria. *Microbiologica*; **14**: 357–362.

Adesiyun AA, Lenz W, Schaal KP. (1992). Production of toxic shock syndrome toxin-1 (TSST-1) by *Staphylococcus aureus* strains isolated from humans, animals and foods in Nigeria. *Microbiologica*; **15**: 125–133.

Adjei O, Brenya RC. (1997). Secondary bacterial infection in Ghanaian patients with scabies. *E Afr Med J*; **74**: 729–731.

Amir M, Paul J, Batchelor B et al. (1995). Nasopharyngeal carriage of *Staphylococcus aureus* and carriage of tetracycline-resistant strains associated with HIV-seropositivity. *Eur J Clin Microbiol Infect Dis*; **14**: 34–40.

Angwafo FF, Sosso AM, Muna WF, Edzoa T, Juimo AG. (1996). Prostatic abscesses in sub-Saharan Africa: a hospital-based experience from Cameroon. *Eur Urol*; **30**: 28–33.

Ansalonl L, Acaye GL, Re MC. (1996). High HIV seroprevalence among patients with pyomyositis in northern Uganda. *Trop Med Int Health*; **1**: 210–212.

Archibald LK, Gill GV, Abbas Z. (1997). Fatal hand sepsis in Tanzanian diabetic patients. *Diabet Med*; **14**: 607–610.

Gebre-Selassie S. (1998). Asymptomatic bacteriuria in pregnancy: epidemiological, clinical and microbiological approach. *Ethiop Med J*; **36**: 185–192.

Hayanga A, Okello A, Hussein R, Nyong'o A. (1997). Experience with methicillin resistant *Staphylococcus aureus* at the Nairobi Hospital. *E Afr Med J*; **74**: 203–204.

Hodes RM. (1993). Endocarditis in Ethiopia. Analysis of 51 cases from Addis Ababa. *Trop Geogr Med*; **45**: 70–72.

Kotisso B, Aseffa A. (1998). Surgical wound infection in a teaching hospital in Ethiopia. *E Afr Med J*; **75**: 402–405.

Musa HA, Shears P, Khagali A. (1999). First report of MRSA from hospitalized patients in Sudan [letter]. *J Hosp Infect*; **42**: 74.

Okoro BA, Ohaegbulam SC. (1995). Experience with ventriculo peritoneal shunts at the University of Nigeria Teaching Hospital, Enugu. *E Afr Med J*; **72**: 322–324.

Olusanya O, Ogunledun A, Olambiwonnu JA et al. (1991). Carriage of *Staphylococcus aureus* among hospital personnel in a Nigerian hospital environment. *Cent Afr J Med*; **37**: 83–87.

Ombui JN, Arimi SM, Kayihura M. (1992). Raw milk as a source of enterotoxigenic *Staphylococcus aureus* and enterotoxins in consumer milk [see comments]. *E Afr Med J*; **69**: 123–125.

Selassie FG. (1995). Tropical pyomyositis in Gondar, Ethiopia. *Trop Geogr Med*; **47**: 200–202.

Smith C, Arregui LM, Promnitz DA, Feldman C. (1991). Septic shock in the Intensive Care Unit, Hillbrow Hospital, Johannesburg. *S Afr Med J*; **80**: s181–s184.

39 *Neisseria meningitidis*

The problem in Africa

Neisseria meningitidis (the meningococcus) is an important cause of meningitis and septicaemia world-wide but infection with this organism is especially prevalent in the countries of the Sahel and sub-Sahel – the African meningitis belt (Lapeyssonnie, 1963) (Fig. 39.1). In this region of Africa, massive epidemics of meningococcal disease have occurred every 5–10 years throughout the past 100 years (Fig. 39.2) (Greenwood, 1999). Why this should be the case is still not certain. Climate is almost certainly important as epidemics rarely spread from the sub-Sahel into neighbouring forested and more humid regions. Furthermore, epidemics occur predominantly in the dry season when absolute humidity is very low (Fig. 39.3). It is possible that the hot, dry and dusty climate characteristic of the harmattan[1] season impairs the local defences of the nasopharynx and predisposes to invasive meningococcal disease.

African epidemics of meningococcal disease may be massive. In 1996, at least 100 000 cases and 10 000 deaths were reported in Nigeria alone; the true incidence is likely to have been two or three times more than this.

The meningococcus

N. meningitidis is a gram-negative diplococcus that is susceptible to a high environmental temperature so that samples collected in the field must be kept cool but not frozen. Meningococci will survive for several days if inoculated into transport medium. Meningococci grow readily on blood agar and chocolate agar plates, producing characteristic colonies. Isolation of meningococci from nasopharyngeal swabs is facilitated by growth on a selective medium containing vancomycin, which inhibits the growth of other bacteria. Meningococci are oxidase-positive and can be differentiated from other less pathogenic *Neisseria* by sugar reactions.

Meningococci possess an outer polysaccharide capsule (Fig. 39.4). At least ten chemically distinct polysaccharide capsules have been described, the commonest of which are designated as groups A,B,C, X,Y,Z W135 and 29e. Differentiation of meningococci according to their capsular group is important because of the link between serogroup and epidemiological characteristics – for example, most large epidemics are caused by bacteria that belong to serogroups A or C. Meningococci can also be typed on the basis of their outer membrane proteins, their lipopolysaccharide or by direct sequencing of a number of genes (multilocus sequence typing)(MLST). Such studies have shown that epidemics are usually caused by meningococci that are genetically closely related, for example the major epidemics seen in Africa during the late 1980s and 1990s were caused by a group of closely related bacteria characterized as clone ET111–1. Molecular typing of meningococci allows the micro-evolution of meningococci to be studied (Morelli et al. 1997) and the spread of the meningococcus from country to country to be followed. There is good evidence that the meningococci responsible for the African epidemics of the late 1980s travelled to Africa from Mecca with returning pilgrims.

Epidemiology

Meningococci are usually spread from person to person by respiratory droplets; rarely sexual transmission occurs. Asymptomatic nasopharyngeal carriage of meningococci is common, especially among those who live in poor

1 The harmattan is a dry wind which blows from the North East across West Africa from about November–February, and brings a fine dust.

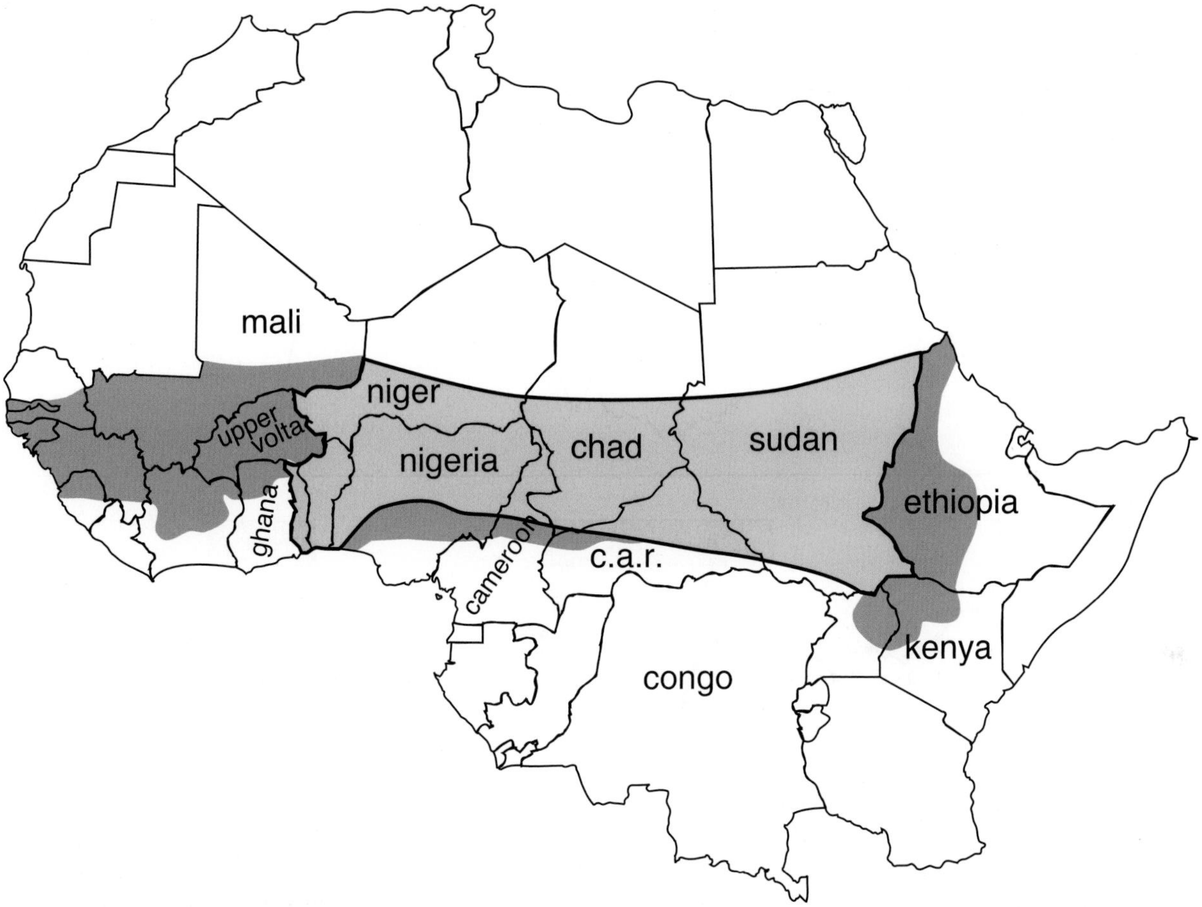

Fig. 39.1. The African meningitis belt. The pale area indicates the belt as first defined by Lapeyssonnie (1963). The darker areas indicate regions to the west and the east of the original belt where typical epidemics of meningococcal disease are now known to occur.

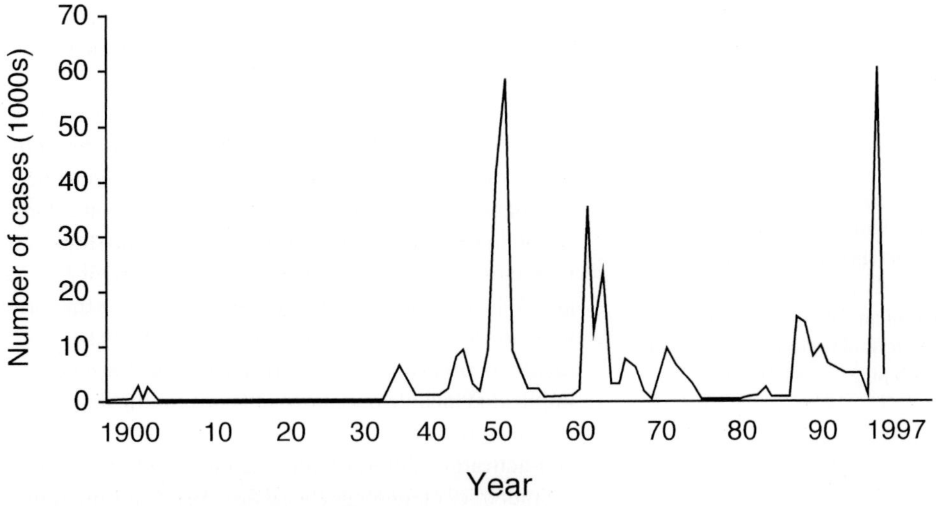

Fig. 39.2. Cases of meningococcal meningitis in Nigeria indicating the periodicity and size of epidemics (based on data obtained from the World Health Organization).

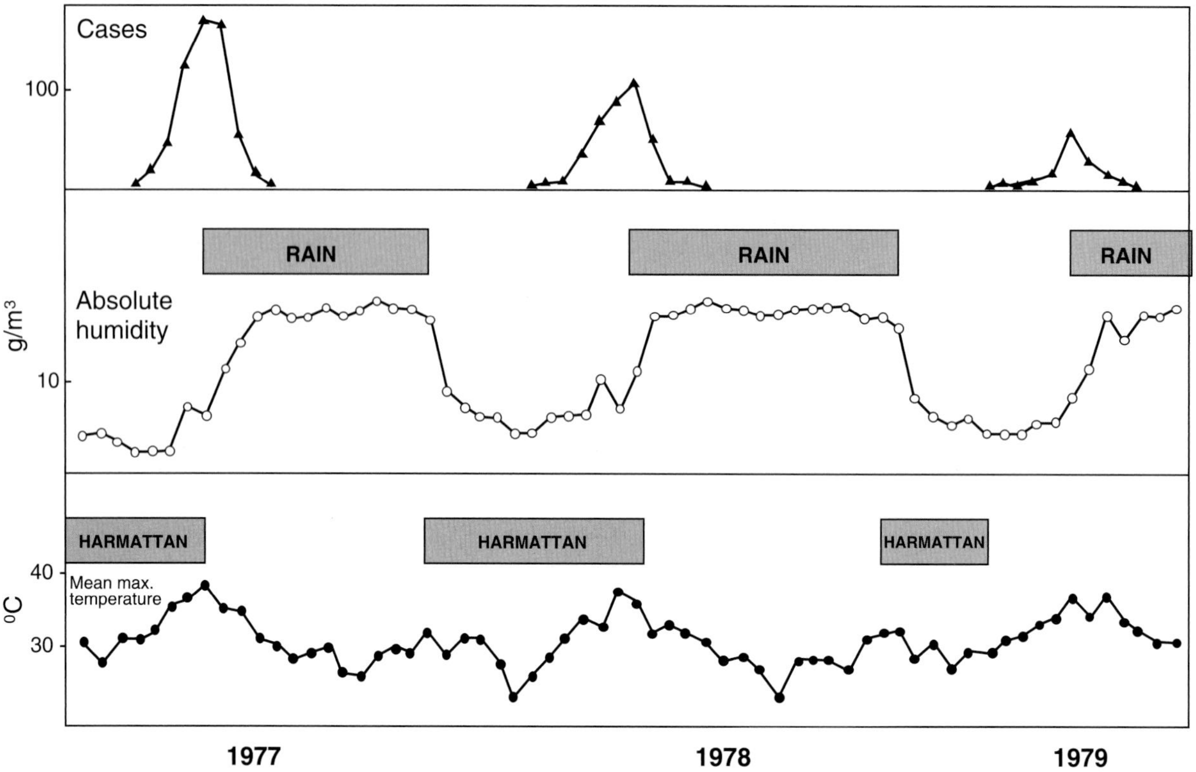

Fig. 39.3. The relationship of epidemic meningococcal disease to climatic variables in northern Nigeria (Greenwood et al., 1979).

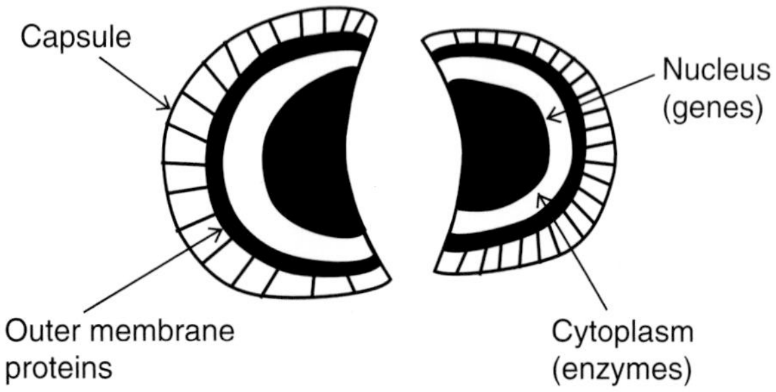

Fig. 39.4. Schematic representation of the meningococcus. Meningococci are frequently typed on the basis of the chemical structure of their capsular polysaccharide and outer membrane proteins. Thus a meningococcus designated B15:Pl.16 has a serogroup B capsule, a type 15 class 2/3 outer membrane protein and a type 16 outer membrane protein. Alternative typing methods are based on electrophoresis of bacterial enzymes (ET) or sequencing of several house-keeping genes (MLST).

social circumstances. Nasopharyngeal carriage of the outbreak strain usually increases during epidemics but it is not possible to predict epidemics on the basis of changes in the carriage rate. The proportion of new infections that results in clinical illness, as opposed to asymptomatic carriage, is usually small, perhaps as low as 1: 1000, but this ratio may increase during epidemics when attack rates as high as 1: 10 of the population have been recorded. Secondary cases may occur among the close contacts of cases. Why a minority of individuals develops severe disease when exposed to a strain of meningococcus that produces asymptomatic nasopharyngeal colonization in the majority of exposed subjects is not fully understood. Both environmental and host genetic factors are likely to be involved. There is some evidence that prior infection with influenza increases susceptibility to meningococcal disease. Genetic factors that have been implicated include mutations in genes coding for complement components, tumour necrosis factor, plasminogen-activator-inhibitor 1 and mannose binding protein.

Epidemics of meningococcal disease occur from time to time throughout Africa but it is only in the meningitis belt that they occur frequently and on a massive scale.

These epidemics have specific characteristics which are shown in the Box.

Features of epidemics of meningococcal disease in the African meningitis belt

Epidemics of meningococcal disease occur from time to time throughout Africa but in countries of the Sahel and sub-Sahel they show characteristic clinical features. These include the following.

- Epidemics occur every 5–10 years.
- Epidemics may be very large and attack rates very high.
- Epidemics nearly always start in the dry season, dying down in the rainy season.
- Epidemics affect all age groups with a peak in those aged 5–14 years.
- Epidemics are usually caused by meningococci belonging to serogroup A; less frequently epidemics are caused by serogroup C meningococci or a combination of group A and group C bacteria. However, in 2002 a large epidemic in Burkina Faso was caused by meningococci belonging to serogroup W135, the first time this has been recorded in Africa raising the possibility of further W135 outbacks in other countries (Deosa & Koama, 2002).

If an epidemic could be predicted, the health authorities could initiate control measures before the outbreak establishes its hold. Predicting epidemics is difficult but some success has been obtained in countries of the meningitis belt using the weekly incidence of cases to define a threshold value above which an epidemic is likely to occur. Initially, this threshold was set at an incidence of 15 cases per week averaged over a period of 2 weeks in an area of at least 40 km × 40 km (Moore et al., 1992). Recently, WHO has issued some new guidelines for epidemic prediction which are more flexible than previous versions and which can be used in small populations (World Health Organization, 2000) (Box). Epidemic prediction requires the accurate documentation of cases of meningitis seen at peripheral centres and the rapid transfer of this information to a co-ordinating centre; this is difficult to achieve in some of the more remote regions of the Sahel.

Control

Control of an outbreak

An epidemic of meningococcal disease can be a frightening experience as it can progress with great rapidity, causing panic in the community and overwhelming the clinical services. Thus, it is essential that in areas where epidemics are likely to occur, procedures for dealing with such an emergency are established in advance. Some of the steps that need to be taken in dealing with an epidemic are summarized in the Box and described in more detail in a WHO report (World Health Organization, 1998).

In the past, chemoprophylaxis with sulphonamides was used to control epidemics of meningococcal disease in Africa. Sulphonamides eliminated carriage and thus interrupted transmission. However, most meningococci are now resistant to sulphonamides and alternatives such as minocyline, rifampicin or ciprofloxacin are too costly for mass administration. Furthermore, there are concerns about the widespread use of rifampicin in communities where tuberculosis is prevalent. Thus, chemoprophylaxis is not recommended for the control of large epidemics in

Prediction of an epidemic

Accurate surveillance of the incidence of cases of meningococcal disease can help to predict an epidemic. Recently WHO has published new guidelines. Two thresholds are proposed – an alert threshold and an epidemic threshold.

	Size of population under surveillance <30 000	>30 000
Alert threshold	• 2 cases in a week • increase in cases over numbers in previous years	5 cases/100 000 population/week
Epidemic threshold	• 5 cases in a week • doubling in cases over a 3-week period, e.g. week 1 – 1 case, week 2 – 2 cases week 3 – 4 cases	15 cases/100 000 population/ week *or* 10 cases/100 000 population/week **if** (a) no epidemic for 3 years and vaccination coverage <80%. (b) threshold crossed early in the dry season.

Crossing the alert threshold should instigate enhanced surveillance and initiation of steps for dealing with a possible epidemic, crossing the epidemic threshold should initiate vaccination.
(WHO, 2000)

> **Managing an epidemic**
> In areas where epidemics of meningococcal disease are frequent, an emergency procedure for dealing with epidemics should be in place. Once surveillance suggests that an epidemic is occurring, a number of steps should be started as soon as possible – speed is essential as epidemics can spread with great rapidity.
> - Activate the emergency procedure and call-up epidemic management committee.
> - Inform the local population through press, radio etc.
> - Notify national and international authorities.
> - Confirm the aetiology of the outbreak and determine the serogroup and antibiotic sensitivity of the causative meningococcus.
> - Ensure the peripheral health centres in the epidemic area have adequate supplies of antibiotics including Tifomycine®.
> - Establish temporary treatment centres if needed.
> - Obtain vaccine and syringes if epidemic is due to a group A or group C meningococcus and initiate vaccination of the affected population. If vaccine supplies are limited vaccination of children and young adults should be given preference.
>
> A new grouping of WHO, NGOs and vaccine manufacturers – the International Co-ordinating Group (ICG) has been established to facilitate rapid dispatch of vaccines and syringes from central stores in Europe to areas where an epidemic has been documented.

Africa. However, rifampicin (600 mg b.d. for 2 days for an adult and 10 mg/kg b.d for 2 days for a child) is sometimes used in the control of small, localized outbreaks.

It has been shown on many occasions during the past 30 years that mass vaccination with a meningococcal polysaccharide vaccine halts epidemics of group A and group C meningococcal disease. However, vaccination often takes place only after an epidemic has become well established and after many deaths have already occurred. The international community has recently taken steps to reduce the time between notification of an epidemic and the start of a mass vaccination campaign (see the Box). Because of the recent occurrence of W135 outbacks a trivalent A.C. W135 polysaccharide vaccine is being developed.

Primary prevention

Epidemic meningococcal disease is a disease of poverty which has largely disappeared from the wealthy countries of the world, so improvement of social conditions in Africa should reduce the frequency of epidemics. However, in the meantime, routine vaccination of the population before an epidemic offers the best prospect for controlling this disease.

The meningococcal polysaccharide vaccines that are highly effective in halting epidemics provide only short lasting protection in young children (Reingold et al. 1985), they do not induce immunological memory and they have little or no effect on nasopharyngeal carriage. Nevertheless, it has been suggested that a programme of routine immunization with four doses of group A meningococcal polysaccharide vaccine given during the first 5 years of life should be introduced in countries of the African meningitis belt, in combination with a programme of catch up vaccination in adults (Robbins et al., 1997). Vaccination on a regular basis outside the routine EPI schedule would be difficult and there are concerns about the safety of repeated injections of polysaccharide, especially group C polysaccharide, in young children. Nevertheless, this approach has the advantage that it could be implemented immediately with a cheap and safe vaccine.

The development of polysaccharide/protein conjugate vaccines (see Chapter 8) provides an alternative and, ultimately, a more promising approach to the prevention of epidemic meningococcal disease. These vaccines are immunogenic in very young children, induce immunological memory, providing long-term protection, and they will probably reduce carriage, providing herd protection (Campagne et al., 2000). A group C meningococcal conjugate vaccine has recently been introduced into the EPI programme of the UK and initial results suggest that it has been highly effective, providing 80–90 per cent protection. No group A meningococcal conjugate vaccine is yet commercially available.

However, work is now under way to develop a group A conjugate vaccine for Africa through a public/private partnership (p. 528).

Pathogenesis and pathology

In some patients with invasive meningococcal disease, bacterial multiplication within the circulation results in a severe systemic illness (acute meningococcaemia) with few localizing features. However, in the majority of patients, the systemic phase of the infection is transitory and illness results only when bacteria localize at a peripheral site, most frequently the meninges. Rarely, a chronic septicaemic illness occurs (chronic meningococcaemia) which is characterized by recurrent episodes of fever, rash and splenomegaly.

Multiplication of bacteria in the circulation leads to the release of endotoxin which activates cytokine, complement and clotting pathways producing shock and bleeding (Pathan et al., 2000). Release of endotoxin by bacteria

Table 39.1. Clinical features of invasive meningococcal disease

Feature	Acute meningococcaemia	Meningitis
Symptoms		
Duration	Often <1 day	2–3 days
Fever	++	++
Malaise	++	++
Headache	+	+++
Neck pain	±	+++
Photophobia	±	++
Diarrhoea	+	−
Signs		
Stiff neck	±	+++
Impaired consciousness	++	++
Shock	++	−
Renal failure	++	±
Petechiae	++	++
Bleeding	++	−
Laboratory findings		
Positive blood culture	++	+
Positive CSF culture	−	++

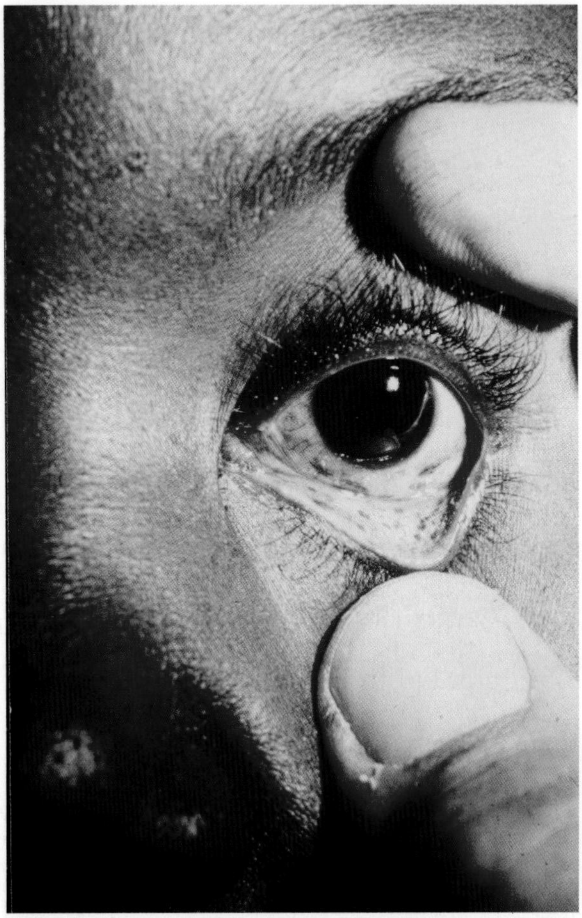

Fig. 39.5. Conjunctival petechiae in a patient with meningococcal septicaemia (copyright D. A. Warrell).

in the subarachnoid space contributes to inflammation of the meninges through similar processes. Raised levels of pro-inflammatory cytokines, such as tumour necrosis factor (TNF), are found in blood and CSF of patients with invasive meningococcal disease, reflecting these changes.

The pathological changes found in patients who have died of acute bacterial meningitis are described in Chapter 16. Multiple haemorrhages may be found in patients who have died from meningococcal septicaemia including haemorrhages into the adrenals. These were once given prominence as adrenal insufficiency was thought to play an important part in the shock seen in patients with this condition (Waterhouse–Friedrichsen syndrome). This is no longer believed to be the case.

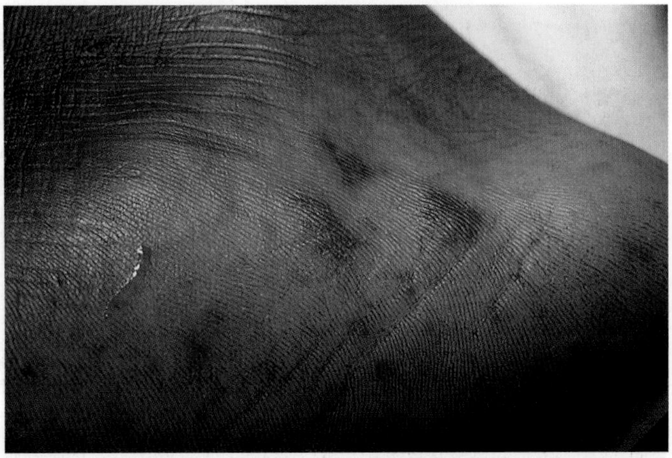

Fig. 39.6. Petechiae on the foot of a patient with acute meningococcaemia.

Clinical features

Acute meningococcaemia

The initial symptoms of meningococcal septicaemia include fever, headache, malaise and diarrhoea (Table 39.1). A non-blanching, macular/papular rash may be present but this is difficult to see in a patient with a dark skin. Petechiae may be present (Figs. 39.5 and 39.6)

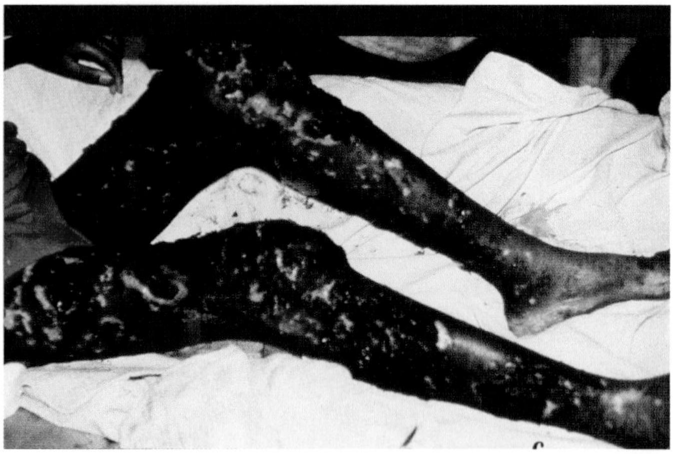

Fig. 39.7. Extensive skin necrosis in acute meningococcaemia.

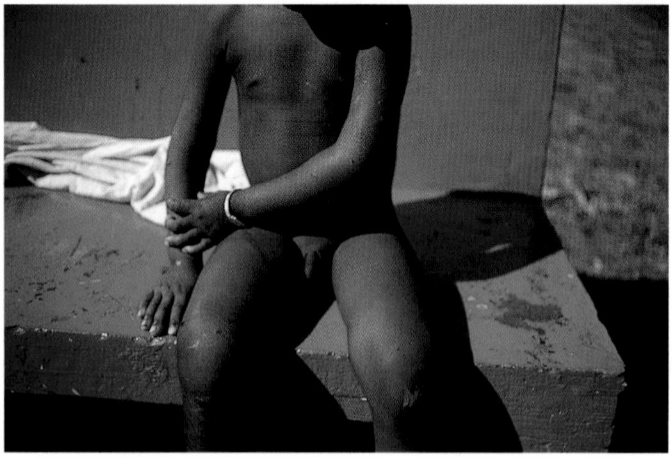

Fig. 39.8. Arthritis of the knee occurring seven days after the onset of meningococcal meningitis when the patient was recovering.

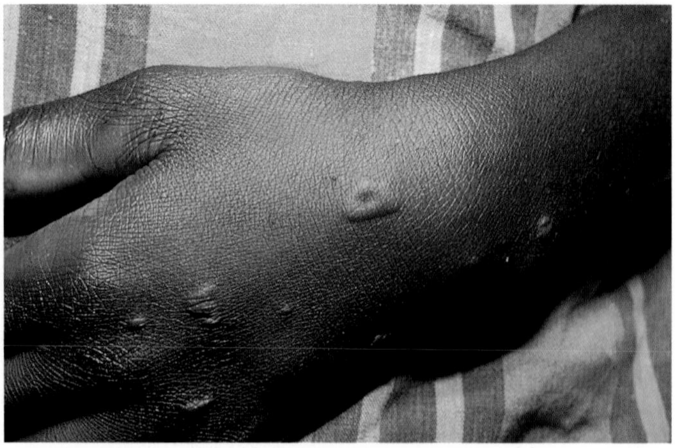

Fig. 39.9. Vasculitic skin lesions on the hand of a child recovering from meningococcal meningitis.

which, in a dark-skinned subject, are detected most easily in the conjunctivae or on the soft palate. Patients with acute meningococcaemia may be hypotensive on presentation and they may also be confused or drowsy.

Laboratory examination usually shows a moderate leukocytosis. Thrombocytopenia is frequently present and there may be other laboratory features of disseminated intravascular coagulation.

Acute meningococcaemia can progress with frightening rapidity and patients may die from shock within a few hours of the first appearance of symptoms. Survivors of the initial phase of the illness often have a stormy course. Renal and/or myocardial failure may occur and damage to larger vessels can lead to extensive tissue necrosis (Fig. 39.7), gangrene and loss of an extremity. Some patients with meningococcal septicaemia or meningitis develop arthritis, cutaneous vasculitis, conjunctivitis or pericarditis a few days after the onset of their illness when their general condition is improving (Figs. 39.8 and 39.9). These complications are caused by the formation of antigen/antibody complexes at sites where bacteria have localized; they usually resolve spontaneously.

Overall mortality from acute meningococcaemia is high. In rural areas of Africa, many patients with this condition die before they reach a health facility. Mortality among those who reach hospital is often 30 per cent or more and may be even higher in those who present in coma or shock (Lewis, 1979).

Meningococcal meningitis

Patients with meningococcal meningitis present with the characteristic clinical and laboratory features of acute bacterial meningitis are shown in Table 39.1. Petechiae may be present. The outcome of patients with meningococcal meningitis is much better than that of patients with meningococcal septicaemia or other forms of acute bacterial meningitis and most patients make an uneventful recovery. About 5–10 per cent develop transitory allergic complications and a similar percentage have persistent neurological sequelae, especially deafness (Smith et al., 1988). Herpes simplex reactivation is common during the recovery period. The overall mortality rate of meningococcal meningitis is about 10 per cent.

Diagnosis

Clinical diagnosis

Diagnosis of a sporadic case of acute meningococcaemia is difficult as initial symptoms and signs are non-specific and similar to those of many other acute infections including malaria. During an epidemic, meningococcaemia should be suspected in any febrile patient or patient with severe diarrhoea, especially if petechiae are present. Clinical diagnosis of bacterial meningitis in adults and older children is usually straightforward, but infants or the elderly may not show the classical signs of meningococcal irritation (Chapter 16). Detection of petechiae in a patient with acute bacterial meningitis suggests, but does not prove, a meningococcal aetiology.

Laboratory diagnosis

A microbiological diagnosis of acute meningococcaemia is usually made on the basis of a positive blood culture. Meningococci can be cultured from petechiae. Isolation of a meningococcus from a throat swab suggests, but does not prove, that this bacterium was the cause of the patient's illness.

Diagnosis of meningococcal meningitis is made by the isolation of a meningococcus from the cerebrospinal fluid (CSF). Demonstration of gram-negative diplococci in a CSF deposit or a positive antigen test makes the diagnosis highly likely. The antibiotic sensitivity pattern and serogroup of the meningococcus should be determined whenever possible. Meningococci are susceptible to many antibiotics so that even a single treatment may render the blood or CSF sterile. In these circumstances, indirect tests such as the latex test for the detection of polysaccharide antigen or a PCR test for bacterial DNA are especially helpful. Such tests can be done on stored samples and so they are particularly useful in the investigation of epidemics that occur in situations where bacterial culture is difficult or impossible.

Treatment

General care and management of shock

Effective management of patients with meningococcal septicaemia requires a high level of expertise and technical support. Whenever possible, patients should be managed in intensive care facilities. General measures include careful management of fluid balance and nursing care for an unconscious patient. Shock is often a prominent feature of acute meningococcaemia and it may be difficult to sustain blood pressure. Treat hypotension initially with an infusion of colloid solution such as 4.5 per cent albumin (20 ml/kg) or plasma. It may be necessary to repeat this, but there is a danger of fluid overload and the development of pulmonary oedema. Whenever possible, fluid replacement should be guided by measurement of the central venous pressure. Give oxygen to patients who are severely shocked. If colloid infusion does not restore blood pressure, a dopamine infusion (5 μg/kg/min) should be tried.

Corticosteroids

Administration of large doses of corticosteroids used to be recommended treatment for patients with acute meningococcaemia, but there is little evidence that this had any effect, and it is no longer recommended. Most patients have normal or raised glucocorticosteroid levels but some physicians still recommend administration of physiological doses of corticosteroids. The question of whether or not dexamethasone should be given to patients with acute bacterial meningitis to reduce the incidence of neurological sequelae is discussed in Chapter 16. So far, there is no evidence that this practice is beneficial in meningococcal meningitis.

Antibiotics

Crystalline penicillin given intravenously or intramuscularly in large doses (2–4 mega units 6-hourly for adults, 1–2 mega units 6-hourly for children) for 5 days is the recommended treatment for meningococcal infection. Chloramphenicol (500 mg/6-hourly for an adult; 25 mg/kg 6-hourly for a child) is an effective alternative treatment for subjects who are allergic to penicillin. Initially, chloramphenicol should be given parenterally but it can be given orally as soon as a patient can take medication by mouth. During epidemics, when an individual hospital may see up to a hundred cases of meningococcal disease a day, administration of parenteral penicillin four- or six-hourly may be beyond the resources of the clinical services. In these circumstances, an oily preparation of chloramphenicol (Tifomycine) may be life-saving. This is given as a single injection on admission (3 g for an adult; 0.1 g/kg for children) with a second injection 24 or 48 hours later if a patient is not improving. Several studies have shown that the outcome of patients treated with Tifomycine is comparable to that achieved with longer courses of other antibiotics (Table 39.2) (Lewis et al. 1998; Greenwood, 1999).

Neither penicillin nor chloramphenicol eliminates nasopharyngeal carriage of meningococci; some physicians recommend the administration of rifampicin at the time of a patient's discharge from hospital to protect their close contacts.

Table 39.2. Trials of Tifomycine in the treatment of meningitis in Africa

Year	Country	Type of meningitis	Number of cases	Mortality % Tifomycine®	Penicillin/ampicillin	Cephalosporin
1972/74	Senegal	Meningococcal	68	7		
	Burkina Faso	Other	65	6		
1978	Nigeria	Meningococcal	131	2	5	
1979	Nigeria	Meningococcal	86	6		
1989/90	Mali	All causes	528	28	25	
	Niger					
1991/92	Mali	All causes	300	22		19
	Niger					

Source: From Greenwood (1999).

The future

At present cases of meningococcal disease can be treated safely in Africa with either penicillin or chloramphenicol. However, it is uncertain for how long these drugs will remain effective, and the report of chloramphenicol resistant meningococci in Vietnam (Galimand, 1998) is a matter for considerable concern as these bacteria could spread to Africa. It is, therefore, very important that the anti-microbial sensitivity pattern of meningococci in the African meningitis belt is kept under close surveillance.

A number of new approaches to the treatment of acute meningococcaemia have recently been reported which are directed at inhibiting the inflammatory and other physiological changes induced by endotoxin (Pathan et al. 2000). These include trials of anti-endotoxin antibodies, human bactericidal permeability increasing protein (an anti-cytokine) and protein C concentrate (an anti-thrombotic). Encouraging results have been obtained but none of these compounds is yet recommended for routine use and they are likely to be expensive.

The best hope for preventing epidemics of meningococcal disease lies in vaccination. Introduction of a group A + C conjugate vaccine, perhaps in combination with other antigens, into the routine EPI programme in combination with a programme of catch-up vaccination of the older population should provide an effective way of preventing epidemics. Unfortunately, although a group C conjugate vaccine is now in routine use in the UK no group A or group A + C conjugate vaccines are available. Because these vaccines would find their main use in some of the poorest countries of Africa, manufacturers have not given priority to the development of these vaccines. Fortunately, thanks to increasing support from the international community, in particular from the Bill and Melinda Gates Foundation, there is now a good chance that a group A, conjugate vaccine will be developed through a public/private partnership, the Meningitis Vaccine Programme (MUP), and that funds will be made available to ensure that it can be used in the areas where it is needed most – the meningitis belt of Africa.

References

Campagne G, Garba A, Fabre P et al. (2000). Safety and immunogenicity of three doses of a *Neisseria meningitidis* A + C diphtheria conjugate vaccine in infants from Niger. *Pediat Infect Dis J*; **19**: 144–150.

Decosas J, Koama J-B T. (2002). Chronicle of an outbreak foretold: meningococcal meningitis W135 in Burkina Faso. *Lancet Infect Dis*; **ii**: 763–765.

Galimand M, Gerbaud G, Guibourdenche M, Riou J-Y, Courvalin P. (1998). High-level chloramphenicol resistance in *Neisseria meningitidis*. *N Engl J Med*; **339**: 868–874.

Greenwood BM. (1999). Meningococcal meningitis in Africa. *Trans Roy Soc Trop Med Hyg*; **93**: 341–353.

Greenwood BM, Bradley AK, Cleland PG et al. (1979). An epidemic of meningococcal infection at Zaria, Northern Nigeria. 1. General epidemiological features. *Trans Roy Soc Trop Med Hyg*; **73**: 557–562.

Lapeyssonnie L. (1963). La méningite cérébrospinale en Afrique. *Bull Wld Hlth Org*; **28**: 3–114.

Lewis LS. (1979). Prognostic factors in acute meningococcaemia. *Arch Dis Childh*; **54**: 44–48.

Lewis RF, Dorlencourt F, Pinel J. (1998). Long-acting oily chloramphenicol for meningococcal meningitis. *Lancet*; **352**: 823.

Morelli G, Malorny B, Müller K et al. (1997). Clonal descent and microevolution of *Neisseria meningitidis* during 30 years of epidemic spread. *Mol Microbiol*; **25**: 1047–1064.

Moore PS, Plikaytis BD, Bolan GA et al. (1992). Detection of men-

ingitis epidemics in Africa: a population-based analysis. *Int J Epidemiol*; **21**: 155–162.
Pathan N, Nadel S, Levin M. (2000). Pathophysiology and management of meningococcal septicaemia. *J Roy Coll Phys*; **34**: 436–444.
Reingold AL, Broome CV, Hightower AW et al. (1985). Age-specific differences in duration of clinical protection with meningococcal A polysaccharide vaccine. *Lancet*; **ii**: 114–118.
Robbins JB, Towne DW, Gotschlich EC, Schneerson R. (1997). 'Love's labours lost': failure to implement mass vaccination against group A meningococal meningitis in sub-Saharan Africa. *Lancet*; **350**: 880–882.
Smith AW, Bradley AK, Wall RA et al. (1988). Sequelae of epidemic meningococcal meningitis in Africa. *Trans Roy Soc Trop Med Hyg*; **82**: 312–320.
World Health Organization. (1998). *Control of Epidemic Meningococcal Disease: WHO Practical Guidelines*, 2nd edn. Geneva: World Health Organization.
World Health Organization. (2000). Detecting meningococcal meningitis epidemics in highly-endemic African countries. *Wkly Epidemiol Rec*; **38**: 306–309.

40 *Haemophilus influenzae*

The problem in Africa

Haemophilus influenzae is a major cause of mucosal and invasive illness in African children, most of whom from an early age carry one or more species of *H. influenzae* in their oropharynx (Mulholland et al., 1999). Usually these are non-encapsulated (non-typable) strains, but 5–20 per cent of young African children carry capsulated strains of *H. influenzae* type b (Hib)(Adegbola et al., 1998). Hib is an important cause of meningitis and pneumonia throughout Africa, which can now be prevented through vaccination.

Most cases of invasive disease (meningitis and pneumonia) occur in children under the age of one year. The annual incidence of Hib meningitis in Africa is 200–250 per 100 000 children under 12 months (Adegbola et al., 1996; Bijlmer et al., 1990; Hussey et al., 1994; Cadoz et al., 1981). In The Gambia, vaccination against Hib prevented 20 per cent of radiologically severe pneumonia (Mulholland et al., 1997). The burden of Hib pneumonia is about four times that of Hib meningitis (Mulholland et al., 1999). As a result of this work, it has been estimated that 1–1.5 per cent of African children experience an episode of Hib meningitis or Hib pneumonia in the first year of life.

The organism

H. influenzae is a gram-negative cocco-bacillus. It may be surrounded by a polysaccharide capsule (encapsulated) or not (non-encapsulated or non-typable). Most invasive disease is caused by encapsulated strains, while non-encapsulated strains tend to cause mucosal infections such as otitis media and lower respiratory tract infections. There are six serotypes of encapsulated *H. influenzae*, classified by the serological response to their polysaccharide capsule, but 95 per cent of invasive disease caused by *H. influenzae* is due to serotype b or Hib (Bijlmer, 1994).

Clinical manifestations of Hib

Meningitis

Meningitis due to Hib is similar to acute meningitis caused by other bacteria, for example *S. pneumoniae, N. meningitidis* (Chapter 16). Children present with fever, drowsiness or unconsciousness, vomiting, convulsions, a bulging fontanelle, a stiff neck and sometimes features of septicaemia and shock. The prognosis in Hib meningitis is better than that of pneumococcal meningitis, but the outcome in African children is worse than in industrialized countries. In published series the case-fatality rate of Hib meningitis is 16–40 per cent, with around a third of survivors exhibiting signs of neurological sequelae (Bijlmer, 1994; Nottidge, 1985; Adegbola et al., 1996; Goetghebeur et al., 2000). By comparison, series of Hib meningitis from industrialized countries before Hib vaccines were introduced typically reported case-fatality rates less than 5 per cent (Gilbert et al., 1995).

It is not clear why the outcome should be worse in African children. Delayed presentation and younger age may play a part, but case control studies have failed to provide strong support for this (Goetghebeur et al., 2000). Some have suggested that the poor prognosis is due to a generally low standard of medical care, but high case-fatality rates are also seen in reputable units providing good quality care (E. Molyneux, personal communication). In Africa a substantial proportion of young children do not have access to even basic medical care (UNICEF, 1996). For these children the case-fatality rate of bacterial meningitis from any cause can be assumed to be close to 100 per cent.

Pneumonia

Hib pneumonia cannot be distinguished clinically from pneumococcal pneumonia (see Chapters 18, 19). It can be severe, causing serious illness and profound radiological changes, and may lead to complications such as pleural effusion or empyema (Mulholland et al., 1997; Riley & Bracken, 1965; Honig et al., 1973).

Septicaemia

Hib is an important cause of septicaemia, bone, joint and soft tissue infections.

- Consider Hib in any young child who presents with evidence of severe bacterial infection. It is a rare cause of bacterial pericarditis.

Clinical manifestations of non-encapsulated *H. Influenzae* infection

The role of non-encapsulated or non-typable *H. influenzae* as a cause of disease in African children is unclear. Globally, these organisms are important causes of otitis media, and this is presumably true in Africa, although studies to confirm this are lacking.

The importance of non-typeable *H. influenzae* as a cause of pneumonia is controversial. Lung aspirate studies in Papua New Guinea, and blood culture studies from Pakistan suggest that non-typable *H. influenzae* is a major contributor to the overall burden of childhood pneumonia, but these findings have not been reproduced in lung aspirate studies from Africa (Falade et al., 1997).

Diagnosis

The organism

The principle is to identify Hib in the CSF:
- culture of CSF
- latex agglutination kit, simple but less specific (Fig. 40.1): not readily available
- gram stain of CSF.

CSF changes

Cells – increased in most cases, but many appear clear to the naked eye. Glucose and protein are routine.

Blood culture

This is fundamental, and significantly improves the management of severely ill children with septicaemia or severe pneumonia.

Management of Hib meningitis

See also Chapter 16.

Antibiotic therapy

Accurate antimicrobial treatment depends on culture and sensitivity results. It is becoming more and more important to determine antimicrobial resistance to commonly available antibiotics. If this cannot be done, empirical therapy must be given. For childhood meningitis or proven

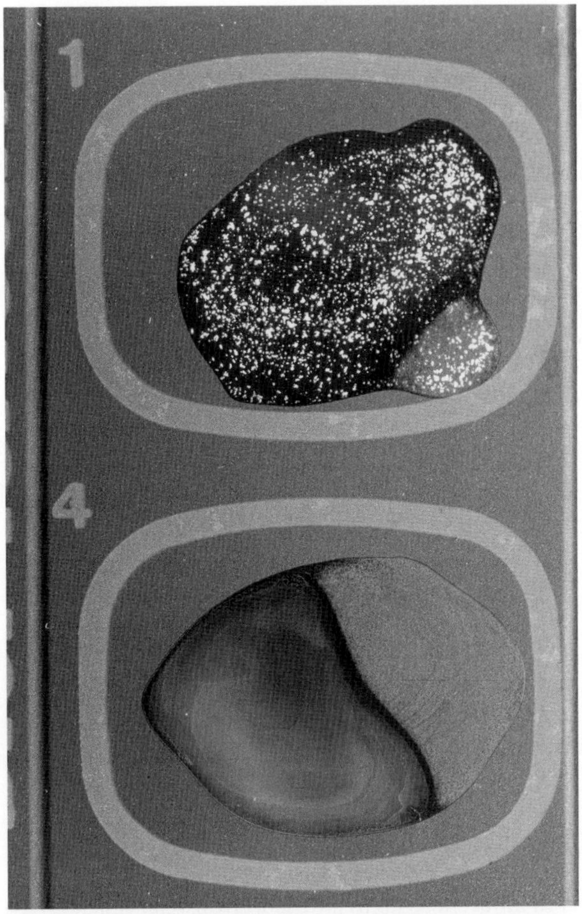

Fig. 40.1. The latex agglutination test for the detection of Hib antigen in CSF. The slide above shows agglutination, that below is the negative control.

Table 40.1. Essential elements in the management of bacterial meningitis in African children.

	Recommended	Alternative
Antibiotics	• Ceftriaxone 50 mg/kg twice daily x 10 days, i.m. or i.v. • Cefotaxime 50 mg/kg 6 hourly for 10 days, i.m. or i.v.	• Penicillin 100,000 IU/kg 6-hourly i.m. or i.v. + chloramphenicol 25 mg/kg 6-hourly i.m. or i.v.[a] • Ampicillin 50 mg/kg 6-hourly i.m. or i.v. + chloramphenicol 25 mg/kg 6-hourly i.m. or i.v.
Fluids Correct under- or over-hydration (see text) (Total i.v. or oral fluid – 80 ml/kg/ 24 hours)	*Enteral* • Oral rehydration solution (ORS) initially if under-hydration • Nasogastric milk feeds if conscious state poor, breast or oral feeds if conscious	*Intravenous* • Normal saline +5% dextrose or normal saline +10% dextrose in very young infants *i.v. fluid is usually not necessary and involves significant risks* *Hypotonic solutions are dangerous and should not be used*
Manage convulsions[b]	• Rectal diazepam 0.5 mg/kg • i.v. diazepam 0.2–0.3 mg/kg	• Rectal paraldehyde 0.3–0.4 ml/kg • i.m. paraldehyde 0.2 ml/kg

Notes:
In addition to the elements listed, good nursing care is essential, particularly if the child is unconscious. As associated pneumonia is common, oxygen may be required.
[a] Oral chloramphenicol may be used after at least 72 hours of parenteral therapy if a child's condition is good, but where there are concerns about absorption, especially in malnourished children, this should be avoided.
[b] If convulsions persist maintenance anticonvulsant therapy with phenytoin or phenobarbitone is indicated. Care should be taken with repeated doses of diazepam which might cause apnoea.

Hib meningitis, give a third-generation cephalosporin when available, either ceftriaxone (50 mg/kg 12-hourly) or cefotaxime (50 mg/kg 6-hourly).

The efficacy of the alternatives, penicillin and chloramphenicol or ampicillin and chloramphenicol, depends on local patterns of susceptibility. Nineteen per cent of Hib isolates from meningitis cases in Malawi were resistant to chloramphenicol, while 20 per cent of pneumococcal isolates were resistant to penicillin.

Supportive treatment

- Do not restrict fluids, as the risks of exacerbating dehydration outweigh risks of the syndrome of inappropriate ADH secretion. In the early stages and in unconscious children great care must be taken with fluid management.
- Give fluid at maintenance levels (80–100 ml/kg/day). Acceptable fluids are listed in Table 40.1. It is dangerous to give large volumes of hypotonic intravenous fluid (such as ¼ or ½ normal saline, even with added dextrose) to children with meningitis as this may exacerbate cerebral oedema.
- If intravenous fluids are used, give 0.9 per cent sodium chloride (isotonic or normal saline) with added (5–10%) dextrose, as hypoglycaemia occurs in 20–30 per cent of infants with meningitis, at presentation or during the first 72 hours of treatment.

Fluid management in meningitis

Some children with bacterial meningitis have hypovolaemia because of vomiting, poor feeding, or systemic sepsis, and others have mild fluid overload and hyponatraemia due to inappropriately increased antidiuretic hormone (ADH) activity. In meningitis, dehydration or fluid overload is associated with higher mortality. For most children moderate fluid restriction is unnecessary and extreme fluid restriction is harmful. But, if 100 per cent of normal maintenance fluids is given intravenously, especially hypotonic fluid, this leads to fluid overload and facial oedema in up to one quarter of children with bacterial meningitis. This is associated with a worse outcome, predominantly because of cerebral oedema, but increased lung water will also worsen hypoxaemia. Correction of dehydration is essential but avoid over-hydration.

- Give children with no signs of dehydration a total of 70–80 per cent of normal maintenance fluid volumes for the first 48 hours. Some of this fluid intake can be enteral feeds, when it is safe to give them. Advise mothers not to breast-feed children who are deeply unconscious, in severe respiratory distress, or having frequent vomiting or convulsions. If children are stable but still have reduced consciousness, milk feeding, to provide a source of hydration and nutrition, can be given via a nasogastric tube, with the child nursed on their side (see Box).

Fluid in meningitis
Mortality is higher if the child is
- Overloaded
- Dehydrated

Clinical dehydration

- Give children who present with clinical signs of dehydration, particularly sunken eyes or poor skin turgor, 20 ml/kg of 0.9 per cent sodium chloride as an initial intravenous bolus, and then 100 per cent of normal maintenance fluid volumes, or more if signs of dehydration persist. If an intravenous cannula cannot be inserted, or ward supervision is not sufficient accurately to control infusion rates or care for the drip, rehydration using a nasogastric tube is appropriate.

Clinical fluid overload

Children with meningitis may develop signs of fluid overload, particularly eyelid oedema, or signs of increased intracranial pressure, such as a bulging fontanelle, papilloedema, or deteriorating conscious state.

- Immediately restrict fluids to 50 per cent of normal maintenance fluids.
- Nurse at 30° head up.
- Closely monitor airway, breathing and circulation.

Serum sodium

Measure this, if possible, as soon as the child arrives in hospital. Children who have hyponatraemia ($[Na^+] < 130$ mmol/l), without signs of dehydration, or with signs of fluid overload, are likely to have inappropriately increased ADH activity. For these children, initial fluid restriction to 60 per cent of maintenance volumes using a combination of isotonic saline and milk feeding is appropriate. More fluid can be allowed after the first 48 hours, or earlier if any signs of dehydration (including significant weight loss) develop.

- Monitor all children with meningitis regularly for alterations in conscious state, and signs of dehydration, fluid overload, or hypoxia.

Corticosteroids

See Chapter 16. The value of steroids in childhood meningitis has not been proven in developing countries. There is no evidence that dexamethasone 0.4 mg/kg 12-hourly for 48 hours gives any advantage. Among 170 cases of Hib meningitis in Malawi, the mortality was 51 per cent and 39 per cent, while neurological sequelae were found in 26 per cent and 41 per cent, in the steroid and placebo groups respectively (Molyneux et al., 2002).

Management of other Hib infections

The management of young children presenting with severe pneumonia, empyema, osteomyelitis or septic arthritis should take into account the possibility that these conditions may be caused by Hib. Where possible, this should be confirmed by obtaining fluid for culture from the site of infection. If Hib cannot be excluded the initial management should include an antibiotic active against Hib such as a third generation cephalosporin, chloramphenicol or ampicillin.

Prevention

Vaccination

The only practical means of preventing Hib disease is by vaccination. Before 1990 Hib was the most important cause of severe bacterial infection in children in most developed countries. The licensure in 1990 of the first protein–polysaccharide conjugate vaccines suitable for use in young infants was a dramatic event in public health that rapidly led to the virtual disappearance of invasive Hib disease in industrialized countries (Adams et al., 1993), but few countries in Africa are vaccinating children against Hib.

Four different types of Hib conjugate are available (see Table 40.2). The vaccines contain different antigens, and their immunogenicities and efficacies also differ. Only PRP-T has been demonstrated to be effective in Africa (Mulholland et al., 1997).

Primary series without booster

Although the manufacturers recommend the use of their vaccines as a primary series followed by a booster, Hib vaccine (PRP-T) has been introduced in the Gambia as a primary series at 2, 3 and 4 months of age without a booster dose. Careful follow-up has revealed no evidence of late cases (Adegbola et al., 1999). It can be concluded that, in Africa, where most disease occurs in the first year of life, the primary series is all that is required. A similar schedule is used in the United Kingdom without evidence of late vaccine failure.

Table 40.2. Types of conjugate Hib vaccine available

Generic name[a]	Protein carrier	Formulation	Dosage schedule[d]	Comments
PRP-T[b]	Tetanus toxoid	Lyophilized	3 doses in infancy with DTP	Can be reconstituted saline diluted with DTP from the same procedure
HbOC or PRP-CRM	CRM197 mutant diphtheria toxin	Liquid formulation	3 doses in infancy with DTP	
PRP-OMP[c]	Group B meningococcus outer membrane protein	Lyophilized	2 doses in infancy with DTP	Produces antibody response after first dose

Notes:

[a] A fourth Hib vaccine, PRP-D (diphtheria toxoid conjugate) is available in some countries, but it is not effective in infants and therefore not suitable for Africa.

[b] Combination formulations exist with DTP and hepatitis B.

[c] Exists as a combination with hepatitis B vaccine.

[d] For all vaccines manufacturers recommend a booster dose at 12–18 months, but this is not necessary in Africa as most disease is in infancy.

Future directions

GAVI

In 1999 the Global Alliance for Vaccines and Immunization (GAVI) was formed by WHO, UNICEF, major financial donors and pharmaceutical manufacturers to replace the children's vaccine initiative (CVI). The basic principle behind GAVI is that all children have the right to lifesaving vaccines regardless of the economic status of their country or their family. In keeping with this principle GAVI has focused its support on the world's poorest countries and is encouraging them to introduce new vaccines, particularly hepatitis B and Hib, once they achieve adequate coverage with routine EPI vaccines. The GAVI fund, combined with the continuing decline in Hib vaccine prices, should help to make Hib vaccine part of a revitalized immunization programme for Africa during the first decade of the twenty-first century – but is there an adequate infrastructure to give it to children?

HIV

The HIV pandemic in sub-Saharan Africa has affected almost every aspect of health services delivery. South African children with HIV are at higher risk of Hib disease, and the HIV pandemic is increasing the burden of Hib disease in Africa (p. 232).

Microbial resistance

Resistance of Hib isolates to first line antibiotics, particularly ampicillin and chloramphenicol, is increasing. This is most important for the management of meningitis and underlines the need to move to third-generation cephalosporins for the treatment of meningitis in African children.

References

Adams WG, Deaver KA, Cochi SL et al. (1993). Decline of childhood *Haemophilus influenzae* type b (Hib) disease in the Hib vaccine era. *JAMA*; **269**: 221–226.

Adegbola RA, Mulholland EK, Falade AG et al. (1996). *Haemophilus influenzae* type b disease in the Western Region of The Gambia: background surveillance for a vaccine efficacy trial. *Ann Trop Paediatr*; **16**: 103–111.

Adegbola RA, Mulholland EK, Secka O et al. (1998). Vaccination with *Haemophilus influenzae* type b conjugate vaccine reduces oropharyngeal carriage of *Haemophilus influenzae* type b among Gambian children. *J Infect Dis*; **177**: 1758–1761.

Adegbola RA, Usen SO, Weber M et al. (1999). Reduction in the incidence of *Haemophilus influenzae* type b (Hib) meningitis in The Gambia, West Africa after the introduction of a Hib conjugate vaccine. *Lancet*; **354**: 1091.

Bijlmer HA. (1994). Epidemiology of *Haemophilus influenzae* invasive disease in developing countries and intervention strategies. In: Ellis RW, Granoff DM, eds. *Development and Uses of Haemophilus b conjugate vaccines*, ed. RW Ellis, DM Granoff, pp. 247–264. New York: Marcel Dekker.

Bijlmer HA, van Alphen L, Greenwood BM et al. (1990). The epidemiology of *Haemophilus influenzae* meningitis in children under 5 years of age in The Gambia, West Africa. *J Infect Dis*; **161**: 1210–1215.

Cadoz M, Denis F, Diop Mar I et al. (1981). Etude epidemiologique des cas de meningites purulentes hopitalises a Dakar pendant la decennie 1970–1979. *Bull WHO*; **59**: 575–584.

Falade AG, Mulholland EK, Adegbola RA et al. (1997). Bacterial isolates from blood and lung aspirate cultures in Gambian children with lobar pneumonia. *Ann Trop Paediatr*, **17**: 315–319.

Goetghebuer T, West TE, Wermenbol V et al. (2000). Outcome of meningitis caused by Streptococcus pneumoniae and Haemophilus influenzae type b in The Gambia. *Trop Med Int Hlth*; **5**: 207–213.

Gilbert GL, Johnson PD, Clements DA. (1995). Clinical manifestations and outcome of *Haemophilus influenzae* type b disease. *J Paediatr Child Hlth*; **31**: 99–104.

Honig PJ, Pasquariello PS, Stool SE. (1973). *H. influenzae* pneumonia in infants and children. *J Pediatr*, **83**: 215–219.

Hussey G, Hitchcock J, Schaaf H et al. (1994). The epidemiology of invasive *Haemophilus influenzae* infections in Cape Town, South Africa. *Ann Trop Paediatr*, **14**: 97–103.

Madhi SA, Peterson K, Madhi A et al. (2000). Increased disease burden and antibiotic resistance of bacteria causing severe community-acquired lower respiratory tract infections in human immunodeficiency virus type 1-infected children. *Clin Infect Dis*; **31**: 170–176.

Molyneux EM, Walsg AL, Forsyth H et al. (2002). Dexamethasone treatment in childhood bacterial meningitis in Malawi: a randomised control trial. *Lancet*; **360**: 211–218.

Mulholland EK, Hilton S, Adegbola RA et al. (1997). Randomized trial of *Haemophilus influenzae* type b-tetanus protein conjugate vaccine for prevention of pneumonia and meningitis in Gambian infants. *Lancet*, **349**: 1191–1197.

Mulholland EK, Levine O, Nohynek H et al. (1999). The evaluation of vaccines for the prevention of pneumonia in children in developing countries. *Epidemiol Rev*; **21**: 1–13.

Mulholland EK, Ogunlesi O, Adegbola RA et al. (1999). The aetiology of serious infections in young Gambian infants. *Pediatr Infect Dis J*; **18**: S35–S41.

Nottidge VA. (1985). *Haemophilus influenzae* meningitis: a 5 year study in Ibadan, Nigeria, *J Infect*, **11**: 109–117.

Riley HD, Bracken EC. (1965). Empyema due to *Haemophilus influenzae* in infants and children. *Am J Dis Child*; **110**: 24–28.

Shann F. (1999). Haemophilus influenzae pneumonia: type b or non-type b? *Lancet*; **354**: 1488–1490.

UNICEF (1996). *State of the World's Children*. New York.

41 Tetanus

Tetanus is caused by toxins produced by *Clostridium tetani* and is characterized by increased muscular tone and spasms. It is commonly known throughout Africa as 'lockjaw', since spasms of the masseter muscles prevent the mouth from opening. Although it occurs in two different clinical situations, neonates (neonatal tetanus) and older children and adults (non-neonatal tetanus), the pathophysiology is similar.

The problem in Africa

Tetanus was first described in Egypt over 3000 years ago. Although vaccination has been available for over 80 years, it remains an important cause of mortality in Africa. Neonates account for over 40 per cent of the patients admitted to hospital with tetanus in some areas, and they have the highest mortality rates. Despite an international resolution to eliminate neonatal tetanus (NNT) by 1995, the World Health Organization (WHO) estimates in 1997 there were 95 000 cases. In 1997 the mortality rates varied from 0.3/1000 live births in Egypt to 15.0 in Somalia.

Non-neonatal tetanus remains an important cause of admission to hospitals in some areas. In a study of three Tanzanian hospitals during 1993–1995, tetanus was responsible for 0.6–2.6 per cent of the deaths in adults (Chandramohan et al., 1998), but data are lacking from other parts of Africa.

Organism

Clostridium tetani is an anaerobic, spore forming gram-positive bacillus. The bacteria are widely distributed in the environment (e.g. soil, house dust), and the intestinal flora of domestic animals and humans. The drumstick shaped endospores are produced after the older organisms lose their flagella. The spores are extremely stable and can remain viable for decades. They are killed by autoclaving at 120 °C, 15 lb/in^2 for 15 minutes or soaking in 2 per cent glutaraldehyde or 1 per cent aqueous iodine for a few hours, although boiling for 15 minutes will kill most spores.

Pathogenesis

The endospores only germinate in relatively hypoxic tissue, such as necrotic or ischaemic tissue, or tissue surrounding a foreign body. As *C. tetani* grows it produces at least two exotoxins, tetanospasmin and tetanolysin. The role of tetanolysin in human tetanus is unclear, but it may promote growth of *C. tetani* or contribute to the autonomic dysfunction.

Tetanospasmin causes the clinical manifestations of tetanus by inhibiting neurotransmitter release from a pre-synaptic terminal of nerves. The gene of the toxin is encoded by a plasmid; strains of *C. tetani* that lack the plasmid do not cause tetanus. Tetanospasmin is synthesised as a single polypeptide, which is homologous to the botulinum neurotoxins. The polypeptide undergoes post-translational cleavage into two disulphide linked fragments, the light (L) and heavy (H) chains. The carboxyl terminal portion of the H chain (H_C) mediates attachment to gangliosides on peripheral nerves, after which the entire toxin molecule enters into pre-synaptic cells via the H_N fragment. After entry into the peripheral nervous system (Fig. 41.1), the toxin moves by retrograde axonal transport and trans-synaptic spread to the central nervous system (CNS).

The L chain, a metalloprotease, cleaves synaptobrevin, a compound essential for the fusion of synaptic vesicles

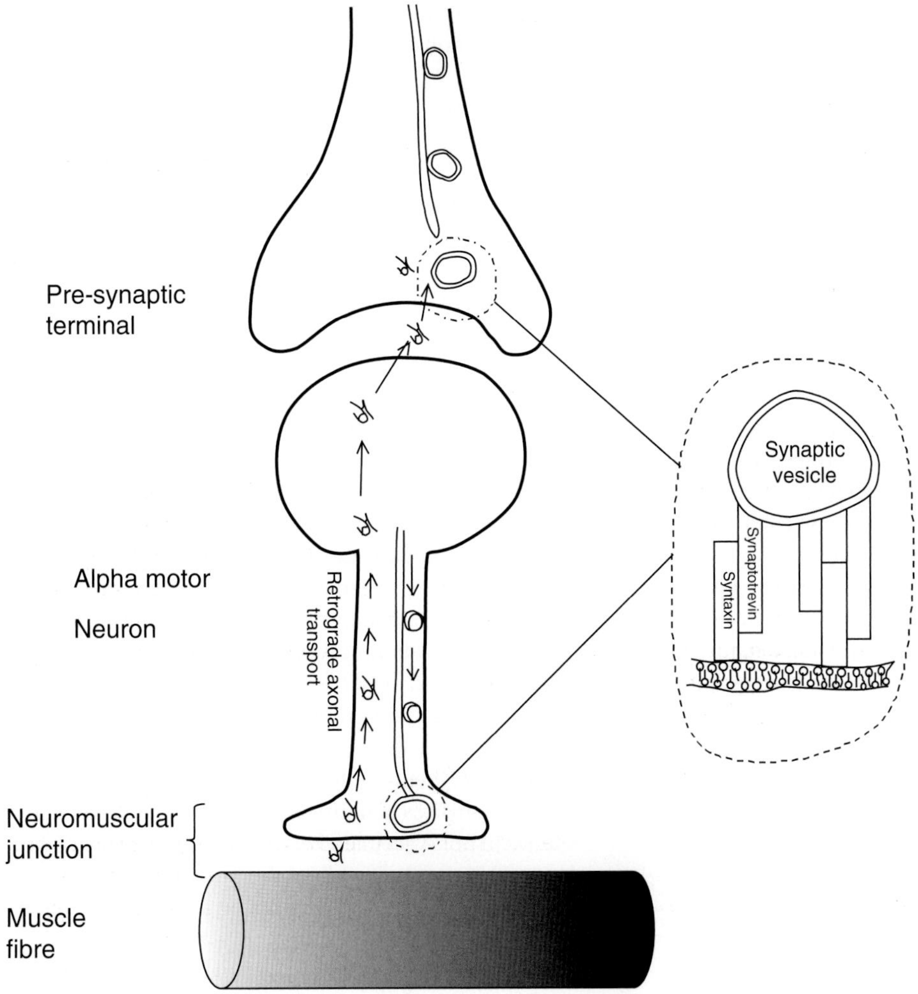

Fig. 41.1. Tetanospasmin diffuses from the site of injury, entering alpha motor neurons through the neuromuscular junction (NMJ). It prevents some transmission at the NMJ by preventing the release of acetylcholine. Of greater clinical significance is that the toxin travels up the alpha motor neuron, passes trans-synaptically into pre-synpatic inhibitory neurons, where it prevents the binding of vesicles containing glycine or gamma-amino butyric acid. The lack of inhibition increases the firing rate in the alpha motor neurons, causing muscle rigidity. (Adapted from Bleck and Brauner, 1997.)

with the presynaptic membrane, thus preventing release of the vesicle's contents, the inhibitory neurotransmitter γ-aminobutyric acid (GABA), into the synaptic cleft. The lack of inhibitory control on the alpha motor neurones promotes sustained excitatory discharge causing the motor spasms. The toxin exerts its effects on muscles, neuromuscular junctions, peripheral nerves, spinal cord and the brainstem.

Autonomic dysfunction with labile hypertension, tachycardia, tachyarrhythmias, vasoconstriction and sweating is common in severe cases. Profound bradycardia and hypotension may also occur and are often pre-terminal events. Noradrenaline levels are markedly raised particularly in response to stimulation.

Epidemiology

Tetanus occurs throughout Africa, the incidence determined by the effectiveness of the vaccination programmes and by traditional practices. In particular, there is an inverse relationship between the number of pregnant women vaccinated with at least two doses of tetanus toxoid (TT) and NNT. In Africa, only 46 per cent (range

10–100%) of pregnant women have had at least two doses of TT (WHO, 2001).

Community surveys in the 1980s estimated that NNT occurred in 8 per 1000 and 18 per 1000 live births in Kenya and Ivory Coast, respectively, and contributed up to 60 per cent of the neonatal deaths in these communities. From 1990 to 1997, the WHO estimated that NNT deaths per 1000 live births decreased by 7 per cent, with the greatest reductions in Ghana (−62%), Kenya (−57%) and Eritrea (−53%). However, in some countries, e.g. Democratic Republic of Congo (+8%), Mali (+22%), Senegal (+4%), there has been an increase (WHO, 2001). In 1988, the Egyptian Ministry of Health initiated an aggressive programme to eliminate NNT, which included annual TT vaccination campaigns during 1988–1993, targeting pregnant women, and supplementary campaigns during 1992–1994 targeting all women of child-bearing age, in districts where NNT rates were highest. This programme produced an 85 per cent decline in reported cases during 1988–1994 (CDC, 1996).

Risk factors associated with the development of NNT include lack of prenatal immunization, delivery at home, with an unskilled birth attendant, who arrived after the birth, and did not wash her hands (Davies-Adetugbo et al., 1998). Other studies have found an increased risk associated with male infants, unhygienic cord cutting and application of potentially infectious substances to the umbilical stump (Bjerregaard et al., 1993).

Recent data on the epidemiology of tetanus in older children and adults in Africa are limited.

Control/prevention

Tetanus toxoid for vaccination has been available since 1923, and has almost eliminated tetanus from many countries. It is produced by formaldehyde treatment of the toxin. Its immunogenicity is improved by absorption with aluminium hydroxide; it has a failure rate of only 4 per 100 million in immunocompetent individuals.

Vaccination schedules of children vary across Africa, but in most countries 3 doses are given in conjunction with diphtheria and pertussis vaccination, between 6 weeks and 3 months of age. Serum antitoxin levels above 0.01units/ml are considered protective, although cases have been reported in patients with protective serum antibody levels. A protective antibody level is attained after the second dose, but a third dose ensures longer lasting immunity. A booster dose is often administered 3 years after the primary vaccination schedule. In order to maintain adequate levels of protection, additional booster doses should be administered every 10 years, or if the vaccination status is unknown at the time of the injury.

Pregnant women should be immunized to prevent NNT. Two or three doses of absorbed toxin should be administered, with the last dose at least 1 month prior to delivery. Maternal anti-tetanus antibodies are passively transferred to the fetus and persist long enough to protect the baby for the first few months of life.

The evidence that malaria and human immunodeficiency virus (HIV) interfere with the transfer of tetanus antibodies to the fetus is conflicting. Some studies have reported a reduction in antibodies in the babies of HIV-infected women, although the concentrations were greater than 0.01 i.u./ml. Other studies have not confirmed these findings. Similarly in women with malaria-infected placentae, some studies have reported a reduction in antibody transfer, with some babies having concentrations less than 0.01 i.u./ml (de Moraes-Pinto et al., 1998).

Reactions to tetanus toxoid are estimated to be 1 in 50000 injections, most commonly local tenderness, oedema, flu-like illness and low-grade fever. Severe reactions such as the Guillian–Barré syndrome and acute relapsing polyneuropathy are rare.

For prophylaxis of injuries likely to be associated with tetanus in non-vaccinated persons, 1500–3000 i.u. equine or 500 i.u. (8 i.u./kg in children) human anti-tetanus immunoglobulin should be given, in addition to a course of tetanus toxoid.

Clinical features

In NNT the route of entry is the umbilical cord (cutting with unsterile instruments, use of substances e.g. animal faeces applied to the cord). In non-neonatal tetanus, wounds on the lower limbs include jiggers (*Tunga penetrans*), compound fractures, post-partum or post-abortion infections of the uterus, and non-sterile intramuscular injections. It can also follow procedures such as scarification, earpiercing, circumcision, dental procedures, toothpicks, or infections, e.g. otitis media, Guinea worm (Dracunculiasis) ulcers or from a decubitus ulcer. In one-third of all patients no route of entry can be identified.

After the organism has gained entry to the body, the period to the development of the first symptom (incubation period) can be as short as 24 hours or as long as many months. This period is determined by the distance the toxin must travel within the nervous system, and may

Table 41.1. Scale used in older children and adults with tetanus

Grade	
I (mild)	Mild to moderate trismus, general spastisticity No respiratory embarrassment, spasms
II (moderate)	Moderate trismus, well-marked rigidity Mild to moderate spasms Respiratory embarrassment with respiratory rate >30/min Mild dysphagia
III (severe)	Severe trismus, generalized spasticity Prolonged spasms, often spontaneous Respiratory impairment: RR >40/min, apnoeic spells Severe dysphagia
IV (very severe)	Grade III + Autonomic dysfunction with hypertension (either persistent or with bradycardia), hypotension or cardiac arrhthymias

Source: From Uwadia (1994).

be related to the quantity of toxin released. The incubation period and interval between the first symptom and the start of spasms (period of onset) are important prognostically, since the shorter these periods, the more severe the disease.

There are a number of scores (Phillips, 1967; Bollot et al., 1975; Uwadia, 1994), used for monitoring the severity during the course of the illness, but they have not been rigorously tested (Table 41.1).

Neonatal tetanus

Neonates with tetanus present a median 6 (range 3–10) days after birth with refusal to feed, mainly due to difficulty in opening the mouth. Thereafter, sucking stops, and 'risus sardonicus' may develop. The hands often become clenched, the feet dorsiflexed, with increased tone, progressing to rigidity and opisthotonus (Fig. 41.2). Spasms of the limbs develop early, but become generalized, occurring spontaneously or provoked by touching the body, sound or light.

Mortality is high, with 65 per cent (range 34–90%) neonates dying in Africa in hospitals that lack facilities for ventilation . If ventilation and intensive care can be given, the mortality decreases to 22 per cent, although the infants require ventilation for 23 (17–60) days and intensive care for 35 (13–87) days (Jeena et al., 1997). Factors associated with a poor prognosis include onset of symptoms within the first 6 days of life, low birthweight (especially <2.5 kg) and recurrent apnoea.

Twenty to forty per cent of neonates who survive have evidence of brain damage, manifesting as microcephaly, mild neurological, developmental and behavioural problems (Barlow et al., 2001).

Non-neonatal tetanus

In children and adults the incubation period is usually 4 days to 3 weeks after the insult (if remembered). The inability to open the mouth fully owing to rigidity of the masseters (trismus or lockjaw), is often the first symptom. Pain, headache, stiffness, rigidity, opisthotonus, laryngeal obstruction and spasms may follow. The spasms may be precipitated by stimuli such as noise, touch, and/or bright light, but also occur spontaneously. They are most prominent in the first 2 weeks and are very painful. Dysphagia and dysphasia can occur. Autonomic dysfunction (labile blood pressure especially hypertension, tachyarhythmias, hyperpyrexia and hypersalivation) usually starts some days after the spasms and reaches a peak during the second week of the disease. The condition tends to improve thereafter, but the rigidity may last beyond the duration of both spasms and autonomic disturbance, for up to 6 weeks.

Tetanus can be localized at the site of injury causing local rigidity and pain. This form has the lowest mortality, although cephalic tetanus (in which the cranial nerves,

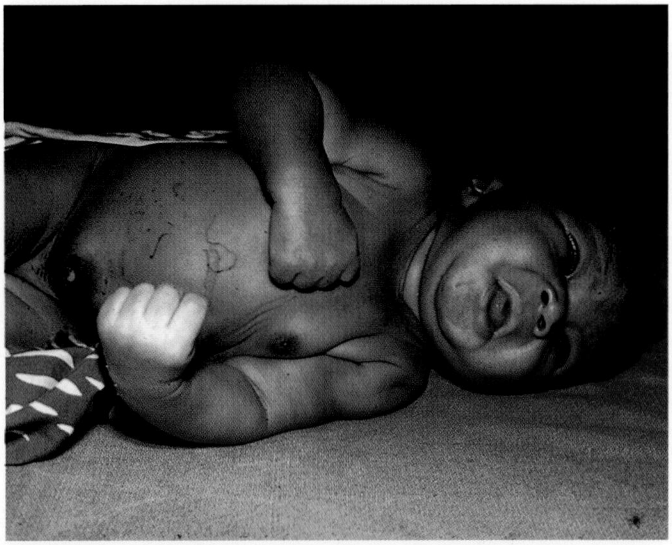

Fig. 41.2. Risus sardonicus and fist clenching in a neonate with tetanus (C.R.J.C. Newton).

especially nerve VII are affected) is a local form with a higher mortality.

Mortality in Africa ranges from 20 to 50 per cent, the lower mortalities occur in hospitals that can perform tracheostomies and/or provide ventilation. The commonest causes of death are respiratory failure (secondary to uncontrolled spasms), autonomic dysfunction, and septicaemia. Most patients who survive have no sequelae, but some are left with contractures, chest deformities, seizures, myoclonus, or the consequences of hypoxia. There is little information on follow-up of patients after tetanus, particularly with regard to cognitive function.

Diagnosis

Tetanus is a clinical diagnosis. *C. tetani* is difficult to culture, a positive result does not indicate that the organism contains the toxin-producing plasmid, and *C. tetani* may be present without disease in patients with protective immunity.

The differential diagnosis includes strychnine poisoning, drug-induced dystonic reactions (phenothiazines), rabies, orofacial infection and hysteria. Patients who present with stiff necks are often thought to have meningitis.

In neonates, birth asphyxia, hypocalcaemic tetany and seizures can sometimes cause confusion.

Management

The main aim of management is to support the patient during the time it takes for the toxin to be bound to the vesicles, and new vesicles to be produced. The principles are similar, although they depend upon the facilities available (Table 41.2). There are differences between the management of neonates (Table 41.3) and adults (Table 41.4).

Nursing care

Good quality nursing is likely to be important in the management of tetanus, although no trials have been performed. The care consists of:

- reduction in stimuli (nursing in a quiet, darkened environment, limiting physical contact with the patient),
- adequate fluids (since fluid loss is increased by profuse sweating and frequent spasms)
- nutrition – the muscle spasms increase the metabolic rate

Table 41.2. Management by level of health care

Level of Health Care	
Health Centre	Clean cord Start antibiotics Insert nasogastric tube Single dose of sedation Transfer to DGH
District General Hospital	As above + Titration of sedative drugs Intravenous fluids Human anti-tetanus toxin Transfer to secondary hospital for ventilation if available
Secondary hospital	As above + Paralysis and ventilation Parenteral nutrition

Table 41.3. Management of neonatal tetanus

Nursing	• Darkened, quiet room/ incubator • Nasogastric feeds with expressed breast milk
Antibiotics	• Benzylpenicillin (25 000 i.u./kg 8-hourly i.v.) + Gentamicin (for aspiration) ***or*** • Metronidazole (7.5 mg/kg 8-hourly)
Antitoxin	• Human anti-tetanus toxin (500 i.u.)
Sedation	• Diazepam (0.1–0.25 mg/kg i.v. or p.r.) ***and/or*** • Phenobarbitone (15 mg/kg loading dose, 5–8 mg/kg maintenance) ***and/or*** • Chlorpromazine (0.5 mg/kg/dose 4–6-hourly orally or i.m.)
Ventilation	• Indications: – Spasms producing hypoxia – Prolonged spasms causing apnoea and bradycardia • Intermittent positive pressure ventilation • Alloferin (0.1–0.2 mg/kg/dose) prn
Fluids	• 150–200 ml/kg/day during period with severe spasms
Vaccination	• Tetanus toxoid 0.5 ml i.m. or deep subcutaneous injection

Scores of activity are useful in monitoring the course of the illness and titration of the sedation (Table 41.1).

Treat the infection

Benzylpenicillin is most often used to kill *C. tetani.* Theoretically, it may aggravate the condition, as the β-lactam ring is similar to GABA and thus it may act as a

Table 41.4. Management of tetanus in children and adults

Nursing	• Darkened, quiet room • Nasogastric feeds with increased calories • Parenteral nutrition
Antibiotics	• Metronidazole for 7–10 days – Children: 10 mg/kg 6-hourly i.v. – Adults: 400 mg PR 6-hourly, or 500 mg i.v. 6-hourly ***or*** • Benzylpenicillin for 7–10 days – Children: 100 000 IU/kg/day i.m. or i.v. – Adults: 100 000–200 000 IU/kg/day i.m. or i.v.
Antitoxin	• Human: 5000–8000 IU ***or*** • Equine: 500–1000 IU/kg
Sedation	• Diazepam – Children: 0.1–0.25 mg/kg i.v. or p.r. – Adults: 5 mg increments to control spasms • Chlorpromazine – Children: 0.5 mg/kg/dose 4–6-hourly p.o., i.m. or i.v. – Adults: 25–50 mg i.m., p.o. 6-hourly
Tracheostomy	• Indications: – Moderate to severe tetanus
Ventilation	• Indications: – Spasms producing hypoxia – Prolonged spasms causing apnoea and bradycardia • Intermittent positive pressure ventilation.
Autonomic dysfunction	• Labetolol 0.25–1.0 mg/min • Morphine 0.5–1.0 mg/kg/hr
Vaccination	• Tetanus toxoid 0.5 ml i.m. or deep subcutaneous injection

competitive anatagonist to GABA. Penicillin can cause hyperexcitability of the CNS, and thus could synergize the action of the toxin in blocking transmitter release at GABA neurones.

Metronidazole is a safe alternative, but the rectal suppositories and intravenous preparation are much more expensive. It is rapidly bioavailable when administered per rectum. Compared to penicillin it is associated with a reduction in the requirements of sedation and muscular relaxants in patients. In some, but not all studies it is associated with a reduction in mortality (Farrar et al., 2000).

Antimicrobial sensitivity patterns of clinical isolates of *C. tetani* are often unknown. Erythromycin, tetracycline, vancomycin, clindamycin, doxycycline and chloramphenicol have been used as alternatives to penicillin and metronidazole.

Neutralize the toxin

Tetanus immunoglobulin shortens the course and may reduce the severity of tetanus. There are three types: equine, bovine and human. The equine form has a half-life of only 2 days, and is associated with a higher incidence of anaphylaxis (up to 20%); but since it is cheaper, it is used more widely than the human form. The human antiserum is isolated from a pool of plasma derived from healthy human tetanus immune donors, and has a half-life of 25–32 days.

Although antiserum neutralizes only the circulating and unbound toxin (demonstrated in the serum of only 10% of cases at presentation and in 4% of cerebrospinal fluid) it should be administered to all patients with tetanus. It is unclear if there is an advantage in administering antiserum at the site of entry. The intrathecal administration of antitetanus immunoglobulin has not been shown to benefit either neonates or older patients.

The side effects of immunoglobulin include:

- local reactions (which occur in 5% of patients)
- acute anaphylactic reactions (which occur in 1 in 200 000 patients)
- delayed serum sickness.

Immediate reactions can be reduced by the concurrent administration of an antihistamine, e.g. promethazine.

Immunize with tetanus toxoid

Give a tetanus toxoid booster, or a full course to those not previously immunized – so-called active-passive immunization. Passive immunization with antiserum induces short-term immunity, whilst active immunization with toxoid induces long-term humoral and cellular immunity. As the former is declining the latter appears, avoiding a window of non-protection. The toxoid competes with the toxin for ganglioside receptors and prevents wild type toxin binding. The toxoid and the human (or equine) anti-tetanus immunoglobulin should be administered at different sites on the body to prevent interaction at the injection site. If both are to be administered together no more than 1000 i.u. human or 5000 i.u. equine should be administered, since higher doses can neutralize the immunogenicity of the toxoid.

Control spasms and reduce respiratory complications

The control of spasms ranges from sedation (to reduce the effect of stimuli) and muscle relaxants to paralysis and ventilation.

Sedation is useful for controlling spasms and rigidity. Benzodiazepines are commonly used as a sedative and muscle relaxant, as they compete with an endogenous inhibitor at the $GABA_A$ receptor. Diazepam is most widely used, since it is cheap, has a wide margin of safety and can be given orally, rectally or intravenously. However it has a long cumulative half-life (72 hours) and in the doses required to control spasms commonly causes respiratory depression and coma. Titration of the dose is difficult. Midazolam and propofol have been used, but these are often not available or not affordable in regions where tetanus is seen frequently.

Phenobarbitone and phenothiazines are commonly used as sedatives (Masawe, 1973), despite the lack of controlled trials. Many centres use a combination of diazepam, phenobarbitone and chlorpromazine rotated as frequently as 3-hourly (Masawe, 1973), despite the pharmacokinetics of these drugs. Phenobarbitone, starting with a loading dose, then administered once daily, is probably sufficient. Chlorpromazine acts on the reticular activating system, where in moderate doses it can reduce muscle spasm, but high doses may aggravate the condition.

Paralysis and ventilation significantly improves the outcome of tetanus, but the facilities for ventilation are rarely available in Africa. Pancuronium and tubocurarine, long-acting muscular relaxants, are most often used. However, since pancuronium inhibits catecholamine reuptake, it could worsen autonomic instability in severely affected patients. Other muscular relaxants that have been used include alloferin (used in neonates), alcuronium, vecuronium (fewer cardiovascular side effects, but short acting), rocuronium (expensive).

Ventilation is necessary when the patient is paralysed with the above drugs. Intermittent positive pressure ventilation with positive end expiratory pressure is often required. Other modes of respiratory support, e.g. continuous positive airway pressure, may be useful when the sedation has been reduced, since they optimize the respiratory pattern, minimize muscle wastage and reduce the likelihood of acquired critical illness neuropathy or myopathy.

Death from laryngeal spasm can be prevented by elective tracheostomy in older children and adults, with insertion of a cuffed tube. They are not indicated in neonates, since they may cause complications, including haemorrhage, creation of a false passage, surgical emphysema and haematoma leading to asphyxia and tracheal stenosis. Tracheostomies can be used for ventilation and suction, and are associated with a significant reduction in mortality. If a tracheostomy has not been performed, insertion of a trocar and cannula or wide bore needle through the cricothyroid membrane may be life-saving in patients with laryngeal spasm (since endotracheal intubation is almost impossible). Oxygen can be delivered under pressure, although a wider bore may be needed for adequate gas exchange.

Control cardiovascular instability

Autonomic disturbances are difficult to control. Adrenoceptor blocking drugs, such as propanolol, betanidine or labetolol do not reduce mortality. Esmolol, an ultra-short acting β-blocker may have advantages over other drugs, but it is very expensive. Morphine is found to be useful by some authors. Oral clonidine and epidural or spinal bupivacaine may also be useful, but these treatments have not been properly assessed. Blockade of the parasympathetic nervous system with high doses of atropine has been suggested.

Provide fluids and calories

Tetanus leads to an increase in energy and fluid requirements (muscular contractions, excessive sweating and sepsis). Weight loss is almost inevitable. Enteral feeding should be started as soon as possible, but can be difficult if spasms are uncontrolled. Parenteral feeding is rarely available and associated with many complications. Percutaneous endoscopic gastrostomy may be useful.

Prevent or treat other complications

Other common complications of tetanus are often attributable to prolonged periods in intensive care or to the force of the spasms. They include:

(a) secondary infections, most commonly in the respiratory tract, urinary tract (catheterization) or wound sepsis
(b) thromboembolic complications, which can be prevented by compression stockings, subcutaneous heparin and physiotherapy
(c) rhabdomyolysis, this rarely causes renal failure.
(d) vertebral compression fractures, especially in older patients.

Other treatments

Magnesium sulphate was found to be a useful adjunct to sedation and to decrease the need for ventilation (Attygalle & Rodrigo, 1997). It also helps to control autonomic disturbances (Lipman et al., 1987). However, it decreases tidal volume, and increases secretions. Its role in the management of tetanus is not yet established.

Pyridoxine, which enhances the production of GABA, and corticosteroids have been claimed to reduce the mortality in NNT and non-neonatal tetanus respectively, but neither of these compounds was subjected to proper randomized controlled trials.

Unsolved problems

Tetanus is a preventable disease, but will continue to occur in Africa until the logistics of vaccine delivery are improved. Vaccination programmes targeting pregnant women and children can significantly reduce the incidence of tetanus. Changes in birth practices may also help.

The development of tetanus in the presence of apparently adequate serum antibody levels still needs to be investigated. In particular factors that impair maternal transfer of antibodies should be defined more clearly. The cause of death is often unclear, particularly in neonates. Regimens that are used for sedation, particularly in unventilated patients, require further examination. The use of magnesium sulphate and other drugs to prevent the need for ventilation, and improve autonomic stability need to be subjected to more rigorous investigation. The cognitive consequences of tetanus need to be defined more clearly.

References

Attygalle D, Rodrigo N. (1997). Magnesium sulphate for control of spasms in severe tetanus. Can we avoid sedation and artificial ventilation? *Anaesthesia*; **52**: 956–962.

Barlow, J, Mung'ala-Odera V, Gona J, Newton CRJC. (2001). Brain damage after neonatal tetanus in a rural Kenyan hospital. *Trop Med Int Health*; **6**: 1–4.

Bjerregaard P, Steinglass R, Mutie DM, Kimani G, Mjomba M, Orinda V. (1993). Neonatal tetanus mortality in coastal Kenya: a community survey. *Int J Epidemiol*; **22**: 163–169.

Bleck TP, Brauner JS. (1997). *Tetanus in Infections of the Central Nervous System*, 2nd edn, ed. WM Scheld, RJ Whitely & DT Durack. Philadelphia: Lippincourt Raven Publishers.

Bollot JF, Rey M, Stelman C. (1975). Les facteurs de gravite du tetanus etude preliminaire pour l'establissement d'une classification internationale de type prognostique. In *Proceedings 4th International Conference onTetanus*, Dakar, 317. Foundation Merieux, Lyons.

CDC. (1996). Progress toward elimination of neonatal tetanus – Egypt, 1988–1994. *JAMA*; **275**: 679–680.

Chandramohan D, Maude GH, Rodrigues LC, Hayes RJ. (1998). Verbal autopsies for adult deaths: their development and validation in a multicentre study. *Trop Med Int Health*; **3**: 436–446.

Davies-Adetugbo AA, Torimiro SE, Ako-Nai KA. (1998). Prognostic factors in neonatal tetanus. *Trop Med Int Health*; **3**: 9–13.

de Moraes-Pinto MI, Verhoeff F, Chimsuku L, Milligan PJ, Wesumperuma L, Broadhead RL, Brabin BJ, Johnson PM, Hart CA. (1998). Placental antibody transfer: influence of maternal HIV infection and placental malaria. *Arch Dis Child Fetal Neonatal Ed*; **79**: F202–F205.

Farrar JJ, Yen LM, Cook T, Fairweather N, Binh N, Parry J, Parry CM. (2000). Tetanus. *J Neurol Neurosurg Psychiatry*, **69**: 292–301.

Jeena PM, Coovadia HM, Gouws E. (1997). Risk factors for neonatal tetanus in KwaZulu-Natal. *S Afr Med J*; **87**: 46–48.

Lipman J, James MF, Erskine J, Plit ML, Eidelman J, Esser JD. (1987). Autonomic dysfunction in severe tetanus: magnesium sulfate as an adjunct to deep sedation. *Crit Care Med*; **15**: 987–988.

Masawe AE. (1973). An approach to prognosis and treatment of tetanus: with special reference to tetanus in Kampala-Uganda. *E Afr Med J*, **50**: 727–737.

Phillips LA. (1967). A classification of tetanus. *Lancet*; **i**:. 1216–1217.

Uwadia FE. (1996). Tetanus. In *Oxford Textbook of Medicine*, 3rd. edn. ed. DJ Weatherall, JGG Ledingham, DA Warrell. Oxford: Oxford University Press.

WHO (2001). Neonatal tetanus progress towards the global elimination of neonatal tetanus, 1990–1997. http: //www.who.int/vaccines-diseases/diseases/NeonatalTetanus.shtml

42 Pertussis

Pertussis ('whooping cough') is a highly infectious acute respiratory disease that mainly affects children. The causative organism is usually *Bordetella pertussis* with a minority of cases caused by *Bordetella parapertussis.* Based on mathematical models, the World Health Organization estimates that 20–40 million cases of pertussis occur world-wide each year (90% in developing countries), resulting in 200 000–400 000 deaths, most in young infants (WHO, 1999). Pertussis can affect all age groups but presents as a more severe disease with a higher mortality in infancy and early childhood (Miller & Fletcher, 1976; Stojanov et al., 2000).

Table 42.1. Incidence of pertussis reported in Africa and USA (prior to introduction of widespread vaccination)

Regions studied	Incidence (per 100 000 population/yr)
Kenya (Muller et al., 1984) 1974–81	1628*
Sudan (Abdalla et al., 1998) 1977–79	268
South Africa (Strebel et al., 1991) 1988–89	187
USA (Madson, 1925) 1932–41	157

Notes:
* denominator refers to children under 15 years of age.

The problem in Africa

Data are scarce on the epidemiology of pertussis in Africa: most studies describe isolated pertussis epidemics (Abdalla et al., 1998; Strebel et al., 1991; Bwibo, 1971; Morley et al., 1966; Muller et al., 1984). Pertussis-specific mortality rates in Africa appear to be comparable to those of industrialized countries before widespread vaccination programmes were introduced. However, reported incidences of pertussis disease in African studies are greater than those seen in the USA in the pre-vaccine era (Table 42.1). It is likely that this is a better indication of the true situation, and that both pertussis and pertussis mortality are greater in Africa. The increased incidence in Africa can be attributed to higher pertussis attack rates associated with overcrowding and more intense exposure in African populations (Aaby, 1992). In Guinea Bissau, where traditional housing increases the effect of crowding, epidemics in the pre-vaccine era resulted in very high mortality rates.

Persisting pertussis

In spite of widespread use of pertussis vaccines, pertussis continues to persist in Africa (Stroffolini et al., 1991). This is partly due to the extreme variability in vaccine uptake, with coverage less than 20% in many areas (Abdalla et al., 1998; Voorhoeve et al., 1978) but it is also likely that there is a reservoir of infection. Subclinical infection has been identified in vaccinated individuals and it is unclear what contribution this makes to the circulation of the organism (Ramkissoon et al., 1995). In addition, the young adult population is likely to be increasingly important as a pertussis reservoir due to the waning of vaccine-induced immunity (Nelson, 1978). The presence of a pertussis reservoir in young adults, combined with poor trans-placental passive immunity, will increase the number of young African infants at risk from pertussis in coming years (Mulholland, 1995) (Fig. 42.1).

Clinical manifestations

Classical picture

The incubation period for pertussis is usually 6 to 12 days following exposure. Classically the infection presents with coryzal symptoms and a progressively worsening cough. The cough increases in severity, developing into paroxysms of intractable coughing, frequently resulting in cyanosis or vomiting. This is followed by a loud inspiratory whoop as the exhausted child gasps for breath. The paroxysmal phase can last up to 6 weeks and is followed by a convalescent phase characterized by a reduction in the severity and frequency of cough and paroxysms. The clinical presentation of pertussis is age dependent and variable. Immunized individuals develop a milder less protracted illness, while adults may simply present with a prolonged, troublesome cough.

Infants

In infancy the clinical signs differ and the disease is associated with a high mortality. The catarrhal symptoms are minimal and the whoop is often absent. Infants tend to have periods of apnoea and cyanosis rather than the classical paroxysms, and they may present with seizures secondary to apnoea (Fig. 42.2).

Physical examination at presentation may reveal periorbital oedema, subconjunctival haemorrhages and petechiae on the upper body.

- Respiratory findings are often absent.
- Malnutrition is commonly seen in infected infants as a result of inadequate food intake during a prolonged illness. This can be exacerbated by
- post-tussive vomiting which may lead to dehydration and/or aspiration.
- Secondary pneumonia and otitis media are frequent.
- Prolonged apnoea can result in hypoxic encephalopathy and seizures.

Table 42.2. Complications of pertussis infection in childhood

Malnutrition
Infection
• Pneumonia
• Otitis media
• Reactivation of latent tuberculosis
Apnoea
• Seizures
• Hypoxic encephalopathy
Sequelae of forceful coughing
• Subconjunctival haemorrhage
• Petechiae on upper body
• Epistaxis
• Intracranial haemorrhage
• Pneumothorax
• Subcutaneous emphysema
• Umbilical and inguinal hernia

- Physical sequelae of forceful coughing and paroxysms may also be present (Table 42.2).

Diagnosis

Clinical

- Consider pertussis when a child presents with a prolonged respiratory tract infection. In children presenting with a classical history of pertussis diagnosis is not difficult.

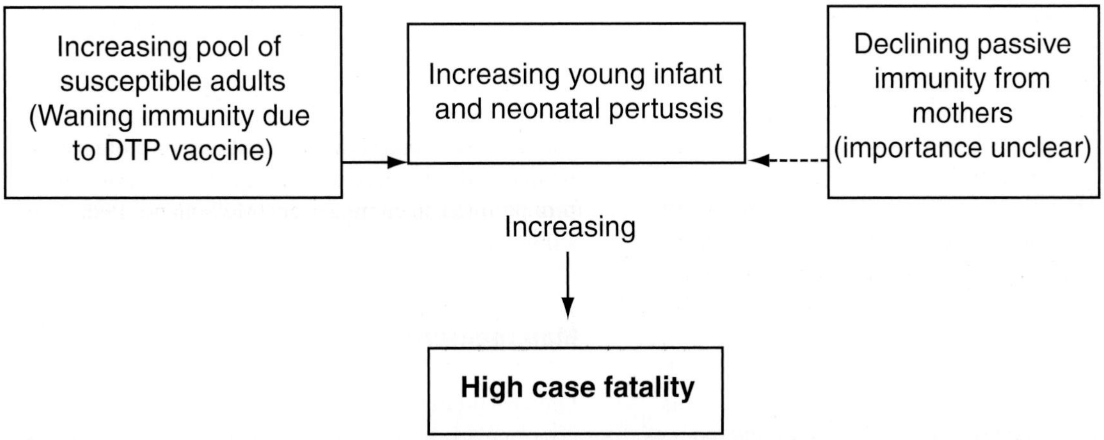

Fig. 42.1. Factors increasing cases of young infant and neonatal pertussis. (The importance of declining passive maternal immunity is unclear as maternal immunity did not adequately protect young infants in the pre-vaccine era.)

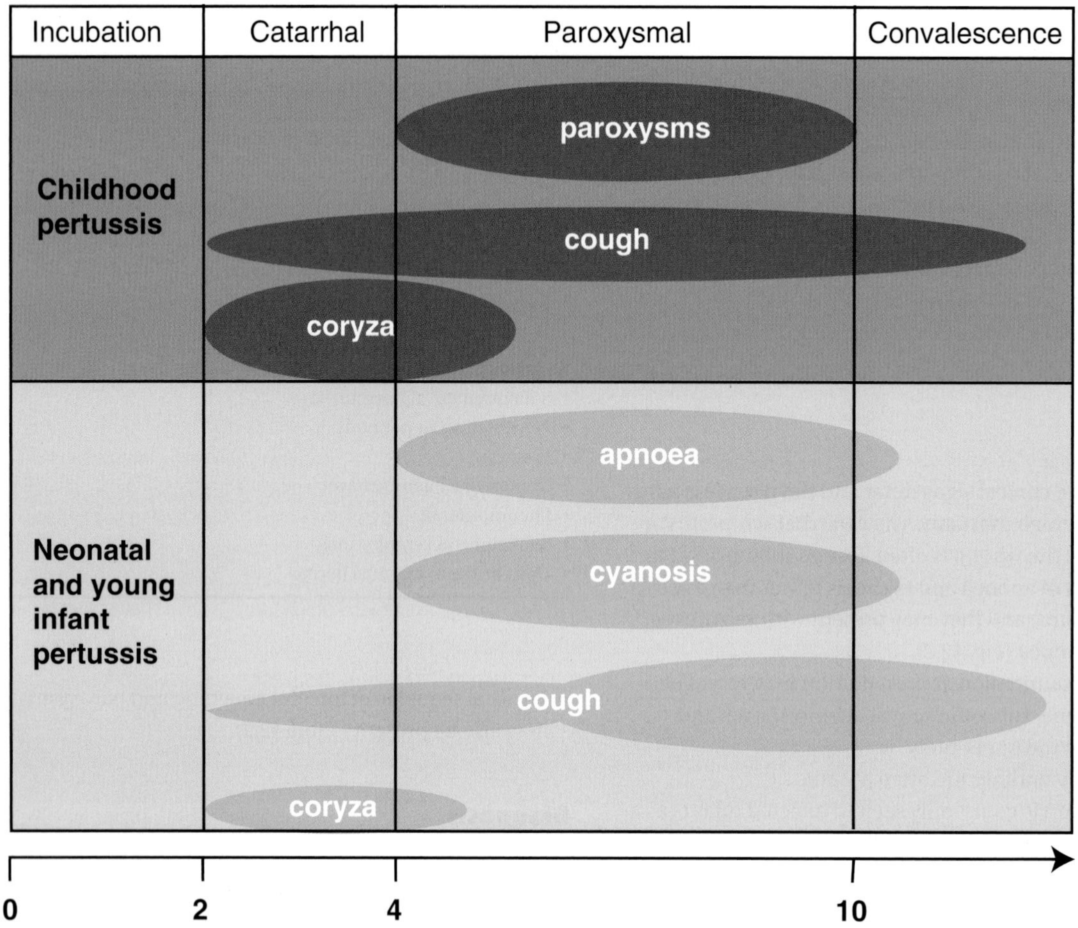

Fig. 42.2. Clinical phases of pertussis in childhood and infancy. (Adapted from Morley, 1973.)

- Be very careful with neonates and young infants as they may appear clinically well on initial examination even with severe pertussis.
- A history of incomplete immunization or exposure to a pertussis contact within 28 days of symptoms developing should raise suspicions.

Laboratory

Laboratory investigations can aid diagnosis, but their value depends on the timing of patient presentation.

Nasal swab

The first three weeks of infection have the highest yield of *B. pertussis* culture from per-nasal swab. However, this can be hindered by prior antibiotic therapy and requires specific swabs and media for culture.

Blood

Lymphocytosis is common from the end of the catarrhal phase through the paroxysmal phase, and this can be useful for the diagnosis (Muller et al., 1984).

Serological evidence of pertussis requires a documented rise in IgA or IgG antibodies to pertussis toxin or filamentous haemagglutinin, a cell surface protein on *B. pertussis*. Ideally, this requires acute and convalescent sera although diagnosis is often made on a high titre from a single sample.

Management

Effective prompt care depends on early diagnosis, which is particularly important in neonates and young infants. Therefore, health care workers and the general public must be aware of pertussis and alert if a child is sick.

Most children with pertussis can be satisfactorily managed at home with general supportive measures. However, young infants with suspected pertussis, and older children with prolonged cyanosis are better managed in hospital, where they can be closely observed and where measures to limit coughing, offer respiratory support and provide adequate nutrition can be undertaken. Coughing may be exacerbated by over-zealous pharyngeal suction or when a nasopharyngeal catheter is introduced, so limit these procedures strictly! If oxygen is required, it can be delivered perfectly adequately with nasal prongs rather than a nasopharyngeal catheter.

- Encourage breast feeding and food by mouth.
- Regular nasogastric feeds can be used in infants unable to drink, although coughing may be made worse when a nasogastric tube is inserted at first.
- Rarely, intravenous fluids may be needed for a short time if respiratory distress is severe or vomiting is excessive, but avoid this if possible.
- Erythromycin by mouth to an infected person reduces *B. pertussis* carriage and the period of infectivity and so limits the spread of the disease (Bergquist et al., 1987).
- Treat cases complicated by pneumonia with a broad spectrum antibiotic such as chloramphenicol or cotrimoxazole (Hoppe et al., 1989).
- Give a dose of DTP vaccine to any inadequately immunized children who have been in contact with a case of pertussis.

Vaccines

History

The effectiveness of whole cell pertussis vaccines has been demonstrated since the 1920s (Madson, 1925). Initial vaccines varied in efficacy so that an international standard was introduced in 1964. The triple antigen vaccine, which has been used throughout the world, consists of diphtheria and tetanus toxoid in combination with cellular components of pertussis. In 1966, aluminium salts were added as adjuvants, in an attempt to increase vaccine potency and lessen reactogenicity. After cellular pertussis vaccine was introduced in industrialized countries, the notifications of pertussis (Black, 1997) fell dramatically.

Adverse effects

Adverse effects associated with the whole cell vaccine include redness at the injection site, fever, persistent crying, drowsiness and fretfulness. Less common adverse neurological effects include hypotonic-hyporesponsive episodes and convulsions (Cody et al., 1981). Once the disease began to disappear in developed countries the public became increasingly concerned about adverse effects and this affected vaccination rates in some countries. Reduced vaccine uptake in the UK in the 1970s was followed by resurgence of pertussis, providing powerful evidence of the role of the pertussis vaccine in pertussis control (Pollard, 1980).

Because of continuing unease about the safety and reactogenicity of whole cell vaccines, a number of acellular vaccines have been developed. These contain 1–5 of the major pertussis antigens. They have similar adverse effects to the whole cell vaccines, but they occur less frequently (Cherry, 1997). They have similar efficacy to the effective whole cell vaccines, but the duration of the protection they confer is unknown. It is possible that several doses may be required through adulthood.

Unsolved problems

Waning vaccination rates over the past 10 years are likely to result in an increase in the number of cases of pertussis seen in Africa in the future. This increase will be superimposed on increasingly unstable epidemiology as waning vaccine-derived immunity leaves an increasing number of young adults susceptible to pertussis.

There is a real possibility that rates of pertussis in young African infants may increase substantially, and it is imperative that all health workers are alert to this possibility. In general, if vaccination rates increase so that more children complete the scheduled three doses of pertussis vaccine, the morbidity of pertussis will be reduced but pertussis will continue to circulate in well-immunized populations (Halperin et al., 1989; Christie et al., 1994).

Early recognition, improved diagnosis and improved case management of pertussis must be a high priority (see Box).

PERTUSSIS VACCINATION
an increased coverage, which includes isolated communites
is essential.
IT WILL REDUCE
the morbidity of pertussis in children.

In order to achieve a true reduction in childhood pertussis rates in Africa, immunization coverage must increase and vaccination programmes must reach the many isolated communities with poor vaccine coverage, where pertussis continues to circulate freely.

Theoretically, further reductions in neonatal and young infant pertussis may be possible by reducing the adult pertussis reservoir. This may be achieved by targeting susceptible young adults for booster vaccinations.

References

Aaby P. (1992). Overcrowding and intensive exposure. Major determinants of variation in measles mortality in Africa. *Mortality and Society in Sub-Saharan Africa*, pp. 319–348. Oxford: Clarendon Press.

Abdalla BA, Salih MA, Yousif EA et al. (1998). Whooping cough in Sudanese children. *East Afr Med J*; **75**: 353–357.

Bergquist S, Bernander S, Dahnsjo H et al. (1987). Erythromycin in the treatment of pertussis: a study of bacteriologic and clinical effects. *Pediatr Infect Dis J*; **6**: 458–461.

Black S. (1997). Epidemiology of pertussis. *Pediatr Infect Dis J*; **16**: S85–S89.

Bwibo N. (1971). Whooping cough in Uganda. *Scand J Infect Dis*; **3**: 41–43.

Cherry JD. (1997). Comparative efficacy of acellular pertussis vaccines: an analysis of recent trials. *Pediatr Infect Dis J*; **16**: S90–S96.

Christie CDC, Marx ML, Marchant CD et al. (1994). Resurgence of disease in a highly immunized population of children. *N Engl J Med*; **331**: 16–21.

Cody CL, Baraff LJ, Cherry JD et al. (1981). Nature and rates of adverse reactions associated with DTP and DT immunizations in infants and children. *Pediatrics*; **68**: 650–660.

Halperin SA, Bortolussi R, Maclean D et al. (1989). Persistence of pertussis in an immunized population: results of the Nova Scotia Enhanced Pertussis Surveillance Program. *J Pediatr*; **155**: 686–693.

Hoppe JE, Halm U, Hagedorn HJ et al. (1989). Comparison of erythromycin ethylsuccinate and cotrimoxazole for treatment of pertussis. *Infection*; 17: 227–231.

Madson T. (1925). Whooping cough: its bacteriology, diagnosis, prevention and treatment. *Boston Med Surg J*; **192**: 50–60.

Miller CL Fletcher WB. (1976). Severity of notified whooping cough. *Br Med J*; **1**:117–119.

Morley D. (1973). *Paediatric Priorities in the Developing World.* Butterworth Press.

Morley D, Woodland M, Martin WJ. (1966). Whooping cough in Nigerian Children. *Trop Geogr Med*; **18**: 169–182.

Mulholland K. (1995). Measles and pertussis in developing countries with good vaccine coverage. *Lancet*; **345**: 305–307.

Muller AS, Leeuwenburg J, Voorhoeve AM. (1984). Pertussis in a rural area of Kenya: epidemiology and results of a vaccine trial. *Bull WHO*; **62**: 899–908.

Nelson JD. (1978). The changing epidemiology of pertussis in young infants. *Am J Dis Child*; **132**: 371–373.

Pollard R. (1980). Relation between vaccination and notification rates for whooping cough in England and Wales. *Lancet*; **ii**: 1180–1182.

Ramkissoon A, Coovadia HM, Loening WEK. (1995). Subclinical pertussis in incompletely vaccinated and unvaccinated infants. *S Afr Med J*; **85**: 662–667.

Stojanov S, Liese J, Belohradsky BH. (2000). Hospitalization and complications in children under 2 years of age with *Bordetella pertussis* infection. *J Infect Dis*; **182**: 174–179.

Strebel P, Hussey G, Metcalf C, et al. (1991). An outbreak of whooping cough in a highly vaccinated urban community. *J Trop Pediatr*; **37**: 71–76.

Stroffolini T, Giammanco A, Chiarini A et al. (1991). Seroepidemiology of pertussis infection in an urban childhood population in Cameroon. *Eur J Epidemiol*; **7**: 64–67.

Voorhoeve AM, Muller AS, Schulpen TWJ,'t Mannetje W, Van Rens M. (1978). Machakos project studies: the epidemiology of pertussis. *Trop Geogr Med*; **30**: 125–139.

World Health Organization. (1999); *Wkly Epidemiol Rec*; **74**: 137–144.

43

Diphtheria

The problem in Africa

Classical faucial diphtheria, complicated by myocarditis and neuropathy, is not a common problem in Africa, but it does occur, and sporadic epidemics have been described (van Geldermalsen & Wenning, 1993; Loevinsohn, 1990). Diphtheritic ulcers of the skin, which usually occur on the legs, are more common, and occur sporadically.

The organism

Corynebacterium diphtheriae is a club-shaped gram-positive rod. Toxigenic strains cause necrosis of the mucosal epithelium of the nasopharynx. This, combined with an acute inflammatory exudate, gives rise to the classical diphtheritic membrane, which can lead to obstruction of the airway. *C. diphtheriae* secretes an exotoxin, which enters the circulation and may cause myocarditis or peripheral neuropathy.

Epidemiology

C. diphtheriae has no animal reservoir but it may be carried in the throat and on the skin. Spread of infection is by direct contact, droplet infection and fomites which may infect milk. Non-toxigenic strains are harmless, and may be isolated from the upper respiratory tract or skin.

Control and prevention

Vaccination with toxoid (toxin rendered safe by heat and formalin treatment) reduces carriage of the toxigenic form of the organism and also the incidence and severity of disease. Three doses of diphtheria toxoid are given in infancy, combined with tetanus toxoid and pertussis vaccine (DPT or triple vaccine). Natural immunity continues to be generated by non-toxigenic strains in the community (Kurtzhals et al., 1997).

Clinical features

Classical diphtheria

C. diphtheriae is not an invasive organism. Respiratory tract disease occurs at the anterior nares, fauces, larynx or large airways 2–4 days after colonization. Faucial infection (posterior mouth and proximal pharynx) is the most common and is characterized by an abrupt onset of sore throat, low grade fever, malaise and the characteristic adherent whitish-grey membrane on the tonsils (this appearance led to the name 'diphtheria' which is a term derived from the Greek word for leather). The membrane can become extensive and occlude the airway. Toxic effects are produced when the diphteria exotoxin enters host cells by specific receptors and kills the cell by altering protein synthesis. These effects are dose dependent and occur in proportion to the amount of local disease. Cardiac toxicity (myocarditis) with arrhythmias and heart failure, and neurologic toxicity with cranial and somatic nerve paralysis carry a very high mortality (Salih et al., 1981).

Diphtheritic skin lesions

Skin lesions vary greatly. They may start as a small vesicle, which ulcerates rapidly, and can be indistinguishable from streptococcal pyoderma. It is usually on the leg, single, well demarcated and very vascular, bleeding easily. A grey membranous exudate may be seen, which is shed leaving a shallow ulcer, which may be slow to heal, and can give rise to a typical tropical ulcer.

Diagnosis and treatment

Classical faucial diphtheria can be diagnosed clinically. The organism can be isolated from fragments of diphtheritic membrane using special media, but swabbing of the throat must only be attempted with caution because bleeding can result. Skin lesions are diagnosed by isolation of the organism.

Treatment

The aim is to neutralize the exotoxin, to kill residual organisms and to minimize the established effects of pharyngeal palsy or myocardial failure. Give diphtheria antitoxin 20 000–40 000 units intramuscularly (i.m.)or intravenously, and procaine penicillin 1.2 million units i.m. daily, or erythromycin 2 g daily, for 10 days.

References

CDC. (2000). *Diphtheria*. CDC website. 2000. http: //www.cdc.gov/health/diseases.htm.

Kurtzhals JA, Kjeldsen K, Hey AS, Okong'o-Odera EA, Heron I. (1997). Immunity to tetanus and diphtheria in rural Africa. *Am J Trop Med Hyg*; **56**: 576–579.

Loevinsohn BP. (1990). The changing age structure of diphtheria patients: evidence for the effectiveness of EPI in the Sudan. *Bull Wld Hlth Org*; **68**: 353–357.

Salih MA, Suliman GI, Hassan HS. (1981). Complications of diphtheria seen during the 1978 outbreak in Khartoum. *Ann Trop Paediatr*; **1**: 97–101.

van Geldermalsen AA, Wenning U. (1993). A diphtheria epidemic in Lesotho, 1989. Did vaccination increase the population's susceptibility? *Ann Trop Paediatr*; **13**: 13–19.

Rickettsial infections

44

Rickettsioses are among the oldest recognized infectious diseases (Raoult & Roux, 1997). Epidemic typhus is suspected to have been responsible for the plague in Athens during the fifth century BC and the disease was differentiated from typhoid in the sixteenth century. In 1928, Nicolle demonstrated that epidemic typhus was transmitted by the body louse. In 1910, the first cases of the tick-borne Mediterranean spotted fever were reported in Tunis by Conor and Bruch and the role of *Rhipicephalus sanguineus*, the brown dog tick, in the transmission of the disease was established in 1930. Rickettsioses, however, have also recently been presented as a model of emerging diseases. Of the 12 currently recognized tick-borne human rickettsioses throughout the world, 7 have been described since 1991, including *Rickettsia africae*, the agent of African tick-bite fever (Kelly et al., 1996; Raoult & Roux, 1997; Parola & Raoult., 2001).

The organisms

Rickettsioses are caused by bacteria of the order Rickettsiales. These organisms were first described as short, gram-negative rods that retained basic fuchsin when stained by the method of Gimenez (Raoult & Roux, 1997). Recent developments in molecular taxonomic methods, however, have resulted in the reclassification of the rickettsiae. For example, the Rochalimaea, united within the genus Bartonella, and Coxiella were removed from the order Rickettsiales and the classification of this order continues to be modified as new data become available. Human rickettsioses occurring in Africa include those caused by bacteria of the genus *Rickettsia* which is sub-divided into:

(i) the typhus group including *Rickettsia typhi*, the agent of murine typhus, and *R. prowazekii*, the agent of epidemic typhus, and

(ii) the spotted fever group including *R. conorii*, the agent of Mediterranean spotted fever, *R. africae* the agent of African tick-bite fever and more than 20 other species (pathogenic or of unknown pathogenicity) throughout the world.

Because Q fever caused by *Coxiella burnetii* and infections due to *Bartonella* spp., particularly trench fever, have been called 'rickettsioses' for a long time, they will also be described in this chapter.

Bacteria of the genus Rickettsia are strict intracellular, short (0.8 –2 μm long and 0.3–0.5 μm in diameter) gram-negative rods, which retain basic fuchsin when stained by the method of Gimenez. In the laboratory they can be grown in live organisms (animals, embryonated eggs) or cell cultures (VERO, L929, HEL or MRC5 cells). They live within the cytoplasm of host cells but are not enclosed in a vacuole. Their genome is small (1 to 1.6 Mb) and is contained in a single circular chromosome (Raoult & Roux, 1997).

Rickettsia species are associated with arthropods which may act as vectors, reservoirs, and/or amplifiers of the organisms. Ixodids (hard ticks) are the main vectors and/or reservoirs of spotted fever group rickettsiae, while in the typhus group rickettsiae lice and fleas are the vectors of *Rickettsia prowazekii* and *Rickettsia typhi*, respectively. With the exception of *Rickettsia prowazekii*, most rickettsiae do not normally infect humans during their natural cycles between their arthropod and vertebrate hosts.

In the human host, pathogenic rickettsiae multiply in endothelial cells causing a vasculitis, which is responsible for the clinical and laboratory abnormalities that occur in rickettsioses (Raoult & Roux, 1997). In natural vertebrate hosts, though, infections may result in a rickettsaemia which enables further arthropod vectors to become infected and for the natural cycle to be perpetuated.

Of the rickettsial protein antigens, two high molecular mass surface proteins (rOmpA and rOmpB) contain species-specific epitopes which provide the basis for rickettsial serotyping using comparative micro-immunofluorescence which remains the reference method for the identification of rickettsiae (Lascola & Raoult, 1997). The main problem with this serological identification is the need for reference sera. Each time a new isolate is tested, it must be screened against anti-sera to all known rickettsiae, which is time consuming and the required anti-sera can be only be produced in specialized laboratories.

Sequence analysis of polymerase chain reaction (PCR) products is currently the most rapid, convenient and sensitive technique for the detection and identification of rickettsiae. Several rickettsial genes have been used for the study of the phylogeny of the rickettsiae, the identification of new isolates and to diagnose and describe emerging diseases (Lascola & Raoult, 1997). With this technique numerous samples, including blood, skin biopsies and arthropods can be used for the detection and identification of rickettsiae. Thus, any laboratory with facilities for molecular methods and access to sequence databases is able to detect and identify all known species of the genus Rickettsia.

The development of these molecular methods has greatly facilitated collaborative research between rickettsial reference laboratories and laboratories in countries with less developed facilities for research. For example, we could confirm the presence of *Rickettsia prowazekii*, the agent of epidemic typhus, in lice collected from refugees in Burundi and sent to Marseille in plastic containers at room temperature and humidity (Roux et al., 1999).

Tick-borne rickettsioses in Africa

Tick-borne rickettsioses were first described in Africa at the beginning of the twentieth century and it is now known that at least two human tick-borne rickettsioses occur on the continent:

- Mediterranean spotted fever caused by *Rickettsia conorii* and
- African tick-bite fever caused by *Rickettsia africae*.

Mediterranean spotted fever was first reported by Conor and Bruch in Tunisia in 1910 and subsequently found to be caused by *Rickettsia conorii* and transmitted by the brown dog tick *Rhipicephalus sanguineus*. This potentially severe disease was sometimes also referred to as 'boutonneuse fever' because of the papular rash seen with the disease.

Tick-borne diseases of humans were also described in southern Africa in the early twentieth century, and there was debate as to whether these were cases of Mediterranean spotted fever. In the 1930s in South Africa, Pijper described African tick-bite fever as a rural disease occurring in people having contact with cattle ticks, particularly *Amblyomma* spp. The disease was far milder than Mediterranean spotted fever and was not associated with skin rash or complications. On the basis of this clinical and epidemiological data, Pijper considered African tick-bite fever to be distinct from Mediterranean spotted fever. His results were not generally accepted, and for the next 60 years, both Mediterranean spotted fever and African tick-bite fever were erroneously attributed to infections with *Rickettsia conorii*.

In 1990, Kelly et al. isolated rickettsial strains from *Amblyomma hebraeum* ticks in Zimbabwe and demonstrated them to be distinct from *Rickettsia conorii* and indistinguishable from an isolate obtained from an *Amblyomma variegatum* in Ethiopia. In 1992, a rickettsia was isolated from a patient suffering from African tick-bite fever in Zimbabwe and was found to be indistinguishable from the isolates from *A. hebraeum* ticks. This was subsequently characterized as a distinct species of the spotted fever group rickettsiae, named *Rickettsia africae* (Kelly et al., 1996), and African tick-bite fever is now known to be a distinct spotted fever group rickettsiosis.

Mediterranean spotted fever

Epidemiology

The disease is caused by *Rickettsia conorii*, a spotted fever group rickettsia which is transmitted by the brown dog tick, *Rhipicephalus sanguineus*, in Europe and North Africa. The yellow dog tick, *Haemaphysalis leachi*, and *Rhipicephalus simus* have been suspected as vectors in southern Africa, but no isolate is currently available from these ticks. Ticks are known to be reservoirs of spotted fever group rickettsioses, maintaining the infection by transstadial (i.e., passage of bacteria from stage to stage, from larvae to nymphs and then to adults) and transovarial (from one generation to the next via the female ovaries) transmission. Rickettsiae infect and multiply in almost all the organs of ticks, in particular the salivary glands, which enables them to be transmitted to vertebrate hosts during feeding. Humans do not appear to be natural reservoirs of spotted fever group rickettsiae, as many ticks do not feed readily on humans, who are only rickettseamic for relatively short periods (Raoult & Roux, 1997).

In Africa, *Rickettsia conorii* is found in the Mediterranean area (Algeria, Morocco, Libya and Egypt) and has also been isolated or detected in Kenya, Central African Republic, Zimbabwe and South Africa. It probably also occurs in other African countries where dogs and the reservoir ticks are prevalent. Infection of humans in sub-Saharan Africa with *Rickettsia conorii* appears to be rare, however, as the vector ticks are relatively host-specific and rarely feed on humans. Moreover, the prevalence of infected ticks is generally low (under 10%). In the Mediterranean area, the disease occurs in late spring and summer, particularly in August when there is increased activity of immature forms of the ticks. These are far smaller than adults and are usually not observed.

Clinical features

The mean incubation period of Mediterranean spotted fever is about 6 days. The onset of signs is abrupt and, typically, patients have high fever (>39 °C), malaise, chills, headache, myalgia, arthralgia and a unique eschar (the 'tache noire') at the tick-bite site (about 75% of the cases). On about day 3 or 4 of the illness, a rash appears (97%) on the body and generalizes in 1 to 3 days to include the hands and feet. It is papular rather than macular and may be purpuric (10%). Mildly affected patients may recover spontaneously after 2 or 3 weeks. With appropriate antibiotic therapy defervescence usually occurs in 2 to 3 days. Severe forms of the disease occur in 6 per cent of patients, particularly in elderly people, and include neurological, renal, and cardiac or vascular complications. The mortality rate may be as high as 2.5 per cent (Raoult & Roux, 1997).

African tick-bite fever

Epidemiology

African tick-bite fever is a tick-borne disease caused by *Rickettsia africae*, a member of the spotted fever group rickettsiae. In southern Africa the vector of the disease is *Amblyomma hebraeum*, a tick of large ruminants and wildlife species that is prevalent in many rural areas. *Rickettsia africae* is transmitted transtadially and transovarially by *Amblyomma hebraeum* and all feeding stages of the tick can transmit the infection to susceptible hosts (Fig. 44.1). As up to 100 per cent of these ticks in an area may be infected with *Rickettsia africae*, and the tick also feeds readily on humans, cases of African tick-bite fever often occur in clusters and patients often present with multiple inoculation eschars (Raoult et al., 2001a).

Rickettsia africae has been detected in *Amblyomma variegatum* from the Central African Republic, Mali, Niger, Burundi and Ethiopia (Parola et al., 2001) and in *Amblyomma lepidum* from the Sudan (Parola et al., 2001). Recently, we documented cases in tourists returning from numerous countries including those in western and eastern Africa (Raoult et al., 2001a) and the geographical distribution of African tick-bite fever appears to parallel that of Amblyomma ticks, the vectors and reservoirs of *Rickettsia africae*. African tick-bite fever is also endemic

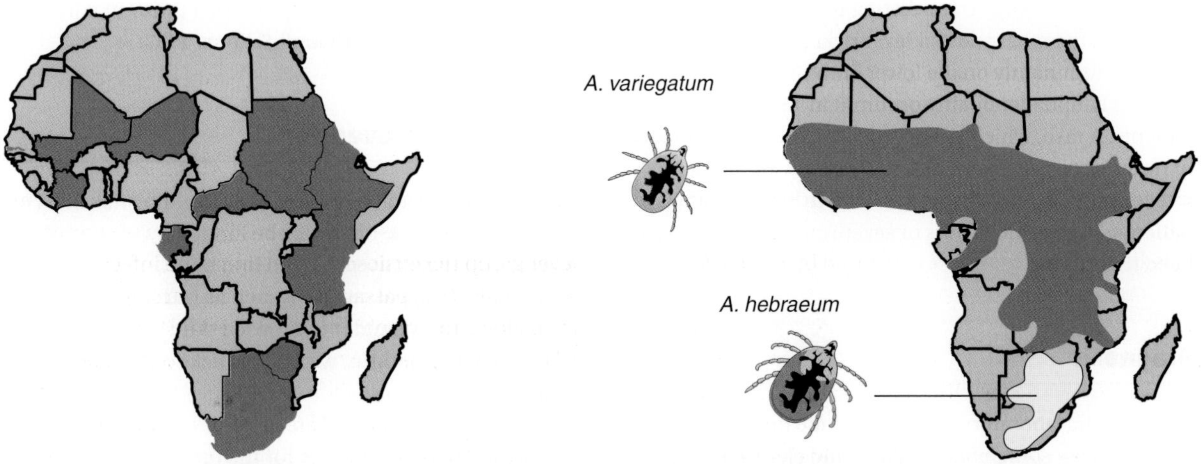

Fig. 44.1. Geographical distribution of African tick-bite fever (left) according to detection and/or isolation of *Rickettsia africae* from patients or ticks, and geographical distribution of the major potential vectors (right), *Amblyomma hebraeum* and *Amblyomma variegatum*.

in the West Indies, where *Amblyomma variegatum* was introduced during the eighteenth or nineteenth century on cattle shipped from Senegal to Guadeloupe (Parola et al., 1998a, 1999).

Serosurveys in Africa have shown high prevalences (30 – 80%) of antibodies to spotted fever group rickettsiae. These high rates of infection may be explained by the high prevalences (30 – 100%) of *Rickettsia africae* infection in *Amblyomma* species (Parola et al., 2001), the wide distribution of these ticks in Africa and the fact that Amblyomma are well known to feed readily on humans. Despite the apparent very high prevalence of African tick-bite fever in native Africans the disease is most commonly recognized in Europeans and tourists. Serological evidence indicates the infection is often acquired at an early age, and at this time it may be less severe with patients not presenting for medical treatment. It might also be that African tick-bite fever is often misdiagnosed as one of the other common febrile diseases in Africa, such as malaria (Raoult et al., 2001a).

Clinical features

More than 100 cases of African tick-bite fever have now been diagnosed in our laboratory, all in people returning from Africa, and particularly those who have been on safari in southern Africa (Raoult et al., 2001a). Tick-bites or tick contact was reported by 44 per cent of the patients and the mean incubation period to onset of signs was 6.6 (+/− 3) days. Fever occurred in 88 per cent of the patients and clinical signs were generally mild. Specific features of the disease include its occurrence in groups of people (74%) and the high prevalence of multiple inoculation eschars (55%), which distinguishes African tick-bite fever from the other spotted fever rickettsioses. Eschars were predominantly on the lower limbs (62%) and regional lymphadenopathy occurred in 43 per cent of patients. A rash, which is usually considered the hallmark of rickettsioses, is infrequent in patients with African tick-bite fever (49%) and may be vesicular in 50 per cent of patients. To date, no deaths or severe complications have been reported.

Diagnosis

Non-specific laboratory findings include thrombocytopenia, leukocyte count abnormalities and elevated hepatic enzyme levels.

Serology is the most available and simplest diagnostic test for the diagnosis of tick-borne rickettsioses (Lascola & Raoult, 1997). Immunofluorescence is the reference method and should be used to detect rising antibody titres with acute and convalescent sera. A major limitation to the test is serological cross-reactivity; generally it is not possible to differentiate between immune responses to the different spotted fever rickettsiae, including *Rickettsia conorii* and *Rickettsia africae.* Western blot immunoassays, particularly with sera that has been cross-adsorbed, can be used to determine the rickettsia species causing an immune response, but the technique is only available in specialized laboratories.

Rickettsiae may be isolated from blood, skin biopsies or ticks using cell culture. The centrifugation shell-vial technique using HEL fibroblasts is the reference method, but this is usually only performed in reference laboratories. Immunodetection methods may also be used to identify rickettsiae in biopsy specimens and arthropods.

Molecular methods based on PCR have enabled the development of useful, sensitive and rapid tools to detect and identify rickettsiae in blood, skin biopsies (the 'tache noire' being the most useful specimen) and even ticks. Primers amplifying sequences of several rickettsial genes can be used and any laboratory with facilities for molecular methods and access to sequence databases can identify rickettsiae.

Treatment

Empirical treatment is usually started before laboratory confirmation of the diagnosis. The treatment of choice of both Mediterranean spotted fever and African tick-bite fever is 200 mg doxycycline daily for 1–7 days depending on the severity of the disease. In children and pregnant women, josamycin (50 mg/kg/day or 3 g/day in adults) can be used for 8 days (Raoult & Roux, 1997).

Control and prevention

These diseases can be prevented by avoiding tick bites in infested areas. Tick-bites may be limited by:

- wearing long trousers tucked into boots.
- applying a topical repellent such as DEET (N,N-Diethyl-m-toluamide) to exposed skin
- applying permethrin, which kills ticks on contact, to clothes.

People staying in infested areas should be advised to check their bodies routinely for the presence of attached ticks. The immature stages of ticks may be only the size of a pin-head and these may attach at sites which are difficult to examine, in particular the scalp and the anogenital areas. Any tick found attached should be removed immediately using blunt, rounded forceps.

Louse-borne rickettsiosis: epidemic typhus

Epidemic typhus may have been responsible for the plague described in Athens in the fifth century BC. The disease was certainly recognized during the sixteenth century when the presence of an exanthem allowed its distinction from typhoid. Nicole subsequently demonstrated it was transmitted by the body louse and, for this discovery, he was awarded the Nobel prize (Raoult & Roux, 1999).

The problem in Africa

Body lice thrive during times of war, conflict, famine and natural catastrophes and it is at these times that epidemic typhus can cause severe morbidity and mortality. As Zinsser stated (1935), epidemic typhus probably caused more deaths than all the wars in human history. The disease re-emerged during World War I, and during the revolution in Russia there were 25 million cases with 3 million deaths. During World War II, typhus was prevalent in Northern Africa and in southern, central and eastern Europe.

Foci remained in the cooler mountainous countries in northern, north-eastern and central Africa. Only a few cases were recorded from these sites, however, and in the 1980s the WHO ceased monitoring the disease in most countries. In 1995 it was suspected to be endemic only in Ethiopia, but it dramatically re-emerged in 1997, with more than 100 000 cases during the civil war in Burundi (Raoult et al., 1998; Raoult & Roux, 1999).

A case was recently reported in North Africa (Niang et al., 1999). Epidemic typhus remains a potential major health risk in Africa, particularly in refugee camps in the cooler mountainous areas.

Epidemiology

Epidemic typhus is caused by *Rickettsia prowazekii*, which belongs to the typhus group of the genus *Rickettsia*. It is transmitted to humans by the body louse *Pediculus humanus humanus* (or *Pediculus humanus corporis*), which lives in clothes and thrives in cold climates under conditions of poor hygiene (Raoult & Roux, 1999) (Fig. 44.2). The body louse becomes infected with *Rickettsia prowazekii* while feeding on rickettsaemic patients. Within 5 to 7 days massive quantities of rickettsiae are discharged in the faeces of lice and may remain infective for up to 100 days. *Rickettsia prowazekii* is transmitted to humans when the infected faeces of lice contaminate their feeding sites, or when conjunctivae or mucous membranes are exposed to the crushed bodies or faeces of infected lice. Transmission might also result from the inhalation of infected faeces and this is thought to be the main route of infection for health workers attending patients.

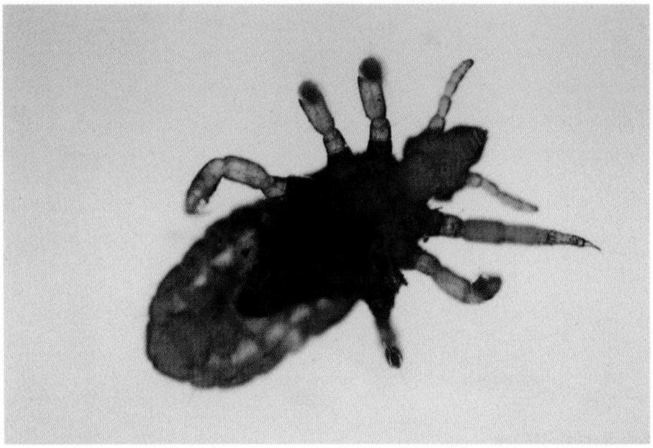

Fig. 44.2. The human body louse, *Pediculus humanus humanus* (= *Pediculus humanus corporis*).

Infected lice always die within 1 to 2 weeks; humans are the major reservoir of infection. People who survive epidemic typhus remain infected with *Rickettsia prowazekii* for life and when stressed they may suffer from a milder form of typhus, the Brill–Zinsser disease. People with Brill–Zinsser disease may be the source of a new epidemic if they become infested with body lice (Raoult & Roux, 1999).

Clinical features

The incubation period is 10–14 days. Patients develop malaise and vague symptoms before the abrupt onset of fever (100%), headache (100%) and myalgia (70–100%). In a recent investigation in Burundi, a crouching attitude due to myalgia, named 'sutama', was reported (Raoult et al., 1998). Other frequently observed signs are nausea or vomiting (42–56%), coughing (38–70%) and abnormalities of central nervous system function ranging from confusion to stupor (18–80%) and coma (4%) (Raoult et al., 1998). Diarrhoea, pulmonary involvement, myocarditis, splenomegaly and conjunctivitis may also occur. Most patients develop a skin rash that classically begins on the

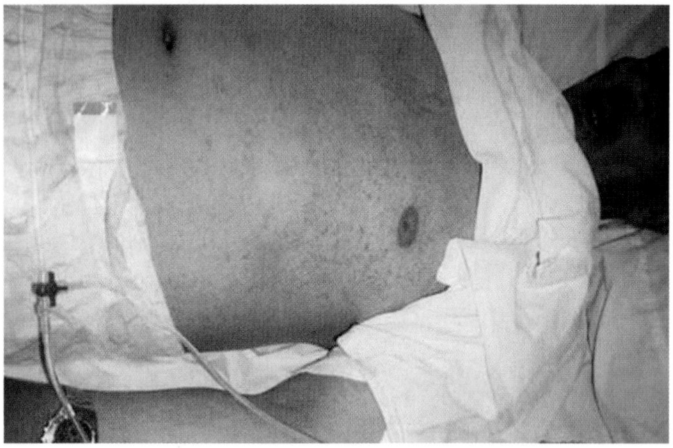

Fig. 44.3. The rash in epidemic typhus.

trunk and spreads to the limbs. It may be macular, maculo-papular or petechial and may be difficult to see in pigmented skins (Fig. 44.3). Gangrene of the distal extremities may occur in severe cases. Without treatment mortality rates are 10–30 per cent, depending on the presence of other underlying conditions and the nutritional status of patients. The recrudescence of epidemic typhus, Brill–Zinsser disease, can appear many years after the acute disease and is milder (Raoult & Roux, 1999).

Diagnosis

Thrombocytopenia and hepatic abnormalities may occur, particularly in severe cases. The diagnosis of typhus is based on serology, with indirect immunofluorescence being the reference method (Lascola et al., 1997). Serology, however, does not enable patients with epidemic typhus to be differentiated from those with murine typhus caused by *Rickettsia typhi* unless cross-absorption and/or Western-blotting are performed (Lascola et al., 2000). In specialized laboratories the disease may be diagnosed using shell-vial tissue culture (see tick-borne rickettsioses) or with molecular tools (Birg et al., 1999). Lice can be also used as epidemiologic diagnostic tools: *Rickettsia prowazekii* was detected in lice collected from refugees in Burundi and sent to our laboratory in Marseille in plastic boxes at room temperature and humidity (Roux et al., 1999).

Treatment

Any patient suspected to have epidemic typhus must be treated empirically with a tetracycline. A single 200 mg dose of oral doxycycline usually leads to defervescence within 48 hours. Chloramphenicol may also be used.

Control and prevention

Louse eradication is the most important preventive measure and is essential in the control of outbreaks. Since body lice live only in clothing, where they also lay their eggs, the simplest method of delousing is to remove and destroy all clothing. Thoroughly washing and boiling clothes can also be effective. Dusting of all clothing with 10 per cent DDT, 1 per cent malathion, or 1 per cent permethrin (as in the protocol of the World Health Organization) is also a rapid and effective method of killing body lice and reduces the risk of reinfestation (Raoult & Roux, 1999). Protective vaccines have been developed, but they have not been widely used because effective antibiotic treatments are readily available. Vaccination is currently reserved for workers in laboratories which handle potentially infected specimens.

Flea-borne rickettsiosis: murine typhus

Murine (flea-borne) typhus is one of the oldest recognized arthropod-borne zoonoses. It was reported in Mexico in 1570 by Bravo and described clinically in a grain silo worker in Australia in 1923. The disease was recognized to be distinct from epidemic typhus in the 1920s. The causative organism was named *Rickettsia mooseri*, later changed to *Rickettsia typhi*.

The problem in Africa

Although murine typhus has a worldwide distribution, it is often unrecognized and documented cases are rarely reported, particularly in tropical countries. Information on the prevalence of murine typhus in humans is based principally on serosurveys, but also on some case series and case reports in tourists (Parola et al., 1998b). Generally, the prevalence of the disease is higher in coastal areas where rats are more prevalent (Fig. 44.4).

Epidemiology

Murine typhus is caused by *Rickettsia typhi*, formerly *Rickettsia mooseri*, which belongs to the typhus group of the genus Rickettsia. The main vector is the rat flea

Xenopsylla cheopis and rodents, mainly *Rattus norvegicus* and *Rattus rattus*, act as reservoirs. The classical cycle of infection is rat to rat flea to rat; *Rickettsia typhi* is only rarely transmitted transovarially in fleas. Infections in rats are not fatal and rickettsemia persists from day-7 to day-12 after inoculation. Although fleas remain infected for life, their lifespan is not shortened by the infection. Rickettsiae are excreted in the faeces where they remain viable for several years. Humans become infected when flea faeces containing *Rickettsia typhi* contaminate disrupted skin, or are inhaled. Rarely, infections may result from flea bites (Azad et al., 1997; Raoult & Roux, 1997).

Clinical features

Murine typhus is a mild disease with non-specific signs. The incubation period is 7 to 14 days and at presentation the classical triad of fever, headache and skin rash is observed in less than 15 per cent of cases. Later in the disease fever and headache occur more frequently, but a rash is present in less than 50 per cent of patients and is often transient or difficult to see. Nausea, vomiting, abdominal pain, diarrhoea, jaundice, confusion and seizures have been reported. Fewer than 50 per cent of patients report exposure to fleas or flea hosts. In untreated patients the illness lasts for 7 to 14 days, after which there is usually a rapid recovery (Raoult & Roux, 1997; Parola et al., 1998b).

Diagnosis

Common laboratory abnormalities are leukocytosis or mild leukopenia, anaemia and thrombocytopenia. Hyponatraemia, hypoalbuminaemia and hepatic and renal abnormalities may also be seen. The diagnosis of murine typhus is based on serology; immunofluorescence is the reference method (Lascola et al., 1997). Cross-absorption of sera and Western-blotting can be used to differentiate infections with *Rickettsia typhi* and *Rickettsia prowazekii* (Lascola et al., 2000). Molecular tools and tissue cultures using the shell-vial technique may be used to diagnose infections in specialized laboratories (see tick-borne rickettsioses).

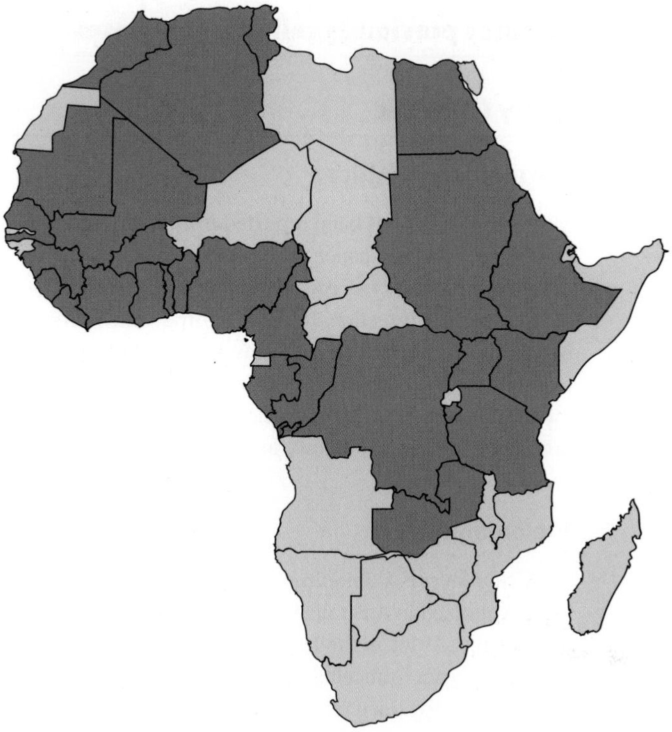

Fig. 44.4. Documented risk areas of murine typhus in Africa according to seroepidemiologic studies, case series or imported cases in travellers. (Cowan, 1997; Anstey et al. 1997; Parola et al., 1998; Okabayashi et al., 1999.)

Treatment

The treatment of choice is a single 200 mg dose of oral doxycycline, which usually leads to defervescence within 72 hours.

Control and prevention

People may protect themselves against fleas with topical DEET (*N*,*N*-diethyl-*m*-toluamide), a repellent applied to exposed skin. Rat flea populations can be controlled by dusting rat passageways with insecticides, and houses can be made less attractive to rats by improving hygiene and limiting access to areas below the floors. Eradicating rats will also decrease flea populations but it is essential to first control rat flea populations. Otherwise, in the absence of rats, their fleas will be forced to feed on alternative hosts which might result in outbreaks of *Rickettsia typhi* infections in local people.

Diseases previously called 'rickettioses'

Query (Q) fever

The problem in Africa

Although Q fever has been reported from many African countries, the significance of the disease is probably underestimated, as few countries have laboratories able to diagnose the infection. In West, Central, and Southern Africa, seroprevalences in humans are highest (up to 40%) in countries with large numbers of domestic ruminants, including Mali, Burkina Faso, Nigeria, the Central-African Republic, Zambia, Zimbabwe and South Africa.

The organism

Query (Q) fever is a ubiquitous zoonotic disease that was first recognized in Australia by Derrick in 1935, and described in Africa in the 1950s. It is caused by *Coxiella burnetii*, a strict intracellular gram-negative bacterium that has recently been removed from the order Rickettsiales because of its distinct genotype. *C. burnetii* is characterised by its antigenic phase variation (Maurin & Raoult, 1999) and lives in the phagosome of host cells, but can also survive in the environment under very harsh conditions.

Epidemiology

Infections are usually acquired by inhaling or ingesting virulent organisms from infected mammals, in particular goats, sheep and cats. Although *Coxiella burnetii* causes little, if any, disease in domestic animals, it multiplies and reaches high concentrations in their placentas, and aerosols generated during parturition are particularly infective (Maurin & Raoult, 1999). Although *Coxiella burnetii* has been found to infect ticks, their role in human infections is probably minimal. The faeces of infected ticks, however, have high concentrations of viable organisms which may persist for long periods in the environment. Thus ticks may play a role in the dissemination of *Coxiella burnetii.*

Clinical features

There are distinctly different clinical features in the acute and chronic forms of Q fever. The acute disease is usually mild and up to half of infected people may be asymptomatic. A self-limited febrile syndrome or 'pseudo-flu' occurs most frequently in symptomatic patients, but in more serious cases there might be hepatitis, pneumonitis and prolonged fever.

Chronic Q fever may present as endocarditis in patients with underlying valvulopathies or, more rarely, as vascular aneurysms, graft infections, chronic bone infections, or pseudotumours of the lung (Raoult et al., 2000).

Diagnosis

The diagnosis is usually serological, with immunofluorescence being the reference method. The presence of phase I and phase II antibodies enable the acute and chronic forms of the disease to be distinguished. Molecular methods and cell culture systems (see tick-borne rickettsioses) may be used for diagnosis but this is only possible in specialized laboratories.

Treatment and prevention

A 2-week regimen of doxycycline is recommended for the treatment of acute Q fever (Maurin & Raoult, 1999). Fluoroquinolones are also effective. Treatment with macrolides and co-trimoxazole is not always effective, and currently there is no regimen that can be recommended for children and pregnant women. The prognosis for patients with chronic Q fever has recently been improved with the use of long-term treatment with combinations of doxycycline with chloroquine, but there is no broadly accepted treatment regimen for this condition (Maurin & Raoult, 1999). Effective vaccines are only available in Australia.

Bartonella infections

Bartonella are gram-negative, fastidious aerobic rod-shaped bacteria that grow in axenic medium and/or blood-enriched agar. Species previously known as Rochalimaea have been renamed Bartonella and the genus has been removed from the order Rickettsiales (Maurin et al., 1997). Currently, only *Bartonella henselae* (Kelly et al., 1998) and *Bartonella quintana* (Raoult et al., 1998; Roux et al., 1999) have been reported to occur in Africa. *Bartonella henselae* is an agent of cat scratch disease and may also cause bacillary angiomatosis, peliosis, endocarditis, bacteraemia, lymphadenitis and neurological signs in HIV-infected patients (Maurin et al., 1997). *Bartonella quintana* is the agent of trench fever and may also cause bacillary angiomatosis and hepatic peliosis in immunocompromised people. Of these diseases, only cat scratch disease and bacillary angiomatosis have been reported in Africa (Kelly et al., 1998).

Trench fever

Bartonella quintana is transmitted by the human body louse, *Pediculus humanus humanus* (see epidemic typhus) and causes trench fever, also known as five-day or quintan fever due to the cyclical nature of the disease. The disease occurred in more than 1 million Allied troops during World War I, but nowadays it is reported in urban homeless populations and chronic alcoholics from developed countries (Brouqui et al., 1999). Clinical signs are non-specific and complications of chronic infection include endocarditis. Infections can be diagnosed with blood cultures, serology and molecular methods. Tetracyclines and aminoglycosides have been proposed for treatment while controlling lice is the best way of preventing infections.

Cat scratch disease

Bartonella henselae is one agent of cat scratch disease, which occurs world-wide, particularly in children. Cats are the main reservoirs of *Bartonella henselae* and the organism is transmitted to people with scratches or bites, but also by cat fleas. It has been isolated in wild felines including in Africa. Usually there is no significant lesion at the inoculation site but regional lymphadenopathy is a hallmark of the disease. The enlarged lymph nodes may become tender and sometimes suppurate. The lymphadenopathy may be accompanied by mild clinical signs and usually regresses spontaneously within a few weeks. The disease responds poorly to antibiotic therapy although aminoglycosides have been suggested for patients with suppurative complications (Maurin et al., 1997).

Bacillary angiomatosis

Bacillary angiomatosis is a vascular proliferative disease that usually involves the skin, but may disseminate to other organs. Cutaneous lesions appear as small red/purple papules which enlarge to form nodules (sometimes confused with Kaposi's sarcoma). The disease was first described in HIV-infected patients and organ transplant recipients, but may occur in immunocompetent patients. In patients with non-cutaneous bacillary angiomatosis (bone, heart, spleen, liver, lymph nodes), a variety of non-specific symptoms may occur, including fever, chills, weight loss and vomiting (Maurin et al., 1997). Three cases have been reported in Southern Africa (Kelly et al., 1998).

Unsolved problems

In general little is known about the rickettsioses in Africa and much of the information on the epidemiology of the diseases has been obtained in first-world laboratories that promote international co-operation and have well developed facilities. Similarly, data on the clinical aspects of these diseases have often been derived from infected visitors to the continent returning to their homes in developed countries. It is hoped that as health workers in Africa become increasingly aware of rickettsioses, the regional epidemiology and clinical features in local populations will be better described.

Apart from the conditions described above, other rickettsioses might also occur in Africa. *Rickettsia mongolotimonae* is an emerging pathogen that was first isolated from an *Hyalomma asiaticum* collected in Inner Mongolia, China. Later this spotted fever group Rickettsia was established as a human pathogen when it was found in five clinical patients in southern France (Raoult et al., 1996; Fournier et al., 2000; Raoult, personal communication). Although the vector of *Rickettsia mongolotimonae* is unknown in France, the organism has been identified in *Hyalomma truncatum* from Niger. These ticks are widely distributed in Africa; perhaps infections with *Rickettsia mongolotimonae* should be considered as a potential cause of fever in patients in Africa.

Other spotted fever group rickettsiae of unknown pathogenicity have been found in African ticks. *Rickettsia aeschlimannii* has been found in Morocco, Zimbabwe, Mali and Niger, and *Rickettsia massiliae* in ticks from the Central African Republic and Mali (Parola et al., 2001). The significance of these organisms has yet to be determined, but it should be remembered that a number of *Rickettsiae* currently known as human pathogens were first described as 'organisms of unknown pathogenicity'.

Rickettsia felis (formerly the ELB agent), is an emerging pathogen which until recently had only been found in the New world (Raoult et al., 2001b). It is a spotted fever group Rickettsia which was first detected in cat fleas, *Ctenocephalides felis*, in 1990 and later in *Pulex irritans* in 1997. We have found this agent in a flea from Addis Ababa, Ethiopia, and it appears likely that *Rickettsia felis* is widely distributed.

Finally, ehrlichioses caused by rickettsiae in the genus

Ehrlichia, which originally contained only veterinary pathogens, have recently been recognized as emerging human diseases. The organisms involved are *Ehrlichia chaffeensis* (the agent of human monocytic ehrlichiosis) and *Ehrlichia ewingii* in the USA, and the agent of human granulocytic ehrlichiosis in the USA and Europe (Parola & Raoult, 2001). In 1992, a survey for antibodies to *Ehrlichia chaffeensis* in human sera from eight African countries indicated that human ehrlichioses might occur on the continent. More recently, however, serological cross-reactivity has been found between the agents of human ehrlichioses and the ehrlichia of veterinary importance which are widely distributed in Africa. To date, then, there is no definitive evidence for the presence of human ehrlichioses in Africa (Parola & Raoult, 2001). Much work remains to be done in Africa before the true picture of the rickettsioses on the continent can emerge.

References

Azad AF, Radulovič S, Higgins JA, Noden BH, Troyer JM. (1997). Flea-borne rickettsioses: ecologic considerations. *Emerg Infect Dis*; **3**: 319–327.

Birg ML, La Scola B, Roux V, Brouqui P, Raoult D. (1999). Isolation of *Rickettsia prowazekii* from blood by shell vial cell culture. *J Clin Microbiol*; **37**: 3722–3724.

Brouqui P, Lascola B, Roux V, Raoult D. (1999). Chronic *Bartonella quintana* bacteremia in homeless patients. *N Engl J Med*; **340**: 186–189.

Fournier PE, Tissot-Dupont H, Gallais H, Raoult D. (2000). *Rickettsia mongolotimonae*: a rare pathogen in France. *Emerg Infect Dis*; **6**: 290–292.

Kelly PJ, Matthewman LA, Beati L et al. (1992). African tick-bite fever – a new spotted fever group rickettsiosis under an old name. *Lancet*; **340**: 982–983.

Kelly PJ, Beati L, Mason PR, Matthewman LA, Roux V, Raoult D. (1996). *Rickettsia africae* sp nov, the etiological agent of African tick bite fever. *Int J Syst Bact*; **46**: 611–614.

Kelly PJ, Rooney JJA, Morsten J, Regnery R. (1998). *Bartonella henselae* isolated from cats in Zimbabwe. *Lancet*; **351**: 1706.

Lascola B, Raoult D. (1997). Laboratory diagnosis of rickettsioses: current approaches to diagnosis of old and new rickettsial diseases. *J Clin Microbiol*; **35**: 2715–2727.

Lascola B, Rydkina L, Ndihokubwayo JB, Vene S, Raoult D. (2000). Serological differentiation of murine typhus and epidemic typhus using cross-adsorption and Western blotting. *Clin Diagn Lab Immunol*; **7**: 612–616.

Maurin M, Birtles R, Raoult D. (1997). Current knowledge of *Bartonella* species. *Eur J Clin Microbiol Infect Dis*; **16**: 487–506.

Maurin M, Raoult D. (1996). *Bartonella (Rochalimaea) quintana* infections. *Clin Microbiol Rev*; **9**: 273–292.

Maurin M, Raoult D. (1999). Q fever. *Clin Microbiol Rev*; **12**:518–553.

Niang M, Brouqui P, Raoult D. (1999). Epidemic typhus imported from Algeria. *Emerg Infect Dis*; **5**: 716–718.

Parola P, Raoult D. (2001). Tick-borne bacterial diseases in humans, an emerging infectious threat. *Clin Infect Dis*; **32**: 897–928.

Parola P, Jourdan J, Raoult D. (1998a). Tick-borne infection caused by *Rickettsia africae* in West Indies. *N Engl J Med*; **338**: 1391.

Parola P, Vogelaers D, Roure C, Janbon F, Raoult D. (1998b). Imported murine typhus in travelers returning from Indonesia. *Emerg Inf Dis*; **4**: 677–680.

Parola P, Vestris G, Martinez D, Brochier B, Roux V, Raoult D. (1999). Tick-borne rickettsiosis in Guadeloupe, The French West Indies: isolation of *Rickettsia africae* from *Amblyomma variegatum* ticks and serosurvey in humans, cattle and goats. *Am J Trop Med Hyg*; **60**: 883–887.

Parola P, Inokuma H, Camicas JL, Brouqui P, Raoult D. (2001). Detection and identification of spotted fever group *Rickettsiae* and *Ehrlichiae* in African ticks. *Emerg Inf Dis*: *in press.*

Raoult D, Roux V. (1997). Rickettsioses as paradigms of new or emerging infectious diseases. *Clin Microbiol Rev*; **10**: 694–719.

Raoult D, Roux V. (1999). The body louse as a vector of reemerging human diseases. *Clin Infect Dis*; **29**: 888–911.

Raoult D, Brouqui P, Roux V. (1996) A new spotted-fever-group Rickettsiosis. *Lancet*; **348**: 412.

Raoult D, Roux V, Ndihokubwayo JB et al. (1997). Jail fever (epidemic typhus) outbreak in Burundi. *Emerg Infect Dis*; **3**: 357–359.

Raoult D, Ndihokubwayo JB et al. (1998). Outbreak of epidemic typhus associated with trench fever in Burundi. *Lancet*; **352** 353–358.

Raoult D, Tissot-Dupont H, Foucault C et al. (2000). Q fever 1985–1998. Clinical and epidemiologic features of 1,383 infections. *Medicine*; **79**: 109–123.

Raoult D, Fournier PE, Fenollar F et al. (2001a). *Rickettsia africae*: a common tick-transmitted pathogen for travelers to sub-Saharian Africa. A report of 119 cases. *N Engl J Med*: *in press.*

Raoult D, La Scola B, Enea M et al. (2001b). A flea-asociated rickettsia pathogenic from humans. *Emerg Infect Dis*; **7**: 73–81.

Roux V, Raoult D. (1999). Body lice as tools for diagnosis and surveillance of reemerging diseases. *J Clin Microbiol*; **37**: 596–599.

Zinsser H. (1935). *Rats, Lice and History*. London: Broadway House.

Relapsing fevers

45

The relapsing fevers are acute infections caused by spirochaetes of the genus Borrelia. There are two epidemiological forms: louse-borne relapsing fever, which can be epidemic, is transmitted only between humans by the body louse, whereas tick-borne relapsing fever is a zoonosis and does not appear in epidemics.

LOUSE-BORNE RELAPSING FEVER (LBRF)

The problem in Africa

Louse-borne relapsing fever is endemic in the highlands of Ethiopia, the Sudan, and Rwanda. In Ethiopia, the main endemic focus of the disease, over 10 000 cases are reported annually. LBRF caused large world-wide epidemics that affected several million people following the two World Wars (Bryceson et al., 1970). Localized epidemics still occur; the latest in 1991, at the end of the civil war in Ethiopia (Sundens & Haimanot, 1993). Untreated mortality is high, exceeding 40 per cent in some epidemics; treatment reduces mortality to 1–5 per cent. When refugees are on the move, whether from war or disaster, and are forced to live in a wretched state, this ancient scourge could easily strike such vulnerable people again.

The organism and its vector

A single organism, *Borrelia recurrentis,* causes LBRF. Borreliae are slender, actively motile, microaerophilic organisms. They are 10–20 microns long, and 0.2–0.5 wide, with 4–10 loose coils. Electron microscopic studies show that the organism contains 9–11 periplasmic flagellae. *Borrelia recurrentis* was considered non-cultivable in vitro, but it has recently been grown and propagated in artificial media (Cutler et al., 1997). It contains a variable lipoprotein, structurally homologous to murein lipoprotein of *Escherichia coli* (Scragg et al., 2000), and it is this which induces tumour necrosis factor in the reaction to treatment (Vidal et al., 1998). The organism is extremely sensitive to tetracycline, penicillin, chloramphenicol and erythromycin.

The human is the only reservoir of louse-borne relapsing fever.

The body louse *Pediculus humanus* transmits LBRF. Lice become infected when they feed on an infected person. The ingested spirochaetes enter the gut and cross the epithelium into the haemolymph, where they multiply. The spirochaetes are transmitted to another person when an infected louse is crushed onto the skin: they enter the circulation through abrasions in the skin. There is then an incubation period of 5–10 days, when they multiply and cause a high level of spirochaetaemia.

Epidemiology

Louse-borne relapsing fever is a classic disease of poverty, overcrowding, poor personal hygiene and infestation with lice. Up to 60 per cent of the inhabitants of the highlands of Ethiopia may harbour lice (Shold, 1978). They bathe and wash their clothing less frequently, and use more bedding because the highlands are cold at night; these factors favour transmission of the disease, which occurs mainly among migrant labourers, prisoners and the poor (see Fig. 45.1).

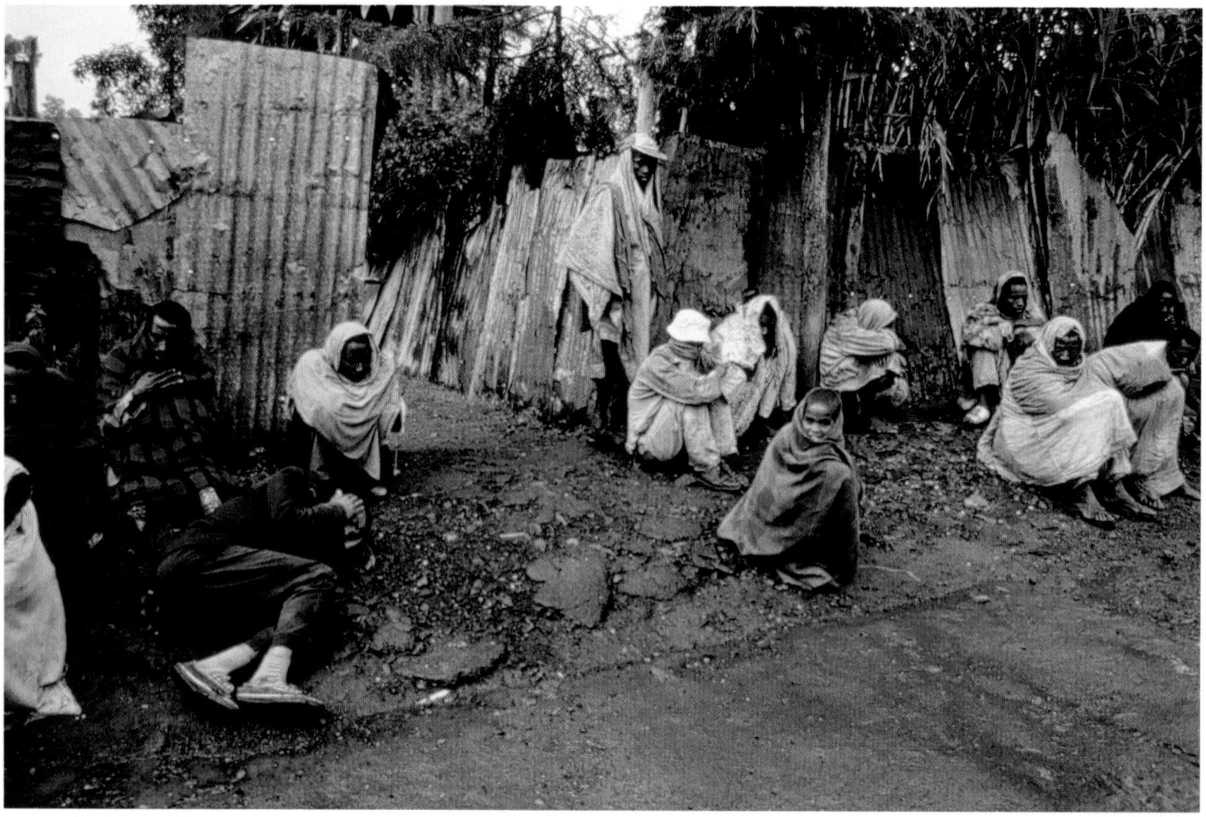

Fig. 45.1. Those at risk: poor people, crowded and wrapped against the cold of the rainy season in Addis Ababa. (Photo Daniel Fekade.)

Seasonal variation

The disease is transmitted throughout the year, but there is an increase in the number of cases during the rainy season between June to September. The reason for this change with the seasons is not understood.

Prevention and control

If the poor could have better housing and a reliable safe water supply with better personal hygiene, the cycle of transmission would be broken. Insecticides like DDT are effective in killing lice. Delousing measures are important to control epidemic outbreaks. It is often necessary to shave the hair of a heavily infected person and either to destroy or to powder badly infested clothes thoroughly with DDT.

Clinical features

The incubation period ranges from 5–10 days. Patients develop a high fever abruptly, accompanied by headache, a dry cough, and aches and pains in the back and the joints.

The temperature comes down by crisis. Spirochaetes are cleared from the circulation in 3–5 days, due to the production of opsonizing antibodies. Four to seven days after the fever has disappeared, a repeat wave of spirochaetaemia with a new antigenic variant occurs, so that clinical symptoms recur (Barbour, 1990). There will be three to five relapses: successive relapses tend to be clinically milder.

The spectrum of clinical signs

The range of clinical signs is wide: no system is unaffected.

A typical severe case

The dominant signs are:
- high fever
- bleeding with epistaxis, a purpuric rash – often with buccal and subconjunctival haemorrhages;
- jaundice and hepatomegaly (in up to 65 per cent) and splenomegaly (in 70 per cent);

- cardiovascular signs: tachycardia, a third heart sound, evidence of pulmonary oedema and a prolonged QTc in the electrocardiogram (Parry et al., 1970);
- neurological changes, with a confusional state, meningism and focal neurological signs. Fatal intracranial bleeding has been found at autopsy (Ahmed et al., 1980).

The spectrum of signs in each system varies from evidence of slight dysfunction – for example, the patient has no jaundice (over 60 per cent) but there is evidence of some hepatocellular damage (in 75 per cent) in a raised aminotransferase. Some patients have a palpable spleen and a fever and no other signs: others bleed extensively and are deeply jaundiced. While the blood urea is raised in 80 per cent of patients, acute renal failure is rare.

Platelet counts are normal or low, but they can decrease to very low counts during the first 24 hours after treatment, and then increase gradually and so regain normal levels by 5–7 days (Perine et al., 1971).

Pregnancy

The pregnant mother is at high risk of losing her baby, whether or not she has a reaction to treatment. Abortion and stillbirth occur in up to 40 per cent of patients, if infection is acquired during pregnancy.

Diagnosis

Borrelia are readily stained by aniline dyes such as Giemsa and Wright stain. Diagnosis is commonly confirmed by the demonstration of spirochaetes on a Leishman-stained peripheral blood film (Fig. 45.2). The differential diagnosis in Africa includes any cause of fever with jaundice and bleeding: it will depend on the place, the season and the prevalent local infections. These may include malaria, louse-borne typhus, viral haemorrhagic fevers, acute hepatic necrosis of whatever cause, and sometimes typhoid. But spirochaetes are not found in a blood film in any of these infections. A blood film is obligatory to confirm a diagnosis in an endemic area.

Treatment

The principles are:

(i) to eradicate the spirochaetes with an appropriate antibiotic;
(ii) to restore body fluids to normal and to maintain them during the reaction;

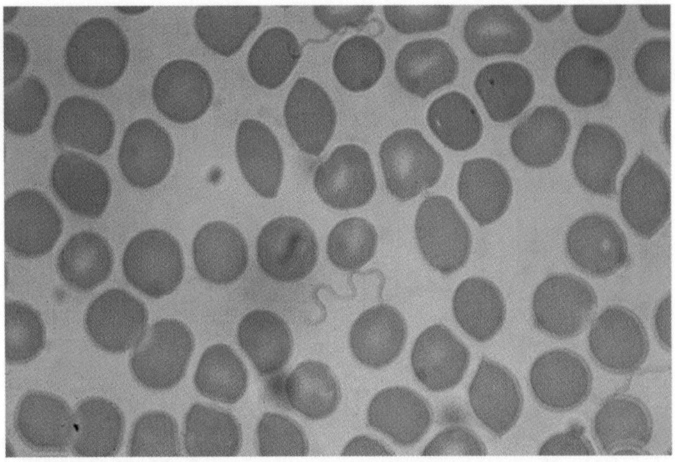

Fig. 45.2. Thin blood film to show many spirochaetes: note, although the film is technically poor, the spirochaetes are easily seen.

(iii) to maintain blood pressure and circulation during the reaction;
(iv) to treat any associated complication.

Antibiotics

A number of antibiotics including tetracycline, penicillin, chloramphenicol and erythromycin are effective treatment of louse-borne relapsing fever (Perine & Teklu, 1983). However, antibiotic treatment is complicated by the severe and life-threatening Jarisch–Herxheimer reaction.

Single dose penicillin is associated with less frequent reactions, but may fail to clear spirochaetes in up to 20 per cent of cases and is associated with frequent relapses. While tetracycline treatment very rarely fails to eradicate the spirochaetes, it is accompanied by a higher incidence of severe reactions.

Since a severe reaction is associated with a significant mortality, and since relapses are clinically mild and are easy to treat, single dose procaine penicillin 400 000–600 000 units intramuscularly, followed by tetracycline 500 mg by mouth for 2 days is the recommended treatment (Salih & Mustafa, 1978; Gebrehiwot & Fiseha, 1992; Seboxa & Rahlenbeck, 1995).

Action in an epidemic

During an epidemic and in areas where medical resources are poor, a single oral dose of doxycycline, 100 mg, is effective treatment. Erythromycin 500 mg, as a single dose, is effective treatment during pregnancy and childhood.

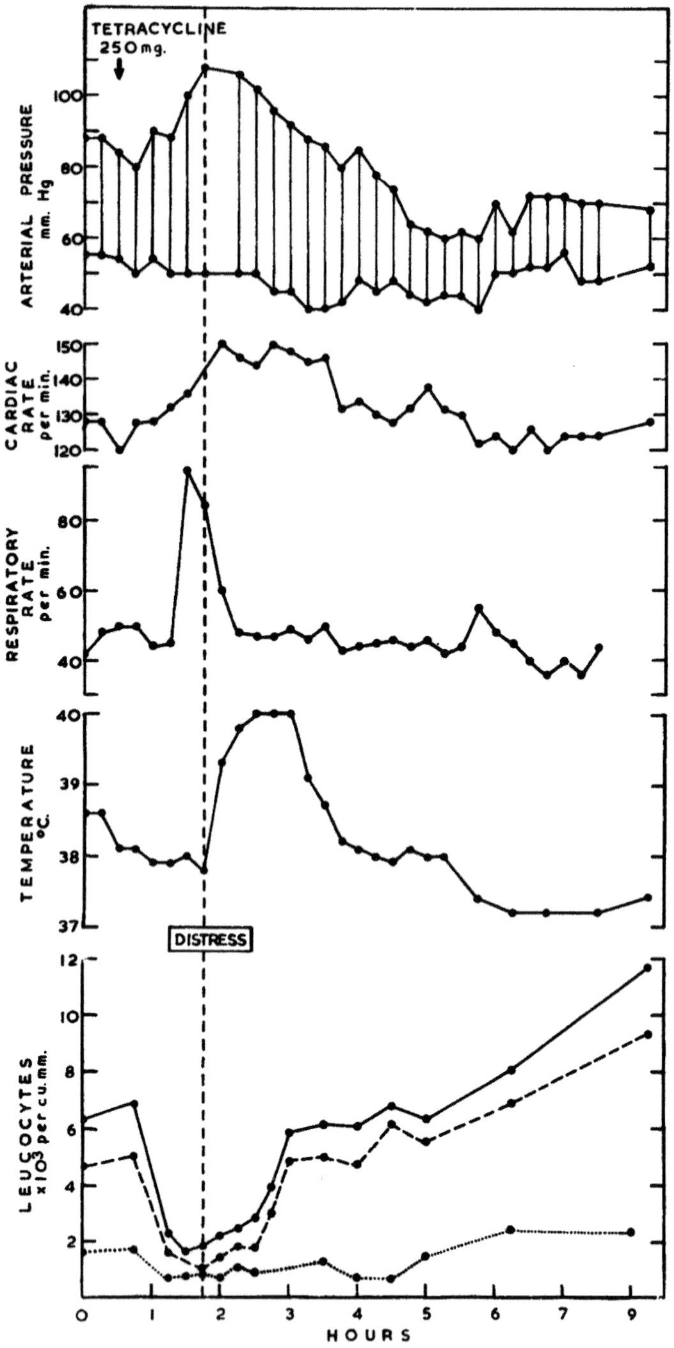

Fig. 45.3. The physiological changes of the Jarisch–Herxheimer reaction: note the abrupt rise of temperature, arterial pressure and respiratory rate as spirochaetes disappear and the low arterial pressure during the flush phase (from Schofield T.P.C. (1968) *Lancet*: **i**: 58–62).

General care

In very ill patients:

- set up an intravenous line, and infuse isotonic saline.
- monitor the blood pressure after the antibiotic has been given, as often as staffing will allow, but particularly during the flush phase of the reaction, as it can fall very low during this phase.
- keep the patient lying down during the reaction until the blood pressure is normal again.
- do not forget to de-louse the patient: for this, DDT is excellent. Often the clothes of the really poor have to be destroyed, because they are so infected and so ragged. Find means to supply them with clean and louse-free clothes.

Reaction to treatment

A reaction occurs following treatment in 35–100 per cent of patients. It is distressing to the patient and is associated with a 5 per cent mortality.

Physiological changes

The reaction begins 60–90 minutes after tetracycline or penicillin has been given. The clinical and pathophysiological characteristics of the reaction are shown in Fig. 45.3 (Schofield et al., 1968). The reaction has four phases, which can be clearly recognized.

The prodromal phase
The chills phase, during which the temperature, blood pressure, pulse and respiratory rate rise abruptly: for example the temperature may rise to over 40 °C and the respiratory rate to around 80/min.
The flush phase, when blood pressure falls dramatically.
The phase of defervescence, which lasts up to 24 hours.

Haematological changes

The white cell count falls dramatically at the peak of the reaction, and returns to its pretreatment levels at about 12 hours. While neutrophils disappear rapidly from the blood, stained blood films show fewer and fewer spirochaetes also. The lowest neutrophil counts (as few as 600×10^9/l) are seen at the peak of the fever when the spirochaetes disappear.

Cytokine profile during the reaction

There is a marked but transient rise in levels of circulating TNF, IL-6, and IL-8 at the peak of the reaction. Their plasma levels can rise to six or eight times their level on admission before treatment (Fig. 45.4; Negussie et al., 1992), but they fall again to their admission levels by 12 hours, as the vigorous clinical symptoms abate. The stimulus for the reaction has been studied intensively. A variable lipoprotein, homologous to the murein lipoprotein of *E.coli,* is the major TNF-inducing factor in louse-borne relapsing fever (Vidal et al., 1998; Scragg et al., 2000).

Pharmacological modulation of the reaction

Corticosteroids

In a small-uncontrolled trial hydrocortisone reduced fever, but failed to prevent the reaction (Warrell et al., 1970).

Opiate antagonists

In a randomized controlled clinical trial, meptazinol, an opiate antagonist, reduced the clinical severity of the reaction compared to naloxone and placebo, but did not prevent it (Teklu et al.,1983).

TNF inhibitors

In an open label study, pretreatment with pentoxyfilline, a weak inhibitor of TNF synthesis, failed to prevent the reaction or associated cytokine release (Remick et al., 1996). But, in a randomized placebo-controlled trial, pretreatment with an ovine polyclonal anti-TNF antibody significantly reduced the incidence of the reaction from 90 per cent in controls to 45 per cent in the treated (Fekade et al., 1996). Another important result from this study was that there was no delay in clearance of spirochaetes in patients treated with anti-TNF antibody. Sadly, this form of treatment is neither available nor affordable, except in highly advanced units.

Unsolved problems

Further research is necessary to understand the seasonal variation and the persistence of isolated endemic foci in East and Central Africa. Based on our current understanding of the pathophysiology of the reaction, new approaches for the prevention of the reaction need to be studied. Work on the reaction has a wider interest than the impact on the disease itself. Because of the predictable course and similarity in the pathophysiology and cytokine profile between the reaction and the systemic

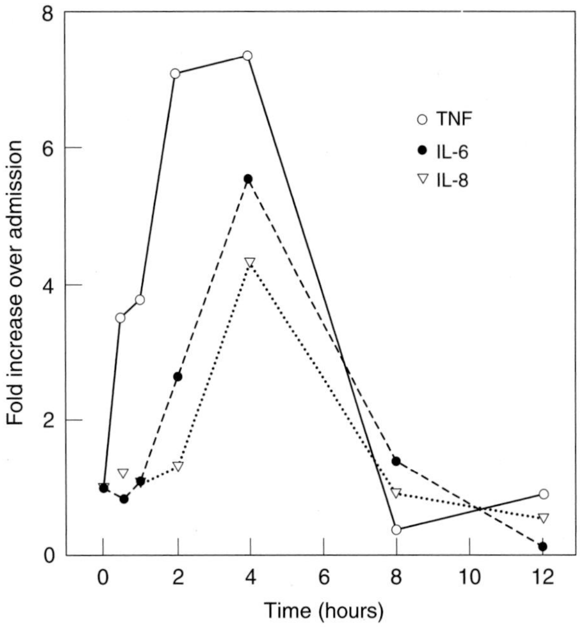

Fig. 45.4. The cytokine changes during the reaction (after Negussie et al., 1992).

inflammatory response syndrome – SIRS, it is a useful human model of the cytokine cascade.

TICK-BORNE RELAPSING FEVER

The problem in Africa

Tick-borne (endemic) relapsing fever is widely distributed in different foci around the world. The disease is endemic in parts of East and Central Africa, while it occurs sporadically in other places. The epidemiology is dependent on the tick vector, the natural host (often a wild rodent), and the possibility of contact between man and the vector. At a hospital in southern Congo, over 7 per cent of new outpatients were found to be infected with the *Borrellia duttoni* (Dupont et al., 1997).

Epidemiology

Organism, vector and life cycle

Several different *Borrelia* species cause tick-borne relapsing fever. In Africa *Borrelia duttoni, and Borrelia croicuidare* are the predominant species. Soft-bodied ticks of the genus Ornithodoros transmit the organisms. There is high tick–Borrelia specificity. Ticks remain infected for several years, and can transmit the infection to their offspring. In Africa three Ornithodoros–Borrelia complexes are found. *O. mobuta* and *B. duttoni* are the most important, but in parts of East Africa and in West Africa and the Mediterranean, *O. erraticus* and *B. hispanica* and *B. croicuidare* are important. *O. mobuta is* secondarily adapted to human dwellings, where it lives in cracks and holes of walls, so that the traditionally built mud and wattle huts are ideal for it. *0. erraticus* lives in rodent burrows in the savanna and semi-desert areas of Africa.

Prevention

The principle is to break transmission between the tick and the human victim

Houses

If the inside and the floor of huts are sprayed with a residual insecticide ticks can be controlled for 2 years. Lambda-cyhalothrin eradicated ticks in villages in central Tanzania, where TBRF is an important cause of morbidity and mortality (Talbert et al., 1998).

Individuals

There is no short cut to picking off each tick. Tick repellents, such as 5 per cent dimethylphthalate, can help to prevent infection in someone vulnerable on account of work in an endemic area.

Clinical features

These are the same as in louse-borne relapsing fever. The disease tends to be clinically milder, and is associated with less frequent reactions, but neurological manifestations are more frequent, with meningeal signs, a mild CSF lymphocytic pleocytosis, and a raised CSF protein in 50–100 per cent of patients. Spirochaetes have also been found in the CSF. Cranial neuritis, mainly facial palsy, is reported in up to a third of patients. Abortion, and even maternal death, are feared in infected pregnant women (Dupont et al., 1997).

Treatment

In general, one or two doses of procaine penicillin or tetracycline have been less efficacious and have been associated with more frequent relapses in tick-borne than in louse-borne relapsing fever. Relapses probably occur because the spirochaete is sequestered in small intracerebral blood vessels. However, higher doses and a longer duration of treatment have prevented relapses and eradicated residual brain infection.

For an adult, give procaine penicillin 800 000 units daily intramuscularly, or tetracycline 500 mg by mouth every 6 hours for 5 days.

References

Ahmed MAM, Abdel Wahab SM, Abdel Malik MO, et al. (1980). Louse-borne relapsing fever in the Sudan a historical review and a clinico-pathological study. *Trop Geogr Med*; **32**: 106–111.

Barbour A. (1990). Antigenic variation of a relapsing fever *Borrelia* species. *Ann Rev Microbiol*; **44**: 155–171.

Bryceson ADM, Parry EHO, Perine PL et al. (1970). Louse borne relapsing fever: a clinical and laboratory study of 62 cases in Ethiopia and reconsideration of the literature. *Quart J Med*; **39**: 129–170.

Cooper PJ, Fekade D, Remick DG et al. (2000). Recombinant human interleukin-10 fails to alter proinflammatory cytokine production or physiologic changes associated with Jarisch–Herxheimer reaction. *J infect Dis*; **181**: 203–309.

Cutler SJ, Moss J, Fukunaga M et al. (1997). *Borrelia recurrentis*. Characterization and comparison with relpasing-fever, Lyme-associated, and other *Borrelia* spp. *Int J Syst Bact*; **47**: 958–968.

Dupont HT, LaScola B, Williams R et al. (1997). A focus of tick-borne relapsing fever in southern Zaire. *Clin Infect Dis*; **25**: 139–144.

Fekade D, Knox K, Hussein K et al. (1996). Prevention of Jarisch–Herxheimer reactions by treatment with antibodies against tumor necrosis factor alpha. *N Engl J Med*; **335**: 311–315.

Negussie Y, Remick DG, DeForge LE et al. (1992). Detection of plasma tumor necrosis factor, Interleukins 6, and 8 during the Jarisch–Herxheimer reaction of relapsing fever. *J Exp Med*; **175**: 1207–1212.

Parry EHO, Warrell DA, Perine PL et al. (1976). Some effects of louse-borne relapsing fever onthe function of the heart. *Am J Med*; **49**: 472–479.

Perine PL, Kidan TG, Warrell DA et al. (1971). Bleeding in louse-borne relapsing fever. *Trans Roy Soc Trop Med Hyg*; **65**: 782–787.

Perine PL, Teklu B. (1983). Antibiotic treatment of louse borne relapsing fever in Ethiopia. A report of 377 cases. *Am J Trop Med Hyg*; **32**: 1096–1100.

Remick DG, Negussie Y, Fekade D et al. (1996). Pentoxifylline fails to prevent the Jarisch Herxheimer reaction or associated cytokine release. *J Infect Dis*; **174**: 627–630.

Salih SY, Mustafa D. (1977). Louse-borne relapsing fever: II. Combined penicillin and tetracycline therapy in 160 Sudanese patients. *Trans Roy Soc Trop Med Hyg*; **71**: 49–51.

Schofield T.P.C., Talbot JM, Bryceson ADM et al. (1968).

Leucopenia and fever in the 'Jarisch–Herxheimer' reaction of louse-borne relapsing fever *Lancet*; **i**: 58–62.
Scragg I G, Kwiatowski D, Vidal V et al. (2000). Structural characterisation of the inflammatory moiety of a variable major lipoprotein of *Borrelia recurrentis. J Biol Chem*; **275**: 937–941.
Seboxa T, Rahlenbeck SI. (1995). Treatment of louse-borne relapsing fever with low dose penicillin or tetracycline: a clinical trail. *Scand J Infect Dis*; **27**: 29–31.
Shold LL. (1978). The epidemiology of human pediculosis in Ethiopia. PhD dissertation, Department of Medicine, Colorado State University, Fort Collins, 277pp.
Sundens KO, Haimonot AT. (1993). Epidemic louse-borne relapsing fever in Ethiopia. *Lancet*; **302**: 1213–1215.
Talbert A, Nyange A, Molteni F. (1998). Spraying tick-infested houses with lambda-cyhalothrin reduces the incidence of tick-borne relapsing fever in children under five years old. *Trans Roy Soc Trop Med Hyg*; **92**: 251–253.
Teklu B, Habte-Michael A, Warrell DA. et al. (1983). Meptazinol diminishes the Jarisch–Herxheimer reaction of relapsing fever. *Lancet*; **1**: 835–839.
Vidal V, Scragg IG, Cutler SJ et al. (1998). Variable major lipoprotein is a principal TNF-inducing factor of louse-borne relapsing fever. *Nature*; **4**: 1416–1420.
Warrell DA, Pope HM, Parry EHO et al. (1970). Cardio respiratory disturbances associated with infective fever in man: studies of Ethiopian louse borne relapsing fever. *Clin Science*; **39**: 123–145.

46 Yaws and endemic syphilis

YAWS

Yaws (also known as *Framboesia tropica*, Buba, Bomba or Pian) is an infectious disease caused by *Treponema pallidum pertenue*, affecting skin and bone. Its distribution in Africa is limited to the hot and humid forest areas near the Equator, where little clothing is worn and hygiene is generally poor. Children between age 2 and 10 are predominantly affected in endemic areas.

The problem in Africa

In 1948, the World Health Organization, in collaboration with UNICEF and many national governments, launched a global initiative to combat yaws. During many large-scale campaigns, millions of individuals were given penicillin monostearate by injection in an attempt to eradicate the disease. Although these campaigns dramatically reduced the numbers of affected individuals, and also the number of countries where the disease prevailed, resurgence in several African areas has been reported in the 1980s (Agadzi et al., 1983; Baudon & Houssou, 1984; N'Da, 1985; Omar, 1986; Ziefer et al., 1985). Cases have continued to be reported in the 1990s from various regions in the tropical rain forest zone of Africa (Herve et al., 1992; Edorh et al., 1994; Akogun, 1999). Yaws may heal without medical intervention, and we suspect that many cases never report to hospital. We have seen children with yaws in the community that never brought their disease to the attention of health professionals.

In most areas, late stages and extensive presentations of the disease appear to be less common than in the 1950s, but in some resurgent areas, late and extensive lesions have begun to reappear (Edorh et al., 1994). In the Central African Republic, yaws has remained highly prevalent among the Pygmies (Widy-Wirski et al., 1980). Some researchers believe that the disease has again spread from this tribe to other populations throughout the region and indeed, into a number of West African countries (Widy-Wirski, 1985; Toure, 1985; Herve et al., 1992).

Micro-organism and host immune defence

Treponema pallidum pertenue is the cause of yaws. Its morphology and serology are indistinguishable (Noordhoek et al., 1990) from *T. pallidum pallidum*, which causes syphilis (both endemic and venereal). Only by sequencing the genome of the different species has it been possible to separate the different species of *Treponema* (Noordhoek et al., 1989; Weinstock et al., 1998; Stamm et al., 1998). The micro-organism is thin and motile, measuring 0.15 μm in diameter and 6–50 μm in length. In a darkfield microscope, 6–14 spirals can be observed; the viable organisms make spinning and corkscrew movements, flexing in the middle. The outer membrane is made up of phospholipids with very scant proteins. Immune recognition by their human hosts is difficult, as antibodies only recognize non-surface exposed proteins (Radolf et al., 1989, 1995). In an animal model, *T. pallidum pertenue* is unable to enter the internal organs, and to pass the blood–brain barrier and the placenta, unlike *T. pallidum pallidum* which may cause aortitis, neuro-syphilis and congenital syphilis (Wicher et al., 2000). High serum antibody levels are found after infection with treponemes, but these antibodies are not protective. They are directed against proteins of the core of the spirochaete, while the outer membrane protects the treponeme from opsonization by host antibodies (Cox et al., 1992). Animal studies suggest that T-cells play a role in host defence (Liu et al., 1990).

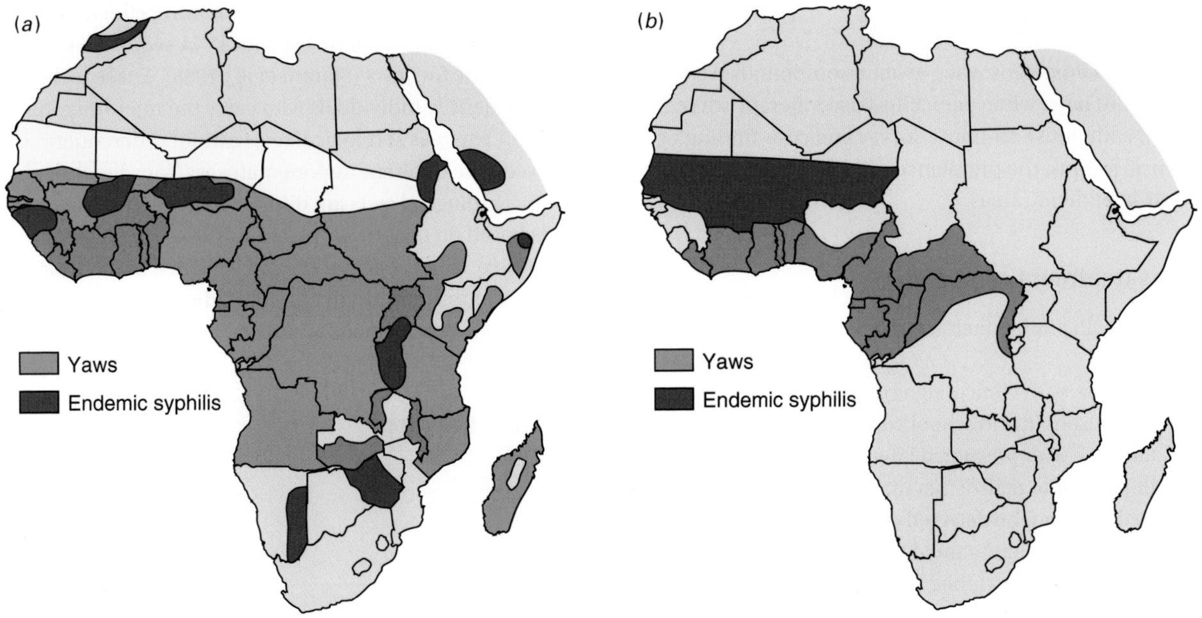

Fig. 46.1. Prevalence of yaws and endemic syphilis (*a*) before and (*b*) after the mass campaigns in the 1950s.

Epidemiology

Yaws is predominantly a disease of the forest and wet savannah, because *T. pallidum pertenue* needs a hot humid environment (Fig. 46.1).

Prevalence

There have been striking fluctuations in the prevalence of the disease over the last decades in various regions of Africa. After initial reduction in numbers of infected individuals, it has become clear that eradication is far more difficult that initially expected. Persistence of endemic foci, e.g. among the Pygmies, have caused the eradication programs to fail (Widy-Wirski, 1985). In Papua New Guinea, mass treatment with long-acting penicillin was less effective than initially believed (Backhouse et al., 1998). Because serological tests remain positive for a long time, assessments using blood tests may be unable to detect rapid changes in epidemiology. On the other hand, many more individuals appear to be infected as assessed by serological testing than can be clinically detected with yaws. Yaws predominantly affects children, typically between age 2 and 10 years.

Transmission

Close personal contact, particularly between children who play together, is probably the essential factor in transmission. Poor hygienic conditions facilitate the spread of the disease, especially when water for bathing and washing of clothes is scant. The organism is unable to penetrate the intact skin, but it readily attacks abrasions and scratches in the skin. Once a person has developed a primary ('mother yaw') lesion, it spreads because of the itch it causes, by scratching, subsequently affecting other parts of the body. Compared to lesions of endemic syphilis, the causative organisms of yaws are found in the epidermal layer of the skin in the lesions (Engelkens et al., 1993). This might explain why yaws is more contagious than endemic syphilis. Transmission is highest in the rainy season.

Non-human reservoir

T. pallidum pertenue has been isolated from Cynomolgus monkeys, but it is unclear whether the animal reservoir plays any role in the transmission and resurgence of yaws among humans.

Prevention

The principles are to identify the people affected, to break the transmission of yaws among them with penicillin, treating not only the index patient, but also all household and school contacts; and then to follow up the communities treated.

Definition of the problem

The early campaigns when arsenic compounds were used failed, but later, when penicillin-based therapy was combined with house-to-house survey and case-finding by clinical lesions, the prevalence of yaws decreased dramatically in endemic areas.

Mass treatment campaigns

The following individuals should be included in penicillin treatment:
(i) all those with clinical signs of yaws;
(ii) all household and school contacts;
(iii) all those with presumed latent infection.
It is important to realize that many more people are infected than can be detected clinically, and therefore, a great deal of publicity should be given to a campaign. Health education by public health workers is essential, and the support of officials and traditional leaders in the community, should be maintained.

Follow-up of mass campaigns

The prevalence of active yaws lesions has consistently been found to have fallen dramatically after a mass campaign (Edorh et al., 1994; Toure, 1985; Ziefer et al., 1985; Herve et al., 1992; Akogun, 1999). In Zaire – now called Congo – a survey revealed a prevalence of 7.9 per cent in 1981. Benzathine penicillin mass treatment was given to all cases and contacts, and the prevalence had dropped to 2.5 per cent in 1982 (Ziefer et al., 1985). Follow-up after the mass campaigns in the 1950s has shown resurgence of yaws in many areas. In some areas, yaws has apparently vanished. In other areas, however, where the disease has allegedly disappeared, occasional surveys still detect important numbers of patients, as in the mid-Hawal river valley, Gardika area, in Nigeria (Akogun, 1999). Endemic foci of transmission may easily persist among populations that are deprived of health services, like the Pygmy population in the Central African Republic (Widy-Wirski, 1985) and in Zaire (Ziefer et al., 1985). One recent report from Karkar Island, Papua New Guinea, suggested that mass campaigns may have reduced effectiveness because of reduced sensitivity to penicillin (Backhouse et al., 1998) but others have not confirmed this. In fact, all investigators agree that penicillin is a highly effective therapy.

Future preventive campaigns

New diagnostic tools based on molecular biological techniques are now available (Perine et al., 1985). Dried blood drop specimens may be collected on nitrocellulose filter paper, which may later be used for DNA sequence detection specific for yaws (Stamm et al., 1998). These techniques identify individuals who carry the micro-organism directly, whereas serological tests cannot differentiate between the different treponematoses (Noordhoek et al., 1990). Serological tests are difficult to interpret, and the tests based on genetic amplification are complicated and expensive. Clinical detection and vigilance by all health workers at the community level will therefore remain of paramount importance.

Clinical features

Early

Skin

A primary, small papule, which is commonly on the legs, appears first. Crops of infectious papillomata, which are often itchy, and contain large numbers of spirochaetes, follow it (Fig 46. 2). The initial lesion – referred to as the 'mother yaw' – may heal leaving a depigmented scar, or persist for months, and ulcerate. Scratching of this lesion may carry the micro-organisms to other parts of the body surface where skin lesions may become infected. These secondary lesions often appear as small berries – hence the name framboesia – which means raspberry. These secondary lesions may appear in crops, sometimes weeks or months after the mother yaw has healed. Secondary yaws, with macular and papular lesions, may appear everywhere. Lesions may also appear on the palmar or plantar skin, and may be a diffuse non-ulcerative dermatitis, papilloma, or a hyperkeratotic lesion. If the soles of the feet are affected, healing may be slow and walking painful. This may result in a typical sideways crab-like gait referred to as '*crab yaws*'. Regional lymph nodes may become tender and swollen.

Bone

Periosteal swelling results in pain, which is usually worse at night. A symmetrical hypertrophic periostitis affects metacarpals and the two proximal phalanges; the terminal phalanges are spared. Dactylitis and swelling of the ulna may occasionally be seen. Involvement of the long bones of the leg may result in the typical '*sabre shin*', which can also be detected on a radiograph of the tibia. In rare cases, hypertrophic osteitis of the nose and paranasal sinuses may result in a typical swelling of the face at both sides of the nose, referred to as '*goundou*' (Fig. 46.3).

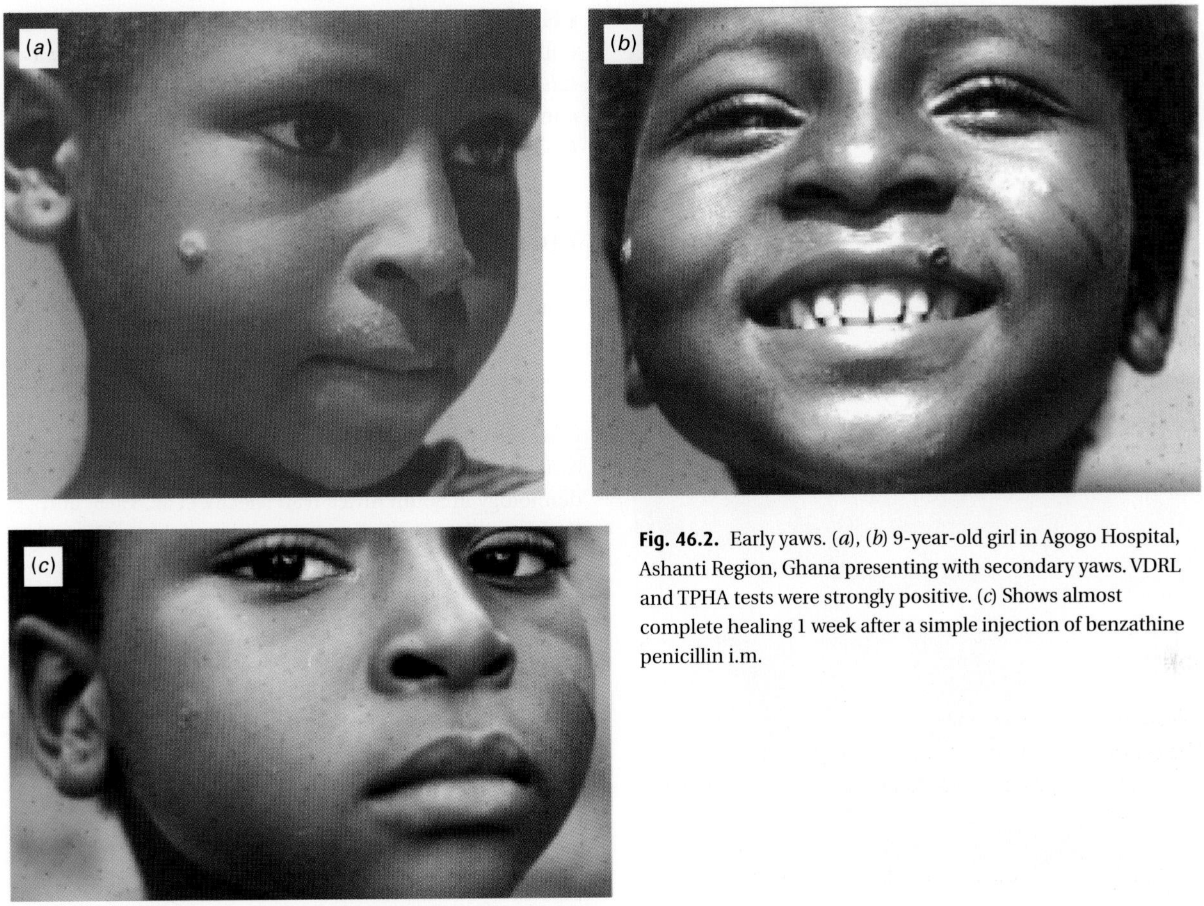

Fig. 46.2. Early yaws. (*a*), (*b*) 9-year-old girl in Agogo Hospital, Ashanti Region, Ghana presenting with secondary yaws. VDRL and TPHA tests were strongly positive. (*c*) Shows almost complete healing 1 week after a simple injection of benzathine penicillin i.m.

Late

Tertiary lesions typically appear years after infection. Necrotic skin lesions and gummata in bone may cause disabling deformities. The face may show conspicuous stigmatizing lesions such as goundou or a collapse of the nose bridge (saddle nose deformity) resulting from destruction of bone and cartilage (see Fig. 46.3). Plantar hyperkeratosis may persist and may be severe. Periarticular nodes, often at the knees, may be seen.

Clinical diagnosis

Clinical detection is easy in areas where the disease is common, and a clinical diagnosis is usually sufficient. The differential diagnosis of skin lesions on the foot may include tungiasis; hand and foot lesions may be mistaken for syphilis or scabies. Ulcerative and gummatous lesions of the feet may be confused with tropical ulcer, dracunculiasis, leishmaniasis, leprosy or Buruli ulcer. Juxta-articular nodes should be differentiated from the nodules of onchocerciasis. Dactylitis may also be caused by sickle cell disease or tuberculosis.

Laboratory diagnosis

Spirochaetes can be seen by dark-field microscopy in exudate from the lesions, especially if they are ulcerative, but the diagnosis is usually confirmed serologically. There are two different types of serological test.

Non-treponemal tests that detect antibodies directed to cardiolipin, which is a component of many tissues and organs, such as the VDRL (Venereal Disease Research Laboratory) and the RPR (rapid plasma reagin) tests. False-positive tests may occur in patients with chronic diseases such as rheumatoid arthritis; infectious conditions such as infective endocarditis, tuberculosis, HIV, and malaria; and in pregnancy.

The treponemal serological tests (*T. pallidum* haemagglutination or TPHA; and the fluorescent treponemal

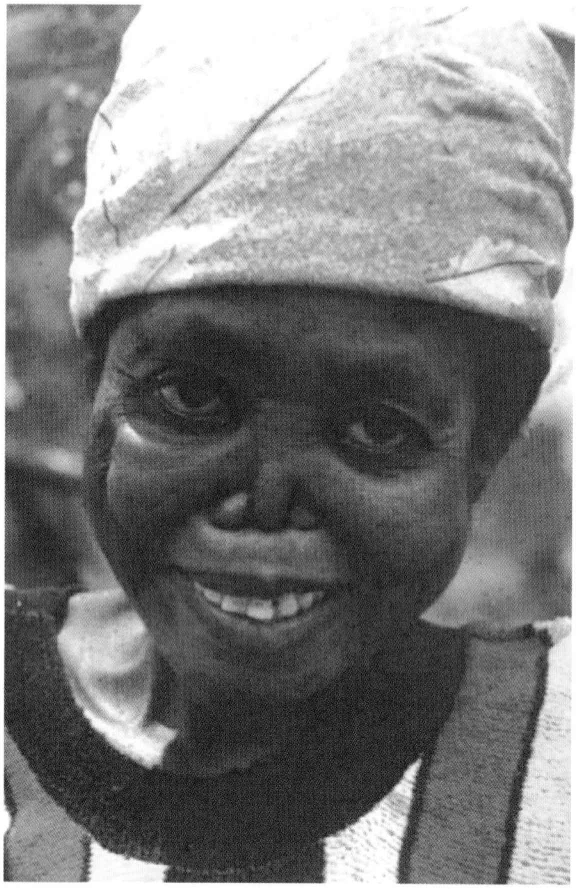

Fig. 46.3. Late yaws; saddle nose deformity and goundou. Figure shows a 60-year-old woman who presented with tuberculosis to the Agogo Hospital, Ashanti Region in Ghana. She had had yaws during childhood, and had developed a collapsed nose (saddle nose deformity) and swelling of the face at both sides of the nose, compatible with hypertrophic osteitis (*goundou*).

antibody absorption, or FTA-ABS) are specific for treponematoses, but cannot differentiate between yaws and syphilis. Once positive, they usually remain so for life.

Treatment

The principle is to produce a treponemicidal blood concentration of penicillin for at least 10 days in patients with early lesions. Most lesions heal within 2–3 weeks after a single dose of 3–4 mega units of benzathine penicillin or penicillin aluminium monostearate. In late lesions, repeated daily doses of procaine penicillin may be needed.

ENDEMIC SYPHILIS

Endemic syphilis is caused by *Treponema pallidum pallidum*. It occurs in arid, dry savannah areas, predominantly in the Sahel zone of Africa. It also occurs on the Arabian peninsula, where the disease is known as Bejel.

The problem in Africa

This non-venereal infection is prevalent in Chad, Niger (Julvez et al., 1998), Burkina Faso (Baudon et al., 1985), Mali (Autier et al., 1989), Mauritania (Lepers et al., 1988) and Senegal (Ridet et al., 1979; Antal & Causse, 1985). After mass campaigns, the disease has disappeared from African countries south of the Equator, although the epidemiology in South Africa (van Niekirk et al., 1985) and Botswana (Wiis & Sheller, 1995) is uncertain (see Fig. 46.1).

Organism

T. pallidum pallidum is the cause. Although there are wide differences in transmission, biological behaviour, and age distribution, the organism is indistinguishable from the treponeme that causes sexually transmitted syphilis.

Epidemiology

The tribal groups of the sahel savannah include the semi-nomadic Touareg, who move to and from the desert, the pastoral Peuls (Fulani), and more settled agricultural groups (Basset et al., 1969; Bourdillon et al., 1981). Some Touareg groups like the poor Bouzou lead a life with very poor hygiene, and they are worst affected. Lesions cluster among people from the same family, and breast-feeding infants may be infected by their mothers. The disease chiefly affects children and adolescents, but among the Touareg, adults are also affected.

Transmission

Cases in the same family and among children suggest that the organism is transmitted directly by close person-to-person contact, and perhaps also indirectly from a drinking vessel such as a porous calabash.

Seasonal change

The lesions of the Touareg are most florid during the short rainy season, and either disappear or improve spontaneously during the dry season. Among the Peuls, who often find pasture in the wetter valleys, and among the agricultural tribes, lesions are more florid, particularly in children, and persist during the dry season.

Clinics and mass campaigns

The pattern of lesions of the Touareg may be partly explained by special clinics, which operate during their annual gatherings in August, at Ingall in Niger. Mass treatment campaigns have been carried out, e.g. in Burkina Faso.

Prevalence and follow-up

As in yaws, many more individuals are treponeme seropositive than have clinically detectable lesions (Baudon et al., 1985; Gazin & Meynard, 1988) which are therefore not a good index of the prevalence of infection. In several regions (e.g. Senegal), increasing numbers of cases have been detected in recent years (Julvez et al., 1998).

Prevention

Mass treatment is the main control strategy. It is possible that the control of endemic syphilis leaves populations more susceptible to venereal syphilis. Follow-up surveillance after mass campaigns is essential, but difficult to achieve in nomadic and pastoral tribes.

Clinical features

The disease affects the skin, especially in the peri-oral and perineal regions; and bone. The disease is generally milder than venereally transmitted syphilis, and neurosyphilis is said not to occur.

Children

The characteristic early lesion is a slightly raised mucous plaque, commonly on the inside of the lips or in the oral cavity. These ulcers may be painful and interfere with feeding. In the ano-genital region, moist condylomata are seen. Angular stomatitis also occurs. In later life scars may be seen in those places.

Adults

(i) Early lesions are more florid after puberty. There are papular mucocutaneous lesions, significantly different from those of children. These can be hypertrophied and macerated; the skin of the genital region, axillae, and under the breast is affected.
(ii) Late mutilating lesions (gummata), which penetrate the bones of the face and nose, may be seen.

Diagnosis

As for yaws.

Treatment

The aim is to produce a high treponemicidal blood level of penicillin for about 3 weeks, as for yaws, but the timing of the dosage depends as much on the patient's nomadic habits as on his clinical lesions.

References

Agadzi VK, Aboagye-Atta Y, Nelson JW, Perine PL, Hopkins DR. (1983). Resurgence of yaws in Ghana. *Lancet*; **ii**: 389–390.

Akogun OB (1999) Yaws and syphilis in the Garkida area of Nigeria. *Zentralbl Bakteriol*; **289**: 101–107.

Antal GM, Causse G. (1985). The control of endemic treponematoses. *Rev Infect Dis*; **7**: S220–S226.

Autier P, Delcambe JF, Sangare D et al. (1989). Etudes sérologiques et cliniques sur la tréponematose endemique en République du Mali. *Ann Soc Belg Med Trop*; **69**: 319–329.

Backhouse JL, Hudson BJ, Hamilton PA, Nesteroff SI. (1998). Failure of penicillin treatment of yaws on Karkar Island, Papua New Guinea. *Am J Trop Med Hyg*; **59**: 388–392.

Basset A, Maleville J, Basset M. (1969). Aspects de la syphilis endémique des Touareg du Niger. *Bull Soc Pathol Exot Filiales*; **62**: 80–92.

Baudon D, Houssou B. (1984). Le niveau de l'endémie pianique dans le sud du Benin en 1982. *Ann Soc Belg Med Trop*; **64**: 397–402.

Baudon D, Saliou P, Bibane L, Buisson Y. (1985). La syphilis endémique dans une region sahélienne du Burkina-Faso. Enquête sero-clinique. *Bull Soc Pathol Exot Filiales*; **78**: 555–562.

Bourdillon F, Monjour L, Druilhe P et al. (1981). La syphilis endémique en Haute-Volta. Un aspect particulier du profil épidémiologique. *Bull Soc Pathol Exot Filiales*; **74**: 375–381.

Cox DL, Chang P, McDowall AW, Radolf JD. (1992). The outer membrane, not a coat of host proteins, limits antigenicity of virulent *Treponema pallidum*. *Infect Immun*; **60**: 1076–1083.

Edorh AA, Siamevi EK, Adanlete FA et al. (1994). Résurgence de l'endémie pianique au Togo. Cause et approche d'éradication. *Bull Soc Pathol Exot*; **87**: 17–18.

Engelkens HJ, ten Kate FJ, Judanarso J et al. (1993). The localisation of treponemes and characterisation of the inflammatory infiltrate in skin biopsies from patients with primary or secondary syphilis, or early infectious yaws. *Genitourin Med*; **69**: 102–107.

Gazin P, Meynard D (1988). Enquête clinique et sérologique sur le bejel au nord du Burkina Faso. *Bull Soc Pathol Exot Filiales*; **81**: 827–831.

Herve V, Kassa KE, Normand P, Georges A, Mathiot C, Martin P. (1992). Résurgence du pian en République centrafricaine. Rôle de la population pygmée comme reservoir de virus. *Bull Soc Pathol Exot*; **85**: 342–346.

Julvez J, Michault A, Kerdelhue V. (1998). Etude sérologique des tréponematoses non véneriennes chez l'enfant à Niamey, Niger. *Med Trop (Mars)*; **58**: 38–40.

Lepers JP, Billon C, Pesce JL, Rollin PE, Saint-Martin J. (1988). Etude sero-épidémiologique en Mauritanie (1985–1986): fréquence des tréponematoses, du virus de l'hepatite B, du virus VIH et des fièvres hémorragiques virales. *Bull Soc Pathol Exot Filiales*; **81**: 24–31.

Liu H, Steiner BM, Alder JD, Baertschy DK, Schell RF. (1990). Immune T cells sorted by flow cytometry confer protection against infection with *Treponema pallidum* subsp. *pertenue* in hamsters. *Infect Immun*; **58**: 1685–1690.

N'Da K (1985) Some epidemiologic aspects of yaws in the Ivory Coast. *Rev Infect Dis*; **7**: S237–S238.

Noordhoek GT, Hermans PW, Paul AN, Schouls LM, van der Sluis JJ, van Embden JD. (1989). *Treponema pallidum* subspecies *pallidum* (Nichols) and *Treponema pallidum* subspecies *pertenue* (CDC 2575) differ in at least one nucleotide: comparison of two homologous antigens. *Microb Pathog*; **6**: 29–42.

Noordhoek GT, Cockayne A, Schouls LM, Meloen RH, Stolz E, van Embden JD. (1990). A new attempt to distinguish serologically the subspecies of *Treponema pallidum* causing syphilis and yaws. *J Clin Microbiol*; **28**: 1600–1607.

Omar MA. (1986). Yaws assessment in Somalia. *Southeast Asian J Trop Med Public Health*; **17**: 66–69.

Perine PL, Nelson JW, Lewis JO et al. (1985). New technologies for use in the surveillance and control of yaws. *Rev Infect Dis*; **7**: S295–S299.

Radolf JD, Norgard MV, Schulz WW. (1989). Outer membrane ultrastructure explains the limited antigenicity of virulent *Treponema pallidum*. *Proc Natl Acad Sci USA*; **86**: 2051–2055.

Radolf JD, Robinson EJ, Bourell KW et al. (1995). Characterization of outer membranes isolated from *Treponema pallidum*, the syphilis spirochete. *Infect Immun*; **63**: 4244–4252.

Radolf JD. (1995). *Treponema pallidum* and the quest for outer membrane proteins. *Mol Microbiol*; **16**: 1067–1073.

Ridet J, Grab B, Costa JD, Akribas A, Causse G. (1979). Etude séro-épidemiologique sur l'endemicité tréponemique au Senegal. *Bull Wld Hlth Org*; **57**: 315–327.

Stamm LV, Greene SR, Bergen HL, Hardham JM, Barnes NY. (1998). Identification and sequence analysis of *Treponema pallidum* tprJ, a member of a polymorphic multigene family. *FEMS Microbiol Lett*; **169**: 155–163.

Toure IM. (1985). Endemic treponematoses in Togo and other west African states. *Rev Infect Dis*; **7**: S242–S244.

van Niekerk CH, van Niekerk LC, van den EJ. (1985). Positiewe serologiese toetse vir sifilis by swart laerskoolkinders van Bloemfontein. 'n Loodsstudie. *S Afr Med J*; **67**: 90–91.

Weinstock GM, Hardham JM, McLeod MP, Sodergren EJ, Norris SJ. (1998). The genome of *Treponema pallidum*: new light on the agent of syphilis. *FEMS Microbiol Rev*; **22**: 323–332.

Wicher K, Wicher V, Abbruscato F, Baughn RE. (2000). *Treponema pallidum* subsp. *pertenue* displays pathogenic properties different from those of *T. pallidum* subsp. *pallidum*. *Infect Immu*; **68**: 3219–3225.

Wiis J, Sheller JP. (1995). Treponemal infektion blandt born i Ramotswa, Botswana. Et serologisk studie. *Ugeskr Laeger*; **157**: 4134–4136.

Widy-Wirski R. (1985). Surveillance and control of resurgent yaws in the African region. *Rev Infect Dis*; **7**: S227–S232.

Widy-Wirski R, D'Costa J, Meheus A. (1980). Prévalence du pian chez les pygmées en Centrafrique. *Ann Soc Belg Med Trop*; **60**: 61–67.

Ziefer A, Lanoie LO, Meyers WM, Vanderpas J, Charon F, Connor DH. (1985). Studies on a focus of yaws in Ubangi, Zaire. *Trop Med Parasitol*; **36**: 63–71.

Leprosy

47

The problem in Africa

Leprosy is a chronic disease that may result in deformity and social stigma, creating problems for patients and their families. Africa is the second most affected region world-wide after India (WHO, 2000). In 1999 11 African countries still had more than one leprosy patient per 10 000 population.

In many countries leprosy work is being integrated into general health services, so all medical professionals need to be aware of the signs and symptoms of leprosy. Since new patients may have nerve function impairment at diagnosis, every health professional should know how to manage nerve impairment caused by leprosy (Rijk et al., 1994).

The organism

Leprosy is caused by *Mycobacterium leprae*, an acid-fast intracellular organism not yet cultivated in vitro. The organism was first identified in the nodules of lepromatous leprosy patients by Hansen in 1873. *M. leprae* parasitizes skin macrophages and peripheral nerve Schwann cells.

M. leprae can be grown in the mouse footpad, but growth is slow, taking over 6 months to produce significant yields. The nine-banded armadillo is susceptible to *M. leprae* infection, and develops disease with widespread bacterial multiplication. The armadillo and mouse models of *M. leprae* infection have been useful for producing *M. leprae* for biological studies and studying drug sensitivity patterns (Hastings, 1985).

M. leprae is a stable, hardy organism withstanding drying for up to 5 months. It has a doubling time of 12 days (compared with 20 minutes for E. coli). The optimum growth temperature is 27–30 °C, which is consistent with the clinical observation of maximal *M. leprae* growth at cool superficial sites (skin, nasal mucosa and peripheral nerves). *M. leprae* is a single species with isolates having similar biological characteristics and identical genotypes (using restriction fragment polymorphism analysis) irrespective of the type of leprosy, race or geographic origin of the isolates (Hastings, 1985).

M. leprae posses a complex cell wall comprising lipids and carbohydrates. *M. leprae* synthesizes a species-specific phenolic glycolipid (PGL) and lipoarabinomannan. Numerous protein antigens have been identified as important immune targets using antibody and T-cell screening.

The recent sequencing of the *M.leprae* genome has yielded surprises. The genome is small (3.27 Mb) and shows extreme reductive evolution. Less than half the genome contains functional genes, and many pseudogenes are present. 165 genes are unique to *M. leprae*, and functions can be attributed to 29 of them. Analysis of these unique proteins will be critical for developing new diagnostic tests. Comparison of biosynthetic pathways with *M. tuberculosis* is giving new insights into *M. leprae* metabolism. For lipolysis *M. leprae* has only 2 genes (*M. tuberculosis* has 22). *M. leprae* has also lost many genes for carbon catabolism and many carbon sources (e.g. acetate and galactose) are unavailable to it. This gene loss leaves *M. leprae* unable to respond to different environments and explains the impossibility of growing the organism in vitro (Cole et al., 2001).

Epidemiology

In 2000 there were 64 000 patients on treatment for leprosy in Africa, of whom 55 635 were newly registered cases. The overall prevalence is 8.6 per 10 000 population. (WHO, 2000). The highest prevalence in Africa is in Madagascar, at 7.7 per 10 000 population. Madagascar, Ethiopia, Mozambique, Congo, Tanzania and Guinea are the 6 African countries in the top 11 high prevalence countries world-wide (WHO, 2000).

Improved coverage of leprosy services and multi-drug therapy has increased the number of newly diagnosed, treated and cured cases. Leprosy Elimination Campaigns (LEC) aim to detect hidden cases and treat them with multi-drug therapy (MDT); when such campaigns were conducted in Nigeria, Madagascar and Guinea, the number of newly detected cases doubled (WHO, 1997).

Although prevalence has fallen, the incidence of leprosy has not declined in the last decade, indicating that transmission continues. New cases can be expected for the next decade and beyond.

Risk factors

Age and sex are important determinants of leprosy risk. In most countries male: female ratios are similar until puberty. After this age there is an excess of male cases, sometimes reaching a ratio of 2:1 (male:female). In Ethiopia and elsewhere the highest prevalence is seen in the 15–34 year age group. In Malawi a poor standard of housing and lack of schooling were found to be risk factors for leprosy. Studies in Malawi and Uganda have shown that BCG vaccination decreases the risk of leprosy (Pönnighaus et al., 1994).

HIV and leprosy

Early in the HIV/AIDS epidemic, it was suggested that HIV infection might be a risk factor for leprosy (Turk & Rees, 1988) but studies in Mali, Uganda and Ethiopia have not confirmed this (Lucas, 1993; Lienhardt et al., 1996; Kawuma et al., 1994; Gebre et al., 2000).

HIV infection may predispose to leprosy reactions. In a Ugandan study there were more Type 1 reactions and episodes of neuritis in seropositive patients. (Bwire & Kawuma, 1994). In an Ethiopian study there was a significant association between HIV seropositivity and Erythema Nodosum Leprosum (ENL) reactions, but only twenty HIV-positive cases were studied (Gebre et al., 2000).

Unusual presentation of leprosy in HIV seropositives has been reported (Kennedy et al., 1990; Thappa et al., 1996; Almedia et al., 1994). It remains important to continue monitoring for possible interactions between HIV and leprosy.

Transmission

The nasal mucosa is the main route for exit of *M. leprae* and the nasal secretions of untreated lepromatous cases contain many organisms. Studies detecting *M. leprae* DNA by the polymerase chain reaction (PCR) in nasal secretions have shown that *M. leprae* DNA is carried by normal individuals and contacts in leprosy endemic countries (in Ethiopia 6 per cent of the population) (Cree & Smith, 1998). These individuals may transmit the infection.

Transmission studies are difficult in leprosy because of the unique biology of the organism and the long incubation period of disease. Leprosy has an insidious onset, and the source of the infection in an infected individual is rarely identified.

Pathogenesis

In leprosy the clinical features are determined by the host immune response. There are four aspects of leprosy pathogenesis:

- the spectrum of immune response
- the bacterial load
- immune mediated reactions and
- nerve damage.

The typical leprosy lesion is granulomatous inflammation in skin and nerve.

Spectrum of disease

Most individuals exposed to *M.leprae* do not develop leprosy; they will have sub-clinical infection and presumably develop protective immunity. It is not clear why some develop disease and most do not. There are no tests available for measuring protective immunity.

In those who do develop disease a spectrum of immune responses are seen. At one end of the spectrum is tuberculoid leprosy (TT), characterized by strong cell-mediated immunity (CMI) towards *M. leprae*. These patients have few hypopigmented, anaesthetic lesions. At the other pole is lepromatous leprosy (LL), which is characterized by the absence of a CMI response. These patients have numerous lesions and high bacillary loads. Most patients have features between these two extreme groups (Fig. 47.1, Table 47.1) (Ridley, 1988).

Table 47.1. Major clinical features of the disease spectrum in leprosy

	Classification				
	TT	BT	BB	BL	LL
Clinical features					
Skin					
Infiltrated lesions	Defined plaques, diffuse thickening	Irregular plaques	Polymorphic	Papules, nodules	Diffuse thickening
	Healing centres	Partially raised edges,	'Punched out centres'		
Macular lesions	Single, small	Several, any size,	Multiple, all sizes	Innumerable, small	Innumerable, confluent
		'Geographic'	Bizarre		
Nerve					
Peripheral nerve	Solitary, enlarged	Several nerves	Many nerves	Late neural thickening	Slow, symmetrical loss
	Nerves	Asymmetrical	Asymmetrical pattern	Asymmetrical anaesthesia and paresis	Glove and stocking anaesthesia
Microbiology					
Bacterial index	0–1	0–2	2–3	1–4	4–6
Histology					
Lymphocytes	+	++	+/−	++	+/−
Macrophages	−	−	+/−	−	−
Epithelioid cells	++	+/−	−	−	−
Antibody, anti-*M.leprae*	−/+	−/++	+	++	++

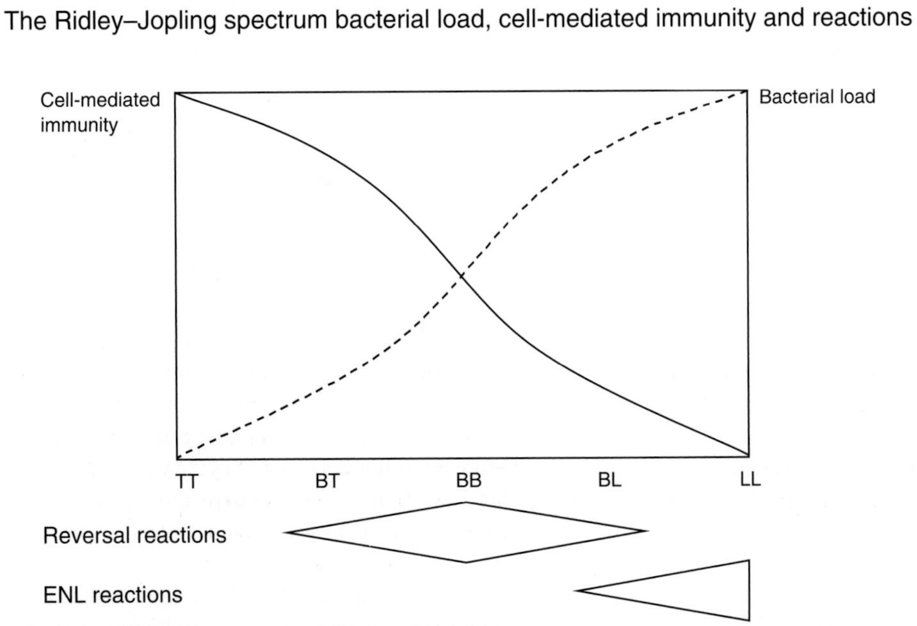

Fig. 47.1. The spectrum of immunological responses to *M. leprae* and its relationship to clinical features of leprosy.

Reactions

Leprosy reactions are superimposed on the spectrum described above. Borderline (BT, BB, BL) patients are immunologically unstable and are at risk of reversal (Type1) reactions. These are delayed hyper-sensitivity reactions against *M.leprae* antigens in skin and nerve. They are characterized by enhanced T cell proliferation towards *M. leprae* antigens, increased numbers of CD4+ cells in granulomas, and local over-production of cytokines such as IFN-γ, IL-12, iNOS and TNFα (Yamamura et al., 1992). Although the end result is the elimination of mycobacteria, this is only achieved at the expense of severe local tissue damage particularly in nerves (Khanolkar-Young et al., 1995).

Type 2 reactions, erythema nodosum leprosum (ENL) are partly due to immune complex deposition and occur in BL and LL patients who produce antibodies and have a large antigen load. Local vasculitis is present. Lesions contain immunoglobulin, complement, polymorphs and immune complexes. There is also enhanced T-cell activity with increased CD8 cells, increased circulating interleukin-2 receptors and high levels of circulating TNF-α.

The frequency of ENL reaction has decreased from 50 per cent to 15 per cent in LL patients since the introduction of multiple drug treatment (MDT). In Ethiopia ENL is unusual, occurring only in 12 per cent of LL and 3.6 per cent of BL patients (Saunderson & Gronen, 2000).

Nerve involvement in leprosy

Nerve involvement is important in leprosy; in Ethiopia 55 per cent patients had some degree of nerve function impairment (NFI) at diagnosis (Rijk et al., 1994, Saunderson & Gronen, 2000). In tuberculoid leprosy perineural inflammation and granulomas are found. In lepromatous leprosy nerves contain large numbers of bacilli. In borderline leprosy the combination of intraneural bacilli and cell-mediated immunity produces widespread damage. In leprosy reactions the nerve suddenly becomes oedematous due to inflammation, giving little time for the perineurium to expand. The tight perineurium causes intraneural ischemia, and transient paralysis of nerves (Turk et al., 1993).

Clinical features

Patients commonly present with skin lesions, weakness or numbness due to a peripheral nerve lesion or a burn or ulcer in an anaesthetic hand or foot. Borderline patients may present in reaction with nerve pain, sudden palsy, multiple new skin lesions, pain in the eye, or a systemic febrile illness.

Presenting symptoms

Skin lesions

The type of skin lesion depends on the type of leprosy. Patients may have hypopigmented patches, papules or nodules. Lesions may be single or multiple. At the tuberculoid end of the spectrum lesions are anaesthetic.

Loss of nerve function

Single or multiple nerves can be affected, resulting in loss of function. This results in weakness or paralysis of hands and feet. Patients may present with clawed hands, foot drop or impaired eyelid closure. These patients complain that they cannot work, eat with their hands or walk.

Acute erythematous skin lesion

Patients may present in reaction with new acute skin lesions. If a patient presents in reaction the main complaint may be pain. When a multibacillary patient develops ENL the first presentation may be fever and pain.

Nasal discharge and blockage

Lepromatous patients may have nasal blockage and discharge due to invasion of the nasal mucosa by *M. leprae*.

Ulceration on hands and feet

This is usually a late presentation and is due to anesthesia.

Delay in diagnosis can result in permanent nerve damage. In Nigeria 68 per cent of patients had delays of more than one year before starting treatment (Weg et al., 1998). In Ethiopia 77 per cent of patients delayed a year or more before attending a leprosy clinic (Assefa et al., 2000). In the Nigerian study 37 per cent of patients consulted folk healers while 32 per cent went to the leprosy service. Those who went to folk healers were not advised to attend leprosy clinics. Ex-leprosy patients may have a role in advising new patients to attend leprosy clinics (Assefa et al., 2000). Health education for the public and for traditional healers, with emphasis on the early symptoms and signs of leprosy, is important in promoting the early diagnosis of leprosy.

Classification of leprosy

Patients are classified according to clinical findings in skin, nerves and other organs (Table 47.1).

Classifying patients according to the Ridley–Jopling scale given below is clinically useful. Borderline tuberculoid leprosy may be associated with rapid, severe nerve damage while lepromatous disease is associated with chronicity and long-term complications. Borderline disease is unstable and may be complicated by reactions. There is also a simpler field classification of paucibacillary(few)/multibacillary(many) (Table 47.2) based solely on the number of bacilli in skin lesions. This classification is useful for guiding the length of treatment in the field.

Indeterminate leprosy

Indeterminate leprosy is the early form of leprosy. It is commonly seen in children. The lesions consist of one or two hypopigmented macules with ill-defined margins. The lesion is not anaesthetic. The surface is smooth. The skin biopsy may show a lymphocytic infiltrate without granuloma formation. Most heal without treatment but 25 per cent may progress to established leprosy.

Nerves

No nerve enlargement

Slit skin smears (SSS)

Negative

Tuberculoid leprosy (TT)

Tuberculoid leprosy is one of the stable polar forms of leprosy.

Skin

There is usually one lesion, which may be a macule, a plaque, or have raised margins (Fig. 47.2). The lesion has a well-defined margin, is anaesthetic and hypopigmented. Both sweating and hair are lost. The surface is dry and rough.

Nerves

A single nerve involved.

Slit skin smears

Negative

Borderline tuberculoid (BT)

Skin

Individual lesions are similar to TT lesions. However there are multiple lesions (Fig. 47.3). The margins may be ill-defined. The surface is less dry and less hairless. There may be central healing, and satellite lesions are also common in this group.

Nerves

Multiple nerves may be involved.

Slit skin smears

Negative or 1+ (See Table 47.2).

Borderline borderline (BB)

This is an unstable type of leprosy which soon moves down to BL or upgrades to BT.

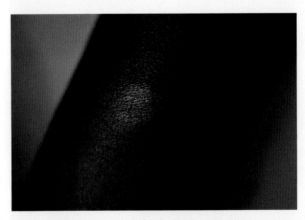

Fig. 47.2. TT leprosy. A single hypopigmented anaesthetic patch with an active, inflamed edge. (Reproduced with permission from Diana Lockwood.)

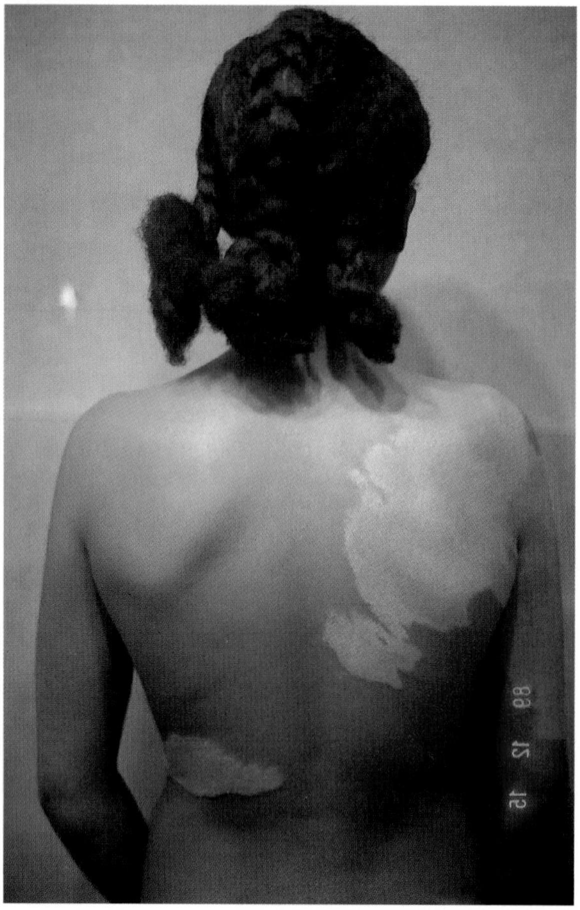

Fig. 47.3. BT leprosy. Hypopigmented anaesthetic patches on the trunk and arm. Slit skin smears negative (Martin Dietz).

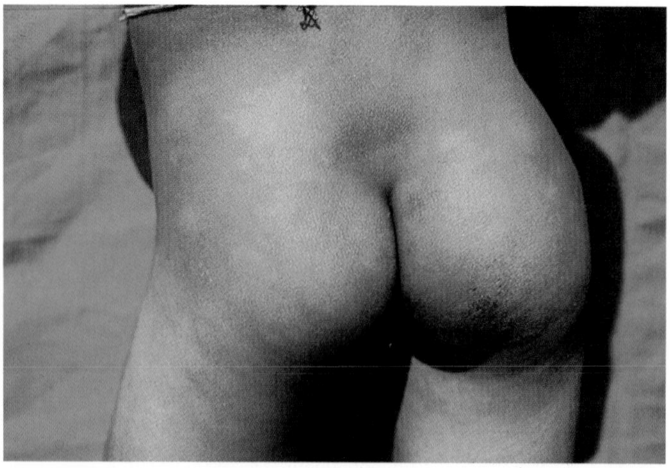

Fig. 47.4. BL leprosy. Multiple non-anaesthetic plaques and infiltration (Diana Lockwood).

Table 47.2. Bacterial Index

Score	Bacilli per field
6+	Many clumps (1000) in an average field
5+	100–1000 bacilli in an average field
4+	10–100 bacilli in an average field
3+	1–10 bacilli in an average field
2+	1–10 bacilli in 10 fields
1+	1–10 bacilli in 100 fields

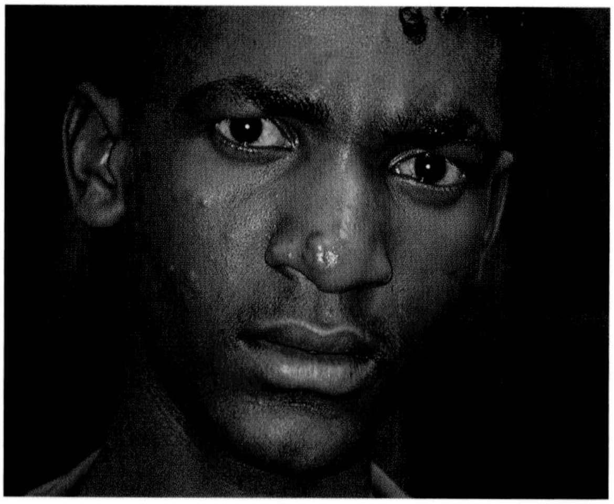

Fig. 47.5. BL leprosy. A young man with papules and nodules on his face. This could have been mistaken for acne if the whole body had not been examined, and similar lesions found in other areas (Martin Dietz).

Skin

There are multiple plaque lesions with punched out centers. Lesions are usually erythematous and may be bilateral and symmetrical. Sensory loss is variable.

Nerves

Multiple nerves can be involved.

Slit skin smears

+ to +++.

Borderline lepromatous leprosy (BL)

Skin

There may be erythematous macules, papules or nodules of variable size (Figs. 47.4, 47.5). The lesions are symmetrical and multiple. There is only slight loss of sensation.

Nerves

There is multiple asymmetrical nerve enlargement.

Slit skin smears

++ to ++++.

Lepromatous leprosy (LL)

Skin

Multiple, uncountable lesions which may be macules, papules or nodules (Figs. 47.6, 47.7). Early LL disease presents with ill-defined macules, which are not anaesthetic. Lepromatous nodules are skin coloured, non-tender soft papules occurring anywhere on the body in a symmetrical distribution. The nasal mucosa, larynx, and palate can be involved with infiltration and lepromatous nodules. Even normal-looking skin between the nodules is involved and infiltrated.

Nerves

Multiple nerves can be enlarged and involvement is symmetrical.

Slit skin smears

+++ to ++++++.

Nerve damage in leprosy

Damage to peripheral nerve trunks produces characteristic signs with sensory loss and dysfunction of the muscles supplied by peripheral nerves. The sensory function is the earliest affected in leprosy, and sensory impairment can occur alone without motor involvement (Hastings, 1985). Autonomic nerve damage results in dryness of the hands and feet. The ulnar, median, radial, common peroneal and posterior tibial nerves are most commonly involved.

Acute neuritis also occurs with sudden development of nerve tenderness, pain and loss of function. Nerve function may also be lost without nerve pains or tenderness (silent neuropathy). Thus it is vital to check nerve func-

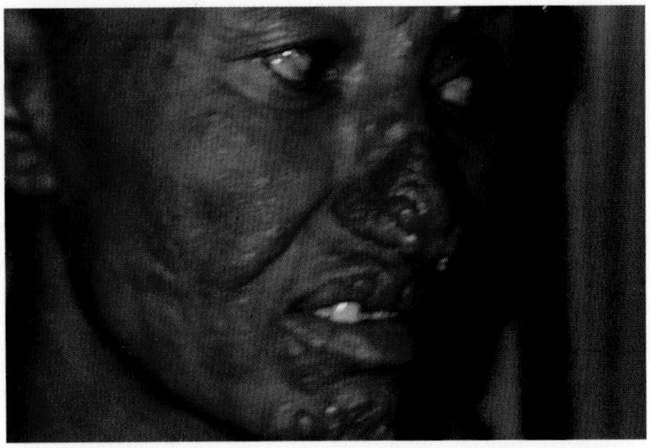

Fig. 47.6. LL leprosy. Elderly lady with typical facial features of lepromatous leprosy: infiltration, thickening of the nasolabial folds, nodules on the face and madarosis (loss of eyebrows) (Martin Dietz).

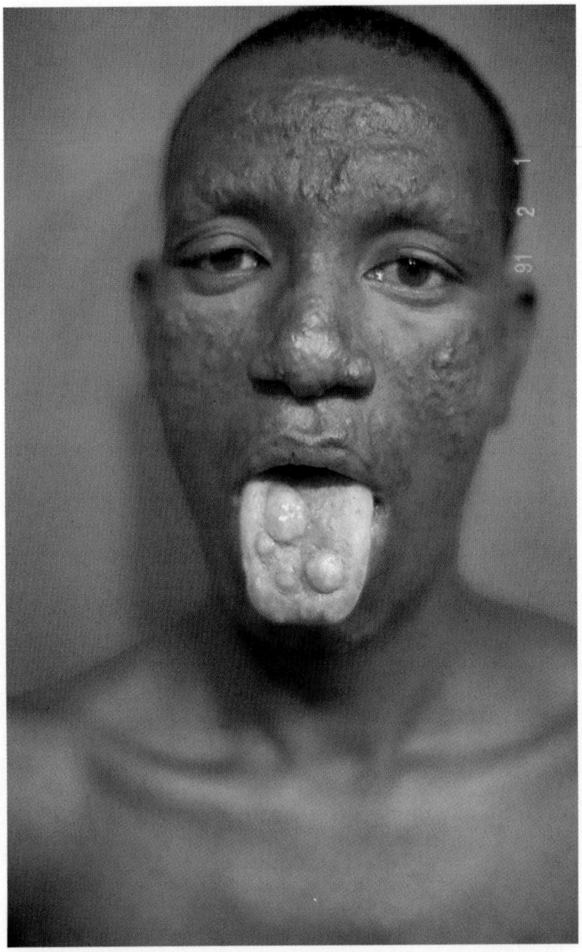

Fig. 47.7. LL leprosy. Papules and nodules on face and tongue (Martin Dietz).

Table 47.3. Nerve examination in leprosy

Nerve	Site palpated	Muscle to test (VMT)	Area of sensory testing (ST)
Ulnar	Olecranon groove	First dorsal interosseus, abducter digiti minimi (index finger out)	Three points, on pulp of little finger, and on the fifth metacarpophalangial (MCP) joint, and three points on the hypothenar eminence.
Median	Wrist (flexure)	Abductor pollicis brevis, opponens pollicis (thumb up)	Four points, on the pulp of thumb, on the palm over the second MCP joint, the tip of the index and middle finger
Radial	Humerus at deltoid insertion	Extensor carpi ulnaris, extensor digitorum communis (wrist up)	
Common peroneal	At the neck of fibula	Peroneal muscle, dorsiflexors of feet (Dorsiflexion of the feet, eversion of feet)	Peroneal
Posterior tibial	Behind medial maleollus	Intrinsic muscles of the feet (clawing of toes)	10 points are examined on sole, on tip of each toe, on the plantar skin over the first and fifth metacarpophalangial joints, lateral border of sole, heel
Facial nerve		Orbicularis oculi muscle (eye closure)	
Trigeminal nerve		–	Cornea, conjunctiva and face

tion on every clinic visit so that loss of function can be detected early.

Nerve trunks are palpated at the sites shown in Table 47.3 and in Fig. 47.8. Note the size of the nerve, the consistency and tenderness. Nerves are normally palpable and subtle enlargement may only be detected by experienced observers. Nerve function is assessed by sensory and motor testing

Sensory testing

It is important to detect and monitor sensory loss both in skin lesions and in regions supplied by peripheral nerves. This can be done using a ball-point pen or nylon monofilaments. Table 47.3 and Fig. 47.8 give the areas that should be tested for each nerve.

Motor testing

This is easily done by systematically evaluating the function of small muscles of the hands and feet (Table 47.3).

Eye involvement in leprosy

Leprosy is a common cause of blindness. Eye involvement in leprosy is due to structural and immunological problems. The structural problems include impaired eyelid closure due to malfunction of the orbicularis oculi muscle, and loss of corneal sensation. These two factors interact to produce exposure keratitis (Figs. 47.9, 47.10). The immunological problems affecting the eye manifest as iritis and episcleritis in ENL.

Diagnosis of leprosy

The diagnosis is essentially clinical, based on finding one or more of the cardinal signs of leprosy. Histological examination of a skin or nerve biopsy may be needed in difficult cases. Serological and PCR-based diagnostic tests are not yet clinically useful.

Cardinal signs of leprosy

A typical skin lesion with loss of sensation

To check sensation first explain to the patient what you are doing. Ask the patient to close their eyes. Then touch the normal skin and make the patient understand how it feels, and then check the normal and the abnormal skin by turn and tell the patient to point when they feel. If there is definite loss of sensation one can diagnose leprosy.

An enlarged peripheral nerve

Leprosy is the most important cause of thickened peripheral nerves. Other causes such as amyloid are exceedingly rare. In an Ethiopian study 84 per cent of new leprosy cases had nerve enlargement (Saunderson & Gronen, 2000).

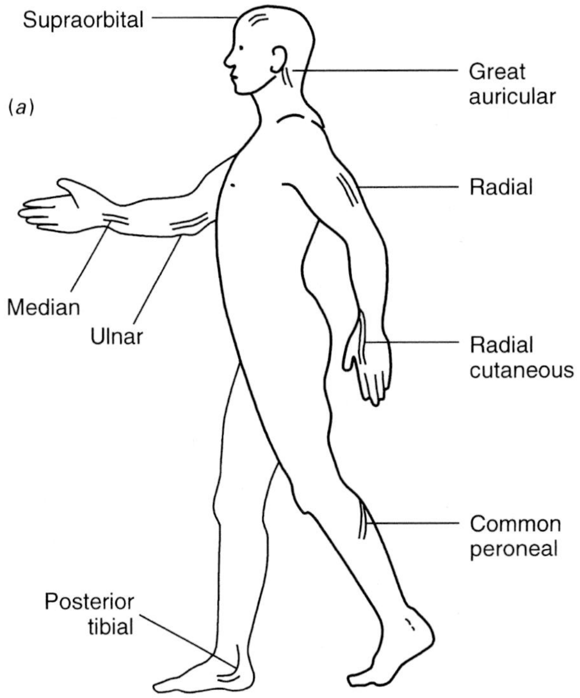

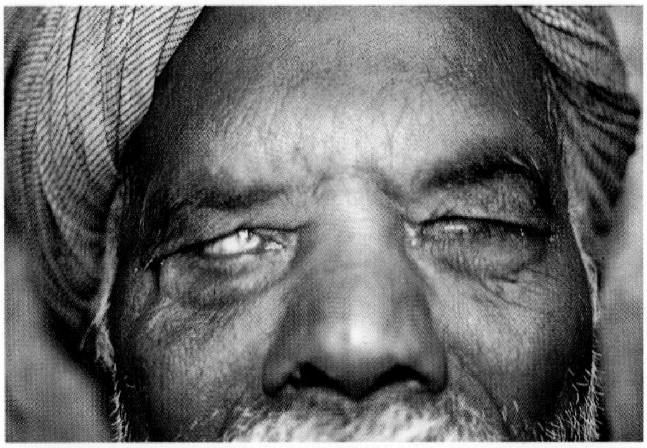

Fig. 47.9. Lagophthalmos – inability to close the eye (Diana Lockwood).

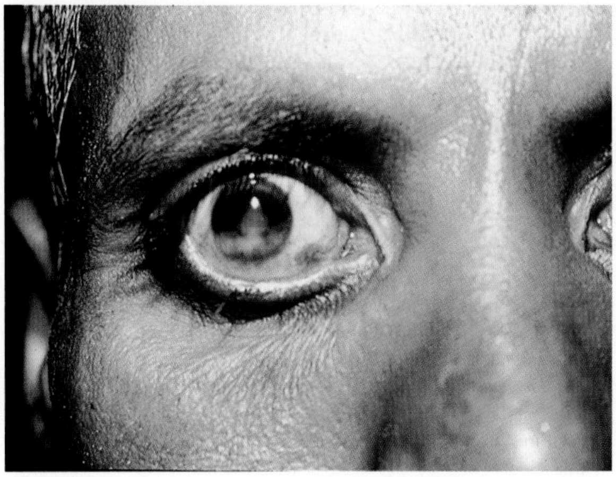

Fig. 47.10. Exposure keratitis secondary to lagophthalmos (Diana Lockwood).

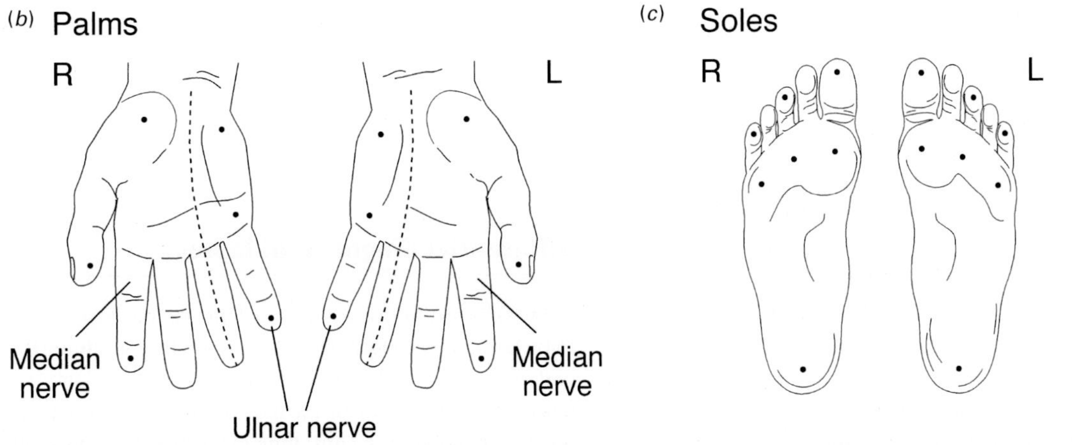

Fig. 47.8. (*a*) The sites of predilection at which the peripheral nerves are most commonly enlarged and palpable in leprosy. (*b*) Points to test sensation on palms and soles.

Table 47.4. Differential diagnosis of macules

Disease	Lesion	Diagnostic points
Pityriasi alba	Hypopigmented macule	Has scales on surface, seen in children, not anaesthetic
Vitiligo	Hypopigmented macule, asymptomatic	Normal skin texture, not anaesthetic, leprosy lesion does not become depigmented
Naevus anemicus	Hypopigmented macule	Present since birth, normal skin texture, no anaesthesia
Pityriasis versicolor	Hypopigmented macule on neck and chest	Has powdery scale on surface, no anaesthesia, microscopy will show sporea and hyphae
Post-inflammatory	Hypopigmented macule	History of previous lesion on the site, normal texture, no anaesthesia hypopigmentation

Notes:
All these lesions may appear similar to tuberculoid and borderline tuberculoid lesions.

Table 47.5. Differential diagnosis of plaques

Disease	Lesion	Diagnostic points
Pityriasis rosea	Multiple plaque lesions on the trunk and upper arm	Itchy, has herald patch, has scales on surface
Secondary syphilis	Multiple non-itchy plaque	May be history of primary chancre palms and soles
Psoriasis	Multiple erythematous plaque	Recurrence is common, abundant scales on surface
Tinea corporis	Well-defined plaque	Vesicles and papules in margins, not anaesthetic, skin scrapings show fungal filaments
Skin tuberculosis	Chronic plaque lesion, papules or nodules, can cause deformity on nose or other site	Usually distinguished by skin biopsy, showing tuberculoid granuloma, without nerve involvement
Granuloma multiforme	Well-defined plaque	Not anaesthetic, histology from skin biopsy will show granuloma without dermal nerve involvement

Notes:
All these may appear similar to borderline tuberculoid and borderline lepromatous lesions.

Acid-fast bacilli in a skin smear

Slit skin smears are made from six sites: ear lobe, forehead, buttock, arm and knee and suspect lesions. A skin fold is cleaned with alcohol, then pinched between index finger and thumb to reduce blood flow. An incision is made with a sterile scalpel blade, the blade is turned through 90 degrees and scraped. The tissue is smeared on the slide. The slide is stained by the Ziehl–Neelsen method and slides are examined using a 100 × oil immersion lens. Grading of smears is explained in Table 47.1

In one analysis of 594 Ethiopian patients, clinical examination and slit skin smears identified 584 cases (Saunderson & Gronen, 2000). The remaining ten cases required biopsy because there were hypopigmented patches without loss of sensation.

Leprosy should not be diagnosed in the absence of cardinal signs. The diagnosis of leprosy still causes many social problems for the patient and his/her family. If you are in doubt, you should keep the patient under observation.

Differential diagnosis of leprosy

Many skin conditions can mimic leprosy. It is important to be familiar with local skin colour and its variations. In endemic countries health workers tend to over-diagnose leprosy, while in countries where leprosy is not endemic the health worker may not think of leprosy. The common differential diagnoses of leprosy are listed in Tables 47.4, 47.5, 47.6.

Table 47.6. Differential diagnosis of papules and nodules

	Papules and nodules	
Disease	Lesion	Diagnostic points
Diffuse cutaneous leishmaniasis	Multiple asymptomatic nodules	Skin between the nodules is normal, SSS negative, smear for *Leishmania donovani* bodies positive
Neurofibroma	Skin coloured asymptomatic papule and nodule	Nodules are reducible, café-au-lait spots may be seen, SSS is negative
Sarcoidosis	Asymptotic papules and nodules, erythematous nodules on shin	SSS negative, biopsy of skin shows granuloma with scanty lymphocyte and dermal nerves not involved
Molluscum contagiosum	Asymptomatic papules and nodules	Umblicated at the centre of nodules, SSS is negative

Notes:
All these may be confused with borderline lepromatous and lepromatous disease.

Table 47.7. Drugs used in multi-drug therapy

Drugs	Characteristic	Mechanism of action	Side effect
Rifampicin	Potent bactericidal drug	Inhibits DNA-dependent RNA polymerase of micro-organism, interferes with bacterial RNA synthesis	Hepatotoxicity rare at this dosage, 'flu-like syndrome after monthly dose
Dapsone	Sulfone group, 4,4-diaminodiphenylsulfone, weakly bactericidal	Inhibition of dihydropterate synthetase pathway	Haemolytic anaemia exfoliative dermatitis
Clofazimine	Rimino-phenazine dye, bacteriostatic drug, has long half-life of up to 70 days	Mechanism of action unknown	Gastrointestinal symptoms, sometimes serious, pigmentation and dryness of skin are common problems

Management of leprosy

The treatment of leprosy has six main components:

- chemotherapy
- patient education
- management of reactions and neuritis
- prevention of disability
- management of ulcers and
- social and psychological support.

Chemotherapy

All leprosy patients should be given an appropriate multi-drug combination to kill mycobacteria and prevent the emergence of resistant organisms. Multi-drug therapy (MDT) has rifampicin as the key agent, combined with either dapsone alone or dapsone and clofazimine. The characteristics of these drugs are detailed in Table 47.7.

The monthly dose of rifampicin and clofazimine should be supervised by a health worker to make sure the drug is taken.

MDT has been widely implemented, and more than 10 million people have been successfully treated (WHO, 2000). Skin lesions start to improve within weeks of starting MDT, but up to 50 per cent of lesions will not have resolved at the completion of MDT. Patients may not be happy at having their treatment stopped and health workers need to explain that resolution of skin lesions occurs over several years.

Table 47.8 gives the drug doses and duration for MDT. Patients should be warned that rifampicin will turn their urine, sweat and tears pink for 48 hours post-dose. Clofazimine skin pigmentation is troublesome in light coloured skins. Patients can be reassured that the pigmentation will fade after stopping MDT. Other toxic side effects are rare.

Table 47.8. Modified WHO recommended multi-drug therapy regimens

Type of leprosy	Drug treatment: Monthly supervised	Drug treatment: Daily self-administered	Duration of treatment
Paucibacillary	Rifampicin 600 mg	Dapsone 100 mg	6 months
Multibacillary	Rifampicin 600 mg	Clofazimine 50 mg	12 months
	Clofazimine 300 mg	Dapsone 100 mg	
Paucibacillary single lesion	Rifampicin 600 mg, ofloxacin 400 mg, minocycline 100 mg		Single dose

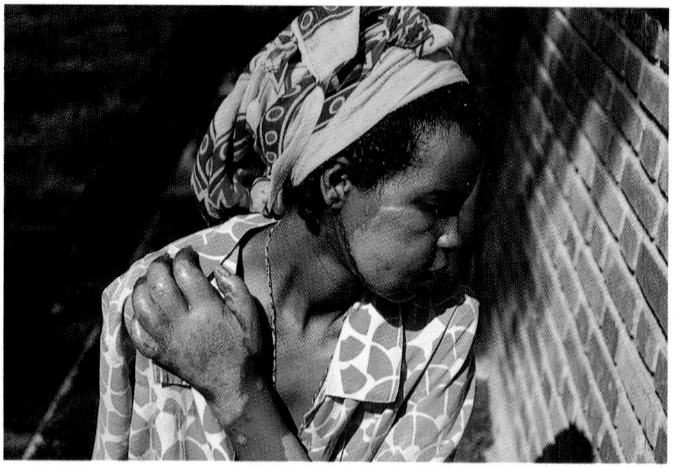

Fig. 47.11. BL leprosy with type 1 reversal reaction. Erythematous plaque on face and hands. This patient delivered 4 months previously, and also had severe neuritis causing clawing of the hand (Martin Dietz).

WHO studies have reported a cumulative relapse rate of 1.1 per cent for paucibacillary leprosy and 0.8 per cent for multibacillary leprosy at 9 years after completion of MDT.

The duration of MDT was recently shortened to 1 year on the recommendation of the WHO expert committee (WHO, 1997). This recommendation was not based on clinical trials, and there are concerns that patients with a high bacterial load are being undertreated. Data from Senegal and India (Jamet et al., 1995; Girdhar et al., 2000) shows that patients with a high initial bacterial load (BL >4+) treated for two years with rifampicin, clofazimine and dapsone have a high relapse rate (in India 8/100 person years with 2 years of MDT) whereas patients treated to smear negativity had a relapse rate of 2/100 person years (Ji, 2001). These patients may form a sub group who need treatment until their skin smears are negative.

Patient education

Many patients are worried and depressed by the diagnosis of leprosy, so it is the duty of the health worker to explain the treatment and the importance of compliance with MDT. Patients with anaesthetic hands and feet need education to prevent injury and disability. Patients need to be warned about reactions that may occur soon after starting treatment.

Most people have erroneous concepts about leprosy, fearing that it is hereditary or due to a divine curse. They can be reassured that within a few days of starting treatment they are non-infectious and will not transmit leprosy by touch, sex or other daily activities. They should also be taught about the early symptoms and signs of reaction so that they can seek medical help promptly.

Leprosy reactions

Type I (reversal reaction)

Clinical features

Reversal reactions are seen in borderline patients, particularly after starting treatment and, in women, after parturition. Reversal reactions may occur before, during or after MDT. In Ethiopia 22 per cent of BL patients develop reversal reactions. The patient with reversal reaction has skin lesion and/or neuritis with little systemic upset. The hands and feet may be severely oedematous.

Skin

The lesions are inflamed. Macular lesions become erythematous plaques (Figs. 47.11, 47.12). This may be difficult to appreciate in dark skin. The lesion will be tender on gentle tapping or it can even be painful. If the reaction is severe, lesions can ulcerate.

Nerves
Nerves are frequently involved in RR. The nerves are enlarged and tender. Loss of function (motor and sensory) occurs. Nerve abscess can occur in severe cases.

Patients may experience more than one reaction and reactions can occcur up to 7 years after stopping MDT.

Management of Type I reaction (reversal reaction)

The management of type 1 reaction requires the use of anti-inflammatory drugs.

General treatment
The patient with reaction needs rest, analgesics and may need admission.

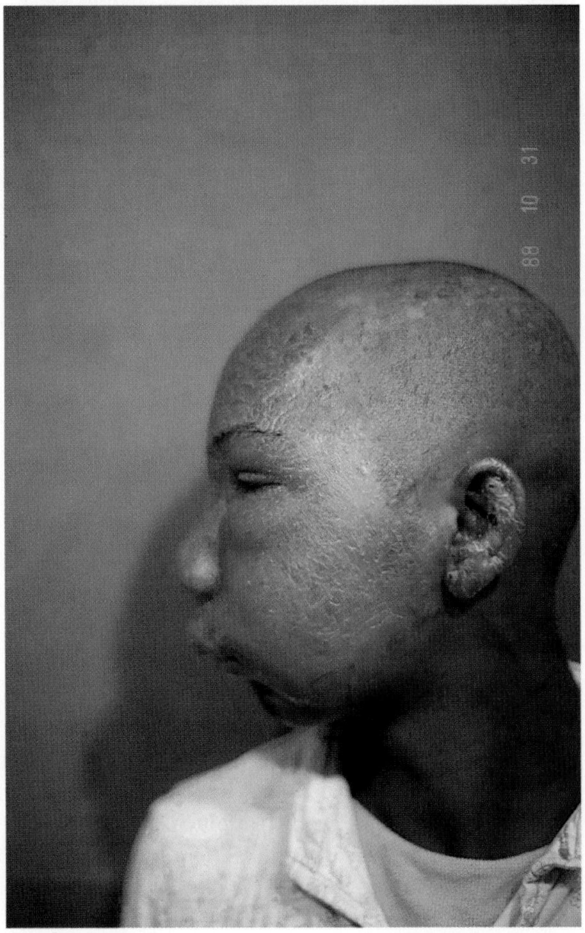

Fig. 47.12. BT leprosy with type 1 reversal reaction. Swollen face with a tender erythematous skin lesion. The ears are similarly affected. An enlarged greater auricular nerve is visible (Martin Dietz.).

Corticosteroids
Corticosteroids are the drug of choice in management of reversal reaction.

The main effect of corticosteroids is to suppress the T-cell driven inflammatory response to *M. leprae* antigen within skin and nerves. Corticosteroids reduce oedema in the skin and nerves and there will be rapid improvement (few days). Prednisolone is widely used with an initial dose of 40 mg in most cases but severe reactions may require 60 mg. The initial dose can be given for the first two weeks and then gradually tapered by 5 mg every 4 weeks depending on the patient's response. Patients are monitored by checking sensory testing and voluntary muscle testing. The total duration of steroid treatment is 6 months though BL patients may require a longer course. In field management the dose of steroid is fixed for easier prescribing by paramedical workers.

New silent neuropathy should be treated in the same way as reversal reactions. The response to steroids depends on the severity of inflammation and the length of time before treatment is started. Other immunosuppressive drugs such as cyclosporin are currently being evaluated for their effectiveness in treating reactions.

Type II (Erythema nodosum leprosum)

ENL occurs in BL and LL patients. The patients may have severe generalized symptoms and signs with severe malaise, pain, headache, anorexia, and high fever. The hands and feet may swell up.

Skin
ENL nodules are seen on the skin. These are multiple dome shaped, tender subcutaneous nodules found particularly on the extremities and face. Crops of nodules occur, new ones appearing as old ones subside. The lesions leave hyperpigmentation when they heal. The nodules can develop into pustules and may ulcerate. ENL can be chronic with nodules persisting for months.

Nerves
Neuritis can occur in ENL but is usually less severe than that seen in RR.

Other organ involvement

Eye
The first sign of ENL may be a red eye. Iritis and episcleritis are common.

Testes

The testes become swollen, tender and painful. This can result in testicular atrophy.

Joints

Can be swollen and tender

Kidney

Proteinurea occurs.

This is a difficult condition to treat and frequently requires treatment with high dose steroids. ENL frequently recurs, sometimes over up to 7 years. This makes it a very difficult condition for both patients and their doctors.

Mild ENL (few erythema nodosum nodules without nerve or other organ involvement) is managed with non-steroidal anti-inflammatory drugs, such as aspirin 400 mg every 6 hours or indomethacin 50 mg 8-hourly

ENL with widespread skin lesions, neuritis, orchitis and iritis should be treated with high dose prednisolone. Prednisolone 40 mg to 60 mg or more is started and tapered down as rapidly as possible. One aims to stop steroid treatment within 2–4 weeks but often this is not possible as lesions flare up when the steroid dose is reduced.

Thalidomide is effective in treating acute and severe recurrent ENL with a rapid response (8–48 hours). The dose is 10 to 15 mg per kg, decreasing to maintenance dose of 100 mg daily (Lockwood & Sinha, 1996). It is very effective for ENL involving skin and the testis, but is not very effective in neuritis. It is teratogenic so it cannot be used in women of childbearing age. Its use is frequently restricted to inpatients only.

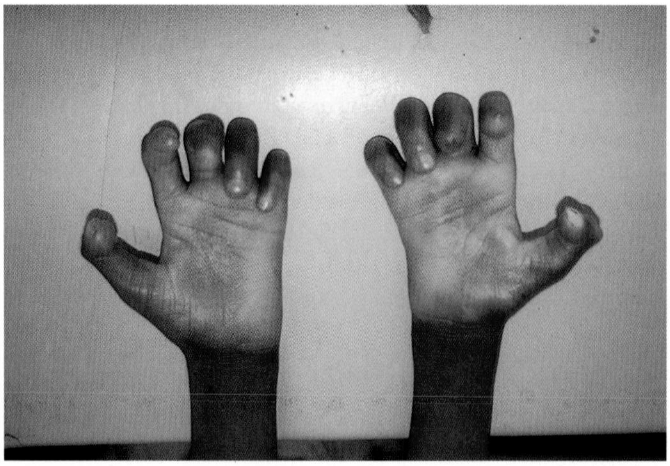

Fig. 47.13. Nerve damage: bilateral ulnar and median nerve damage with wasting of the small muscles of the hand and clawing of the fingers (Diana Lockwood).

Clofazimine

This is helpful in maintenance therapy of ENL when the acute phase has settled. The initial dose given is 300 mg daily which is then reduced by 100 mg every 2 months.

Both reversal reactions and ENL can present after MDT.

Prevention of disability

The aim is:

- to prevent new disabilities or deformities
- to prevent worsening of existing disabilities and deformities.

The patient and the health worker should work together to achieve this goal. At-risk patients (those with disability, MB patients, pregnant women) should be identified and their neurological status recorded with muscle and sensory testing for hands, feet and eyes.

The key points in training patients to prevent disability are shown in the box:

1. Teach patient to recognize early signs of inflammation, loss of sensation and muscle weakness.
2. Protect insensitive hands and feet from injury.
3. Advice on skin care. This includes soaking of hands and feet, oiling and shaving off dry skin.
4. Wear protective footwear and if possible provide proper footwear with soft insole and firm outer sole.
5. Patients are encouraged to do these things on their own (self-care).
6. The training should include monitoring of what the patient is doing (Srinivasan, 1993).

Patients can be encouraged to have self-care groups and to practise what they have been taught with each other.

Management of ulcers

Peripheral nerve damage in leprosy results in loss of sensation and paralysis of nerves (Fig. 47.13). The loss of protective sensation results in injury to hands and feet, since the patient loses sensation such as touch, pain, pressure and temperature. Muscle paralysis alters stress on the hands and feet (Kazen, 1999).

Ulcers occur as a result of:

(i) Repetitive moderate stress. Because of loss of sensation the patient over uses the feet or hands.
(ii) Trauma.
(iii) Pressure causing ischaemia, e.g. from tight shoes.

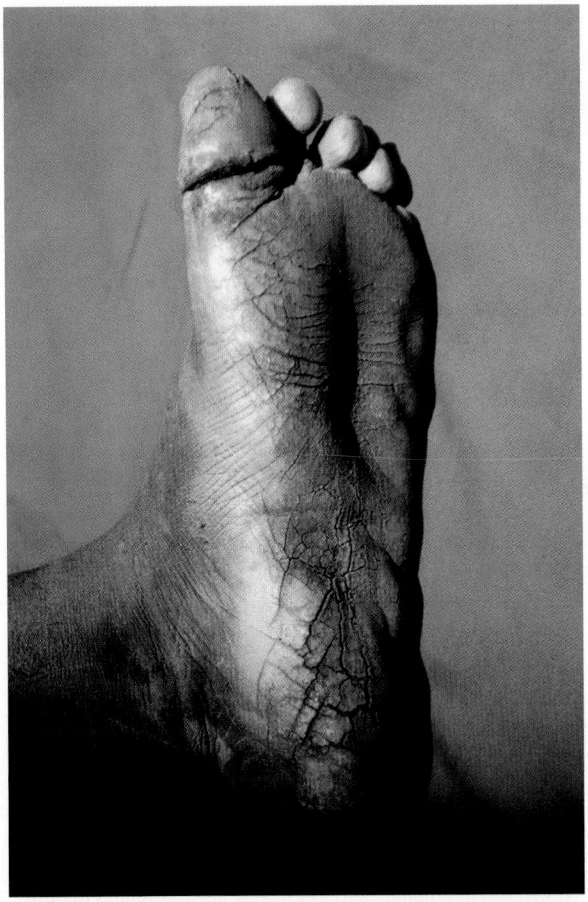

Fig. 47.14. Sole of foot to show fissure, already ulcerated, around base of great toe. Note the cracked skin of the heel, liable to trauma and thus to ulcerate in an anaesthetic foot.

(iv) Burns, especially on hands because of loss of protective sensation.

There are two types of ulcer: superficial (Fig. 47.14), which involves the skin and subcutis, and deep, which can involve bone joints, fascia and tendons. Osteomyelitis may be revealed if a deep ulcer is probed.

The important steps in ulcer management are the following:

(i) Immobilization – the affected part should not be used.
(ii) Surgical – removal of dead tissue by wide excision if the ulcer is deep.
(iii) Plan to avoid subsequent trauma by restoring weight-bearing surface.
(iv) Identify the cause of the ulcer; if the cause is not avoided the ulcer will recur (Kazen, 1999).

The surgical management of ulcer should be undertaken close to the patient's home except when very specialized procedures are needed.

Prevention is the key to a successful ulcer management.

Rehabilitation

The most important objective of treating a leprosy patient is to keep the patient physically and socially active. Many leprosy patients are displaced and are beggars in towns. The health worker should work hard to keep the patient in his own environment. Treatment for leprosy should be available to patients in their own area. For this to take place all levels of health workers should be aware of leprosy, so training is important.

Leprosy and women

Women often have lower social and economic status than men in African communities and are often less educated. They may be less aware of the cause, symptoms, signs and consequences of the disease. They may also be dependent on men to seek medical help. Stigma may be more severe in women than in men (Shale, 2000). Reactions and neuritis may occur in the post-partum period, worsening disability (Lockwood & Sinha, 1999). Health education should focus on women, but the whole community should be aware of these problems since decision making often lies in the hands of men (Shale, 2000).

Vaccination in leprosy

The substantial cross-reactivity between BCG and *M. leprae* has been exploited in attempts to develop a vaccine against leprosy. Trials of BCG as a vaccine against leprosy in Uganda, New Guinea, Burma and South India showed it to confer statistically significant but variable protection, ranging from 80 per cent in Uganda to 20 per cent in Burma. A case control study in Venezuela showed BCG vaccination to give 56 per cent protection to the household contacts of leprosy patients. Combining BCG and killed *M. leprae* has been tried, but in both a large population-based trial in Malawi and an immunoprophylactic trial in Venezuela there was no advantage for BCG plus *M. leprae* over BCG alone.

References

Almedia AM, Roselino AM et al. (1994). Leprosy and HIV infection. *Int J Lep*, **62**: 133–135.

Assefa A, Nash J et al. (2000). Patterns of health seeking behavior amongst leprosy patients in former Shoa province, Ethiopia. *Ethiop J Health Dev*; **14**: 43–47.

Bwire R, Kawuma HJS. (1994). Type one reaction in leprosy, neuritis and steroid therapy: the impact of the human immunodeficiency virus. *Trans Roy Soc Trop Med Hyg*; **88**: 315–316.

Cole ST et al. (2001). Massive gene decay in the leprosy bacillus. *Nature*; **409**: 1007–1011.

Cree IA, Smith WC. (1998). Leprosy transmission and mucosal immunity: toward eradication? *Lepr Rev*; **69**: 112–121.

Gebre S, Saunderson P, Messele T, Byass P. (2000). The effect of HIV status on the clinical picture of leprosy: a prospective study in *Ethiopia. Lepr Rev*; **71**: 338–343.

Girdhar BK, Girdhar A et al. (2000). Relapses in multibacillary leprosy patients: effect of length of therapy. *Lepr Rev*; **71**: 144–153.

Hastings RC. (1985). Microbiology of leprosy. In *Leprosy*, ed. RJW Rees *Med Tropics*; 31–52. Edinburgh: Churchill-Livingstone.

Jamet P, Ji B, Marchoux Chemotherapy Study Group. (1995). Relapse after long-term follow-up of multibacillary patients treated by WHO Multidrug regimen. *Int J Lepr*; **63**: 195–201.

Ji B. (2001). Does there exist a subgroup of MB patients at greater risk of relapse after MDT? *Lepr Rev*; **72**: 3–8.

Kawuma JS, Bwire R, Adatu-Engwau F. (1994). Leprosy and infection with human immunodeficency virus in Uganda; Case-control study. *Int J Lep*; **62**: 521–526.

Kazen R. (1999). Management of plantar ulcer in leprosy. *Lepr Rev*; **70**: 63–69.

Kennedy C et al. (1990). Leprosy and human immunodeficiency virus infection. A closer look at the lesion. *Int J Lep*; **29**: 139–140.

Khanolkar-Young S, Rayment N et al. (1995). Tumour necrosis factor-alpha (TNF-α) synthesis is associated with the skin and peripheral nerve pathology of leprosy reversal reaction. *Clin Exp Immunol*; **99**: 196–202.

Lienhardt C, Kamate B, Jamet P et al. (1996). Effect of HIV infection on leprosy: a three-year survey in Bamako, Mali. *Int J Lep*; **64**: 383–391.

Lockwood D. (1996). The management of erythema nodosum leprosum: current and future options. *Lepr Rev*; **67**:253–259.

Lockwood DN, Sinha HH. (1999). Pregnancy and leprosy: a comprehensive literature review. *Int J Lepr Other Mycobact Dis*; **67**: 6–12.

Lucas S. (1993). Human immunodeficiency virus and leprosy. *Lepr Rev*; **64**: 97–103.

Naafs B. (1996). Treatment of reactions and nerve damage. *Int. Lepr*; **64**: s21–s28.

Pönnighaus JM, Fine PEM et al. (1994). Incidence rate of leprosy in Karonga district, Northern Malawi: Patterns by age, sex, BCG status and classification. *Int J Lep*; **62**: 345–352.

Pönnighaus JM, Fine PEM et al. (1994). Extended schooling and good housing conditions are associated with reduced risk of leprosy in rural Malawi. *Int J Lep*; **62**: 345–352.

Ridley D S. (1988). The leprosy bacillus. In *Pathogenesis of Leprosy and Related Diseases*, ed PP Wright pp. 39–42,45–60.

Rijk AJ, Shibru Gebre, Byass P, Birhanu T. (1994). Field evaluation of WHO-MDT of fixed duration at ALERT, Ethiopia: the AMFES project-I. MDT course completion, case-holding and another score of disability grading. *Lepr Rev*; **65**: 305–319.

Saunderson P, Gronen G. (2000). Which physical signs help most in diagnosis of leprosy? A proposal based on experience in the AMFES project, ALERT, Ethiopia. *Lepr Rev*; **71**: 285–308.

Saunderson P, Gebre S, Byass P. (2000a). The pattern of leprosy related neuropathy in the AMFES patients in Ethiopia: incidence and risk factors and outcome. *Lepr Rev*; **71**: 285–308.

Saunderson P, Gebre S, Byass P. (2000b). Reversal reaction in the skin lesions of AMFES patients: incidence and risk factors. *Lepr Rev*; **71**: 309–317.

Saunderson P, Gebre S, Byass P. (2000c). ENL reactions in the multibacillary cases of the AMFES cohort in central Ethiopia: Incidence and risk factors. *Lepr Rev*; **71**: 318–324.

Shale M. (2000). Women with leprosy a women with leprosy is in double jeopardy. *Lepr Rev*; **71**: 5–17.

Srinivasan H. (1993). *Prevention of Disabilities in Patients with Leprosy. A Practical Guide.* Geneva: WHO.

Thappa DM, Rao MV, Gharami R. (1996). Impact of HIV infection on leprosy. *Ind J Lepr*; **68**: 255–256.

Turk JL, Rees RJW. (1988). AIDS and leprosy. *Lepr Rev*; **59**: 193–194.

Turk JL, Curtis J, Blaquiere G. (1993). Immunopathology of nerve involvement in leprosy. *Lepr Rev*; **64**: 1–6.

Weg NVG, Post EB et al. (1998). Explanatory models and help-seeking behavior of leprosy patients in Adamawa state, Nigeria. *Lep Rev*; **69**: 382–389.

World Health Organization. (1997a). Global case detection trend in leprosy. *Wkly Epidemiol Rec*; **24**: 165–172.

World Health Organization. (1997b). Leprosy elimination campaigns – reaching every patient in every village. *Wkly Epidemiol Rec*; **72**: 165–172.

World Health Organization. (1997). Shortening duration of treatment of multibacillary leprosy. *Wkly Epidemiol Rec*; **72**: 125–128.

World Health Organization. (2000). Leprosy – Global situation. *Wkly Epidemiol Rec*; **28**: 226–231.

Yamamura M, Wang XH et al. (1992). Cytokine patterns of immunologically mediated tissue damage. *J Immunol*; **149**: 1470–1475.

Cholera

48

The problem in Africa

Cholera, caused by *Vibrio cholerae*, is an ancient disease with its traditional 'heartland' in the Ganges delta on the Indian subcontinent, where it was described as early as the fifteenth century. There are reports of a cholera-like illness in Africa in the seventeenth century.

Six pandemics of classical cholera occurred from 1817 until 1960, affecting Asia, the Middle East, Europe and the Americas. The emergence of the new 'El Tor' biotype in Indonesia in 1961 led to the present seventh pandemic of cholera, which spread world-wide and arrived in Africa in 1970. Cholera has since been epidemic throughout Africa and endemic in some areas. Larger outbreaks have often been related to war, the displacement and migration of peoples, refugee camps, famine, and flooding. 120 000–150 000 cases of cholera are reported annually, of which 80 per cent are from Africa. The overall case-fatality rate remains disappointingly high (4–5%), and very high case-fatality rates (20%) have also been reported from Africa (Anonymous, 1998).

The organism

Vibrio cholerae is a small, comma-shaped, motile gram-negative bacillus. It grows best in alkaline media, in the presence of bile salts, and at 30–40 °C. It is killed above 50 °C. It grows well in saline conditions, and survives for months in sea water and for weeks if frozen. A high infecting dose of 10^8 organisms is required to cause disease. Individuals with achlorhydria are more susceptible to cholera.

Two biotypes of *V. cholerae* are described. The more recent 'El Tor' differs from 'classical' in being haemolytic, and resistant to polymyxin B. It persists longer in the environment than classical cholera, and a greater proportion of those infected are asymptomatic, which may be why it has replaced the classical biotype in most parts of the world.

Both classical and El Tor *V. cholerae* are divided into three serotypes (Ogawa, Inaba, Hikojima) by antisera to the O antigen. *V. cholerae* that do not react with the O antisera are referred to as 'non-O1', and do not usually cause epidemic diarrhoea. A new and important exception to this rule is the O139 'Bengal' strain of *V. cholerae*, which is genetically related to El Tor, but does not react with standard O antisera. *V. cholerae* O139 emerged in 1992 in Bangladesh, causes severe epidemic diarrhoea, and has spread within Asia. The *V. cholerae* genome has recently been completely sequenced.

Cholera toxin

The clinical features of cholera are caused by a chromosomally encoded heat-labile protein enterotoxin, which is secreted following colonization of the small bowel by *V. cholerae*. It is composed of five identical 'B' 11.5 kDa protein subunits arranged circularly around the enzymatically active 'A' subunit, which can be separated into two proteins (A_1 22 kDa, A_2 5 kDa). The B sub-unit binds specifically to the lipid GM1 ganglioside receptor on enterocytes, and the A_1 sub-unit activates adenylate cyclase, increasing intracellular cAMP. This inhibits absorption and stimulates secretion of large amounts of sodium chloride and bicarbonate, resulting in copious secretory diarrhoea, which is isotonic and has a low protein content (see Chapter 20).

Epidemiology

Cholera is a water-borne disease, and is usually transmitted by contaminated drinking water. Immediate household

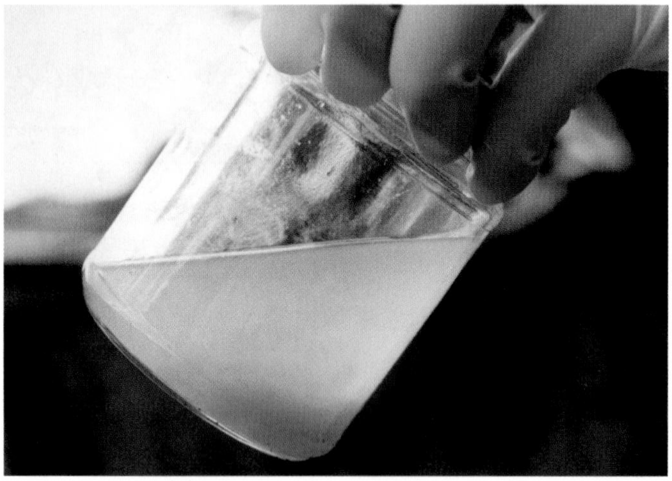

Fig. 48.1. Rice-water stool in cholera. Note the watery nature, and the presence of white/yellow sediment.

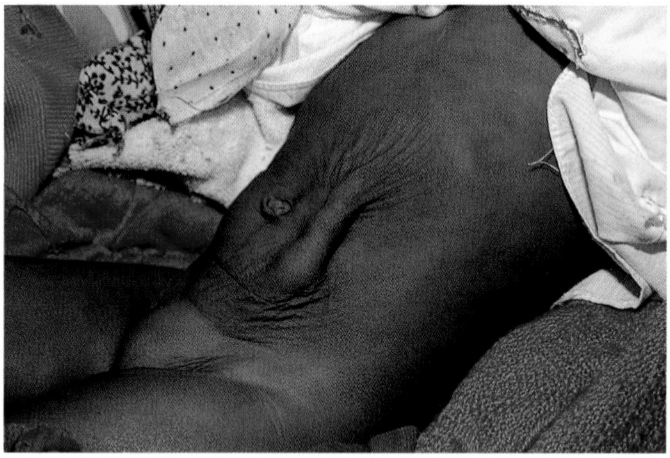

Fig. 48.2. Severe dehydration in cholera shown by skin folds on abdominal wall associated with decreased skin turgor.

contacts of cases are at greatest risk of cholera. During an El Tor outbreak there are many sub-clinically infected people, and social activities involving travel and gatherings, particularly funerals during an outbreak, may be an important factor facilitating the spread of cholera.

In endemic areas there is acquired immunity among adults, and most cases occur in children under 10 years. In Africa, however, cholera is mainly epidemic, and all ages are affected. Cholera is seen in children under 2, but is rare in neonates. There is presently no evidence that it is commoner or more severe in HIV-infected patients.

The reservoir for cholera between epidemics is not clear, but may be in an ecological niche involving surface water, or in the rare long-term human carriers. There are no known animal hosts or vectors for cholera.

Clinical features

The stool

Cholera usually presents with the sudden onset of painless, profuse diarrhoea which becomes progressively less faecal and more watery until it resembles 'rice water', being nearly clear with a white or yellow cloudy sediment (see Fig. 48.1). The patient passes large and frequent volumes of this watery stool, which has very little odour.

Shock and dehydration

Although many cases have a moderate, mild or subclinical illness, the disease can progress to death within hours, and extreme dehydration and hypovolaemic shock occur with frightening rapidity. The patient is hypotensive, with low volume or impalpable peripheral pulses, and in severe cases virtually inaudible heart sounds. A dramatic loss of skin turgor causes sunken eyes, shrivelled 'washerwoman's hands', and a dough-like consistency of the abdomen (Fig. 48.2).

Abdominal features

Vomiting is often present from early in the illness, contributing to fluid and electrolyte losses, and if severe makes oral rehydration difficult or impossible. Ileus is common, is related to electrolyte imbalance, and resolves with successful intravenous rehydration and electrolyte repletion. Occasionally, patients present with ileus at the outset, so that small bowel secretions are pooled and rapid collapse may occur with little or no diarrhoea. This is called 'cholera sicca', and is a dangerous presentation because the volume of fluid lost may be greatly underestimated.

Abdominal pain is not usually present early on, but may develop after some hours, and is sometimes severe. The abdomen is not usually tender. Anuria may occur and urine output should be carefully monitored.

General features

The patient may become mentally 'detached' and unresponsive, but is rarely truly unconscious. The core rectal temperature may be raised, but the peripheries remain cold and clammy. After 2–3 days or during recovery, a late febrile state known as 'cholera typhoid' has been described.

Hypoglycaemia

The most important, reversible biochemical complication of cholera is hypoglycaemia, and loss of consciousness or fits should be assumed to be due to this complication and treated presumptively if glucose measurement is not possible.

Give an immediate bolus of glucose (10 ml of 50% dextrose), followed by the addition of glucose to intravenous fluids.

Electrolyte imbalance and renal function

Electrolyte imbalances and acidosis may also present with altered consciousness or fits. Most cholera outbreaks are successfully managed in situations where it is not possible to measure electrolytes, and hypokalaemia, hyponatraemia or hypernatraemia are gradually reversed with oral replacement fluid or intravenous fluid replacement. Hyperkalaemia is rare even in the presence of anuria. Marked uraemia is common, and may be aggravated by inappropriate use of drugs before rehydration. It is often reversible without dialysis.

Complications

Complications include abortion in pregnant women, aspiration pneumonia as a result of prolonged vomiting, cholecystitis, and stroke or myocardial infarction secondary to critical hypoperfusion in patients with vascular disease.

Diagnosis

Clinical diagnosis

The diagnosis of cholera is clinical, and can be made equally effectively at all levels of heath care. Start treatment immediately, and prepare to manage an outbreak.

Laboratory diagnosis

Laboratory identification is helpful to confirm an outbreak for surveillance and epidemiological purposes, and to provide information about antibiotic sensitivity. Laboratory diagnosis is by identification of motile vibrios in a stool preparation on dark field or phase microscopy, which are immobilised using specific multivalent antisera (Benenson et al., 1964). A slide agglutination method can be used for rapid provisional diagnosis in the field. The O139 Bengal strain is not agglutinated by standard antisera. *V. cholerae* can be grown from stool or rectal swab, may be transported in Cary Blair or TTP media, and grown on several media including MacConkey's and TCBS.

Treatment

The three important elements of cholera treatment are:

- Immediate rehydration
- Maintenance fluids
- Antibiotic treatment.

Rehydration

Prompt and adequate rehydration is crucial to successful treatment of cholera, and should never be delayed.

Oral Replacement Therapy (ORT) (see Chapter 20)
Mild and moderate cases can be rehydrated orally. Use an ORT with a high sodium content (WHO formula). In order to ensure compliance, it must be emphasized that ORT is highly effective in rehydration, but does NOT reduce the volume or duration of diarrhoea. Some newer cereal-based low-osmolarity ORT formulations shorten diarrhoea by 30–50 per cent (Pizarro et al., 1991). If home-made ORT/SSS is used, the addition of fruit juice, coconut milk or bananas to the regimen will replace potassium losses. During an outbreak, water used to reconstitute ORT should be adequately treated or sterilized (see below).

Intravenous fluids
If dehydration is severe (over 5%), if stool output is more than 10 per cent of body weight in 24 hours, or if vomiting, ileus or reduced consciousness prevent oral rehydration, parenteral fluids (Ringer's lactate) should be used. Initial rehydration should be immediate, and completed within the first 1–2 hours.

Venous access in severe cases

Venous access is often difficult in the most severe cases. Sometimes the dehydrated patient's blood is so viscous, and the blood volume so low, that when a needle is introduced into a vein, little or no blood appears.

Be persistent and do not give up – rehydration can be successful even if pulses are very weak, heart sounds inaudible, and the patient appears near-terminal. An initial temporary line is needed to quickly administer the first 1–2 litres of fluid. Sterilize the skin, and insert the cannula in either:

(i) the femoral vein (just medial to the femoral arterial pulse)
(ii) the external jugular vein (prop the foot of the bed, or place the patient on a slope, with the head slightly down).

After the first few litres have been given, a more stable peripheral site (e.g. antecubital fossa) can usually be secured. Internal jugular access is effective, but is often dangerously time-consuming and has too great a risk of complications to be used in the field.

Maintenance fluids

Maintenance fluid requirement may be substantial while diarrhoea continues, and can be met using intravenous fluids, ORT or a combination. The maintenance requirement is ideally assessed using a 'cholera cot' which allows faecal losses to be collected and measured before being safely disposed of. The volume lost in each 24 hours should be replaced with the addition of 500 ml in each 24-hour period. Maintenance requirements can also be successfully estimated and titrated against the clinical state of hydration and the urine output, if cholera cots are not available.

Antibiotic treatment

Antibiotics are useful in cholera, as they shorten the duration of diarrhoea, which reduces the requirement for intravenous fluids, and shorten the excretion of *vibrios* in the stool which helps to prevent spread.

Antibiotics are usually given orally after initial rehydration, when the patient is no longer vomiting. They are *not* part of the emergency treatment of cholera.

Choice of antibiotic will depend on local sensitivity. There is most experience with tetracycline (Greenough et al., 1964). The dose of tetracycline is 500 mg four times daily by mouth for 3 days. There is increasing resistance to tetracycline and other effective regimens include: chloramphenicol 500 mg q.i.d., orally or i.v., for 3 days; cotrimoxazole 2 tablets b.i.d. for 4 days; doxycycline 300 mg as a single oral dose (Alam et al., 1990); erythromycin 500 mg t.i.d. for 3 days. Fluoroquinolones (given for 3 days) are also highly effective.

Mortality

The mortality from cholera in the early twentieth century was 50–70 per cent. With the use of ORT, the mortality of a well-managed outbreak should now be less than 1 per cent in adults, but slightly higher in children. The overall case-fatality rate reported from Africa over the last decade has been 4–5 per cent.

Management of a cholera outbreak

During an outbreak, the priorities are to manage the logistics of mass treatment in the community and in treatment centres, and to prevent the further spread of cholera. No disease is a better example of a team effort than cholera. The most junior health worker, or even previously untrained volunteers can be trained to monitor intravenous fluids, measure fluid losses and give ORT.

Community

Local health workers should urgently educate the local community in how to mix and give clean ORT, and in the importance of handwashing and simple hygiene. The use of soap in households has repeatedly been shown to be important (Peterson et al., 1998). Radio may be an effective medium for these messages.

Sterilizing water for ORT by boiling is effective, but it uses precious costly fuel. Simple acidifying agents such as lime juice in food and water ('a lime in a litre') may help sterility (Rowe et al., 1998; Rodrigues et al., 1997). Sunlight sterilization of water (Jorgensen & Nohr, 1995), and bleach treatment (Daniels et al., 1999) are also effective.

Water sources should be examined, and wells in affected areas may be treated with chlorination (1–2 parts in 5 million) or potassium permanganate (1:500 000). Funerals of people dying of the disease have been linked to the further spread of cholera, both because handling of the body may be followed by food preparation, and because of travel into surrounding areas by the family and guests (Gunnlaugsson et al., 1998). It is advisable that relatives do not handle the body, that the body be disinfected, or that burial is supervised and takes place in a designated area. Meals at funerals should also be discouraged. This is not easy to enforce in some cultures, and requires education and co-operation.

Treatment centres

Establish treatment centres with 24-hour staffing where access by severely ill patients is realistic. Infected patients should not travel long distances to find treatment, because this will disseminate cholera and delay treatment. Large volumes of rehydration fluids, cannulae, tubing, and temporary beds or cots will be required.

Protection of staff and carers

Contamination of the treatment centre can be minimized, and staff can be protected by prominent handwashing facilities including dipping hands in disinfectant, and by sterilization of all stool, vomitus, contaminated sheets and other clinical material by chlorination in clearly labelled large vats, before they are handled or disposed of.

Antibiotic treatment of cases will decrease environmental contamination and reduce the risk for household contacts. Prophylactic antibiotic treatment of close contacts may be useful in crowded or endemic situations (De et al., 1976), but mass chemotherapy is not effective. Vaccination has no role in an acute outbreak.

Prevention of cholera

The long-term control of cholera, as of other diarrhoeal diseases, depends on the supply of clean safe water, and provision of adequate sewage and surface water drainage, particularly in areas of crowded, poor or temporary housing. Surveillance and prompt reporting will help to anticipate and contain an outbreak, and allow adequate planning for treatment measures. Present vaccines are relatively ineffective with short-lived protection, do not prevent the spread of disease, and are not cost effective in Africa. Newer genetically modified live oral vaccines are under development and show promise.

References

Alam AM, Alam NH, Sack DA. (1990). Randomised double blind trial of single dose doxycycline for treating cholera in adults. *Br Med J*; **300**: 1619.

Benenson AS, Islam MR, Greenough WBI. (1964). Rapid identification of Vibrio cholerae by darkfield microscopy. *Bull Wld Hlth Org*; **30**: 827.

Daniels NA, Simons SL, Rodrigues A et al. (1999). First do no harm: making oral rehydration solution safer in a cholera epidemic. *Am J Trop Med Hyg*; **60**: 1051–1055.

De S, Chaudhuri A, Dutta P. (1976). *Bull Wld Hlth Org*; **54**: 177.

Greenough WBI, Rosenberg IS, Gordon RS. (1964). Tetracycline in the treatment of cholera. *Lancet*; **1**: 355.

Gunnlaugsson G, Einarsdottir J, Angulo FJ et al. (1998). Funerals during the 1994 cholera epidemic in Guinea-Bissau, West Africa: the need for disinfection of bodies of persons dying of cholera. *Epidemiol Infect*; **120**: 7–15.

Jorgensen AJ, Nohr K. (1995). Cholera: water pasteurization using solar energy. *Trop Doct*; **25**: 175.

Peterson EA, Roberts L, Toole MJ, Peterson DE. (1998). The effect of soap distribution on diarrhoea: Nyamithuthu Refugee Camp. *Int J Epidemiol*; **27**: 520–524.

Pizarro D, Posada G, Sandi L, Moran JR. (1991). Rice-based oral electrolyte solutions for the management of infantile diarrhoea. *N Engl J Med*; **324**: 517.

Rodrigues A, Brun H, Sandstrom A. (1997). Risk factors for cholera infection in the initial phase of an epidemic in Guinea-Bissau: protection by lime juice. *Am J Trop Med Hyg*; **57**: 601–604.

Rowe AK, Angulo FJ, Tauxe RV. (1998). A lime in a litre rapidly kills toxogenic *Vibrio cholerae* O1. *Trop Doct*; **28**: 247–248.

WHO (1998). Cholera in 1997. *Wkly Epidemiol Rec*; **73**: 201–208.

49 Typhoid and other salmonella infections

The problem in Africa

Salmonella infections are common everywhere in Africa. The WHO estimates that 12.5 million cases of typhoid fever occur annually world-wide. Most cases are in Asia, but typhoid remains endemic in much of Africa, and epidemics are also reported. Whenever an African patient has few signs, yet is ill with a fever, typhoid is high on the list of differential diagnoses.

Invasive non-typhoid salmonella (NTS) infections, a long-standing cause of illness and death in African infants and children, have increased dramatically among both adults and children as a result of the HIV epidemic. Salmonellae are isolated from the blood of hospital patients in Africa more commonly than any other organism, with the possible exception of *Strep. pneumoniae.*

The organism

Salmonellae are gram-negative, motile, facultatively anaerobic bacilli, which produce acid on glucose fermentation, reduce nitrates and do not ferment lactose. They can be grown on selective media such as MacConkey, salmonella–Shigella or Brilliant Green.

Under the new classification, the species *Salmonella enterica* covers all medically important salmonellae. Agglutination of O (somatic) antigens with specific antisera is used to define salmonella serogroups A to E, and more extensive agglutination reactions of both O and H (flagellar) antigens can be used to classify salmonellae into over 2000 serotypes (e.g. typhi, typhimurium, enteritidis). *S. typhi* and *S. paratyphi* C also carry abundant Vi antigen, a polymer of *N*-acetylgalactosaminouronic acid. Salmonellae can be further distinguished within serotypes by pulsed field gel electrophoresis, bacteriophage and plasmid typing for epidemiological purposes.

Epidemiology

Salmonellae have a world-wide distribution, and affect many vertebrates including mammals, reptiles and birds. Different serotypes show different degrees of host restriction, and cause a variety of clinical syndromes in humans.

(i) The **'typhoid'** serotypes (*S. typhi, S. paratyphi*), only infect humans, and cause typhoid fever, a distinctive severe systemic disease.
(ii) The **'non-typhoid'** salmonella serotypes (NTS), such as *S. typhimurium* and *S. enteritidis*, typically have a broad vertebrate host range, and cause a variety of clinical syndromes in humans. These include diarrhoea, bacteraemia, and metastatic infection of bone, joints and other organs. The clinical features of these two groupings will be considered separately below.

TYPHOID FEVER

Epidemiology

Typhoid fever (also called 'enteric fever') is a major health problem in Africa, SE Asia, the Indian subcontinent, and South America. It is caused most commonly by *S. typhi;* infections with *S. paratyphi* A, B and C are less common and cause milder disease.

The peak age incidence is 10–25 years. The infection is transmitted from a case or a convalescent or asymptomatic carrier, usually by ingestion of food or drink contaminated with excreta. There is often a seasonal pattern in endemic areas, with transmission starting at the end of the dry season when water is sparse and sanitation may be poor, and continuing into the rains, when infected water may be easily dispersed. A relatively high inoculum (10^5 organisms or more) is needed to overcome the barrier imposed by low gastric pH, at least in immunocompetent subjects. If gastric acid is reduced, for example by smoking cannabis, a lower infecting dose is required.

Schistosomiasis

Patients with schistosomiasis can develop persistent systemic typhoid fever which will not respond to antibiotics until the schistosomiasis has also been treated. This is because the salmonella bacterium uses the tegument or cuticle of the adult helminth as a 'sanctuary site'. In addition, patients with urinary schistosomiasis can become chronic asymptomatic urinary carriers of *S. typhi*.

Sickle cell homozygotes

These patients are at risk of chronic salmonella osteomyelitis

Drug resistance

Mortality is higher in multi-drug resistant outbreaks.

HIV/AIDS

There is presently little information to suggest that HIV/AIDS causes an increased susceptibility to typhoid fever, but some reports show increased mortality from typhoid fever in those with AIDS.

Pathogenesis (see Fig. 49.1)

Following oral ingestion, salmonellae must survive the acidic barrier in the stomach and then colonize the small intestine. This primary phase of small bowel infection is rapid and causes no more than a mild transient enterocolitis in a few cases. After invading and crossing the gut epithelial cells, the bacteria are taken up by phagocytic mononuclear cells which lie on the basal surface of the gut epithelium, and are transported to the Peyer's patches and other local mucosa-associated lymphoid tissue (MALT) of the small bowel.

The infection disseminates from the small bowel, via the lymphatics, to the blood and reticuloendothelial system including the bone marrow, spleen and liver, where a chronic infection is established. Salmonellae survive well inside macrophages in vitro, and probably also 'hide' intracellularly in tissue macrophages in these organs. During the bacteraemic phase, organisms are also seeded to other sites, especially damaged or abnormal tissue in the renal tract, endothelium, bone and joints, where metastatic infections may arise.

Organisms reach and persist in the gall bladder and re-enter the gut in bile, setting up a later secondary small bowel infection. Unlike the mild primary infection, this causes severe Peyer's patch inflammation, which is the basis of the abdominal symptoms and late complications that occur in some cases of typhoid fever.

Clinical features

The incubation period ranges from 5 to 21 days, depending on age, immune status, gastric acidity and infecting dose. The patient occasionally describes transient mild diarrhoea, corresponding to the primary phase of bowel colonization. This resolves, but is followed by a week of rising fever with bacteraemia, as systemic and secondary small bowel infections are established. The patient usually presents at this stage.

Fever is almost always present, and usually high (38.5–40 °C). Most patients complain of a headache, and many of cough and abdominal pain or discomfort. Some complain of constipation or diarrhoea. Listlessness and apathy in a febrile patient suggest typhoid.

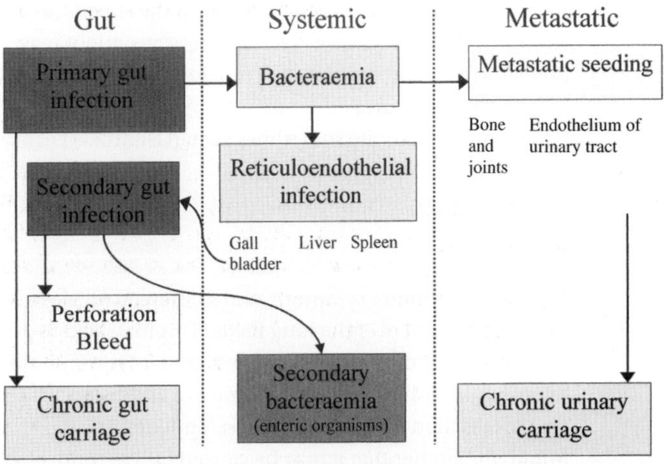

Fig. 49.1. Scheme to illustrate the pathogenesis of typhoid fever.

Cardiovascular features

A lower pulse is sometimes seen than would be expected with a high fever. This 'relative bradycardia' is not diagnostically reliable as it occurs in less than 50 per cent of cases of typhoid. If the patient has tachycardia over 120 bpm and a low blood pressure, look for signs of perforation or bleeding from the gut, secondary bacterial sepsis, or rarely acute myocarditis. Acute myocarditis is seen in 1 per cent of cases, and the features are tachycardia, a gallop rhythm, an enlarged heart and sometimes heart failure and pulmonary oedema.

The abdomen

Patients often present with little or no apparent gastrointestinal involvement. Diarrhoea and vomiting may be present, especially in children, while constipation is seen in approximately 30 per cent of adult cases.

Abdominal distension with ileus is common as typhoid progresses, and the abdomen becomes tender to deep palpation. Peritonism is found following perforation, and another pointer to this may be a rising pulse, and high white cell count.

Splenomegaly is found in 30–70 per cent of cases, and hepatomegaly, which may be tender, in 40 per cent. Jaundice, secondary to hepatic inflammation and congestion, is less common. Pain and tenderness may localize to the right upper quadrant in the rare complication of cholangitis.

Neuropsychiatric

Headache is very common, and other neuropsychiatric features occur in 5–15 per cent of cases. These may include confusion, agitation, 'picking' at the sheets, posturing, or florid psychosis. Alternatively, the patient may appear listless and depressed. A proximal myopathy, poly- or mono-neuropathy, and extrapyramidal Parkinsonian signs are sometimes seen (Osuntokun et al., 1972).

Respiratory

Cough is a common symptom, and scattered crackles are frequently heard over the lung fields. This may lead to a mistaken diagnosis of primary pneumonia. True typhoid pneumonia with consolidation is rare in adults, occurring in less than 3 per cent of cases; if pneumonia is found, remember that it may be caused by a second pathogen.

Renal

Proteinuria is found in up to 50 per cent of cases. Renal failure may occur, caused by an acute reversible nephritic syndrome, especially in those with associated schistosomiasis. Nephrotic syndrome is also a rare complication of typhoid fever. Haemolysis in G6PD deficient patients may cause renal failure.

Skin and muculoskeletal

So-called 'rose spots' appear reddish-maroon in dark skin. They are transient and maculopapular, blanch on pressure, and are seen in 10–20 per cent of cases at most. Joint pains or myalgia are reported in 15 per cent of uncomplicated cases. Remember also the risk of bone infarction and osteomyelitis in patients with sickle-cell disease.

Diagnosis

The initial diagnosis is made on clinical grounds. At rural or district centres where culture facilities are not available, an improvement following a trial of treatment (see below) is the best diagnostic test.

A definitive diagnosis is made by isolating *S. typhi* or *S. paratyphi* from appropriate clinical specimens. Bone marrow, blood and intestinal secretions have the highest yield. Blood culture alone has about 70 per cent sensitivity in the early stages, but becomes less sensitive after the second week as bacteraemia subsides. Separation of the mononuclear fraction of blood by centrifugation for culture improves the speed of diagnosis but not the sensitivity (Rubin et al., 1990). Bone marrow culture has 90 per cent sensitivity, even if there has been prior antibiotic use, but the procedure is relatively invasive and inconvenient. Intestinal secretions can be cultured non-invasively using a 'hairy string' capsule to sample duodenal secretions. The use of blood culture combined with hairy string culture can give a yield close to that of bone marrow culture. Stool culture may be positive in weeks 2 and 3, but is not diagnostic in an endemic area, since asymptomatic carriage is common. Urine cultures are positive in a minority of cases (Fig. 49.2).

The Widal test detects agglutinating antibodies against the O and H antigens. These start to rise after 2 weeks. Only a pair of acute and convalescent samples showing a four-fold rise in antibodies is significant. Since a single high titre value is of no value for diagnosis in an endemic area, the Widal test cannot be used for diagnosis at presentation.

Other investigations

Full blood count may show anaemia and thrombocytopenia. The white cell count is usually low but may be raised in early presentation or following complications. Elevated liver and muscle enzymes are common, as is mild proteinuria, but renal function is rarely impaired. Chest X-ray is not always necessary and is usually normal, but rarely shows signs of myocarditis or pneumonia. Free gas will be seen under the diaphragm on an erect CXR if there has been perforation.

CSF is usually normal despite the high frequency of neuropsychiatric symptoms. Encephalitis with pleocytosis is occasionally seen, and typhoid meningitis with neutrophils in the CSF is even more rare. If the CSF is abnormal, carefully consider the possibility of a different or an additional diagnosis.

Complications

Small bowel complications

The secondary small bowel infection by *S. typhi* causes intense local inflammation, and 'microperforation' can lead to late, secondary bacteraemia and peritonitis caused by 'leaking' of other enteric flora. The patient deteriorates, with recurrence of fever and abdominal pain, and this should be a signal to broaden antibiotic cover. As Peyer's patch infection becomes established, ulceration and necrosis lead to the complications of profuse ileocaecal bleeding or perforation in 3–10 per cent of hospitalized cases. Prompt surgery (segmental bowel resection) after rapid resuscitation of the patient is life-saving.

Other complications

Rarer complications include splenic or liver abscess, cholangitis, pneumonia, pancreatitis, endocarditis, pericarditis, myocarditis,and orchitis. The classical description of a 'third week of complications' is now often modified in timing and presentation by early administration of antibiotics.

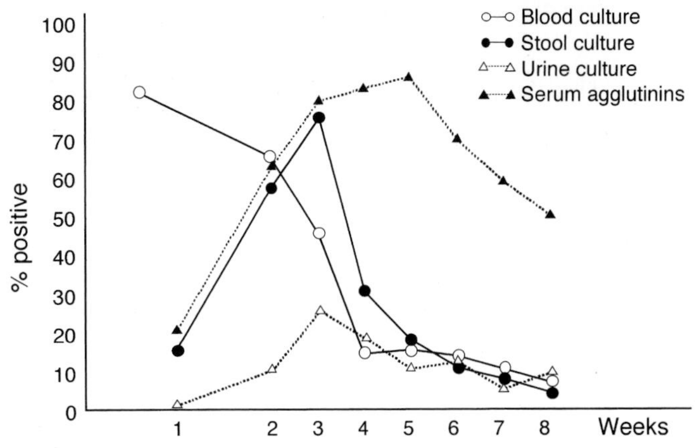

Fig. 49.2. Presence of *S. typhi* in blood, urine, and stool, and rise of antibodies after ingestion of the organism.

Chronic carriage

One to six per cent of cases develop asymptomatic chronic carriage of *S. typhi*, defined as positive stool or urine cultures for more than a year. The stool and urine may be negative immediately after treatment, but become positive at follow-up after some weeks. Biliary abnormalities such as gallstones and urinary abnormalities such *Schistosoma haematobium* or renal stones are risk factors for developing the carrier state. Chronic carriers have high titres of antibodies to the Vi antigen, and this can help to distinguish carriage from acute disease. The main importance of chronic carriage is that it permits the spread of typhoid within a community, particularly if the patient handles or prepares food, or lives in crowded conditions with poor water supply and sanitation.

Mortality of typhoid fever

Mortality from typhoid fever in the pre-antibiotic era was 15–20 per cent, attributable to overwhelming sepsis and complications. Treated promptly, mortality can now be as low as 1–3 per cent, but remains higher in some parts of Africa, and in susceptible patients (see above). Symptomatic relapse may occur in 10–25 per cent of immunologically competent subjects after apparently successful treatment with chloramphenicol, and re-treatment with the same agent is usually successful. The effect of HIV/AIDS on the relapse rate of typhoid fever is unknown.

Treatment of typhoid fever

Chloramphenicol

Chloramphenicol has been used since 1948, and remains effective, available and affordable treatment for typhoid fever in most of Africa. It produces a clinical response within 2–3 days, reduces the duration of fever to 3–6 days, and reduces mortality to as low as 1 per cent if given early.

The dose of chloramphenicol is 500 mg four times daily for 14 days, by mouth. In severe cases, a higher initial dose of 750 mg q.i.d. can be used until the temperature comes down, after which 500 mg q.i.d. can be used for the remainder of the 14-day course. The total dose should not exceed 42 g.

Bioavailability of chloramphenicol is greatest, and serum concentration is highest following oral administration. Give chloramphenicol intravenously only if there is vomiting or reduced consciousness. The intramuscular route should not be used. A longer treatment course does not prevent complications or chronic carriage, but a shorter course leads to more frequent relapses.

Other antibiotics

Amoxicillin and co-trimoxazole are alternatives to chloramphenicol, and have approximately equal efficacy. The dose of amoxycillin is 1 g four times daily for 14 days, and of co-trimoxazole is 2 tablets (equivalent to trimethoprim 160 mg, sulphamethoxazole 800 mg) twice daily for 14 days.

Multi-drug resistance

Plasmid-borne resistance to chloramphenicol, ampicillin and co-trimoxazole, known as multi-drug resistance (MDR) is now widespread in parts of Asia. It is not yet common in Africa, but has been reported in South Africa and Egypt (Rowe et al., 1997). Where there is MDR typhoid, the most useful drugs are quinolones (ciprofloxacin, ofloxacin). They produce a rapid clinical response, have high efficacy in infections with MDR strains of S. typhi, and result in low relapse and carriage rates, as they are bactericidal and concentrated intracellularly and in the bile.

MDR typhoid will present a problem if it occurs at health centres and district hospitals where these drugs are not available, and full doses of chloramphenicol must therefore continue to be used in these settings.

If MDR typhoid is seen in the setting of a specialist referral hospital, standard treatment is with oral ciprofloxacin 500 mg b.d. for 7–10 days or ofloxacin 400 mg b.d. for 7–10 days (Alam et al., 1995). 'Short course' quinolone treatment for 3–5 days has, however, been shown to be equally effective in areas with no ciprofloxacin resistance, as is presently the case in Africa (Tran et al., 1995). This reduced course will save valuable resources. Full course treatment is necessary if nalidixic resistance is seen, as this is an early warning of emerging ciprofloxacin resistance.

Third-generation cephalosporins (ceftriaxone 2 g q.i.d. for 7 days) are also effective if available, and should be given parenterally. A shorter ceftriaxone course of 3–5 days is less effective than a quinolone (Smith et al., 1994). First- and second-generation cephalosporins are not effective and should not be used.

Adjunctive treatment

High-dose dexamethasone as an adjunct to chloramphenicol treatment has been shown to reduce mortality in very severe typhoid with shock and reduced consciousness (Hoffman et al., 1984), and dexamethasone 3 mg/kg has been recommended in these severe cases (McGowan et al., 1992). But in Africa where HIV/AIDS is now so common, it is very important to first consider whether the patient might have a dual infection such as TB, which could be made worse by steroid treatment. Additional treatment cover may be wise.

Treatment of chronic carriage

Chronic carriage of *S. typhi* can been treated with high dose amoxycillin or ampicillin (4–6 g/day) with partial success. Cholecystectomy is also needed if the gall bladder is damaged. Longer courses of quinolones (e.g. ciprofloxacin 500 mg b.d. for 14 days, norfloxacin 400 mg b.d. for 28 days) may be successful in eradicating chronic carriage in up to 80–90 per cent of cases. Cotrimoxazole is excreted in the urine, and may be useful to eradicate urinary carriage.

Chronic carriers with schistosomiasis should also be treated with praziquantel (see Chapter 25)

NON-TYPHOID SALMONELLA (NTS) INFECTIONS

Epidemiology

Since 1990, there has been a dramatic increase in severe, recurrent invasive NTS infections in African adults, accompanying the HIV/AIDS epidemic. Three cases of recurrent NTS bacteraemia in AIDS were reported from Central Africa in 1983. Blood culture series from Kenya, Cote-d'Ivoire, Tanzania and Malawi have shown NTS to be the commonest cause of adult bacteraemia in the 1990s, with an overwhelming association with HIV infection (Gilks et al., 1990; Gordon et al., 2001; Archibald et al., 1998) (Fig. 49.3).

Invasive NTS infections have been a long-standing problem in African children, and there is an association with malaria and anaemia in children (Mabey et al., 1987). Transmission among children is increased in hot and rainy seasons, and a similar pattern seems to be preserved in African adults with HIV/AIDS.

Studies in the USA have shown that salmonella infections at all sites are increased in adults with HIV/AIDS, and that bacteraemia occurs 200 times more frequently in AIDS patients than in the general population (Gruenewald et al., 1992). In Europe and North America, most cases of non-typhoid salmonellosis arise from contamination of the food chain as a result of the wide host range of these serotypes. Eggs and poultry are most commonly involved, but unpasteurised milk, cheese, fresh vegetables and even rattlesnake meat have been implicated (Hohmann, 2001). The role of contaminated foods or animals is not clear in Africa. Chronic carriage by humans is not thought to play a substantial role in transmission of NTS, but person-to-person faeco-oral transmission is important in outbreaks especially in families with children. It seems likely that the chain of transmission to adults with HIV/AIDS in Africa may also involve children in a household.

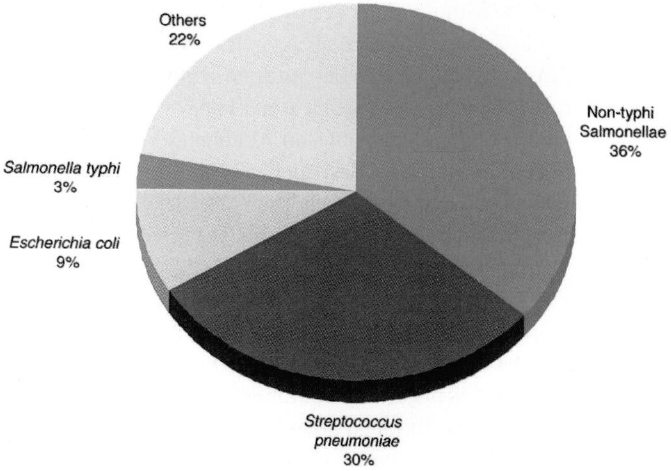

Fig. 49.3. Causes of adult bacteraemia in Malawi, 1998 (449 cases).

Clinical presentations of NTS infection

The NTS serotypes cause a range of clinical syndromes, some of which may affect particular groups of susceptible patients. These are described below.

Gastroenteritis in immunocompetent adults

Salmonella gastroenteritis in immunocompetent individuals is clinically similar to that caused by other bacterial pathogens. Nausea, vomiting, diarrhoea and abdominal cramps with high continuous fever occur 24–48 hours after ingestion of contaminated food or water. Diarrhoea may be profuse, and sometimes bloody. Systemic symptoms and malaise are common. The illness is usually self-limiting and resolves after 4–10 days, and mortality is low (0.5%). Ninety per cent of survivors have cleared salmonella from the stool by 3 months, but stool carriage and relapse may be increased following antibiotic treatment.

NTS bacteraemia

Transient bacteraemia is seen in 1–4 per cent of cases of salmonella gastroenteritis in immunocompetent populations, and acute mortality overall is low. This may, however, allow seeding of organisms to remote sites where structural abnormalities of the endothelium, the urinary tract, and bones can harbour metastatic complications as described below. NTS bacteraemia is commoner and has a higher mortality in the elderly, and in those with underlying conditions such as malignancy, lymphoma or autoimmune disease. NTS bacteraemia is common in HIV-infected adults, results in very high mortality and recurrence rates, and is discussed separately below.

NTS bacteraemia and HIV/AIDS

NTS bacteraemia, most commonly caused by *S. typhimurium* and *S. enteritidis*, is a common and devastating illness in African adults with HIV/AIDS. It usually occurs once patients have advanced HIV disease, and is an AIDS-defining condition.

Presentation

Forty per cent of cases present with acute diarrhoea and fever. Abdominal pain or discomfort is common, and occasionally the presentation closely mimics typhoid fever. The clinical picture may, however, be of fever and malaise without diarrhoea or any other obvious focus (20% of cases), simulating malaria.

As in typhoid, cough is a common symptom (40% of cases). Up to 35 per cent of cases also have crackles, consolidation or pulmonary effusion. Although NTS salmonella pneumonia has been described in HIV, co-infection with a second pathogen (especially TB or *Streptococcus pneumoniae*) is the commonest explanation for findings in the chest. Investigations for TB should be thorough, and treatment may need to be broadened to cover these pathogens.

Splenomegaly occurs in 40 per cent of cases, and may be a useful pointer to the diagnosis, especially if a malaria blood film is negative. Hepatomegaly is seen in 20 per cent of cases. Although other focal NTS infections (bone, CNS, joints) have been reported in HIV, this is not very common (Sperber and Schleupner, 1987). Anaemia and leukopenia are common, and are poor prognostic indicators (Galofre et al., 1993).

Diagnosis of NTS bacteraemia

As with typhoid, it is not possible to make a definitive diagnosis without blood cultures. A trial of treatment is therefore the best diagnostic tool in rural or district settings. Unfortunately, clinical diagnosis and management is made much more difficult by the wide range of presentations, particularly when signs are found in the chest. A chest focus may obscure or divert attention from the diagnosis of NTS bacteraemia. Remember that an enlarged spleen in this setting should always arouse suspicion of salmonella bacteraemia.Where blood culture facilities are available, diagnosis is straightforward, and will also guide antibiotic treatment (see below).

Mortality and recurrence in HIV/AIDS

Acute mortality is very high, being reported as 40–90% despite antibiotic treatment (Gilks et al., 1990; Gordon et al., 2001). The reasons for this very high mortality are not clear, but may include the advanced stage of HIV disease, and the presence of co-infections.

Among HIV-positive survivors of NTS bacteraemia, recurrence of bacteraemia occurred in 39 per cent of Malawian adults within 1–6 months of chloramphenicol treatment. Recurrence can also follow ciprofloxacin treatment. Recurrence usually represents a relapse with the same organism that caused the first bacteraemia, but the clinical picture of relapse does not necessarily mimic the original presentation, and may be a milder illness. Retreatment for 4–6 weeks with the same agent is often successful in treating an episode of relapse, but multiple later relapses may still occur.

NTS vascular infection

Salmonellae infect structurally damaged endothelial arterial sites, such as atherosclerotic plaques or aneurysms, and this is clinically suggested by persistent fever and high-grade bacteraemia following salmonella gastroenteritis. This is probably rarer in Africa than in America or Europe, where vascular disease is more common. Many sites can be involved, and local erosion may lead to additional complications. For example, erosion from an infected aortic aneurysm may cause back pain and vertebral osteomyelitis, or it may lead to aorto-duodenal fistula causing catastrophic GI bleeding. Vascular prostheses and grafts are at particularly high risk of infection. Endocarditis, by contrast, is rare following salmonella bacteraemia. Salmonella aortic infection has a high mortality, and antibiotic treatment alone is not effective. Joint medical and surgical management is needed for successful management, but is often not technically feasible in Africa. Additional long-term suppressive antibiotic therapy is also required.

NTS osteomyelitis

Salmonella osteomyelitis occurs by haematogenous spread, and is seen particularly in association with sickle cell disease and other haemoglobinopathies. The presentation of osteomyelitis may mimic a sickle cell crisis, so that diagnosis is difficult. Malignancy, and other causes of immunosuppression can also predispose to osteomyelitis, and bony abnormalities or trauma can provide a site for an infective focus. Only half of these cases give a history of diarrhoeal illness. Blood culture is positive in 70 per cent of cases. Seventy-five per cent of cases are cured by prolonged antibiotic treatment. The remainder may relapse and develop chronic osteomyelitis.

NTS reactive arthritis

Sterile reactive arthritis involving multiple joints follows 2 per cent of cases of salmonella gastroenteritis, and is commoner in HLA B27 positive individuals. About 1–2 weeks after the onset of diarrhoea, the patient presents with joint symptoms ranging from mild arthralgia to severe, prolonged but non-destructive arthritis. The knee, ankle, wrist and sacroiliac joints are most commonly involved. The features of Reiter's syndrome (conjunctivitis, urethritis) may also be seen. Treatment is symptomatic with a careful explanation to the patient of their illness and the use of non-steroidal anti-inflammatory drugs. Antibiotics are not helpful.

NTS septic arthritis

More rarely, septic arthritis may occur. This is often accompanied by osteomyelitis, and the risk factors are similar (see above). The knee, hip and shoulder are most commonly affected. Antibiotic treatment and, if necessary, repeated needle aspiration of the joints is successful in 80 per cent of cases, and surgery is often not required.

NTS and schistosomiasis

NTS bacteraemia may be persistent or recurrent in the presence of schistosomal infection. This association has been shown in children in Africa (Gendrel et al., 1993), and probably also occurs in adults. Treat concurrent schistosomiasis with praziquantel.

Other localized NTS infections

Other rare sites for extraintestinal metastatic NTS infections include pericarditis, pancreatitis, spontaneous peritonitis, skin abcess at the site of trauma, mastitis, thyroiditis, meningitis, pneumonia and empyema (Cohen et al., 1987). Sites should be drained or debrided where possible, and antibiotic treatment for 4–6 weeks is usually necessary.

Treatment of NTS infections

Treatment of salmonella gastroenteritis

Simple non-invasive salmonella gastroenteritis is usually a self-limiting illness lasting 4–10 days, and the main priority is rehydration and fluid maintenance. Antibiotics should NOT normally be used, as they are not effective, and may increase the rate of chronic carriage of salmonella (Nelson et al., 1980). The exceptions to this are:

(i) patients with severe illness (see section on acute diarrhoea);

(ii) patients at special risk for bacteraemia (elderly or immunosuppressed patients including those with known HIV);

(iii) patients with a known risk-factor for metastatic infection (haemoglobinopathy, structurally damaged bone, abnormal renal tract, schistosomiasis);

(iv) There is very widespread resistance to commonly available antibiotics among NTS in Africa (Dougle et al., 1997), and the choice of agent for treating NTS infections will depend on local resistance patterns. Ampicillin or co-trimoxazole can be used for 3–7 days. If antibiotic resistance is broad, the best treatment is ciprofloxacin (Dryden et al., 1996), at a dose of 500 mg b.d. for 5 days.

Treatment of NTS bacteraemia in HIV/AIDS

There are no trials of treatment in Africa to guide treatment of NTS bacteraemia in HIV-infected patients. Because it is a serious illness with high mortality and recurrence rate, treatment should probably be similar to that for typhoid fever (see above). The optimal treatment is therefore chloramphenicol 500 mg four times daily for 14 days or ciprofloxacin 500 mg twice daily for 10 days. Equivalent 14-day courses of amoxycillin or co-trimoxazole would also be appropriate if the organism is sensitive.

Continuous long-term suppressive treatment for 6 months or more might prevent recurrences of bacteraemia, but in the case of chloramphenicol this carries the risk of dose-related bone-marrow suppression, and in the case of ciprofloxacin would be prohibitively expensive in most settings. Longer treatment might be appropriate with amoxycillin or cotrimoxazole, if the organism is sensitive.

Prophylaxis against NTS bacteraemia

Prophylaxis with co-trimoxazole (2 tablets daily) has been shown to be partially effective in preventing NTS bacteraemia and enteritis in HIV-positive adults in Abidjan, where there is little resistance to this antibiotic (Wiktor et al., 1999; Anglaret et al., 1999). Unfortunately, this may not apply in the many areas of Africa where co-trimoxazole resistance among NTS is more common.

Control and prevention of salmonella infections

Community

Typhoid is transmitted from acute cases or asymptomatic carriers, usually by sewage contamination of food or water. The main reservoirs of NTS in Africa are unknown, but spread by contaminated food and water is also likely. Until food handling and hygiene are improved, water treatment is efficient, and access to clean water is the rule, transmission will continue. Follow-up, tracing and treatment of chronic urinary or faecal carriers, who may live in crowded situations with poor sanitation, should also help to prevent transmission in the community.

Vaccine

Three typhoid vaccines are available; a phenol inactivated parenteral vaccine, a live attenuated oral vaccine (Ty21a) and a purified Vi capsular polysaccharide vaccine. Multiple doses are required to achieve approximately 70 per cent efficacy for 3–5 years, and none are in routine use in endemic areas. Vaccination is, however, useful to protect some groups who are at increased risk from typhoid, such as sickle cell homozygotes (see below). The live Ty21a vaccine has markedly fewer side effects than the older parenteral vaccine, but is not recommended for children or immunosuppressed adults, including those with HIV.

References

Alam MM, Haq SA, Das KK. (1995). Efficacy of ciprofloxacin in enteric fever: comparison of treatment in sensitive and multidrug resistant Salmonella. *Am J Trop Med Hyg*; **53**: 306.

Anglaret X, Chene G, Attia A et al. (1999). Early chemoprophylaxis with trimethoprim-sulphamethoxazole for HIV-1 infected adults in Abidjan, Cote d'Ivoire: a randomised trial. *Lancet*; **353**: 1463–1468.

Archibald LK, den Dulk MO, Pallangyo KJ, Reller LB. (1998). Fatal Mycobacterium tuberculosis bloodstream infections in febrile hospitalised adults in Dar es Salaam, Tanzania. *Clin Infect Dis*; **26**: 290–296.

Cohen JI, Bartlett JA, Corey GR. (1987). Extra-intestinal manifestations of Salmonella infections. *Medicine*; **66**: 349–388.

Dougle ML, Hendriks ER, Sanders EJ, Dorigo-Zetsma JW. (1997). Laboratory investigations in the diagnosis of septicaemia and malaria. *E Afr Med J*; **74**: 353–356.

Dryden M, Gabb R, Wright S. (1996). Empirical treatment of severe acute community-acquired gastroenteritis with ciprofloxacin. *Clin Infect Dis*; **22**: 1019–1025.

Galofre J, Moreno A, Mensa J et al. (1993). Analysis of factors influencing the outcome and development of septic metastasis or relapse in salmonella bacteraemia. *Clin Infect Dis*; **18**: 873–878.

Gendrel D, Kombila M, Beaudoin-Leblevec G, Richard-Lenoble D. (1993). Nontyphoidal Salmonella septicaemia in Gabonese children infected with *Schistosoma intercalatum*. *Clin Infect Dis*; **18**: 103–105.

Gilks CF, Brindle RJ, Otieno LS et al. (1990). Life-threatening bacteraemia in HIV-1 seropositive adults admitted to hospital in Nairobi, Kenya. *Lancet*; **336**: 545–549.

Gordon MA, Walsh AL, Chaponda M et al. (2001). Bacteraemia and mortality among adult medical admissions in Malawi – predominance of non-typhi salmonellae and *Streptococcus pneumoniae*. *J Infect*; **42**: 44–49.

Gruenewald R, Blum S, Chan J. (1992). Relationship between human immunodeficiency virus infection and Salmonellosis in 20- to 59-year-old residents of New York City. *Clin Infect Dis*; **18**: 358–363.

Hoffman S, Punjabi NH, Kumala S. (1984). Reduction of mortality in chloramphenicol-treated severe typhoid by high dose dexamethasone. *N Engl J Med*; **310**: 82–88.

Hohmann EL. (2001). Nontyphoidal salmonellosis. *Clin Infect Dis*; **32**: 263–269.

Mabey DCW, Brown A, Greenwood BM. (1987). *Plasmodium falciparum* malaria and Salmonella infections in Gambian children. *J Infect Dis*; **155**: 1319–1321.

McGowan JE, Chesney PJ, Crossley K, LaForce FM. (1992). Guidelines for the use of systemic glucocorticoids in the management of selected infections. *J Infect Dis*; **165**: 1–13.

Nelson JD, Kusmiesz HJLH, Woodman E. (1980). Treatment of Salmonella gastroenteritis with ampicillin, amoxicillin or placebo. *Pediatrics*; **65**: 1125–1130.

Osuntokun, BO, Bademosi O, Ogunremik, Wright SG. (1972). Neuropsychiatric manifestations of typhoid fever in 959 patients *Arch Neurol*; **27**: 7–13.

Rowe B, Ward LR, Threlfall EJ. (1997). Multidrug resistant *Salmonella typhi*: a worldwide epidemic. *Clin Infect Dis*; **24**: S106–S109.

Rubin FA, Mcwhirter PD, Burr D et al. (1990). Rapid diagnosis of typhoid fever through identification of *Salmonella typhi* within 18 hours of specimen acquisition by culture of the mononuclear cell-platelet fraction of blood. *J Clin Microbiol*; **28**: 825–827.

Smith MD, Duong NM, Hoa NT et al. (1994). Comparison of ofloxacin and ceftriaxone for short-course treatment of enteric fever. *Antimicrob Agents Chemother*; **38**: 1716–1720.

Sperber SJ, Schleupner CJ. (1987). Salmonellosis during infection with Human Immunodeficiency Virus. *Rev Infect Dis*; **9**: 925–934.

Tran TH, Bethell DB, Nguyen TT et al. (1995). Short course of ofloxacin for treatment of multidrug-resistant typhoid. *Clin Infect Dis*; **20**: 917–923.

Wiktor SZ, Sassan-Morokro M, Grant AD et al. (1999). Efficacy of trimethoprim-sulphamethoxazole prophylaxis to decrease morbidity and mortality in HIV-1 infected patients with tuberculosis in Abidjan, Cote d'Ivoire: a randomised controlled trial. *Lancet*; **353**: 1469–1475.

Shigella infection

50

The problem in Africa

The causes of dysentery (bloody infective diarrhoea) in Africa are bacillary (most commonly Shigella, but also Salmonella, Campylobacter and enterohaemorrhagic *E. coli*), and amoebic (*Entamoeba histolytica*). *Shigella* is present throughout Africa, is isolated from the stool in 10–20 per cent of cases of diarrhoea overall, and is the main bacterial cause of bloody diarrhoea. Epidemics of dysentery are widespread, and account for substantial mortality (Birmingham et al., 1997). Enterohaemorrhagic *E. coli* (EHEC) O157 is also an emerging cause of bloody diarrhoea in some parts of Africa.

The organism

Shigella are gram-negative rods, and are members of the enterobacteriacae family. They are microbiologically similar to *E.coli*, but differ by being non-motile, and non-lactose fermenting. They are identified from stool after growth on selective media. Serological and biochemical testing divides Shigella into four groups: A (*S. dysenteriae*), *B (S. flexneri*), C (*S. boydii*), and D (*S. sonnei*).

Pathogenesis

A tiny infecting dose of 200 organisms causes disease, and this explains why Shigella dysentery is highly communicable, with direct transmission from person to person and a high attack rate. Shigella organisms readily invade the epithelial cells lining the colon, where they multiply, spread from cell to cell, and cause extensive superficial destruction leading to bloody diarrhoea. There is rarely penetration beyond the mucosa, and invasive disease with positive blood cultures is rare, despite the presence of high fever in many cases. Children and people with HIV are at higher risk of bacteraemia.

The 'Shiga' toxin inhibits protein synthesis by inactivating the 60S ribosomal subunit, leading to mucosal damage, electrolyte and fluid loss. A similar toxin is produced by EHEC.

Epidemiology

Humans are the only natural host of Shigella. Shigella transmission is usually greatest in the hot season, and is probably facilitated by flies (Chavasse et al., 1999).

Compared to organisms such as salmonella or *E.coli*, spread of Shigella is more often caused by direct person-to-person spread, and less often by contaminated water or food, but both modes of transmission are important.

Shigella outbreaks are a major problem in institutions such as prisons, in overcrowded situations including refugee camps, and where sanitation is poor. The attack rate following a single case in a household is 20–40 per cent. Acute cases shed the largest numbers of organisms, and lower numbers are found in the stool for 1–4 weeks. Chronic carriage of Shigella is rare; unlike salmonella carriers, Shigella carriers are often intermittently symptomatic with diarrhoea. Carriage can be successfully treated with antibiotics, but often clears spontaneously after 6–12 months.

Clinical features

Shigella infection is initially indistinguishable from other infectious diarrhoeas, with fever, abdominal pain and passage of large volumes of stool, which may be watery in the first few days. Over the next 2–3 days, however, the stool becomes much more frequent but of small volume, and mucoid (50%) or bloody (40%). Urgency, tenesmus and rectal 'burning'are also typical.

On examination, 30–40 per cent of cases are febrile, and the temperature may exceed 40 °C. The abdomen may be tender, especially over the lower quadrants. If sigmoidoscopy is performed, a friable rectal mucosa is seen, with mucus, blood and frank ulceration in some cases. The illness usually lasts 1 week in mild cases, but 2–4 weeks in more severe cases, and relapses are common. The organism is usually cleared from the stool after 4 weeks.

Complications

Severe dehydration occurs, but is not common in Shigella infection. Altered consciousness and seizures may be seen, particularly in children. Ileus, toxic dilatation of the colon or perforation may occur in up to 10 per cent of hospitalized cases, and may be precipitated by anti-motility drugs. Haemolytic–uraemic syndrome may occur, particularly in children (Bhimma et al., 1997), and a severe leukaemoid reaction has been described. Post-diarrhoeal arthritis or Reiter's syndrome may occur after 2–4 weeks.

Mortality is very low in well-treated healthy adults. Reported mortality in Africa varies widely, but may be over 10 per cent in hospitalized patients during outbreaks if circumstances are adverse. Mortality and complications are increased by malnutrition, in young children and in elderly patients, and if the organism is resistant to available antibiotics (Legros et al., 1999). The mortality and complication rate from *S. dysenteriae* is higher than that caused by other Shigella types. Shigella infections are increased in HIV/AIDS, but the effect of HIV on mortality from Shigella infection has not been described.

Diagnosis

The clinical picture (fever, frequent small volume bloody diarrhoea, abdominal pain) is often most helpful in suggesting the diagnosis. Microscopy of a fresh stool specimen stained with methylene blue is useful to establish the presence of numerous leukocytes indicating an exudative bacillary bowel infection, and an iodine stain helps to distinguish bacillary from amoebic dysentery. These findings are sufficient to warrant the use of empirical antibiotics. If stool culture is available, it is best performed on fresh material taken early in the course of disease, when many organisms are shed. The number of viable organisms in the stool falls dramatically in the later stages of disease, or if the stool is left to stand before being plated for culture. Blood tests are not usually helpful, and blood culture is very rarely positive.

Treatment

Because the diarrhoea is usually frequent but of small volume, profound fluid and electrolyte loss are not common, and patients can often be managed with ORT (see Chapter 20). Intravenous fluids are required in more severe cases. Do not give anti-diarrhoeal drugs such as opiates, lomotil and loperamide, as they may precipitate toxic megacolon.

Antibiotics are useful in the treatment of Shigella dysentery, as they reduce mortality, shorten the illness and reduce the excretion of organisms. Co-trimoxazole and ampicillin (but *not* amoxycillin) are effective, but resistant strains are highly prevalent throughout Africa. Resistance to nalidixic acid is less extensive in Africa, and this is the cheapest and most effective antibiotic in some areas (Aseffa et al., 1997; Karas et al., 1999; Legros et al., 1998; Obi et al., 1998). Fluoroquinolones are also effective but more expensive. Up-to-date knowledge of local resistance patterns is essential for rational prescribing (Musa et al., 1997).

References

Aseffa A, Gedlu E, Asmelash T. (1997). Antibiotic resistance of prevalent Salmonella and Shigella strains in northwest Ethiopia. *E Afr Med J*; **74**: 708–713.

Bhimma R, Rollins NC, Coovadia HM, Adhikari M. (1997). Post-dysenteric hemolytic uremic syndrome in children during an epidemic of Shigella dysentery in Kwazulu/Natal. *Pediatr Nephrol*; **11**: 560–564.

Birmingham ME, Lee LA, Ntakibirora M, Bizimana F, Deming MS. (1997). A household survey of dysentery in Burundi: implications for the current pandemic in sub-Saharan Africa. *Bull Wld Hlth Org*; **75**: 45–53.

Chavasse DC, Shier RP, Murphy OA Huttly, SR, Cousens SN, Akhtar T. (1999). Impact of fly control on childhood diarrhoea in Pakistan: community-randomised trial. *Lancet*; **353**: 22–25.

Karas JA, Pillay DG, Naicker T, Sturm AW. (1999). Laboratory surveillance of *Shigella dysenteriae* type 1 in KwaZulu-Natal. *S Afr Med J*; **89**: 59–63.

Legros D, Ochola D, Lwanga N, Guma G. (1998). Antibiotic sensitivity of endemic Shigella in Mbarara, Uganda. *E Afr Med J*; **75**: 160–161.

Legros D, Paquet C, Dorlencourt F, Saoult E. (1999). Risk factors for death in hospitalized dysentery patients in Rwanda. *Trop Med Int Health*; **4**: 428–432.

Musa HA, Hassan HS, Shears P. (1997). Occurrence in Sudan of *Shigella dysenteriae* type 1 with transferable antimicrobial resistance. *Ann Trop Med Parasitol*; **91**: 669–671.

Obi CL, Coker AO, Epoke J, Ndip RN. (1998). Distributional patterns of bacterial diarrhoeagenic agents and antibiograms of isolates from diarrhoeaic and non-diarrhoeaic patients in urban and rural areas of Nigeria. *Cent Afr J Med*; **44**: 223–229.

51 Brucellosis

The problem in Africa

Brucellosis is a zoonosis (an infection of humans from an animal reservoir) caused by *Brucella* species, which is usually contracted from infected camels, cows, goats, sheep or pigs. The disease is found world-wide, but serological studies have suggested especially high prevalences among animal herders in the Sahel region and the Horn of Africa (Gavazzi et al., 1997).

The pattern of disease varies, depending on animal husbandry methods and dietary habits. Cattle are the main source of infection among cattle herders who often drink raw milk. Goats and sheep are the main source where milk is seldom drunk and small ruminants are kept within the compound. In South Africa, children who had drunk unpasteurized milk developed brucellosis (Hendricks et al., 1995).

Accurate diagnosis of infection due to Brucella is not possible in most African settings, because microbiological and serological testing is not widely available. Thus, brucellosis often goes unrecognized and is treated as other diseases or as 'fever of unknown origin'. The true incidence has been estimated to be between 10 and 25 times higher than officially reported figures indicate, and the WHO considers that brucellosis in humans and animals is increasing in many parts of Africa.

The organism

Brucellae are small gram-negative coccobacilli, which are often located intracellularly in macrophages. Four species affect humans:

Brucella melitensis: found in sheep, goats and camels. This is the most virulent and invasive species.

Brucella abortus: found in cattle and camels

Brucella suis: found in pigs and cattle

Brucella canis: found in dogs. This is the least common human infection.

Brucellae are found infecting many wild animals, but these are not important reservoirs for human transmission.

Pathogenesis

Brucellae may invade the human body via the mucosal lining of the mouth, nose, conjunctiva, or intestine, via the respiratory tract or through breaks in the skin surface. They can survive and multiply within mononuclear phagocytes, by mechanisms which include the inhibition of phago-lysosome fusion. They multiply in local lymph nodes and then become disseminated via the bloodstream to lymphoid tissues: the spleen, liver, bone marrow and lymph nodes (Young, 1995).

The host response is the formation of granulomas, which may caseate and heal with fibrosis and calcification. The antibody response is important in protection from re-infection; however, control and resolution of infection depends on cellular immune mechanisms. Although brucellosis causes abortion in domestic animals, this is not a prime feature of the human infection, because human fetal and placental tissues do not contain the carbohydrate erythritol, which favours growth of Brucellae in these tissues in animal hosts.

Epidemiology

The main source of infection is raw milk or cheese from infected animals. The second source of infection is direct contact with infected animals, and their tissues and body fluids: blood, urine, vaginal discharges, aborted fetuses and placentas.

Animal herders, and those involved in slaughtering or processing meat are at risk. Farmers, veterinary service workers, abattoir workers and butchers may be exposed to infection at work. Human-to-human transmission is rare, but can occur via blood transfusion or sexual contact.

Prevention and control

There is no effective vaccine for human brucellosis, and prevention in humans depends on:

- control of the disease in the domestic animals
- avoiding the consumption of raw milk and raw milk products.

Vaccination of animals against *Brucella abortus*/*Brucella melitensis* and heat treatment of milk and milk products (pasteurization) have greatly reduced the incidence in some developed countries, but are not routinely practised in endemic areas in Africa, where local customs, traditional habits and beliefs, and lack of resources may impede their wide acceptance or application.

Clinical features

Brucellosis is usually a systemic infection, characterized by fever, fatigue and other symptoms that may occur or recur over weeks, months or years. Bacteria may also lodge in one site and result in organ-specific illness, such as endocarditis, meningitis, pneumonitis, osteitis, spondylitis or orchitis.

Acute brucellosis

The usual incubation period of acute brucellosis is 2–4 weeks, but can be several months. Infection may be mild or unnoticed, and a majority of patients recover completely within 3–6 months without treatment. The disease may start suddenly, with fever, chills and sweats; or slowly with headaches, malaise and marked fatigue, with absent or intermittent fever. Musculoskeletal symptoms and depression are common. Gastrointestinal symptoms include anorexia, nausea, vomiting, abdominal pain, diarrhoea and constipation. Haematuria and cough may be reported. Enlarged cervical and axillary lymph nodes, liver and spleen may be found.

Differential diagnosis

Because none of these signs or symptoms is specific to brucellosis, the differential diagnosis is wide. It includes malaria, typhoid, typhus, relapsing fever, viral infections such as influenza, tuberculosis, autoimmune disease such as systemic lupus erythematosus, and lymphoma.

Always consider brucellosis as a cause of 'pyrexia of unknown origin', particularly if risk factors are present. The combination of numerous symptoms and few abnormal physical signs could lead to patients with brucellosis being misdiagnosed as having psychosomatic illness or depression. Always consider brucellosis in patients at risk.

Sub-acute localized disease

If the initial disease is unrecognized or undertreated, the disease may become localized. Granulomas and vasculitis can affect any organ system. The commonest manifestations are bone and joint disease, meningitis and orchitis. Endocarditis, though uncommon, is important as a cause of death.

Bone or joint involvement has been reported in 20–40 per cent of published cases, with a predilection for vertebrae. Sacroiliitis and spondylitis (with suppuration and paraspinal abscess formation) are most common, presenting with back pain and fever. Osteitis and or osteomyelitis involving the shafts of long bones and suppurative arthritis of joints, especially the hips, knees or ankles may occur. While tuberculosis chiefly infects cervical and thoracic vertebrae, brucellosis characteristically infects lumbar vertebrae.

Invasion of the *CNS* usually presents as acute or chronic meningitis. Encephalitis, psychosis, depression, meningovascular disease, and polyradiculopathy have also been described. Myelitis and myelopathy may occur, and spinal abscess formation may lead to cord compression, or a cauda equina syndrome. Peripheral neuropathy affecting motor and sensory nerves, or single or multiple nerve roots, has been described, presumably due to granuloma formation or vasculitis

Orchitis and epididymo-orchitis may occur, with associated signs of systemic infection. More rarely the kidney is affected: interstitial nephritis, glomerulonephritis and pyelonephritis with renal abscesses have all been reported.

Endocarditis, although reported in less than 2 per cent of cases, is the commonest cause of death in brucellosis. The aortic valve is most commonly affected. Myocarditis and pericarditis may also occur.

Respiratory symptoms, usually cough, occur in up to 25 per cent of patients. Bronchitis, lung abscess, hilar lymphadenopathy and effusions may occur. Granulomas of the liver are common; they heal with fibrosis and calcification and do not lead to cirrhosis. Transient skin manifestations include rashes, papules, erythema nodosum and vasculitis.

Differential diagnosis of localized brucellosis

Tuberculosis, lymphoma, autoimmune disease and vasculitis, pyogenic infections and other forms of bone and joint disease may resemble localized brucellosis.

Chronic brucellosis

Brucellae have been isolated from human tissues many years after infection. 'Chronic brucellosis' refers to chronic ill-health, associated with the recurrence or persistence of systemic or local symptoms of brucellosis for a year or more. In both east and west Africa, some of these patients present with massive splenomegaly like hyperreactive malarial splenomegaly (HMS) (Chapter 78) which resolves when the brucellae are treated with antibiotics (Cox, 1966; Onyemelukwe, 1988).

HIV and brucellosis

It might be expected that African HIV-infected subjects would experience an increased incidence of brucellosis, in common with other intracellular bacterial infections such as tuberculosis or salmonellosis in which cell mediated immunity is important in host defence. Though Brucella infection has been reported in HIV-infected subjects in Africa, an increased incidence has not yet been established.

Laboratory diagnosis

The only way to make a certain diagnosis of brucellosis is to isolate Brucellae from blood, bone marrow, pus or other body fluids. In acute brucellosis bone marrow cultures have been found to be more sensitive than blood cultures, and remain positive for longer. If isolation facilities are available, it is important to inform the laboratory that brucellosis is suspected, as the cultures may take up to six weeks to become positive (Gotuzzo et al., 1986).

Serology

Serological methods, commonly a tube agglutination IgG test may be available in some centres. A four-fold rise in titre or a single titre of 1 in 80 or higher indicate brucellosis. False negative results may be due to a 'prozone' effect, in which the agglutination reaction is blocked at low dilutions and only detected when higher dilutions are made.

Other investigations

The FBC is usually normal, but anaemia, a low white cell count, or a mild lymphocytosis may be found. The ESR is usually raised in acute brucellosis. Liver transaminases may be raised. A chest X-ray is usually normal but may show interstitial infiltration in the perihilar or peribronchial regions. X-rays are more helpful in detecting bone lesions: blurring of articular margins and widening of the sacro-iliac space in sacroiliitis, and epiphysitis with destruction of vertebrae and narrowing of the intervertebral disc space in spondylitis.

Treatment

- Use two or more antibiotics in combination, because there is a high relapse rate with single agent treatment (Hall, 1990). Tetracyclines are effective. Doxycycline is usually preferred because it can be administered once or twice daily dosage.
- Treat acute brucellosis with doxycycline 200 mg daily and rifampicin 600–900 mg daily for 4–6 weeks. Aminoglycosides can be used as an alternative to rifampicin, or added to rifampicin/doxycycline in severe cases, but have the disadvantage of requiring intramuscular administration. Streptomycin 1 g twice daily or gentamicin 240 mg daily i.m. should be given for 2–3 weeks, and doxycycline is continued for 6–12 weeks.
- Treat pregnant women and children under 8 years of age with co-trimoxazole rather than doxycycline; trimethoprim/sulphamethoxazole 160 mg/800mg twice daily in adults, 4/20 mg/kg twice daily in children. Combine this with either with rifampicin 600–900 mg daily (10–20 mg/kg daily) or an intramuscular aminoglycoside.

Patients with bone involvement, neurobrucellosis or endocarditis may need longer courses of treatment (2–3 months), according to the outcome. Abscesses may require surgical drainage.

Unsolved problems

The epidemiology of brucellosis in Africa is not well described, since it cannot be confidently diagnosed clinically, and few laboratories can diagnose it. There is a need for cheap alternatives to rifampicin and streptomycin for the treatment of brucellosis, since widespread use of these drugs will encourage the spread of resistant tuberculosis.

References

Cox PSV. (1966). Brucellosis: a survey in South Karamoja. *E Afr Med J*; **43**: 43.

Gavazzi G, Prigent D, Baudet JM et al. (1997). Epidemiological aspects of 42 cases of human brucellosis in the Republic of Djibouti. *Med Trop (Mars)*; **57**: 365–368.

Gotuzzo E, Carrillo C, Guerra J et al. (1986). An evaluation of diagnostic methods for brucellosis – the value of bone marrow culture. *J Infect Dis*; **153**: 122–125.

Hall WH. (1990). Modern chemotherapy for brucellosis in humans. *Rev Infect Dis*; **12**: 1066–1099.

Hendricks MK, Perez EM, Burger PJ et al. (1995). Brucellosis in childhood in the Western Cape. *S Afr Med J*; **85**: 176–178.

Onyemelukwe GC. (1989). Brucellosis in Northern Nigerians. *W Afr J Med*; **8**: 234–240.

WHO factsheet on Brucellosis: http//www.who.int/infofs/en/fact173.html.

Young EJ. (1995). An overview of human brucellosis. *Clin Infects Dis*; **21**: 238–290.

52 Leptospirosis

Leptospirosis is a zoonosis (an infection of humans from an animal reservoir host) caused by *Leptospira interrogans*. *Leptospira* spp. may be excreted in the urine by over 160 different kinds of mammals, birds and reptiles, and can survive in fresh water for several weeks. Humans are usually infected by fresh water contact.

The problem in Africa

Leptospirosis is found world-wide, except in desert and permafrost regions, and exposure is common in much of sub-Saharan Africa. Thirty-nine per cent of rural Ghanaian farmers and plantation workers were seropositive in one study (Hogerzeil et al., 1986a, b). It is an acute febrile illness, which is frequently mild or asymptomatic. Occasionally, it has severe manifestations, the most life-threatening of which is renal failure. Although its epidemiology has not been well documented in Africa, leptospirosis is probably a significant cause of febrile illness, particularly in the rainy season when fresh water exposure is greatest.

The organism

Leptospires are fine spiral bacteria, which often appear as rods hooked at both ends under dark ground microscopy. There are over 200 serovars in the *Leptospira interrogans* complex. Human infections have been caused by many serovars including *Leptospira hardjo*, which is excreted by cattle, *Leptospira canicola* by dogs, and *Leptospira pomona* by pigs. The most important cause of human infection is probably *Leptospira icterohaemorrhagiae*, whose host is the brown rat *Rattus norvegicus*.

Epidemiology

Leptospires replicate in the renal tubules of infected animals after primary infection, and are excreted for months. The main source of human infection is exposure to fresh water contaminated with rat urine. Leptospires can penetrate intact skin, though the presence of cuts or abrasions probably facilitates transmission. Cultivators of rice and sugar cane, miners, meat and fish processors, rubbish collectors, outdoor labourers and soldiers under wet tropical field conditions are at risk. Tourists who use rivers or lakes for recreations, such as canoeing or white-water rafting, can become infected. Human-to-human transmission is very rare.

Pathogenesis

Following penetration of skin or mucosal surface, leptospires multiply in the blood and cause general symptoms after a few days. From day 7 they localize in kidney, liver, heart, brain and muscle, where they cause local inflammation, necrosis and capillary leakage. In the liver, centrilobular necrosis, and in the kidney tubular necrosis may result. With recovery, leptospires are cleared from these sites, but they may persist in brain and kidney and are commonly excreted in urine for up to 2 months.

Prevention and control

Because it is not possible to eliminate animal reservoirs, elimination of leptospirosis is not a realistic hope or goal. Protective clothing, covering cuts or abrasions with waterproof dressings and sterilizing drinking water may all reduce risk. In China, vaccines for humans have been made from local serovars, but evidence of effectiveness is lacking, and the approach is not likely to be generally effective because of the diversity of serovars. Cattle have been vaccinated against *L. hardjo*, and dogs against *L. canicola* in developed countries, but vaccines are unlikely to be available to control human disease in Africa. Where the risk of leptospirosis is high and unavoidable, for example, during military campaigns, 200 mg of doxycycline weekly is effective as prophylaxis.

Clinical features

The usual incubation period of leptospirosis is 7–14 days (range 2–21 days). Most infections are mild (Hogerzeil et al., 1986b) so that the individuals do not seek hospital care for their fever headache and muscle pains, which may last for 3–5 days. A specific diagnosis is rarely made in these cases.

In more severe cases one or more of the following syndromes may occur:

- an influenza-like illness
- a pyrexia of uncertain origin (PUO)
- jaundice
- renal failure
- aseptic meningitis.

Any combination or all of the above may be present. The pattern of disease is not related to the infecting serovar. The illness may be biphasic, with a first phase of acute fever, chills, headache, myalgia, and often conjunctival suffusion with subconjunctival haemorrhages; followed by 1 or 2 days of remission, and then a second phase of meningeal or hepatorenal manifestations and bleeding into the skin, mucous membranes and lungs (Heron et al., 1997).

In severe cases the first and second phases may merge together in a severe toxic illness with acute liver failure, acute renal failure and extensive bleeding. Mortality is high in these cases.

In Africa the differential diagnosis of leptospirosis includes

- Malaria
- Typhoid
- Relapsing fever
- Meningococcal sepsis
- Typhus
- Hantavirus infection
- Dengue
- Sandfly fever
- Yellow fever and other viral haemorrhagic fevers
- Viral hepatitis.

Suspect leptospirosis in a patient who seems to have viral hepatitis, but also has red or white cell casts in the urine, conjunctival suffusion or prominent muscle pain and tenderness. The combination of petechiae and meningitis may simulate meningococcal disease. Bleeding and renal failure may simulate haemolytic uraemic syndrome, but that is usually associated with dysentery caused by *Shigella* or *E. coli O157*. Leptospirosis may resemble viral meningitis or encephalitis: in the rainy season consider it as a possible diagnosis in febrile subjects whose blood film for malaria is negative.

Diagnosis

Red and white cell casts and protein may be found in the urine, and a full blood count will usually show leukocytosis and thrombocytopenia. Liver enzymes may be raised, and when meningitis is present the CSF cell count is increased, with neutrophils early in the illness and lymphocytes later, but no bacterial growth. Renal failure is characteristically due to acute tubular necrosis. It may be possible to visualize leptospires by dark ground microscopy of centrifuged blood or urine, but this is difficult. In a few centres antibody detection methods such as ELISA or slide agglutination tests may be available to confirm the diagnosis, but in most African settings a presumptive diagnosis will be made on clinical suspicion supported by the few specific features above.

Treatment

Penicillin and related beta-lactam antibiotics such as ampicillin are effective against leptospirosis. Tetracyclines such as doxycycline are also effective, but chloramphenicol and most cephalosporins are not (Takafuji et al., 1984).

For mild disease, give oral doxycycline 100 mg b.d. for 7 days; for moderate/severe disease give i.v. benzylpenicillin 2 MU 6-hourly for 7 days. A Jarisch–Herxheimer reaction may occur 1–2 hours after the first dose. In penicillin-allergic subjects and those in whom doxycycline is contraindicated (pregnant women and children under 8) erythromycin is an effective alternative. Treatment is probably beneficial at all stages of the illness. Severely ill patients may require intensive supportive treatment and dialysis if available.

References

De Geus A. (1977). Clinical leptospirosis in Kenya. *E Afr Med J*; **54**: 115–132.

Heron LG, Reiss-Levy EA, Jacques TC et al. (1997). Leptospirosis presenting as a haemorrhagic fever in a traveller from Africa. *Med J Aust*; **167**: 477–479.

Hogerzeil HV, Terpstra WJ, De Geus A et al. (1986a). Leptospirosis in rural Ghana. *Trop Geogr Med*; **38**: 162–166.

Hogerzeil HV, Terpstra WJ, De Geus A et al. (1986a). Leptospirosis in rural Ghana: Part 2, Current leptospirosis. *Trop Geogr. Med*; **38**: 408–414.

Takafuji ET, Kirkpatrick JW, Miller RN et al. (1984). An efficacy trial of doxycycline prophylaxis against leptospirosis. *N Engl Med J*; **310**: 497–500.

53

Plague

The problem in Africa

Plague remains endemic in several parts of Africa, in southern, eastern and northern parts of the continent (Fig. 53.1). Its incidence in Africa has probably declined over the last century (Davis, 1953), but it is unlikely ever to be eliminated, and there may even be a mild upsurge at present. Africa currently has 67 per cent of the world's human plague, with an estimated 1000 cases per year, and a reported case-fatality rate of around 10 per cent in treated cases (Kilonzo, 1999). Table 53.1 gives recent official WHO data on plague, an international notifiable disease, but this should be interpreted with caution. Good epidemiological studies consistently show that individual cases of plague are missed and that, conversely, during epidemics it is over-diagnosed. The main thing to take from the table is the very uneven distribution throughout the continent, and over time.

The importance of plague does not lie in the fact it is common (it is not), but that it is essential not to miss it when it occurs. This is for the sake of the individual, for health care workers caring for the patient, and for public health reasons. Plague, with its overtones of the Black Death decimating populations in major pandemics, has induced mass panic when potential outbreaks are announced. This panic, which has serious implications for public health, is partially justified. Untreated, even the mildest (bubonic) form has a mortality of over 50 per cent, and untreated pneumonic plague is almost 100 per cent fatal.

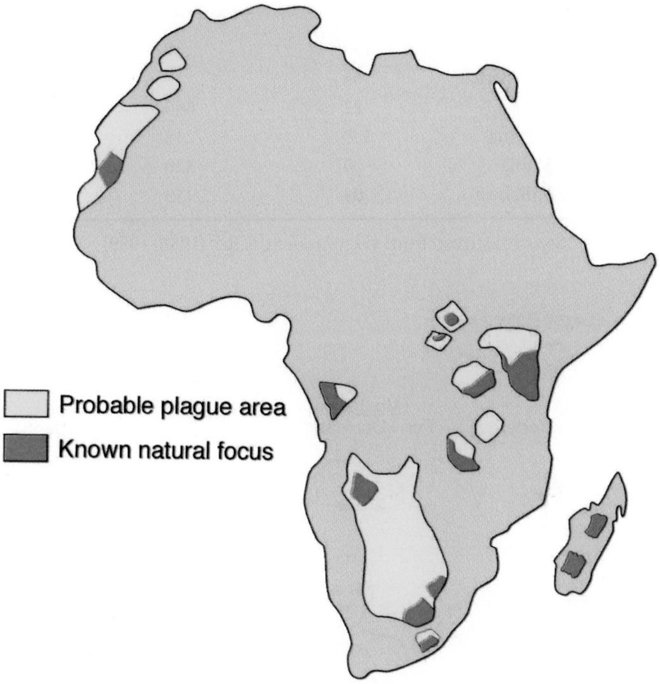

Fig. 53.1. The enzootic foci of plague in Africa.

Organism, hosts and vectors

Plague is a bacterial zoonosis which occasionally spreads to man. It has interconnected planes or cycles (Fig. 53.2), and it is when any component or stage in these cycles is disturbed, by war, internally displaced people or natural disasters, that an outbreak is liable to occur. The cause, *Yersinia pestis,* is a gram-negative coccobacillus which is non-motile, non-lactose fermenting and grows on a variety of media including unenriched agar and blood agar. It does not generally survive for long outside its mammalian hosts or flea vectors, and rapidly dies at temperatures above 40 °C.

The major hosts of importance in Africa are swamp and field rats (*Mastomys natalensis* and *Rattus rattus*),

Table 53.1. Cases of human plague reported to the WHO 1954–98

	1954–1974	1975–1998	Total
Angola	0	76	76
Botswana	0	173	173
Burkina Faso	1	0	1
Cameroon	1	0	1
D.R. Congo	474	2812	3286
Guinea	52	0	52
Kenya	129	442	571
Lesotho	131	8	139
Libya	16	38	54
Madagascar	460	6194	6624
Malawi	30	591	621
Mozambique	0	1165	1165
Namibia	194	0	194
South Africa	64	19	83
Uganda	22	660	682
Tanzania	566	7248	7814
Zambia	0	320	320
Zimbabwe	84	439	523

Source: Derived from *Wkly Epidemiol Rec* (1956–1999).

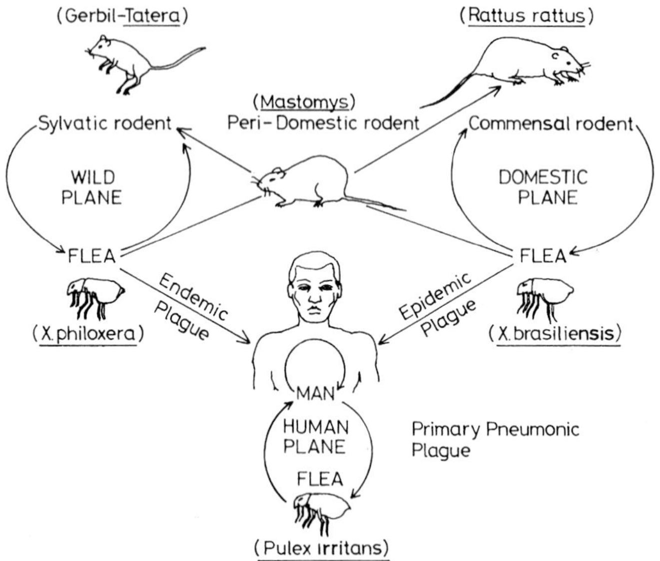

Fig. 53.2. The interconnected cycles or planes of plague.

multimammate mice, grass mice and gerbils, with transmission to man via fleas. Rodents and their fleas are not the only potential source of infection, however, and plague has been identified in over 200 species of mammal and more than 150 species of flea. Plague can also be passed on by handling infected animals, and between humans by body lice, whilst pneumonic plague can be transmitted from person to person directly.

Control and prevention

The public health aspects of managing plague are challenging. Where potential outbreaks are announced mass panic can set in, with populations fleeing in every direction, potentially including cases of pneumonic plague. Plague is an international notifiable disease. This means that all proven cases must be reported to the WHO in Geneva, either directly or via the central government health authorities. Isolated cases of bubonic or septicaemic plague in known endemic areas usually have no public health significance beyond that. The problem comes where several cases of plague are found in areas not known to be endemic, or primary pneumonic plague is diagnosed. These could mark the start of an outbreak, but are highly unlikely to do so; the authors of the WHO Plague Manual state that 'the possibility of outbreaks of anthroponotic and primary pneumonic plague . . . has been reduced nearly to zero' (WHO Expert Panel on Plague, 1999).

There is a balance to be struck between identifying a potential epidemic early enough to deal with it effectively, and, on the other hand, not creating what may be a major false alarm. Individual clinicians should not have to make that decision, but it is important that central health authorities are informed at the earliest possible opportunity if unexpected cases of plague are diagnosed. Effective control measures do exist – a combination of rat-control, anti-flea measures and prophylaxis are all effective, and with widely available drugs and recent advances in rapid bedside diagnosis even a significant outbreak should be containable.

Pathophysiology

The pathophysiology of the disease is not fully understood, but is probably largely endotoxin mediated. *Y. pestis* has several proteins capable of initiating gram-negative shock and disseminated intravascular coagulation including pH6 antigen (Lindler et al., 1990) *Yersinia* outer-membrane proteins (Yops) and lipopolysaccharide endotoxins. *Y. pestis* also produces an exotoxin which is probably important in rodent, but not human, disease.

Clinical presentation

There are three classical and sometimes overlapping presentations of plague; bubonic, septicaemic and pneumonic. Other localized forms, including meningitic plague, also occur. The symptoms common to all from the largest reported series are a relatively rapid onset of fever, headache, chills, myalgia, prostration, malaise and gastrointestinal symptoms. This non-specific presentation clearly has a very wide differential diagnosis. The incubation period for plague is generally 2–3 days, although up to 8 days is considered possible. If the last potential plague contact is more than 8 days ago the diagnosis is highly unlikely.

Bubonic plague is the most common form, and is due to flea-transmitted plague or handling infected animals. It is also the only form where a clinician is likely to guess the diagnosis on clinical grounds alone. Lymph nodes draining the site of the infected bite become enlarged and tender, usually within a day or two of the initial non-specific symptoms (Butler et al., 1974). Case series report generally tender nodes ranging in size from a few millimetres to a hen's egg. They are non-fluctuant, and seldom contain pus. The commonest site is the groin (following flea bites to the leg), followed by the axilla (especially after handling infected animals), and then the cervical chain. Single buboes are the norm, and multiple enlarged lymph nodes in several sites should raise doubts about the diagnosis, although this may be seen following haematogenous spread. The site of the infected bite may ulcerate, but this is rare.

Septicaemic plague may present following inadequate treatment of bubonic plague, or as a primary presenting disease. Where it is the primary presentation clinical diagnosis is difficult. The diagnosis can only be made by isolating *Y. pestis* from the blood of the infected individual. The presentation of septicaemic plague can be similar to severe gram-negative sepsis caused by other organisms, with multiple organ failure (including adult respiratory distress syndrome), disseminated intravascular coagulation and death. Septicaemic plague can also seed to local sites, causing secondary plague pneumonia, or more rarely meningitis, endophthalmitis and localized abscesses in liver, spleen, kidneys and lungs.

Secondary pneumonic plague is a complication of septicaemic plague with the lungs infected by haematogenous spread. In addition to the generalized symptoms of plague patients may have cough, dyspnoea and haemoptysis, usually with thick sputum. Radiography shows patchy shadowing or a diffuse pneumonic process. The mortality from pneumonic plague is high, and those who recover may be left with extensive lung damage.

Secondary pneumonic plague is moderately infectious, and patients infected by droplet transmission usually develop primary pneumonic plague. Whilst secondary pneumonic plague is a late stage disease, when patients are usually very ill, with a weak cough reflex and thick sputum which probably reduces transmission, primary pneumonic plague patients are infectious early in the disease, and produce a thin sputum which aerosolizes easily. Once an outbreak of primary pneumonic plague occurs, it can potentially move rapidly through a community without the need for flea vectors, although the attack rate is probably less than 10 per cent of those exposed (Ratsitorahina et al., 2000).

Laboratory diagnosis

The clinical diagnosis of non-bubonic plague is difficult. Even bubonic plague with its presentation of systemic infection and enlarged painful lymph nodes has a wide differential. Because of its public health importance, if plague is suspected, try to make a firm aetiological diagnosis.

'Basic' investigations are of limited use. Severe plague is usually associated with a significant neutrophilia, and platelets are often reduced. There are three methods of making a relatively firm diagnosis of plague which are clinically useful; microscopy, culture and immunological methods. In addition there are PCR-based methods and serological assays, but these have proved insensitive and unhelpful in the field (Rahalison et al., 2000).

Microscopy is relatively non-specific, but is available in almost all hospitals. It is also quick. In suspected cases of bubonic plague, aspirate the bubo. Conventional practice is to use a 10 ml syringe with 1 ml of sterile normal saline, and insert and withdraw several times whilst aspirating until the aspirate becomes blood-tinged. Plague buboes do not contain pus, and it may be necessary to inject some of the saline and immediately re-aspirate. Perform a gram stain and, if possible, set up cultures of the aspirated material. Gram stain may reveal gram-negative coccobacilli and bacilli 1–2 μm long.

Simple blood microscopy (gram stain) may show plague bacilli in cases of septicaemic plague; this indicates a poor prognosis. In pneumonic plague the sputum smear usually contains pus and occasionally plague bacilli (sensitivity less than 10%).

Culture of specimens and more specific staining will improve both sensitivity and specificity of diagnosis.

Y. pestis grows readily on blood agar and MacConkey plates, and in broth. Wayson stain, which shows *Y. pestis* as light blue bacilli with blue polar bodies on a pink background, is ideal for microscopy both of direct specimens and of cultured isolates.

Immunological methods

F1 antigen capture rapid immunogold dipsticks look promising, and are likely to be helpful in endemic areas and during outbreaks. Field trials suggest they are 100 per cent specific, 100 per cent sensitive for bubo aspirates and 50 per cent sensitive for serum against a gold standard of culture (Chanteau et al., 2000). They are even more helpful in cases of pneumonic plague, since they are ten times as sensitive as microscopy and 3 times as sensitive as culture (Ratsitorahina et al., 2000). It is unlikely that these will be available in most hospitals in Africa, but if outbreaks occur dipsticks should prove an invaluable tool, and obtaining them should be a priority for international organizations. A few strains of plague are F1 antigen-negative, so the method cannot be completely relied upon.

Treatment and follow-up

Plague can progress rapidly. If there are strong clinical reasons for suspecting it, start treatment immediately, before laboratory confirmation. Antibiotic and supportive treatment are both important.

Antibiotics

Streptomycin is the traditional antibiotic drug of choice, and works well in clinical studies. Tetracycline, trimethoprim-sulphamethoxazole and chloramphenicol are also effective in clinical studies. Gentamicin can probably be substituted for streptomycin and doxycycline for tetracycline, although there is less clinical experience with these drugs.

Cephalosporins and quinolones, which are not available in many hospitals for cost reasons, are effective in vitro, but less good in vivo. Penicillins have reasonable activity in vitro, but relatively little in vivo, at least in animal studies, and should not be used.

Drug regimens, which follow, are based on what has worked in clinical series, but there are few good published clinical trials comparing different regimens. Optimal drug combinations, duration of treatment and dosing have not been determined.

Treatment regimens

Streptomycin at a dose of 30 mg/kg/day in two divided doses intramuscularly for 10 days has been the most widely used treatment for plague for over 40 years (Butler et al., 1976). Case series from India suggest a mortality of 10 per cent in those treated with streptomycin, compared to 21 per cent in those treated with sulphonamides. Drug resistance is currently rare – a study of 156 strains found only two resistant to streptomycin. Nevertheless, adding tetracycline to streptomycin is often advocated, despite no evidence that the combination is better.

Multi-drug resistant *Y. pestis* mediated by plasmid has been reported in Africa, but the antibiotic selection pressure on the organism is very small, and there is no reason to anticipate it will spread (Galimand et al., 1997).

Where streptomycin is not available, the following combinations are probably as effective:

Gentamicin 3 mg/kg/day in divided doses 8-hourly intravenous or intramuscular.

Tetracycline 2–4 g/day in 4 divided doses or doxycycline 200 mg a day.

Chloramphenicol 4 g/day (60 mg/kg/day) in divided doses, following a loading dose of 25 mg/kg.

Although 10 days' treatment is usually recommended for all drugs, it is reasonable to continue treatment for 3 days after the patient becomes afebrile if this is longer. Relapse after treatment is rare.

Because streptomycin does not penetrate the CNS well, treat meningitic plague with chloramphenicol.

Patients usually start to improve within 2–3 days of starting treatment, although buboes may continue to grow, and remain swollen and tender for several weeks after successful treatment.

Supportive treatment for gram-negative shock and all the complications of multi-organ failure may be needed. There is no evidence that steroids have any part to play, although this has not been tested formally.

Prophylaxis and protection of health-care workers

Pure bubonic or septicaemic plague is not highly infectious, but it is conventional practice to offer close or household contacts chemoprophylaxis for 7 days after their last exposure. All contacts (including casual contacts) of those with pneumonic plague, and their health-care workers, should receive chemoprophylaxis for 7 days after exposure with tetracycline 250 mg four times a day or doxycycline 100 mg a day. Babies and pregnant women in the first trimester are given amoxycillin. Older children under 9 years should take co-trimoxazole.

Isolate and, if possile, barrier nurse all cases of pneumonic plague. All carers should wear masks, and gloves if handling specimens. For those in regular contact with plague, and during epidemics, there is a formalin-inactivated vaccine, but it has not been well evaluated (Jefferson et al., 2000). It may be partially effective against flea-borne plague, but has not been demonstrated to protect against pneumonic plague. In cases of pneumonic plague there is probably a place for giving carers prophylactic doxycycline/tetracycline.

Unsolved problems

There have been rapid strides forward recently in diagnosis, but this has not been matched by research into better treatments. The optimal drug or combination of antibiotics, dose, route of administration, duration of treatment and additional treatments remain to be determined. The current regimens are based on reports of what has worked in relatively small series rather than any clinical trials. Given the mortality from plague there may well be room for improvement, and clinical trials using current regimens as a gold standard are a clear priority in research into plague.

Further information

The latest edition of the *Plague Manual* from the WHO may be obtained from the WHO, or for those with internet access, can be downloaded from www.who.int/csr/resources/publications.

References

Butler T, Bell WR, Nguyen NL, Nguyen DT, Arnold K. (1974). *Yersinia pestis* infection in Vietnam. I. Clinical and hematologic aspects, *J Infect Dis*; vol. **129**, Suppl-84.

Butler T, Levin J, Linh NN, Chau DM, Adickman M, Arnold K. (1976). *Yersinia pestis* infection in Vietnam. II. Quantiative blood cultures and detection of endotoxin in the cerebrospinal fluid of patients with meningitis, *J Infect Dis*; **133**: 493–499.

Chanteau S, Rahalison L, Ratsitorahina M. et al. (2000). Early diagnosis of bubonic plague using F1 antigen capture ELISA assay and rapid immunogold dipstick, *Int J Med Microbiol*; **290**: 279–283.

Davis DH. (1953). Plague in Africa from 1935–1949. *Bull Wld Hlth Org*; **9**: 665.

Galimand M, Guiyoule A, Gerbaud G et al. (1997). Multidrug resistance in Yersinia pestis mediated by a transferable plasmid. *N Engl J Med*; **337**: 677–680.

Jefferson T, Demicheli V, Pratt M. (2000). Vaccines for preventing plague. *Cochrane Database Syst Rev*; 2, CD000976.

Kilonzo BS. (1999). Plague epidemiology and control in eastern and southern Africa during the period 1978–1997. *Cent Afr J Med*; **45**: 70–76.

Lindler LE, Klempner MS, Straley SC. (1990). *Yersinia pestis* pH 6 antigen: genetic, biochemical, and virulence characterization of a protein involved in the pathogenesis of bubonic plague. *Infect Immun*; **58**: 2569–2577.

Rahalison L, Vololonirina E, Ratsitorahina M, Chanteau S. (2000). Diagnosis of bubonic plague by PCR in Madagascar under field conditions. *J Clin Microbiol*; **38**: 260–263.

Ratsitorahina M, Chanteau S, Rahalison L, Ratsifasoamanana L, Boisier P. (2000). Epidemiological and diagnostic aspects of the outbreak of pneumonic plague in Madagascar. *Lancet*; **355**: 111–113.

WHO Expert Panel on Plague. (1999). *Plague Manual: Epidemiology, Distribution, Surveillance and Control.* World Health Organization, CSR/EDC/99.2.

54 Anthrax

Anthrax is a widespread zoonosis transmitted from animals (mainly herbivores) to humans. The disease was well known to the ancient Greeks and Romans and widespread in Europe in the past century. Robert Koch discovered the transmission cycle at the end of the nineteenth Century (Dubovsky, 1982). Since then anthrax has been successfully controlled in Europe and the USA; only two cases of cutaneous anthrax were reported in the USA between 1992 and 2000 (CDC, 2000). Interest in *Bacillus anthracis* has recently risen focused on the danger of its being used in biological warfare (Morgan, 2000).

The problem in Africa

In Africa anthrax is a common infection of animals, both domestic and wild, and sporadic outbreaks of human anthrax are common in many parts of the continent. Every clinician practising in Africa needs to have a basic knowledge of the epidemiology and clinical picture of anthrax.

Outbreaks of anthrax have been reported from Zambia, Zimbabwe (Davies, 1982), Tanzania, Kenya and South Africa (WHO, 1994), Ghana (Opare et al., 2000), Burkina Faso (Coulibaly & Yameogo, 2000) and Guinea Bissau (De Ridders, 1994). In The Gambia, human anthrax is endemic occurring every dry season in a specific region (Heyworth et al., 1975).

The organism

Anthrax is caused by *Bacillus anthracis*, a gram-positive encapsulated, non-motile, aerobic bacterium that forms spores, which can survive in dry ground for many years.

Epidemiology

All animals are susceptible to *Bacillus anthracis*, but the disease is most prevalent and severe in domestic and wild herbivores, which ingest spores while grazing. Infection leads to severe disease, with overwhelming bacteraemia and usually death of the animal. Carcasses and secretions from dead or dying animals, such as blood or faeces, are a source of infection. Vultures or biting flies transmit the bacillus from infected to uninfected areas (Fig. 54.1).

Spores can survive in the ground long after a dead animal has been removed or buried, becoming a source of infection for farmers cultivating their fields or for other animals. Investigations in South Africa revealed infected bone diggings in Krueger National Park which dated back more than 200 years (WHO, 1994). Traditionally, we differentiate agricultural and industrial cases of anthrax, the former being acquired through contact with animals or carcasses, the latter acquired through industrial contact with animal skin (leather), meat, hair or wool.

In Africa, transmission from human to human has also been reported in an endemic region of The Gambia, where fibrous vegetables used for washing were found to be contaminated with *B. anthracis* leading to infection of other family members (Heyworth et al., 1975).

Incidence

It is difficult to determine incidence rates of anthrax due to incomplete reporting systems both for human and veterinary cases. Estimates range from 20 000 to 100 000 cases/year world-wide (Harrison, 1999). No recent incidence figures are available for Africa, but sporadic outbreaks are common, such as the one reported in Ethiopia in July 2000 (WHO, homepage).

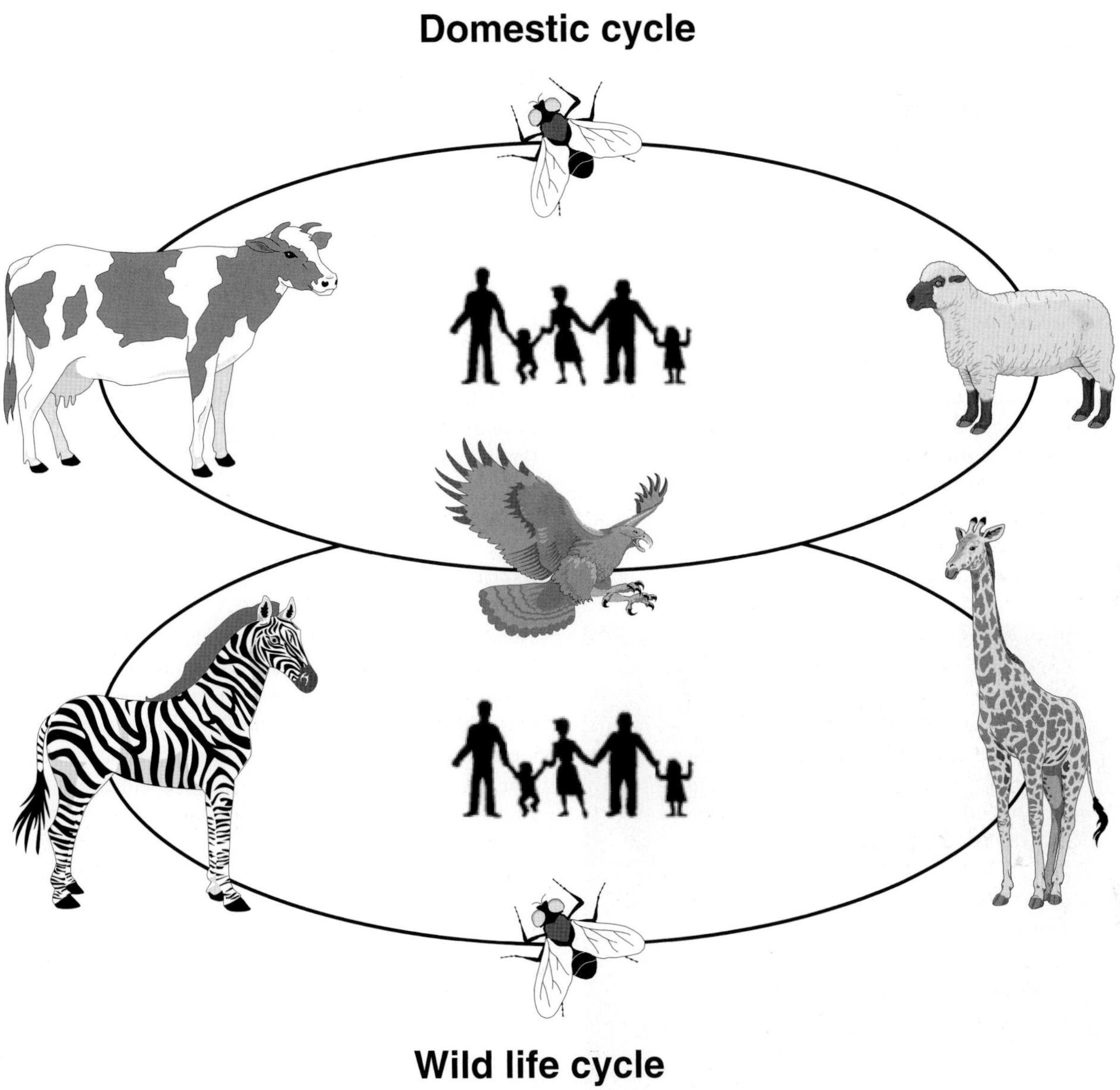

Fig. 54.1. Transmission cycle of *Bacillus anthracis.*

Seasonal variation

Overall infection with *Bacillus anthracis* is reported mainly in the dry seasons, especially after some years of drought, except for Kenya where it is more common in unusually wet years (WHO, 1994; Seboxa & Goldhagen, 1988). Clinical data from The Gambia show a clustering of cases during the end of the dry season in an area where anthrax is endemic, and well known to the local population as 'fonyo' or 'fayo' (something that 'flies on you') (Heyworth et al., 1975; Schneider, 1997).

Pathogenesis

Bacillus anthracis is an extracellular pathogen that can invade the bloodstream quickly and multiply rapidly. The main cause of pathology is a capsular polypeptide and the anthrax toxin. This was discovered in studies where sterile blood from infected guinea pigs killed the recipients. The anthrax toxin consists of three proteins called the protective antigen (PA), the oedema factor (EF) and the lethal factor (LF). The PA binds to the cell and serves as a receptor for EF and LF. The biological effects of EF include oedema formation and the inhibition of polymorphonuclear leukocyte functions. LF leads to cell death by unknown mechanisms (Harrison, 1999).

Clinical features

There are three clinical forms of human anthrax. The most common form is

Cutaneous anthrax

A skin lesion develops 1 to 6 days after infection with *Bacillus anthracis*: Initially a red macula forms followed by a papule and a ring of vesicles leading to the typical black eschar surrounded by multiple vesicles that may develop into pustules. This lesion is accompanied by various degrees of oedema from mild to severe (Fig. 54.2). As the disease progresses the central lesion dries out and necrosis may lead to skin defects. Several cases of ocular anthrax were seen by the author, leading to the defects of the eyelids, requiring plastic surgery but without any effect on the vision after the oedema and necrosis had subsided.

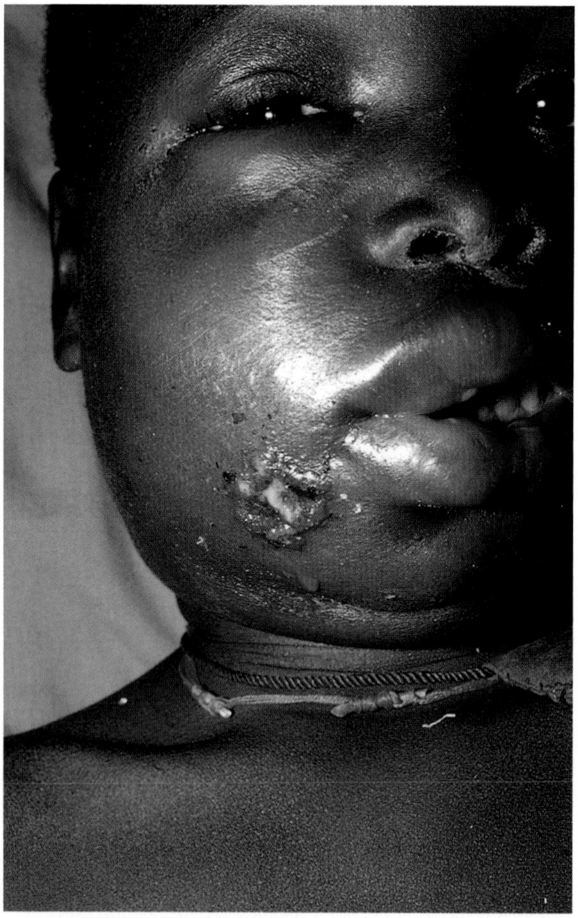

Fig. 54.2. Anthrax of face. (M. Weber)

The distribution of the lesions on the body varies. Reports from Zimbabwe show that lesions in children are more likely to be on the head, neck or face, whereas adults are more likely to acquire lesions on the extremities. In The Gambia 63 per cent of lesions were on the head and neck, 21 per cent on the trunk and 16 per cent on the extremities (Heyworth et al., 1975).

Ten to twenty per cent of untreated cutaneous infections lead to bacteriaemia and subsequent death (Harrison, 1999). Data from an outbreak in Ethiopia show a case-fatality rate of 11 per cent (Seboxa & Goldhagen, 1988). In The Gambia case-fatality rates were lower in treated patients (2 deaths in over 400 cases) (Heyworth et al., 1975).

Diagnosis

The diagnosis can usually be made clinically. Consider anthrax when typical skin lesions occur in endemic regions, or when people are exposed to animals or carcasses possibly infected with *Bacillus anthracis*. Anthrax must be distinguished from staphylococcal infections that can lead to a similar central necrosis. Tularaemia, plague and orf should also be considered.

Gastrointestinal anthrax

This form of anthrax is rare but often fatal. Several cases often present at the same time, having eaten the same dead animal. Symptoms include nausea, fever, abdominal cramps and anorexia with or without bloody diarrhoea. The disease usually quickly progresses leading to shock, paralytic ileus and death. Mortality rates are high. In the Gambia among 448 cases of anthrax investigated 2 had intestinal anthrax and both died (Heyworth et al., 1975). Oropharyngeal anthrax with fever, sore throat and regional lymphadenopathy has been reported. The primary lesion is usually found on the tonsils.

Inhalation anthrax

This form of anthrax, also known as 'wool sorters' disease', is rare. It presents initially as an acute respiratory tract infection, followed by a rapid onset of hypoxia, dyspnoea, fever and shock nearly always leading to death. X-ray evidence will show a widened mediastinum representing a haemorrhagic mediastinitis.

Diagnosis

The diagnosis of anthrax is based on:
(i) clinical signs and symptoms;
(ii) a high level of suspicion especially in endemic areas;
(iii) laboratory investigations, which may include:
- isolation of *Bacillus anthracis* by culture from a clinical specimen (vesicular lesions, blood or discharges)
- demonstration of *B.anthracis* in a clinical specimen by microscopic examination of stained smears (gram staining) (vesicular fluid, blood, CSF, pleural fluid, stools)
- positive serology (Elisa, Western blot, toxin detection, chromatographic assay, fluorescent antibody test (FAT)) (WHO homepage: A22 Anthrax).

It may not be possible to demonstrate *B.anthracis* in clinical specimens if the patient has been treated with antibiotics previously.

In practical terms in many rural African hospitals, it may not be possible to culture *B. anthracis* or use serological markers, but a simple microscope with gram or Giemsa staining will reveal typical gram-positive bacilli.

Management of anthrax

Cutaneous anthrax

Mild cases

Lesions with little oedema, which are not located on the face or neck.

These can be treated as outpatients with:

Procaine Penicillin 2 million IU i.m. daily for 5 days
Cover lesions where necessary and avoid any surgical intervention.

Moderate cases

Lesions with moderate oedema possibly located on the face or neck.

Inpatient management:

Benzylpenicillin 2 million IU i.m. or i.v. 6-hourly until oedema is reduced (usually at least 48 hours), then procaine penicillin or oral penicillin for 7–10 days.
Check BP 2–4-hourly initially to recognize any systemic reaction

Severe cases

Lesions with severe oedema, especially around face and neck; or a drop in BP, dizziness or early signs of shock.

Inpatient management and careful monitoring of vital signs:

Benzylpenicillin 2 million IU i.m. or i.v. 4-hourly until patient is stable and oedema is reduced (usually at least 24–48 hours), then benzyl penicillin 2 million IU i.m. or i.v. 6-hourly for 48 hours followed by i.m. procaine penicillin or oral penicillin for 7–10 days

Anthrax in children

Children with anthrax should always be admitted and treated with

Benzylpenicillin 50 000 IU/kg 6-hourly i.m.

In severe cases

Benzylpenicillin 100 000 IU/kg 4–6-hourly i.v.

In case of penicillin allergy the following drugs can be used:

Erythromycin 500 mg q.i.d. for 5–7 days
or tetracycline 500 mg q.i.d. for 5–7 days (not for children or pregnant mothers)
or chloramphenicol 500 mg q.i.d. for 5–7 days
or cripofloxacin 500 mg b.d. (rarely available in rural settings in Africa)

Management of systemic anthrax

As severe cutaneous anthrax and in addition:

- Streptomycin 1 g i.m. daily for 5–7 days for adults
- Or chloramphenicol 500 mg q.i.d. in case of anthrax meningitis
- i.v. fluids: 500 ml 0.9% saline or Ringer lactate solution every 4–6 hours
- Exact fluid balances
- Transfusion of fresh blood in case of disseminated intravascular coagulation.

Caution: Never attempt to incise or aspirate anthrax lesions.

Table 54.1. Control and prevention of anthrax

1. Surveillance of Anthrax cases (WHO: outbreak@who.ch)
- Livestock (unexplained sudden livestock deaths)
- Case reporting from high-risk groups such as slaughter house workers, shepherds, veterinarians, wool workers, etc.
- Clinical case reporting for any case of anthrax
- Necessary laboratory investigations and follow-up of all clinical cases

2. Additional measures: (WHO, 1994 #166)
- Disposal of carcasses and subsequent disinfection and decontamination
- Burning of carcasses and burying (long-term contamination?)
- Prohibition of selling meat from an animal that died of an undiagnosed cause
- Quarantine of an infected area and vaccination of all domestic animals within the affected area until 3 months after the last reported case
- Education campaigns for affected population about the danger of consuming or handling uninspected meat.

Control and prevention of anthrax

Anthrax can be controlled where there is good collaboration between clinicians, public health officials and veterinary staff for the surveillance of cases and appropriate disposal and disinfection of infected areas, and the vaccination is available for animals (Table 54.1).

Unsolved problems

1. What are the reasons for the development of severe disease? Host factors, or the virulence of the bacillus and toxin production?
2. Oedema can be severe in cutaneous anthrax. Is there a role for the use of antitoxin (passive immunization) to control oedema and/or systemic reactions?
3. Is there a role for systemic hydrocortisone in the management of severe anthrax?
4. Should a preventive vaccine for the general population be considered in endemic areas?

References

CDC (2000). Human ingestion of *Bacillus anthracis* – contaminated meat – Minnesota August 2000. *Morb Mortality Wkly Rep*; **284**: 813–816.

Charatan F. (2000). Fears over anthrax vaccination driving away US reservists. *Br Med J*; **321**: 980.

Coulibaly N, Yameogo K. (2000). Prevalence and control of zoonotic diseases: collaboration between public health workers and verterinarians. *Acta Tropica*; **76**: 53–57.

Davies J. (1982). A major epidemic of Anthrax in Zimbabwe. *Cent Afr J Med*; **28**: 291–298.

De Ridders J. (1994). An epidemic in Guinea Bissau. *Trop Doctor*; **24**: 32.

Dubovsky H. (1982). Robert Koch (1843 – 1910) – the man and his work.' *S Afr Medical Journal*; **17 Nov** (Special Issue): 3–5.

Heyworth B, Ropp M, Voos VG et al. (1975). Anthrax in The Gambia: an epidemiological study. *Br Med J*; **4**: 79–82.

Morgan M. (2000). Anthrax. An old disease returns as a bioterrorism weapon. *N J Med*; **97**: 35–41.

Opare C, Nsiira A, Awumbilla B et al. (2000). Human behavioural factors implicated in outbreaks of human anthrax in the Tamale municipality of northern Ghana. *Acta Trop*; **76**: 49–52.

Schneider G. (1997). *WEC International, Annual Medical Report 1996*. Banjul, WEC International.

Seboxa T, Goldhagen J. (1988). Anthrax in Ethiopia. *Trop Geogr Med*; **41**: 108–112.

Steele J. (2000). Book review: anthrax: the investigation of a deadly outbreak *N Engl J Med*; **342**: 1373.

WHO (1994). Anthrax control and research, with special reference to national programme development in Africa: Memorandum from a WHO meeting. *Bull WHO*; **72**: 13–22.

Fungi

55 Fungal infections

The problem in Africa

Fungi are important plant and animal pathogens. They are also found as saprophytes on organic (e.g. soil) and non-organic (e.g. buildings) surfaces. Fungi occur throughout the many climatic conditions found in Africa. There are two principal fungal cell forms known as the yeasts and moulds. Yeasts are single cells which reproduce by a process of budding to give rise to single daughter cells. Mycelial or mould fungi form chains of cells. The dimorphic fungi may exist in either yeast or mycelial phase at different stages of their life cycles.

Because fungi are ubiquitous they can cause diseases in different ways, through the production of toxins or mycotoxins, the possession of sensitizing antigens (allergens) or the invasion of tissue. This chapter will be mainly concerned with invasive fungal disease. In Africa, though, allergic fungal disease and toxicosis due to fungi, such as *Aspergillus flavus*, contaminating stored foodstuffs (aflatoxicosis) are recognized diseases in some areas. The common invasive fungal diseases are shown in Table 55.1. They include the ringworm or dermatophyte infections as well as candidosis amongst the superficial infections and systemic mycoses such as cryptococcosis, commonly associated with AIDS, as well as rarer diseases, e.g. African or large form histoplasmosis. These main invasive fungal infections are known as the superficial, subcutaneous or systemic mycoses.

Table 55.1. Classification of mycoses

Superficial mycoses
Dermatophytosis (ringworm)
Superficial candidosis (oral, vaginal, cutaneous)
Diseases due to *Malassezia*–pityriasis versicolor, *Malassezia* folliculitis, seborrhoeic dermatitis
Onychomycosis
Rare, e.g. white piedra
Otomycosis, keratomycosis (corneal infection)
Sub-cutaneous mycoses
Mycetoma
Chromoblastomycosis
Phaeohyphomycosis
Sporotrichosis
Others: infection due to *Conidiobolus* and *Basidiobolus* (Lobomycosis)
Systemic mycoses
Endemic infections
Histoplasmosis
African histoplasmosis
Blastomycosis
(Coccidioidomycosis, paracoccidioidomycosis and infections due to *Penicillium marneffei*)
Opportunist infections
Deep or systemic candidosis
Aspergillosis
Cryptococcosis
Others, e.g. *Fusarium*, *Trichosporon* infections

Superficial mycoses

Superficial infections caused by fungi are common in all environments, but are more prevalent in tropical climates. Climate, humidity of the skin surface and the Pco_2 concentration may all affect the expression of these diseases. The main superficial infections are dermatophytosis or ringworm (Verhagen, 1973), superficial candidosis (Samaranayake & MacFarlane, 1990) and pityriasis (tinea) versicolor. However, other conditions such as foot infections caused by *Scytalidium dimidiatum* as well as the hair shaft infections, white and black piedra, and tinea nigra are also seen. *Scytalidium* infections, in particular, are common although frequently they pass unrecognized in the tropics. Otomycosis, a superficial fungal infection of the external auditory meatus, is also common. The superficial mycoses affecting the skin are discussed in detail in Chapter 93.

Subcutaneous mycoses

Subcutaneous fungal infections are sporadic diseases which are mainly confined to the tropics and subtropics. These infections are generally caused by direct introduction of organisms through the skin into the dermis or subcutaneous tissues and for this reason they are often called 'mycoses of implantation'.

Mycetoma

Mycetoma (madura foot) is a chronic subcutaneous infection caused by actinomycetes (actinomycetomas) or fungi (eumycetomas). The organisms form into aggregates (or grains) which are surrounded by foci of acute inflammation, leading to the development of draining sinuses opening onto the overlying skin (Mahgoub & Murray, 1973). Mycetomas have been described from all over Africa but Sudan, Senegal and parts of South Africa appear to have the highest incidences. The main causes of mycetoma seen throughout the continent are shown in Table 55.2. In most African countries *Madurella mycetomatis* is the most common cause. The colour of grains provides a clue to the diagnosis and can, in many instances, serve to distinguish between the more readily treatable actinomycetomas and the eumycetomas (Mariat et al., 1973).

Table 55.2. Mycetomas in Africa

Organism	Fungus or actinomycete	Grain colour	Geography
Madurella mycetomatis	Fungus	Brown	Throughout Africa
Leptosphaeria senegalensis	Fungus	Brown	Around Sahara
Exophiala jeanselemi	Fungus	Brown	Locally rare
Pyrenochaeta romeroi	Fungus	Brown	Locally rare
Scedosporium apiospermum	Fungus	White/yellow	Locally rare
Streptomyces somaliensis	Actino	White/yellow	Around Sahara
Actinomadura madurae	Actino	White/yellow	Sudan, East Africa
A.pelletieri	Actino	Red	Locally rare
Nocardia species	Actino	Not seen	Locally rare

Individual cases caused by other agents such as *Aspergillus nidulans*, *Acremonium* or *Fusarium* species are occasionally found in Africa.

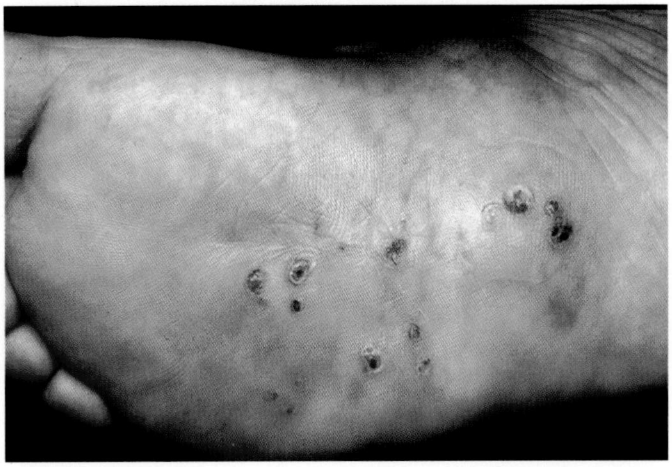

Fig. 55.1. Mycetoma due to *Madurella mycetomatis* involving the foot.

Clinical features

Mycetoma usually occurs on exposed sites, e.g. feet or hands, and is more common in males than females (Mahe et al., 1996). It affects otherwise healthy individuals. Infection follows implantation of plant material, e.g. a thorn, or soil, often years before clinical presentation. The earliest sign of a mycetoma is a small symptomless subcutaneous nodule (Fahal et al., 1998). Later sinuses appear on its upper surface (Fig 55.1). Chronically discharging sinuses may be formed in well-established lesions. Radiological changes include cortical thinning or hypertrophy, periosteal proliferation and lytic lesions.

Laboratory diagnosis

Confirming the diagnosis depends on extracting grains (Palestine & Rogers, 1983), which are often to be found in new sinuses where there is a small collection of pus beneath the skin surface, using a sterile needle. Once removed grains can be examined with direct microscopy or submitted for culture and histopathology. All organisms producing dark or black grains are fungi, whereas red grains are only produced by actinomycetes. In addition direct microscopy of grains in 10–20 per cent KOH may serve to separate fungi from actinomycetes (Fig. 55.2). The hyphal elements can be seen under ×40 magnification and if no filaments can be seen the organisms are likely to be actinomycetes. The simple process of direct microscopy can thereby lead to a decision on treatment before cultures or histopathology are available. The histopathological appearances are sometimes typical of each organism even in haematoxylin and eosin

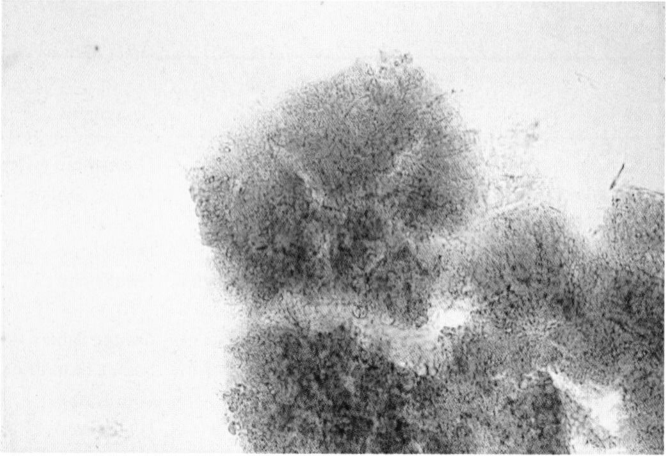

Fig. 55.2. Black grain (direct microscopy in 10% potassium hydroxide).

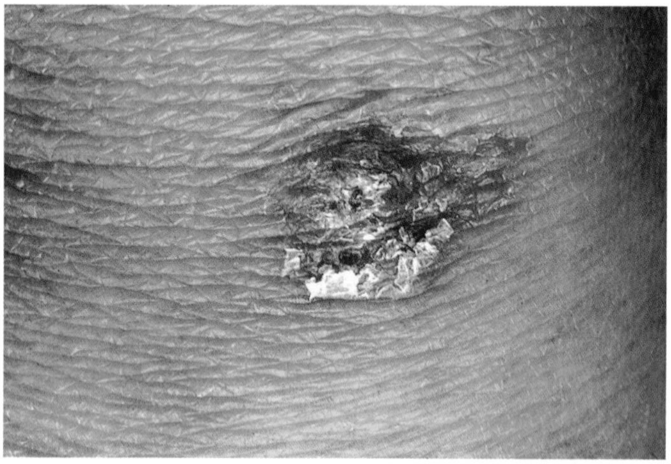

Fig. 55.3. Chromoblastomycosis showing verrucous and plaque-like changes.

(HE) stained sections. Grains can be cultured on a variety of media and the appearances of the fungi or actinomycetes isolated is typical, although their identification requires a specialist laboratory (McGinnins, 1996).

Management

The treatment of actinomycetoma (Mahgoub, 1976; Palestine & Rogers, 1983) includes a variety of antibiotics such as sulphonamides and sulphones or cotrimoxazole plus rifampicin or even streptomycin. Two drugs are given for at least 3 months and then the primary antibiotic is continued. Alternative antibiotics include amikacin, ciprofloxacin and imipenem for difficult cases. The response rates are variable but generally over 80 per cent should respond. Infections due to *Streptomyces somaliensis* are often difficult to eradicate.

Medical treatment of eumycetomas is notoriously difficult. About 40–50 per cent of infections due to *Madurella mycetomatis* respond to ketoconazole 200–400 mg daily. Although surgery remains an option, the most effective surgical approach is amputation. However, any decision should be taken with great care if the patient is not incapacitated by the infection, which is often the case, as removal of a limb severely restricts ability to earn a living. The long-term use of some antifungals such as itraconazole, terbinafine or griseofulvin may slow the disease process, allowing the patient to continue to earn a livelihood, and is an alternative option.

Initiating treatment for mycetoma (Box)

Obtain grains from sinuses and determine by colour and size of filaments whether this is due to fungus or bacteria. In Africa the commonest cause of dark grains is *Madurella mycetomatis*

If fungal (eumycetoma)	If bacterial (actinomycetoma)
Initial treatment. Try ketoconazole 400 mg daily – alternatives griseofulvin, itraconazole	Initial treatment – rifampicin plus cotrimoxazole. Alternatives streptomycin plus dapsone.

Chromoblastomycosis

Chromoblastomycosis (chromomycosis) is a chronic infection caused by pigmented fungi which form into specialized cells, muriform or sclerotic cells, in tissue (Bayles, 1989; Elgart, 1996). The main causes are *Fonsecaea pedrosoi, Cladophialophora carrionii* and *Phialophora verrucosa*. The organisms which cause this infection are found in the natural environment in plant debris or forest detritus. The disease is most prevalent on the east coast of southern Africa, and Madagascar (Esterre et al., 1997) but can occur elsewhere in the continent.

Clinical features

The early lesions are small nodules or papules which slowly enlarge (Banks, 1985; Esterre, 1996).They become raised and warty and adjacent nodules amalgamate to form a complex of hypertrophic growth or plaques with central atrophy (Fig. 55.3). Long-standing lesions can cause considerable deformity mimicking elephantiasis and, rarely, squamous carcinomas can develop in the site of infection. The hands and feet are the main sites affected.

Laboratory diagnosis

Chromoblastomycosis can be diagnosed by direct microscopy, histopathology and culture. The pigmented muriform cells with transverse septa can be seen in potassium hydroxide-treated scrapings from the surface of lesions or histology of biopsy material; their presence is diagnostic. Although the organisms grow readily on conventional mycological media they are black moulds which are difficult to identify. At present identification of the species of fungal agent does not provide any additional information of use in the management of individual cases.

Management

The commonly used drugs are itraconazole (100–400 mg daily), terbinafine 250 mg daily or flucytosine 150 mg/kg; the latter dose is for a patient with normal renal function. Thiabendazole is an alternative. A combination of flucytosine and itraconazole or even amphotericin B is probably most successful in late and extensive cases. A further approach to therapy is the use of local heat applied from heat-retaining gels or pocket hand-warmers. While early lesions can be treated completely with chemotherapy, it is less successful in extensive or late cases. It is also important to biopsy areas of lesions which show rapid or exuberant growth in view of the risk of squamous carcinoma.

Sporotrichosis

Sporotrichosis (de Albornoz, 1989), the infection caused by the dimorphic fungal pathogen *Sporothrix schenckii,* occurs throughout Africa but is usually sporadic, and not common (Vismer & Hull, 1997). In South Africa contamination of pit props has been associated with infection in mine workers (Quintal, 2000).

Clinical features

The main forms of cutaneous sporotrichosis (Kauffman 1999) are:

- the fixed type, which presents with solitary ulcerated granulomas on exposed sites, including the face
- the lymphangitic type, where a primary nodule or ulcer is followed by secondary nodular lesions along the course of local lymphatics.

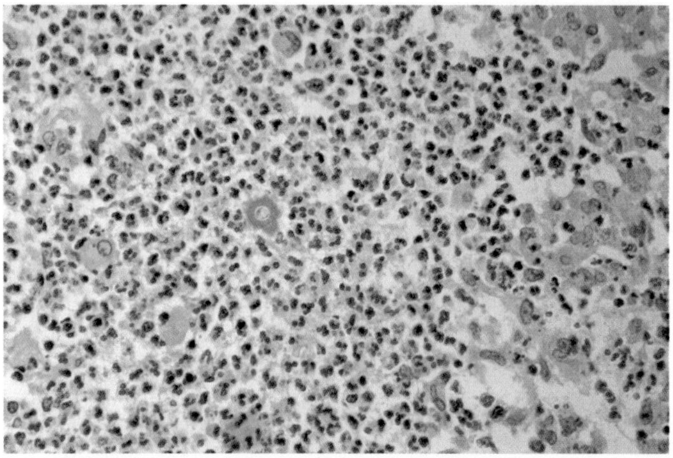

Fig. 55. 4. Cutaneous sporotrichosis. High power view of skin showing an abscess, the centre of which contains a round yeast form of fungus surrounded by pink material. (H&E stain) (by Courtesy of the Wellcome Trust.)

Other forms of infection may mimic chronic leg ulcers and lupus vulgaris. Disseminated deep lesions of sporotrichosis may affect other body sites such as the joints, lungs and meninges (Brian & Strom, 1978). In patients with AIDS these infections may spread to involve multiple skin sites with large numbers of ulcers or nodules (Bibler et al., 1986).

The differential diagnosis of the lymphangitic type includes *Mycobacterium marinum* infection and cutaneous leishmaniasis.

Laboratory diagnosis

In contrast to the other subcutaneous mycoses, culture from biopsies or curettings is the best way of confirming the diagnosis of sporotrichosis. *Sporothrix schenckii* grows well on Sabouraud's agar and forms characteristic spores (Kauffman, 1999). The histopathology shows a mixed granulomatous and polymorphonuclear response (Fig. 55.4). Organisms are scattered very sparsely in this infiltrate and may be absent, although some are surrounded by a refractile eosinophilic halo called an asteroid body.

Management

The main treatment for sporotrichosis is potassium iodide made up in a saturated solution. The starting dose is 1–2 ml given three times daily and increased drop by drop to a maximum of 4–6 ml three times a day. The slow increase is necessary because of the unpleasant taste and the possibility of symptoms of iodism: nausea, dry mouth, altered taste, swollen salivary glands. The normal duration of therapy is at least 2 months and often up to 4 months. Alternatives are itraconazole in doses of 100–200 mg daily or terbinafine 250 mg daily. Both are highly effective but it is not possible to reduce the duration of therapy using these anti-fungal drugs.

Differential diagnosis of nodules spreading along the course of a lymphatic (Box)

Sporotrichosis	Mycobacterial infection	Cutaneous leishmaniasis
Nodules are often soft and may ulcerate. Rarely a history of injury but patient may be handling plant materials	Patient usually has a history of contact with fish – either in a tank, at sea or in artificial lakes. Usual cause *Mycobacterium marinum*	Uncommon on feet. May recall insect bite.

Value of laboratory diagnostic measures in subcutaneous fungal infections

	Mycetoma	Chromoblastomycosis	Sporotrichosis
Direct microscopy	Very useful – can provide information on diagnosis and treatment options	Very useful and diagnostic	Rarely helpful – few organisms
Culture	Useful – but difficult to identify	Difficult to identify	Best method of confirming diagnosis
Histology	Very useful – cannot always identify the cause	Very useful	Often not helpful – few organisms
Serology	There are no commercially available serodiagnostic kits		

Subcutaneous zygomycosis

Subcutaneous zygomycosis due to *Conidiobolus* (conidiobolomycosis, rhinoentomophthoromycosis) is uncommon (Baker et al., 1962) but is found in different tropical areas of Africa. The causative organism is usually *C. coronatus*. The focus of infection is within the nasal cavity and the infection spreads from the inferior turbinates to involve the subcutaneous tissues of the face and neck with a hard painless swelling. The deformity may be grotesque (Fig. 55.5). This infection is seen mainly in adults. Subcutaneous zygomycosis is also caused by *Basidiobolus* (subcutaneous phycomycosis, basidiobolomycosis). The usual cause of this infection is *B. haptosporus*. The site of infection is usually confined to the limb girdles or proximal limbs. It is mainly seen in Central, East and West Africa and chiefly affects children. The swelling is deforming and has a woody consistency.

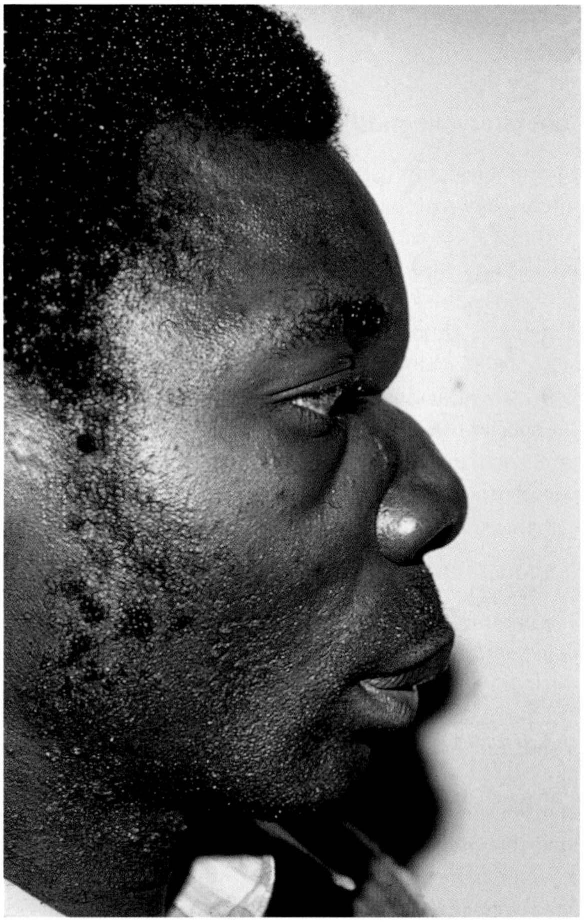

Fig. 55.5. Subcutaneous zygomycosis due to *Conidiobolus coronatus*.

The treatment of both diseases is either itraconazole or ketoconazole, although saturated potassium iodide solution is an alternative.

Systemic mycoses

The systemic mycoses are infections caused by fungi which have the capacity to invade deep organs. In some cases the entry point is through the respiratory tract from where the infection can spread to other sites. In other cases the organisms gain direct entry to the blood stream, for example through an intravenous cannula or through skin. Some, often referred to as the endemic mycoses, affect both healthy and immunocompromised individuals, while others are opportunistic infections which occur in patients with some underlying predisposition. The endemic mycoses are not common in Africa, but African or large form histoplasmosis is only found in Africa. Some of the other systemic mycoses, notably cryptococcosis, nocardiosis and histoplasmosis are particularly associated with AIDS.

Endemic systemic mycoses

The main endemic mycoses are histoplasmosis (small and large forms), and blastomycosis. The usual route of entry of these organisms is the lung, although direct implantation into the skin is also possible. The majority of people exposed to infection are merely sensitized to the organism and develop delayed-type hypersensitivity to the fungus, detected on intradermal testing with an appropriate antigen. However, localized pulmonary and disseminated forms also occur.

Different clinical forms of endemic systemic mycoses

- Asymptomatic – patients develop positive skin test (DTH)
- acute pulmonary – usually follows massive exposure to organisms – symptoms suggestive of immune complex disease, e,g, arthritis, uveitis
- chronic pulmonary – either lung nodules (inactive) or progressive inflammation or cavitation (active)
- disseminated – spread outside lung. Rapid extrapulmonary spread may be associated with immunological impairment, e.g. AIDS
- primary cutaneous – infection acquired by inoculation, e.g. in laboratory.

Histoplasmosis

The classification of human histoplasmosis is complicated by the existence of two different variants caused by *Histoplasma* species which are culturally, but not genetically, indistinguishable. Both show distinct clinical features and both occur in Africa.

The first, sometimes called classical or small form histoplasmosis, is caused by *H. capsulatum* var. *capsulatum* (Goodwin et al., 1981). This is a dimorphic fungus which, at room temperature, produces chains of cells or hyphae; but in tissue or at higher temperatures, or in naturally occurring or experimental infections, forms single cells or yeasts. The disease is endemic throughout much of the world, with the exception of Europe, and presents with pulmonary and disseminated infection affecting the lungs, reticuloendothelial system and mucosal surfaces. The yeast forms seen in tissue are small (2–4 μm in diameter).

The second form, African or large-form histoplasmosis, caused by *H. capsulatum* var. *duboisii*, only occurs in Africa (Drouhet, 1989; Cockshott & Lucas, 1968). The yeasts found in tissue are large (12–20 μm) and are often located in giant cells. The main signs of infection follow dissemination to lymph nodes, skin and bones. The organisms isolated from both are identical in culture and are regarded as variants of a single species, *H. capsulatum*.

Histoplasmosis (classical or small form histoplasmosis)

Histoplasmosis is an infection caused by the dimorphic fungus, *H. capsulatum* var. *capsulatum*. The organism can be found in soil but is most easily isolated from areas where large numbers of birds or bats have roosted, including barns, caves and under the eaves of houses. The endemic areas include parts of the USA, West Indies, Central and South America, Africa, India and the Far East. The prevalence of exposure is best estimated by skin testing. There have been few such studies in Africa and where this has been done, e.g. Kenya, usually fewer than 20 per cent of the population are positive. Skin testing does not distinguish between exposure to classical and African histoplasmosis.

It is thought that the excreta of birds and bats provides the necessary conditions for growth of organisms present in the environment, although bats may be infected as well. Exposure in man is usually sporadic, although occasionally the disease occurs in clusters suggesting exposure to a common source such as a cave. Defence against *H. capsulatum* is largely mediated by T-lymphocytes. The infection may therefore be prolonged or widely disseminated in individuals with defective T-lymphocyte-mediated responses, including patients with AIDS.

Clinical features

The majority of patients who acquire histoplasmosis remain asymptomatic, the only sign of past exposure being a positive intradermal histoplasmin test which is read after 48 hours. Some exposed individuals develop a localized pulmonary nodule which remains asymptomatic but may be detected by X-ray or CT scan.

The acute pulmonary form of histoplasmosis often follows exposure to a site such as a cave containing large numbers of *Histoplasma* spores. Patients develop an acute febrile illness 10–14 days after exposure. There is cough, chest pain, joint pains and, in some cases, a skin rash such as erythema multiforme. Radiologically, there is often diffuse mottling of the lung fields and in some cases hilar enlargement. Normally, spontaneous recovery occurs and no specific treatment is given. However, rarely in some patients the disease progresses directly from this primary infection and dissemination to other organs occurs.

In chronic pulmonary disease there is focal consolidation and cavitation, usually affecting one or both apices and these can be detected on X-ray or CT scan. The pattern of infection closely resembles pulmonary tuberculosis. The main symptoms, such as cough, chest pain and haemoptysis, are also similar. In the early stages there may be partial recovery but later in established cases there is slow progression of the inflammatory mass which can encroach on other lung areas. This form of histoplasmosis is not often seen in Africa.

Acute disseminated histoplasmosis is often widely spread and affects the bone marrow and lymph glands as well as the liver and spleen (Goodwin et al., 1980). Patients present with fever, weight loss, malaise and hepatosplenomegaly. There may be evidence of bruising and purpura. Diffuse pulmonary infiltrates and small skin papules and ulcers can also occur. This type of histoplasmosis will progress to death unless treated. Acute forms of disseminated histoplasmosis are seen in patients with AIDS (Barton et al., 1984; Manfredi et al., 1984). In the latter groups the symptoms may be non-specific (weight loss and fever), although some clues such as hepatosplenomegaly or multiple skin lesions (nodules, papules, ulcers) may be seen. A more chronic type of disseminated histoplasmosis is seen in otherwise healthy individuals. These patients usually present with either oral ulceration or hypoadrenalism. Chronic disseminated histoplasmosis may present years after the patient has left an endemic area. The oral ulcers are persistent and painful. Laryngeal involvement, meningitis and endocarditis can also occur.

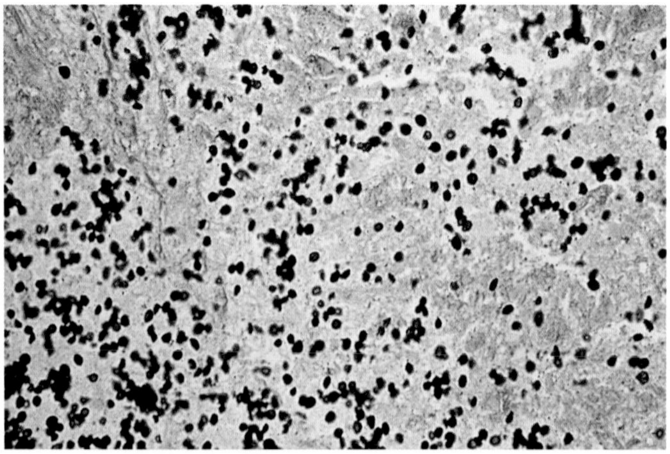

Fig. 55.6. Histoplasmosis – scattered yeasts in a lung biopsy (×240) Methenamine silver stain.

Laboratory diagnosis

The organisms of *H. capsulatum* are very small and difficult to visualize by direct microscopy, but they can sometimes be seen in bone marrow or blood smears stained with Giemsa stain. Very rarely small forms of either *Blastomyces* or *Cryptococcus* may be mistaken for *Histoplasma*. *H. capsulatum* can be grown readily from sputum or other sources such as bone marrow in appropriate cases. Blood cultures are sometimes positive in patients with AIDS.

The organisms grow as moulds at room temperature and have to be converted into yeast phase at 37 °C. As this process is slow a more rapid test involving the detection of antigen leached from culture plates flooded overnight with sterile medium, the exoantigen test, is available. Serology has a useful role in diagnosis. New tests of particular value in patients with AIDS have been developed for the detection of circulating *Histoplasma* antigen, either cell wall polysaccharide or a cytoplasmic glycoprotein, but are not widely available. Histopathology is also useful in diagnosis. The organisms of *Histoplasma capsulatum* are small oval yeasts up to 5 μm in diameter (Fig. 55.6). They are usually found intracellularly in macrophages.

Management

Asymptomatic histoplasmosis does not require therapy. Anti-fungal therapy is also usually withheld in acute pulmonary forms (Lortholary et al., 1999), although supportive treatment such as bed-rest and fluids may be given where necessary. The true value of anti-fungal drugs in acute pulmonary disease is not known, although itraconazole would be a possible choice. Chronic pulmonary histoplasmosis and chronic disseminated histoplasmosis are usually treated with either ketoconazole or itraconazole.

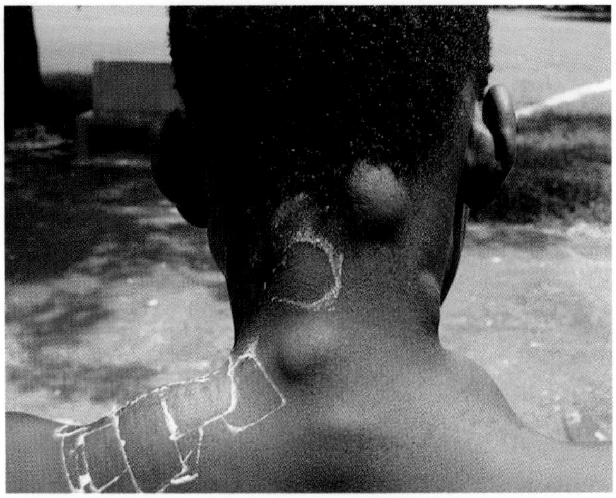

Fig. 55.7. African histoplasmosis – lymph node involvement (copyright D. Mabey).

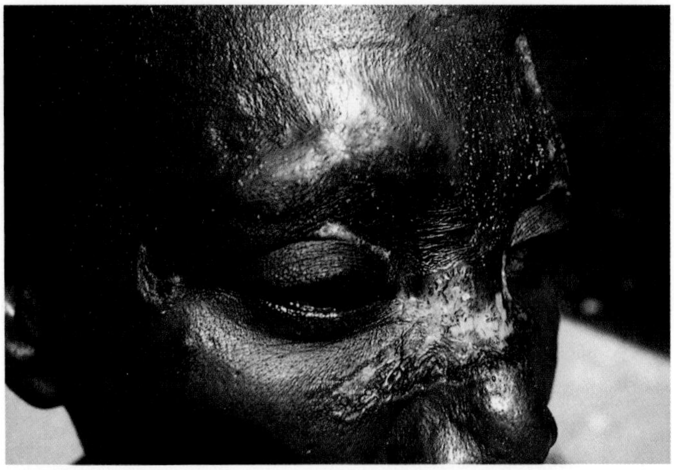

Fig. 55.8. African histoplasmosis – extensive local skin lesion (copyright D. Mabey).

Fluconazole is also active in this infection but it has not been compared with itraconazole.

Itraconazole (200–400 mg daily) can also be given in more rapidly disseminating types of infection. An alternative is amphotericin B (0.6–1.0 mg/kg intravenous daily) in the disseminated types. Amphotericin B is also appropriate in the first stage of treatment of AIDS patients, i.e. for an initial 2–3 weeks. Thereafter it is necessary to use long-term suppressive therapy with itraconazole after induction of remission, otherwise relapse will occur. There is some evidence to suggest that long-term suppressive treatment may not be necessary if patients are receiving highly active antiretroviral therapy (HAART).

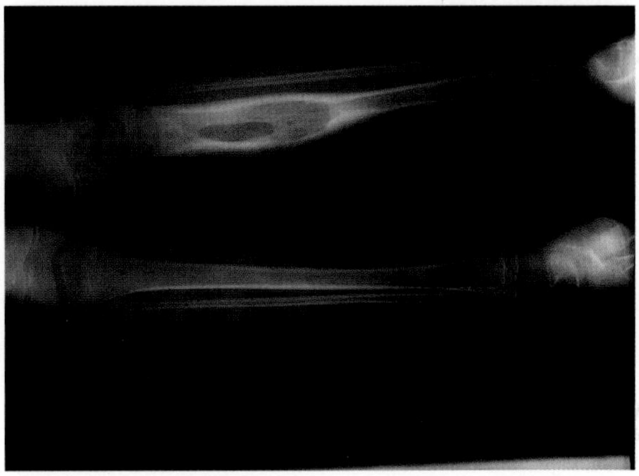

Fig. 55.9. African histoplasmosis – osteomyelitis of the tibia (copyright D. Mabey).

African histoplasmosis

African histoplasmosis, as the name suggests, is confined to Africa. It is caused by *H. capsulatum* var. *duboisii*, which resembles the other small form variant but develops into larger yeasts in tissue. The infection is not common but occurs sporadically in Central and West Africa, south of the Sahara and north of the Zambezi river. The natural source of this fungus is unknown. It is thought that, as with the other type of histoplasmosis, invasive spores gain entry through the lungs.

The patient usually presents with focal extra-pulmonary disease affecting the skin, bone or a lymph gland (Figs 55.7, 55.8, 55.9) (Cockshott & Lucas, 1968). Subcutaneous 'cold abscesses' may be seen (Fig. 55.10). Alternatively multiple sites may be affected, including the gastrointestinal tract, lungs and other mucosal surfaces (Sanguino et al., 1996). This form is more rapidly progressive.

African histoplasmosis is diagnosed by the presence of large oval yeasts (8–14 μm) seen by direct microscopy or histopathological examination of biopsied lesions. The organism can be isolated in culture (see above). Conventional histoplasma serology is generally negative. Unlike small form histoplasmosis, African histoplasmosis is not often seen in AIDS patients.

The main treatments are itraconazole, ketoconazole or amphotericin B. Sulphonamides have also been used in some cases where there has been limited spread.

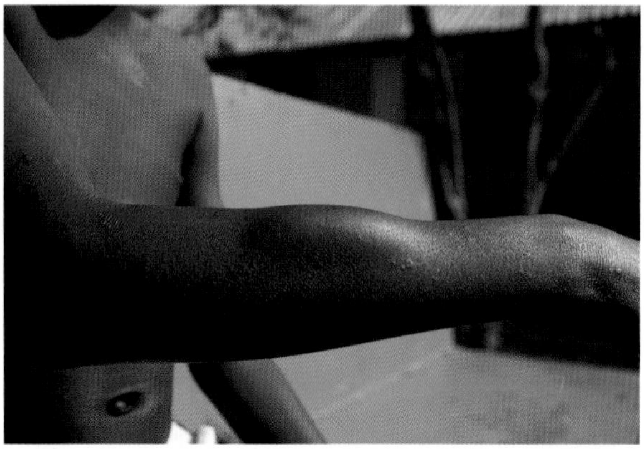

Fig. 55.10. African histoplasmosis – subcutaneous cold abscess (copyright D. Mabey).

Blastomycosis

Blastomycosis is a systemic fungal infection caused by *Blastomyces dermatitidis*, a dimorphic pathogen (Sarosi & Davies, 1979). The disease is mainly found in the USA and Canada but cases have also been seen in Africa, India and the Middle East. As with histoplasmosis the main portal of entry is via the respiratory tract. *Blastomyces dermatitidis* has only occasionally been isolated from the natural environment, usually in North America and in sites where there is a risk of flooding, such as river banks (Klein et al., 1986). The organism has not been isolated from such sources in Africa and its ecological niche there is unknown. Cases have been described in a variety of African countries from the north coast (e.g. Algeria) to Namibia (Emerson et al., 1984). The largest number of cases have been seen in Zimbabwe. In Africa the principal signs of the disease are those of disseminated infection affecting the bone or skin.

Clinical features

The clinical features of infection are similar to those of histoplasmosis. The chronic pulmonary type of blastomycosis presents with focal consolidation and cavitation in the chest with symptoms of cough, fever and weight loss. This may be confused radiologically with pulmonary tuberculosis. Unlike histoplasmosis this may co-exist with disseminated lesions of blastomycosis. The main sites of dissemination are the skin and bones. Skin lesions may be ulcers, cold abscesses, granulomas or crusted plaques which heal with scar formation. The bones involved are principally axial skeletal bones, such as vertebrae, and spinal cord compression may occur. Dissemination also occurs in the immunocompromised patient (Recht et al., 1982).

Laboratory diagnosis

The diagnosis is based on direct microscopy of smears taken from suitable sites as well as sputum and culture. *B. dermatitidis* is a dimorphic fungus which grows as a mould at room temperature but as a yeast at 37 °C. Histological changes of blastomycosis are typical as the yeasts bud on a characteristic broad-base. Serological tests are not widely available.

Management

Blastomycosis is treated with either itraconazole (200–400 mg daily) or ketoconazole (200–400 mg daily). Intravenous amphotericin B is an alternative (0.6–1.0 mg/kg daily).

Diagnosis of yeasts in tissue sections (Box)

Feature	Organism
Capsule present (Mucicarmine stain)	*Cryptococcus*
Small round to oval yeasts in macrophages	*Histoplasma capsulatum* – rarely small forms of *Cryptococcus* or *Blastomyces* can mimic
Yeasts with large broad-based budding	*Blastomyces*
Medium-sized yeasts in giant cells	*Histoplasma duboisii* (rarely *Blastomyces)*
Yeasts plus hyphae	*Candida albicans*

Systemic opportunistic pathogens

In industrialized countries opportunistic fungi are a major problem in severely ill patients (Hay, 1989; Warnock & Richardson, 1989), particularly those with neutropenia and those receiving solid organ or bone marrow transplants. They are also seen in intensive care units. In addition to these, some infections such as cryptococcosis occur in patients with AIDS. In Africa less attention has been paid to opportunists such as candidosis and aspergillosis; by contrast, cryptococcosis is recognized to be a common and increasingly important problem everywhere.

Aspergillosis is a disease caused by species of the genus *Aspergillus*, principally *A. fumigatus*, *A. flavus* and *A. niger*. There are a number of different clinical syndromes caused by these fungi which occur in both temperate and tropical climates (Rowe-Jones, 1992). A form of aspergillosis seen regularly in Africa is the development of a fungus ball in patients with pre-existing pulmonary cavitation, usually secondary to tuberculosis. This colonizing ball may elicit an inflammatory response and in a minority of patients (15%) causes haemoptysis, which may be severe enough to be life-threatening.

A slowly progressive form of aspergillosis seen in Africa is invasive paranasal *Aspergillus* granuloma (Veress et al., 1973), affecting the sinuses, orbit and brain. It is seen mainly in East Africa, e.g. particularly Sudan, and the Middle East and, in most patients, is caused by *A. flavus*. The patient presents with headache, nasal obstruction and orbital swelling with, in some cases, proptosis. In later stages invasion of the brain may ensue. On radiography a mass can be seen in the maxillary or ethmoid sinsuses with erosion of the bones of the base of the skull and orbit. These changes can be confirmed with computerized tomography. The main histological change is a hard progressive granulomatous mass with fibrosis. Scattered and atypical fungal fragments can be seen within giant cells, using a methenamine silver or periodic acid Schiff stain, and the organism can be isolated in culture. Serology (immunodiffusion) is often positive.

The main treatment for paranasal *Aspergillus* granuloma is surgical removal of as much of the tumour as is possible, followed by long-term therapy with itraconazole (200–400 mg daily). This may have to be extended for 6–24 months and, if available, serology is a helpful way of monitoring. An alternative therapeutic option is amphotericin B but long-term therapy is not possible with this drug.

Mucormycosis

Fungi belonging to the genera *Absidia, Rhizopus* and *Rhizomucor*, and less commonly other groups, may cause an aggressive paranasal, pulmonary or disseminated infection in predisposed groups such as diabetic or neutropenic patients (Bahadur et al., 1983). This infection, known as mucormycosis, is seen in temperate as well as tropical countries and may be rapidly fatal unless there is prompt surgical intervention and treatment with intravenous amphotericin B. It may also present with orbital cellulitis or as a necrotizing wound infection. In malnourished children it may cause a necrotizing gastrointestinal infection. Treatment with amphotericin B combined, where possible, with surgical debridement offers the best chance of recovery. The new lipid associated amphotericins (liposomal, or in colloidal dispersion) are particularly useful in such cases as they can be given in high doses without compromising renal function, but are very expensive.

Cryptococcosis

Cryptococcosis is the systemic infection caused by an encapsulated yeast, *Cryptococcus neoformans*. Its distribution is worldwide and it generally presents with meningitis or some other manifestation of extrapulmonary dissemination. While it may cause disease in otherwise healthy individuals, it is also a pathogen of patients with defective T-lymphocyte function, such as those with AIDS, lymphoma or patients receiving corticosteroid therapy. In many countries it is the commonest systemic fungal infection in AIDS patients (Table 55.3).

There are two variants of *C. neoformans: C. neoformans* var. *neoformans* and *C. neoformans* var. *gattii*. (Bennett et al., 1977; Boekhout et al., 1997). The *neoformans* variety causes disease in immunocompromised patients including those with AIDS (Dupont, 1989), and is found in most countries. Its ecological niche appears to be soil or areas where there are large amounts of pigeon excreta, from which this fungus can be isolated. The presumed route of entry is via inhalation. The *gattii* form is seen mainly in tropical areas in otherwise healthy individuals. It has been reported from Africa (Odhiambo et al., 1983), the Far East, Papua New Guinea and Australia.

There is evidence, from the use of experimental skin test reagents, that subclinical exposure may occur in the general population, as with other systemic mycoses such as histoplasmosis. Infection rates in the tropics are not known. In Zaire about 12 per cent of those with AIDS were found to have circulating cryptococcal antigen (Swinne & de Vroey, 1982), indicating active infection, and cryptococcal infection is also common in Zambia. However, in AIDS patients in Ghana the incidence is lower (Frimpong & Lartey 1997).

Clinical features

Cryptococcal infection may present with respiratory signs and symptoms-cough, chest pain and fever. However, pulmonary lesions are more often present as an incidental (Domoua et al., 1997), and symptomless, finding in a

Table 55.3. Cryptococcosis in Africa – differences between AIDS and non-AIDS patients

	AIDS	Non-AIDS
Organism	*C.neoformans* var *neoformans*	*C.neoformans* var *gattii* in many
Pulmonary lesions	Present in many cases	Common – may present with large areas of consolidation
Blood cultures	Often positive	Rarely positive
Serology	Higher titres in serum than CSF	In the presence of meningitis higher titres in CSF than serum
Antigen titres	Often higher than 1: 1000	Usually less than 1:100
Treatment	Initial treatment with amphotericin B ± flucytosine followed by long-term suppression with fluconazole	Most: amphotericin B + flucytosine. Isolated cutaneous forms – fluconazole

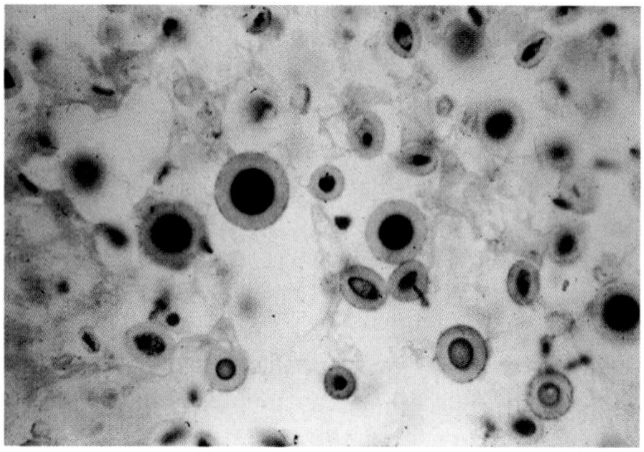

Fig. 55.11. *Crypococcus neoformans:* high power view of a CSF preparation encapsulated yeast organism, India-ink stain. (Courtesy of the Wellcome Trust.)

patient with other manifestations of cryptococcosis. The main clinical form of this infection in the non-AIDS patient is meningitis, although headache and neck stiffness may not be severe; but other signs such as confusion, drowsiness, photophobia and cranial nerve palsies may be seen. Other signs of dissemination such as papular or ulcerative skin lesions, lytic bone deposits and prostatitis may be found. In patients with AIDS the symptoms of meningitis are often minimal and fever may be the main clinical sign of infection, together with headache, malaise and tiredness. Skin lesions occur in about 15 per cent of patients and range in clinical appearance from small umbilicated papules to ulcers, abscesses and cellulitis.

Laboratory diagnosis

The laboratory diagnosis of cryptococcosis depends on the demonstration of the organism(s) by staining smears, CSF or sputum with Indian ink or nigrosin (Odhiambo et al., 1997). The capsule surrounding the organism displaces the particles in these dense stains leaving a clear halo around a central fungal cell (Fig 55.11): this is typical of *Cryptococcus.* The organism can be cultured readily on conventional mycological media such as Sabouraud's agar, although it may take 3–12 days for the yeasts to be recognizable. Sources of culture material include: CSF, sputum and biopsies. In patients with AIDS, blood cultures may also be positive.

The quickest method of diagnosis is the antigen detection test, using antibody-sensitized latex particles or an ELISA. It is used to detect capsular antigen in serum or CSF. The test is specific and gives a positive result in 30 minutes. It can also be used to follow the course of therapy. Biopsy material shows the large yeast cells using periodic acid-Schiff or Grocott stains; the mucicarmine stain is specific for the cryptococcal capsular polysaccharide, which it stains pink.

The main therapy in the non-AIDS patient is a combination of intravenous amphotericin B (0.4–0.8 mg/kg daily) and flucytosine (120–150 mg/kg daily divided in four doses). The response in most patients is good but therapy may have to be continued for 4–6 weeks, and sometimes longer. The treatment of the AIDS patient is more complex. Few treatments can produce permanent recovery and the usual strategy is to start with a period of induction therapy followed by long-term suppression to prevent relapse. The most frequent choice is an initial period of amphotericin (0.4–0.8 mg/kg daily), with or without flucytosine, for 2 weeks, followed by long-term daily suppressive therapy with fluconazole (200–400 mg) or itraconazole (200–300 mg). Fluconazole may also be used to produce remission on its own, although the correct dose is not clearly established.

Summary of treatment of cryptococcosis in AIDS

- Initiate treatment with **amphotericin** B 0.4–0.8 mg/kg/d ± **flucytosine (5FC)** 120–150 mg/kg/d in four divided doses. Check renal function and full blood

picture through treatment and, if using 5FC, reduce dose if creatinine rises
- Follow initial therapy with **fluconazole** 400 mg daily orally.

References

Bahadur S, Ghosh P, Chopra P et al. (1983). Rhinocerebral phycomycosis. *J Laryngol Otol*; **97**: 267–270.

Baker RD, Seabury JH, Schneidau JD. (1962). Subcutaneous and cutaneous mucormycosis and subcutaneous phycomycosis. *Lab Invest*; **11**: 1091–1102.

Banks IS, Palmieri JR, Lanoie L, Connor DH, Meyers WM. (1985). Chromomycosis in Zaire. *Int J Dermatol*; **24**: 302–307.

Barton EN, Roberts L, Ince WE et al. (1988). Cutaneous histoplasmosis in the acquired immunodeficiency syndrome: a report of three cases from Trinidad. *Trop Geogr Med*; **40**: 153–157.

Bayles MAH. (1989). Chromomycosis. *Baillière's Clin Trop Med Commun Dis*; **4**: 45–70.

Bennett JE, Kwon-Chung KJ, Howard DH. (1977). Epidemiologic differences among serotypes of *Cryptococcus neoformans. Am J Epidermiol*; **10**: 582–586.

Bibler MR, Luber HJ, Clueck HI et al. (1986). Disseminated sporotrichosis in a patient with HIV infection after treatment for acquired factor VIII inhibitor. *J Am Med Assoc*; **256**: 3125–3126.

Boekhout T, van Belkum A, Leenders AC et al. (1997). Molecular typing of *Cryptococcus neoformans*: taxonomic and epidemiological aspects. *Int J Syst Bacteriol*; **47**: 432–442.

Brian M, Strom R. (1978). Multiarticular sporotrichosis. *J Am Med Assoc*; **240**: 556–557.

Cockshott WP, Lucas AO. (1964). *Histoplasmosis duboisii. Quart. J. Med.*; **130**: 223–238.

de Albornoz MCB. (1989). Sporotrichosis. *Baillière's Clin Trop Med Commun Dis*; **4**: 71–96.

Domoua KG, N'Dhatz MN et al. (1994). Pulmonary cryptococcosis: an uncommon opportunistic infection in AIDS on the Ivory Coast. *Rev Pneumol Clin*; **50**: 184–185.

Drouhet E. (1989). African histoplasmosis. *Baillière's Clin Trop Med Commun Dis*; **4**: 221–247.

Dupont B. (1989). Cryptococcosis. *Baillière's Clin Trop Med Commun Dis*; **4**: 113–124.

Elgart GW. (1996). Chromoblastomycosis. *Dermatol Clin*; **14**: 77–83.

Emerson PA, Higgins E, Branfoot A. (1984). North American blastomycosis in Africans. *Br J Dis Chest*; **78**: 286–291.

Esterre P, Andriantsimahavandy A, Ramarcel ER, Pecarrere JL. (1996). Forty years of chromoblastomycosis in Madagascar: a review. *Am J Trop Med Hyg*; **55**: 45–7.

Esterre P, Andriantsimahavandy A, Raharisolo C. (1997). Natural history of chromo-blastomycosis in Madagascar and the Indian Ocean. *Bull Soc Pathol Exot*; **90**: 312–317.

Fahal AH, el Hassan AM, Abdelalla AO, Sheik HE. (1998). Cystic mycetoma: an unusual clinical presentation of Madurella mycetomatis infection. *Trans Roy Soc Trop Med Hyg*; **92**: 66–67.

Frimpong EH, Lartey RA. (1998). Study of the aetiologic agents of meningitis in Kumasi, Ghana, with special reference to *Cryptococcal neoformans. E Af Med J*; **75**: 516–519.

Goodwin RA, Shapiro JL, Thurman GH et al. (1980). Disseminated histoplasmosis. *Medicine*; **59**: 1–33.

Goodwin RA, Loyd JE, DesPrez RM. (1981). Histoplasmosis in normal hosts. *Medicine*; **60**: 231–266.

Hay RJ. (1989). Opportunistic fungal infection in the tropics. *Ballière's Clin Trop Med Commun Dis*; **4**: 249–267.

Kauffman CA. (1999). Sporotrichosis. *Clin Infect Dis*. **29**: 231–236.

Klein BS, Vergeront JM, Weeks RJ et al. (1986). Isolation of *Blastomyces dermatitidis* in soil associated with a large outbreak of blastomycosis in Wisconsin. *N Engl J Med*; **314**: 529–534.

Lortholary O. Denning DW, Dupont B. (1999). Endemic mycoses: a treatment update. *J Antimicrob Chemother*; **43**: 321–331.

McGinnis MR. (1996). Mycetoma. *Dermatol Clin*; **14**: 97–104.

Mahe A, Develoux M, Lienhardt C, Keita S, Bobin P. (1976). Mycetomas in Mali: causative agents and geographic distribution. *Am J Trop Med Hyg*; **54**: 77–79.

Mahgoub ES. (1976). Medical management of mycetoma. *Bull Wld Hlth Org*; **54**: 303–310.

Mahgoub ES, Murray IG. (1973). *Mycetoma*. London: Heinemann.

Manfredi R, Mazzoni A, Nanetti A, Chiodo F. (1994). Histoplasmosis capsulati and duboisii in Europe: the impact of the HIV pandemic, travel and immigration. *Eur J Epidemiol*; **10**: 675–681.

Mariat F, Destombes P, Segretain G. (1977). The mycetomas: clinical features, pathology, etiology and epidemiology. *Contrib Microbiol Immunol*; **4**: 1–39.

Odhiambo FA. Murage EM. Ngare W. Ndinya-Achola JO. (1997). Detection rate of Cryptococcus neoformans in cerebrospinal fluid specimens at Kenyatta National Hospital, Nairobi. *E Afr Med J*; **74**: 576–578.

Palestine RF, Rogers RS. (1982). Diagnosis and treatment of mycetoma. *J Am Acad Dermatol*; **6**: 107–111.

Quintal D. (2000). Sporotrichosis infection on mines of the Witwatersrand. *J Cutan Med Surg*; **4**: 51–54.

Recht LD, Davies SF, Eckman MR et al. (1982). Blastomycosis in immunosuppressed patients. *Am Rev Respir Dis*; **125**: 359–362.

Rowe-Jones J. (1993). Paranasal aspergillosis – a spectrum of disease. *J Laryngol Otol*; **107**: 773–774.

Samaranayake LP, MacFarlane TW (eds). (1990). *Oral Candidosis*. London: Wright.

Sanguino JC, Rodrigues B, Baptista A, Quina M. (1996). Focal lesion of African histoplasmosis presenting as a malignant gastric ulcer. *Hepato-Gastroenterol*; **43**: 771–775.

Sarosi GA, Davies SF. (1979). Blastomycosis. *Am Rev Respir Dis*; **120**: 911–938.

Swinne D, de Vroey C. (1987). Epidémiologie de la cryptococcose. *Rev Iberica Micol*; **4**: 77–83.

Veress B, Malik OA, El Tayeb AA et al. (1973). Further observations on the primary paranasal aspergillus granuloma in the Sudan. *Am J Trop Med Hyg*; **22**: 765–772.

Verhagen AR. (1973). Distribution of dermatophytes causing tinea capitis in Africa. *Trop Geogr Med*; **26**: 101–120.

Vismer HF, Hull PR. (1997). Prevalence, epidemiology and geographical distribution of *Sporothrix schenckii* infections in Gauteng, South Africa. *Mycopathol*; **137**: 137–143.

Warnock D, Richardson MD (eds). (1989). *Fungal Infections in the Compromised Patient.* Chichester: Wiley.

Viruses

56 Measles

The problem in Africa

About 1 million children die of measles each year. The problem is worst in sub-Saharan Africa, which has the highest incidence, the highest mortality and the lowest vaccine coverage in the world.

Massive urban migration and civil wars have swollen cities and refugee camps where mortality from measles due to crowding and intense exposure has risen as high as 30 per cent. The synergistic effect of HIV infection on the spread and severity of measles needs urgent definition.

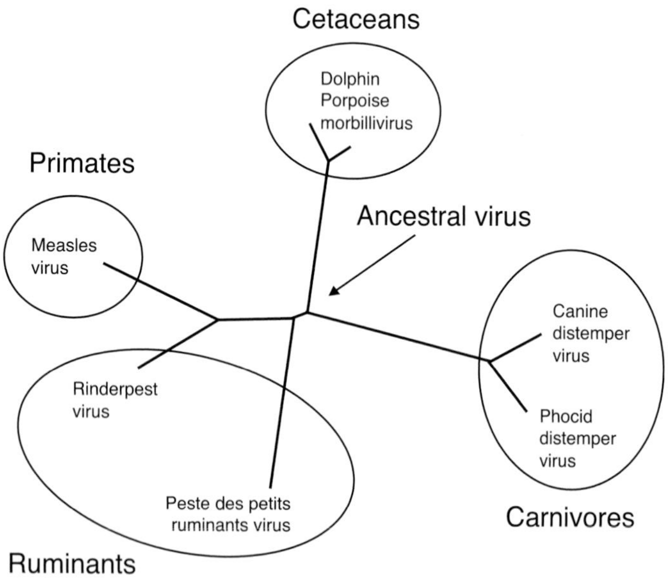

Fig. 56.1. Genetic relationships between morbilliviruses based on comparison of the nucleotide sequence of the N genes. Measles and rinderpest viruses are most closely related. (Barrett, 1999.)

The organism

Measles mainly infects man but may have originated as a zoonosis for it is closely related to animal viruses such as rinderpest and is able to cross species to infect other primates and on occasion dogs (Fig. 56.1). It contains a single strand of RNA, which is highly pleomorphic, ranging from 100 to 300 nm in diameter (Fig 56.2). The virus propagates by budding from the cell membrane, from which it acquires an envelope. The membrane of infected cells and the virion envelope contain two surface glycoproteins, the haemagglutinin (H) and fusion (F) proteins, and a non-glycosylated matrix (M) protein, which forms the inner layer. The H protein, which allows the attachment of the virus to cells, via either the CD_{46} or the CD*w* 150 receptors, is the main target for neutralizing antibodies; the F protein is responsible for fusion and syncytium formation of infected cells.

CD_{46} is a membrane protein, which together with five other proteins, protects cells from complement activation and lysis. The CD_w 150 receptor (also known as the signalling lymphocyte-activator molecule or SLAM) is expressed on immature lymphocytes and on memory T-cells, and is rapidly induced on T- and B-cells after immune activation (Tatsuo et al., 2000). The internal components or nucleocapsid consist of RNA, the nucleoprotein (N), which is the major protein, the phosphoprotein (P) and the large protein (L). The F protein is remarkably stable, the H protein shows minor antigenic variation but the N protein, which contains a variable region in the C terminus, is highly divergent among different strains of virus. Genetic analysis of H and N genes has allowed molecular surveillance of measles virus suggesting that the majority of cases in highly vaccinated countries like the USA are the result of importation of the virus.

Table 56.1. Measles case-fatality rates (CFR) in African communities[a]

	CFR (%)	
	0–4 Years	All ages
Rural		
Guinea Bissau	34	24
Gambia	22	ND[c]
Senegal	20	13
Nigeria	7	ND
Kenya[b]	8	6
Urban		
Guinea Bissau	21	17
Guinea Bissau[b]	15	14
Zaire[b]	6	ND

Notes:
[a] case-fatality rate in hospitalized cases in England was 0.02%.
[b] these partially immunized populations had a lower mortality.
[c] no data.
Source: From Aaby (1988).

Epidemiology

Measles is one of the most infectious of all micro-organisms. Its reproductive rate (*R*o), the average number of new infections originating from an index case, is 15 in unvaccinated populations. Measles tends to occur in epidemics, which originate in rapidly growing cities with high birth and migration rates, and spreads to the countryside (Strebel & Cochi, 2001).

In Africa, measles rivals malaria as a cause of death. It is a droplet-borne infection, which thrives at low humidity (Fig. 56.3). Thus, it spreads during the dry season when Africans are wont to travel, resulting in devastating outbreaks with a peculiarly high morbidity and mortality compared to industrialized countries (Table 56.1). A number of theories have been advanced to explain this phenomenon.

Increased viral virulence

There is no evidence to support this. The virus is relatively stable. Various subtypes have been described according to variation in the nucleoprotein but these do not relate to virulence. When imported from Africa to other countries, the African strains have not caused particularly severe disease.

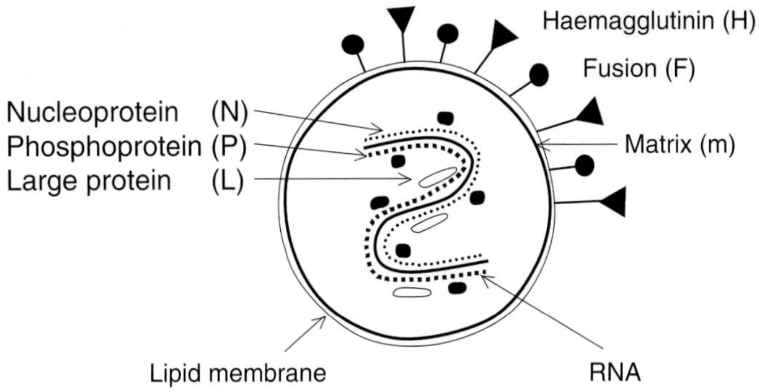

Fig. 56.2. The measles virion and its proteins.

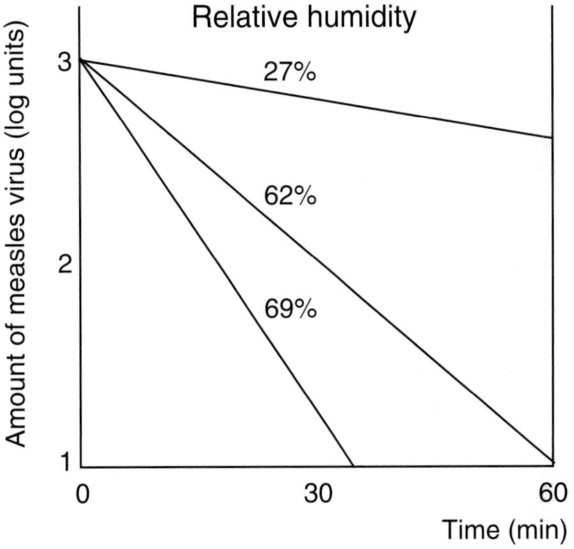

Fig. 56.3. Survival of measles virus in droplets at varying relative humidities of air kept at 20 °C. The virus survives best in dry air (de Jong, 1965).

Malnutrition

There is good evidence that measles is worse in severely malnourished children and that the infection can cause severe malnutrition (Morley, 1969). However, prospective community-based studies such as that in Guinea Bissau have not supported the notion that preceding under-nutrition is the underlying cause of severe measles (Aaby, 1988).

Intense exposure due to overcrowding

This is the most plausible theory. Studies in Senegal and Guinea Bissau have shown that mortality is clearly

Table 56.2. Case-fatality rate (CFR) of measles infection by age and type of exposure, Bandim, Guinea Bissau, 1979

Age (Months)	CFR (%) (deaths/no. ill)		
		Houses with multiple cases	
	Isolated cases	Index cases	Secondary cases
0–5	0% (0/1)	–	24% (4/17)
5–11	14% (1/7)	0% (0/15)	42% (11/26)
12–23	11% (2/19)	21% (3/14)	33% (14/43)
24–35	0% (0/10)	14% (2/14)	38% (14/37)
36–59	0% (0/10)	5% (2/38)	13% (5/39)
60+	33% (1/3)	6% (2/36)	0% (0/50)
Total	8% (4/50)	8% (9/117)	23% (48/212)

Source: From Aaby (1988).

Table 56.3. Measles case fatality ratio Niakhar, Senegal 1983–90

Age (years)	1983–86[a]	1987–90[b]
<1	19/165 (12.0%)	1/43 (2%)
1–2	58/480 (12.0%)	5/67 (6%)
3–4	16/321 (5.0%)	0/63 (0%)
5–9	5/407 (1.0%)	3/251 (1%)
Total	98/1373 (7.1%)	9/424 (2.1%)

Notes:
[a] low vaccine coverage.
[b] high vaccine coverage; no vaccinated cases died.
Source: Samb et al. (1997).

related to the sequence of infections in overcrowded compounds. The first case, who usually contracts measles outside the house, has mild disease whereas severity and mortality increases with each wave of infection in the compound (Table 56.2). Exposure to a large dose of virus during close contact with a severe case results in a large dose of virus and severe disease. The chance of dying is dependent on the severity of disease in the preceding case. Strangely, transmission of measles from one sex to the other has been found to increase mortality two- to three-fold compared to transmission from the same sex. The exceptionally high mortality found in West Africa is likely to be due to the very large polygamous and extended families, which increase the risk of intense exposure to measles and to secondary infections (Aaby & Samb, 1994).

Age of infection

Mortality is highest in the second half of infancy and in early childhood (Tables 56.2 and 56.3). Age of infection varies according to locality (Fig. 56.4); 20 per cent to 40 per cent of children with measles in the cities of Africa are infected before they are due for vaccination (Fig. 56.5).

Traditional practices and beliefs

In most cultures, measles has a specific local name and is a much-feared disease. Popular understanding is centered around the rash, which if it stays in the body will lead to severe disease. Therapeutic practices such as rubbing the skin with palm oil or kerosene are aimed at eliciting the rash quickly.

In West Africa, it is believed that cold keeps the rash within the body so the child will be covered with warm sand or blankets and is not washed or given cold water to drink (Aaby & Samb, 1994). Measles is still a major cause of blindness in Africa (SteinKuller et al., 1999); the use of traditional eye medicines made from roots or herbs aggravate the damage caused by measles and allow secondary infections such as herpes simplex virus or *Staphylococcus aureus* to flourish.

Lack of vaccination

Unimmunized children have more severe measles with a three- to five-fold higher mortality than vaccinated children. In a rural area of Senegal following a major increase in vaccine coverage, measles incidence declined by 69 per cent and the risk of dying by 91 per cent (Table 56.3). Children infected by an immunized case tended to have a lower case-fatality ratio than those infected by an unimmunized index case and generated fewer secondary cases. Measles immunization directly lowers mortality by reducing incidence and indirectly through increasing age at infection, lessening the severity of infection and by changing the transmission pattern (Samb et al., 1997).

HIV infection

Mortality from measles is increased two- to three-fold in HIV-infected children (Moss et al., 2002). They are ill for longer, excrete more virus and are probably more infectious (Permar et al., 2001). However, as in the severely malnourished, the rash may not appear (Smythe et al., 1971). Thus, measles may masquerade as a respiratory infection without a rash in children with AIDS.

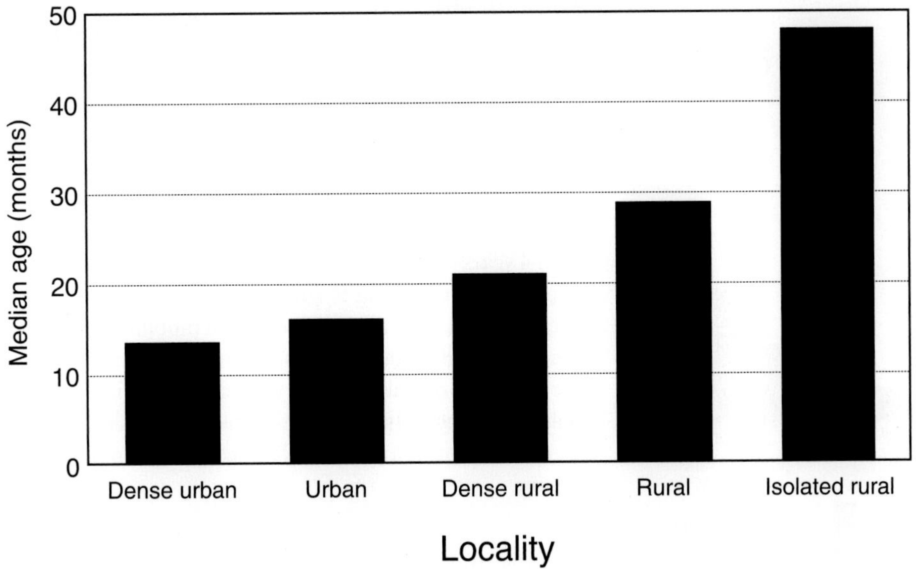

Fig. 56.4. Median age of measles by locality in West Africa. Age of infection is lower in urban than in rural areas. (After Walsh, 1983.)

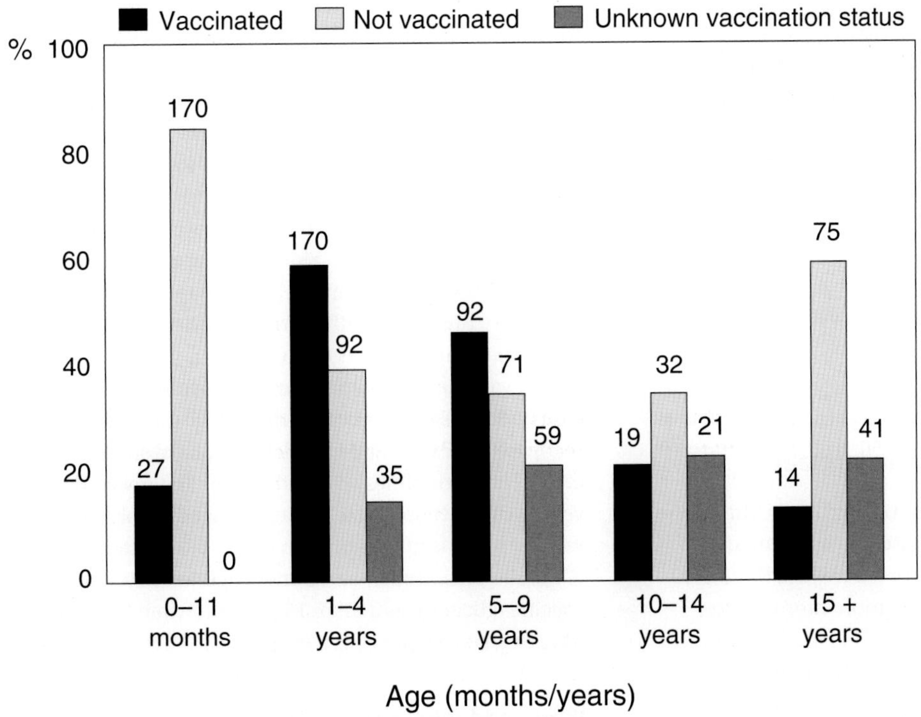

Fig. 56.5. Proportion, by age group, of previously vaccinated individuals who contracted measles during an outbreak in The Gambia 1996/1997. Sixty per cent of children aged 1–9 years had been vaccinated; 20% of all cases were less than 1 year of age. Number of cases in each category are shown above bars.

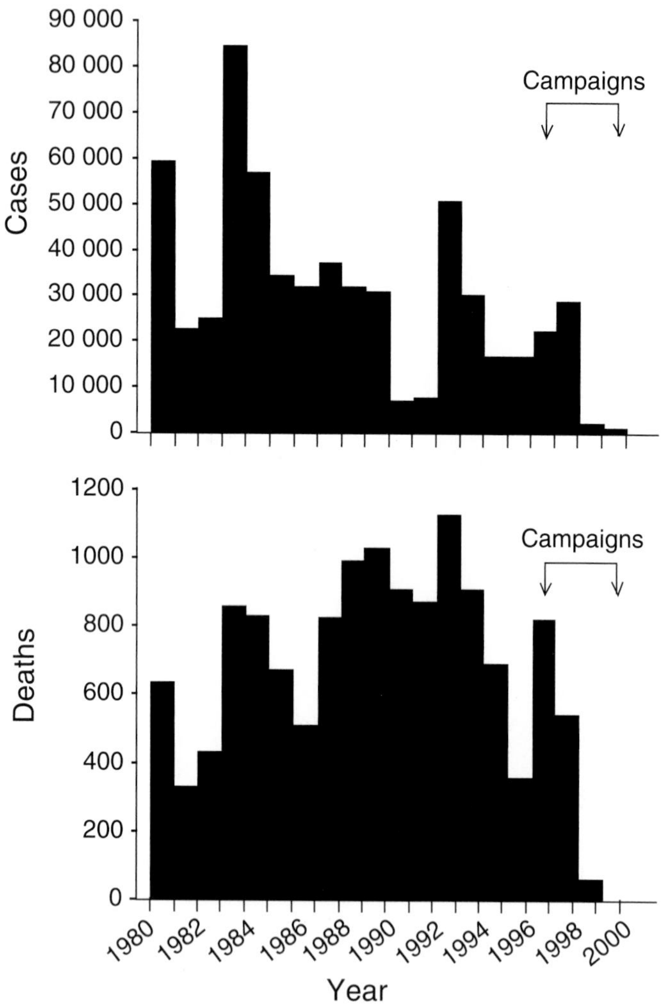

Fig. 56.6. Reported measles cases and deaths by year, in seven Southern African countries, 1983–2000. Mass campaigns drastically lowered number of cases and deaths (Beillik et al, 2002).

Increased delayed long-term mortality

This has been much debated. Undoubtedly, the brunt of disease is borne in the first 6 weeks of the infection. However, early studies described a two- to three-fold increase in mortality up to 6 or more months after measles (Aaby & Clements 1989; Hull et al., 1983), which has been ascribed to persisting malnutrition (Morley, 1969) coupled with immunosuppression (Dossetor et al., 1977). Recent studies in less severely affected, partially vaccinated, populations have failed to document this phenomenon (Akramuzzaman et al., 2000).

Prevention

The vaccine prevents or attenuates measles and, if applied widely and for long enough, may temporarily eliminate the virus. Using a strategy of high routine vaccination coverage and catch-up and follow-up campaigns, a block of seven South African countries have been able to reduce the number of measles cases from 60 000 to 117 over 4 years (Fig. 56.6). Unfortunately, such efforts are expensive and difficult to sustain for most African governments do not have the political will to mobilize enough resources to maintain adequate routine immunization services. The overall coverage of measles vaccine in sub-Saharan Africa is the lowest in the world; measles, despite a good vaccine, remains largely uncontrolled in the region.

The vaccine

Several strains of the wild type of virus have been attenuated by repeated passage in chick embryo fibroblasts or other cells. Different countries use these strains as vaccines, the most popular being the Schwartz and the Moraten strains. The Edmonton–Zagreb strain, which was passaged in human lung fibroblasts, is less easily neutralized by measles antibody and has proved very successful as a booster vaccine when given as an aerosol (Dilraj et al., 2000).

Measles vaccines are given at a dose of 1500–5000 plaque forming units by subcutaneous injection. The virus multiplies in the child and reproduces a mild subclinical attack of measles which confers immunity of variable duration (see below). Side effects are few and seldom serious: most children have mild fever about 10 days later, a few have high fever with febrile convulsions. The rash, if it is seen, is mild and passes quickly.

New vaccine formulations are much more resistant to heat and even when reconstituted prove potent after being left for 7 days at 24 °C. However, local storage conditions are sometimes so bad that even the freeze-dried vaccine has deteriorated. In Lagos, Nigeria, only 1 of 14 vaccine vials used in suburban clinics was potent (Omilabu et al., 1999). In another Nigerian city, Kano, vaccine efficacy was a mere 15 per cent when it should have been 85–90 per cent (Hargreaves, 2002).

When and whom to vaccinate

- All children except a few seriously ill (see below) should be vaccinated as soon as maternal passively transferred antibody has disappeared from their blood. This is

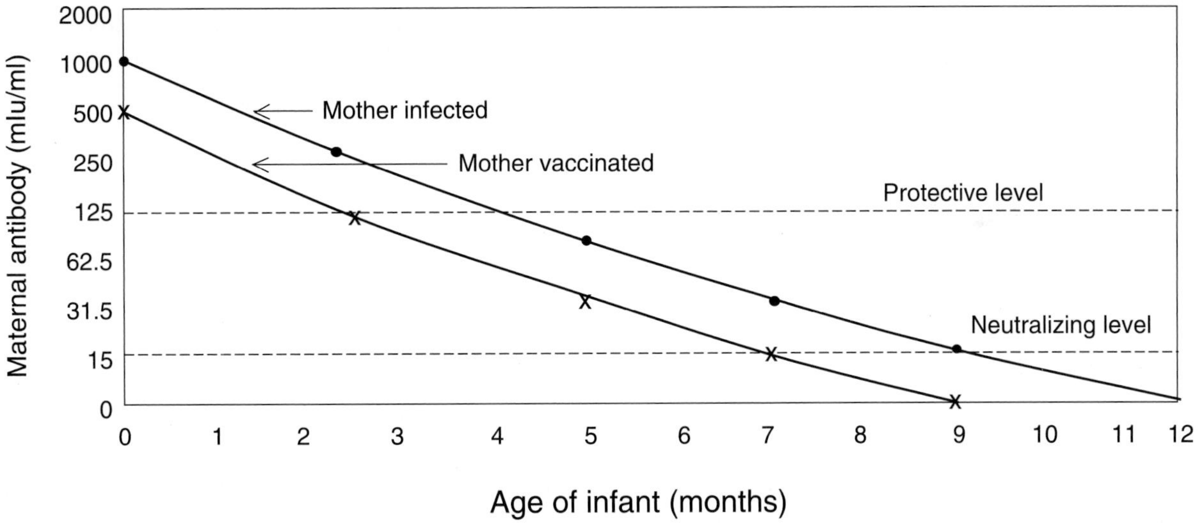

Fig. 56.7. Schematic view of decay of maternal measles antibody concentrations in children according to whether mother had measles or had been vaccinated. X antibody level ≥125 m i.u./ml prevents disease; a level ≥15 m i.u./ml neutralizes the vaccine. Arrows denote age at which infant is susceptible to measles.

easier said than done for the concentration of maternal antibody and the age at which the child is susceptible varies according to whether the mother had measles or was vaccinated (Fig. 56.7). If the child is vaccinated too young the vaccine will be neutralized by maternal antibody and the response will be poor; if too late, measles will strike before the child is vaccinated (Fig. 56.8).

- In practice, vaccinate at 9 months of age.
- As this may already be too late (Fig. 56.4) in cities with poor coverage or during large outbreaks, a two dose regimen at 6 and 9 months of age may be recommended.
- In countries attempting to eliminate measles, a more radical strategy is recommended (Beillik et al., 2002):
  (a) high routine coverage at 9 months of age,
  (b) a nationwide catch-up campaign among all children 9 months to 14 years of age
  (c) follow-up campaigns every 3–4 years among children 9 months to 4 years.

Sick children, either infected or malnourished, are at great risk of contracting measles when they attend clinics or hospitals, or are admitted to the wards. Live vaccines must be given to them in the outpatient clinic and on the wards if they have not had measles unless they have:

- nutritional oedema
- AIDS
- cancer
- treatment with immunosuppressive drugs
- primary immunodeficiencies.

Give such children gammaglobulin 2 ml, wait 1 month, and in those that have recovered use the live vaccine. Children with asymptomatic HIV infection (but not AIDS) should be given the live vaccine though they do not respond as well as normal children and antibody levels decline more rapidly (Moss et al., 1999).

Failure of vaccination

Vaccination against measles has failed in many countries; vaccine efficacy is low, around 70 per cent, and seldom reaches the desired target of 85–90 per cent. The reasons for this failure are seldom publicized for they are symptoms of poor health planning, lack of political will to implement primary health care and failure to maintain the cold chain (Hargreaves, 2002; McBean et al., 1976).

There are more subtle reasons for failure. In countries such as The Gambia, even though coverage is high and the cold chain is intact, a high proportion of children with measles aged 1–9 years have been vaccinated (Fig. 56.5). The causes of vaccine failure are:

(a) the vaccine given at 9 months is partially neutralized by maternal antibody (Fig. 56.7). The optimal age for a high and durable response is probably 15 months when no trace of maternal antibody is present.

(b) Antibody following vaccination decays rapidly as the result of early immunization and of other infections such as malaria which increase immunoglobulin turnover (Cohen et al., 1961; Whittle et al., 1999).

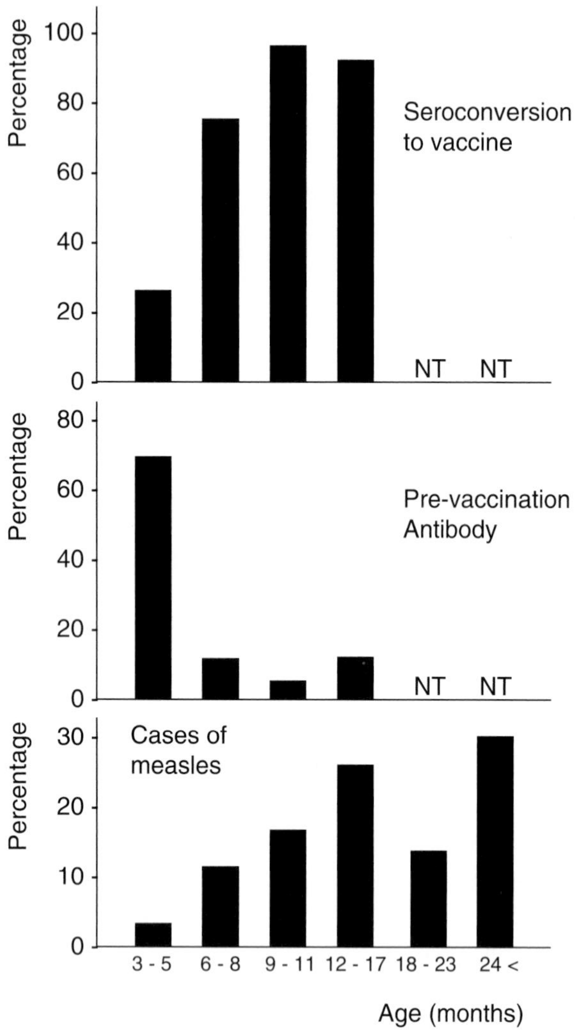

Fig. 56.8. Relationship between age of infection, maternal transmission of measles antibody, and response to vaccination among children in northern Nigeria. n.t. = not tested. (From Greenwood & Whittle, 1981.)

(c) Lack of circulating measles to boost immunity. Subclinical measles which is common in vaccinated children in areas where measles is rife boosts antibody levels thus preventing clinical measles (Table 56.4). Paradoxically, if vaccine coverage is high, measles no longer circulates freely, boosting is then uncommon and vaccine-induced immunity wanes (Whittle et al., 1999).

The future

Measles will be difficult and expensive to control in the large, poor crowded cities of Africa unless a new vaccine

Table 56.4. Geometric mean antibody titres at exposure and 1 month and 6 months after exposure for children with clinical measles, subclinical measles, and no measles

	Log$_2$ geometric mean titre [number of children]		
	At exposure	1 month after exposure	6 months after exposure
Measles	0.8 [21]	8.2 [21]	8.8 [16]
Subclinical cases	3.0 [43]	8.5 [43]	5.8 [29]
No measles	5.5 [59]	5.4 [59]	5.8 [42]

Source: From Whittle et al. (1999).

is available to protect young infants. Large numbers of susceptible children are born or brought into the community; there is ample time for infection between the loss of protective maternal antibody and the time of vaccination at 9 months (Fig. 56.7). Attempts to vaccinate earlier with a high dose of vaccine resulted in an unexpected increase in female mortality 1 to 3 years after vaccination (Aaby et al., 1993). The explanation is complicated: it seems that measles vaccine has a beneficial non-specific effect on the immune system which is particularly advantageous to girls living in areas where mortality from infectious diseases is high. The effect is not obtained by a high dose vaccine hence a relative increase in mortality (Aaby et al., 1995). Scientists are developing new vaccines using recombinant vector technologies such as DNA encoding measles genes or modified vaccinia viruses that express the H and F proteins that immunize at an early age in the presence of maternal antibody. Recombinant vaccines have been highly successful in protecting monkeys from measles (Stittelaar et al., 2000) and in preventing rinderpest in cows. They have yet to be used in man.

Pathogenesis and the immune response

The course of infection and the immune response to this invasion are shown in Fig. 56.9. The measles virus is spread to susceptible contacts in droplets during sneezing and coughing.

Day 0

First the virus infects and multiplies in the epithelium of the upper respiratory tract or the conjunctivae, then it spreads to the local lymph nodes. Four to six days later, the virus is found in the reticuloendothelial tissue of the liver and the spleen after spread via the blood. Here, and

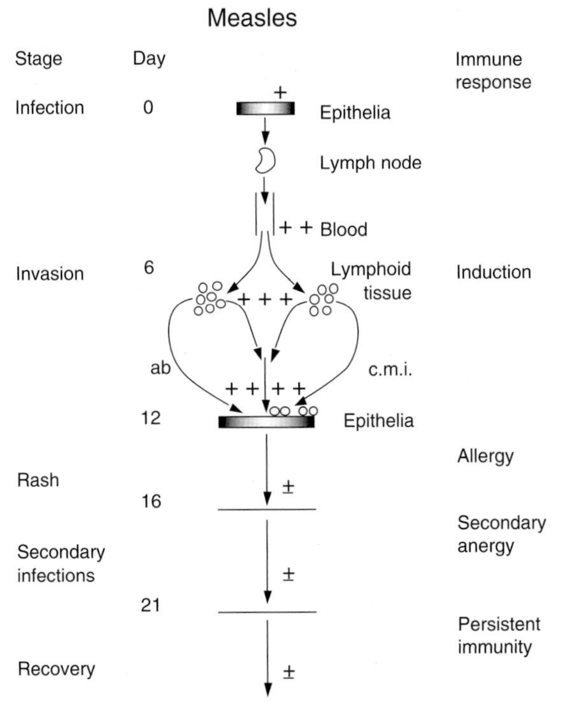

Fig. 56.9. Pathogenesis of measles: + denotes amount of virus, c.m.i. = cell-mediated immunity, ab = antibody.

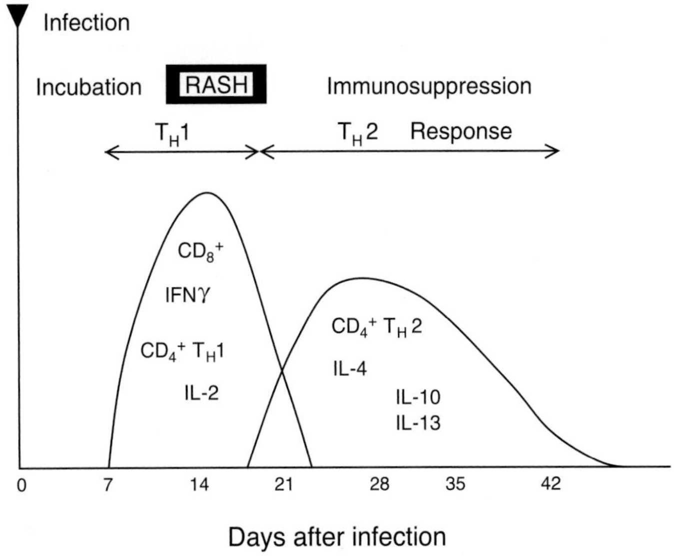

Fig. 56.10. Schematic view of T-cell and cytokine responses during measles (adapted from Griffin et al., 1994.) CD_8^+ cytotoxic T-lymphocytes and CD_4^+ type 1 helper T-lymphocytes control viral replication during incubation and at time of rash; CD_4^+ type 2 helper T-lymphocytes proliferate and produce type 2 cytokines later and are associated with immunosuppression. (T_H1 = T-helper type 1 lymphocytes; T_H2 = T-helper type 2 lymphocytes, IFNγ = gamma-interferon, IL = interleukin).

in the lymph nodes, it multiplies, causing fusion of cells to form giant cells with many nuclei. Viral antigens, presented by dendritic cells which are also infected by the virus, now induce the immune response.

First, natural killer cells and cytotoxic T-cells mount a cell-mediated reaction that contains the virus and limits its spread within cells. The response is augmented by type 1 cytokines, gamma-interferon and 1L-2, produced by T helper type 1 lymphocytes (T_H1). Later type 2 cytokines, 1L-4, 1L-10 and 1L-13, produced by T helper type 2 lymphocytes (T_H2) prime B cells to make IgM and then IgG antibody (Fig. 56.10). The first antibody to appear is to the nucleoprotein antigen. The second, which is largely responsible for neutralization of the virus, is to the haemagglutinin. Finally, antibody to the fusion glycoprotein appears in a low titre. This antibody stops cell-to-cell spread of the virus.

Day 8

By this time, the measles virus is carried either free or in circulating mononuclear cells by the blood to the target tissues – the epithelium of eye, lung and gut. Once again, the virus multiplies causing the prodrome, which is clinically evident around days 12–14 with fever, a runny nose, and Koplik's spots. These are small irregular spots, of a bright red colour in the centre of which is a minute bluish speck. The specks are foci where the virus has multiplied. At this stage, the patient is most infectious and virus may be isolated or viral RNA detected by the reverse transcriptase polymerase chain reaction (RT-PCR) from nasopharyngeal secretions. Antigen and virus can be detected by immunofluorescent techniques in the characteristic giant cells of the buccal mucosa, in epithelial cells and in monocytes and T- and B-cells in the blood.

Day 14–16

The rash, appearing around this time, is in reality the sign of a strong and complicated allergic reaction to measles virus in the epithelia of skin, gut and lung. Histological examination shows virus in the epidermis, corium, and capillary endothelia, mononuclear cell infiltration and the occasional giant cell. The extent and severity of the rash, provided the immune response is normal, will be determined by the number of target cells infected.

Day 17 or 18

Two or three days after the start of the rash, virus can no longer be cultured from the epithelia for infected cells have been disrupted and the free virus neutralized by antibody. The patient is now markedly immunosuppressed and susceptible to secondary infections of the eye, mouth gut and lung.

The mechanisms of immunosuppression are complex. The cytotoxic T-cell response which is exuberant results in destruction of infected T-cells and dendritic cells leading to their depletion, deficient antigen processing and generalized immunosuppression. IL-12, a crucial cytokine for the development of T_H1 and delayed hypersensitivity responses, is down-regulated; infection of CD_W 150 positive lymphocytes results in suppression of lymphoproliferation and in cell death. Thus, the T_H1 response is ultimately damped resulting in a skewing towards a T_H2 cytokine response and susceptibility to intracellular and other pathogens (Fig. 56.10).

Pathogenesis in the malnourished and in the HIV-infected

Measles in moderately to severely malnourished children and in children with symptomatic HIV infection is more severe and more prolonged, and secondary infections more frequent. Experimental data suggest that cells of these patients are more readily infected during the induction phase and that viraemia is heavy. A vigorous immune response, except in those who are grossly immunodeficient, generates a severe and widespread rash which is followed by prolonged immunosuppression (Whittle et al., 1980). Virus persists in lymphocytes and epithelial cells for 30 days or longer after the start of the rash (Dossetor et al., 1977; Permar et al., 2001).

Secondary infections with, for example, *Streptococcus pneumoniae* or latent infections such as herpes simplex or *Mycobacterium tuberculosis* recrudesce causing further immunosuppression and death of the child (Fig. 56.11).

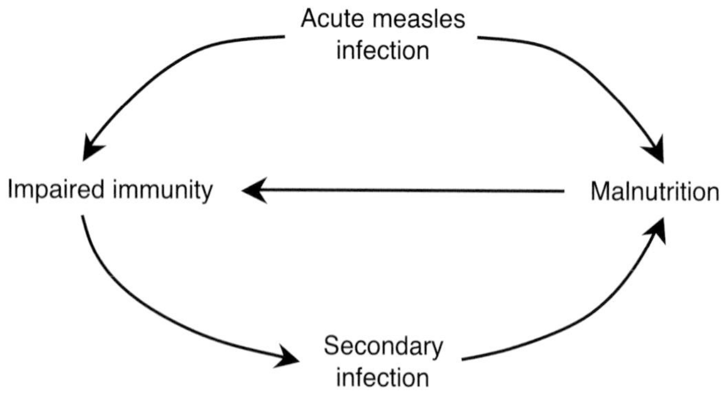

Fig. 56.11. Relationship between measles, malnutrition and immunosuppression (Greenwood, 1996).

Serum antibody concentrations are normal but secretory IgA antibody is deficient (Chandra, 1975). Such children may remain infective longer and shed more virus than normal children with measles. Some severely malnourished children (Smythe et al; 1971), and some with AIDS, are so immunosuppressed that they raise no rash and, like children with leukaemia (Enders et al; 1959) or those with primary T-cell immunodeficiency (Burnet, 1968), die of giant cell pneumonia caused by occult measles.

Clinical features and complications

There is a spectrum of severity that ranges from mild in the privileged and well nourished to severe in the blatantly malnourished or immunosuppressed. However, the rule is not inviolate and other factors such as the age and dose of infection are probably as important in determining the severity of disease. Measles, often severe, occasionally infects unvaccinated young adults or individuals who have lived in isolated communities. Figure 56.12 shows the clinical features and when they are found; Table 56.5 gives the frequency of these features in hospitalized children with or without HIV infection.

Prodrome (day 10–14)

Diagnosis is often missed at this stage when fever, sometimes complicated by convulsions, is the main feature (see Box).

> *In an endemic area,* **always consider mesles in a child with fever,**
> **look for** the other signs of the prodrome:
> - a runny nose,
> - mild conjunctivitiis,
> - red mucosa,
> - Koplik's spots,
> - doarrhoea.
>
> **Ask about** measles in the neighbourhood
> **Ask whether** the child has been vaccinated.

A useful diagnostic test is to scrape the buccal mucosa with a wooden spatula, place the scraping on a microscopic slide, stain with Leishman's stain and examine under high power of the microscope. Giant cells, diagnostic of measles, will be seen (Lightwood, 1970). The prodrome is prolonged in severe cases and reduced in vaccinated children or in individuals with modified measles due to maternal antibodies or prophylactic use of immunoglobulin.

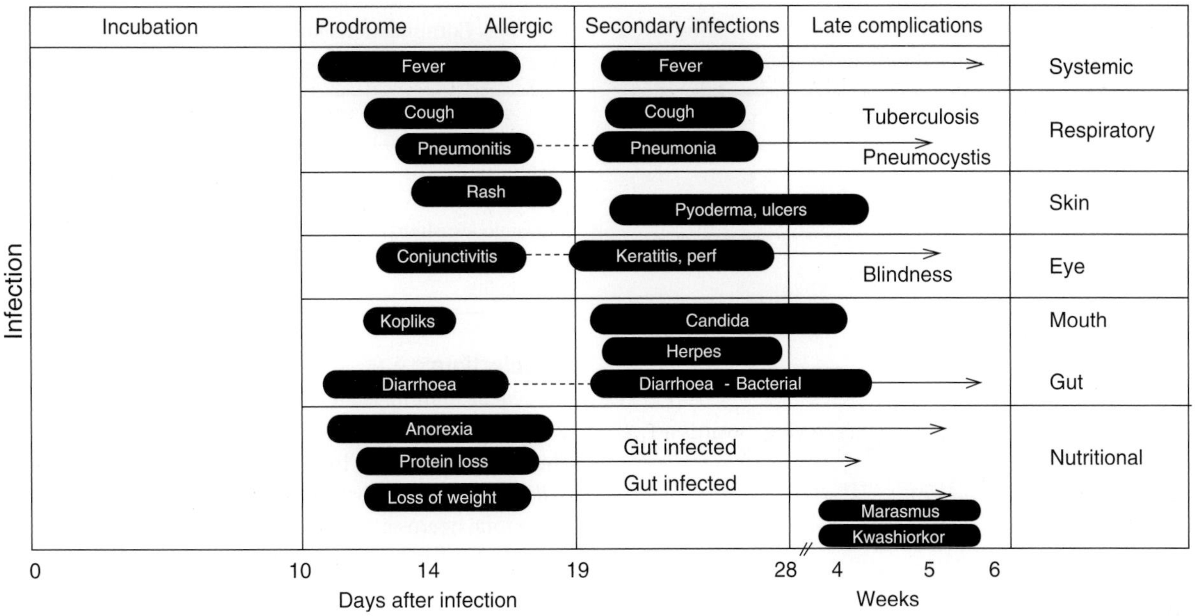

Fig. 56.12. Clinical features of measles and its complications.

The rash (day 14–18)

This, the cardinal sign of the allergic reaction, starts as discrete morbilliform spots on the upper part of the face progressing over the days to the shoulders, trunk and limbs (Fig. 56.13 (*a*)). In Africa, in severe cases, it is often red, confluent, raised, very extensive and sometimes accompanied by bleeding into the skin and even the gut. Later, the rash darkens to black, then the skin peels causing extensive desquamation (Fig. 56.13(*b*)). Other epithelial surfaces are inflamed, the severity matching that of the rash, these are:

Laryngo-tracheo-bronchitis

The child with hoarse cough and difficulty of inspiration requires admission.

Pneumonitis

The bronchioles and alveoli are inflamed by the allergic reaction. Crepitations are heard in all areas of the lungs. Admit the child to hospital if there is a cyanosis or subcutaneous emphysema, best felt in the suproclavicular fossa. The percentage oxygen saturation is a useful index of severity.

Enteritis

Diarrhoea may be profuse resulting in malabsorption of food and water. Protein loss from the inflamed gut accompanies the diarrhoea (Fig. 56.14), which coupled with profound anorexia and malabsorption, precipitates severe weight loss and, at times kwashiorkor. The mouth is painful and inflamed which multiplies the misery and adds to the anorexia of the child who at this stage may even refuse to suck the breast.

Acute encephalitis

This is a rare but serious sign.

Secondary Infections (day 19–30)

The virus has now been eradicated from most tissues by the immune response, but, as a consequence, the patient is left severely immunosuppressed and is susceptible to infections of lung, gut and eye.

Pneumonia

This causes most deaths (Table 56.6), and is heralded by a rise in fever, leukocytosis and respiratory difficulty. The causative organisms have been little studied and so are largely unknown. Common infections such as *Streptococcus pneumoniae*, *Staphylococcus aureus* or *Haemophilius influenzae* are most likely but measles itself or secondary viral infections may be responsible, as herpes simplex and adenovirus have been cultured from the lungs of children dying after measles (Kipps & Kaschula, 1976). Twenty per cent of children with herpes simplex ulceration of the mouth had bronchopneumonia, which was associated with laryngotracheitis. A variety of other organisms such as gram-negative bacteria, cytomegalovirus, fungi, *Mycobacterium tuberculosis* and *Pneumocystis carinii* should be considered as potential pathogens of the lung after immunosuppression due to measles.

Table 56.5. Clinical features of HIV-infected and uninfected children with measles in a Zambian Hospital, 1998–2000

Clinical feature	HIV-infected (n=117) %	HIV-uninfected (n=521) %
Age (months)		
<9	32[a]	22
9–23	30	38
24–59	21	19
>60	17	21
Vaccinated: yes	80	75
no[b]	20	25
Previous hospitalization	49[a]	28
Rash		
morbilliform	69[a]	78
desquamative	30	23
none	3	4
Wasted	19[a]	10
Thrush	35[a]	17
Stridor	7[a]	2
Pneumonia	71	69
Diarrhoea	65	58
median (interquartile range) days in ward	3[a] (2–6)	3 (2–4)
Deaths	9.4[a]	4.0

Notes:
[a] % significantly different.
[b] children not vaccinated against measles were more likely to have thrush, diarrhoea and/or pneumonia even after adjusting for age, gender and HIV infection.
Source: From Moss (2002).

Stomatitis and enteritis

Chronic diarrhoea and a sore mouth are common complications of measles. Candida infection, easily identified in the mouth, infects the small bowel and sometimes spreads to the anus. Diarrhoea can be dramatically improved by treatment with nystatin. Children with diarrhoea after measles have the small bowel superinfected with bacteroides spp., *E. coli, Pseudomonas* and *Staph. aureus*, and may lose large amounts of protein from their gut (Dossetor & Whittle, 1975).

Deep ulcers, caused by herpes simplex erode the corners of the mouth, the lips, the gums and even the palate and nasal bones: these are seen, in the second and third weeks after the rash, in about 10 per cent of patients, most of whom are malnourished. The children are ill, miserable, in great pain and refuse to eat: cancrum oris develops in a few.

Table 56.6. Complications and mortality in patients with measles in hospital, Northern Nigeria, July–December 1978

	Number	Died
Pneumonia	169	32
Gastroenteritis	65	9
Marasmic-kwashiorkor or kwashiorkor	25	6
Laryngo-tracheo-bronchitis	21	4
Encephalitis	10	4

Eye infections

Corneal ulceration, leading to impaired vision or blindness is common after measles, especially in the malnourished. The appearance varies from superficial punctuate keratitis to deep stromal ulcers which erode through the cornea to cause total necrosis. Ulcers are often asymmetrical, unilateral and dendritic in appearance. In Northern Nigeria herpes simplex was found in 47% of active corneal ulcers after measles, and measles virus in 12 per cent: the children usually had evidence of oral herpes (Whittle et al., 1979).

Skin and other infections

Pyoderma is common after measles. In malnourished patients deep-eroding ulcers may bore through the skin and sometimes bone, in the head and other sites. Otitis media is common; the micro-organisms causing this and other infections are unknown. Latent tuberculosis may be reactivated by measles: it should be suspected when a chronic cough with sputum develops.

Malnutrition

Most children lose weight during an attack of measles and may take many weeks to regain it. Those who are originally underweight lose most weight because they have severe measles, prolonged anorexia, much protein loss from the gut and frequent secondary infections, which lead to kwashiorkor or marasmic-kwashiorkor often (Fig. 56.11). Measles lowers plasma vitamin A levels markedly.

Persistence of infection

Measles virus persists for longer than realized: it can be cultured from blood 7–10 days after the rash has appeared. Kenyan children with severe skin staining after measles excreted giant cells, an indication of persistent measles infection, for an average of 12 days after the rash. They were markedly underweight and had many complications of measles (Scheifele and Forbes, 1972). Measles virus can be frequently detected by RT–PCR 30 to 60 days after the onset of the rash in children with HIV and measles infection (Permar et al., 2001).

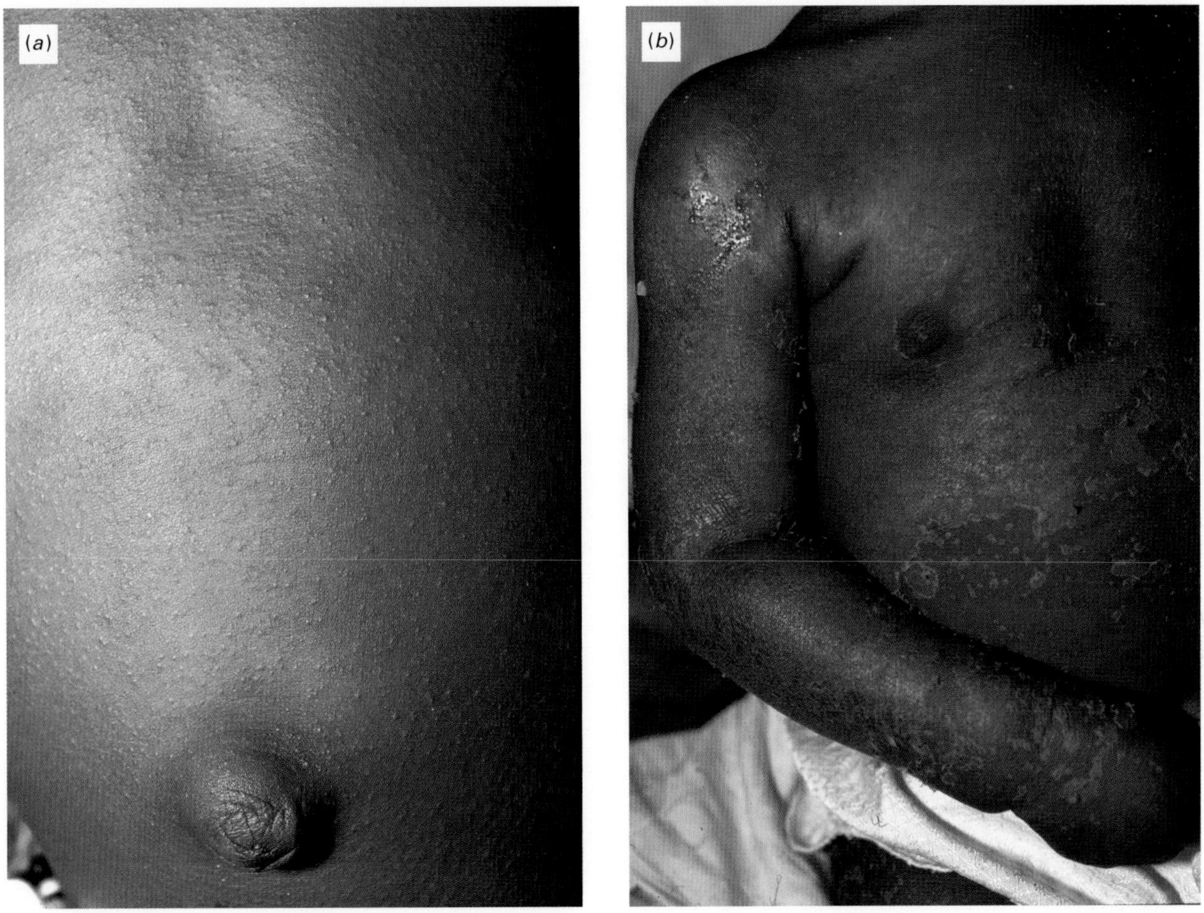

Fig. 56.13. (*a*) Early measles rash in a Gambian child. (*b*) Desquamating rash in a Gambian child (both courtesy of Dr Martin Weber).

Giant-cell pneumonia

Children with leukaemia and sometimes those with kwashiorkor or AIDS may have persistent uncontrolled measles which causes a lethal giant-cell pneumonia.

Subacute sclerosing panencephaltis (SSPE)

Subacute sclerosing panencephalitis is a rare complication of measles. Five or six years after measles the child starts to behave abnormally, and has convulsions and disturbances of motor function characterized by myoclonic jerking. Eventually, the child dies 1 to 3 years later of progressive cerebral deterioration. Measles virus is found in the brain at autopsy.

Multiple sclerosis, autism, Crohn's disease

There is no convincing evidence that measles virus or immune response to it have a causative role in these diseases. The alleged association between Measles, Mumps and Rubella (MMR) vaccine, autism and Crohn's disease was based on weak science and has now been convincingly refuted by larger and stronger epidemiological studies. Subsequent molecular studies have been unable to confirm the original finding of measles virus and genomic RNA in the diseased bowel of Crohn's disease (Afzal et al., 2000).

Treatment and prognosis

There is no specific treatment for the virus but intelligent management in outpatients and the ward will reduce morbidity and mortality.

Outpatients

The acute attack is often best managed here.

- Explain to the mother:
  (a) the nature of the infection
  (b) the necessity to continue breast-feeding
  (c) the necessity of adequate hydration
  (d) the necessity of returning in 1 week, or sooner should the child deteriorate.

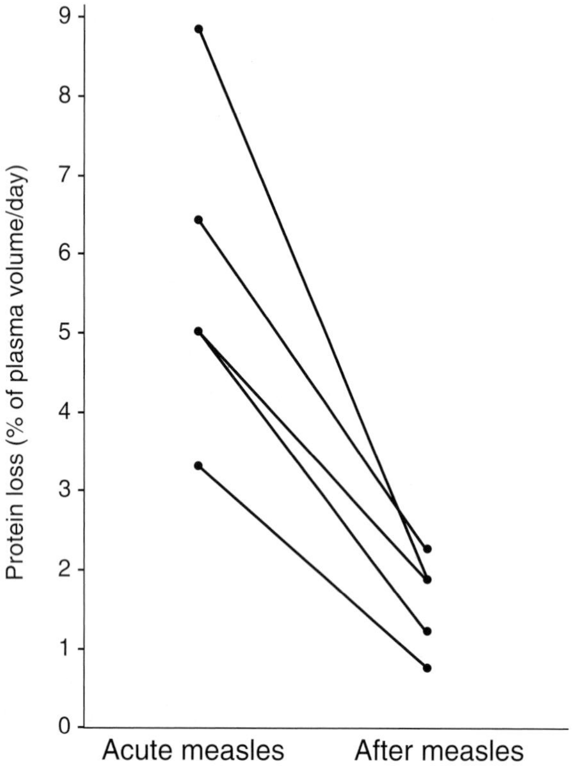

Fig. 56.14. Protein loss from the gut in acute measles and on recovery. Mean loss is equivalent to 20% of a child's normal protein intake. (From Dossetor & Whittle, 1975.)

- Give antibiotic eye ointment routinely, and show the mother how to use it.
- Consider giving a course of cotrimoxazole to those with moderate or severe measles, though there is only weak evidence that this prevents secondary pneumonia (Samb et al., 1995).
- Secondary pneumonia, due to bacteria or other viruses is commonly seen in the second week. Give a broad-spectrum antibiotic, co-trimoxazole or ampicillin.
- Treat thrush, with or without persistent diarrhoea, with nystatin and if diarrhoea persists, give metronidazole.
- Treat mouth ulcers with paracetamol and a single dose of benzathine penicillin.

WHO (2000) recommends vitamin A for all children with measles (see Table 56.8 for dosage). There is no proof that vitamin A supplementation before measles influences the incidence or severity of measles in West Africa. In a community-based double-blind placebo-controlled trial of vitamin A supplementation in rural northern Ghana measles case-fatality rate was 15.4% and 14.5% in the supplemented and placebo groups, respectively (Dollimore et al., 1997).

Inpatients

The following clinical features indicate severe disease which usually needs treatment in hospital. This is particularly true if the child is underweight or frankly malnourished (see Box).

> **Clinical features of severe measles**
> 1. a rash that darkens or desquamates in large plaques;
> 2. signs of laryngeal obstruction;
> 3. marked dehydration, blood in the stool or more than five stools a day;
> 4. convulsions or loss of consciousness;
> 5. corneal ulceration;
> 6. severe secondary pneumonia.

Some children, despite all efforts, die of pneumonia and malnutrition; the prognosis is related to weight on admission, for children may lose 10–15% of their weight before arriving at hospital.

Table 56.7. Mortality and morbidity in 189 children with measles according to whether they have received vitamin A or not

Characteristic	No vitamin A (n=97)	%	Vitamin A[a] (n=92)	%
Death	10	10.3	2	2.1
Pneumonia (days)				
Duration[b]	12.4		6.5	
≥10	29	29.8	12	10.8
Diarrhoea (days)				
Duration[b]	8.5		5.6	
≥10	21	21.6	8	8.6
Croup	27	27.8	13	14.1
Herpes stomatitis	9	0.9	2	0.2
Adverse outcome[c]	52	53	25	27.1
Hospital stay (days)[b]	15.2		10.5	

Notes:
[a] all differences significantly less in Vit A group ($P \leq 0.05$) except herpes stomatitis (P=0.06).
[b] mean duration in days; all other values are numbers of patients.
[c] defined as death, pneumonia ≥10 days' duration, diarrhoea ≥10 days' duration, post-measles croup or transfer for intensive care.
Source: From Hussey and Klein (1990).

- Hydrate the child orally or intravenously.
- Treat pneumonia with parenteral antibiotics (preferably after a chest radiograph).
- Treat lobar pneumonia with benzylpenicillin; bronchopneumonia with gentamicin and flucloxacillin or chloramphenicol.
- Eye ulcers should, if possible, be seen by an ophthalmologist. If you suspect herpes, send a scraping from the ulcer to the laboratory, and give a course of acyclovir (see Box).
- Give systemic antibiotics and vitamin A capsules, for there is convincing evidence of its efficacy in hospitalized patients (Table 56.7); dosage is shown in Table 56.8.
- Feeding is difficult, for children with measles are anorexic and refuse to eat; tube feed with a skimmed milk preparation or a lactose-free liquid diet if diarrhoea is precipitated by lactose.

Table 56.8. Dosage of vitamin A

	dosage[a]
Mild or moderate measles	
Day 1	
<6 months of age	50000 i.u.
6–12 months of age	100000 i.u.
>12 months	200000 i.u.
Day 2	repeat above
Severe measles or malnourished	
Day 14–21	repeat above[b]

Notes:
[a] The oil-based preparation is usually given orally.
[b] If child is severely anorexic or has oedematous malnutrition or septic shock give intramuscularly.
Source: From WHO (2000).

Treatment of corneal ulcers associated with measles:

1. Vitamin A – oral
2. Corneal infections should be managed, where possible, by ophthalmologists or appropriately trained eye care professionals.
3. Corneal scrapes should be taken where there are facilities to perform microscopy and bacterial culture.
4. Intensive topical treatment with either:
   a. Quinolone (ofloxacin 0.3% or ciprofloxacin 0.3%) eye drops
   OR
   b. Fortified gentamicin 1.5% and cefuroxime 5% eye drops

   The frequency of the instillation of drops is tailored to the severity of the infection and the response to treatment. For a severe corneal ulcer it is usual to commence with hourly treatment (day and night). The condition of the cornea and its response to treatment needs to be regularly monitored (daily and as the situation improves the frequency of the drops can be reduced.)
5. If a herpetic infection is suspected: aciclovir 3% eye ointment, five times a day.
6. For particularly severe infections or those associated with the use of traditional eye remedies consider gonococcal or fungal infections.

Unsolved problems

1. Levels of maternal antibody are variable. If it is absent, the infant is unprotected before 9 months of age. If it is present, the vaccine is partially neutralized leading to low level immunity. New vaccines are sorely needed. They need to be effective in early infancy in areas of Africa where measles is hyperendemic and infants are at great risk of infection.
2. The relative merits of vaccination by subcutaneous or aerosol route need defining. An aerosol might raise a greater and more durable immune response particularly in those already vaccinated or in those with maternal antibody, but safety needs to be fully established and more practical means of delivering the aerosol invented.
3. Bronchopneumonia is still a major cause of death following measles, particularly in the malnourished and HIV-infected. More clinical and post-mortem research is needed to identify the causative organisms before rational treatment can be given.
4. Research is needed to explain the non-specific beneficial effects of measles vaccines (see the Box).

Can measles be eradicated? **Yes,**

- if sufficient money and effort is applied to elimination strategies on a continent-wide basis. **But,**
- In practice, this is unlikely and may be thwarted by the growing number of HIV-infected children who:
  1. are poorly responsive to the vaccine,
  2. are highly susceptible to measles,
  3. may harbour occult infections, which spread the virus.

References

Aaby P. (1998). Malnutrition and overcrowding – exposure in severe measles infection; a review of community studies. *Rev Infect Dis*; **10**: 478–491.

Aaby P, Samb B. (1994). Measles and its control: dogmas and new perspectives in *Health and Disease in Developing Countries*, ed. KS Lankinen, S Bergstrom, PH Makela, M Peltola, pp. 163–176. London: The Macmillan Press Limited.

Aaby P, Clements CJ. (1989). Measles immunization research: a review. *Bull Wld Hlth Org*; **67**: 443–448.

Aaby P, Knudsen K, Whittle H et al. (1993). Long term survival after Edmonston–Zagreb measles vaccination: increased female mortality. *J Pediatric*; **122**: 904–908.

Aaby P, Samb B, Simondon F, Seck AMC, Knudsen K, Whittle H. (1995). Non-specific beneficial effect of measles immunization: analysis of mortality studies from developing countries. *Br Med J*; **311**: 481–485.

Adu FD, Ikusika A, Omotade. (1997). Measles outbreak in Ibadan: Clinical serological and virological identification of affected children in selected hospitals. *J Infect*; **35**: 241–245.

Afzal MA, Minor PD, Schild GC. (2000). Clinical safety issues of measles, mumps and rubella vaccines. *Bull Wld Hlth Org*; **78**: 199–204.

Akramuzzaman SM, Cutts FT, Wheeler JG, Hossain MJ. (2000). Increased childhood morbidity after measles is short-term in urban Bangladesh. *J Epidemiol*; **151**: 723–735.

Atabani S, Byrnes AA, Jaye A et al. (2001). Natural measles causes prolonged suppression of interleukin-12 production. *J Infect Dis*; **184**: 1–9.

Barrett T. (1999). Morbillivirus infections, with special emphasis on morbillivirus of carnivores. *Vet Microbiol*; **69**: 3–13.

Beillik R, Madema S, Taole A et al. (2002). First 5 years of measles elimination in southern Africa: 1996–2000. *Lancet*; **359**: 1564–1568.

Burnet FM. (1968). Measles as an index of immunological function. *Lancet*; **ii**: 610–613.

Chandra RK. (1975). Reduced secretory antibody response to live attenuated measles and poliovirus vaccines in malnutrition. *Br Med J*; **2**: 583–585.

Cohen S, McGregor IA, Carrington S. (1961). γ-globulin and acquired immunity to human malaria. *Nature*; **192**: 733–737.

de Jong HG. (1965). Survival of measles virus at various humidities of air. *Virus Forschung*; **16**: 97–102.

Dilraj A, Cutts FG, de Castro JF et al. (2000). Response to different measles vaccine strains given by aerosol and subcutaneous route to schoolchildren: a randomised trial. *Lancet*; **355**: 798–803.

Dollimore N, Cutts, Birika FN, Ross DA, Morris SS, Smith PG. (1997). Measles incidence, case fatality, and delayed mortality in children with or without vit A supplementation in rural Ghana. *Am J Epidemiol*; **146**: 646–654.

Dossetor, JFB, Whittle HC. (1975). Protein-losing enteropathy and malabsorption in acute measles enteritis. Br Med J; 2: 592–593.

Dosseter J, Whittle HC, Greenwood BM. (1977). Persistent measles infection in malnourished children. *Br Med J*; **1**: 1633–1635.

Enders JF, Mc Carthy K, Mitas A, Cheatham WJ. (1959). Isolation of measles viruses at autopsy in cases of giant cell pneumonia without a rash. *N Engl J Med*; **261**: 875–881.

Fayet MT, Gilles HM. (1981). Studies with combined meningococcal vaccines. I: A combined meningococcal, measles and tetanus vaccine. *Ann Trop Med Parasitol*; XXXXXX

Garenne M, Aaby P. (1996). Pattern of exposure and measles mortality in Senegal. *J Infect Dis*; **161**: 1088–1094.

Greenwood BM. (1996). The host's response to infection. In *Oxford Textbook of Medicine*, ed. DJ Weatherall, JGG Ledingham, DA Warrell, p. 282. Oxford: Oxford University Press.

Greenwood BM, Whittle HC. (1981). *Immunology of Medicine in the Tropics*. London: Arnold.

Griffin D. (2001). Measles. in *Fields Virology*, ed. DM Knipe, PM Howley, pp. 1401–1442. Philadelphia: Lippincott, Williams, Wilkins.

Griffin DE, Ward BJ, Esolen LM. (1994). Pathogenesis of measles virus infection, an hypothesis for the altered immune responses. *J Infect Dis*; **170**: s24–s31.

Hargreaves S. (2002). Time to right the wrongs: improving basic health care in Nigeria. *Lancet*; **359**: 2030–2035.

Hull HF, Williams PJ, Oldfield F. (1983). Measles mortality and vaccine efficacy in rural West Africa. *Lancet*; **i**: 972–975.

Hussey GD, Klein M. (1990). A randomised, controlled trial of vitamin A in children with severe measles. *N Engl J Med*; **323**: 160–164.

Kipps A, Kaschula ROC. (1976). Virus pneumonia following measles. *S Afr Med J*; **50**: 1083–1088.

Lightwood R. (1970). Epithelial giant cells in measles as an aid in diagnosis. *J Pediat*; **77**: 59–64.

McBean AM, Foster SO, Herrmann KL, Gateff C. (1976). Evaluation of a mass measles immunization campaign in Yaounde, Cameroun. *Trans Roy Soc Trop Med Hyg*; **70**: 206–212.

Morley D. (1969). Severe measles in the tropics. *Br Med J*; **1**: 297–300; 363–365.

Moss WG, Cutts F, Griffin DE. (1999). Implications of the human immunodeficiency virus epidemic for control and eradication of measles. *Clin Infect Dis*; **29**: 106–112.

Moss WJ, Monze M, Ryon JJ, Quinn TC, Griffin DE, Cutts F. (2002). Prospective study of measles in hospitalized, HIV-infected and uninfected children in Zambia. *Clin Infect Dis*; **35**: 189–196.

Omilabu SA, Oyefolu AO, Ojo OO, Audu RA. (1999). Potency status and efficacy of measles vaccine administered in Nigeria: a case study of three EPI centres in Lagos, Nigeria. *Afr J Med Sci*; **28**: 209–212.

Permar SR, Moss WJ, Ryon JJ et al. (2001). Prolonged measles virus shedding in Human Immunodeficiency Virus – infected children, detected by Reverse Transcriptase – Polymerase Chain Reaction. *J Infect Dis*; **183**: 532–538.

Samb B, Simondon F, Aaby P, Whittle H, Seck AMC. (1995). Prophylactic use of antibiotics and reduced case fatality in measles infection. *Pediatr Infect Dis J*; **14**: 695–696.

Samb B, Aaby P, Whittle H, Seck AM, Simondon F. (1997). Decline in measles case fatality ratio after introduction of measles immunization in rural Senegal. *Am J Epidemiol*; **145**: 51–57.

Scheifele DW, Forbes CE. (1972). Prolonged giant cell excretion in African measles. *Pediatrics*; **50**: 867–873.

Smythe PM, Breton-Stiles GG, Grace HJ et al. (1971). Thymolymphatic deficiency and depression of cell-mediated immunity in protein calorie malnutrition. *Lancet*; **ii**: 939–943.

Steinkuller PG, Du L, Gilbert C, Foster A, Collins ML, Coats DK. (1999). Childhood blindness. *J AAPOS*; **1**: 26–32.

Stitterlaar KJ, Wyatt LS, de Swart RK et al. (2000). Protective immunity in macaques vaccinated with a modified vaccinia virus Ankara-based measles virus vaccine in the presence of passively acquired antibodies. *J Virol*; **74**; 4236–4243.

Strebel PM, Cochi SL. (2001). Waving goodbye to measles. *Nature*; **414**: 695–696.

Tatsuo H, Ono M, Tanaka K, Yanagi Y. (2000). SLAM (CDw 150) is a cellular receptor for measles virus. *Nature*, **406**, 893–897.

Whittle HC, Aaby P, Samb B, Jensen H, Bennett J, Simonden F. (1999). Effect of subclinical infection on maintaining immunity against measles in vaccinated children in West Africa. *Lancet*; **353**: 98–101.

Walshe JA (1983). Selective primary health care: strategies for control of disease in the developing world. IV Measles. *Rev Infect Dis*; **5**: 330–340.

Whittle HC, Smith SJ, Kogbe OI, Dossetor J, Duggan M. (1979). Severe ulcerative herpes of mouth and eye following measles. *Trans Roy Soc Trop Med Hyg*; **73**: 66–69.

Whittle HC, Mee J, Werblinska J, Yankubu A, Onuora C, Gomwalk N. (1980). Immunity to measles in malnourished children. *Clin Exp Immunol*; 42: 144–151.

World Health Organization. (2000). *Management of the Child with a Serious Infection or Severe Malnutrition*. Geneva: World Health Organization.

57 Dengue

The problem in Africa

The descriptions from China in AD 992 of a disease 'water poison' characterized by rash, fever, arthralgia, haemorrhage and associated with flying insects and water may account for the very first descriptions of dengue. By the eighteenth century there are good descriptions of an illness compatible with dengue from Asia, North America and Africa, suggesting that, by this time, there was widespread geographical spread of the disease. *The Oxford English Dictionary* claims that the term dengue originated from the Swahili phrase *Ka dinga pepo* (a sudden cramp-like seizure from an evil spirit or plague) and suggests that the disease crossed from Africa to the Caribbean during the mass forced migration of people during the eighteenth century. Other sources claim it to be derived from a Spanish description *quebranta huesos* (break bone fever). There were epidemics described throughout the eighteenth and nineteenth centuries in Africa (Egypt, Senegal, Libya, Kenya, and Tanzania) Asia, and the Americas (Gubler, 1998b).

There is very little systematic surveillance data for dengue in Africa and it is unclear how much of a problem dengue currently is, or could become in the future, across the continent. Since the 1980s reports of epidemic dengue have increased dramatically. There have been reports of limited outbreaks in West Africa, Seychelles, Kenya, Sudan, Dijbouti, Somalia, and Saudi Arabia. To date, epidemic dengue haemorrhagic fever (DHF) has not been reported in Africa but clinical cases compatible with DHF have been reported from Mozambique, Dijbouti, and Saudi Arabia (for review see Gubler, 1998b).

Many of the features probably necessary for dengue to become established in Africa now exist. The virus has been isolated from most regions of the continent, the major vector, *Aedes aegypti*, is present and other potential vectors (*Ae. luteocephalus*, *Ae. africanus*, and *Ae. opok*) are available to transmit the virus. There has also been increasing urbanization and migration by large numbers of people into these rapidly growing cities. Population growth and concentration in large unplanned cities has led to an explosion in the vector population throughout the Asian region. With urbanization often comes poor housing and waste disposal. This all provides an excellent habitat for the principal vector *Ae. aegypti*.

Organism, life cycle, vector/intermediate host, and host

Dengue is the most widely distributed mosquito-borne viral infection of humans, affecting an estimated 100 million people world-wide each year, with 40 per cent (2.5 billion) of the world's population estimated to be at risk of infection. It is endemic in parts of Asia and the Americas, and has been increasingly reported from many tropical countries in recent years. It has been classified by the World Health Organization (WHO) into dengue Fever (DF), dengue haemorrhagic fever (DHF) and dengue shock syndrome (DSS) (Table 57.1). It is amongst the leading causes of paediatric hospitalization in Asia, with up to 500 000 cases reported annually to the WHO. Once shock becomes established, mortality rates of 12–40 per cent have been reported.

The dengue virus is a single-stranded positive sense RNA virus of approximately 11 kb in length and encodes three structural and seven non-structural genes. It is a member of the *Flavivirus* genus, which also includes the yellow fever, Japanese Encephalitis, West Nile, and Hepatitis C. There is considerable genetic diversity in the dengue virus family with four serotypes (Den-I, Den-II, Den-III and Dev-IV), all of which may produce either a

Table 57.1. WHO definitions of dengue severity

Grade of severity	Platelet (lowest) Per μl	Plasma leakage	Circulatory collapse	Other
Dengue fever	Variable	Absent	Absent	Tourniquet test variable. Haemorrhage may be present
Dengue haemorrhagic fever Grade I	<100 000	Present	Absent	Positive tourniquet test No haemorrhage
Dengue haemorrhagic fever Grade II	<100 000	Present	Absent	Positive tourniquet test Haemorrhage
Dengue haemorrhagic fever Grade III (DSS)	<100 000	Present	Pulse pressure <20 mmHg	Variable tourniquet test Haemorrhage
Dengue haemorrhagic fever Grade IV (DSS)	<100 000	Present	Absent blood pressure	Variable tourniquet test Haemorrhage

non-specific febrile illness, dengue fever (DF), or may result in the more severe manifestation of DHF and DSS.

The dengue viruses are transmitted from viraemic to susceptible hosts by mosquitoes of the subgenus *Stegomyia*, the major global vector is *Aedes aegypti*, although other species may be more important in restricted geographical areas. *Ae. aegypti* lays individual eggs in the damp walls of artificial and natural water containers and these eggs can remain viable for months. The adult mosquito is strongly anthropophilic, prefers resting in sheltered dark areas inside houses and has a diurnal feeding pattern, usually peaking in the mid-morning and late afternoon. The female will usually feed twice during a single gonotrophic cycle, and their average lifespan is 8–14 days.

Control and prevention

There is no vaccine currently available and no specific anti-viral treatment for dengue and so control of the vector remains the most important factor in preventing and reducing the transmission intensity of the virus. Larval source reduction is an effective approach but requires a major investment either in trained professional inspectors or direct involvement by the community involved. Lavicides, biological control methods (larvivorous fish or crustacean larval predators) and insecticides and indoor spraying have all been tried with some success. *Ae. aegypti* is a day-biting mosquito and bed nets have traditionally not been thought of as a useful addition to the protection against dengue. However, there is some biting activity in the hours before dawn, and after dark and, in countries where afternoon rests or siesta are part of the lifestyle, bed nets may make a valuable contribution to protection.

Pathophysiology and epidemiology

DHF is characterized by increased vascular permeability and plasma leakage, thrombocytopenia and haemorrhage, and the degree of each of these parameters usually correlates with clinically graded disease severity. Mild DHF (DHF grades I and II) is normally characterized by only mild haemorrhage as indicated by spontaneous petechiae and a positive tourniquet test, while bruising, often at injection sites, purpura and other haemorrhage manifestations are usually present in the more severe grades of DHF, Grade III and IV.

Vascular permeability is the most important parameter determining DHF severity and precipitates dengue shock syndrome (DSS) (DHF-III and DHF-IV) through circulatory failure (reduced pulse-pressure and hypotension) (WHO, 1997, 1999). The capillary leak predisposes to pulmonary oedema, pleural effusion, and ascites as well as intravascular compromise and haemoconcentration.

The most widely cited hypotheses to explain the vascular leak and haemorrhage is increased viral replication due to enhanced infection of monocytes in the presence of pre-existing anti-dengue antibodies at sub-neutralizing levels – antibody dependent immune enhancement (Halstead, 1988). This theory, which has strong epidemiological and in vitro experimental evidence to support it, argues that, in the primary asymptomatic dengue infection, the moderate viraemia is well controlled. The host immune system develops long-lasting immunity to the

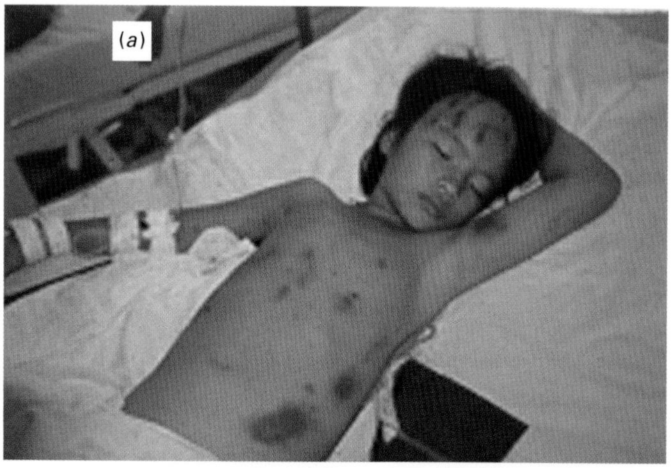

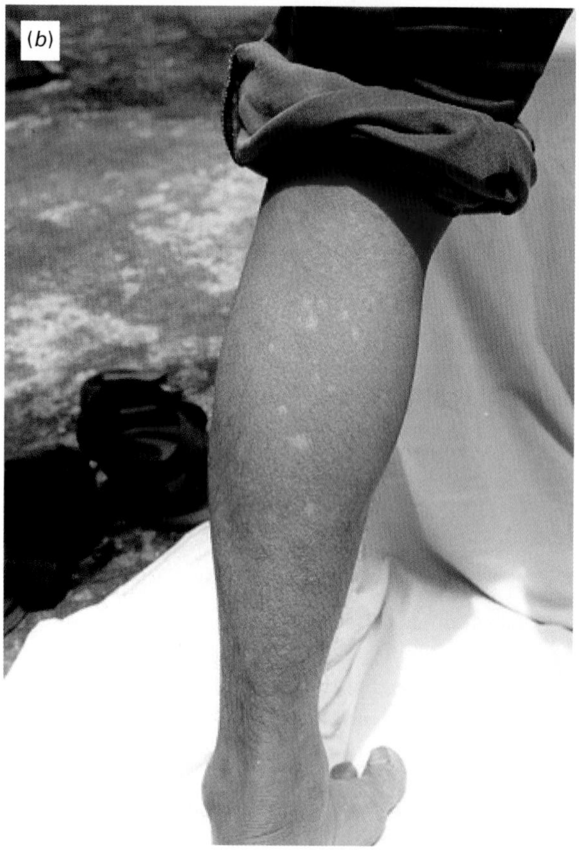

Fig. 57.1. (*a*) Characteristic haemorrhagic manifestations in dengue haemorrhagic fever. Venous access is often very difficult and multiple sites may be needed. Haemorrhage typically appears at these injection sites.
(*b*) The rash during the recovery phase. There is extensive red confluent rash surrounding discrete islands of normal skin.

serotype of the infecting strain and short-lived cross-protection against heterologous serotypes. However, after a few months, the levels of cross-protective antibody directed against the heterologous serotypes fall below neutralizing levels and from this stage onward infection with a second heterologous strain may result in increased viral uptake via Fcγ receptors into monocytes and enhanced viral replication. However, severe disease has been reported during apparently primary infections and, clearly, not all secondary infection leads to severe disease so other theories (viral and host genetic factors) have been put forward to try and explain the complex epidemiological and immunopathogenetic features. (Kurane & Ennis, 1998; Rico-Hesse et al., 1997; Watts et al., 1999; Green et al., 1999; Sudiro et al., 2001).

Clinical features and diagnosis

Dengue fever (DF) is a mild, self-limited febrile episode that is associated with a rash. It usually begins with fever, respiratory symptoms (sore throat, coryza, and cough), anorexia, nausea, vomiting and headache. Back pain, myalgias, arthralgias and conjunctivitis may also occur. The initial fever usually resolves within a week, and a few days later a generalized morbilliform or maculopapular rash may develop (Fig. 57.1(*b*)). Fever may return with the rash. DHF has been classified into four grades of severity by the WHO (Table 57.1); grades I and II have only mild capillary leak, insufficient to result in the development of shock and are differentiated by the absence (grade I) or presence (grade II) of spontaneous bleeding; in grade III circulatory failure occurs, manifested by a rapid and weak pulse with narrowing of the pulse pressure to $\leq$20 mm Hg; in grade IV shock is severe with no detectable pulse or blood pressure. DHF grades III and IV are collectively referred to as dengue shock syndrome (DSS) (approximately 25% of cases) characterized by severe hypovolemia and shock. Petechiae and bleeding at injection sites are characteristic (Fig. 57.1(*a*)). Severe bleeding including intracerebral haemorrhage usually associated with multi-organ dysfunction is rare but often fatal. Mortality rates vary from 1 per cent to 5 per cent, although much higher rates have been reported. Complications include severe bleeding, pleural effusions, shock, pneumonia, liver dysfunction or failure, encephalopathy, and pulmonary haemorrhage. The differential diagnosis is extensive and will vary depending where the patient is seen but would include in Africa; malaria, typhoid, leptospirosis, septicaemia, other viral haemorrhagic fevers (Ebola, Lassa fever, etc), Chikungunya, West Nile fever, O'nyong-nyong fever, and Rift Valley fever (usually without a rash).

A pulse pressure of less than 20 mmHg is one of the earliest manifestations of shock, prior to the development of systolic hypotension. The mainstay of treatment is prompt, vigorous but careful fluid resuscitation. If appropriate volume resuscitation is instituted at an early stage shock is usually reversible; in certain very severe cases, and in those inadequately resuscitated, patients may progress to irreversible shock and death. Very careful clinical judgement is required throughout the patient's stay in hospital to maintain an effective circulation whilst assiduously avoiding fluid overload. Very close attention and regular review (every 15–30 minutes during episodes of shock) of the haematocrit, pulse pressure and peripheral perfusion is essential (Dung et al., 1999; Nhan et al., 2001). For patients with DSS the WHO recommends immediate volume replacement with isotonic crystalloid solutions, followed by the use of plasma or colloid solutions, specifically dextrans, for profound or continuing shock (WHO, 1997, 1999).

Thrombocytopenia is universal in DHF and platelet function is also abnormal. Mild prolongation of the prothrombin and partial thromboplastin times with reduced fibrinogen levels is common, but fibrin degradation products have not been found to be elevated to a degree consistent with classical disseminated intravascular coagulation. Patients with DSS have significant abnormalities in all the major pathways of the coagulation cascade (Wills, 2002).

The diagnosis is a clinical one with supportive laboratory tests. Proof of a dengue infection depends on confirmatory dengue serology and viral isolation if available. Serological confirmation of acute dengue infection relies on the demonstration of specific IgM and IgG antibodies against dengue in the serum of patients. Ideally, acute and convalescent sera should be tested but as this is not always possible guidelines have been established to allow diagnoses to be made on the basis of single samples.

Viral isolation is performed by culturing patients' serum with *Aedes albopictus* C6/36 cell monolayers and virus infection of C6/36 cells was confirmed by immunofluorescent assay (IFA) using a flavivirus-specific monoclonal antibody (MAb). Dengue virus RNA can also be amplified by reverse transcriptase nested PCR from serum (Lanciotti et al., 1992).

Clinical aligorithms for the assessment and management of DHF and DSS are outlined in Tables 57.2 and 57.3.

Table 57.2. Clinical algorithms – assessment

A. In the history ask about the onset, pattern, and degree of the fever. Risk factors include recent travel to an area with endemic dengue fever. Note any respiratory symptoms: cough, sore throat, fast or difficult breathing, and chest indrawing (retractions). Assess GI symptoms, anorexia, nausea, vomiting, diarrhoea, abdominal pain, blood in stools, and jaundice and renal symptoms, decreased urinary frequency, flank pain, lower abdominal pain. Ask about headache, retro-orbital pain, arthralgia, myalgias and back pain. Assess alterations in the mental status and normal level of activity: playfulness, weakness, irritability, feeding and sleeping patterns, responsiveness.

B. On physical examination, look for findings that suggests progression to haemorrhagic fever and shock syndrome. These include spontaneous petechiae and bruising (Fig. 57.1), too weak to feed, unresponsive, irritability. The tourniquet test may be useful early in the disease. Also look for dehydration and poor perfusion: skin turgor, moist mucous membranes, colour and warmth of the extremities and capillary refill time (>2 seconds is abnormal), low blood pressure, narrowing of the pulse pressure to 20 mm Hg or less. Examine carefully for petechiae, purpura, haemoptysis, bloody vomits, bloody stools and rash.

C. In DHF and DSS the most common laboratory findings are haemoconcentration (an increase of 20% in the haematocrit), thrombocytopenia, increase in prothrombin time, and abnormalities in fibrinogen and other coagulation factors. Liver function may be impaired, virus isolation and serologic tests are confirmatory. Leukopenia and neutropenia are characteristic findings.

D. Hospitalize patients with moderate or severe signs. The shock should be managed with very careful fluid (i.v.) replacement with an isotonic fluid (Ringer's lactate or normal saline) in the first instance to stabilize the circulation. In patients with severe shock rescusitation should be started at 10–20 ml/kg/h i.v. If no improvement in clinical state (perfusion, pulse pressure, or haematocrit) within 1 hour consider changing to a colloid solution. To prevent fluid overload the rate of infusion should be reduced to 1–5 ml/kg/h maintenance fluid as soon as the condition stabilizes.

E. In very severe cases fluid replacement should be monitored by hourly haematocrit, urine output and if possible a central line. If, on admission the pulse pressure is <10 mmHg one should consider initial rescusitation with a colloid solution starting at <10 ml/kg/h. Consider blood transfusions if the haematocrit is falling without improvement in haemodynamic profile and consider ocult GI blood loss and fresh frozen plasma to correct severe anaemia and replace clotting factors. Systemic steroids do not affect outcome. Diuretics may be required in the recovery phase to prevent sustained fluid overload.

Table 57.3. Clinical algorithms – treatment

Dengue haemorrhagic fever Grade I and II
Bleeding tendency, thrombocytopenia, Raised haematocrit
If unable to tolerate oral fluids or haematocrit >20% above expected
Start IV Crystalloid 1–3 ml/kg/h. Review after 2 hours.

- **Improvement**
  (Vital signs and urine output stable)
  Maintenance i.v. fluids 1–3 ml/kg/h
  - **Continued improvement**
    Stop i.v. fluids at 24 hours
- **No improvement**
  (Perfusion/Pulse pressure/haematocrit)
  Increase i.v. crystalloid 10 ml/kg/h. Review at 1 hour
  - **No improvement**
    DHF Grade III/IV
    See below
  - **Improvement**
    Reduce i.v. fluids
    3–6 ml/kg/h
    - **Continued improvement**
      Stop i.v. fluids at 36 hours

Dengue haemorrhagic fever Grade III and IV
Start i.v. therapy 10–20 ml/kg/h crystalloid.
Review BP, RR, PR hourly and haematocrit 2-hourly

- **Improvement**
  (Perfusion/pulse pressure/haematocrit)
  Reduce i.v. fluids over the next 6 hours
  10 then 5 then 3 ml/kg/h
  - **Continued improvement**
    Maintain intravenous access
    Stop i.v. fluids at 48 hours
- **No improvement**
  (Perfusion/pulse pressure/haematocrit)
  Colloid 10 ml/kg/h
  Review after 1 hour
  - **No improvement**
    Oxygen, intensive care
    Central venous line
    Inotropes/ventilation
    Transfusion
  - **Improvement**
    Reduce i.v. colloid
    3–6 ml/kg/h
    For 2–4 hours
    - **Continued improvement**
      Crystalloid 3–6 ml/kg/h
      Maintain intravenous access
      Stop i.v. fluids at 48 hours
      +/− diuretics in recovery phase

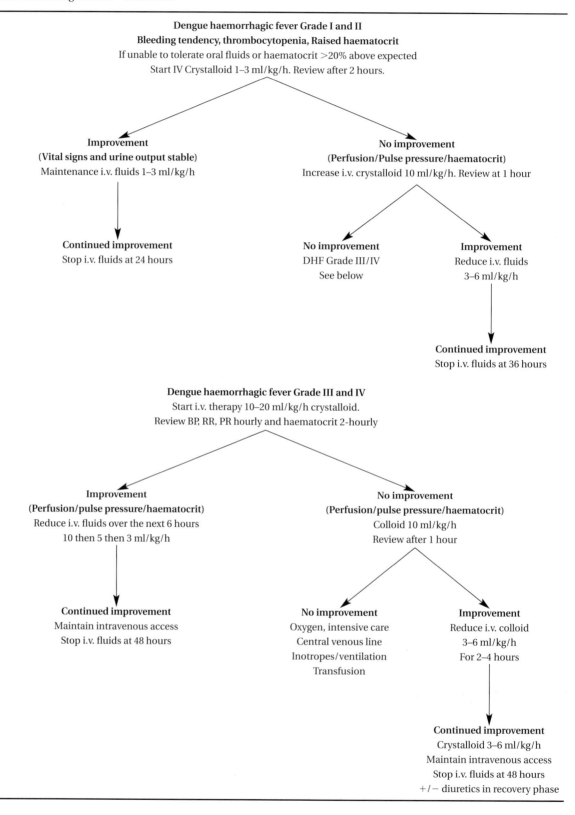

Unsolved problems

There is almost no systematic data on the epidemiology of dengue in Africa, although isolated case reports and surveys suggest that it may be important. Certainly the conditions needed to facilitate the spread of dengue exist in many areas of the continent. A better understanding of the burden of the disease and epidemiology of dengue in Africa would be very important.

There has been progress in our understanding of the pathogenesis of dengue over the last few years. However, we still do not have clear evidence based treatment guidelines, and we do not have a clear understanding of the role of the virus, the host's immune response and the complex epidemiology in the basic pathology underlying the disease. Control of the vector is difficult and there is no vaccine currently available. There remain many unanswered questions.

The relative importance and interaction between the virus and the host immune system is central to an understanding of the pathology. The virus is constantly evolving and inter- and intraserotype recombination among dengue viruses could mean that humans are being exposed to increasingly diverse viral strains, some of which may evade immunity in previously exposed populations. Increasing genetic diversity also has major implications for vaccine design, and the likelihood of a vaccine providing effective protection. There are concerns that, if a tetravalent vaccine does not produce good long-term protection against all four serotypes it runs the risk of precipitating an increase in DHF via antibody-dependent immune enhancement (Worobey et al., 1999).

The importance of the host genetic make-up, in particular the HLA system, and the role of CD4+ and CD8+ in protection against, and development of, DHF, has been less well studied. Further studies of CD8+T−cell responses to natural infection are required to assess the role of cell-mediated immunity in dengue. These issues have particular relevance to dengue vaccine design. The critical question is whether protective responses can be induced without predisposing a minority to more severe disease.

Dengue has emerged as a major global problem. There is a need for a further understanding of the vector, the virus and the host response to infection. The epidemiology of the disease, what happens during the inter-epidemic periods and what factors lead to the disease becoming established endemically in a region need further study. It is heartening to see the lead the WHO has taken in bringing dengue into the TDR cluster of diseases. The hope is that this will lead to a greater awareness of the disease and the likely impact it will have in the coming years.

References

Bhamarapravati N, Yoksan S. (1997). Live attenuated tetravalent dengue vaccine. In *Dengue and Dengue Haemorrhagic Fever*, ed. DJ Gubler, G Kuno, pp. 367–377. New York: CAB International.

Chiewslip P, McNair Scott R, Bhamarapravati N. (1981). Histocompatibility antigens and dengue haemorrhagic fever. *Am J Trop Med Hyg*; **30**: 1100–1105.

Dung NM, Day NPJ, Tam DTH et al. (1999). Fluid replacement in dengue shock syndrome: a randomised double blind comparison of four intravenous fluid regimens. *Clin Infect Dis*; **29**: 787–799.

Green S, Vaughn DW, Kalayanarooj S et al. (1999). Elevated plasma interleukin-10 levels in acute dengue correlate with disease severity. *J Med Virol*; **59**: 329–334.

Gubler DJ. (1998a). Dengue and dengue haemorrhagic fever. *Clin Microbiol Rev*; **11**: 480–496.

Gubler DJ. (1998b). Dengue and dengue hemorrhagic fever: its history and resurgence as a global health problem. In *Dengue and Dengue Hemorrhagic Fever*, ed. DJ Gubler, G Kuno, pp. 1–23. New York: CAB International.

Guzman MG, Kouri GP, Bravo J, Soler M, Vazquez S, Morier L. (1990). Dengue hemorrhagic fever in Cuba, 1981: a retrospective seroepidemiologic study. *Am J Trop Med Hyg*; **42**: 179–184.

Guzman MG, Kouri G, Valdes L et al. Epidemiologic studies on Dengue in Santiago de Cuba, 1997. *Am J Epidemiol*; **152**: 793–799.

Halstead SB. (1988). Pathogenesis of dengue: challenges to molecular biology. *Science*; **239**: 476–481.

Innis BL, Nisalak A, Nimmannitya S et al. (1989). An enzyme-linked immunosorbent assay to characterize dengue infections where dengue and Japanese encephalitis co-circulate. *Am J Trop Med Hyg*; **40**: 418–427.

Kouri G, Guzman MG, Bravo JR, Triana C. (1989). Dengue haemorrhagic fever/dengue shock syndrome: lessons from the Cuban epidemic 1981. *Bull Wld Hlth Org*; **67**: 375–380.

Kurane I, Ennis FA. (1998). Immunopathogenesis of dengue virus infections. Dengue and dengue hemorrhagic fever: its history and resurgence as a global health problem. In *Dengue and Dengue Hemorrhagic Fever*, ed DJ Gubler, G Kung. pp. 273–291. New York: CAB International.

Lanciotti RS, Calisher CH, Gubler DJ, Chang G-J, Vorndam AV. (1992). Rapid detection and typing of dengue viruses from clinical samples by using reverse transcriptase-polymerase chain reaction. *J Clin Microbiol*; **30**: 545–551.

Nam VS, Yen NT, Kay BH, Marten GG, Reid JW. (1998). Eradication of *Aedes aegypti* from a village in Vietnam, using copepods and community participation. *Am J Trop Med Hyg*; **59**: 657–660.

Nhan NT, Kneen R, My NV et al. (2001). Acute management of dengue shock syndrome: a randomised double blind comparison of dextran 70, gelatin, lactated ringer's and normal saline for the first hour. *Clin Inf Dis*; **32**: 204–213.

Rico-Hesse R, Harrison LM, Salas RA et al. (1997). Origins of dengue type 2 viruses associated with increased pathogenicity in Thailand. *Virology*; **230**: 244–251.

Rigau-Perez JG, Clark GC, Gubler DJ, Reiter P, Sanders EJ, Vorndam AV. (1998). Dengue and dengue haemorrhagic fever. *Lancet*; **352**: 971–977.

Rodier GR, Gubler DJ, Cope SE et al. (1996). Epidemic dengue 2 in the city of Djibouti 1991–1992. *Trans Roy Soc Trop Med Hyg*; **90**: 237–240.

Sudiro TM, Zivny J, Ishiko H et al. (2001). Analysis of plasma viral RNA levels during acute dengue virus infection using quantitative competitor reverse transcription-polymerase chain reaction. *J Med Virol*; **63**: 29–34.

Tassniyom S, Vasanawathana S, Chirawarkul A, Rojanasuphot F. (1993). Failure of high dose methylpredisolone in established dengue shock syndrome: a placebo controlled, double-blind study. *Paediatrics*; **92**: 111–115.

Watts DM, Porter KR, Putvatana P et al. (1999). Failure of secondary infection with American genotype dengue 2 to cause dengue haemorrhagic fever. *Lancet*; **354**: 1431–1434.

WHO (1997). *Dengue Haemorrhagic Fever: Diagnosis, Treatment, Control.* Geneva: World Health Organization.

WHO (1999). *Guidelines for Treatment of Dengue Fever/Dengue Haemorrhagic Fever in Small Hospitals.* New Delhi: Regional Office for South-East Asia, World Health Organization.

Wills B, Oragui E, Dung NM, Loan HT, Farrar J, Levin M. (2002). Coagulation abnormalities in dengue haemorrhagic fever: serial investigations in 167 Vietnamese children with dengue shock syndrome. *Clin Infect Dis*; **35**: 277–285.

Worobey M, Rambaut A, Holmes EC. (1999). Widespread intra-serotype recombination in natural populations of dengue virus. *Proc Natl Acad Sci USA*; **96**: 7352–7357.

58

Viral haemorrhagic fevers: yellow fever, Lassa fever, Rift Valley fever, Ebola/Marburg fever and Crimean–Congo fever

Viral haemorrhagic fever (VHF) is an imprecisely defined clinical syndrome, the hallmarks of which are high fever, bleeding tendency and shock. It can be caused by several viruses, whose natural reservoirs are animals or insects, and is characterized by loss of plasma from small blood vessels ('capillary leakage') and bleeding. Liver involvement is common, leading to jaundice. Clinically, these infections can be confused with severe malaria, typhoid fever, shigellosis ('diarrhée rouge'), leptospirosis, rickettsial diseases, viral hepatitis, meningococcocaemia and gram-negative sepsis. Some viruses can be easily spread between humans, especially in the hospital setting.

The problem in Africa

Yellow fever (YF) is the prototypic viral haemorrhagic fever and remains a constant threat for much of sub-Saharan Africa, where it is endemic. Presently, 34 countries, with a combined population of 250 million are at risk. WHO (1998a,b) estimates that up to 200 000 cases of YF with 30 000 deaths occur annually in Africa. Because of low immunization coverage of the susceptible populations, the number of YF cases is increasing, as is the risk of large urban epidemics.

Other VHFs have probably also been endemic for thousands of years but have 'emerged' or 're-emerged' in the public's perception only since the 1960s. This is partly due to increased contact between humans and the animal or insect reservoirs, and partly due to increased awareness of these diseases and improved diagnostic methods.

VHFs cause relatively few deaths, but are feared for their tendency to cause epidemics and their potential for direct human-to-human transmission. Several thousand cases of VHFs are estimated to occur in Africa each year, with a mortality ranging from 1 per cent to 90 per cent, depending on the infecting virus. With rapid ecological change on the one hand, and political and social destabilization leading to population movements on the other, the two main factors which bring humans into closer contact with the reservoirs of VHFs will continue to give rise to outbreaks.

Epidemiology

The enveloped RNA-viruses which cause VHFs belong to four different families: Flaviviruses, Filoviruses, Arenaviruses and Bunyaviruses. VHFs are anthropozoonoses. The viruses are maintained endemically in nature, with animals or insects serving as natural reservoirs. To date, neither the natural reservoir nor the vector of Filoviruses has been identified. Table 58.1 gives an overview of the ecology and epidemiology of these viruses.

Transmission of viruses

The viruses can be transmitted:

- through the excreta of their natural animal reservoir to human (Lassa);
- through bites of insects which function as reservoirs and/or vectors (yellow fever, Rift Valley, Crimean-Congo);
- through contact with the blood of an infected animal (Rift Valley, Crimean-Congo, Ebola/Marburg);
- directly from human to human (all, except yellow fever).

Person-to-person transmission occurs through close contact with body fluids. The infectivity of some VHFs, notably Ebola, Marburg and Crimean-Congo is quite high, so that family members caring for a sick relative or preparing a corpse for burial are easily infected. Explosive

Table 58.1. Epidemiology of VHFs

Disease	Reservoir	Vector	Distribution	Clinical cases/year[a]	Risk factors for transmission	Lethality[b]
YF	Mosquitoes	Mosquitoes	Sub-Saharan Africa	200 000	Not vaccinated. Sporadic cases originate in jungle, outbreaks in semi-humid savannah	10–50%
LF	Rodent	Rodent	West Africa	150 000	Contact with rodents and their excreta	10–20%
CCHF	Ticks (birds? hares?)	Ticks	Sub-Saharan Africa	>100	Contact with blood of diseased animals (ruminants)	10–40%
RVF	Mosquitoes	Mosquitoes	Sub-Saharan Africa	20–100 000[c]	Epizootics of ruminants. Contact with animal blood	1–50%[d]
EHF, MHF	Unknown	Unknown	West, Central, East Africa	5–300[c]	Contact with dead of diseased monkeys[c]	50–90%

Notes:
LF: Lassa fever, CCHF: Congo–Crimean haemorrhagic fever, RVF: Rift Valley fever, EHF, MHF: Ebola, Marburg haemorrhagic fevers.
[a] Estimation by WHO and others.
[b] For clinically ill patients. The majority of YF, RVF and LF cases are clinically mild or inapparent.
[c] Higher figure for epidemics only.
[d] Higher figure for haemorrhagic cases only.
[e] Ebola virus: Chimpanzees. Marburg virus: Green monkeys (*Cercopithecus aethiops*).

nosocomial outbreaks occur because of the poor standards of hygiene in many regional hospitals, where needles are reused without proper sterilization, and gloves are not available. There is no clear epidemiological evidence that VHFs are transmitted between humans in the form of aerosols. Simple 'barrier nursing' techniques (wearing a gown, gloves, a mask and goggles) effectively protect from direct contact with the infectious droplets a patient may produce during coughing, vomiting, defecating, bleeding, etc.

Pathogenesis

All viruses have a broad tissue tropism and they can be isolated from many organs, with especially high titres found in liver, spleen and kidney. All infections involve the liver, but the degree of damage may range from only focal lesions to massive necrosis. Interestingly, there is no or very little inflammatory, neutrophilic infiltration of infected organs. Because all HF viruses infect monocytes/macrophages and endothelial cells, it is presently proposed that the release of cytokines from infected macrophages (TNFα, IL6 and others), altered responses of infected endothelial cells to these cytokines and other biochemical abnormalities lead to plasma leakage, disseminated intravascular coagulopathy, decreased thrombocyte aggregation, and bleeding. Cytokine release would also explain the 'flu-like' early stages of VHFs and the severe wasting seen within a few days in Filovirus infections (TNFα). Both Ebola and Rift Valley fever virus recently have been shown effectively to block the interferon type I response of infected cells, thus allowing unchecked replication of the virus early in the course of infection.

Neurological symptoms are common both in the acute and convalescent stage and present in some VHF as disease specific signs. However, major destruction of structures of the CNS are not observed on autopsy.

In some VHFs (Lassa, Ebola, Marburg) the immune response is presumably strongly T-cell based, since neutralizing antibodies appear late and only at low titres. In others (yellow fever and Rift Valley fever) the appearance of neutralizing antibodies limits viral replication. The 17D vaccine against yellow fever is one of the most successful live attenuated vaccines ever produced and raises neutralizing antibodies which confer protection for at least 10 years. Because of their virulence, live attenuation has not been attempted for the other VHF viruses (except Rift Valley). Traditional vaccines using killed virus induce antibodies but do not protect laboratory animals against viral challenge. Recently, experimental vaccination with biotechnologically generated viral DNA, followed by a boost with a genetically engineered adenovirus expressing the proteins of VHF viruses, has shown promising results.

Clinical presentation

After variable incubation periods (Table 58.2), the onset of VHFs is non-specific with fever, myalgia, arthralgia and

Table 58.2. Pathogenetic and laboratory findings in VHFs[a]

VHF	Incubation period	Clinical disease course	Principal pathology	WBC	Proteinuria	AST, ALT	Haemostasis	Bleeding
YF	2–5 days	5–12 days	Liver, kidney	↓	+++	500–>2000	Tc↓ DIC	25–50%, M, S
LF	7–16 (21) days	7–17 days	Liver, placenta	n–↑	++	100–1500	Tc↓	15–20%, M
CCHF	2–5 days	5–8 days	Liver	↓	+	400–>2000	Tc↓ DIC	20–30%, M, S
RVF	2–6 days	5–8 (21) days	Liver, brain, retina	↓	+	100–1500	Tc↓ DIC	1%, M, S, R
E/MHF	5–12 (21) days	5–9 days	Liver	↓, AL	++	100–1500	Tc↓ DIC	<50%, M, S

Notes:
[a] For clinically ill cases.
Tc: thrombocytes. DIC: disseminated intravascular coagulopathy. M: muscosal, S: skin, R: retinal. AL: atypical lymphocytes, ALT: alanine aminotransferase; AST: aspartate aminotransferase, E/MHF: Ebola/Marburg haemorrhagic fever.

headache. The majority of Yellow fever and Rift Valley fever infections, and probably as many as 75 per cent of Lassa virus infections are only mildly symptomatic or asymptomatic. The onset of symptoms may be very abrupt as in RVF and CCHF.

- Fever is usually high and unremitting.
- Conjunctival injection is common.
- Gastrointestinal symptoms: vomiting and diarrhoea may occur; abdominal pain has been sufficiently severe to cause laparotomy.
- A rash may appear in some VHFs, through capillary dilatation leading to erythema of the upper trunk, or petechial, as in Ebola and Marburg disease.
- Bradycardia is often noticeable.
- Later features: hepatitis, proteinuria, plasma leakage, oedema, bleeding and encephalopathy develop in some patients, usually during the second week of illness.

Capillary leak is often heralded by petechiae on the trunk and in the oropharynx, followed by bleeding from the gums, vagina, lower GI tract and kidneys.

Management

Therapy with a nucleoside analogue (Ribavirin), which reduces synthesis of all messenger RNA in infected and uninfected cells, has been well evaluated for Lassa fever. Experimental and anecdotal data indicate that it might also be effective in Rift Valley fever and Crimean–Congo fever. Plasma from presumably immune or convalescent persons usually contains low titres of neutralizing antibody, so that immune therapy has produced mostly negative or equivocal results and is therefore not recommended.

General care

With good supportive care, fluid control and antibiotic coverage if necessary, the mortality of VHF infections can be reduced. Nosocomial transmission can be prevented by strict barrier nursing (Table 58.3, Fig. 58.1) together with special disinfection and burial procedures.

Other techniques

Advanced life support, haemodialysis and surgical interventions will require higher levels of protection for the staff, e.g. HEPA-filter respirators, but these medical interventions are normally not available where VHF outbreaks occur.

Recovery period

Patients usually suffer from prolonged periods of asthenia during recovery and may shed infectious virus in urine and semen for some weeks in the case of Ebola/Marburg and Lassa virus infections.

Diagnosis

Presumptive diagnosis

Suspect VHF in a patient who:

- lives in or comes within the incubation period from a known VHF-endemic area
- presents with otherwise unexplained high fever, oedema, haemorrhagic diathesis, jaundice, CNS symptoms
- reports contact with another VHF patient or a known VHF-vector.

Haemorrhagic fever is primarily a clinical diagnosis, but for public health reasons, rapid laboratory confirmation of

Table 58.3. Principles of barrier nursing (WHO guidelines)

Protective clothing	Double gloves, (single use) gown, plastic apron, mask (P3 protection preferable), goggles. Disinfect within isolation area or destroy (single use material)	
Hand washing	After each patient contact or contact with infected material. Rinse in disinfectant, then wash with soap and water. Disinfectant/washing facilities must be located just outside isolation rooms.	
Instruments	Individual thermometer for each patient, keep in receptacle with disinfectant. Disinfect stethoscope and sleeve of sphygmomanometer between each use. Place all reusable instruments in disinfecting fluid after use.	
Bed covering and linen	Use of plastic sheet to cover and protect entire mattress is essential. Disinfect after discharge or death of the patient. Place bedding and linen in plastic bag for sterilization (soak in disinfectant, boil or autoclave)	
Food	Food should be supplied by hospital, not by relatives. Each patient must have own eating utensils. Wash and disinfect in isolation area, dispose of uneaten food.	
Charts and records	Keep outside isolation area	
Methods of disinfection	Household beach:	VHF-viruses are killed by 1 min exposure to 1:10 solution, or 10 min exposure to 1:100 solution
	Heat–sterilization:	If autoclave not available, boil at 100 °C for 20 min

a suspected VHF is mandatory. During the first week of clinical illness, virus is easily detected by cell culture, viral antigen by ELISA and viral RNA by polymerase chain reaction, but all methods require specialized laboratories.

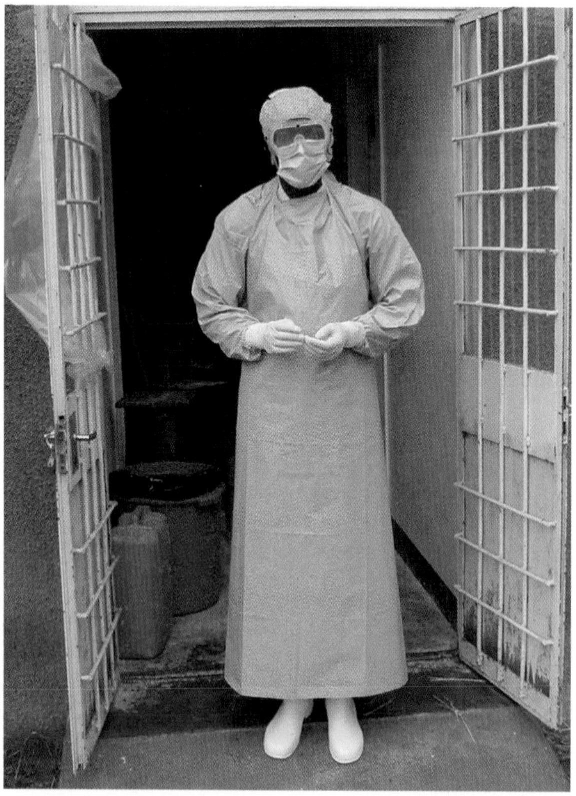

Fig. 58.1. Protective clothing in Uganda: health worker in full protective clothing in Mbarara during the Ebola outbreak.

Blood samples have to be handled and shipped to a reference laboratory using special precautions (triple packaging: a leakproof primary, leakproof secondary and robust outer container, with absorbent material between) and have to be inactivated for performing routine laboratory tests (Table 58.4).

If the patient dies in the second week, antiviral antibodies often remain undetectable or very low. Otherwise IgM and IgG antibodies can be detected by ELISA or immunofluorescence, preferably in paired serum samples. Detection of IgM antibodies in a single serum sample is sufficient for the presumptive diagnosis of yellow fever.

Management of VHFs

First line

- Isolate the patient, protect staff, give basic supportive care.
- Notify local health authorities early.
- Enquire about similar cases – ongoing epidemic?

Supportive care

In case of limited facilities, give:

- oral rehydration for dehydration
- paracetamol for fever
- diazepam for restlessness.

Table 58.4. Inactivation of blood/serum from VHF patients for laboratory analysis

Material	Examination	Inactivation
Blood	Thick film	Add formalin to a final concentration of 1% to solution used for lysis of erythrocytes
Blood	Thin film	Methanol fixation
Blood	Leukocyte count	1:100 in 3% acetic acid, 15 min room temperature
Serum/plasma	Serological tests	Heat for 60 min at 60 °C[a] 0.25% β – propiolactone (final concentration), 30 min 37 °C
Serum/plasma	Clinical chemistry	heat for 60 min at 60 °C[b] 0.25% β – propiolactone (final concentration), 30 min 37 °C[c] 0.1% Triton X-100 (final concentration), 60 min room temp[d]

Notes:
[a] Loss of reactivity. Heating at 56 °C for 1 hour preserves antibodies better but leaves sample with residual infectivity. Only recommended if sample can safely be handled under biological safety level 2 conditions (laminar air flow).
[b] No influence on sodium, potassium, magnesium, urea, creatinine, urate, bilirubin, glucose, C-reactive protein (CRP). Bicarbonate, aspartate aminotransferase (AST), calcium, phosphate, albumin, total protein reduced. Alkaline phosphate (ALP), alanine aminotransferase(ALT), gamma glutamyl transpeptidase (GGT), creatine kinase (CK) cannot be measured.
[c] Liver enzyme values reduced by 20%. pH and bicarbonate not useful.
[d] Influence on clinical chemistry not evaluated.

Treat concurrent malaria and bacterial infections with locally recommended drugs

Careful maintenance of hydration and management of shock, cerebral oedema, renal failure and hypoxia are important.

Keep injections and parenteral interventions to a minimum to avoid bleeding. Replacement of coagulation factors, e.g. with fresh blood, and of platelets may be of value.

Prevention of VHFs

Since 1991, yellow fever vaccination has been recommended for the Expanded Program of Immunization (EPI), but only 17 African countries have adopted this policy. Monitoring of the different risk factors which lead to transmission of the other viruses causing VHFs is a Public Health task (see respective chapters). Control of CCHF and RVF is a veterinary problem. Lassa fever can be prevented through reducing contact between rodents and humans (food storage, destruction of rodents). Since the natural reservoir of filoviruses remains unknown, avoidance of contact with dead and diseased monkeys and control of monkey sellers remain the only feasible options.

Timely implementation of relatively simple hygiene measures (Table 58.3) when dealing with suspected VHF cases is the most important action to prevent nosocomial spread. This requires a high level of suspicion on the part of the primary physician practising in a VHF-endemic region, and the necessary equipment to be kept in stock. Equally important is a functional communication system which channels the report of suspected VHF cases through the national health system to WHO.

YELLOW FEVER

Clinical case definition for suspected yellow fever (WHO):
An illness characterized by acute onset of fever followed by jaundice within 2 weeks of onset of first symptoms *and* one of the following: (i) bleeding from nose, gums, skin or GI tract or (ii) death within 3 weeks of onset of illness.

Historical perspective

The first clinical description of YF in Africa (Senegal) dates back to the end of the eighteenth century. However, the slave trade had brought the virus and its vector, *Aedes aegypti*, to South America where epidemics were recorded as early as the seventeenth century. The first theory of mosquito transmission of yellow fever was published in 1881 by the Cuban physician C.J. Finlay and was later proven by Walter Reed by experimental transmisson of the virus from mosquitoes to humans (1900). Using immune serum, M. Theiler developed a mouse protection assay in 1931, which became the basis for the development of a vaccine.

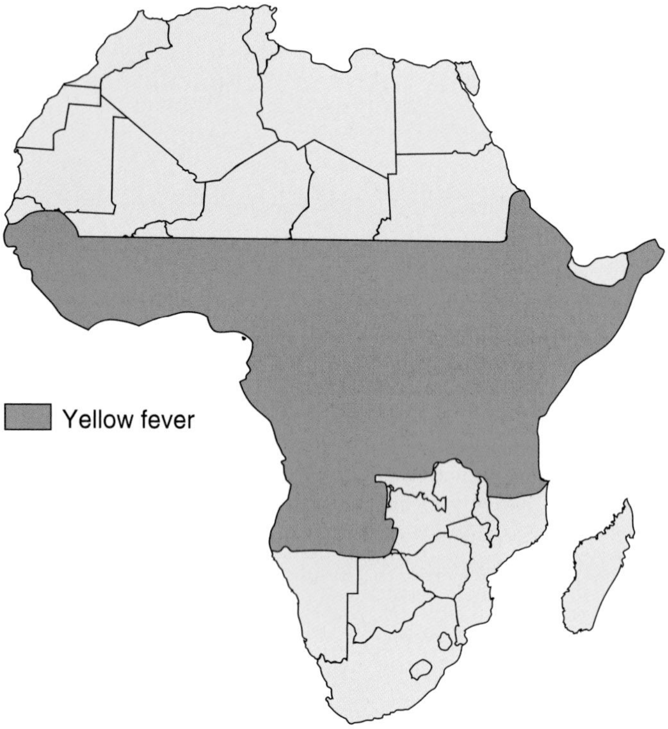

Fig. 58.2. Distribution of yellow fever in Africa.

Subsequently, two live attenuated vaccines were developed, the 'French neurotropic vaccine' and the '17D vaccine'.

After administering more than 40 million doses of the French vaccine until the 1950s, yellow fever activity in the francophone parts of West Africa dropped considerably. However, because it caused encephalitis in 0.3 per cent of children under the age of 10, vaccination with the French neurotropic vaccine was stopped in 1980. The 17D vaccine, which was derived at the Rockefeller Laboratories, New York, through 176 serial passages of a yellow fever isolate named 'Asibi' (Ghana, 1927), was found to be very efficacious and exceptionally safe in studies in South America. It is today the only type of YF vaccine produced. Approximately 100 million doses of vaccine are produced annually under the control of WHO. This is far from sufficient if YF should re-emerge in large epidemics in South America or Africa.

Epidemiology

The problem in Africa

Yellow fever is endemic in sub-saharan Africa south of 15° northern latitude and north of 10° southern latitude (Fig. 58.2). Thirty-four countries with an estimated population of 510 million people are located in this area. Approximately 250 million people live in high-risk countries for yellow fever, which are defined by WHO as countries with 'large epidemics in recent years, high number of reported cases, highly populated, poor EPI and weak infrastructure'. Medium-risk countries are those with epidemics/reported cases in the past, including countries that have included YF into EPI; lower-risk countries have not reported epidemics, or at least not in the last 20 years. Eighty-three per cent of the population from the high- and medium-risk countries live in Cameroon, Ghana, Côte d'Ivoire, Nigeria and Senegal. Africa has seen a steady increase of cases and the re-occurrence of epidemics since the 1980s.

During YF epidemics the incidence of infection may be as high as 20 per cent and the incidence of disease 3 per cent. In the past 25 years major epidemics have occurred in Ethiopia 1960–62 (100 000 cases), Senegal 1965 (10 000 cases), the Gambia 1978 (8500 cases) and Nigeria 1986–91 (>100 000 cases). Endemic YF and small outbreaks occur throughout much of Africa, but in the absence of epidemics, YF cases are usually substantially underreported. Thorough epidemiologic and virologic studies have shown that, even during outbreaks, the ratio of actual to reported cases varies from 3: 1 to 250: 1.

According to WHO estimates, up to 200 000 cases and 30 000 deaths may occur each year in sub-Saharan Africa. The range of yellow fever cases has expanded in recent years. Gabon and Liberia, which experienced outbreaks in 1994/95 had previously not reported any cases of yellow fever since the 1950s and 1960s, respectively. Sierra Leone reported its first outbreak since 1975. In 2000, the Republic of Guinea experienced its first major epidemic (>800 cases/290 deaths). In 1992 Kenya reported its first outbreak of yellow fever since 1950 and has consistently reported cases each year since then. Thus yellow fever may be expanding its range to include previously unaffected areas.

Ecological patterns

Yellow fever is a truly re-emerging disease. In Africa, it occurs in three ecologically different settings (Fig. 58.3).

Rainforest – jungle YF

In the rainforest, the virus is en- and epizootically transmitted between monkeys by *Aedes africanus*, a tree-hole breeding mosquito adapted to feeding on monkeys. The virus is transovarially passed on to the next generation, therefore the mosquito must be regarded as the true reservoir. Humans working in the forest are occasionally bitten and infected ('jungle yellow fever').

Savannah/forest – intermediate YF

Increased transmission occurs on the border between forest and moist-savannah and within the savannah, especially where monkeys are numerous. There, the virus is transmitted enzootically between monkeys by tree-hole breeding *Ae. furcifer* and *Ae. luteocephalus*. However, because these mosquitoes additionally feed on humans, the virus also causes endemic yellow fever in the savannah ('intermediate yellow fever'). Depending on the density of the mosquito and monkey populations, this ecology often gives rise to small or large outbreaks occurring simultaneously in many separate villages. The savannah is therefore called the 'zone of emergence'.

Urban YF

In the presence of *Ae. aegypti*, a day-biting mosquito well adapted to feeding on humans and breeding in artificial containers, human-to-human transmission can give rise to epidemics. If patients seek treatment in villages or towns with a susceptible (non-vaccinated) population, where *Ae. aegypti* is present (Breteau index >50, see below), devastating epidemics of 'urban' yellow fever can occur. *Ae. aegypti* breeds in many types of artificially made containers (e.g. discarded cans, flower dishes, tyres, uncovered containers for drinking water) and the extent of infestation with this mosquito is graded by counting the number of containers with larvae of *Ae. aegypti* detected per 100 houses/premises ('Breteau-Index').

Immunity

Immunity against YF increases with age in endemic regions, and children are at greatest risk of infection. Antibody and T-cell-mediated immunity against other flaviviruses circulating in the same geographic region (e.g. Dengue, Zika) may play a role by partially cross-protecting against YF virus.

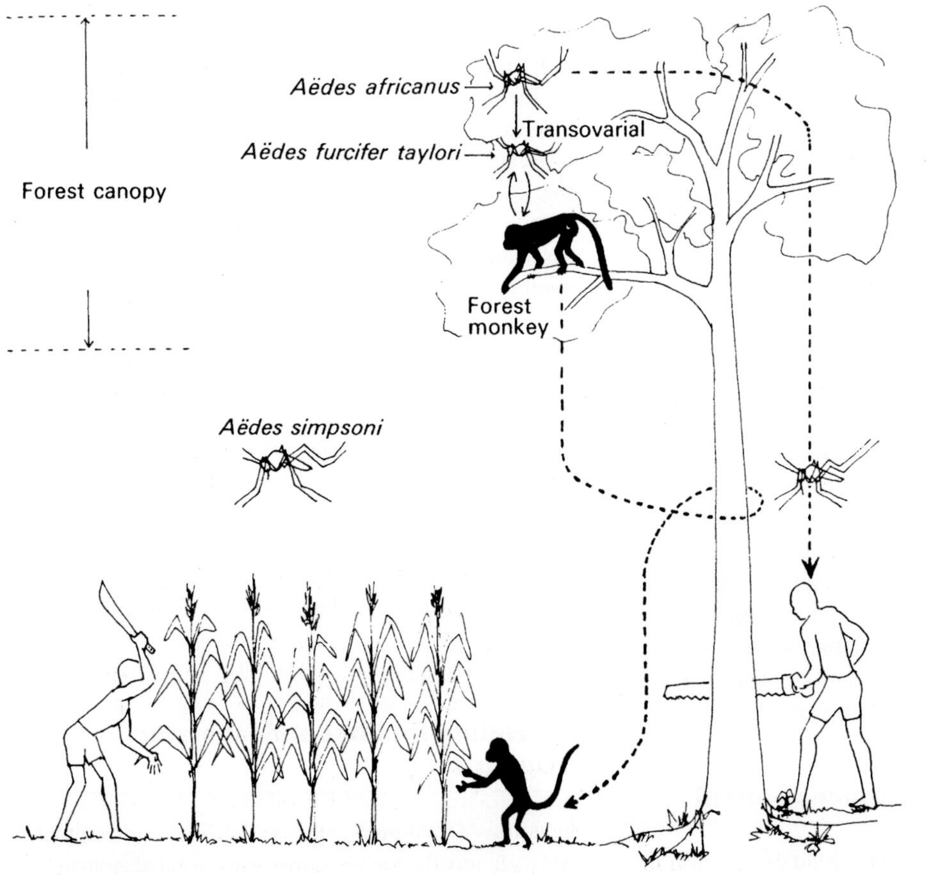

Fig. 58.3. Forest and savannah yellow fever transmission.

Reasons for the resurgence of yellow fever in Africa include:
- low immunization coverage
- increasing settlement of forested areas
- substandard water systems (breeding sites for mosquitoes)
- increase in distribution and density of mosquito vectors
- widespread international air travel.

The virus

Whereas until recently only two genotypes (genetically distinct variants) of yellow fever had been identified in Africa, new sequence data reveal the existence of five genotypes (Central/East Africa, East Africa, Angola, West Africa I, West Africa II). Most genotypes are highly homogeneous but the YF strains belonging to the West Africa I genotype show higher genetic variation, probably due to regular human epidemics. There is no evidence that the 17D vaccine does not offer protection against all genotypes of YF.

Pathogenesis

Severe yellow fever is characterized by combined hepatic and renal dysfunction, haemorrhage and circulatory shock. Initially, the virus replicates in the regional lymph nodes and spreads via the bloodstream to liver, spleen, bone marrow and myocardium. The Kupffer cells of the liver are infected first, thereafter the hepatocytes in the midzone of the liver lobule. Eosinophilic degeneration ('Councilman bodies') of these cells probably represents apoptosis and is characteristic of the infection, as well as vacuolar fatty changes and minimal mononuclear infiltration. Serum transaminases and bilirubin are raised. Prolonged prothrombin, partial thromboplastin and clotting time, and thrombocytopenia are all responsible for the observed haemorrhages. A subset of patients develops disseminated intravascular coagulopathy (DIC).

Haemorrhages are found on mucosal surfaces of the gastrointestinal tract, the abdominal and pleural serosa and in the brain, where oedema is also present. Some degree of renal failure is present in all severe infections, the underlying pathology of which is characterized by acute tubular necrosis and fatty change. Kidney damage results in low urine output and uraemia. The myocardial fibres show cloudy swelling and fatty degeneration.

Clinical presentation and management

The incubation period is 3 to 6 days. Mild disease occurs in 80–90 per cent of infections with sudden onset of fever and headaches, myalgia and lassitude, lasting for 2–4 days. Mild YF resembles influenza, except that coryzal symptoms are lacking. Ten to twenty per cent of patients develop the classical symptoms of yellow fever characterized by three distinct clinical periods.

The infectious period is characterized by abrupt onset of high fever (40 °C), chills, headache, generalized myalgias, lumbosacral pain, nausea with vomiting, and dizziness. Minor bleeding from the nose and gums may occur. Young children may have febrile convulsions. The patient presents with congestion of conjunctivae and face, a centrally white-furred tongue with bright reddening at the edges and the tip, and a pulse slow in relation to the fever (Faget's sign). During this phase, which lasts several days, virus can be isolated from the blood.

Period of remission

On the third day of illness the fever may fall, and the patient either enters the period of remission or, in the malignant form, massive haemorrhages, delirium and anuria may occur. Remission lasts several hours to several days.

Period of intoxication

The illness reappears after the remission and progresses during the period of intoxication, which is the most variable, lasting up to 2 weeks. The 'classic' symptoms are fever, slow pulse, prostration, epigastric pain and vomiting, jaundice and haemorrhages. Haematemesis ('black vomit') is more characteristic than jaundice and is often associated with a fatal outcome. Other manifestations of haemorrhage are epistaxis, petechiae, ecchymoses, melaena, uterine haemorrhages and bleeding from needle puncture sites. Despite albuminuria occurring in 90 per cent of patients, ascites and oedema are not reported.

The case-fatality rate in severe cases is as high as 50 per cent. Most patients die 7–10 days after onset of illness. Hypothermia, hypotension, coma, delirium and intractable hiccups are terminal events. Convalescence is prolonged. Late deaths from arrhythmias and heart failure have been reported and bacterial pneumonia may occur. The liver recovers completely without developing cirrhosis.

Laboratory findings and laboratory diagnosis

Leukopenia is common early in the disease (down to 2000 cells/μl), mostly due to neutropenia. Total leukocyte counts return to normal by the tenth day, but in fatal cases there may be terminal leukocytosis. Platelet numbers are depressed. Albuminuria is in the range of 3–20 g/l. Hepatic transaminases may be grossly elevated and total and conjugated bilirubin rise simultaneously. Hypoglycaemia and hyperkalaemia occur preterminally. The CSF shows increased pressure and elevated protein, but no cells. The electrocardiogram may show ST segment or T-wave abnormalities.

At present, there are 15 laboratories in Africa that have the facilities and expertise to diagnose yellow fever. The IgM-ELISA is the most widely used serologic test, because IgM antibody appears early in the course of infection. Yellow fever is diagnosed presumptively on the basis of one single positive IgM result; however, confirmation depends on detection of a four-fold rise of antibody titre in paired serum samples (second sample 10–14 days later). Virus isolation (inoculation of serum on AP61 insect cells) is possible only for a few days during the infectious period and requires biological safety equipment. The polymerase chain reaction (PCR) for detection of viral RNA is of limited value and less sensitive than the IgM test. However, isolation and characterization of YF virus from at least a few patients is highly desirable during suspected outbreaks, because other flaviviruses circulating in the same geographic region (e.g. dengue) may give rise to false-positive or doubtful antibody test results. Post-mortem transdermal needle biopsy of the liver is a convenient way to diagnose YF (immuno-) histopathologically, but hepatic biopsy during the acute illness is contraindicated because of bleeding complications.

Management

There is no specific treatment for yellow fever. Good supportive care is important (see above). Intravenous cimetidine has been used to reduce the risk of gastric haemorrhage.

Prevention and control

Bed net

The acutely ill patient should be placed under a bednet to prevent contact with mosquito vectors.

Vaccination

The currently available live attenuated yellow fever vaccine 17D is very safe, protects over 95 per cent of recipients and confers immunity for at least 10 years. Contraindications to routine vaccination include age <9 months (most encephalitis cases reported in children aged <4 months), pregnancy (some studies suggest a small increase of spontaneous abortions in early pregnancy), and clinically manifest immunosuppression. During YF epidemics these precautions may be modified if the risk of YF outweighs the risk of vaccination.

Because the vaccine is propagated in chick embryos, persons with known egg allergy should be tested before vaccination.

Vaccination and HIV

Asymptomatic HIV patients can be safely vaccinated. From the very few good data available on vaccination of HIV-infected persons it seems that the vaccine induces neutralizing antibodies and does not cause serious side effects.

Two strategies

There are two strategies for YF prevention and control.

For outbreak prevention

YF immunization is given routinely as part of EPI or in mass immunization campaigns.

For outbreak control

Countries rely on surveillance to detect YF cases and then perform mass immunizations in response to the outbreak. As of May 1996, YF immunization coverage data had been reported to WHO by 16 African countries, 11 of them during 1994–1995. Coverage levels ranged from 1 per cent to 87 per cent, with only three countries, Burkina Faso (55 per cent), the Central African Republic (52 per cent) and the Gambia (87 per cent) exceeding 50 per cent coverage. Depending on vector biting rate and vector competence, the prevalence of immunity in humans to prevent an epidemic has been estimated as being between 60 and 90 per cent.

LASSA FEVER

Lassa fever should be suspected in a patient:
- living in or coming within the incubation period (7–21 days) from rural areas in Sierra Leone, Liberia, Nigeria or the Republic of Guinea
- presenting with otherwise unexplained high fever (>38.5 °C), pharyngitis with dry cough and chest pain or abdominal pain and diarrhoea, facial oedema, mucosal bleeding, CNS symptoms. Thirty per cent of convalescent patients have acute hearing loss.

Epidemiology

The problem in Africa

The Lassa virus is confined to sub-saharan Africa (McCormick et al 1987a,b). Clinical cases occur regularly in rural areas of Nigeria, Liberia, Sierra Leone and the Republic of Guinea. Serological evidence of Lassa virus infection has been reported from Senegal, Ghana and Ivory Coast. Lassa or Lassa-like viruses are very likely to exist in small endemic foci in many other West African countries, too. Lassa-like viruses with unknown pathogenicity for man have been isolated from rodents in the Central African Republic and Mozambique.

Three hundred thousand to 500 000 infections are estimated to occur annually in West Africa, resulting in approximately 150 000 clinical cases, which range from flu-like illness to haemorrhagic fever, and approximately 5000 deaths. Seventy-five per cent of all Lassa virus infections are believed to be asymptomatic in endemic areas. The overall mortality is 1–5 per cent.

An antibody prevalence of up to 50 per cent may be found in people living in hyperendemic areas. Lassa fever accounts for up to 15 per cent of all medical admissions in selected hospitals in eastern Sierra Leone.

The reservoir

Reservoir hosts include several subspecies of a ubiquitous African small rodent, the multimammate rat (*Mastomys natalensis*), which live in and around human habitations. Infection of rodents is very focal; in one village 30 per cent of rodents may be infected, in the neighbouring village none.

Transmission

Rodents, which are infected in utero, become chronic carriers of the virus and shed it all their lives in urine and saliva. People become infected by ingestion of foodstuff contaminated with rodent excreta, by inhaling small, urine-contaminated dust particles, to which the virus has dried, and by direct handling of infected rodents. In some forest areas rodents are hunted and eaten, which poses a great risk for infection.

Human-to-human transmission does not seem to play a major role in the community. Lassa fever is notorious for hospital outbreaks, when it is mainly transmitted during procedures involving intimate contact with blood and through improperly sterilized instruments. Lassa fever patients are not infectious during the incubation period and quite close contact with body fluids is required to transmit Lassa virus from a clinically ill patient to another person. However, airborne transmission, most likely through direct contact with droplets produced during heavy coughing (*Lassa pneumonitis*), has been reported in a few instances.

Transmission of Lassa fever may also occur in a quasi-epidemic fashion in rural areas due to increased rodent-to-human contact because of fluctuations in rodent density, human population movements (new susceptibles) or harvest activities.

Pathogenesis and specific clinical presentation

Prodromal phase

After an incubation period of 7 to 16 days, Lassa fever has an insidious onset and flu-like prodrome (fever, rigors, headache, muscle and backache, malaise).

Pharyngitis

The development a few days later of a severe, exudative (or ulcerative) pharyngitis is quite typical, if encountered in combination with high (or spiking) fever (to 40 °C), adominal pain, vomiting, transient diarrhoea, retrosternal pain and dry cough. The yellow and white patches of exudate and shallow ulcers over the fauces, soft palate and tonsils can easily be confused with streptococcal pharyngitis, infectious mononucleosis or diphtheria. The pharyngitis may be severe enough to prevent the patient from swallowing his own saliva. In Lassa endemic areas, the combination of fever, pharyngitis, retrosternal pain and proteinuria has a positive predictive value for Lassa fever of 81 per cent (specificity 89 per cent, sensitivity 46 per cent).

Blood and urine changes

Lassa fever is the only HF in which the number of thrombocytes is not significantly depressed. Other haematological findings include a mean WBC count of 6×10^9/l on admission, an early lymphopenia, a relative neutrophilia and immature forms of leukocytes. Urinalysis reveals proteinuria, which is often massive. The parameters of haemostasis are normal or only slightly depressed, whereas thrombocyte aggregation is severely impaired.

Most patients (75 per cent) start to recover during the second week, but 30 per cent of these develop a uni- or bilateral auditory deficit, which remains permanent in half of the cases.

Increased capillary permeability

Those who deteriorate suffer from severe vomiting and show evidence of diffusely increased capillary permeability, which manifests itself in swelling of the eyelids, face and neck. Effusions into serous cavities, cerebral and pulmonary oedema and albuminuria lead to loss of circulating volume and result in hypotension, renal failure and death.

Bleeding, mostly confined to external and internal mucosal surfaces, occurs in 10–20 per cent. Neurological symptoms (encephalopathy and encephalitis) occur infrequently. High viral titre in serum ($>10^4$/ml), markedly raised liver enzymes and bleeding carry a poor prognosis. High neutrophil counts ($>30\times10^9$/l) may be observed in these patients. Mortality of patients in hospital is 10–15 per cent, but 20 per cent in the first and 30 per cent in the second trimester of pregnancy. Fetal loss occurs in 87 per cent of pregnant women with Lassa fever.

Viraemia is prolonged (up to 4 weeks) in the presence of high titres of non-neutralizing antibodies. Viruria during the acute phase of the disease is not the rule, however, infectious virus has been recovered from urine as long as 3 months after onset of disease.

Specific treatment and prophylaxis

The guanosine analogue ribavirin has been shown to reduce mortality five- to ten-fold if given intravenously within the first 6 days of clinical illness. Loading dose is 30 mg/kg, followed by 16 mg/kg every 6 hours for 4 days and then 8 mg/kg every 8 hours for 6 more days. Side effects are reversible anaemia and rigors, if the drug is infused too quickly. There is no convincing evidence that oral ribavirin delays or prevents Lassa fever after exposure to the virus and it is therefore not generally recommended as post-exposure prophylaxis. However, it may be considered for high-risk contacts of Lassa fever patients.

In pregnant women with Lassa fever, spontaneous or therapeutic abortion resulted in a four-fold reduction of mortality.

Public health measures to reduce human-rodent contact are of vital importance, as well as immediately installing barrier nursing techniques in cases of suspected Lassa fever.

RIFT VALLEY FEVER

The problem in Africa

Rift Valley fever virus is prevalent throughout Africa. Epizootics (epidemics among animals) affecting livestock have occurred most frequently in Kenya, Tanzania, Uganda, Zimbabwe, Zambia and South Africa, but the virus has also been isolated in other sub-saharan countries – Mauretania, Senegal, Guinea, Burkina Faso, Nigeria, CAR, Namibia, South Africa, Sudan, DRC (Wilson et al., 1994). Serological evidence of the virus is found in many other countries. In contrast, epidemics of severe human disease have been reported to date only from Egypt, Mauretania, Madagascar and East Africa. Rift Valley fever virus was recently exported with non-quarantined livestock from East Africa to Saudi Arabia and Yemen.

Epidemiology

The natural reservoirs and vectors are Culicine and Anopheline mosquitoes, which pass the virus transovarially to their offspring. Virus can survive in dried mosquito eggs deposited in 'dambos'; these are low lying areas of perpetual flooding. New generations of infected mosquitoes may hatch even after several years from these infected eggs. Virus activity thus coincides with rainfall and mosquito density (Fontenille et al., 1998).

In endemic foci, Rift Valley fever virus causes disease and abortion in small ruminants, particularly sheep. Between epizootics, RVF antibody prevalences of 10–20 per cent are found within herds. Longitudinal studies show seroconversion rates of about 5 per cent per year. Human cases are usually linked to periods of intense epizootics, when many mosquitoes of different species become infected and the cattle serve as amplifier for the virus. Introduction of the virus into susceptible populations is also important. Major epidemics have occurred in Egypt (1977–1978, 18 000 cases/598 deaths), Mauretania (1987, 1998), Madagascar (1991), Somalia/Kenya (1997–1998, 89 000 cases/200 deaths) and Saudi Arabia/Yemen (2000, 857 cases/119 deaths in Saudi Arabia).

Between epidemics, higher seroprevalences (20 per cent) are found in the age groups which have been exposed to the virus during past epidemics, whereas non-exposed age groups show rates of less than 5 per cent. IgM antibodies indicative of recent infection are found in high-risk populations such as abattoir and livestock workers, who therefore constitute a good sentinel group for the monitoring of RVF. A very significant risk factor for seropositivity among semi-nomadic people is caring for sick animals, independent of sex and age group. Under non-epizootic conditions, contact with sick animals is probably the major risk factor for human transmission, rather than mosquito transmission. Rodents have also been found seropositive for RVF antibodies and the species *Mastomys* and *Arvicanthis* may be involved in an enzootic cycle of the virus.

Pathogenesis and specific clinical presentation

In animals

RVF virus causes severe disease in cattle, sheep, camels and goats, with sheep being most and goats least susceptible. Disease is characterized by fever, hyperactivity, mucoid or bloody nasal discharges, vomiting, bloody diarrhoea, external haemorrhage and clinical manifestations of nervous disorders. Ninety per cent of lambs infected with RFV will die, whereas mortality amongst adult sheep may be as low as 10 per cent. The abortion rate amongst pregnant, infected ewes is almost 100 per cent. Equines and pigs are refractory to disease and infection is usually asymptomatic in camels, except for abortions. Epizootics tend to manifest themselves as a wave of unexplained abortion among livestock.

In humans

After an incubation period of 2 to 6 days, the onset of disease is sudden. Mild disease is characterized by an influenza-like illness with high fever (often saddleback-type), headache, myalgia and backache (Gear, 1989). The patient may also develop neck stiffness, photophobia and vomiting, thus giving the impression of meningitis. The viraemia is brief, and the patient makes a full recovery after the disease has run its course of 5 to 8 days. Haematological findings include an initially normal leukocyte count, followed by leukopenia and neutropenia with increase in band forms.

While the majority of infections are asymptomatic or mild, severe disease manifests itself as encephalitis (<1 per cent), retinitis (0.5–2 per cent) or haemorrhagic fever (<1 per cent). Severe liver involvement (jaundice) and haemorrhagic complications (purpuric rash, vomiting of blood, melaena, gum bleeding) may develop 2 to 4 days after the onset of symptoms. The patient is often afebrile when severe complications develop. Case fatality rates of up to 50 per cent have been reported for severe cases.

Meningoencephalitic complications (neurological symptoms, elevated CSF lymphocyte count) and ocular involvement (retinal lesions) develop 1 to 3 weeks after the onset of fever and can have permanent sequelae. The retinal lesions (extensive vasculitis accompanied by white macular lesions) are specific for Rift Valley fever. There is presently no evidence that RVF infection causes abortion in humans.

Specific treatment and prophylaxis

Most RVF cases are mild and do not require treatment. Ribavirin (see Lassa fever) has been shown to inhibit viral replication experimentally but has not yet been investigated in humans. A formalin-inactivated and a live-attenuated vaccine ('MP-12') are available for veterinary use.

EBOLA AND MARBURG HAEMORRHAGIC FEVERS (EHF, MHF)

Epidemiology

Outbreaks of Ebola fever have occurred in Sudan (1976, 1979), Zaire/DRC (1976, 1977, 1995 – see *J Infect Dis* 1999 **179**, Suppl. 1 ix–xvi, 1–288), Côte d'Ivoire (1994), Gabon (1994, 1995, 1996, 1999) and most recently in Uganda, chiefly in the north (2000). Ebola virus, strain Reston, was imported on several occasions with wild-caught monkeys (*Macaca fascicularis*) from Mindanao, Republic of the Philippines, to USA and Italy (1989–1996), but appears not to be pathogenic for humans.

Marburg virus was imported with monkeys (*Cercopithecus aethiops*) from Uganda to Germany in 1967. Three sporadic cases of Marburg virus infection have been reported in Zimbabwe and Kenya (1975, 1980, 1987). Marburg virus appeared recently in the Democratic Republic of Congo (1999), were it caused its first, still ongoing, outbreak.

Ebola and Marburg viruses (family *filoviruses*) have caused over 1400 human haemorrhagic fever cases with a mortality ranging from 20–80 per cent. Despite intensive research, it has not been possible to identify the natural reservoirs or vectors of the viruses. Primates and other monkeys are victims of the viruses themselves; therefore they are not the reservoir, but may transmit the infection to humans. Contact with dead chimpanzees found in the rainforest transmitted Ebola virus in Côte d'Ivoire (Tai forest) and in Gabon where the chimp's meat was used for food.

Contact with bats was reported for the Ebola and Marburg index cases of the Sudan and DRC epidemics, respectively. Bats can be experimentally infected with Ebola virus. Since they excrete the virus in body fluids and do not develop disease, they are high on the list as potential reservoirs. Asymptomatic Ebola infections have recently clearly been documented in humans during the Gabon epidemics, but are thought to be uncommon.

Filoviruses are transmitted through direct skin or mucous membrane contact with virus-infected body fluids such as blood, saliva, vomitus, faeces and possibly sweat. There is no evidence that close personal contact with a non-febrile, non-symptomatic, Ebola-infected individual during the incubation period results in transmission. The viruses have been shown to be present in the genital secretions of convalescent patients several weeks after illness and sexual transmission during convalescence has been documented for Marburg virus.

Household contacts have been responsible for up to 20 per cent of transmission and up to five generations of infection. Previous epidemics in Africa have resulted largely from secondary spread to health care workers and family contacts caring for the ill. Nosocomial spread through improperly sterilized reusable syringes caused explosive Ebola epidemics in Sudan and Zaire. The mortality among surgical staff operating on VHF patients is also exceptionally high. Nursing activities and preparing the corpse for burial carry a high risk of infection, as do burial practices which include touching the corpse and collectively washing hands in a common bowl thereafter. There is no convincing epidemiological evidence that Ebola or Marburg viruses are transmitted as true, small particle aerosols between humans, but direct mucosal exposure to droplets generated by a patient during coughing poses a high risk of infection.

Clinical features

Marburg and Ebola viruses cause identical clinical disease. After an incubation period of 5 to 12 days, the onset is sudden with fever, headache, myalgia, sore throat, and extreme fatigue. Early signs also include conjunctivitis and bradycardia. Severe nausea, vomiting, abdominal pain and profuse watery diarrhoea are commonly observed. A perifollicular, non-itching, maculopapular rash frequently appears around day 5 on the trunk, back and shoulders, spreading to the face and limbs and becoming confluent. It may be difficult to see and has a measles-like appearance on dark skin. The rash fades in 3–10 days and is followed by desquamation in survivors.

In about half of the patients haemorrhagic manifestations occur between the fifth and seventh day, including epistaxis, gum-bleeding, haematemesis, melaena, petechiae, ecchymoses, haemorrhages from needle sticks and postmortem evidence of visceral haemorrhagic effusions. Dehydration and prostration are frequent, the patients show the ghost-like facial expression typical of the disease.

During the first week the temperature remains high around 40 °C, falling by lysis during the second week, to rise again between days 12 and 14. Other clinical signs during the second week include hepatosplenomegaly, oedema, orchitis, scrotal or labial reddening, myocarditis and pancreatitis. A poor prognosis is marked by haemorrhagic signs, oliguria or anuria, chest pain, shock, tachypnoea and neurological symptoms (sudden hearing loss, blindness, painful paraesthesia, intractable hiccups). Death in shock usually occurs 6 to 9 days after onset of clinical disease (range 1–21 days). Abortion is a common consequence of infection.

Laboratory investigations

Haematological studies reveal early leukopenia, thrombocytopenia accompanied by abnormal platelet aggregation, subsequent relative neutrophilia and the appearance of atypical lymphocytes. Liver enzymes are elevated, alkaline phosphatase and bilirubin levels are usually normal or only slightly elevated.

Recovery

Recovery from Marburg and Ebola disease is prolonged (5 weeks or more) with arthralgia/persistent arthritis, ocular disease (ocular pain, photophobia, hyperlacrimation, loss of visual acuity, uveitis), hearing loss and orchitis occurring as late manifestations. Marburg virus has been isolated from the anterior chamber of the eye and from seminal fluid 7 weeks after onset of clinical disease and there has been a documented case of sexual transmission. The shedding of EBO–RNA has been detectable in semen/vaginal fluid by polymerase chain reaction (PCR) for months, but not by virus isolation. Patients should therefore refrain from unprotected sex during early convalescence.

Viral antigen post-mortem

In fatal cases there are disseminated deposits of viral antigen in different organs, including the sweat glands and the skin. This may explain the risk involved in touching corpses for burial preparations. A diagnostic immunohistochemical test has been devised based on a post-mortem skin-snip of the neck region, which can be fixed in formalin and sent to specialized laboratories.

Specific treatment and prophylaxis

There is no specific treatment for filovirus infections. Because lesions are widespread and the immune response is ineffective, it seems questionable whether good supportive care alone will have any major effect on the clinical outcome. Despite good clinical care being delivered to the majority of patients during the Ebola outbreak in Uganda (2000), the overall mortality was around 50 per cent.

Prevention

Barrier nursing
In cases of suspected Ebola or Marburg fever, more than with any other VHF,
Immediately install barrier nursing techniques

Sufficient skin, mucous membrane and respiratory protection (sufficiently large goggles or face shields, P3-masks or respirators, gowns, gloves, aprons, rubber boots) are necessary (Fig. 58.1). Very thorough training of the staff, not too long shifts on the Ebola ward and sufficient resting time are all extremely important to avoid infections (Bitekyerezo et al., 2002). The rate of nosocomial infection of hospital staff during the last Ebola epidemic in Gulu, Uganda was high, despite timely installing of barrier nursing measures and sufficient supply of protective materials. There were 29 infections leading to 17 deaths, including the medical superintendent of St Mary's hospital, Dr Matthew Lukwiya, who was prepared to stay at his post, and played an important role in fighting the epidemic. Diminished concentration of overworked staff most probably leads to self-inoculation with the virus, e.g. when wiping sweat off the forehead or eyes with contaminated gloves. Because the goggles used as eye protection tended to fog, many nurses reportedly did not use them regularly. Fine droplets of blood sprayed during coughing on the conjunctiva might have been an important mode of transmission. Any persons with close contact to EHF/MHF patients, their body fluids or contaminated materials without barrier nursing attire should be kept under strict surveillance for 3 weeks (temperature check twice daily, hospitalization and isolation if fever >38.8 °C/101 °F). Patients dying of EHF/MHF should be rapidly buried using special precautions.

Since the natural reservoir of filovirus infections remains unknown, avoidance of contact with dead and diseased monkeys and control of monkey sellers remain the only feasible options for prevention.

CRIMEAN-CONGO HAEMORRHAGIC FEVER (CCHF)

Epidemiology

CCHF occurs throughout Africa, the Middle East and in parts of Asia and Eastern Europe. It is an uncommon, sporadic illness, but it is feared for causing nosocomial outbreaks. Airborne spread, however, is not observed. Approximately ten haemorrhagic cases are diagnosed annually in South Africa.

The distribution of the virus parallels that of its vector and presumed reservoir, hard (ixodid) ticks of several genera. *Amblyomma*, *Rhipicephalus* and *Hylalomma* species are important vectors in Africa, the latter being most efficient transmitters of CCHF and most important vectors for humans. The ticks parasitize a variety of wild and domestic animals (sheep, goats, cattle, camels), including birds, which apparently do not develop clinical disease. Antibody prevalences ranging from 28 per cent to 45 per cent have been found in cattle from Zimbabwe and South Africa. Prevalences of 1 to 20 per cent in semi-nomadic tribes and up to 70 per cent in their sheep were reported in Senegal (Mariner et al., 1995).

Transmission of the virus to humans takes place through bites of infected ticks, through contact with blood of infected animals, or nosocomially through contact with infected body fluids. Despite high antibody prevalences in domestic animals, human infection is relatively infrequent, suggesting inefficient transmission of the virus or low virus prevalence in ticks. Activities involving contact with animals and their ticks (sheep shearing, milking, etc.) carry a risk of infection and abattoir workers are at increased risk.

Pathogenesis and specific clinical presentation

Apparently CCHF virus infection causes severe disease only in humans, who are accidental dead-end hosts for the virus. The illness-to-infection ratio after an infected tick-bite is not known, but is probably high. Viraemia is highest during the first 3 days of clinical onset and may persist into the second week.

After an incubation period of 2 to 5 days, the onset of disease is abrupt with severe headache, high fever, chills, myalgia and joint pains. Conjunctivitis, flushing of the face, petechiae on the palate, vomiting and occasionally diarrhoea are observed. Hepatomegaly occurs in half the patients, respiratory signs are unusual. Haemorrhagic manifestations usually begin on the fourth day with petechiae on the oral mucosa and skin (developing to ecchymoses), epistaxis, gingival bleeding, haematemisis, melaena and haematuria. Up to 25 per cent of patients develop neurological abnormalities, suggestive of encephalopathy.

Laboratory findings show a WBC count as low as $1.0 \times 10^9/l$, severe thrombocytopenia, prolonged PTT, raised AST and proteinuria. Uraemia and oliguria are uncommon. Generalized hepatorenal and cardiac failure may be observed in the terminal stages. Death is attributed to shock (partly because of DIC and bleeding into inner organs) or intercurrent infection. The pathology closely resembles that caused by filovirus infections. Convalescence may be prolonged and sequelae include transient alopecia and mono- or polyneuritis. Mortality varies from 9 to 50 per cent.

Specific treatment and prophylaxis

Prompt installation of barrier nursing is mandatory if CCHF is suspected and therapy is largely supportive. A few case reports suggest ribavirin may be beneficial (Fisher-Hoch et al., 1995), if administered early in the course of the disease (for regimen, see Lassa fever). Post-exposure prophylaxis with oral ribavirin should be considered for high-risk contacts of CCHF patients.

Avoiding tick bites (repellents, protective clothing, etc.) and de-ticking cattle through mass-treatment with 2 per cent hypochlorite ('cattle dip') are important prophylactic measures.

References and resources

Yellow fever

World Health Organization (1998a). 'Yellow fever'. WHO document: WHO/EPI/GEN/98.11.

World Health Organization (1998b). 'District guidelines for yellow fever surveillance'. WHO document: WHO/EPI/GEN/98.09. Both documents are available from the Global Programme for Vaccines and Immunization, World Health Organization, 20 avenue Appia, CH-1211 Geneva 27, Switzerland. Fax. ++41 22 791 4193/4192; E-mail gpv@who.ch, or on the INTERNET: http://www.who.ch/gov-documents/

Lassa fever

McCormick JB, Webb PA, Krebs JW et al. (1987a). A prospective study of the epidemiology and ecology of Lassa fever. *J Infect Dis*; **155**: 437–444.

McCormick JB, King IJ, Webb PA et al. (1987b). A case-control study of the clinical diagnosis and course of Lassa fever. *J Infect Dis*; **155**: 445–455.

The Centers for Disease Control (CDC), Special Pathogen Branch, Atlanta, USA, has produced a video on Lassa fever in Sierra Leone. This is available online on the INTERNET at http://www.cdc.gov/ncidod/dvrd/spb/mnpages/lassavideo.htm. Also available online is a Lassa fever slide set at: http://www.cdc.gov/ncidod/dvrd/spb/mnpages/lassaslides.htm

Rift Valley fever

Fontenille D, Traore-Lamizana M, Diallo M et al. (1998). New vectors of Rift Valley fever in West Africa. *Emerg Infect Dis*; **4**: 289–293.

Gear JH. (1989). Clinical aspects of African viral hemorrhagic fevers. *Rev Infect Dis*; S777–82.

Wilson ML, Chapman LE, Hall DB et al. (1994). Rift Valley fever in rural northern Senegal: human risk factors and potential vectors. *Am J Trop Med Hyg*; **50**: 663–675.

Ebola fever

Bitekyerezo M, Kyobutungi C, Kizza R et al. (2002). The outbreak and control of Ebola viral haemorrhagic fever in a Ugandan Medical School. *Trop Doct*; **32**: 10–15.

Journal of Infectious Diseases; **179**: Suppl. 1, February 1999. This is a special edition reporting all epidemiological, clinical, virological and laboratory data collected during the Ebola outbreak in Kikwit, DRC, 1995. This journal is also available for free on the INTERNET at: www.journals.uchicago.edu/JID/journal/contents/v179nS1.html

WHO guidelines for epidemic preparedness and response: Ebola Haemorrhagic Fever (EHF). (WHO Document: WHO/EMC/DIS/97.7). Available from the Division of Emerging and Other Communicable Diseases (EMC), World Health Organization, 20 avenue Appia, CH-1211 Geneva 27, Switzerland. Tel. ++41 22 791 2109; Fax. ++41 22 791 4893; E-mail: outbreakemc@who.ch, or on the INTERNET at http://www.who.int/emc

CCHF

Fisher-Hoch SP, Khan JA, Rehman S et al. (1995). Crimean Congo-haemorrhagic fever treated with oral ribavirin (1995). *Lancet*; 472–475.

Mariner JC, Morrill J, Ksiazek TG. (1995). Antibodies to hemorrhagic fever viruses in domestic livestock in Niger: Rift Valley fever and Crimean-Congo hemorrhagic fever (1995). *Am J Trop Med Hyg*; **53**: 217–221.

59 Respiratory syncytial virus (RSV)

The respiratory syncytial virus (RSV) is the most important cause of acute lower respiratory tract infection in young children world-wide (Sumoes, 1999; Weber et al., 1998a). Between a quarter and half of admissions to hospitals with ARI are due to RSV (Fig. 59.1).

Severe infections are most common in the first year of life, and it causes a characteristic disease entity called 'bronchiolitis'. RSV was identified first in 1956 in a group of chimpanzees and accordingly called chimpanzee coryza agent (CCA) but was already suspected to be a mainly human pathogen. Further studies from all continents found RSV or serum antibodies against RSV wherever these were sought (Weber et al., 1998a).

The organism

Respiratory syncytial virus is a RNA virus in the family of viruses called Paramyxoviridae, and in the genus Pneumovirus. It is related to measles and the parainfluenzaviruses, other important causes of acute respiratory tract infections (Fig. 59.2).

RSV is predominantly a human virus. RSV has also been recovered from chimpanzees, cattle, goats, and sheep, but these are not believed to play an important role in transmission. Two groups of RSV strains have been identified using monoclonal antibodies, which are called group A and group B. In most outbreaks, both types co-circulate, and the outbreaks are composed of different RSV strains (Cane et al., 1999). The appearance of different strains in an outbreak in the Gambia is shown in Fig. 59.3.

Transmission occurs mainly from older children, who infect young infants. These manifest the most severe symptoms, and are the ones who usually require hospitalization. The incubation period of illness from RSV has been reported as being between 2 and 8 days, most commonly between 4 and 6 days (Simoes, 1999).

Epidemiology

Seasonality

RSV infection is strongly seasonal in most settings (Selwyn, 1990; Weber et al., 1998a), and outbreaks occur regularly every year. In temperate and Mediterranean climates, outbreaks occur mainly during the winter months, extending into spring. This temperature-dependent pattern appears to be independent of the rainfall pattern. In Africa, such temperature-dependant RSV outbreaks are seen north of the Sahara and in South Africa. In areas with tropical or subtropical climates and seasonal rainfall, as is the case in most of Africa, RSV outbreaks are associated frequently with the rainy season, and not with the colder season. The peak of RSV transmission is usually 1 to 2 months after the onset of the rains. Fig. 59.4 shows the seasonality of RSV infections in The Gambia.

Outbreaks are usually sharp in onset and last between 2 and 5 months.

Age distribution

The peak incidence of hospitalized cases of RSV is in the age group 2 to 5 months, with some variation between years (Selwyn, 1990). Figure 59.5 shows the age distribution of hospitalized cases in The Gambia over a period of 4 years.

Serological studies suggest that about half of all children are infected during the first year of exposure, and that almost all have been infected after the second outbreak that they encountered (Glezen et al., 1986). Reinfection with RSV is common. RSV spreads effectively within families. Studies correlating RSV outbreaks with excess deaths from respiratory infections indicate that RSV might be as important a cause of increased mortality in elderly people as influenza.

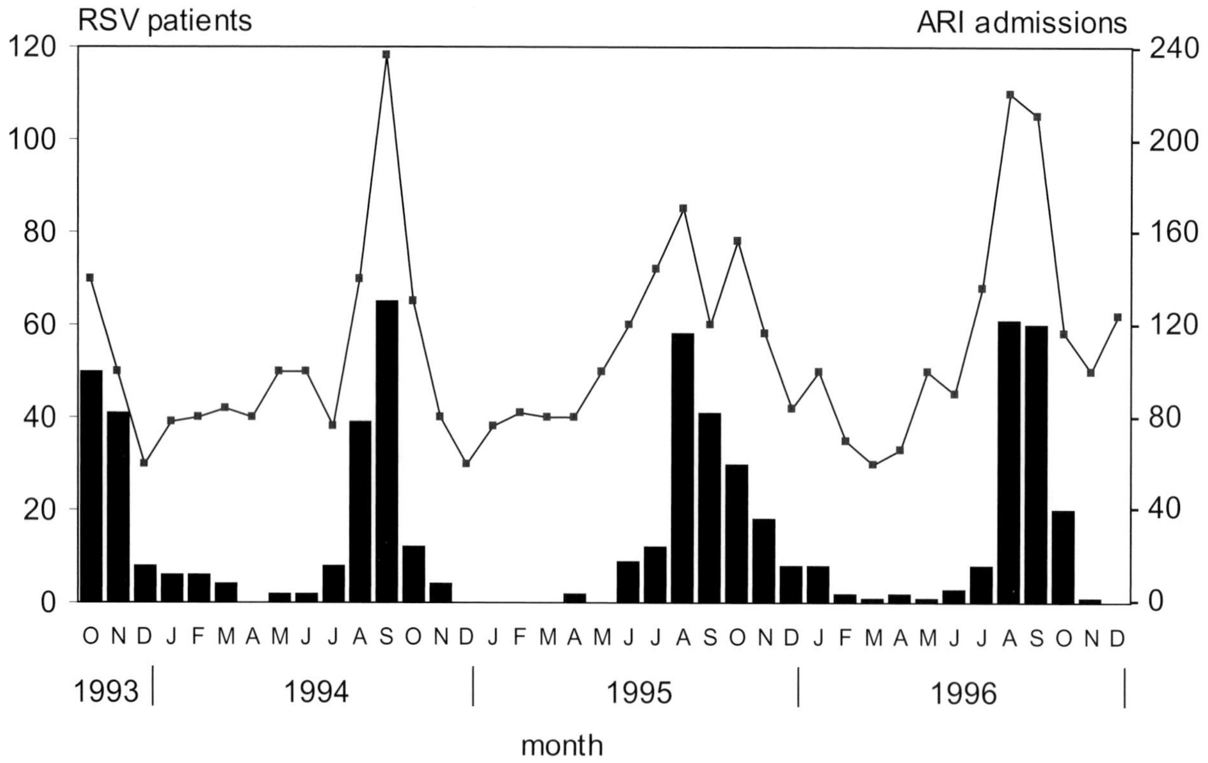

Fig. 59.1. Monthly number of RSV cases and of children less than 2 years of age with acute respiratory infection admitted to three hospitals in The Gambia over the period from October 1993 to December 1996. The seasonality of admissions follows the seasonality of RSV. Line graph represents ARI admissions; bars are the RSV cases (Weber et al., 1998a).

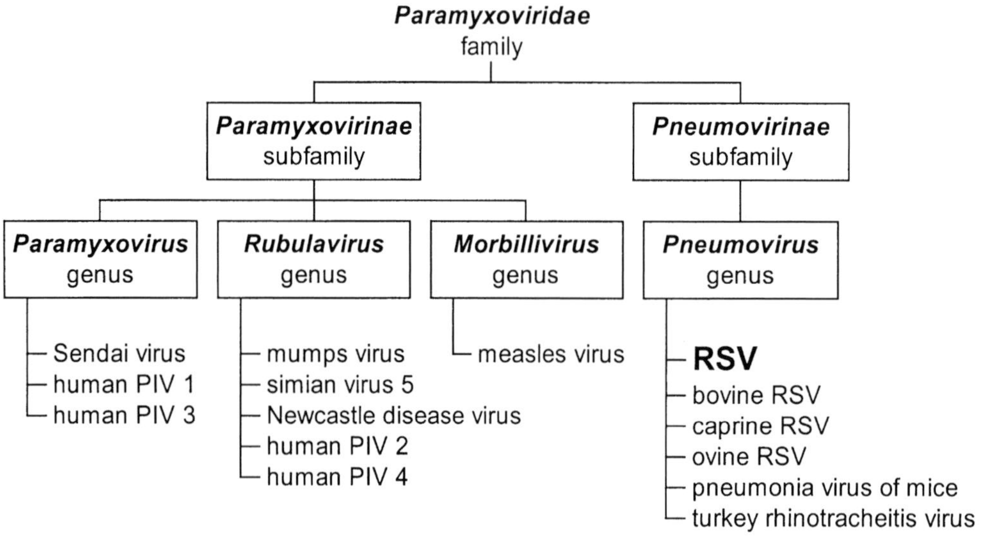

Fig. 59.2. Relationship of viruses in the family *Paramyxoviridae.* Note: Caprine and ovine RSV are possibly only subgroups of bovine RSV rather then distinct viruses. PIV: Parainfluenza virus.

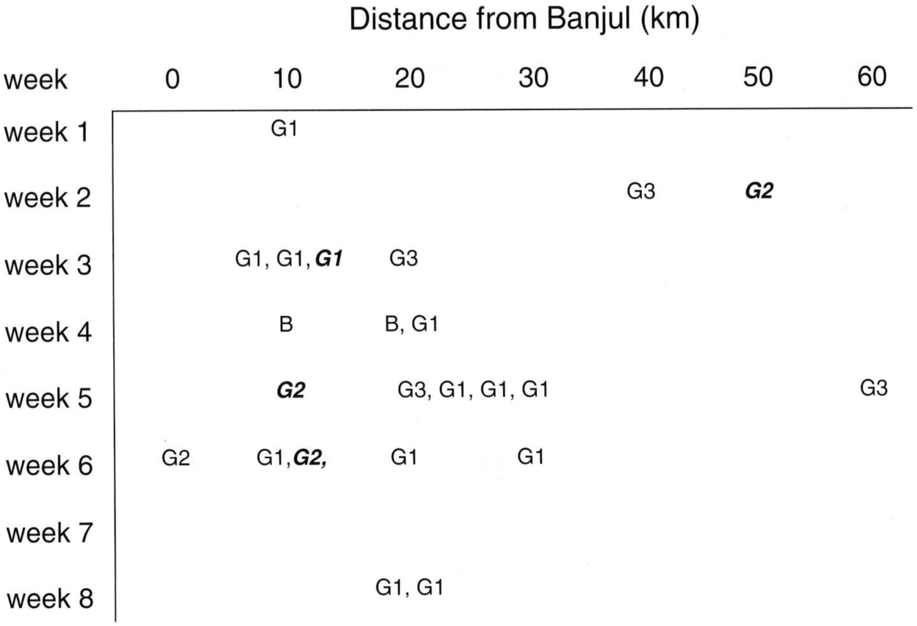

Fig. 59.3. The appearance of RSV cases in an outbreak in the Gambia in 1993 by week of outbreak and distance from the capital Banjul. The outbreak was composed of at least four different RSV strains, three of which belonged to subtype A (indicated as G1–3) and one to subtype B. Secondary cases (found on the compounds of index cases) are indicated in bold and italics.

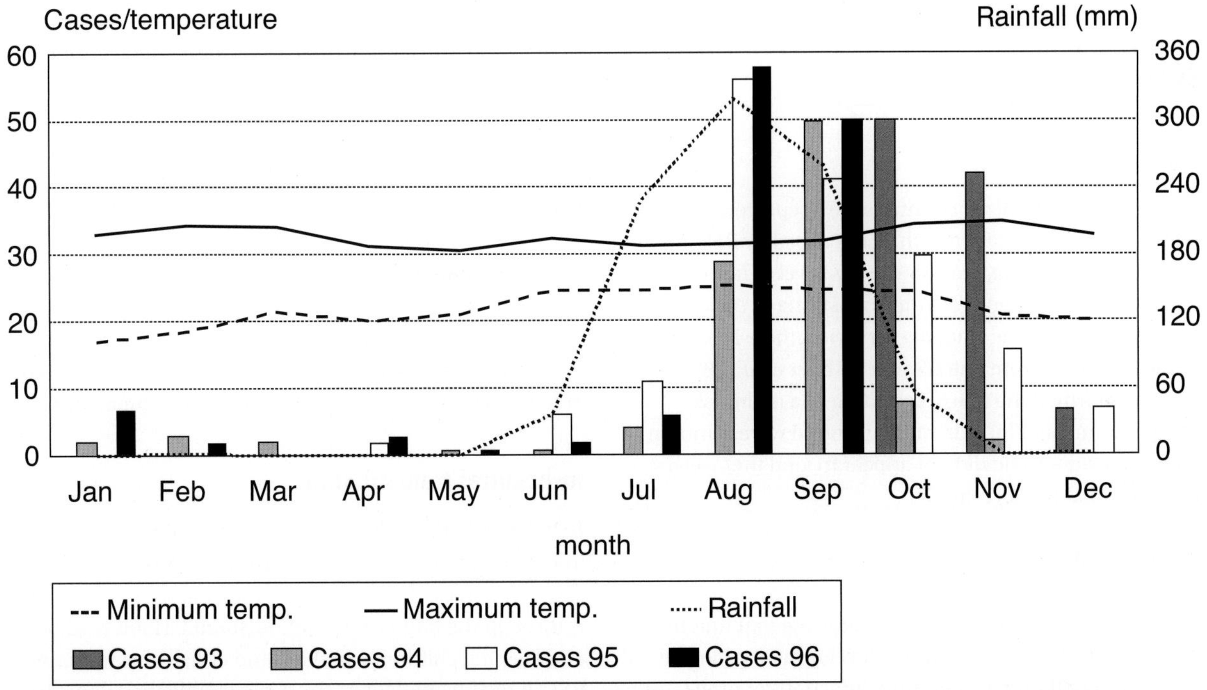

Fig. 59.4. Seasonality of RSV infection in The Gambia (Weber et al., 1998b).

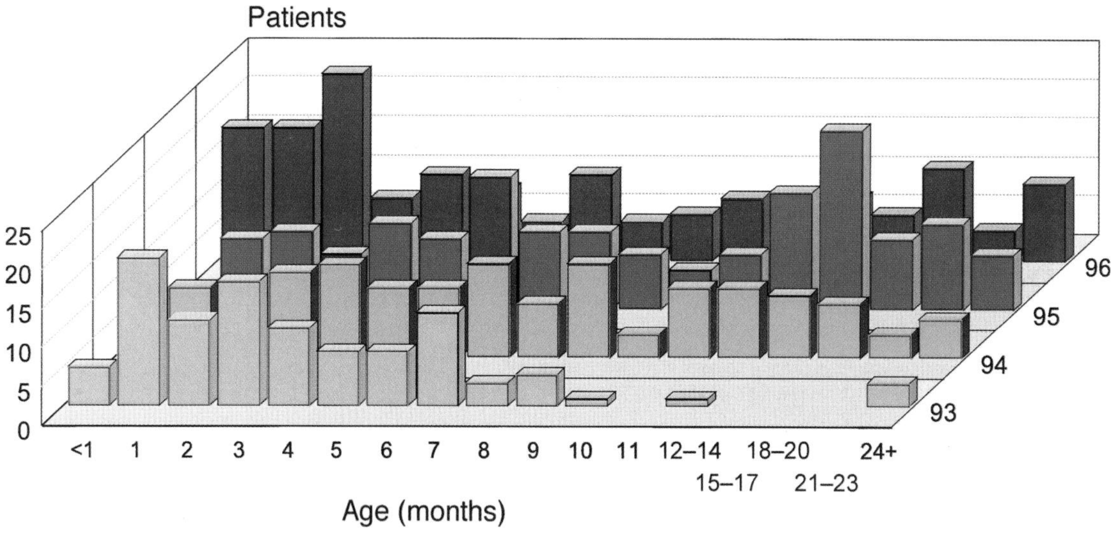

Fig. 59.5. Age distribution of the children seen during four sequential RSV outbreaks in The Gambia from 1993 to 1996 (Weber et al., 1998b).

Sex distribution

Boys are more commonly affected by severe disease, on average two-thirds of hospitalized children are male (Weber et al., 1998a). This male preponderance corresponds to the generally higher incidence of ARI of any aetiology in boys. However, in mild disease the distribution between sexes is equal.

Control and prevention

Risk factors

Studies in industrialized countries have reported that risk factors for hospitalization with ALRI caused by RSV are lack of breast feeding, crowding, a low level of maternal education, the presence of atopy or asthma in the parents, and parental smoking. In Africa, there is only one published study from The Gambia (Weber et al., 1999a), which confirmed the role of crowding as a main risk factor, but most of the other factors found were minor in their importance and did not appear to lend themselves to public health interventions.

Malnutrition

Most of the children hospitalized with RSV are not visibly malnourished, and several studies indicate that malnutrition is less of a risk factor for the development of severe RSV infection than for respiratory infections of other aetiologies.

Prevention

Prevention of RSV infection through vaccination has been hampered by a disastrous experience with a formalin inactivated vaccine in the 1960s which enhanced disease in vaccinated children and led to increased morbidity and also mortality. Further efforts to develop a vaccine were aimed first at understanding the mechanism of immune enhancement, but even today this is not completely understood. Development of a live attenuated vaccine was thus considered a safer approach, but the vaccine candidates were either over-attenuated and did not result in protection, or still caused lower respiratory infection. Another approach has been the development of vaccines based on purified subunits of the virus such as the F protein or a chimeric FG protein. There are some promising candidates, but currently, no vaccine is available for use in children (Piedra, 2000).

Immunoglobulin with a high titre of anti-RSV antibody is effective at preventing severe RSV infection in children at high risk but its cost prevents more widespread use.

In-hospital transmission

RSV is easily transmitted from child to child through infected secretions. As droplets from the nose fly only short distances, the main risk of transmission in hospital is through the hands of health personnel. Hand washing and keeping children with RSV, and at risk of contracting RSV in the hospital for as short as possible time contribute to a reduction of hospital acquired infections.

Clinical features

The first infection of an infant with RSV is almost always apparent, but clinical features vary between a runny nose and severe pneumonia. Children who develop a lower respiratory illness may do so again in the following years, but these episodes are generally less severe. The most common manifestation of RSV–ALRI is pneumonia, the ratio between cases of pneumonia and bronchiolitis ranges between 7: 1 and 1: 1. The clinical signs of bronchiolitis are expiratory wheeze, hyperinflation of the lung, and fine crepitations on auscultation. Often the signs of both entities overlap, and pneumonia appears to be a continuum of bronchiolitis (Fig. 59.6).

Pathological changes in the lungs of children who have died of RSV bronchiolitis include a peri-bronchiolar mononuclear infiltration, necrosis of the epithelium of the small airways, plugging of the lumina of the small airways, and hyperinflation and atelectasis. The most common signs of RSV–ALRI are cough (97–100 per cent), rhinitis (56–82 per cent), dyspnoea (50–78 per cent), rhonchi (59–78 per cent), wheeze (45–76 per cent) and crepitations (27–72 per cent) Table 59.1 shows the frequency of selected clinical signs in inpatients and outpatients in the Gambia. Fever is less common in younger children than in older ones. Clinical assessment of children is directed mainly at the detection of hypoxaemia (Fig. 59.7).

Useful signs indicating possible hypoxaemia are inability to feed, severe respiratory distress with signs such as head nodding, and cyanosis (Usen et al., 1999). Younger children become hypoxaemic more frequently than older ones. However, all these signs have limited sensitivity and specificity, so, where available, a pulse oximeter should be used in the assessment of children with RSV–ALRI. Hypoxaemia in RSV infection is probably due to a low ventilation-perfusion ratio rather than to shunting through unventilated lung. Most children admitted to hospital improve sufficiently within 4 to 7 days to be discharged, but inflammation in the lung may persist longer with abnormalities in gas exchange and wheezing.

Bacterial co-infections

Of major clinical importance is the frequency of bacterial co-infections in children with RSV, as this determines the need for antibiotic therapy. Most published studies looking at this issue were small, and found bacteria only occasionally. In The Gambia, bacteria were found in 3.5 per cent of 255 children (Weber et al., 1998b). All these children had a high temperature on admission. The only large study with a high bacterial isolation rate was one conducted in Pakistan, in which bacteria were found in

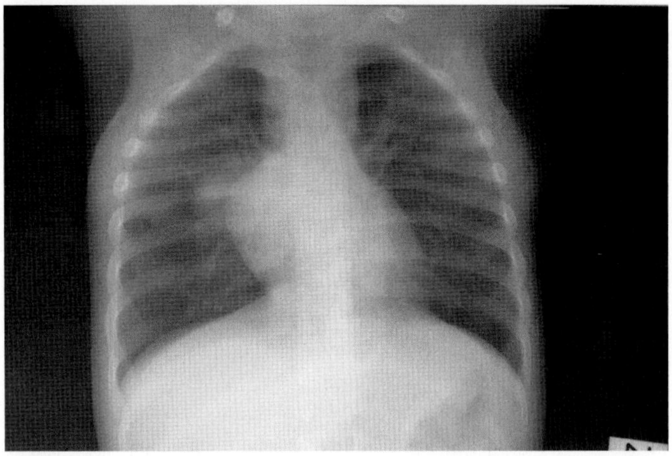

Fig. 59.6. A chest radiograph of an infant with bronchiolitis. Note the features of hyperinflation: a small heart, horizontal ribs, herniation of the lung over the mediastinum, and flattened diaphragms. There are also some patchy infiltrates of the lung parenchymum.

31% of all cases of RSV infection (Ghafoor et al., 1990). In most studies, *S. pneumoniae* was the most frequently isolated organism, followed by *H. influenzae.*

Diagnosis

The suspicion of RSV infection is high, if children present with bronchiolitis during the RSV season. The diagnosis can be confirmed by viral culture, or by the detection of RSV antigen in nasal secretion by immunofluorescence (Fig. 59.8) or antigen detection Elisa.

The latter are available commercially, and can be done by personnel with limited training. However, as the consequences of a positive test result are limited, these tests will not be done routinely in countries with limited resources.

Treatment and follow-up

Treatment of RSV infection is largely supportive, aimed at mechanically clearing secretions obstructing the airways and maintaining nutritional and fluid status and oxygenation (WHO, 2000). The main issue is the risk of concomitant bacterial infection, which is still unresolved, as indicated above. Therefore, for the classification of severity, the WHO algorithm for pneumonia is used (see page xx). No distinction is made between the treatment of RSV pneumonia and bronchiolitis. Children with fast breathing

Table 59.1. Comparison of physical findings in inpatients and outpatients with RSV disease in The Gambia (n=519, percentages in brackets) (Weber et al., 1998b)

Sign	Categories	Inpatients (n=472)	Outpatients (n=47)	P-value
Nasal flaring	present	191 (40%)	22 (47%)	0.47
Lower chest wall indrawing	moderate or severe	241 (51%)	16 (34%)	0.03
Grunting	present	130 (28%)	9 (19%)	0.28
Crepitations	present	379 (80%)	19 (40%)	<0.0001
Wheezing	present	182 (39%)	35 (75%)	<0.0001
Rhonchi	present	163 (35%)	30 (64%)	0.0001
Wheezes *or* rhonchi	present	240 (47%)	40 (85%)	0.0001
Respiratory rate	mean (SD)	65.7 (14.9)	55.6 (11.2)	<0.0001
Temperature	mean (SD)	38.1 (0.96)	38.1 (0.86)	0.6
SaO_2	median (25%, 75%)	95 (92,98)	98 (96,99)	<0.0001
Heart rate	mean (SD)	157 (18.4)	153 (18.9)	0.22

who have no danger signs and are able to feed receive an oral antibiotic. Children with lower chest wall indrawing, or with danger signs are admitted for inpatient treatment with an injectable antibiotic.

Children under 2 months of age who are irritable, unable to feed, or dyspnoeic, would fulfil the criteria for neonatal sepsis and accordingly be treated as inpatients with a combination of crystalline penicillin and gentamicin.

Children who are hypoxaemic receive supplemental oxygen. As the main abnormality in the affected lungs is a mismatch of ventilation and perfusion, relatively low concentrations of inspired oxygen are usually sufficient. This can be achieved with nasal prongs or nasal cannulae and low oxygen flow rates, typically 1 l/min (Fig. 59.9).

Bronchodilators play a limited role in the treatment of RSV bronchiolitis. They appear to be least useful in younger children. Some authorities recommend a trial of bronchodilator therapy and to continue with this treatment if there is clinical improvement after the application. Steroids do not appear to be useful. Specific antiviral

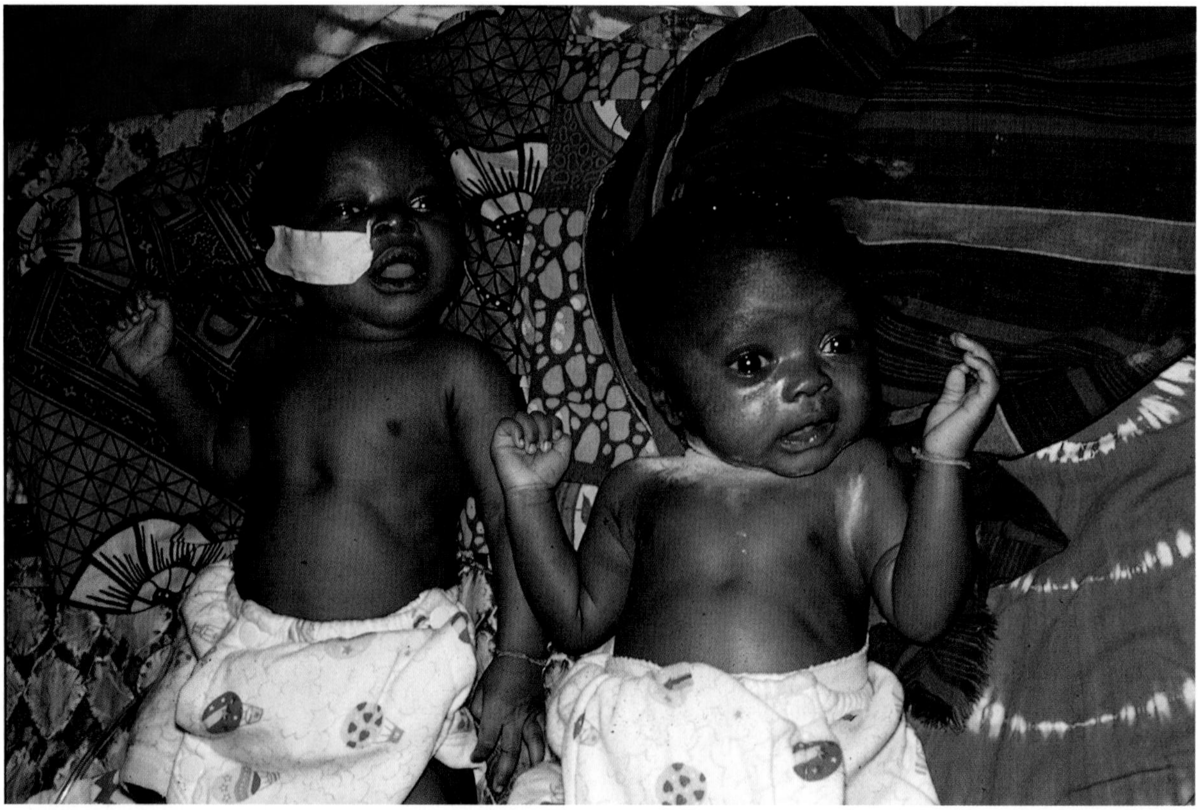

Fig. 59.7. 6-week-old twins with bronchiolitis caused by RSV. Both show marked lower chest wall indrawing, the twin on the left receives oxygen by nasopharyngeal catheter because of hypoxaemia.

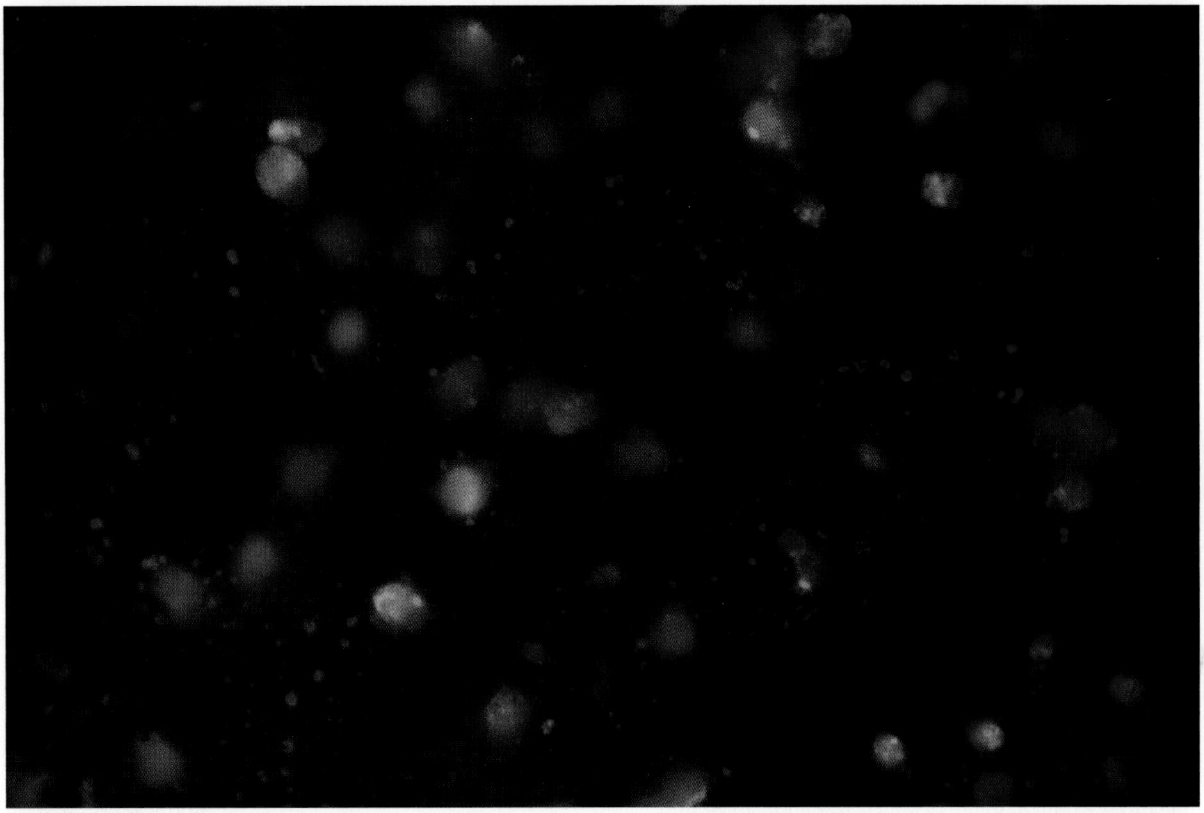

Fig. 59.8. Fluorescence-microphotograph of nasal secretions. The nuclei of epithelial cells obtained by a nasopharyngeal aspirate are stained red, and RSV antigen on the cell surface is stained with fluorescence-conjugated specific antibodies, resulting in a bright green pattern.

treatment with ribavirin may be beneficial in high risk children, but its cost–benefit ratio is low.

One important factor is nutritional support. As children with severe RSV infection have an increased work of breathing, and might be unable to feed, they need to be monitored closely. If there is concern about their ability to suck, the mother should express breast milk and feed by cup, or by nasogastric tube. If a nasogastric tube is passed, care has to be taken to clear nasal secretions, and if both a nasogastric tube and a nasal oxygen catheter are passed, both should be passed through the same nostril to minimize airways obstruction (Fig. 59.10).

Follow-up is done according to the ALRI guidelines (see p. 366): children not admitted should be seen after 2 days, and the mother should be told to seek care earlier if the child becomes sicker or is unable to feed.

Mortality

The mortality of children admitted to hospital with RSV–ALRI is low, approximately 1–3 per cent of hospital

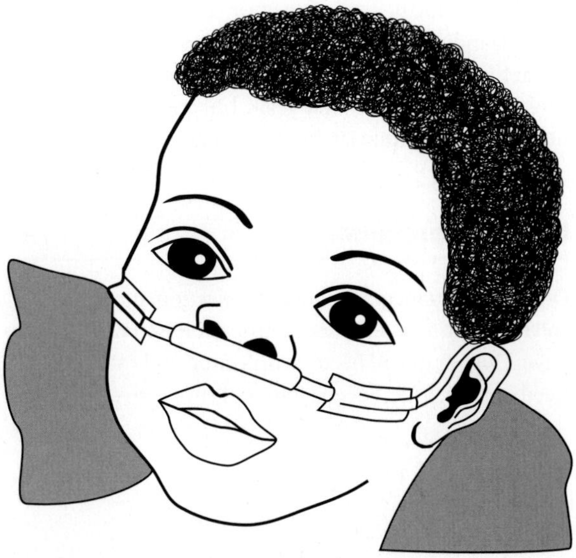

Fig. 59.9. A child receiving oxygen with nasal prongs.

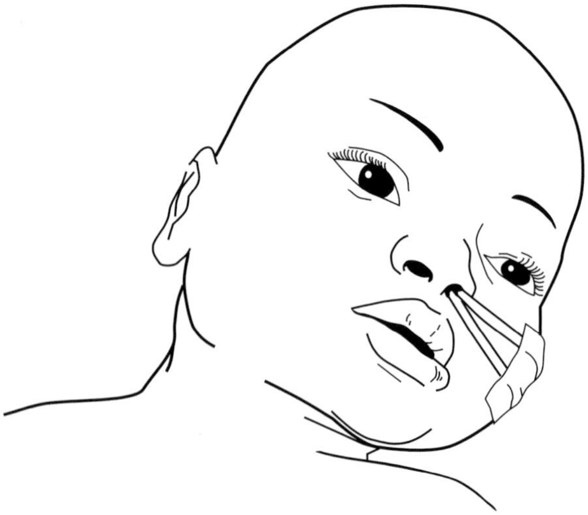

Fig. 59.10. Child with nasogastric tube and nasal oxygen catheter in recommended position (through the same nostril) to minimize obstruction of the nasal airways.

admissions die, mostly those with an underlying illness, such as congenital heart disease or bronchopulmonary dysplasia. However, where oxygen is not routinely available, or routine monitoring of inpatients to detect complications or the inability to feed is not done, mortality may be considerably higher. The impact of RSV on mortality in the community is unknown.

Further wheezing

In developed countries, there is debate about whether RSV triggers further episodes of wheezing. Data from the Gambia indicate that children with severe RSV infection are at higher risk to be admitted again with respiratory problems over the next few years, but appear to have no higher risk of asthma later (Weber et al., 1999b).

Unsolved problems

On the case management of RSV infection, the unresolved question is whether in Africa children with RSV have a higher rate of bacterial infection and routinely need an antibiotic. Several issues of supportive care need investigations, such as how much fluid to give to children with RSV infection, how best to feed children with respiratory distress, and whether paracetamol is useful in febrile children with RSV (Weber, 2000). Once a vaccine becomes available, the benefit of this vaccine needs to be determined in Africa.

References

Cane PA, Weber M, Sanneh M et al. (1999). Molecular epidemiology of respiratory syncytial virus in The Gambia. *Epidemiol Infect*; **122**: 155–160.

Ghafoor A, Nomani NK, Ishaq Z et al. (1990). Diagnoses of acute lower respiratory tract infections in children in Rawalpindi and Islamabad, Pakistan. *Rev Infect Dis*; **12** Suppl 8: S907–S914.

Glezen WP, Taber LH, Frank AL, Kasel JA (1986). Risk of primary infection and reinfection with respiratory syncytial virus. *Am J Dis Child*; **140**: 543–546.

Piedra PA (2000). Respiratory syncytial virus vaccines: recent developments. *Pediat Infect Dis J*; **19**, 805–808.

Selwyn BJ (1990). The epidemiology of acute respiratory tract infection in young children: comparison of findings from several developing countries. Coordinated Data Group of BOSTID Researchers. *Rev Infect Dis*; **12** Suppl 8: S870–S888.

Simoes EA (1999). Respiratory syncytial virus infection. *Lancet*; **354**: 847–852.

Usen S, Weber M, Mulholland K et al. (1999). Clinical predictors of hypoxaemia in Gambian children with acute lower respiratory tract infection: prospective cohort study. *Br Med J*; **318**: 86–91.

Weber M (2000). Open questions in the case management of sick children. *Trans Roy Soc Trop Med Hyg*; **94**: 14–16.

Weber MW, Dackour R, Usen S et al. (1998b). The clinical spectrum of RSV disease in The Gambia. *Pediat Infect Dis J*; **17**: 224–230.

Weber MW, Milligan P, Giadom B et al. (1999b). Respiratory illness after severe respiratory syncytial virus disease in infancy in The Gambia. *J Pediat*; **135**; 683–688.

Weber MW, Milligan P, Hilton S et al. (1999a). Risk factors for severe RSV infection leading to hospital admission in children in The Gambia. *Int J Epidemiol*; **28**: 157–162.

Weber MW, Mulholland EK, Greenwood BM (1998a). Respiratory syncytial virus infection in tropical and developing countries. *Trop Med International Health*; **3**: 268–280.

WHO (2000). Management of the Child with a Serious Infection or Severe Malnutrition. Geneva: World Health Organization.

Epstein–Barr Virus

60

The Epstein–Barr Virus (EBV) was discovered in the cells of a Burkitt's lymphoma (BL) (Epstein et al., 1964), which is the commonest childhood cancer in Africa. Here the virus infects at an early age resulting in persistent sub-clinical infection; in affluent countries infection may be later causing infectious mononucleosis. In malarious areas of Africa and Papua New Guinea EBV is linked to a high incidence of BL of 1 in 1000 children. In South China, North Africa and the highlands of Kenya the virus is associated with carcinoma of the nasopharynx and in patients with AIDS it causes lymphoproliferative disease and B-cell tumours (Epstein & Crawford, 1996).

The virus

EBV is a member of the hepesvirus family. The viral genome consists of a linear DNA molecule that encodes nearly 100 viral proteins, which is encased in a nucleocapsid wrapped in a viral envelope. It infects B-cells and squamous epithelial cells by binding to a receptor, the CD21 molecule (or C3d complement receptor), resulting in lytic infection and shedding of virus or latent infection and persistence (Cohen, 200). The proteins, or antigens, expressed by the virus in either the lytic or latent phases of infection are summarized in Table 60.1. Antibodies to these antigens, which are important in diagnosis, vary according to the type of infection. However the cellular immune response is more important for control of the infection. Thus CD8 HLA restricted cytotoxic T-cells, and to a lesser extent CD4 cytotoxic T-cells and natural killer cells, limit the primary infection and drive it to latency where it is held in B-cells. Reactivation to the lytic form with production of virus occurs when the cellular immune system is damaged as in AIDS or when temporarily deranged as in malaria (Cohen, 2000; Thorley-Lawson, 2001).

The problem in Africa

In Africa, EBV infection, which is spread by droplets and kissing, occurs at an early age and is symptomless (Biggar et al., 1978a, b). Like many other infections such as hepatitis B virus and cytomegalovirus, the main route of transmission is horizontal, usually between siblings. In the western world where crowding is less and hygiene better, up to 50 per cent of children may remain uninfected until they are teenagers. When they become infected through kissing, half may become ill with a febrile illness called infections mononucleosis or glandular fever. Active infection is diagnosed by the presence of serum IgM anti-VCA antibodies and past infection by serum IgG anti-VCA antibody (Henle & Henle, 1979).

Prevention

There is currently no practical means of preventing infection. In the future a vaccine might be useful for children in areas with a high incidence of Burkitt's lymphoma (equatorial Africa) or nasopharyngeal carcinoma (southern China), for uninfected adolescents, and for patients undergoing transplantation surgery. A phase I trial of vaccinia virus expressing EBV glycoprotein 350 has been successfully completed in Chinese children.

Clinical syndromes

Infectious mononucleosis

EBV infection in adolescents and young adults is characterized by fever, lymphadenopathy and pharyngitis. The syndrome is seldom seen in Africa for most children are already sub-clinically infected by the age of 5 years. The

Table 60.1. Expression of EBV proteins during lytic and latent infection and in various diseases

	Lytic proteins		Latent proteins					
	EA	VCA	EBNA1	EBNA2	EBNA3	LMP1	LMP2	EBER
Acute infection	+	+	+	+	+	+	+	+
Healthy carrier	(±)	(±)	(±)	−	−	−	+	+
Burkitt's lymphoma	+	+	+	−	−	−	−	+
Nasopharyngeal carcinoma	+	+	+	−	−	+	+	+
Lymphoproliferative disease	+	+	+	+	+	+	+	+

Notes:
EA denotes early antigen, VCA denotes viral capsid antigen.
EBNA Epstein–Barr virus nuclear antigen, LMP latent membrane protein.
EBER Epstein–Barr virus-encoded RNA. A plus indicates that the gene and protein is exposed, a minus sign that they are not and a plus minus sign in brackets that they are expressed in a few cells, which are in the lytic phase.

infection causes a leukocytosis, with an increase in mononuclear cells and atypical lymphocytes, which are activated T-cells. Activation and infection of B-cells results in a polyclonal antibody response including a rise in heterophile antibodies. The illness is over in one or two weeks but in one in 2000 cases it persists as a chronic active infection causing fever and lassitude. The detection of IgM anti-VCA antibodies in serum, or of EBV DNA in tissues confirms the diagnosis (Cohen, 2000).

Burkitt's lymphoma

Dennis Burkitt, a surgeon working in Uganda, first described this common tumour of African children in the late 1950s (Burkitt, 1958). He noted its geographical restriction to low-lying areas and postulated that it was caused by an arthropod-borne virus. In 1964 Epstein, Achong and Barr discovered a virus, subsequently named after them, by electron microscopy of cells from a Burkitt's tumour. The virus has oncogenic potential for it is able to immortalize cultured B-cells and is now accepted as a necessary but not sufficient factor in the genesis of a variety of B-cell lymphomas. Additional co-factors are required for each type of lymphoma, malaria being most important for Burkitt's lymphoma (Burkitt, 1969; see Table 60.2). Repeated attacks of malaria diminish T-cell control of EBV infected B-cells allowing them to grow abnormally fast, thus increasing the chances of chromosomal rearrangements (Whittle et al., 1984).

The lymphoma cell is a B-cell immortalized by EBV which contains a translocation involving chromosomes 8 and 14, 2 or 22 (Lenoir, 1986). These rearrangements result in the displacement of the c-myc oncogene from chromosome 8 alongside the immunoglobulin heavy chain locus (chromosome 14) or light chain locus (chromosome 2 or 22). The resulting deregulation leads to malignant change with very rapid growth of a clone of tumour cells that usually arises in the jaw or abdomen. The malignant cells are infected with EBV that only expresses EBV latent protein EBNA1, thus allowing the cell to evade immune recognition and destruction by cytotoxic T-cells (see Table 60.1). Epidemiological evidence from a malarious region of Uganda supports the role of EBV in the genesis of the tumour, for children who later developed the tumour had anti-VCA IgG antibodies eight to ten times higher than age and sex matched controls and also had higher levels of anti-EA antibodies (de-The et al., 1978). The findings suggest a high level of EBV replication, which may have been due to repeated bouts of malaria. (For clinical details of Burkitt's lymphoma see Chapter 90.)

Nasopharyngeal carcinoma

This tumour, which is also associated with EBV infection, occurs across North Africa, down through the Sudan and into the highlands of Kenya. The age distribution in Africa is bimodal: the first peak involves children and adolescents, the second elderly adults. The tumour arises in the nasopharynx where it causes local obstruction and later erodes into the skull with destruction of cranial nerves. It spreads to cervical lymph nodes and, in the end, to bones, liver and lungs.

This anaplastic carcinoma contains EBV genomes which express various proteins (Table 60.2). In South China, which has a very high incidence, the tumour is four times more frequent in people with the HLA haplotype A2 BW36. Here, there is strong epidemiological evidence that traditional herbal medicines, taken as snuff, and salted fish, which contains nitrosamines, act as co-factors (Ito, 1986; Table 58.1). The genetic and environmental factors at work in Africa are unknown. The diagnosis is made by histology coupled with raised serum

Table 60.2. Co-factors for EBV-associated tumours or disease

Co-factor	Burkitt's lymphoma	Nasopharyngeal carcinoma	Lymphoproliferative disease
Other infections	Malaria suppresses cellular immunity to EBV and enhances growth of viral lymphomas in mice. BL is frequent in hyperendemic areas and age distribution follows peak incidence of malaria	No	HIV leads to immunosuppression and high EBV viral load with an increase in lymphomas and oral hairy leucoplakia
Genetic susceptibility	No	HLA A2 BW36	X-linked lympho-proliferative disease
Tumour-promoting agents	No	Herbal medicines containing phorbolester, salt fish with nitrosamines	No

IgA anti-VCA and EA antibodies. Radiotherapy is the treatment of choice.

Lymphoproliferative disease

Congenital or acquired immunodeficiency is associated with EBV-driven lymphoproliferative disease (Purtilo, 1980). Patients with X-linked lymphoproliferative disease, a rare inherited disease of males, lack a functional lymphocyte activation molecule which impairs the normal interaction of T- and B-cells, thus allowing the virus to grow undetected in B cells. Immunosuppressed patients undergoing transplant surgery or patients with AIDS have impaired T-cell immunity to EBV and other viruses, resulting in 10 to 20 times as many EBV-infected B-cells and higher EBV antibody levels than normal (Birx et al., 1986). Those with AIDS are prone to develop oral hairy leukoplakia, which is a raised, white, corrugated plaque of hyperplastic epithelial cells on the oral mucosa. They are also prone to develop a variety of EBV-associated lymphomas ranging from the Burkitt type with c-myc translocations to large cell lymphomas and immunoblastic lymphomas which invade the central nervous system. Lymphoid intestinal pneumonitis, due to infiltration of the alveolar septa by plasma cells containing EBV DNA, occurs in HIV-infected children and occasionally in adults.

Lymphoproliferative disease is only likely in late stage HIV disease. Most patients with AIDS in Africa die of other common infections before lymphoproliferative disease is apparent (see Chapter 13).

References

Biggar J, Henle W, Fleisher G, Böcker J, Lennette ET, Henle G (1978). Primary Epstein–Barr virus infections in African infants. I. Decline of maternal antibodies and time of infection. *Int J Cancer*, **22**: 239–243.

Biggar J, Henle W, Fleisher G, Böcker J, Lennette ET, Henle G (1978). Primary Epstein–Barr virus infections in African infants. II. Clinical and serological observations during seroconversion. *Int J Cancer*, **22**: 244–250.

Birx DL, Redfield RR, Tosato G (1986). Defective regulation of Epstein-Barr virus infection in patients with acquired immunodeficiency syndrome (AIDS) or AIDS-related disorders. *New Engl J Med*; **314**: 874–879.

Burkitt D (1958). A sarcoma involving the jaw in African children. *Br J Surgery*, **46**: 218-223.

Burkitt DP (1969). Etiology of Burkitt's lymphoma – an alternative hypothesis to a vectored virus. *J Nat Cancer Inst*; **42**: 19–28.

Cohen JI (2000). Epstein–Barr infection. *New Engl J Med*; **343**: 481–492.

de-Thé G, Gesar A, Day NE et al (1978). Epidemiological evidence for casual relationship between Epstein–Barr virus and Burkitt's lymphoma from Ugandan prospective study. *Nature*; **274**: 756–761.

Epstein MA, Achong BA, Barr YM (1964). Virus particles in cultured lymphoblasts from Burkitt's lymphoma. *Lancet* **i**: 702–703.

Epstein MA and Crawford DH (1996). The Epstein–Barr virus. In *Oxford Textbook of Medicine*, ed. DJ Weatherall, JGG Ledingham, DA Warrell. pp. 352–357. Oxford: Oxford University Press.

Henle W, Henle G (1979). Sero-epidemiology of the virus. In The Epstein-Barr virus, ed. MA Epstein and BG Achong, pp 62–73. Berlin: Springer-Verlag.

Lenoir GM (1986). Role of the virus, chromosomed translocations and cellular oncogenes in the aetiology of Burkitts' lymphoma. *In the Epstein–Barr Virus: Recent Advances*, ed. MA Epstein, BG Achong, pp. 183–205. London: William Heinemann.

Purtilo D (1980). Epstein–Barr-virus induced oncogenesis in immune deficient individuals. *Lancet*; **i**: 300–303.

Thorley-Lawson DA (2001). Epstein–Barr virus: exploiting the immune system. *Nat Revs: Immunol*; **1**: 75–82.

Whittle HC, Brown J, Marsh K et al. (1984). T-cell control of Epstein–Barr-virus-infected B cells is lost during *P. falciparum* malaria. *Nat*; **312**: 449–450.

61 Influenza

The problem in Africa

Epidemics of influenza are well recognized in Africa and can be due to strains of influenza virus not previously encountered, so that the population is non-immune and is therefore highly susceptible. For example, the 1998 epidemic in South Africa, which was clinically very severe, was due to just such a virus, the A/Sydney/6/97-like H3N2 strain (Besselaar et al., 1999). Similarly, the sporadic cases and those infected during the months of peak incidence in Dakar were also due to an unfamiliar strain (Dosseh et al., 2000). Now that HIV infection is so transforming the picture of the infectious diseases of the continent, it is sobering to record that the mortality of HIV+ children with viral-associated (including influenza A and B) severe lower respiratory tract infection was higher than in HIV− children (Madhi et al., 2000). In contrast to colder northern countries, many young children become infected.

The virus and its effects

The virus is a myxovirus and has two antigenic substances on its surface, the haemagglutinin (H) and neuraminidase (N) so that variant strains are described according to H/N composition. Influenza A virus is capable of substantial antigenic variation, probably in birds harbouring the virus, to produce new strains to which whole populations are not immune. The haemagglutinin specifically reacts with receptor substance (sialic acid groupings on a glycoprotein) on the epithelial cells of the respiratory tract where it destroys the mucociliary defensive apparatus. The tract is supremely vulnerable therefore to other micro-organisms: *Strep. pneumoniae* and *Staph. aureus* each account for about one-third of cases of post-influenzal pneumonia and *Haemophilus influenzae* for over 10 per cent.

The virus can infect the central nervous system and skeletal and cardiac muscle.

Transmission

The virus is transmitted in a small-particle aerosol, and it survives best in a low humidity and low temperature. The harmattan of West Africa, the dry season of the higher altitudes of East Africa, and the cold of the desert or the cold dry months of south and central Africa, are thus ideal for its transmission. A seasonal pandemic can be disastrous, particularly as the mucociliary apparatus of the bronchial tree is less efficient when the humidity is low. The seasonal peak in Dakar appears to be the warmer wetter months.

Antibody response

Haemagglutination–agglutinating antibodies appear in the second week and reach a peak at about the fourth week of the illness. They persist for a much shorter time in a tropical community, possibly due to the more rapid turnover of IgG as a result of repeated subsequent infections.

Vaccination

Vaccination against the prevalent global virus strain is given in industrialized countries to vulnerable people – the old, the immunosuppressed and those with chronic cardiac or respiratory disease. In Africa, this is not yet a priority: moreover the shorter duration of acquired immunity after natural infection could make an immunization programme relatively ineffective. It will only be possible to produce appropriate vaccines for use in Africa if international co-operation in sharing data about, and surveillance of, influenzal strains becomes established.

Clinical features

Two to 3 days after infection, fever, malaise, headache, and muscular aches and pains begin relatively suddenly. The nose is congested, it streams clear liquid mucus, which may quickly become purulent: the patient coughs and feels awful. Such upper respiratory symptoms are not dominant in malaria, while the abrupt start is not usual in typhoid. In an epidemic the diagnosis should be easy – at other times the muscle aches are characteristic. The patient gets better quickly, but easy fatiguability and depression may prolong recovery.

The dreaded superinfection of acute viral or bacterial pneumonia starts suddenly with tachypnoea, cough and cyanosis: the patient looks very ill and there are crackles all over the chest. The respiratory epithelium is necrotic – so that haemoptysis is common: in fatal cases a hyaline membrane is seen in the alveoli.

Treatment

The only treatment is vigorous antibiotic treatment of a superinfection.

References

Besselaar TG, Schoub BD, Blackburn NK. (1999). Impact of the introduction of A/Sydney/5/97 H3N2 influenza virus into South Africa. *J Med Virol*; **59**: 561–568.

Dosseh A, Ndiaye K, Spiegel A et al. (2000). Epidemiological and virological influenza survey in Dakar, Senegal: 1996–1998. *Am J Trop Med Hyg*; **62**: 639–644.

Madhi SA, Schoub B, Simmank K et al. (2000). Increased burden of respiratory viral associated severe lower respiratory tract infections in children infected with human immunodeficiency virus type-1. *J Pediatr*; **137**: 78–84.

Mulholland EK, Ogunlesi OO, Adegbola RA et al. (1999). Etiology of serious infections in young Gambian infants. *Pediatr Infect Dis J*; **18**: S35–S41.

62

Varicella (chickenpox) and herpes zoster

Varicella (chickenpox) is an acute highly infectious disease, with outbreaks in schools and emergency settings. The public health impact of herpes zoster (reactivated varicella infection) has increased in areas of Africa with high HIV prevalence.

Organism

Both conditions are caused by infection with varicella-zoster virus, an α-herpes virus. Humans are the only reservoir. Primary infection results in varicella. The virus then establishes latency in dorsal root ganglia, maintained by specific cell-mediated immunity. Zoster occurs if latent virus reactivates.

Varicella is highly infectious, from 1–2 days before rash onset until all scabs have formed. New cases arise from droplet or aerosol transmission from varicella cases, or close contact with varicella or zoster cases. The incubation period of varicella is 10–21 days.

Epidemiology

In temperate countries, varicella occurs in early childhood, with almost universal immunity by adolescence. Some tropical countries have a later average age at onset, and a higher proportion of susceptible adults. The reasons for this are unknown. Zoster predominantly affects older individuals, as specific cell-mediated immunity wanes. The lifetime risk of zoster is 10–20 per cent, but is higher in immunosuppressed individuals; more than 90 per cent of adults with zoster in some African settings are HIV-infected. Zoster occurs in immunocompetent children who were exposed to varicella in utero or in the first year of life.

Clinical features (Fig. 62.1)

Varicella is usually mild in children, but may be severe in adults and the immunosuppressed. Prodrome comprises 1–2 days of malaise and mild fever. The rash is densest on

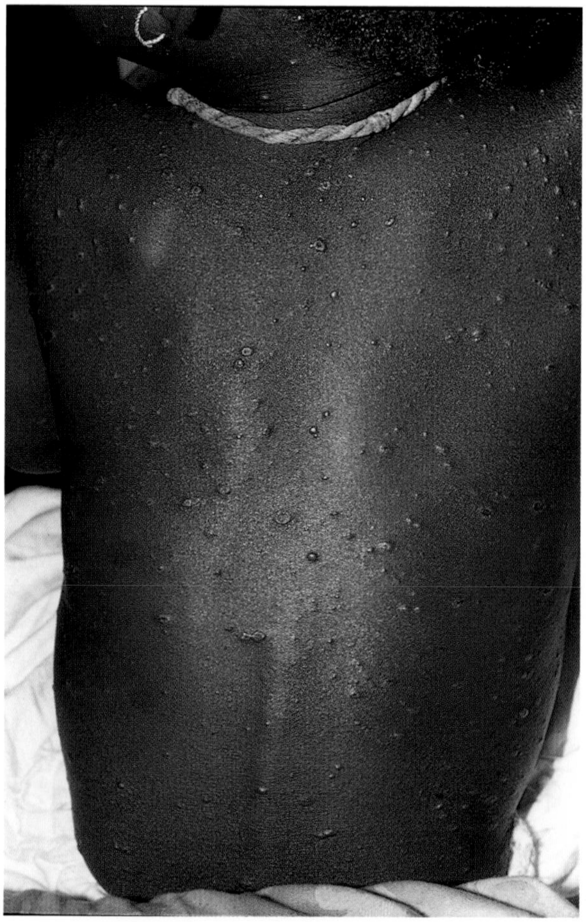

Fig. 62.1. Typical rash of chicken pox on the back.

the trunk; successive crops of itchy maculopapules evolve into vesicles, pustules and scabs, and several stages are seen simultaneously. Complications include bacterial superinfection of vesicles, pneumonia (in up to 10% of adults), and more rarely neurological complications (meningoencephalitis, cerebellar ataxia or transverse myelitis) or haemorrhagic disorders. Immunosuppressed individuals may develop disseminated infection, with fatality rates of 7–17 per cent without treatment. Immunity is usually lifelong.

Neonates whose mothers contracted varicella 5 days before to 2 days after delivery may develop severe generalized varicella, with up to 30 per cent mortality. One per cent of infections in the first 20 weeks of pregnancy result in congenital varicella syndrome, comprising congenital limb hypoplasia, dermatomal skin scarring, microphthalmia and microcephaly.

The unilateral vesicular scabbing rash of zoster is in the distribution of the affected dermatome, most commonly thoracic or ophthalmic. It is usually accompanied by severe pain and paraesthesia, and lasts 1–2 weeks. Complications include post-herpetic neuralgia (in 10% of patients), ocular damage (2%), motor deficits (1%), and rarely contralateral hemiplegia or meningoencephalitis. Immunosuppressed patients have a higher risk of disseminated rash, complications and recurrent zoster.

Diagnosis

Varicella and zoster are usually diagnosed clinically. Latex agglutination tests can detect rise in serum antibody, and immunofluorescence used to detect viral antigen in scrapings of the base of lesions. Viral isolation is insensitive, but polymerase chain reaction can detect viral DNA in vesicular fluid if facilities are available.

Treatment

Supportive treatment is given for uncomplicated varicella. Aspirin should be avoided, as this may precipitate Reye's syndrome. Acyclovir is used for systemic complications or in the immunosuppressed, but is expensive.

Analgesia is given for zoster. Acyclovir, valacyclovir or famcyclovir may limit neuralgia and prevent dissemination in the immunosuppressed if available and given within 72 hours of rash onset. Low-dose tricyclic antidepressants may relieve post-herpetic neuralgia.

Prevention/control

Varicella cases should be excluded from school or workplace until scabbed, and should avoid susceptible pregnant women, babies and the immunosuppressed. Varicella-zoster immune globulin (if available) prevents or modifies disease in high-risk susceptibles if given within 96 hours of exposure.

Live attenuated varicella virus vaccine may not be a priority for national immunization programmes in developing countries. Inadequate coverage could increase the age at infection, resulting in more severe disease, and vaccination may result in disseminated varicella in severely immunosuppressed individuals.

References

Arvin A. (1996). Varciella-zoster virus. *Clin Microbiol Rev*; **9**: 361–381.

Colebunders R, Mann JM, Francis H. et al (1988). Herpes zoster in African patients: a clinical predictor of human immunodeficiency virus infection. *J Infect Dis*; **157**: 314–318.

World Health Organization (unpublished). The WHO Position Paper on Varicella Vaccines. http: //www.who.int/vaccines-diseases/diseases/PP_Varicella.htm

63 Monkeypox

Monkeypox

Monkeypox is a sporadic zoonosis of Western/Central Africa, identified in humans in 1970. Smallpox vaccination used to provide some protection, but susceptibility to monkeypox has risen since eradication of smallpox and cessation of vaccination.

Organism

Monkeypox virus is an orthopox virus. Reservoir hosts include squirrels and primates. Primary transmission to humans occurs after handling infected animals, and secondary person-to-person transmission occurs via direct contact or aerosol.

Epidemiology

Most cases occur among children in villages near tropical rain forests. Between 1970 and 1986, 404 cases were reported from seven West or Central African countries, including 338 from the Democratic Republic of the Congo (DRC). Of these, 72 per cent were attributed to animal contact, and spread from secondary cases was limited. A 1996–1998 outbreak in the DRC included more than 800 suspected cases, with retrospective serological analysis demonstrating both monkeypox and chickenpox. Monkeypox cases were milder than previously, more adults were infected, and more than 70 per cent of cases were attributed to person-to-person transmission. Transmissibility appeared unchanged, with secondary household attack rates of 8 per cent. The changing epidemiology may result from increasing adult susceptibility, as smallpox vaccine-induced cross-immunity wanes.

Clinical features

The prodrome of pyrexia, headache, prostration and cervical lymphadenopathy lasts 1–3 days. Subsequent rash is densest on the face and limbs, and evolves through macular, vesicular, pustular and scabbing stages. In most individuals the rash emerges over 1–2 days and evolves at the same rate. Illness lasts 2–4 weeks, but is milder and atypical in those vaccinated against smallpox. Complications include secondary bacterial skin infection, bronchopneumonia or diarrhoea (12 per cent and 7 per cent of unvaccinated cases), and septicaemia or encephalitis (less than 1 per cent of cases). Case-fatality rates were 10 per cent in unvaccinated children before 1996, and 1 per cent subsequently.

Diagnosis

Table 63.1 contrasts the typical clinical presentations of monkeypox and varicella. Specific ELISA or Western Blot tests detect rising monkeypox antibody titres, and viral culture and polymerase chain reaction are used in collaborating centres to detect virus or viral DNA.

Treatment

Treatment is symptomatic. The World Health Organization (WHO) has called for field trials of cidofovir, an anti-orthopoxviral drug.

Prevention/control

Cases should be isolated. Education focuses on decreasing animal contacts. Smallpox vaccination may result in generalized vaccinia in HIV-infected individuals, and WHO does not currently recommend re-establishing vaccination in monkeypox-endemic areas. However, strengthening of monkeypox surveillance systems is needed.

References

Heymann DL, Szczeniowski M, Esteves K. (1998). Re-emergence of monkeypox in Africa: a review of the past six years. *Brit Med Bull;* **54**: 693–702.

Jezek Z, Szczeniowski M, Paluku, KM, Mutombo M. (1987). Human monkeypox: clinical features of 282 patients. *J Infect Dis*; **156**: 293–298.

World Health Organization.(1999). Technical Advisory Group on Human Monkeypox. Report of a WHO Meeting (11–12 January 1999) (WHO/CDX/CSR/APH/99.5). Geneva: WHO.

Table 63.1. Differences in typical clinical presentation of monkeypox vs. chickenpox

Clinical feature	Monkeypox	Chickenpox
Prodrome	Fever/malaise severe	Fever/malaise slight or absent
Lymphadenopathy	Marked	Mild/absent
Rash distribution	Centrifugal (densest on face, limbs)	Centripetal (densest on trunk)
Rash evolution	Usually all appears within 1–2 days – vesicles and scabs not seen simultaneously	Appears successively – vesicles and scabs seen simultaneously

64 Poliomyelitis

The problem in Africa

In the first half of the twentieth century, it was accepted that polio occurred at lower rates in Africa than in industrialized countries. In the 1970s, studies in many African countries showed that post-polio lameness occurred at the same rate as Europe and America in the pre-vaccine era (Nicholas et al., 1977; Mabey, 1981). As a result, polio was included in the basic course of vaccines recommended by the Expanded Programme on Immunization (EPI). From the mid-1970s to 1990, the effectiveness of national immunization programmes was improved throughout Africa and the rest of the world. The achievements of immunization programmes were not uniform, however. The majority of countries that were unable to immunize even half of their children in the 1980s and 1990s were in Africa.

Increasing global immunization coverage resulted in decreased levels of disease, setting the stage for a global polio eradication initiative. When the initiative began, polio was highly endemic in virtually all of sub-Saharan Africa with the exception of selected small countries and some countries in Southern Africa. By the year 2000, polio was absent from Southern and East Africa and parts of West Africa. It remains endemic in Central Africa and the Horn of Africa and in some areas of West Africa, particularly Nigeria. Armed conflict is a significant challenge to the eradication initiative. Intensification of the eradication initiative should lead to eradication of the disease from the African continent and the world in the next few years.

Causative agent

Polio is caused by three closely related enteroviruses: poliovirus types 1, 2 and 3. The naturally occurring viruses are designated as wild viruses. Type 1 poliovirus produces the highest rate of paralysis and is most often associated with epidemics. Type 3 poliovirus has proved to be the most difficult virus to eradicate. Type 2 poliovirus has presumably been eradicated with the last isolation occurring in India in 1999.

Epidemiology

Acute polio is primarily a disease of young children (Otten et al., 1992). Two-thirds to three-quarters of cases are less than 3 years of age and more than 90 per cent of cases are less than 5 years of age. Faecal–oral transmission predominates. Respiratory transmission been postulated to be important in areas with very high levels of sanitation. Food- and water-borne transmission may occur when food or water supplies are contaminated. Flies can serve as vectors through passive transfer of infectious faecal matter. The incubation period for polio is 5–35 days.

Polio is a seasonal disease in temperate climates with epidemics occurring in late summer. In tropical climates, cases occur more uniformly through the year, but cases peak during the hot, rainy season. Humans are the only natural host of polio. Higher primates can be infected in the laboratory, but transmission is not sustained in the wild. Polioviruses can persist for several months in surface water or sewage.

The risk of paralysis during polio infection is increased by a number of factors including strenuous exercise during the prodrome, intramuscular injections in the 2–4 weeks prior to the onset of illness, tonsillectomy and pregnancy. During polio outbreaks, do not give an intramuscular injection unless it is essential.

Prevention

Polio has been preventable for nearly half a century. The first inactivated polio vaccine (IPV) was released in 1955. Live oral, attenuated oral polio vaccine (OPV) became available in the early 1960s. Higher potency IPV became available in the 1980s. Both IPV and OPV are highly effective, but the choice of vaccine will depend both on a country's polio status and the national health priorities.

IPV is a trivalent, injectable vaccine prepared from killed wild polioviruses. IPV produces high levels of humoral immunity, blocking spread of poliovirus into the central nervous system. IPV, therefore, provides excellent individual protection against paralytic polio. However, IPV does not produce significant levels of secretory immunity, particularly in the intestines, the primary site of viral replication. Because faecal–oral spread predominates in developing countries, it is doubtful that global eradication could be achieved with IPV. The immune response to IPV is sub-optimal when these doses are administered at 6, 10 and 14 weeks in the EPI schedule (WHO, 1997). The need for booster doses of IPV at older ages is not clear, but immunity is long-lasting. A major benefit of IPV is the absence of vaccine-associated paralytic polio (VAPP).

OPV is a trivalent, orally administered vaccine that contains live, attenuated polioviruses. The vaccine viruses multiply in the intestines, producing high levels of both humoral and secretory immunity. Because OPV provides excellent individual protection against polio and superior population immunity, OPV is the only vaccine recommended by WHO for use in the eradication initiative.

Three doses of OPV in infancy are the basic course of vaccination recommended by the Expanded Programme on Immunization. While two doses of OPV will protect more than 90 per cent of children in the USA, three doses of OPV are only 70–80 per cent effective in tropical countries when given in the EPI schedule (Deming, Jaiteh et al., 1992, 1997). The primary reason for reduced immunogenicity is the high levels of maternal antibody prevalent in polio-endemic countries(WHO, 1997), but a seasonal effect is also important (Deming et al., 1997). Diarrhoea also reduces the immune response to OPV. Those presenting to immunization clinics with diarrhoea should receive OPV, but the dose should be repeated when the child is healthy. Some countries have recommended a fourth dose of OPV administered at birth.

The major disadvantage of OPV is VAPP, which results from the reversion of vaccine virus to neurovirulence. Although non-immune contacts may contract VAPP, the majority of cases occur among recent vaccinees. The highest risk is associated with the first dose where 1 case occurs for every 700 000 births. Persons with congenital and acquired B-cell immunodeficiency are at increased risk of VAPP. There is no increased risk of VAPP associated with human immunodeficiency virus infection.

Pathogenesis

Poliomyelitis is a viral infection of the central nervous system, characterized by the acute onset of flaccid paralysis. In approximately 1 in every 200 infections, poliovirus spreads from the intestines and regional lymph nodes to the central nervous system. There, it selectively destroys anterior horn cells, producing paralysis of the affected muscles. Polio paralysis is permanent, although some improvement in function may be seen.

Clinical description

The vast majority (90–95 per cent) of poliovirus infections are either asymptomatic or sub-clinical. Abortive poliomyelitis occurs in 4–8 per cent of infections and is indistinguishable from many other viral infections. It is characterized by 2–3 days of fever, headache, sore throat, anorexia, vomiting, abdominal pain and listlessness. Non-paralytic polio has the same symptoms as abortive polio, but they are more severe and meningeal irritation is present. Non-paralytic polio is clinically indistinguishable from aseptic meningitis caused by other enteroviruses.

Spinal paralytic polio occurs in less than 1 in 200 poliovirus infections. A biphasic course of illness, with minor and major phases, occurs in one-third of childhood cases. The minor phase, coinciding with viraemia, lasts 1–3 days and is similar to abortive poliomyelitis. The patient then appears to recover for 2–5 days before the abrupt onset of the major illness, characterized by fever, headache, malaise, vomiting and neck stiffness. Meningismus and severe myalgias are usually present for 1–2 days before the onset of weakness and paralysis. Involuntary muscle spasms may occur and muscular fasiculations may be observed. The onset of paralysis is rapid, sometimes progressing to quadriplegia over several hours. Fever is present at the onset of paralysis. The progression of paralysis is normally complete by 72 hours, ending as the patient becomes afebrile. The paralysis is usually asymmetrical. Any combination of muscles may be affected. Proximal muscles tend to be affected more often than distal. The legs are more often affected than the arms (Fig. 64.1). Isolated facial palsy may occur, but is unusual. Sensory impairment is rare in polio.

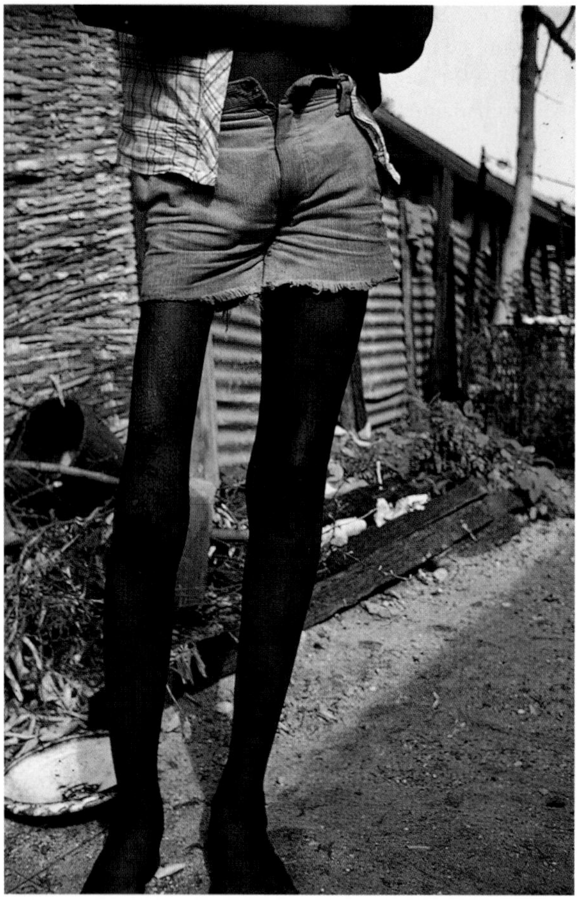

Fig. 64.1. Wasted limb of a boy from old polio (D. Mabey).

Bulbar paralytic polio occurs when the muscle groups: innervated by the cranial nerves are involved. The result is dysphagia, nasal speech and dyspnoea. Patients are anxious and agitated because of their inability to swallow and impaired breathing. Bulbar polio occurs in 5–35 per cent of cases and is more common in adults. Pure bulbar polio is uncommon; most cases have mixed spinal and bulbar involvement.

Polio encephalitis is rare and is manifest by confusion and disturbances of consciousness. It may be associated with seizures and spastic paralysis. Gastrointestinal complications may include haemorrhage, paralytic ileus and gastric dilation. Urinary stones may occur in patients on prolonged bed rest.

Diagnosis

The differential diagnosis of paralytic polio includes any cause of acute flaccid paralysis (AFP) (Marx et al., 2000). A thorough history, including an immunization history, and clinical examination is essential for proper diagnosis. AFP may occur in the course of: acute myelopathy (space occupying lesions producing spinal block and transverse myelopathy which are, in turn associated with a number of infections including rabies, hepatitis A, and parasitic lesions of the brain and spinal cord including schistosomiasis, cystercercosis, echinococcosis and Taenia infestations); peripheral neuropathy (Guillain–Barré syndrome (GBS), acute demyelinating neuropathy, post-rabies vaccine, neuropathies in the course of infectious diseases – diphtheria, Lyme borreliosis, rabies, neuropathies produced by heavy metals or biological toxins); systemic illnesses (acute intermittent porphyria, critical illness neuropathy); disorders of neuromuscular transmission (myasthenia gravis, snake bite, botulism, insecticide intoxication, tick paralysis); and disorders of the muscle (polymyositis, trichinosis, hypokalemic and hyperkalemic paralysis, including familial periodic paralysis).

Other paralytic syndromes may be mistaken for AFP including acute onset spastic paraparesis associated with tropical myeloneuropathies. These include konzo in the Congo, the Central African Republic, Mozambique and Tanzania, which is linked with bitter cassava consumption. Lathyrism associated with excess ingestion of certain flowering peas in times of famine is endemic in Ethiopia.

GBS causes half of non-polio AFP cases in children. GBS is an ascending, symmetrical paralysis with progression over 1–2 weeks. Polio is characterized by rapid onset of an asymmetrical paralysis accompanied by fever. Paralysis is complete by 2–3 days and there is no sensory deficit. CSF examination in GBS will normally demonstrate high protein and low cell counts while a pleocytosis will be found in polio. Most GBS cases will have significant recovery over several months while polio paralysis is permanent.

Poliomyelitis caused by wild polioviruses must also be distinguished from poliomyelitis syndromes caused by other enteroviruses and vaccine-associated paralytic polio. Both are clinically identical to wild virus poliomyelitis. Paralysis caused by non-polio enteroviruses is more likely to resolve over time.

Where immunization levels are low, polio is the most common cause of AFP and clinical diagnosis is sufficient. As eradication approaches, other causes of paralysis must be reliably distinguished from polio. Because there is no pathognomonic clinical finding to absolutely distinguish polio from other causes of AFP, particularly vaccine-associated polio and polio syndromes caused by other enteroviruses, virological investigation of all possible polio cases is necessary (Hull & Dowdle, 1997). All cases of acute-onset, flaccid paralysis under 15 years of age should be reported to the National Ministry of Health.

Two stool specimens should be collected at least 24 hours apart. Ideally, stool specimens are at least 10 grams, the size of an adult thumb. Since the titre of excreted virus is highest at the onset of illness and falls over time, specimens should be collected within 14 days of the onset of paralysis. To preserve the viability of the virus, specimens should be refrigerated during storage and transport. Viral cultures of spinal fluid or throat are insensitive for polio diagnosis. Serologic testing done in a reliable virology laboratory can support the diagnosis, but the results are often difficult to interpret. Importantly, serologic testing cannot distinguish between wild and vaccine virus infections.

Treatment

There is no cure for polio. Treatment of polio cases is supportive, based on the symptoms and extent of the disease. Non-paralytic forms can be treated outside the hospital with bed rest and analgesics. Exertion should be avoided for several weeks after illness.

Patients with acute paralytic poliomyelitis should be hospitalized and placed on bed rest to limit extension of paralysis. Hot, moist packs should be applied to the affected muscles to relieve pain and spasms. Analgesics are also used for pain relief. Sedatives may be needed, but should be used cautiously to prevent respiratory compromise. Polio cases should be kept well hydrated to reduce the risk of urinary stone formation.

In bulbar polio, the airway must be kept clear of secretions. Paralysis of the respiratory muscles may necessitate mechanical ventilation, if available. Weakness or paralysis of the bladder may require catherization. Physical therapy should be initiated as soon as possible after the paralysis is complete. Good rehabilitation services will allow most polio cases to lead useful, productive lives.

The global polio eradication initiative

In 1988, The World Health Organization committed to eradicating polio world-wide, defined as both the elimination of clinical cases of polio and ending transmission of wild polioviruses. Eradication is achieved through the use of mass immunization campaigns, and intensive disease surveillance (Hull et al., 1994).

National immunization days

Because the immune response is sub-optimal in tropical zones and many developing countries are able to immunize only 50–80 per cent of infants, polio cannot be eradicated world-wide with routine immunization alone. Mass immunization campaigns, called NIDs in most countries, are used to boost individual immunity, immunize a higher percentage of the population and suppress wild poliovirus circulation (Birmingham et al., 1997a). Two doses of OPV are given annually to all children less than 5 years of age. In countries where routine immunization coverage is low and birth rates and population density are high, additional NIDs doses are needed. All children are immunized, regardless of prior immunization status. NIDs are normally conducted during the cool, dry season, both because of easier access to the population and improved immune response to OPV. Particular attention must be paid to reaching minorities and economically disadvantaged populations, migrants, nomads and residents of remote areas. Oral vitamin A supplements can be successfully added to NIDs to reduce the morbidity and mortality of measles (Ching et al., 2000; Goodman et al., 2000).

Acute flaccid paralysis surveillance

Any eradication initiative must have a highly sensitive surveillance system to document progress, identify the final chains of transmission and document the absence of disease after eradication has been achieved (Birmingham et al., 1997b). Because polio lacks a clinical finding equivalent to the pathognomonic rash used in the smallpox eradication effort, virological confirmation of polio cases must be employed. All AFP cases less than 15 years of age must be considered as possible polio cases and reported to the Ministry of Health for virological investigation (Hull & Dowdle, 1997).

Progress towards eradication

In 1988, polio was a disease of global concern. An estimated 350 000 cases occurred in more than 100 countries on all the major continents. By the end of the year 2000, polio had been eradicated from North and South America, Europe and much of Africa, Asia and the Middle East. Poliovirus transmission was concentrated in South Asia (Afghanistan, India and Pakistan), the horn of Africa (Ethiopia, Somalia and Sudan), West Africa (Nigeria and Niger), Central Africa (Angola). WHO estimates that less than 1000 cases occurred in the year 2001. Intensified eradication efforts in these remaining countries means that global eradication is likely to be achieved in the very near future. War and civil unrest are a continuing challenge for the eradication initiative (Biellik et al., 1997; elZein et al., 1997; Valente et al., 2000). Truces for polio immunization have been successfully implemented in many countries (Tangermann et al., 2000).

Post-eradication era

The polio eradication initiative will not end with the last case of polio. Because more than 99 per cent of poliovirus infections are non-paralytic, intensive AFP surveillance must continue for at least 3 years after the last wild poliovirus is identified. At that time, Regional and Global commissions will certify that polio has been eradicated (Hull 2001).

After eradication, wild polioviruses will no longer exist in nature. However, many laboratories have stocks of wild virus that must either be destroyed or contained to prevent an inadvertent release after immunization has stopped (Wood et al., 2000). WHO and national ministries of health are inventorying laboratory stocks of polioviruses to be contained after eradication is certified. Few laboratories in developing countries have wild polioviruses, so concern is focused on the industrialized countries.

The ultimate aim of the polio eradication initiative is to stop immunization against polio. Stopping all immunization will save more than US$1.5 billion annually, forever. Two major issues must be addressed to define a strategy for stopping immunization. They are the potential emergence of feral polioviruses – vaccine viruses that have mutated back to neurovirulent forms – and persisting vaccine virus infection of immunodeficient persons. Feral polioviruses circulated in Egypt in the 1980s and caused an outbreak of polio on the island of Hispaniola in 2000–1 (WHO, 2000; Kew et al., 2002). In both instances, these viruses appeared when immunization coverage was low and disappeared with effective NIDs. Chronic poliovirus infection has been recognized for many years, but several recently identified cases have been infected for more than a decade. In the interim, all countries must maintain high immunization coverage until the use of all OPV is stopped. The feasibility and effectiveness of using IPV globally for an interim period remain uncertain.

References

Biellik RJ, T Allies, Woodfill CJ et al. (1997). Polio outbreaks in Namibia, 1993–1995: lessons learned. *J Infect Dis*; **175**: S30–S36.

Birmingham ME, Aylward RB, Cochi SL et al. (1997). National immunization days: state of the art. *J Infect Dis*; **175**: S183–S188.

Birmingham ME, Linkins RW, Hull BP et al. (1997). Poliomyelitis surveillance: the compass for eradication. *J Infect Dis*; **175**: S146–S150.

Ching P, Birmingham M, Goodman T et al. (2000). Childhood mortality impact and costs of integrating vitamin A supplementation into immunization campaigns. *Am J Public Hlth*; **90**: 1526–1529.

Deming MS, Jaiteh KO, Otten MW Jr et al. (1992). Epidemic poliomyelitis in The Gambia following the control of poliomyelitis as an endemic disease. II. Clinical efficacy of trivalent oral polio vaccine. *Am J Epidemiol*; **135**: 393–408.

Deming, MS, Linkins RW, Jaitch KO et al. (1997). The clinical efficacy of trivalent oral polio vaccine in The Gambia by season of vaccine administration. *J Infect Dis*; **175**: S254–S257.

elZein HA, Birmingham ME, Karrar ZA et al. (1997). Poliomyelitis outbreak and subsequent progress towards poliomyelitis eradication in Sudan. *Lancet*; **350**: 715–716.

Goodman, T, Dalmiya N, de Benoist B et al. (2000). Polio as a platform: using national immunization days to deliver vitamin A supplements. *Bull Wld Hlth Org*; **78**: 305–314.

Hull BP; Dowdle WR (1997). Poliovirus surveillance: building the global Polio Laboratory Network. *J Infect Dis*; **175**: S113–S116.

Hull HF (2001). The future of polio eradication. *Lancet Infect Dis*; **1**: 299–303.

Hull HF, Ward NA, Hull BP et al. (1994). Paralytic poliomyelitis: seasoned strategies, disappearing disease. *Lancet*; **343**: 1331–1337.

Kew O, Morris-Glasgow V, Landaverde M et al. (2002). Outbreak of poliomyelitis in Hispaniola associated with circulating type 1 vaccine-derived poliovirus. *Science*; **296**: 356–359.

Mabey DC (1981). Paralytic poliomyelitis in The Gambia: lameness in urban children. *Ann Trop Paediatr*; **1**: 45–49.

Marx A, Glass JD, Sutter RW (2000). Differential diagnosis of acute flaccid paralysis and its role in poliomyelitis surveillance. *Epidemiol Rev*; **22**: 298–316.

Nicholas DD, Kratzer JH, Ofosu-Amaah J et al. (1977). Outside Europe. Is poliomyelitis a serious problem in developing countries? – the Danfa experience. *Br Med J*; **1**: 1009–1012.

Otten M W, Jr, Deming MS, Jaiteh KQ et al. (1992). Epidemic poliomyelitis in The Gambia following the control of poliomyelitis as an endemic disease. I. Descriptive findings. *Am J Epidemiol*; **135**: 381–392.

Tangermann RH, Hull HF, Jafari H et al. (2000). Eradication of poliomyelitis in countries affected by conflict. *Bull Wld Hlth Org*; **78**: 330–338.

Valente F, Otten M, Balbina F et al. (2000). Massive outbreak of poliomyelitis casued by type-3 wild poliovirus in Angola in 1999. *Bull Wld Hlth Org*; **78**: 339–346.

WHO (1997). Combined immunization of infants with oral and inactivated poliovirus vaccines: results of a randomized trial in The Gambia, Oman, and Thailand. WHO Collaborative Study Group on Oral and Inactivated Poliovirus Vaccines. *J Infect Dis*; S215–S227.

WHO (2000). Poliomyelitis, Dominican Republic and Haiti. *Wkly Epidemiol Rec*; **75**: 397–399.

WHO (2001). Circulation of a type 2 vaccine-derived poliovirus, Egypt. *Wkly Epidemiol Rec*; **76**: 27–29.

Wood DJ, Sutter RW, Dowdle WR (2000). Stopping poliovirus vaccination after eradication: issues and challenges. *Bull Wld Hlth Org*; **78**: 347–357.

65 Rubella

The public health importance of rubella relates to its effects in pregnant women, which can lead to spontaneous abortion, stillbirth, or delivery of an infant with congenital malformations. The risk of congenital rubella is highest following maternal infection in the first trimester, with up to 85 per cent of infants affected. The risk declines with infection later in pregnancy, and congenital rubella is rare if maternal infection occurs after 20 weeks. Manifestations of congenital rubella syndrome (CRS) may include eye defects (cataract, glaucoma, retinopathy), deafness, cardiovascular defects (patent ductus arteriosus, ventricular septal defect, pulmonary stenosis, etc.), neurological problems (mental retardation, microcephaly, encephalitis), low birthweight, involvement of the liver, spleen, bones, or endocrine organs. Clinical signs of CRS, especially deafness, may not manifest for several years. The long-term disability due to CRS represents a serious burden for patients, their families, and society.

The problem in Africa

There are an estimated 110 000 new cases of CRS in developing countries each year, including 25 000 on the African continent (Cutts & Vynnycky, 1999).

A limited number of special studies on CRS have been reported from Africa. In Ghana, 18 cases of CRS were identified following an outbreak in 1995, yielding an incidence of 0.8 CRS cases per 1000 live births (Lawn et al., 2000). In Uganda, 7 per cent of 348 children with congenital cataracts had other clinical signs of CRS, including heart disease, deafness, and/or retinopathy (Waddell, 1998). In Tanzania, 10 per cent of 20 patients with congenital cataract in 1980–81 and 12 per cent of 24 patients with congenital heart disease in 1985–86 had additional CRS-compatible defects (Maselle et al., 1988).

There has been sustained interest in serological studies to assess rubella immunity in Africa. Several authors have previously reviewed African serological data (Mingle, 1985; Gomwalk & Ahmad, 1989; Cutts et al., 1997).

Between the 1970s and mid-2000, the scientific literature reports 60 rubella serosurveys conducted in Africa. Results of these studies should be interpreted with caution due to differences in sampling methods and laboratory assays.

Forty-seven serosurveys have assessed rubella immunity among African women in 27 countries. Rates of rubella susceptibility (absence of rubella IgG antibody) vary widely, with 13 serosurveys (28 per cent) showing $\geq$20 per cent of women susceptible, 17 serosurveys (36 per cent) with 10–19 per cent susceptible, and 17 serosurveys (36 per cent) with $<$10 per cent. The risk of CRS is highest in countries with high susceptibility rates among women of child-bearing age. African countries with very high susceptibility rates (20 per cent or higher) include Algeria (rural areas), Angola, Cote d`Ivoire, Gabon, Ghana, Morocco, Niger, Nigeria (4 surveys), Togo, and Tunisia (Fig. 65.1). Although low susceptibility rates have been reported in some countries, these may reflect a recent rubella outbreak or local variation, and extrapolating from such studies may mask a significant national benefit from the introduction of rubella vaccine (WHO, 2000).

Eleven serosurveys provide data on rubella virus circulation in younger age groups. In three countries (Eritrea, Ethiopia, and The Gambia), serosurveys show a rubella seroprevalence of about 95 per cent by 10 years of age, suggesting a relatively low risk of infection in adult women. In eight countries (Angola, Burkina Faso, Cote d'Ivoire, Libya, Nigeria, Somalia, South Africa, and Tunisia) surveys show a seroprevalence of 65–78 per cent by 10 years of age, consistent with higher risks of infection in adult women.

Organism, life cycle, host

Rubella virus, a togavirus, is found world-wide. Humans are the only natural host. Rubella virus is transmitted by droplets or direct contact. The incubation period ranges from 12 to 23 days. The virus replicates in the nasopharyngeal mucosa and local lymph nodes; viraemia occurs 5–7 days after exposure. In pregnant women, the virus infects the placenta and the developing fetus. Rubella virus can be found in the nasopharynx of persons with clinical disease from 1 week before to 2 weeks after rash onset. Patients with subclinical disease are also infectious. Infants with congenital rubella shed rubella virus in urine and nasopharyngeal secretions (60 per cent of infants shed virus during the first 4 months of life, dropping to 10 per cent by age 9–11 months).

Epidemiology

Although the incidence of CRS has not been studied in every country, there are sufficient data to state that rates of CRS in developing countries are as high as those reported from industrialized countries before the introduction of rubella vaccine (Cutts et al., 1997). During endemic periods the rate of CRS ranges from 0.1 to 0.2 per 1000 live births, but during epidemics, which occur every 4–7 years, the CRS rate rises to 0.6 to 4.1 per 1000 live births.

Immunity is acquired after natural infection or immunization. It is usually permanent after natural infection and thought to be long term, probably lifelong, after immunization. Infants of immune mothers are protected by transplacental antibody, but this wanes so that nearly all infants are susceptible by 9 months of age (Kebede et al., 2000).

Control/prevention

Live attenuated rubella vaccine has been available since 1969; the RA27/3 strain is the main vaccine used around the world (Robertson et al., 1997). More than 95 per cent of persons seroconvert after a single vaccine dose. The vaccine virus is heat and light sensitive, and rubella vaccine requires cold chain storage in the same manner as measles vaccine. Rubella vaccine is available as single antigen rubella vaccine, measles–rubella (MR) vaccine, or measles–mumps–rubella (MMR) vaccine.

Rubella vaccine is usually administered to young children at age 12–15 months, although excellent seroconversion rates are also achieved at 9 months. The vaccine may also be administered to adolescents and adults. Rubella vaccine should be avoided in pregnancy because of the theoretical but never demonstrated teratogenic risk. No cases of CRS have been reported in more than 1000 susceptible women who inadvertently received rubella vaccine early in pregnancy (WHO, 2000). Consequently, there is no need to screen women for pregnancy before rubella vaccination. However, if pregnancy is planned, an interval of 1 month should be observed after immunization. Rubella vaccination during pregnancy is not an indication for abortion.

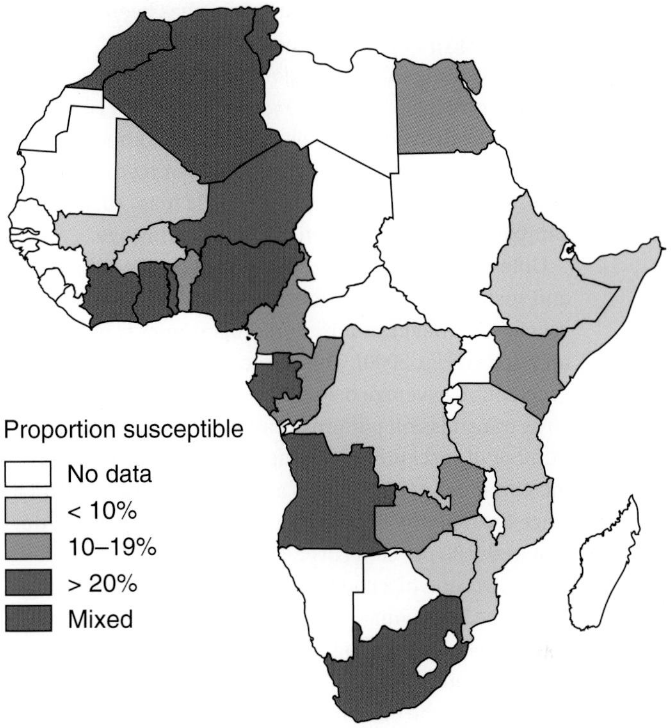

Fig. 65.1. Rubella susceptibility among women of child-bearing age.

Rubella vaccines should not be given to persons with advanced immunodeficiency disorders; however, asymptomatic HIV-positive individuals can receive rubella vaccine (WHO, 2000). Common adverse events include low grade fever, rash, lymphadenopathy, and myalgia. Joint symptoms tend to be rare in children and men, but transient arthralgias are reported in up to 25 per cent of women.

Rubella vaccine is increasingly being introduced around the world. Based on data reported to WHO as of July 2000, 114 countries (53 per cent) were using rubella vaccine in their national immunization programmes. On the African continent, rubella vaccine has been introduced in Egypt, Mauritius and Seychelles.

In preventing CRS, the major target group for vaccination is women of child-bearing age. This group can be reached by delivery of rubella vaccine to women post-partum, women in the workplace, and/or teenage schoolgirls. Some countries have used rubella mass vaccination campaigns to reach women of child-bearing age.

Unless high coverage (>80 per cent) can be achieved and sustained on a long-term basis, adding rubella vaccine to child immunization programmes is not recommended (WHO, 2000). This is because childhood rubella vaccination coverage below 80 per cent can interfere with virus transmission patterns, leading to an increased number of susceptibles among adults, and thereby an increased risk of CRS. This is an important issue in Africa since the majority of countries have not yet achieved the required >80 per cent coverage level.

The decision of a country to introduce rubella vaccine should be based on:

- the level of susceptibility in women of child-bearing age
- the burden of disease due to CRS
- strength of the basic immunization programme as indicated by routine measles vaccine coverage, which should be >80 per cent for several years before childhood rubella immunization is considered
- infrastructure and resources for child and adult immunization programmes
- assurance of injection safety and
- other disease priorities.

Some countries with limited resources may place higher priority on other diseases such as neonatal tetanus. A few countries with low susceptibility rates among women of childbearing age (<10 per cent), a high seroprevalence among children by age 10 years (95 per cent or higher), also reflected in low incidence of CRS, may be well advised not to start on any large scale vaccination against rubella.

Diagnosis/clinical features

Acquired (post-natal) rubella causes mild fever and maculopapular rash, often with occipital and post-auricular lymphadenopathy. Mild rashes may be difficult to identify on black skin. Moreover, up to half of acquired rubella infections occur without a rash. Arthralgia/arthritis is common in women. The differential diagnosis includes measles, dengue, parvovirus B-19, and human herpesvirus-6. Laboratory confirmation of acquired rubella is usually carried out with an IgM ELISA test on a blood specimen obtained within one month after rash onset.

Congenital rubella syndrome (CRS) should be suspected when an infant presents with heart disease and/or suspicion of deafness and/or one or more of the following eye signs: cataract, diminished vision, nystagmus, squint, microphthalmus, or congenital glaucoma. The WHO-recommended definition for clinically confirmed CRS is: an infant in whom a qualified physician detects two of the complications listed in group (a) or one in (a) and one in (b).

Group (a) cataract(s), congenital glaucoma, congenital heart disease, loss of hearing, pigmentary retinopathy.

Group (b) purpura, splenomegaly, microcephaly, mental retardation, meningocephalitis, radiolucent bone disease, jaundice with onset within 24 hours after birth. The WHO-recommended definition for laboratory-confirmed CRS is an infant with clinically confirmed CRS who has a positive blood test for rubella-specific IgM. Further guidance on CRS and rubella surveillance is provided in WHO guidelines (Cutts et al., 1999).

Treatment and follow-up

Treatment is symptomatic. Pregnant women infected in the first trimester should be given culturally appropriate counselling, which may include the option of abortion in some countries. Post-exposure treatment with IgG for pregnant women exposed to rubella in the first trimester is not generally recommended. The efficacy of this treatment is not certain, and infants with CRS have been born to women given IgG soon after rubella exposure.

Unsolved problems

There is growing interest in global elimination of both measles and rubella. As of mid-2000, specific regional elimination targets for one or both diseases have been set in the Americas, the Eastern Mediterrean, and Europe. There is the expectation that other regions, including Africa, will move towards accelerated measles and rubella control; however, many issues are still unresolved. Reaching women as a target group for rubella vaccine is challenging and the risk posed by childhood rubella immunization coverage <80 per cent complicates control strategies. Further assessments are needed to consider the feasibility of attaining and sustaining high rubella immunization coverage with different potential vaccination strategies, particularly in countries where measles immunization coverage is low. Efforts are under way with assistance from WHO and other agencies to establish a global measles/rubella laboratory network.

Research is on-going to establish new methods for testing rubella immunity, and one promising area involves tests based on saliva specimens. A global collection of rubella virus strains is needed to enable molecular research.

Studies on the medical, social, and educational costs of caring for individuals with CRS would be useful, as this will permit cost–benefit assessments relevant to the introduction of rubella vaccine.

References

Cutts FT, Robertson SE, Diaz-Ortega JL, Samuel R. (1997). Control of rubella and congenital rubella syndrome (CRS) in developing countries, part 1: burden of disease from CRS. *Bull Wld Hlth Org*; **75**: 55–68.

Cutts FT, Best J, Siqueira MM, Engstrom K, Robertson SE. (1999). Guidelines for surveillance of congenital rubella syndrome and rubella. *Document WHO/V&B/99.22*. Geneva: World Health Organization.

Cutts FT, Vynnycky E. (1999). Modelling the incidence of congenital rubella syndrome in developing countries. *Int J Epidemiol*; **28**: 1176–1184.

Gomwalk NE, Ahmad AA. (1989). Prevalence of rubella antibodies on the African continent. *Rev Infect Dis*; **11**: 116–121.

Kebede S, Nokes DJ, Cutts FT, Nigatu W, Sanderson F, Beyene H. (2000). Maternal rubella-specific antibody prevalence in Ethiopian infants. *Trans Roy Soc Trop Med Hyg*; **94**: 333–340.

Lawn JE, Reef S, Baffoe-Bonnie B, Adadevoh S, Caul EO, Griffin GE. (2000). Unseen blindness, unheard deafness, and unrecorded death and disability: congenital rubella in Kumasi, Ghana. *Am J Publ Hlth*; **90**: 1555–1561.

Masella SY, Haukenes G, Rutahindurwa A. (1999). Preliminary observations on rubella infection in Tanzania and the challenge for its control. *E Afr Med J*; **65**: 319–324.

Mingle JAA. (1985). Frequency of rubella antibodies in the population of some tropical African countries. *Rev Infect Dis*; **7**: S68–S71.

Robertson SE, Cutts FT, Samuel R, Diaz-Ortega JL. (1997). Control of rubella and congenital rubella syndrome (CRS) in developing countries, part 2: vaccination against rubella. *Bull Wld Hlth Org*; **75**: 69–80.

Waddell KM. (1998). Childhood blindness and low vision in Uganda. *Eye*; **12**: 184–192.

WHO. (2000). Rubella vaccines: WHO position paper. *Wkly Epidemiol Rec*; **75**: 161–169.

66 Mumps

Mumps is an acute systemic infection caused by a paramyxovirus. Mumps most commonly causes inflammation of the salivary glands, parotitis. The disease is usually mild, but it is more likely to be severe in adults.

The problem in Africa

Few studies have addressed mumps infection in Africa. One serosurvey in Eritrea found rates of mumps seropositivity differed widely among various adult populations, most likely reflecting degree of exposure: 85 per cent in female sexworkers, 46 per cent in pregnant women in an urban area, and 29 per cent in an isolated tribal group (Tolfvenstam et al., 2000).

Organism, life cycle, host

Humans are the only natural hosts for mumps virus, which is spread by droplets or by direct contact with saliva of an infected person. Virus has been cultured from saliva from 7 days before until 9 days after parotid swelling. The incubation period averages 16–18 days, range 2–4 weeks. Infection is asymptomatic in one-third of cases; asymptomatic cases may be infectious. Immunity develops after both symptomatic and asymptomatic infections and is generally life-long.

Clinical diagnosis is obvious in patients with parotitis. Mumps infection can be confirmed by the presence of mumps IgM antibody in a serum sample obtained within 30 days after infection, a four-fold rise in mumps IgG antibody titer in acute and convalescent sera, or virus culture. Urine or saliva specimens for culture should be obtained within 7 days after onset of parotitis.

Epidemiology

In countries where there is no vaccination against mumps, the disease incidence remains high (above 100 per 100 000 population), with epidemic peaks every 2–5 years, and the age group 5–9 years consistently the most affected. Historical records as far back as the eighteenth century document mumps epidemics world-wide, with greater frequency in crowded environments, such as schools, orphanages and military bases. Infants are protected by transplacental antibody; however, this wanes during the first months of life and most children are susceptible by 9 months of age.

Control/prevention

At least eight strains of mumps virus are in use throughout the world to produce live attenuated mumps vaccine. Rates of adverse reactions differ among the strains and policy makers considering introduction of mumps vaccine need to take this into consideration (Galazka et al., 1997). Sero-response is >90 per cent to a single dose of mumps vaccine and antibody is thought to be life-long. In a clinical trial in South Africa the sero-conversion rate to a dose of Jeryl Lynn strain mumps vaccine was 98% among 146 children aged 9 months compared with 100 per cent among 52 children aged 15 months (Schoub et al., 1990).

Based on data reported to the World Health Organization as of July 2000, 102 countries/areas (48 per cent) are using mumps vaccine in their national immunization programme; most administer the triple-antigen measles–mumps–rubella (MMR) vaccine at 12–15 months of age. On the African continent, mumps vaccine is administered routinely to children in Egypt, Mauritius and Seychelles.

Diagnosis/clinical features

Non-specific prodromal symptoms include low-grade fever, anorexia, malaise and headache. The disease may vary from a mild upper respiratory illness to widespread systemic involvement. Classic mumps is characterized by enlargement of the parotid and other salivary glands, with pain on eating. Parotitis is bilateral in three-quarters of cases; other salivary glands are involved in 10 per cent of cases (Fig. 66.1).

In post-pubertal men with mumps, about one-quarter develop orchitis; testicular atrophy occurs in about one-third of these individuals, but sterility is rare. Mumps orchitis appears to be a risk factor for testicular cancer, though not a major one. Among women who acquire mumps in the first 12 weeks of pregnancy, more than one-quarter suffer spontaneous abortion. However, studies have not demonstrated an increased incidence of congenital malformations following maternal mumps infection during pregnancy.

Sensorineural deafness is a well-recognized complication of mumps, especially in children. It may have sudden onset and is not related to the occurrence of meningitis. Mumps virus has been found in the perilymph. A study from Tanzania found mumps as the aetiology of permanent deafness in 15 per cent of 354 students at a school for the deaf (Minja, 1998).

Up to 10 per cent of mumps patients develop aseptic meningitis, but this usually resolves without sequelae. In countries where mumps vaccine is not widely used, mumps is one of the major causes of aseptic meningitis. A 2-year review in Cairo, Egypt found that mumps was the most important aetiology of aseptic meningitis (Abdel Wahab et al., 1969). A 9-year review in Cape Town, South Africa showed that, for 3406 meningitis patients with an established viral aetiology, 9 per cent were due to mumps (McIntyre & Keen, 1993). Mumps meningitis appears within a few days of parotid swelling, though half of mumps meningitis patients do not have any parotid swelling. Symptoms of meningitis include severe headache aggravated by movement, photophobia, and neck stiffness. As with other types of aseptic meningitis, the CSF shows pleocytosis, increased protein and normal or low glucose. Patients recover from mumps meningitis without complications, but many require hospitalization during the course of the illness.

A less common but more serious neurological complication is encephalitis, which can result in death or disability. Mumps encephalitis is a rare event (1 in 6000 to 1 in 300 mumps cases), which occurs more often in males. Symptoms of encephalitis range from mild alterations of consciousness to coma and death.

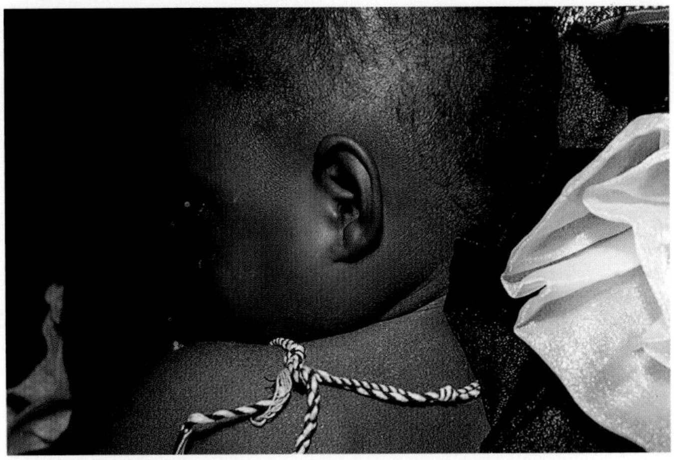

Fig. 66.1. Typical parotid swelling in a child with mumps (M. Weber).

Pancreatitis is seen in about 4 per cent of mumps cases. It has been suggested that mumps virus can trigger the onset of insulin-dependent diabetes mellitus; however, this remains unproven. A variety of other clinical symptoms are seen with mumps, including mild renal function abnormalities and transient ECG changes.

Treatment and follow-up

Treatment is symptomatic with supportive measures. For fever and pain, paracetamol or salicylates may be used. Orchitis can be extremely painful: bedrest, scrotal support, cold packs, and stronger analgesics may be needed. Parenteral fluids may be indicated for patients with persistent vomiting due to pancreatitis.

Unsolved problems

More data are needed on the disease burden due to mumps, especially in developing countries. Such assessments should include information on the costs due to mumps, including hospitalization, rehabilitation and days lost from school and work. It is thought that mumps has the potential to be eradicated through vaccination, although there are no specific regional or global initiatives.

References

Abdel Wahab KSE, El-Masry NA, Ismail M et al. (1969). A study of viral etiology of aseptic meningitis and encephalitis in Cairo. *J Egypt Pub Hlth Assoc*; **44**: 309–325.

Galazka AM, Robertson SE, Kraigher A. (1999). Mumps and mumps vaccine: a global review. *Bull Wld Hlth Org*; **77**: 3–14.
McIntrye JP, Keen GA. (1993). Laboratory surveillance of viral meningitis by examination of cerebrospinal fluid in Cape Town, 1981–9. *Epidemiol Infect*; **111**: 357–371.
Minja BM. (1998). Aetiology of deafness among children at the Buguruni School for the Deaf in Dar es Salaam, Tanzania. *Int J Pediat Otorhinolaryngol*; **42**: 225–231.
Schoub BD, Johnson S, McAnerney JM et al. (1990). Measles, mumps and rubella immunization at nine months in a developing country. *Pediat Infect Dis J*; **9**: 263–267.
Tolfvenstam T, Enbom M, Ghebrekidan H et al. (2000). Seroprevalence of viral childhood infections in Eritrea. *J Clin Virol*; **16**: 49–54.

Hepatitis viruses

67

Acute hepatitis is an illness usually beginning with fever. After 1–3 days the person develops yellowness of the sclera of the eye and mucosae – jaundice. This usually lasts a few days but may persist for months in some people. The illness is often associated with marked tiredness. 99 per cent of people make a full recovery. However, rarely liver failure develops which is virtually uniformly fatal without liver transplantation. For a fuller description see Chapter 80. This illness has multiple causes but probably the most common are the group of viruses known as the hepatitis viruses. These are given letters to identify them: A, B, C, D and E. Yellow fever virus is another important cause of hepatitis in Africa but is discussed elsewhere (Chapter 58). Occasionally, herpes viruses – cytomegalovirus and Epstein–Barr virus – may cause mild hepatitis.

It is impossible to know from examining the patient which virus is causing their hepatitis. Serological tests (see below) are needed which are expensive and many of which are only available in specialist laboratories.

Although the hepatitis viruses all have a letter of the alphabet they are completely different structurally and come from different families of viruses. They share this name simply because they all infect liver cells – hepatocytes. The best way to think of them is by route of transmission and whether or not they lead to chronic infection. This puts them into two groups.

Hepatitis A and E are both transmitted by the faecal–oral route. Neither of them causes a chronic infection and therefore neither of them causes chronic liver disease. Hepatitis B, D and C are all transmitted by contaminated needles, sexual intercourse and intimate contact. They can all lead to persistent infection and chronic liver disease.

Enteric transmission

Hepatitis A

Agent

This is a picornavirus.

Transmission

It is spread by faecal–oral contamination. This can take two forms. First by hand-to-mouth contact with faecal material – this is usually in small children in unhygienic conditions. Secondly, by contamination of foodstuff. Sealife that filters its food – such as clams and mussels – can become particularly heavily contaminated.

Infection and disease

The major determinant of whether infection causes disease, or not, is the age at which it occurs. If people are infected young – under 5 years of age, there is virtually no disease. In adolescence and adult life, infection produces disease in between one-third and two-thirds of infections. At these ages the quantity of virus (dose) swallowed probably plays an important role in determining whether disease results. In addition, the age at which people get disease is related to severity – so the proportion of people with liver failure who need hospital treatment is greater in older age groups.

Global epidemiology

WHO divides the world into three zones for hepatitis A:

- the endemic zone where transmission is at a high level at a young age so that, by the age of 15 years, more than 90 per cent of the population have been infected and are immune. In this zone there is very little disease resulting from hepatitis A, although it is circulating constantly in the childhood population;

- the intermediate zone where only perhaps half the population are exposed to infection under the age of 15 years. In this situation there are major epidemics of adult hepatitis every few years;
- the hypoendemic zone is where there is very limited circulation of virus and little disease. Here disease is largely related to travel to an intermediate or endemic zone with just very occasional epidemics of infection in children.

African epidemiology (Fig. 67.1)

The whole of Africa is defined as an endemic area. Studies in many countries have shown that 95 per cent of the young adult population have antibody to hepatitis A virus, indicating immunity. However, many of these studies are quite old and the situation in some urban centres has changed. There may well be relatively weathy urban families who have grown up with a good piped water supply who have been protected against childhood infection. This may lead to the appearance of adult hepatitis A over the next few years.

Control (Balayan et al., 1995)

It is a paradox that improving water supplies and hygiene causes the age at infection with this virus to rise and there is then more disease. This continues until the level of sanitation and hygiene reaches a level where circulation of the virus is interrupted. In countries with the intermediate epidemic pattern and in travellers from hypoendemic areas to countries with infection, vaccination is recommended. There are two main vaccines. One is a killed vaccine produced by a commercial vaccine manufacturer that is widely used in Europe and America. It is highly effective and provides more than 90 per cent protection after just one dose. Protection is likely to last at least 10 years. The other is a live attentuated vaccine made in China. This also appears to be effective and may lead to longer immunity. Neither vaccine is necessary in Africa since children are naturally immunized without disease. However, this requires careful monitoring and use of the vaccine may become necessary as hygienic conditions improve.

Hepatitis E

Agent

This is related to the caliciviruses.

Transmission

Faecal-oral, but has been particularly associated with heavy faecal contamination of the water supply. It has been particularly associated with flooding and storms. It tends to occur in epidemics (Isaacson et al., 2000).

Infection and disease

The surprising and important thing about this virus is that disease occurs in adults, and it is particularly severe in pregnant women. If it affects the woman in the first 3 months of pregnancy, the fetus is usually lost. In the last 3 months of pregnancy there is a very high mortality rate in the woman. The reasons for this are not clear but are presumably related to the immune changes that occur during pregnancy.

Global epidemiology

The disease occurs most commonly in a relatively narrow belt around the tropics. There are certain areas – such as the Kashmir valley and the island of Kalimantan that have regular epidemics on a 7–10 year cycle. In other populations epidemics only occur at the time of flooding – in places such as Mexico. Refugee camps are particularly likely to be affected.

African epidemiology

Sporadic cases are seen in West Africa – for example, physicians reported seeing probable cases in Kumasi in Ghana regularly. However, outbreaks have been seen in association with refugee camps – particularly camps for Somali people in northern Kenya. Some recent work suggests that the virus frequently infects cattle in these areas and this may be the source in times of disrupted sanitation.

Control

Safe water supply is the best means of prevention. There is no effective treatment. It is hoped that a vaccine will be available in the near future.

Blood-borne transmission

Hepatitis B

Agent

This is a hepadnavirus. It is a DNA virus. There are similar viruses that affect woodchucks, Pekin ducks and ground squirrels.

Transmission

This occurs by one of four routes: perinatal, child-to-child, sexual or iatrogenic.

Perinatal transmission occurs from mothers who are infectious to their babies around the time of birth.

Child-to-child transmission occurs between an infectious and a susceptible child – usually at home and usually between brothers or sisters. The exact route of transmission is not know but may involve biting, kissing, sharing cups and spoons or open skin wounds.

Sexual transmission occurs from an infectious person to a susceptible one during unprotected sexual intercourse.

Iatrogenic transmission is mostly related to unsafe injections – where the needle is contaminated by infectious blood or body fluids. Blood transfusion was an important source of infection until screening of donated blood was introduced.

Infection and disease

The critical aspect of infection with this virus is that, in a proportion of patients, it leads to a persistent infection – the 'carrier state'. People who have a persistent infection are known as 'carriers'. These people may, or may not, be infectious. In general, the younger they are, and therefore the more recently infected, the more infectious they are. These aspects are reflected in serological markers of infection with the virus.

Hepatitis B surface antigen (HbsAg) which is part of the coat of the virus is produced in great excess when the liver is infected. This excess circulates in the blood and can be measured. It is found at the time of acute infection and in carriers. The definition of a carrier is a person who is positive for HbsAg on two occasions at least 6 months apart. This excludes the possibility that it is an acute infection.

Hepatitis B e antigen is a part of the core of the virus that is found when there is circulating virus in the blood stream. It is closely associated with being infectious.

Hepatitis B core antibody is produced by an infection and lasts for many years. The core antigen cannot be found outside the liver, but the presence of this antibody circulating in the blood is a useful indication that the person has been infected by the virus. It does not tell you when, unless the IgM antibody is found positive indicating a recent infection.

Hepatitis B surface antibody is produced in response not only to infection but to vaccination. The hepatitis B vaccine is made from purified hepatitis B surface antigen. It does not contain core or e antigen. A vaccinated individual who has never been infected would be positive for surface antibody alone.

Infection has two important outcomes. The first is acute hepatitis. The second is being a carrier of the virus. Age affects these two things in different ways. Carriage is more common the younger the age at infection. Perinatal transmission from an e antigen-positive mother leads to the child being a carrier in 90 per cent of transmissions. If infection occurs between the age of 1 and 5, 20–30 per cent of infections result in carriage. After that age only 5 per cent of infections end in carriage. In contrast, acute hepatitis is rare in children and becomes increasingly frequent in adolescence and adult life. Even then only perhaps one-third of infections result in clinical acute hepatitis.

Carriage is not only important because carriers are infectious. It is important to the individual because they are at increased risk of chronic liver disease – cirrhosis, and of primary liver cancer. A carrier is about ten times more likely to develop cirrhosis and 50 times more likely to get primary liver cancer, than somebody who is not a carrier. Ten per cent of the adult male African population die from complications of hepatitis B carriage.

Global epidemiology

The world can be divided geographically on the basis of the proportion of the adult population who are carriers. Low endemic areas are those where less than 1 per cent of adults are carriers (most of western Europe and north America). Intermediate areas are those with carriage rates between 1 and 5 per cent (north Africa, eastern Europe, India) and holoendemic areas are those with adult rates >5 per cent (sub-Saharan Africa, China). In low endemicity areas transmission is largely by sex or intravenous drug use. In intermediate and high endemicity areas it is by these routes + child-to-child and perinatal transmission. The critical difference lies between China and Africa. In China perinatal transmission plays a much greater role than in Africa. In China appoximately 15 per cent of adult women are carriers of the virus and about

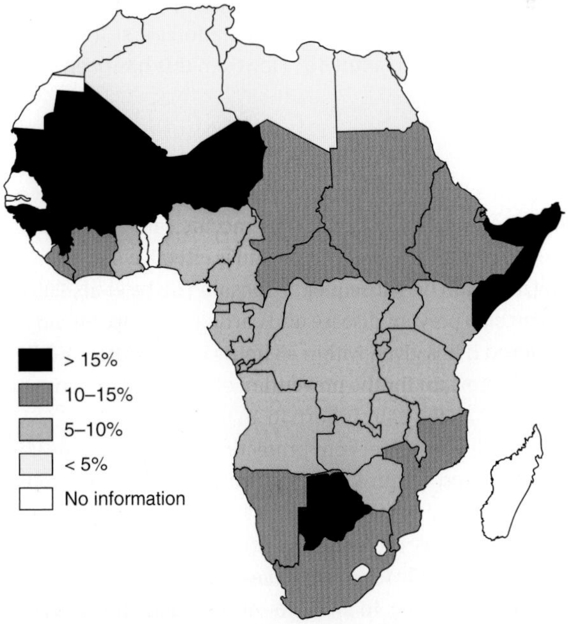

Fig. 67.1. Prevalence of HB$_5$AG in adult males.

half of these are also e antigen-positive, i.e. infectious. In parts of Africa (see below) the proportion of African women who are carriers is similar but only a tenth of them are infectious. Thus in China around 40 per cent of carriers may be due to perinatal transmission. In Africa this proportion is estimated to be around 10 per cent.

African epidemiology

Child-to-child transmission dominates the pattern of hepatitis B infection. Cross-sectional surveys of the population clearly show that infection predominantly occurs before the age of 10 years. Perinatal infection is unusual as referred to above. However, there is quite marked geographical variation in the pattern of infection. Figure 67.1 shows the proportion of adults who are carriers of hepatitis B virus by country. This is based on both published and unpublished surveys. There is a clear pattern with high rates of carriage across the Sahel south of the Sahara and across the Namib and Kalahari deserts in southern Africa. North of the Sahara carriage is much less common and Central and East Africa also have lower rates. This implies that childhood transmission is particularly associated with the desert zones. The exact mechanism of transmission between children is unknown. Studies in West Africa have clearly shown that it tends to occur at home and is from older infectious carrier siblings. Studies of possible insect vectors have not shown any association. Transmission in childhood is more frequent in rural than in urban areas (Barin et al., 1981; Van Mayans et al., 1990).

In the lower prevalence areas of Africa – central, east and northern – there is a possibility of sexual transmission since around half of the population are still susceptible to infection in adult life. However, this has been studied little.

Control

Hepatitis B vaccine is purified surface antigen. It is given by intramuscular injection. The vaccine can be given from the moment of birth onwards and is effective in preventing infection on subsequent exposure (Tsebe et al., 2001). It can also prevent disease and carriage in those already exposed if it is given within 48 hours of exposure. This is very important for the prevention of perinatal infection. It means that, if a baby is born to an infectious carrier mother, it gets 90 per cent protection against carriage if it is vaccinated within 48 hours of birth. This is clearly most important in countries such as China where perinatal infection is very important. In Africa a dose at birth is not currently feasible for most babies since the majority are delivered at home. In those countries where the vaccine has been introduced it has been at the same time as DPT, e.g. 6, 10 and 14 weeks of age. This ensures that the baby is fully protected by 6 months of age. This vaccine schedule has been highly effective at almost eliminating hepatitis B infection from villages where it has been vigorously applied. It has also been shown to be a very cost-effective health intervention for Africa (Hall et al., 1993). It is hoped that, over the next few years, most countries will introduce it as recommended by the WHO. Since the high risk of becoming a carrier is limited to childhood, it is probably unnecessary to give booster doses of vaccine later in life but further study is needed to assess this.

Hepatitis D

Agent

The agent of hepatitis D is a very unusual single strand of RNA without a coat.

Transmission

The virus is highly unusual in that it needs the presence of hepatitis B virus in order to survive. It uses the coat of hepatitis B as its own since it does not have one. This means that it can only infect people who are already hepatitis B carriers (superinfection) or be transmitted simultaneously with hepatitis B virus (co-infection). Transmission can clearly occur by contaminated needles since this infection has been found in intravenous drug users. Sexual transmission does not appear to be at all common. The infection did not spread in the male homosexual community in the USA before hepatitis B vaccination became available although there were many HBV carriers. Transmission in the Amazon appears to include child-to-child transmission – it is unclear what the mechanism of this is.

Infection and disease

The pattern of disease resulting from infection is dependent on whether it superinfects a carrier or co-infects. Around 50–70 per cent of co- or super-infections result in clinical acute hepatitis. Fulminant disease occurs in 10 per cent of co-infections and 20 per cent of superinfections. Subsequent chronic infection with HDV produces a marked increase in the risk of chronic liver disease – particularly as a superinfection. HDV is not an independent cause of primary liver cancer.

Global epidemiology

The major focus of hepatitis D or delta hepatitis is amongst the indigenous tribes of the Amazon basin. There infection occurs predominantly in late childhood and adolescence by mechanisms that have not been defined. Intravenous drug users in Europe – particularly in Italy – have been the other major focus of infection.

African epidemiology

The infection occurs in Africa but it is very patchily distributed. In one village there will be none despite high rates of HBV carriage and in the next 20 per cent of carriers will be infected. The full extent of hepatitis D has not been documented on the continent.

Control

Since the virus requires hepatitis B to survive, control of HBV will control delta hepatitis. However there are still over 100 million carriers in the world who are potentially susceptible to super-infection with delta hepatitis. There are therefore attempts to make a vaccine but none is currently available.

Hepatitis C

Agent

This virus is in the flavivirus group. It is a RNA virus.

Transmission

Injections are the common mode of transmission of this virus. Whether it can be transmitted sexually is controversial, but it is likely that it does happen for the short period after infection when there are high levels of virus circulating in the blood stream. The virus can also be transmitted perinatally. However, this only occurs in about 10–20 per cent of deliveries to HCV carrier mothers although it can be higher in women who are intravenous drug users – for reasons that are not known.

Infection and disease

A very high proportion of infections result in persistent infection, at least 80 per cent and quite possibly more. The virus constantly mutates in much the same way as HIV allowing it to evade the immune response. Infection rarely leads to acute hepatitis. However, persistent infection can lead to cirrhosis and primary liver cancer. The exact size of this risk is still unclear. However, it is clear that alcohol is an important factor in accelerating the liver damage.

Global epidemiology

Infection in childhood is rare and perinatal infection is uncommon. Most infections occur in adult life as a result of intravenous drug use or accidental infection related to medical procedures. Carriage rates around the world vary from 0.1–1 per cent in the general population. The infection appears to have become common during the 1960s when the illicit use of intravenous drugs became widespread in Europe and America. Amongst intravenous drug users up to 80 per cent have been found infected. The one general population rate comparable to this is in Egypt – see below.

African epidemiology

As many as 40 per cent of adult Egyptians are infected in some areas. This is clearly due to the transmission of the infection by contaminated needles during mass treatment of schistosomiasis–bilharzia. Elsewhere on the continent infection appears to be at a low level of around 1 per cent of the general population. Some studies are difficult to interpret as the tests for HCV are subject to cross-reactions.

Control

There is no vaccine. It is likely to be some time before one becomes available because of the high rate of mutation in the virus. Control is dependent on assuring safe injections. This needs to include all parts of the medical services but also the traditional medical sector where injections are commonly given. The safe disposal of needles is particularly important.

Chronic liver disease and primary liver cancer

As discussed in Chapter 80, these two conditions are major causes of illness and death in Africa. Hepatitis B and C viruses cause in excess of 80 per cent of the disease burden. Hepatitis B vaccination and safe injection are the two major public health interventions to reduce these in Africa.

References

Balayan MS, Chunsutiwat S, Flehmig B et al. (1995). Public health control of hepatitis A: memorandum from a WHO meeting. *Bull Wld Hlth Org*; **73**: 15–20.

Barin F, Perrin J, Chotard J et al. (1981). Cross sectional and longitudinal epidemiology of hepatitis B in Senegal *Prog Med Virol*; **41**: 83–87.

Hall AJ, Robertson RL, Crivella PE et al. (1993). Cost-effectiveness of hepatitis B vaccine in The Gambia. *Trans Roy Soc Trop Med Hyg*; **87**: 333–336.

Isaacson M, Frean J, He J, Seriwatana J, Innis BL. (2000). An outbreak of hepatitis E in Northern Namibia, 1983. *Am J Trop Med Hyg*; **62**: 619–625.

Tsebe KV, Burnett RJ, Jlungwani NP, Sibara MM, Venter PA, Mphahlele MJ. (2001). The first five years of universal hepatitis B vaccination in South Africa: evidence for elimination of HbsAg carriage in under 5 years olds. *Vaccine*; **19**: 3919–3926.

Vall Mayans M, Hall AJ, Inskip HM et al. (1990). Risk factors for transmission of hepatitis B virus to Gambian children *Lancet*; **336**; 1107–1109.

68 Rabies

Rabies is a viral zoonosis of mammals, which is occasionally transmitted to the human, usually through the bite of an infected dog.

The problem in Africa

Rabies has probably existed in parts of Africa for centuries. It was reported by European travellers to Ethiopia and Southern Africa in the eighteenth and early nineteenth centuries. Among the Bantu of South Africa, rabies in spotted genets led to the belief that these animals had poisonous saliva (Synman, 1940). Rabies has long been familiar to the Ndebele people of Zimbabwe and to the inhabitants of South Kavirondo in Kenya (Hudson, 1944). The infection was reintroduced by dogs imported by the European settlers.

The risk of rabies is now present in all mainland African countries, including Madagascar. In 1998 only Libya and some African islands reported no cases of rabies. Human rabies is grossly underreported in Africa. In 1998, only 204 cases were notified to WHO (WHO, 2000), 91 per cent of which had been diagnosed clinically and 79 per cent were attributable to dog bites. The largest number, 43, occurred in Ethiopia. Table 68.1 gives the numbers of human deaths in 9 African countries.

Table 68.1. Human deaths from rabies reported in nine African countries

Country	Average (maximum) number of human deaths per year	Period
Madagascar	16	1996–1998
Mozambique	18 (92) (increasing)	
Malawi	30–40 (increasing)	1992–1996
South Africa	21 (26)	1992–1996
Sudan	23	1992–1998
Tanzania	29 (58)	1992–1996
Uganda	25	1992–1995
Zambia	55 (118)	1992–1996
Zimbabwe	3 (6)	1992–1996

Sources: WHO, 1998; South Eastern and Eastern African Rabies Group, 2000.

Rabies and rabies-like viruses

Rabies is caused by a bullet-shaped RNA virus, one of the Rhabdoviridae or rod-shaped viruses. Rabies virus is a member of the Lyssavirus genus (rabies and rabies-like viruses), four of which (classical rabies, Mokola, Duvenhage and Lagos bat virus) occur in Africa. All four have been identified in Zimbabwe and South Africa. Lagos bat virus does not cause disease in humans.

The term 'street' virus refers to virus isolated from naturally infected animals, such as the mad dogs in the streets of Paris used by Louis Pasteur in his classical studies. Street virus was attenuated (weakened) by repeated infection (passage) in rabbits, yielding 'fixed' virus which has a shortened, predictable incubation period and has been used experimentally and for vaccine production.

Epidemiology

Animal vectors and reservoirs

Any warm-blooded animal (mammal or bird) can be infected with rabies, but in practice only mammals, principally carnivores, are important hosts. The principal

Table 68.2. Examples of rabies reservoir species

Country	Reservoir species
North Africa	Domestic dog, jackal, fox, wolf
East and West Africa	Domestic dog
Southern Africa	
Zimbabwe	Black-backed jackal
Zambia, Malawi, Mozambique	Domestic dog
Namibia	Kudu antelope
South Africa	Yellow mongoose, black-backed jackal, bat-eared fox
Kwazulu Natal	Domestic dog

Source: From WHO (1998).

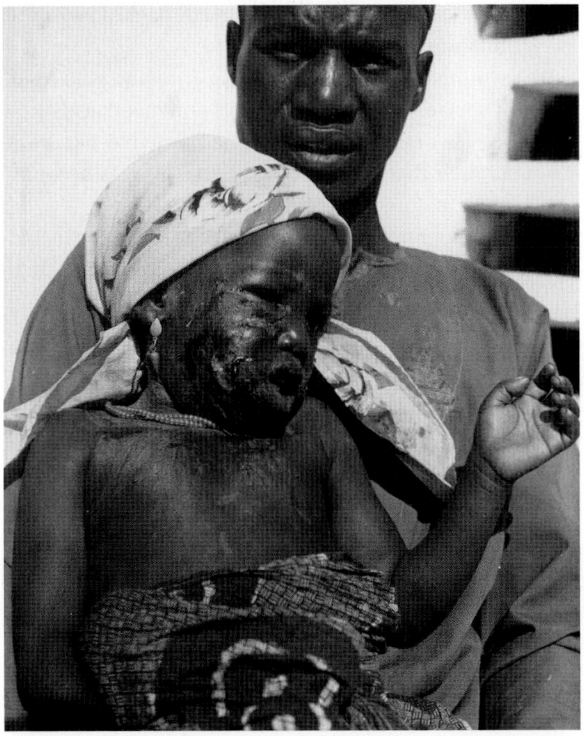

Fig. 68.1. Severe facial bites inflicted by a rabid dog in a Nigerian girl. Children are particularly vulnerable to such attacks. Copyright © D. A. Warrell.

reservoir species, which vary in different parts of Africa, are shown in Table 68.2. In the late 1970s and early 1980s, 30 000 Kudu antelopes died of rabies in Namibia. In March 2001 there was a recurrence of this epizootic in Okahandja and Omaruru Districts of western Namibia with 200 deaths. In the 1990s, several packs of African wild dogs were killed by rabies in the Serengeti area. In

Table 68.3. Incidence of dog bite in three African cities

	Incidence of bites per 100 000 population per year	Percentage of bite victims aged less than 20	M:F ratio
Accra, Ghana (Belcher et al., 1976)	670	65	1: 1
Ibadan, Nigeria (Kale, 1977)	250	75	1.3: 1
Zaria, Nigeria	?	57	3.45: 1

this same region, 37 per cent of spotted hyenas were found to have serological evidence of past rabies infection while 45 per cent were excreting the virus intermittently in their saliva. The strain of virus was peculiar to this species (East et al., 2001). In June 2002, an epizootic of rabies broke out in Kerio Valley, Marakawet District, Kenya, among domestic dogs that had been abandoned by their owners and become feral (Promed).

It has been suggested that rodents, such as ground squirrels in northern Nigeria and gerbils in Egypt, might be reservoirs of rabies. However, there is no convincing evidence for this (McMillan & Boulger, 1960).

Domestic animals

Throughout Africa, the domestic dog is the single most important reservoir species and is everywhere the most important vector of rabies to the human. In 1998, more than 50 per cent of all cases of rabies diagnosed in mammals in Africa were in domestic dogs, while 26 per cent were in domestic ruminants (WHO, 2000).

Dog bite is common in Africa (Fig. 68.1). Table 68.3 shows the incidence of bites severe enough to make people go to hospital. Young males are the most likely to be bitten by rabid dogs. In Accra, half the patients admitted with rabies were less than 20 years old and there were 2.5 times as many males as females (Belcher et al., 1976).

Seasonal variation

In Accra, there is a peak of canine rabies in September, shortly following a period of increased fighting and mating amongst the dogs. The peak incidence of human rabies occurs in December (Belcher et al., 1976).

Economic burden

Rabies among domestic animals, especially cattle (Elegbe & Banejee, 1970), can impose an economic burden, but this is insignificant compared with the fear experienced by human victims of dog bites and their relatives.

Prevention

The prognosis of human rabies is so appalling that every community must attempt to control the disease in animal reservoirs and vectors, to give effective protection to those particularly at risk and to treat those who have been bitten by mammals.

General control measures

(i) Educate the population, including young children, about the dangers of mammal bites and rabies (Fig. 68.2).
(ii) Improve facilities for post-exposure treatment of people bitten by animals and provide pre-exposure vaccination for those at high risk (see below).
(iii) Reduce the urban dog (and cat) reservoir through door-to-door campaigns to vaccinate all owned dogs and cats (Wandeler & Bingham, 2000). The keeping of these animals may be limited by licensing and their owners encouraged, as far as possible, to keep their dogs within the compound and to muzzle them if they are aggressive. Co-ordinated mass vaccination campaigns have proved effective in large cities of South America and in Yemen. To be effective, at least 70 per cent of the total dog population must be vaccinated. Stray dogs are much more of a problem. It is difficult to control their numbers, but it may prove possible to immunize them against rabies, using oral vaccines in bait (see below).
(iv) Reduce the wild mammal reservoir, not by killing, which is an ineffective, short-lived and cruel policy, but by immunization, using live-attenuated or recombinant vaccines distributed in bait. This technique was being pioneered in black-backed jackals in Zimbabwe.
(v) Discourage people from keeping attractive wild reservoir species, such as mongooses and meerkats (suricates), as pets. Children must be warned to avoid wild mammals that seem to be friendly: this may be a presenting feature of rabies!
(vi) Control of imported mammals and statutory vaccination and quarantine may be effective in islands (such as Hawaii, Japan and the British Isles) in maintaining a rabies-free status.

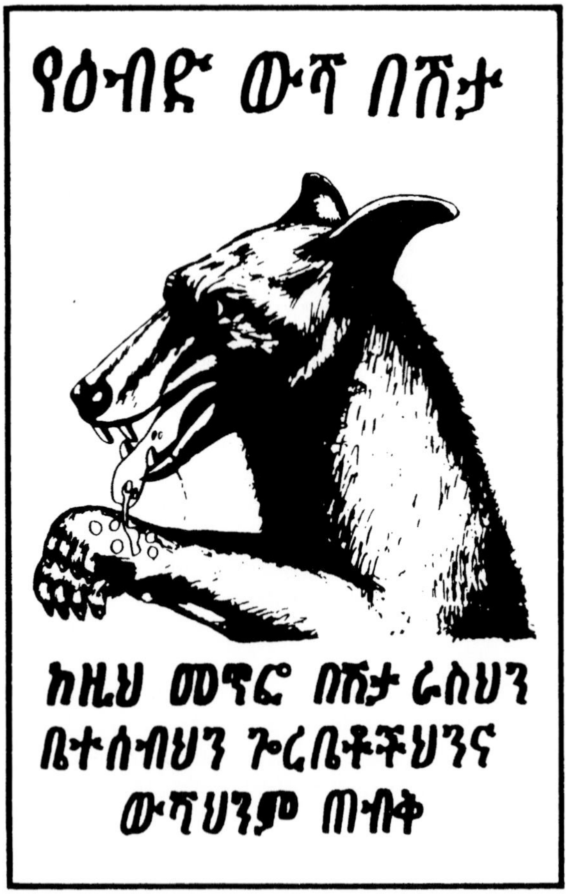

Fig. 68.2. Ethiopian rabies poster. The caption reads: protect yourself, your family, your neighbours and your dog from this central nervous system disease. Copyright © D. A. Warrell.

Simple preventive methods including loudspeaker van publicity, provision of a weekly dog vaccination clinic and collection of stray and unlicensed dogs were tried in the Kaneshire District of Accra in 1972, and resulted in a significant fall in the need for anti-rabies vaccine (Engmann & Engmann, 1973).

Protection of the individual

Pre-exposure vaccination

Veterinary workers, dog catchers, zoologists and other field workers and laboratory workers who are particularly exposed to the risk of rabies can be protected by vaccination. The safest and most potent vaccines are human diploid cell vaccine (HDCV), purified vero cell vaccine (PVRV) and purified chicken embryo cell vaccine (PCECV). Three doses are given on day 0, 3 and 28 (or 21). The dose is 1 vial intramuscularly into the deltoid (or the anterolateral thigh in children), or 0.1 ml intradermally. The small dose of 0.1 ml is adequate only if the injection is truly intradermal, rather than subcutaneous or intramuscular (Fig. 68.3). Chloroquine, in the dose used for malaria prophylaxis, can reduce the immune response to intradermal rabies vaccination. A single booster dose, 1–2

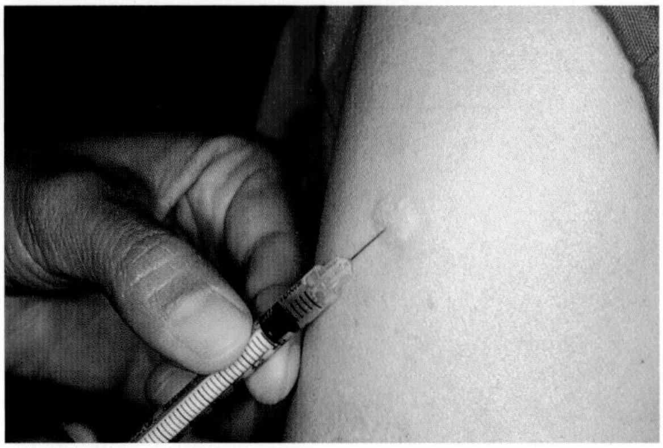

Fig. 68.3. Correct technique of intradermal injection. A small papule (area of peau d'orange) is raised at the site of the injection (as in the case of BCG vaccination). Copyright © D. A. Warrell.

years after the primary course, results in persistence of neutralizing antibody for five years or more. The neutralizing antibody response need not be checked unless immunosuppression is suspected or the vaccinee is at continuing high risk (as in the case of rabies laboratory staff).

Post-exposure treatment

Emergency treatment of dog and other mammal bites (including human bites)

Urgent, energetic and thorough cleaning of the wound is essential. This may require general anaesthesia in a child or someone with severe multiple bites. The wound should be scrubbed with soap or detergent under a running tap, for at least 5 minutes. Foreign bodies, tooth fragments and dead tissue should be removed. After washing away the cleansing agent with plain water, apply antiseptics such as alcohol (40–70 per cent) or tincture or aqueous solution of iodine (1 per cent) which kill rabies virus. Quaternary ammonium compounds (cetrimide, benzalkonium) are neutralized by soap and hydrogen peroxide is ineffective. Avoid suturing as this may inoculate virus deeper into the wound. Many other pathogens, apart from rabies virus, can be transmitted by mammal bites, notably *Clostridium tetani* and *Pasteurella multocida* (see Table 1, Chapter 92 Injuries and envenoming caused by animals). Human bites are usually complicated by infection with *Staphylococcus aureus*, streptococci and anaerobic organisms.

Specific anti-rabies treatment

The decision whether to give specific post-exposure treatment with anti-rabies vaccine and rabies immune globulin is based on the severity of the bite wound, species of biting mammal, and level of suspicion that it was rabid (Table 68.4). The appearance and behaviour of a domestic dog responsible for biting someone, and the circumstances of the bite, may influence the decision whether or not to go ahead with specific anti-rabies treatment. If the dog has been reliably vaccinated against rabies within the past year (preferably with a certificate to prove it) and if the bite was obviously provoked by the animal's being molested or its territory or puppies threatened, the likelihood of rabies is reduced. However, if there has been a recent change in behaviour, the animal is obviously unwell with paralysis of the neck and hindquarters, drooling, dysphagia and an altered bark, there is a high risk of rabies. Urgent examination by a veterinarian may be appropriate. The circumstances may justify the veterinarian's putting down the animal immediately if it is possible to test its brain for rabies (see below). Severe or multiple bites (especially facial) and bites by wild carnivores should always be regarded as rabid, until proved otherwise. Even if weeks have passed since the bite, vaccine and rabies immunoglobulin should be given. However, once undeniable symptoms of rabies encephalitis have developed (see below), it is too late for pre-exposure treatment.

Table 68.4. Specific post-exposure prophylaxis for use in a rabies endemic area[a] following contact with a domestic or wild rabies vector species, whether or not the animal is available for observation or diagnostic tests

Minor exposure
(including licks of broken skin, scratches or abrasions without bleeding)
- Start vaccine immediately
- Stop treatment if animal remains healthy for 10 days
- Stop treatment if animal's brain proves negative for rabies by appropriate laboratory tests

Major exposure
(including licks of mucosa, minor bites on arms, trunk or legs, or major bites – multiple or on face, head, fingers or neck)
- Immediate rabies immune globulin and vaccine
- Stop treatment if domestic cat or dog remains healthy for 10 days
- Stop treatment if animal's brain proves negative for rabies by appropriate laboratory tests

Note:
[a] This scheme is a simplification of the WHO recommendations on rabies post-exposure treatment (WHO, 1997).

Rabies vaccines available in Africa (Table 68.5)

Only nervous tissue vaccines are manufactured in Africa (for example, in Ethiopia, Nigeria, Tunisia and Sudan).

Table 68.5. Rabies vaccines available in Africa

Vaccine	Manufacturer	Daily dose	Route	Course (Fig. 68.5)
Tissue culture vaccines				
Purified vero cell vaccine	Aventis Pasteur	) see Fig. 68.5) 0.5 ml	i.d. i.m.	see Fig. 68.5 days 0, 3, 7, 14 and 28
Human diploid cell vaccine	Aventis Pasteur	) see Fig. 68.5) 1.0 ml	i.d. i.m.	see Fig. 68.5 days 0, 3, 7, 14 and 28
Purified chicken embryo cell vaccine	Chiron	) see Fig. 68.5) 1.0 ml	i.d. i.m.	see Fig. 68.5 days 0, 3, 7, 14 and 28
Nervous tissue vaccines[a]				
Semple and Fermi type 5 per cent brain suspension	various African	2–4 ml	s.c.	10–21 daily injections with boosters
Suckling mouse brain vaccine	various African	2 ml	s.c.	7 daily injections with boosters

Note:
[a] To be used only if tissue culture vaccines are not available.

Tissue culture vaccines are imported. Because of problems with potency and safety, there is a global initiative to replace nervous tissue vaccines (Semple and Fermi vaccines consisting of sheep or goat brain and suckling mouse brain vaccine) as soon as possible. The economic problem of using relatively costly tissue culture vaccines manufactured in Europe has been partly overcome by the development of highly effective, economical, multi-site intradermal regimens which are now recommended by WHO (WHO, 1997). When the bitten patient first comes for treatment, the contents of a whole vial of tissue culture vaccine are drawn up into a 1 ml insulin or Mantoux syringe and, using a fine (25) gauge needle, the contents of the vial are divided, roughly equally, between 8 different sites (Fig. 68.4) and given by intradermal injection. This method ensures optimal speed and magnitude of antibody response. At the next visit, 1 week later, half a vial of vaccine is divided equally among four intradermal sites. There are two further visits for single site intradermal injections of one-tenth of the volume of the whole vial, on days 28 and 90. An alternative intradermal regimen, also recommended by WHO, involves the injection of one-fifth of the vial at each of two intradermal sites on days 0, 3 and 7, followed by two further single site intradermal injections on days 28 and 90 (WHO, 1997).

The standard regimen for using tissue culture vaccines is to inject a whole vial intramuscularly into the deltoid on days 0, 3, 7, 14 and 28 but this requires 60 per cent more vaccine than the 8-site and 2-site intradermal regimens and one more hospital visit than the 8-site regimen. The 8-site intradermal regimen has two other very important advantages for use in Africa. If compliance is poor and the patient fails to return after the visits on day 0 or day 7, this regimen is still likely to give a good neutralizing antibody response. The high and rapidly developing antibody response to the 8-site regimen is specially important when, as is usually the case in Africa, rabies immunoglobulin is not available to provide immediate neutralization of virus.

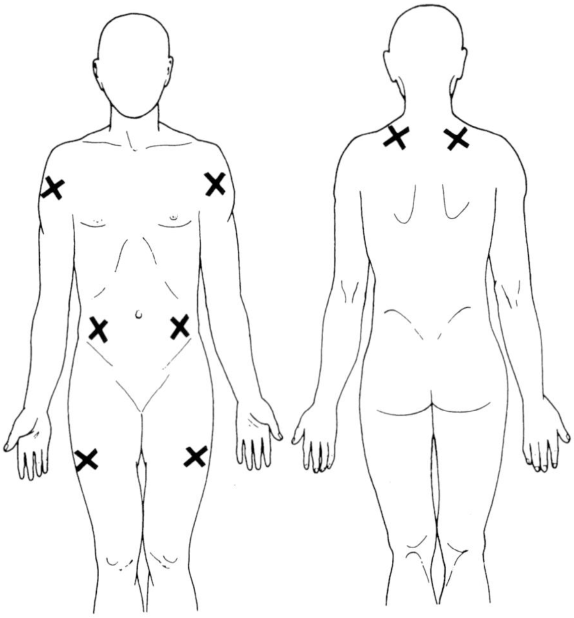

Fig. 68.4. Sites for intradermal injection using the 8-site intradermal regimen. (see Fig. 68.5). Copyright © D. A. Warrell.

Nervous tissue vaccines are no longer recommended unless tissue culture vaccine is not available. Because of the risk of serious side effects from nervous tissue vaccines, it is important to make a careful assessment of the risk of rabies exposure before starting vaccination.

Complications of anti-rabies vaccine

Modern tissue culture vaccines (HDCS, PVRV, PCEC) cause only mild local and rare feverish reactions which are unimportant. However, the old-fashioned nervous tissue vaccines can cause serious allergic complications involving the nervous system. Various types of ascending and transverse myelitis, meningoencephalitis or polyneuritis, especially Guillain–Barré syndrome, may develop 3 days or longer (usually about 2 weeks) after the first injection of vaccine. The overall incidence is up to 1 in 200 courses of sheep brain Semple-type vaccine, with an average case-fatality of about 3 per cent; and between 1 in 7865 to 1 in 27 000 courses of suckling mouse brain vaccine, with a 22 per cent case-fatality. Most reactions to Semple vaccine affect the central nervous system, whereas at least 70 per cent of those following suckling mouse brain vaccine involve the peripheral nervous system.

Rabies immuneglobulin

Immuneglobulin of human or animal origin, if available, is given immediately after vaccination when the patient first comes for treatment. It is infiltrated around the wound. If the wounds are numerous and large, the rabies immuneglobulin can be diluted two- to three-fold with saline. Any residual material is injected intramuscularly, distant from the sites of vaccination.

Complications of rabies immune globulin

Passive immunization with equine or caprine rabies immune globulin results in serum sickness in 1–6 per cent of cases. Intradermal hypersensitivity tests are not predictive of reactions and should not be used. At the time of treatment, epinephrine (adrenaline) (0.1 per cent solution for intramuscular injection) must always be available to treat anaphylaxis. Human rabies immune globulin does not cause reactions.

Practical problems associated with post-exposure prophylaxis

Apart from the enormous problems of cost, supply, distribution and cool storage of rabies vaccine and rabies immune globulin in Africa, there is the difficulty of persuading patients to return to hospital to complete the full course of vaccination. In this situation, the concept of 8-site intradermal immunization on day 0 is particularly important. For the patient who has travelled a long distance to reach hospital, the alternatives are either to stay near the hospital at least for the first week of the course, or to be referred to a local dispensary with a letter of instructions and the necessary supplies of vaccine. Among a group of patients attending University College Hospital, Ibadan, almost 40 per cent defaulted before completing the course (Kale, 1977).

Effectiveness of post-exposure treatment (Fig. 68.5)

Deaths from rabies have occurred despite vaccine treatment. These are attributable to the use of low-potency nervous-tissue vaccines, delay in starting vaccination, an incomplete vaccine course, omission of passive immunization, failure to infiltrate rabies immuneglobulin around the wound, injection of vaccine into the buttock (where it is less immunogenic), or, increasingly, decreased immune responsiveness of the vaccinee, resulting from immunosuppression, such as from HIV/AIDS. It seems likely that vaccine-induced immunity would be less effective in neutralizing Mokola and Duvenhage viruses than classical rabies virus. It is appropriate to double the initial dose of vaccine or divide the first dose of cell culture vaccine between eight sites intradermally if post-exposure treatment has been delayed by more than a few days after exposure, if no rabies immuneglobulin is available for severe bites, the patient is immunocompromised or a rabies-related virus infection is suspected.

Pathogenesis of rabies encephalomyelitis

Rabies virus inoculated through the skin by a bite multiplies locally in muscle fibres, possibly for days or weeks. Virus particles then enter nerve fibres, by binding with acetylcholine receptors at the neuromuscular junction or with other receptors, and are then carried in the axoplasm, to reach the spinal cord and brain. In the central nervous system there is multiplication and dispersion of virus by inter-neuronal spread, producing the encephalomyelitis which is the clinical disease known as rabies. Virus is then disseminated centrifugally, via neurones, to a variety of tissues and organs, including skeletal and heart muscle, skin (where it can be detected by immunofluorescence – see below). It also reaches the salivary and lacrimal glands from which it is shed to infect a new host.

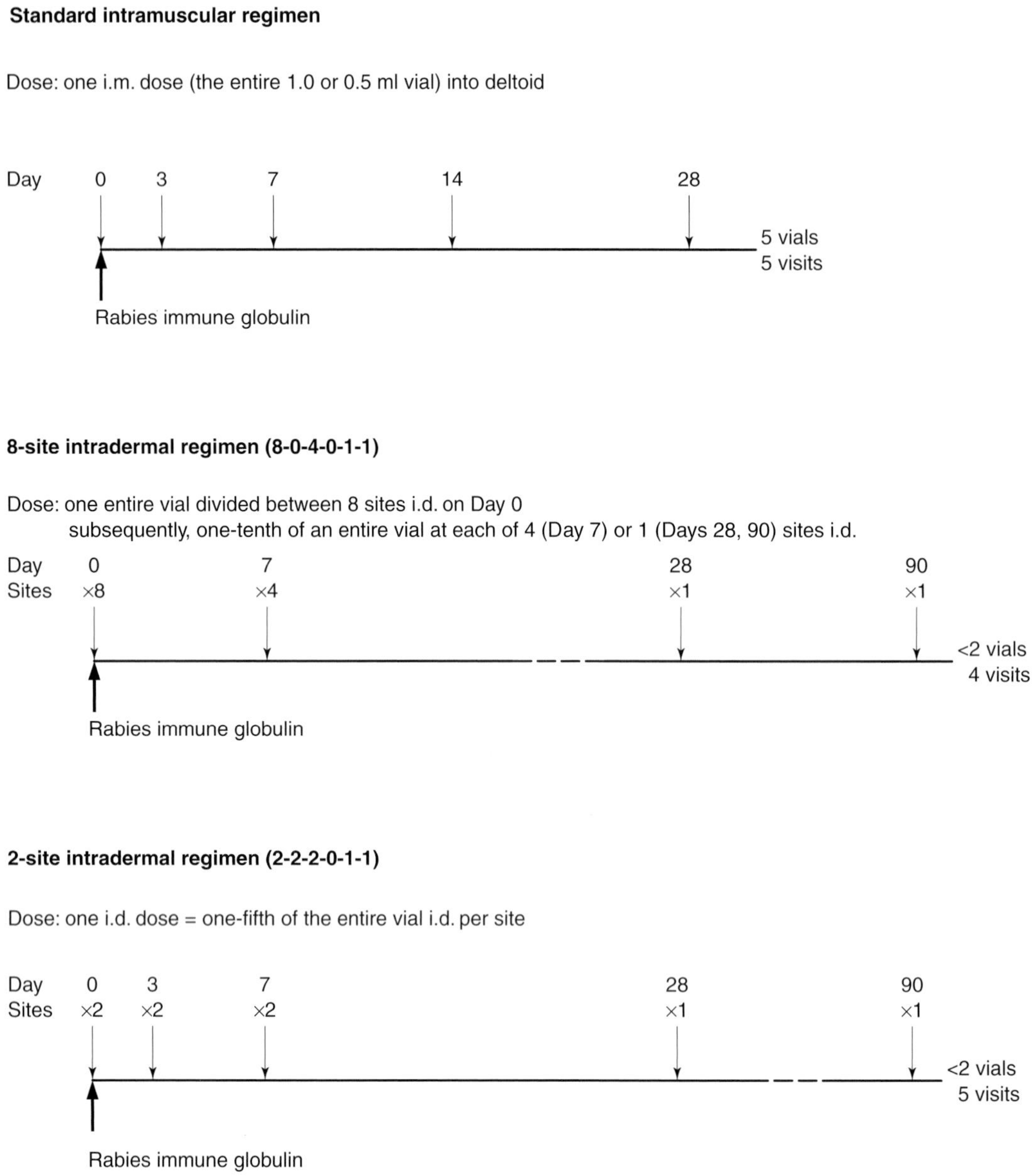

Fig. 68.5. Regimens for administering post-exposure prophylaxis using tissue culture vaccines. Standard intramuscular regimen and two economical multi-site intradermal regimens. (World Health Organization, 1997.)

Clinical features

Signs of rabies in mammals

In dogs, signs of rabies usually develop 3–12 weeks (extreme range 5 days to 14 months) after exposure to infection (a bite by a rabid mammal). The first symptom is intense irritation at the site of the infective bite, followed by a change in behaviour, loss of appetite and inability to drink. Despite the popular idea of the 'mad' rabid dog, only 25 per cent develop furious rabies.

Furious rabies is the more familiar but less common form. The dog is restless and aggressive, travels long distances, attacks other animals, humans and inanimate objects. It shows dysphagia and has an altered bark and paralysis of the jaw, neck and hind limbs. It hypersalivates, trembles, snaps at imaginary objects and develops pica (abnormal appetite) so that it swallows sticks and stones.

Dumb rabies is the less familiar but more common presentation which is less likely to be suspected. The dog becomes apathetic, it lies around, cowers under the furniture and is usually not aggressive. The owner may think that a bone has lodged in its throat and may attempt to extract it manually!

The rabid dog's saliva is infective for a few days before the start of symptoms and it usually dies within the next 5 days. Survival for longer than 10 days virtually excludes rabies but, very rarely, dogs may recover, develop asymptomatic infections, or even a healthy carrier state in which virus is excreted in the saliva. 'Oulou fato', a form of paralytic canine rabies in which symptoms were mild, was first recognized in French West Africa at the beginning of the twentieth century. More recently, healthy dogs with rabies in their saliva were discovered in Ethiopia (Fekadu, 1975).

Among other mammalian species, cats and horses are more likely to show furious features, while cattle and other domestic ungulates are more likely to develop paralytic symptoms. Wild mammals may show abnormal tameness or abnormal aggression.

Laboratory diagnosis

Brain or spinal cord from the mammal suspected of being rabid is examined by immunofluorescence. Rabies antigen is detected in brain smears using an antibody conjugate which fluoresces in ultraviolet light. This takes only about 3 hours and is highly specific. Negri bodies are much less specific than immunofluorescence. They are cytoplasmic intraneuronal inclusion bodies which stain purplish with Seller's stain. Viral isolation is the most accurate test, but takes up to 3 weeks by intracerebral inoculation of suckling mice, or about 4 days in murine neuroblastoma cell culture.

Rabies in man

Route of infection

Rabies virus cannot penetrate intact skin. Infection is usually the result of a mammal bite, but is also possible if saliva contaminates damaged skin or even intact mucous membranes. On very rare occasions, virus has been inhaled as an aerosol. Those who handle infected material should be careful to avoid accidents with contaminated knives and needles, should always wear gloves and should avoid creating infective aerosols.

Human-to-human spread

This is always a theoretical danger to those close to the patient; for saliva, tears, respiratory secretions and urine contain virus, and patients with rabies may cough, spit and even bite. However, transmission of rabies from one person to another has been proved only in a group of patients who received infected corneal transplant grafts. Transmission by breast milk and transplacentally has been proved in animals but not in humans. A number of women with rabies encephalitis have been delivered of healthy babies.

Clinical features (Warrell, 1976; Warrell et al., 1976; Warrell & Warrell, 1995)

The incubation period is usually between 20 and 90 days (extreme range 4 days to 19 years). It tends to be shorter after bites on the face (average 35 days) than after those on the limbs (average 52 days).

Risk of rabies infection

Even the very severe exposure associated with wolf bites involving the head does not lead inevitably to rabies encephalitis. In this case, about 50–60 per cent of the victims will develop rabies if they are not given post-exposure treatment. With lesser bites, the risk is around 10–40 per cent. However, modern post-exposure treatment, instituted on the day of the bite, can reduce the risk to virtually zero.

Symptoms

Itching, other paraesthesiae or pain at the site of the healed bite wound are the only early symptoms which suggests rabies. Non-specific prodromal symptoms include fever, headache and anxiety. As in animals, the disease in humans may follow a furious or paralytic course. Furious rabies is the commoner form in man. Hydrophobia is the most characteristic feature. Attempts to drink water provoke jerky spasms of the inspiratory muscles associated with a profound and inexplicable terror (Fig. 68.6). Eventually, the sight, sound or mere mention of water may induce the hydrophobic response. The spasms may progress to opisthotonos (as in tetanus), generalized convulsions and sudden death from respiratory and cardiac arrest. Aerophobia is a similar reflex provoked by a draught of air on the skin. Patients suffer periodic attacks of intense excitation during which they are agitated, hallucinated, noisy and even violent (Fig. 68.7). Other common features are hypersalivation, cranial nerve palsies, dysphagia, hyperpyrexia, cardiac arrhythmias, fluctuations in blood pressure and psychiatric disturbances. After a few days of furious symptoms they lapse into coma and generalized flaccid paralysis. Survival beyond a week is unlikely without intensive care.

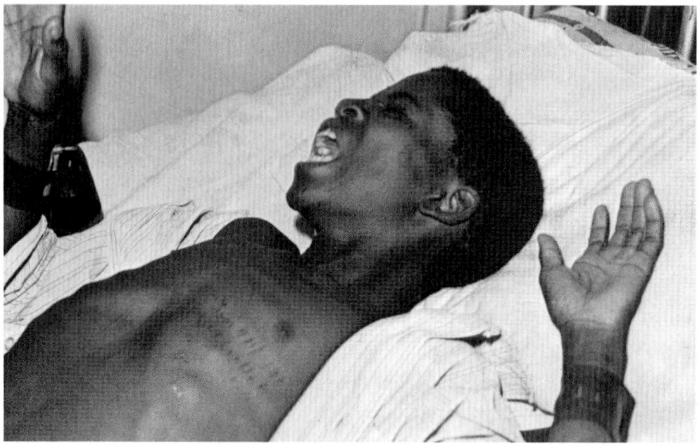

Fig. 68.6. Nigerian boy with hydrophobic spasm induced by an attempt to drink. Copyright © D. A. Warrell.

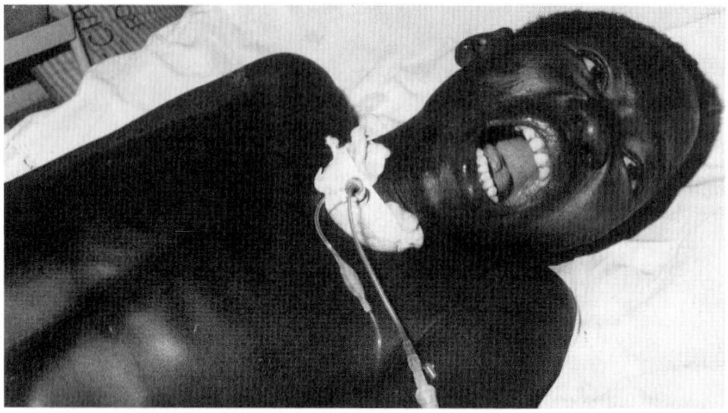

Fig. 68.7. Intermittent excitement, agitation and hallucination in a Nigerian patient with furious rabies. Copyright © D. A. Warrell.

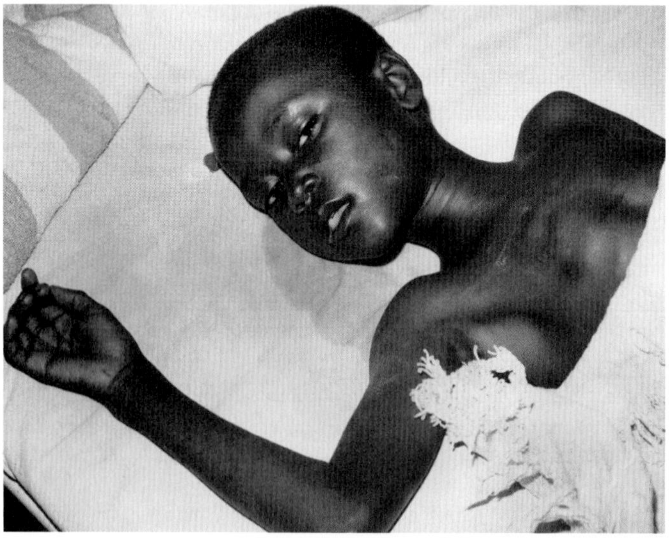

Fig. 68.8. Nigerian boy with paralytic rabies showing generalized flaccid paralysis with dysphagia (note pool of saliva on the sheet). Copyright © D. A. Warrell.

Paralytic or dumb rabies

After the usual prodromal symptoms, such as fever, headache and local paraesthesiae, flaccid paralysis develops, usually in the bitten limb, and ascends with pain and fasciculation in the affected muscles and mild sensory disturbances, resulting in paraplegia, sphincter involvement and, finally, fatal paralysis of the muscles of swallowing and breathing (Fig. 68.8). Hydrophobia is unusual. Even without intensive care, these patients have survived for up to 30 days.

Differential diagnosis

Rabies should be suspected whenever a patient develops severe neurological symptoms after being bitten by a mammal in a rabies-endemic area. Some patients forget that they have been bitten. Hydrophobia is pathognomonic of rabies and may be the only abnormal physical sign. It can be provoked by asking the patient to swallow or by allowing a draft of air to blow across their face. Tetanus, which can also follow an animal bite, is distinguished by its shorter incubation period (usually less than 15 days), the presence of trismus, the persistence of muscle rigidity between spasms, the absence of meningoencephalitis (cerebrospinal fluid is universally normal), and the better prognosis. Delirium tremens and intoxications by plants (especially Solanaceae) and drugs (especially metamphetamine) may cause some of the features of rabies. Paralytic rabies can be confused with other causes of ascending paralysis, especially the post-vaccinal encephalomyelitis complicating the use of nervous-tissue rabies vaccines. In poliomyelitis, objective sensory disturbances are absent.

Laboratory diagnosis

During life, rabies antigen can be detected in nerve twiglets in hair follicles using immunofluorescence in rapidly frozen skin punch biopsy specimens (Bryceson et al., 1975). Corneal impression smears are usually falsely negative. The use of PCR tests on saliva, cerebrospinal fluid and other samples is being evaluated. Rabies virus may be isolated from saliva, brain, cerebrospinal fluid and, very rarely, urine during the first week of illness. Rabies neutralizing antibodies may be detectable in serum and cerebrospinal fluid after the eighth day of illness in unvaccinated patients.

Treatment of rabies encephalitis

The principles are to relieve pain and anxiety. Life can be prolonged by protecting the airway with a cuffed tracheostomy and by controlling convulsions, cerebral oedema and cardiac arrhythmias. However, in view of the disappointing results of intensive care and the problems of funding such heroic efforts in developing countries, the emphasis should be on heavy sedation and adequate analgesia.

Medical attendants and relatives must be protected from infection by saliva and other secretions by wearing masks, goggles, gowns and gloves. With this protective clothing and normal barrier nursing procedures, there is no risk of person-to-person infection. However, those who have had close contact with patients should be offered post-exposure treatment.

References

Belcher DW, Wurapa FK, Atuora DOC et al (1976). Endemic rabies in Ghana. Epidemiology and control measures. *Am J Trop Med Hyg*; **25**: 724–729.

Bryceson ADM, Greenwood BM, Warrell DA, Davidson N McD, Pope HM, Lawrie J. (1975). Demonstration during life of rabies antigen in humans. *J Infect Dis*; **131**: 71–74.

East ML, Hofer H, Cox JH, Wulle V, Wiik H, Pitra C. (2001). Regular exposure to rabies virus and lack of symptomatic disease in Serengeti spotted hyenas. *Proc Natl Acad Sci*; **98**: 15026–15031.

Elegbe SO, Banerjee AK. (1970). A case report of rabies in the bovine in the northwestern State of Nigeria. *Bull Epizootic Dis Africa*; **18**: 57–62.

Engmann HM, Engmann N-L. (1973). Dog menace in Accra: some reflections and exhortations regarding corrective measures in the Kaneshie suburban region. *Ghana Med J*; **12**: 227–231.

Fekadu M. (1972). Atypical rabies in dogs in Ethiopia. *Ethiop Med J*; **10**: 79–86.

Fekadu M, Shaddock JH, Baer GM. (1982). Excretion of rabies virus in the saliva of dogs. *J Infect Dis*; **145**: 715–719.

Hudson JR. (1944). A short note on the history of rabies in Kenya. *E Afr Med J*; **21**: 322–327.

Kale OO. (1977). Epidemiology and treatment of dog bites in Ibadan: a 12-year retrospective study of cases seen at the University College Hospital, Ibadan (1962–1973). *Afr J Med Sci*; **6**: 133–140.

McMillan B, Boulger LR. (1960). The susceptibility of the ground squirrel *Xerus (uxerus) erythropus* Geoffroy 1803 to rabies street virus and its potentiality as a reservoir of rabies in northern Nigeria. *Ann Trop Med & Parasitol*; **54**: 165–171.

South Eastern and Eastern African Rabies Group (2000). Proceedings of the Southern and Eastern African Rabies Group/World Health Organisation meeting. Entebbe, Uganda, 29–31 March 1999. Edition Fondation Marcel Mérieux, Lyon, France.

Synman PJ. (1940). The study and control of the vectors of rabies in South Africa. *Ondersterpoort J Veterin Sci*; **15**: 9–140.

Wandeler AI, Bingham J. (2000). Dogs and rabies. In Dogs, Zoonoses and Public health, (ed CNL Macpherson et al.) pp. 63–90. Wallingford, UK: CABI Publishing.

Warrell DA. (1976). The clinical picture of rabies in man. *Trans Roy Soc Trop Med Hyg*; **70**: 188–195.

Warrell MJ, Warrell DA. (1995). Rhabdovirus infections of man. In *Handbook of Infectious Diseases* Vol III *Exotic Viral Infections*, ed JS Porterfield, DAJ Tyrrell, pp. 343–383. London: Chapman & Hall.

Warrell DA, Davidson N McD, Pope HM et al. (1976). Pathophysiologic studies in human rabies. *Am J Med*; **60**: 180–190.

World Health Organization (1997). WHO Recommendations on rabies post-exposure treatment and the correct technique of intradermal immunisation against rabies. WHO/EMC/ZOO.96.6 (website) WHO Geneva.

World Health Organization (1998). Report of visits to South Africa, Zimbabwe, Mozambique, Malawi, Zambia from 30 September to 9 November 1997 and to Uganda and Tanzania from 24 November to 15 December 1997 in relation to rabies by Dr Arthur King, Addlestone, Surrey, UK. ZDI/98.5, WHO Geneva.

World Health Organization (2000). World Survey of Rabies No 34 for the year 1998. WHO/CDS/CSR/APH/99.6. WHO Geneva.

Part III

Non-communicable diseases

69

The growing importance of non-communicable disease

Introduction

This chapter provides an introduction to the current and growing importance of non-communicable diseases as a cause of ill health and death in Africa. The term 'non-communicable diseases' covers a very wide variety of conditions, such as cardiovascular diseases and diabetes, cancers, haemoglobinopathies, mental health disorders, and musculoskeletal disorders. This chapter aims to provide a framework for considering the current and future of chronic disease patterns in Africa, and a description of those patterns. This includes consideration of the economic and demographic determinants that underlie such trends and are likely to lead to non-communicable diseases replacing communicable diseases as the major health problems throughout Africa in the first part of the twenty-first century.

Distinction between non-communicable and communicable diseases

The terms 'non-communicable diseases' (NCDs) and 'communicable diseases' imply that it is possible to make a clear distinction between diseases that are caused by an infective agent and those that are not. This distinction often cannot be maintained. Many conditions classified as NCDs have been shown to be at least partly caused or triggered by an infective agent. Examples include certain cancers (such as liver and cervical cancers), certain arthropathies, and some types of epilepsy. Infective agents have been implicated as causes or triggers in several other 'non-communicable' diseases, such as coronary heart disease and type 1 diabetes (Couper, 2001; Mehta et al., 1998). Thus, although we use the 'non-communicable' vs. 'communicable' disease classification in this chapter, we acknowledge some of its inconsistencies. However, it remains in widespread use, and much of the data available on disease patterns in Africa is presented in this format. In addition, a substantial proportion of the diseases considered under this heading share a relatively small number of risk factors (illustrated in Fig. 69.1), and this fact increases the usefulness of the category.

Current importance of NCDs in Africa

Global overview of burden of NCDs

Non-communicable diseases are already the commonest cause of death world-wide. The Global Burden of Disease Study (hereafter abbreviated to 'GBDS') estimates that NCDs were responsible for 56 per cent of all deaths and over 40 per cent of global disability in 2000 (Murray & Lopez, 1996). However, the proportion of deaths from NCDs varies from 86 per cent of all deaths in developed regions to 47 per cent in developing regions. Nevertheless, because of the greater numbers of people living there, the majority of people who die from, or are disabled by, NCDs are from the developing rather than the developed world. The burden of disease from NCDs is predicted to grow sizeably in developing countries in the future (see Fig. 69.2); (Murray & Lopez, 1996).

Overview of the data available from Africa

The overriding problem facing those attempting to assess the burden of non-communicable diseases in Africa is the dearth of accurate and representative mortality and morbidity data, especially in adults. In deriving its estimates

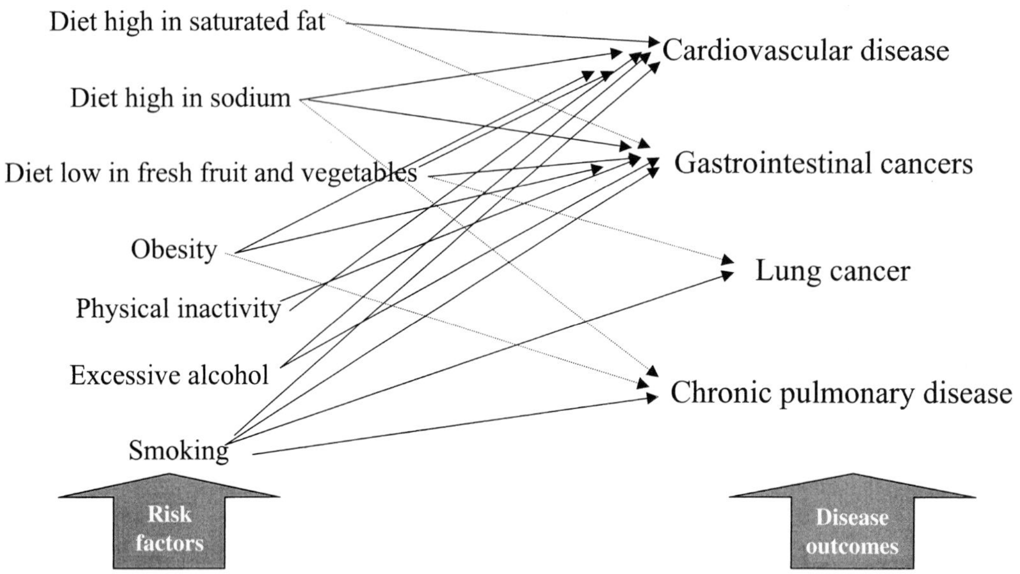

Fig. 69.1. Schematic illustration of the common risk factors for some common non-communicable diseases. Dashed lines represent less well-established relationships.

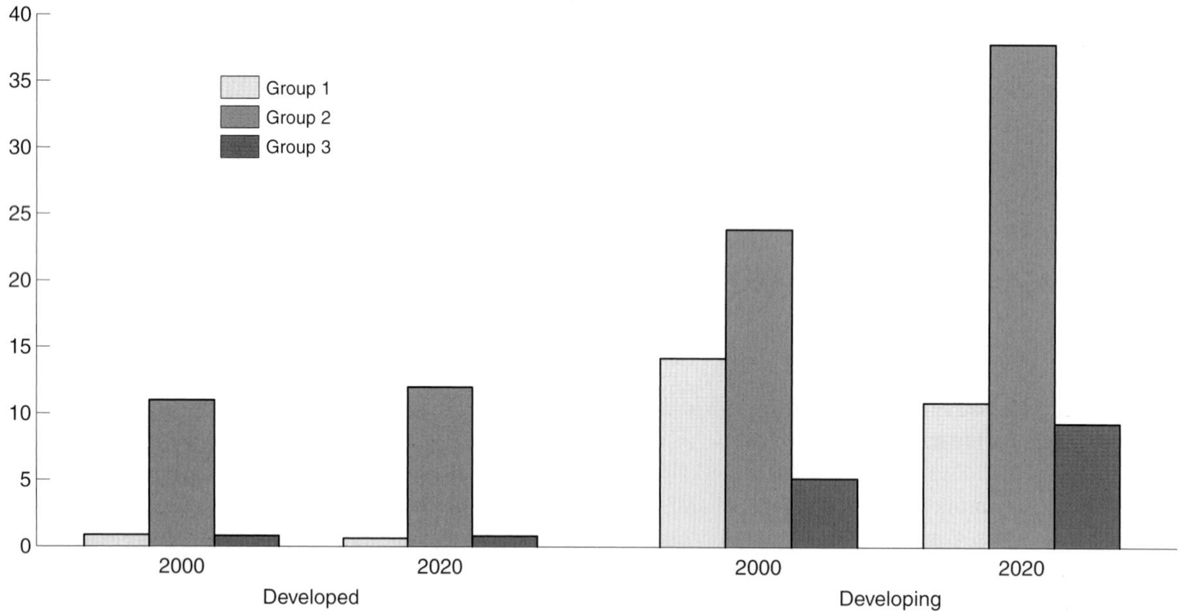

Group 1 = communicable and infectious causes; Group 2 = non-communicable causes; Group 3 = external causes

Fig. 69.2. Estimated and predicted number of deaths (in millions) by major cause in developed and developing regions in 2000 and 2020. (From Murray and Lopez, 1996.)

for Africa (particularly sub-Saharan Africa), the Global Burden of Disease Study relied mainly on models based on data of proportionate mortality and disease patterns from other parts of the world. These estimates have been criticized because of their reliance on assumptions and poor data (Cooper et al., 1998). They are used here as providing the most plausible estimates of current NCD burden throughout Africa, though this description will be supplemented with data from two countries at opposite ends of the economic spectrum in Africa from which rea-

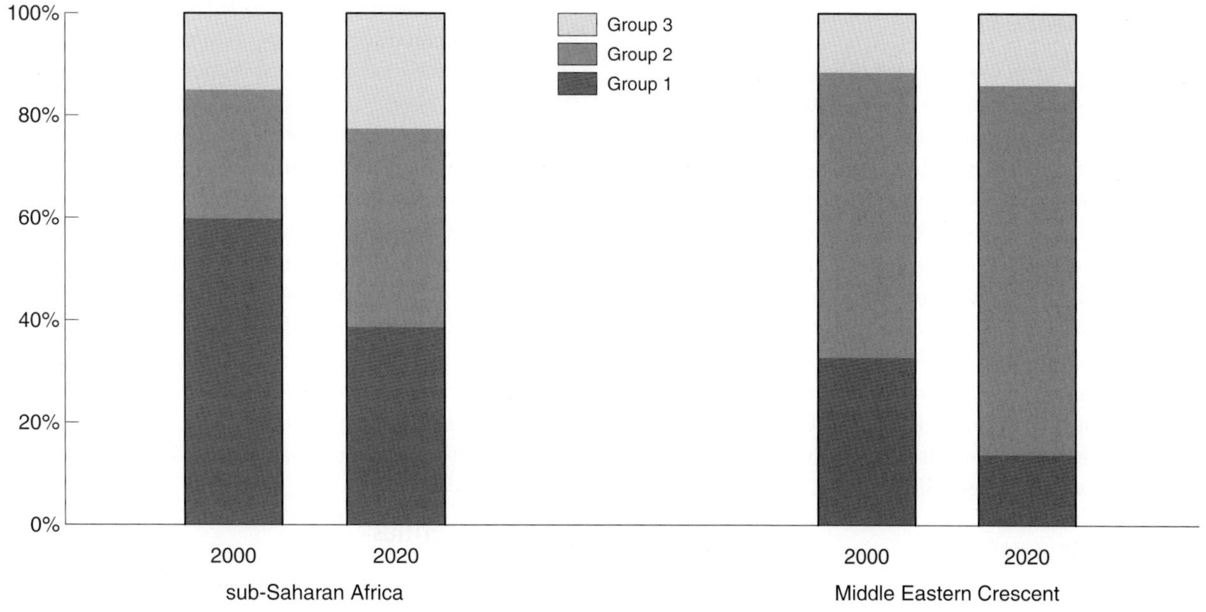

Group 1 = communicable and infectious causes; Group 2 = non-communicable causes; Group 3 = external causes

Fig. 69.3. Estimated and predicated percentage of deaths by major cause in Africa.

sonably detailed and timely data exist – Mauritius and Tanzania.

Overview from the Global Burden of Disease Study

Fig. 69.3 shows the proportion of deaths by major cause for all NCD deaths. The GBDS (Murray & Lopez, 1996) estimates that NCDs were responsible for 26 per cent (2.4 million) of all deaths in sub-Saharan Africa in 2000, including over 60 per cent of deaths in those over 30 years old. The greatest number of these (44% or 1.03 million deaths) was attributed to cardiovascular diseases. In contrast to all other regions, cerebrovascular disease (21% of all NCD deaths) rather than ischaemic heart disease (11%) was the most common single cause of NCD mortality. Malignant neoplasms were estimated to be responsible for 23 per cent of NCD deaths in 2000; however, cancers typically associated with other NCD risk factors (e.g. lung and colon carcinomas) were less common than those associated with infections, such as liver and cervical cancers.

GBDS makes estimates for North Africa as part of the 'Middle Eastern Crescent', a region that also includes countries between Turkey and Iran. It is estimated that NCDs accounted for 55 per cent of all deaths here in 2000. The most important cause of death was cardiovascular diseases (62% of all NCD deaths). The largest single cause was ischaemic heart disease, which accounted for 30 per cent of all NCD deaths, followed by cerebrovascular disease (10%). Unlike in sub-Saharan Africa, lung cancer was by far the commonest fatal malignancy, responsible for 20 per cent of all cancer deaths.

Despite accounting for a lower proportion of overall mortality, the risk of developing certain NCDs is often higher in Africa than in developed regions. For instance, estimated cerebrovascular mortality rates in males and females aged 45–59 years in sub-Saharan Africa were 157.6 and 210.3 per 100 000 people respectively. These are far in excess of the equivalent estimated age-specific rates for established market economies (EME) – 36.4 and 22.2 per 100 000 people respectively.

Finally, one of the great strengths of the GBDS was its attempt to produce estimates of morbidity as well as mortality and to combine the estimates of morbidity and mortality into a single figure – known as the disability adjusted life year or DALY. Such figures highlight the huge importance of some causes of morbidity that are relatively unimportant causes of mortality, such as mental health problems and arthropathies. For example, the study estimated that in 2000 these disorders would account for 5.0 and 10.6 per cent of DALYs in sub-Saharan Africa and the Middle Eastern Crescent, respectively, but only 0.5 and 1.3 per cent of deaths, respectively.

Data from Tanzania

The estimates from the GBDS for sub-Saharan Africa suggest a high (compared to established market economies) probability of death from NCDs, but low contribution of these conditions to the overall burden of disease. Real data from one of Africa's poorest countries, Tanzania, support this picture. Fig. 69.4(*a*), (*b*) present age-adjusted mortality rates from the Tanzanian demographic surveillance system of the Adult Morbidity and Mortality Project (Kitange et al., 1996) for the age group 15 to 59 years. Rates of death from NCDs are higher in the three Tanzanian areas than in established market economies although the proportion of deaths due to NCDs is much smaller. Death rates from stroke are several fold higher. For example, annual age-adjusted rates per 100 000 in people aged 15–64 living in Dar es Salaam were 65 in men and 88 in women respectively as compared with England and Wales (1993) rates of 10.8 for men and 8.6 for women (Walker et al., 2000).

Survey data from Tanzania have demonstrated marked differences between urban and rural areas in the prevalence of certain risk factors. Figure 69.5 shows differences in the prevalence of overweight, hypertension and diabetes between an area of Dar es Salaam and Hai (near Mount Kilimanjaro) (Aspray et al., 2000; Edwards et al., 2000). A country like Tanzania can be described accurately as having 'the worst of both worlds', i.e. continuing high levels of communicable diseases, and high and increasing levels of NCDs, particularly in urban areas. Indeed, this is likely to be the pattern in most sub-Saharan Africa countries.

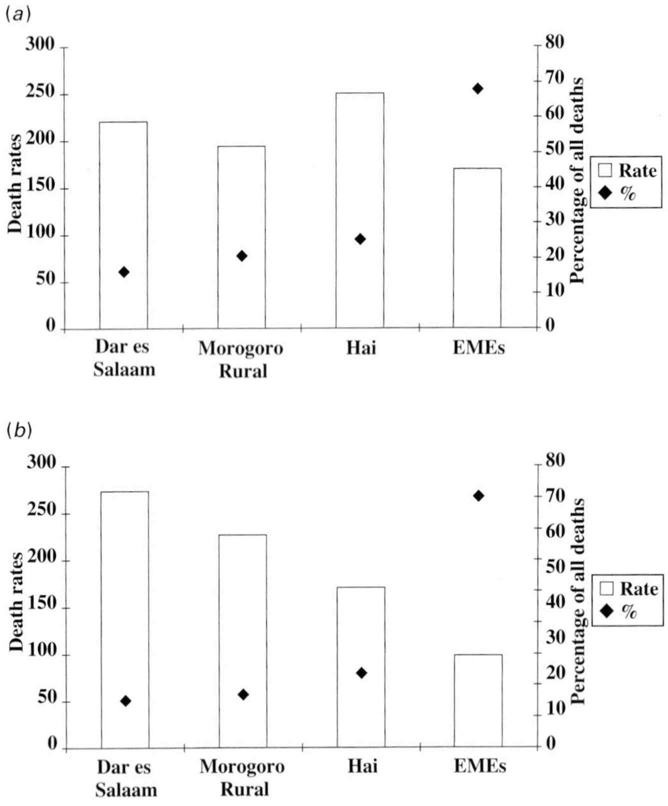

Fig. 69.4. (*a*) Rates of death (per 100000 per year) from NCDs in three areas of Tanzania, and in established market economies (EMEs); as well as percentages of total deaths due to NCDs. Men 15–59 yrs. Rates age adjusted to the New World population. (*b*) Rates of death (per 100000 per year) from NCDs in three areas of Tanzania, and in established market economies (EMEs); as well as percentages of total deaths due to NCDs. Women 15–59 yrs. Rates age adjusted to the New World population.

Data for Mauritius

Mauritius contains a multi-ethnic population of African, European, Indian and Chinese origin. Since the 1940s the country has experienced rapid economic growth, and it now has the second highest Gross National Income per capita in Africa (after Seychelles). During this time the population has undergone a demographic transition with sharp falls in crude death rates followed by falls in birth rates (Cader Kalla, 1995). Infectious diseases fell dramatically over this time and there have been increases in both age-specific and proportionate prevalence and mortality from common NCDs, particularly cardiovascular disease and diabetes. For example, between 1976 and 1995 deaths from infectious disease fell from 56 to 14 per 100 000 population whilst deaths from cardiovascular disease rose from 233 to 321 per 100 000 (figures taken from WHO Statistics Annuals). Diabetes affects over 10 per cent of the adult population. Similar prevalence has been found in all ethnic groups on the island, including Chinese, Creole (mixed African, European and Indian origin) and South Asian origin populations (Dowse et al., 1990).

Conclusions on the current importance of NCDs in Africa

It is clear that, even in the poorest countries of Africa, the burden of NCDs is already substantial. These conditions typically affect economically active adults and make significant demands on health care resources. Nevertheless, their impact in the majority of countries is still dwarfed by the huge burden of infectious disease. However, this pattern of disease is likely to change in the future, and both the absolute and relative importance of NCDs in Africa will overtake that of infectious diseases in the next 20 to 30 years.

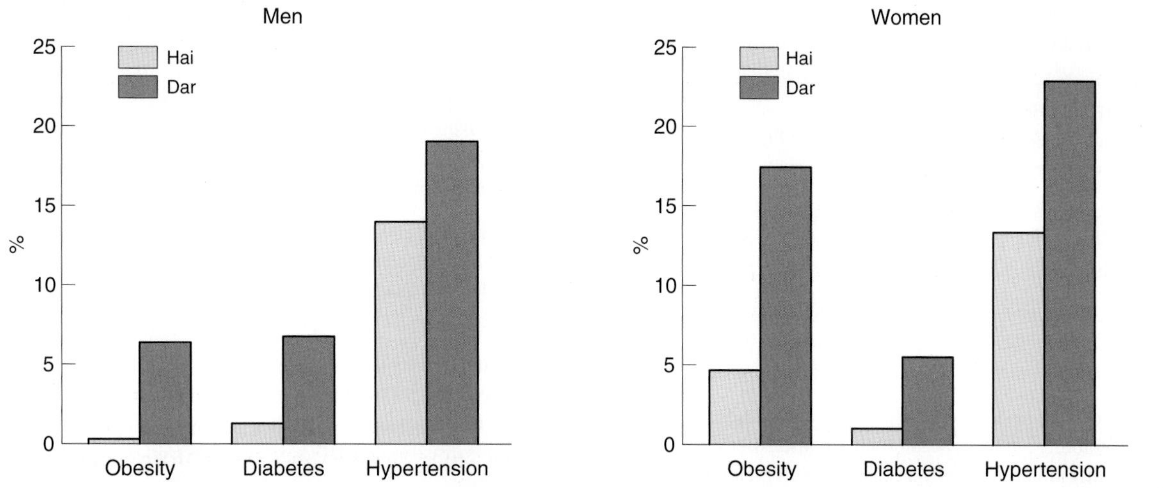

Obesity = BMI >30 kg m^{-2}; diabetes = fasting capillary glucose 6.1 mmol l^{-1}; hypertension = BP >160/95 mmHg

Fig. 69.5. Prevalence of obesity, diabetes and hypertension in a rural (Hai) and urban (Dar es Salaam) area of Tanzania in ages 15 years and over in 1996/7. Figures age adjusted to the New World population.

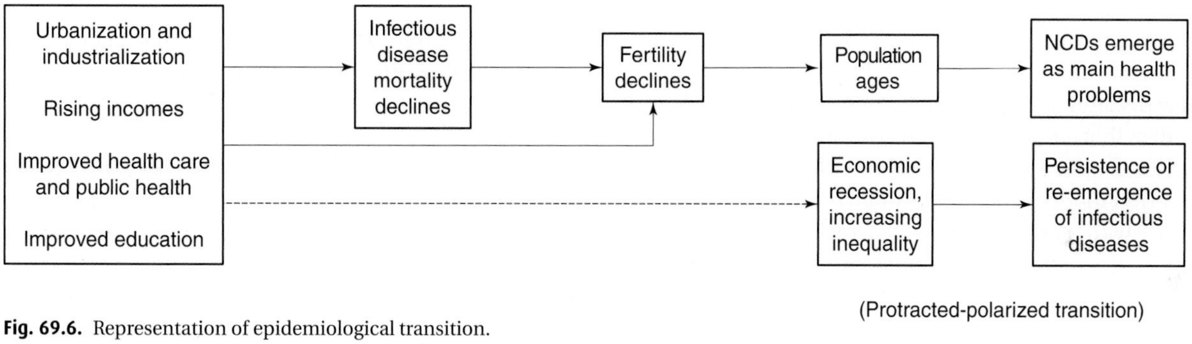

Fig. 69.6. Representation of epidemiological transition.

Future importance of non-communicable disease in Africa

The theory of the epidemiological transition provides a framework for considering changing disease patterns, and the determinants of those patterns, within populations. The theory and its relevance to predicting future disease patterns in Africa is described below.

Epidemiological transition in Africa

The theory of epidemiological transition was developed in order to provide an overall framework for considering changes in population fertility and mortality (demographic change), the relationship of these to disease patterns, and the relationship of both of these to economic, social and technological changes (Omran, 1971). The relationships between these various factors are summarized in Fig. 69.6.

A variety of economic and social factors drive this process. They include rising incomes, industrialization and urbanization, improved access to education (particularly for women), and public and personal health measures. The relative importance of these has differed over time and between populations. Collectively, these types of changes are often referred to as the 'modernization complex'.

Falling mortality, particularly in infants and young children, and falling fertility lead to a greater proportion of the population being made up of people in older age groups. Over time, the population age structure moves from the 'pyramid' still seen in low income countries today to the 'stack' seen in most rich countries. As the population becomes older, they develop the chronic diseases associated with ageing. It is therefore the increasing proportion of adults in the population that is the major reason why NCDs progressively become the predominant health problems within such a population. Omran identified three broad mortality patterns as stages of this process, and Olshansky and Ault (1986) added a fourth (see Box).

Mortality patterns

The age of pestilence and famine, with a high fluctuating mortality that prevents sustained population growth;

The age of receding pandemics, when mortality declines progressively and the rate of decline accelerates as epidemic peaks disappear;

The age of degenerative diseases, with a continuing mortality decline towards stability at a relatively low level; NCDs becoming the main health problems within a population.

The age of delayed degenerative diseases, the change from NCDs afflicting adults between their 30s and 50s, to predominantly afflicting elderly adults, between their 60s and 80s. This is now the case for most populations living in western European and North American countries.

Four main models of epidemiological transition have been described. These are summarized in the Box in next column. These models describe different rates of moving through the stages described above, ranging from one or more centuries in the classical model to a few decades in the accelerated model. The models also reflect that some populations continue to have high levels of infectious disease even as NCDs emerge (the delayed model), and that in some populations (usually those with marked economic inequality) subgroups are at different stages (the polarized model) (Omran, 1971). As will be apparent from the descriptions in the previous section, both the delayed and the polarized models are particularly apt for many parts of Africa today.

The theory of epidemiological transition is sometimes mistaken as providing a set of laws for predicting the future. It does not. It provides a useful framework for considering the interrelationships between demography, disease patterns and social and economic conditions. The nature and relative importance of these relationships are likely to differ between populations and over time. New and unforeseen factors complicate efforts to extrapolate from the experience of other populations that have gone through the epidemiological transition (Caldwell, 2001; Mackenbach, 1994). The HIV pandemic, resistance to anti-malarial drugs, the fragile and inequitable nature of economic growth, and the ravages of armed conflict are but four examples of major unpredictable determinants of disease patterns affecting populations in Africa. While acknowledging the uncertainties of predicting future disease patterns, the next section describes the projections of the GBDS, and considers the major forces that are likely to affect future disease patterns.

Models of epidemiological transition

The classical or western model
A gradual progressive decline from high to low mortality and fertility taking place over several centuries. This accompanied the process of modernization in most western European and North American societies.

The accelerated model
A much faster decline in mortality and fertility than in the classical model, taking placed over decades rather than centuries. Examples include Japan, Mauritius and the Seychelles.

The contemporary or delayed model
The recent and yet to be completed transition in many low-income countries, often with a high burden from old and new infectious diseases (e.g. HIV), while NCDs gain increasing importance.

The polarized model
Different sections of the population at different stages of the transition, strongly related to both economic inequity and different levels of urbanization within those populations.

Predictions of the future importance of NCDs in Africa

The Global Burden of Disease Study estimates that by 2020, NCDs will account for almost 40 per cent of deaths in sub-Saharan Africa. Figure 69.3 shows the proportion of deaths by major disease groups in 2000 and those predicted for 2020 in sub-Saharan Africa and the Middle Eastern Crescent. At present communicable, childhood and maternal diseases (Group 1) account for the majority of deaths but by 2020 NCDs (Group 2) will be responsible for an equal proportion of total mortality in the region. In the Middle Eastern Crescent, NCDs will be responsible for 63 per cent of all deaths in 2020 from an estimated contribution of 55 per cent in 2000. Similar proportionate increases will occur in all the major NCD groups.

These estimates are largely based on extrapolations from the historical experience of countries with full vital registration between 1950 and 1990. Although such an approach is necessary because of the lack of reliable long-term data from Africa itself, it may underestimate the future importance of NCDs. For example, Africa may not follow the same pattern of gradually rising prevalence of NCD risk factors. Below are discussed some of the major forces that will shape future disease patterns in Africa, making reference to possible differences in their evolution between different African countries and that experienced by countries going through the epidemiological transition since the mid-twentieth century.

The major forces driving the epidemiological transition in Africa

Demographic change

It is estimated that the total African population has been increasing by at least 2–3 per cent per year for the past decade(World Bank, 2000). In addition, as infant death rates and birth rates fall, an increasing proportion of the African population will consist of elderly people. This is illustrated in Fig. 69.7, which shows the annual predicted population increase by age group, showing the greatest increases in adults and elderly.

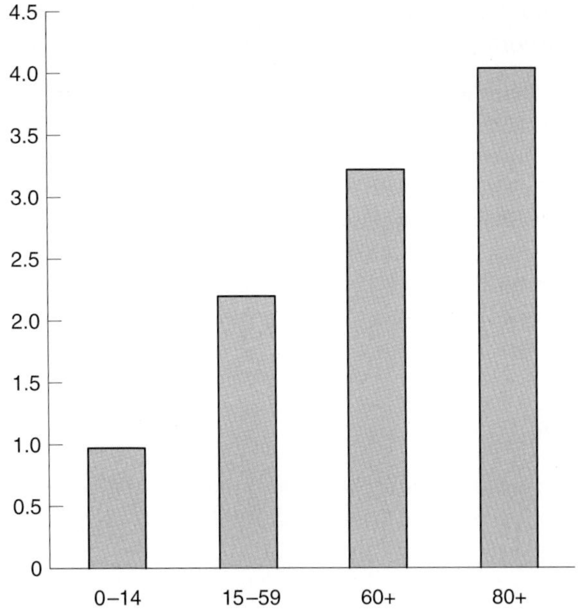

Fig. 69.7. Predicted annual percentage increase in population size, 2000 to 2050, in Africa by age group.

Changing living conditions and lifestyles

Two major changes suggest that the prevalence of risk factors typically associated with an increased risk of NCDs (especially cardiovascular disease and some cancers) will rise substantially in African societies in the near future. These are the rapid urbanization of the continent, and the activities of multinational corporations promoting tobacco use and some foodstuffs (see Box below).

> **The forces of epidemiological transition**
> Urbanization
> Globalization
> Tobacco
> Nutritional change

Urbanization

Urban living tends to be associated with a series of NCD risk factors, including aspects of diet, e.g. high fat and sodium intakes, low levels of physical activity, excess body fat, alcohol excess, and tobacco smoking. There are data, from several parts of Africa that demonstrate that such risk factors are commoner in urban than rural areas in Africa. For example, data from Tanzania found that urban dwellers were significantly more likely to be overweight, less physically active, and to have substantially higher prevalence of diabetes and hypertension than rural counterparts (as shown in Fig. 69.5) (Aspray et al., 2000; Edwards et al., 2000). A study of rural to urban migrants in Kenya demonstrated marked and sustained increases in blood pressure associated with migration (Poulter et al., 1990). In addition to these known risk factors for NCDs, other aspects of urban living more difficult to assess (such as greater levels of insecurity and lower social support) may also contribute to NCD risk.

Although Africa is the least urbanized continent, with an estimated 34 per cent of people in sub-Saharan Africa living in cities or towns, urbanization here is progressing at a more rapid pace than anywhere else on Earth (United Nations, 2000). Estimates suggest that, between 1970 and 1995, the average African country's urban population grew by 5.2 per cent per annum. However, this was not accompanied by economic growth and during this period Africa's gross national income declined by 0.7 per cent per year. This phenomenon is almost unique, even across other poor countries. It implies that urbanization has been occurring without generating additional resources and employment opportunities. The results of this are that an increasing proportion of the African population is exposed to the worst aspects of urban living without access to its benefits. The effect of this combination of urbanization and lack of economic growth on future NCD burden is not clear, but may suggest a greater burden than found in countries where urbanization and economic growth went together.

Globalization and the activities of multinational corporations

The term 'globalization' refers to the process through which the world is becoming increasingly interconnected and interdependent – economically and culturally. The overall health benefits of this process are fiercely debated but remain largely under-researched. Nevertheless, even the most optimistic view acknowledges that it is likely that any benefits will be accompanied by public health dangers, notably increasing exposure of populations to risk factors for common NCDs.

Tobacco

The best example of globalization that is detrimental to health is provided by the tobacco industry. The limited smoking data currently available from Africa suggest that, in general, both smoking prevalence and per capita consumption in the Africa Region are lower than in other regions, with generally around 20 to 30 per cent of the adult male population smoking and 5 per cent or less of the female population (WHO, 1997). According to the historical experience of the UK population, which forms the basis of the GBDS predictions of future tobacco consumption in the Africa, these prevalences will rise only slowly over the next 20–30 years (Murray & Lopez, 1996). However, the activities of the tobacco industry and the presence of an enormous and highly susceptible youth market (almost 50% of African residents are under 15 years old) suggest that more rapid rises in tobacco consumption are likely. There is no doubt that the tobacco industry is actively seeking to substantially increase cigarette sales in Africa and other developing regions, as markets in developed regions come under pressure (see Fig. 69.8). Lobbying African governments is an important part of their strategy, both to undermine the tobacco control activities of the WHO, and to exploit some countries' economic reliance on tobacco as a cash crop (WHO, 2000; Bettcher et al., 2001).

In recognition of the global health impact of tobacco, the WHO launched the Tobacco Free Initiative and has been taking the lead in developing the world's first global tobacco control treaty – the Framework Convention on Tobacco Control.

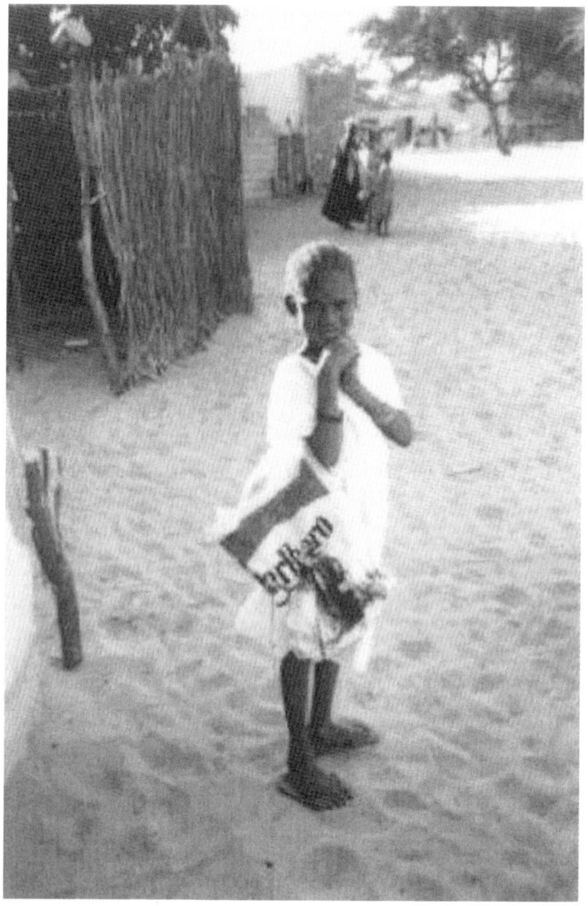

Fig. 69.8. Covert tobacco promotion in Africa. (Photograph by Anna White.)

Nutritional changes

Globalization has had far-reaching effects on food consumption around the world. The marketing and increasing availability of fast foods and fats (particularly cooking oils) has led to striking increases in average daily fat intake in certain developing regions. This phenomenon has been described as the 'nutritional transition' and now occurs at lower levels of gross national income than previously, again casting doubt on the comparability of historical trends in 'western' countries to current circumstances in African settings (Drewnowski & Popkin, 1997). In Africa, the data are scanty, but evidence from South Africa has demonstrated a progressive shift from a traditional high-carbohydrate diet to a higher fat content, 'western' diet over the last few decades in communities of low socio-economic status(Bourne et al., 1993). Genetically modified food technology offers opportunities for more reliable crop yields, but also presents opportunities for multi-national food corporations to increase their control over food production in ways that may discourage African farmers from cultivating traditional foodstuffs in favour of crops for which there is mass global demand (George, 1990).

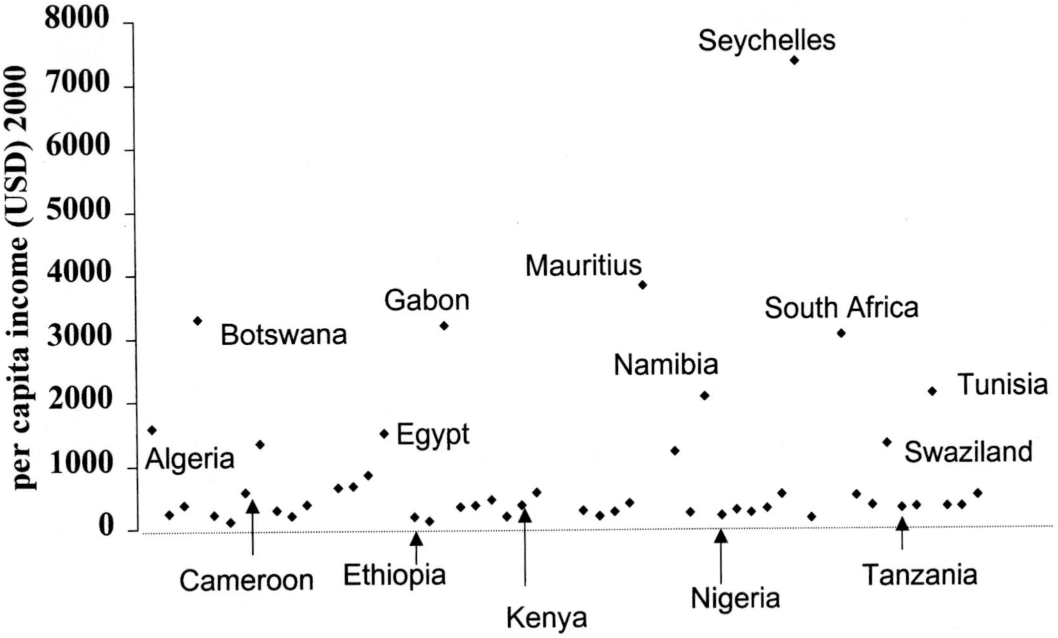

Fig. 69.9. Estimated per capita (USD) income for 49 African countries. (From World Bank, 2000.)

Socio-economic conditions

Socio-economic conditions are one of the most fundamental determinants of health and disease patterns, and this is recognized in the theory of epidemiological transition. They vary widely across Africa: in general health and disease patterns are predictable from them, for example, the predominance of NCDs in the wealthiest African countries of Mauritius and Seychelles, compared to the picture found Tanzania and other very poor countries of sub-Saharan Africa.

Africa has the least favourable economic markers of any continent and contains two-thirds of the poorest countries in the world. However, economic circumstances are far from uniform and both between, and within, countries there is much variation. Figure 69.9 shows the estimated gross national income (GNI) per capita in 49 countries in Africa. There are roughly three groups of countries – the poorest, whose GNIs are less than \$500 per year (such as Tanzania, Ethiopia and Sierra Leone); the wealthiest, with GNIs greater than \$1500 per year, (such as Mauritius, Gabon and South Africa); and in-between these, a diverse group including Côte d'Ivoire, Swaziland and most of the North African countries (WHO, 2000).

Within countries in Africa, there is little information on the prevalence and mortality of NCDs according to socio-economic status. The limited available data suggest that the common impression that NCDs in developing regions are problems of the small minority of affluent residents, and not important for the majority of the (poor) population, is simplistic. Data from other developing regions suggest a mixed picture with certain diseases and risk factors (diabetes and obesity) more common in the rich and better educated, while others (hypertension) are at least equally prevalent in the poorer and least educated (Gupta et al., 1994; Singh et al., 1998). Arguably NCDs are better understood as diseases of urbanization rather than affluence.

Conclusions – future importance of NCDs in Africa

The burden of NCDs in Africa is already substantial. This will increase significantly in the future, principally as a result of demographic change, although the uncertainties posed by the unfolding of the HIV pandemic mean that any predictions must be tentative. Other factors, leading to changes in lifestyles and exposure to common NCD risk factors may accelerate this process, and these conditions are likely to overtake infectious diseases as the leading problems on the continent within the first part of the twenty-first century. Exposure to factors influencing this transition will differ between African countries and within populations, with the underlying socio-economic circumstances being the main determinants of these differences.

Challenges posed by the increasing importance of NCDs in Africa

The rising importance of NCDs in Africa poses substantial challenges to health care policy makers, providers and researchers. These challenges fall under the broad headings of prevention, control and surveillance (Unwin et al., 2001).

Prevention

As illustrated in Fig. 69.1 most NCDs are believed to arise from a 'common soil' of risk factors. There is no reason to believe that the major risk factors for conditions such as diabetes, cardiovascular disease, and chronic lung disease in western European or North American countries are different in African populations. Nevertheless, the social, cultural and economic conditions that produce the risk factors are certainly different, and it is also likely that there will be differences in genetic susceptibility to some conditions. This implies that new research into determinants and risk factors is desirable in Africa. It also suggests that there may be great difficulties in transferring health promotion interventions designed in western Europe and North America to African settings. It has been argued that efforts should focus on the creation of conducive environments, including perhaps fiscal and taxation policies for the control of major risk factors such as tobacco and some foodstuffs (Ebrahim & Davey Smith, 2001).

Control

The limited systematic evidence available on the quality of care suggests that the present management of NCDs in Africa could be much improved (Levitt et al., 1996; Unwin et al., 1999). Health workers should:

- identify the resources which are currently used on ineffective and inefficient practices.
- use these resources more effectively and efficiently.
- develop robust methods for the rapid evaluation of the quality of care for major NCDs, in order to provide useful information to health care planners and policy makers.
- develop interventions, in a rigorous manner, which are locally appropriate (giving consideration to specific local factors that influence the access to, and use of, effective health care), and accompanied by appropriate staff training.

Examples include the design and implementation of protocols for the management of common NCDs at primary health care level.

Surveillance – addressing the need for better data

The coverage of vital registration systems is far too low in the vast majority of sub-Saharan African countries to provide useful data on the burden of NCDs. In order for the priority given to different health interventions within a population to reflect the relative burden of diseases, this lack of data needs to be addressed. A major challenge is to do this within available resources, both local and from external agencies.

Useful data on the current burden (disease prevalence) and likely future burden of major NCDs (through measuring the prevalence of risk factors), can be collected with limited financial resources. At the time of writing the WHO is promoting a stepwise approach to collecting such data using a standard approach. The idea is that the lower 'steps' will be affordable by most developing countries, with more detailed data collected as resources allow.

Conclusions

Although in most parts of Africa communicable diseases continue to be the major burden, NCDs nonetheless contribute substantially to the overall burden at age specific rates that are often several fold higher than those in developed countries.

The challenge to health policy makers, providers and researchers, is to address the current and future burden of NCDs, while at the same time addressing that of communicable diseases. Failure to do this will leave the emergence and prevention of NCD risk factors outside the control of health care systems, and the running and growth of health services for NCDs largely undirected by issues of clinical need and cost-effectiveness.

References

Aspray TJ, Mugusi F, Rashid S et al. (2000). Rural and urban differences in diabetes prevalence in Tanzania: the role of obesity, physical inactivity and urban living. *Trans Roy Soc Trop Med Hyg*; **94**: 637–644.

Bettcher D, Subramanian C, Guidon E et al. (2001). *Confronting the Tobacco Epidemic in an area of Trade Liberalisation.* Geneva: World Health Organization.

Bourne L, Langenhoven M, Steyn K et al. (1993). Nutrient intake in the urban African population of the Cape Peninsula, South Africa. The BRISK Study. *Centr Afr Med J*; **40**: 140–148.

Cader Kalla A. (1995). Health transition in Mauritius: characteristics and trends. *Health Place*; **1**: 227–234.

Caldwell J. (2001). Population health in transition. *Bull Wld Hlth Org*; **79**: 159–160.

Cooper RS, Osotimehin B, Kaufman JS et al. (1998). Disease burden in sub-Saharan Africa: what should we conclude in the absence of data? *Lancet*; **351**: 208–210.

Couper JJ. (2001). Environmental triggers of type 1 diabetes. *J Paed Child Hlth*; **37**: 218–220.

Dowse G, Gareeboo H, Zimmet P et al. (1990). High prevalence of NIDDM and impaired glucose tolerance in Indian, Creole and Chinese Mauritians. *Diabetes*; **39**: 390–396.

Drewnowski A, Popkin BM. (1997). The nutrition transition: new trends in the global diet. *Nutr Rev*; **55**: 31–43.

Ebrahim S, Davey Smith G. (2001). Exporting failure? Coronary heart disease and stroke in developing countries. *Int J Epidem*; **30**: 201–205.

Edwards R, Unwin N, Mugusi F et al. (2000). Hypertension prevalence and care in an urban and rural area of Tanzania. *J Hypertens*; **18**: 145–152.

George S. (1990). *Ill Fares the Land: Essays on Food, Hunger and Power*. London: Penguin.

Gupta R, Gupta V, Ahluwalia N. (1994). Education status, coronary heart disease and coronary risk factor prevalence in a rural population of India. *Br Med J*; **309**: 1332–1336.

Kitange HM, Machibya H, Black J et al. (1996). The outlook for survivors of childhood in sub-Saharan Africa: adult mortality in Tanzania. *Br Med J*; **312**: 216–220.

Levitt NS, Zwarenstein MF, Doepfmer S et al. (1996). Public sector primary care of diabetics—a record review of quality of care in Cape Town. *S Afr Med J*; **86**: 1013–1017.

Mackenbach JP. (1994). The epidemiologic transition theory. *J Epidem Comm Hlth*; **48**: 329–331.

Mehta JL, Saldeen TG, Rand K. (1998). Interactive role of infection, inflammation and traditional risk factors in atherosclerosis and coronary artery disease. *J Am Coll Cardiol*; **31**: 1217–1225.

Murray C, Lopez A. (1996). *The Global Burden of Disease: A Comprehensive Assessment of Mortality and Disability from Diseases, Injuries, and Risk Factors in 1990 and Projected to 2020*, Vol 1. Geneva: World Health Organization.

Olshansky SJ, Ault AB.(1986). The fourth stage of the epidemiologic transition: the age of delayed degenerative diseases. *Milbank Quart*; **64**: 355–391.

Omran AR. (1971). The epidemiologic transition. A theory of the epidemiology of population change. *Milbank Memor Fund Quart*; **49**: 509–538.

Poulter NR, Khaw KT, Hopwood BEC et al. (1990). The Kenyan Luo migration study: observations on the initiaion of a rise of blood pressure. *Br Med J*; **300**: 967–973.

Singh R, Niaz M, Thakur A et al. (1998). Social class and coronary artery disease in an urban population of North India in the Indian Lifestyle and Heart Study. *Int J Cardiol*; **64**: 195–203.

The World Bank. (2000). *World Development Indicators 2000*. New York: World Bank.

United Nations. (2000). *World Urbanization Prospects: The 1999 revision*. New York: United Nations.

Unwin N, Mugusi F, Aspray T et al. (1999). Tackling the emerging pandemic of non-communicable diseases in sub-Saharan Africa: the essential NCD health intervention project. *Publ Hlth*; **113**: 141–146.

Unwin N, Setel P, Rashid S et al. (2001). Non-communicable diseases in sub-Saharan Africa: where do they feature in the health research agenda? *Bull Wld Hlth Org*; **79**: 947–953.

Walker RW, McLarty DG, Kitange HM et al. (2000). Stroke mortality in urban and rural Tanzania. *Lancet*; **355**: 1684–1687.

WHO (1997). *Tobacco or Health: A Global Status Report*. Geneva: World Health Organisation.

WHO (2000). *Tobacco Company Strategies to Undermine Tobacco Control Activities at the World Health Organisation*. Report of the committee of experts on tobacco industry documents. Geneva: World Health Organisation.

70

Diabetes mellitus

Diabetes mellitus is a chronic metabolic disease characterized by hyperglycaemia resulting from defects in insulin secretion, insulin action or both. If the chronic hyperglycaemia is uncontrolled, diabetes is associated with long-term damage, particular dysfunction and failure of the eyes, heart and blood vessels, nerves and kidneys. In 1901 Albert Cook, a medical missionary in Uganda, reported that 'diabetes is rather uncommon and very fatal . . .' (Cook, 1901). Over the next 50–60 years diabetes continued to be regarded as rare in sub-Saharan Africa, although in North Africa it was probably more widely recognized. Presently, the continent is entering a diabetes epidemic.

Classification of diabetes

Type 1 and type 2 diabetes

The classification of diabetes has evolved over the years and recently a World Health Organization (WHO, 1999) Consultation has classified diabetes into four main types (see Box below). More details on the classification of diabetes can be obtained from the reports of these consultations. People with type 1 diabetes have beta cell destruction, which ultimately leads to diabetes in which insulin is required for survival in order to prevent the development of ketoacidosis, coma and death. While type 1 disease is characterized by the presence of glutamic acid decarboxylase (GAD) and islet cell antibodies (which identify the autoimmune process that leads to beta cell destruction), in some subjects no evidence of autoimmune disorder is present and these are classified as 'type 1 idiopathic'. On the other hand, people with type 2 diabetes frequently are initially, and often throughout their lifetime, resistant to the action of insulin, and these individuals do not need insulin treatment to survive. In most cases, the molecular and metabolic causation of this type of diabetes is not known.

Types of diabetes

Type 1 diabetes	Results from autoimmune destruction of the pancreatic beta cells. Insulin is required for survival.
Type 2 diabetes	Is characterized by insulin resistance and/or abnormal insulin secretion, either of which may predominate, but both of which are usually present. It is the most common type of diabetes.
Other specific types of diabetes	Are less common and include genetic disorders, infections, diseases of the exocrine pancreas, endocrinopathies or due to drugs.
Gestational diabetes	Appearing for the first time in pregnancy.

Other types of diabetes

Other specific types of diabetes also exist.

- Several forms of diabetes are associated with monogenetic defects in beta cell function. These forms of diabetes are frequently characterized by the onset of mild hyperglycaemia at an early age (generally before 25 years). They are usually inherited in an autosomal dominant pattern. These forms of diabetes were formally referred to as 'maturity-onset diabetes of the young' (MODY) and have impaired insulin secretion with minimal or no defect in insulin action.
- There are many unusual causes of diabetes which result from genetically determined abnormalities of insulin action. The metabolic abnormalities associated with mutations of the insulin receptor may range from

hyperinsulinaemia and modest hyperglycaemia to frank diabetes. Some individuals with these mutations may have acanthosis nigricans. Women may be virilized and have enlarged, cystic ovaries.

- Acquired disease processes of the exocrine pancreas including pancreatitis, trauma, infection, pancreatic carcinoma, fibro-calculous pancreatopathy, pancreatic fibrosis and calcium stones in the exocrine ducts and pancreatectomy.
- Several hormones, e.g. growth hormone, cortisol, glucagon, adrenaline, antagonize insulin action. Excess amounts of these hormones can cause diabetes, e.g. acromegaly, Cushing's syndrome, glucagonoma and pheochromocytoma.
- Many drugs can impair insulin secretion and some toxins such as vacor (a rat poison) and pentamidine can permanently destroy pancreatic beta cells.
- Certain viruses including congenital rubella, coxsackie B virus, cytomegalovirus, adenovirus and mumps have been associated with beta cell destruction.
- Uncommon forms of immune-mediated diabetes exist.
- Other genetic syndromes sometimes associated with diabetes – the chromosomal abnormalities of Down's syndrome, Klinefelter's syndrome and Turner's syndrome.

Tropical diabetic syndrome

A clinical syndrome of diabetes occurs in young malnourished subjects in African countries and other developing parts of the world, which is different from the usual clinical presentations of type 1 and type 2 diabetes in developed nations, and also from that of 'fibrocalculous' pancreatic diabetes. The onset of diabetes in these individuals is early, usually below the age of 30 years. They require high doses of insulin (>1.5 U/kg per day) to obtain adequate glycaemic control but they are not ketosis prone even if insulin is withdrawn. They have a low body mass index (BMI), usually below 17.0, with other clinical features of malnutrition and often growth retardation. There is absence of imaging evidence of pancreatic calculi or ductal dilatation. This syndrome has been called by several names, e.g. protein-deficient pancreatic diabetes, protein-deficient diabetes mellitus and recently, malnutrition-modulated diabetes mellitus (MMDM).

Fibrocalculous pancreatic diabetes (FCPD) is now recognized as a specific type of diabetes (WHO, 1999). It is highly prevalent in developing countries of the tropical belt and is characterized by chronic calculous pancreatopathy not due to alcoholism or other recognized ascribable causes such as hyperparathyroidism. Fibrocalculous pancreatic diabetes is usually seen in young and malnourished individuals in their twenties, though sometimes also in middle age. It is rare in children and adolescents. The degree of hyperglycaemia varies from severe to mild with or without ketosis. Gastrointestinal symptoms occurring as recurrent abdominal pains and steatorrhoea, are a consequence of pancreatic exocrine damage. The disease is associated with an increased risk of pancreatic carcinoma. The diagnosis of FCPD is based on the demonstration of large multiple and intraductal pancreatic calculi in the presence of diabetes. Marked ductal dilatation and fibrosis are usual, but inflammatory changes are uncommon. Exocrine pancreatic function tests when performed are invariably abnormal.

Non-diabetic hyperglycaemia (lesser degrees of abnormal glucose levels) form part of the classification of diabetes. Impaired glucose tolerance (IGT) refers to a metabolic state intermediate between normal glucose homeostasis and diabetes, and impaired fasting glycaemia (IFG), implies raised fasting levels of glucose (WHO, 1999). IGT and IFG are risk categories, and they represent a risk of 25 to 50 per cent of developing diabetes in the next 10 years. However, they are amenable to lifestyle interventions. IGT is often associated with the so-called 'metabolic syndrome' – a cluster of type 2 diabetes or IGT with several other major cardiovascular disease risk factors including central obesity, dyslipidaemia, hypertension, insulin resistance and microalbuminuria.

Diagnosis of diabetes

In the majority of people presenting with the classical symptoms of diabetes (e.g. increased thirst and urine volume, unexplained weight loss and, in severe cases, drowsiness and coma), the diagnosis of diabetes is straightforward. However, it may pose a problem for those with a minor degree of hyperglycaemia, and in asymptomatic subjects. In these circumstances, two abnormal results on separate occasions are needed to make the diagnosis. If such samples fail to confirm the diagnosis, it will usually be advisable to maintain surveillance with periodic retesting until the diagnostic situation becomes clear. The clinician should take into consideration additional risk factors for diabetes before deciding on a diagnostic or therapeutic course of action. The diagnostic values for diabetes are shown in Table 70.1. The cut-off points are based on the risk of subsequently developing the specific complications of diabetes such as retinopathy and neuropathy (WHO, 1999).

Epidemiology of type 1 diabetes

Clinical characteristics

Clinically, the features of type 1 diabetes are well known. Patients present at a young age (usually their teens or twenties) with rapid onset of severe symptoms, in particular weight loss, thirst and polyuria. Blood glucose levels are high and ketones often present in the urine. If treatment is delayed, ketoacidosis (DKA) and death may follow. The response to insulin therapy is dramatic and gratifying.

Aetiological factors

Clinically, therefore, type 1 diabetes is similar to elsewhere in the world, though the symptoms, signs and outcome may differ quantitatively because of delayed presentation and inadequate management systems. Aetiological characteristics in Africa (McLarty et al., 1997) can be considered as follows.

- **Genetic factors** There are strong HLA associations with type 1 diabetes. Several HLA antigens are involved, but 90 per cent of patients have one or both of HLA-DR3 and HLA-DR4. HLA analysis is difficult in most parts of Africa, but some studies have been performed, including in South Africa, Sudan, Ethiopia, Algeria and Nigeria (Motala et al., 2000; Magzoub et al., 1991). Though there are some local variations, the overall HLA pattern seems to be similar to that found in other parts of the world.
- **Immunological factors** The main markers of immune islet cell attack are islet cell antibodies (ICA) and glutamic acid decarboxylase antibodies (anti-GAD). These substances are found in most Caucasian type 1 diabetic patients at diagnosis, but levels gradually decline afterwards with time. Interpretation of ICA and anti-GAD levels in type 1 diabetes is very dependent on duration of disease, and this may explain the variable results found in the limited African studies so far carried out. However, more recent work does support the significantly greater presence of these immune markers in type 1 as compared to type 2 diabetes (Motala et al., 1999, 2000), and as with HLA antigens, it seems likely that the role of immune factors in the pathogenesis of type 1 diabetes may be similar to elsewhere.
- **Environmental factors** An environmental 'trigger' factor for the onset of type 1 diabetes has long been sought. Its existence is supported by the well-known seasonality of presentation in Europe, and viral infection (perhaps of the Coxsackie group) is considered a likely candidate. An apparent association between viral hepatitis and type 1 diabetes has been reported from Nigeria (Oli & Nwokolo, 1979), and also a seasonality of presentation in Tanzania (with most cases presenting between August and November) (McLarty et al., 1989). It would therefore seem likely that potential viral triggers operate also in Africa.
- **Beta cell function** Type 1 diabetes is of course characterized by absent or negligible endogenous insulin production. For patients on insulin treatment, this is best assessed by serum levels of C-peptide (which is produced in the beta cell by pro-insulin cleavage, in equimolar amounts to insulin). Again, such investigations are often difficult, but available studies suggest that patients with clinically typical type 1 diabetes do have low or undetectable C-peptide levels and are therefore

Table 70.1. Values for the diagnosis of diabetes and other categories of hyperglycaemia

	Glucose concentration (mmol/l)		
	Whole blood		Plasma
	Venous	Capillary	Venous
Diabetes			
Fasting	6.1 and above	6.1 and above	7.0 and above
or			
2 hour post-glucose load	10.0 and above	11.1 and above	11.1 and above
or both			
Impaired glucose tolerance			
Fasting	less than 6.1	less than 6.1	less than 7.0
and			
2 hour post-glucose load	6.7–9.9	7.8–11.0	7.8–11.0
Impaired fasting glucose			
Fasting	5.6–6.0	5.6–6.0	6.1–6.9
2 hour (if measured)	less than 6.7	less than 7.8	less than 7.8

Notes:
For epidemiological or population screening purposes, the 2 h value after 75 g oral glucose may be used alone. For clinical purposes the diagnosis of diabetes should always be confirmed by repeating the test on another day unless there is unequivocal hyperglycaemia with acute metabolic decompensation or obvious symptoms.
Source: WHO (1999).

truly insulin deficient (Motala et al., 2000; Gill & Huddle, 1991).

Difficulties in categorizing type 1 diabetes

Misclassification of patients as 'type 1' is probably relatively common, as insulin treatment is not the same as insulin dependence. A study of all patients on insulin treatment at the Diabetic Clinic at Baragwanath Hospital in Soweto, South Africa, showed a bimodal distribution of diabetes onset, with younger (15–25 years) and older (40–50 years) peaks (Gill & Hudddle, 1991) (see Fig. 70.1). C-peptide studies showed significant endogenous insulin reserves in the older group, but negligible reserves in the younger patients. The older group were also of higher body mass index (BMI) and were on lower doses of insulin. The strong suggestion was that they were type 2 rather than type 1 diabetic patients. Many of them, however, had been recorded as having an onset in 'coma', or 'needing I/V insulin'. It may well be that they presented severely hyperglycaemic with significant infections (perhaps even hyperosmolar non-ketotic coma), but not in true ketoacidosis. Initial insulin treatment (which may have been reasonable temporarily) was maintained, and the 'type 1' label given.

Incidence of African type 1 diabetes

Investigating the incidence of type 1 diabetes accurately in Africa is difficult. As discussed above, even accurate diagnosis of the type 1 syndrome may be difficult. Also, type 1 diabetes is considerably rarer than type 2 disease, and very large populations need to be surveyed. To assess incidence, the population surveyed should also be accurately known, and this is in itself difficult as censuses in Africa are rare and migration in and out of study areas

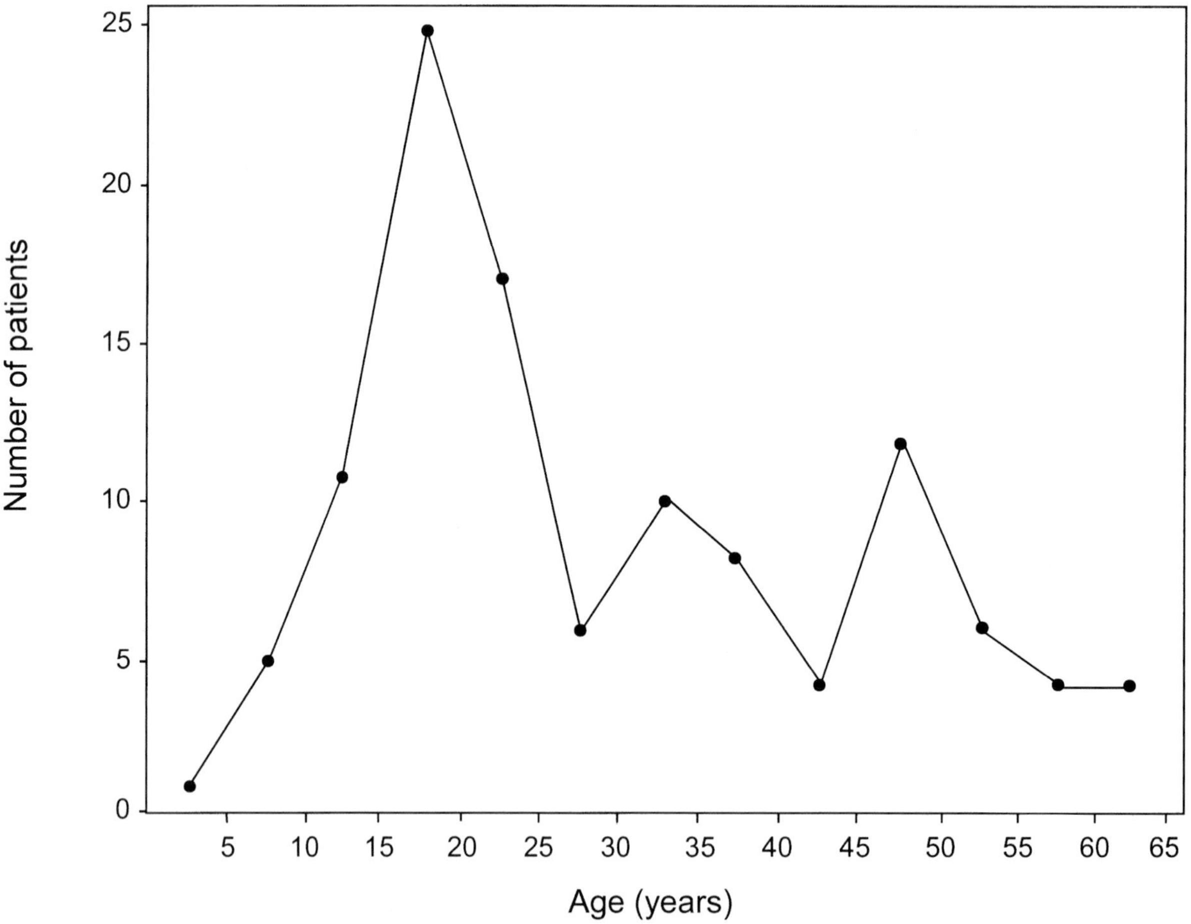

Fig. 70.1. Age frequency graph of insulin-treated diabetic patients at Baragwanath Hospital in Soweto, South Africa. (After Gill & Huddle, 1991.)

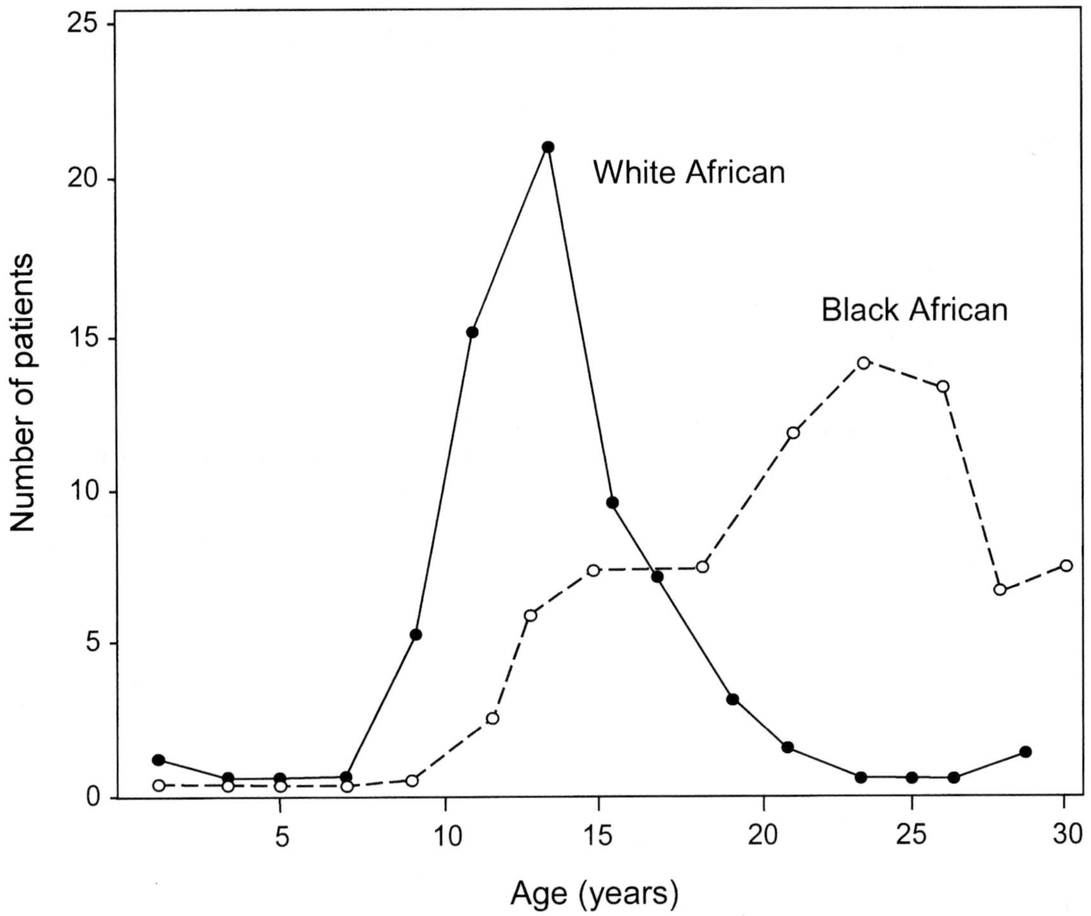

Fig. 70.2. Peak age of onset of type 1 diabetes in white and black Africans in Johannesburg, South Africa. Black Africans have an onset about a decade later than white Africans. (After Kalk et al., 1993.)

common. A final, and very important problem, is that type 1 diabetes is a fatal disease without treatment, and it is likely that many patients die before reaching medical services. A possible answer to this problem is the 'verbal autopsy' technique, but this is a fairly recent epidemiological advance, and has potential problems of accuracy. Whatever the problems, common clinical experience in Africa is that diabetic patients below the age of 15 years (at least known to hospital clinics) are uncommon.

Not surprisingly, therefore, there have only been few studies attempting to assess the incidence of type 1 diabetes in Africa. In Sudan, North Africa, Elamin and colleagues in 1989 reported a survey of nearly 43 000 school children (aged 7–11 years). This was really an untimed prevalence study, and the finding was that 0.95 per 1000 (95 per 100 000) had type 1 diabetes (Elamin et al., 1989). A Tanzanian study reported in 1993 did measure true incidence, which was 1.4 per 100 000 per year (Swai et al., 1993). The authors accepted that deaths before admission artificially reduced their figure (McLarty et al., 1997), but felt that even taking account of this, rates were below those encountered in the west.

The discrepancy between these two studies may be explained by ethnic differences (they come from very different parts of the African continent), and perhaps design problems. The question of whether type 1 diabetes is truly rarer in Africa than elsewhere remains unsettled, and more detailed surveys are needed. The reason why type 1 diabetes appears rare, however, may be because its peak age of onset is a decade later than in western areas. A fascinating study from Johannesburg, South Africa, compared age of onset of type 1 diabetes in white and black Africans (Kalk et al., 1993). The peak age of onset was about 13 years in the white South Africans (similar to in Europe), but was about aged 23 years in the black South Africans (see Fig. 70.2). The reasons for this observation are obscure, though it has been suggested that prolonged breast feeding (common in Africa) may perhaps be reducing the incidence, and delaying the onset of type 1 diabetes. Early introduction of cow's milk protein does seem to be a risk factor for the later development of type 1 diabetes, possibly because bovine albumin can raise antibodies in neonates which mimic islet cell antibodies and attack pancreatic beta cells (Harrison, 1996). This is speculative, and much still remains unknown about the pathogenesis and epidemiology of type 1 diabetes in Africa.

Epidemiology of type 2 diabetes

Clinical characteristics

Most patients present with the classical symptoms of diabetes including polyuria, polydipsia and polyphagia. Additionally, some patients present with sepsis or diabetic coma (hyperosmolar non-ketotic states). A minority are asymptomatic and are therefore identified at screening. The patients usually do not seek early medical attention because of the insidious nature of the disease and therefore may present at diagnosis with features of diabetic complications including visual difficulties from retinopathy, pain and/or tingling in the feet from neuropathy, foot ulceration, and stroke. Serious infection may be a presenting feature of diabetes (including occasional rarities such as mucormycosis). Some elderly type 2 patients present with hyperosmolar non-ketotic coma, which has a high mortality (see Box).

Presenting features of type 2 diabetes in Africa

Fatigue	Hyperosmolar non-ketotic coma
Thirst	Impotence
Polyuria	Cataracts
Weight loss	Large vessel disease
Blurred vision	Neuropathic symptoms
Infections	Cranial nerve lesions

Prevalence and incidence

Though diabetes was considered a rare medical condition in Africa, epidemiological studies carried out in the last decade of the twentieth century have provided evidence of a different picture. There is a global trend towards increased incidence and prevalence of diabetes in African populations (Sobngwi et al., 2001). Indeed, Africa is experiencing the most rapid demographic and epidemiological transition of world history (Mosley et al., 1993). It is characterized by a tremendous rise in the burden of non-communicable diseases (NCDs), underlined by the increasing life expectancy and lifestyle changes, resulting from the reduction in infectious diseases and increased fertility, as well as westernization.

Almost all the reports published between 1959 and 1985 showed a prevalence of diabetes below 1.4 per cent, except those from South Africa where higher prevalences were reported. Comparison between countries is however difficult due to differences in diagnostic methods and criteria. Over the past 20 years, the availability of uniform diagnostic criteria has allowed across-country comparison. Epidemiological studies carried out during this period show the rising prevalence of diabetes all over Africa (Table 70.2). The global estimates of the number of people with diabetes in Africa was approximately 3 million in 1994, but is due to experience a two- to three-fold increase by the year 2010 (Amos et al., 1997). The highest prevalence is found in populations of Indian origin, followed by Black populations and finally Caucasians. Among the population of Indian origin of South Africa and Tanzania, the prevalence is between 12 and 13 per cent (Ramaiya et al., 1991). The prevalence in blacks follows a westernization gradient, with that of rural Africa generally below 1 per cent, but urban Africa between 1 and 6 per cent. The black populations of the Caribbean have a 10–13 per cent prevalence, and African Americans between 12 and 15 per cent or higher. The prevalence of diabetes in Caucasians of Africa is comparable or higher than their European counterparts, between 6 and 10 per cent (Rotimi et al., 2001).

The majority of patients (70–90%) present with typical type 2 diabetes, but up to 25 per cent of patients with diabetes are diagnosed with type 1 diabetes (Papoz et al., 1998). A proportion of patients present with 'tropical' diabetes (about 1%), or with ketosis-prone atypical diabetes (about 10–15%).

Risk factors

The acquisition of economic development in many countries in sub-Saharan Africa has led to increased life expectancy, lifestyle modifications and increased risk factor levels for type 2 diabetes. The identified risk factors are not markedly different from those reported in other populations and may be classified as non-modifiable and modifiable risk factors. Age and ethnicity are the main non-modifiable determinants of diabetes prevalence in Africa as confirmed by the increasing prevalence with age, and the difference between Indian, Black and Caucasians in South Africa. Indians have the highest predisposition and are followed by Blacks and Caucasians (Omar et al., 1993; Levitt et al., 1999).

Table 70.2. Prevalence of type 2 diabetes in Africa

Year	Sample Country	Author	Site	Size	Prevalence (%) (WHO, 1980/85)	Prevalence (%) (WHO, 1999)
Central and West Africa						
1987	Mali	Fisch et al.	R	7472	0.9	–
1987	Togo	Teuscher et al.	R	1381	0.0	–
1988	Nigeria	Ohwovoriolet et al.	U	1627	1.7	–
1989	Nigeria	Erasmus et al.	U+R	2800	1.4	–
1997	Cameroon	Mbanya et al.	U		2.8	2.5
			R		1.1	1.1
1997	Nigeria	Owoaje et al.	U	247	2.8	
1997	Sierra Leone	Ceesay et al.	U	501	2.4	–
East and South Africa						
1984	Tanzania	Ahren & Corrigan	U+R	3145	0.7	–
1989	Tanzania	McLarty et al.	R	6097	1.1	–
1996	Sudan	Elbagir et al.	U+R	1284	3.4	–
1998	Sudan	Elbagir et al.	R	724	10.4	–
South African Republic						
1993	Cape	Levitt et al.	U	729	8.0	–
1993	Durban	Omar et al.	U	479	5.3	–
1995	Orange Free State	Mollentze et al.	U	758	6.0	–
1999	Cape	Levitt et al.	PU	974	10.8	–
2001	Transkei	Erasmus et al.	PU	374	5.1	–
Northern Africa						
1988	Tunisia	Papoz et al.	U	3826	3.8	–
1995	Egypt	Herman et al.	U	6052	9.3	–
1996	Mauritania	Ducorps et al.	U	744	2.6	–
2001	Algeria	Malek et al.	U	1457	8.2	8.8
Migrants						
1991	Tanzania	Ramaiya et al.	A+H	1147	9.8	–
1990	Tanzania	Swai et al.	A+M	1049	7.1	–

Notes:
For site of survey: U = urban.
R = rural.
PU = peri-urban.
A = Asian.
H = Hindu.
M = Muslim.

Among the modifiable risk factors, residence seems a major determinant, since urban residents have a 1.5- to 4-fold higher prevalence of diabetes compared to their rural counterpart. This is attributable to lifestyle changes associated with urbanization and westernization. Urban lifestyle in Africa is characterized by changes in dietary habits involving an increase in consumption of refined sugars and saturated fat, and a reduction in fibre intake (Mennen et al., 2000). Moreover, there is a reduction in physical activity associated with urban lifestyle. Rural populations rely upon walking for transport and often have intense agricultural activities as their main occupation. Rural dwellers therefore have a high physical activity and related energy expenditure compared to urban subjects, thus explaining the higher rates of obesity in the cities – at least four times higher in urban areas compared to rural (Aspray et al., 2000). The population of Africa is predominantly rural but the 1995–2000 urban growth rate was estimated at 4.3 per cent (compared to 0.5% in Europe). Thus, more than 70 per cent of the population of Africa will be urban residents by 2025 (UNPF, 2000). A tremendous increase in the prevalence of diabetes attributable to rapid urbanization is therefore expected. Additionally, life expectancy at birth is also rapidly increasing. For example, in 1960 it was around 35 years in Cameroon, but was raised to approximately 55 years in 1990. An increased diabetes prevalence simply due to the change in the age structure of the population is therefore expected. It is understandable why, by the year 2025, the majority of the world diabetes population will be in the developing countries. These estimates and projections should, however, be modulated by considering the HIV infection pandemic.

An intriguing potential explanation for the rapid increase in type 2 diabetes being seen in Africa and other parts of the developing world, is the 'thrifty genotype' theory. It is suggested that in poor, rural, subsistence zones, type 2 diabetes may have a survival advantage (the 'thrifty gene'). Partially reduced insulin secretion may allow infrequent food intake to be stored rather than rapidly metabolized. However, the process of urbanization and westernization are associated with increased calorie intake and reduced exercise – leading to insulin resistance. The 'thrifty gene' in this situation is overwhelmed and overt type 2 diabetes results (Zimmet & Lefebvre, 1996). Risk factors for type 2 diabetes are summarized in the Box below.

Risk factors for type 2 diabetes
- Age
- Ethnicity
- Positive family history
- Obesity
- Physical inactivity
- Urbanization
- Westernized diets

Gestational diabetes

Epidemiology

Gestational diabetes mellitus (GDM) is, as the name suggests, diabetes which arises in pregnancy. It also reverts to metabolic and clinical normality post-partum, though there is a considerable risk of later type 2 diabetes (WHO, 1999). GDM must therefore be distinguished from existing diabetes in women who become pregnant. Such diabetes is usually (but not always) of the type 1 variety. The particular importance of GDM is that it is associated with a poor pregnancy outcome, especially if unrecognized and untreated. Particular adverse effects include foetal macrosomia, eclampsia, intrauterine growth retardation, birth difficulties, neonatal hypoglycaemia and respiratory distress. There is evidence that the outcome of diabetic pregnancy in Africa is considerably worse than in western countries (Lutale et al., 1991; Huddle et al., 1993). Congenital abnormalities are a feature of existing prepartum diabetes rather than GDM, as the latter develops late in pregnancy, after the first trimester (when organogenesis occurs).

Risk factors

There are a number of risk factors for GDM, and these are shown below. They are important, as such risk factors can be used to identify women suitable for screening for diabetes during pregnancy (Box).

Risk factors for gestational diabetes
- Increased maternal age
- Past large babies (>4 kg)
- Obesity
- Previous gestational diabetes
- Family history of diabetes
- Poor obstetric history
- Glycosuria
- Ethnicity (e.g. Asian origin)

Diagnosis

Criteria for diagnosing GDM are highly controversial (Jovanovic & Pettitt, 2001). The basic difficulty is that glucose tolerance normally alters during pregnancy, making standard diagnostic criteria at least theoretically unsuitable. However, there is no agreement as to what other criteria are ideal. A reasonable compromise proposed by the World Health Organization (WHO, 1999) is to use non-pregnant criteria, but to include those with IGT ('impaired glucose tolerance'), as having gestational diabetes. The appropriate blood or plasma glucose levels have been given earlier in this chapter. GDM develops almost always between 24 and 28 weeks of gestation and is usually asymptomatic. For these reasons, some form of screening system for GDM is ideally required.

Screening

The traditional time for GDM screening is 28 weeks. Before this, the diagnostic yield is low (i.e. cases will be missed), and after this there will be little available time for treatment to improve outcome. Unselected screening is inappropriate unless resources are good, and the incidence of GDM especially high. There is little useful information on the epidemiology of GDM in an African setting, though it is certainly common (Lutale et al., 1991; Huddle et al., 1993), but with resource restrictions, a 'selective, risk-based' strategy is reasonable. This should be adapted from Table 71.1 as shown in the Box.

Screening for GDM – High risk women

Age >35 years
Obese (BMI >30.0 kg m^{-2})
Past babies >4 kg
Previous GDM
Family history of diabetes
Mid-trimester glycosuria
Past poor obstetric history
Symptoms of thirst/polyuria

Ideally, all women falling into these categories at 28 weeks gestation should have a standard 75 g oral glucose tolerance test (GTT). This is clearly impractical in many parts of Africa, and compromise options will be discussed later.

Management

Once diagnosed, all women should receive basic diabetic education, and dietary advice (restriction of refined carbohydrate in particular). Home blood glucose monitoring is unlikely to be feasible, and if possible a blood glucose level should be performed at each visit to the Antenatal Clinic. Surveillance of the pregnancy should be especially close. Blood glucose levels of 4 to 7 mmol/l should be aimed for. Poor obstetric progress, hypertension, or excessive hyperglycaemia are indications for admission to hospital. Standard advice (and current western practice) is to move directly from diet to insulin if blood glucose levels are not adequately controlled. This remains current practice in most parts of Africa also, but it should be remembered that extensive experience in Cape Town, South Africa, has demonstrated the safety of oral hypoglycaemic agents in pregnancy (Coetzee & Jackson, 1980). A recent report from Europe has confirmed this (Hellmuth et al., 2000). This report showed a slight excess of pre-eclampsia and an increase in peri-natal mortality in those treated with metformin, but sulphonylureas appeared quite safe (the drugs used were tolbutamide and glibenclamide). Sulphonylureas (but not metformin) can therefore, on present evidence, be recommended for gestational diabetic patients who have failed on diet alone, and where insulin treatment is likely to be difficult. Post-delivery all treatment can be stopped, as GDM will almost certainly remit. Ideally, a GTT at 6 weeks should be performed. If not possible, then a fasting (preferably) or a random blood glucose level will suffice.

GDM in resource-poor settings

It will be appreciated from the above that the ideal modern diagnosis, screening and treatment of GDM is fairly cost and labour intensive. Where resources are highly limited, it may be a reasonable option to ignore the potential problem and concentrate on more pressing needs. An alternative may be to assume that those with risk factors may have GDM, and give them dietary advice and close surveillance obstetrically, without confirmation of diagnosis. If blood glucose measurement is possible, then a measurement at 28 weeks is reasonable – preferably fasting. The cut-off for blood glucose (most commonly measured in Africa) is over 6.0 mmol/l (equivalent to a fasting plasma glucose of over 7.0 mmol/l). A random glucose estimation will be less sensitive, but is easier to obtain – the same cut-off level should be used as this will be approximately equivalent to IGT on a glucose tolerance test. If possible, two separate tests should be abnormal before the diagnosis is made.

From a therapeutic point of view, simple diet is appropriate initially, and it is recommended that oral agents should be the next step – they are safe and now evidence-based, and much cheaper and easier to use than insulin. Traditional tolbutamide is probably safest (start at 500 mg twice daily, and increase to 1 g twice or three times daily). If not available then glibenclamide is satisfactory – 5 mg daily initially, increasing to twice or three times daily. Beyond this, hospitalization for insulin treatment will be needed. In all cases there needs to be close antenatal care. Early induction of labour at 36 to 38 weeks may be necessary, and a higher than normal caesarean section rate is to be expected.

Management of diabetes in Africa

The effective management of diabetes can reduce mortality and morbidity from diabetic complications. In Africa, socioeconomic considerations dictate that costs should be kept to a minimum. For this reason, the aim should be to control plasma glucose with the least expensive but effective (and not necessarily latest) anti-diabetic drugs. The goals for management should be set for each individual based on the patient's clinical status, social/psychological/cultural and financial background, and willingness to participate actively in self-care.

Delivery of diabetes care in Africa

Most patients in Africa seek health care at primary health care clinics. These clinics in most areas are village dispensaries that are very sparsely equipped and poorly staffed (Amoah et al., 1998; Levitt et al., 1996). In some of the large cities, there are specialized diabetes clinics that are too expensive for the ordinary person. It is against this background of poor accessibility to proper health care and lack of government commitment to NCDs (because of the unfinished agenda of communicable diseases and the AIDS epidemic) that diabetes care is delivered in most African countries. People with diabetes travel long distances to seek appropriate care from specialists who work mostly in large teaching hospitals. Type 2 diabetes can usually be well managed in primary health care settings with properly trained staff with some expertise in diabetes, using approved treatment protocols and algorithms (see Chapter 75). Type 1 diabetes, however, should be reserved for hospitals with a doctor who has some competence in diabetes management.

Dietary and lifestyle modifications

Diet and other lifestyle factors form the basis of treatment of diabetes – especially type 2 disease. The traditional African diet, rich in staples consisting of cereals (rice, cornmeal or flour, sorghum and millet, roots and tubers (yams, plantains, potatoes and cassava), accompanying meat, fish or vegetables, is ideal for patients with diabetes. This traditional diet, which is mainly high in starch and dietary fibre and low in fat and sugar, is for the most part, similar to the WHO, American Diabetes Association, and Diabetes UK dietary recommendations for people with diabetes. Thus, with slight modifications and without fear of making changes to entrenched eating habits, it is relatively easy to draw up dietary guidelines for patients with diabetes in Africa. However, the urban city dwellers have absorbed westernized lifestyle cultures, and their dietary habits are more European or American than African. In such patients, the recommendations of expert groups from Europe and America on low-fat, high carbohydrate, etc. are applicable.

The diversity and complexity of diets in Africa makes it impossible to prescribe a standard diet for the management of people with diabetes living in the region. The situation is worsened by the lack of dieticians in most health institutions. The nurse or doctor (with little training in dietetics) is therefore responsible for supervising the diet of patients. Whatever the individual patient's dietary targets, successful implementation depends on the acceptability of the prescribed diet and on continuous counselling.

Insulin therapy in Africa

Insulin availability

Chronic insulin shortage is serious and widespread in Africa (Alberti, 1994; McLarty et al., 1994; Mbanya, 1997). The exact burden of poor access to insulin in Africa is still unknown, but it is certainly extensive. In the 1997 *International Diabetes Federation's Task Force on Insulin* survey of 25 sub-Saharan African countries, insulin was often unavailable in half the large city hospitals, and only five countries reported regular insulin availability in rural areas (IDF Task Force, 1997). Supply of insulin in most developing countries depends on where the patient lives (presence of a health centre where insulin is constantly stocked), and the affordability of insulin.

The reasons for this chronic lack of access to insulin are many. In some countries, insulin preparations, a life-saving drug, are not included on the national formulary and are therefore not available on a regular and uninterrupted basis. Lack of medical insurance or free health means that the patient has to pay for drugs including insulin. Where there has been an introduction of 'cost-sharing', this has still meant a considerable financial burden on patients and their families. In fact, the cost of outpatient health care for type 1 diabetes in Tanzania was estimated to have been US$229 per person per year, of which some two-thirds (US$156) was the cost of insulin (Chale et al., 1992). This is equivalent to about 6 months of a family's income in most developing countries. Because of this, patients often adhere to treatment very poorly, as most patients cannot afford the prescriptions. Many patients are therefore lost to follow-up, and are sometimes seen again with diabetic complications.

Use of insulin

Insulin therapy is mandatory for all patients with type 1 diabetes, and it should also be used in patients with type 2 diabetes if hyperglycaemia persists despite maximum doses of oral anti-diabetic agents. There is now convincing evidence favouring the early use of insulin in type 2 diabetic patients. It can also be used in combination with oral agents, and is usually most appropriate treatment in the presence of severe hepatic or renal diseases. Type 2 patients may also temporarily require insulin when severely ill, or when undergoing major surgery. There is

Table 70.3. Characteristics of the main insulin preparations available in Africa

Insulin type	Synonyms	Approximate timing of effect (hours)		
		Onset	Peak	Duration
Short-acting insulin	Regular Soluble	0.25–1	1.5–4	5–9
Intermediate-acting insulin				
– NPH	Isophane	0.5–2	3–6	8–14
– Lente	Insulin–zinc suspension (mixed)	1–3	3–10	7–24
Long-acting insulin	Ultralente; insulin zinc suspension (crystalline)	2–4	4–12	8–36
Pre-mixed 30/70		0.1–1	3–13	12–20
Pre-mixed 50/50		0.1–1	3–12	12–20

Notes:
Pre-mixed insulins are available as a mixture of soluble and intermediate-acting insulin in various proportions.

however, evidence of over-prescription of insulin in Africa, despite the chronic lack of access to the drug. Part of this over-prescription is due to lack of adequately trained diabetes staff who misdiagnose type 2 diabetes as type 1 diabetes because of the often relatively acute presentation.

The characteristics of the main insulin preparations available in Africa are given in Table 70.3. There are different species of insulins available, i.e. human, porcine, bovine and insulin analogues. In the African context, there is no practical advantage in using a specific species of insulin. The recently introduced insulin analogues are produced by genetic engineering – substituting or adding amino acid residues of the insulin simply by changing the nucleic acid sequence of the insulin gene. Soluble or 'regular' insulin should be given about 30 minutes before meals, while the recently commercialized insulin analogues can be given just before the meal. Whenever possible, it is now advisable to give multiple insulin injections per day, combining regular insulin before each main meal plus intermediate-acting insulin either before dinner or bedtime. However, care should be taken to monitor patients for hypoglycaemia, which is more frequent with this regimen. Twice daily insulin, combining soluble and intermediate-acting insulin in the morning and evening, is still the norm in Africa. It is advisable not to use ultralente insulin because of the potential risks of hypoglycaemia. Although there is now a tendency to make available only U100 insulin preparations, it should be noted that U40 and U80 insulins are still available in several countries in the region.

Insulin may lose some of its potency if it is stored for long periods at very high temperatures. This effect, however, is of exaggerated importance clinically, as under most African climatic conditions there is little loss of activity. It is sensible, however, to advise patients without refrigeration facilities to keep their insulin vials in a cool place. Popular storage places throughout Africa include holes in the ground, or in porous clay pots half-filled with soil or sand and water (Gill, 2000).

A final problem with insulin therapy which deserves mention, is that of the fast of Ramadan. Africa has large numbers of Muslims, and though a diagnosis of diabetes allows exemption from Ramadan fasting, many patients will want to participate. The fast is from sunrise to sunset, with food taken immediately before and afterwards. For those on twice daily insulin systems, the doses can be reversed, with the usual morning insulin taken with the post-sunset meal, and the usual evening insulin taken with the pre-sunrise meal. Some reduction in doses may be needed. Similar principles can be applied to those on oral agent treatment. In general, and considering the large number of Muslim diabetic patients who undertake the Ramadan fast, there are remarkably few glycaemic problems (Lakhdar, 2000).

Oral therapy

Each patient with type 2 diabetes should be seen as an individual. Until recently, only sulphonylureas and metformin were available, but now drugs can potentially be chosen to attempt to correct the major metabolic defect in an individual patient (Table 70.4 and Fig. 70.3). The most widely used sulphonylureas in Africa are chlorpropamide, tolbutamide and glibenclamide, probably because they are cheap and easily available. Chlorpropamide has the longest elimination half-life of all sulphonylureas and therefore it is particularly prone to cause severe hypoglycaemia. In view of this and the availability of cheap generic forms of glibenclamide, chlorpropamide should also fall out of use in Africa as in western countries.

A simple algorithm using a stepwise approach for the management of type 2 diabetes in Cameroon is shown in Fig. 70.4. Start patients on an oral agent at the lowest possible dose increasing progressively at 2–4 weekly intervals. A second class of compatible and synergistic oral agent if required using the same protocol should be added (Fig. 70.4).

Table 70.4. Oral hypoglycaemic agents in use in Africa

	Duration of action (h)	Tablet size	Daily dose	Comments
First-generation sulphonylureas				
Chlorpropamide	24–72	250	100–500	Cheap but can cause severe hypoglycaemia. Should be used with extreme caution
Tolbutamide	6–10	500	500–2000	
Second-generation sulphonylureas				
Gliclazide	6–12	80	80–320	For once or twice daily dosing. Effective when there is endogenous insulin secretion. Can cause hypoglycaemia.
Glipizide	16–24	5	2.5–20	
Glibenclamide	12–24	5	2.5–20	
Glimepiride	12–24	2	2–8	Once daily dosing
Biguanides				
Metformin	12–24	500/850	500–2550	Twice daily dosing. Useful in overweight patients.
Alpha-glucosidase inhibitors				
Acarbose	8–12	50	150–300	Taken three times daily with meals. Can cause flatulence.
Insulin sensitizers				
Rosiglitazone	24	4	4–8	Taken once daily at breakfast in combination with insulin
Pioglitazone	24	15	15–20	Sulphonylureas or metformin
Insulin secretagogues				
Repaglinide	0.5–4	0.5	4–12	Taken before each meal. Can cause hypoglycaemia

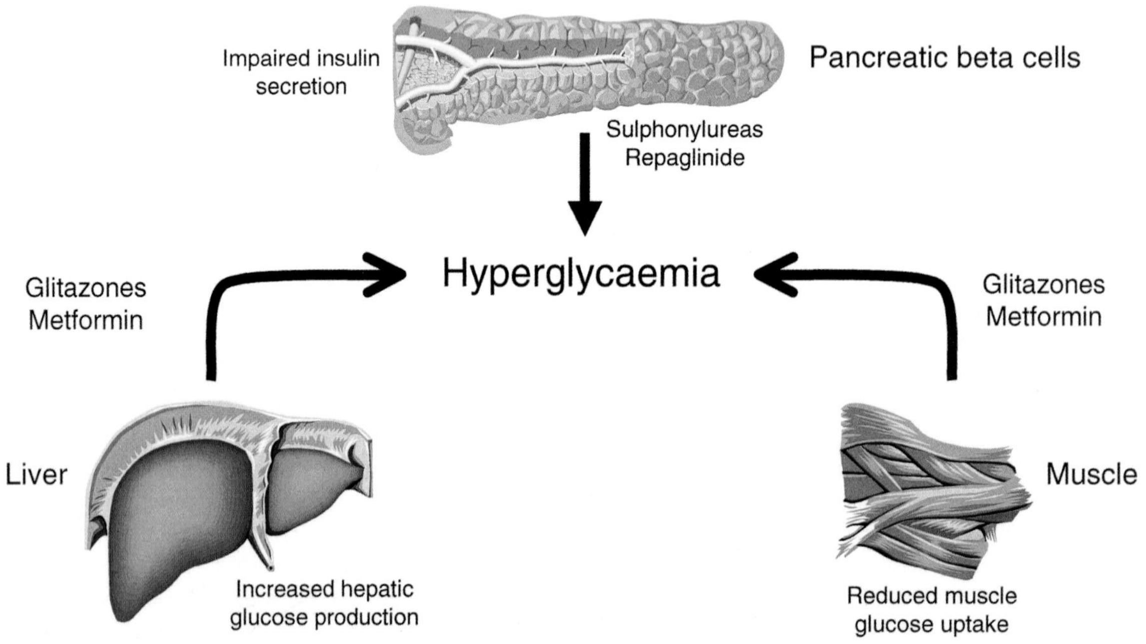

Fig. 70.3. Site of action of oral hypoglycaemic agents.

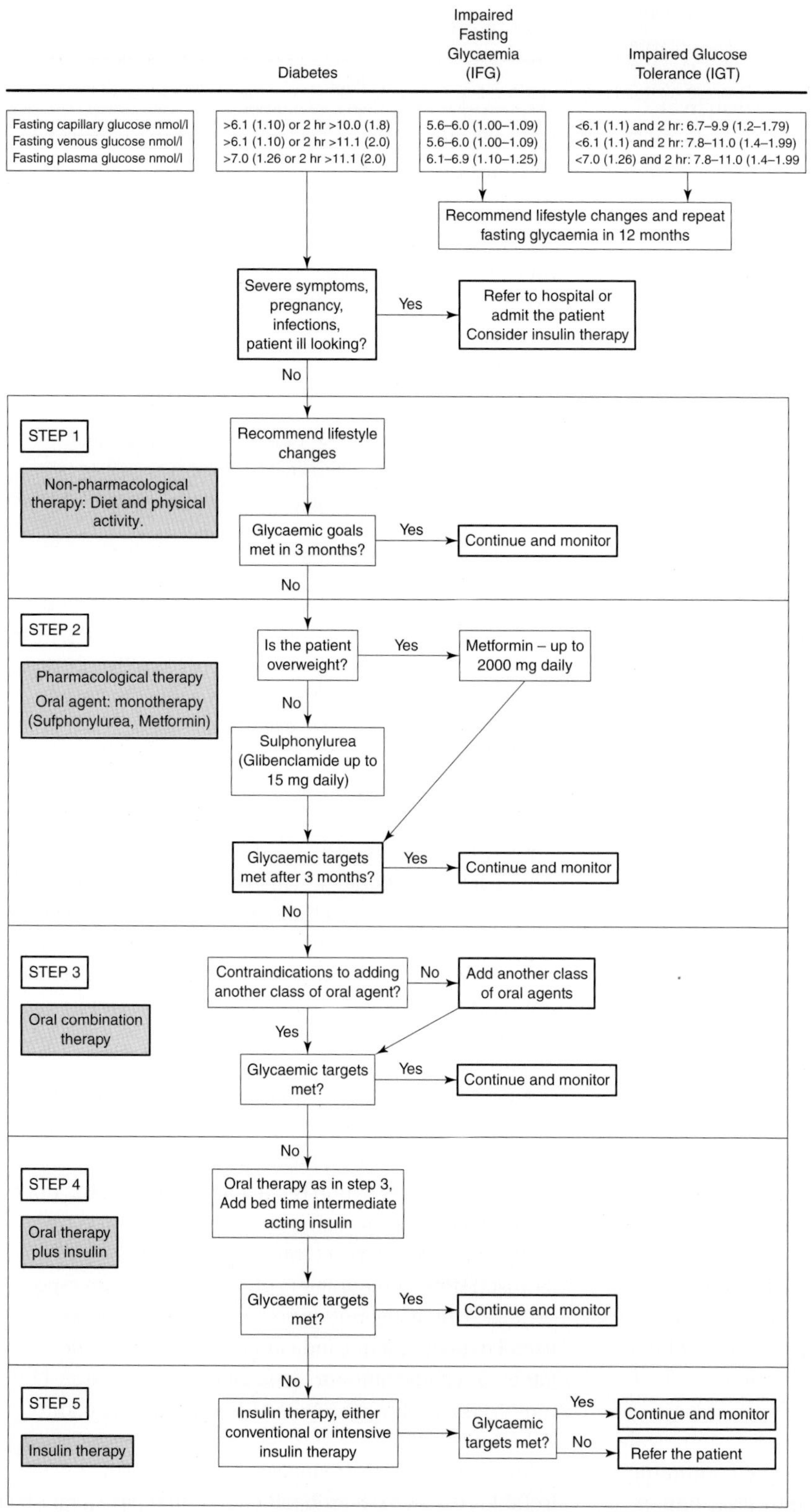
Diabetes
Impaired Fasting Glycaemia (IFG)
Impaired Glucose Tolerance (IGT)
Fasting capillary glucose nmol/l
Fasting venous glucose nmol/l
Fasting plasma glucose nmol/l
>6.1 (1.10) or 2 hr >10.0 (1.8)
>6.1 (1.10) or 2 hr >11.1 (2.0)
>7.0 (1.26 or 2 hr >11.1 (2.0)
5.6–6.0 (1.00–1.09)
5.6–6.0 (1.00–1.09)
6.1–6.9 (1.10–1.25)
<6.1 (1.1) and 2 hr: 6.7–9.9 (1.2–1.79)
<6.1 (1.1) and 2 hr: 7.8–11.0 (1.4–1.99)
<7.0 (1.26) and 2 hr: 7.8–11.0 (1.4–1.99
Recommend lifestyle changes and repeat fasting glycaemia in 12 months
Severe symptoms, pregnancy, infections, patient ill looking?
Yes
Refer to hospital or admit the patient Consider insulin therapy
No
STEP 1
Non-pharmacological therapy: Diet and physical activity.
Recommend lifestyle changes
Glycaemic goals met in 3 months?
Yes
Continue and monitor
No
STEP 2
Pharmacological therapy Oral agent: monotherapy (Sufphonylurea, Metformin)
Is the patient overweight?
Yes
Metformin – up to 2000 mg daily
No
Sulphonylurea (Glibenclamide up to 15 mg daily)
Glycaemic targets met after 3 months?
Yes
Continue and monitor
No
STEP 3
Oral combination therapy
Contraindications to adding another class of oral agent?
No
Add another class of oral agents
Yes
Glycaemic targets met?
Yes
Continue and monitor
No
STEP 4
Oral therapy plus insulin
Oral therapy as in step 3, Add bed time intermediate acting insulin
Glycaemic targets met?
Yes
Continue and monitor
No
STEP 5
Insulin therapy
Insulin therapy, either conventional or intensive insulin therapy
Glycaemic targets met?
Yes
Continue and monitor
No
Refer the patient

Fig. 70.4. Algorithm for the management of type 2 diabetes in Cameroon. Note that a similar though simpler algorithm from rural South Africa is shown on p. 831 (Figure 2, Chapter 75).

The following approaches may be helpful in instituting insulin therapy in type 2 diabetes when there is a primary or secondary failure of oral therapy:

- a single injection of intermediate-acting insulin at bedtime plus oral agents (preferably with metformin)
- conventional insulin therapy – 2 injections per day, combining short and intermediate acting insulin
- intensive insulin therapy – 3 to 4 injections per day (usually short-acting insulin before each meal plus intermediate-acting insulin in the evening).

As insulin analogues become widely available, their use may improve metabolic control in type 2 patients, because of their inherent properties of reducing either fasting or post-prandial hyperglycaemia.

Diabetes education

Knowledge about diabetes is integral to successful management, and diabetes education is the cornerstone of successful diabetes treatment. This is especially true in a continent where diabetes is believed to be caused by supernatural forces and evil spirits. The lack of diabetes educators in most African countries, scarcity of diabetes specialists and multidisciplinary support teams, low patient educational levels, with frequent illiteracy, poor treatment adherence, adverse cultural beliefs, and a lack of reliable and affordable supplies of medication and monitoring equipment, all combine to limit the achievement of good diabetes education. Through the Panafrican Diabetes Educators' Group, the chronic lack of diabetes educators is being addressed in the region. Nevertheless, even where there is a complete lack of diabetes educators, it is often possible to identify nursing staff with interest and experience in diabetes, and who are good communicators. Such nurses can lead a programme of both educating patients and 'educating the educators'.

Diabetes education should be done in a holistic manner to empower people affected with diabetes (patients, relatives, etc.) with knowledge, skills, and motivation for self-care, with freedom of choice and responsibility (Tshabalala, 2001). The education can be started informally either at the out-patient clinics or on admission to hospital, as well as during urine or blood glucose testing, and when giving medication. Encourage patients to join existing diabetes associations or help in creating one. Diabetes education involving the patient, family, healthcare staff and community should be considered as an integral and vitally important component of diabetes treatment especially in Africa.

Table 70.5. Targets for the management of diabetes

	Poor	Acceptable	Good
Urine glucose	>0.5% (++)	<0.5% (+)	Negative
FPG (mmol/l)	>7.0	6.1 to 6.9	>5.0 to <6.1
2-hr post-prandial plasma glucose	>10.0	<10.0	4.5 to 7.8
HbA1c (%)	>7.5	<7.5	<6.5
BMI (kg/m^2)			
Females	>30	<27	20–25
Males	>30	<26	19–24

Notes:
FPG: Fasting plasma glucose. Glucose values are in mmol/l.
Source: Adapted from Mbanya et al. (1996).

Monitoring of diabetes

The monitoring of blood glucose is considered beneficial for achieving and maintaining near normal blood glucose levels and for providing feedback to the health care provider. It also may assist the patient in adjusting insulin doses with diet and physical activity. Language and financial barriers however hinder self-monitoring of blood glucose in Africa.

Although blood glucose testing is more accurate than urine testing, and is generally preferred, urine testing is still a useful additional tool in diabetes management in Africa. In Ethiopia, Feleke and Abdulkadir tested the reliability of urine glucose testing to monitor diabetic control and concluded that urine glucose testing provides reliable information for diabetic patients who cannot afford the cost of blood glucose monitoring (Feleke & Abdulkadir, 1998).

The ideal clinic laboratory test of glycaemic control is, of course, the glycosylated haemoglobin (HbA_{1c}). This test however is expensive and technically difficult. Fructosamine estimation is cheaper and easier, but does not correlate well enough with HbA_{1c} levels. A recent study from South Africa (Rotchford et al., 2002) has assessed simpler parameters of control in resource-poor settings. Urinary symptoms (especially nocturia) are useful hyperglycaemic indicators. In type 2 diabetic patients, a clinic random blood glucose level of over 14.0 mmol/l is strongly predictive of poor glycaemic control (HbA_{1c} over 8.0%).

Ideal targets for the management of diabetes are shown in Table 70.5. At each visit, patients should have a physical examination, urinalysis for glucose and proteins, fasting capillary blood glucose, blood pressure, pulse, weight, and BMI, as well as patient education (empowerment) on diabetes and lifestyle changes. Risk factors should be monitored regularly and blood pressure should be maintained below 130/80 mmHg if possible. At least twice yearly ideally, they should have their feet examined, glycosylated haemoglobin assessment if possible, and a discussion of diet. Annually, fundoscopy, cardiovascular and renal assessments, neurological examination, lipid profiles and investigations for other diabetic complications should be carried out whenever possible. The management of diabetes poses a serious challenge in Africa because of the inadequate health care system and cost of medication – especially insulin. There is an urgent need for public health intervention to reduce the burden and risks factors of diabetes in Africa.

Complications of diabetes in Africa

Chronic complications

Spectrum and prevalence of complications

The seriousness of diabetes is largely due to its associated complications which can be disabling, and even fatal. Prevalence studies on complications reported up to the early 1990s gave very variable figures. These have been reviewed by Rolfe (1997), and include figures ranging from 9 to16 per cent for cataract, retinopathy 7 to 52 per cent, neuropathy 6 to 47 per cent, nephropathy 6 to 30 per cent, and macroangiopathy 1 to 5 per cent. The variations are due to diagnostic criteria problems, local and geographical factors, type of diabetes, and variation in duration of diabetes. Since 1995, however, a number of more vigorous and well-conducted studies have taken place, giving a much clearer picture of complication prevalence, and these are summarized in Table 70.6. It can be seen that there is generally less wide a range between these various studies, and also that the figures themselves are substantial.

Glycaemic control and diabetic complications

Since the 1990s, convincing evidence has demonstrated a close link between long-term blood glucose control and the occurrence of specific diabetic complications. The Diabetes Control and Complications Trial (DCCT) was a US study of nearly 1500 type 1 diabetic patients, randomised to 'tight' and 'routine' control (DCCT, 1993). The HbA_{1c} levels in the two groups were 7.0 per cent and 9.0 per cent respectively, and the reduction in new complications was dramatic, ranging from 39 to 76 per cent (see Table 70.7). More recently, the United Kingdom

Table 70.6. Diabetic complication prevalence rates reported in Africa from 1995

Complication	Country	Prevalence %	Type of DM	Year
Retinopathy	Sudan	43	1	1995[a]
	South Africa	52	1	1995[b]
	Burkina Faso	16	1+2	1996[c]
	South Africa	55	1+2	1997[d]
	Cameroon	37	1+2	1999[e]
	Libya	30	2	1999[f]
Neuropathy	Sudan	37	1	1995[a]
	South Africa	42	1	1995[b]
	Burkina Faso	35	1+2	1996[c]
	Uganda	46	1+2	1996[g]
	South Africa	28	1+2	1997[d]
	Libya	46	2	1997[f]
Nephropathy	Sudan	22	1	1995[a]
	South Africa	28	1	1995[b]
	Burkina Faso	25	1+2	1996[c]
	Uganda	17	1+2	1996[g]
	Libya	25	2	1999[f]
Microalbuminuria	Ethiopia	33	1	1997[h]
	South Africa	37	1+2	1997[d]
	Cameroon	53	1+2	1999[e]
	Ethiopia	36	2	1997[h]
Foot ulcer	Uganda	4	1+2	1996[g]
Impotence	Uganda	22	1+2	1996[g]
Stroke	Sudan	5	1	1995[a]
PVD	Sudan	10	1	1995[a]
IHD	Uganda	5	1+2	1996[g]

Notes:
1. PVD = peripheral vascular disease.
2. IHD = ischaemic heart disease.
2. References as follows: [a] Elbagir et al. (1995); [b] Gill et al. (1995); [c] Drabo et al. (1996); [d] Levitt et al. (1997); [e] Sobngwi et al. (1999); [f] Kadiki et al. (1999); [g] Nambuya et al. (1996); [h] Rahlenbeck et al. (1997).

Table 70.7. Percentage reduction in appearance of new complications in 'tightly' controlled (HbA_{1c} mean 7.0%) patients in type 1 and type 2 diabetes

	Type 1 diabetes (DCCT, 1993)[a]	Type 2 diabetes (UKPDS, 1998)[b]
Retinopathy	76%	21%
Neuropathy	60%	40%
Nephropathy	54%	34%
Microalbuminuria	39%	30%

Notes:
[a] 9 year follow-up, groups had HbA_{1c} levels of 7.0% and 9.0%.
[b] 10 year follow-up, groups had HbA_{1c} levels of 7.0% and 8.0%.

Prospective Diabetes Study (UKPDS) reported on 10 year follow-up in a cohort of nearly 4000 type 2 diabetic patients. They were also randomized to 'tight' (if necessary using insulin) and 'standard' control, with mean HbA_{1c} levels of 7.0 per cent and 8.0 per cent, respectively. The results are also shown in Table 70.7, and reductions of 21–40 per cent were shown (UKPDS, 1998).

In both these studies 'tight' control was however associated with increased hypoglycaemia and weight gain; and was also labour intensive and expensive. Both studies also failed to demonstrate significant reductions in large vessel disease (though significance was almost reached in UKPDS). Despite these issues, both these truly 'landmark' studies have shown the need for optimal glycaemic control in all diabetic patients. In resource-poor areas of Africa, however, it has to be accepted that this will be difficult and hypoglycaemic risks may be a significant problem.

Table 70.8. Classification of diabetic retinopathy

Background	Microaneurysms Dot haemorrhages Blot haemorrhages Exudates Macular oedema
Pre-proliferative	Venous beading Cotton wool spots IRMAs
Proliferative	Neovascularization Retinal haemorrhage
Advanced	Retinal detachment Rubeosis iridis Glaucoma

Notes:
IRMA = intraretinal microvascular abnormality.

Cataract

Diabetic patients frequently suffer cataract in later years, but cataract can also occur in younger diabetic patients, often surprisingly quickly. This has a different appearance, and is often called a 'snowstorm' cataract. Though theoretically simple to treat surgically, diabetic cataracts are an important cause of diabetes-related blindness, because of lack of adequate surgical facilities (and spectacles) in many regions. Indeed, in Africa cataract causes blindness in diabetes more frequently than retinopathy (Rolfe, 1997).

Retinopathy

The classification of the various types of retinopathic changes is shown in Table 70.8. Adequate diabetic eye examination is not easy – it requires visual acuity testing with a Snellen chart in a well-lit room, repeat acuity testing through a pinhole if initial acuity is reduced, dilatation of the pupil with an effective short-acting mydriatic (e.g. 0.5% or 1.0% tropicaimide), and thorough examination with an ophthalmoscope in a darkened room. Unfortunately, there is often little point in undertaking this, as effective therapy (essentially laser treatment) is rarely available. This shortage of laser facilities has hampered both the treatment of, and research into, diabetic retinopathy in Africa. Nevertheless, laser treatment is increasingly available, and the indications for referral should be –

- All proliferative retinopathy
- All pre-proliferative retinopathy
- Advanced background retinopathy
- Any retinopathy involving the macula
- Any unexplained deterioration in visual acuity (in case of macular oedema)

It should be remembered that the non-laser strategy of improved glycaemic control will reduce retinopathy risk, and retard the progression of established retinopathy. There is also some evidence that ACE inhibitor treatment may help in established proliferative retinopathy.

Nephropathy

Diabetic renal disease is being increasingly encountered in African diabetic practice (Table 70.6), probably related to increased diagnostic awareness, and also because longer duration patients are being increasingly seen (Gill et al. 1995). Nephropathy rarely occurs without co-existing retinopathy, and its occurrence is similarly strongly related to disease duration and glycaemic control. The initial indication clinically is proteinuria on urine dipstix testing, which is initially intermittent and later persistent (indicating a urinary protein excretia of over 300 mg/litre). It is important at this stage to exclude other causes of proteinuria (e.g. urinary tract infection schistosomiasis, genital conditions etc) and to treat these appropriately. As nephropathy advances, protein excretion increases and hypertension develops. Later biochemical renal function deteriorates, and eventually end-stage disease is reached with fatal results, unless renal transplantation or dialysis is possible. The time taken for progression is variable, but frequently quite prolonged (often several years). During this period, progression can be greatly slowed by vigorous anti-hypertensive treatment aiming for blood-pressure (BP) levels of ideally below 130/85. ACE inhibitors are the best evidence-based drugs, but they are expensive and not widely available. Any other anti-hypertensive drugs will still be highly beneficial, as long as strict BP targets are achieved. Improved glycaemic control is also beneficial, but this is often hard to achieve, and is less important than good BP control.

Over the last 10–15 years there has been considerable interest in the earliest phase of nephropathy, known as 'microalbuminuria'. This refers to levels of albumin excretia which are abnormal, but below the level of albustix detection (equivalent of urinary albumin levels of about 30–300 mg/l, requiring specialist laboratory assay). If possible, the 'albumin-creatinine ratio' (ACR) on an early morning specimen should be determined, and in resource-rich countries this is now part of the 'annual screen' of all diabetic patients. Microalbuminuria is common (Table 70.6) and represents a stage of diabetic renal disease which is amenable to treatment, and even possibly reversal, with ACE inhibition therapy (even in normotensive patients); though if hypertension is present and ACE inhibitors are not available, other anti-hypertensive drugs are well-worthwhile. Again, improved glycaemic control will help, and smoking should be discouraged.

Neuropathy

Neuropathy is one of the commonest diabetic complications (Table 70.6) and though most patients are only mildly affected, it can be severe and highly debilitating. There are many neuropathic syndromes encountered, though the commonest by far is a peripheral sensory neuropathy usually affecting the feet and lower legs. All the other types of neuropathy may be encountered in Africa however, including the rarer varieties such as amyotrophy and autonomic neuropathy. There are several potential diagnostic pitfalls amongst these less common forms of neuropathy, e.g. thigh weakness (amyotrophy); diplopia, foot drop etc (mononeuritis); 'band-like' unilateral chest or abdominal pain (radiculopathy); and vomiting, diarrhoea, postural hypotension, bladder disturbance, or impotence (autonomic neuropathy). Severe generalized neuropathy can also be associated with marked weight loss (so-called 'diabetic neuropathic cachexia') (see Box).

Syndromes of diabetic neuropathy

Peripheral sensory neuropathy
Sensorimotor neuropathy
Pure motor neuropathy, e.g. amyotrophy
Single peripheral nerves (mononeuritis), e.g. cranial VI
common peroneal
Radiculopathy
Autonomic neuropathy
Diabetic neuropathic cachexia

In areas where alcohol abuse and/or vitamin B malnutrition occur, it may be difficult to be sure whether sensory neuropathy in a diabetic patient is due to these other factors or to diabetes alone. In such cases it may be reasonable to give B vitamins and advise alcohol moderation. For diabetic neuropathy itself there is no specific treatment other than attempting to improve blood glucose control. There may, however, be a number of useful supportive management strategies. These include physiotherapy in amyotrophy, foot splints for a common peroneal nerve palsy, and temporary occlusion of the affected eyes in third or sixth cranial nerve palsies to suppress diplopia. A variety of treatments may help specific types of autonomic neuropathy – for example metroclopromide for vomiting, and for diarrhoea either loperamide or antibiotics (as there is often associated bacterial bowel overgrowth). Fludrocortisone or indomethacin (or other NSAIDs) may cause mild fluid retention, and help postural hypotension. Erectile dysfunction will be discussed later.

Most diabetic neuropathy is not associated with pain, but in a minority there is distressing painful dysaesthesia, classically worse at night and disturbing sleep. This responds poorly to standard analgesics, but can usually be helped by regular tricyclic drugs, for example imipramine or amitryptilline 25 mg at night, increasing up to100 mg daily (ether split, or all at night, depending on symptoms). Other potentially useful drugs for painful neuropathy include carbamazepine, valproate, mexilitine, gabapentin, and topical capsaicin cream. The prognosis of diabetic neuropathy may sometimes be surprisingly good. Mononeuritis syndromes and amyotrophy for example usually resolve completely over a period of months. Other types, however (notably the painful and autonomic sub-groups) tend to continue indefinitely, and remain management challenges.

Macrovascular disease

Coronary artery disease is generally rare in sub-Saharan Africa (Rolfe, 1997), though it is encountered somewhat more frequently in Ethiopia (Lester & Keen, 1988). Peripheral vascular disease (PVD) follows a similar pattern. Cerebral artherosclerotic disease (CVD) is probably more common, though there is little detailed information on this. The future with regard to diabetic macroangiopathy however is far from certain. As African societies increasingly urbanize and westernize, arteriosclerotic disease is likely to increase, and indeed is already emerging. For example, at Baragwanath Hospital in Soweto, South Africa, in the early 1990s a myocardial infarct (MI) in a black African patient was rare. Less than

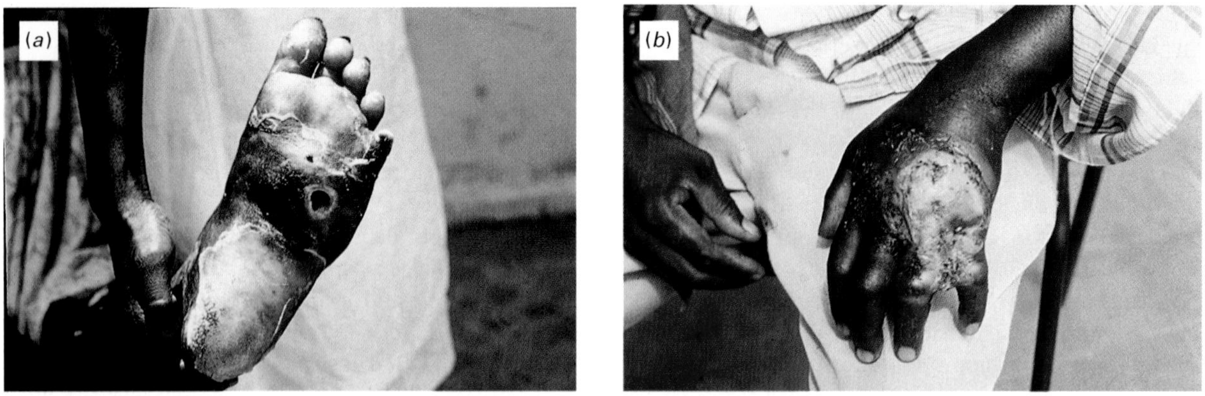

Fig. 70.5. Advanced limb sepsis in African diabetic patients. (*a*) An infected neuropathic foot ulcer, and (*b*) deep palmar hand sepsis. (Reproduced with permission of FSG Publications.)

10 years later, the hospital has its own dedicated coronary care unit. The implications are clear!

Foot and hand ulceration

In Africa, where lower limb atherosclerosis is relatively rare, diabetic foot ulceration usually occurs as a consequence of neuropathy, trauma and infection. When delayed presentation to hospital is added, foot sepsis is often deep and advanced, and the lower limb may not be salvageable (see Fig. 70.5). Even with amputation, inpatient mortality of African patients with advanced diabetic foot sepsis is high, e.g. 33 per cent in one series from Nigeria (Dagogo-Jack, 1991).

Though hospital-presenting diabetic foot ulceration is devastating, there is some evidence that overall rates of diabetic foot ulceration are lower in Africa than in Europe and North America. This may be due to the protective effect of much thicker skin on the sole of the African foot (from barefoot walking), but also to more beneficial foot pressure profiles related to lesser joint contractures of the forefoot (Benbow & Gill, 1998; Dagogo-Jack, 1991). These reasons may explain why neuropathic foot ulcers in black diabetic patients occur on various sites of the dorsum and lateral aspects of the foot, whereas in white patients the major sites by far are over the first or fifth metatarsal heads on the plantar surface.

Serious foot ulceration requires intravenous broad-spectrum antibiotics, and often early surgical intervention. Less urgent foot ulcers should be reviewed frequently on an out or inpatient basis, as necessary; and managed according to the principles of treatment outlined in Table 70.9. All diabetic foot ulcers must be taken seriously – trivial ulcers can progress rapidly to life-threatening septic limbs. A study from Ethiopia has shown that the long-term outlook of diabetic African amputees is very poor, and that few have good life quality due to difficulty in obtaining adequate artificial limbs (Lester, 1995).

A poorly recognized variant of diabetic limb sepsis is ulceration and infection of the hand. This complication is now virtually exclusively associated with the tropics, and though less common than foot ulceration, the clinical scenario is very stereotyped and has led to the term 'Tropical Diabetic Hand Syndrome' (Gill et al., 1998). Patients are often male, and their diabetes is usually neglected and poorly controlled. Trivial trauma, sometimes on a background of upper limb neuropathy, leads to infection, ulceration and deep sepsis. Delayed hospital presentation, sometimes due to treatment by traditional healers and herbalists, results in a classical 'diabetic hand' (Fig. 70.5). Despite early surgery and vigorous antibiotic treatment, some degree of upper limb amputation is often needed, and mortality is also relatively high.

Erectile dysfunction

Partial or complete erectile impotence in diabetic patients has traditionally been considered a complication of autonomic neuropathy, but in practice can be multifactorial. Psychological factors, including depression, may be important, as well as drug treatment (especially anti-hypertensive drugs), alcohol excess, vascular factors and occasionally hormonal disorders (primary or secondary testosterone deficiency, and hyperprolactinaemia). Erectile impotence of some degree is common in diabetic males (see box below) – one Zambian study showed that 44 per cent of diabetic men had some degree of erectile dysfunction, compared with 22 per cent of non-diabetic controls (Rolfe, 1988).

Table 70.9. Principles of managing diabetic foot ulceration

Pressure relief	– Vitally important	
	– Adhesive pads round ulcer	
	– Scotchcast boot	
	– Plaster of paris cast	
Debridement	– Remove callus	
	– Deslough if necessary	
Antibiotics	– Broad spectrum	
	– Consider also metronidazole	
	– Ensure *staph* and *strep* covered	
Dressings	– Ensure non-adhesive	
	– Vaseline-impregnated gauze useful	
	– 'Natural' dressings helpful	
	– For example	– honey
		– sugar paste
		– papaya
Education	– General self-footcare	
	– Sensible shoes	
	– Early self-referral	

Assessing the diabetic patient with erectile impotence

- Check drug therapy (especially for hypertension)
- Look for features of depression, anxiety, etc.
- Take alcohol history and look for features of chronic liver disease
- Examine for peripheral neuropathy
- Simple autonomic tests (e.g. heart rate changes on Valsalva, hand grip, etc.)
- Examine peripheral circulation
- Examine external genitalia, and secondary sexual characteristics
- If possible measure testosterone, FHS/LH and prolactin

The most important potentially treatable causes are depression, drugs and alcohol. Unfortunately, in many cases, curative treatment is not possible; and other therapies are unlikely to be available. These include the recently introduced oral preparation sildafenil ('Viagra'), and suction-pump devices. Other more complex strategies include intra-urethral prostaglandins ('Muse') and intra-cavernosal injections of prostaglandins or papaverine.

Cheiroarthropathy

One of the most fascinating – though not at all dangerous – diabetic complications is 'cheiroarthropathy', sometimes known as 'limited joint mobility' or 'pseudo-sclerodema'. In its simplest form this causes contractures of the fingers, demonstrated by a positive 'prayer sign' (see Fig. 70.6).

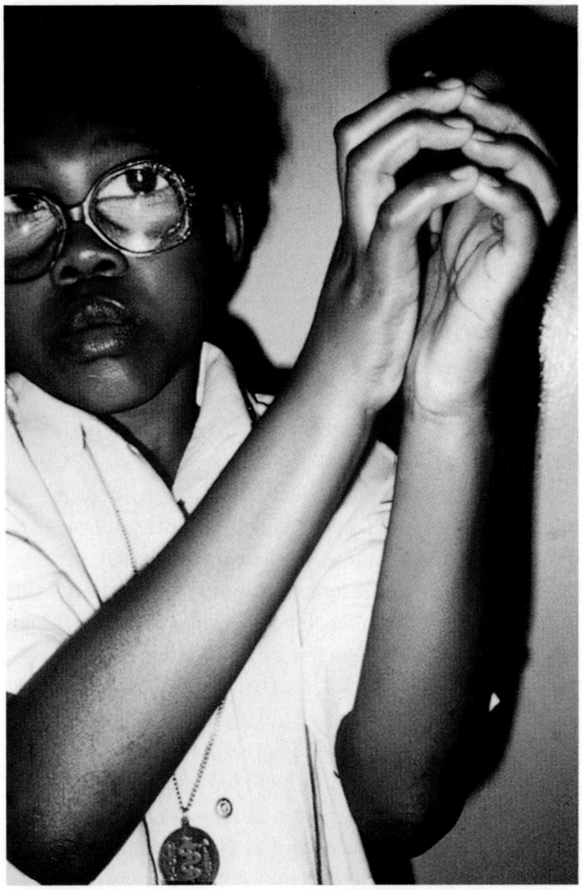

Fig. 70.6. A South African type 1 diabetic patient, demonstrating the 'Prayer Sign' of diabetic cheiroarthropathy.

This is seen in about one-third of type 1 diabetic patients, and is associated with duration of disease, glycaemic control, and the presence of microvascular complications (Huddle & Gill, 1994). It is also seen in type 2 patients, but may be harder to diagnose accurately as a number of these patients may also have osteoarthrosis.

Diabetic cheiroarthropathy is due to glycosylated collagen in the connective tissue around joints. The glucose-complexing process alters the physical characteristics of collagen leading to peri-articular stiffness, and often stretching of the skin over the finger joints (so-called 'pseudosclerodema'). Sometimes larger joints can be involved. The condition is normally quite asymptomatic and the patient is usually unaware of it. There are, however, more symptomatic-related disorders – notably frozen shoulder and Dupuytren's contracture, both of which are seen more commonly in diabetes, and which are probably also related to collagen glycosylation.

Protein glycosylation also damages the basement membranes of retinal and glomerular cells, and may be at least part of the basic pathological process leading to diabetic microangiopathic complications (Stannaway & Gill, 2000). Stiff fingers in diabetic patients may therefore be an intriguing external marker of the presence of (or high risk of) widespread microangiopathic disease.

Hypertension

In all geographical areas, hypertension is more common amongst diabetic patients compared with non-diabetic controls. The reasons are not entirely clear, but are at least in part due to the over-representation of obesity and renal disease in diabetes. Crude prevalence rates of hypertension in diabetes of course vary, but in most parts of Africa are at least 30 per cent (Mugusi et al., 1995), with rates higher in urban areas. Additionally, current figures are serious underestimates, as they are mostly based on now outdated WHO criteria for hypertension (BP levels of over 160/85). Hypertension in diabetes carries particularly high risks, and current evidence-based targets for type 2 diabetes in Europe are BP levels of below 145/80. The large British UKPDS study showed greatly improved outcome in patients treated to achieve BP levels of this or below (UKPDS, 1998). The benefits included a 32 per cent reduction in diabetes-related deaths, 37 per cent reduction in microvascular complications, and 44 per cent reduction in stroke. Though these figures may not be entirely relevant to Africa (where coronary artery disease is much less frequent), there is sufficient evidence to recommend vigorous BP control for all diabetic patients in Africa.

This information is of great importance to African diabetes practice. Improving blood glucose control is often extremely difficult, but hypertension treatment is achievable. The UKPDS showed that no particular anti-hypertensive drug was more beneficial than another, which means that simple and available drugs can be used in Africa – for example low-dose thiazides (which have no adverse metabolic effects), methyldopa, hydrallazine, reserpine, etc. Strict BP targets (as above) should be aimed for, and protocols should be locally designed so that adequate doses of drugs are used (often at least two drugs are needed). Nurse-led treatment is often the most effective strategy for managing diabetic hypertension (see Chapter 75 on the delivery of non-communicable disease care).

Diabetic dyslipidaemia

The major dyslipidaemia of diabetes occurs in the type 2 syndrome, and involves moderate elevation of total and LDL cholesterol, raised trigylceride levels and low HDL cholesterol. There is also evidence that 'diabetic' LDL cholesterol is potentially more atherogenic than equivalent amounts in non-diabetic subjects. Though diabetic dyslipidaemia is of major importance in western countries, and requires vigorous treatment, its relevance in Africa is far less certain. Arteriosclerotic disease is uncommon in most parts of the continent, and lipid levels are also generally much lower. For these reasons, lipid screening in most African diabetic clinics is not practised. An additional factor is that adequate treatment of lipid disorders is expensive; involving expert dietetic advice, and often treatment with statin and/or fibrate drugs. It should, however, be emphasized that the future is less certain As African communities continue to urbanize and westernize, it is unlikely to be long before diabetes-related lipid disorders need adding to the agenda for African health workers involved with diabetes care.

Acute complications

Hypoglycaemia

Pathophysiology

Hypoglycaemia in non-diabetic patients can be a manifestation of hypoadrenalism, severe liver disease, alcohol excess, and rarely insulinoma. Diabetes however is the most frequent cause by far, though hypoglycaemia is really a complication of its treatment rather than the disease itself. It occurs when circulating insulin levels are excessive in relation to carbohydrate intake, and therefore is related only to insulin or sulphonylurea treatment.

Frequency

Hypoglycaemia is the commonest acute complication of diabetes. Mild (self-treatable) 'hypos' occur in virtually all patients on insulin, and severe attacks (requiring external assistance for reversal) occur in Europe in about 10 per cent of the insulin-treated population every year. There is no accurate information from Africa, but rates are likely to be at least as high as those from Europe. Certainly, diabetic hypoglycaemia is a frequent cause of casualty department attendance and medical admission in Africa (Lester, 1997).

Causes and presentation

The commonest cause of diabetic hypoglycaemia is inadequate food intake; other factors include inappropriate treatment, alcohol excess and gastrio–intestinal disorders (Gill & Huddle, 1993; Lester, 1997). Though sulphonylureas are a rare cause of severe hypoglycaemia in western diabetic practice, in Africa they are a relatively common cause – a third of diabetic hypoglycaemia admissions in one study from South Africa, for example (Gill & Huddle, 1993). Any sulphonylurea can cause hypoglycaemia, but the long-acting drug chlorpropamide is especially problematic. Glibenclamide (especially in the elderly) is also prone to cause hypoglycaemia. Gliclazide and glipizide are safer, but if available tolbutamide is safest. The symptoms and presentation of hypoglycaemia are very variable. It must be considered in any comatose or semi-conscious patient, and an immediate bedside blood glucose strip performed. Other presentations include confused or drunken-like behaviour. Mild attacks generally have more typical symptoms and signs, such as hunger, faintness, sweating, pallor and tremulousness.

Mortality and outcome

Prompt and adequate treatment is important, as severe hypoglycaemia can cause death, or recovery with permanent brain damage. Recurrent attacks can also be associated with long-term decline in cognitive function. Mortality figures of up to 20 per cent have been reported in the past from Africa, but this has improved in the last decade and is now probably below 5 per cent in most areas (Gill & Huddle,1993). This is, however, still in excess of western rates.

Management (Table 70.10)

Mild hypos are treated with oral fast-acting carbohydrate (foods containing glucose or sucrose, e.g. cola, sugar in water, jam, chocolate). After recovery, longer-acting carbohydrate should be given, e.g. bread, biscuits, porridge, banana. Management of severe hypoglycaemia, associated with coma or precoma (Lester, 1997) is shown in Table 70.10. Of particular importance is the need for prolonged intravenous glucose after recovery in the case of sulphonylurea or alcohol-associated hypoglycaemia. This is because hypoglycaemia can recur after initial treatment in these cases.

> **Key educational points for preventing hypoglycaemia**
> (after Lester, 1993)
> - Importance of regular food intake
> - Understanding carbohydrate-containing foods
> - What to do if food is short
> - Recognizing the symptoms of hypoglycaemia
> - If on insulin, carry fast-acting carbohydrate
> - Carry some identification of diabetes
> - Let family and workmates know about hypos

Prevention

Most diabetic hypoglycaemia is potentially preventable, and the key factors in patient education are shown in the

Table 70.10. Management of diabetic hypoglycaemic coma or pre-coma

Give i.v. glucose 20–30 g (e.g. 200–300 ml of 10% dextrose, 100–150 ml 20% dextrose, or 40–60 ml 50% dextrose).[a]
On recovery, give a long-acting carbohydrate snack.
Attempt to identify the cause of hypoglycaemia and correct it.
If hypoglycaemia is due to sulphonylureas, or if alcohol is strongly implicated, also put up a slow dextrose drip (5–10%) for 12–14 hours.

Notes:
[a] If i.v. access is impossible, consider nasogastric or rectal glucose; or, if available, glucagon 1 mg i.m. A last resort may be adrenaline 1 ml of 1/1000 strength (adult dose).

Education of doctors and other health carers must also not be forgotten (Box, Column 1). Protocols for the correct management of hypoglycaemia should be displayed in casualty departments and/or admission wards. The prescribing of insulin and sulphonylureas should also be undertaken carefully, and the patient's social and economic situation must be taken into account. For example, it is no use prescribing twice-daily insulin if the patient can only eat once daily!

Ketoacidosis

Pathophysiology

Diabetic ketoacidosis (DKA) is a state of serious metabolic decompensation due mainly to severe insulin deficiency. It is therefore almost always a complication of type 1 diabetes, though it can occasionally occur in type 2 disease (usually in lean individuals with severe infection or other intercurrent illness). Insulin deficiency increases hepatic glucose output but inhibits peripheral glucose uptake. Unrestrained lipolysis occurs, with fatty acids diverted to the formation of ketone bodies (beta-hydroxy butyrate and acetoacetate). The process is often triggered and exacerbated by infection, where the associated rise in counter-regulatory hormones (e.g. cortisol, catecholamines, growth hormone) antagonize insulin, and worsen effective insulin deficiency.

Frequency

Exact incidence figures for DKA in Africa are not known, but the condition is certainly a common cause of diabetes-related hospitalization throughout the continent. Thus, reported percentage figures of DKA patients compared with all diabetic admissions, include 28 per cent in Senegal (Lester, 1997), 55 per cent in Sudan (Ahmed &

Table 70.11. Precipitating factors for DKA in Africa

•	Shortage of insulin	
•	Poor adherence to treatment	
•	Infection	– malaria
		– chest
		– gastrointestinal
		– foot
		– hand
•	Stroke	
•	Myocardial infarction[a]	

Notes:
[a] Still rare in sub-Saharan Africa, but an occasional precipitant in north Africa.
Source: After Lester (1997); Zouvaris et al. (1997); Ahmed & Abdella (1999).

Abdella, 1999), 18% in Ethiopia (Seyoum et al., 1998) and 10 per cent in South Africa (Zouvaris et al., 1997).

Causes and presentation

Precipitating factors for DKA are shown in Table 70.11. Sadly, simple lack of insulin is still a common factor. Others include poor compliance with treatment, and a variety of infections. DKA may be the first presentation of type 1 diabetes – nearly a quarter of patients in one study (Zouvaris et al., 1997). Clinically, patients classically present with vomiting, abdominal pains, collapse, dehydration and hyperventilation ('Kussmaul's respiration'). Milder forms of DKA occur however, and the condition should be considered in any ill diabetic patient. Classically the blood pH is <7.25, serum bicarbonate <15 mmol/l, blood glucose >25 mmol/l, and the urine strongly positive for ketones. Milder biochemical abnormalities may, however, still indicate DKA. There is even a rare 'euglycaemic' form where the blood glucose level is below 15 mmol/l.

In resource-poor settings, blood gas and serum urea and electrolyte measurements may be impossible. Sometimes, even an urgent blood glucose is difficult. Here, close attention needs to be paid to clinical features, and a finger-prick blood glucose strip level, together with strong ketouria, is sufficient to make the diagnosis. If urine is not obtainable, centrifuged plasma can be tested for ketones with a urine 'Acetest' tablet or 'Ketostix' strip.

Outcome and mortality

Mortality rates for DKA in western countries are generally below 5 per cent. Rates in Africa vary geographically, but are substantially higher, generally in the region of 10–20%, though sometimes much more. Vigorous and efficient treatment, however, can improve these figures, for example, rates of death below 10 per cent have been reported from Addis Ababa, Ethiopia (Lester, 1997); and below 5 per cent in Tripoli, Libya (Lakhdar & Elhabroush, 1999). Factors influencing a poor outcome of DKA in Africa are shown in Box.

Factors leading to high mortality rates of DKA in Africa
- Lack of insulin
- Patient educational failure
- Delayed presentation to hospital
- Delayed diagnosis ('doctor educational failure')
- Inappropriate treatment
- Overwhelming infection

Simple lack of insulin is a major and often insurmountable problem. Delayed presentation to hospital is important and may be due to long travelling distances, or patients seeking help from traditional practitioners. Diagnostic delays can also occur in health clinics and wards, often due to the possibility of diabetes or DKA not being considered. The abdominal pain of ketosis may be misinterpreted as an abdominal emergency or gastroenteritis (especially when vomiting is a prominent symptom). Sometimes the precipitating infection is diagnosed, but DKA not considered as a complication. All of these delays can be literally fatal (Rwiza et al., 1986). Even when diagnosed, sub-optimal management systems can contribute to poor outcome. There are thus educational issues involving both patients and health care workers, and these will be discussed further under the topic of prevention.

Management

The major principles of DKA management are prompt diagnosis and adequate fluid and insulin treatment. In addition, potassium (K) will need to be replaced and any underlying precipitating infection must be treated promptly. A standard 'first world' protocol for DKA treatment in common use in Europe is shown in Table 70.12. Low doses of intravenous insulin by infusion are given, along with saline replacement and vigorous potassium treatment (there is always a large potassium deficit in DKA). Potassium should not be given initially as there is often hyperkalaemia due to acidosis, though levels fall rapidly after treatment begins. Bicarbonate is rarely needed and can be hazardous. Close monitoring by both doctors and nurses is needed, especially early on. Later, when the patient is improved and blood glucose has fallen below 15 mmol/l, the insulin and fluid regime can be changed to 'GKI' (glucose – potassium – insulin infusion). This is a useful system for maintaining fluid and

Table 70.12. Management of ketoacidosis (a) with full drugs, equipment and support

1. Fluids	500 ml 0.9% ('normal') saline quickly, then 500 ml hourly for 4–6 hours
2. Insulin	Soluble insulin 50 units in 50 ml 0.9%/saline in a 50 ml i.v. syringe driver (1 ml = 1 unit). Start at 4–6 units/h.
3. Potassium	If initial K level not high, start KCl added to saline at 10–30 mmol/h. Adjust according to U&E.
4. Bicarbonate	Use only if pH <6.90 and patient very ill. Give 50 mmol dilute (not 8.4%) $NaHCO_3$ slowly.
5. Monitoring	Initial blood gases, BG and U&E. Hourly bedside BG monitoring. Lab BG and U&E 2–4-hourly.
6. Support	Nasogastric tube and urinary catheter if patient comatose. Consider antibiotics. CVP line and plasma expanders if shocked.
7. Later	When BG <15 mmol/l and patient improved stop i.v. insulin and saline, and convert to 'GKI' infusion[a] 100 ml/h, altering insulin and KCl content according to lab monitoring. When patient able to eat, revert to s.c insulin.

Notes:

[a] GKI infusion is 500 ml 10% dextrose with 20 units soluble insulin and 20 units KCl.

Table 70.13. Management of ketoacidosis (b) in resource-poor settings

1. Fluids	0.9% saline as in Table 70.12. If not available use Hartman's, Ringer's or Darrow's solutions. In PHC clinics, awaiting transfer to hospital, give s.c. or rectal fluid (at slower rate).
2. Insulin	Soluble 20 units i.m. stat, and 10 units i.m. hourly. If no soluble, use lente or isophane 20 units i.m. stat, and 15 units i.m. hourly.
3. Potassium	None for first hour, then 20 mmol/h × 3 hours, and 10 mmol/h × 2 hours
4. Bicarbonate	Only if patient very ill and not improving. Give 50 mmol $NaHCO_3$ (preferably not 8.4%) slowly i.v. Repeat if necessary once only.
5. Monitoring	Hourly bedside BG by reagent strip. 4-hourly urine ketones.
6. Support	If comatose, nasogastric tube and urinary catheter. Consider malaria, urine and chest infection; and treat if any suspicion.
7. Later	When BG <15 mmol/l convert i.v. fluids to 5% dextrose 500 ml 2-hourly for 4 to 6 hours, then 500 ml 4-hourly. Continue i.m. insulin. When patient can eat and is improved, change to s.c. insulin.

potassium replacement, and delivering glucose and insulin smoothly. The amount of potassium chloride (KCl) and insulin in the infusion can be adjusted according to BG and plasma K levels. Later, the i.v. treatment can be discontinued and the patient returned to food and subcutaneous insulin (Krentz & Nattrass, 1997).

This system is of course relatively 'high-tech', and for many parts of Africa will be inappropriate. Nevertheless, successful adaptations can be made, and these are outlined in Table 70.13. The protocol here assumes that there is no laboratory support, and even gives alternatives when there is no 0.9 per cent saline or soluble insulin! The 'hourly-intramuscular' insulin system is simple and effective. It was described by Alberti and colleagues 30 years ago, and is very appropriate to many African settings (Alberti et al., 1973). Even intermediate-acting insulins such as lente (when soluble insulins are not available), have been used in DKA successfully (Haile, 2000).

Prevention

Many episodes of DKA are potentially preventable, and patient education is the key. Vital messages are for patients to take insulin injections regularly, and not to stop them when ill and anorexic. They must also be encouraged to seek prompt medical advice if severe hyperglycaemic symptoms, and/or infective illnesses develop. As well as patient education, as previously mentioned, it is also important to educate health care workers on the prompt diagnosis and adequate treatment of DKA. Simple, locally appropriate protocols of management should be developed and widely distributed. In particular, they should be displayed on the wall of admission wards, casualty departments etc.

The effect of combined patient and doctor education has been demonstrated in a study from Soweto, South Africa in the 1980s (Huddle & Gill, 1988). Over a 5-year period, these strategies reduced the mortality of hyperglycaemic emergencies (mostly DKA) from 25 per cent to 10 per cent.

Hyperosmolar non-ketotic coma (HNK)

Pathophysiology

Hyperosmolar non-ketotic coma ('HNK' or 'HONK') is an unusual acute complication of type 2 (not type 1) diabetes. The word 'coma' is inaccurate as few patients are truly comatose. It is characterized by severe hyperglycaemia and dehydration without ketosis. Like DKA it is often precipitated by infection, and counter-regulatory hormones antagonize insulin and lead to marked hyperglycaemia. As type 2 diabetic patients have residual insulin secretion however, ketone production remains suppressed.

Frequency

The exact incidence of HNK is unknown, but in a reported series of patients from Baragwanath Hospital, Soweto, HNK made up 12 per cent of all acute diabetic hyperglycaemic emergencies (Rolfe et al., 1995). This figure is perhaps a little higher than western experiences, but exact comparisons have not been carried out.

Causes and presentation

As mentioned, infection (often chest or urinary tract) is a common precipitant. Diuretic treatment is also a trigger, presumably by causing dehydration. Patients virtually always have type 2 disease, and may be known diagnoses, or can be new presentations with HNK. They are usually late-middle aged or elderly (50–70 years). Clinically, patients present ill and comatose or semi-comatose, as well as severely dehydrated and often hypotensive. Blood glucose is usually well in excess of 30 mmol/l – in the South African series the mean was 50.2 mmol/l (Rolfe et al., 1995). Plasma urea and sodium levels are often elevated, due to dehydration; but arterial blood gases are normal and urinalysis shows absent or only mild ketonuria. As the name HNK suggests, plasma osmolality is raised (to above 340 mOsmol/kg). This does not need to be measured however, as it can be calculated if plasma sodium and urea, as well as blood glucose, are known (see Box).

Calculated plasma osmolality $= 2\ (Na + K) + U + G$
Na = sodium
K = potassium
U = urea
G = glucose
(all values must be in mmol/l)

In the absence of biochemical support, the diagnosis must be made from the clinical presentation, extreme hyperglycaemia, and absence of ketosis.

Outcome and mortality

HNK is a serious complication with a higher mortality than DKA. The South African series had a mortality of 7 out of 16 cases (44%), and causes of death included infection and stroke (Rolfe et al., 1995). Thrombotic complications are common in HNK, presumably due to extreme dehydration. HNK patients are generally much older than those with DKA, and this also predisposes to a poorer outcome.

Table 70.14. Managing hyperosmolar non-ketotic diabetic coma (HNK)

Management is essentially the same as for DKA (see Tables 70.12 and 70.13) except:
Larger fluid volumes are needed but because of advanced age, rate of replacement should be slower.
Use 0.9% saline, but if patient is hypernatraemic (Na >150 mmol/l), 'half-normal' (0.45%) saline should be used if available, until plasma Na <150 mmol/l.
Bicarbonate is never needed.
Less vigorous potassium replacement is required.
Use the same insulin system, but patients are more insulin-sensitive, and dose may be able to be later reduced.
Always use s.c. heparin 5000 units 8 hourly for the first 2–3 days.

Management

The basic treatment of HNK is as for DKA (see Tables 70.12 and 70.13), but with some important differences (Table 70.14). The fluid deficit is greater, so the total fluid replaced needs to be more, but it must be given carefully, as the patients are relatively old and may be sensitive to fluid overload. Because of the lack of acidosis bicarbonate is never needed, and potassium replacement can be a little less vigorous. Absence of ketosis makes patients more insulin sensitive, so sometimes smaller amounts of insulin are needed. As with DKA, one should aim for slow and steady correction of hyperglycaemia, rather than fast and precipitous drops. An important difference with DKA is that there is evidence that heparin improves outcome, presumably by reducing thrombotic deaths. It is not known whether 'full' or 'low dose' regimens should be used. In the interests of safety and simplicity a lower dose system is reasonable (Table 70.14).

Prevention

As with DKA, patient education is important. Training health care workers, and the development and distribution of protocols are also vital strategies. The outcome of this serious complication is, however, likely to remain high.

Outcome and mortality of diabetes in Africa

There have been relatively few structured mortality studies from Africa, making quantification of outcome difficult. However, a major study from Zimbabwe in 1980 (Castle & Wicks, 1980) recorded follow-up of 107 newly diagnosed diabetic patients (both type 1 and type 2). There was an 8 per cent inpatient mortality, and the survivors were followed for 6 years, with a high mortality of 41 per cent amongst those originally discharged alive. Most deaths were due to infection, hyperglycaemic emergencies (ketoacidosis and non-ketotic coma), or hypoglycaemia. Particular risk factors for an adverse outcome were male sex, alcohol abuse, and insulin treatment.

A further outcome study from sub-Saharan Africa was reported from Tanzania in 1990. A cohort of 1250 newly diagnosed patients were followed from 1981 to 1987, and actuarial 5-year survival rates were calculated (Swai et al., 1990; McLarty et al., 1990). For those not on insulin, 82 per cent survived 5 years, but the figure was only 60 per cent for the group on insulin treatment. Once again, the causes of death were predominantly metabolic and infective. The authors concluded that in Africa 'diabetes was a serious disease with a poor prognosis'. One reviewer also observed that the Tanzanian study indicated that 5 years from diagnosis, 40 per cent of those on insulin would die, whereas in Europe 40 per cent of similar patients would survive more than 40 years (Gill, 1997; Deckert et al., 1978).

There is some evidence, however, that, at least in some parts of Africa, the prognosis of diabetes is improving. Figures reported from Ethiopia (Lester, 1991, 1993, 1996) for example are considerably better than the Zimbabwean and Tanzanian data. Though metabolic emergencies were still the major cause of death, there was substantial mortality from renal failure (presumably diabetic nephropathy) and large vessel disease. A cohort of type 1 diabetic patients followed in Soweto, South Africa, has also shown relatively prolonged survival (Gill et al., 1995). At 10 years follow-up (mean diabetes duration 14 years), only 16 per cent had died. This figure was still in excess of western rates, though this was entirely due to nephropathy deaths (a complication still mostly untreatable in Africa).

There are obviously many factors that will affect mortality patterns amongst diabetic patients in different parts of Africa. These will include provision of medical care, and supply of insulin and other treatment modalities; as well as a variety of social, cultural and ethnic factors. As diabetes duration slowly extends, this in itself contributes to changing patterns of mortality (see Box) with diabetic nephropathy and macroangiopathy rapidly emerging in many areas. Large vessel disease is likely to accelerate in prevalence also because of western influences, e.g. smoking, obesity, reduced exercise and high-fat diets.

Mortality causes amongst African diabetic patients

Traditional	Emerging
• Infection	• Nephropathy
• Hypoglycaemia	• Stroke
• Ketoacidosis	• Coronary artery disease
• Hyperosmolar coma	

Improving African diabetes outcome significantly in the next 10–20 years will be a major challenge to health carers, and will require optimal treatment of diabetic complications, as well as control of the disease itself.

Conclusions

It is clear that diabetes is a common and complex condition, which is difficult to manage successfully even with adequate numbers of trained staff, and full provision of medicines and equipment. In most parts of Africa, such facilities are rarely available, and diabetes care becomes a challenging and potentially overwhelming task. Nevertheless, there are important elements of overall diabetes care which can be provided in even the most resource-poor areas, and can contribute greatly to patient control and well-being. These are as follows.

Organization of care

An efficiently organized system of care is vital. Care organization for non-communicable diseases (NCDs) in general is discussed in detail in Chapter 75. Devolved care to primary health care clinics in the patient locality is an important principle with central services at the district hospital for more difficult problems, and for those needing admission. A specific doctor in each district should take responsibility for diabetes care organization – possibly together with other NCDs such as asthma and hypertension.

Delivery of care

Even well-organized care will fail if it is not correctly delivered. Good care delivery requires communication with staff so they understand, accept and are trained for their role in diabetes care.

Patient education

It is widely accepted that patient education is a vital part of the overall 'package' of care for the diabetic patient. Again, the nurse is the most appropriate person to deliver such education, and sessions can be with an individual patient or in groups. Simple messages should promote disease understanding and self-care.

Staff training

If clinical care is to be efficient, and patient education is to be informed and appropriate, then a system of staff training needs to be in place. This is sometimes known as 'educating the educators' and should be organized by the doctor locally responsible for diabetes care. Training sessions can take many forms – for example an annual 'diabetes update day' (or half-day), monthly seminars, etc.

Patient empowerment

As mentioned, one of the functions of diabetes patient education is to allow patients to take control of, and to care for their own disease. This is known as 'empowerment', and should be a major aim of diabetes care. It can take the form of avoiding hypoglycaemia or managing intercurrent illness; and also ensuring that foot and blood pressure checks are carried out at clinic visits. The formation of patient organizations for people with diabetes has also proved successful in many areas (Dagogo-Jack, 1997).

References

Ahmed AM, Abdella ME. (1999). Diabetic ketoacidosis in the Sudan. *Pract Diabetes Dig*; **16**: 117–118.

Ahren B, Corrigan CB. (1984). Prevalence of diabetes mellitus in north-western Tanzania. *Diabetologia*; **26**: 333–336.

Alberti KGMM. (1994). Insulin-dependent diabetes: a lethal disease in the developing world. *Br Med J*; **309**: 754–755.

Alberti KGMM, Hockaday TDR, Turner RC. (1973). Small doses of intramuscular insulin in the treatment of diabetic coma. *Lancet*; **2**: 551–522.

Amoah AG, Owusu SK, Saunders JT et al. (1998). Facilities and resources for diabetes care at regional health facilities in southern Ghana. *Diabetes Res Clin Pract*; **42**: 123–130.

Amos AF, McCarty DJ, Zimmet P. (1997). The rising global burden of diabetes and its complications: estimates and projections to the year 2010. *Diabetic Med*; **14**, S1–S85.

Aspray TJ, Mugusi F, Rashid S et al. (2000). Rural and urban differences in diabetes prevalence in Tanzania: the role of obesity, physical inactivity and urban living. *Trans Roy Soc Trop Med Hyg*; **94**: 637–644.

Benbow S, Gill GV. (1998). Diabetic foot ulceration in developed and developing countries. *Int Diabetes Dig*; **8**: 8–10.

Castle WN, Wicks ACB. (1980). Follow-up of 93 newly diagnosed African diabetics for 6 years. *Diabetologia*; **18**: 121–123.

Ceesay MM, Morgan MW, Kamanda MO, Willoughby VR, Lisk DR. (1997). Prevalence of diabetes in rural and urban populations in southern Sierra Leone: a preliminary survey. *Trop Med Int Hlth*; **2**: 272–277.

Chale SS, Swai ABM, Mujinja PGM, McLarty DG. (1992). Must diabetes be a fatal disease in Africa? Study of costs of treatment. *Br Med J*; **304**: 1215–1218.

Coetzee EJ, Jackson WPU. (1980). Pregnancy in established non-insulin dependent diabetes – a 5 year study at Groote Schuur Hospital. *S Afr Med J*; **60**: 275–279.

Coleman R, Gill G, Wilkinson D. (1998). Non-communicable disease management in resource-poor settings: a primary care model from rural South Africa. *Bull Wld Hlth Org*; **76**: 633–640.

Cook, AR. (1901). Notes on the diseases met with in Uganda, central Africa. *J Trop Med*; **4**: 175–178.

Dagogo-Jack S. (1991). Pattern of diabetic foot ulcers in Port Harcourt, Nigeria. *Pract Diabetes Dig*; **2**: 75–78.

Dagogo-Jack S. (1997). Diabetes patient associations in Africa – the Nigerian experience. In *Diabetes in Africa*, eds GV Gill, J-C Mbanya, KGMM Alberti. pp 281–287. Cambridge, UK: FSG Communications Ltd.

Deckert T, Poulsen JE, Larsen M. (1978). Prognosis of diabetics with diabetes onset before the age of thirty-one. I Survival, causes of death, and complications. *Diabetologia*; **14**: 363–370.

Diabetes Control and Complications Trial (DCCT) Research Group. (1993). The effects of intensive treatment of diabetes on the development and progression of long-term complications in insulin-dependent diabetes mellitus. *N Engl J Med*; **329**: 977–986.

Drabo PPY, Kabore J, Lengani A. (1996). Complications of diabetes mellitus at the Hospital Center of Ouagadougou. *Bull Soc Pathol Exot*; **89**: 191–195.

Ducorps M, Baleynaud S, Mayaudon H, Castagne C, Bauduceau B. (1996). A prevalence survey of diabetes in Mauritania. *Diabetes Care*; **19**: 761–763.

Elamin A, Omer MJ, Hofvander Y, Tuvemo T. (1989). Prevalence of IDDM in schoolchildren in Khartoum, Sudan. *Diabetes Care*; **12**: 430–432.

Elbagir MN, Eltom MA, Mahadi EO, Berne C. (1995). Pattern of long-term complications in Sudanese insulin-treated diabetic patients. *Diabetes Res Clin Pract*; **30**: 59–67.

Elbagir MN, Eltom MA, Elmahadi EM, Kadam IM, Berne C. (1996). A population-based study of the prevalence of diabetes and impaired glucose tolerance in adults in northern Sudan. *Diabetes Care*; **19**: 1126–1128.

Elbagir MN, Eltom MA, Elmahadi EM, Kadam IM, Berne C. (1998). A high prevalence of diabetes mellitus and impaired glucose tolerance in the Danagla community in northern Sudan. *Diabet Med*; **15**: 165–169.

Erasmus RT, Fakeye T, Olukoga O et al. (1989). Prevalence of diabetes mellitus in a Nigerian population. *Trans Roy Soc Trop Med Hyg*; **83**: 417–418.

Erasmus RT, Blanco-Blanco E, Okesina AB, Matsha T, Gqweta Z, Mesa JA. (2001). Prevalence of diabetes mellitus and impaired glucose tolerance in factory workers from Transkei, South Africa. *S Afr Med J*; **91**: 157–160.

Feleke Y, Abdulkadir J. (1998). Urine glucose testing: another look at its relevance when blood glucose monitoring is unaffordable. *Ethiop Med J*; **36**: 93–99.

Fisch A, Pichard E, Prazuck T, Leblanc H, Sidibe Y, Brucker G. (1987). Prevalence and risk factors of diabetes mellitus in the rural region of Mali (West Africa): a practical approach. *Diabetologia*; **30**: 859–862.

Gill GV. (1997). Outcome of diabetes in Africa. In *Diabetes in Africa* eds GV Gill, J-C Mbanya, KGMM Alberti. pp 65–71. Cambridge, UK: FSG Communications Ltd.

Gill GV. (2000). Stability of insulin in tropical countries. *Trop Med Int Health*; **5**: 666–667.

Gill GV, Huddle KR. (1991). Patterns of insulin dependence in an African diabetic clinic. *Quart J Med*; **294**: 829–835.

Gill GV, Huddle KR. (1993). Hypoglycaemic admissions among diabetic patients in Soweto, South Africa. *Diabet Med*; **10**: 181–183.

Gill GV, Huddle KR, Rolfe M. (1995). Mortality and outcome of insulin-dependent diabetes in Soweto, South Africa. *Diabet Med*; **12**: 546–550.

Gill GV, Famuyiwa OO, Rolfe M, Archibald LK. (1998). Tropical diabetic hand syndrome. *Lancet*; **351**: 113–114.

Haile S. (2000). Management of diabetic ketoacidosis with lente insulin. *Diabetes Int*; **10**: 61.

Harrison LC. (1996). Cow's milk and IDDM. *Lancet*; **348**: 905–906.

Hellmuth E, Damm P, Molsted-Pedersen L. (2000). Oral hypoglycaemic agents in 118 diabetic pregnancies. *Diabet Med*; **17**: 507–511.

Herman WH, Ali MA, Aubert RE et al. (1995). Diabetes mellitus in Egypt: risk factors and prevalence. *Diabet Med*; **12**: 1126–1131.

Huddle KR, Gill GV. (1989). Reducing acute hyperglycaemic mortality in African diabetic patients. *Diabet Med*; **6**: 64–66.

Huddle KRL, Gill GV. (1994). Diabetes – a Soweto perspective. In *Baragwanath Hospital – 50 Years, a Medical Miscellany*, eds KRL Huddle, A Dubb. pp 69–82. Publ Baragwanath Hospital, Johannesburg.

Huddle KR, England M, Nagar A. (1993). Outcome of pregnancy in diabetic women in Soweto, South Africa 1983–1992. *Diabetic Med*; **10**: 290–294.

IDF Task Force. (1997). *Access to Insulin, a Report on the IDF Insulin Task Force on Insulin 1994–1997*. Brussels: International Diabetes Federation.

Jovanovic L, Pettitt D. (2001). Is gestational diabetes important, and worth screening for? In *Difficult Diabetes*, ed. GV Gill, JC Pickup, G Williams. pp. 36–52. Oxford: Blackwell Science.

Kadiki OA, Roaed RB. (1999). Epidemiological and clinical patterns of diabetes mellitus in Benghazi, Libyan Arab Jamahiriya. *E Medit Hlth J*; **5**: 6–13.

Kalk WJ, Huddle KRL, Raal FJ. (1993). The age of onset of insulin-dependent diabetes mellitus in Africans in South Africa. *Postgrad Med J*; **69**: 552–556.

Krentz AJ, Nattrass M. (1997). Acute metabolic complications of diabetes mellitus: diabetic ketoacidosis, hyperosmolar non-ketotic syndrome and lactic acidosis. In *Textbook of Diabetes*, ed. JC Pickup, G Williams.Oxford, UK: Blackwell Science; 39.1–39.23.

Lakhdar A. (2000). Diabetes mellitus and the fast of Ramadan. *Diabetes Int*; **10**: 9–10.

Lakhdar AA, Elhabroush S. (1999). Characteristics and outcome of ketoacidosis in Libyan diabetic patients. *Pract Diabetes Int*; **16**: 161–173.

Lester FT. (1991). Clinical status of Ethiopian diabetic patients after 20 years of diabetes. *Diabet Med*; **8**: 272–276.

Lester FT. (1993). Clinical features, complications and mortality in type 2 (non-insulin dependent) diabetic patients in Addis Ababa, Ethiopia, 1976–1990. *Ethiop Med J*; **31**: 109–126.

Lester FT. (1995). Amputations in patients attending a diabetic clinic in Addis Ababa, Ethiopia. *Ethiop Med J*; **33**: 15–20.

Lester FT. (1996). Mortality during eight years in a cohort of middle-aged Ethiopian diabetic patients. *Int Diabetes Dig*; **7**: 11–17.

Lester FT. (1997). Acute metabolic complications of diabetes. In *Diabetes in Africa*, ed. GV Gill, J-C Mbanya, KGMM Alberti. pp 35–42. Cambridge, UK: FSG Communications Ltd.

Lester FT, Keen H. (1988). Macrovascular disease in middle-aged diabetic patients in Addis Ababa, Ethiopia. *Diabetologia*; **31**: 361–367.

Levitt NS, Zwarenstein MF, Doepfmer S, Bawa AA, Katzenellenbogen J, Bradshaw D. (1996). Public sector primary care of diabetics—a record review of quality of care in Cape Town. *S Afr Med J*; **86**: 1013–1017.

Levitt NS, Bradshaw D, Zwarenstein MF, Bawa AA, Maphumolo S. (1997). Audit of public sector primary diabetes care in Cape Town, South Africa: high prevalence of complications in uncontrolled hyperglycaemia and hypertension. *Diabet Med*; **14**: 1073–1077.

Levitt NS, Steyn K, Lambert EV et al. (1999). Modifiable risk factors for Type 2 diabetes mellitus in a peri-urban community in South Africa. *Diabet Med*; **16**: 946–950.

Lutale JK, Justesen A, Lema RSM, Swai ABM, McLarty DG. (1991). Outcome of pregnancy in diabetic patients in Dar es Salaam, Tanzania. *Diabet Med*; **8**: 881–884.

Magzoub MM, Stephens HA, Gale EA, Bottazzo GF. (1991). Analysis of HLA-DR and -DQ gene polymorphism in Sudanese patients with type 1 (insulin-dependent) diabetes. *Immunogenetics* 1991; **34**: 366–371.

Malek R, Belateche F, Laouamri S et al. (2001). Prevalence of type 2 diabetes mellitus and glucose intolerance in the Setif area (Algeria). *Diabetes Metab*; **27**: 164–171.

Mbanya JC. (2000). Insulin treatment in Type 1 diabetes in the developing countries. *Int Diabetes Monitor*; **12**: 4–6.

Mbanya JC, Bonnici F, Nagati K. (eds.) (1996). *Consensus Guidelines for the Management of Non-Insulin Dependent Diabetes Mellitus in Africa*. Greece: Novo Nordisk A/S Vouliagmeni.

Mbanya JC, Ngogang J, Salah JN, Minkoulou E, Balkau B. (1997). Prevalence of NIDDM and impaired glucose tolerance in a rural and an urban population in Cameroon. *Diabetologia*; **40**: 824–829.

McLarty DG, Swai AB, Kitange HM et al. (1989a). Prevalence of diabetes and impaired glucose tolerance in rural Tanzania. *Lancet*; **1**: 871–875.

McLarty DG, Yusafai A, Swai ABM. (1989b). Seasonal incidence of diabetes mellitus in tropical Africa. *Diabet Med*; **6**: 762–765.

McLarty DG, Kinabo L, Swai AB. (1990). Diabetes in tropical

Africa: a prospective study, 1981–7. II. Course and prognosis. *Br Med J*; **300**: 1107–1110.

McLarty DG, Swai ABM, Alberti KGMM. (1994). Insulin availability in Africa: an insoluble problem? *Int Diabetes Dig*; **5**: 15–17.

McLarty D, Pollitt C, Swai A, Alberti KGMM. (1997). Epidemiology of diabetes in Africa. In *Diabetes in Africa*, eds GV Gill, J-C Mbanya, KGMM Alberti. pp. 1–17. Cambridge, UK: FSG Communications Ltd.

Mennen LI, Mbanya JC, Cade J et al. (2000). The habitual diet in rural and urban Cameroon. *Eur J Clin Nutr*; **54**: 150–154.

Mosley WH, Bobadilla JL, Jamison DT. (1993). The health transition: implications for health policy in developing countries. In *Disease Control Priorities in Developing Countries*, ed. DT Jamison, WH Mosley. New York: Oxford University Press.

Motala AA, Juta S, Pirie FJ, Omar MAK, Ojwong P. (1999). The role of glutamate decarboxylase (GAD) antibodies in South African black and Indian subjects. *S Afr Med J*; **89**: 461.

Motala AA, Omar MAK, Pirie FJ. (2000). Type 1 diabetes mellitus in Africa: epidemiology and pathogenesis. *Diabetes Int*; **10**: 44–47.

Mugusi F, Ramaiya KL, Chale S et al. (1995). Blood pressure changes in diabetes in urban Tanzania. *Acta Diabetol*; **32**: 28–31.

Nambuya AP, Otim MA, Whitehead H et al. (1996). The presentation of newly-diagnosed diabetic patients in Uganda. *Quart J Med*; **89**: 705–711.

Ohwovoriole AE, Kuti JA, Kabiawu SI. (1988). Casual blood glucose levels and prevalence of undiscovered diabetes mellitus in Lagos Metropolis Nigerians. *Diabetes Res Clin Pract*; **4**: 153–158.

Oli JM, Nwokolo C. (1979). Diabetes after infectious hepatitis – a follow-up study. *Br Med J*; **i**: 926–927.

Omar MA, Seedat MA, Dyer RB et al. (1994). South African Indians show a high prevalence of NIDDM and bimodality in plasma glucose distribution patterns. *Diabetes Care*; **17**: 70–74.

Owoaje EE, Rotimi CN, Kaufman JS, Tracy J, Cooper RS. (1997). Prevalence of adult diabetes in Ibadan, Nigeria. *E Afr Med J*; **74**: 299–302.

Papoz L, Ben Khalifa F, Eschwege E, Ben Ayed H. (1988). Diabetes mellitus in Tunisia: description in urban and rural populations. *Int J Epidemiol*; **17**: 419–422.

Papoz L, Delcourt C, Ponton-Sanchez A et al. (1998). Clinical classification of diabetes in tropical west Africa. *Diabetes Res Clin Pract*; **39**: 219–227.

Rahlenbeck SI, Gewbre-Yohannes A. (1997). Prevalence and epidemiology of micro- and macroalbuminuria in Ethiopian diabetic patients. *J Diabetes Comp*; **11**: 343–349.

Ramaiya KL, Swai AB, McLarty DG, Bhopal RS, Alberti KGMM.(1991a). Prevalences of diabetes and cardiovascular disease risk factors in Hindu Indian subcommunities in Tanzania. *Br Med J*; **303**: 271–276.

Ramaiya KL, Swai AB, McLarty DG, Alberti KGMM.(1991b). Impaired glucose tolerance and diabetes mellitus in Hindu Indian immigrants in Dar es Salaam. *Diabet Med*; **8**: 738–744.

Rolfe M.(1988). The neurology of diabetes mellitus in central Africa. *Diabet Med*; **5**: 399–401.

Rolfe M. (1997). Chronic complications of diabetes in Africa. In *Diabetes in Africa, ed.* GV Gill, J-C Mbanya, KGMM Alberti. pp. 43–50. Cambridge, UK: FSG Communications Ltd.

Rolfe M, Ephraim GG, Lincoln DC, Huddle KRL. (1995). Hyperosmolar non-ketotic diabetic coma as a cause of emergency hyperglycaemic admission to Baragwanath Hospital. *S Afr Med J*; **85**: 173–176.

Rotchford AP, Rotchford K, Machattie T, Gill GV. (2002). Assessing diabetic control – reliability of methods available in resource poor settings. *Diabet Med*; **19**: 195–200.

Rotimi CN, Dunston GM, Berg K et al. (2001). In search of susceptibility genes for type 2 diabetes in West Africa: the design and results of the first phase of the AADM study. *Ann Epidemiol*; **11**: 51–58.

Rwiza HT, Swai ABM, McLarty DG. (1986). Failure to diagnose diabetic ketoacidosis in Tanzania. *Diabet Med*; **3**: 181–183.

Seyoum B, Egziabher FG, Abdulkadir J, Alemayehu B. (1998). The occurrence of diabetic ketoacidosis in Ethiopia. *Int Diabetes Dig*; **9**: 38–39.

Sobngwi E, Mbanya J-C, Moukouri EN, Ngu KB. (1999). Microalbuminuria and retinopathy in a diabetic population of Cameroon. *Diabet Res Clin Pract*; **44**: 191–196.

Sobngwi E, Mauvais-Jarvis E, Vexiau P, Mbanya JC, Gautier JF (2001). Diabetes in Africans. Part 1: Epidemiology and clinical specificities. *Diabetes Metab*; **27**: 628–634.

Stannaway SERS, Gill GV. (2000). Protein glycosylation in diabetes mellitus: biochemical and chemical considerations. *Pract Diabetes Int*; **17**: 21–25.

Swai ABM, Lutale J, McLarty DG. (1990a). Diabetes in tropical Africa: a prospective study 1981–7. I Characteristics of newly presenting patients in Dar es Salaam, Tanzania 1981–7. *Br Med J*; **300**: 1103–1107.

Swai AB, McLarty DG, Sherrif F et al. (1990b). Diabetes and impaired glucose tolerance in an Asian community in Tanzania. *Diabetes Res Clin Pract*; **8**: 227–234.

Swai ABM, Lutale J, McLarty DG. (1993). Prospective study of incidence of juvenile diabetes mellitus over 10 years in Dar es Salaam, Tanzania. *Br Med J*; **306**: 1570–1572.

Teuscher T, Baillod P, Rosman JB, Teuscher A. (1987). Absence of diabetes in a rural West African population with a high carbohydrate/cassava diet. *Lancet*; **1**: 765–768.

Tshabalala G. (2001). Diabetic education in an African setting – focus on South Africa. *Diabetes Int*; **11**: 43–44.

United Kingdom Prospective Diabetes Study (UKPDS) Group. (1998a). Intensive blood-glucose control with sulphonylureas or insulin compared with conventional treatment and risk of complications in patients with type 2 diabetes (UKPDS 33). *Lancet*; **352**: 837–853.

United Kingdom Prospective Diabetes Study (UKPDS) Group. (1998b). Tight blood pressure control and risk of macrovascular and microvascular complications in type 2 diabetes: UKPDS 38. *Br Med J*; **317**: 703–720.

United Nations Population Fund. (2000). *State of World Population*. New York, USA.

van der Sande MA, Milligan PJ, Nyan OA et al. (2000). Blood pressure patterns and cardiovascular risk factors in rural and urban Gambian communities. *J Hum Hypertens*; **14**: 489–496.

WHO (1999). *Definition, Diagnosis and Classification of Diabetes Mellitus and its Complications. Part 1: Diagnosis and Classification of Diabetes Mellitus*. Geneva: World Health Organisation.

Zimmet P, Lefebvre P. (1996). The global NIDDM epidemic. *Diabetologia*; **39**: 1247–1248.

Zouvaris M, Pieterse AC, Seftel HC, Joffe BI. (1997). Clinical characteristics and outcomes of hyperglycaemic emergencies in Johannesburg, Africa. *Diabet Med*; **14**: 603–606.

Note The International Diabetes Federation (IDF) has a useful website (www.idf.org/home/index.cfm?node=1)

71 Asthma

Introduction

Asthma (Greek: 'panting') is an imprecisely defined syndrome of intermittent reversible airways obstruction. Patients experience episodic wheezing, cough and shortness of breath that may be severe. The condition is found world-wide but has a higher prevalence in the western world than in Africa. In the last decades the prevalence in both Africa and the developed countries is increasing (ISAAC Steering Committee, 1998). Genetic and environmental factors have a complex interaction in the pathogenesis and epidemiology of this disease.

Epidemiology and the problem in Africa

In Africa, asthma used to be an uncommon condition. Data from before 1990 show prevalence rates of 0.1–4 per cent (Table 71.1).

In economically developed countries the prevalence of asthma is typically between 5 and 10 per cent. At present, the prevalence of asthma is increasing both in western countries and in Africa. There are relatively few studies of the prevalence of asthma in Africa. The increase in Africa in the urban areas is obvious. There are substantial geographical variations. More 'westernized' urban regions have higher prevalence of asthma as compared to rural areas, where the disease is still rare (Yermaneberhan et al., 1997; Ng'ang'a et al., 1998; Yobo et al., 1997; Keeley et al., 1991; van Niekerk et al., 1979; Godfrey, 1975). Asthma prevalence in various regions over the years is outlined in Table 71.1.

Several hypotheses have been proposed to explain why asthma is increasing:

Allergen exposure

It has been suggested that increasing exposure to the house dust mite and possibly other allergens is responsible for the rising prevalence of asthma (ISAAC Steering Committee, 1998; Van Walraven et al., 2001).

The hygiene hypothesis

In this hypothesis children who are exposed to infections at an earlier stage of live divert their immune system into Th1 rather than Th2 immunity (see Chapter 6). Therefore, asthma in these children is less prevalent. This theory finds support in some epidemiological data: asthma appears to occur less frequently in the youngest of large families and in lower class families. Other data suggest that measles infection (Shaheen et al., 1996), other childhood infections (Alm et al., 1999) and exposure to farm animals (von Ehrenstein et al., 2000) protects against the development of asthma. More recently, exciting support is found in data suggesting that early BCG vaccination may prevent the development of atopy and maybe asthma (Aaby et al., 2000).

Parasite infection

The prevalence of infestation with intestinal parasites is much higher in Africa. Exposure to parasites may protect against asthma as suggested by studies in Gabon and the Gambia (van den Biggelaar et al., 2000, Nyan et al., 2001). Helminths stimulate strongly a Th2-response and cause therefore an opposite response as in the hygiene hypothesis. Either IgE receptor saturation or increased protective IgG4 or interleukin-10 production is a possible explanation. In the urban environment a more hygienic lifestyle leads to less parasitic infestations.

Diet and obesity

A western diet may be responsible for a higher asthma prevalence. This hypothesis could explain the increase of

Table 71.1. Prevalence of asthma in sub-Saharan Africa

Country	Asthma prevalence (%)	Year	Reference
The Gambia		2000	Van Walraven et al. (2001)
Tanzania (semi-rural)	3.5	1999	Sunyer et al. (2000)
Kenya (rural)	13.2	1997	Ng'ang'a et al. (1998)
South Africa	7–16	1996	ISAAC (1998)
Kenya (rural)	5	1996	ISAAC (1998)
Kenya (urban)	20	1996	ISAAC (1998)
Nigeria	11	1996	ISAAC (1998)
Ethiopia	2–12	1996	ISAAC (1998)
Ethiopia (rural)	1.3	1996	Yemaneberhan et al. (1997)
Ethiopia (urban)	3.6	1996	Yemaneberhan et al. (1997)
Ghana (urban)	2.2(poor)–4.7(rich)	1996	Yobo et al. (1997)
Ghana (rural)	1.4	1996	Yobo et al. (1997)
Zimbabwe (urban)	3.1–5.8	1990	Keeley et al. (1991)
Zimbabwe (rural)	0.1	1990	Keeley et al. (1991)
South Africa (rural)	0.14	1978	Van Niekerk et al. (1997)
South Africa (urban)	3.17	1978	Van Niekerk et al. (1997)
The Gambia	0	1974	Godfrey (1975)

asthma in urban compared to the rural communities in Africa and the higher incidence in the obese.

Atmospheric pollution

Pollution in the air may increase symptoms in asthma but have not been proven to cause asthma. The urban–rural discrepancy in the prevalence of asthma has been used as a supportive argument in favour of this theory. However, in the UK the pollution level has been falling in the last few years while asthma prevalence is increasing. Furthermore, the highest asthma prevalences in the world have been recorded in the least polluted areas such as New Zealand.

Pathogenesis

Key abnormalities in asthma (Busse & Lemanske, 2001)

Three pathophysiological features combine to cause the clinical syndrome of asthma. These features are all found in the medium-sized airways and are:

Table 71.2. Causes and exacerbating factors in asthma

Causes	
Genetic factors	**Inflammatory stimuli**
Atopy	Fumes, smoke and irritants
Gender	Allergens
Bronchial hyper-responsiveness	Anaphylaxis
	Viral infections
Environmental factors	
Allergen exposure	**Diurnal variation in airway diameter**
house dust mite	
tree and grass pollen	
Bermuda grass	**Drugs**
Kikuyu grass	Beta blockers
corn pollen	Non-steroidal anti-inflammatory drugs
flower pollen	
cat and dog dander	
feather	**Fog and cold air**
bat guano	
cockroach	**Exercise**
Occupational exposure (200 agents)	
High molecular weight agents	**Emotion**
animal proteins (flour, mites, bird dust)	
hardwood sawdust	
Low molecular weight agents	
isocyanates (varnish and car spraying)	
glutaraldehyde (cleaning endoscopes)	
Immunological history (early exposure to infection possibly protective)	
Smoking and passive smoking	
Cooking in unventilated huts	
Sleeping in kitchen areas	
Kerosene fuel use	

- mucosal inflammation and oedema
- bronchial hyper-responsiveness
- smooth muscle contraction.

Mucosal inflammation

Mucosal inflammation in asthma is characterized by increased numbers of lymphocytes, eosinophils and mast cells in the airway lining, with mucosal oedema and increased production of mucus. Inflammation can be caused by allergens and occupational sensitizers, and perpetuated by the exacerbating stimuli listed in Table 71.2.

Bronchial hyper-responsiveness (BHR)

BHR means that the airways have an abnormal constrictive response to stimuli such as irritant fumes, smoke,

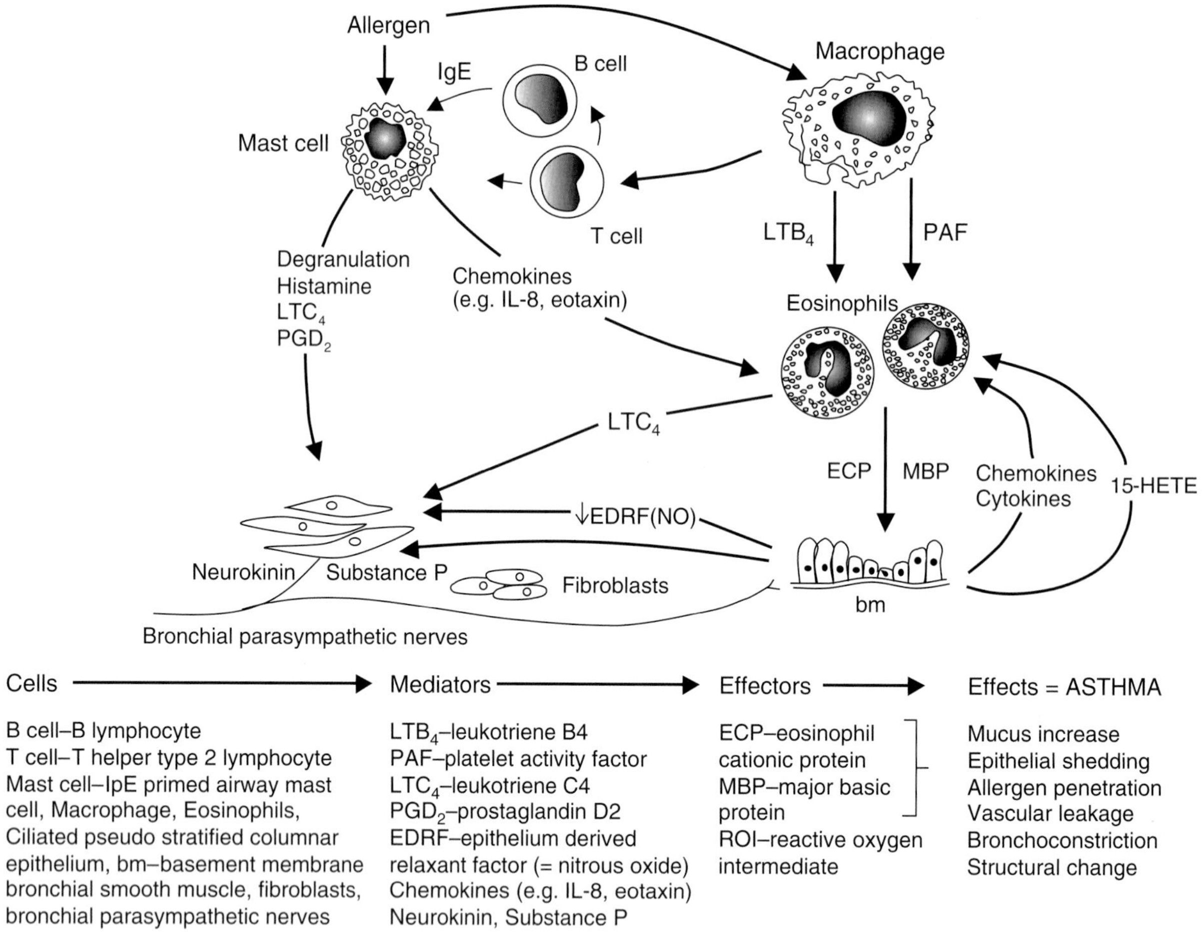

Fig. 71.1. Pathological mechanisms in asthma.

cold and exercise. It can be measured by giving patients low-dose inhaled histamine or methacholine in a respiratory function laboratory. BHR alone is not sufficient for a diagnosis of asthma. Mucosal inflammation causes an increase in baseline BHR, which in a non-asthmatic person may cause wheezing during a viral infection, but in an asthmatic patient may precipitate a serious attack.

Smooth muscle contraction

This is controlled by parasympathetic nerves, which produce a bronchoconstriction opposed by the directly acting bronchodilator effect of circulating adrenaline. Airway diameter is normally smallest when asleep at night and largest when exercising in the day (diurnal variation). Asthma is therefore often most troublesome at night due to the normal underlying diurnal variation. Smooth muscle contraction can occur by neural mechanisms involving the parasympathetic nerves, or as a result of local inflammation affecting muscle function.

The complex interactions at the cellular level in asthma are the subject of much active research. A simplified summary is presented diagrammatically in Fig. 71.1.

Causes of asthma and mechanisms of their effect

The important genetic and environmental factors causing asthma are listed in Table 71.2 and discussed below with reference to the key features of inflammation, bronchial hyper-responsiveness and smooth muscle contraction.

Genetic factors

Atopy

Atopy is a genetic predisposition to develop IgE-mediated allergy to common environmental materials. Atopic individuals may experience some or all of the triad of hayfever (seasonal allergic rhinitis, usually in response to grass and tree pollens), eczema and asthma, as well as having an increased tendency to develop allergy at work. They have increased total IgE and specific IgE to common allergens, and may have increased numbers of circulating eosinophils and airway mast cells. Atopy does not necessarily lead to clinical problems. Many people with raised IgE or positive skin tests have no evidence of asthma, hay fever and allergic rhinitis (Sunyer et al., 2000). The most common allergens to which atopic individuals are sensitive are the proteins of the house dust mite (*Dermatophagoides pterronysimus*), which, as the name suggests, ingests human skin scales. Similar levels of specific IgE to house dust mite have been found in community surveys in Nigeria and Australia (Faniran et al., 1999). The common allergens known in the western world are also troublesome in Africa. However, allergens such as cockroach proteins may contribute specifically to the development of asthma in Africa (Rosenstreich et al., 1997). Other allergens reported specifically in Africa include Bermuda grass (Kambarami et al., 1999), corn and flower pollens (Green & Luyt, 1997; Awotedu et al., 1992), threshing products (Yemaneberhan et al., 1997), Kikuyu grass (Potter et al., 1993), and bat guano (el-Ansary et al., 1987).

Gender

Gender is important. Male children have smaller airways and increased atopy and are therefore more likely to experience symptoms. Over the age of 40, atopy becomes less important and asthma is more common in women.

Bronchial hyper-responsiveness (BHR)

BHR is found in 20 per cent of the whole population, but only about one-third of people with BHR will have asthma. BHR depends on genetic factors, increases with age and is more common in women. The regulation of this response is poorly understood but is known to be dependent on both neural and local mechanisms.

Environmental factors

Allergen inhalation

Allergen inhalation, such as exposure to pollen in an atopic patient, can incite an asthmatic response in a number of ways. Allergens cause an IgE-mediated response which causes an early mast cell degranulation with the multiple secondary effects. Later activation of T-helper 2 lymphocytes contributes to inflammatory response (see Chapter 6).This mucosal inflammation is characterized by lymphocyte and eosinophil infiltration and mucosal oedema as well as increased mucus production and smooth muscle contraction.

Occupational sensitizers

Over 200 agents are described as causes of occupational asthma. High molecular weight agents, e.g. flour dust, animal allergens, act in the manner described above for environmental allergens and typically evoke an immediate response. Low molecular weight agents, e.g. platinum salts, may bind to a tissue protein to form a conjugate that can then elicit an IgE-dependent allergic response. Alternatively, some low molecular weight agents, e.g. isocyanates, cause asthma by non-IgE-related mechanism: this is usually a delayed response and may involve a T-lymphocyte or neurogenic inflammatory mechanism. Up to 20 per cent of exposed workers may develop asthma if ventilation is poor in a workplace using known sensitizers (Rees et al., 1998; Mengesha & Bekele, 1998; Deschamps et al., 1998). Domestic consumption of refined fossil fuels, e.g. kerosene, has been shown to increase the risk of allergic sensitization (Venn et al., 2001).

Cold air and exercise

The inhalation of cold air or a short period of physical exercise can provoke an asthma attack in patients with bronchial hyper-responsiveness. The mechanism is thought to involve smooth muscle contraction following airway drying and changes in lung fluid osmolality. There is no specific inflammatory response.

Drugs

The two most important classes of drugs that can cause asthma are beta-blockers and non-steroidal anti-inflammatory drugs (NSAIDs).

Beta-blockers

Stimulation of airway smooth muscle by beta-2-adrenoceptors can be blocked by the use of beta-blocking drugs used in hypertension. These drugs may cause sudden severe bronchoconstriction. Beta-blockers should not be used in asthma patients.

Non-steroidal anti-inflammatory drugs (NSAIDs)

NSAIDs can precipitate severe asthma in susceptible patients. NSAIDs must therefore be prescribed with caution in asthma patients. More specific NSAIDs have been developed to avoid this problem but are not yet in widespread use.

Emotion

Intense emotional outbursts can precipitate asthma attacks in some patients, presumably via a neural mechanism. More importantly, asthma attacks themselves cause severe anxiety and so calm confident management is very important.

Infections

Many viral infections cause wheezy bronchitis in children due to airway inflammation, in turn leading to asthma in susceptible patients. In adults, viral infections may precipitate asthma attacks, but allergic rhinitis produced by allergen exposure can produce similar upper respiratory symptoms and diagnostic confusion. Bacterial infection frequently causes wheezing in the context of chronic lung disease, but organisms have not been isolated in repeated studies of patients with simple acute asthma attacks, and trials of antibiotics have failed to alter outcome. Bacterial infection is therefore not considered to be an important trigger of asthma attacks, nor an inducer of asthma.

Smoking and air pollution

Cigarette smoking causes increased airway inflammation, increased susceptibility to viral infections and increased bronchial response to allergen. Studies of specific air pollutants such as sulphur dioxide indicate a link between pollution, respiratory symptoms and emergency admissions. This is thought to relate to an irritant effect on bronchial responsiveness but allergen absorption through inflamed mucosa may also be a factor. Large-scale allergen spills, e.g. soya flour, have resulted in 'epidemic' asthma by IgE-dependent mechanisms.

Diet

Specific food allergens can precipitate wheezing as part of a general allergic response. Peanuts and shellfish are some of the most common food allergens. Food-induced asthma appears to be much less common in Africa than in industrialized countries.

Clinical symptoms and signs of asthma

Wheezing, cough and shortness of breath are the most common symptoms of asthma. Wheezing, mainly expiratory, may be an audible sound or a sensation felt in the chest. Patients may attribute the sensation to an abnormality in the throat. Cough is paroxysmal, involuntary and productive of a small volume of sticky sputum. It is typically worst at night or in the early morning and wakes the patient from sleep. Repeated severe coughing bouts can produce vomiting and cracked ribs. Shortness of breath (dyspnoea) felt by asthma patients is different from that of normal exertion. It is a 'tightness' that is not painful but is very uncomfortable and is accompanied by a sensation of not being able to get enough air into the chest. The dyspnoea occurs at rest, is worse at night and can be exacerbated by minimal exercise.

Patterns of presentation

Asthma is a widely varied syndrome that can develop at any age but several patterns can be distinguished. It is useful to classify patients according to severity, immunological status (atopic/non-atopic), and the presence or absence of an extrinsic stimulus.

Acute severe asthma

This is a medical emergency and prompt management is essential. Clinical signs indicating a severe attack are summarized below. Patients with acute severe asthma have often had a delayed presentation for treatment or

Features of severe and life-threatening asthma – the presence of any of this list should cause immediate concern.

In severe asthma the patient:
- is unable to speak in sentences
- has a respiratory rate of more than 25/minute
- has a pulse of greater than 110/min
- has a peak flow of less than 50% of predicted best.

The condition is immediately life-threatening if the patient:
- has a silent chest, cyanosis or feeble respiratory effort
- has bradycardia or hypotension
- is exhausted, confused or unconscious.

The patient should be treated with the following.

Immediately:
- oxygen (4–10 l/min)
- salbutamol 5 mg via nebulizer or spacer, if available
- prednisolone tablets 60 mg or intravenous hydrocortisone 300 mg
- no sedatives of any kind
- CXR to exclude pneumothorax
- i.v. aminophylline 250 mg over 20 minutes if not on oral aminophylline

Subsequently:
- continue oxygen and steroids
- nebulized or inhaled via spacer salbutamol 5 mg and ipratropium bromide 500 μg every 6 hours with nebulized salbutamol 2.5 mg up to every 20 minutes in-between
- aminophylline infusion (1 g over 24 hours).

If not successful:
- intubate.

previous poor management. In Africa, management is often hampered by lack of available drugs, lack of oxygen, and lack of monitoring equipment. In Lagos 49 per cent of asthma deaths were attributed to delay in seeking medical help (Bandele, 1996).

Atopic asthma

The presentation of atopic asthma is classically described as nocturnal cough and wheezing at a young age among patients with a history of allergy. In Africa, the presentation is often later, at 10 to 15 years old. A history of infantile eczema is common – 50 per cent of infants with severe eczema later develop asthma. Hay fever is closely associated with asthma but only 10 per cent of patients with hay fever progress to develop asthma. Common allergens, e.g. house dust and pollen, precipitate attacks and patients' response to treatment is good.

Occupational asthma

Patients with no history of allergy may develop shortness of breath and wheeze related to work. The history may sometimes be difficult to elicit because allergen exposure can result in early, late or dual responses as described above. Workers exposed to an allergen causing an immediate response give a clear history of shortness of breath at work that recovers quickly on leaving work and at the weekends. Workers with delayed responses, however, may have less obvious histories and may take up to 10 days to experience an improvement of symptoms after leaving the workplace. Increasing industrialization and poor work conditions make occupational asthma a real threat to respiratory health in African cities in the future.

Late onset asthma

This pattern describes patients who develop wheezing and shortness of breath for the first time as adults. These patients have no history of allergy, a relatively insidious onset of disease and a poor response to inhaled therapy. It is important to exclude patients in whom a history of allergy has merely not been recognized, as these patients will respond well to inhaled therapy.

Other asthmatic syndromes

Significant respiratory impairment can follow irritant exposure. The reactive airways dysfunction syndrome describes patients with persistent wheezing following a major respiratory insult. The initial insult, e.g. inhalation of acid fumes, usually results in several weeks of severe illness requiring hospital admission, with the asthma-like syndrome following a protracted course for years after this insult. Chronic exposure to irritant stimuli causes cough and airways irritation, but not asthma.

Infection with *Aspergillus fumigatus* can cause a syndrome of difficult asthma (allergic bronchopulmonary aspergillosis, ABPA). This is a syndrome caused by a mixed immunological (IgE, IgG, and cellular) response. The airways are colonized by fungus and thus show chronic inflammation. ABPA is characterized by sudden exacerbations, which may be countered by a short course of high dose oral steroids. The syndrome has usually a poor response to treatment and often needs regular oral steroids.

Clinical signs

The characteristic signs of asthma are increased respiratory rate, prolonged expiratory phase and wheeze. However, asthma is an episodic condition and the examination may be entirely normal. The distinct features on examination in acute severe asthma are summarized in the summary box. Patients with chronic asthma and COPD may have an over-inflated 'barrel-chest' deformity (p. 920).

Investigation

Asthma is often a difficult disease to investigate or manage in rural Africa (Unwin et al., 1999). In the economically developed countries allergic investigations such as skin prick tests and serum allergen specific IgE are useful. In Africa, such tests are less useful (Sunyer et al., 2000; Selassie et al., 2000). In practice, a careful history and sometimes a trial of allergen avoidance has to suffice.

Respiratory function testing

When available, this should be carried out.

Spirometry

This will demonstrate airways obstruction. An FEV1 less than 80 per cent of predicted for age and height, or an FEV1/FVC ratio of less than 75 per cent indicates obstruction. For a diagnosis of asthma, this obstruction should be either variable over time or reversible with pharmacological agents (2 puffs salbutamol and repeat assessment after 30 min).

Peak flow rate

The low cost and portability of the mini peak flow meter have made serial measurements of the peak expiratory flow rate (PEFR) popular. The serial record is valuable in determining the pattern of disease and the response to treatment especially inhaled steroids. Early morning dipping is characteristic of atopic asthma and work-relatedness of occupational asthma. Exercise testing can give similar information if FEV1 measurement is available. After 5 minutes of brisk exercise, the normal response is a 5 per cent increase in FEV1. A decrease of 15 per cent is strongly suggestive of asthma. Inhalation challenge with allergen is potentially dangerous and should not be attempted, but a trial return to work monitored with serial PEFR measurement is useful.

Differential diagnosis

Whilst asthma is an easy diagnosis in a typical case, there may be difficulty when there is co-existing lung disease. The main differential in an African setting is as follows.

Wheezy bronchitis

This is a common clinical picture in children suffering from viral respiratory infection, including measles. The cough and wheeze sounds like asthma, but there is little response to bronchodilators and the condition is self-limiting with supportive measures, including antibiotics if secondary bacterial infection is present (see Chapter 77).

Chronic obstructive pulmonary disease (COPD)

With the increase in smoking throughout Africa, due to intensive promotion by tobacco companies, comes the inevitable increase in chronic lung disease. Many cases are mistakenly labelled as asthma, and sometimes receive costly and/or potentially harmful treatment (such as oral steroids) for years without significant benefit. It is important to carry out lung function testing with measurement of bronchodilator response to delineate asthma from COPD. A short trial of oral steroids is recommended in some cases to help distinguish the two. A typical trial would be prednisolone 30 mg daily for 3 weeks with objective measurements of pulmonary function before and after, taking a >15 per cent rise in FEV1 or PEFR as a positive indication of asthma.

Tropical eosinophilia

This is less common in Africa than in some parts of India. Intense blood and sputum eosinophilia, with soft fleeting chest X-ray changes and clinical wheezing, cough and fever may be confused with asthma. Symptoms are worse at night. Microfilariae may be found in lung biopsies, though not in blood, and serological tests for filariasis are positive. The condition is self-limiting, though sometimes it may persist for years.

Helminth infection

Brief wheeziness may occur when the larvae of certain parasites migrate through the lungs. The most common in Africa are hookworm and ascaris (Chapter 30).

Management and treatment (for acute severe asthma see emergencies)

Preferred management

The modern mainstays of therapy for asthma are inhaled steroids and bronchodilators (Lalloo et al., 2000; Motala et al., 2000) but, as these are often not available, alternatives are discussed later.

Allergen avoidance

Where a specific allergen is identified, either at home or at work, it should be avoided – advice which may be difficult or impossible to follow. In cases of atopic asthma, it is worth avoiding excessive soft furnishings, using foam rather than feather pillows and trying to avoid heavy concentrations of house dust. These changes are unlikely to control symptoms completely but will make therapy more straightforward. For occupational sensitizers, the diagnosis should be as certain as possible because proper allergen avoidance will demand a change of workplace.

Inhaled therapy

Inhaled steroids (beclomethasone, budesonide, fluticasone) are delivered by metered dose inhaler (MDI), dry powder device, CFC-free device, or nebulizer. Asthma is an inflammatory condition and inhaled steroid is appropriate in all but the mildest cases, most of which do not present to hospital in Africa. Unfortunately, all forms of inhaled steroid are expensive and in many health facilities throughout Africa they are not available.

The management of asthma can be described at three levels (see Box).

General principles of management

- Give inhaled steroids in sufficient dose to minimize the use of bronchodilators.
- Use a step-up and step-down approach
- Ensure active patient involvement.

Use of metered dose inhalers (MDIs)

MDI medication is often wasted because poor technique causes the medication to be deposited in the throat where

Asthma management

Management at referral centre level (preferred management everywhere)

Move through the following as severity increases:

Bronchodilators, e.g. salbutamol 2 puffs of 100 μg, as required for symptomatic wheeze. If more than three times a week, add regular inhaled steroids, e.g. beclomethasone 2 puffs of 250 μg twice daily, via a spacer

Regular long-acting bronchodilators (aminophylline 250–400 mg twice daily, salmeterol 50 μg twice daily)

Regular oral steroids

Step down when possible

Double the dose of inhaled steroid during exacerbations

Management at district hospital level

Occasional bronchodilators, e.g. salbutamol 2 puffs of 100 μg

Inhaled steroids are often scarce or not available. Patients who are thought to be compliant and have sufficient understanding of the disease can be selected for the available inhaled steroids.

Regular bronchodilators (aminophylline 250–400 mg twice daily, salmeterol 50 μg twice daily)

Regular oral steroids

Step down when possible

Management at health centre level

This is the most difficult setting for managing asthma.

Inhalers (steroids or bronchodilators) are often scarce or not available. Patients who are thought to be compliant and have sufficient understanding of the disease can be selected for the available inhalers

Regular oral bronchodilators, e.g. aminophylline 250–400 mg twice daily or salbutamol 5 mg twice daily

Short course of steroids in case of exacerbations

Regular oral steroids

Step down when possible

it is swallowed. The box lists the important steps in ensuring that inhaled medication is taken correctly.

- Where possible, prescribe an inhaled steroid twice daily via a spacer from the start (Zar et al., 1999).
- Maintain this dose until intermittent bronchodilator therapy is required no more than three times per week.
- Then reduce the dose incrementally ensuring that the patient remains symptom free and does not need to increase their use of bronchodilator.
- Double the dose of inhaled steroid during exacerbations.
- Explain to the patient that the steroid is the 'preventer' of symptoms and the bronchodilator is merely a 'reliever'.

Correct use of MDI medication

Note: All MDI medication should ideally be taken using a spacer.

- Shake the MDI
- Insert the MDI into the spacer or into a hole cut into the bottom of a plastic bottle (see Fig. 71.2)
- Put one puff into the spacer or bottle
- Put the spacer mouthpiece or bottle neck between the lips
- Breathe in deeply and slowly (30 seconds)
- Hold your breath for 10 seconds at full inspiration
- Take a second breath in the same way

Repeat the process for further puffs of medication

If a spacer is unavailable

- Shake the MDI
- Place the mouthpiece between the lips
- Breathe out steadily
- Fire the inhaler while taking a long slow (30 seconds) breath in
- Hold the breath at full inspiration for 10 seconds.

As first aid out of hospital in an emergency

- Put 10–20 puffs of bronchodilator into the spacer and breath continuously through the spacer.
- Get to hospital very urgently

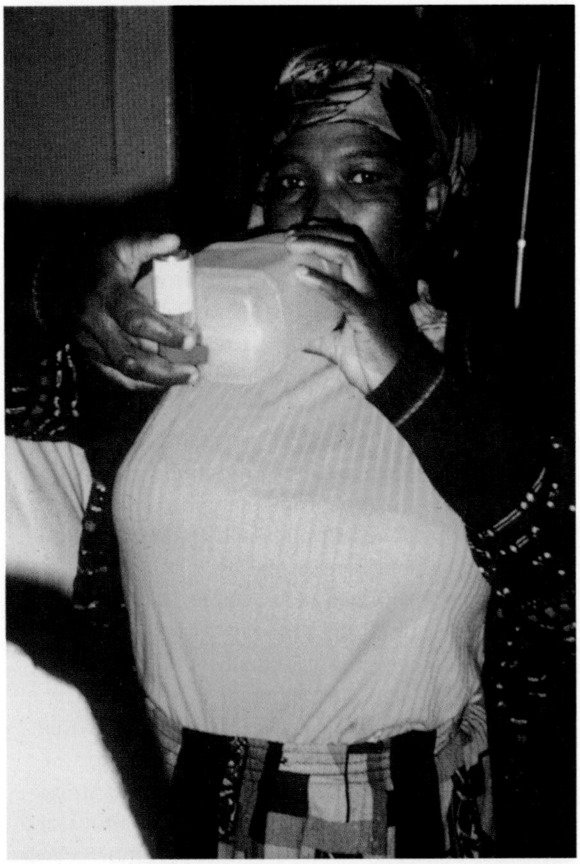

Fig. 71.2. Spacer made from a plastic milk bottle.

Inhaled bronchodilators

These are beta-adrenergic (salbutamol, terbutaline, fenoterol) or anticholinergic (ipratropium bromide). Again, delivery mechanisms make all of these treatments expensive. Generic salbutamol by MDI and spacer is the cheapest and most effective. However, even the cheapest canisters are not available for routine use and should only be used in selected and compliant patients with the inhalation technique carefully checked. Two puffs will relieve moderate symptoms. This dose can be increased as needed but tremor and tachycardia will occur at higher doses. Long-acting bronchodilators (salmeterol and formoterol) are a significant advance in the control of nocturnal symptoms where they can be afforded. Muscle cramp is a common side effect, which tends to persist.

Cromoglycate and nedocromil are primarily used for exercise-induced asthma and asthma in children in the western countries. They do not offer a good alternative to inhaled steroid as a symptom preventer.

Leukotriene antagonists (montelukast, zafirilukast) block the action of LTD4 at the receptor and have been recently introduced as an adjunct to conventional inhaled therapy. They are very expensive and their place in asthma treatment is yet to be established. They do not offer an appropriate first-line oral alternative to inhaled therapy.

Alternative asthma management when inhalers are not available

Theophylline

Oral bronchodilators of the phosphodiesterase class are cheap and moderately effective alternatives. Give a long-acting preparation of theophylline or aminophylline twice daily starting at a low dose and titrating up according to tolerance. Theophyllines have a narrow therapeutic range, and common side effects are gastric irritation, nausea and palpitations. These drugs undergo hepatic metabolism and so alcohol and rifampicin increase clearance. Inhibitors of hepatic metabolism such as erythromycin and cimetidine increase toxicity.

Oral beta agonists such as salbutamol and terbutaline have systemic side effects, especially anxiety and tremor, but are used if there are no alternatives.

Oral steroids can be life saving. Unfortunately, they have serious long-term side effects and should be used only during asthma exacerbations and for the shortest possible period afterwards. Most importantly in Africa, the use of oral steroids may make patients more susceptible to infections, particularly overwhelming tuberculosis and bacterial infections, helminth infections, viral infections (herpes zoster) and possibly the more severe manifestations of malaria. Particularly in areas with a high prevalence of HIV, oral steroids should be used with great caution and for short periods only. Prolonged use of oral steroid causes Cushing's syndrome with obesity, osteoporosis, muscle weakness and diabetes. If using oral steroid, start at 30 to 40 mg prednisolone daily for 4 to 14 days. Give clear warnings to the patient regarding the risk of infection.

Patients with late-onset asthma who require frequent repeated courses of oral prednisolone may be better managed with low dose maintenance therapy with oral steroids. Aim for the lowest possible dose (5–10 mg prednisolone daily).

Chapter 75 of this book presents simple-to-follow management plans for several common non-communicable diseases in a rural African setting. The suggested plan for asthma management is on page 833, and should be read in conjunction with the management set out in the above paragraphs.

Asthma, pregnancy and breast-feeding

Asthma will not change in 50 per cent of women when pregnant – of the remainder, half will get better and half worse. Well-controlled asthma has no adverse effect on the outcome of pregnancy. Inhaled therapy is not toxic to the fetus. Oral steroids have rarely caused both maternal and fetal hypoadrenalism, easily avoided by gradual weaning from high doses. Theophylline can cause irritability in breast-fed infants. In summary, it is better to risk these minor drug-related side effects than to under-treat asthma.

Prognosis

Mild and moderate childhood asthma resolves at puberty to recur in 50 per cent of adults. Severe early childhood asthma, early eczema, a family history of atopy, failure of resolution at puberty and smoking are predictive of continuing adult symptoms. Atopic asthma starting in adulthood is less likely to resolve. Occupational asthma has a poor prognosis unless early removal from allergen exposure is achieved. Poorly treated, occupational asthma may progress to fixed obstructive airways disease. Adult (late-onset) asthma with no extrinsic cause is poorly responsive to therapy and does not typically resolve. Patients surviving a severe asthma attack are at increased risk of further severe attacks and death.

Unsolved problems

There are two major problems in Africa.

1. How can we prevent the increase in asthma prevalence that was so marked in Europe during the economic development of the twentieth century?
2. How can modern effective treatment for asthma be made available to all patients within the limited health budget of most modern African states?

References

Aaby P, Shaheen SO, Heyes CB et al. (2000). Early BCG vaccination and reduction in atopy in Guinea-Bissau. *Clin Exp Allergy*; **30**: 644–650.

Alm JS, Swartz J, Lilja G et al. (1999). Atopy in children of families with an anthroposophic lifestyle. *Lancet*; **353**: 1485–1488.

Awotedu AA, Ooyejide C, Ogunlesi A, Onadeko BO. (1992). Skin sensitivity patterns to inhalant allergens in Nigerian asthmatic patients. *Centr Afr J Med*; **38**: 187–191.

Bandele, E.O. (1996). A ten-year review of asthma deaths at the Lagos University Teaching Hospital. *Afr J Med Med Sci*; **25**: 389–392.

Deschamps, F., Sow, M.L., Prevost, A et al. (1998). Prevalence of respiratory symptoms and increased specific IgE levels in West-African workers exposed to isocyanates. *J Toxicol Environ Health*; **54**: 335–342.

el-Ansary EH, Tee RD, Gordon DJ, Taylor AJ. (1987). Respiratory allergy to inhaled bat guano. *Lancet*; **8528**: 316–318.

Faniran AO, Peat JK, Woolcock AJ (1999). Prevalence of atopy, asthma symptoms and diagnosis, and the management of asthma: comparison of an affluent and a non-affluent country. *Thorax*; **54**: 606–610.

Godfrey RC. (1975). Asthma and IgE levels in rural and urban communities of the Gambia. *Clin Allergy*; **5**: 201–207.

Green R, Luyt D. (1997). Clinical characteristics of childhood asthmatics in Johannesburg. *S Afr Med J*; **87**: 878–882.

International Study of Asthma and Allergies in Childhood (ISAAC) Steering Committee. (1998). Worldwide variation in prevalence of symptoms of asthma, allergic rhinoconjunctivitis, and atopic eczema: ISAAC. *Lancet*; **351**: 1225–1232.

Kambarami RA, Marechera F, Sinbanda EN, Chitiyo ME. (1999). Aero-allergen sensitisation amongst atopic Zimbabwean children. *Centr Afr J Med*; **45**: 144–147.

Keeley DJ, Neill P, Gallivan S. (1991). Comparison of the prevalence of reversible airways obstruction in rural and urban Zimbabwean children. *Thorax*; **46**: 549–553.

Lalloo, U.G., Bateman, E.D., Feldman, C et al. (2000). Guideline for the management of chronic asthma in adults—2000 update. South African Pulmonology Society Adult Asthma Working Group. *S Afr Med J*; **90**: 540–552.

Mengesha YA, Bekele A. (1998). Relative chronic effects of different occupational dusts on respiratory indices and health of workers in three Ethiopian factories. *Am J Ind Med*; **34**: 373–380.

Motala C, Kling S, Gie R et al. (2000). Guideline for the management of chronic asthma in children – 2000 update. Allergy Society of South Africa Working Group. *S Afr Med J*; **90**: 524–528, 530, 532.

Ng'ang'a LW, Odhiambo JA, Mungai MW et al. (1998). Prevalence of exercise induces bronchospasm in Kenyan school children: an urban-rural comparison. *Thorax*; **53**: 919–926.

Nyan OA, Walraven GEL, Banya WAS et al. (2001). Atopy, intestinal parasite infection and total serum IgE in rural and urban adult Gambian communities. *Clin Exp Allergy*; **31**: 1672–1678.

Potter PC, Mather S, Lockey P et al. (1993). IgE specific immune responses to an African grass (Kikuyu, Pennisetum clandestinum). *Clin Exp Allergy*; **23**: 581–586.

Rees D, Nelson G, Kielkowski D, Wasserfall C, da Costa A.(1998). Respiratory health and immunological profile of poultry workers. *S Afr Med J*; **88**: 1110–1117.

Rosenstreich DL, Eggleston P, Kattam M et al. (1997). The role of cockroach allergy and exposure to cockroach allergen in causing morbidity among inner-city children with asthma. *N Engl J Med*; **336**: 1356–1363.

Selassie FG, Stevens RH, Cullinan P et al. (2000). Total and specific IgE (house dust mite and intestinal helminths) in asthmatics and controls from Gondar, Ethiopia. *Clin Exp Allergy*; **30**: 356–358.

Shaheen SO, Aaby P, Hall AJ et al. (1996). Measles and atopy in Guinea-Bissau. *Lancet*; **347**: 1792–1796.

Sunyer J, Toreregrosa J, Anto JM et al. (2000). The association between atopy and asthma in a semirural area of Tanzania (East Africa). *Allergy*; **55**: 762–766.

Unwin N, Mugusi F, Aspray T et al. (1999). Tackling the emerging pandemic of non-communicable diseases in sub-Saharan Africa: the essential NCD health intervention project [In Process Citation]. *Publ Hlth*; **113**: 141–146.

van den Biggelaar AHJ, van Ree R, Rodrigues LC et al. (2000). Decreased atopy in children infected with Schistosoma haematobium: a role for parasite-induced interleukin-10. *Lancet*; **356**: 1723–1727.

van Niekerk CH, Weinberg EG, Shore SC et al. (1979). Prevalence of asthma: a comparative study of urban and rural Xhosa children. *Clin Allergy*; **9**: 319–314.

van Walraven GEL, Nyan OA, van der Sande MAB et al. (2001). Asthma, smoking and chronic cough in rural and urban adult communities in The Gambia. *Clin Exp Allergy*; **31**: 1679–1685.

Venn AJ, Yemaneberhan H, Bekele Z, Lewis SA, Parry E. Brittan J. (2001). Increased risk of allergy associated with the use of kerosene fuel in the home. *Am J Respir Crit Care Med*; **164**: 1660–1664.

von Ehrenstein OS, Von Mutius E, Illi S et al. (2000). Reduced risk of hay fever and asthma among children of farmers. *Clin Exp Allergy*; **30**: 187–193.

Yemaneberhan H, Bekele Z, Venn A. (1997). Prevalence of wheeze and asthma and relation to atopy in urban and rural Ethiopia. *Lancet*; **350**: 85–90.

Yobo AEO, Custovic A, Taggart SC et al. (1997). Exercise induced bronchospasm in Ghana: differences in prevalence between urban and rural schoolchildren. *Thorax*; **52**: 161–165.

Zar HJ, Brown G, Donson H, Brathwaite N, Mann MD, Weinberg EG (1999). Home-made spacers for bronchodilator therapy in children with acute asthma: a randomised trial. *Lancet*; **354**: 979–982.

Suggested further reading

Respiratory Medicine. (1995). 2nd edition. London: W B Saunders Co. Ltd.

Busse WW, Lemanske RF Jr. (2001). Asthma. *N Eng J Med*, **344**: 350–362.

Drazen J.M. (2000). Asthma and related titles. *In Up to Date 8.3.* Washington, USA: Up to Date Inc., or at www.uptodate.com.

72

Hypertension in Africa

The problem in Africa

The Global Burden of Disease study estimated that, in 1990, non-communicable diseases (NCDs) contributed 14 per cent of the total burden of disease in sub-Saharan Africa (30% for adults aged 15–59 years). By 2020, these figures are likely approximately to double (Murray & Lopez, 1996). Much of the burden of disease from NCDs is due to hypertension, and this burden is increasing (Cooper et al.,1998).

Hypertension has not always been a major health problem in Africa. Early studies found a very low prevalence of hypertension: for example, Donnison (1929) found no cases of hypertension or arteriosclerosis among 1800 admissions to a rural Kenyan hospital. Hypertension remains rare in most remote or nomadic tribes and in rural, pastoral or subsistence agricultural communities (Pauletto et al., 1994). Making valid comparisons of hypertension prevalence over time and between populations is difficult due to differing definitions of hypertension and population age structures. However, most recent studies using a cut-off point of 160/95 mm Hg report a prevalence of between 5 and 15 per cent, often higher in urban than rural areas (Astagneau et al., 1992; Cooper et al., 1997a; Steyn et al., 1996; Swai et al., 1993; van der Sande et al., 2000). Some recent studies have found much higher prevalences: for example, 29 per cent rural, and 31 per cent urban in South Africa (Mollentze et al., 1995); a male/female prevalence of 16.4 per cent and 12.1 per cent (urban) and 5.4 per cent and 5.9 per cent (rural) in Cameroon (Mbanya et al. 1998); and an age-standardized prevalence of hypertension of 18 per cent for men and 22 per cent for women in Dar es Salaam, and 13 per cent for both men and women in a rural area of Tanzania (Edwards et al., 2000).

A 1991 meta-analysis (Wilson et al., 1991) compared mean systolic blood pressures (BP) in 40–49-year-old people from sub-Saharan Africa, the West Indies and the USA. There was a clear gradient, with the lowest systolic blood pressure in East African populations, intermediate levels in other sub-Saharan African populations and the highest levels in the West Indies and USA. However, in the 1997 Tanzanian study (Edwards et al., 2000) the mean systolic blood pressure in men aged 40–49 years in Dar es Salaam (136 mm Hg) was higher than in all the urban sub-Saharan African populations (mean 131 mm Hg) in the previous study, and similar to that in urban populations in the USA and West Indies (mean 135 mm Hg).

What is hypertension?

In any population, systolic and diastolic blood pressures are approximately normally distributed. 'Hypertension' is usually defined in relation to a BP cut-off point – for example, 140 mm Hg systolic or 90 mm Hg diastolic. An individual above the chosen level is defined as 'hypertensive' and in need of treatment to reduce their blood pressure and risk of hypertensive complications.

The cut-off point is to some extent arbitrary, as the risk of complications from hypertension increases continuously throughout blood pressure range. A complexity is added by the observation that the risk of hypertensive complications varies between and within populations, with age, sex, and the presence or absence of risk factors such as smoking and diabetes. Hence, of two patients from the same population and with the same BP level but with different other risk factors, only one may require treatment. Thus the definition of hypertension is somewhat blurred, and indeed has changed over time. However, the key points are shown in the Box:

> **Risks of hypertension**
> - The risk of hypertensive complications increases continuously throughout the BP range.
> - Numerous rigorously conducted randomized controlled trials have shown that the treatment of hypertension is effective in reducing the incidence of, and mortality from, hypertensive complications such as stroke and heart disease.

The physiology of blood pressure control

Blood pressure is the pressure of blood within the arterial system. Systolic pressure is the peak pressure occurring during left ventricular contraction, and diastolic pressure is the pressure during left ventricular relaxation. It is maintained by vascular tone and an intact aortic valve. Pulse pressure is the difference between systolic and diastolic pressures, and mean arterial pressure is a time-weighted measure equal to the sum of the diastolic pressure and one-third of the pulse pressure. The arterial BP is determined by the product of the cardiac output and the total peripheral resistance of the circulation; so that, if either increases, BP will rise.

> BP = cardiac output × peripheral resistance

Arterioles and peripheral resistance

Arterioles make the largest contribution to total peripheral resistance, because their combined cross-sectional area is smaller than the large arteries or capillary beds. For an individual arteriole, resistance to blood flow is determined by its lumen size, length and the viscosity of the blood (largely determined by haematocrit). The walls of the arteries, arterioles, larger venules and veins contain smooth muscle innervated by sympathetic nerve fibres. Increased activity in these fibres increases muscle tone. Contraction of arteriolar wall smooth muscle reduces lumen size, increasing peripheral resistance and blood pressure.

Cardiac output

Cardiac output is the volume of blood in litres per minute pumped by the heart. At rest, it is around 5 litres/minute and can increase to 25 litres/minute during vigorous exercise. Cardiac output is the product of heart rate and left ventricular stroke volume, and approximately equals venous return. Thus it is also determined by the intravascular volume. Breathing, gravity and the pumping action of skeletal muscles can all influence venous return and hence cardiac output.

Heart rate

The heart rate is regulated by the action of autonomic nerves on the pacemaker cells of the sinoatrial node. Parasympathetic stimulation decreases (negative chronotropy) and sympathetic stimulation increases (positive chronotropy) the heart rate. Circulating adrenal medullary catecholamines (adrenaline and noradrenaline) also increase heart rate. These, and sympathetic stimulation, increase the force of contraction during systole for any given end-diastolic volume (positive inotropy).

Homeostatic mechanisms in blood pressure regulation

A range of homeostatic mechanisms maintain blood pressure within a narrow range under normal conditions. Intrinsic mechanisms include autoregulation of blood flow within vascular beds. For example, vasoconstriction results from smooth muscle contraction in response to stretching of the vessel wall. Vasodilatation occurs in response to tissue metabolites and local vasoactive substances, such as nitric oxide, released in response to a variety of stimuli. Extrinsic regulation of plasma volume occurs through neural mechanisms and hormonal systems.

Short-term regulation of blood pressure

Neural mechanisms are largely responsible for this. A rise in BP results in increased firing of the baroreceptor afferents in the aortic arch and the carotid sinuses. This activates the parasympathetic nervous system and causes a reflex slowing of the heart, peripheral vasodilatation and a fall in blood pressure. Autonomic nerve fibres and hormones exert extrinsic control over the heart (see above) and circulation in response to information arising from cardiovascular receptors. Activity in the sympathetic nervous system raises blood pressure through vasoconstriction which increases peripheral resistance, and through an increased heart rate and strength of cardiac contraction; so that the cardiac output rises.

Long-term regulation of blood pressure

Hormonal mechanisms involved in longer-term regulation of blood pressure include the renin–angiotensinogen–angiotensin–aldosterone system (RAAS) (see Fig. 72.1), anti-diuretic hormone (ADH), and atrial natriuretic peptide (ANP). These largely act, directly or indirectly, through regulation of fluid volume by the kidneys.

The kidneys and blood pressure

The kidneys have an enormous capacity to conserve sodium, retaining as much as 98 per cent of sodium

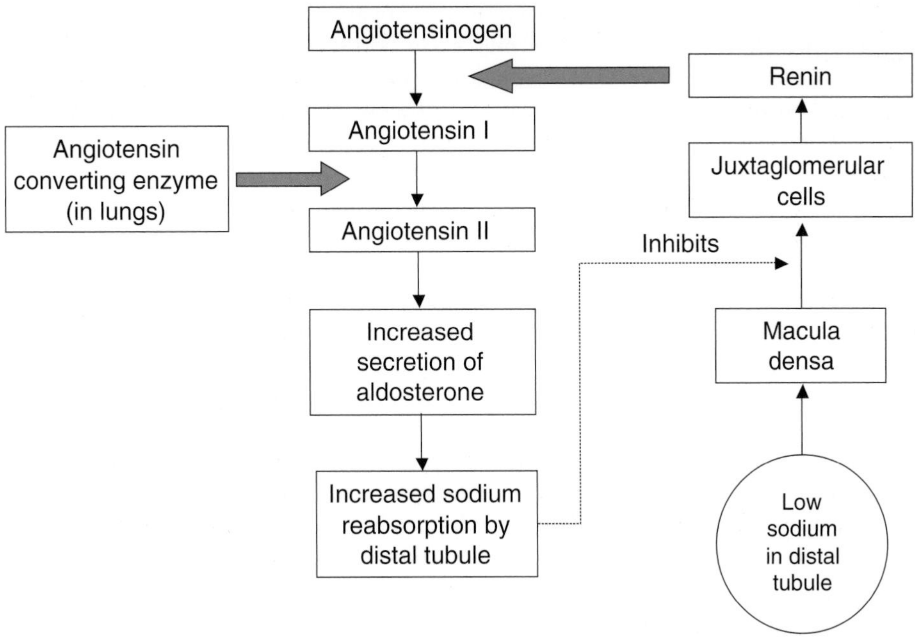

Fig. 72.1. Renin–angiotensinogen–angiotensin–aldosterone system.

passing through the renal circulation. Sodium reabsorption is under the control of the RAAS system (Fig. 72.1). When the blood pressure (and hence renal perfusion pressure) drops, renin is released. Renin increases the conversion of angiotensinogen to angiotensin I, which in turn is converted to angiotensin II in the lungs. This immediately raises BP through vasoconstriction, and also promotes sodium and fluid retention by stimulating the production of aldosterone in the adrenal cortex. The opposite sequence occurs with sodium and fluid overload. The action of renin is inhibited by ANP, released in response to increased atrial volume.

The RAAS is a relatively slow-acting mechanism, since increased aldosterone secretion requires the synthesis of new proteins. Its effects start at 1 hour and reach a peak after about 24 hours.

Anti-diuretic hormone

Urine osmolality is modulated by the secretion of ADH (arginine vasopressin, or AVP). During dehydration, ADH secretion is increased and water is reabsorbed by the collecting ducts so that a small volume of concentrated urine is produced. During overhydration, the opposite occurs.

The aetiology of hypertension

About 95 per cent of hypertension is of unknown aetiology and is termed 'essential hypertension'. There are many theories about, and postulated contributory factors which influence the level of blood pressure in individuals and populations. In all except some isolated, traditional pastoral communities, systolic BP tends to rise progressively throughout childhood, adolescence and adulthood, to reach an average value of about 140 mm Hg by the seventh or eighth decade. Diastolic blood pressure does not rise as steeply and tends to remain flat, or to decline after the fifth decade; so that, with advancing age, pulse pressure widens and isolated increases of systolic pressures become more common.

Genetic factors

Some rare forms of hypertension, such as Liddle's syndrome, are clearly genetic in origin. Essential hypertension develops in individuals due to behavioural or environmental factors acting on a genetic predisposition. Evidence for the genetic basis of essential hypertension comes from a variety of studies. There is greater concordance of hypertension in monozygotic twins compared to non-twin siblings, and siblings are more likely to be concordant for hypertension than their parents. The marked correlation of blood pressure, even between siblings or twins living apart, suggests concordance is not due only to shared environmental exposures (Bouchard et al., 1980). Twin studies in Los Angeles, Barbados and Dominica suggest that inherited factors are the major reasons for individual differences in blood pressure for African Americans (Grim et al., 1995).

Genetic factors probably account for 25–40 per cent of the variability in blood pressure between individuals. Inheritance is polygenic, with at least 10–15 genes involved. Genes coding for angiotensinogen and others influencing renal function and sodium metabolism are likely candidates. However, genetic factors are unlikely to explain the large variations in hypertension and blood pressure distributions between populations (Cruickshank et al., 2001). Rapid changes in BP distributions over time, and in individual BP levels in response to migration (Poulter et al., 1990), suggest that behavioural and environmental factors are strong determinants at individual and population levels.

Fetal origins hypothesis (early life influences)

Exposures in fetal life and infancy may influence the development of adult diseases including hypertension, cardiovascular diseases and their risk factors. According to the fetal origins hypothesis, metabolic and physiological parameters in adult life may be programmed by adverse influences, particularly undernutrition, during critical periods of early development (Barker, 1995). Numerous well-conducted studies in many different populations around the world have found that possible markers of poor fetal nutrition, such as low birthweight and increased placental size, are related inversely to blood pressure throughout life, with the exception of the period of rapid growth during adolescence (Law & Shiell, 1996). The mechanisms are unclear. One hypothesis is that excess glucocorticoid hormones during pregnancy cause intrauterine growth retardation and programme raised blood pressure. Another postulates that poor fetal nutrition reduces arterial elasticity (Barker, 1995). An inverse relation between blood pressure and birthweight has been demonstrated in African children in Soweto (Levitt et al., 1999), in Zimbabwe (Woelk et al., 1997) and in Zaire (Longo-Mbenza et al., 1999). Since the prevalence of low birthweight and poor nutrition during pregnancy is common in sub-Saharan Africa, this is a potentially important mechanism in the causation of hypertension.

Salt intake and sodium/fluid retention

Long-term exposure to large sodium loads may cause a sustained rise in intravascular volume and hence blood pressure. Increased salt intake is associated with higher blood pressure in individuals and populations, and a higher rate of BP increase with age (Elliot et al., 1996). Populations with a salt intake of lower than 50 mmol per day appear not to suffer from primary hypertension (Kaplan, 1993). People of African origin seem to be particularly sensitive to salt intake and exhibit enhanced salt retention. This is due to reduced excretion of sodium loads, increased blood volume and lower plasma renin levels (Seedat, 1999). One hypothesis states that enhanced salt retention is caused by an inherited defect in sodium handling – a physiological adaptation to living in hot and humid climates; and that in black Americans this was amplified by selective survival of individuals with an enhanced ability to conserve salt during the Atlantic voyages of the slave trade (Grim et al., 1995). Interestingly, individuals from indigenous populations in areas of Africa with a natural abundance of salt, such as The Gambia and Senegal, tend to retain a salt load less well than people in salt-poor areas (Akinkugbe, 1989). Others, however, dispute the 'slavery hypothesis' (Curtin, 1992). For example, Africans who have moved to Europe more recently also have higher blood pressure than white people. The finding that rural Zulus have a higher plasma renin activity than urban Zulus suggests that environmental influences are also important (Hoosen et al., 1985).

A potassium-deficient diet is another possible aetiological factor for hypertension in Africa. An increased dietary sodium to potassium ratio was implicated in causing the rise in blood pressure observed following rural to urban migration in Kenya (Poulter et al., 1990).

Environment and habits

Epidemiological studies from throughout the world, including Africa, have demonstrated that the following lifestyle or behavioural factors are important in the aetiology of hypertension (JNC VI, 1997):

- high body weight and central obesity
- high sodium intake
- excessive alcohol consumption
- insufficient physical activity.

These provide an important focus for prevention and treatment of hypertension.

Obesity and Body Mass Index (BMI)

Of the modifiable risk factors, obesity or high BMI is most strongly associated with hypertension in African studies, at a population level (Cooper et al., 1997) and in individuals (Astagneau et al.,1992; Mufunda et al., 2000; Steyn et al., 1996; van der Sande et al., 2000).

Urban migrants – why does blood pressure increase?

One suggestion is that urban: rural differences in hypertension in African populations may be due to chronic physical or mental stress, for example, associated with an urban lifestyle (Bogin, 1988). This may cause excessive sympathetic nervous system activity and a sustained rise in blood pressure. One African rural to urban migration study has demonstrated rapid increases in BP following migration. The authors suggested that an interaction between environmental stress, increased weight and increased dietary sodium intake may initiate the rise in blood pressure (Poulter et al, 1990). However, specific evidence for stress as a cause of hypertension is generally weaker than for other risk factors (JNC VI, 1997).

Secondary hypertension

In about 5 per cent of patients with hypertension, there is an underlying cause. These causes can be grouped as follows:

- Renal disease, e.g. chronic pyelonephritis, chronic glomerulonephritis, polycystic kidneys
- Reno-vascular disease, e.g. renal artery stenosis
- Endocrine conditions (rare), e.g. phaeochromocytoma, Conn's syndrome, Cushing's syndrome, secondary hyperaldosteronism, acromegaly.
- Coarctation of the aorta (rare)
- Drugs, e.g. steroids, non-steroidal anti-inflammatory drugs, oral contraceptives

Pathology of hypertension

Small arterioles

Mild to moderate hypertension causes hypertrophy of smooth muscle in small arterioles. Subsequent degenerative changes lead to hyaline deposition and a decrease in lumen size resulting in reduced blood supply to the kidneys, heart and brain. In patients with lipid abnormalities, accelerated endothelial atherosclerotic disease occurs, so that lipids are more easily deposited within the vascular wall.

Malignant hypertension

The hallmark of malignant hypertension is fibrinoid necrosis, with fibrin deposition in small arterioles, intravascular thrombosis, reduced numbers of small vessels in vascular networks (microvascular rarefaction), and reorganization of wall structure. This causes more severe tissue ischaemia so that the patients may present with hypertensive encephalopathy and multifocal neurological deficits.

Central arteries

Stiffening of the central arteries (the thoraco-abdominal aorta and its main branches) leads to increased systolic and pulse pressure, and diminished capacity for coronary perfusion. The aortic diameter also increases. Hypertensive patients with wide pulse pressures and isolated systolic hypertension (ISH) have a particularly poor prognosis. Hypertensive thickening of the carotid and more peripheral artery walls is associated with increased risk of myocardial and cerebral infarction.

Left ventricle

Sustained hypertension leads to left ventricular hypertrophy (LVH) with enlarged cardiac myocytes and increased deposition of extracellular collagen matrix. The left ventricle becomes less compliant. Unless hypertension is treated, LVH may result in congestive cardiac failure.

Complications of hypertension ('target organ damage')

Hypertension can lead to:

- stroke
- cardiac failure
- renal failure
- coronary artery disease.

The size of the risk was demonstrated in a pooled analysis of nine prospective observational studies of over 400 000 adults without cardiovascular disease at base line (MacMahon et al., 1990). The incidence of coronary heart disease was nearly five times higher, and the risk of stroke over ten times higher, among the highest (mean diastolic BP 105 mm Hg) compared with the lowest BP strata (mean diastolic BP 76 mm Hg). A 7.5 mm Hg lower diastolic pressure was associated with a 29 per cent lower risk of coronary heart disease and 46 per cent lower risk of stroke.

Systolic and diastolic pressures are independent predictors of risk of complications, and isolated systolic hypertension is also associated with an increased risk of stroke (Staessen et al., 1992). Cardiovascular and renal risk increases progressively through the entire range of blood pressure with no evidence of a threshold (MacMahon et al., 1990). The risk of complications is greatly increased by the presence of other risk factors such as diabetes, pre-existing cardiovascular disease and smoking.

Frequency of complications in black populations

The frequency of hypertensive complications differs between ethnic groups and is higher in black populations in the US and UK. For example, compared to the general population, African Americans have an 80 per cent higher stroke rate, 50 per cent higher heart disease rate and 320 per cent higher rate of end-stage renal disease (JNC VI, 1997). However, these results may not be generalizable to indigenous African populations. The higher rate of complications in black people may reflect the earlier onset and greater severity of hypertension (Cooper & Liao, 1992). Another possible explanation is an absence or reduction of the usual nocturnal dip in blood pressure. This has been associated with increased renal and cardiovascular complications (Profant & Dimsdale, 1999).

Mortality related to hypertension

There is little prognostic data for hypertension from Africa. In a cohort study from Oyo State, Nigeria, a 20 mmHg increase in diastolic BP was associated with a 60 per cent increased risk of death over a 2-year period (Kaufman et al., 1996). Without treatment, malignant hypertension has a mortality of almost 100 per cent within 2 years.

Renal disease

Renal complications are particularly common in Africa (Mensah et al., 1994). In South Africa, hypertension causes 35 per cent of end stage renal disease (ESRD) in black people but only 4 per cent in white people (Veriava et al., 1990).

Heart disease

Although ischaemic heart disease (IHD) is rare in Africa, LVH and congestive heart failure (CHF) are common (Mensah et al., 1994).

Cerebrovascular disease

Unexpectedly high cerebrovascular mortality is emerging in sub-Saharan Africa (Bradshaw et al., 1995; Walker et al., 2000). Untreated hypertension is the most important treatable risk factor in African patients with stroke, and chronic hypertension is present in up to 60–80 per cent of such patients (Mensah et al., 1994).

Management of hypertension

Most patients in Africa are likely to be treated at the primary care level, because hypertension is so prevalent and resources for health care are so limited. Many community-based studies from around the world have found that hypertension is poorly detected and treated (Fuentes et al., 2000). The 'rule of halves' is often quoted. This states that of all patients with high blood pressure, only about a half are detected. Of those detected only half are treated, and of treated hypertensives only half are controlled. The rule of halves (or worse) has been confirmed in population-based studies from Senegal, Zaire, South Africa, Tanzania, Cameroon and Ghana (Astagneau et al., 1992; Edwards et al., 2000; Mbanya et al., 1998; M'Buyamba-Kabangu et al., 1986; Mollentze et al., 1995; Pobee, 1993; Steyn et al., 1996).

Do patients take prescribed treatment?

Poor adherence to treatment and loss to follow-up or non-attendance undermines good hypertension control (Kital & Irwig, 1979; Saunders et al., 1982). In a hypertensive control programme in Ghana, default rates after 4 years among hypertensive patients were 62 per cent among civil servants and 38 per cent from the general population (Pobee, 1993).

Organization of hypertension care

Good hypertension care depends on good organization and delivery of health care. One cost-effective and sustainable method of delivering hypertension care is through nurse-led systems in primary health care settings. Such an approach using clinical protocols has been shown to be effective in South Africa (Coleman et al., 1998). Ensuring that care is easily accessible is important to reduce loss to follow-up. Accessibility is best achieved by organizing follow-up at local health centres near patients' homes. This will minimize costs related to travel and drugs. Some essential requirements for the delivery of care and some interventions to improve and maintain the quality of care are described in the Box.

The rationale for treatment

The aim of hypertension management is to reduce the risk of complications, and BP control is a major component of this. Drug treatment of hypertension is highly effective – stroke is reduced by 38–42 per cent, coronary events by 14–16 per cent and cardiovascular mortality by

Achieving high-quality hypertension care

Essential requirements for the delivery of hypertension care	Examples of interventions to improve the quality of hypertension care
Accessible health care facilities	Structured clinical records
Functioning diagnostic equipment	Staff training
Sufficient trained staff	Management guidelines and protocols
Affordable and sustainable source of essential drugs	Audit (structured monitoring and feedback of the quality of care)
Referral centre for difficult clinical cases and emergencies	Patient education and empowerment/ Patient held records
	Structured annual reviews
	Call and recall (for non-attenders) systems
	Dedicated hypertension/chronic diseases clinics and staff

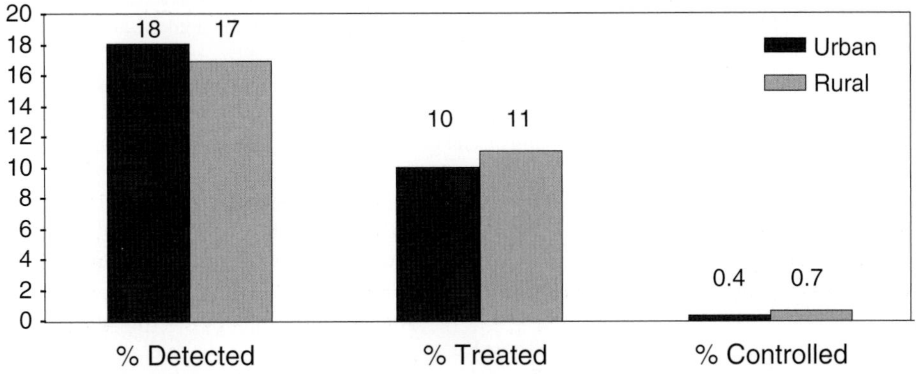

Fig. 72.2. Hypertension detection, treatment and control in rural and urban Tanzania. Hypertension defined as BP ≥ 140/90 Hg or on current anti-hypertensive treatment, control = BP < 140/90 mm Hg (Edwards et al., 2000).

about 21 per cent (Collins et al., 1990; Gueyffier et al., 1997). However, hypertension is not an isolated condition, and management will also depend on whether other risk factors for cardiovascular complications, such as diabetes and smoking, are present. Management should involve interventions to control BP and to reduce cardiovascular risk.

Major components of care

These include:

- screening and detection
- diagnosis
- clinical evaluation and investigation
- initial and continuing treatment
- follow-up and review.

Screening and detection (Fig. 72.2)

Unless all adults in a population have their BP measured regularly, most hypertensive patients will remain undetected. Awareness of hypertension among patients identified as hypertensive in recent population-based surveys from Africa vary from 11 per cent in a rural population in Cameroon (Mbanya et al., 1998) to 61 per cent in an urban population in South Africa (Steyn et al., 1996). To treat a small proportion of hypertensive patients in primary and secondary care, while most patients remain untreated, and at high risk of complications, in the community, makes little sense.

To ensure that hypertension is detected, adults should have their BP measurements regularly – at least once every 5 years. In adults with high normal readings (over 130/85 mm Hg) or previous raised readings, monitoring of BP every year is advised (Ramsey et al., 1999), though it may be difficult to follow up these patients. The best way to achieve good BP monitoring in a population is unclear. There is little evidence that expensive organized population screening is more effective than opportunistic measurements ('case-finding') of blood pressure of patients attending clinics for other reasons (Ebrahim, 1998).

Diagnosis

Clinical features of hypertension

Hypertension is generally symptomless but may present with symptoms and signs relating to underlying causes in secondary hypertension (see below), or due to cardiovascular or renal complications. Malignant hypertension may present with headache and multiple neurological symptoms and signs.

Definition of hypertension

The WHO has produced a definition and classification of hypertension (Guidelines Subcommittee of the WHO, 1999). These and other recent guidelines generally use a cut-off point of 140/90 mmHg to define hypertension and as a target level below which hypertension is defined as 'controlled' in previously diagnosed hypertensive patients (Guidelines Subcommittee of the WHO, 1999; JNC VI, 1997; Ramsey et al., 1999). This cut-off point is derived from the findings of recent clinical trials, notably the 'HOT' trial (Hansson et al., 1998), which demonstrated treatment benefit for blood pressures between 140 and 160 mmHg systolic, with an optimum target blood pressure for the best clinical outcome at about 139/83 mmHg.

Risk in different populations

The relative reduction in risk appears constant in different populations and throughout the BP distribution. However, the absolute benefit is greatest in patients or populations at greatest risk of complications, and so is greatest for patients with higher levels of blood pressure and patients with higher cardiovascular risk.

What cut-off point is realistic for Africa?

The cut-off point chosen should reflect a feasible and sustainable level of hypertension treatment in the community. This will depend on: local availability of clinics, equipment, trained staff and drugs; the burden of disease due to hypertension-related complications; and the cost-effectiveness and priority of hypertension management compared to interventions for other conditions. Given current resources and priorities in Africa, and the levels of absolute and relative risk of cardiovascular complications, a realistic threshold for treatment may be 160 mm Hg systolic blood pressure (Cooper et al., 1998).

Blood pressure measurement

Blood pressure should be measured correctly as recommended in established guidelines (see Box). Currently, the gold standard method for clinical practice remains the mercury sphygmomanometer. Except in the case of malignant hypertension, the diagnosis of hypertension should be based on readings repeated over a period of weeks or months. The number of readings and the time period depends on the grade of hypertension. For mild hypertension, monthly readings over 4 to 6 months are appropriate, while for severe hypertension two to three visits over a 1- to 2-week period is more sensible.

Blood pressure measurement

- Use a properly calibrated and maintained device.
- Measure BP sitting except for the elderly or diabetics (standing).
- Explain procedure to patient.
- Remove tight clothing and support arm at level of heart.
- Use appropriate cuff size (smaller for children, larger for fat arms).
- Place cuff 2–3 cm above position of maximum pulsation of brachial artery.
- Inflate cuff to 30mm Hg above point where brachial artery pulsation disappears.
- Place stethoscope over brachial artery.
- Deflate cuff at 2 mm Hg/second.
- Systolic blood pressure = point at which tapping sounds first appear.
- Diastolic BP = point at which tapping sounds disappear (Phase V).
- Take at least two measurements per visit, record BP in both arms at first visit if evidence of peripheral vascular disease.

Ambulatory blood pressure measurement

There is increasing interest in using non-invasive devices to measure BP levels away from the clinic setting – 'ambulatory blood pressure' measurement. Ambulatory BP readings are about 12/7mm Hg lower than clinic readings (Ramsey et al., 1999), and measured over the daytime or 24-hour periods, may better predict target organ damage than clinic BP measurement. The method is also used to diagnose 'white coat hypertension', when blood pressure is excessively elevated compared to levels measured away from the clinic. This should be excluded in patients with resistant hypertension, despite multiple drug treatments. However, the role of ambulatory measurement in clinical practice is not agreed and, due to the cost of the equipment, it is unlikely to be feasible in routine clinical practice in Africa. Investigation for white coat hypertension is not indicated in patients with multiple risk factors for cardiovascular complications or existing target organ damage, since treatment will be required whatever the findings.

Clinical evaluation and investigation

There are six objectives of the clinical evaluation and investigation of hypertensive patients:

- confirmation of diagnosis and level of BP
- investigation of secondary causes of hypertension
- diagnosis of target-organ damage and associated clinical conditions
- assessment of risk factors for hypertensive complications
- identification of contraindications to drug treatments
- identification of patients requiring referral for further investigation or specialist management.

The assessment of hypertensive patients is summarized in Table 72.1.

Investigation of secondary hypertension

Secondary hypertension occurs in about 5 per cent of patients. Abnormal results from the medical history, examination and screening tests for newly diagnosed hypertensive patients (see Table 72.1), will usually suggest when secondary hypertension is a possibility. Other situations in which there should be a heightened suspicion are malignant or accelerated phase hypertension, and treatment resistant (more than three drugs) hypertension in young patients (especially less than 25 years).

Further investigations will be determined by the possible diagnoses. Specialist endocrine investigations will be required to diagnose conditions such as Conn's syndromes and phaeochromocytoma. Abdominal ultrasound will detect hydronephrosis, polycystic kidneys or diminished renal size; but is not usually sensitive enough to detect renal artery stenosis, for which the definitive test remains renal arteriography. Ultrasound may show adrenal tumours though CT scanning is more sensitive.

Initial and continuing treatment

Goals of treatment

The aim of hypertension treatment is to reduce the risk of morbidity and mortality from the complications of hypertension (principally stroke, renal failure and cardiovascular disease). This is achieved through lowering BP and also controlling other factors which contribute to the risk of cardiovascular complications. Hence, decisions about the initiation of treatment should be based on BP level and an assessment of other factors contributing to the risk of hypertensive complications.

Stratification by risk of hypertensive complications

Decisions about when to introduce treatment for hypertension should be based on the overall level of cardiovascular risk, not BP levels alone. Recent clinical guidelines have provided clinical algorithms to guide hypertension management. Some require extensive investigations, and the use of cardiovascular risk assessment tables or computer programmes (e.g. Ramsey et al., 1999). This approach is probably unrealistic in most settings in Africa. An alternative risk stratification method, based on WHO guidelines, is shown in Table 72.2. In practice, it will rarely be possible to measure serum lipid levels. However, given the current rarity of hyperlipidaemia in African populations (Oelofse et al., 1996; Swai et al., 1993), this will not usually result in an underestimate of cardiovascular risk.

Non-pharmacological treatment

Numerous recent trials have confirmed that non-pharmacological treatments (NPT) are effective in reducing blood pressure, enhancing the action of anti-hypertensive drugs and reducing the requirement for anti-hypertensive drugs (Ramsey et al., 1999). It is also assumed, though unproven, that NPTs will be effective at reducing cardiovascular complications of hypertension. All hypertensive patients should receive non-pharmacological treatment and advice. Recommended NPTs are summarized in the Box.

Non-pharmacological treatments for hypertension

- *Weight reduction:* In overweight hypertensives, advise at least 5 kg weight loss – 5 kg weight loss reduces BP by 12.5/7.5 mmHg.
- *Salt reduction:* Advise reducing salt intake, e.g. no added salt in cooking or at the table. Reducing salt consumption from 10 to 5 grams per day lowers BP by 5/3 mmHg
- *Reduced alcohol consumption:* Advise heavy drinkers to cut down to maximum of 21 units per week in men and 14 units per week for women following binge drinking.
- *Increased physical activity:* If no regular physical activity, advise regular dynamic exercise as appropriate to the age and fitness of the patient.
- *Increased fruit and vegetable consumption:* if consumption low, advise increased consumption – an increase in fruit and vegetables from two to seven portions per day lowers BP by 7/3 mmHg.
- *Smoking cessation:* among hypertensive patients who smoke, smoking is the most important risk factor for cardiovascular complications. Ask all hypertensive patients regularly about smoking, and strongly advise smokers to stop.

Initiation of drug treatment

The decision on when to initiate treatment is summarized in Fig. 72.3. In clinical practice this means that, after initial clinical evaluation and confirmation of the diagnosis, the following courses of action are advised.

Table 72.1. Clinical assessment of hypertensive patients

	Confirmation of diagnosis and level of blood pressure	Identification of secondary causes	Assessment of target organ damage or associated clinical conditions	Assessment of contributory factors and risk factors for hypertensive complications	Identification of contra-indications to anti-hypertensive drugs
History	• Previous history of hypertension – duration and level, current and previous treatments and response • Symptoms of malignant hypertension – nausea and vomiting, headaches, fits, visual disturbances	• Family history of HT or renal disease • Past history of renal disease • Symptoms of phaeochromocytoma (e.g. paroxysms of sweating and palpitations) • Symptoms of endocrine causes, e.g. weakness and tetany in Conn's syndrome, weight gain in Cushing's syndrome • Drug history, e.g. oral contraceptive pill, NSAIDS, steroids	• History or symptoms of stroke, TIA, angina, myocardial infarction, heart failure or peripheral vascular disease • History of renal disease	• Family history of premature (<65 years) cardiovascular disease • History of diabetes • Alcohol intake • Tobacco smoking • Added salt in cooking and at the table • Physical activity	• History of gout, asthma, COPD, • Pregnancy
Clinical examination	• BP measurement – 2× per visit over 4–6 weeks to confirm diagnosis (see above) • Fundi for evidence of retinopathy	• Delayed or absent femoral pulses (coarctation) • Renal bruits (renal artery stenosis) • Palpable kidneys (polycystic kidneys) • Cushingoid, acromegalic or hypothyroid stigmata	• Full cardiovascular examination including pulses, bruits, LVH, heart failure and fundi • Neurological examination for stroke	• Height and weight – BMI	• Heart block • Pregnancy
Investigation	• Ambulatory BP if feasible and indicated (see above)	• Urinalysis (haematuria and proteinuria in renal disease) • Urea and electrolytes (abnormal in renal disease and Conn's syndrome) CXR (coarctation – rib notching) • Specialist investigations for endocrine and renal causes	• Urinalysis • ECG (LVH, IHD, arrhythmias) • CXR (LVH, CHF) • Echocardiography and other specialist cardiovascular investigations	• Urinalysis (Diabetes) • Fasting blood sugar (Diabetes) • Blood lipids	• ECG • Pregnancy test

Note:
It is accepted that a number of the investigations mentioned may not be available in an African setting.

1. Patient with Grade 3 hypertension or evidence of target organ damage (or an associated clinical condition) should start drug treatment immediately.
2. Patients with Grade 1 or 2 hypertension, and three or more risk factors, should start drug treatment immediately.
3. Patients with Grade 2 hypertension and less than three risk factors, or Grade 1 hypertension and one or two other risk factors should be monitored on non-pharmacological treatment for 3 to 6 months, and drug treatment started only if blood pressure is persistently over 140/90 mm Hg.
4. Patients with Grade 1 hypertension and no other risk factors should be monitored for 6 to12 months on non-pharmacological treatment, and drug treatment started only if the mean BP is over 150/95 mm Hg.

These thresholds could be modified to reflect local availability of anti-hypertensive drugs – for example, by increasing the thresholds to ≥150/95 mm Hg and ≥160/100 mm Hg for groups 3 and 4, respectively.

Table 72.2. Risk stratification of hypertensive patients

	Grade of hypertension		
	Grade 1 (140–159/90–99 mmHg)	Grade 2 (160–179/ 100–109 mmHg)	Grade 3 (≥180/110 mmHg)
No risk factors[a]	Low risk	Medium risk	High risk
1–2 risk factors[a]	Medium risk	Medium risk	Very high risk
≥3 risk factors or target organ damage[b] or diabetes	High risk	High risk	Very high risk
Associated clinical condition[c]	Very high risk	Very high risk	Very high risk

Notes:

[a] Risk factors = Men >55 yrs, women >65 years, current smoker, family history of premature cardiovascular disease, total cholesterol >6.5 mmol/l.

[b] Target organ damage = LVH, Renal impairment (proteinuria or raised creatinine), Grade 2 retinopathy.

[c] Associated Clinical Conditions = Stroke, TIA, angina, myocardial infarction, congestive heart failure, chronic renal failure or diabetic nephropathy, grade 3 or 4 hypertensive retinopathy.

Choice of anti-hypertensive drug treatment

Each class of anti-hypertensive drug has compelling indications for use and also clear contraindications. These are summarized in Table 72.3 (adapted from the British Hypertension Society Guidelines) (Ramsey et al., 1999).

Clinical trials of anti-hypertensive drugs have mostly involved European and American populations. Most show drug classes to be equally effective. However, evidence of effectiveness in preventing long-term complications such as stroke and heart disease is strongest for beta-blockers and thiazide diuretics (Psaty et al., 1997), although similar evidence is now accumulating for angiotensin converting enzyme inhibitors (ACE) and calcium antagonists (Blood Pressure Lowering Treatment Trialists Collaboration, 2000). Thiazides and beta-blockers are cheap and cost-effective. Therefore, most treatment guidelines recommend initial treatment with drugs from these classes.

A consistent finding from trials including black hypertensive patients is that monotherapy with beta-blockers or ACE is relatively ineffective in lowering BP levels, whereas thiazides, calcium antagonists, and alpha-blockers are highly effective anti-hypertensive treatments. The reduced effect of beta-blockers and ACEs in black people is abolished by the addition of a low-dose thiazide. These findings have been replicated to some extent in African studies (Gibbs et al., 1999; Seedat, 1999). Other possible drugs for use in African populations include methyldopa, hydralazine, low-dose reserpine and combined alpha-and beta-blockers such as labetalol. The place of newer drugs such as angiotensin II receptor antagonists is uncertain.

The choice of drug depends on availability and cost. Generic drugs, particularly thiazides and reserpine, are usually much the cheapest. Based on the above evidence, initial therapy should probably be a thiazide diuretic or, if resources allow, a calcium antagonist. If control is not achieved with a low dose of the first drug, there are several possible strategies for achieving an effective treatment regime.

These strategies can be continued if control is not achieved with two drugs. Whatever strategy is used, the following principles should be followed. (Also, see the box).

Strategies for achieving hypertension control

- **Titrate up** the dose of the initial drug in accordance with the manufacturers instructions – best used if a response occurs and the drug is tolerated, but blood pressure is still not controlled. Do not titrate up doses of thiazides.
- **Add** a low dose of an additional drug (and then titrate up if necessary) – best used where hypertension is severe or complicated, particularly if a partial response occurred to the previous regime.
- **Substitute** a different drug – best used if there has been no or minimal response to the first drug and the hypertension is mild and uncomplicated.

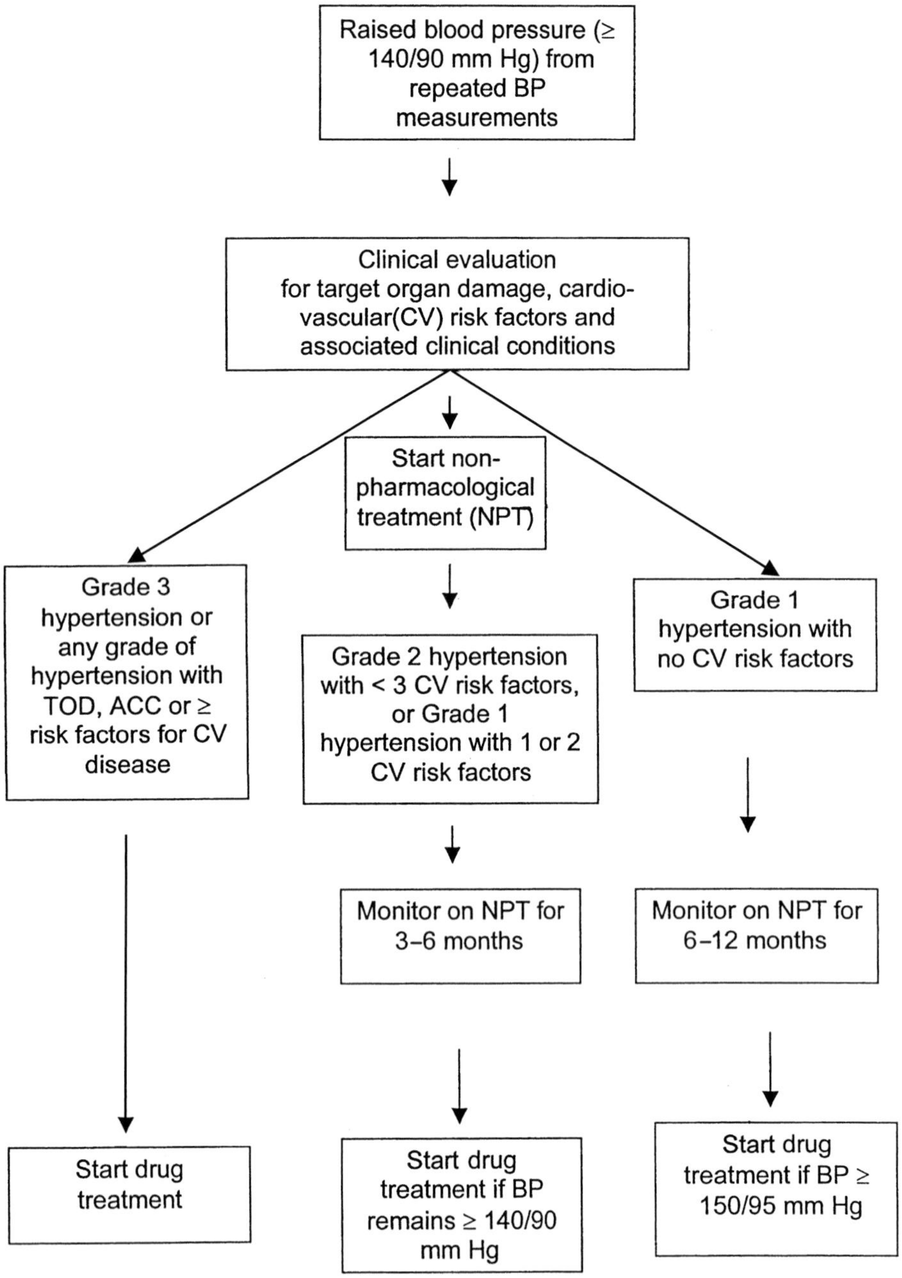

Fig. 72.3. Initiation of treatment in hypertension.

- To minimize side effects, aim to control BP with the lowest possible dose of each drug.
- After each change of drug therapy wait at least 4 weeks to allow the full response to develop (unless rapid control is required).
- Sub-maximal doses of two drugs often result in greater blood pressure reductions than maximal dose of a single drug
- Over two-thirds of hypertensive patients will require at least two drugs to achieve control and more than a third will need three or more drugs (Hansson et al., 1998).

Other drug treatments

Recent clinical trials have found that 75 mg aspirin per day reduces cardiovascular events in selected hypertensive patients (Hansson et al., 1998). However, the margin

Table 72.3. Major anti-hypertensive drugs

Class of drug	Example with typical and max dose per day	Main mechanism(s) of action	Specific indications (Possible and compelling)	Contraindications (Possible and compelling)	Common and important side effects
Alpha-blockers	Prazosin 1 mg t.d.s. (max 20 mg daily)	Vasodilator	Dyslipidaemia Prostatism	Postural hypotension Urinary incontinence Aortic stenosis	OH[a] Headache Fatigue
ACE-inhibitors	Captopril 12.5 mg b.d. (max 50 mg b.d.)	Vasodilator	LV dysfunction Type 1 diabetic nephropathy Heart failure Chronic renal disease[b] Type 2 diabetic nephropathy	Renal impairment[a] PVD[c] Aortic stenosis Pregnancy Hyperkalaemia Renovascular disease	OH[a] Dry cough Renal impairment Hyperkalaemia
Angiotensin II-antagonists	Losartan 50 mg o.d. (max 100 mg o.d.)	Vasodilator	As above and ACE inhibitor induced cough	As above	OH[a] Renal impairment Hyperkalaemia
Beta-blockers	Propranolol (non-selective) 80 mg b.d. (max 160 mg b.d.) Atenolol (cardio-selective) 25 mg b.d. (max 100 mg o.d.)	↓ Cardiac output (↓contractility and bradycardia)	Pregnancy Heart failure[d] History of myocardial infarction Angina	Uncontrolled heart failure[d] Dyslipidaemia Severe PVD Asthma/COPD Heart block/ bradycardia	Heart failure Bradycardia Bronchospasm Exacerbation of PVD
Calcium antagonists (dihydropyridine)	Nifedipine 20 mg b.d. (max 30 mgs t.d.s.)	↓ Cardiac output (↓contractility) Vasodilator	Elderly with isolated systolic hypertension, angina	Unstable angina Severe aortic stenosi	Ankle oedema Flushing Headache
Calcium antagonists (rate-limiting)	Verapamil 40 mg t.d.s. (max 480 mg daily) Diltiazem 60 mg t.d.s. (max 360 mg daily)	As above and slows heart rate	Angina	Combination with Beta-blocker Heart block Heart failure	As above plus bradycardia Heart block Heart failure
Hydralazine	25 mg bd (max 50 mg b.d.)	Vasodilator	Heart failure (with a long acting nitrate) Hypertensive crisis (including pregnancy related)	SLE Porphyria Severe tachycardia High output heart failure	Tachycardia and fluid retention when used alone SLE (long-term treatment) OH[a]
Methyldopa	Methyldopa 250 mg 2–3 times daily (max 1 g t.d.s.)	Centrally acting	Safe in pregnancy	History of depression Active liver disease Phaeochromocytoma Porphyria	Positive direct Coomb's test in up to 20% (may effect blood cross matching) Depression OH[a] Abnormal LFTs
Reserpine (low dose only)	0.625 mg q.d.s. (max 0.5 mg daily)	Centrally acting and vasodilator	Cheap	History of depression Active depression or recent electro-convulsive therapy Active peptic ulcer or ulcerative colitis	CNS symptoms – depression and anxiety GI symptoms

Table 72.3 (*cont.*)

Class of drug	Example with typical and max dose per day	Main mechanism(s) of action	Specific indications (Possible and compelling)	Contraindications (Possible and compelling)	Common and important side effects
Thiazides	Bendrofluazide 2.5 mg o.d., hydrochlorothiazide 25 mg o.d. (do not increase dose – minimal further BP decrease but increased side effects)	Diuretic	Elderly	Dyslipidaemia Gout Severe hypokalaemia or hyponatraemia	Impaired glucose tolerance and hyperglycaemia Hyponatraemia Hypokalaemia Dyslipidaemia

Notes:

[a] Most anti-hypertensive drugs can cause OH but this is commonest in the elderly and with vasodilators. The first dose should be small and taken lying down or at bedtime.

[b] ACE inhibitors may be *beneficial* in chronic renal failure but should only be used with caution, close supervision and specialist advice when there is established and significant renal impairment.

[c] Caution with ACE inhibitors and angiotensin II antagonists in peripheral vascular disease because of association with renovascular disease.

[d] Beta-blockers may worsen heart failure, but in specialist hands may be used to treat heart failure.

Abbreviations: COPD, chronic obstructive pulmonary disease; ISH, Isolated systolic hypertension; OH, orthostatic hypotension; PVD, peripheral vascular disease.

between benefits and harm was narrow, and this may be particularly true in populations with a high prevalence of haemorrhagic stroke. Current advice is that aspirin use should be restricted to hypertensive patients with existing cardiovascular disease, or are at very high risk of cardiovascular complications (Ramsay et al., 1999). If used, aspirin should not be initiated until BP levels are below 150/90 mm Hg.

Another emerging issue is the treatment of hyperlipidaemia in hypertensive patients, with lipid lowering agents such as statins (HMG CoA reductase inhibitors).

However, this is not an important issue in Africa as hyperlipidaemia is rare in African populations, and lipid-lowering drugs and lipid-testing facilities are expensive and rarely available.

Education of patients

Hypertension is a chronic disease generally requiring life-long monitoring and treatment. Convincing a patient to take one or more drugs for the rest of their life, particularly when they are symptom-free is difficult. Hence, to achieve good long-term adherence to treatment and care, health care staff must give clear explanations of the nature of hypertension, the need for treatment and the risks of non-treatment. Encourage your patients to ask questions about their condition and its treatment and wherever possible involve them in making decisions about management of their hypertension. The Box shows the main points to be explained at diagnosis and during follow-up visits.

Education of patients – main components

- Hypertension usually requires lifelong treatment (it cannot be cured).
- High blood pressure increases the risk of serious diseases like stroke. That risk is reduced or abolished by treatment.
- Treatment is by drugs and non-pharmacological treatments to lower blood pressure and reduce the risk of complications.
- Adherence to treatment (including tablets every day) is vital.
- Ensure that patients understand: why they need treatment, what treatment can prevent, how it will be given, the need for ongoing follow-up.

In patients with uncontrolled hypertension, check how much they understand about hypertension, the reasons for treatment and their adherence with treatment. If patients decide not to take anti-hypertensive drugs, their choice should be respected, though it must be an informed choice made only after the risks of hypertension and benefits of treatment have been described fully.

Stopping and stepping down treatment

Hypertension treatment is usually for life. However, for patients with prolonged optimal control and where cardiovascular risk has been reduced successfully, stepping down or even stopping treatment should be considered. If drug treatment is stopped, non-pharmacological interventions should be maintained and annual BP monitoring continued for life.

Follow-up and review

Follow-up is vital to ensure that treatment is maintained, BP control monitored, and hypertensive complications detected. This is best achieved with regular appointments and a system for recall and follow-up of non-attenders.

Frequency of follow-up will depend on the severity of hypertension and the stability of the current treatment regime. Well-controlled hypertensive patients with no complications should be seen every 3 to 6 months. Newly diagnosed patients just starting treatment, poorly controlled patients, and patients whose regime has recently changed should be seen every 4–6 weeks. Follow-up visits should usually involve the following:

- BP and weight measurement
- check on other risk factors for cardiovascular complications
- enquiry about general health, and specifically about side effects of, and adherence with, treatment
- reinforcement of education about hypertension, and non-pharmacological treatments
- annual urinalysis for proteinuria and glycosuria.

Where health care is fragmented, the best way to maintain a continuous clinical record may be through patient-held records (Saunders et al., 1991) – see Fig. 72.4.

Referral criteria

In sub-Saharan Africa, most hypertension care can be delivered through primary health care clinics (PHC). However, some patients will require referral to hospitals. The main indications are summarized in the Box.

> **Possible criteria for referral to specialist care**
> - Urgent treatment required, e.g. malignant or very severe (>220/120 mm Hg) hypertension.
> - Investigation of possible secondary hypertension e.g. symptoms/signs of underlying cause, treatment resistant hypertension, worsening hypertension, young age of onset (<20–30 years).
> - Treatment ineffective or not tolerated
> - Complicated hypertension e.g. pregnancy, renal disease.

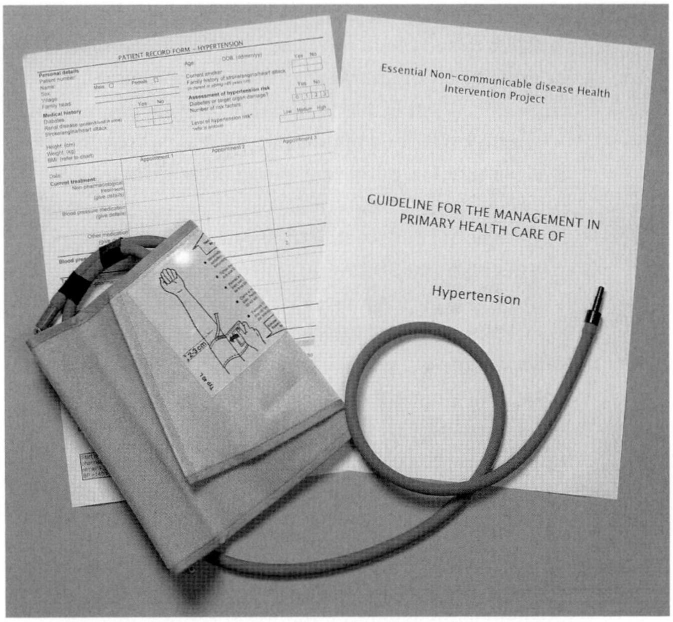

Fig. 72.4. Guidelines for treatment and patient record cards. Good organization of care systems is essential in community hypertension management.

Other issues

Malignant hypertension

A hypertensive emergency is defined as a case in which cardiovascular and/or neurological decompensation has occurred, and includes hypertensive encephalopathy, heart failure and pre-eclampsia. In a specialist unit, immediate intravenous treatment, e.g. sodium nitroprusside, nicardipine or glyceryl trinitrate, may be given. Intramuscular hydralazine is also effective. But in practice, these drugs are available rarely in Africa and oral methyldopa **with a** thiazide diuretic is used commonly. Look for secondary causes of hypertension, which are more common in patients with malignant hypertension. Hypertensive 'urgencies' are cases where there is evidence of accelerated microvascular damage, i.e. retinal or renal, but where decompensation has not yet occurred. Start oral treatment and aim to lower BP over hours to days. See 'Emergencies', Chapter 97. Never use immediate-release nifedipine due to its unpredictable absorption and the risk of dangerously rapid falls in blood pressure. Nifedine slow release, however, 10–20 mg is effective.

Hypertension in pregnancy

Hypertension complicates up to 10 per cent of pregnancies. It is usually divided into chronic hypertension and pre-eclampsia. Pre-eclampsia is a multi-system disorder in which raised blood pressure is only one component. It is defined as proteinuria (over 300 mg/24 hours) occurring with a diastolic blood pressure of over 90 mm Hg on two occasions over 4 hours apart, or a single reading of over 110 mm Hg, or a rise of blood pressure of over 30/15 mm Hg from first trimester levels. Pre-eclampsia requires urgent referral and treatment. It can occur superimposed on a background of chronic hypertension.

Chronic hypertension is defined as a blood pressure greater than 140/90 mm Hg before 20 weeks' gestation. Newly diagnosed chronic hypertension is most often idiopathic, but clinical evaluation is required to exclude secondary causes. Thresholds for treatment are uncertain, though there is a general consensus that levels over 170/110 mm Hg should certainly be treated. Many physicians treat at levels over 140/90 mm Hg.

For chronic hypertension in pregnancy, the drug of choice is methyldopa. It has been extensively used in pregnant women without reports of serious adverse effects to the fetus (Kyle, 1979). Second-line agents include calcium antagonists, labetalol and hydralazine. ACE inhibitors and angiotensin II receptor antagonists are contraindicated due to associations with fetal growth retardation and malformations. Women already on these drugs who plan to become, or become, pregnant should switch to other anti-hypertensives. Thiazides are often advised against on theoretical grounds that they may further decrease the reduced circulatory volume found in pre-eclampsia. However, they are effective in reducing the risk of pre-eclampsia, and there is no reason to discontinue low-dose thiazides in women with pre-existing hypertension (Ramsey et al., 1999).

Hypertension in the elderly

Treatment of elderly patients aged less than 80 years, with a BP over 160/90 mm Hg is highly effective. Risk of cardiovascular complications is particularly high in these patients, so the absolute benefits of treatment are higher than for younger hypertensive patients. For BP levels of 140–159/<90 mm Hg in patients under 80 years, there is no clear evidence to guide treatment decisions. Treatment of patients with target organ damage or cardiovascular complications is almost certainly justified.

Decisions about treatment for uncomplicated patients with this level of BP or any patient aged above 80 years with hypertension, should take into account the availability of resources, and the relative priority and cost-effectiveness of hypertension treatment in these patients. If treatment is contemplated, a clinical decision is needed for each patient after assessing the likely benefits and harm from treatment, taking into account current fitness and quality of life. Side effects such as postural hypotension are more common. Low-dose thiazides are the treatment of choice in the elderly. Dihydropyridine calcium antagonists are a reasonable alternative (Ramsey et al., 1999).

Hypertension in diabetes

Diabetic patients have a greatly increased risk of hypertension. Hypertension in such patients is particularly important as it causes a vast increase in the risk of the microvascular and macrovascular complications of diabetes (UKPDS, 1998), and there is compelling evidence that vigorous treatment is highly effective in preventing these complications.

Evidence from the HOT study and UKPDS trial strongly support a threshold for starting treatment of 140/85 mm Hg and a more stringent target blood pressure of 130/80 mm Hg (Hansson et al, 1998; UKPDS, 1998). A threshold of 125/75 mm Hg in the presence of proteinuria greater than 1gm/24 hrs is advised. To achieve these targets, combination drug treatment will usually be required. There is no clear evidence as to which is the most effective treatment, though low-dose thiazides, β-blockers, dihydropyridine calcium antagonists and ACE inhibitors are safe and effective. In Type I diabetic nephropathy, ACE inhibitor treatment slows the progression of renal disease (Lewis et al., 1993), so these are the drugs of choice. Aspirin and statin treatment should be considered.

Hypertension and renal disease

Hypertension is a cause and a consequence of renal disease. Uncontrolled hypertension causes progression in established renal impairment. Hence, as in diabetes, tight control is vital. Treatment of patients with chronic renal impairment should be initiated if the BP is over 140/90 mm Hg, and the target BP should be 130/85 mm Hg or below (125/75 mm Hg in the presence of proteinuria over 1 g/24 h). The treatment of choice is uncertain (Ramsey et al., 1999). Salt restriction is likely to be particularly effective. Thiazides may be ineffective in the presence of renal impairment. ACE inhibitors can be renoprotective, particularly in the presence of marked proteinuria (over 3 g/day) or rapidly progressive renal failure. However, they must be used with care in severe renal impairment and may worsen renal impairment in the presence of renovascular disease. Aspirin and statin treatment should be considered.

Hypertension prevention and control: the high risk and population approaches

A hypertension prevention and control strategy focusing on very high risk individuals through the detection, treatment and control of hypertension, will reduce the rate of cardiovascular complications in such patients, and hence reduce morbidity and mortality in the population. The strategy will be efficient because it will focus interventions on individuals with the greatest capacity to benefit. For example, in the MRFIT trial, the 5 per cent of subjects with Grade 2 and 3 hypertension accounted for almost a quarter of the population with excess risk of cardiovascular events. However, nearly 80 per cent of hypertensive subjects had Grade 1 hypertension. These patients had a much lower risk of cardiovascular events, but still accounted for about 43 per cent of the overall population excess risk and nearly two-thirds of the hypertension-related population excess risk. Even so, in absolute numbers, because cardiovascular risk is continuously related to BP levels, and most people are not classified as hypertensive, most cardiovascular events occur in people with BP levels considered 'normal'.

This observation has prompted some commentators to argue that the high risk approach is a conservative strategy, which will not affect the overall population BP distribution or reduce the incidence of new cases of hypertension. Instead they argue for a population-based approach to prevention of cardiovascular disease (Rose, 1985). This approach aims to reduce the overall population risk by shifting the blood pressure distribution for the whole population downwards. For example, a downward shift of about 2 mm Hg in BP distribution in the general population in the USA should result in an annual reduction of stroke, coronary heart disease and all cause mortality of 6 per cent, 4 per cent and 3 per cent, respectively (Stamler, 1991). This is a more radical strategy, requiring health promotion and preventive interventions that target the whole population – not just high risk individuals arbitrarily labelled as hypertensive. Many public health specialists would argue that a combination of both approaches is required, so that individuals at highest risk receive the necessary treatment, whilst in the longer term more radical measures act to reduce the prevalence of hypertension in the population.

Future challenges

Hypertension poses numerous challenges in sub-Saharan Africa. However, to pick out just two; perhaps the biggest challenges facing researchers, health care staff, planners and policy makers are as follows.

1. To develop strategies to ensure that the vast body of evidence about how hypertension should be managed is implemented in everyday clinical practice in resource-poor primary care settings.
2. To develop effective health promotion and preventive interventions and strategies to prevent the predicted increase in the burden of disease due to hypertension and related non-communicable diseases.

References

Abson CCCP, Levy LM, Eyherabide G. (1981). Once daily atenolol in hypertensive Zimbabwean blacks. A double-blind trial using two different doses. *S Afr Med J*; **60**: 47–48.

Akinkugbe, OO. (1980). Current aspects of high blood pressure research in Africa. *Clin Cardiol*; **12**: 87–90.

Astagneau P, Lang T, Delarocque E, Jeanee E, Salem G. (1992). Arterial hypertension in urban Africa: an epidemiological study on a representative sample of Dakar inhabitants in Senegal. *J Hypertens*; **10**: 1095–1101.

Barker DJP. (1995). Fetal origins of coronary heart disease. *Br Med J*; **311**: 171–174.

Bianchi S, Bigazzi R, Baldari G, Sgherri, G, Campese VM. (1994). Diurnal variations of blood pressure and microalbuminuria in essential hypertension. *Am J Hypertens*; **7**: 23–29.

Blood Pressure Lowering Treatment Trialists Collaboration. (2000). Effect of ACE inhibitors, calcium antagonists, and other blood-pressure lowering drugs: results of prospectively designed overviews of randomised trials. *Lancet*; **356**: 1955–1964.

Bogin B. (1988). Rural to urban migration. In *Biological aspects of Human Migration, Cambridge Studies in Biological Anthropology*, ed. CGN Mascie-Taylor & GW Lasker. Cambridge: Cambridge University Press.

Bosman AR, Goldberg B, Mckechnie JK, Offermeier J, Oosthuizen OJ. (1977). South African multicentre study of metoprolol and propanolol in essential hypertension. *S Afr Med J*; **51**: 57–61.

Bouchard TJJ, Lykken DT, McGue M, Segal NL, Tellegen A. (1980). Sources of human psychological differences: the Minnesota Study of Twins Reared Apart. *Science*; **250**: 223–228.

Bradshaw D, Bourne D, Schneider M, Sayed R. (1995). Mortality patterns of chronic diseases of lifestyle in South Africa. In *Chronic Diseases of Lifestyle in South Africa*, ed. J Fourie & K Steyn. Cape Town: Medical Research Council.

Coleman R, Gill G, Wilkinson D. (1998). Noncommunicable disease management in resource-poor settings: a primary care model from rural South Africa. *Bull Wld Hlth Org*; **76**: 633–640.

Collins R, Peto R, MacMahon S et al. (1990). Blood pressure, stroke, and coronary heart disease. Part 2. Short-term reductions in blood pressure: overview of randomised drug trials in their epidemiological context. *Lancet*; **335**: 827–838.

Cooper RS, Rotimi CN, Kaufman JS, Muna WF, Mensah GA. (1998). Hypertension treatment and control in sub-Saharan Africa: the epidemiological basis for policy. *Br Med J*; **316**: 614–617.

Cooper RS, Rotimi CN, Ataman SL et al. (1997). The prevalence of hypertension in seven populations of West African origin. *Am J Public Hlth*; **87**: 160–168.

Cooper RS, Rotimi C. (1997). Hypertension in blacks. *Am J Hypertens*; **10**: 804–812.

Cooper RS, Liao Y. (1992). Is hypertension among blacks more severe or simply more common. *Circulation*; **85**: 12.

Cruickshank JK, Mbanya J-C, Wilkes R et al. (2001). Sick genes, sick individuals or sick populations with chronic disease? The emergence of diabetes and high blood pressure in African-origin populations. *Int J Epidemiol*; **30**: 111–117.

Curtin PD. (1992). The slavery hypothesis for hypertension among African Americans: the historical evidence. *Am. J. Public Hlth*; **82**: 1681–1686.

Donnison CP. (1929). Blood pressure in the African native. *Lancet*; 1: 6–7.

Ebrahim S. (1998). Detection, adherence and control of hypertension for the prevention of stroke: a systematic review. *Hlth Technol Assessm*; **2**.

Edwards R, Unwin N, Mugusi F et al. (2000). Hypertension prevalence and care in an urban and rural area of Tanzania. *J Hypertens*; **18**: 145–152.

Elliot P, Stamler J, Nichols R et al. (1996). Intersalt revisited: further analyses of 24 hour sodium excretion and blood pressure within and across populations. Intersalt Cooperative Research Group. *Br Med J*; **312**: 1249–1253.

Fuentes R, Llmaniemi N, Laurikainen E, Tuomilehto J, Nissinen A. (2000). Hypertension in developing economies: a review of population-based studies carried out from 1980 to 1998. *J Hypertens*; **18**: 521–529.

Gibbs CR, Beevers DG, Lip GYH. (1999). The management of hypertensive disease in black patients. *Quart J Med*; **92**: 187–192.

Grim CE, Henry JP, Myers H. (1995). High blood pressure in blacks: salt, slavery, survival, stress and racism. In *Hypertension*, ed. JH Laragh & BA Brenner, pp. 171–207. New York: Raven Press.

Gueyffier F, Boutitie F, Boissel JP et al. (1997). Effect of antihypertensive drug treatment on cardiovascular outcomes in women and men. A meta-analysis of individual patient data from randomised, controlled trials. The INDANA Investigators. *Ann Intern Med*; **126**: 761–767.

Guidelines Subcommittee of the World Health Organisation – International Society of Hypertension Mild Hypertension Liaison Committee. (1999). World Health Organization – International Society of Hypertension Guidelines for the Management of Hypertension. *J Hypertens*; **17**: 151–183.

Hansson L, Zanchetti A, Carruthers SG et al. (1998). Effects of intensive blood-pressure lowering and low-dose aspirin in patients with hypertension: principal results of the Hypertension Optimal Treatment (HOT) randomised trial. HOT Study Group. *Lancet*; **351**: 1755–1762.

Hoosen S, Seedat YK, Bhigjee AI, Neerahoo RM. (1985). A study of urinary sodium and potassium excretion rates among urban and rural Zulus and Indians. *J Hypertens* 1985; **68**: 351–358.

Intersalt Co-op Research Group. (1988). Intersalt: an international study of electrolyte excretion and blood pressure: results for 24 hour urinary sodium and potassium excretion. *Br Med J*; **297**: 319–328.

Joint National Committee on Prevention, Detection, Evaluation, and Treatment of High Blood Pressure (JNC VI). (1997). The sixth report of the Joint National Committee on the Prevention, Detection, Evaluation, and Treatment of High Blood Pressure. *Arch Intern Med;* **153**: 154–183.

Kaplan NM. (1993). Salt and blood pressure. In *Hypertension Primer*, ed JL Izzo & HR Black, pp. 167–169. Dallas: American Heart Association.

Kaufman JS, Rotimi CN, Brieger WR et al. (1996). The mortality risk associated with hypertension: preliminary results of a prospective study in rural Nigeria. *J Hum Hypertens*; **10**: 461–464.

Kital I, Irwig L. (1979). Hypertension in urban black outpatients. *S Afr Med J*; **55**: 241–244.

Kyle PM. (1979). Comparative risk-benefit assessment of drugs used in the management of hypertension in pregnancy. *Drug Safety*; **7**: 223–234.

Law C, A Shiell. (1996). Is blood pressure inversely related to birth weight? The strength of evidence from a systematic review of the literature. *J Hypertens*; **14**: 935–940.

Levitt NS, Steyn K, De Wet T et al. (1999). An inverse relation between blood pressure and birth weight among 5 year old children from Soweto, South Africa. *J Epidemiol Commun Hlth*; **53**: 264–268.

Lewis EJ, Hunsideer LG, Bain RP, Rohde RD; for the Collaborative Study Group. (1993). The effect of angiotensin-converting-enzyme inhibition on diabetic nephropathy. *New Engl J Med*; **329**: 1456–1462.

Longo-Mbenza B, Ngiyulu R, Bayekula M et al. (1999). Low birth weight and risk of hypertension in African school children. *J Cardiovasc Risk*; **6**: 311–314.

MacMahon S, Peto R, Cutler J et al. (1990). Blood pressure, stroke, and coronary heart disease. Part 1, prolonged differences in blood pressure: prospective observational studies corrected for the regression dilution bias. *Lancet*; **335**: 765–774.

M'Buyamba-Kabangu J, Fagard R, Lijnen P et al. (1986). Epidemiological Study of Blood Pressure and hypertension in a sample of urban Bantu of Zaire. *J Hypertens*; **4**: 485–491.

M'Buyamba-Kabangu JR, Fagard R, Lijnen P et al. (1988). Intracellular sodium and the response to nitrendipine or atenolol in African blacks. *Hypertension*; **11**: 100–105.

Mbanya J, Minkoulou E, Salah J, Balkau B. (1998). The prevalence of hypertension in rural and urban Cameroon. *Int J Epidemiol*; **27**: 181–185.

Mensah GA, Barkey NL, Cooper RS. (1994). Spectrum of hypertensive target organ damage in Africa: a review of published studies. *J Hum Hypertens*; **8**: 799–808.

Mollentze W, Moore A, Steyn AJ et al. (1995). Coronary heart disease risk factors in a rural and urban Orange Free State black population. *S Afr Med J*; **85**: 90–97.

Mufunda J, Scott LJ, Chifamba J et al. (2000). Correlates of blood pressure in an urban Zimbabwean population and comparison to other populations of African origin. *J Hum Hypertens*; **14**: 65–73.

Murray C, Lopez A., eds. (1996). *Global Burden of Disease.* Geneva: World Health Organization.

Nissinen A, Bothig S, Granroth H, Lopez AD. (1988). Hypertension in developing countries. *Wld Hlth Stat Quart*; **41**: 141–154.

Oelofse A, Josste PL, Steyn K et al. (1996). The lipid and lipoprotein profile of the urban black population of the Cape Peninsula – the BRISK study. *S Afr Med J*; **86**: 162–166.

Opie L. (1995). Hypertension. In *Chronic Diseases of Lifestyle in South Africa*, ed J Fourie & K Steyn. Cape Town: Medical Research Council.

Pauletto P, Caroli M, Pessina AC, Dal Palu C. (1994). Hypertension prevalence and age-related changes of blood pressure in semi-nomadic and urban Oromos of Ethiopia. *Eur J Epidemi*; **10**: 159–164.

Pobee JOM. (1993). Community-based high blood pressure programs in sub-Saharan Africa. *Ethnicity Dis*; **3**: S38–S45.

Poulter NR, Khaw KT, Hopwood BEC et al. (1990). The Kenya Luo migration study: observations on the initiation of a rise in blood pressure. *Br Med J*; **300**: 967–972.

Profant J, Dimsdale JE. (1999). Race and diurnal blood pressure patterns. A review and meta-analysis. *Hypertension*; **33**: 1099–1104.

Psaty BM, Smith NL, Siscovick DS et al. (1997). Health outcomes associated with antihypertensive therapies used as first-line agents: a systematic review and meta-analysis. *J Am Med Assoc*; **277**: 739–745.

Ramsey LE, Williams B, Johnstone GD et al. (1999). Guidelines for the management of hypertension: report of the third working party of the British Hypertension Society. *J Hum Hypertens*; **13**: 569–592.

Rose G. (1985). 'Sick individuals and sick populations.' *Int Epidemiol*; **14**: 32–38.

Saunders L, Irwig L, Wilson T. (1982). Hypertension management and patient compliance at a Soweto polyclinic. *S Afr Med J*; **61**: 147–151.

Saunders LD, Irwig LM, Gear JS, Ramushu DL. (1991). A randomised controlled trial of compliance improving strategies in Soweto hypertensives. *Med Care*; **29**: 669–678.

Seedat YK. (1974). The clinical pattern of hypertension in the South African black population. A study of 1000 patients. *N Z Med J*; **79**: 946–951.

Seedat YK. (1980). Trial of atenolol and chlorothalidone in black Africans. *Br Med J*; **281**: 1241–1243.

Seedat YK. (1999). Hypertension in black South Africans. *J Hum Hypertens*; **13**: 97–103.

Staessen J, Amery A, Birkenhager W et al. (1992). Syst-Eur – a multicentre trial on the treatment of isolated systolic hypertension in the elderly: first interim report. *J Cardiovasc Pharmacol*; **19**: 120–125.

Stamler R. (1991). Implications of the INTERSALT study. *Hypertension*; **17**: 116–120.

Steyn K, Fourie J, Lombard C, Katzenellenbogen J, Bourne L, Jooste P. (1996). Hypertension in the black community of the Cape Peninsula, South Africa. *Ea Afr Med J*; **73**: 758–763.

Swai AB, McLarty DG, Kitange HM et al. (1993). Low prevalence of risk factors for coronary heart disease in rural Tanzania. *Int J Epidemiol*; **22**: 651–659.

United Kingdom Prospective Diabetes Study Group. (UKPDS) (1998). Tight blood pressure control and risk of macrovascular and microvascular complications in type 2 diabetes. *Br Med J*; **317**: 703–713.

van der Sande MAB, Milligan, PJM, Nyan OA et al. (2000). Blood pressure patterns and cardiovascular risk factors in rural and urban Gambian communities. *J Hum Hypertens*; **14**: 489–496.

Veriava Y, du Toit E, Lawleym CG, Milne FJ, Reinach SG. (1990). Hypertension as a cause of end-stage renal failure in South Africa. *J Hum Hypertens*; **4**: 379–383.

Walker RW, McLarty DG, Kitange HM, Whiting D, Masuki G, Mtasiwa DM. (2000). Stroke mortality in urban and rural Tanzania. *Lancet*; **355**: 1684–1687.

Wilson TW, Hollifield LR, Grim CE. (1991). Systolic blood pressure levels in black populations in sub-Sahara Africa, the West Indies, and the United States: a meta-analysis. *Hypertension*; **18**: 187–191.

Woelk G, Emmanuel I, Weis N et al. (1997). Birthweight and blood pressure among children in Harare, Zimbabwe. *Arch Dis Child*; **79**: F119–F122.

73 Stroke

The World Health Organization's (WHO) definition of stroke is *rapidly developing clinical signs of focal (or global) disturbance of cerebral function with symptoms lasting 24 hours or longer or leading to death with no apparent cause other than that of vascular origin* (WHO MONICA Project,1988). It is also commonly referred to as cerebrovascular accident (CVA). Stroke is not a diagnosis but a clinical syndrome. In developed countries it is due to cerebral infarction in 85 per cent, primary intracerebral haemorrhage (PICH) in 10 per cent, sub-arachnoid haemorrhage (SAH) in 5 per cent, and cerebral venous thrombosis in less than 1 per cent. Although SAH is included in the WHO definition of stroke, it is a distinct epidemiological entity with different risk factors, different age distribution and considerably different outcome.

Clinical assessment

History

Sudden onset

The patient usually has a focal neurological deficit, which in most cases reaches its maximum deficit over seconds or minutes. It is not possible clinically to distinguish reliably between PICH and infarction although headache, coma at onset and vomiting are more common in haemorrhage.

Slowly progressive

If the symptoms and signs develop slowly, a space occupying lesion, e.g. cerebral tumour, is possible, although rarely propagation of thrombus may cause ischaemic stroke to progress in a stepwise manner.

Sudden headache

SAH characteristically presents with a sudden onset of severe generalized headache associated with neck stiffness, whereas in meningitis there is a longer history of headache and fever. Focal deficits occur if there is associated bleeding into the brain (intracerebral haemorrhage) or when there is vasospasm with secondary ischaemia. It may present with collapse, coma or sudden death.

Examination

- Assess the patient's level of consciousness.
- Define the probable site of the lesion.
- Look for neck stiffness – sub-arachnoid haemorrhage (SAH) or meningitis.
- Examine for signs of risk factors – atrial fibrillation, mitral valve disease, infective endocarditis, sepsis, otitis media, obesity, hypertension.
- Palpate and auscultate arterial pulses in the neck and arms (tropical aortitis or atherosclerosis); auscultate the skull (arteriovenous malformation (AVM)).
- Is the patient pregnant?

Clinical classification of the site and size of stroke is possible. In the Bamford classification, strokes are classified as total anterior circulation stroke (TACS), partial anterior circulation stroke (PACS), lacunar stroke (LACS), and posterior circulation stroke (POCS) according to clinical findings (Anonymous, 1996). This can guide investigations into the cause of stroke, e.g. no indication for carotid ultrasound in POCS, and is very helpful in determining prognosis (see Table 73.1).

Pathological mechanisms

Cerebral infarction

This is due to embolism or thrombosis. The heart is a common source for emboli, usually in patients with atrial

Table 73.1. Clinical classification of stroke

Classification of stroke	Clinical features
Total anterior circulation stroke (TACS)	Unilateral weakness (and/or sensory deficit) of face, arm and leg Homonymous hemianopia Higher cerebral dysfunction (dysphasia, visuospatial disorder)
Partial anterior circulation stroke (PACS)	Unilateral weakness (and/or sensory deficit) of face, arm or leg Homonymous hemianopia or higher cerebral dysfunction
Lacunar stroke (LACS)	Unilateral weakness (and/or sensory deficit) of face and arm, arm and leg or all three Ataxic hemiparesis No evidence higher cerebral dysfunction
Posterior circulation stroke (POCS)	Cerebellar or brainstem syndromes Loss of consciousness Isolated homonymous hemianopia

Notes:
The replacement of S by I denotes that the stroke is secondary to an infarct (e.g. TACI = total anterior circulation infarct).
The classification is based on the physical signs at initial presentation.

fibrillation (AF). Atherosclerosis in the major vessels supplying the brain is the other main source of cerebral embolism. An embolus is usually a platelet aggregate or thrombus formed on atherosclerotic plaques, but occasionally comprises cholesterol and other atherosclerotic debris. Rupture of a plaque exposes the intensely thrombogenic lipid core of the plaque to blood, thus activating the clotting cascade to cause thrombosis. Symptomatic athersclerosis is most common at the carotid artery bifurcation, but it can also arise in the aorta, carotid syphon, common carotid artery and vertebral and basilar arteries.

Dissection of the vertebral or carotid artery accounts for about 5 per cent of ischaemic stroke and transient ischaemic attack (TIA) in those under 60 years. Suspect dissection if there is localized pain in the neck or ipsilateral Horner's syndrome, and if there is a history of recent neck trauma (which may be minor) days or weeks before the onset of stroke, although this is not always the case.

Occlusion of a major vessel may cause symptoms to progress over minutes or a few hours. Patients in whom occlusion develops slowly, so that a good collateral blood supply develops, may have no symptoms. If the collaterals are inadequate, 'borderzone' infarction occurs.

Stroke after carotid occlusion is often caused by embolism to the middle cerebral artery from thrombus in the stump of the occluded carotid. Middle cerebral artery occlusion can be due to localized intracranial atherosclerosis, but is usually the result of cerebral embolism. Occlusion of small penetrating arterioles, usually secondary to hypertension or diabetes, leads to small infarcts – termed lacunar infarcts – in the subcortical white matter, internal capsule, basal ganglia or pons.

Subarachnoid haemorrhage

Rupture of an aneurysm in one of the arteries at the base of the brain is the most common cause, but it can occur from an AVM, as a result of trauma, or spontaneously. Cerebral vasospasm causes delayed cerebral infarction 4–14 days after onset in 30 per cent of patients, and recurrent haemorrhage and hydrocephalus are other complications.

Intracerebral haemorrhage

This characteristically occurs in the basal ganglia, brain stem or cerebellum, and results from a sudden rupture of small, deep perforating arteries, secondary to degeneration of the vessel wall or microaneurysms, caused by chronic hypertension. In the elderly, however, more superficial haemorrhages may occur related to cerebral amyloid angiopathy. Bleeding disorders, such as uncontrolled anticoagulation, are a possible cause. There may be underlying aneurysms and AVMs (possibly causing cranial bruits), and 10 per cent are found to have underlying neoplasms.

Cerebral venous thrombosis

This is due to thrombosis in the lateral or sagittal sinus, or small cortical veins and usually occurs as a complication of dehydration, sepsis or hypercoagulable states – particularly during pregnancy and also in the puerperium. There may be raised intracranial pressure with headache and papilloedema, and in more severe cases seizures, confusion and coma can occur progressing to death if untreated. In cortical venous occlusion there are focal symptoms and signs. On computerized tomography (CT) the infarcts do not appear wedge-shaped, like those with arterial infarction, and they are often haemorrhagic.

Transient ischaemic attacks

Transient ischaemic attack (TIA) has the same definition as stroke except that the symptoms and signs resolve within 24 hours. Most patients recover within 30 minutes, and if a dense deficit lasts more than 1 hour, then full recovery within 24 hours is unusual. CT shows that as many as 20 per cent of patients sustain a small infarct, particularly if the symptoms last more than 30 minutes. A patient with a TIA has about 5–10 times the risk of stroke, but conversely only 15% of CVAs are preceded by a TIA. Many middle-aged and elderly patients without a history of stroke or TIA have small infarcts, lacunes or patchy ischaemic periventricular imaging abnormalities (leukoaraiosis) on CT or magnetic resonance imaging (MRI).

Focal epilepsy can cause transient focal neurological symptoms, as does migraine (symptoms usually progress over 10–30 minutes), but a good history should prevent misdiagnosis. Transient global amnesia causes loss of recent memory, without other cognitive impairment, lasting 30 minutes to several hours, and has a good prognosis. Vertigo and dizziness alone are rarely due to a TIA. Hypoglycaemia may cause transient hemiparesis.

Rare causes of stroke

Abnormalities that promote thrombosis include polycythaemia, thrombocythaemia and anti-cardiolipin antibodies. Thrombophilia is more commonly associated with cerebral venous thrombosis than arterial stroke. Severe systemic hypotension or cardiac arrest usually results in diffuse cerebral damage, but can occasionally cause focal infarction in the 'watershed' areas between the territories of the major cerebral arteries. Migraine is a rare cause of cerebral infarction, but remember that stroke itself may often cause a migraine-like headache. Vasculitis is a rare cause of both haemorrhagic and ischaemic stroke. This is due to conditions such as systemic lupus erythematosus, polyarteritis nodosa and giant cell arteritis, which also usually cause systemic symptoms. Cerebral infarction in HIV-infected individuals is not common in the absence of cerebral non-HIV infection, lymphoma or embolic sources (Connor et al., 2000 (see the Box).

Important conditions in stroke differential diagnosis

Malignancy – primary and secondary
Subdural haematoma

Infections important in Africa

HIV-positive – consider CNS infection, e.g. toxoplasma, CMV: also consider lymphoma.
Syphilis
Cerebral abscess
Cerebral cysticercosis
Tuberculoma
Echinococcus cysts

Investigation

Radiological

This is possible only in tertiary referral hospitals, where it may confirm the diagnosis, establish the underlying pathology, identify the size and site of the lesion and establish the aetiological mechanism. CT or MRI will establish the pathological diagnosis (infarction or haemorrhage) and exclude other conditions that may mimic stroke, e.g. sub-dural haematoma or intracranial tumour. The site of the infarction may give clues to the pathogenesis; for example, multiple cortical infarcts in different territories suggest emboli from the heart. In SAH, subarachnoid blood may be demonstrated. Urgent scanning is particularly important if the patient has the following, as all may indicate a surgically treatable condition:

- progressive or fluctuating symptoms
- drowsiness or coma
- brainstem symptoms or signs
- papilloedema
- neck stiffness or fever
- severe headache
- deterioration unexpectedly.

CT appearance

A haemorrhage is seen within a few minutes as an area of increased attenuation, but after a few weeks becomes cystic and of low attenuation. After 2 weeks it may be impossible to distinguish infarct from haemorrhage. The appearances of an infarct change over the first few weeks, and not all infarcts show up on CT scan (see Figs 73.1 and 73.2). MRI is more sensitive to small areas of ischaemia, and can detect the traces of old haemorrhage (haemosiderin deposits) indefinitely.

Advanced techniques

Carotid ultrasonography using duplex imaging and colour-coded doppler measurement of blood flow velocity can identify internal carotid artery stenosis, occlusion, and dissection. It is only indicated if there has been a definite symptomatic carotid territory event leading to TIA or non-disabling stroke, and there is a potential for referral for carotid endarterectomy if a significant stenosis is found.

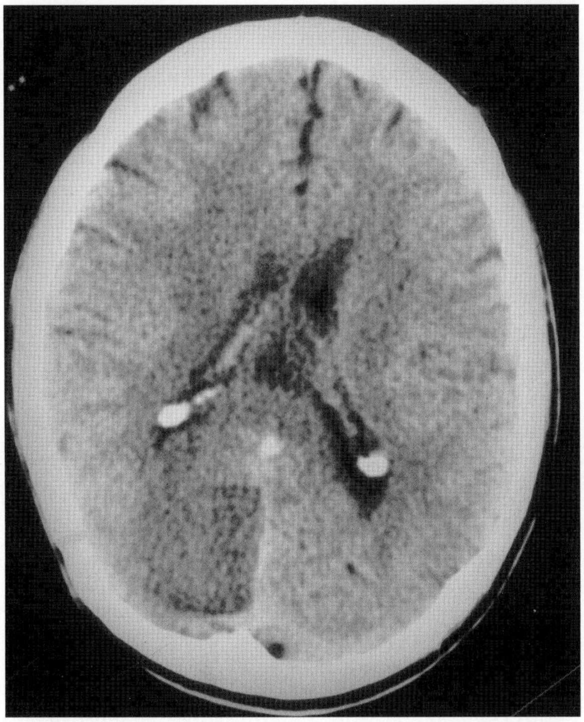

Fig. 73.1. Computerized tomogram (CT) showing a right posterior cerebral infarction.

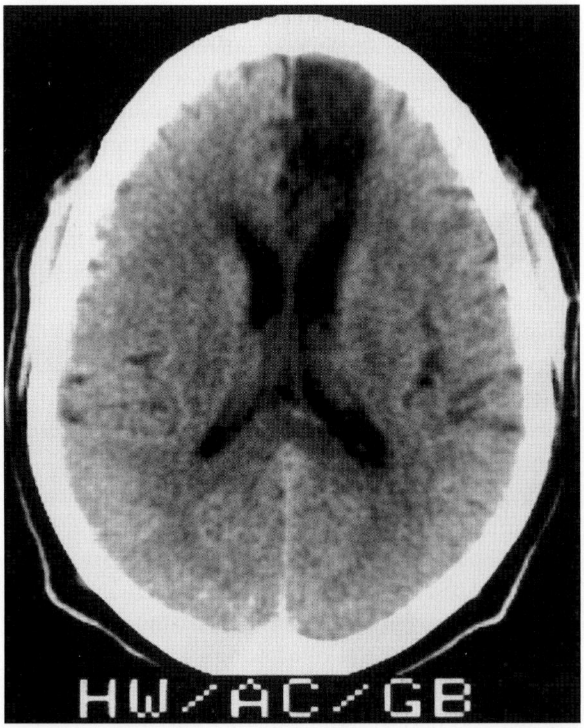

Fig. 73.2. CT brain scan showing cerebral infarction in the left anterior cerebral artery territory.

Investigations in acute stroke

Essential	
Full blood count	Polycythaemia ↑ WCC may suggest infection Thrombocythaemia (increased risk of infarction) thrombocytopenia (increased risk of haemorrhage)
ESR	↑ may indicate infection or vasculitis
Urea and electrolytes	Dehydration
Fasting blood glucose	Often raised initially: if persists – diabetes
Syphilis serology	Meningo-vascular neurosyphilis
ECG	Atrial fibrillation
Possible (depending on indications and facilities available)	
CT head scan (MRI)	Confirm diagnosis. Haemorrhage or infarction
CXR	Possible aspiration pneumonia
Carotid Doppler ultrasound	Only if potential referral for carotid endarterectomy
Echocardiogram	If suspect cardioembolic source
Clotting screen	In PICH
Blood cultures	If suspect bacterial endocarditis
Thrombophilia screen	Young patients without identifiable risk factors
Fasting lipids	
Lumbar puncture	SAH (xanthochromia), meningitis or encephalitis. See Neurology chapter for precautions

Laboratory investigations

These are summarized below. There is considerable debate about cholesterol and the risk of stroke, but raised cholesterol would appear to increase slightly the risk of ischaemic stroke (see the Box).

Cardiac investigations

An ECG will define AF, and an echocardiogram may demonstrate thrombus in the heart. Transoesophageal echocardiography (TOE) can be used to identify an atrial abnormality or patent foramen ovale, and can also identify ulcerated aortic atherosclerosis or dissection.

Treatment

Nursing care

Good care is fundamental.

- Make certain that the family acts to help.

Aspirin

Consensus guidelines have recently been agreed in the UK (Anonymous, 2000). As soon as the diagnosis of ischaemic stroke is confirmed, give aspirin 300 mg, and give it daily thereafter, but reduce to 75 mg after 2 weeks, as secondary prophylaxis. The International Stroke Trial Collaborative Group (IST, 1997) showed that aspirin in the first 10 days following stroke reduced mortality by 1 per cent.

Anticoagulants

There is no evidence to support the use of anticoagulants for the treatment of acute stroke and they cause a significant excess of extracranial and intracranial bleeds. Anticoagulation is commonly undertaken for basilar artery thrombosis, carotid artery dissection and patients with left ventricular thrombus with acute stroke, although there is no strong evidence for this. Although heparin does prevent deep vein thrombosis (DVT), the risk of fatal pulmonary embolism is lower than the risk of intracranial haemorrhage, and therefore physical methods of preventing DVT, such as support stockings and early mobilization, are preferable.

Hypertension

Treat hypertension cautiously as a reduction in blood pressure may lower cerebral blood flow in the regions surrounding an infarct below a critical level at which ischaemic brain damage will occur.

Metabolic disorder

Hypoxia, hyperglycaemia, sepsis and pyrexia can all lead to a worse outcome and are all amenable to treatment. Trials of intravenous magnesium, and tight glucose control in acute stroke, are in progress. Nimodipine (a calcium antagonist) prevents ischaemic brain damage and reduces the numbers who remain disabled after SAH, but has no apparent benefit in acute ischaemic stroke or PICH.

Neurosurgery

This has little to offer patients with stroke disease, with occasional exceptions. Evacuation of a cerebellar haematoma is life saving. Evacuation of supratentorial haematomas should only be considered in younger patients with deteriorating consciousness. Neurosurgery is beneficial for obstructive hydrocephalus following stroke. In SAH from a ruptured aneurysm early intervention aims to clip or coil the aneurysm to prevent rebleeding.

Secondary prevention

In the UK Oxfordshire Community Stroke Project (OCSP) the average risk of recurrent stroke in 675 patients following their first-ever stroke was 13 per cent in the first year and 4 per cent in subsequent years. In those that survived, the risk of recurrence was 30 per cent by 5 years (Burn et al., 1994). There are no comparable studies from Africa.

Thrombolysis

Intravenous thrombolytic therapy with recombinant tissue plasminogen activator (rtPA) gives clear benefit when given within 3 hours of the first symptom in patients with cerebral infarction without extensive early CT signs. (Number needed to treat to prevent one death or disability = 9.) This is applicable in only a very small proportion of stroke patients and is not applicable in Africa at the present time.

Drug treatment

Control of blood pressure following stroke, in those diagnosed to be hypertensive after 1 week, is very important for secondary prevention. Indeed, recent evidence from 2 trials of ACE inhibitors (perindopril and ramipril) demonstrated a 25–30% reduction in further CVA, regardless of starting blood pressure, for both infarction and haemorrhage. Aspirin (75 mg) has a clear benefit in preventing recurrent stroke, and a combination of aspirin and modified-release dipyridamole 200 mg b.d. has been shown to be about twice as effective as either agent alone in reducing recurrent stroke. In patients intolerant of aspirin, clopidogrel is of proven benefit, although it is a lot more expensive than aspirin. Do not give aspirin in the primary prevention of stroke as side effects outweigh benefits.

Atrial fibrillation

Treatment should be with warfarin (currently impracticable in most parts of Africa), with a target International Normalized Ratio (INR) of 2.5, as prophylaxis, or 300 mg of aspirin, if warfarin is contraindicated. Warfarin and aspirin should only be used together in exceptional circumstances. To minimize the risks of cerebral haemorrhage, warfarin should not normally be commenced, or recommenced, for 2 weeks following a stroke.

Statin therapy for raised cholesterol levels has been shown to prevent stroke in patients with ischaemic heart disease and also in patients with a history of cerebrovascular disease. These drugs are very expensive and hypercholesterolaemia is not generally a problem in Africa.

Carotid endarterectomy

Severe carotid stenosis is very rare in Africa and so the great individual benefit which can follow endarterectomy, in preventing stroke in symptomatic patients with recent TIA or stroke, and severe stenosis (>70%) of the internal carotid artery on the affected side, is of academic interest only.

Complications after stroke

Immobility

- Pressure sores
- Shoulder pain.

Brain damage

- Cerebral oedema – a sudden decline after 24–48 hours
- Spontaneous haemorrhagic transformation of an infarct – worsening of symptoms
- Communication problems.

Thrombembolism

- DVT leading to pulmonary emboli.

Emotions

- Anxiety, depression, emotional lability.

Swallowing problems occur in half the patients in the first 2–3 days (particularly in posterior circulation infarcts which generally have a good long-term outcome) and may cause aspiration pneumonia. Patients may be fed by nasogastric tube, but after 2 weeks percutaneous endoscopic gastrostomy (PEG tube) is preferred, if this is available.

Nursing care is supremely important. Where nurses are few, and the family is inexperienced, pressure sores, particularly in incontinent people, are liable to occur early.

Rehabilitation

The aim of rehabilitation is to improve quality of life by reducing emotional, functional, cognitive, physical and communication disorders.

Specialized stroke units can reduce mortality (Langhorne et al., 1993) and morbidity following stroke by about 28 per cent, at whatever age or whatever severity. The ideal is to have a co-ordinated expert interdisciplinary team, including physiotherapy, occupational therapy, speech and language therapy, medical and nursing staff, with regular team meetings.

Community-based rehabilitation services play a key role following discharge. The emotional impact of stroke can include anger, denial, anxiety, depression, emotionalism and post-traumatic stress disorder, all of which are associated with worse outcomes (see the Box).

Checklist for action post-stroke

Nursing

Good nursing care with frequent turning of comatose patients to prevent pressure sores.
Early physiotherapy.
Occupational and speech and language therapy, where available.
Teach family good nursing care/manual handling techniques before discharge home.

General care

Swallowing screen at admission and repeated as necessary.
Be aware of possible aspiration pneumonia in patients with swallowing problems.
Intravenous or subcutaneous fluids to maintain hydration if necessary.
Treat pyrexia and hyperglycaemia as necessary.
Monitor blood pressure regularly.

Drugs

Aspirin 300 mg for first 2 weeks (then 75 mg daily) if infarct confirmed.
Warfarin commenced/recommenced at week 2 if patient has atrial fibrillation, or aspirin 300 mg long term).
Anti-hypertensive treatment if BP still elevated after 1 week (DO NOT try to reduce BP rapidly)

Follow-up

Address individual risk factors and start secondary prevention.

African stroke studies

'When all possible causes had been considered, there still remained a bafflingly large number of younger patients, for whom there was no detectable explanation for the ictus which struck them down but seldom killed them' (Billinghurst, 1970). What was true in the 1960s is still true today.

Table 73.2. Aetiology of stroke in Africa

Author	Publication	Country	Type of study	Number of strokes	Number of CT scans	PICH (%)	Infarct (%) [emboli][a]
Matenga et al.	1986	Zimbabwe	Prospective	93	80	31	69
Rosman	1986	RSA	Prospective	116	92	33	67 [14]
Joubert	1991	RSA	Prospective	250	250	29	71 [24]
Nyame et al.	1998	Ghana	Retrospective	907	907	60	40

Notes:
[a] As percentage of total number of strokes.

Mortality – verbal autopsy

Most of the limited information for Africa is based on verbal autopsy, which relies on an interview with relations and/or carers after death, to ascribe the likely cause of death. In a South African rural subdistrict, 5 per cent of deaths were attributable to stroke (Kahn & Tollman, 1999). In Tanzania mortality was highest in a relatively affluent rural area and lowest in a poor rural area (Walker et al., 2000a). Age-adjusted mortality rates for those aged 15–64 years were significantly higher in all 3 areas where they were measured than in similar UK data, but mortality rose with age, as in industrialized countries (Bonita & Beaglehole, 1992).

Incidence

The incidence of all three main pathological types of stroke, cerebral infarction, PICH and SAH, increases with age. Many cases of stroke in Africa are not recorded because they have no contact with organized medical services and a truly community-based, incidence study has yet to be done.

Prevalence

As hospital-based studies reflect only those people who manage to reach hospital, they do not necessarily give an accurate picture of disability from stroke within the community. We have very little idea about the burden of disability relating to stroke in sub-Saharan Africa, but prevalence per 100 000 has varied from 15 in central Ethiopia (Tekle-Haimanot et al., 1990) to 58 in Southern Nigeria (Osuntokun et al., 1987), and 73 in Northern Tanzania (Walker et al., 2000b).

Trends with time

In most developed countries there has been a gradual decline in stroke mortality rates. In Accra, however, there was a dramatic increase in the number of cases of CVA from the 1960s, 1976–1983, to the 1990s (Nyame et al., 1994), but these data were collected at different times by different people and for different reasons and are therefore difficult to compare.

Aetiology

Clinical scales are of some value in differentiating strokes caused by haemorrhage from those caused by infarction (Sandercock et al., 1985; Poungvarin et al., 1991), and they can be useful to identify patients at low risk of haemorrhage (Celani et al., 1994), though this still leaves many strokes in which it is difficult to be certain of aetiology. While there are few CT scanners in sub-Saharan Africa, data from the few reported series are summarized in Table 73.2.

It has been suggested that PICH causes a higher proportion of strokes in Zimbabwe than in industrialized countries (Matenga et al., 1986), though patients with primary intracranial haemorrhage have more severe strokes and are more likely to go to hospital; in Ghana (Nyame et al 1998) at a tertiary referral hospital all patients were included who had been referred for a CT head scan with a diagnosis of CVA or stroke, so there is likely to be considerable selection bias.

Differential diagnosis

Data from sub-Saharan Africa (Aiyesimoju et al., 1983; Matenga et al., 1986; Nyame et al., 1998; Rosman, 1986) are similar to those from industrialized countries where about 5 per cent of patients presenting with 'stroke' have a space occupying lesion such as subdural haematoma, tumour or cerebral abscess. Cerebral malaria may cause focal neurological deficits similar to a stroke.

Autopsy studies

Information is scarce. In Ghana (Anim & Kofi, 1989) significant atherosclerotic lesions in the cerebral vessels were found in 11 per cent of hypertensive, and 2 per cent of normotensive, patients but amongst the hypertensives those with cerebral haemorrhage did not have more severe atherosclerosis. Nigerians had least atherosclerosis of all groups in a large comparative USA and West African study (Resch et al., 1970; Williams et al., 1975).

Characteristics of patients in African stroke studies

Age

The mean age of stroke patients in African reports is under 60 years (usually 55 to 60), and the peak decade for stroke is the sixth, with no major difference between males and females.

Sex

Up to twice as many males as females are represented in hospital studies in Africa, possibly because women are less likely than men to go to hospital, but there may also be a sex difference in incidence (Osuntokun, 1994). Patterns may be changing: thus, for 273 'first-ever' strokes in Harare (Matenga, 1997), the age-specific crude incidence rates for women were consistently higher at all age groups except for the 45–54 year group. The overall male to female crude ratio was 1 to 1.1. In Accra, whereas in the 1960s males outnumbered females by 2: 1, approximately equal numbers were admitted in the years 1990–1993 (Nyame et al., 1994).

Risk factors

Hypertension

The level of both systolic and diastolic blood pressure (BP) is important as a risk factor for stroke (Shaper et al., 1991). In many African studies it is difficult to be certain how important hypertension is (Walker 1994), because

1. The BP may be raised within the first few days after a stroke as a normal physiological response.
2. The BP history of those who die early may not be known.
3. End organ damage – ECG criteria for LV hypertrophy, hypertensive retinal changes, and renal damage – may not have been recorded.

In spite of these 'difficulties', rates are between 30 and 70 per cent for cohorts of stroke patients, and there is no doubt whatever that treatment of hypertension reduces risk of stroke (Collins et al., 1990), so that an average reduction of BP by 8.5 mmHg reduces the incidence of stroke by 42 per cent.

History of cerebrovascular disease

The percentage of people with a first stroke who give a past history of TIA in African studies varies from 0 to 11 per cent, and of previous stroke from 4 to 10 per cent (Bahemuka, 1985; Abebe & Haimenot, 1990; Joubert, 1991; Nwosu et al., 1992).

Carotid stenosis

No atherosclerotic changes were found in stroke patients in Lusaka, Zambia (Umerah, 1980). In the 30 patients from the Medunsa Stroke Data Bank (MSDB) who came to autopsy (Joubert et al., 1990), the maximum degree of atherosclerotic stenosis of the extracranial carotid arteries was only 22 per cent.

Coronary artery disease (CAD)

While this is a very common risk factor in stroke patients in industrialized countries, it is very rare in Africa (Matenga et al., 1986; Rosman, 1986; Bahemuka, 1985). The prevalence of CAD in African stroke patients may, however, be higher: Joubert and McClean (2000) found resting ECG evidence of myocardial ischaemia in 15 per cent.

Cardiac embolic source

Emboli secondary to rheumatic heart disease are often proposed as the cause of stroke in young people in sub-Saharan Africa. In the only African study in which patients were investigated prospectively with echocardiography, 24 per cent had a definite embolic source (Joubert et al., 1989). Rates elsewhere have varied from 3–15 per cent (Osuntokun et al., 1979; Matenga et al., 1986; Rosman, 1986; Abebe & Haimanot, 1990; Nwosu et al., 1992).

Rates of AF have been reported rarely but range from 5 to 10 per cent of patients, whose strokes were generally

Table 73.3. Main risk factors for stroke

Risk factor	Cerebral infarction	Intracerebral haemorrhage	Sub-arachnoid haemorrhage
Greater age	++	++	+
Hypertension	++	++	+
Ischaemic heart disease	++	0	0
Atrial fibrillation	++	0	0
Diabetes mellitus	++	0	0
Peripheral vascular disease	++	0	0
Raised haematocrit	+	0	0
High cholesterol	+	0	0
Low cholesterol	0	+	0
High plasma fibrinogen	+	0	0
Smoking	++	+	++
Alcohol	–	++	+
Obesity	+	+	?
Transient ischaemic attack	++	0	0

Notes:
++, strong association; + moderate association; 0, no association; -, protective in moderation.

classified as embolic. AF increases with age in industrialized countries, and it is not therefore surprising that it seems to be less common in African studies.

Diabetes

People with diabetes have double the risk of stroke compared to non-diabetic subjects (Kannel & McGee, 1979), as demonstrated in Lagos by Danesi et al. (1983). Blood glucose may be raised, probably because of a stress response, immediately after stroke in non-diabetic as well as diabetic patients (Stout, 1989) and this appears to affect outcome adversely. Most African studies report rates of diabetes of between 5 and 10 per cent, of whom half were known to be diabetic.

Smoking

Smoking is a strong risk factor for SAH and for cerebral infarction, but not for PICH. It is an increasing problem in Africa.

Pregnancy and oral contraceptives

There is a slightly increased risk of stroke in pregnancy and the puerperium, and a very slightly increased risk from the oral contraceptive (OC), particularly older higher oestrogen pills. This becomes more important in conjunction with other risk factors such as smoking.

Sickle cell disease

Homozygous sickle cell disease (SCD) can cause stroke (including cerebral infarction, cerebral haemorrhage and subarachnoid haemorrhage) in children, but it is rare as a cause of stroke in adults (Osuntokun, 1994).

Meningovascular neurosyphilis

In sub-Saharan Africa the prevalence of positive syphilis serology among the general population is between 5 and 15 per cent, so that positive syphilis serology in a patient presenting with stroke may be coincidental. If the cerebral spinal fluid (CSF) is also positive, the stroke *may* be due to syphilis, but this is rare, whether in Ethiopia (Abebe & Haimanot, 1990) or Sierra Leone (Lisk, 1993).

Stroke in young adults

Sickle cell disease, idiopathic tropical aortitis and embolism secondary to rheumatic heart disease with atrial fibrillation are possible causes.

Socio-economic group

There is conflicting evidence on the relationship between socio-economic group and stroke in Africa, whether an increased risk in the higher socio-economic groups (Osuntokun et al., 1969), or in the lower (Dada et al., 1969; Danesi et al. 1983) – the pattern in industrialized countries. Table 73.3 summarizes the effect of the major risk factors and other variables on different types of stroke.

Outcome and prognosis

More patients with SAH or PICH die within 30 days than do those with cerebral infarction, but outcome is slightly better at 1 year in survivors of a haemorrhage. Overall 25 to 30 per cent remain significantly disabled and dependent on others. Lacunar infarction has a better prognosis, while total anterior cerebral infarction (TACI) has a very poor outcome. Greater age, coma at onset, and persistent neglect predict a poor outcome. Recovery is fastest in the early stages, most occurs in the first month; but further recovery, particularly functional, may continue for more than one year. Over 50 demographic, radiological, neurophysiological and neurological determinants are claimed individually, or in combination, to predict stroke outcome, but the accuracy of these predictions is very variable. Table 73.4 reviews the major published African

Table 73.4. Case-fatality in African stroke studies

Author	Publication year	Country	Study type	Number of cases	Mortality
Prospective					
Rosman	1986	South Africa	CT scans	116	34% at 1 month (22% for infarction and 58% for PICH)
Joubert	1991	South Africa	CT scans	304	33% at 1 month
Longo-Mbenza et al.	1999	Congo	Some CTs	1032	58% in hospital (62% for infarction and 38% for PICH)
Matenga	1997	Zimbabwe	No CT scans	273	35% in 1 week (40% for females and 31% for males)
Retrospective					
Nyame et al.	1994	Ghana	Hospital admissions data		42–50%
Zabsonre et al.	1997	Burkina Faso	Hospital admissions	193	32% in hospital (NB 22 = TIAs)
Bahemuka	1985	Kenya	Hospital admissions	207	19% at 100 days (data on 188)

mortality studies, all of which are based on in-hospital data.

Prospective african studies

A 1-month mortality of 33 per cent of the 304 strokes was reported by the South African MSDB study (Joubert, 1991), but no breakdown into haemorrhage and infarction was given. In the Pretoria study (Rosman, 1986), the overall mortality at 1 month was 34 per cent (22 per cent for cerebral infarction and 58 per cent for PICH), but the method of follow-up and the place of death (hospital or home) were not recorded. In Kinshasa, 58 per cent of 1032 (ischaemic 49 per cent and haemorrhagic 51 per cent) stroke patients died in hospital (Longo-Mbenza et al., 1999) and, of these, 62 per cent had had an ischaemic stroke, and 38 per cent a haemorrhagic stroke. In Harare, 35 per cent of patients with a first-ever stroke died within the first week (Matenga, 1997). The Gambia mortality study showed that 65 per cent of these deaths were due to complications of 'decubitus'.

Retrospective case note reviews

With retrospective studies often not all records can be traced, and those that can may have incomplete information. Such studies are also restricted to looking at in-hospital mortality. The clinical diagnosis of haemorrhage and infarction is likely to be even less accurate than for prospective studies without CT scans. Often only positive findings are documented in notes and if, for instance, history of alcohol is not recorded, it is often assumed that patients were non-drinkers. There will be subjective variations between the different doctors writing in the notes. Therefore, the inferences and conclusions from these papers need to be considered carefully with these thoughts in mind. A study from Accra (Nyame et al. 1994) looking at stroke admissions from the early 1960s to the early 1990s found a dramatic increase in both admissions and case-fatality for the early 1990s. CVA was the leading cause of death in adults accounting for 17.2 per cent of deaths on the medical wards and case-fatality ranged from 42 per cent to 50 per cent over the time period.

None of the above studies looked at mortality in relation to time to admission to hospital which is very important. For various reasons (including distance from hospital, access to transport, ability to afford hospital fees and local beliefs), it is likely that there is greater delay in patients reaching hospital in Africa (particularly in rural areas) than in industrialized countries. Many studies, both prospective and retrospective, are from tertiary referral hospitals, so that time to admission is likely to be longer than in other hospitals. Patients dying early from their stroke, or making a rapid recovery, are less likely to be admitted.

Morbidity

While good mortality data are scarce, good morbidity data are even harder to find. Of the 318 patients in the prospective Ibadan Stroke Register (Osuntokun et al., 1979), 207 were alive at 3 weeks, of whom most were living with their families. Relating to follow-up, there were major problems with incorrect addresses, and many patients did not return to the clinics for evaluation.

Important areas for future research

There is a great need for the following areas to be studied:

- Stroke incidence – a community based incidence study would add to knowledge gained from prevalence and mortality studies.
- Are haemorrhagic strokes more common as has been suggested by hospital-based studies utilizing CT scans?
- What is the relative importance of the different risk factors for stroke in Africa?
- Where should patients be treated and which patients may benefit from attending hospital?
- Is community-based rehabilitation the most cost-effective form of rehabilitation and, if so, what is the best model?

There is no doubt that the problem of stroke in Africa is going to increase dramatically over the next few years. It is important that cost-effective prevention programmes are designed and implemented and cost-effective rehabilitation programmes are developed.

References

Anonymous. (1996). Where is the lesion? In *Stroke. A Practical Guide to Management*, ed. CP Warlow, MS Dennis, J van Gijn et al., pp. 80–145. Oxford: Blackwell Science.

Anonymous. (2000). *Consensus Statement on Stroke Treatment and Service Delivery.* Edinburgh: Royal College of Physicians of Edinburgh.

Abebe M, Haimanot RT. (1990). Cerebrovascular accidents in Ethiopia. *Ethiop Med J*; **28**: 53–61.

Aiyesimoju AB, Osuntokun BO, Adeuja AOG, Olumide, A., Ogunseyinde, AO. (1983). Misdiagnosis of stroke. *Afr J Med Sci*; **12**: 107–112.

Anim JI, Kofi AD. (1989). Hypertension, cerebral vascular changes and stroke in Ghana: cerebral atherosclerosis and stroke. *E Afr Med J*; **66**: 468–475.

Bahemuka M. (1985). Cerebrovascular accidents in 207 Kenyans: general peculiarities and prognosis of stroke in an urban medical centre. *E Afr Med J*; **62**: 315–322.

Billinghurst JR. (1970). The pattern of adult neurological admissions to Mulago hospital, Kampala (June, 1966 to May, 1968). *E Afr Med J*; **47**: 653–663.

Bonita R, Beaglehole R. (1992). Stroke mortality. In *Population Based Studies of Stroke*, ed. JP Whisnant, pp. 1–30. Publ Butterworths.

Burn J, Dennis M, Bamford J, Sandercock P, Wade D, Warlow C. (1994). Long-term risk of recurrent stroke after a first-ever stroke. *Stroke*; **25**: 333–337.

Celani MG, Righetti E, Migliacci R.et al. (1994). Comparability and validity of two clinical scores in the early differential diagnosis of acute stroke. *Br Med J*; **308**: 1674–1676.

Collins R, Peto R, MacMahon S et al. (1990). Blood pressure, stroke, and coronary heart disease. Part 2, short-term reductions in blood pressure: overview of randomised drug trials in their epidemiological context. *Lancet*; **335**: 827–838.

Connor MD, Lammie GA, Bell JE et al. (2000). Cerebral infarction in adult AIDS patients. Observations from the Edinburgh HIV Autopsy Cohort. *Stroke*; **31**: 2117–2126.

Dada TO, Johnson FA, Araba AB. (1969). Cerebrovascular accidents in Nigerians – a review of 205 cases. *W Afr Med J*; **18**: 95–108.

Danesi MA, Oyenola YA, Ontiri AS. (1983). Risk factors associated with cerebrovascular accidents in Nigerians (a case control study). *E Afr Med J*; **60**: 190–195.

Joubert G, McLean CA, Reid et al. (2000). Ischemic heart disease in black South African stroke patients. *Stroke*; **31**: 1294–1298.

Joubert J. (1991). The Medunsa stroke data bank: an analysis of 304 patients seen between 1986 and 1987. *S Afr Med J*; **80**: 567–570.

Joubert J, Van Gelder AL, Darazs B, Pilloy WJ. (1989). The cardiovascular status of the black stroke patient. *S Afr Med J*; **76:** 657–664.

Joubert J, Lemmer LB, Fourie PA, Vangelder AL, Daraz B. (1990). Are clinical differences between black and white stroke patients caused by variations in the atherosclerotic involvement of the arterial tree? *S Afr Med J*; **77**: 248–251.

Kahn K, Tollman SM. (1999). Stroke in rural South Africa – contributing to the little known about a big problem. *S Afr Med J*; **89**: 63–65.

Kannel WB, McGee DL. (1979). Diabetes and cardiovascular disease. The Framingham Study. *J Am Med Assoc*; **241**: 2035–2038.

Langhorne P, Williams BO, Gilchrist W, Howie K. (1993). Do stroke units save lives? *Lancet*; **342**: 395–398.

Lisk DR (1993). Stroke risk factors in an African population: a report from Sierra Leone. *Stroke*; **24**: 139–140.

Longo-Mbenza B, Phanzu-Mbete LB, M'Buyamba-Kabangu JR et al. (1999). Haematocrit and stroke in black Africans under tropical climate and meteorological influence. *Ann Méd Interne*; **150**: 171–177.

Matenga J. (1997). Stroke incidence rates among black residents of Harare – a prospective community-based study. *S Afr Med J*; **87**: 606–609.

Matenga J, Kitai I, Levy L. (1986). Strokes among black people in Harare, Zimbabwe: results of computed tomography and associated risk factors. *Br Med J*; **292**: 1649–1651.

Nwosu CM, Nwabueze AC, Ikeh VO. (1992). Stroke at the prime of life: a study of Nigerian Africans between the ages of 16 and 45 years. *E Afr Med J*; **69**: 384–390.

Nyame PK, Bonsu-Bruce N, Amoah AGB. et al. (1994). Current trends in the incidence of cerebrovascular accidents in Accra. *W Afr J Med*; **13**: 183–186.

Nyame PK, Jumah KB, Adjei S. (1998). Computerised tomographic scan of the head in evaluation of stroke in Ghanaians. *E Afr Med J*; **75**: 637–639.

Osuntokun BO, Odeku EL, Adeloye RBA. (1969). Cerebrovascular accidents in Nigerians: a study of 348 patients. *W Afr J Med*; **18**: 160–173.

Osuntokun BO, Bademosi O, Akinkugbe OO, Oyediran ABO, Carlisle R. (1979). Incidence of stroke in an African city: results from the stroke registry at Ibadan, Nigeria, 1973–1975. *Stroke*; **10**: 205–207.

Osuntokun BO, Adeuja AOG, Schoenberg BS et al. (1987). Neurological disorders in Nigerian Africans: a community-based study. *Acta Neurol Scand*; **75**: 13–21.

Osuntokun BO. (1994). Epidemiology of stroke in blacks in Africa. *Hypertens Res*; **17**: S1–S10.

Poungvarin N, Viriyavejakal A, Komontri C. (1991). Siriraj stroke score and validation study to distinguish supratentorial intracerebral haemorrhage from infarction. *Br Med J*; **302**: 1565–1567.

Resch JA, Williams AO, Lemercier G, Lowenson B. (1970). Comparative autopsy studies on cerebral atherosclerosis in Nigerian and Senegal negroes, American negroes and caucasians. *Atherosclerosis*; **12**: 401–407.

Rosman KD. (1986). The epidemiology of stroke in an urban black population. *Stroke*; **17**: 667–669.

Sandercock P, Molyneux A, Warlow C. (1985). Value of computerised tomography in patients with stroke: the Oxfordshire Community Stroke Project. *Br Med J*; **290**: 193–197.

Shaper AG, Phillips AN, Pocock SJ, Walker M, Macfarlane PW. (1991). Risk factors for stroke in middle aged British men. *Br Med J*; **302**: 1111–1115.

Stout RW. (1989). Hyperglycaemia and stroke. *Quart J Med*; **73**: 997–1004.

Tekle-Haimanot R, Abebe M, Gebre-Mariam A. et al. (1990). Community-based study of neurological disorders in rural central Ethiopia. *Neuroepidemiology*; **9**: 263–277.

Umerah BC. (1980). Angiography of stroke in central Africa. *Am J Roentgenol*; **134**: 963–965.

Walker, R. (1994). Hypertension and stroke in sub-saharan Africa. *Trans Roy Soc Trop Med Hyg*; **88**: 609–611.

Walker RW, McLarty DG, Kitange, HM et al. (2000a). Stroke mortality in urban and rural Tanzania. *Lancet*; **355**: 1684–1687.

Walker RW, McLarty DG, Masuki G. et al. (2000b). Age specific prevalence of impairment and disability relating to hemiplegic stroke in the Hai District of Northern Tanzania. *J Neurol Neurosurg Psychiatry*; **68**: 744–749.

WHO MONICA Project. (1988). Monitoring trends and determinants in cardiovascular disease: a major international collaboration. *J Clin Epidemiol*; **41**: 105–114.

Williams AO, Loewenson RB, Lippert DM, Resch JA. (1975). Cerebral atherosclerosis and its relationship to selected diseases in Nigerians: a pathological study. *Stroke*; **6**: 395–401.

Zabsonre P, Yameogo A, Millogo A, Dyemkouma FX, Durand G. (1997). Risk and severity factors in cerebrovascular accidents in west african Blacks of Burkina Faso. *Méd Trop*; **57**: 147–152.

74 Epilepsy

Epilepsy is common and affects all age groups. Untreated epileptic seizures lead to injury and a social stigma with deep effects. In rural areas where open fires are used for cooking, epilepsy is classically associated with burns (Fig. 74.1). Frequent seizures have a detrimental effect on education, employment and marital life. Poorly controlled seizures are also associated with increased mortality.

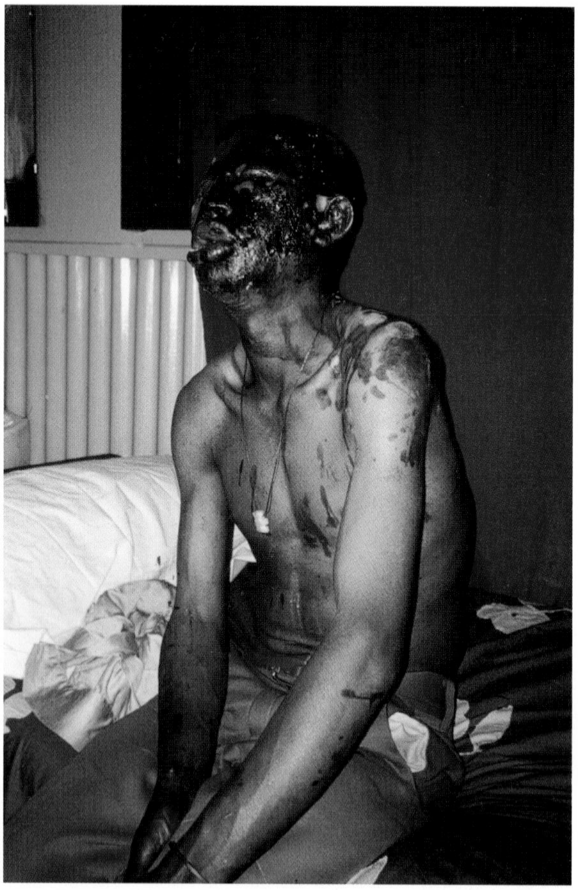

Fig. 74.1. Severe burns to the face caused by a fall into an open fire used for cooking.

Inexpensive treatment exists and is effective in about 70 per cent of patients, but most people with epilepsy living in sub-Saharan Africa (up to 98 per cent in some areas) are not receiving treatment. Inaccessibility of medical treatment, shortage of drugs, lack of awareness of the existence of medical treatment and cultural factors contribute to this 'treatment gap'.

Studies of epilepsy in sub-Saharan Africa have often been limited by lack of consistent definition of terms and classification. In this chapter, therefore, definitions and classification are addressed in detail.

> The diagnosis of epilepsy is clinical and based on the history from the patient and more importantly from a witness. EEG is not necessary to make a diagnosis of epilepsy. The most common differential diagnoses are syncope and non-epileptic seizures (pseudoseizures).

Definitions

Epileptic seizures

Epileptic seizures are the clinical manifestation of an abnormal and excessive discharge of a group of neurons in the brain. The nature of an epileptic seizure is determined by the anatomical localization and spread of the abnormal neuronal discharge, and may involve transient alteration of consciousness, motor, sensory, autonomic or psychic events. Epileptic seizures occur as the result of a wide variety of cerebral and systemic disorders. They may be provoked (acute symptomatic seizures) or unprovoked.

Provoked seizures

Provoked or acute symptomatic seizures occur during, or are closely associated with, an acute cerebral or systemic insult such as cerebral infection, head injury, stroke, metabolic disturbance or alcohol withdrawal. They may be an isolated event, or recurrent if the underlying acute disorder recurs.

Febrile seizures

These are a special form of provoked seizure occurring in childhood after the age of one month and usually before the age of 6 years. They are associated with a febrile illness not caused by CNS infection and do not meet criteria for other acute symptomatic seizures.

Unprovoked seizures

Unprovoked seizures may be a late consequence of an antecedent condition such as cerebral infection, stroke and head injury (remote symptomatic seizures) or there may be no clear antecedent aetiology (idiopathic and cryptogenic).

Idiopathic

This term refers to certain partial and generalized epilepsy syndromes with particular clinical and EEG characteristics, and should not be used for seizures without obvious cause.

Cryptogenic

This term refers to unprovoked seizures for which there is no obvious cause, and includes seizures that do not satisfy the criteria for the symptomatic or idiopathic categories.

Epilepsy

Recurrent, i.e. two or more, unprovoked seizures constitute a diagnosis of epilepsy and are the subject of this chapter (Commission on Epidemiology and Prognosis, ILAE, 1993).

Classification

Classification of the epilepsies and epileptic syndromes

Epilepsy is best viewed, not as a single condition, but as a symptom of cerebral disorder. The international classification of the epilepsies and epilepsy syndromes (Commission on Classification and Terminology, ILAE, 1989) incorporates anatomical, aetiological and syndromic features. This classification is complex and includes many rare syndromes. It also relies on the availability of EEG and neuroimaging, and is difficult to apply outside well resourced specialist clinics.

Table 74.1. Classification by seizure type

I. Partial (focal) seizures
A. Simple partial seizures
B. Complex partial seizures
C. Partial seizures evolving to secondarily generalized seizures.
II. Generalized seizures
A. Absence seizures
B. Myoclonic seizures
C. Clonic seizures
D. Tonic seizures
E. Tonic–clonic seizures
F. Atonic seizures
III. Unclassified epileptic seizures

Source: Adapted from International League Against Epilepsy classification of seizure type, Commission on Classification and Terminology of the ILAE, 1981.

Classification by seizure type

Another method of classification proposed by the International League Against Epilepsy (ILAE) is based on seizure type (Commission on Classification and Terminology, ILAE, 1981). This classification relies on clinical and EEG criteria, and is easier to apply (Table 74.1). A modification allows classification of seizures on purely clinical grounds and is suitable when facilities for investigation are limited (Commission on Epidemiology and Prognosis, ILAE, 1993). Seizures are divided into two main categories, partial and generalized.

Partial seizures

A seizure should be classified as partial when there is either clinical or EEG evidence of partial (focal) onset.

Partial seizures are divided into three categories:

- Simple partial seizures, in which there is no alteration of consciousness.
- Complex partial seizures, in which there is alteration or loss of consciousness.
- Secondarily generalized seizures, which evolve from either simple or complex partial seizures.

Simple partial seizures may evolve into complex partial seizures, and either may evolve into a secondarily generalized seizure (usually a tonic–clonic seizure). An aura or warning before a complex partial or secondarily generalized seizure is, in fact, a simple partial seizure.

Simple partial seizures

The clinical manifestations of simple partial seizures depend on the anatomical localization of the discharge in the brain and may be motor, e.g. focal jerking or posturing, somatosensory, e.g. focal numbness or paraesthesia, special sensory, e.g. visual, auditory, olfactory or gustatory hallucination, autonomic, e.g. rising epigastric sensation or psychic, e.g. déjà-vu.

Complex partial seizures

Complex partial seizures may begin with an aura, typically lasting seconds, before consciousness is affected, or may start abruptly. The altered consciousness is characterized by a blank stare. This may be accompanied by automatisms, which may be:

- verbal, e.g. humming, whistling or meaningless words
- orofacial, e.g. lip smacking or chewing
- manual, e.g. fiddling, tapping or more complex such as removal of items of clothing
- ambulatory, e.g. wandering or circling.

Complex partial seizures typically last 1 or 2 minutes and are followed by a period of confusion and drowsiness lasting up to 15 minutes.

Secondarily generalized seizures

Secondarily generalized seizures usually take the form of a tonic–clonic seizure. Atonic, tonic and clonic seizures occur less frequently. If the seizure spread is rapid, there may be no obvious partial onset. Partial onset can, however, be assumed if the patient also has simple or complex partial seizures which occur independently or if there are focal epileptiform discharges on the EEG.

Generalized seizures

Generalized seizures are characterized by widespread involvement of both cerebral hemispheres from the onset. Typically, the seizure starts with abrupt alteration of consciousness without warning. EEG discharges are bilateral, grossly synchronous and symmetrical over both cerebral hemispheres. Generalized seizures are divided into six categories, of which tonic–clonic, absence and myoclonic seizures are most common.

Generalized tonic–clonic seizures

Generalized tonic–clonic seizures (GTCS) usually begin with sudden loss of consciousness, sometimes accompanied by a scream, and the patient falls to the ground. Occasionally GTCS are preceded by increasing myoclonic jerks. If there is an aura, the seizure should be classified as partial (secondarily generalized).

Loss of consciousness is followed by the tonic phase with clenching of the jaw and stiffness of the limbs. Respiration ceases and cyanosis is common.

This is succeeded by the clonic phase, which is characterized by jerking of the limbs and facial muscles. Breathing is stertorous and saliva may froth from the mouth. If the tongue is bitten, the saliva may be blood-stained. At the end of the clonic phase there may be incontinence. Although the duration of the tonic and clonic phases varies, in most seizures the tonic–clonic phase lasts less than 5 minutes.

During the final phase the patient is unconscious with flaccid muscles. Consciousness is slowly regained, but invariably the patient is confused and drowsy and will often need to sleep. On waking, there may be headache and muscle soreness.

Absence seizures

Absence seizures (previously known as petit mal) occur without warning and are characterized by arrest of activity and a blank stare. Muscle tone is preserved and the patient does not fall. The eyes may deviate upwards with flickering of the eyelids. More than 80 per cent of attacks last less than 10 seconds. Minor automatisms are seen in more prolonged attacks. Recovery is rapid without drowsiness or confusion, and the patient will typically resume normal activity as if nothing has happened. Absence seizures can often be precipitated by hyperventilation.

The most useful clinical features in distinguishing absence from complex partial seizures are:

- duration of 10 seconds or less
- lack of aura
- rapid return to full consciousness.

> Misclassification of partial seizures as generalized seizures is common. If there is an aura before a tonic–clonic seizure, the seizure should be classified as partial (secondarily generalized). Do not confuse absence seizures with complex partial seizures; lack of aura, duration of 10 seconds or less and rapid return to full consciousness are the most useful clinical features in making this distinction.

Myoclonic seizures

Myoclonic seizures are characterized by a brief twitch or jerk of the limbs which may occur singly or repetitively and is often asymmetrical. Recovery is immediate and alteration of consciousness may not be obvious.

Tonic, clonic and atonic seizures

- Tonic seizures – generalized tonic contraction with loss of consciousness and no clonic phase
- Clonic seizures – loss of consciousness and generalized clonic jerking, not preceded by a tonic phase
- Atonic seizures – loss of consciousness with loss of muscle tone.

Recovery from these three seizure types tends to be more rapid than that following a GTCS. These seizures are usually seen in diffuse cerebral disorders often associated with learning disability, but may also be seen as a result of a partial response to treatment.

Unclassifiable seizures

A third category, unclassifiable seizures, is included in the classification of seizure type, and describes those seizures which do not conform to the descriptions of partial and generalized seizures outlined above.

Accurate classification of seizures depends on a detailed description of the attacks and to some extent will be influenced by the level of experience of the person taking the history. Cultural factors and language may make it difficult to obtain a clear description of the attacks, and an aura or partial onset can easily be overlooked by the patient or their family, so that partial seizures are incorrectly classified as generalized seizures. If an EEG is not available, this will also lead to underdiagnosis of partial seizures.

Epidemiology

Methodological considerations

The epidemiology of epilepsy provides a description of epilepsy within the community. The incidence of epilepsy is usually expressed as the number of new cases per 100000 population per year. The prevalence gives an estimate of the number of people at any one time with active epilepsy. Determination of both incidence and prevalence may be difficult (Sander & Shorvon, 1987), because of:

- the differing definitions of epilepsy used by different researchers
- the problems in making a diagnosis of epilepsy
- the difficulty of identifying those with epilepsy.

The problem of definition

Epilepsy is defined as 'the tendency to recurrent, unprovoked seizures', but differing criteria have been used by different authors in assessing incidence and prevalence. Some studies have deemed single seizures to be 'epilepsy', while others have included seizures provoked by fever or alcohol, and those occurring in the context of acute illness. The question of definition is also important in determining prevalence. The term 'people with epilepsy' could include all those who have ever had a seizure (or at least two unprovoked seizures). However, it may be limited to those with active epilepsy – defined, for example, as those who have had either a seizure, or have taken anti-epileptic drugs to prevent seizures, in the last 2 (or sometimes 5) years.

The problem of diagnosis

The diagnosis of epilepsy can be difficult. It relies on a clinical description, which may not be available if no witnesses are present. Minor seizures may be difficult to recognize and may be misdiagnosed as sensory symptoms or panic attacks, and the differential diagnosis is wide. The diagnosis is often suspected but not proven for a considerable length of time. In sub-Saharan Africa, people whose seizures do not amount to tonic–clonic seizures are unlikely to seek help, particularly where medical facilities are not readily accessible, through cost or distance, and so the statistics are skewed towards those with severe epilepsy.

The problem of identification

It is often difficult to identify people with epilepsy in epidemiological studies. Questionnaires and community studies may be viewed with suspicion and symptoms of epilepsy denied, particularly where the diagnosis carries a major stigma. The accuracy of results obtained depends on the sensitivity and specificity of the method used. These will vary for different seizure types: surveys designed to identify tonic–clonic seizures, by asking about specific symptoms, are likely to be poor at detecting partial seizures. Studies from a hospital or clinic will probably be more accurate diagnostically, but will be biased towards people with severe epilepsy. As many patients may particularly seek traditional healers, hospital-based studies seriously underestimate the prevalence of epilepsy. In retrospective studies seizures may be 'forgotten', particularly where stigma or other social disadvantage is attached. Some studies have used other methods, such as that of notification by a 'key informant' within the village (Feksi et al., 1991), but it seems likely that this too underestimates the true prevalence of epilepsy.

The prevalence of epilepsy

In the industrialized countries, the prevalence of epilepsy has been estimated as between 4 and 10/1000

Table 74.2. Epidemiological studies of epilepsy

Study	Location	Methodology	Case definition	Results
Osuntokun et al. (1987)	Nigeria	Door-to-door survey	Two or more unprovoked seizures in last 2 years (or last 5 yrs if on treatment)	Prevalence: 5.3/1000
Tekle-Haimanot et al. (1997)	Ethiopia	Door-to-door survey	Two or more unprovoked seizures	Incidence: 64/100 000
Kaamugisha & Feksi (1988)	Kenya	(i) Random cluster survey method (ii) Key informants in the community	Two or more unprovoked seizures, with at least 1 seizure within 1 year if untreated or within 5 years if on treatment	(i) Random cluster method – prevalence 18.2/1000 (ii) Key informant method – prevalence 3.6/1000
Younis (1983)	Sudan	Cases identified in schools, hospitals and doctors' private clinics	Recurrent major seizures	Prevalence: 0.9/1000.
Izuora & Azubuike (1977)	Nigeria	Survey of 200 mothers about occurrence and frequency of convulsions in 763 children in their families	Two or more non-febrile seizures	Prevalence: 14/1000
Debrock et al. (2000)	Benin	(i) Door-to-door cross-sectional study, (ii) key informants, and evaluation of medical records		Overall prevalence: 21.1/1000, or 35.1/1000 after application of the capture-recapture method.
Rwiza et al. (1992)	Tanzania	Random cluster sample survey	Two or more unprovoked seizures with at least 1 seizure within 2 years or receiving treatment	Overall prevalence of active epilepsy 10.2/1000. Incidence: 73.3/100 000

(Sander & Shorvon, 1987), whereas in Africa, where the population is generally younger, and more likely to be poor and rural, estimates of prevalence are often higher, reflecting these factors and a greater likelihood of epilepsy occurring as a result of infection. Differing methods for estimating prevalence profoundly affect the prevalence rate, which has varied from 0.9/1000 in Sudan (Younis, 1983) to 18.2/1000, in Kenya, which Kaamugisha and Feksi (1988) obtained through a 'random cluster survey method' in which people living adjacent to children randomly picked from those attending a certain school were surveyed. However, when these authors used a 'key informant' method, in which responsible people from within the community were used to identify those with epilepsy, a prevalence rate of 3.6/1000 was obtained.

The incidence of epilepsy

The incidence of epilepsy lies between 20/100 000 and 70/100 000 per annum in richer northern countries. Few incidence studies have been carried out in Africa: a mobile population, the lack of medical records, the difficulties of a precise diagnosis, and the fact that many people with epilepsy will not seek medical help or will be treated by a traditional healer, make such studies difficult. In Tanzania Rwiza et al (1992) found an annual incidence of 73.3/100 000; while in Ethiopia Tekle-Haimanot et al (1997) carried out a door-to-door survey of people previously assessed 3½ years earlier, and found an annual incidence of epilepsy of 64/100 000. These figures seem to corroborate suggestions of an increased incidence of epilepsy in developing countries. Table 74.2 shows the results of a number of epidemiological surveys carried out in Africa.

Seizure type

The proportion of patients with partial and generalized seizures varies considerably between studies. Tekle-Haimanot et al. (1997) found that only 20 per cent of patients had seizures with evidence of partial onset, whereas in Nigeria, Osuntokun et al. (1987) found 52 per cent. Few studies in sub-Saharan Africa have used EEG

Table 74.3. Aetiology of Epilepsy

	Location	Perinatal insult	Head injury	Cerebral infection	Tumour	Stroke	Other	Total
Danesi (1983)	Nigeria	3	7	2	1	1		14
Osuntokun et al. (1987)	Nigeria	2	6		1	2		11
Feksi et al. (1991)	Kenya	6	4	8			2	20
Rwiza et al. (1992)	Tanzania	1	1	8	0.5	0.5	1	12
Tekle-Haimanot et al. (1997)	Ethiopia	6	6	1		1		14

Notes:
Expressed as percentage of patients in each study with symptomatic epilepsy with an identifiable aetiology.

and the differences in the proportion of patients with partial seizures are most likely due to differences in the methods of case ascertainment.

The causes of epilepsy

Identifying the aetiology

Neuroimaging

The proportion of patients with epilepsy in whom a cause is identified depends partly on the use and availability of investigations, particularly neuroimaging (CT or MRI). There are approximately 30 CT scanners and even fewer MRI scanners in sub-Saharan Africa for a population of greater than 500 million. The vast majority of people with epilepsy will, therefore, not have access to neuroimaging. If neuroimaging is not available, the aetiology is less likely to be identified and in particular certain aetiologies such as cerebral tumours will be under-represented.

The clinical history

Without neuroimaging, aetiology is inferred from the history and, as with classification of seizure type, the quality of the history is crucial. Cultural factors may make it difficult to obtain an adequate history and in rural areas previous medical records may not be available, reducing further the proportion of patients in whom a clear aetiology is identified.

Community studies

Community-based studies of epilepsy performed in Nigeria, Tanzania and Ethiopia found a clear aetiology in 11–14 per cent of patients (Osuntokun et al., 1987; Rwiza et al., 1992; Tekle-Haimanot et al., 1997). In more selected patient groups in a community programme in Kenya (Feksi et al., 1991) and in a hospital clinic in Nigeria (Danesi, 1983), a clear aetiology was identified in 14 and 20 per cent (Table 74.3). Neuroimaging was not used in any of these studies.

Compared with a population-based study in the UK (Sander et al., 1990), the studies from sub-Saharan Africa generally report cerebral infection, head injury and perinatal factors more frequently, and stroke and cerebral tumours less frequently.

Cerebral infection

In studies from sub-Saharan Africa a history of previous cerebral infection has been found in 1–8 per cent of cases of epilepsy (Table 74.3). Any infection with cerebral involvement may cause acute symptomatic seizures. The incidence of epilepsy after many of the infections prevalent in sub-Saharan Africa is, however, unknown: case-control studies are needed. Most cerebral infections which lead to epilepsy cause partial seizures.

Bacterial infections

Bacterial meningitis carries a 10 per cent risk of subsequent epilepsy if seizures occur acutely and a 3 per cent risk if there are no acute seizures. Up to 70 per cent of survivors of acute bacterial cerebral abscess develop partial epilepsy, which is often unresponsive to treatment. The incidence of epilepsy following subdural empyema is less well established.

Tuberculosis

Epilepsy is seen in 8–14 per cent of patients after TB meningitis, and seizures are a common manifestation of cerebral tuberculoma (Senanayake & Roman, 1993) (Fig. 74.2).

Viral infections

Twenty-five per cent of patients with viral encephalitis who have seizures acutely and 10 per cent of those who do not have seizures acutely develop epilepsy.

Subacute sclerosing panencephalitis (SSPE)
SSPE causes generalized tonic–clonic and myoclonic seizures and is seen more frequently in countries where there is not widespread vaccination against measles.

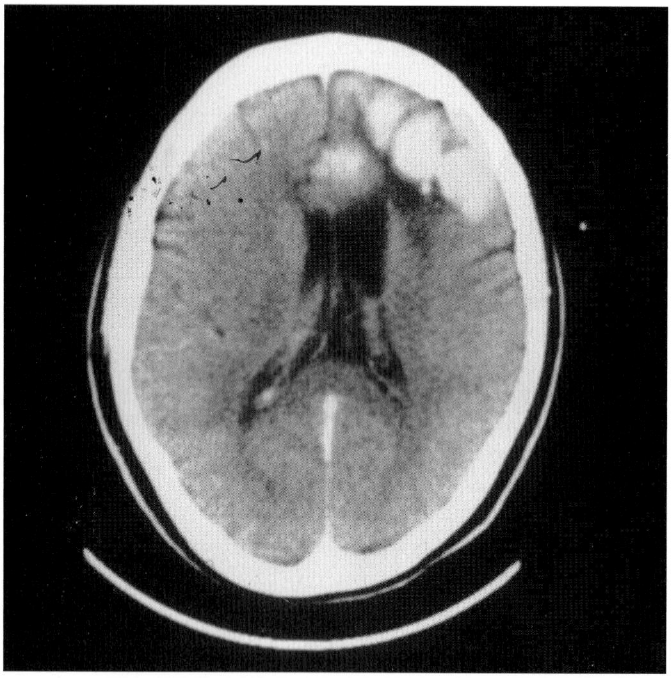

Fig. 74.2. Tuberculoma; contrast-enhanced CT brain scan showing four enhancing lesions in the left frontal region.

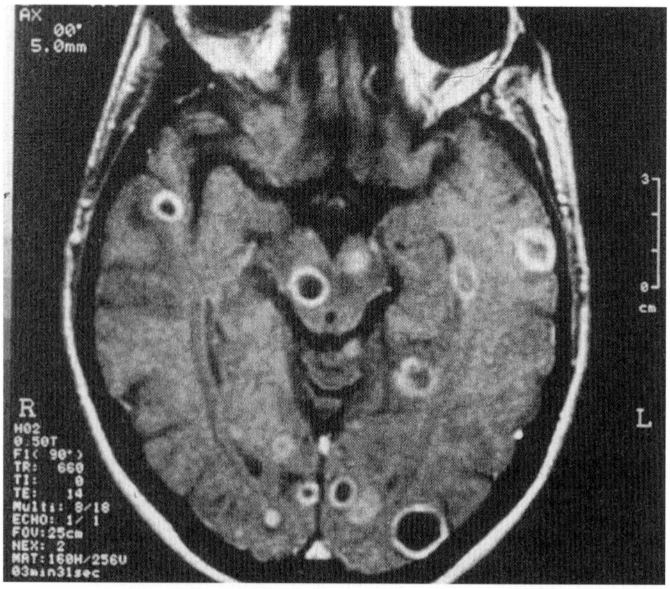

Fig. 74.3. Neurocysticercosis.

HIV
HIV infection may cause epilepsy through direct invasion of the brain, and seizures may be the presenting feature. The seizures tend to be generalized tonic–clonic or myoclonic. Seizures may also occur as a consequence of opportunistic infections such as cerebral toxoplasmosis, cryptococcal meningitis and tuberculosis, and are usually partial. Up to 60 per cent of HIV-positive patients experience seizures, and HIV infection is likely to be an increasingly important cause of epilepsy (Adamolekun, 1995)

Parasitic infections

Neurocysticercosis
Cysticercosis is the commonest parasitic infection of the brain and epilepsy is the commonest manifestation of neurocysticercosis (Commission on Tropical Diseases, ILAE, 1994). Although about 90 per cent with active disease have seizures, most patients with epilepsy have inactive disease with single or multiple cerebral calcifications (Fig. 74.3). There is scant evidence that it is a significant cause of epilepsy in Africa, although in South Africa it is important – 28 per cent of 578 patients with epilepsy had evidence of cysticercosis on CT of the brain (van As & Joubert, 1991). It is, however, difficult to be certain that this was the cause of the epilepsy in all these cases because neurocysticercosis can be asymptomatic and there was no control group.

Other studies have relied on detection of cysticercal antigen in serum using an ELISA. In a random sample of 5264 subjects in Northern Togo, 2.4 per cent had evidence of cysticercosis. Eighty-eight had epilepsy and in this group, 39 per cent had evidence of cysticercosis (Dumas et al., 1989). Studies in Burundi (Newell et al., 1997) and Central African Republic (Druet-Cabanac et al., 1999) have failed to demonstrate a link between serological evidence of cysticercosis and epilepsy.

In regions where consumption of pork is restricted and there are very few pigs, e.g. Ethiopia, it is unlikely that neurocysticercosis is responsible for many cases of epilepsy.

Malaria
Although malaria with cerebral involvement is associated with acute symptomatic seizures, it is not known whether the incidence of epilepsy is increased in patients who have a previous history of cerebral malaria (Commission on Tropical Diseases, ILAE, 1994).

Malaria with or without cerebral involvement is a common cause of seizures in children in sub-Saharan

Africa. A study of acute paediatric admissions to the university hospital in Ibadan, Nigeria found malaria parasitaemia in 45 per cent of those presenting with fever and seizures (Familusi & Sinnette, 1971)). In children admitted to a district hospital in Kenya, malaria was associated with 69 per cent of admissions with seizures (Waruiru et al., 1996), but only 25 per cent of these had evidence of cerebral involvement. Of the remainder some may have had febrile seizures, but in 54 per cent the seizures were not related to fever.

The incidence of epilepsy following acute symptomatic seizures associated with malaria in childhood is not known, but indirect evidence suggests that the incidence may be increased. Firstly, it has been reported from Nigeria that up to 30 per cent of children with febrile seizures develop recurrent unprovoked seizures within 5 years (Osuntokun, 1983)). In the UK only 3 per cent of children with febrile seizures develop epilepsy (Verity & Golding, 1991). The majority of what are referred to as febrile seizures in the literature from sub-Saharan Africa are associated with malaria. Although many of these so-called febrile seizures would be more appropriately classified as acute symptomatic seizures, it does suggest that there may be link between malaria in childhood and subsequent epilepsy. Secondly, neurological morbidity in children following acute symptomatic seizures associated with malaria is relatively high, 8 per cent in the study from Ibadan, Nigeria (Familusi & Sinnette, 1971), and the underlying cerebral damage is likely to increase the risk of epilepsy. Prospective studies are, however, needed to confirm whether there is a significant association between malaria in childhood and epilepsy.

Onchocerciasis
Several studies from Uganda have shown a correlation between the prevalence of epilepsy and the endemicity of onchocerciasis (Kipp et al., 1994; Kaiser et al., 1996), and seizures have been better controlled after treatment with ivermectin (Kipp et al., 1992). However, in a case-control study in Central African Republic, epilepsy was not shown to be associated with onchocerciasis (Druet-Cabanac et al., 1999).

Other parasites
Although seizures may be a manifestation of meningoencephalitis during the acute phase of some parasitic infections, including sleeping sickness, schistosomiasis and Loa-loa, the risk of subsequently developing epilepsy is not known. Cerebral hydatid disease is now thought to be a rare cause of seizures.

Head Injury

Head injury is reported as an aetiological factor in 1–7 per cent of cases of epilepsy (Table 74.3), but different criteria are used for what constitutes a significant head injury, so studies are not comparable. A large community-based study (Annegers et al., 1998) showed cumulative risk at 5 years of developing epilepsy following:

- severe head injury (loss of consciousness or amnesia of 24 hours or longer, brain contusion, or subdural haematoma) – 10 per cent
- moderate head injury (loss of consciousness or amnesia of more than 30 minutes but less than 24 hours, or skull fracture) – 1–2 per cent
- mild head injury (loss of consciousness or amnesia lasting less than 30 minutes) – <1 per cent.

Perinatal factors

It is often assumed that poor perinatal care will result in a high frequency of epilepsy, but this is not proven. It is possible that in Africa those with severe cerebral damage and with the greatest risk of epilepsy, do not survive. One to six per cent of cases of epilepsy have been attributed to perinatal factors (Table 74.3). Prenatal infection and developmental malformations of the brain are likely to be relevant as well as birth trauma and hypoxia. Detailed knowledge of birth history and obstetric records is often not available, and cerebral palsy and learning disability have been used as markers of perinatal factors. In a community study performed in a rural area of central Ethiopia, learning disability was found in 7.9 per cent of patients with epilepsy (Tekle-Haimanot et al., 1990).

Stroke

As life expectancy increases, it is likely that stroke will become a more important cause of epilepsy in sub-Saharan Africa (Chapter 73), but to date only 1–2 per cent of cases of epilepsy have been attributed to stroke (Table 74.3). In a case-control study performed in a hospital clinic population in Nigeria stroke was not significantly associated with epilepsy (Ogunniyi et al., 1987).

Tumours

Seizures are the presenting feature in about 40 per cent of patients with cerebral tumours, and, where neuroimaging is possible, about 6 per cent of patients with newly diagnosed epilepsy are found to have a tumour (Sander et al., 1990). With low-grade tumours seizures may be present for many years before other features develop. In sub-Saharan Africa cerebral tumours are reported in no more than 1 per cent of patients with epilepsy (Table 74.3). A study with cerebral angiography in Nigeria found tumours in 4 per cent of a group of patients with epilepsy (Osuntokun & Odeku, 1970).

Genetic causes of epilepsy

A family history of epilepsy is reported by up to 33 per cent of patients in sub-Saharan Africa (Druet-Cabanac et al., 1999). In a community-based study in rural Ethiopia, 32 per cent of patients with epilepsy had a relative who had one or more seizures and 12 per cent had affected first degree relatives (Tekle-Haimanot et al., 1990).

In isolated communities specific diseases may be an important cause of epilepsy. Examples include Grand Bassa county in Liberia (Goudsmit et al., 1983) and the Wapogoro people in a rural area of Tanzania (Jilek-Aall et al., 1979). In both cases possible inherited neurodegenerative disorders, known locally as *See-ee* in Grand Bassa County and *Kifafa* amongst the Wapogoro people seem to explain some of the highest local prevalences of epilepsy reported in Africa.

In addition to these rare genetic causes of epilepsy, there is a genetic contribution to more common cases of symptomatic epilepsy. For example, the risk of epilepsy following a head injury is greater in those with a family history of epilepsy than those without.

There is a strong genetic component to the idiopathic epilepsies, both generalized and partial. Most families with idiopathic epilepsies exhibit complex inheritance. There is increasing evidence that idiopathic generalized epilepsies are due to disorders of ion channel function.

With advances in molecular biology, increasingly cases previously classified as cryptogenic are found to have genetic causes.

Diagnosis

There is no short cut – as the diagnosis of epilepsy is *clinical, take a detailed, careful history* from the patient and more importantly from a witness, and always ask about:

- a warning or aura
- the details of the attack
- what the patient feels or does after the attack is over.

Remember that the epilepsy may be the first symptom of a systemic disease: therefore, after taking a full history, do a careful full examination and then examine the central nervous system carefully.

The most important differential diagnoses are syncope and non-epileptic seizures ('pseudoseizures'). During a syncopal attack brief stiffening and a few myoclonic jerks are not uncommon, but loss of consciousness is typically brief and the circumstances of the attack, prodromal symptoms, speed of recovery and lack of significant confusion usually allow syncope to be differentiated from epileptic seizures (see the Box).

Syncope

- Syncope is the most common cause of loss of awareness and must be differentiated from epileptic seizures.
- Ask about the circumstances of the episode and the precipitating factors, e.g. prolonged standing especially in hot, crowded areas, emotional and painful stimuli.
- Ask about prodromal symptoms (light headedness, nausea, dimming of vision).
- Recovery of consciousness is rapid when supine.
- There may be mild disorientation after regaining consciousness but not prolonged confusion.

Non-epileptic seizures or pseudoseizures have a psychological basis. In the UK 10–15 per cent of patients referred to specialist epilepsy clinics with apparent refractory seizures have non-epileptic seizures. The extent of the problem in sub-Saharan Africa is not known, but clinical experience suggests that it exists and that some of those responding to exorcism may fall into this category.

Investigation

Investigations are not necessary for a diagnosis of epilepsy, but, when a provisional cause has been suggested by the history and examination, specific tests may help to classify the seizure disorder and determine the aetiology.

Electroencephalography (EEG)

EEG is not necessary to make a diagnosis of epilepsy, and in most rural areas will not be available.When available, EEG, if it shows epileptiform discharges, will support a clinical diagnosis of epilepsy, but a routine EEG recording will be normal in approximately 40 per cent of patients with a definite clinical diagnosis of epilepsy. Although the yield can be increased to about 80 per cent by performing the EEG under conditions of sleep deprivation or during drug-induced sleep, a normal EEG does not rule out a diagnosis of epilepsy.

An abnormal EEG, as well as supporting a clinical diagnosis of epilepsy, may assist classification and help to distinguish between partial and generalized seizure disorders (Fig. 74.4).

Neuroimaging

The purpose of neuroimaging is to determine the cause of the epilepsy. Plain X-rays of the skull are of little value and radiological investigation is only indicated in advanced centres where CT or MRI are available. MRI will identify structural abnormalities in a much a higher proportion of patients with epilepsy than CT.

Counselling and education

Stigma and traditional beliefs

There is a stigma to epilepsy in many societies in sub-Saharan Africa, often the result of ignorance and superstition. Although 74 per cent of patients in one community in Ethiopia said that they did not know the cause of seizures, 17 per cent thought they were due to evil spirits (Tekle-Haimanot et al., 1990), while in other countries epilepsy is commonly believed to be due to supernatural causes (Jilek-Aall, 1999). There is also often a fear that epilepsy is contagious. Most patients seek help from traditional healers, because they are unaware of medical treatment or believe in supernatural causes. In Nigeria more than 90 per cent of patients in a hospital clinic had previously tried traditional medicine or spiritual healing (Danesi & Adetunji, 1994). There are regional differences, but herbal remedies, holy water and amulets are among the more common treatments.

Involving the patient

As with any chronic disease, success in the treatment of epilepsy is some extent depends on the patient understanding the nature of their condition and being willing to take part in its management. Once a diagnosis has been established and before any treatment is started, it is important to discuss in simple terms the nature of the epilepsy and its causes. Use the health team to educate and reassure patients, their families and, whenever possible, the wider community that epilepsy is not contagious.

Seizures provoked by various specific circumstances

Seizures may be provoked by specific circumstances. Discuss, and when it is possible counsel the patient accordingly.

Febrile seizures occurring in children must be differentiated from epilepsy and the parents advised about cooling the child. Some patients have seizures precipitated by sleep deprivation. Electroencephalographic studies suggest that seizures provoked by light – photosensitivity – are uncommon in black Africans, in contrast to their commonness in white people (Mundy-Castle et al, 1953; Danesi, 1988).

Advice to the family

Always give basic advice to the patient's family on management of the patient during a seizure, to reduce the risk of injury. Discuss the aims and limitations of treatment, and the importance of treatment being taken regularly and conscientiously, particularly with certain drugs because of the risk of status epilepticus if they are withdrawn abruptly. Always warn your patients of potential adverse effects.

Pregnancy

Advise women that epilepsy and its treatment do not preclude a successful pregnancy. Anti-epileptic drugs increase the risk of fetal malformation by about 3 per cent for each drug taken: therefore, to reduce the risk, treat women who are likely to become pregnant with a single anti-epileptic drug in as small a dose as possible necessary to achieve control. Folic acid 5 mg/day taken before conception and during the first trimester may minimize the risk of spina bifida. In women who are currently taking hepatic enzyme-inducing drugs, such as phenobarbitone and phenytoin, oral vitamin K 20 mg/day during the last month of pregnancy may reduce the risk of haemorrhagic disease of the newborn.

Breast-feeding is not contraindicated and the risk of a child developing epilepsy is on average only about 6 per cent.

Principles of treatment (see the Box)

Duration

Regular medication for a long time is almost invariable (at least 2 years for adults and one year for children):

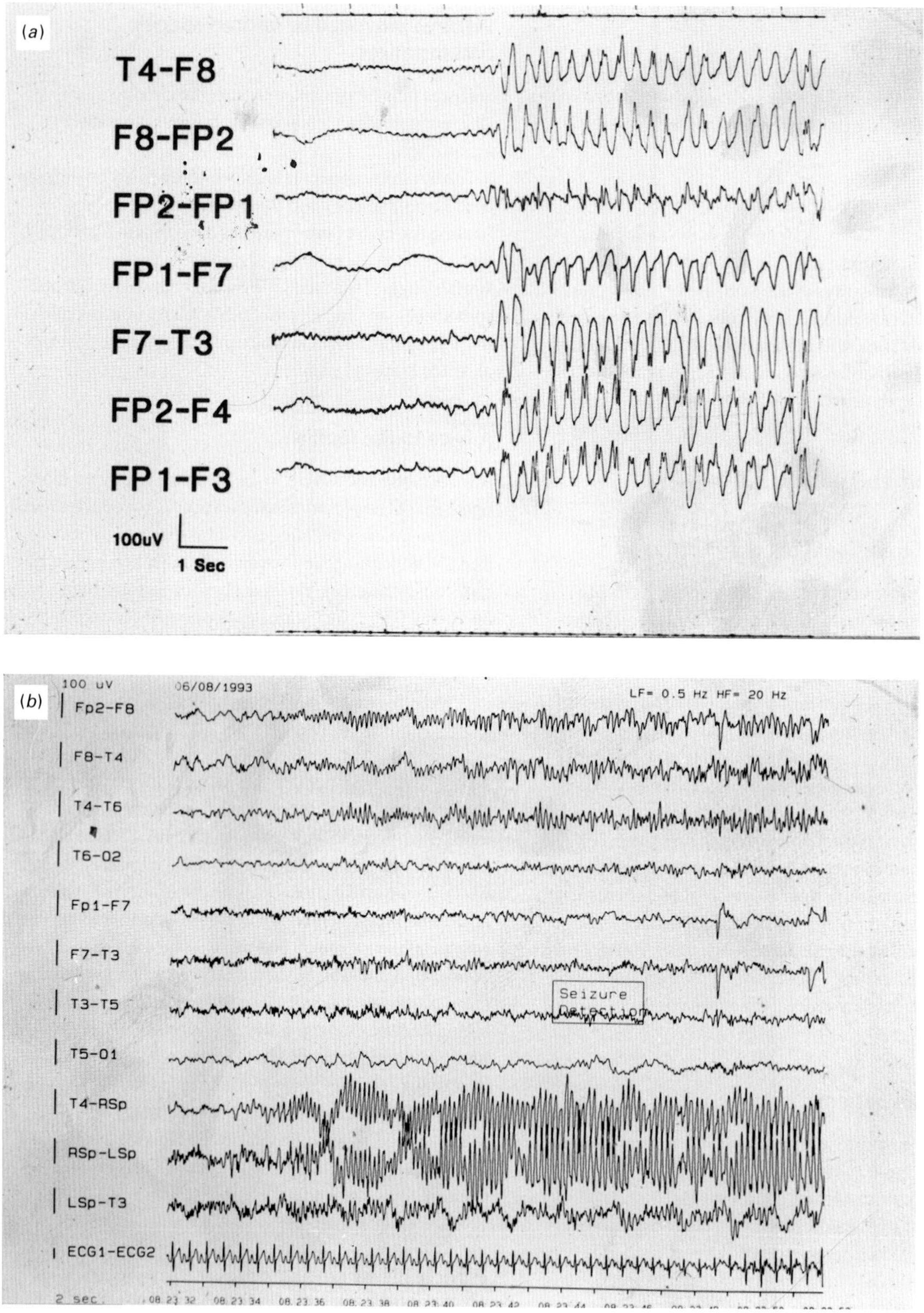

Fig. 74.4. (*a*) Generalized seizure; EEG showing a burst of 3 Hz generalized spike and wave activity arising from a normal background. (*b*) Partial seizure: EEG showing the onset of rhythmic seizure activity in the right temporal region, maximal in the right sphenoidal channel (T4-RSp and RSp-LSp).

The aim of treatment
- to prevent the recurrence of seizures
- to avoid the mortality, morbidity and psychosocial effects associated with seizures
- to achieve a long-term remission and eventual withdrawal of treatment.

treatment is directed at the seizures themselves, since the cause of epilepsy in most people is not known.

Diagnosis

Do not start anti-epileptic drugs unless the diagnosis is certain: they may cause significant adverse effects, including acute idiosyncratic reactions, toxicity, teratogenicity, and chronic adverse reactions.

Decision to treat – consider:

- the frequency and severity of the seizures
- costs: many drugs are expensive and can account for a considerable proportion of the family income.
- constant supply of drugs: the risk of withdrawal seizures is a major consideration (particularly in the case of phenobarbitone) if supplies of the drug cannot be guaranteed.

The economic realities

Phenobarbitone

In many developing countries phenobarbitone represents the only regularly available anti-epileptic drug, and, as the cheapest drug, it is recommended by the World Health Organization. It is appropriate treatment for generalized tonic–clonic seizures and seizures of partial onset.

Other drugs

Phenytoin is the second most readily available drug, followed by *carbamazepine*: these have a similar spectrum of action.

Sodium valproate would be the drug of choice in patients with idiopathic generalized epilepsy, in which generalized tonic–clonic seizures may be accompanied by absence and myoclonic seizures, but its cost is prohibitive, just like the cost of carbamazepine – usually 15–30 times greater than phenobarbitone.

Recently developed

Prohibitive cost excludes recently developed anti-epileptic drugs such as lamotrigine and topiramate (both active in generalized tonic–clonic seizures and seizures of partial onset), gabapentin, tiagabine, oxcarbazepine, vigabatrin and levetiracetam. None of the recently developed drugs have been shown to be any more effective than the older drugs, but some may be better tolerated.

Dosage of drugs

Ideally, medication used for the treatment of epilepsy should be started at a low dose and gradually increased, either until the seizures are controlled or until toxic effects develop. However, in rural areas where medical contact is infrequent so that regular monitoring of the patient does not occur, it is often preferable to increase the medication according to a set protocol until a standard, moderate dose is achieved. Only if the patient is intolerant of the drug, or if it is ineffective, should a second drug appropriate to the seizure type be introduced: in this case, discontinue the initial drug. Where a patient proves to have epilepsy resistant to drug treatment, *do not* continue to increase their anti-epileptic drugs, regardless of adverse effects (see the Box).

Discuss the aims and limitations of treatment with the patient, and the importance of *following advice about treatment.* Emphasise that this is particularly important with phenobarbitone because of the risk of withdrawal seizures if it is stopped abruptly.

Anti-epileptic drugs

Phenobarbitone

Phenobarbitone is cheap and generally the most readily available anti-epileptic drug in sub-Saharan Africa. It is effective in the treatment of both generalized tonic clonic–seizures and seizures of partial onset.

Mode of action

It acts at the $GABA_A$ receptor, where it enhances GABA binding, thereby increasing inhibitory neurotransmission. It is available in tablet form and as a preparation for intravenous (or intramuscular) use.

Properties and dosage

The half-life is long (50–160 hours) so that it will take approximately three weeks before a steady state is reached. About 90 per cent of an oral dose is absorbed. The usual starting dose is 30–60 mg/day for adults, the effective daily dose in adults being about 60 to 180 mg, given as a single dose. Metabolism is largely by conjugation in the liver, and phenobarbitone induces the microsomal P450 system, so that the clearance of certain drugs including isoniazid is increased.

Adverse effects

The most common are sedation in adults, and behavioural difficulties, particularly hyperactivity, in children. (It is also excreted in breast milk, and sedation may occur in the babies of mothers taking phenobarbitone.) Other adverse effects include a decrease in serum and red cell folate levels, occasional osteomalacia, Dupuytren's contracture, and hypersensitivity reactions especially rash or fever. Aplastic anaemia, agranulocytosis, jaundice and hepatitis are very rare. Teratogenicity may occur, though no more frequently than with other commonly used anti-epileptic drugs. Symptoms of toxicity include ataxia, dysarthria, drowsiness and coma.

Withdrawal seizures

A major disadvantage of using phenobarbitone in situations in which the supply may not be guaranteed is the risk of withdrawal seizures, especially if sudden withdrawal occurs. Planned withdrawal of phenobarbitone in patients who have been seizure-free (preferably for at least 2 years) should take place over a period of several months (see the Box).

> **Phenobarbitone**
> Often phenobarbitone is the only regularly available anti-epileptic drug and is recommended by the World Health Organization. It is an appropriate treatment for generalized tonic-clonic and partial seizures. The usual starting dose is 30–60mg/day for adults, the effective daily dose in most cases being 60–180mg/day as a single daily dose.

Phenytoin

Phenytoin is useful in the treatment of generalized tonic–clonic seizures and seizures of partial onset, but may exacerbate absence seizures in idiopathic generalized epilepsy.

Mode of action

Phenytoin has its main action as an anti-epileptic drug by virtue of its sodium-channel blocking properties.

Properties and dosage

It is available both orally (with about 90 per cent absorption) and as a preparation for intravenous use: do not give it by intramuscular injection since its absorption by this route is slow and unpredictable. The half-life of phenytoin is about 24 hours, but varies according to the blood level, since it exhibits non-linear pharmacokinetics. Therefore, when the blood level approaches the therapeutic range, a small increment in dose can lead to a large increase in plasma level and resultant toxicity. Measurement of drug levels may be helpful (McFadyen et al., 1990), but in practice, dosage is usually guided by the clinical response. The starting dose in adults is usually 200–300 mg daily, and the usual maintenance dose in adults about 250–400 mg daily, occasionally more.

Like phenobarbitone, phenytoin induces hepatic microsomal enzymes and hence interacts with a variety of other medications.

Adverse effects

Toxic effects usually take the form of ataxia, visual disturbance, nystagmus, lethargy and headache. Other adverse effects are facial changes including gum hypertrophy, impairment of cognitive function, cerebellar atrophy, low serum folate levels, and rarely, osteomalacia. Idiosyncratic reactions include skin rash, hepatitis, blood dyscrasias, and a lupus-like syndrome. Teratogenic effects, which may affect around 3 per cent of babies, include cardiac abnormalities, cleft lip and palate, and microcephaly.

Carbamazepine

Mode of action

Carbamazepine, like phenytoin, is a sodium-channel blocking agent, and has a similar spectrum of action.

Properties and dosage

It is available orally (and as suppositories, though the latter are unlikely to be readily available in developing countries), but not in injectable form. The usual daily dose in adults is 400–1600 mg. In order to avoid adverse effects, particularly nausea, dizziness and ataxia, start the drug at a dose of 100–200 mg daily and increase the dose by 200 mg at intervals of two weeks.

Carbamazepine is metabolized predominantly by oxidation to carbamazepine-10,11-epoxide, which itself has anti-convulsant properties in animals. Because of hepatic enzyme induction by carbamazepine, autoinduction occurs, by which the clearance of carbamazepine is increased in patients taking the drug over a period of time. As a result of this phenomenon, blood levels may fall within the first 20–30 days. As an enzyme-inducing drug, carbamazepine also interacts with a number of other drugs.

Adverse effects

These include idiosyncratic reactions, particularly skin rash, and occasionally lymphadenopathy, hepatomegaly, vasculitis, and blood dyscrasias. Leukopenia, usually mild, may occur, as may hyponatraemia. Common toxic effects are nausea, ataxia, dizziness, blurred vision, fatigue and headache. It is teratogenic to around 3 per cent of babies, whose mothers take the drug.

Sodium valproate

Valproic acid is a branched chain fatty acid which is a broad-spectrum anti-epileptic drug, and is effective both in seizures of partial onset and generalized seizures (including absences and myoclonus).

Mode of action

Its precise mode of action is unknown, although it is thought to act at GABA receptors.

Properties and dosage

It is available orally and as an intravenous preparation. The usual starting dose in adults is 600 mg daily in divided doses, unless a slow-release preparation is available. This is a therapeutic dose in some patients, although doses up to 2.5 g daily may be required. Metabolism occurs within the liver. However, unlike phenobarbitone, phenytoin and carbamazepine, valproate does not induce liver enzymes.

Adverse effects

In adults these include nausea, weight gain, hair loss, and dose-related tremor. The most serious adverse effect of sodium valproate in children is hepatotoxicity, which is most common in children, particularly those with mental retardation, under the age of 2 years, especially when taking polytherapy. Pancreatitis, thrombocytopenia, and rarely stupor and coma develop as a result of hyperammonaemia. Teratogenicity not infrequently takes the form of neural tube defects, and these are particularly common in women taking doses of >1000 mg per day.

> **Drug-resistant seizures**
> Where a patient proves to have epilepsy resistant to drug treatment, attempts to improve seizure control must be balanced against the increased incidence of drug related adverse effects at higher doses. The temptation to continue increasing anti-epileptic drugs regardless of adverse effects should be resisted.

Prognosis

There has long been debate as to whether 'seizures beget seizures' as postulated by Gowers (Shorvon, 1987; Reynolds, 1987). If this were the case, one might expect that delaying the introduction of medication, as may be inevitable where there is poor access to medical care or a shortage of medication, would lead to a poorer prognosis for seizure control. In practice, throughout Africa, a significant proportion of patients receiving treatment do obtain good seizure control, the figures for complete remission being little short of those seen in developed countries.

Results of treatment in Africa

In a clinic established in rural Tanzania by Jilek-Aall and Rwiza (1992), using phenobarbitone for treatment, 52.4 per cent of patients achieved complete seizure suppression, while 36 per cent experienced a reduction in seizure frequency. In a study by Feksi et al. (1991) in rural and semi-urban Kenya, 302 patients were treated with either carbamazepine or phenobarbitone. Of the 249 patients who completed the study, 53 per cent became seizure-free in the second 6 months, and 79 per cent experienced at least a 50 per cent reduction in seizures. Watts (1990) treated people with epilepsy attending a clinic in Malawi with phenobarbitone as first-line drug, using phenytoin in those with resistant seizures. She reported that 56 per cent of patients followed up for 6 to 11 months became seizure-free, the figure falling to 40 per cent for patients treated for a year: in only 15 per cent was control 'unsatisfactory'. Kaiser et al. (1998) obtained similar success rates in a study in a rural district in Uganda, patients being treated with phenobarbitone. Approximately 35 per cent of patients who took drugs conscientiously became seizure-free in the first 6 months of treatment, and around 80 per cent showed at least a 50 per cent reduction in seizures (those who did not follow treatment and those lost to follow-up, constituting 20 per cent of the total, were excluded from analysis). In contrast, Ogunniyi et al. (1998), studying the effectiveness of anti-convulsant therapy in the treatment of epilepsy in Nigeria, usually with phenobarbitone but occasionally with phenytoin or carbamazepine, found that complete seizure control occurred in only 17 per cent, although a further 50 per cent experienced a reduction in seizures of at least 50 per cent. However, this study was carried out at University College Hospital, Ibadan, and it is possible therefore that the patients were more likely to have severe epilepsy which had failed to respond to simple treatment within the community. Factors associated with good control were infrequent seizures and monotherapy: duration of seizures and absence of aetiological factors were not correlated with good control.

Lifetime prognosis

The picture is considerably bleaker. In Jilek-Aall's study, after 30 years, only 36 (21.9 per cent) of the 164 patients were known to be alive, while 110 (67.1 per cent) were known to have died, the mortality rate being twice that of the general rural Tanzanian population of similar age. In more than 50 per cent of patients, the death was epilepsy related – status epilepticus, drowning, burns, and death directly due to a seizure. Epilepsy-related deaths were proportionately higher after drug supply was stopped and among patients who were receiving drugs irregularly or who had only partial seizure control, but the mortality rate was greater than for people without epilepsy even when patients were receiving medication.

Surgical treatment

Where facilities are advanced and cost is no barrier, surgical treatment has become increasingly popular in patients with intractable epilepsy in whom the epileptogenic focus can be readily identified and is in a position in which it can be safely resected.

Treatment of status epilepticus

Status epilepticus is usually defined as the occurrence of serial seizures without recovery of consciousness between, or a single seizure lasting for longer than 30 minutes. It may occur as the presenting feature of epilepsy, or in people with established epilepsy. In the latter it may occur due to abrupt withdrawal of medication, as the result of intercurrent illness, due to the underlying disease itself, or for no apparent reason. Not infrequently it is preceded by an increase in seizure frequency occurring over hours to days, and treatment at this stage, for example with diazepam, may prevent the development of status.

Speed is of the essence in the treatment of status epilepticus. If tonic–clonic status persists beyond an hour or so, compensatory physiological mechanisms begin to fail, and the prognosis for recovery after status epilepticus is affected mainly by the duration of the status and the underlying cause. Treatment will vary according to the facilities available. It includes supportive measures, and treatment of the underlying cause, including reinstatement of the patient's usual anti-epileptic medication, if necessary by nasogastric tube, when this has been discontinued. Fever and hypoglycaemia should also be treated. If available diazepam 10–20 mg may be given by slow intravenous injection, followed by intravenous phenytoin 15 mg/kg given by slow infusion at a rate of not more than 50 mg/minute. Where facilities for intravenous injection are not available, diazepam may be given by the rectal route, and phenytoin by nasogastric tube, although intravenous injection is preferred. Loading with phenytoin should be followed by a maintenance dose of 200–300 mg per day orally or via nasogastric tube. Intravenous phenobarbitone (10 mg/kg at a rate not exceeding 100 mg/minute) is an alternative in patients already receiving phenytoin but not phenobarbitone.

Eighty percent of patients will respond to treatment with a benzodiazepine followed by phenytoin or phenobarbitone. If seizures continue the outlook will be poor unless there are facilities for general anaesthesia. When available general anaesthesia with thiopentone or propofol and EEG monitoring is indicated (see the Box).

Tonic–clonic status epilepticus

- Diazepam 10–20 mg given by slow intravenous injection followed by intravenous phenytoin 15 mg/kg given by intravenous infusion diluted in normal saline at a rate of not more than 50mg/min is recommended for the treatment of tonic–clonic status epilepticus.
- Where facilities for intravenous treatment are not available, diazepam may be given rectally and phenytoin by nasogastric tube.
- Follow loading with phenytoin by a maintenance dose of 200–300 mg per day orally or via a nasogastric tube.

Models of epilepsy care

Currently most people with epilepsy in sub-Saharan Africa are not receiving treatment, because of:

- lack of awareness of the existence of anti-epileptic drug treatment
- lack of access to medical facilities
- lack of availability of drugs.

Hospital base and mobile clinics

In an attempt to overcome some of these problems Watts (1989) set up a hospital-based treatment service in Malawi with mobile clinics to improve accessibility. Education of both patients and their communities was an integral part of the programme. This model proved effective and there was a rapid increase in the number of people attending the clinics and receiving treatment. The model was subsequently adopted in other areas of Malawi.

Community health workers

A similar community-based programme has been described in Kenya (Feksi et al., 1991). Community health workers were trained to identify cases, provide counselling, education and follow-up. In another study, devolvement of responsibility was taken a step further by employing community assistants to distribute treatment (Kaiser et al., 1998). Whilst this appeared to be successful, the lack of contact with medical personnel could be a disadvantage for those patients with incomplete seizure control or those experiencing adverse effects. In addition such a strategy may present difficulties in countries where phenobarbitone is a controlled drug.

Epilepsy in primary care

Where resources are limited existing primary health-care infrastructure originally developed for the management of communicable disorders has been successfully used to treat non-communicable disorders such as epilepsy. In northern Ethiopia nurse-led clinics were established in rural health centres to follow up patients with epilepsy. Large numbers of previously untreated patients were identified and started on treatment with phenobarbitone (Berhanu et al., 2002). A similar approach was used in a poor area of rural South Africa for a range of non-communicable diseases including epilepsy (Coleman et al., 1998).

Supply of drugs

A survey of anti-epileptic treatment in Cameroon showed that, whilst some pharmacies stocked a variety of anti-epileptic drugs including some of the newer drugs, phenobarbitone was the only drug that was regularly delivered to pharmacies and stocks of other drugs frequently ran out (Preux et al., 2000). This experience is common to other countries in sub-Saharan Africa, and phenobarbitone has been the mainstay of treatment in the programmes described. Unfortunately, the quality of the drugs cannot always be relied on. Variability in the efficacy of drugs from different sources is often suspected. A study in Nigeria found that mechanisms for quality assurance were inadequate and substandard drugs were often sold by pharmacies (Taylor et al., 2001).

The challenge

Treatment programmes such as those described above are not widespread and reach only a small proportion of people with epilepsy who could benefit from treatment. In order to improve this treatment gap, the treatment of epilepsy needs to be given greater priority at a national level. Governments, therefore, will need to be persuaded by evidence of the cost-effectiveness of treatment. The World Health Organization and the ILAE have embarked on a number of practical demonstration studies to evaluate community-based treatment programmes (Pal et al., 1999). Other studies under way in Tanzania and Cameroon are also designed to provide costed and evaluated treatment packages (Unwin et al., 1999). It is hoped that the results of such studies will serve as the basis for improvement of the plight of those suffering from epilepsy and other chronic non-communicable diseases in sub-Saharan Africa.

References

Adamolekun B. (1995). The aetiologies of epilepsy in tropical Africa. *Trop Geogr Med*; **47**: 115–117.

Annegers JF, Hauser WA, Coan SP et al. (1998). A population-based study of seizures after traumatic brain injuries. *N Engl J Med*; **338**: 20–24.

Berhanu S, Alemu S, Asmera J et al. (2002). Primary care treatment of epilepsy in rural Ethiopia. *Ethiop J Health Dev*; **16:** 235–240.

Birbeck GL. (2000). Seizures in rural Zambia. *Epilepsia*; **41**: 277–281.

Coleman R, Gill G, Wilkinson D. (1998). Noncommunicable disease management in resource-poor settings: a primary care model from rural South Africa. *Bull Wld Hlth Org*; **76**: 633–640.

Commission on Classification and Terminology of the International League Against Epilepsy. (1981). Proposal for revised clinical and electroencephalographic classification of epileptic seizures. *Epilepsia*; **22**: 489–501.

Commission on Classification and Terminology of the International League Against Epilepsy. (1989). Proposal for revised classification of epilepsies and epileptic syndromes. *Epilepsia*; **30**: 389–399.

Commission on Epidemiology and Prognosis, International League Against Epilepsy. (1993). Guidelines for epidemiologic studies on epilepsy. *Epilepsia*; **34**: 592–596.

Commission on Tropical Diseases of the International League Against Epilepsy. (1994). Relationship between epilepsy and tropical diseases. *Epilepsia*; **35**: 89–93.

Danesi MA. (1983). Acquired aetiological factors in Nigerian epileptics (an investigation of 378 patients). *Trop Geog Med*; **35**: 293–297.

Danesi MA. (1988). Electroencephalographic manifestations of grand mal epilepsy in Africans: observation of relative rarity of interictal abnormalities. *Epilepsia*; **29**: 446–450.

Danesi MA, Adetunji JB. (1994). Use of alternative medicine by patients with epilepsy: a survey of 265 epileptic patients in a developing country. *Epilepsia*; **35**: 344–351.

Debrock C, Preux PM, Houinato D et al. (2000). Estimation of the prevalence of epilepsy in the Benin region of Zinvie using the capture-recapture method. *Int J Epidemiol*; **29**: 330–335.

Druet-Cabanac M, Preux P-M, Bouteille B et al. (1999). Onchocerciasis and epilepsy: a matched case control study in the Central African Republic. *Am J Epidemiol*; **149**: 565–570.

Dumas M, Grunitzky E, Deniau M et al. (1989). Epidemiological study of neuro-cysticercosis in northern Togo (West Africa). *Acta Leiden*; **57**: 191–196.

Familusi JB, Sinnette CH. (1971). Febrile convulsions in Ibadan children. *Afr J Med Sci*; **2**: 135–149.

Feksi AT, Kaamugisha J, Gatiti S et al. (1991a). A comprehensive community epilepsy programme: the Nakuru project. *Epilepsy Res*; **8**: 252–259.

Feksi AT, Kaamugisha J, Sander JWAS et al. for ICBERG (International Community-based Epilepsy Research Group). (1991b). Comprehensive primary health care antiepileptic drug treatment programme in rural and semi-urban Kenya. *Lancet*; **337**: 406–409.

Goudsmit J, van der Waals FW, Gajdusek DC. (1983). Epilepsy in the Gbawein and Wroughbarh clan of Grand Bassa County, Liberia; the endemic occurrence of 'See-ee' in the native population. *Neuroepidemiology*; **2**: 24–34.

Izuora GI, Azubuike JC. (1977). Prevalence of seizure disorders in Nigerian Children around Enugu (a preliminary report). *Centr Afr J Med*; **54**: 80–83.

Jilek-Aall L, Jilek W, Miller JR. (1979). Clinical and genetic aspects of seizure disorders prevalent in an isolated African population. *Epilepsia*; **20**: 613–622.

Jilek-Aall L, Rwiza HT. (1992). Prognosis of epilepsy in a rural African community: a 30-year follow-up of 164 patients in an outpatient clinic in rural Tanzania. *Epilepsia*; **33**: 645–650.

Jilek-Aall L. (1990). Morbus sacer in Africa: some religious aspects of epilepsy in traditional cultures. *Epilepsia*; **40**: 382–386.

Kaamugisha J, Feksi AT. (1998). Determining the prevalence of epilepsy in the semi-urban population of Nakuru, Kenya, comparing two independent methods not apparently used before in epilepsy studies. *Neuroepidemiology*; **7**: 115–121.

Kaiser C, Kipp W, Asaba G et al. (1996). The prevalence of epilepsy follows the distribution of onchocerciasis in west Ugandan focus. *Bull Wld Hlth Org*; **74**: 361–367.

Kaiser C, Asaba G, Mugisa C et al. (1998). Antiepileptic drug treatment in rural Africa: involving the community. *Trop Doct*; **28**: 73–77.

Kipp W, Burnham G, Kamugisha J. (1992). Improvement in seizures after ivermectin. *Lancet*; **340**: 789–790.

Kipp W, Kasoro S, Burnham G. (1994). Onchocerciasis and epilepsy in Uganda. *Lancet*; **343**: 183–184.

McFadyen ML, Miller R, Juta M et al. (1990). The relevance of a First-World therapeutic drug monitoring service to the treatment of epilepsy in Third-World conditions. *S Afr Med J*; **78**: 587–590.

Mundy-Castle AC, McKiever BL, Prinsloo T. (1953). A comparative study of the electroencephalograms of normal Africans and Europeans of Southern Africa. *Electroencephalogr Clin Neurophysiol*; **5**: 533–543.

Newell E, Vyungimana F, Geerts S et al. (1997). Prevalence of cysticercosis in epileptics and members of their families in Burundi. *Trans Roy Soc Trop Med Hyg*; **91**: 389–391.

Ogunniyi A, Osuntokun BO. (1991). Effectiveness of anticonvulsant therapy in the epilepsies in Nigerian Africans. *E Afr Med J*; **68**: 707– 713.

Ogunniyi A, Osuntokun BO, Bademosi O et al. (1987). Risk factors for epilepsy: case-control study in Nigerians. *Epilepsia*; **28**: 280–285.

Ogunniyi A, Oluwole OSA, Osuntokun BO. (1998). Two-year remission in Nigerian epileptics. *E Afr Med J*; **75**: 392–335.

Osuntokun BO. (1983). Malaria and the nervous system. *Afr J Med Sci*; **12**: 165–172.

Osuntokun BO, Adeuja AOG, Nottidge VA et al. (1987). Prevalence of the epilepsies in Nigerian Africans: a community-based study. *Epilepsia*; **28**: 272–279.

Pal DK, Nandy S, Sander JWAS. (1999). Towards a coherent public health analysis for epilepsy. *Lancet*; **353**: 1817–1818.

Preux P-M, Tiemagni F, Fodzo L et al. (2000). Antiepileptic therapies in the Mifi Province in Cameroon. *Epilepsia*; **41**: 432–439.

Reynolds EH. (1987). Early treatment and prognosis of epilepsy. *Epilepsia*; **28**: 97–106.

Rwiza HT, Kilonzo GP, Haule J et al. (1992). Prevalence and incidence of epilepsy in Ulanga, a rural Tanzanian district: a community-based study. *Epilepsia*; **33**: 1051–1056.

Sander JWAS, Shorvon SD. (1987). Incidence and prevalence studies in epilepsy and their methodological problems: a review. *J Neurol Neurosurg Psychiatry*; **50**: 829–839.

Sander JWAS, Hart YM, Johnson AL, et al. (1990). National General Practice Study of Epilepsy: newly diagnosed epileptic seizures in a general population. *Lancet*; **336**: 1267–1271.

Senanayake N, Roman GC. (1993). Epidemiology of epilepsy in developing countries. *Bull Wld Hlth Org*; **71**: 247–258.

Shorvon SD. (1987). Do anticonvulsants influence the natural history of epilepsy? In *More Dilemmas in the Management of the Neurological Patient*, ed. C Warlow, J Garfield, pp. 8–13. Edinburgh: Churchill Livingstone.

Shorvon SD, Farmer PJ. (1988). Epilepsy in developing countries: a review of epidemiological, sociocultural and treatment aspects. *Epilepsia*; **29**: S36–S54.

Sridharan R, Radhakrishnan K, Ashok PP et al.(1986). Epidemiological and clinical study of epilepsy in Benghazi, Libya. *Epilepsia*; **27**: 60–65.

Taylor RB, Shakoor O, Behrens RH et al. (2001). Pharmacopoeial quality of drugs supplied by Nigerian pharmacies. *Lancet*; **357**: 1933–1936.

Tekle-Haimanot R, Forsgren L, Abebe M et al. (1990). Clinical and electroencephalographic characteristics of epilepsy in rural Ethiopia: a community based study. *Epilepsy Res*; **7**: 230–239.

Tekle-Haimanot R, Forsgren L, Ekstedt J. (1997). Incidence of epilepsy in rural central Ethiopia. *Epilepsia*; **38**: 541–546.

Unwin N, Mugusi F, Aspray T et al. (1999). Tackling the emerging pandemic of non-communicable diseases in sub-Saharan Africa: the essential NCD health intervention project. *Publ Hlth*; **113**: 141–146.

Verity CM, Golding J. (1991). Risk of epilepsy after febrile convulsions: a national cohort study. *Br Med J*; **303**: 1373–1376.

van As AD, Joubert J. (1991). Neurocysticercosis in 578 black epileptic patients. *S Afr Med J*; **80**: 327–328.

Waruiru CM, Newton CR, Forster D et al. (1996). Epileptic seizures and malaria in Kenyan children. *Trans Roy Soc Trop Med Hyg*; **90**: 152–155.

Watts AE. (1989). A model for managing epilepsy in a rural community in Africa. *Br Med J*; **298**: 805–807.

Watts AE. (1990). Treating epilepsy in Malawi: lessons learned. *Trop Doct*; **20**: 52–55.

Younis YO. (1983). Epidemiology of epilepsy among school populations in Khartoum Province, Sudan. *J Trop Med Hyg*; **86**: 213–216.

75 Organization of non-communicable disease care

The problem in Africa

Across Africa, practioners are aware of the large and growing burden of non-communicable diseases (NCDs), including diabetes, hypertension, asthma, epilepsy and others. In most settings the the burden of infectious diseases including malaria, tuberculosis, respiratory tract infections and HIV/AIDS seems to be larger than the burden of NCDs. Infectious diseases are typically acute and present urgently, making themof much more immediate concern to the doctor, nurse or medical assistant. NCDs, on the other hand, may be asymptomatic (hypertension, diabetes), highly stigmatized and as such partly hidden (epilepsy), or associated with seemingly hopeless clinical presentations (severe heart failure and stroke). As such, historically the level of priority given to NCDs has been very low.

The inevitable outcome of this is typically a low profile for NCD care and their neglect, even at the district hospital level. In Hlabisa hospital and health district in rural KwaZulu–Natal, South Africa in the 1990s the large numbers of people with NCDs in the district were managed in an unstructured and unsatisfactory way. Care of these patients was a low priority for medical staff and the result was inadequate control and poor health outcomes.

These observations are far from unique and indeed the limited literature on NCDs in Africa suggests that low priority, neglect, low levels of detection and diagnosis, low levels of control and hence poor health outcomes are usual (Zimmet & Lefebvre, 1996; Beavers & Prince, 1991).

In this chapter we report on how we developed a structured and simple approach to the care of people with NCDs in the Hlabisa health district, using all the resources available in the district, and the impact this had on disease control.

The setting

Hlabisa health district is located in KwaZulu–Natal province, South Africa and has a population of approximately 250 000 people. The large majority of the residents are Zulu speaking and most people live in scattered rural homesteads, although there is one large peri-urban area. Income and sustenance are mainly derived from subsistence farming, pension remittances, and migrant labour in major cities and mining areas.

The literacy rate in KwaZulu–Natal is 69 per cent and the life expectancy was 63 years before the explosive HIV epidemic that is common across South Africa. A 400-bed district hospital and 12 village clinics provide government health services across the district. The village clinics and associated mobile clinic services offer a primary care service. Nurses staff these clinics, and a doctor visits once per month but does not travel with the mobile service.

Nurses in the outpatient department of the district hospital provide primary care to the community living in the vicinity of the hospital. Primary care clinics thus include the village clinics, mobile clinics, and the hospital outpatient department. The only laboratory facilities are at the hospital.

Pre-intervention NCD care

Before we restructured the care of people with NCDs in Hlabisa, patients could attend whichever primary care clinic they chose, subject to a government charge of R3 (US$ 0.75) per consultation, which also covered investigations and drugs. Early in 1993, NCD management was reassessed and discussions were held with patients and health workers. Rational structure was lacking, leaving primary care nurses without guidelines or support. There were no management protocols or an established referral structure, which led to poor levels of disease control, erratic drug ordering, and unnecessary referral from village and mobile clinics to the district hospital. This situation was inconvenient for patients, wasteful of resources and demotivated clinic staff.

Typical examples

Hypertension

Typically, when a patient with hypertension had been identified at a village clinic, she or he might, or might not be referred to the hospital for assessment and initiation of therapy by a doctor. The doctor would choose a drug according to his or her personal preference with little consideration for effectiveness, cost, patient tolerance, the Essentials Drug List, or what the pharmacy had in stock. The patient would receive little or no education about their condition other than to 'take these tablets'. With no structure to follow-up, non-adherence was understandably common and the patient might be seen several months later, with uncontrolled hypertension, for example, and be scolded by the nurse and doctor and sent away with more pills. Even worse, he or she might present with a stroke or as sudden death secondary to uncontrolled hypertension.

Diabetes

The same problems might occur with a diabetic patient, only this time random blood glucose levels would be checked in the laboratory at monthly follow-up visits, adding to time and expense and yielding little if any useful information.

The general outpatient department

Patients with NCDs were managed routinely through this department where 100–200 patients might be seen each day, many with acute medical emergencies. Often, patients with NCDs were considered (at best) as unimportant, and (at worst) a hindrance to the day's work.

The faults defined

Our assessment of the service demonstrated the following:

- No structured record of the number of patients with NCDs attending the service, their disease profile, or any basic demographic details. As such, any rational health system planning was impossible.
- No defined diagnostic criteria or agreed management protocols. Therefore hypertension and diabetes, for example, might be defined differently by different doctors, and management plans would vary according to the practitioner.
- Patients seemed almost universally unaware of what conditions they suffered from, and what symptoms related to poor control.
- Drug dispensing was often inconvenient so that patients had to travel long distances from home to clinics or hospital, and at unnecessarily frequent intervals (often monthly).
- Review of control, adherence and side effects was almost always irregular (Coleman et al., 1998).

Developing a solution

Our first response was to set objectives to define what we hoped to achieve. These were to describe the demographics of patients with NCDs; to develop diagnostic and treatment algorithms that enable nurses to manage most patients with NCDs; to transfer patients to their local village clinic for continued NCD care whenever feasible; and to improve patient-reported adherence to treatment. Following on from our established experience and success with community-based tuberculosis control in Hlabisa (Wilkinson, 1994), we agreed to adopt the following principles (see the Box).

Planning community NCD care

- Keep the new programme simple.
- Focus on using nurses as the primary care givers as they are the more stable workforce, and are drawn from the community.
- Use standardized protocols of management that are evidence-based and adjusted to local circumstances.
- Take a pragmatic and public health approach to the problem, recognizing that we could have the greatest impact overall by having a modest effect on the largest number of people possible.

We therefore planned the following four components to our intervention programme which responded directly to the four major issues identified during our assessment of the service (see the Box on the next page).

A new service structure

While wanting to improve radically the management and care of our patients with NCDs we did not necessarily want to radically change the organization and structure of

Essentials of an NCD service

- Create a clinic-held card register with demographic, diagnostic and management details.
- Develop diagnostic and management protocols with treatment algorithms, and train primary care nurses in their use.
- Incorporate education and self-care into management protocols.
- Prioritize patient convenience, introduce repeat prescriptions, rationalize drug ordering, monitor adherence and side effects.

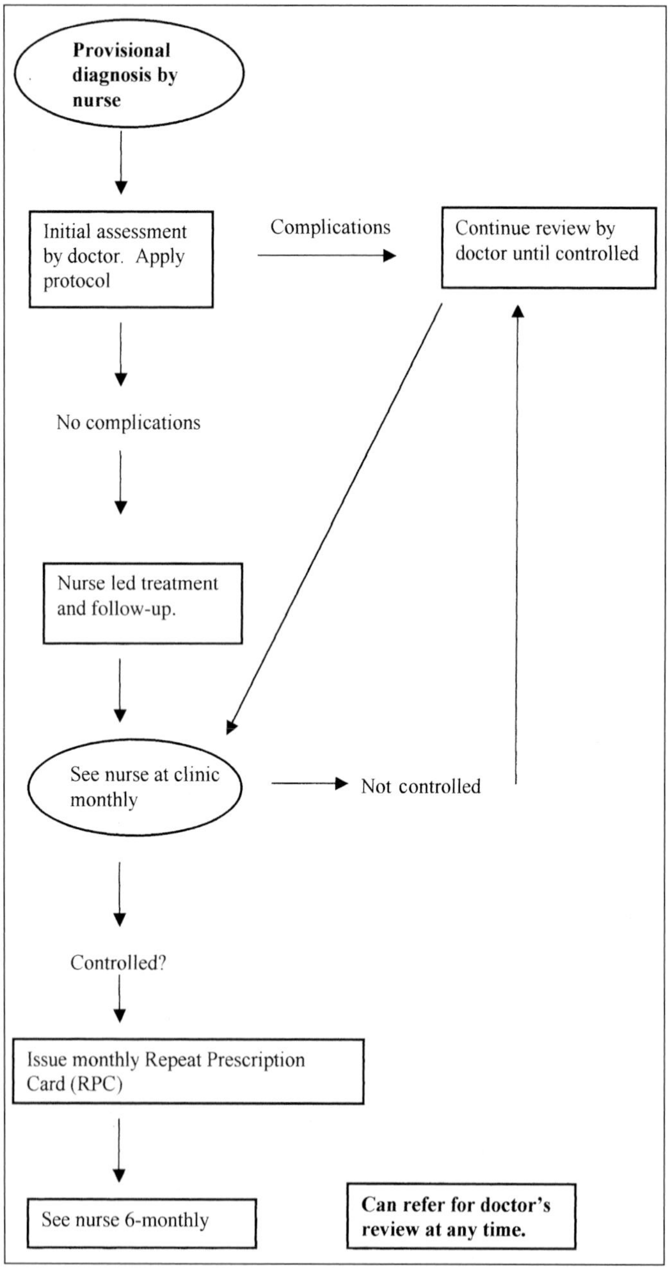

Fig. 75.1. General clinic model. This shows the pathway of care followed by clinic nurses undertaking NCD care.

the health system. This would have been difficult, if not impossible, and might not have produced the outcome we sought. So, we looked for ways of readjusting work practices in the clinics and the hospitals, and always aimed to make life easier for doctors and nurses, as well as patients; reasoning that, if we achieved this, change was likely to be much easier to achieve.

How the service operated

The model we developed was designed to be suitable for use at any of the primary care clinics. Protocols were devised so that nurses could provisionally diagnose patients with a new NCD, decide upon initial management, alter treatment in non-complex cases and identify patients requiring referral to hospital. Each newly diagnosed NCD patient was to be seen by a doctor at a primary care clinic for confirmation of diagnosis and detection of complications. Patients with complex conditions continued to be reviewed by a doctor until control was achieved, whereupon they were referred back to nursing staff for management. Optimal control of a NCD was defined clinically, also taking into consideration patient self-reported treatment adherence and treatment side effects. When optimal control was achieved, a repeat prescription card was started, which allowed monthly collection of treatment from any primary care clinic for 6 months without further clinical review. Collection of medicines could be delegated by the patient to a neighbour or family member. After 6 months of repeat prescriptions the patient was reviewed by a nurse and, depending on whether the control criteria were satisfied, the repeat prescription card was reissued or the treatment modified according to the protocol.

Management protocols

Management protocols rationalize care and are believed to reduce morbidity in primary care clinics. The protocols we devised were based on available evidence and modified by clinical experience and the local setting. Our aim was to provide a clear description of the essential aspects of diagnosis, monitoring and treatment adherence for each major NCD. Except for hypertension (where control was assessed by blood pressure), monitoring was based on the patient's reported symptoms. The basic model care pathway is shown in Fig. 75.1 and all the specific disease protocols were based on this. These specific protocols were for type 2 diabetes treated with diet or oral agents (Fig. 75.2), hypertension (Fig. 75.3) and asthma (Fig. 75.4).

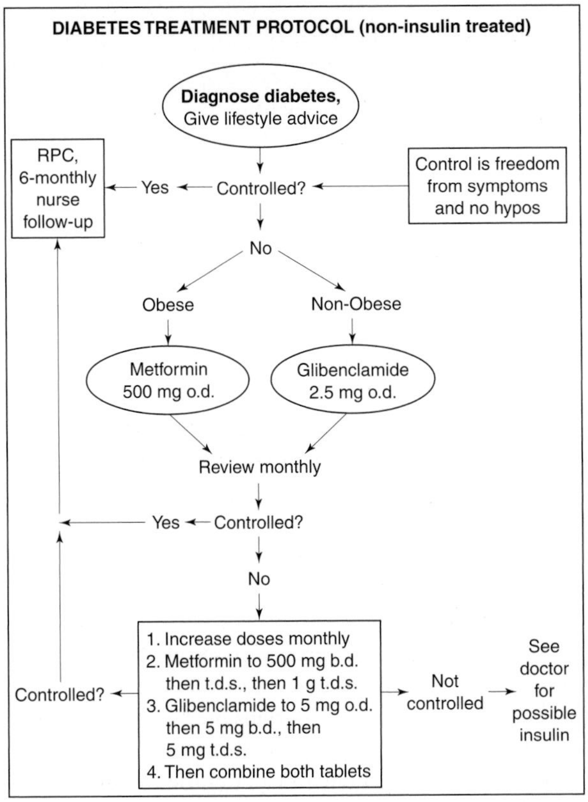

Fig. 75.2. Diabetes treatment protocol. Diagnosis of diabetes was in accordance with WHO criteria. Disease control was defined as freedom from symptoms of hyper and hypoglycaemia, as reported by patients. This strategy was a practical response to the unavailability of glucose self-monitoring facilities, the dubious value of clinic random blood glucose measurements, inflexible or erratic diets, and the real possibility of potentially fatal hypoglycaemia related to insulin or sulphonylurea drugs. Education and lifestyle advice were provided, and drugs given in increasing doses, followed by additional drugs as necessary. If this approach failed to achieve control, insulin could then by initiated by a doctor. Note that a similar and slightly more detailed protocol is shown on p. 751 (Figure 4, Chapter 70) as used in Cameroon.

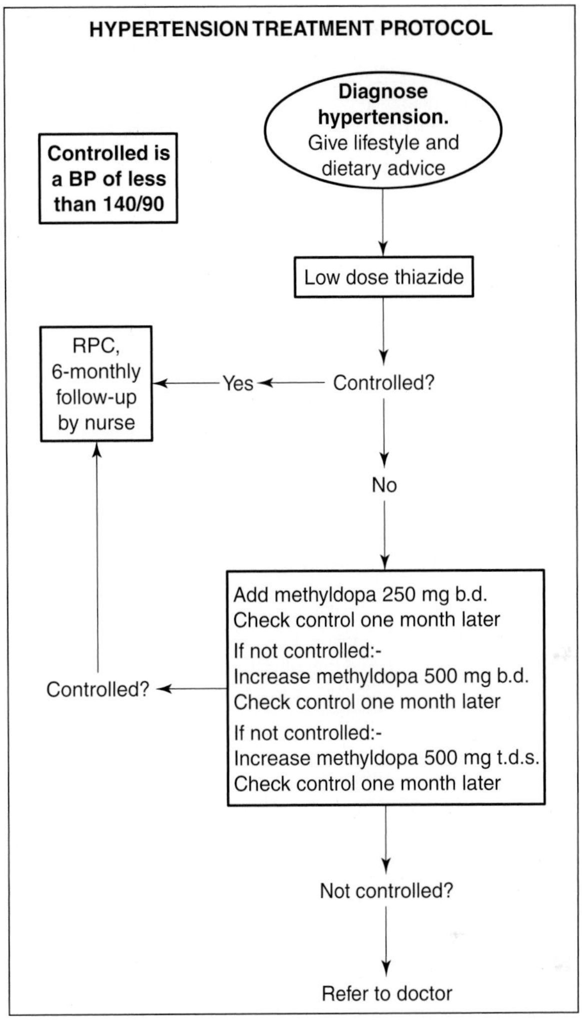

Fig. 75.3. Hypertension treatment protocol. Diagnostic criteria were based on national and WHO guidelines, emphasizing measurement technique and the need for repeated high blood pressure readings before diagnosis and treatment. Lifestyle and dietary advice were given, and the first-line drug was a low-dose thiazide, to which increasing doses of methyldopa could be added. The drug cascade follows other schedules of hypertension treatment, and is sensitive to the poor anti-hypertensive action of beta-blockers in black Africans, as well as to the expense and poor availability of ACE inhibitors and calcium channel blockers.

The use of drugs

The drugs used in the treatment algorithms were all on the provincial Essential Drugs List and were approved for prescription by nurses. Other drugs, prescribed by the doctor, could be dispensed in primary care clinics under special circumstances. Senior nurses were qualified to modify treatment of hypertension, asthma and non-insulin treated diabetes. Treatment for epilepsy and insulin-treated diabetes was prescribed and altered by the doctor until control was achieved, when nurses continued disease monitoring.

The diagnosis of epilepsy was entirely clinical, and control was judged by seizure frequency, with 'acceptable' control being defined by the patient or carer. Home fit charts were successfully introduced. Treatment was adjusted by a doctor to achieve control (hopefully 'fit-free'). Phenytoin was the drug of choice in adults and carbamazepine in children (many of whom had previously received phenobarbitone).

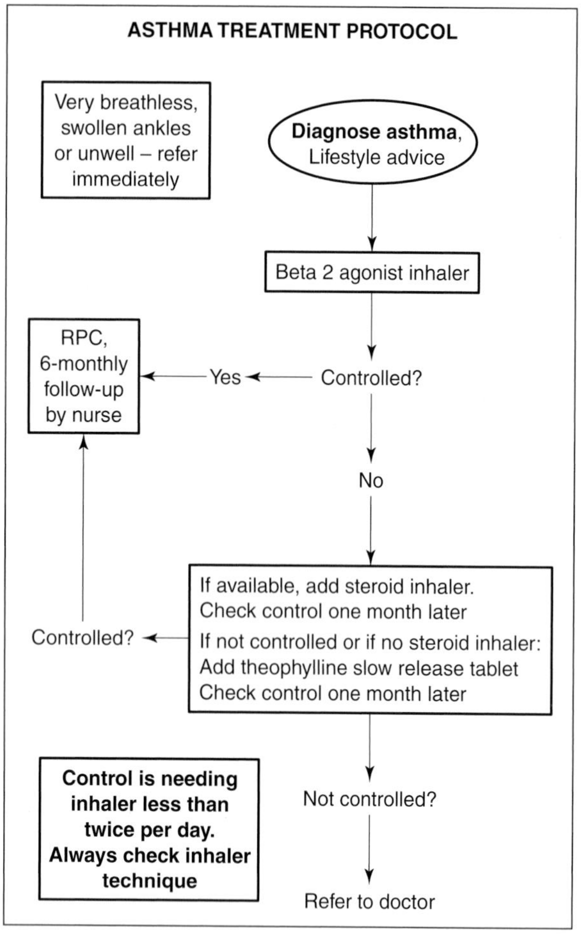

Fig. 75.4. **Asthma treatment protocol**. Diagnosis of asthma was clinical, based on a history of wheeze or nocturnal cough with clinically detected bronchospasm. Control was defined as freedom from nocturnal symptoms and daytime activity unrestricted by breathlessness. Education and encouragement with inhaler technique were emphasised. The additive treatment cascade followed standard guidelines, i.e. salbutamol inhaler, steroid inhaler, and oral theophylline. A spacer was 'home-made' using a plastic cup or bottle, a system which has been shown to be as effective as expensive proprietary spacers (Kerac, Montgomery & Johnson, 1998).

Evaluation and impact

Although simply adjusting service procedures can bring benefits and make things easier for patients and staff, we wanted to have a greater impact than this and so we developed a careful evaluation framework.

District NCD service records were reviewed 2 years after the service had been established. We extracted demographic and diagnostic details from all 1343 patients registered with a NCD and have reported these findings

Table 75.1. Levels of disease control by nurses and doctors

	Control achieved by:		
protocol	Nurse and input	Doctor's controlled	Total
Hypertension	113 (68%)	20 (12%)	133 (80%)
Non-insulin treated diabetes	23 (82%)	0 (0%)	23 (82%)
Asthma	26 (84%)	3 (10%)	29 (94%)

(Coleman et al., 1998). To assess the extent to which the programme's objectives were achieved, we extracted details on clinical management from the records of a random 448 patients.

Management by nurses

At the time of the audit, nurses working alone (using the protocols we had established) had achieved control of 68 per cent of patients with hypertension, 82 per cent of those with non-insulin treated diabetes, and 84 per cent of those with asthma (Table 75.1). Control (by nurse and doctor) was achieved in 80 per cent of epileptic patients and 83 per cent of patients with insulin-treated diabetes and their care was then continued by nurses.

At the patients' most recent clinic visit, nurses were effectively managing the condition of 92 per cent of patients with hypertension, 96 per cent of patients with non-insulin treated diabetes, and 97 per cent of patients with asthma, as many were still working their way through the protocols and had not reached a definite end point.

Adherence

Adherence was assessed by self-reporting of medicines by the patient. Maintenance of adherence was facilitated through the use of repeat prescription cards and transfer of patients to their local village or mobile clinic when appropriate. Of those patients for whom the hospital was the local clinic, and who had attended for more than 1 month, correct adherence was described by 79 per cent at their first visit. This had improved significantly to 87 per cent at their most recent visit.

The new service structure was also effective in shifting the management of patients to their nearest primary care facility. During the 2 years following establishment of the NCD service, 79 per cent of patients from a distant clinic area had their management transferred from hospital back to their local clinic. Similarly, 83 per cent of patients who used the hospital as their local clinic had qualified for a repeat prescription card, indicating control and adherence and simplification of their care.

Lessons learned and lessons for consideration

Our experience and results show that appropriate management of patients with NCDs can be achieved in a relatively resource-poor situation by making the most effective use of available primary care services. Nursing staff used practical stepwise diagnostic and treatment protocols, and managed to control most patients with hypertension, non-insulin treated diabetes, and asthma (Table 75.1). Because drug treatment and collection were simplified and the use of laboratory facilities was rationalized, patients could be conveniently managed at local village clinics. When they were helped to understand and accept the medication prescribed, many more patients adhered to their treatment. These principles can be adopted in any African setting.

Providing management at local clinics is particularly important, as many patients have limited access to transport and little spare time in their daily routine. This also helps reduce congestion in specialist clinics, so that patients with complex conditions can be managed more efficiently.

Methods to improve adherence

Adherence to treatment is a particular issue for patients with NCDs and clinic staff. Since it is difficult to sustain motivation for treatment, especially for asymptomatic conditions, how can patients with NCDs be helped to adhere to treatment? Methods include identifying side effects, educating patients in the need for long-term management, simplifying treatment and involving the patient in agreeing to an acceptable drug regimen: these strategies significantly improved adherence in our patients.

The only available method of measuring adherence at clinics in resource-poor areas is patient-reported treatment taking, although this may result in over-estimation. Reporting by patients is a low-technology approach which reinforces health education by emphasizing the contribution of patients and nurses in establishing treatment. We observed that most patients' conditions were controlled, and that most qualified for a repeat prescription card. Obviously, control requires adherence first.

Nurses are central for NCD care

Effective management of the increasing number of patients with NCDs in Africa can really only be provided by nurses and other paramedical staff. Where resources are scarce, poor urban and rural people can have access to care if health care is decentralized to primary care settings (see Fig. 75.5). The use of practical, evidence-based clinical protocols makes the best use of the resources, so that convenient and effective treatment is a reality.

Slowly, a few models for NCD management in different settings in Africa are emerging (Gill, 1979; Kaiser et al., 1998; Unwin et al., 1999), and it is from these, and from further experimentation and exploration, that progress in pragmatic and effective NCD management and control in Africa will occur.

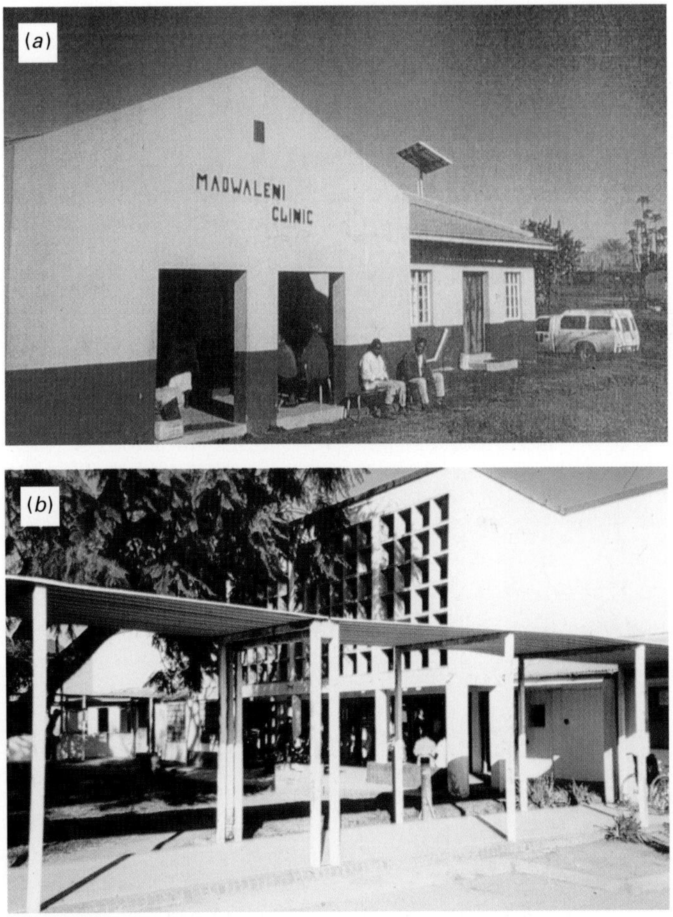

Fig. 75.5. Central and Peripheral Services for NCD Care. This is a major principle for effective management provision. (*a*) One of the local primary health care clinics in the district. (*b*) The central 'Chronic Disease' clinic at Hlabisa Hospital in Kwazulu–Natal.

References

Beavers DG, Prince JS. (1991). Hypertension: an emerging problem in tropical countries. *Trans Roy Soc Trop Med & Hyg*; **85**: 324–326.

Coleman R, Wilkinson D, Gill G. (1998). Non-communicable disease management in resource-poor settings: a primary care model from rural South Africa. *Bull Wld Hlth Org*; **76**: 633–640.

Gill GV. (1979). An asthma clinic for provincial tropical hospitals. *Trop Doctor*; **9**: 155–157.

Kaiser C, Asaba G, Mugisa C et al. (1998). Antiepileptic drug treatment in rural Africa: involving the community. *Trop Doctor*; **28**: 73–77.

Kerac M, Montgomery H, Johnson N. (1998). A low cost spacer device used for asthma treatment in a Calcutta street clinic to improve efficacy of metered dose inhalers. *Trop Doctor*; **28**: 228–229.

Unwin N, Mugusi F, Aspray T et al. (1999). Tackling the emerging pandemic of non-communicable diseases in sub-Saharan Africa: the essential NCD health intervention project. *Public Hlth*; **113**: 141–146.

Wilkinson D. (1994). High-compliance tuberculosis treatment programme in a rural community. *Lancet*; **343**: 647–648.

Zimmet P, Lefebvre P. (1996). The global NIDDM epidemic: treating the disease and ignoring the symptom. *Diabetalogia*; **39**: 1247–1248.

Part IV

Diseases of body systems

The heart

76

The problem in Africa

Patterns of disease are changing in Africa. Not only does HIV dominate hospital practice in many countries, but urban life and its attendant obesity, lack of exercise and smoking, together with diabetes and hypertension, are responsible for a new pattern of urban disease, which includes coronary arterial disease. But this is still a rare disease because rural people lack its risk factors, whether in Tanzania (Swai et al., 1993), north west Ethiopia (Gebre-Yohannes et al., 1998) or north east Nigeria (Okesina et al., 1999). Hypertension, however, particularly complicated by stroke, is a great problem and accounts for up to 20 per cent of patients with cardiac failure (Amoah et al., 2000), which is significant in the small ageing population (Lodenyo et al., 1997).

Rheumatic heart disease still disables young patients and contributes the highest proportion of cases of cardiac failure in many countries. It is difficult to get patients to take or to attend for prophylaxis of rheumatic fever and to ensure that cardiac patients adhere to their prescribed treatment.

Finally, the response to beta-blockers, angiotensin-converting enzyme inhibitors, and angiotensin II receptor antagonists, unless combined with a diuretic, is poor in African in contrast to Caucasian or Asian people (Seedat, 2000).

The history

Environment and origin of patient

Always ask yourself – why should this patient (man or woman, occupation, culture and habits) from this place (geographical region and its crops) fall ill in this way (cardiac disease) at this time (seasonal factors, pregnancy)? Relate the diagnosis to the context of the patient so that treatment can take account of the patient's work, their attitude to their disease, their ability to pay for drugs and the distance of their home from the clinic.

Symptoms

Swelling

Swelling (oedema) in the legs, face and arms, or around the sacral region of those who have been sitting down, is one of the commonest symptoms in cardiac failure. When it is generalized, the term anasarca may be used.

Oedema is usually first noticed in the feet at the end of the day: later it becomes more widespread, and does not vary during the day. Although a swollen face is classically seen in renal disease, it is also found in Africa when oedema is substantial. Some cases of endomyocardial fibrosis (EMF) have swelling of the face early in their illness.

Breathlessness

In a number of languages in Africa the distinction between pain in the chest and breathlessness is scarcely recognized, and so it is easy to think a patient has chest pain, if a direct question is asked, when the real problem is breathlessness. This is the most common symptom and is found in all with cardiac failure. They have breathlessness (dyspnoea) on exertion, at rest, or when lying down (orthopnoea), or in paroxysms during the night, which wake them from sleep and get better when they stand up (paroxysmal nocturnal dyspnoea).

- Relate breathlessness to everyday tasks: is the patient able to walk uphill or only on the flat, does she become breathless doing simple household tasks, has her breathlessness made it impossible for her to carry water or to go to the market?

- Can the patient lie down flat without becoming short of breath and distressed?
- Is her sleep disturbed by attacks of breathlessness?

Cough

Cough at first produces no sputum but, as pulmonary venous congestion increases there is whitish sputum, which may be flecked with blood and frothy when pulmonary oedema is established. Cough only on lying is an early symptom of pulmonary venous congestion.

Palpitation

The patient may complain of rapid beating of the heart (palpitation)(p. 845), or episodes of fainting (syncope), (p. 1121), caused by an acute fall in cardiac output.

Physical signs

General

- Look for signs of any associated disease or deficiency, which may be secondary to cardiac disease, for example a protein-losing enteropathy secondary to heart failure.

Wasting and anaemia

Severe long-standing heart disease may be associated with wasting (p. 853):

- Look for pallor of tongue and conjunctivae – anaemia may precipitate cardiac failure.

Cyanosis (see also p. 895)

Central cyanosis

When there is 5 g or more of deoxygenated haemoglobin in the blood, cyanosis can be detected in the tongue, mucosae of the mouth, and nail beds, and the vessels of the conjunctivae are obvious (conjunctival injection). In anaemic patients it may not be seen in spite of their having a disease which would normally produce cyanosis, because they have too low a haemoglobin to allow 5 g to be deoxygenated. It is caused by:

- reduced pulmonary oxygen uptake (p. 890)
- right to left shunting of blood, in the heart (tetralogy of Fallot; R to L shunts with pulmonary hypertension, pulmonary arterio-venous anastomoses), and in the lung (consolidation – lobar pneumonia; collapse – from whatever cause).

Peripheral cyanosis

When the fingers and hands, the toes, the ear lobes and the nose appear cyanosed, and yet the tongue (and other places where central cyanosis is found) are not cyanosed, the patient is said to have peripheral cyanosis. It is less easily detected in deeply pigmented than in white skin. The mechanism is a greatly increased extraction of oxygen from blood which is flowing sluggishly through the peripheral vessels as a result of a diminished cardiac output. As blood flow is reduced, the cyanosed digits or nose are cold, and superficial veins are empty.

The hands

Cold, cyanosed fingers and hands and empty veins indicate a low cardiac output, whereas warm hands and full veins are associated with an increased cardiac output. Digital pulses may disappear if occluded by an embolus, and tender nodules in the palm (called Osler's nodes in infective endocarditis), are related to deposition of immune complexes in arterioles.

The finger nails and the nail beds

Contour

Clubbing of the fingers (p. 898) may point to infective endocarditis or sickle cell anaemia: when associated with central cyanosis, it may be due to chronic hypoxic pulmonary disease (which has led to cor pulmonale), suppurative lung disease or congenital cyanotic heart disease.

Consistency

The easily broken and brittle nails of iron deficiency precede koilonychia.

Colour

Distinguish the opaque white nails (leukonychia) of chronic hypoalbuminaemia from anaemic pallor.

Splinter haemorrhages

Small linear haemorrhages in the long axis of the nail are seen in infective endocarditis (p. 878) but are more commonly due to trauma: they also occur in chronic bronchitis.

The arterial pulse

The arterial pulse is a vital sign in patients with a reduced blood volume, whether due to fluid or blood loss, and is very important in the clinical diagnosis of heart disease.

Rate

- Count the pulse over at least 30 seconds and, when the rhythm is irregular, count the heart rate by auscultation. This may reveal a pulse 'deficit', the arterial pulse has fewer palpable beats than are heard, because beats of low stroke volume are impalpable.

Rhythm

- Analyse any irregularity of rhythm. Is it regular, for example, with respiratory movements (sinus arrhythmia), or with every alternate beat, as when a ventricular ectopic beat follows a normal beat and causes 'coupled' beats (pulsus bigeminus)?

The term 'irregularly irregular' is used sometimes to describe an arterial pulse in which the rhythm is irregular and the irregularity has no consistent pattern. It is characteristic of atrial fibrillation, but may be found if there are multiple ventricular ectopic beats.

Volume or pulse pressure

If the stroke volume is low, the pulse pressure is small, and the arterial pulse is scarcely palpable. Avoid using adjectives like 'thready'; instead, describe the volume and pulse pressure and record the arterial pressure.

If the cardiac output and stroke volume are high, the arterial pulse is easily palpable: when there is widespread peripheral arteriolar dilatation, the pulse will 'collapse' quickly to a low pressure and its wave will change.

Pulse wave

This is determined by:

- the stroke volume
- the anatomy of the aortic valve
- the calibre of the systemic arterioles – constricted or dilated.

The small volume pulse and collapsing pulse are important: others are uncommon.

Collapsing pulse

High fever and severe anaemia cause arteriolar dilatation and a low peripheral resistance so that the pulse tends to 'collapse' to the low level of the diastolic pressure.

Aortic incompetence allows blood to regurgitate into the left ventricle and so the arterial pressure falls quickly to a low level. If the left ventricular end-diastolic pressure

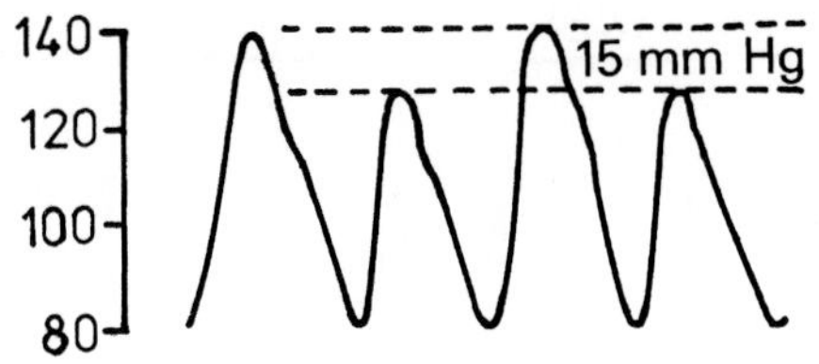

Fig. 76.1. Pulsus alternans.

rises and systolic power falls (left ventricular failure), the amplitude of the pulse is reduced and in severe failure it may not even be felt to 'collapse'.

Arterio-venous anastomoses cause a similar rapid fall in diastolic pressure, whether they are single (patent ductus arteriosus or traumatic arterio-venous fistula), or small and multiple (as in the uterus during pregnancy, or in widespread Kaposi's sarcoma).

Other abnormalities of the arterial pulse

Pulsus alternans

This is found in left ventricular failure: alternate beats are strong and weak (Fig. 76.1). It is best detected with a sphygmomanometer: alternate beats, at a rate of exactly half the ventricular rate are heard first. Then, as the blood pressure cuff is slowly deflated and the column of mercury falls, a level of pressure is reached at which the rate abruptly doubles, so that all the beats are now heard. The difference between the first level and the second is the number of mm Hg of alternans.

Pulsus paradoxus

During normal inspiration intra-thoracic pressure falls, the lung expands, and blood pools in the pulmonary vessels; less blood enters the left ventricle, stroke volume falls, and arterial blood pressure decreases by about 3–10 mm Hg. When the decline in the blood pressure is greater than 10 mm Hg, pulsus paradoxus is said to exist. In severe cases the peripheral pulse may be impalpable on inspiration (Fig. 76.2).

This pulse is found in acute cardiac tamponade, constrictive pericarditis and restrictive heart disease(EMF), and in severe asthma.

Unequal pulses

- Palpate the brachial pulse in each arm at the same time: if it is not felt in one arm, while it is normal in the other, it may be occluded by an embolus, by primary disease of the great vessels, or by occlusive pressure of a rib or intra-thoracic tumour.

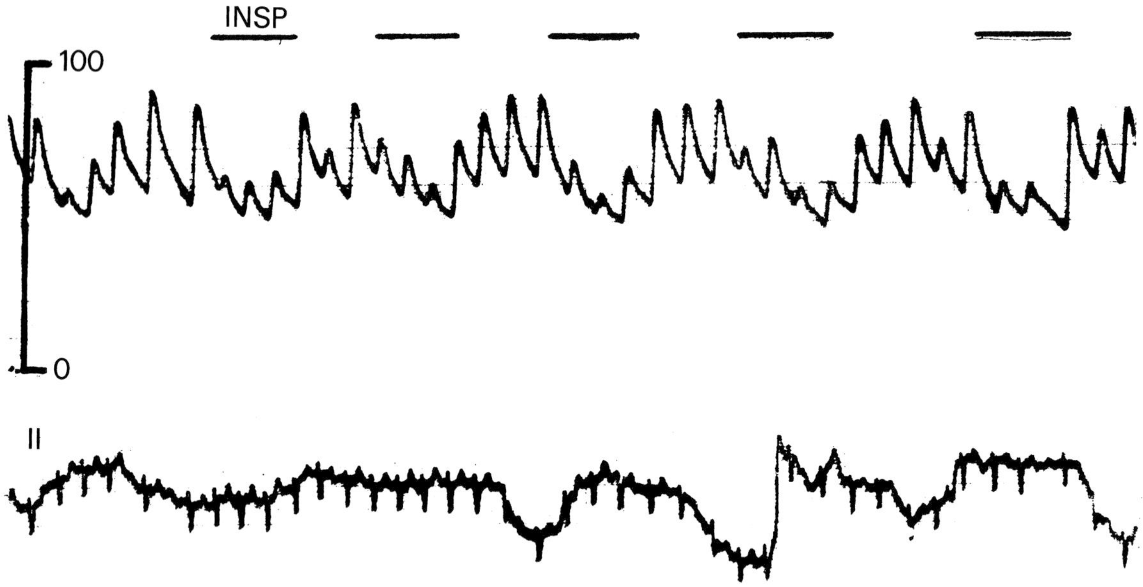

Fig. 76.2. Pulsus paradoxus: from a patient with EMF (INSP = inspiration).

Taking the blood pressure

The cuff must be of the right size for the arm circumference (i.e. 20 per cent greater than the diameter of the arm): a cuff that is too small will give a falsely high pressure, whereas a large cuff gives a low reading (See Chapter 72 box p. 786).

Take the blood pressure with the subject lying and standing, comfortable, and rested. Apply the cuff snugly with its inflatable bag positioned over the brachial artery. Inflate the cuff and palpate the artery to determine the pressure which obliterates the arterial pressure. For auscultation, deflate the cuff and then reinflate it to 20–30 mm Hg above the pressure determined by palpation, then deflate it slowly at a rate of 2–3 mm Hg per second. The systolic pressure is the level at which the first tapping Korotkov's sounds are heard (phase I): the diastolic pressure is the level at which abrupt muffling of the sounds occurs (phase IV): the pressure at which the sounds disappear is phase V.

The difference between the systolic and the diastolic pressure is the pulse pressure. The mean pressure can be estimated as one-third of the pulse pressure plus the diastolic blood pressure.

In surveys of arterial blood pressure in the community, two further precautions can avoid bias in the collection of data: the subjects are rested for 10 minutes before the pressure is taken, and random zero machines are used so that an observer's digit preference and expectation can be discounted.

The jugular venous pulse

Think of the internal jugular vein as a manometer continuous with the right atrium. The height of the jugular venous pressure, measured from the sternal angle, depends on:

The right atrial pressure

This is governed by the diastolic pressure within the right ventricle, the integrity of the tricuspid valve and the movements of the atrioventricular ring.

The total blood volume

The normal pulse

The internal jugular vein is best examined (not the external jugular) when the patient is in a good light, their head and shoulders supported at any angle which brings the vein into view; this may be at 45 or 90 degrees if the pressure is very high – there is no special value in 45 degrees!

If the jugular vein is full and does not pulsate, it is obstructed, commonly in the superior mediastinum.

- Time the jugular venous pulse wave(s) on one side of the neck in relation to the carotid pulse, which is palpated on the other side.

The venous pulse is not normally seen in health unless the patient lies down nearly flat. It may be visible in

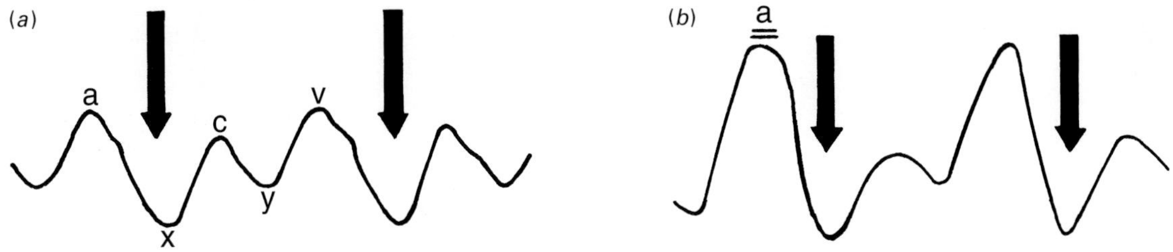

Fig. 76.3. (*a*) The normal jugular pulse: the normal *a* wave precedes the palpable arterial pulse (shown by vertical arrow): it is followed by the *x* descent, the *v* wave and the *y* descent. (*b*) Jugular venous pulse to show a large *a* wave, as in pulmonary hypertension and cor pulmonale. It can be timed just before the carotid pulse is felt in the neck.

patients with massive ascites due to upward displacement of the diaphragm and obstruction of venous return to the heart.

The normal jugular venous pulse wave consists of three positive pulse waves (*a, c,* and *v* waves) and two negative waves (*x* and *y* descents) (Fig. 76.3(*a*)).

The *a* wave is due to right atrial contraction which transmits pressure back to the jugular vein to produce a positive wave.

The *x* descent is produced by atrial relaxation and a fall in atrial pressure as the tricuspid valve and the base of the right ventricle move downwards during ventricular systole.

The *v* wave is produced in systole when the tricuspid valve is closed and blood from the systemic veins fills the right atrium. At the peak of the *v* wave the tricuspid valve opens and blood flows from the right atrium into the right ventricle so that the pressure drops quickly in the right atrium and the *y* descent is formed.

The *c* wave is not important, is often not seen, and need not be looked for.

Distinction of jugular from arterial pulse

Manoeuvres which affect the jugular, but not the arterial, pulse are used to distinguish one from the other: thus,

(i) Coughing, or pressure on the abdomen or liver.
(ii) Respiration. During inspiration the JVP falls in normal people, but rises if the heart is constricted or if there is tricuspid regurgitation.
(iii) Posture. The JVP appears to rise in the neck as the patient lies down, but its vertical height in relation to the heart does not change.
(iv) Firm pressure at the root of the neck will obliterate a venous but not an arterial pulse.

Note that:

(v) a jugular pulse is palpable if its pressure is high.
(vi) a jugular pulse may have a single giant systolic wave. (These signs, (v) and (vi), do not therefore distinguish it from the arterial pulse.) If it is necessary to check that a raised venous pressure is not being missed, press lightly with a finger at the base of the external jugular vein: if the jugular pressure is normal, the distended vein empties rapidly when the finger is released. Never assume that the JVP is normal until it has been seen.

Common abnormalities

Abnormal *a* wave:

This immediately precedes the carotid pulse – against which it should be timed by palpation. It can be seen as a sharp flick (*a* wave and *x* descent) in the venous pulse above the clavicle in any disease in which the right atrium contracts at an increased pressure to fill an abnormal right ventricle, for example cor pulmonale. The *a* wave is absent in atrial fibrillation because it depends on normal atrial systole (Fig. 76.3(*b*)).

Systolic wave

This is synchronous with the carotid pulse and occurs when the tricuspid valve is incompetent. It is the only certain sign of tricuspid incompetence and occurs in no other disorder. Blood regurgitates during ventricular systole from the ventricle to the atrium and jugular veins: a big swelling pulse wave can therefore be seen, which is often 10 cm or more above the sternal angle (Fig. 76.4).

Dominant *y* descent with *a* and *v* waves

This is the distinctive pulse of cardiac constriction. The high pressure in the right atrium falls abruptly when the tricuspid valve opens (*y* descent) but rises again quickly because the ventricle resists further filling. The atrium must contract at a high pressure to fill the resistant constricted ventricle so it produces an exaggerated *a* wave, which is followed by a deep but normal *x* descent because the tricuspid valve is normal (Fig. 76.5).

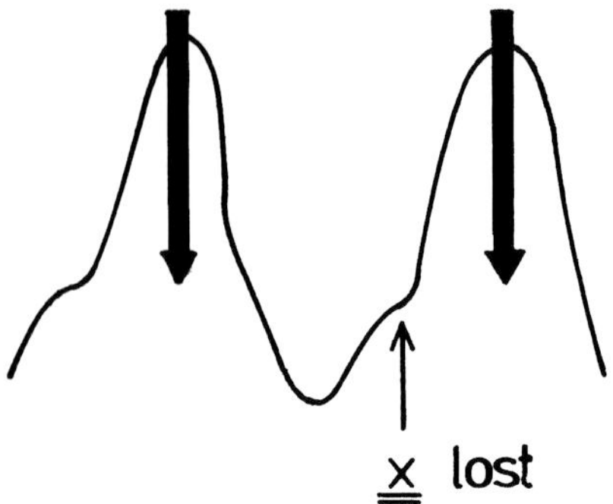

Fig. 76.4. Jugular venous pulse in tricuspid regurgitation: the *x* descent is lost and the systolic wave is synchronous with the carotid pulse.

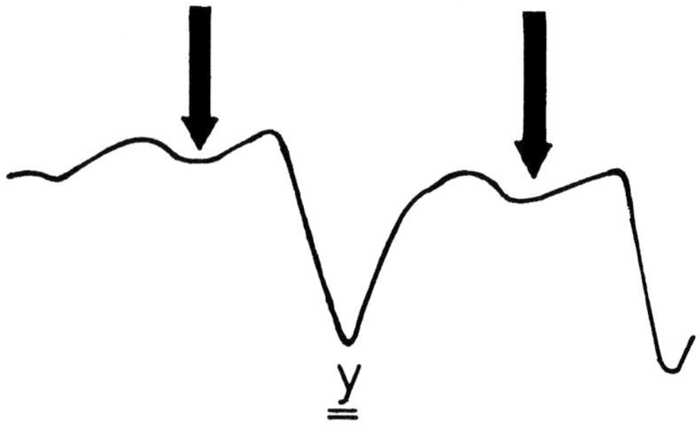

Fig. 76.5. Jugular venous pulse in cardiac constriction – EMF, constrictive pericarditis – note the prominent *y* descent.

Measurement of the jugular venous pressure

The height of the jugular venous pressure can be estimated indirectly. A horizontal line is drawn from the top of the jugular venous pulse to reach a perpendicular line drawn from the sternal angle. The height of the pulse is measured in centimetres from the sternal angle to where the two lines meet. A normal jugular venous pulse should not be above 2–3 cm. The highest pressures are seen in constrictive pericarditis and tricuspid incompetence.

Inspection and palpation of the praecordium

Left sternal border

Left parasternal bulging, and a vigorous left parasternal impulse is seen in children with a large right ventricle. In adults there is usually no praecordial bulging because the ventricle enlarges after the thoracic cage has fully formed. Common causes are pulmonary hypertension secondary to mitral valve disease, or cor pulmonale.

- Look for scarifications at the left border of the sternum: old scars will indicate that the patient has had pulmonary hypertension for a long time.

Right sternal border

A palpable impulse may be due to a displaced heart (pleural effusion), an aortic aneurysm or, very rarely, a subvalvular left ventricular aneurysm.

Apex beat

The normal apex beat is in the left fifth intercostal space in the mid-clavicular line. When the left ventricle becomes large the apex is displaced inferiorly and laterally. It may be diffuse if there is left ventricular volume overload (mitral and aortic regurgitation, or congenital heart disease with a large left to right shunt – ventricular septal defect or patent ductus arteriosus). If the apex beat is localized and/or powerful, left ventricular pressure overload is suspected (hypertension, or rarely aortic stenosis).

Thrill

A praecordial thrill is due to vibrations (caused by turbulence of blood at a valve or a defect in the heart) which are transmitted to the chest wall. Define where a thrill is best felt; and whether it is in systole or diastole, when it means the same as a murmur heard in the same area. A thrill over an artery indicates a stenotic segment or an arterio-venous fistula.

Heart sounds

Concentrate on the first heart sound and then the second heart sound: when you are certain of these, listen to systole and then to diastole (Fig. 76.6).

- Palpate the carotid pulse, which precedes the palpable pulse, to confirm the first sound.

First heart sound

This is due to mitral and tricuspid valve closure. When either valve shuts abruptly at an increased pressure, as in mitral stenosis, it is louder than normal; it is softer if the a–v valve cusps meet at a low pressure, as in some beats in complete heart block, when the first heart sound varies according to the timing of atrial systole: it is soft when atrial systole is early in diastole, and normal when atrial systole is in the normal late diastole.

Second heart sound

The two components are due to aortic and pulmonary valve closure, in that order; they are loud in systemic or

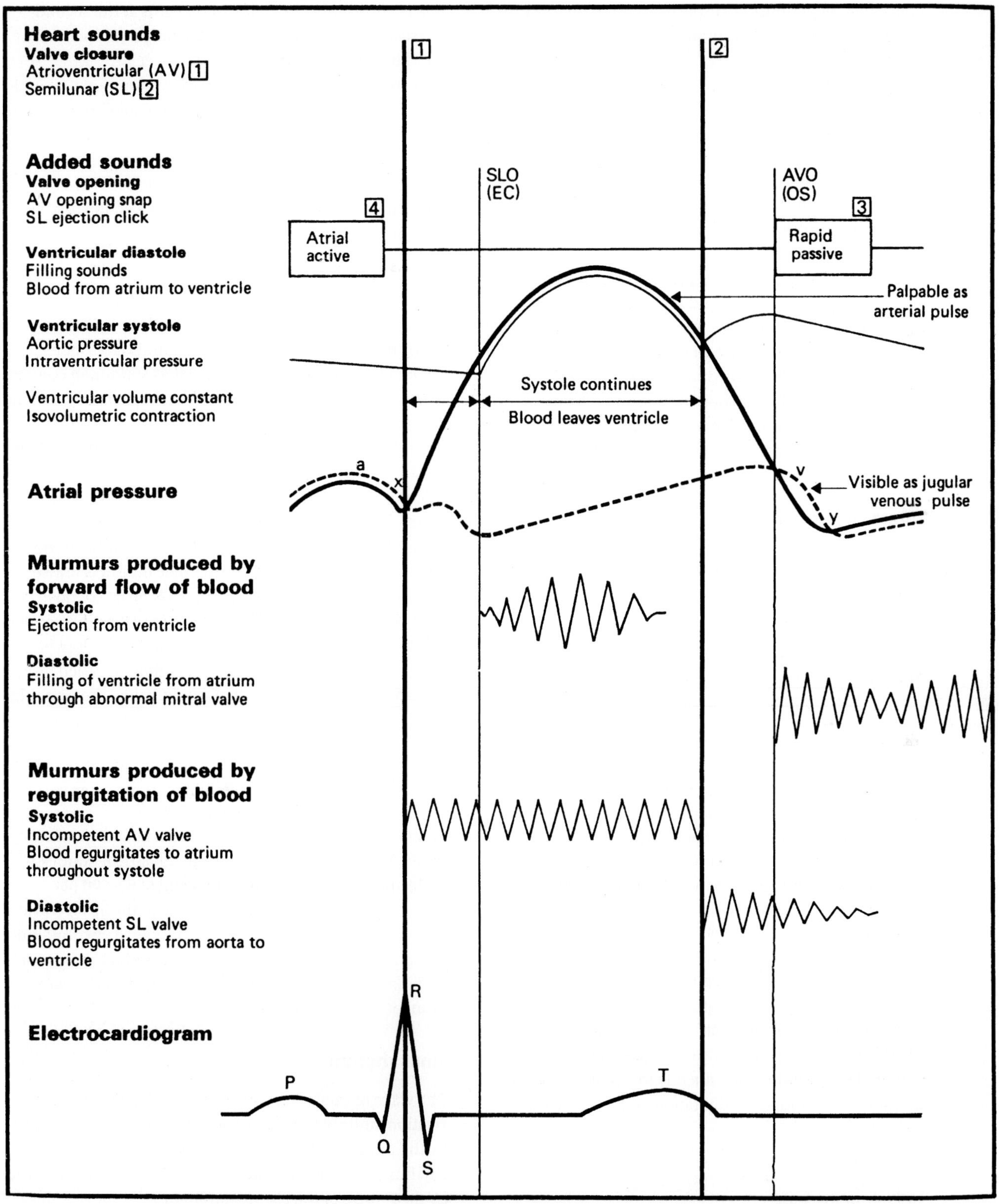
Heart sounds
Valve closure
Atrioventricular (AV) 1
Semilunar (SL) 2
Added sounds
Valve opening
AV opening snap
SL ejection click
Ventricular diastole
Filling sounds
Blood from atrium to ventricle
Ventricular systole
Aortic pressure
Intraventricular pressure
Ventricular volume constant
Isovolumetric contraction
Atrial pressure
Murmurs produced by forward flow of blood
Systolic
Ejection from ventricle
Diastolic
Filling of ventricle from atrium through abnormal mitral valve
Murmurs produced by regurgitation of blood
Systolic
Incompetent AV valve
Blood regurgitates to atrium throughout systole
Diastolic
Incompetent SL valve
Blood regurgitates from aorta to ventricle
Electrocardiogram
1
2
SLO
(EC)
AVO
(OS)
4
3
Atrial active
Rapid passive
Palpable as arterial pulse
Systole continues
Blood leaves ventricle
a
x
v
y
Visible as jugular venous pulse
R
P
T
Q
S

Fig. 76.6. The events of the cardiac cycle.

pulmonary hypertension, respectively. Pulmonary closure is normally delayed by inspiration.

Gallop sounds

Diastolic sounds associated with ventricular filling, the third and fourth heart sounds, are called gallop sounds. They may arise from left or right ventricles.

The third heart sound occurs during rapid passive ventricular filling; the fourth or atrial sound occurs during rapid active ventricular filling produced by atrial systole. At fast heart rates the added diastolic sound and the first and second resemble the gallop of a horse (gallop rhythm). The third heart sound is almost always a sign of ventricular failure. It is a low frequency sound, therefore it will be best heard with the bell of the stethoscope, not the diaphragm. Some healthy young people have a third heart sound. A higher pitched third sound is heard in most patients with cardiac constriction, whether due to EMF or constrictive pericarditis.

Heart murmurs

These arise from turbulence of blood at an orifice, usually but not always when the valve orifice/volume of blood relationship is altered.

Systolic

Ejection

This arises at the aortic and pulmonary (semilunar) valves and cannot therefore begin until the valves open, a little after the first heart sound (Fig. 76.6). The intensity of the murmur rises and falls. It does not usually indicate valve disease and is common in anaemia, pregnancy, or any state when cardiac output is increased. If there is evidence of heart disease, it may indicate semilunar valvular stenosis.

Pansystolic

This murmur arises when an atrioventricular valve is incompetent: it therefore begins at the first heart sound, when systole begins and continues throughout systole while blood regurgitates from ventricle to atrium. Pansystolic murmurs may disappear during the treatment of heart failure if they are due to papillary muscle dysfunction secondary to dilatation of the ventricle.

Diastolic

Early or immediate

This murmur occurs if the aortic (or pulmonary) valve is incompetent. It is high-pitched, becomes softer as diastole proceeds (diminuendo) and begins at the second heart sound. It is caused by regurgitation of blood from aorta to left ventricle.

Aortic incompetence is much more common than pulmonary incompetence. The diagnosis can often be made from its peripheral signs: a collapsing pulse, a wide pulse pressure and vigorous arterial pulsation in the neck, together with signs of a large left ventricle. Patients with aortic incompetence may also have an ejection systolic murmur.

Atrioventricular

Mitral stenosis causes a murmur when blood flows through the valve during ventricular diastole. The murmur can only begin when the mitral valve opens (a distinct interval after the second heart sound), in contrast to the aortic diastolic murmur which begins at the second heart sound. It can also be distinguished from an aortic diastolic murmur because it is a low pitched 'rumble', and because it does not become softer as diastole proceeds: by contrast, in patients with normal sinus rhythm it increases during atrial systole when the atrium forces blood through the mitral valve (the pre-systolic murmur). If mitral stenosis is severe, the cardiac output is low so that the arterial pulse is small, the first heart sound is loud, and the apex beat has an abnormal tapping impulse due to the accentuated first heart sound.

The murmur of mitral stenosis is often preceded by a high-pitched sound, early in diastole, called the 'opening snap', which is produced as the mitral cusps 'snap' open.

The rhythm of the heart

Activation of the cardiac muscle begins in the sino-atrial node (SA node) in the right atrium. Electrical impulses are generated spontaneously at a rate of 60–100 per minute, spread through atrial muscle to the atrioventricular node, and then pass down the Bundle of His, and into its right and left main bundle branches which subdivide and ramify into Purkinje fibres throughout the myocardium of the ventricles.

Sinus rhythm

The wave of excitation causes myocardial fibre depolarization, and rhythmic cardiac contraction at the rate set by the pacemaker cells of the SA node – this is sinus rhythm. Atrial depolarization from the SA node is marked by the P wave of the electrocardiogram.

Atrial contraction at the end of ventricular diastole assists ventricular filling by up to 20 per cent, which may not be clinically important in normal hearts, but in hearts which are only just able to maintain an adequate cardiac output, it may be critical: patients with heart disease often develop their first symptoms of cardiac failure when sinus rhythm changes to atrial fibrillation.

Sinus arrhythmia in young people may produce variations in cardiac rate so that a pathological arrhythmia may be suspected. Watch the respiration to see whether the heart rate increases with each inspiration.

The patient with tachycardia

Sinus tachycardia, a normal physiological response, is by far the most common cause. A good history is essential. Patients with an established tachycardia may have become suddenly conscious of a forceful heart beat, which may be regular or irregular. Ask the patient to choose between a regular and irregular beat which you tap out on the table.

- Fever. A rise of body temperature of 1 °C raises the heart rate by about 18–20 per minute.
- Anxiety.
- Hypovolaemia. The tachycardia with a low stroke output is usually, but by no means always, accompanied by a low blood pressure.
- Myocardial failure, or acute cardiac compression, when the failing heart can only maintain its output through an increase of rate – caused by a rapidly forming pericardial effusion.
- Thyrotoxicosis.

Irregular rhythm

By far the commonest cause is atrial fibrillation, although rarely multiple ventricular ectopic beats may be indistinguishable without an electrocardiogram.

Disorders of rhythm

Paroxysmal supraventricular tachycardia

Paroxysmal supraventricular tachycardias are rapid, regular rhythms arising from an abnormal focus, in the atrium, A–V node or an accessory pathway, as occurs in Wolff-Parkinson–White syndrome.

Clinical features

Paroxysmal atrial tachycardia starts and ends suddenly. Symptoms of regional ischaemia, for example cardiac pain or dizziness and syncope, may occur during an attack owing to the poor perfusion of the coronary or cerebral vessels. The patient may also report polyuria during an episode. The ventricular rate is up to 180 per minute: if the atrial rate is faster than this the ventricle may be unable to respond and A–V block will result. This is common, whether or not there is underlying cardiac disease; it may also follow overdose with digoxin when a variable A–V block is usual.

Management

1. First, treat any obvious cause.
2. Manoeuvres which stimulate the vagus may cut short an attack:
   - cautious carotid sinus massage
   - taking in and holding a deep breath
   - a Valsalva manoeuvre
   - swallowing an ice-cold drink
   - forceful expiration
3. Most attacks stop spontaneously. If manoeuvres are ineffective and the patient is distressed, verapamil, given as an intravenous bolus of 5 mg, repeated after 10 minutes, will abort an attack in up to 90 per cent of cases. Digoxin 0.5 mg, given as an intravenous infusion over 10 minutes, may be used as an alternative. (Where available, intravenous adenosine has been shown to be very effective.)

Atrial fibrillation and atrial flutter

In atrial fibrillation there is no co-ordinated effective contraction of the atrium. The ventricles cannot respond regularly to the very rapid excitation from the atrial focus. Atrial flutter is very similar to atrial fibrillation but, because the abnormal atrial focus has a slower rate, the ventricle may respond regularly and a 2: 1 or 3: 1 A–V block will follow.

Causes

(i) Any form of heart disease – notably rheumatic heart disease, but also right ventricular endomyocardial fibrosis, dilated cardiomyopathy, hypertensive heart disease, and constrictive pericarditis.
(ii) Digoxin overdosage – the rhythm reverts to sinus rhythm when the drug is withdrawn.
(iii) Acute infections – such as typhoid or pneumococcal infection.
(iv) Ischaemic heart disease.
(v) Thyrotoxicosis.

Effects
Atrial function is ineffective, ventricular filling is reduced by about 20 per cent and cardiac output therefore falls; the failing ventricle may depend absolutely on atrial filling if it is to maintain an adequate stroke output. When atrial fibrillation or flutter is associated with a rapid ventricular rate, the diastolic filling time of the ventricle is reduced and stroke output falls further.

Clinical features

Symptoms
When atrial fibrillation starts, the patient may notice a sudden rapid and irregular beat or may become acutely breathless; similarly, symptoms of cardiac failure, particularly breathlessness on effort, may become unexpectedly worse.

Signs
The arterial pulse is irregular in both rhythm and volume, and the volume varies with the length of the preceding ventricular diastole. Some beats produce a very small stroke volume, which cannot be felt in the brachial artery, so there is a pulse deficit. The *a* wave disappears from the jugular venous pulse.

Electrocardiogram
P waves are absent (Fig. 76.7(*a*) and (*b*)).

Treatment
The aims are to slow the ventricular rate and, if possible, to re-establish sinus rhythm.

Digoxin slows conduction of impulses in the Bundle of His so that fewer atrial impulses reach the ventricle. Give the drug in full doses.

If the heart disease is not advanced, electrical direct current counter shock or cardioversion, is a method available in advanced centres.

Heart block

Disordered physiology
The transmission of the electrical impulse from the atrium to the ventricle is delayed or stopped.

First degree
Atrial conduction, and therefore the PR interval of the electrocardiogram, is prolonged. This occurs in all forms of acute carditis and in digoxin overdose.

Second degree
Conduction from atria to ventricles is impaired and leads to intermittent AV block. Two types are recognized; in Mobitz type I block (Wenckebach phenomenon), there is progressive prolongation of the PR interval eventually ending in a blocked atrial impulse. In Mobitz type II block, atrial impulses are regularly blocked from being conducted to the ventricles in a ratio such as 2: 1.

Complete heart block
Atrial beats occur at a rate of 70–80 per minute, while the ventricle beats independently, at a rate of about 40 per minute. There is complete dissociation of atrial and ventricular rhythms. Complete heart block is most often due to degeneration of the conduction system of the heart, or to damage of the AV node in infective endocarditis or cardiac surgery; or it can be congenital.

Diagnosis

Symptoms are caused by inadequate regional perfusion; transient cerebral ischaemia with loss of consciousness, Stokes–Adams attacks, are characteristic of complete heart block.

Signs
There is bradycardia, together with two signs which depend on the timing of the atrial beat. When this is during systole, or in diastole when the tricuspid valve is closed, a cannon wave is produced in the jugular pulse because blood is ejected during atrial contraction back into the jugular vein. When the atrial beat occurs in late diastole, the first heart sound becomes loud, because the cusps of the atrioventricular valves shut briskly. In contrast, the first heart sound is quiet when the atrial beat is elsewhere in the cardiac cycle, a variable first heart sound is, therefore, a characteristic finding in complete heart block.

Treatment

1. The ideal: this is a temporary or permanent pacemaker which gives an artificial electrical impulse to the heart. This is used when the cause of heart block is transient or before a permanent pacemaker can be inserted, which is the definitive long-term treatment of this disorder. In at least ten centres in sub-Saharan countries north of South Africa, pacemakers are being given to patients with symptomatic complete heart block (Mayosi & Millar, 2000). But these devices do not work consistently, and long-term effectiveness cannot be guaranteed.

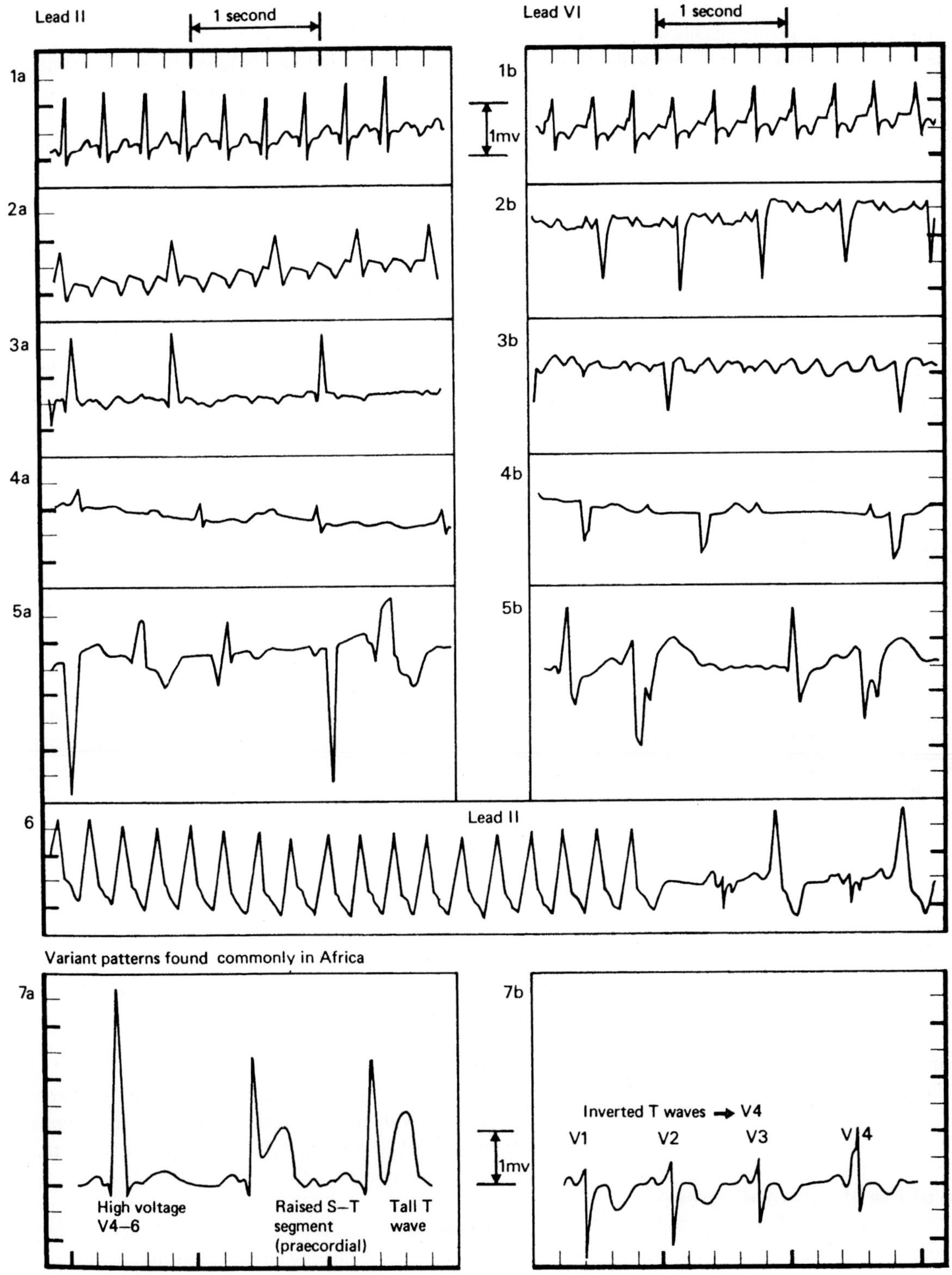

Fig. 76.7. The electrocardiogram (Leads II and VI)

1a and 1b Paroxysmal atrial tachycardia: 2a and 2b Atrial flutter with 2:1 and 3:1 A/V block: 3a and 3b Atrial fibrillation: 4a and 4b Complete heart block: 5a and 5b Coupled beats, due to ventricular ectopic beats: 6and 6b Ventricular tachycardia reverting to coupled ventricular ectopic beats: 7a and 7b African variants.

2.The practicable: often drugs are all that can be given. Give isoprenaline, 10–20 mg sublingually, as often as needed; alternatively, ephedrine, 15–30 mg orally every 2–4 hours, or hydroxyamphetamine, 40–60 mg orally every 2–4 hours. Atropine 1–2 mg every 2–4 hours may also be tried but it is seldom successful.

Prognosis

This depends on the primary disease. In transient/acute carditis, sinus rhythm becomes established when the inflammation subsides, but in older patients, or those with organic heart disease, heart block persists.

Ventricular ectopic beats or extrasystoles

In most patients these do not indicate heart disease: in a patient with established heart disease they probably signify digoxin intoxication or active muscle disease; and in a patient with an acute infection, myocarditis. The patient notices a missed beat which is due to a compensatory pause, because the normal excitation occurs during the refractory period of the ventricle. The ECG shows ectopic beats with bizarre QRS complexes (Fig. 76.7(*a*) and (*b*)). They may be abolished by exercise, or may be produced by exercise in patients with ischaemic heart disease. When an ectopic beat regularly follows a normal sinus beat, there is a pause and a 'coupled beat' rhythm (bigeminy) is produced. The treatment is that of the primary heart disease; in digoxin overdosage, stop the drug and correct a low potassium by oral or possibly intravenous administration.

Ventricular tachycardia

A prolonged run of ventricular ectopic beats is called ventricular tachycardia. Diastole is abruptly shortened so that the cardiac output falls disastrously. Lignocaine, but not the local anaesthetic preparation, is the drug of choice. Give an initial dose as a bolus of 75–100 mg (1–2 mg/kg) intravenously over 1–2 minutes followed by an infusion in isotonic saline thereafter, at a rate of 2–4 mg/min initially dropping after an hour to 1–2 mg/min.

The use of the electrocardiogram

The electrocardiogram (ECG) reflects the spread of electrical depolarization and repolarization of the heart muscle.

Technical details

Paper with 1 mm and 5 mm squares is used, at a standard speed of 25 mm per second, so that each small square (horizontally) represents 0.04 s and each larger square of 5 mm represents 0.2 s. All electrocardiograms are standardized so that 1 mV of electrical force moves the recording stylus vertically 10 mm. Always take a 12-lead ECG.

Interpretation

Arrhythmias

These are discussed above. They are often best analysed from leads II or V_{1-2}.

Left ventricular hypertrophy

A high voltage S wave, in V_1, or V_2, whose deflection when added to the deflection of a high voltage R wave in V_5 or V_6 is 35mm or greater.

Right ventricular hypertrophy

Tall R wave in V_1, with the ratio R: S in V_1 greater than 1.0.

Left atrial enlargement

Broad notched P waves in leads, II, III, and aVF of a duration greater than 2.5 small squares, and biphasic broad P waves in V_1 with broad negative phase.

Right atrial enlargement

Tall, peaked P wave in II, III of a height greater than 2.5 small squares, and large biphasic P in V_1.

Myocarditis

A prolonged PR interval, and QT interval, both corrected for heart rate (QTc), are sometimes accompanied by flat or inverted T waves.

Pericarditis

In some cases of acute pericarditis there is ST segment elevation with upward concavity and PQ interval depression while in chronic pericarditis there is T wave flattening or inversion.

Ischaemia

In chronic myocardial ischaemia there may be variable changes of the ST segments and T waves, but acute myocardial infarction is recognized by changes that include deep Q waves, ST segment elevation with upward convexity (coving) and T wave inversion.

African variants

Electrocardiograms of Africans are similar to those of Caucasians, but four variants from the normal are seen, and have been reported from most African countries. These are shown in Fig. 76.7. Their mechanism is uncertain: the inverted T waves over the right ventricle are sometimes described as persistent infantile pattern.

Echocardiography

This investigation uses ultrasound (U/S) and can give information about semi-solid organs, particularly if they contain fluid or are surrounded by fluid, so that the heart is ideal for this technique. Difficulties can arise, however, from overlying lung or crowding of ribs, because bones and air-containing structures are not suitable for echocardiography.

A good knowledge of the anatomy and pathology of the heart is fundamental, and the user should learn from echocardiographic 'movies and pictures'. The sensitivity of echocardiography depends on the experience of the user, the quality of the medical history and clinical findings, and to a lesser extent on the sophistication of the echo-machine. Even in ideal conditions, echo does not yield a cardiac diagnosis in about 5 per cent of cases, but it is a very useful technique in African practice (Freers et al., 1996).

Technical methods

There are three main methods:

- real time or two-dimensional (2D) echocardiography,
- one-dimensional – time motion or m-mode echocardiography
- doppler echocardiography.

Real time or two-dimensional echocardiography

This 'looks' through intercostal spaces and cuts out a two-dimensional sector-shaped slice of the heart so that heart structures and movements can be seen. A good impression of wall thickness and motion, chamber width and valve structures and movements is obtained from two-dimensional echo (Fig. 76.8).

M-mode echocardiography

One single U/S beam is sent through the heart. All structures traversed are viewed on a time-based axis. Although real-time (2D) echocardiography gives a good general impression of the state and function of the heart, exact

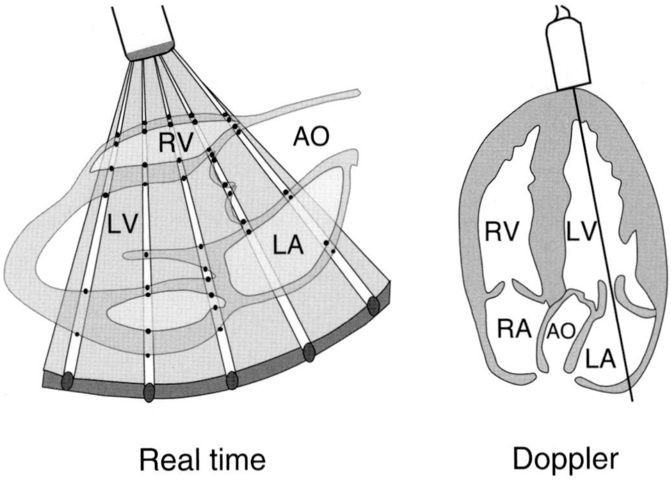

Fig. 76.8. Positions of the transducer in real time and Doppler echocardiography.

measurements of valvular movements, wall thickness and chamber size and their changes in systole and diastole are more accurate in m-mode.

Routine measurements

The **contractility** of the heart is measured as ejection fraction (EF) or as fractional fibre shortening (FS). The formula for cardiac contractility in terms of FS is:

$[(EDD - ESD): EDD] \times 100 = FS\%$
EDD = Left Ventricular End **D**iastolic **D**iameter
ESD = Left Ventricular End **S**ystolic **D**iameter.
Normal range for FS is 25% to 44%. Values below 25% indicate hypo-contractility of the heart and those above 45% signify hyper-contractility.

	range	mean (cm)
Thickness of the Interventricular Septum (IVS)	0.6–1.1	0.9
Thickness of the left ventricular posterior wall (LVPW)	0.6–1.1	0.9
End diastolic diameter (EDD)	3.5–5.7	4.7
Right ventricular diameter (RV)	0.9–2.6	1.76
Diameter of the left atrium (LA)	1.7–4.0	2.77
Diameter of the aortic root (AO)	2.0–3.7	2.7
Aortic cusp separation	1.5–2.6	1.9

Doppler echocardiography

This measures flow phenomena. Here the U/S beam is not reflected by heart structures but by the RBC and WBC of flowing blood. The direction of blood flow can be visualized, in some machines in colour, and the intensity of

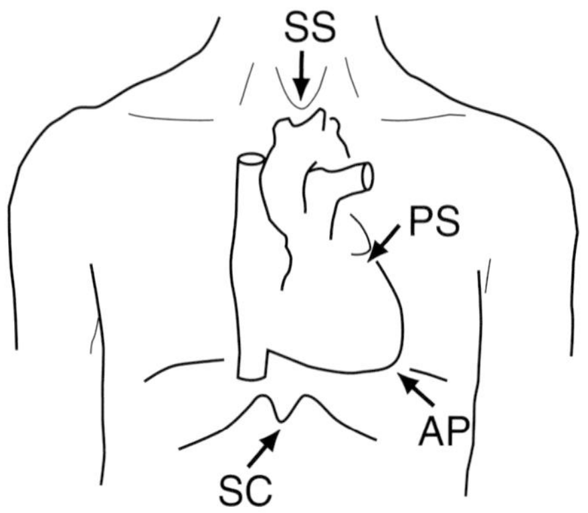

Fig. 76.9. The four standard placements of the echo-probe (transducer) over the heart.

the velocity across the valves can be quantified. Pressure gradients can be estimated.

In m-mode echocardiography most accurate measurements are obtained when the U/S beam meets a structure at an angle of 90° whereas for Doppler echocardiography flow estimations are most accurate when obtained with the U/S beam placed directly in line with the flow (Fig. 76.9).

Positions of the probe

There are four standard placements of the echo-probe (transducer) allowing the following views of the heart:

1. Left parasternal long axis view ('cuts' the heart at length)

1(a) Left parasternal short axis view (this is the same position of the transducer but rotated by 90° and 'cuts' the heart across)

2. Apical view (views from the apex upward and shows all four chambers)
3. Subcostal view (all four chambers are viewed)
4. Suprasternal view (shows the aortic arch) (Fig. 76.9).

If it is difficult to view the heart well because of overlying emphysematous lung, crowding of ribs, thoracic fat or severe kypho-scoliosis, trans-oesophageal echocardiography with a special probe can give an accurate view from behind the heart.

Echocardiographic features of cardiac conditions

Systemic hypertension (HT)

Left ventricular hypertrophy is the most common echo-diagnosis, shown on echo as increased thickness of intraventricular septum (IVS) and left ventricular posterior wall (LVPW). The increased peripheral vascular resistance impedes contractility (FS<25%). Left ventricular dilatation, mitral incompetence (MI) and left atrial dilatation are late consequences of HT and can be verified on echo.

Dilated cardiomyopathy (DCM)

Typical echocardiographic findings are a dilated left ventricle (LVID>56 mm) together with poor contractility (FS <20%, often less than 10%) and the absence of left ventricular hypertrophy (Fig. 76.10(*a*)).

Endomyocardial fibrosis

It has a typical echo-picture (Fig. 76.11).

Other conditions (See pp. 876, 879)

Cardiac failure

Cardiac failure is common in hospital practice. Careful clinical method and simple investigations, ideally with echocardiography, can often identify its cause.

Definition

No single definition is ideal. The clinician must decide on the basis of physical signs whether a patient has cardiac failure: it is a state in which the heart is unable to pump out the blood returned to it from the systemic or pulmonary circulations, and is unable to deliver an adequate amount of oxygenated blood to the tissues.

Disordered physiology

Filling pressure/stroke output relationships

Starling showed that the stroke output of an isolated heart increased as the filling pressure was increased. However, in the failing heart, a filling pressure was reached beyond which the stroke output did not increase further, but rather decreased. Sarnoff, 50 years later, found that, in the intact heart, the stroke output at a known filling pressure could be increased by sympathetic stimulation and digoxin which improved the force of contraction at a given filling pressure. It was therefore assumed that in cardiac failure, the tone (myocardial contractility) of the heart muscle decreases so that, despite an increased filling pressure, the stroke output falls.

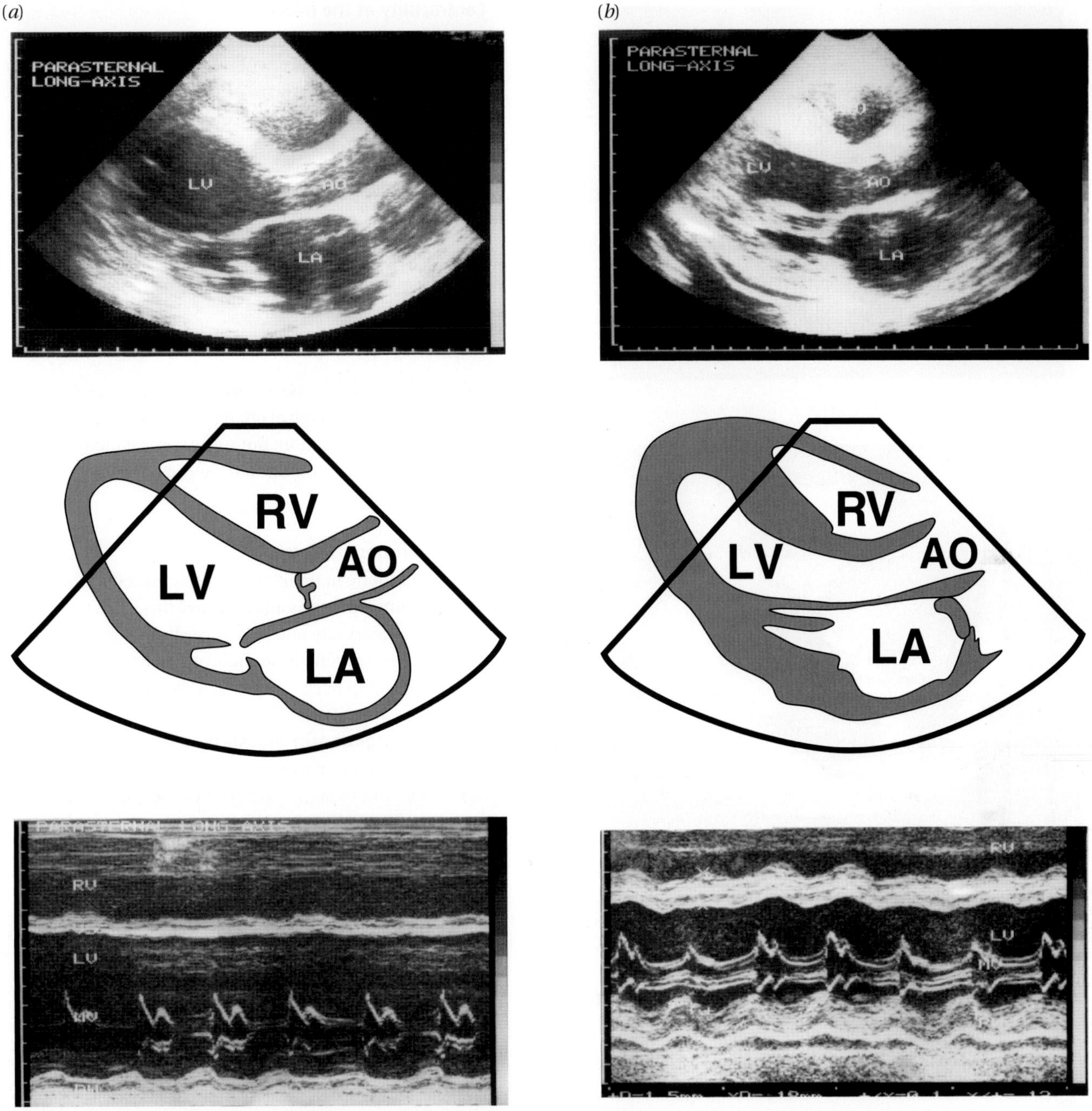

Fig. 76.10. Echocardiography (*a*) The dilated thin-walled left ventricle with reduced contractility in dilated cardiomyopathy. (*b*) The thick-walled concentrically hypertrophied left ventricle with reduced contractility in hypertensive heart disease: contrast the ventricular walls.

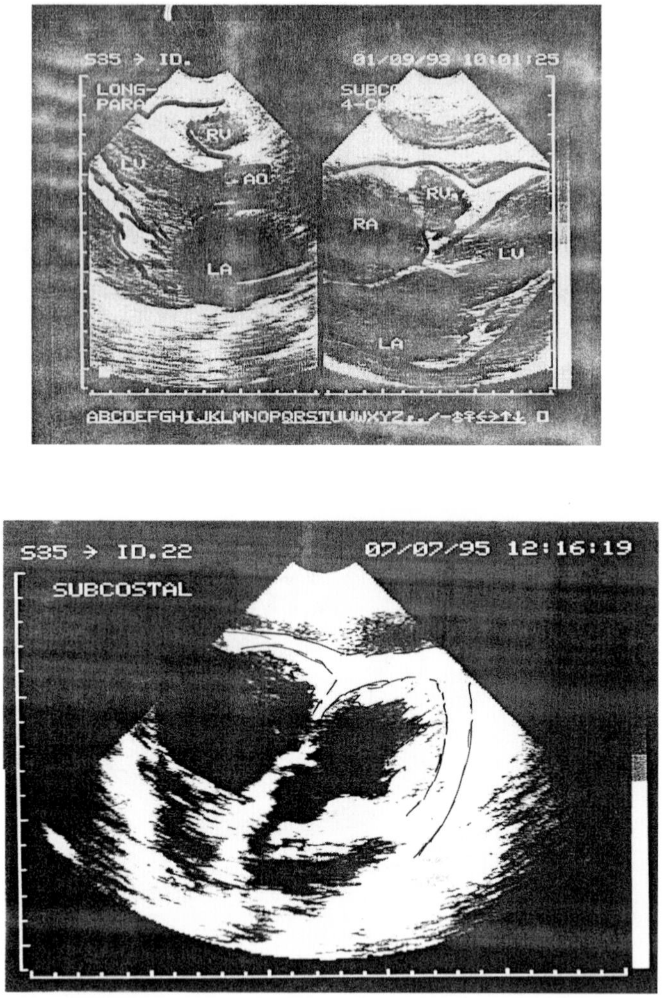

Fig. 76.11. Endomyocardial fibrosis: note the tiny right ventricular and the dilated right atrial cavities in the upper figure and the dense fibrosis at the apices of both ventricles in the lower figure.

Factors affecting cardiac performance and cardiac output

Pre-load

This is the tension on a muscle as it begins to contract. In the intact heart it is the filling pressure or the quantity of blood in the ventricle at the end of diastole (end-diastolic volume).

After-load

This is the resistance against which the heart must pump. Increase in after load or peripheral resistance, whether caused pharmacologically by vasopressor drugs or pathophysiologically by increased angiotensin II secretion in cardiac failure, results in increased contractility.

Contractility of the heart

This describes the ability of the heart to act as a pump. In the hypertrophied heart (without failure), or after $\beta 1$ symphathomimetic agents, cardiac contractility is increased but it is decreased in heart failure, hypoxia, general anaesthesia, or acidosis.

Heart rate

The normal range of heart rate is 60–100 beats per minute: at rates of less than 40 or more than 180 per minute cardiac output drops.

Physiological responses in cardiac failure

If cardiac output is to be restored and maintained, a sequence of physiological changes is necessary to support cardiac function, but these very changes themselves contribute to the cardiac failure becoming more advanced.

Autonomic nervous system

The sympathetic nervous system is activated initially through baroceptor stimulation, and this leads to an increase in heart rate and in myocardial contractility, a positive inotropic effect, so that cardiac work is increased. Vasoconstriction occurs and this increases after load.

The renin–angiotensin–aldosterone system

This is also activated by sustained sympathetic stimulation, leading both to an increased venous tone and thus an increased pre-load, and to an increased arterial tone and after-load.

Angiotensin II leads to an increased secretion of aldosterone, which causes sodium and water to be retained and potassium to be excreted. Pre-load is therefore increased, on account of the inevitable rise in plasma volume, so that cardiac work has to increase further. Ultimately, this retention of sodium and water leads to oedema, because the extracellular fluid volume is significantly increased.

Sustained sympathetic activation, however, leads to venous vasoconstriction, which increases pre-load, and arteriolar vasoconstriction, which increases after-load and still further increases cardiac work. The changes are shown in Fig. 76.12.

Natriuretic peptides

The rise in pre-load raises right atrial pressure and stretches the atrial wall. This leads to the secretion of ANP (atrial natriuretic peptide) which causes sodium to be excreted and vasodilatation. There are two other natriu-

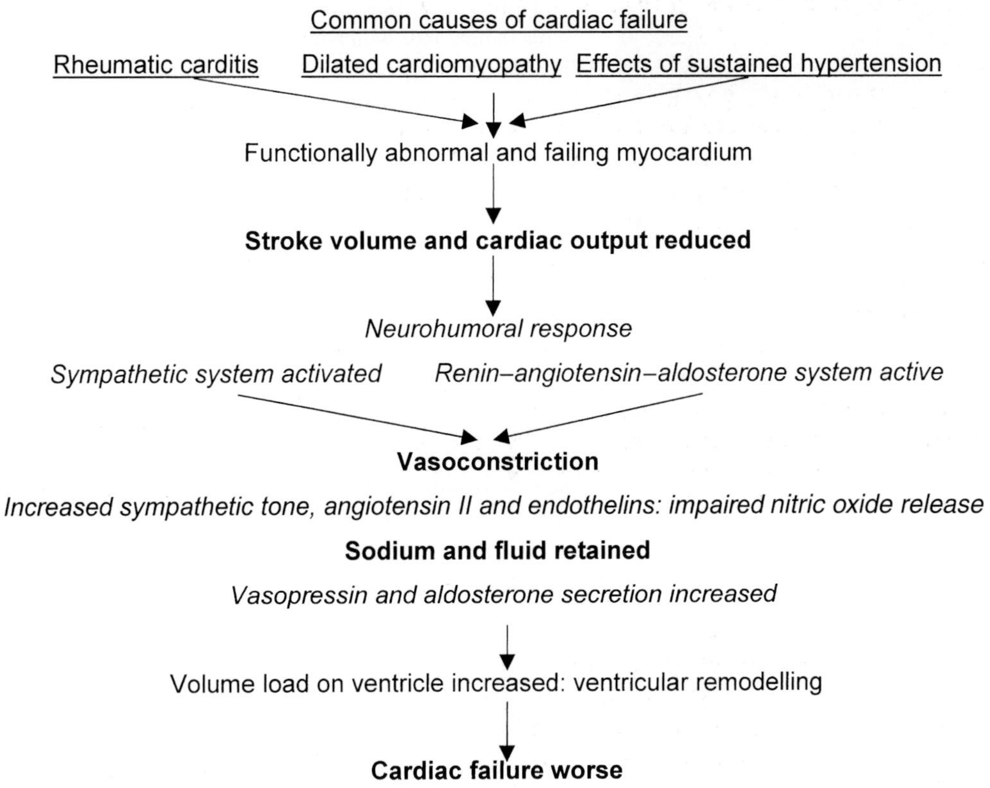

Fig. 76.12. Mechanism of changes in cardiac failure (bold type – physical signs; italic type – mechanisms). (Modified with permission from Jackson et al., 2000.)

retic peptides – brain natriuretic peptide, which has similar effects – and the physiologically much less potent C type natriuretic peptide.

Changes in the myocardium

The increased load on the left ventricle is matched by hypertrophy of its myocytes and also of fibroblasts within the myocardium, which leads to an hypertrophied ventricle, so familiar in the cardiomyopathies of Africa. This remodelling of the myocardium depends on changes in the expression of the genes of the contractile proteins of the myocardium. Increased apoptosis (programmed cell death) and even focal myocardial necrosis also follow sustained sympathetic stimulation.

Changes in the endothelium

Endothelin is a powerful vasoconstrictor and is released by vascular endothelial cells, chiefly in the pulmonary vessels in cardiac failure. Endothelin is also a powerful vasoconstrictor of renal vessels: this activates the renin – angiotensin – aldosterone mechanism, which leads to further sodium and water retention. The normal vasodilatation of vessels is impaired in cardiac failure due to abnormal nitric oxide metabolism.

Changes in skeletal muscle

Chronic cardiac failure leads to reduced skeletal muscle mass and abnormalities in its metabolism and function. The vasoconstriction of cardiac failure is associated with a reduced blood supply to resting and to exercising muscle. These changes are enough to explain the fatigue of patients with cardiac failure.

Changes in nutrition and body mass

The patient with cardiac failure is wasted; severe wasting is called cardiac cachexia and is the result of a reduced muscle mass and:

- malabsorption, particularly in those with a sustainedly high venous pressure in whom a protein-losing enteropathy may also develop
- loss of appetite, often worse in those with hepatic venous congestion

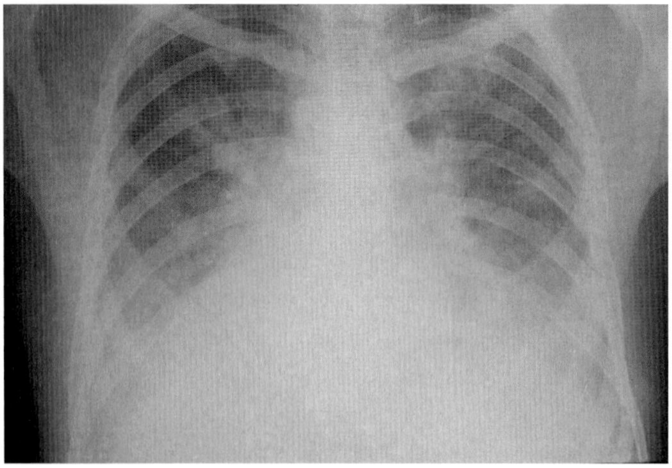

Fig. 76.13. Chest radiograph in pulmonary oedema: note the distended upper lobe veins, the hilar shadowing and the large cardiac shadow.

- the raised basal metabolic rate associated with cardiac failure
- effects of a raised TNF alpha, which has a catabolic effect.

Tissue oxygenation

When stroke output delivers inadequate blood to the tissues, more oxygen must be extracted from arterial blood and this increases the arterio-venous oxygen difference. As the tissues are not adequately perfused, their metabolism changes to anaerobic metabolism, lactic acid accumulates, and a metabolic acidosis develops.

Clinical recognition of cardiac failure

The diagnosis of cardiac failure depends on recognizing a group of symptoms and physical signs, none of which is conclusive in itself. Cardiac failure usually presents with shortness of breath on exertion, orthopnoea, paroxysmal nocturnal dyspnoea, swelling of legs, ascites and easy fatiguability. Two distinct patterns can be distinguished, but in practice these are seldom seen in pure forms.

Systemic venous congestion and oedema

(Predominantly right-sided failure: 'congestive' heart failure). The patient complains of swelling of the legs and abdomen, and is also breathless: there is oedema of legs, and buttocks and sacrum if he is in bed; ascites and a large tender liver, which may be pulsatile; and a raised jugular venous pressure, which may show a prominent systolic wave (tricuspid incompetence).

Pulmonary venous congestion and oedema

(Predominantly left-sided failure). Patients become increasingly breathless even from quite small tasks. They cannot lie down without being very uncomfortable, so they prefer to sit up (Fig. 76.13). At night they can have sudden severe attacks of breathlessness, which wake them up (paroxysmal nocturnal dyspnoea), and force them to sit up or to go out of the house. Their breathing is noisy and often wheezing ('cardiac asthma') and they have an irritating dry cough: later their sputum can be spotted with blood and frothy. They sweat, cannot get comfortable, and think that they are dying. The attack may disappear as quickly as it comes.

Early signs of pulmonary oedema are:
- restlessness,
- a dry cough,
- tachypnoea,
- an inability to lie flat.

Later, widespread crackles may be heard in the chest.

Additional cardiovascular signs

Further evidence is often needed to distinguish cardiac failure from other causes of oedema and breathlessness.

Abnormal heart

It is usual to find clinical or radiological signs of a large heart, or an abnormal valve. Left ventricular disease is shown by signs of abnormal diastolic filling – gallop rhythm, or abnormal systolic work – pulsus alternans (p. 839); the chest radiograph shows enlarged pulmonary veins and shadows due to oedema (Fig. 76.14).

Peripheral vasoconstriction and Inadequate circulation

The signs are also due to inadequate systolic work and sympathetic nervous system stimulation: arterial pulse of small volume and small pulse pressure; cold hands, feet, and nose with constricted veins. Central cyanosis is sometimes seen.

Disordered physiology and clinical picture

Although some symptoms and signs can be explained by disorders of function, the mechanism of others is obscure.

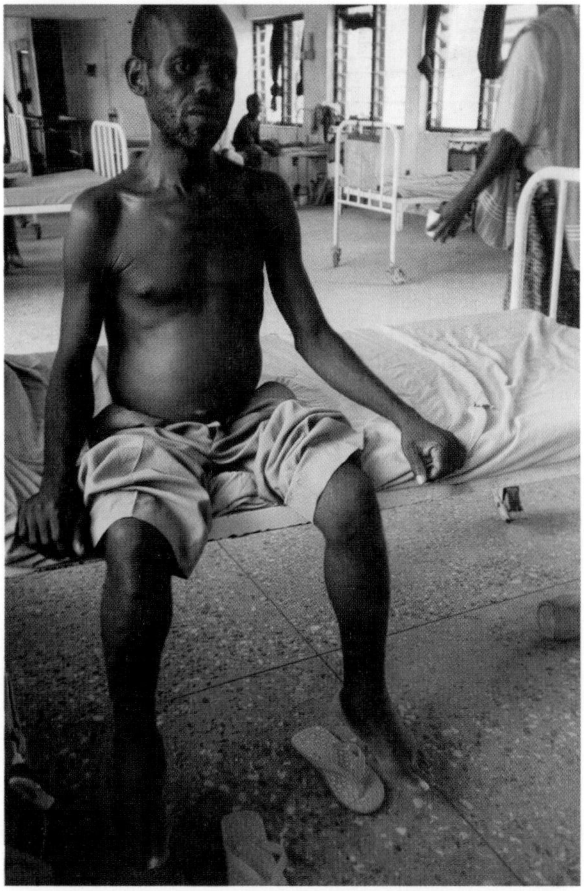

Fig. 76.14. Pulmonary oedema in a patient with dilated cardiomyopathy: the patient was sitting on the edge of his bed, unable to lie flat.

Peripheral oedema and ascites

The extracellular fluid volume, and thus also the plasma volume, is increased, which is probably due to a decreased pressure in the renal artery: stretch receptors elsewhere, e.g. the atria, may also be involved in this response, which causes the kidney to conserve sodium, under the influence of aldosterone and by other mechanisms.

Oedema will form in a patient in cardiac failure if the hydrostatic pressure in the veins exceeds the plasma oncotic pressure and tissue pressure. Oedema thus tends to form in areas with high hydrostatic pressure due to gravity and a low tissue pressure; it is also favoured by a low plasma protein concentration.

Pulmonary oedema

The tissue pressure of the lung is very low and so fluid collects in the alveoli when pulmonary capillary pressure exceeds plasma oncotic pressure. Pulmonary capillary pressure rises with pulmonary venous and left atrial pressures if, owing to obstruction of flow at the mitral valve (mitral stenosis) or failure of the left ventricle, there is a raised filling pressure and incomplete emptying of the left atrium or ventricle.

Raised jugular venous pressure

In cardiac failure a raised jugular venous pressure results from obstruction to emptying of the right atrium secondary to the raised end-diastolic pressure in the right ventricle (the failing ventricle does not empty completely and resists filling because its muscle is stiffer than normal). A raised jugular venous pressure alone is not diagnostic of cardiac failure; it may be seen in hypervolaemia, and in patients with tense ascites as a result of a high intra-abdominal pressure.

A prominent systolic wave is very often seen in Africa in 'congestive cardiac failure' when dilatation of the right ventricle causes malalignment of the papillary muscles of the tricuspid valve and makes it incompetent.

Breathlessness

Breathlessness on exertion

The mechanism is complicated. Neural and humoral stimuli from exercising muscles contribute to the increase in ventilation. Low cardiac output and inefficient distribution of blood flow together with arterial hypoxaemia cause hypoxia in the exercising muscles where acid metabolites such as lactic acid are formed.

Orthopnoea

Pulmonary congestion, due to gravity, in the vessels and interstitial spaces in the dependent parts of the lungs, makes the lungs stiff and difficult to ventilate and narrows or collapses airways.

Paroxysmal nocturnal dyspnoea (p. 837)

Fluid is mobilized from the legs, venous return increases and central blood volume rises. This increased fluid load (pre-load) leads to left ventricular decompensation and acute pulmonary venous congestion. Relief from standing up is due to the fall of central blood volume and the reduction in pre-load to the failing left ventricle.

Hypoxaemia

In cardiac failure, areas of lung, which are relatively well perfused with blood, are underventilated. The gas exchanging parts of the lung may be choked with oedema fluid, airways may be blocked by fluid or collapsed, and areas of lung may be so stiffened by congestion of vessels and interstitial spaces that they are difficult to inflate. The respiratory muscles may become fatigued because they have a poor blood supply: the work of breathing is increased by the increasing rigidity of congested lungs.

Cheyne–Stokes respiration

This is periodic breathing in which progressive hyperventilation is followed by apnoea. Ventilation then builds up again and the cycle is repeated at regular intervals. The greatly prolonged circulation time in severe cardiac failure causes the respiratory centre to be out of phase with the lungs. Patients are often restless or overactive during the ventilatory phase, while they are very quiet indeed during the apnoeic phase.

Posture in cardiac failure

When an individual lies down, the cardiac output increases by about 20 per cent because the venous return and central blood volume increase. In cardiac failure this may so increase venous return (pre-load) that the heart is unable to pump out the returned blood and pulmonary oedema follows.

- Keep patients with left ventricular failure in the most physiologically beneficial position, sitting up, well supported, and with legs down. Beds are less physiologically friendly than armchairs!

Some patients cannot lie down because tense ascites pushes the diaphragm upward.

Diagnosis of cardiac failure

Approach the diagnosis by defining:

- the functional disorder; for example pulmonary venous congestion and oedema, due to left ventricular failure
- the anatomical disorder; for example, left ventricular hypertrophy and mitral incompetence
- the aetiology of the anatomical disorder; for example rheumatic heart disease.

A diagnosis of cardiac failure cannot be made until the heart is found to be abnormal, and there is pulmonary or systemic venous congestion. The common problems are:

(a) unexplained oedema or breathlessness
(b) unexplained cardiac failure in someone known to have cardiac disease.

Problems in diagnosis – has this patient got cardiac failure?

Physical signs of an abnormal heart are usually obvious except in cardiac constriction (chronic constrictive pericarditis or EMF), cardiac compression (acute pericardial effusion), and rarely in patients with severe mitral stenosis.

Systemic venous congestion

In patients with systemic venous congestion, the triad of oedema, ascites and a large tender liver may mimic liver disease. Look for an abnormal heart, and a high venous pressure.

Oedema

Other possible causes are:

- hypoalbuminaemia: look also for silken hair and patchy depigmentation.
- nephrotic syndrome: look for heavy proteinuria; the heart is normal.

Tender liver

The congested liver may be mistaken for a liver abscess, unless the jugular veins are carefully examined. A very high jugular venous pressure is often missed unless the area round the lobe of the ear is examined with a patient sitting or standing up. This is an essential sign in cardiac constriction, or compression due, for example, to tamponade in tuberculous pericardial effusion.

Children with cardiac failure may be thought to have liver disease because a tender liver obscures other signs; the tachycardia of acute rheumatic carditis may be thought to be due to an infection.

Pulmonary venous congestion

Acute breathlessness

The problem is usually one of acute breathlessness.

- Fever and tachypnoea, in someone previously well, are often due to an acute pneumonia: signs of consolidation are not found in the first few days.
- *Pnuemocystis carinii* pneumonia, in patients with immunosuppression due to HIV infection, pulmonary Kaposi's sarcoma, or diffuse pulmonary tuberculosis, may give physical signs like pulmonary congestion, so look for other HIV/AIDS related signs.
- Breathlessness and wheezing, due to bronchial asthma may be a difficult problem: the diagnosis is suspected in the patient who has no other signs or symptoms of cardiac failure, but who has had previous attacks of

breathlessness with wheeze, cough, and mucoid sputum – and who has some residual cough between attacks, which are often worse at certain seasons of the year. Early morning exacerbation of asthma may be mistaken for paroxysmal nocturnal dyspnoea. Physical signs of a grossly over-inflated chest may be found during an asthmatic attack.
- Cor pulmonale associated with chronic airways obstruction with respiratory failure may present in acute cardiac failure. A long history of respiratory symptoms, and signs of chronic airways obstruction with thoracic distortion, are helpful.
- Acute lobar pneumonia sometimes presents as pulmonary oedema.

Other causes of pulmonary oedema include head injury or cerebrovascular accident, acute viral encephalitis, malaria and uraemia.

Management of cardiac failure

Inpatient or outpatient treatment

Systemic oedema and even pulmonary oedema can be treated in the outpatient clinic; when beds are few, admission is necessary if the patient has:

(a) travelled far and has nowhere to stay near the hospital
(b) severe symptoms of breathlessness and cough
(c) any complication of cardiac failure
(d) a disease which demands hospital care, e.g. infective endocarditis.

Principles of treatment

Treatment is designed to:
- reduce the expanded ECF volume (blood and interstitial fluid volumes) and induce a sodium diuresis – by diuretics
- reduce the work of the heart, by after-load and pre-load reduction, by angiotensin-converting enzyme inhibitors and vasodilators
- increase the tone of the cardiac muscle – by digoxin
- correct neurohumoral disturbances with angiotensin-converting enzyme inhibitors and beta-blockers
- correct the underlying cause of cardiac failure, if possible
- eliminate any associated diseases.

Diuretics

Diuretics are used to promote a large flow of urine and thus reduce the expanded plasma and interstitial fluid volume. Powerful oral diuretics may cause potassium and sodium depletion and hypovolaemia.

Thiazide diuretics

These are absorbed rapidly from the gut. They act primarily on the distal renal tubules to increase urinary excretion of sodium, potassium, chloride, and water. Those in common use are, bendrofluazide (5–10 mg orally), chlorothiazide (500 mg –1.5 g orally) and hydrochlorothiazide (25–50 mg orally). Their side effects include hypokalaemia (a potassium supplement may be needed), hyperuricaemia, hyperglycaemia, glycosuria and thrombocytopenia.

Frusemide and other loop diuretics

These are very potent, and may be used orally (onset of action 30 minutes), or intravenously (within minutes) when they can be life-saving. They prevent sodium reabsorption in the ascending limb of the loop of Henle, increase the excretion of potassium and hydrogen ion, and remain effective in renal failure. The initial dose of frusemide is 40–80 mg orally or i.v.; this dose may be increased to 200 mg.

Side effects include hypokalaemia, hypovolaemia, hyperuricaemia, hyperglycaemia, agranulocytosis, and acute hearing loss.

Spironolactone and other postassium-sparing diuretics

Spironolactone has been shown to improve survival in heart failure, when given in doses of 25–50 mg once a day. Other potassium-sparing diuretics, such as amiloride (5–10 mg once a day) and triamterene (50–100 mg twice a day), are often used as adjuncts to the more potent loop diuretics to augment their action. However, in mild to moderate heart failure a combination of hydrochlorothiazide and amiloride may achieve an adequate diuresis. Do not give potassium supplements when using postassium-sparing diuretics, even when thiazides or loop diuretics are concurrently used, because dangerous hyperkalaemia can progressively develop.

Potassium in food

Patients who take diuretics for a long time may lose a lot of potassium in the urine. Those who have renal failure have high plasma levels of K^+ and may be in danger if they ingest excess potassium. Potassium salts are unpleasant and few patients are likely to take them regularly: tropical fruits are an excellent source of available potassium and particularly the banana (Table 76.1).

Table 76.1. Sodium and potassium and caloric values of tropical fruits

	Per 100 g edible portion		
Item	Kilocalories	Sodium (mmol)	Potassium (mmol)
Avacado pear	162	0	7.2
Banana – green, raw	104	0.5	9.7
– green, boiled	104	0.5	4.4
– green, ripe, raw	100	0.5	10.0
Coconut – grated	314	0.8	6.1
– milk	354	0.7	6.5
– water		0.7[a]	4.0[a]
Lime juice – fresh	21	0.01[a]	3.0[a]
Mango – raw	70	0	6.2
Orange	40	0.1	3.0
Paw paw (papaya)	39	0.5	4.3
Pineapple	50	0.5	4.0
Tangerine	43	0.1	4.8
Tomato	15	0.1	6.6

Notes:
[a] Na^+, K^+ concentrations in mmol/100 ml.
Source: From Delapenha & Alleyne (1980).

ACE inhibitors

Captopril, enalapril and other angiotension converting enzyme inhibitors

The ACE inhibitors have been shown to improve survival in heart failure and hence they have become very common in the treatment of heart failure in industrialized countries.

Many patients in Africa are now on ACE inhibitors but cost has prevented their widespread use. Captopril (12.5–25 mg three times a day or 25–50 mg twice a day) has been the earliest ACE inhibitor used for heart failure, but others such as enalapril (5–20 mg once a day) and lisinopril (5–20 mg once a day) are in common use.

The side effects of ACE inhibitors include a persistent cough, metallic taste in the mouth, hyperkalaemia, rash and angioneurotic oedema. These agents must be started with a small dose, such as captopril 6.25 mg or enalapril 2.5 mg because the first dose may cause profound hypotension especially in individuals who have been receiving heavy doses of diuretics.

Digoxin

Digoxin has somewhat lost its position as the most important drug in the treatment of heart failure. But after several years of debate when some people avoided it while others considered it an important drug, most people now accept that digoxin has a place in the treatment of heart failure. It is cheap and is widely available, while other more expensive drugs may well be too costly or unavailable. If heart failure has failed to respond to diuretics alone or in addition to ACE inhibitors, digoxin may rapidly improve symptoms.

Digoxin is also useful in heart failure associated with tachycardia, especially atrial fibrillation, because of its control of ventricular rate. Digoxin is often given orally, when it acts in 1–2 hours. For rapid digitalization 0.5–0.75 mg is given followed by 0.25–0.5 mg every 6–8 hours until a total loading dose of 1–1.25 mg (adults) has been given. More often a dose of 0.25 mg once a day is given without the loading dose. Urgent digitalization is needed in acute pulmonary oedema and atrial fibrillation with a rapid ventricular rate and decompensation.

Digoxin toxicity can be a serious complication, especially in the elderly and in those with renal failure. Apart from poor appetite, nausea and vomiting, serious arrhythmias such as severe bradycardia, supra-ventricular tachycardia and AV block may occur. When these toxic effects are noted, stop digoxin and measure electrolytes, urea and creatinine. Potassium may be given by mouth.

Vasodilators

Vasodilators act on systemic arteries and veins to cause dilatation. A combination of isosorbide dinitrate (10–20 mg three times a day) and hydralazine (25–50 mg two to three times a day) can be used in place of angiotensin converting inhibitors if these are not available.

Prazocin 0.5–5 mg three times a day is another alternative vasodilator treatment.

Beta-blockers

Whilst beta-blockers were previously contraindicated in patients with heart failure, we have gone full circle and now recommend beta-blockers as treatment for heart failure. Most of the research work that has been done with beta-blockers has used agents like metoprolol and more recently carvedilol which are not easily available in most African hospitals and clinics. However, some people have used propranolol, which is more commonly available, for the management of heart failure. Start cautiously with a small dose, for example 5–10 mg, and watch its effect before escalating the dose to more conventional levels, such as 40 mg three times a day. Some patients have got much better when beta-blockers have been added to their treatment for heart failure.

Dobutamine increases cardiac contractility and cardiac output and decreases total peripheral resistance when used in appropriate doses. It may be useful when heart failure is severe and intractable, especially in an intensive care unit, but it is not recommended for long-term use.

Low sodium diet

As sodium is retained in cardiac failure by the action of aldosterone on the distal renal tubule, it is rational to reduce sodium in the diet. In Africa it is seldom practicable to insist on diet which has only 22 mmol sodium: instead, advise your patients to take their food without salt, whether added to the cooking pot or to the plate.

Reducing the work of the heart

Rest, whether in hospital, or at home, reduces cardiac work. For children it may be difficult to ensure adequate rest. Anxiety, particularly in pulmonary oedema, prevents rest, both by the physical activity of restlessness and also by the adrenergic drive.

Morphine is an excellent sedative in pulmonary oedema in a dose of 10–15 mg i.m. or i.v. It also relieves pulmonary congestion by pooling blood due to venodilatation (see Box).

Treatment apparently ineffective

Problems in treatment

- Has the patient received the prescribed drugs, and in the correct dose?
- Have diuretics caused hypokalaemia or hyponatraemia, so that they are no longer effective?
- Is the patient eating salt-rich foods (at home) or brought to hospital by his family?

Problems in diagnosis

- Is the original cardiac diagnosis correct?
- Is there atrial fibrillation with an uncontrolled ventricular rate or some other arrhythmia or heart block?
- Is there infective endocarditis or active rheumatic carditis?

Associated problems

- Consider infections, e.g. acute pneumonia, urinary tract infections or tuberculosis, pregnancy, anaemia, hypoproteinaemia, venous thromboembolism (deep venous thrombosis and pulmonary embolism).

Causes of cardiac failure

In Africa acquired heart disease is by far the most important. In children and younger adults, rheumatic carditis is the major cause. Later, hypertensive heart disease and cardiomyopathy are dominant. The various groups of causes are shown in Table 76.2.

Rheumatic fever (RF) and rheumatic heart disease (RHD)

These are diseases of poverty. The incidence of RF and the prevalence of RHD have been falling consistently in the industrialized countries since the mid nineteenth century, independently of the advent of penicillin: sadly, RF and RHD are still highly prevalent in Africa (Fig. 76.15).

The problem in Africa and risk factors

Prevalence

RHD is by far the most important form of acquired heart disease in Africa, and accounts for over a quarter of all patients with cardiac failure in many countries. It is an uncontrolled killer of children and young adults. In Kampala, the disease is about four or five times less common among the immigrant Rwanda than among the indigenous Baganda (Mayanja-Kizza et al., 2000).

Geography

It is more common in the dry savannah grasslands and highlands (Oyoo et al., 1999), than in the rainforest, probably because *Streptococcus pyogenes* is carried easily in dry air and because the poor are crowded together during the colder seasons.

Age and sex

The disease in Africa causes established valvular disease in children as young as 6 years. As the prevalence is highest in the 10–19-year-olds, it is about three times higher in secondary than in primary school children. At least 10 per cent of patients are less than 10 years old and females are affected more often than males (Chauvet et al., 1989). (Note: estimates of prevalence through surveys of schoolchildren underestimate the prevalence in poor children, who will be absent from school if they are ill, or if they have to look after their younger siblings at home.)

Poverty

The social gradient is well illustrated in Khartoum (Ibrahim-Khalil et al., 1992) and Kinshasa (Longo-Mbenza

Table 76.2. Causes of heart failure, common or increasing in Africa

I. Congenital heart disease
II. Acquired heart disease
  A. Physiological causes: for example arrhythmias, typically in an already abnormal heart.
  B. Anatomical causes

Intrinsic causes – left or right side
Endocardial disease
1. Valvular endocardium
   Acute: – rheumatic fever, infective endocarditis
   Chronic: rheumatic valvular disease, prolapsed mitral valve
2. Mural endocardium: endomyocardial fibrosis

Myocardial disease
1. Acute: infective: rheumatic carditis, typhoid, relapsing fever, septic myocarditis, diphtheria, Coxsackie B infection, HIV
2. Chronic: dilated cardiomyopathy, ischaemic heart disease: toxins, for example, alcohol

Pericardial disease
1. Acute: infective pericarditis with or without effusion, rheumatic fever
2. Chronic: constrictive pericarditis

Extrinsic causes – increased pre-load or after-load
1. Increased peripheral vascular resistance: hypertension
2. Increased pulmonary vascular resistance: cor pulmonale from destructive hypoxic lung disease, schistosomal pulmonary arteriolitis
3. Conditions causing volume overload: renal disease
4. Conditions causing high cardiac output: anaemia, beri-beri, thyrotoxicosis

Notes:
1. Physiological causes operate synergistically with anatomical causes in some disorders: thus:
   (a) Cor pulmonale: pulmonary vasoconstriction-a physiological response to hypoxia, and occlusion of pulmonary vessels (anatomical) in areas of diseased lung.
   (b) Arrhythmias develop in abnormal hearts and can thus precipitate heart failure in subjects whose hearts can cope perfectly well provided atrial filling or ventricular rate are normal.
2. Not every disease is given under the headings shown above but only those which are important in Africa or which are classic examples, for example, diphtheria.
3. Ischaemic heart disease: the myocardial damage may be local (acute infarct) or diffuse (ischaemic fibrosis) and may therefore provoke acute cardiac failure or, as is more usual, chronic failure.

Extrinsic causes
3. The hypervolaemic state of acute glomerulonephritis and of some cases of peripartum cardiac failure causes pulmonary and systemic venous congestion, which resembles cardiac failure but in which the heart can increase its output in response to an increased filling pressure.
4. Beri-beri is uncommon: occasional series are reported (Bouramone & Ekoba, 1975).

et al., 1998) where the prevalence was only 4 in children in the best city schools, but it was 22.2 in children who lived in slums. The poorest people have:
- overcrowded housing
- larger families so that there is often less food for each child
- less access to health care
- less money for treatment.

Prevention and case-finding

Primary prevention against a first attack of rheumatic fever aims to eradicate rheumatogenic streptococci: secondary prevention is designed to prevent re-infection with these organisms and thus a recurrence of rheumatic fever, both in known cases of RHD and in children with undetected RHD. Nurses can be trained and can dramatically improve case detection among schoolchildren (Oli & Porteous, 1999). Other methods of case-finding are very costly.

Recurrences

Carditis is very common in second and subsequent attacks and can lead to death and irreversible cardiac damage (see the Box).

Recurrences – risk factors
- younger age
- poverty
- presence and severity of heart disease
- short interval since last attack
- number of previous attacks
- prevalence of RF in the community.

Primary

Primary prevention depends on economic advance and on the health service:
- social: when will the poor be released from poverty?
- microbiological: eradication of rheumatogenic strains of Group A streptococci.

This demands adequate primary care and resources to train staff to distinguish streptococcal from viral sore throat, which is commonly associated with conjunctivitis and rhinitis which are not features of a streptococcal throat. Similarly, a viral throat does not have a white tonsillar exudate and tender lymphadenopathy.

In a closed community, in which *Strep. pyogenes* infection spreads quickly and causes cases of rheumatic fever, transmission can be stopped by one dose of benzathine penicillin G, 1.2 mega units, to everyone (see the Box).

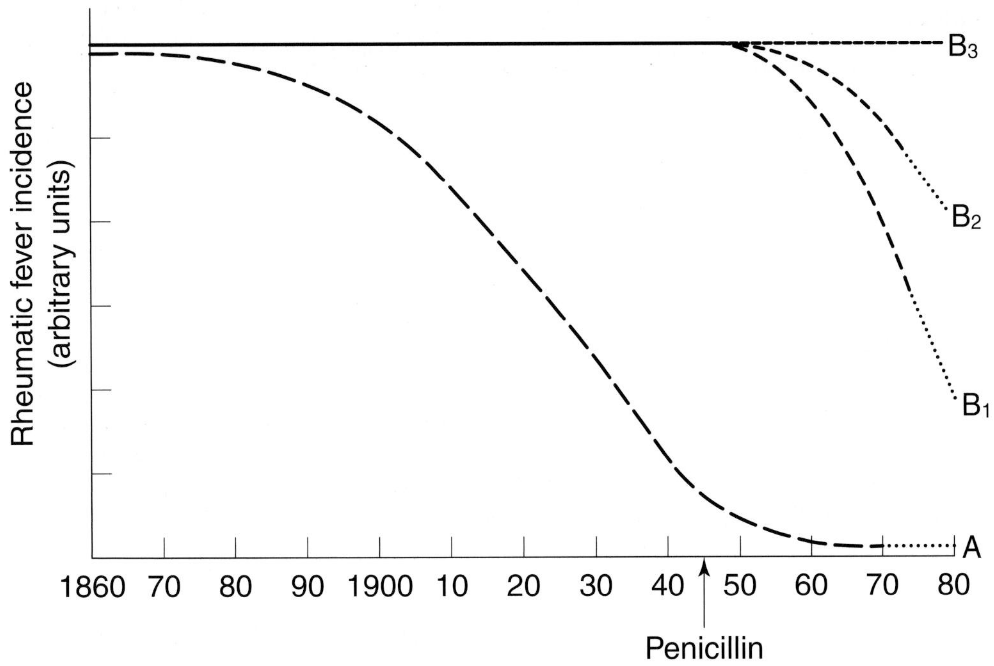

Fig. 76.15. Rheumatic fever: changed and unchanging. Curve A is typical of industrialized countries: curves B1 and B2 represent the changed pattern in some developing countries, while the unchanged B3 represents the pattern in many African countries. (From Strasser, 1978.)

> **Primary prevention**
>
> *Example: Costa Rica (Arguedas & Mohs, 1992).*
>
> Decision: to treat all cases of Group A Streptococcal sore throat with a single dose of benzathine penicillin –
> under age 3 years, 300 000u;
> age 3–5 years, 500 000u;
> over 5 years,1200 000u.
>
> Result: dramatic fall in cases of rheumatic fever
>
> Diagnosis: *symptoms,* sore throat or fever:
> *signs,* halitosis, redness of pharynx, hypertrophy of tonsils, white exudate
> (we would add tender cervical lymphadenopathy).

Secondary prevention

This can only succeed if there is effective primary health care:

- trained health centre and district hospital staff: ideally, close to the patient's home
- effective records, follow-up and a system for finding those who do not return
- community nurses and reliable simple transport (Edginton & Gear, 1982)
- a dedicated and interested health team
- a supply of benzathine penicillin or sulphadiazine
- a policy of exemption from fees for chronic illness in children and adults.

Give benzathine penicillin 1.2 mega units every 3 or 4 weeks, or sulphadiazine 0.5 mg twice daily, to those aged 10 and over, and once daily to those under 10. The age at which prophylaxis can be discontinued depends on the severity of disease and the number of years since the last attack, but assess also the risk factors in your area before you decide about any individual patient (Berrios et al., 1993).

The streptococcus and pathogenesis

After infection of the throat with *Streptococcus pyogenes,* Lancefield group A, of a distinctive rheumatogenic M-protein serotype, the host has an autoimmune response to epitopes in the bacterium that are immunologically cross-reactive with host tissues in synovium, heart, brain and skin (Stollerman, 1997). In severe cases there is fibrinoid necrosis in connective tissue and in the heart, where muscle, valves, and pericardium are affected. This is rheumatic fever: it may lead to established rheumatic heart disease.

Sore throat and streptococci

Twenty per cent of cases of symptomatic sore throat are due to Group A streptococci, but 80 per cent of all cases of Group A streptococcal infections are not symptomatic. Of the 20 symptomatic cases, two may develop RF. Of the asymptomatic cases, one may develop RF, except in an outbreak when the numbers double. Transmission of a rheumatogenic strain is much more likely from a recent carrier than from a chronic carrier.

Morbid anatomy

The typical lesions in the myocardium are Aschoff bodies: platelet thrombi form along the lines of closure of the valve cusps, which become fibrosed and tethered, rigid (incompetent), and stenotic. In South Africa, by contrast, severe mitral incompetence is associated with pliable and unscarred valve leaflets, a dilated mitral annulus, elongated chordae tendineae and anterior leaflet prolapse, and with active carditis (Marcus et al., 1994).

Secondary changes include atrial thrombi, which can cause peripheral emboli, ventricular dilatation and hypertrophy, and atrial fibrillation.

Echocardiography

Two-dimensional echo is ideal in demonstrating ragged, distorted, thickened or calcified valves. Mitral and aortic valves are most commonly affected.

Mitral stenosis (MS)

This has a rather typical echo appearance in two-dimensional and m-mode. The posterior mitral leaflet is usually tethered to the left ventricular posterior wall and is often virtually immobile. The anterior mitral leaflet 'domes' into the left ventricle in atrial systole when blood is pressed by a forceful prolonged atrial contraction through the narrow mitral orifice.

The size of the mitral opening can be measured in two-dimensional left parasternal short axis view: normal mitral valve opening is 4–6 cm^2, it is critical when below 1 cm^2. In pure MS the left atrium is dilated and the left ventricle is small with normal contractility.

Left atrial clots

They are often present and visualized. In the left parasternal long axis m-mode the typical M-shaped mirror like mitral valve image is lost since there is no mid-diastolic pressure equilibrium between left atrium and ventricle. Both mitral leaflets (PML and AML) are partially attached to each other and they move in parallel.

Table 76.3. Duckett Jones criteria, modified 1992, for diagnosis of an initial attack of rheumatic fever (two major criteria, or one major and two minor, *with* evidence of preceding streptococcal infection)

Major		Minor
Carditis	*Clinical*	Arthralgia
Polyarthritis		Fever
Chorea	*Laboratory*	Elevated acute phase reactants
Much less common		ESR
Erythema marginatum		C-reactive protein
Subcutaneous nodules		Prolonged PR interval
Supporting evidence of antecedent Group A streptococcal infection		
Positive throat culture or rapid streptococcal antigen test		
Raised or rising streptococcal antibody titre		

Notes:
These criteria are not easily applied in Africa, where clinical patterns are different, patients present late and laboratory facilities are generally less available, than in a temperate country.
Source: From Recommendations of American Heart Association. *J. Am Med. Assoc.* (1992).

Mitral regurgitation with incompetent valve

This is more of a flow phenomenon than a structural change and it is better demonstrated by Doppler.

Aortic regurgitation with incompetent valve

This flow phenomenon can be quantified by Doppler.

Clinical course

Rheumatic fever

A typical patient has a sore throat and about 2–3 weeks later develops fever, and pain (arthralgia) or painful swelling (arthritis) of the larger joints, which moves from joint to joint. Among patients in Africa there is no typical picture in rheumatic fever, so that the revised modified Jones criteria are of only limited value (Table 76.3).

Acute carditis

Pancarditis, which affects pericardium, myocardium, and endocardium follows arthritis.The clinical features are:

- Tachycardia. Throughout, and sometimes the only manifestation of acute carditis, the child or adolescent has an unexplained and persistent tachycardia, which is disproportionate to the degree of fever.
- Changing heart murmurs: mitral systolic and diastolic

murmurs may come and go: sophisticated analysis of serial echocardiograms may also reveal changing patterns at the mitral valve.
- Pericardial friction rub, if there is acute rheumatic pericarditis.
- Signs of cardiac failure, evidence of heart muscle damage.

Diagnosis
The episode of rheumatic fever may be so mild that it is forgotten: only 25 per cent of patients with established valve disease give a history of an attack of rheumatic fever. Doppler echocardiography may reveal subclinical lesions at the aortic and mitral valves, which are not heard on auscultation. These lesions are not necessarily benign and may still be detected years after the acute episode of RF (Figueroa et al., 2001).

Established valvular disease
Combined mitral valvular stenosis and incompetence is the most common lesion, next is mitral incompetence, and third is pure mitral stenosis, frequent in Senegal and Khartoum (Fig. 76.16). Aortic incompetence and mitral disease is seen in about 10–15 per cent of patients but pure rheumatic aortic incompetence is seen in less than 5 per cent (Serme, 1992).

Pulmonary hypertension, possibly a result of much walking and activity, inevitable for poor people, develops early and is usual in patients with mitral valve disease.

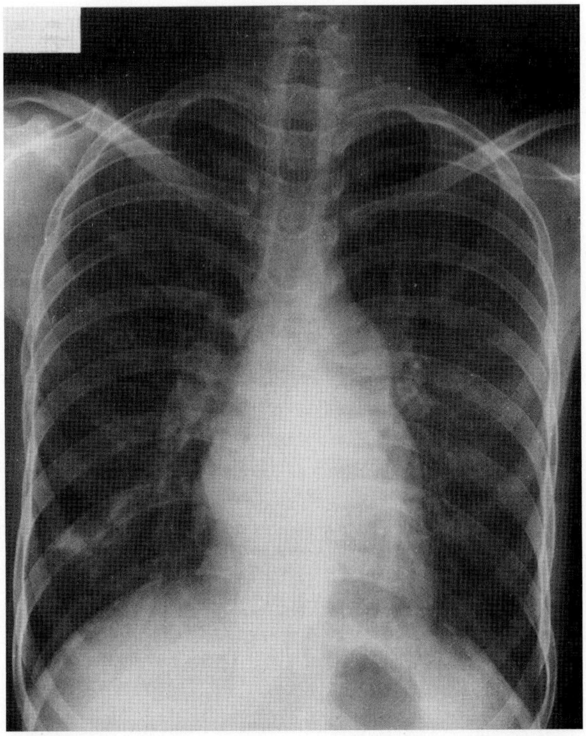

Fig. 76.16. Mitral stenosis and pulmonary hypertension: note the large pulmonary artery and the distinct left atrial shadow.

Prognosis

The prognosis is governed by the anatomical damage to the valve, the rhythm of the heart, the severity of pulmonary hypertension, rheumatic activity in a recurrence, and the major complications – systemic emboli and infective endocarditis.

Diagnosis

Any patient who has valvular disease with mitral stenosis, alone or with some mitral incompetence, or who has mitral and aortic lesions, can be confidently diagnosed as having rheumatic heart disease. Most patients present with cardiac failure; atrial fibrillation is less common in Africa than in industrialized countries probably because many patients are young; systemic emboli or infective endocarditis are major complications.

The diagnosis in those with mitral incompetence alone can be difficult as some patients with EMF or dilated cardiomyopathy may have similar signs: if echocardiography is available, the diagnosis can be quickly established.

Treatment

Rheumatic fever
Rest in bed; aspirin in a dose of 1–1.5 g 4-hourly till joint pains and fever are suppressed; and benzylpenicillin, 250 000 units four times daily or penicillin V 125 mg four times daily, for 7–10 days; followed by long-term prophylaxis. Prednisone, not aspirin, can be used if severe cardiac failure complicates carditis: the initial dose is 10–15 mg four times daily (Barlow et al., 1990).

Chronic rheumatic heart disease
1. Prevent acute streptococcal infection.
2. Manage cardiac failure.
3. Control ventricular rate in atrial fibrillation with digoxin, up to 0.25 mg daily.
4. Relieve mitral stenosis surgically – if pure valvular lesion.
5. Prevent infective endocarditis: early treatment of pelvic infection, and antibiotic prophylaxis for dental care, childbirth or genito-urinary manipulation.

- *Dental procedure:* Benzylpenicillin 2 mega units, plus procaine penicillin 600 000 units, 30 minutes before the procedure, followed by procaine penicillin 600 000 units on the following day; or amoxycillin 3 g orally, 60 minutes before the procedure.
- *Delivery:* When labour begins, give amoxycillin 3 g followed by 500 mg 8-hourly for 2 days: ampicillin is less effective as *Strep. faecalis* is the organism of risk.
- *Genito-urinary manipulations:* Give amoxycillin 3 g before, and proceed as above.

The future

RF and RHD will begin to decline in Africa only when:

- overcrowded housing, limited access to health care, inadequate education and the persistent inability to pay health care charges, have been changed, so that the poor have a better chance;
- an efficient primary health care system is established, so that secondary prophylaxis is successfully given;
- adequate resources for health care are released.

Cardiomyopathy

Definition

Aetiological

Cardiomyopathy (CM): this is defined as myocardial disease of uncertain cause, when all known causes of cardiac failure have been excluded. Thus, for example, the presence of hypertension or of mitral valvular disease exclude a diagnosis of cardiomyopathy.

Physiological and anatomical

There are three distinct types of cardiomyopathy:

1. Dilated or congestive cardiomyopathy (DCM). This is the type commonly seen in Africa. The left ventricle is dilated and hypofunctional and may contain an intraventricular thrombus which may lead to peripheral emboli (Kingue et al., 1999).
2. Hypertrophic cardiomyopathy. This group of disorders is rare in Africa. The dominant abnormality is asymmetrical and abnormal hypertrophy of the left ventricle; hypertrophic obstructive cardiomyopathy (HOCM, pronounced *hokum*) is the most studied condition.
3. Restrictive cardiomyopathy. In this group the dominant physiological defect is restricted diastolic filling of the ventricles, which become abnormally stiff, so that their compliance is reduced, and stroke volume is fixed and limited. Very rare in Africa, its causes include amyloidosis, haemochromatosis, sarcoidosis, and neoplastic infiltration.

Although there is a significant restrictive defect in endomyocardial fibrosis, atrioventricular valvular incompetence and obliteration of the right ventricular cavity may also be found.

The clinical presentation in cardiac failure of these three types may be very similar, but it is important to make a physiological diagnosis because outcome and management differ in the different types.

The problem in Africa

Patients who have cardiac failure of uncertain cause and who become labelled as cases of cardiomyopathy are seen all over the continent: they may account for up to 20 per cent of patients with cardiovascular disease (Hakim & Manyemba, 1998; Amoah & Kallen, 2000). The prevalence varies from country to country, and also within countries: for example, peri-partum cardiac failure (PPCF) is particularly common in just one area in Nigeria (Ford et al., 1998). Why is dilated cardiomyopathy so common? The prevalence in Africa is totally different from what is seen in, for example, Europe, where cardiomyopathy is rare.

Aetiology

Possible factors are:

1. burnt out untreated hypertension. The evidence is persuasive:
   Some patients with cardiac failure and a normal blood pressure have documented evidence of hypertension in the past.
   The blood pressure may rise, after treatment for cardiac failure, to hypertensive levels.
   The aortic diameter in DCM patients is greater than normal but is less than in established hypertensive patients (Falase & Kolawole,1980).
   The age and sex pattern is the same as hypertensive heart failure – male, and in the fifth and sixth decades (Araoye & Olowoyeye, 1984).
2. Viral myocarditis. This may be important in younger individuals, but it is not common, except related to HIV. In Congo, for example, 55 per cent of patients with HIV developed cardiomyopathy over a 7-year follow-up period (Longo-Mbenza et al., 1998).
3. Alcohol. This is well documented, from the palm wine tapper in coastal West Africa to the urban or rural chronic alcoholic (Falase,1979).

4. Poverty. This is a risk factor in Nigeria and Cote d'Ivoire (Malu et al., 1991).
5. Pregnancy and childbirth. Peri-partum cardiomyopathy is described below.
6. Metabolic causes. Iron excess, previously common in South Africa, and referred to as Bantu haemosiderosis, is today an uncommon cause of cardiomyopathy. Its decline may be due to replacement of iron pots for alcoholic beverages by plastic mugs or glass bottles.
7. Beri-beri, due to thiamine deficiency, causes two types of cardiac failure:
   Wet beri-beri: a high output state, with tachycardia and a full arterial pulse.
   Shoshin beri-beri: a shock-like low output state, with lactic acidosis and renal failure, hypoglycaemia and hypothermia, justifiably called pernicious beri-beri.

Clinical features

The clinical problem is cardiac failure, with its characteristic symptoms, but without any obvious cause.

Dilated cardiomyopathy

The signs depend on the stage of the disease, and possibly also on whether the case is one of burnt out hypertension; thus, typically, there is a feebly contracting left ventricle, with a small pulse pressure, small volume arterial pulse, often with pulsus alternans, a low systolic arterial pressure, a weak cardiac impulse displaced down and outwards, distant heart sounds and a third heart sound. There may also be mitral and tricuspid incompetence, due to valvular ring dilatation, atrial fibrillation and evidence of peripheral emboli.

Diagnosis

The problem is a patient with cardiac failure, without obvious valvular disease. When the patient has a murmur, this may disappear after treatment for cardiac failure, whereas it does not change if there is organic valvular disease.

Echocardiography

Provides valuable data about the structure and function of the heart.

Chest radiograph

A large, almost globular, heart shadow is typical. While it may be confused with a pericardial effusion, pulmonary venous congestion, so common in cardiomyopathy, is not seen in pericardial effusion (Fig. 76.17).

Electrocardiogram

There is no specific pattern: some cases have a low voltage with R waves of less than 10 mm in the chest leads.

Prognosis

Most patients with DCM, especially those over 55 years of age, die within 5 years of their first symptom. About 25 per cent improve spontaneously.

The most common cause of death is progressive congestive heart failure or heart rhythm disorders. A persistently low arterial pressure and mitral and/or tricuspid incompetence carry a poor prognosis (Kingue et al., 1999).

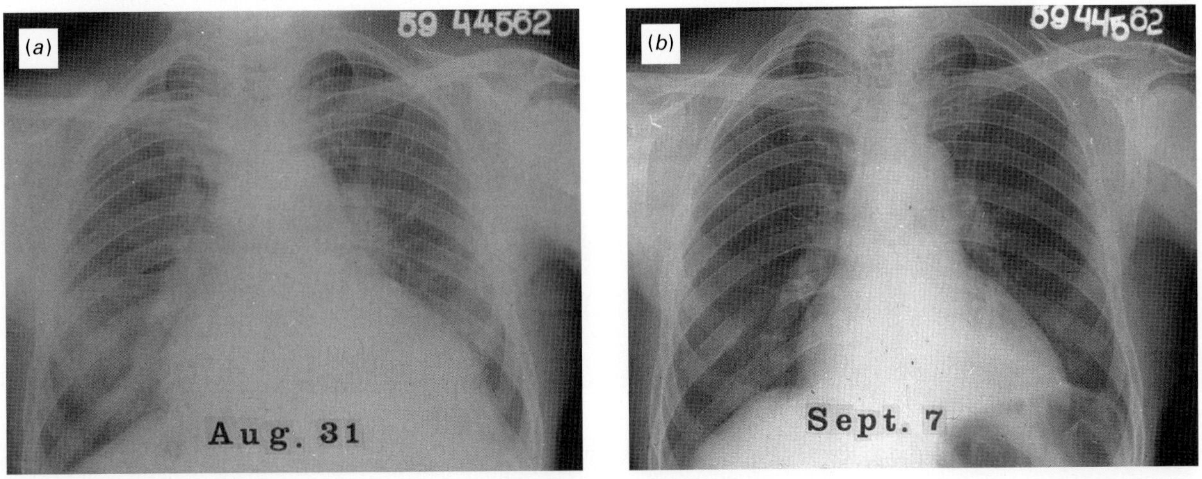

Fig. 76.17. Chest radiograph, pulmonary oedema in dilated cardiomyopathy: the effect of frusemide and digoxin for 1 week (without admission to hospital).

Treatment

The principles are:

- Give standard treatment for cardiac failure.
- *Treat any identifiable cause:* In those rare cases in whom a precipitating cause can be identified, treat it vigorously. For example, alcohol: there can be no compromise: the patient must agree to absolute abstinence from alcohol, and in the rare cases of beri-beri, thiamine in large doses intravenously is essential.

Hypertrophic obstructive cardiomyopathy

Patients with HOCM are often asymptomatic: the first event may also be the last, as sudden death, particularly on exercise, is common. If they have symptoms, patients complain of dyspnoea, retro-sternal chest pain, fatigue, syncope, and the light-headedness of near-syncope. The electrocardiogram has signs of left ventricular hypertrophy, but with unexplained Q-waves not attributable to any focus of myocardial necrosis.

Treatment

Give standard cardiac failure treatment (p. 857). Strenuous exercise and sports are forbidden. Digoxin is contraindicated because the inotropic effect may worsen left ventricular outflow obstruction. Beta-adrenergic blockers may relieve and/or improve angina pectoris, reduce syncopal attacks and decrease cardiac contractility, thus reducing outflow tract obstruction. Verapamil and diltiazem may reduce the stiffness of the ventricle, reduce the elevated diastolic pressures and increase exercise tolerance. Sudden death due to ventricular tachyarrhythmias is a constant threat.

Peripartum cardiac failure (PPCF)

This syndrome, well recognized in South Africa (Desai et al., 1995) and in Niger (Cenac et al., 1998), is the most important cause of cardiac failure among women around Zaria, northern Nigeria (Davidson & Parry, 1979) where it was defined as '*cardiac failure, with symptoms beginning in pregnancy or up to six months post-partum, of up to six months duration, with no history of cardiac failure other than PPCF itself, and with no discernible cause for cardiac failure other than anaemia or hypertension presumed to be acute*'.

Pathogenesis

The traditional habits, which contribute significantly to the pathogenesis of PPCF in Zaria, lead to the mother becoming excessively vasodilated so that she is unable to excrete the added salt load which she takes (Chapter 2). She becomes overloaded with fluid which she retains and may therefore become very oedematous (Sanderson et al., 1979; Marin-Neto et al., 1991). The added heat load of the hot season also contributes and accounts for the syndrome being most common after the hottest time of year. There is some evidence that the women are a potentially hypertensive population, and they also take significantly more salt than women in their villages who have not had PPCF.

Clinical features

The picture is of cardiac failure, with pulmonary and massive systemic oedema, and a blood pressure which may be slightly raised in the acute phase. Rest and diuretics cause a voluminous diuresis. The prognosis is good and women can carry a normal subsequent pregnancy unless there is electrocardiographic evidence of left ventricular hypertrophy, a raised diastolic blood pressure and an increased transverse diameter of the heart (C/T ratio increased). The syndrome recurred in women who had an increased QRS amplitude (33.6, *vs.* no recurrence 28.3) or a slightly increased systolic blood pressure (Ford et al., 1998). Those who had a recurrence of PPCF or of CF unrelated to pregnancy had a bad prognosis.

Comment

PPCF is a heterogeneous syndrome and, although the provoking factors in Zaria may be distinctive, PPCF in all places is characterized by some deaths in the acute phase, episodes of cardiac failure unrelated to pregnancy, the dire outlook if there is a recurrence and the relationship between an enlarged left ventricle and prognosis.

Endomyocardial fibrosis (EMF)

Endomyocardial fibrosis is a disease of uncertain cause in which dense fibrous tissue in the endocardium restricts ventricular diastole and thus distorts the papillary muscles of the atrio-ventricular valves. Its cause is unknown but, as many EMF patients have an eosinophilia at some stage of their illness, cardiac damage by the eosinophil is probably one factor.

The problem in Africa

JNP Davies first defined EMF in Kampala, Uganda. He had found thickened endocardium at the apices of the ventricles in patients dying of heart failure (Davies, 1948) Davies' work was extended in Kampala, Ibadan, Nigeria,

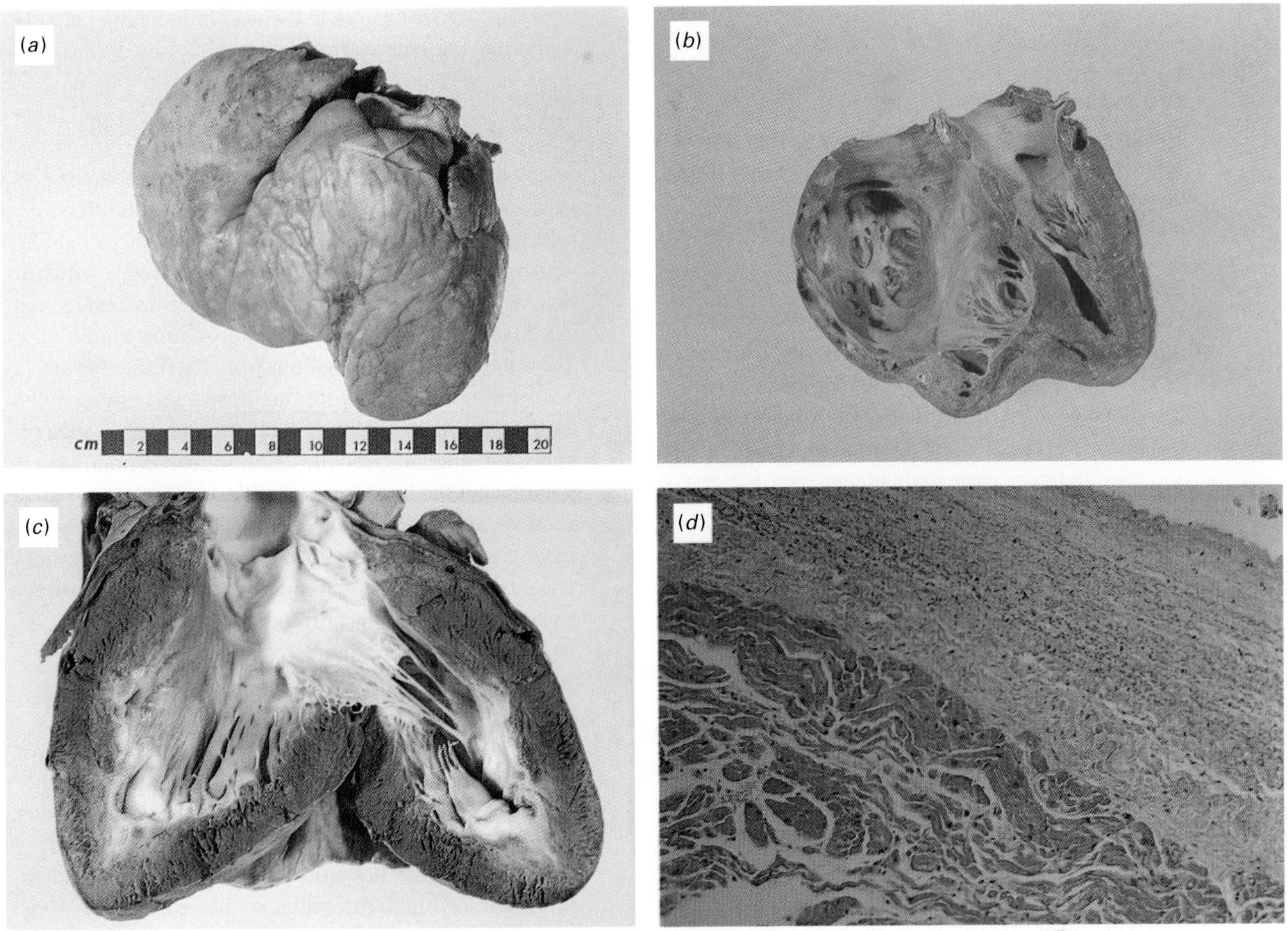

Fig. 76.18. Endomyocardial fibrosis: (*a*) and (*b*) right ventricular disease, note the enormous right atrium and the indentation on the free wall of the right ventricle, the chamber of which is virtually obliterated. (*c*) Left ventricular disease. (*d*) Histology of the endocardium in established chronic disease: note its relative acellularity and the sharp border between the myocardium and the endocardium.

and Abidjan, Cote d'Ivoire (Connor et al., 1967, 1968; Abrahams, 1962; Parry & Abrahams, 1965) (Fig. 76.18(*a*)(*b*)(*c*)(*d*)).

Epidemiology

Geographical distribution

Within Africa, EMF is uncommon outside the wet tropics, so that, despite excellent facilities in the north and south of the continent, it is very rare indeed there. Similarly, while cases are commonly seen in wet Kampala, they are rare in drier and more temperate Nairobi. Similarly, it is found in wetter areas of the tropics, Malaysia, coastal Latin America, and southern India, particularly Kerala. World-wide, EMF is rare, although a histologically similar disorder, Loeffler's endocarditis, is occasionally seen in northern countries.

Ethnic association

In Kampala, the indigenous Baganda have significantly less EMF than the immigrants from neighbouring highland Rwanda and Burundi. Among the Rwandese, a kindred was described in whom EMF was associated with an unusually high incidence of hyper immune malarial splenomegaly (Ziegler & Stuiver, 1972). No other clear ethnic differences have been described (Mayanja-Kizza et al., 2000).

Social background

EMF is dominantly a disease of poorer people (Rutakingirwa et al., 1999). In Uganda, all patients are poor rural people who just subsist and thus eat a poor diet, often with cassava as the sole staple food, with little or no animal protein. But EMF is still being documented in foreigners, who have lived in coastal West Africa, and so it cannot be explained solely on the basis of deprivation.

Age and sex distribution

The peak age incidence of EMF is between 11 and 15 years in both sexes, but females show a second peak between 26 and 30 years. Females are more affected than males with a ratio of approximately 2:1.

Eosinophilia

This is a risk factor for endomyocardial fibrosis (Rutakingirwa et al., 1999), and is reported from East and West Africa. Andy et al. (1998) found a count of 1000×10^9/l in 80 per cent of early cases: the level of eosinophilia was inversely related to the duration of reported illness, and they therefore argue that patients who do not have an eosinophilia are at a late stage of EMF.

Other possible factors

Malaria

EMF in Africa is prevalent where malaria is also prevalent. Although no causal relationship has been established, endocardial thrombi which formed in mice infected with *P. falciparum* and a rebound eosinophilia reported after malarial infection in Thailand suggest that malaria may perhaps have a role in EMF.

Trace elements

In South Kerala, India, clusters of EMF patients were found in areas with high cerium and low magnesium in the soil, without any significant filariasis and eosinophilia. A similar distribution of cerium and magnesium was found in heart muscle tissue of Indian EMF patients, but not in patients in Uganda.

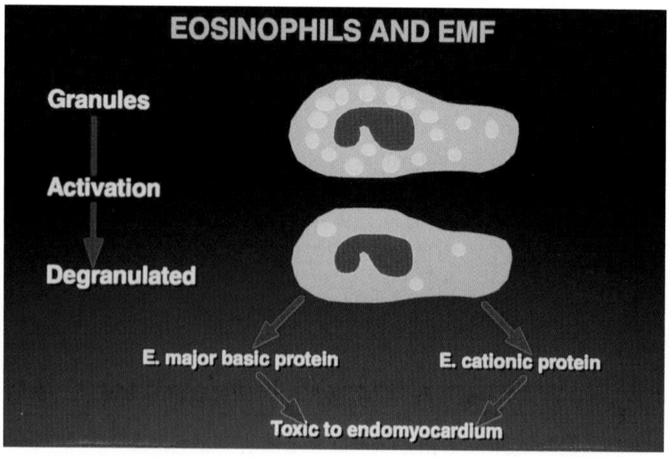

Fig. 76.19. Activation and degranulation of eosinophils release their cationin protein and major basic protein, which are toxic to the myocardium.

What is the significance of the eosinophilia?

Many different parasites have been suggested as the responsible triggers of the eosinophilia. Eosinophils contain major basic protein, cationic protein, protein X, and other substances (Po-Chun Tai et al., 1987), which are released during degranulation and which are toxic to the endo- and myocardium, so that fibrosis and mural thrombosis follow. Eosinophils from EMF patients are morphologically different from those seen in other conditions (Mayanja-Kizza et al., 2000) but the significance of this is not known. The cardiac lesions of eosinophilic leukaemia and the hyper-eosinophilia syndromes are similar to those of EMF (Spry et al., 1982). The probable sequence of events is shown in Fig. 76.19: an unidentified stimulus triggers endocardial inflammation followed by necrosis, thrombosis and finally fibrosis. The resulting fibrosis varies from patient to patient.

Relationship between structure and function

Endocardial fibrosis anchors the papillary muscles

The atrio-ventricular valves are therefore distorted and so become incompetent. In advanced disease of the right ventricle, its cavity is almost obliterated by layers of organized fibrotic mural thrombus, so that the papillary muscles are buried and the tricuspid valve ceases to function. In systole, therefore, there is free regurgitation of blood up the jugular vein, which produces a very high systolic wave in the jugular venous pulse. Regurgitant flow into the inferior vena cava enters the hepatic vein, which leads to systolic pulsatile expansion of the liver, until the liver fibroses as a result of the sustained high hepatic venous pressure.

The left ventricle, as it is a higher pressure chamber, is never obliterated, but the mitral valve becomes incompetent, both because its papillary muscles become anchored in fibrous tissue and because the posterior cusp of the mitral valve becomes stuck by endocardial fibrous tissue. Fibrotic changes appear exclusively in the inflow tracts or apices of the ventricle: the outflow tracts and inter-ventricular septum are spared.

Fibrous tissue restricts ventricular diastole

In both ventricles, fibrous tissue in the endocardium, and patches of fibrosis in the myocardium, stiffen the ventricle so that its compliance is reduced, ventricular diastole and filling are restricted and stroke output falls (Fig. 76.20).

Left, right or bi-ventricular disease

Either left or right ventricle, alone, or both ventricles, can be affected: bi-ventricular EMF is the most common type.

Clinical features

These depend on:
- the activity of the disease
- the stage of the disease
- the anatomical distortion of the heart.

The initial illness

Children or adolescents describe an initial illness with fever, chills and night sweats in nearly 50 per cent. Facial and periorbital swelling and itching of the body, sometimes with urticaria, occur in up to 30 per cent. The patient has cough and breathlessness and may have abdominal swelling: some of the symptoms come and go over a few weeks (Parry & Abrahams, 1965; Andy & Bishara, 1982). This phase may be accompanied by clinical evidence of left- or right-sided EMF. This illness may disappear, or it may lead to rapidly developing cardiac failure and early death, or it may evolve into established and apparently inactive EMF. A small group of the patients of Andy et al. (1998) also had focal neurological symptoms at the beginning of their illness. Histologically there are focal areas of myocardial necrosis and a vigorous inflammatory reaction in the endocardium (Fig. 76.21(*a*) and (*b*)).

Left ventricular disease

There are no specific symptoms beyond the inevitable symptoms and signs of cardiac failure. Abdominal swelling may occur. The signs depend on the degree of mitral valvular incompetence: the pansystolic murmur of mitral regurgitation may be accompanied by a clear third heart sound (restrictive disease).

Right ventricular disease

Abdominal swelling and sometimes a little ankle oedema are dominant. The major signs are ascites, an enlarged liver with systolic pulsation and a very quiet heart, which may be virtually impalpable because its enlargement is due to the aneurysmal right atrium, accompanied by a pericardial effusion. In early cases the murmur of tricuspid regurgitation is heard but this disappears, and the only auscultatory sign may be a third heart sound. Atrial fibrillation is found in those with

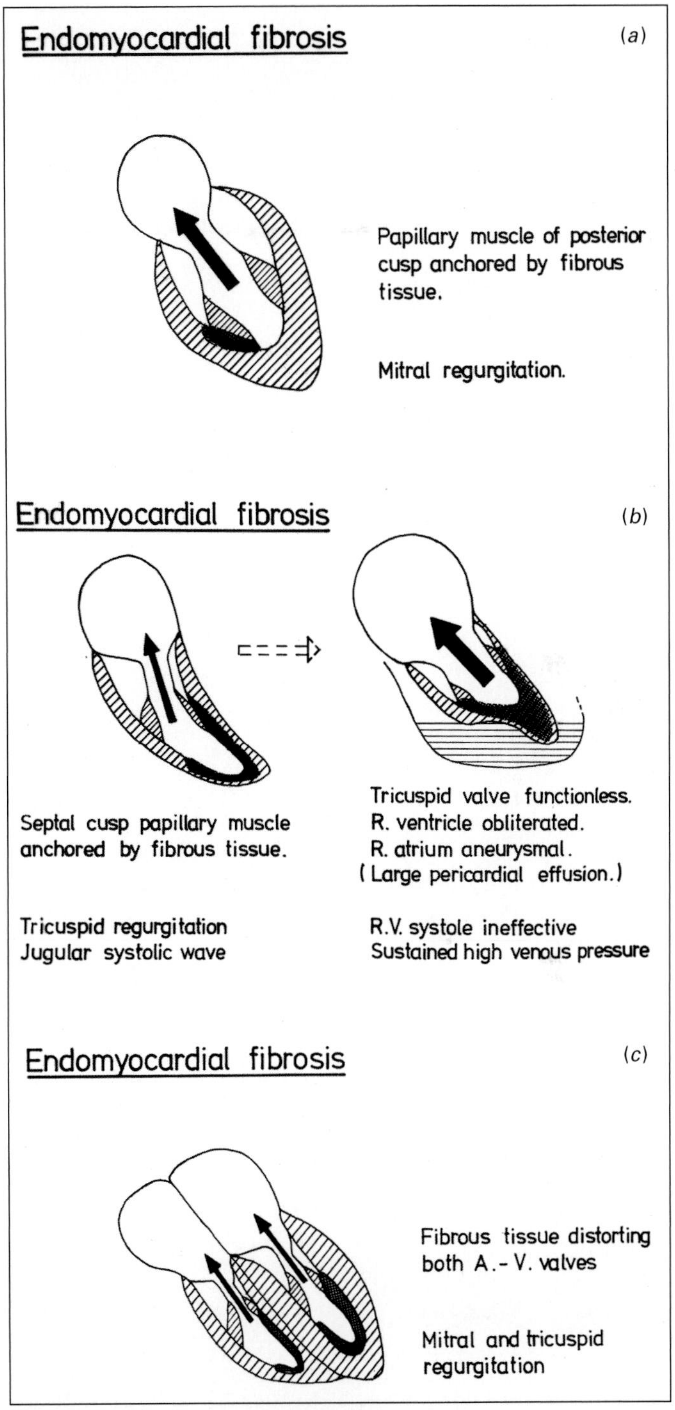

Fig. 76.20. Diagrams to show the effect of EMF on the heart: a restrictive ventricular defect, and fibrosis which leads to atrio-ventricular valvular incompetence.

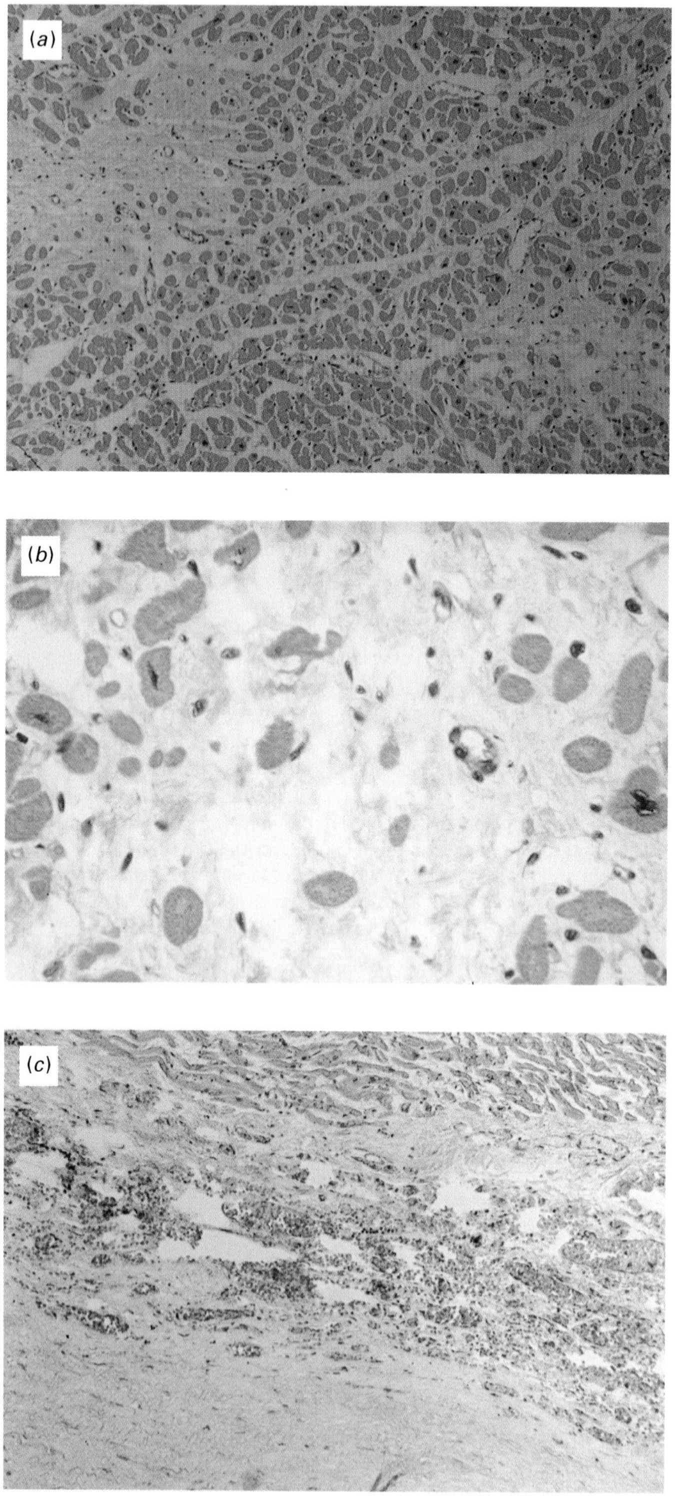

Fig. 76.21. Endomyocardial fibrosis: histological sections in the initial illness. (*a*) Areas of focal necrosis in the myocardium; (*b*) myocardial necrosis ×400; (*c*) acute inflammation in the endocardium.

long-standing disease. The arterial pulse is inevitably of low pulse pressure and volume. A giant systolic wave in the jugular venous pulse is seen in all cases of established right ventricular EMF and many patients also have proptosis. Finger and toe clubbing and central cyanosis may be found in those with massive tense ascites. Cases beginning in childhood have retarded growth, testicular atrophy and failure of male secondary sexual characters (Fig. 76.22).

Ascites

Ascites in EMF also occurs in lone left ventricular disease. In 75 per cent the ascites is an exudate (SG >1.1017, protein >60 g/1) (Freers et al., 1996). This high protein and the peritoneal fibrosis found in EMF, often with infiltrates of lymphocytes and plasma cells, may indicate a generalised process of fibrosis – the 'EMF syndrome', not merely EMF (Freers et al., 2000).

A protein-losing enteropathy has not been demonstrated, but is probable, in those with the sustainedly high venous pressure of right ventricular EMF.

Laboratory investigations

Echocardiography

This technique reliably identifies the site and extent of the lesion: it is almost as accurate as an autopsy. The echocardiographic picture of LV EMF may resemble that of previous infective endocarditis if the posterior mitral leaflet is tethered to the left ventricular posterior wall (Freers et al., 1996).

Electrocardiography (ECG)

This contributes little, except to confirm atrial fibrillation. In cases with a pericardial effusion, low voltage or electrical alternans (varying voltage in each heart cycle) may be found.

Chest radiography

There are no pathognomonic features. An enlarged cardiac silhouette may be due to pericardial effusion, or an enlarged right atrium. Ascites may raise the diaphragm. In left ventricular disease pulmonary venous congestion can be seen.

Blood

Eosinophil counts vary according to the stage of the disease (Andy et al., 1998). In Uganda between 60 and 80 per cent of all EMF patients show eosinophilia of more than 500 × 10^9/l, but this is not related to blood or stool parasitic infections. Eosinophils from EMF patients, particularly those with hypereosinophilia, display distinct abnormalities:

- granules, large, coarse, deeper staining and more compact than normal
- degranulation around the nucleus
- vacuoles between granules (mostly two in number)
- nuclei with three or more equally sized lobes, a normal third lobe is a mere appendix.

Differential diagnosis

Where echocardiography is available, EMF can be differentiated from other causes of gross ascites such as tuberculous peritonitis, advanced hepato-splenic schistosomiasis, liver cirrhosis, or constrictive pericarditis by its pathognomonic changes.

Where this technique is not available, do not rush into a diagnosis, but consider the evidence very carefully and wait to see whether signs change with rest in bed and diuretic treatment, as may happen in rheumatic heart disease or dilated cardiomyopathy. If there is no murmur at mitral or tricuspid valve, the patient may well have constrictive pericarditis.

Treatment

Early illness

Although controlled trials are not available, experience in Uganda, supported by reports from Brazil, show that corticosteroids and immuno-suppressants may have a role in the early illness of EMF especially or perhaps only in patients with hyper-eosinophilia.

Established disease

Traditional treatment with cardiac glycosides and diuretics has little effect, except in those with pulmonary venous congestion.

Right ventricular disease

Ascites is often resistant to treatment. Paracentesis may have to be done to relieve severe abdominal distension, which leads to upward compression of the lungs, but this causes significant loss of protein and the fluid re-accumulates quickly.

Surgery

Surgical excision of fibrotic material and reconstitution of the AV-valve can be done in advanced centres, but only if the primary disease is quiescent.

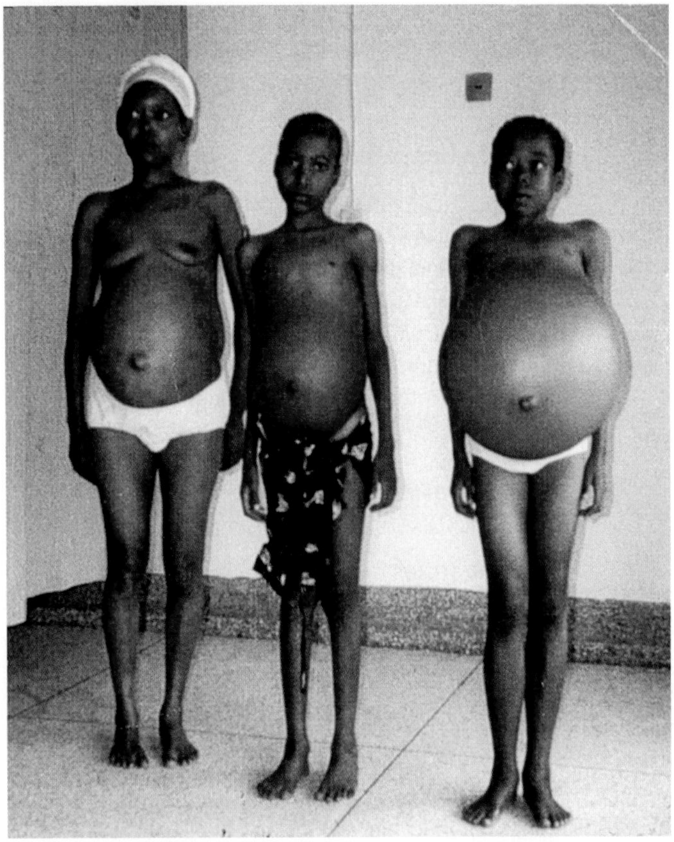

Fig. 76.22. Ugandan patients with right ventricular EMF.

Cor pulmonale

This term denotes right-sided heart disease which results from:

(i) destruction of the gas-exchanging tissue of the lung
(ii) severe chronic airways obstruction
(iii) pulmonary vascular disease, as in schistosomal arteriolar occlusion – very important in Egypt and other schistosomiasis endemic countries in Africa
(iv) chest wall deformities, such as kyphoscoliosis due to tuberculosis
(v) living at high altitudes, possibly a factor in some patients in Ethiopia
(v) rarely in HIV infection (Mehta et al., 2000).

Epidemiology

In some areas of Africa women who have cooked over a fire in a poorly ventilated hut are vulnerable: in Egypt schistosomiasis is the dominant cause; an average of about 7 per cent of cases of cardiac failure are due to cor pulmonale. It may become more common as industrial growth leads to air pollution, and cigarette smoking increases.

Disordered physiology

The work of the right ventricle is increased if the lung tissue and small vessels are destroyed: this leads to arterial hypoxaemia, pulmonary vasoconstriction and a further increase in pulmonary vascular resistance.

Right ventricular hypertrophy and dilatation as well as right atrial dilatation are detectable by two-dimensional echo. Doppler studies can quantify pulmonary artery pressure and thus the severity of cor pulmonale. In cor pulmonale due to schistosomiasis, the echo-probe over the liver can demonstrate Symmer's fibrosis.

Clinical features

(i) Evidence of chest disease (Chapter 77): there are signs either of lung destruction, as in tuberculosis, of severe airways obstruction with distortion of the chest, or of kyphoscoliosis.
(ii) Signs of impaired pulmonary gas exchange: central cyanosis, which may be seen only during exercise, and clubbing of the fingers.
(iii) Signs of pulmonary hypertension: a prominent *a* wave in the jugular pulse; a palpable or loud pulmonary closure sound; and a prominent right ventricle palpable at the left border of the sternum. The electrocardiogram shows varying degrees of *P* pulmonale and RV strain.
(iv) Signs of right heart cardiac failure with systemic congestion: oedema is very commonly found. In advanced cases the dilated right ventricle leads to tricuspid regurgitation.

Course and treatment

The prognosis depends on the primary lung disease. Routine treatment for cardiac failure is needed: digoxin may be ineffective. Respiratory failure, particularly its acute provoking factor, must be carefully managed. Oxygen can significantly lower pulmonary arterial pressure, but must be used cautiously as these patients depend on a hypoxic drive and may develop respiratory failure if the oxygen concentration is too high. Never use morphine as it may depress respiration fatally.

Congenital heart disease

Children with severe defects, like transposition of the great vessels, die very early. Many babies are born and die at home, and nothing is known of their cause of death: others die in infancy from an infection, as they are at high risk.

All common congenital lesions have been reported from Africa.

Clinical picture

The anatomical site of the lesion governs the symptoms and signs. Pulmonary and aortic stenosis cause right or left ventricular hypertrophy. An increased pulmonary blood flow is found if there is a left-to-right shunt through an atrial or ventricular septal defect or through a patent ductus arteriosus. The signs depend on the size and site of the shunt, and, in some children, on the presence of pulmonary hypertension. If there is right-to-left shunting of blood, as in Fallot's tetralogy, the child may squat, and have cyanosis and digital clubbing (Table 76.4).

Anaemia and the heart

The effects of anaemia on the heart are described in detail in Chapter 78. In addition to being important as a cause of severe circulatory congestion, anaemia may aggravate existing heart disease or may unmask clinically inapparent disease.

Patients with severe chronic cardiac failure can often be improved dramatically by slow transfusion of packed red cells, or whole blood if packed cells are unavailable, provided 80–120 mg frusemide are given at the same time to prevent acute hypervolaemia.

Infection of the heart

The heart can be affected in infections directly by the presence of an organism, by the effects of drugs taken in treatment of other conditions such as HIV infection, or indirectly by any component of the host's immune response to the organism. Wherever the infection – endocardium, myocardium, or pericardium – symptoms and signs are caused by:

- anatomical damage to the heart
- effects of cardiac function
- embolic effects
- systemic/immune mediated effects of infection
- conduction defects and arrhythmias.

Table 76.4. Summary of basic changes in congenital heart disease

	Effects	Physical signs	Chest radiograph
Intracardiac shunts signs and effects depend on the volume of shunted blood			
Left-to-right shunt			
Atrial septal defect	Increased pulmonary blood flow	Ejection systolic murmur at left sternal edge Pulmonary closure sound fixed on inspiration	Right atrium enlarged Pulmonary plethora Aorta small
Ventricular septal defect	Increased pulmonary blood flow Left ventricle enlarged if shunt large	Pansystolic murmur at lower left sternal edge	Pulmonary plethora Left ventricle enlarged
Patent ductus arteriosus	Arterial run-off Left ventricle enlarged if shunt large	To-and-fro murmur around pulmonary area Pulse-pressure wide-wave collapsing	Pulmonary plethora Left ventricle enlarged
Right-to-left shunt			
Defects listed above: when the shunt reverses there are signs of severe pulmonary hypertension and a low cardiac output			
Tetralogy of Fallot			
1. Pulmonary stenosis 2. Large ventricular septal defect 3. Right ventricular hypertrophy 4. Over-riding aorta		Cyanosis, clubbing, squatting Systolic murmur over praecordium, often with thrill	Oligaemic lung fields Right ventricle enlarged Sometimes right-sided aortic arch
Valvular stenosis			
Pulmonary	Right ventricular hypertrophy	Pulmonary closure delayed or inaudible Ejection systolic murmur at pulmonary area	Pulmonary oligaemia Right ventricle prominent
Aortic	Left ventricular hypertrophy	Left ventricle enlarged Ejection murmur and delayed or absent aortic closure sound	
Other lesions			
Coarctation of aorta			
Stenotic segment in aorta below site of ductus arteriosus	Hypertension Development of collateral blood supply	Blood pressure in arms raised (not recordable in legs) Delayed or absent femoral pulses Systolic murmur often heard in back	Aortic knuckle absent Left ventricle enlarged Knotches in ribs caused by collateral vessels

In any infection the clinical picture may vary from signs which suggest transient myocarditis (a persistent tachycardia particularly) to those of valvular destruction and multiple emboli or gross heart failure (Fig. 76.23).

Pericardium and pericarditis

Organisms reach the pericardium in bacterial pericarditis from adjacent tissues: lung (*Strep. pneumoniae*), lymph nodes (*M. tuberculosis*), and liver (*E.histolytica*); or from the blood (*Staph. aureus*). Infection of the pericardium alone is rare.

Symptoms and signs and diagnosis

Some signs are caused by the primary infection and its systemic effects: the pericardial signs can be divided into three groups:

- those due to pericardial inflammation
- those due to pericardial effusion
- those due to the effects on cardiac function.

Pericardial inflammation

Pericardial pain

This is retrosternal and may resemble cardiac and pleural pain because the heart, pericardium, and adjacent pleura share a common nerve supply; pain is felt locally or is referred to areas supplied from the same segment. It can be either transverse and retrosternal or localized over the pericardium: but it is not provoked by effort as is ischaemic cardiac pain, and it can be made worse by breathing and coughing, as is pleural pain.

Pericardial rub

This is the only definite diagnostic sign of acute pericardial inflammation: it is a scratching sound which is altered by position, and may appear when the breath is held in full expiration. It is often heard at the lower end of the sternum. It may come and go and, even if a sizeable effusion is present, it may still be heard. If the stethoscope moves over the skin a false 'rub' may be heard (see Box on page 875).

Pericardial effusion

In some patients there are no signs and the diagnosis is only suspected when the cardiac shadow has become unexpectedly enlarged in a chest radiograph: in others the cardiac impulse can scarcely be felt and the heart sounds are much less loud than usual; and in a few, when it accumulates quickly, the effusion causes acute cardiac compression. The diagnosis is confirmed when pericardial fluid is aspirated from the pericardial sac, or by echocardiography.

The echo-diagnosis is easy. In all standard echo-windows the heart is surrounded by fluid.

Empirical estimations of the amount of fluid are possible:

0.5–0.8 cm of fluid	=	approx. 200 ml
0.9–1.4 cm	=	approx. 300–500 ml
1.5–1.8 cm	=	approx. 600–1000 ml

Whereas 'blind' pericardiocentesis is easy in a large pericardial effusion, small effusions are better tapped for safety under echo-guidance, if available (Fig. 76.24).

Effects on cardiac function

1. Chronic constrictive pericarditis.
2. Acute cardiac compression (cardiac tamponade). Dyspnoea and restlessness are caused by a rising pulmonary venous pressure, because venous inflow is impeded; a critical fall in cardiac output may cause a confusional state and syncope. It is recognized by a rapid and rising heart rate, pulsus paradoxus, low arterial pressure, and intense venoconstriction with cold hands and feet; obstruction to venous inflow leads to a quickly rising jugular venous pressure with engorged veins which may eventually lose any visible pulse, and sometimes signs of pulmonary oedema.

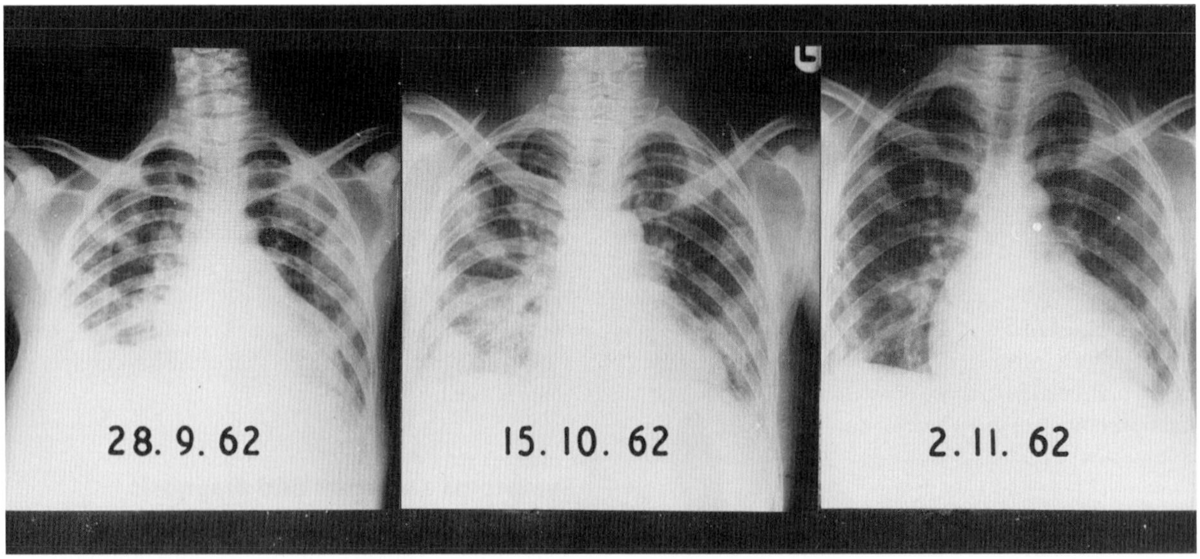

Fig. 76.23. Staphylococcal septicaemia: chest radiograph with initial pulmonary infarcts: there was a right sided endocarditis, and later a pericardial effusion.

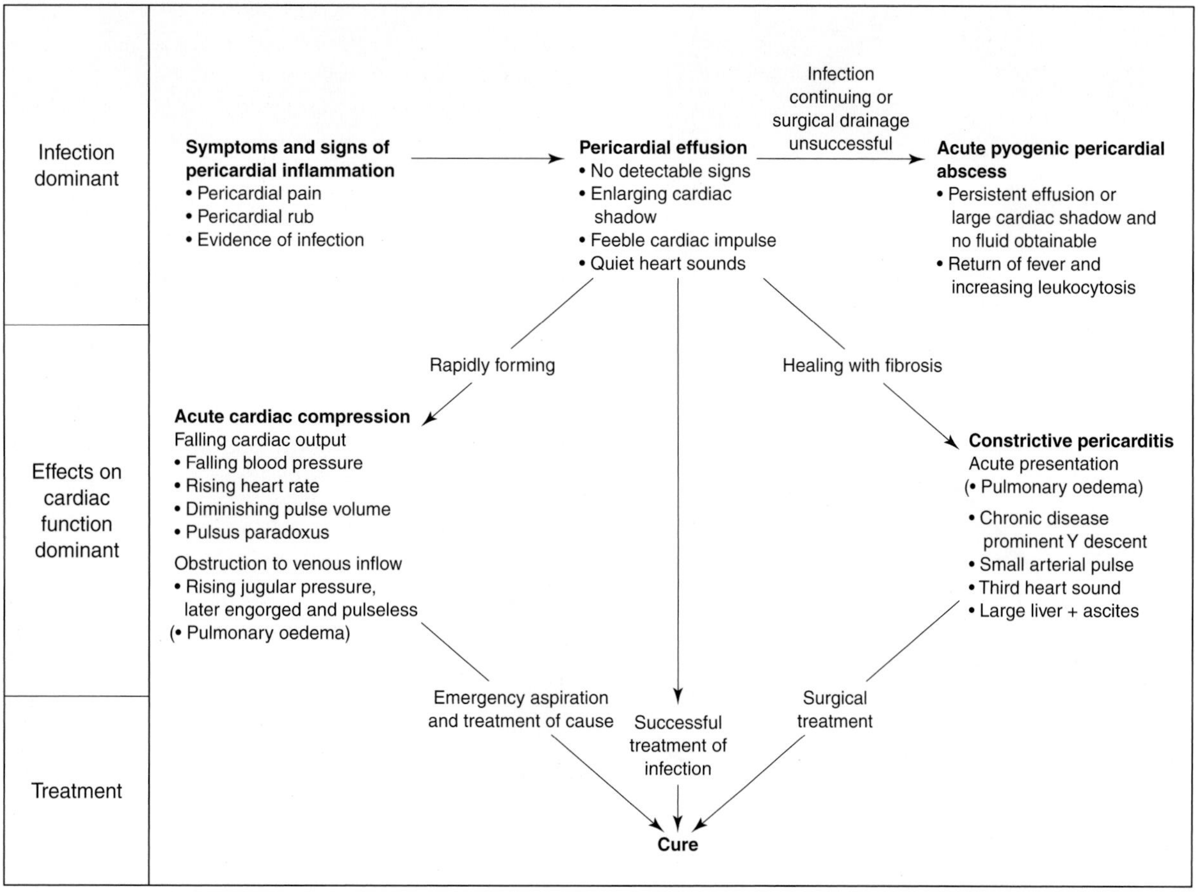

> **Acute cardiac tamponade**
> *Immediate action*: This is a desperate emergency and the pericardial sac must be aspirated at once.

Clinical types of pericarditis

Acute pyogenic effusion

In a patient with pneumonia, suspect a pericardial effusion if breathlessness, cough and a raised respiratory rate persist; if the arterial pressure falls, if the jugular venous pressure rises, and if the cardiac shadow is unexplainably large in the chest radiograph, or enlarging in serial radiographs.

The diagnosis is confirmed when:

- fluid is aspirated from the pericardial sac by the xiphisternal approach, and is shown to contain polymorphoneutrophil cells in abundance, and (if no antibiotics have been given) organisms are detected by gram stain or by culture (Fig. 76.25).
- fluid is demonstrated by echocardiography.

Treatment

The principles are to kill the organism and to prevent thick pus from forming. If thick pus has formed, immediate surgical drainage is essential.

Antibiotics

Cloxacillin in a dose of 500 mg four times a day is needed for a *staphylococcus* and at least 10 mega units of benzyl penicillin for a *pneumococcus*. There is no need to inject antibiotics into the pericardial fluid because the level of penicillin or gentamicin in it after a standard dose exceeds the plasma level at 2 hours in infected patients, and is above the minimum inhibitory concentration throughout. Closed drainage and antibiotics are satisfactory as constrictive pericarditis may develop quickly in some patients with pus in the pericardial sac.

Tuberculous effusion

The incidence of tuberculous pericarditis has increased in Africa as a result of the huge HIV epidemic (Ceglieski et al., 1990; Wragg et al., 2000).

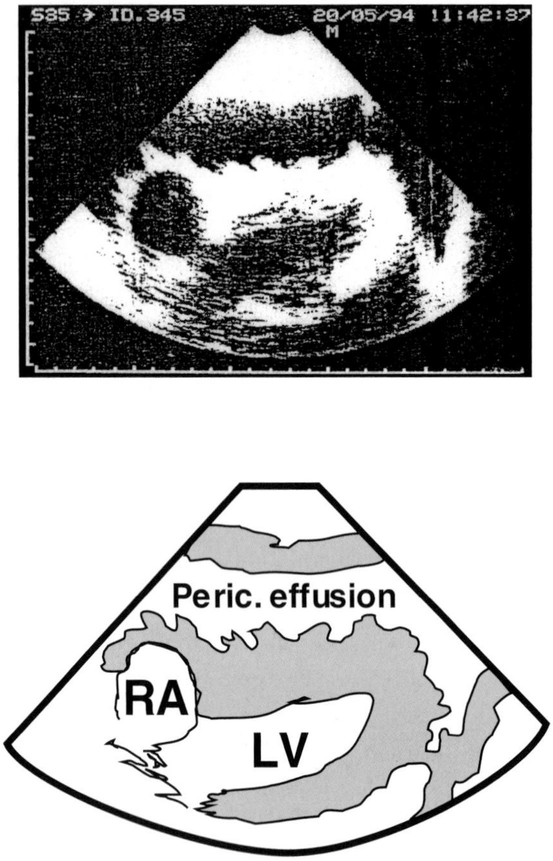

Fig. 76.24. Tuberculous pericarditis: Echocardiogram to show pericardial fluid and fibrinous strands on the surface of the visceral pericardium.

The patient presents with fever, night sweats and fatigue. The pericardial fluid is blood-stained in about 80 per cent of cases: it has a high lymphocyte count and a protein content above 30 g/l. A pleural effusion is found in about 25–30 per cent. There is not a blood polymorphonuclear leukocytosis. Standard treatment for tuberculosis is essential: the effusion will resolve in 80 per cent of patients within 2–3 months: 20 per cent develop subacute constriction and half of this group will require pericardiectomy.

Prednisolone speeds recovery, reduces the risk of death in HIV-negative and HIV-positive cases (Hakim et al., 2000) and the need for pericardiectomy (Strang et al., 1988): an initial dose of 120 mg daily, tapering the dose and stopping in 3–4 weeks, is newly recommended because rifampicin enhances the metabolism of prednisolone (Wragg et al., 2000). A dose of 60 mg initially has been widely used, reducing to 30 mg for weeks 5–8, 15 mg for weeks 9–10 and 5 mg only for week 11.

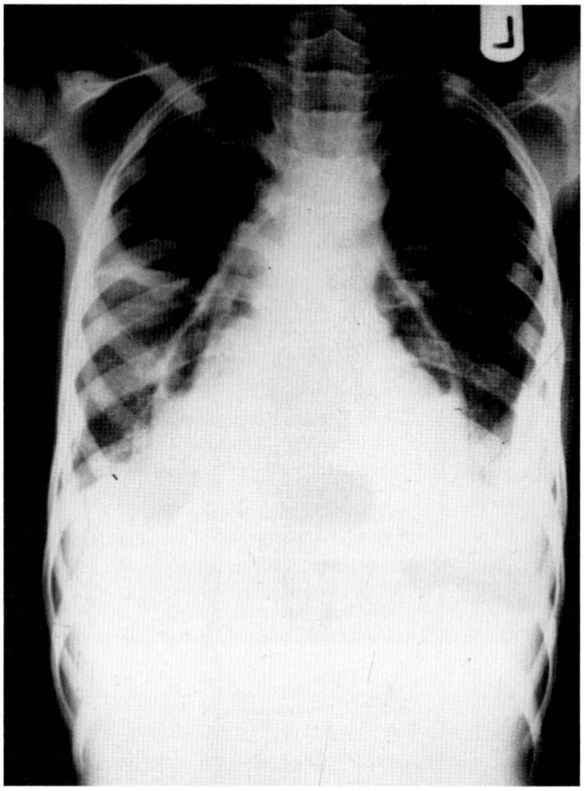

Fig. 76.25. Pyogenic pericarditis: chest radiograph to show air and fluid (pus) in the pericardial sac: note the thick pericardium, thickened with organizing pus.

Other causes of pericarditis

(i) Terminal renal failure.
(ii) Amoebic liver abscess.
(iii) Trauma.
(iv) Cancer metastases.
(v) Viral pericarditis. Fever, pericardial pain, and a pericardial rub, but without evidence of a systemic pyogenic infection or of obstruction to blood flow, are seen. The rub disappears in a few days and no treatment is needed.
(vi) HIV infection. A serous non-infective effusion is common in HIV-infected individuals especially those at an advanced stage of illness. Several other HIV related conditions may be complicated by a pericarditis, with or without effusion, such as Kaposi's sarcoma and cryptococcal infection (Silva-Cardoso et al., 1999).

Right ventricular endomyocardial fibrosis may also cause an effusion, but the history is long and the cardiac signs differ.

Chronic constrictive pericarditis

Nearly all cases are due to tuberculosis, the fibrotic result of an old tuberculous pericardial infection with effusion; pyogenic infections may be responsible in a few cases.

Clinical picture

The symptoms are those of cardiac failure, dominated by swelling of the abdomen, ascites and a large liver, if the disease has been established for a long time. Pulmonary oedema is seen if the constriction is around the left ventricle chiefly.

Signs of cardiac constriction

(i) A low cardiac output. The arterial pulse is of small volume and it becomes still smaller on inspiration (pulsus paradoxus, Fig. 76.2).
(ii) A high venous pressure, which may rise on inspiration; the jugular pulse has prominent x and y descents and is characteristic (Fig. 76.5).
(iii) Rapid limited ventricular filling, with a high-pitched third heart sound (pericardial knock) early in diastole.
(iv) Effects of a high systemic venous pressure – large liver, ascites.

Hypoproteinaemia

This problem is common in active tuberculosis, and is aggravated by the repeated aspiration of a pleural or ascitic fluid, and a protein-losing enteropathy, secondary to the high venous pressure.

Treatment

Surgical excision of the fibrotic pericardium may not relieve the restriction because the fibrous tissue may spread into the subjacent myocardium. Active tuberculosis requires standard chemotherapy. The beneficial effects of added prednisolene have been described above (Strang et al., 1988; Wragg & Strang, 2000).

Myocardium

Local abscess

This is rarely recognized in life when it may complicate a pyaemia, as in staphylococcal pyomyositis.

Diffuse damage

This may be caused either by organisms within the muscle, by their toxins, by pro-inflammatory cytokines, or a dysregulated immune response. In most cases it is not known which mechanism is more important.

Minor histological changes may be seen in the myocardium in many infections, particularly viral infections; clinically recognizable myocarditis is described in the following infections in Africa: bacterial – *N. meningitidis*; *C. diphtheriae*; *S. typhi*: parasitic – *toxoplasmosis*; *Trypanosoma rhodesiense*.

If anyone with an acute infection develops ventricular ectopic beats, signs of unexplained cardiac failure or of an enlarging heart, or if the electrocardiogram shows a prolonged QTc interval, acute myocarditis is probable. The management is as for cardiac failure, but REST is important until all signs have gone because myocarditis is an unstable state. Treatment with steroids has no beneficial effect in acute myocarditis.

Endocardium – infective endocarditis

The terms subacute and acute bacterial endocarditis overlap: it is therefore best to use the general term infective endocarditis and if possible specify the organism.

Source of infection

In a patient with a heart valve previously damaged by rheumatic heart disease the organism is often one of low pathogenicity such as *Strep. viridans*, derived often from the mouth, or after dental extraction.

In contrast, if a septicaemia occurs from a pyogenic focus, whether or not the heart valves were previously damaged, a more virulent pyogenic organism, such as *Strep. pneumoniae* or *Staph. aureus*, is usually responsible. In Africa, post-partum pelvic infection, and an acute pyomyositis are important. In industrialized countries, drug addicts who inject themselves, the aged often after genitourinary procedures, and patients after cardiac surgery are at risk.

Pathogenesis

If there is a high velocity flow between areas of high and low pressure, the jet of blood damages the endothelium where it strikes, and a jet lesion is formed on which bacteria, platelets, fibrin, and cellular elements settle, particularly on a valve already damaged by rheumatic activity, or a congenital defect. When blood is forced through a stenotic valve a lesion may form on the post-stenotic surface. The mechanism of infective endocarditis on a

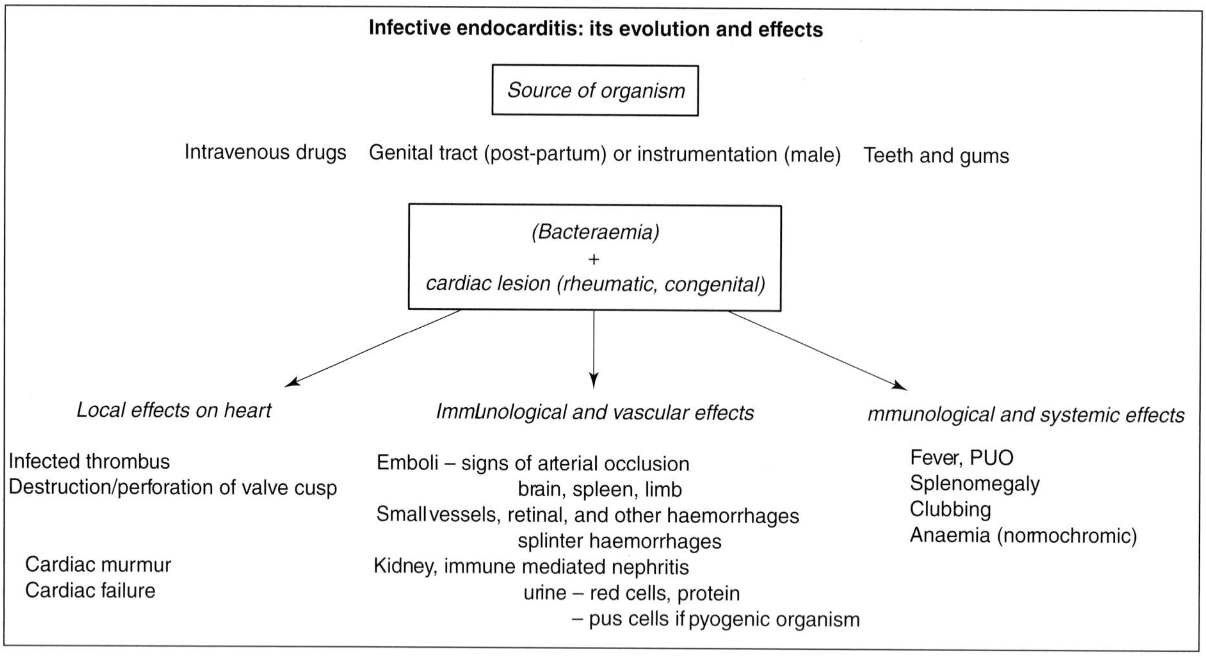
Infective endocarditis: its evolution and effects
Source of organism
Intravenous drugs
Genital tract (post-partum) or instrumentation (male)
Teeth and gums
(Bacteraemia)
+
cardiac lesion (rheumatic, congenital)
Local effects on heart
Immunological and vascular effects
mmunological and systemic effects
Infected thrombus
Destruction/perforation of valve cusp
Cardiac murmur
Cardiac failure
Emboli – signs of arterial occlusion
brain, spleen, limb
Small vessels, retinal, and other haemorrhages
splinter haemorrhages
Kidney, immune mediated nephritis
urine – red cells, protein
– pus cells if pyogenic organism
Fever, PUO
Splenomegaly
Clubbing
Anaemia (normochromic)

normal valve is not clear. Many of the systemic and vascular effects of infective endocarditis are caused by circulating immune complexes with activation of the complement classical pathway (Messias-Reason et al., 2002).

Kidney

In some inadequately treated, or long-standing untreated cases, a glomerulonephritis develops with immunoglobulin deposits along the glomerular basement membrane.

Clinical picture and diagnosis

Suspect infective endocarditis in any patient who has valvular heart disease with signs of local infection, and signs of any of the many effects shown in the box.

The infection has to be distinguished from:

(i) acute rheumatic carditis
(ii) pyogenic infection without endocardial infection
(iii) valvular heart disease with splenomegaly, but without other evidence of the systemic or 'immunological' effects shown above.

Blood culture

A definitive diagnosis is only made if a positive blood culture develops from one of the several specimens taken before treatment. If the diagnosis is strongly suspected and the patient is very ill, take three specimens at 30–60-minute intervals with strict aseptic technique.

Echocardiography

Floating vegetations on affected valves are demonstrable in 50–70 per cent of clinically diagnosed cases. Note, endocardial vegetations are sometimes seen in apparently healthy patients: these vegetations might be healed and sterile remainders of earlier episodes of infective endocarditis (Fig. 76.26).

Treatment

In all patients blood culture is essential before any treatment is given. In practice in Africa it is reasonable in most patients to begin treatment if clinical signs are suggestive because, untreated, the disease is fatal.

As with any infection, the principle is to give the correct antibiotic for as long as is necessary; and as with any heart disease, it is important to control cardiac failure.

If a blood culture is not available, give benzylpenicillin in a total daily dose of 8–16 mega units and gentamicin 1.5 mg/kg twice daily.

Very large doses of penicillin may be needed and should be given in an intravenous infusion but not in 5 per cent dextrose which inactivates the penicillin. Isotonic sodium chloride is best, but do not give more than 500 ml per 24 hours for fear of precipitating or aggravating cardiac failure.

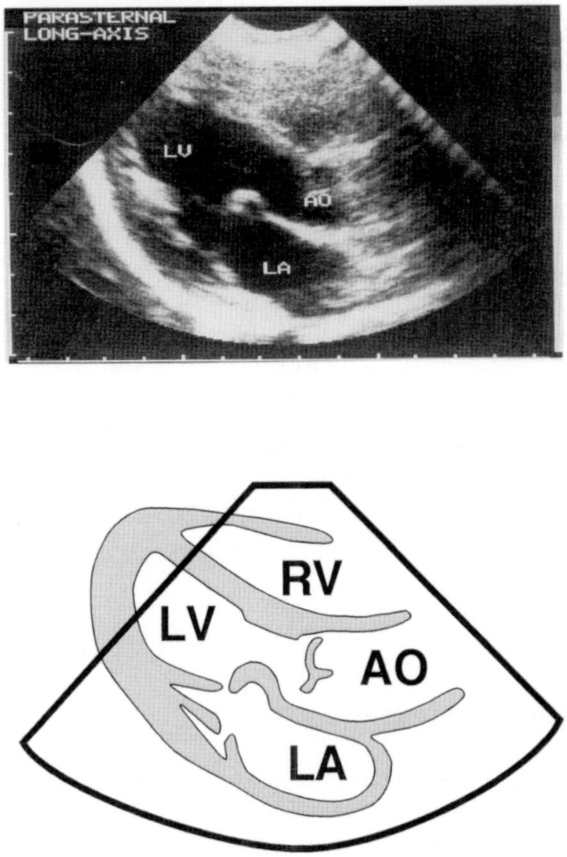

Fig. 76.26. Infective endocarditis: echocardiogram to show floating vegetation on the anterior leaflet of the mitral valve (patient with mitral valve prolapse).

Continue treatment until signs of the infection have gone: this is usually 4–6 weeks.

Annular subvalvular aneurysms of the left ventricle

This rare disease has been seen in Nigeria, Ethiopia and Congo (Abrahams et al., 1962). A curious pouching beneath the aortic or mitral valves forms an aneurysm which may extend inwards into the interventricular septum, upwards into the left atrium, or outwards on to the free border of the left ventricle, easily seen on a chest radiograph (Fig. 76.27). There is not enough evidence to link the disorder with tuberculosis. Patients present with cardiac failure, which may arise suddenly or slowly, mitral or aortic incompetence, systemic emboli from mural thrombi in the aneurysm, or cardiac pain from distortion of the left coronary artery.

DISORDERS OF ARTERIES

Occlusive arterial disease is uncommon in Africa except among the white population of South Africa, but the pattern is changing gradually among urban people with classical risk factors for coronary disease.

Large arteries may be affected by idiopathic 'tropical' aortitis and syphilis; medium-sized arteries are commonly affected by atherosclerosis, or by the giant cell (temporal) arteritis; the arterioles are affected by hypertension and all forms of allergic vasculitis.

Arteries are occluded in three ways.

- By an embolus in the lumen of the vessel: this may arise from left atrial thrombus in rheumatic heart disease, from an infected vegetation in infective endocarditis, from mural thrombus in EMF or intracavitary thrombus in dilated cardiomyopathy.
- By disease primarily of the wall of the vessel, so that the lumen is secondarily affected, as occurs in atherosclerosis. Rarely, a vasospastic alkaloid may lead to occlusion of arterioles, if grain is contaminated with ergot containing fungi. In Ethiopia, wild oats *Avena abyssinica*, infected by the fungus *Claviceps purpurea*, were eaten by people during famine in 1978. Hundreds developed gangrene.
- By pressure from outside the vessel disease: for example by a large benign tumour.

Clinical presentation

Whatever the artery, the symptoms and signs are governed by:

1. the organ or area of tissue supplied by the artery.
2. the balance between tissue needs and tissue arterial perfusion. A stenosed artery may supply adequate blood at rest, but the extra demands of exercise lead to ischaemic pain, typically in cardiac or skeletal muscle, because the vessel cannot accommodate an increased flow. When the exercise stops, the pain is quickly relieved by rest.
3. the speed of arterial occlusion. If this is slow a good collateral circulation can often develop, but if it is abrupt the patient will have sudden severe symptoms. Repetitive minor transient symptoms may precede a major occlusion.

Signs

Changes in the artery

A bruit may be heard over a partially occluded artery, which has no pulsation if it is occluded. Local arteritis causes tenderness, as in giant cell arteritis.

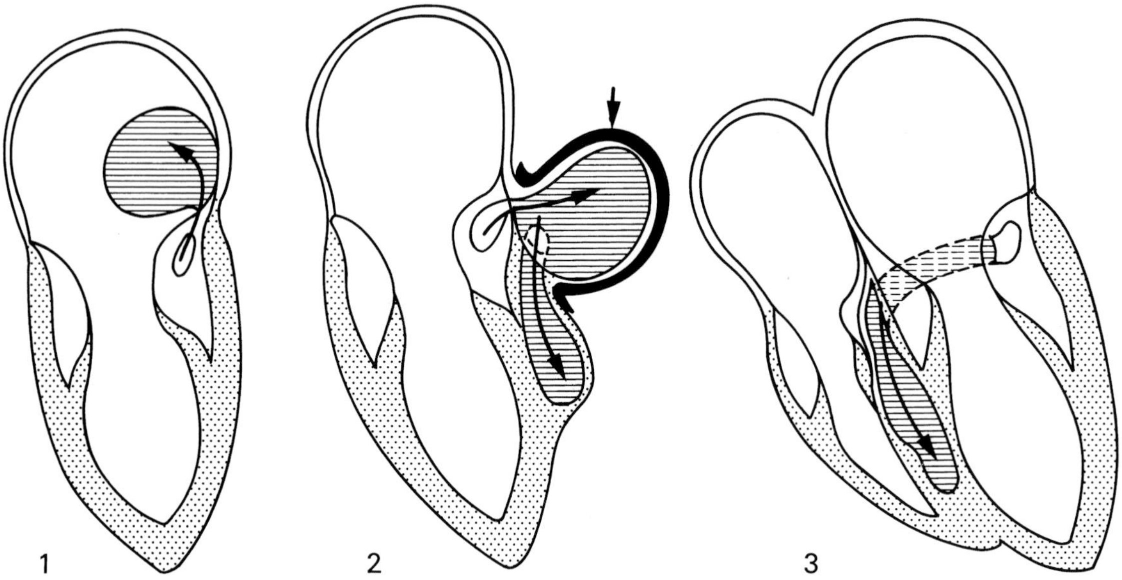

Fig. 76.27. Annular subvalvular aneurysms.

Changes in the tissues

Structural

If, for example, the arteries of the leg are diseased, wounds heal slowly and hairs grow poorly. When a large embolus blocks the iliac or femoral artery, the limb will be cold distal to the block.

If a serous membrane overlies the area of ischaemic tissue, it may secondarily produce signs, as when a pericardial rub is heard if an anterior myocardial infarction is transmural.

Functional

The hemiplegia following cerebral thrombosis or the cardiac failure after coronary thrombosis are examples.

Demonstration of ischaemia

Cause

Angiography can be used to show where an artery is occluded.

Effects

Investigations are useful to confirm tissue necrosis: for example haematuria after renal infarction and raised enzymes or an abnormal ECG after myocardial infarction.

Atherosclerosis

The factors that are responsible for the epidemic of atheromatous disease in industrialized countries – smoking, a diet rich in saturated fat and low in HDL (high density lipoproteins), lack of exercise, diabetes and hypercholesterolaemia – are not yet a problem in Africa.

Pathological changes

Irregularly distributed plaques of lipid, complex carbohydrate, blood, and calcium are laid down on the intima of blood vessels. Plaques may ulcerate, bleed, embolize, act as the source of platelet emboli, or even occlude a vessel. The carotid, vertebrobasilar, coronary, and limb vessels are chiefly affected. In Africa large plaques are uncommon, although fatty streaks and fibrous plaques are seen.

Clinical syndromes

(i) Vertebrobasilar insufficiency and cerebral thrombosis. See Chapter 73, Stroke, and Chapter 86 for neurological disease due to arterial disease.
(ii) Cardiac pain and coronary thrombosis.
(iii) Intermittent claudication and gangrene of the leg. The patient has ischaemic pain in the calf on walking, quickly relieved by rest: risk factors are smoking and diabetes (Adoh et al., 1991).
(iv) Mesenteric artery occlusion – 'intestinal angina' and infarction of the gut.

Coronary arterial disease

This leads to cardiac pain (angina pectoris) or myocardial infarction. The need of the heart for oxygenated blood cannot be met by the flow of blood through narrowed arteries.

Epidemiology

Although risk factors are present among the urban population, particularly when compounded by diabetes mellitus, coronary disease is still rare in sub-Saharan Africa. Rural people eat little saturated fat, smoke few if any cigarettes and have low levels of blood cholesterol: they also take abundant physical exercise.

Cardiac pain

It is a deep pain, characteristically transverse and retrosternal. It may be referred to the distribution of the Tl and T2 dermatome on the inside of the arm, and it may go through to the back or up to the neck. It is typically described as 'pressing' or a 'tightness' in the chest.

Unlike pleural or pericardial pain it is not made worse by breathing. Cardiac pain is usually first noticed when it is provoked by effort ('angina of effort') or emotion. Rest relieves it within minutes. If pain is *not* relieved within a minute or two by rest it is unlikely to be cardiac pain, unless the patient has an acute myocardial infarction when pain persists.

Although cardiac pain in many people is stable over years, it may suddenly become more frequent and is thus provoked by less and less effort: such 'crescendo angina' may herald an imminent acute myocardial infarction.

Angina in a rural African, rarely due to coronary arterial disease, may be caused by a coronary embolus (look for a possible source of emboli), anaemia, or even sickle cell disease.

Myocardial infarction

Symptoms

Prolonged cardiac pain, which is not relieved by rest, is characteristic. Vomiting, nausea and sweating develop in some people.

Old people may have little or no pain and instead present with other symptoms. Some have acute breathlessness due to pulmonary venous congestion, while others complain of dizziness or syncope due to an acute fall in cardiac output which leads to inadequate cerebral perfusion. Sometimes, pericardial or pleural pain mimic myocardial infarction, but in such patients the pain is also altered by respiration.

Signs

The size of the infarct, its effect on the heart, and the associated vasovagal effects govern the signs; thus, there may be a tachycardia and a low arterial pressure, a gallop sound and evidence of systemic and/or pulmonary venous congestion, with sweating and retching. Ventricular ectopic beats are found frequently in the first 48 hours.

Tests

These confirm the damage to the myocardium (serum enzymes) and its site (ECG). A neutrophil leukocytosis develops during the first week.

The enzymes change as follows: increased aspartate aminotransferase AST (formerly glutamic oxaloacetic transaminase), total LDH and LDH isoenzyme 1 (LDH), as well as total creatine phosphokinase (CPK). The most specific of all these for myocardial injury is the CKMB isoenzyme.

Two-dimensional echocardiography is able to visualize areas of reduced or absent myocardial wall motility (dys- or akinesia). Intraventricular thrombus, or paradoxical motility, a sign of a cardiac aneurysm, are well seen on two-dimensional echo.

Management

1. Pain and anxiety. Give morphine, 10 mg or pethidine 50 mg, i.v./i.m. use sparingly.
2. Nitrates or a beta-blocker lower myocardial oxygen consumption: atenolol 50–100 mg daily.
3. Oxygen, and if any signs of cardiac failure, a diuretic, e.g. frusemide 40 mg daily.
4. Vigilance to detect and manage any complication, particularly an arrhythmia, and then to rehabilitate the patient as effectively as possible. When available, electrical defibrillation is needed at once in ventricular fibrillation.

Diseases of the aorta

Atheroma and dissection of the aorta

As aortic atheroma is not severe in Africa, aortic dissection, which begins at an atheromatous plaque and leads to a dissecting aneurysm, is rare: blood, tracking between the coats of the aorta, occludes its branches and causes great pain.

Atheroma and aortic aneurysm

In South African whites, atheroma is responsible overwhelmingly for aortic aneurysm, but more black South

Table 76.5. Idiopathic tropical aortitis/arteritis and syphilis

Syphilis		Idiopathic tropical aortitis/arteritis
Distribution	World-wide	Common in some tropical countries
Cause	*Treponema pailidum*	Unknown: probably not one disease
Age group	Over 35 years	Young people, usually
Effects	Dilatation of aorta	Occlusion and dilatation of arteries
Arteries affected	Thoracic aorta, often ascending aorta	Many: aorta and its branches
Distribution	Continuous	Patchy and segmental
Wall of aorta	Aneurysmal, thin	Thickened, or aneurysmal and thin
Aortic valve	Incompetent, if ascending aorta affected	Very rarely secondarily affected
Histology	Obliterative endarteritis of vasa vasorum with perivascular lymphocytes	Panarteritis: necrosis of elastic tissue of media, adventitial perivascular lymphocytes

Africans are now affected than formerly (Madiba et al., 1999).

Aortitis

Historically, aortitis was due to tertiary syphilis, but this is now less common since penicillin treatment has been widely given for early syphilis (Table 76.5). Dilatation of the ascending aorta stretches the aortic valve ring, so that the valve becomes incompetent.

The treatment is for syphilis, with 1 mega unit procaine penicillin daily for 10 days.

Idiopathic tropical aortitis

An idiopathic aortitis has been defined in Senegal, Ethiopia, Nigeria, and South Africa and very similar cases are seen in West Malaysia (Table 76.5). It is similar to, and is sometimes called Takayasu's disease. This has been linked inconclusively with tuberculosis. Some patients have initial inflammatory phase with arthralgia, myalgia, a neutrophil leukocytosis and raised inflammatory markers such as CRP (Schrire & Asherson, 1964; Seedat, 2000).

Clinical features

These depend on the anatomy of the disease, and its effects on the branches of the aorta, whatever the cause of the aortic disease.

- If the disease affects the ostia of the coronary arteries, it may lead to cardiac pain on effort.
- Disease of the arch may occlude the orifices of its major branches and cause, for example, cerebral ischaemic symptoms, or absent pulses in the arms.
- Disease of the abdominal aorta may occlude a renal artery and lead to hypertension: this is a common presentation in children (Fig. 76.28).
- A large aneurysm anywhere acts as a space-occupying lesion and can cause local pressure, whether on a bronchus (pulmonary collapse), a vertebra (pain in the back), or the great veins (superior mediastinal obstruction).

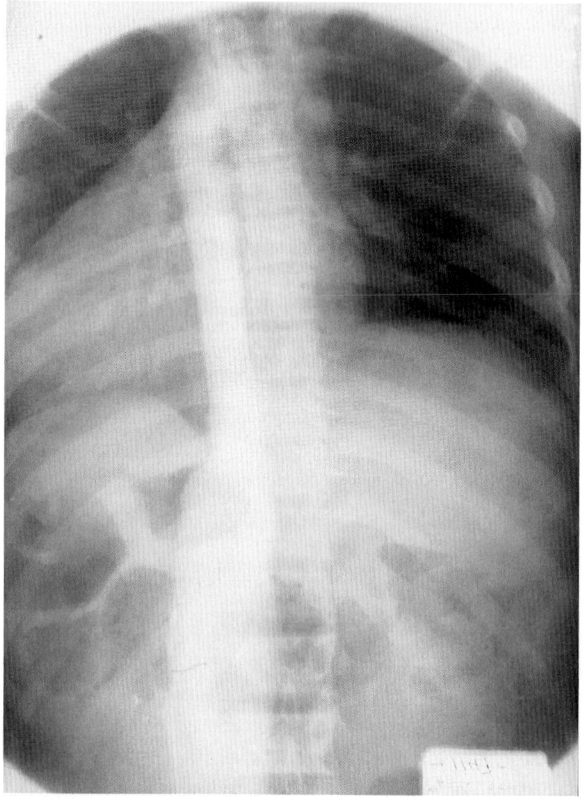

Fig. 76.28. Idiopathic tropical aortitis: aortogram to show dilated aorta in a man who presented with hypertension as a result of left renal artery stenosis.

Diagnosis

The anatomical diagnosis is made from the effects of the arterial disease: a chest radiograph can confirm a thoracic aneurysm.

The aetiological diagnosis is between syphilis and idiopathic aortitis: when there is doubt, biopsy of an artery and negative serology confirm aortitis (Fig. 76.28).

Course and treatment

In South African children with aortic disease, which involved the renal arteries, immunosuppression, aspirin and anti-tuberculosis treatment halted the disease process (Hahn et al., 1998). Prognosis depends on the activity of the disease and the arteries/end organs affected.

DISORDERS OF VEINS

The central problem in Africa is to explain why venous thrombosis, with its sequela of pulmonary embolism, is uncommon.

Superficial thrombophlebitis

This is commonly due to local infection, an intravenous injection, whether in therapy or by a drug addict or an infusion; very rarely, it is due to a carcinoma. The affected vein is tender and warm: for treatment, rest and analgesics alone are needed.

Deep venous thrombosis (DVT)

This is seen more frequently at necropsy than it is detected in life; its provoking factors in African practice are:

- sluggish venous flow: in cardiac failure, immobility after a stroke
- cancer, notably pancreas, stomach, uterus, cervix, and ovary
- increased viscosity of blood–dehydration
- infection – any septicaemia (see peripheral gangrene below)
- the puerperium.

Thrombi form in the deep veins of the calf of the leg, thigh, and pelvis, and, if dislodged, cause pulmonary embolism. It is essential that susceptible patients exercise their calf muscles as a regular discipline to prevent stasis of blood.

Signs

(i) Local inflammation: a local point of tenderness on deep palpation of the calf muscles, or pain if they are gently compressed, or if the foot is dorsiflexed.
(ii) Fever, for which there is no obvious cause.
(iii) Obstruction to venous flow, leading to ankle oedema or an increase in the circumference of the calf, when compared with the other normal side from the same reference point. Therefore, measure the calf in any case in whom a DVT is suspected.

Treatment

Anti-coagulants

Give heparin, 5000 units intravenously as soon as the diagnosis is made: thereafter 500 units per kilogram i.v. in divided doses every 4–6 hours for 7–10 days.

Mobilization

It is essential to get the patient up and moving to prevent further stasis and further thrombi forming.

Pulmonary embolism

When a venous thrombus breaks, an embolus passes to a pulmonary artery, which it occludes.

Large embolus

A major pulmonary artery is blocked, acute cor pulmonale develops (raised *a* wave in jugular pulse, RV gallop sound), the cardiac output falls quickly and the patient may die. ECG shows acute right heart strain.

Recurrent small emboli

In this rare condition, emboli slowly obliterate the pulmonary arterial tree and may only be evident by short episodes of breathlessness. Cor pulmonale follows as the pulmonary vasculature is obliterated, but infarction of the lung is unusual.

Emboli of varying size with pulmonary infarction

The patient develops pleural pain, cough – often with haemoptysis – and a fever, and has a transient shadow at the periphery of the lung in a chest radiograph.

Treatment

(i) Massive embolus (See p. 1346)
(ii) Smaller embolus; heparin 7500 to 10 000 units intravenously every 4–6 h for 48 h (500 U/kg per 24 h), and then subcutaneously for 10 days. Start warfarin on day 7–10, and continue indefinitely if the source or basic cause of emboli cannot be corrected: regulate dose by prothrombin time.

UNUSUAL VASCULAR DISORDERS IN AFRICA

Idiopathic gangrene of the extremities

This has been seen at all ages and in males and females, but it is more common in infants and children. As it is often bilateral, it has also been called 'bilateral symmetrical gangrene'.

Most victims have suggestive evidence of an infection: *S. typhi* and *paratyphi* and *N. meningitidis* have been incriminated. Risk factors are dehydration and malnutrition, which reduce flow and increase viscosity of blood. The syndrome is distinct from ergot or other vasospastic alkaloid poisoning.

Clinical picture

This depends on the primary disease: the child develops sudden fever and malaise, and soon there is often a petechial rash. Larger pulses are palpable. Gangrene develops quickly in the fingers or toes of one or more limbs: the tips of the fingers or toes may be lost.

The nature of the disorder

The syndrome is similar to some cases of severe meningococcal sepsis in which there is rapid depletion of activated protein C, which has anti-coagulant and fibrinolytic properties (Faust et al., 2001). The natural response of the body to restore its disordered haemostatic systems is to activate protein C, but this has a short half-life and so is quickly depleted. The syndrome is best considered as an unusual presentation of an infection, in which the coagulation cascade is activated and in which there may also be local endothelial damage. Aim therefore to define the infection.

Peripheral arteriograms show normal vessels with an irregular lumen, and occlusion of smaller vessels. The histological changes, which resemble those of an arteritis, are not specific. It is not yet known whether the small vascular occlusions in the already gangrenous part of the limb are primary or secondary.

Treatment

- Take blood cultures.
- Treat the primary infection vigorously.
- Restore circulating volume and maintain hydration.
- Look very carefully for changes in signs daily and evidence of further vascular damage.
- Heparin can be tried.

Gangrene associated with tropical phlebitis

Gangrene of the limbs, associated with tropical phlebitis, was described by Gelfand in Zimbabwe and is probably part of the same spectrum of disease as the peripheral gangrene syndrome. There is no seasonal pattern, although patients are often clustered in time.

Pathology

The veins are inflamed, and later thrombosed and occluded. An adjoining artery may also be affected.

Clinical picture

Fever, a painful thrombosed vein, and oedema of the affected limb are seen. The cavernous sinus, the internal jugular vein, or the limb veins have all been affected, but most commonly the femoral veins, on one or both sides. The prognosis is good but gangrene of the hands or feet sometimes follows.

Gangrene associated with acquired haemolytic anaemia

A history of exposure to cold, as the precipitating factor, and high titres of circulating cold agglutinins in the serum have been found. The gangrene has been considered to be due mainly to thrombosis of superficial veins.

Varicose veins

As few people seek treatment, the extent of the problem is not known, but in the countries of the Sahel, and in Tanzania, the prevalence is from 5–10 per cent of the adult population.

References

Abrahams DG. (1962). Endomyocardial fibrosis of the right ventricle *Quart J Med*; **31**: 1–20.

Abrahams DG, Barton J, Cockshott WP et al. (1962). Annular subvalvular left ventricular aneurysms. *Quart J Med*; **31**: 345–360.

Adoh A, Kouassi-Yapo F, N'Dori R et al. (1991). Etiologie des artériopathies des membres inférieurs chez les Noirs Africains à Abidjan. *Cardiol Trop*; **17**: 59–65.

Amoah AG, Kallen C. (2000). Aetiology of heart failure as seen from a National Cardiac Referral Centre in Africa. *Cardiology*; **93**: 11–18.

Andy JJ, Bishara FF. (1982). Obsevations on clinical features of early disease of African endomyocardial fibrosis. *Cardiol Trop*; **8**: 23–33.

Andy JJ, Ogunwo PO, Akpan NA et al. (1998). Helminth associated hypereosinophilia and tropical endomyocardial fibrosis (EMF) in Nigeria *Acta Trop*; **69**: 127–140.

Araoye MA, Olowoyeye O. (1984). The clinical spectrum of hypertensive heart failure: a point score system for solving an old problem. *E Afr Med J*; **61**: 306–315.

Arguedas A, Mohs E. (1992). Prevention of rheumatic fever in Costa Rica. *J Pediatr*; **121**: 569–572.

Barlow JB, Marcus RH, Pocock WA et al. (1990). Mechanisms and management of heart failure in active rheumatic carditis. *S Afr Med J*; **78**: 181–186.

Berrios X, del Campo E, Guzman B et al. (1993). Discontinuing rheumatic fever prophylaxis in selected adolescents and young adults: a prospective study. *Ann Intern Med*; **118**: 401–406.

Bouramonc C, Ekoba J. (1975). Les formes cliniques du béri-béri cardiaque. A propos de 5 observations. *Cardiol Trop*; **1**: 41–48.

Cegielski JP, Rumaiya K, Lallinger GJ et al. (1990). Pericardial disease and human immunodeficiency virus in Dar es Salaam, Tanzania. *Lancet*; **335**: 209–212.

Cenac A, Djibo A. (1998). Postpartum cardiac failure in Sudanese-Sahelian Africa: clinical prevalence in western Niger. *Am J Trop Med Hyg*; **58**: 319–323.

Chauvet J, Kakou Guikahue M, Aka F et al. (1989). La gravité des cardites rheumatismales à Abidjan. A propos de 52 cas à Abidjan chez les enfants de moins de 15 ans. *Cardiol Trop*; **15**: 77–81.

Connor DH, Somers K, Hutt MSR et al. (1967). Endomyocardial fibrosis in Uganda (Davies' disease) Parts I and II. *Am Heart J*; **74**: 687–709 and 1968; **75**: 107–124.

Davidson N Mc D, Parry EHO. (1979). Peripartum cardiac failure. *Quart J Med*; **47**: 431–461.

Davies JNP (1948). Endomyocardial fibrosis. A heart disease of obscure aetiology in Africans. *E Afr Med J*; **25**: 10–16.

Delapenha RA, Alleyne GAO. (1980). The bioavailability of potassium in bananas. *W Ind Med J*; **29**: 117–122.

Desai D, Moodley J, Naidoo D. (1995). Peripartum cardiomyopathy: experiences at King Edward VIII Hospital, Durban, South Africa and a review of the literature. *Trop Doct*; **25**: 118–123.

Edginton ME, Gear JSS. (1982). Rheumatic heart disease in Soweto – a programme for secondary prevention. *S Afr Med J*; **62**: 523–525.

Falase AO. (1979). Heart muscle disease among adult Nigerians: role of nutritional factors in its aetiology. *Eur J Cardiol*; **10**: 197–204.

Falase A O, Kolawole TM. (1980). The radiology of heart muscle disease in adult Africans: further support for hypertension as an aetiological factor. *Cardiol Trop*; **6**: 6–14.

Faust SN, Levin M, Harrison OB et al. (2001). Dysfunction of endothelial protein C activation in severe meningococcal sepsis. *N Engl J Med*; **345**: 408–416.

Figueroa FE, Soledad Fernandez M, Caldes P et al. (2001). Prospective comparison of clinical and echocardiographic diagnosis of rheumatic carditis: long term follow up of patients with subclinical disease *Heart*; **85**: 407–410.

Ford L, Abdullahi A, Anjorin FI et al. (1998). The outcome of peripartum cardiac failure in Zaria, Nigeria. *Quart J Med*; **91**: 93–103.

Freers J, Mugerwa R, Amandua J. (1993). Endomyocardial fibrosis and eosinophilia. *Lancet*; **342**: 1233.

Freers J, Mayanja-Kizza H, Rutakingirwa M et al. (1996a). Endomyocardial fibrosis: why is there striking ascites with little or no peripheral oedema? *Lancet*; **347**: 197.

Freers J, Ziegler J, Mayanja-Kizza H et al. (1996b). Echocardiographic diagnosis of heart disease in Uganda. *Trop Doctor*; **26**: 1–4.

Freers J, Masembe V, Schmauz R et al. (2000). Peritoneal fibrosis and muscle fibrosis are part of the Endomyocardial Fibrosis (EMF) Syndrome. *Lancet*; **355**: 1994.

Gebre-Yohannes A, Rahlenbeck SI. (1998). Coronary heart disease risk factors among blood donors in northwest Ethiopia. *E Afr Med J*; **75**: 485–500.

Hahn D, Thomson PD, Kala U et al. (1998). A review of Takayasu's arteritis in children in Gauteng, South Africa. *Pediatr Nephrol*; **12**: 668–675.

Hakim JG, Manyemba J. (1998). Cardiac disease distribution among patients referred for echocardiography in Harare, Zimbabwe. *Centr Afr J Med*; **44**: 140–144.

Hakim JG, Ternouth I, Mushangi E et al. (2000). Double blind randomized placebo controlled trial of adjunctive prednisolone in the treatment of effusive tuberculous pericarditis in HIV seropositive patients. *Heart*; **84**: 183–188.

Ibrahim-Khalil, Elhag M, Ali E et al. (1992). An epidemiological survey of rheumatic fever and rheumatic heart disease in Sahafa Town, Sudan. *J Epidemiol Commun Hlth*; **46**: 477–499.

Jackson G, Gibbs CR, Davies MK, Lipp GY. (2000). ABC of heart failure. Pathophysiology. *Br Med J*; **320**: 167–170.

Jones T (1992). Criteria. *J Am Med Associ*; **268**: 2069–73.

Kingue S, Kamdajeu R, Ngu BK et al. (1999). Pronostic de la cardiomyopathie dilatée chez le noir africain selon les données échocardiographiques et le degré de l'insuffisance cardiaque *Cardiol Trop*; **25**: 49–53.

Lodenyo HA, McLigeyo S O, Ogola EN (1997). Cardiovascular disease in elderly in-patients at the Kenyatta National Hospital, Nairobi, Kenya. *E Afr Med J*; **74**: 647–651.

Longo-Mbenza B, Bayekula M, Ngiyulu R et al. (1998a). Survey of rheumatic heart disease in schoolchildren of Kinshasa town. *Int J Cardiol*; **63**: 287–294.

Longo-Mbenza B, Seghers KV, Phuati M et al. (1998b). Heart involvement and HIV infection in African patients: determinants of survival. *Int J Cardiol*; **13**: 63–73.

Madiba TE, Mars M, Robbs JV et al. (1999). Aorto-iliac occlusive disease in the different population groups – clinical pattern, risk profile and results of reconstruction. *S Afr Med J*; **89**: 1288–1292.

Malu K, Ticolat R, Renambot I et al. (1991). Enquête épidémiologique sur les myocardopathies chroniques dilatées apparemment primitives: 69 cas. *Cardiol Trop*; **17**: 127–132.

Marcus RH, Sarch P, Pocock W et al. (1994). The spectrum of severe rheumatic valve disease in a developing country. *Ann Intern Med*; **120**: 177–183.

Marin-Neto JA, Maciel BC, Teran Urbanetz LL et al. (1991). High output failure in patients with peripartum cardiomyopathy: a comparative study with dilated cardiomyopathy. *Am Heart J*; **121**: 134–140.

Mayanja-Kizza H, Gerwing E, Rutakingirwa M et al. (2000). Tropical endomyocardial fibrosis in Uganda: the tribal and geographic distribution, and the association with eosinophilia. *Trop Cardiology*; **103**: 45–48.

Mayosi BM, Scott Millar RN, (2000). Permanent cardiac pacing in Africa. *E Afr Med J*; **77**: 339.

Mehta NJ,Khan IA, Mehta RN et al. (2000). HIV-Related pulmonary hypertension: analytic review of 131 cases. *Chest*; **118**: 1133–1141.

Messias-Reason IJ, Hayashi SY, Nisihara RM et al. (2002). Complement activation in infective endocarditis: correlation with extracardiac manifestations and prognosis. *Clin Exp Immunol*; **127**: 310–315.

Okesina AB, Oparinde DP, Akindoyin KA et al. (1999). Prevalence of some risk factors of coronary heart disease in a rural Nigerian population. *E Afr Med J*; **76**: 211–216.

Oli K, Porteous R. (1999). Prevalence of rheumatic heart disease among school children in Addis Ababa. *E Afr Med J*; **76**: 601–605.

Oyoo GO, Ogola EN. (1999). Clinical and socio-demographic aspects of congestive heart failure patients at Kenyatta National Hospital, Nairobi. *E Afr Med J*; **76**: 23–27.

Parry EHO, Abrahams DG. (1965). The natural history of endomyocardial fibrosis. *Quart J Med*; **34**: 383–408.

Po-chun Tai, Spry CJF, Obsen EGJ et al. (1987). Deposits of eosinophil granule proteins in cardiac tissues of patients with endomyocardial fibrosis. *Lancet*; **i**: 643–647.

Rutakingirwa M, Ziegler JL, Newton R et al. (1999). Poverty and eosinophilia are risk factors for endomyocardial fibrosis (EMF) in Uganda. *Trop Med Int Hlth*; **4**: 229–235.

Sanderson JE, Adesanya CO, Anjorin FI et al. (1979). Postpartum cardiac failure – heart failure due to volume overload? *Am Heart J*; **97**: 613–621.

Schrire V, Asherson RA. (1964). Arteritis of the aorta and its major branches. *Quart J Med*; **33**: 439–463.

Seedat YK. (2000). Hypertension in developing nations in sub-Saharan Africa. *J Hum Hypertens*; **14**: 739–747.

Serme D. (1992). Etude épidémiologique, clinique et évolutive de valvulopathies rheumatismales observées à Ouagadougou. *Cardiol Trop*; **18**: 93–99.

Silva-Cardoso J, Moura B, Martins L et al. (1999). Pericardial involvement in human immunodeficiency virus infection *Chest*; **18**: 415–422.

Spry CJF, Davies J, Tai P-C et al. (1982). Clinical features of fifteen patients with the hypereosinophilic syndrome. *Quart J Med*; **52**: 1–22.

Stollerman GH. (1997). Rheumatic fever. *Lancet*; **349**: 935–942.

Strang JIG, Gibson DG, Mitchison DA et al. (1988). Controlled clinical trial of complete open surgical drainage and of prednisolone in treatment of tuberculous pericardial effusion in Transkei. *Lancet*; **ii**: 759–764.

Strang JIG, Gibson DG, Nunn AJ et al. (1987). Controlled trial of prednisolone as adjuvant in treatment of tuberculous constrictive pericarditis in Transkei. *Lancet*; **i**: 1418–1422.

Wragg A, Strang JI. (2000). Tuberculosis pericarditis and HIV infection. *Heart*; **84**: 183–188.

Swai AB, McLarty DG, Kitange HM et al. (1993). Low prevalence of risk factors for coronary heart disease in rural Tanzania. *Int J Epidemiol*; **22**: 651–659.

Strasser T. (1978). Rheumatic fever and rheumatic heart disease in the 1970s. *Wld Hlth Org Bull*, **32**: 18–25.

Ziegler J, Stuiver PC. (1972). Tropical splenomegaly syndrome in a Rwandan kindred in Uganda. *Br Med J*; **3**: 79–82.

The lung

77

The problem in Africa

Respiratory diseases have always caused much disability and death in Africa. The situation now is worse than ever, with the HIV/AIDS pandemic adding a huge additional burden of respiratory disease. Pneumonia and tuberculosis comprise 75–85 per cent of all respiratory cases: bronchial asthma is the third most common. These three major respiratory diseases are described in detail in other chapters: this present chapter describes the underlying anatomy and physiology of the lung and the clinical methods used in diagnosis of respiratory disease. Individual lung diseases are then described, including those associated with HIV/AIDS infection.

The period 1960–90 saw an improvement in mortality rates from respiratory disease but pneumonia and tuberculosis still remained dominant causes of morbidity and mortality. Both have now increased dramatically as the HIV/AIDS pandemic has taken hold across Africa, with soaring mortality rates in every sub-Saharan hospital. It is interesting to look at the pattern of respiratory admissions in five African countries before the HIV/AIDS pandemic (Table 77.1), and to reflect on how much the picture has now changed, with at least 50 per cent of all adult medical hospital admissions in 2002 being due to respiratory complications of AIDS (Buvé et al., 2002).

How the lung works

The respiratory system allows gas exchange between inspired air and blood returning from the tissues. Blood and air are brought into close proximity across the alveolar membrane which separates alveoli and pulmonary capillaries. Several processes are necessary to achieve this contact.

* A substantial portion of this chapter is based on the 2nd edition, where the chapter on lung was written by Bayu Teklu, DA Warrell, and D Femi-Pearse.

Ventilation

Air must be moved in and out of the lungs and distributed through the branching system of airways so that respiratory gases can diffuse in and out of the alveoli. This involves a bellows, the thoracic cage, operated by the respiratory muscles and controlled by the respiratory centres in the medulla.

Pulmonary blood flow

Blood must be distributed through the pulmonary arteries and their branches so that the pulmonary capillary bed is perfused. Perfusion and ventilation must coincide so that gas exchange can take place. The respiratory gases must be combined with blood for transport to the tissues.

Figure 77.1 shows an idealized lung, with normal values for ventilation, perfusion and gas exchange

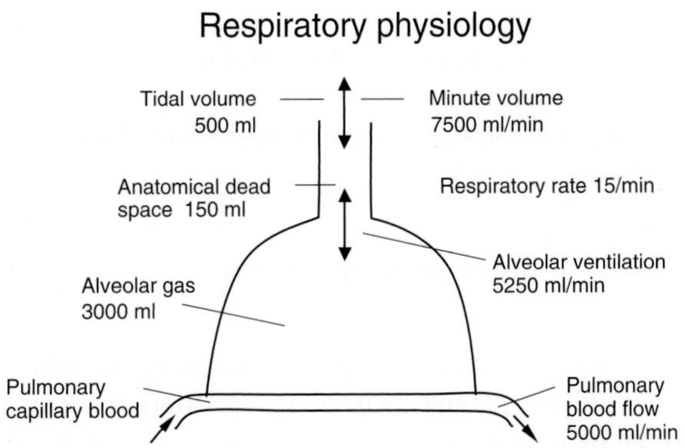

Fig. 77.1. The ideal lung.

Table 77.1. Respiratory admissions to hospital in Africa before the HIV/AIDS pandemic

	Ethiopia	Kenya	Malawi	Nigeria	Uganda
Total medical admissions	2336	2006	2230	1384	5154
Total respiratory disease admissions (% total)	387 (17%)	482 (24%)	494 (22%)	255 (18%)	995 (19%)
Pneumonias	142 (37%)	232 (48%)	384 (78%)	92 (36%)	486 (49%)
Tuberculosis	125 (32%)	126 (26%)		104 (41%)	177 (18%)
Asthma	50 (13%)	47 (10%)	13 (; %)	7 (3%)	68 (7%)
Bronchiectasis	16 (4%)	22 (5%)	8 (2%)	17 (7%)	56 (6%)
Lung abscess	4 (1%)	17 (4%)	10 (2%)	14 (5%)	40 (4%)
Upper respiratory infection	4 (1%)	9 (2%)	16 (3%)		47 (5%)
Acute bronchitis	5 (1%)	18 (4%)			13 (1%)
Chronic bronchitis	5 (1%)		34 (7%)		16 (2%)
Empyema	3 (1%)	2 (0.4%)	6 (1.2%)	8 (3%)	32 (3%)
Lung cancer	10 (3%)	2 (0.4%)	2 (0.4%)	–	
Cor pulmonale	7 (2%)			–	
Sarcoidosis	5 (1%)			–	–
Pulmonary fibrosis	1 (0.25%)	1 (0.2%)		–	10 (1%)
Pleurisy		1 (0.2%)	8(2%)	–	50 (5%)
Pulmonary eosinophilia		6 (1%)		–	
Undiagnosed	10 (3%)			–	
Others				13 (5%)	

Source: From Parry (1982).

The chest bellows

The volume of the thorax is increased by two actions. The ribs move upwards and forwards (pump-handle movement) increasing the front to back diameter of the chest: they also move outwards and upwards (bucket-handle action) increasing the side-to-side diameter. This accounts for one-third of the inspired tidal volume during quiet breathing; the other two-thirds result from the piston-like descent of the diaphragm. During expiration the inspiratory muscles relax, allowing the lungs and thoracic cage to deflate by elastic recoil.

The oxygen consumption of the respiratory muscles increases from 2 ml/min at rest, when about 250 ml/min are being delivered to the body, to 100 ml/min during exercise when 3000 ml/min are going to the remainder of the body.

Control of the respiratory muscles

The depth and frequency of breathing are controlled by the medullary, respiratory centres which direct the respiratory muscles through their innervation. The control of respiration involves:

Changes in blood PO_2, PCO_2 and H^+

Unless the alveoli are sufficiently ventilated to blow off the load of CO_2 produced by metabolism, CO_2 will begin to accumulate in the body and arterial PCO_2 will rise. A rise in PCO_2 (with the related rise in H^+ ions) is detected by central chemoreceptors in the medulla and the ventilatory effort is adjusted accordingly. In contrast, a fall in arterial PO_2 stimulates respiration principally through peripheral chemoreceptors in the carotid bodies. Hypoxia only begins to exert an effect on ventilation when the PO_2 falls below 64 mmHg (8.5 kPa).

Proprioceptive information

Receptors in joints and muscles are important in coordinating the action of the respiratory muscles to product smooth regular breathing, and also the ventilatory response to exercise.

The airways

When the chest cage expands, the lungs must also expand (unless there is a leak into the pleural space). Air is drawn into the respiratory tract. Bulk flow of air reaches as far as the alveolar ducts; the remaining distance to the alveolar gas exchange region is achieved by diffusion. The cross-sectional area of the respiratory tract increases ten-fold from the trachea to the level of the respiratory bronchioles. The surface area of the gas-exchanging respiratory bronchioles and alveoli is enormous – approximately 85 square metres tucked via a myriad of folds into a total volume of only 4 litres. Nearly all the mechanical resistance to breathing is attributable to the resistance to airflow offered by the airways. Airway calibre changes passively with change in lung volume, but it is also determined by the tone of bronchial smooth muscle. Smooth muscle tone is controlled through reflex pathways (vagal constrictor, sympathetic dilator) and the direct action of gases, mediators, and hormones. For example, airway resistance can be increased by suggestion (via the vagus nerve, blocked by atropine) and by inspiring cold or dry air (direct action).

Particles 10–30 microns in radius, which can penetrate the airways, are caught on a carpet of mucus secreted by goblet cells and submucous glands, and carried upwards by ciliary action at a rate of 10–15 mm/min to a level in the trachea whence they can be coughed out. Immunological defences, including secretory IgA, may be involved in inactivating inhaled pathogens.

The alveoli

Gases are exchanged in the alveoli. Figure 77.2 represents the main structural elements in gas exchange, protection against inhaled particles, and the counteracting of surface tension. Alveolar Type I epithelial cells, the interstitial space, and pulmonary capillary endothelial cells constitute the alveolar membrane. Alveolar Type II epithelial cells secrete surfactant (see below), and roving pseudopodial alveolar macrophages and lymphocytes phagocytose tiny inhaled particles (0.3–2 microns radius) or exuded matter.

Alveolar surfactant

The surface tension at the gas–liquid interface inside the alveoli would cause collapse of the alveoli and exudation from the capillaries if it were not for alveolar surfactant. This lipoprotein is secreted by Type II alveolar cells and causes surface tension in the alveoli to decrease during expiration and increase during inspiration. Destruction of the surfactant by breathing a high concentration of oxygen may result in extensive alveolar collapse. Some infants, born before surfactant has begun to be secreted at about the 30th week of pregnancy, have the respiratory distress syndrome of the newborn in which the lungs are very difficult to inflate and an eosinophilic fibrinous exudate is sucked into the alveoli. This exudate led to the descriptive term hyaline membrane disease.

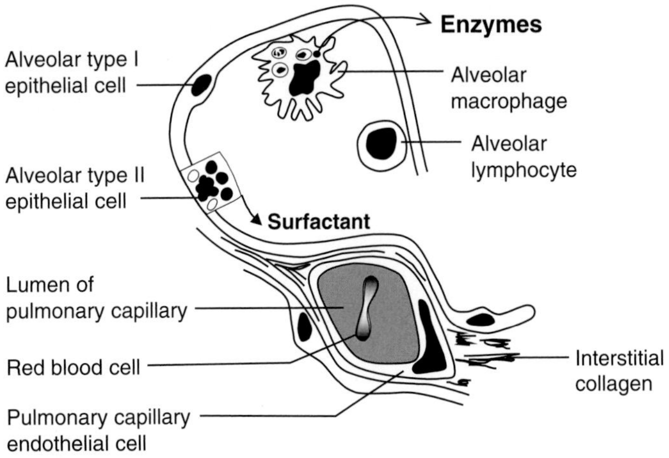

Fig. 77.2. Diagram of the alveolar capillary interface.

Pulmonary blood flow

The pulmonary vascular bed is unique in having to accommodate the entire cardiac output at all times. Large increases in cardiac output (for example, in exercise) produce only slight rises in pulmonary artery pressure, indicating that vascular resistance has fallen. This fall is achieved by opening of previously closed channels (recruitment) and increases in volume of channels which are already opened. This flexibility is lost when areas of the pulmonary vascular bed are destroyed by conditions such as chronic bronchitis and emphysema, extensive pulmonary tuberculosis, and the lung changes associated with mitral stenosis. The normal pulmonary artery pressure has a limited range, but is usually about 26/13 mm Hg with a mean pressure of about 18 mm Hg. The pulmonary vascular resistance is about one-tenth of the systemic vascular resistance. A fall in alveolar PO_2 (for example at high altitude or in respiratory failure) causes pulmonary vasoconstriction and a rise in pulmonary artery pressure. This mechanism, acting regionally, directs blood flow away from poorly ventilated areas.

Distribution of ventilation and perfusion

Ideally, for purposes of gas exchange, blood flow to different areas of the lung should be matched by equivalent alveolar ventilation. When the distributions of ventilation and perfusion do not coincide, gas exchange is impaired, and the compositions of expired gas and arterial blood

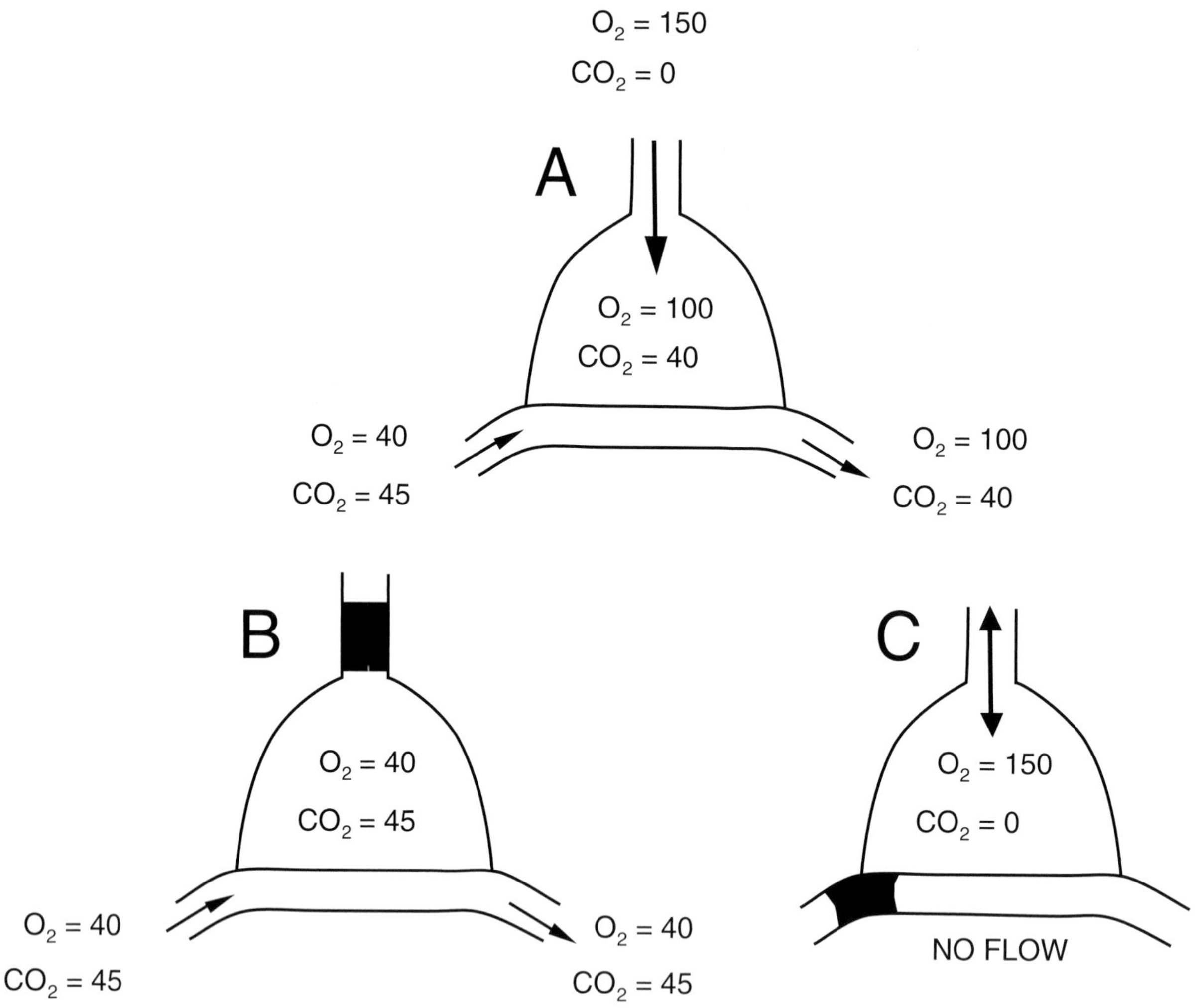

Fig. 77.3. Effect of altered ventilation perfusion ratio. (*a*) shows the ideal relationship between inspired air and perfusing blood. In (*b*) there is a block to ventilation (e.g. by secretion). In (*c*) perfusion is blocked (e.g. by pulmonary embolism). All figures in mm Hg.

are abnormal. Some of the ways in which ventilation and perfusion mismatch can occur are illustrated in Fig. 77.3.

Gas exchange across the alveolar membrane

It was once thought that thickening of the alveolar membrane in disease might, by increasing the barrier to oxygen and carbon dioxide diffusion between alveolar air and pulmonary capillary blood, interfere with gas exchange. In fact respiratory gases are so diffusible that, even in patients with severe pulmonary disease, this happens only on exercise, and in healthy people only when the inspired PO_2 is very low (for example at high altitude, or when anaesthetic or noxious gases are inhaled). By far the most important cause of disturbed pulmonary gas exchange is ventilation/perfusion mismatch. In every disease of the lungs mismatch occurs to some degree.

Oxygen

The terms partial pressure, content, and saturation are all used to describe different facets of oxygen transport.

Partial pressure – PO_2

Inspired air is fully saturated with water vapour by the time it enters the trachea. In a moist gas mixture such as this the partial pressure of a component gas is calculated by multiplying its partial concentration by the total (barometric) pressure after subtracting saturated water vapour pressure. At sea level barometric pressure is 760 mmHg, saturated water vapour pressure is 47 mmHg and oxygen concentration is 20.93%. PO_2 is therefore:

$$\frac{20.93}{100} \times (760-47) = 150 \text{ mmHg (20 kPa)}$$

Content

Liquids in contact with gas mixtures will take up the gases by diffusion until, at equilibrium, the partial pressure of each gas will be the same in both phases. The volume of a gas (in mls at standard temperature pressure, STP) taken up by a given volume (100 ml) of the liquid is known as the content. At a given partial pressure this content depends on the physical solubility of the gas at the prevailing temperature together with any chemical combination between gas and liquid. Equilibrium between alveolar gas and capillary blood is usually achieved by the end of the pulmonary capillary. So, for oxygen, end capillary PO_2 is equal to alveolar PO_2.

The O_2 content of blood consists of physically dissolved O_2 in the plasma and red cells, and chemically combined O_2 in the haemoglobin. For example: physically dissolved O_2 at a body temperature of 37 °C and PO_2 of 100 mmHg = 3 ml per litre blood. Chemically combined O_2 at the same temperature and PO_2 in blood whose haemoglobin concentration is 150 grams per litre = 200 ml per litre.

Saturation

The PO_2 of blood is exerted by physically dissolved oxygen and not by the oxygen in chemical combination with haemoglobin. As the PO_2 in blood increases, more oxygen combines with haemoglobin until eventually at a PO_2 more than 150 mmHg the haemoglobin is saturated with oxygen and no more oxygen can be combined. The relation between per cent saturation of haemoglobin and PO_2 is a complicated one explained by the stepwise combination of oxygen and haem, which results in the familiar oxyhaemoglobin (HbO_2) dissociation curve (Fig. 77.4).

Oxygen saturation at a given PO_2 is independent of haemoglobin concentration but depends on the position of the dissociation curve. The simplest way of describing the position of the curve is the *P*50, the PO_2 at which Hb is 50 per cent saturated. The curve is shifted to the right, with little change in its shape, by increased temperature, PCO_2 (the Bohr effect), hydrogen ion concentration, and 2,3-diphosphoglyceric acid (2,3-DPG) concentration. The effects of 2,3-DPG are of great interest as they may explain shifts to the right in sickle-cell and other anaemias, chronic lung disease, cyanotic heart disease, pregnancy, liver disease, exposure to high altitude, and hyperthyroidism. Carbon monoxide inhalation, for example by tobacco smokers, shifts the curve to the left. A shift to the right reflects decreased affinity of Hb for O_2 (at a given partial pressure), which encourages unloading of oxygen in the tissues. This is advantageous in anaemia and in conditions causing acidosis, such as septicaemia, acute heart failure and respiratory failure.

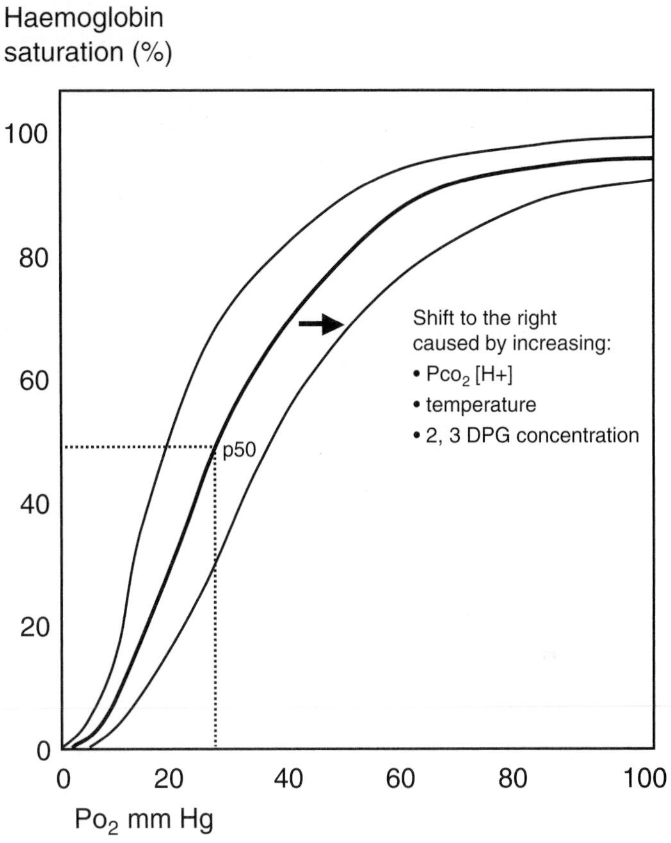

Fig. 77.4. Oxyhaemoglobin dissociation curve.

Carbon dioxide

In contrast CO_2 transport is relatively simple, due to the high solubility of the gas. Large volumes of CO_2, constantly produced from the tissues, are carried dissolved in the plasma or in combination with haemoglobin. The essential reactions are:

$CO_2 + H_2O \rightarrow H_2CO_3$ (reaction catalysed by carbonic anhydrase)

Carbonic acid then dissociates:

$H_2CO_3 \leftrightarrow H^+ + HCO_3^-$

Thus a rise in PCO_2 produces an increase in H^+ and a decrease in pH. This is fundamental to the control of ventilation and acid–base balance.

For further reading on lung function, West's *Respiratory Phsiology, The Essentials*, is recommended (see References).

Symptoms of respiratory disease

Breathlessness (dyspnoea)

The sensation of breathlessness arises when breathing becomes difficult, painful or when the respiratory drive feels excessive. Breathlessness may be caused by various mechanical hindrances to ventilation and by chemical and neural respiratory stimulants; examples of all these are given in Table 77.2.

Diagnosis of breathlessness

History

When breathlessness is a major symptom, it is useful to ask the questions in the Box.

History of breathlessness
When did it start?
How did it start? (suddenly or gradually.)
What was the patient doing when it started (walking, lying down, straining)?
Has it worsened, over a short or long period?
What symptoms are associated with breathlessness (wheeze, cough, haemoptysis, hysterical behaviour)?

It is important to discover whether the breathlessness has progressed over several weeks or months (heart disease, chronic respiratory disease, anaemia), whether it is noticed only during exertion (early stages of heart and lung disease) or also at rest (late stages). Breathlessness made worse by lying flat (orthopnoea) is characteristic of heart failure, but it can also occur in many primarily respiratory diseases. Does it come in attacks with spontaneous recovery especially at night (bronchial asthma and acute pulmonary oedema) and is there is associated wheeze, which the doctor can imitate (bronchial asthma)? Asthmatics may complain of 'tightness' of the chest rather than breathlessness. Local influences must be taken into account. For example, in Malawi, severely dyspnoeic patients often complain of palpitations, but may only later admit to being breathless.

Table 77.2. Causes of breathlessness

Mechanical hindrances (increased work of breathing)
Airflow obstruction – inhaled foreign bodies, bronchial asthma, tumours of larynx or trachea, strangulation
Stiff lungs (reduced compliance) – consolidation, fibrosis, lung entrapment by pleural thickening, pulmonary vascular congestion
Deformed thoracic cage (restricted chest expansion) – kyphoscoliosis, flail chest
Weak respiratory muscles – damage to muscles or nerves (for example, poliomyelitis)
Space-limitation within the thorax – pleural effusion, pneumothorax, distended abdomen (obesity, ascites)
Pleural pain – pleurisy, broken rib

Respiratory stimulants – chemical
Hypoxaemia and hypercapnia – obstructive lung disease
Acidaemia – diabetic keto-acidosis, renal failure, lactic acidosis
Hormones – pregnancy, hepatic coma, catecholamines
Drugs – salicylate overdosage
Anaemia

Respiratory stimulants – neural
1. Pulmonary vascular reflexes – pulmonary oedema, pulmonary embolism
2. Airway reflexes – pneumonia
3. Damage to midbrain and pons – trauma, bleeds, tumours
4. Cerebral cortical overactivity – hysteria and anxiety
5. Fever – via pyrogens and the thermoregulatory centre

Examination

The physical examination of a breathless patient is obviously focused on the respiratory tract, but a full clinical examination is essential because of the wide differential diagnosis given in Table 77.2. The doctor carrying out a physical examination must not forget non-respiratory causes of dyspnoea, which include cardiac disease, anaemia, hyperthyroidism and neurological causes.

Clinical examples of sudden breathlessness

Acute pulmonary oedema

Typically worse at night. The patient is unable to lie down. There may be evidence of heart disease from past history or physical signs.

Bronchial asthma

Typically worse at night or on exertion. Signs of wheeze and airways obstruction but neither signs nor history of heart disease. History of previous similar episodes.

Spontaneous pneumothorax

Comes on suddenly, often during exertion, with unilateral chest pain. Breathlessness is variable: in a fit young person there may be little or none. The chief signs are a normal (or hyper-resonant) percussion note and absent breath sounds on the affected side.

Pulmonary embolism

Begins with sudden chest pain and tightness, often with haemoptysis: signs of acute right heart strain.

The following Box presents a clinical case illustrating difficulties in diagnosing breathlessness.

Clinical example of breathlessness

A young woman of 18 years old was admitted to hospital complaining of general malaise and fever. In the evening the resident was asked to see her, because a nurse observed that she was 'severely breathless and thought that she might be suffering from an asthmatic attack'. The resident examined the patient and saw that she had a decreased conscious level, a respiratory rate of 24 per minute and was taking very deep breaths. The patient's expiratory phase was not prolonged and there were no added sounds on auscultation. Her blood pressure was 75/30 and her temperature was 35.5 °C. On these clinical grounds the resident diagnosed septicaemia. The resident did well in avoiding several potential pitfalls. Firstly, the nurse reported that the patient was breathless which by definition could not be true because the patient was not able to give a history and therefore, could not subjectively complain about breathlessness. Secondly, the nurse suggested the diagnosis of asthma. Again, the resident recognized this to be wrong because of the absence of prolonged expiration and wheezing. Instead, he made the right diagnosis. Later, this young patient was confirmed by blood culture to have a *Salmonella typhimurium* septicaemia. She was also HIV sero-positive. Tragically, she died the next day.

Cough and sputum

Cough is a protective reflex triggered by receptors in the respiratory tract epithelium. The sequence of events is:

(i) deep inspiration
(ii) closure of glottis, apposition of vocal cords, bronchoconstriction
(iii) violent expiration against closed glottis
(iv) sudden opening of glottis and cords releasing a very rapid air flow (960 km/h) through the large airways and clearing large particles trapped in mucus.

Causes of cough

- Inhalation of fumes or particles – tobacco smoke, rock dust, foreign bodies
- Inhalation of allergens – pollens, moulds
- Respiratory tract infections – tracheitis
- Airways invaded by tumour – bronchial carcinoma
- Accumulation of exudate in the airways – pus, mucus, oedema fluid, blood
- Invasion by parasites during migration (Ascaris) or established (Paragonimus, Echinococcus)

Diagnosis of cough

Essential questions about cough are summarized in the Box.

History of cough

When was the onset?
Did it start suddenly after inhaling something, or was it a gradual onset?
Is it getting better or worse?
Is it productive?
Has there been any blood?
Is the sputum clear or coloured?
Are there any accompanying symptoms, such as fever, weight loss, night sweats, wheeze?
Are there any triggering factors such as posture, heartburn (acid reflux), inhalation of specific substances?

Useful pointers

1. For how long has the patient had a cough? This important question often helps to define disease in the setting of a busy polyclinic:
   a few days – acute infection, foreign body
   a few weeks – tuberculosis, cancer
   some years – chronic bronchitis
2. When do the attacks of cough occur, and are they related to a time of day, a season of the year, or work? For example, cough at night with breathlessness and wheeze suggests bronchial asthma or acute pulmonary oedema, whereas attacks at work in a cotton ginnery worker may suggest exposure to a particular dust – byssinosis.
3. Are there any associated allergic manifestations? For example, paroxysmal sneezing, rhinitis, and conjunctival irritation. Asthma itself can present as a cough with few other symptoms
4. Nocturnal cough with heartburn may indicate aspiration – a diagnosis often overlooked

Table 77.3. Common causes of chest pain

Pleuropulmonary disorders	Pleuritic pain Infection Pneumothorax Pulmonary embolism Sickle cell disease Rheumatic pleurisy Mesothelioma Mediastinitis Tracheobronchial pain Tracheobronchitis Malignancy Inhalation trauma
Cardiovascular disorders	Myocardial ischaemia Cardiomyopathy Myocarditis Aortic valve disease Dissection of the aorta Thoracic aneurysm Pericarditis
Gastrointestinal disorders	Reflux oesophagitis Oesophageal motility disorders Peptic ulcer Cholecystitis Pancreatitis Splenic abnormalities
Musculoskeletal disorders	Costochondritis (Tietze's syndrome) Rib fracture Myalgia Malignancy (e.g. Pancoast tumour) Infection (e.g. herpes zoster neuralgia) Nerve compression Spondylitis Sickle cell disease
Skin	Burns Infection (e.g. shingles) Malignancies
Other disorders	Psychiatric Hyperventilation Panic disorders Breast disorders

Sputum

Patients must be asked to describe their sputum, its volume, colour, and consistency. The sputum should be looked at and also examined microscopically with gram stain and Ziehl–Neelsen's stain in all who have had a cough for a month or longer. Sputa in different diseases vary: the list below gives the clinical terms, the patient's descriptions, and their significance.

1. Mucoid: colourless, whitish, jelly-like or frothy (tobacco smoking, chronic bronchitis, bronchial asthma).
2. Purulent: yellow, green, thick, foul smelling or tasting (infection). A blueish tinge may be seen in infection due to *Pseudomonas pyocyanea.*
3. Plugs, casts, spirals: transparent lumps occur in bronchial asthma, and dark hard lumps in allergic aspergillosis.
4. Black: dusts or tobacco tar.
5. Blood-stained: blood may alter sputum so that it appears as:
   (a) pink and frothy – pulmonary oedema;
   (b) red-brown and blood-flecked – pneumococcal pneumonia;
   (c) frankly bloody – pulmonary tuberculosis, paragonimus, pulmonary infarction, bronchial carcinoma, bleeding diathesis (snake bite). Much bright red blood may indicate pulmonary artery erosion by tuberculous granuloma, or ruptured pulmonary veins as in mitral stenosis or bronchiectasis. The fear and stigma of pulmonary tuberculosis may so intimidate a patient who has been coughing blood that he will not admit this symptom at all. Patients with chronic pulmonary suppuration, e.g. bronchiectasis, may complain of foul breath.

Chest pain

There are many causes of chest pain (Table 77.3). As with pain in any part of the body, consider first the anatomical structures at the site of the pain, and the common patterns of pain radiation.

History of chest pain

The Box lists useful questions.

History taking in cases of chest pain

Have you had this pain before?
Where is the pain? Where does it spread?
How did it start?
What makes the pain better or worse?
Is the pain continuous or intermittent? Is it sharp, stabbing or dull?
Are you woken at night by the pain?
Is the pain associated with any other symptoms (breathlessness, cough, sputum)?

Some specific chest pains

Pleural pain

This important and easily recognized type of pain is a localized, usually unilateral pain, often described as being 'sharp' or 'like a needle', which is made worse by taking a deep breath, coughing or twisting the body. This indicates irritation of pain receptors by stretch in the parietal pleura at an area of pleural inflammation overlying infected lung (for example, lobar pneumonia), a broken rib, pericarditis, or pneumothorax.

Retrosternal pain

This is an extremely common and sometimes misleading symptom. It may have the characteristics of cardiac pain (such as radiation to neck, jaws and arms, and association with exertion), but it can also be caused by many different pathologies, including peptic ulcer. Amongst the more common causes in an African setting, pericarditis, pleurisy, sternal trauma, and malignancies must be borne in mind.

Pain with segmental distribution

This arises if nerves to the chest wall are compressed in spinal spondylitis and prolapsed intervertebral disc, or affected by the virus of herpes zoster, when pain precedes the vesicular eruption.

Diaphragmatic irritation

Any inflammatory process adjacent to the diaphragm, whether due to pleurisy associated with pneumonia, hepatic or subphrenic abscess, pericarditis, or perisplenitis, may cause pain to be referred to the shoulder because this has the same segmental nerve supply (C3,4,5) as the central area of the diaphragm.

Examination of the respiratory system

Along with astute history taking, skilled physical examination is still the most important method of clinical diagnosis, particularly in dealing with acute emergencies where facilities such as CT scanning may not be available.

Increased respiratory rate (tachypnoea)

A sustained respiratory rate above 20 per minute in an adult is abnormal. It may be due to high fever alone, or to cardiac and respiratory disease. Sometimes a patient's breaths are so shallow that they are not noticed until dilated nostrils (alae nasi) attract attention.

Exercise tolerance can easily be checked by walking or running with the patient or by getting the patient to run up and down stairs or step on and off a box. Respiratory rate, pulse rate and central cyanosis should be checked before and after the exercise. A portable oximeter, if available, will give invaluable information about the pulse rate and oxygen saturation during this test.

Cyanosis

Cyanosis describes the bluish appearance of tissues whose capillary blood contains an increased amount of deoxygenated haemoglobin (more than 5 grams per cent), or abnormal haemoglobins such as methaemoglobin and sulphaemoglobin.

Peripheral cyanosis

Cyanosis in the exposed extremities is difficult to detect in many African patients, but when it is seen (look at the end of the nose, ears, fingers, toes, and especially the nail beds) it is the result of sluggish blood flow through the capillaries resulting in increased extraction of oxygen by the tissues. Exposure to cold is the commonest cause.

Central cyanosis

This is the only clinical sign of decreased oxygen saturation in the blood and is best looked for in the warm well-perfused central areas such as the tongue and buccal mucosa: a normal subject should be compared at the same time. In Africans the buccal mucosa is often a misleading site in which to look for central cyanosis because of patchy pigmentation. Central cyanosis is not detected until the arterial oxygen saturation is less than 85 per cent (PO_2 about 50 mm Hg), and it can be obscured by thick mucosa and pigmentation. Clinically detectable cyanosis indicates that there are at least 5 grams per 100 ml of deoxygenated haemoglobin in the capillary blood. It follows that clinical cyanosis cannot occur in a severely anaemic patient, whose haemoglobin level may be near or below this figure. Contrariwise a polycythaemic patient with an Hb of say 18 grams per 100 ml may appear markedly cyanosed despite a PO_2 in the normal range (Table 77.4).

Examination of the chest

Inspection

The spine, and the shape of the chest must be examined, because if either is badly deformed respiratory failure

Table 77.4. Causes of central cyanosis

Reduced pulmonary oxygen uptake
This may be due to low PO_2 of inspired air (anaesthesia, or noxious gases, high altitude), reduced total alveolar ventilation (respiratory depression), or ventilation: perfusion mismatch (this arises in many respiratory diseases). In these cases cyanosis may appear only on exercise. It is corrected by breathing a high concentration of oxygen or by voluntary hyperventilation.

Right-to-left shunting of blood
This may occur through regions of lung with no ventilation (collapse, or consolidation in pneumonia); through intracardiac shunts; and through anastomoses between the pulmonary arteries and pulmonary veins. Breathing of oxygen does not usually correct the central cyanosis.

Chemically altered haemoglobins
Methaemoglobin and sulphaemoglobin.

Excessive haemoglobin
Primary and secondary polycythaemia

may follow. The front-to-back diameter should be assessed because it is increased relatively more than the side-to-side diameter in severe airways obstruction. The roundness of the chest wall should be compared on the two sides: a flat area is seen over areas of long-standing contraction due to fibrosis, collapse or surgical resection. The movements of the two sides should be compared

Paradoxical movement, when a section of the chest wall is drawn in during inspiration and pushed out during expiration, is known as flail chest; it is due to fractures in two places of a group of adjacent ribs.

The trachea and mediastinum

The trachea should be gently palpated in the suprasternal notch to find whether it is deviated to the left or right. If it is deviated, immediately define the position of the apex beat, which will be correspondingly displaced if the lower mediastinum is also shifted. In patients with severe airways obstruction the trachea seems to drop into the sternal notch as the accessory muscles contract to pull up the over-inflated thoracic cage during inspiration. The space between the thyroid cartilage and suprasternal notch, which normally admits two or three finger tips, is narrowed. Patients with long-standing emphysema show these signs, often accompanied by 'pursed lip' breathing – a natural method by which pressure inside the airways during expiration can be increased to prevent premature collapse of small airways.

Percussion, palpation, auscultation

The major changes in common disorders are shown in Table 77.5.

Areas of the chest to examine

Both sides should be compared, and the following areas examined:
(i) front – upper lobes
(ii) right axilla – middle lobe
(iii) left axilla – lingula segments of upper lobe
(iv) back – lower lobes.

Percussion over the clavicles is sometimes helpful. A tuberculous cavity or destroyed upper lobe can often be suspected from the simple signs of a flattened upper part of the front of the chest and a dull note to percussion on the clavicle.

Breath sounds

These are high-pitched and so are best heard with the diaphragm. Breath sounds are best heard if the patient is asked to open the mouth and take slow deep breaths. All breath sounds originate in the larynx and large central airways. They are termed bronchial breath sounds, and can easily be heard by placing the stethoscope on the trachea. These coarse sounds are not normally heard peripherally, because the lung tissue acts as an acoustic filter and turns them into rustling distant vesicular sounds. However, when a lobe is consolidated or densely scarred, bronchial breath sounds may be conducted to the stethoscope placed peripherally over the affected part of the lung.

Added sounds

These are described in Table 77.6. For an interesting modern analysis of lung sounds, see Pasterkamp et al., 1997.

Additional helpful signs

Vocal resonance and tactile fremitus

These signs are elicited by asking the patient to say '99' or some equivalent word involving resonant vowel sounds and listening (vocal resonance) or feeling (tactile fremitus) over various parts of the chest. Resonance is conducted through consolidated or densely fibrotic lung and thus increased on auscultation over the affected area.

Table 77.5. Summary of typical signs in some respiratory disorders

	Consolidation (as in lobar pneumonia)	Collapse (due to obstruction of major bronchus)	Pleural effusion	Pneumothorax	Bronchial asthma
Movement of chest wall	Reduced on side affected	Reduced on side affected	Normal or reduced on side affected	Reduced or absent on side affected	Chest hyperexpanded Accessory muscles in use. Laboured
Mediastinal displacement	None	Towards side of lesion	None or towards opposite side if large effusion	None or towards opposite side if tension pneumothorax	None
Percussion note	Dull	Dull	Stony dull	Normal or hyperresonant	Normal
Breath sounds	Bronchial	Diminished or absent	Diminished or absent, occasionally bronchial just above effusion	Very distant or absent	Prolonged expiration, reduced or absent in very severe asthma
Voice sounds	Increased	Reduced or absent	Reduced or absent	Distant or absent	Normal
Added sounds	Crepitations	None	Pleural rub in occasional cases above effusion	None	Polyphonic generalized expiratory wheezing

Tactile fremitus is most useful for detecting pleural effusions – the fluid damps out the resonance and tactile fremitus is thus clearly reduced over the effusion.

Whispering pectoriloquy

This can be detected by asking the patient to whisper. Where there is consolidation or dense fibrosis the whisper is transmitted very distinctly to the stethoscope.

Forced expiratory time (FET)

The patient is asked to take as deep a breath as possible and then to breathe out as quickly as possible, continuing until no more air can be expelled. The expiratory sound is timed while listening over the trachea or sternum. The normal value is 2–3 seconds. An FET of more than 5 seconds suggests significant obstruction (ratio between forced expiratory volume in 1 second and forced vital capacity (FEV1/FVC) less than 65 per cent).

Table 77.6. Added sounds in the diagnosis of chest disease

Sound added	Significance	Example
Heard at the mouth		
Stridor	Large airway obstruction (main bronchi, trachea, larynx)	Foreign body, croup Laryngeal cancer
Audible wheeze	Obstruction in large and medium airways	Bronchial asthma
Heard with stethoscope		
Crepitations (crackles)	Snapping open of small airways, distorted by local disease, or lack of surfactant	Pulmonary oedema Bronchiectasis Pneumonia
Wheeze (rhonchi)	Narrowing of bronchi (exudate, inflammation, or smooth muscle spasm)	Asthma Bronchitis
Pleural rub	Roughening of pleura by inflammation	Pleurisy (pleuritis)

Other useful extra-thoracic signs in respiratory diagnosis

Clubbing of the fingers and toes (Fig. 77.5)

This is first and best seen at the nail fold angles, which become boggy and flat, so that the normal angle is lost. Clubbing is a part of the so-called hypertrophic pulmonary osteo-arthropathy, which in its fully developed state produces not only severe ('drumstick') clubbing but also severe painful arthropathy of wrists and ankles, with periosteal erosions best seen in X-rays of the distal bones of the limbs.

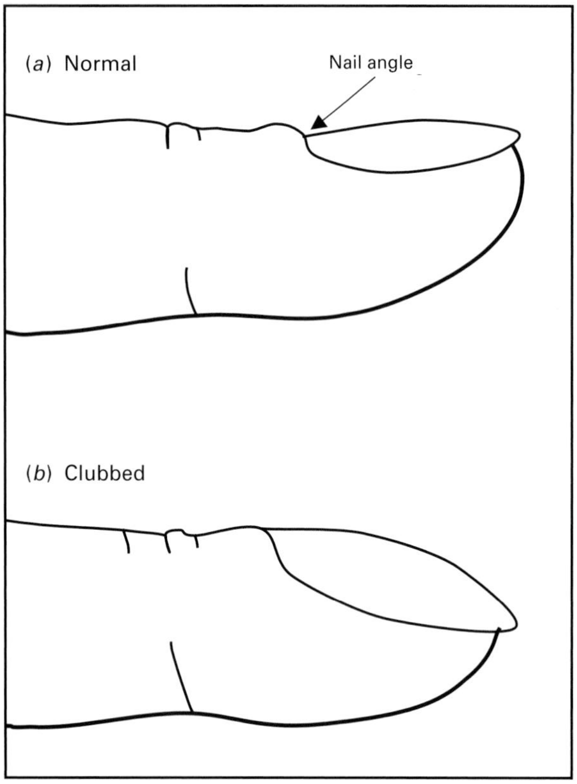

Fig. 77.5. Clubbing.

Table 77.7. Common causes of clubbing

Respiratory
Suppurative intrathoracic conditions:
Lung abscess
Bronchiectasis
Empyaema
Pulmonary fibrosis of any cause
Destructive tuberculosis
Bronchial carcinoma
Lymophocytic interstitial pneumonia (HIV-associated in children)
Gastrointestinal
Severe liver fibrosis
Some malabsorption states
Ulcerative colitis
Cardiac
Infective endocarditis
Cyanotic heart disease, congenital or acquired
Other
Sickle cell disease
Congenital
Traumatic

The mechanism of clubbing is incompletely understood. It is potentially reversible (for example after successful removal of a bronchial carcinoma) and so must be due to circulating humeral factors, perhaps growth hormone (Mito et al., 2001). The common causes of clubbing are in Table 77.7.

Asterixis

This is also called respiratory flap and is similar to the hepatic flap. It is accentuated by dorsiflexing the hands against gentle resistance and waiting for a full minute. A slow irregular flap of the whole hand will be felt at about 20 or fewer flaps per minute. It is caused by CO_2 retention.

Skin

The skin should be inspected for diseases such as Kaposi's sarcoma and wasting. It can be a good indicator of disease (tuberculosis, HIV).

The sputum

This must be carefully examined as part of the examination of the chest.

The cardiovascular system

Not only must signs of pulmonary hypertension and right ventricular failure be looked for, but signs of left ventricular disease also, as the patient with pulmonary oedema may be wrongly thought to have chest disease primarily.

Investigations

Examination of sputum

This gives essential information even when resources are limited. In most cases, expectorated sputum is adequate for examination. However, if the patient is unable to expectorate and the diagnosis is not clear clinically, a transtracheal aspiration is performed. The technique is as follows. The patient who is supine or in a semi-sitting position extends his neck. The skin over the trachea is cleaned thoroughly and the skin over the cricothyroid membrane anaesthetized. A 14-gauge needle is inserted into the trachea. A polyethylene catheter is inserted through the needle into the trachea and the needle then withdrawn. A syringe is attached to the catheter and 5 ml of saline injected rapidly into the trachea. This induces vigorous cough and at this time aspiration is performed. This bronchopulmonary aspirate is good for gram stain and culture is not contaminated by oropharyngeal flora. There is a small risk of bleeding and surgical emphysema following this procedure.

Expectorated sputum should be differentiated from saliva. Saliva contains lots of squamous cells, while sputum will contain many pus cells. Sputum is most useful in patients who have not had antibiotics recently. In those who had even one injection of penicillin, the oropharyngeal flora changes and the gram stain in such cases should be interpreted cautiously.

Macroscopic examination

(already described above)

Microscopic examination

Organisms

(i) Gram stain. To define acute respiratory pathogens, for example, *Streptococcus pneumoniae.*
(ii) Ziehl-Neelsen stain. To demonstrate *Mycobacterium tuberculosis.*
(iii) Ova. Paragonimus, schistosomes, nematodes, or their larvae.
(iv) *Fungal mycelium* can be found, especially if sputum plugs are sectioned, in allergic aspergillosis.

Cells

(i) Polymorphs are seen in pyogenic infections.
(ii) Eosinophils are seen in asthma or pulmonary larva migrans.
(iii) Malignant cells. Sputum cytology, in expert hands, can be used to define squamous cells, oat cells, and adenocarcinomas.

Chest radiography

A chest X-ray is an essential investigation in the diagnosis of many respiratory diseases. Abnormalities in the mediastinum, the heart, the diaphragm, the pleura, the hila, the lungs, the bony structures and the soft tissues can be seen. Normal postero-anterior (or antero-posterior when using a portable X-ray machine) views are sufficient. A lateral view is sometimes needed, particularly for localizing lesions, and for revealing 'hidden' areas behind the heart and the domes of the diaphragms. Figures 77.6 and 77.7 illustrate the value of a lateral chest X-ray.

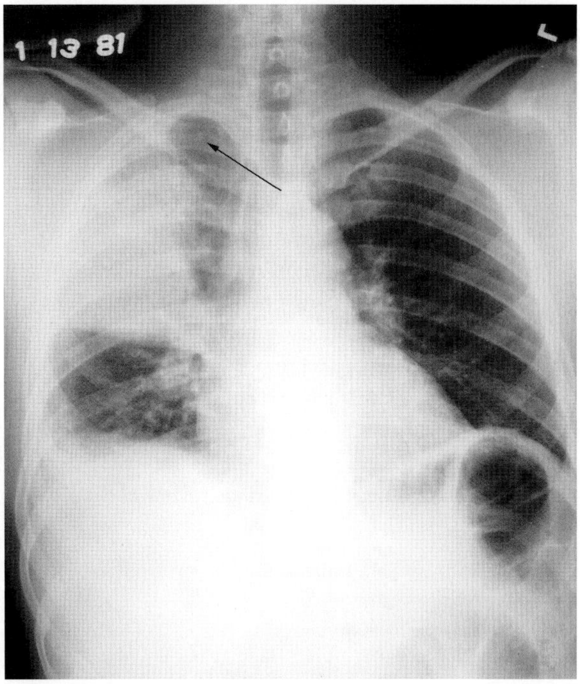

Fig. 77.6. Lobar pneumonia (right upper lobe). Note aerated lung (arrowed) in the right lower lobe, which has expanded up behind the partially collapsed upper lobe.

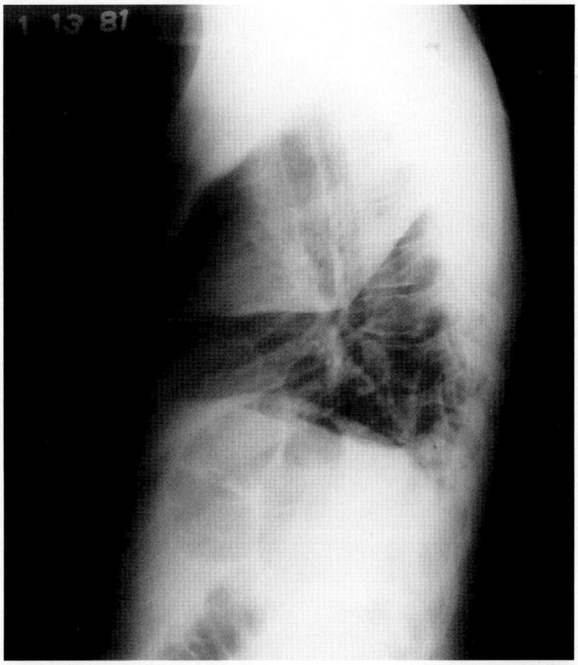

Fig. 77.7. Lateral view of pneumonic consolidation of right upper lobe. Greater and lesser fissures clearly shown.

When reviewing a chest X-ray, always assess the technical quality of the film.

(i) Is it the correct X-ray for the patient (check the name and date)?
(ii) Is the left/right mark correctly set?
(iii) Has the X-ray been taken in full inspiration? X-rays should show the ninth to eleventh rib posteriorly or the seventhth to ninth anteriorly above the diaphragm. Under-expansion may give a false impression of lung densities especially at the lung bases.
(iv) Is there rotation or asymmetry?
(v) What is the technical quality of the image: focus, movement artefact, penetration, is the entire chest on the X-ray?

After this assessment, a systematic review of the X-ray takes place (Fig. 77.8), always following a set pattern so that nothing is overlooked.

An important sign in chest roentgenology is the presence of the silhouette sign. This is the obscuring of normal silhouettes like the cardiac silhouette or the diaphragm because of pathology in the adjacent lung part. Thus a blurred left heart border indicates lingula pathology. Blurring of the right heart border points at middle lobe pathology (Fig. 77.9).

Computed axial tomography (CT scanning)

The advent of the CT scanner has made a profound difference to the accuracy of diagnosis, especially in thoracic medicine. Although CT scanners are still difficult to access in parts of Africa, they will undoubtedly increase, and CT scans are included in the illustrations for this chapter.

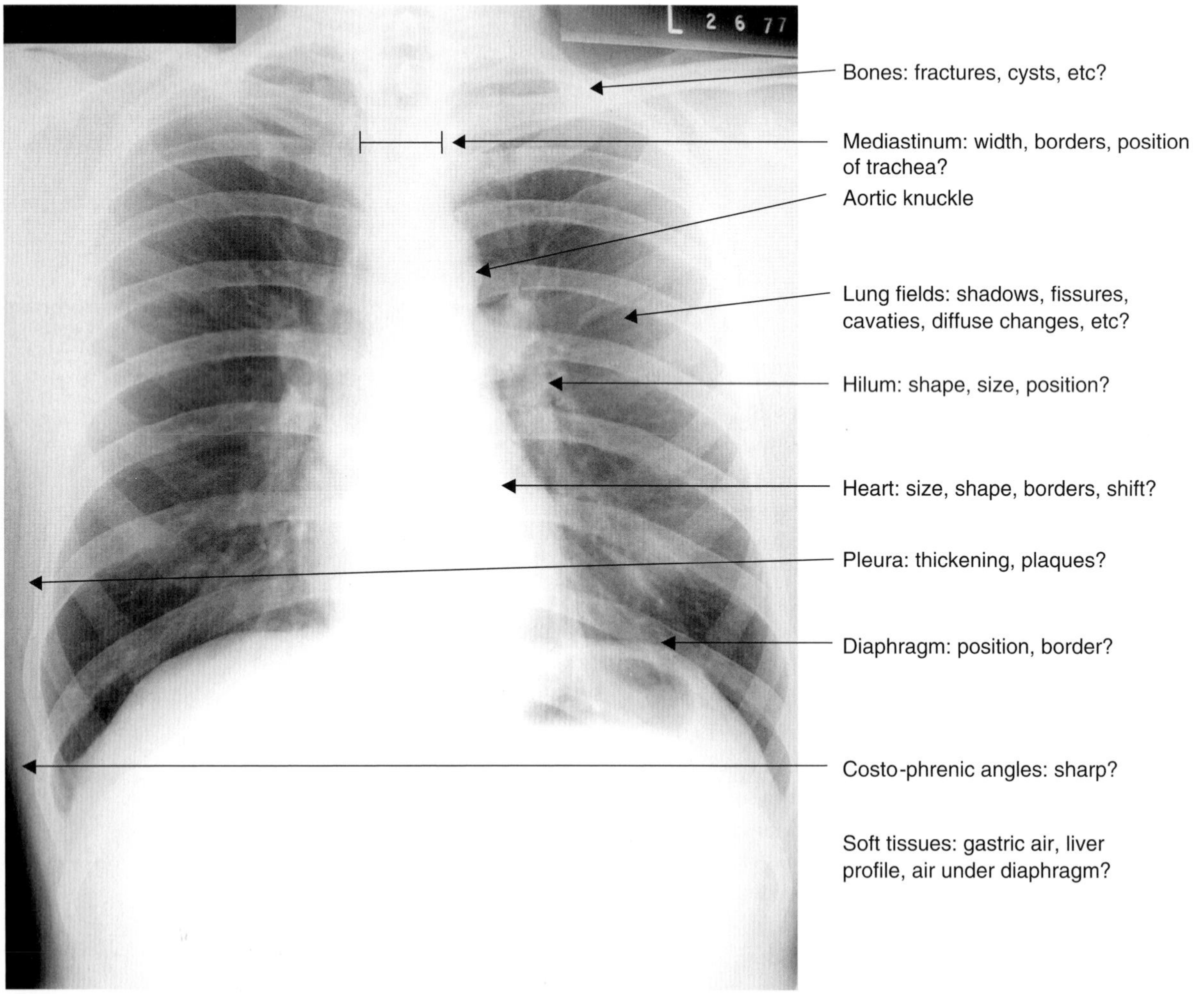

Fig. 77.8. A system for reading a PA chest X-ray.

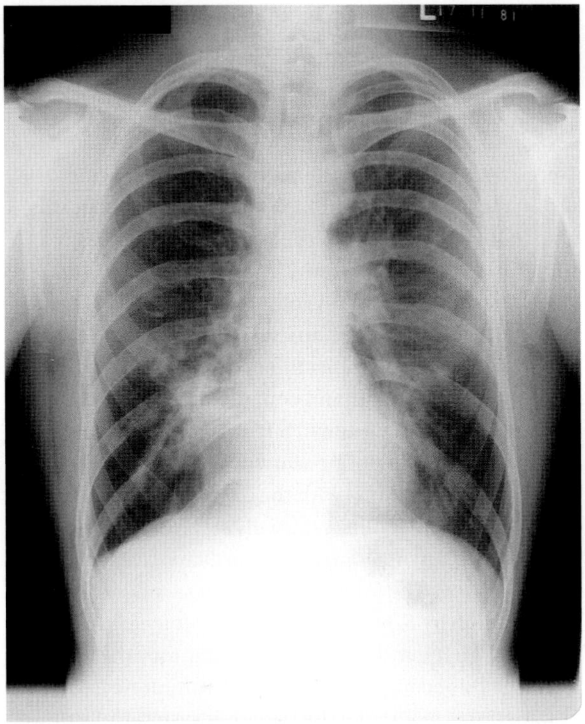

Fig. 77.9. Blurring of the right heart border by overlying middle lobe consolidation.

Bronchoscopy and other invasive diagnostic procedures

Bronchoscopy

There are two techniques: a rigid technique under direct visualization or a flexible technique with fibre-optic visualization, which is now the preferred technique except in the case of foreign bodies – these are still best removed via the rigid bronchoscope, which has a much larger lumen for instrumentation. Bronchoscopy is useful to obtain material for microbiological investigation. Furthermore, it is used to diagnose diseases with endobronchial abnormalities such as bronchial carcinoma or Kaposi's sarcoma.

Other methods to obtain cytological or microbiological material include transthoracic needle biopsy, thoracoscopy, and mediastinoscopy. These are only safely carried out where there are well-developed facilities, including a thoracic surgical service.

Investigation of the pleura

This is covered below under pleural effusions.

Table 77.8. Principal causes of respiratory failure

Low inspired PO_2
high altitude, anaesthesia, noxious gases
Ventilation/perfusion mismatching
Airways obstruction/destruction
foreign body, bronchitis, bronchiolitis, emphysema, bronchiectasis
Damaged gas-exchanging tissue
infections (pneumonia), infiltration, fibrosis
Neural control
Respiratory centres
drugs (morphine, barbiturates), anaesthesia, encephalitis (rabies) trauma, haemorrhage, tumours, primary hypoventilation
Spinal tracts
High cervical dislocation
Inhibitory neurons
tetanus (strychnine)
Anterior horn cells
poliomyelitis
Motor nerves
Guillain–Barré syndrome, Landry's paralysis, diphtheria
Neuro-muscular junction
myasthenia gravis, curariform drugs, snake neurotoxins
Mechanical problems affecting ventilation
Respiratory muscles weakness
poliomyelitis, muscular dystrophy
Thoracic cage deformity
trauma (crush, flail), kyphoscoliosis, Pott's disease
Pleural cavity obliterated
air, effusion, fibrosis
Upper airway obliterated
foreign body, infections (diphtheria, epiglottitis), tumours

Respiratory failure

Respiratory failure is simply defined as inability to keep blood gas tensions within normal limits. When the arterial PCO_2 rises above 50 mmHg (6.5 kPa) or the arterial PO_2 falls below 60 mmHg (10.6 kPa) in a resting patient breathing room air at sea level, respiratory failure is present.

Causes

The many causes of respiratory failure (Table 77.8) fall into four main categories:

(i) Inspiration of air containing reduced oxygen concentration
(ii) Ventilation/perfusion mismatching in the lungs
(iii) Inadequate drive by the respiratory centre or interrupted neural control
(iv) Mechanical impairment of ventilation.

Clinical features of respiratory failure

Symptoms and signs

These are chiefly neurological. Mental confusion, headache, abnormal behaviour, nightmares, drowsiness, and finally unconsciousness and convulsions, are associated with a fall in PO_2 and rise in PCO_2. The patient may or may not feel breathless.

There may be signs due to the primary disease plus neurological signs such as disturbed conscious and depressed reflexes. Coarse flapping tremor of the hands and rarely papilloedema may be present if PCO_2 is raised. Cyanosis should be checked, but is often a difficult sign in Africa.

The plasma bicarbonate may give information about the duration of respiratory failure – a raised level shows that there has been time (days or weeks) for metabolic compensation of respiratory acidosis to take place. Wherever possible, arterial blood gases and continous measurement of oxygen saturation by oximetry provide the surest methods of monitoring the patient in respiratory failure.

Treatment of respiratory failure

The essential components of successful management in all cases are:

- Make an accurate diagnosis of the cause of respiratory failure, and treat it appropriately.
- Whilst making this accurate diagnosis, take whatever emergency measures are necessary to maintain circulating oxygen at a safe level.

For full description of the emergency management of respiratory failure, please refer to the emergency section.

Common respiratory diseases

Introduction

In Africa, respiratory diseases are the most common causes of presentation to health care services. Tuberculosis, pneumonia, and asthma will be discussed in other chapters. Other common respiratory diseases will be described here.

Upper respiratory tract infection (URTI)

Upper respiratory tract infections are very common. They are, in most cases, self-limiting viral infections, but can lead to severe secondary problems in the lower respiratory tract, including bacterial pneumonia.

Rhinitis or the common cold (*coryza*) is an inflammation of the mucosa of the nose. It is in almost all cases viral and caused by droplet infections. It may be associated with pharyngitis and conjuntivitis. Influenza may begin with these symptoms, but with more fever and general prostration. Influenzal tracheo-bronchitis may progress to pneumonia with the danger of serious secondary bacterial infection (especially staphylococcal).

Sinusitis is an infection of the maxillary, frontal or ethmoid sinus. The infection is often a secondary bacterial infection by *S. pneumoniae* or *H. influenzae* following a viral URTI. It may be important to improve the local drainage by decongestive treatment. Antibiotic treatment is sometimes required if the patient is systemically unwell and in pain. Mild sinusitis is self-limiting. Chronic sinusitis may require sinus drainage. Sinusitis may cause a chronic relapsing bronchitis because of the post-nasal drip syndrome, where infectious material from the nasopharynx drips into the lower airways.

Otitis media is an infection of the middle ear due to the same causative organisms as sinusitis. It is treated similarly.

Pharyngitis (sore throat) is an inflammation of the pharynx. The nasopharynx and the tonsils (tonsillitis) can be involved as well. Again, it is mostly viral. The main bacterial cause is *S. pyogenes*. Local abscesses can occur. Complications of streptococcal infections are dealt with in Chapters 36 and 37. Rheumatic fever and its sequelae are described in Chapter 76.

Acute obstructive laryngotracheobronchitis (croup)

The viruses involved are parainfluenza type 1 and 11, respiratory syncytial virus (RSV), adenovirus and influenza A and B. The disease is particularly liable to occur at the beginning of the dry season or at any time when the humidity falls quickly. The disease affects children at any age.

Clinical features

Symptoms start suddenly with an acute upper respiratory infection or coryza. This is rapidly succeeded by cough, inspiratory stridor, severe distress and breathlessness –

demonstrated by increased respiratory rate, use of accessory muscles of respiration, inspiratory stridor, in-drawing of lower intercostal and subcostal areas, cyanosis, and restlessness. Hypoxia is due to ventilation: perfusion mismatch due to inflammatory changes in airways and alveoli. PO_2 is low in most children. The child and his parents become exceedingly alarmed. Treatment is summarized in the Box.

Treatment of croup

There is no time to lose. The most severely ill child may need tracheostomy and intensive care, but this should not be done until the following methods have been tried.

1. Give oxygen in as high a concentration as possible.
2. Antibiotics. A broad-spectrum antibiotic is needed, if the disease persists, to prevent secondary infection with common respiratory pathogens.
3. There is no strong evidence that corticosteroids help during the acute stage, but many experienced paediatricians advise their use.
4. Monitor vital signs carefully: a rising heart rate often indicates increasing hypoxaemia.

Lower respiratory tract infections

Acute bronchitis is often part of a general viral respiratory tract infection. Secondary bacterial infections are mostly due to *S. pneumoniae, H. influenzae, M. catharralis.* In poorly vaccinated populations pertussis due to *Bordetella pertussis* is a problem.

Chronic bronchitis is a part of the syndrome of chronic obstructive pulmonary disease (COPD) dealt with later in this chapter.

Bronchiolitis is an inflammation of the bronchioli. Diffuse bronchiolitis such as bronchiolitis obliterans as part of the diffuse alveolar–interstitial disorders. In small children, it is typically associated with RSV infections (see croup, above).

Pulmonary manifestations of HIV-associated conditions

Respiratory disease is common in patients who are infected with the human immunodeficiency virus (HIV) (Graham et al., 2001). In general, all respiratory diseases that occur in the HIV sero-negative patient also occur in the HIV sero-positive patient. However, these diseases tend to present more seriously and occur more frequently, depending on the severity of suppression of the immune system. Furthermore, in an HIV-positive individual specific diseases can present which are rare or absent in the HIV-negative patient. These diseases can be infectious as well as non-infectious. The risk of developing specific disorders is strongly related to the area of residence, degree of immune suppression, HIV risk group, and use of prophylactic therapies.

Table 77.9. Pulmonary disease in HIV/AIDS

Common
Pulmonary tuberculosis
Bacterial pneumonia
Pulmonary Kaposi's sarcoma
Non-specific interstitial pneumonitis
Cytomegalovirus
Infrequent
Pneumocystis carinii pneumonia
Pulmonary cryptococcosis
Pulmonary nocardiosis
Pulmonary cryptococcosis
Viral pneumonitis
Rare
Mycobacterium avium complex
Pulmonary aspergillosis and candidiasis
Body cavity based lymphoma
T-cell lymphoma

In sub-Saharan Africa the pattern of HIV-related pulmonary disease is different to that encountered in industrialized countries. Several authors emphasize that the prevalence of indigenous pathogens governs this pattern. In particular, *Pneumocystis carinii* pneumonia and infections with *Mycobacterium avium* complex are less common in Africa. Pulmonary tuberculosis and bacterial pneumonia are the most frequent diseases associated with HIV infection (discussed in Chapters 17 and 18). Kaposi's sarcoma and non- specific interstitial pneumonitis are also common (Table 77.9).

Community-acquired pneumonia in the HIV-positive patient

Bacterial pneumonia is frequent in HIV-positive individuals. This is a result of decreased immune protection in the lung. The main reason for this decrease is not known but impaired function of alveolar macrophages, increased $CD8^+$ T-lymphocytes, increased production of cytokines and reduced antigen-specific antibody have been demonstrated (Hirschtick, 1995). Mycobacterial infections increase replication of HIV within lung macrophages.

In general, the clinical picture of pneumonia does not differ from bacterial pneumonia in the HIV-negative person. *Streptococcus pneumoniae* is the leading cause world-wide and particularly in Africa. Pneumococcal pneumonia is often the first presenting disease in HIV infection.

Pulmonary Kaposi's sarcoma

Kaposi's sarcoma (KS) is the most common AIDS associated malignancy in the lung and the third most frequent cause of pulmonary disease in HIV-infected Africans. The reported frequency among HIV-infected patients with pulmonary disease is 8–9 per cent. In HIV-infected patients KS was the cause of 10–45 per cent of pleural effusions (Aboulafia, 2000). There is a strong correlation between cutaneous KS and pulmonary KS: the appearance of respiratory symptoms in patients with cutaneous KS is predictive of pulmonary KS in 21–40 per cent of patients. At necropsy, in 38–75 per cent of cases with cutaneous KS, evidence of intrathoracic KS was found. Nevertheless, cutaneous KS may be absent in some patients. KS is assumed to be a malignancy of a multipotential cell of mesenchymal derivation. Histologically, this gives rise to the typical 'spindle cells' described in KS lesions. The recently discovered Kaposi's sarcoma herpes virus (KSHV or HHV-8) has been identified as the most likely causative agent.

Symptoms

KS is insidious in most cases and is often not symptomatic. It may also be associated with non-specific symptoms such as progressive dyspnoea, non-productive cough, mild haemoptysis, lower chest pain, and fever. The latter is mostly related to a concomitant infection.

Radiology

KS may present with no abnormalities (5–20 per cent). Two major patterns that correspond well with the pathological findings have been described: perihilar linear densities that follow septal lines (40 per cent), and single or multiple macronodular opacities (40 per cent). Either of these patterns can be seen in 70 per cent. In addition, large bilateral pleural effusions have been observed in 7–50 per cent of chest radiographs. (Pleural aspirates are blood-stained in almost all cases.)

Clinical course

Survival time for untreated patients is usually less than 4 months, although patients without symptoms may survive several years. Chemotherapy and/or radiation treatment prolongs this by a mean period of 2–4 weeks. Therefore, treatment is usually palliative. The high cost limits the availability of such treatment in Africa.

Non-specific interstitial pneumonitis

Non-specific interstitial pneumonitis (NSIP) is a poorly understood pulmonary complication of HIV infection. It probably represents a spectrum of lymphoproliferative processes that overlap, rather than a distinct illness. In adults, NSIP seems to be the clinical equivalent of HIV-related lymphoid interstitial pneumonitis (LIP) in children, although the histological appearance differs. HIV itself or a yet-to-be-determined infectious agent may play a causative role. The reported frequency of this condition ranges between 10 and 38 per cent. Clinical presentation and radiographic findings are not specific and a transbronchial biopsy by bronchoscopy or open lung biopsy is required for definitive diagnosis.

Most NSIP presents with a gradual onset of dyspnoea, with or without cough, and chest radiographs showing diffuse infiltrates. Clinically, it can resemble smear-negative tuberculosis or *Pneumocystis carinii* pneumonia but occurs when the CD4 and total lymphocyte counts are still preserved. The pneumonitis resolves spontaneously or responds to steroids, and does not itself lead directly to the patient's death. It does, however, appear to mark a downturn in the course of HIV infection.

Pneumocystis carinii pneumonia

Before the era of highly active antiretroviral therapy *P. carinii* pneumonia (PCP) was the commonest opportunistic infection seen in the lung (>80 per cent in the course of HIV infection) in the developed world. In Africa it is probably less frequent, though considerably underreported (Ruffini & Madhi, 2002; Hargreaves et al., 2001). *P. carinii* has recently been classified as a fungus.

Clinically, PCP presents with a subacute onset of dyspnoea (tachypnoea with a respiratory rate >40), dry cough and fever with a moderate to severe hypoxaemia (SaO_2 typically <85 per cent at rest, falling to <60 per cent on exertion). The fall in oxygen saturation on even trivial exertion is a striking and pathognomonic feature. The chest X-ray shows asymmetric or bilateral infiltrates, but may be normal. No radiographic pattern is pathognomonic. The diagnosis depends on identification of the organism in pulmonary specimen, either via induced sputum (yield 30–85 per cent), via broncho-alveolar lavage (yield over 95 per cent in AIDS), or via biopsy specimens (yield over 95 per cent).

Treatment of PCP is with high dose cotrimoxazole, 120 mg/kg for 3 weeks, together with prednisolone 1mg/kg when there is severe hypoxaemia. Alternatives are pentamidine, dapsone, or clindamycin. Oxygen in high percentage should be given whenever possible.

Others

Incidental reports have been made of pulmonary manifestations of opportunistic infection with more unusual organisms.

- *Nocardia asteroides* presents with one or more nodules/masses, cavitation, consolidation/infiltrates, and pleural thickening. In a post-mortem study in Ivory Coast the prevalence in 247 HIV-positive patients was 4 per cent. Pulmonary nocardiosis is treated with cotrimoxazole 60 mg/kg in two divided doses.
- Infections with *Cryptococcus neoformans* present mostly as meningitis. Nevertheless, pulmonary cryptococcosis can also occur without neurological involvement. It is often in combination with other pulmonary disease such as PTB or KS. In a bronchoscopy study in Rwanda *C. neoformans* was found in 13 per cent of HIV-positive patients with pulmonary disease; in 3.6 per cent the lung was the sole site and there was no meningitis. Treatment is with either fluconazole, itraconazole or amphotericin B.
- *Mycobacterium avium* complex (MAC) is uncommon in sub-Saharan Africa. It is often disseminated at presentation. Because of the limited diagnostic facilities in most district and central hospitals it will probably be missed as it occurs in the occasional patient only.
- *Aspergillus fumigatus* and *Candida albicans* are thought to be less important in HIV. Therefore, HIV-related cases are uncommon. However, they are increasingly reported in association with established AIDS.
- *Histoplasma capsulatum, Blastomyces dermatitidis* and *Coccidioides immitis* have also been described as opportunistic pulmonary infections, but are thought to be very rare or absent in Africa.
- All known viral pneumonias can manifest in the HIV-positive patient. However, cytomegalovirus (CMV) is specifically related to HIV infection and other immunosuppresive states. In almost 100 per cent of the HIV-infected persons evidence of the presence of CMV can be found. The exact role of CMV is still not completely understood. Furthermore, HIV itself can give an acute pneumonitis 1–3 weeks after infection, which is completely reversible.
- Finally, HIV-associated malignancies should be mentioned. Besides pulmonary KS, lymphomas, such as the rare B-cell lymphoma the body cavity based lymphoma (BCBL), and T-cell lymphoproliferative malignancies may occur in the lung (as can leukaemia).

Finally in this section on respiratory complications of HIV, the Box presents a summary of three practical points for clinicians dealing with the ever-growing number of patients.

Practical points in dealing with respiratory complications of HIV

1. There is a strong correlation of cutaneous KS and pulmonary KS: the appearence of respiratory symptoms in patients with cutaneous KS is highly predictive of pulmonary KS.
2. When in presumed smear-negative PTB there is no improvement on anti-tuberculous treatment, non-specific pneumonitis, pulmonary KS or PCP should be considered. Bronchoscopy is indicated, if available.
3. When in doubt: tuberculosis, tuberculosis, tuberculosis.

Pleural disease

The pleura consists of visceral and parietal layers lined with mesothelium richly supplied with blood vessels and lymphatics. The function of the cavity is to allow all regions of the lung to be freely and evenly inflated and deflated during respiration. Air, or any sort of fluid in the cavity, compresses the lung and eventually makes it collapse. Leaks of air into the pleural cavity (pneumothorax), either from the lung and airways or through the chest wall, prevent the development of negative intrapleural pressure which is needed to draw open the lung with each breath.

Pleural effusion

Pathogenesis

Normally, there is only very little fluid in the pleural cavity to act as a lubricant. The accumulation of fluid in the pleural and other body cavities is governed by the same factors that determine the formation of oedema in tissue – capillary permeability; oncotic, hydrostatic, and tissue pressures; and lymphatic drainage. In disease this delicate equilibrium is upset and a pleural effusion develops. The principal mechanisms and causes of pleural effusion are given in Table 77.10. The only primary pleural tumour is the mesothelioma, which is common among asbestos workers in South Africa. Some common secondary tumours, often responsible for pleural effusion, are breast, lung, and ovary (in decreasing order of frequency).

Table 77.10. Pleural effusions

Mechanism	Type of pleural fluid	Clinical examples
Increased capillary permeability	exudate: high protein content (>30 g/1) high specific gravity (>1016) high LDH (>200 IU)	Infection: 1. Tuberculosis 2. Bacterial pneumonias Inflammation: 1. Malignant disease 2. Rheumatic fever 3. Collagen diseases Infarction of the lung
Increased capillary hydrostatic pressure	transudate: low protein content (<30 g/1) low specific gravity(<1016) low LDH (<200 IU)	Cardiac failure, constrictive pericarditis Acute glomerulonephritis Pulmonary vein thrombosis
Decreased plasma oncotic pressure (hypoproteinaemia)	transudate: very low protein content	Hepatic cirrhosis, nephrotic syndrome, protein malnutrition, protein-losing gastro-enteropathy
Decreased lymphatic drainage	transudate: moderate protein content	Infiltration or obliteration of lymphatics by cancer
Leakage into pleural cavity resulting from damage to vessels or viscera, or draining through diaphragmatic lymphatics	blood (haemothorax) pus (empyema) chyle (chylothorax) exudate/transudate	Trauma or malignant invasion of lung, chest wall, great vessels, etc. Pneumothorax Subphrenic abscess, amoebic liver abscess Filariasis, lymphoma, trauma to thoracic duct Miscellaneous conditions, including pancreatitis, hepatic cirrhosis, malignant invasions of pleural lymphatics

Clinical features

Symptoms

Pain from the parietal pleura is usually well localized, but central diaphragmatic pleural pain may be referred to the shoulders or abdomen (where it may be confused with an acute abdomen). Respiration is rapid and shallow because it is painful: large pleural effusions also cause breathlessness.

Signs (Table 77.5)

More than 500 ml free fluid can be detected by clinical signs. Tactile fremitus, percussion note, vocal resonance, and breath sounds are all reduced over an effusion. The earliest signs are usually detected at the base posteriorly. If the effusion is large, dullness extends up into the axilla. A very large effusion may shift the trachea and the heart towards the opposite side, and reduce movements on the affected side.

Radiology

Effusions of more than 250 ml may be seen as blunting of the costophrenic angle in the postero-anterior film (Fig. 77.10), or of the vertebrophrenic angle in the lateral view. The upper limit of the uniform opacity caused by larger effusions curves upwards into the axilla (PA view) (Fig. 77.11) unless there is a hydropneumothorax (Fig. 77.12). Left and right lateral decubitus films may reveal even smaller amounts of fluid and differentiate between pleural fluid, pleural thickening, and encysted (loculated) fluid. Interlobar effusions are detectable only by radiographs.

Pleural biopsy

Pleural biopsy remains a useful diagnostic tool, although it is one that needs skill and repeated practice. The method is described in the next Box.

Complications of biopsy and aspiration

- Pneumothorax
- Haemothorax
- Air embolism if the visceral pleura is punctured or nicked
- Implantation of tumour in the needle track
- Painful mediastinal shift, unilateral pulmonary oedema and circulatory collapse if too much fluid is removed.

Examination of pleural fluid

Appearance

This is often helpful – whether blood-stained, purulent, chylous, etc.

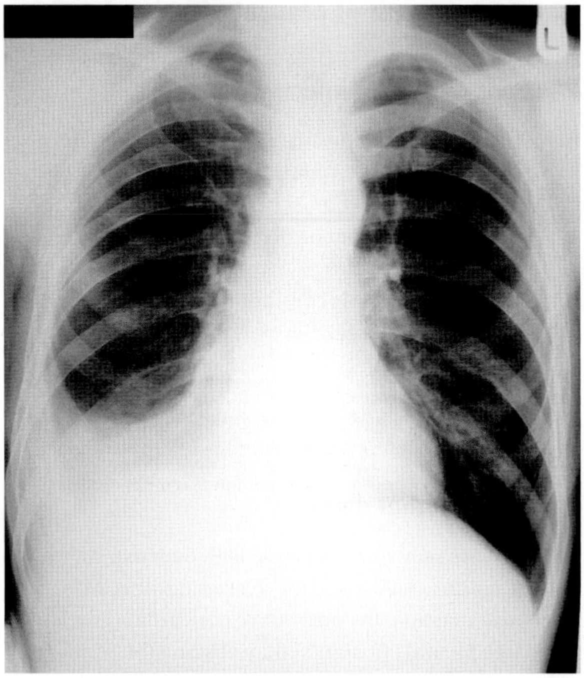

Fig. 77.10. A small right pleural effusion, with underlying collapse of the right middle and lower lobes.

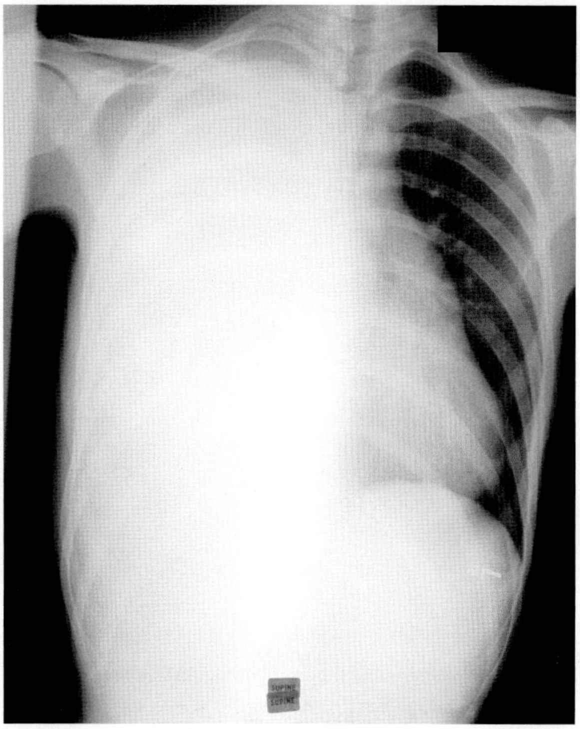

Fig. 77.11. A large right pleural diffusion causing mediastinal shift to the left (adenocarcinoma of lung and pleura).

Pleural biopsy and aspiration

1. First localize the effusion by percussion and radiography. When aspiration is planned, make certain the patient is seated comfortably, leaning forward. Do not attempt a biopsy if there is very little fluid.
2. If the effusion is not loculated, choose a point in the axilla posteriorly which is well above the diaphragm and two intercostal spaces below the determined upper border of the effusion.
3. Infiltrate the skin with local anaesthetic, connect a 3.75 cm 21-gauge needle and, choosing a point immediately above the upper border of the rib, advance the needle gently, aspirate frequently, and introduce more local anaesthetic. The patient feels a sharp pain as the needle penetrates the parietal pleura. Irritation of the visceral pleura often causes coughing. Unless fluid is freely aspirated, another point should be chosen.
4. Having found the site of the effusion, a 5-mm long nick in the skin is made with a scalpel blade and a silk suture placed loosely in place (eventually to close the wound).
5. The Abrams punch biopsy needle, connected to an aspirating syringe with the aperture closed, is introduced, and when the needle is judged to be in the pleural space the aperture is opened and fluid aspirated as required.
6. If the fluid is freely aspirated, it is safe to proceed with pleural biopsy. The notch is directed along the intercostal space (if it is pointed upwards to the lower border of the rib, there is a danger of cutting the intercostal vessels and nerve) and, while tension is applied along the space, the needle is slowly withdrawn until the notch is felt to catch on the pleura. The biopsy is then taken and the needle withdrawn while an assistant tightens the skin suture.
7. Fluid should be aspirated up to a total of 600 ml over 15 minutes or unless the patient becomes distressed. While the needle is in the pleural space, it should not be opened to the air during inspiration, or air will be sucked into the space.
8. A chest radiograph should be taken to check that a pneumothorax has not been induced.

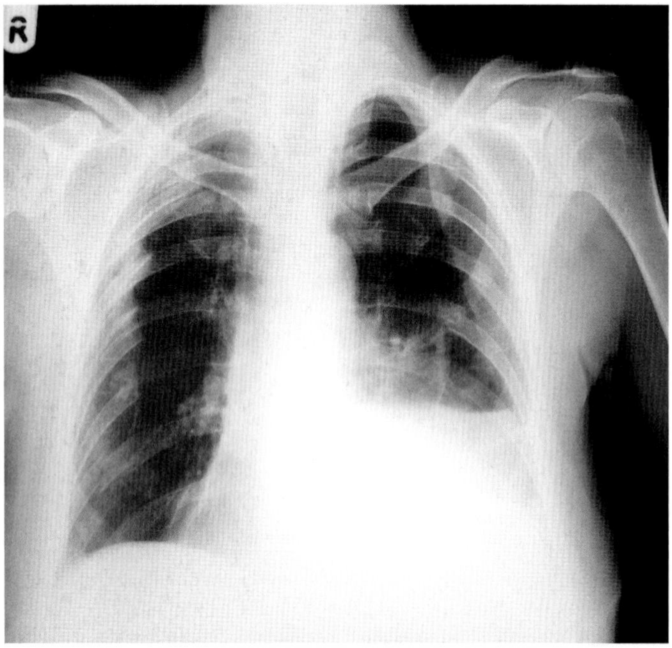

Fig. 77.12. Hydropneumothorax following rib fractures in a road accident.

Smell

Foul smelling fluid suggests anaerobic bacterial infection.

Microscopy

This is essential. Red cells suggest injury, infarct or any cancer, but may be found in tuberculosis; polymorphs denote any acute pyogenic infection (empyema); lymphocytes are found in a chronic effusion, particularly tuberculosis (counts of 50–1000 cells/mm^3); and eosinophils in tuberculosis, parasitic diseases, and asthma. Fluid should be centrifuged and the sediment stained by gram and Ziehl–Neelsen's stains and examined cytologically for malignant cells. Culture for bacteria, tuberculosis or fungi may be appropriate.

Protein content and biochemistry

A fluid which clots contains much protein and is an exudate. Both transudates and exudates are usually pale yellow or brown. The distinction between transudate and exudate is important (Table 77.10). Other biochemical tests are seldom used but include glucose (reduced in tuberculosis, secondary cancer, and rheumatoid pleurisy); amylase (exceeds serum level in pancreatitis); cholesterol (increased in tuberculosis and rheumatoid pleurisy); and triglycerides (raised in chylous fluid).

Important types of pleural effusion in Africa

Effusions related to infection

(i) Pneumonia. An effusion after *Strep. pneumoniae, Staph. aureus,* and *Klebsiella pneumoniae* is quite common. The fluid must be aspirated again and again until none can be detected. Surgical drainage may be necessary.

(ii) Tuberculosis. This is commonly incidental to obvious lung disease. Pleural biopsy is most useful in diagnosis.

(iii) Amoebic liver abscess may cause a small right-sided effusion.

Effusions in other diseases

Effusions are seen in any disease with oedema, such as cardiac failure, cirrhosis of the liver, and sometimes hypoproteinaemia. In constrictive pericarditis and EMF a very large pleural effusion(s) may obscure the primary cardiac disease: this may also happen in Burkitt's lymphoma, or any other cancer including bronchogenic cancer.

Management of recurrent pleural effusions

The commonest causes of recurrent pleural effusions are metastatic cancers, but other common diseases like hepatic cirrhosis can cause persistent effusions. The treatment, therefore, is symptomatic: to reduce pain and discomfort and also relieve respiratory distress. If fluid is drained it usually reaccumulates promptly, and medical pleurodesis should be tried to prevent this. The steps in pleurodesis are in the Box.

Medical pleurodesis

1. Drain the pleural effusion as completely as possible with a pleural drain overnight.
2. Instil an agent designed to cause inflammation in the pleura, causing the 2 layers to adhere permanently together and thus eliminating the pleural space. The agents often used are dextrose (50% solution) and tetracycline (200mg in solution)
3. Leave the pleural drain in situ for another 24 hours, and encourage the patient to lie flat on the affected side after installation to distribute the agent in the pleural cavity.
4. Pain from pleurodesis may be severe. Ensure adequate analgesia.

If medical pleurodesis fails, surgical pleurodesis may be successful. This can either be by talc poudrage through a

Table 77.11. Causes of pneumothorax

- Ruptured apical sub-pleural bleb: the commonest cause of spontaneous pneumothorax in otherwise healthy young men
- Tuberculosis: rupture of a cavity or abscess of the wall of an airway (bronchopleural fistula)
- Pyogenic lung abscess, which may rupture into the pleural cavity (especially staphylococcal lung abscess in children)
- Chronic obstructive bronchitis and emphysema: a large bulla may rupture
- Bronchial asthma
- Chest injuries: fractured ribs especially in road traffic accidents
- Neoplasms, such as primary carcinoma of lung or oesophagus
- Pulmonary fibrosis, pneumoconiosis, or rarely a connective tissue disease

thoracoscope, or by thoracotomy and surgical pleurectomy or pleurodesis.

Pneumothorax

Air may enter the pleural cavity either through a penetrating injury through the chest wall (traumatic pneumothorax) or as a result of rupture of part of the lung or airway (spontaneous pneumothorax) (Table 77.11).

Pathophysiology

Normally, the visceral and parietal layers of the pleura are separated by a thin layer of fluid. Due to its elastic tissue, the lung is trying to shrink while the chest wall is trying to expand like a compressed spring. These two forces create negative pressure in the pleural cavity. Any communication between the pleural cavity and the outside air, or air inside the bronchi, allows air to be sucked in. The lung shrinks and the chest wall expands until the intrapleural pressure is no longer negative. Usually, the communicating hole closes and the trapped air is slowly reabsorbed, but if the hole has a valve action, air drawn into the pleural cavity during inspiration does not escape during expiration, and so accumulates. Intrapleural pressure rises and creates a dangerous tension pneumothorax.

Clinical features

Symptoms

Sudden pleural pain, and breathlessness, which may get quickly worse as air accumulates in the pleural cavity and the lung collapses, are typical. Patients with established lung disease may become severely breathless and develop acute respiratory failure.

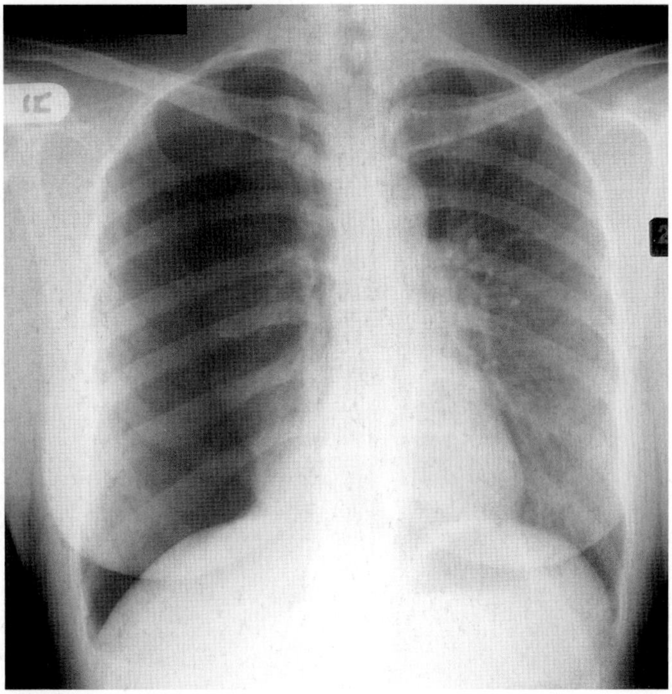

Fig. 77.13. Right pneumothorax, with lung approximately 60% collapsed.

Signs (Table 77.5)

Breathlessness, with absent or diminished breath sounds on one side of the chest, which may be more resonant to percussion than the other side, is characteristic. If a tension pneumothorax develops, the primary disease or injury, for example road accident trauma or pulmonary tuberculosis, may divert attention from the significance of dyspnoea, central cyanosis, low blood pressure, and rapid pulse. Urgent treatment is essential.

Radiology

A minor pneumothorax can be easily overlooked, but usually the PA chest X-ray makes the diagnosis obvious (Figs. 77.13 and 77.14). Watch for signs of mediatinal shift, an indication of a tension pneumothorax, needing urgent action.

Treatment

The urgency and vigour of treatment depend on the underlying lung disease; the size of the pneumothorax;

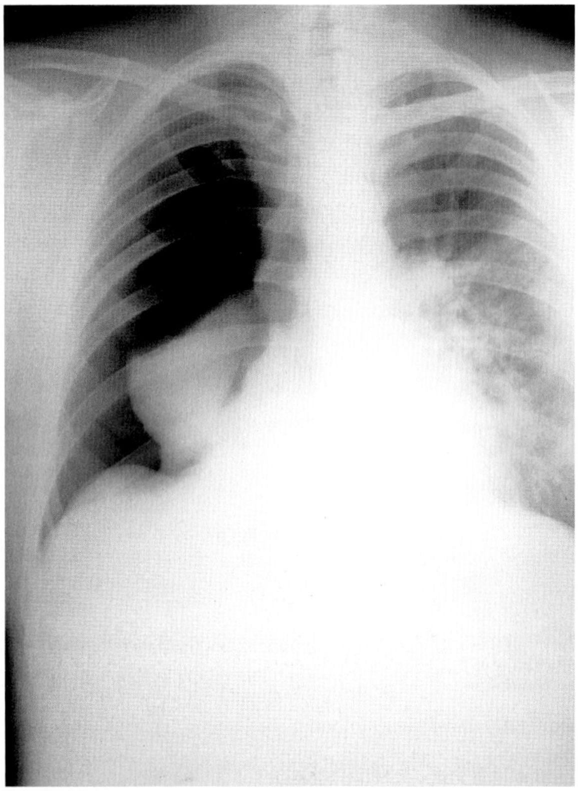

Fig. 77.14. Right pneumothorax, with lung completely collapsed.

whether it is uni- or bilateral; and whether it is open, closed or tension.

A small pneumothorax can safely be left to be reabsorbed unless the patient has old severe lung disease and cannot afford to lose any pulmonary function even for a short time. Tension pneumothorax is always an emergency.

A pneumothorax which involves more than one-third of the area of the thorax (on the PA film) is best treated by continuous suction through an intercostal drain and underwater seal. Recurrent pneumothorax is treated by obliterating the pleural cavity surgically (pleurectomy, decortication), or by exciting fibrosis with an irritant such as talc powder or blood.

Complications

Bleeding, infection, irreversible lung collapse, respiratory failure, cardiac failure, and surgical emphysema, occur acutely; a chronic effusion may be associated with a rigid thickened pleura.

Prognosis

Twenty per cent of spontaneous pneumothoraces recur within a year; some may last for more than three months. In an otherwise healthy individual with pneumothorax, re-expansion of the lung occurs at a rate of 1.25 per cent per day. Full re-expansion may take 3–10 weeks. A follow up chest X-ray is necessary to exclude underlying disease.

Pulmonary embolism

The epidemiology of pulmonary embolism in Africa is unknown. There is no evidence that thrombotic disease is less frequent in Africans as compared to other races. An Ethiopian study showed a comparable prevalence (Gebremedhin & Shamebo, 1998). Venous thrombosis and pulmonary embolism must be in the differential diagnosis of breathless patients, particularly if any of the following risk factors are present:

- recent air travel, or long-distance road journeys
- use of the contraceptive pill, or hormone replacement therapy
- recent surgery
- recent diabetic ketoacidosis
- any debilitating illness with associated inactivity
- any cancer.

Small pulmonary emboli may cause symptoms of pleural pain, dyspnoea and fever. On physical examination there is tachypnoea, cyanosis, tachycardia or sometimes a pleural rub. The diagnosis in primary health facilities is very difficult, and a high index of suspicion is required if cases are not to be missed. Clinical examination in severe cases may reveal signs of acute right heart failure (raised JVP and left parasternal heave), and there will be a sustained tachycardia due to anxiety and hypoxaemia. An ECG may show the S1Q3T3 pattern of acute right ventricular strain.

In fully equipped referral centres the diagnosis is made by ventilation/perfusion scintigraphy, high resolution CT scanning, and/or pulmonary artery angiography.

Treatment

Intravenous heparin should be started when there is strong suspicion of acute pulmonary embolus. Low molecular weight heparin now offers a useful method of anti-coagulation without the need for laboratory monitoring, but it is expensive. Long-term warfarin is given empirically for 3 to 6 months after acute pulmonary embolism, but this can only be done safely if regular laboratory monitoring of INR is available.

Bronchopulmonary suppuration

Lung abscess, empyema, and bronchiectasis are common in Africa as a result of inadequate care of pulmonary infections such as pneumonia.

Lung abscess

This is defined as suppuration and necrosis in the substance of the lung. Table 77.12 gives the common causes.

Clinical features

Lung abscess should be suspected if any patient with pneumonia starts to cough up copious purulent foul-smelling sputum, or develops clubbing of the fingers, or has a renewed high fever. Physical signs are finger clubbing, and (if the abscess is large) dullness to percussion, reduced breath sounds, and crackles.

Radiology

At first, this shows a homogeneous shadow, but a cavity with a fluid level develops quickly when the abscess connects to a bronchus, and may resemble a cavitated tuberculous lesion, carcinoma, or infected pulmonary infarct (Fig. 77.15). Sometimes the abscess is so large that it may resemble a pyopneumothorax, but beware of aspirating the pleural cavity, for fear of creating an empyema which could have been avoided by correct management of a lung abscess.

Treatment

The guiding principles are:

1. To kill the organisms, often a mixed flora, with the appropriate antibiotic, which may have to be given for 4–6 weeks. Give benzylpenicillin 2–4 mega units every 6 h (this dose may have to be given i.v.), or metronidazole 400 mg every 6 h, because anaerobic organisms, indicated by foul smelling pus, are common.
2. To drain pus by postural percussion and coughing.
3. To do a bronchoscopy if a foreign body or cancer is suspected.

If all these methods fail and the abscess does not close, the affected lobe may have to be removed surgically.

Table 77.12. Common causes of lung abscess

1. After aspiration of vomitus in an alcoholic bout (a common weekend problem in new industrial centres such as Harare, Zimbabwe), anaesthesia, inhalation of a foreign body, or aspiration of anything else from the mouth like infected material in sinusitis, dental caries, or pyorrhoea
2. As a complication of pneumonia due to *Staphylococcus aureus* or *Klebsiella pneumoniae*, when abscesses are multiple. *Strep. pneumoniae* is also an important cause of lung abscess, usually a solitary abscess in a lower lobe
3. When an infected pulmonary infarct breaks down
4. When an amoebic liver abscess spreads up through the diaphragm (rare now)
5. When a carcinoma blocks a bronchus

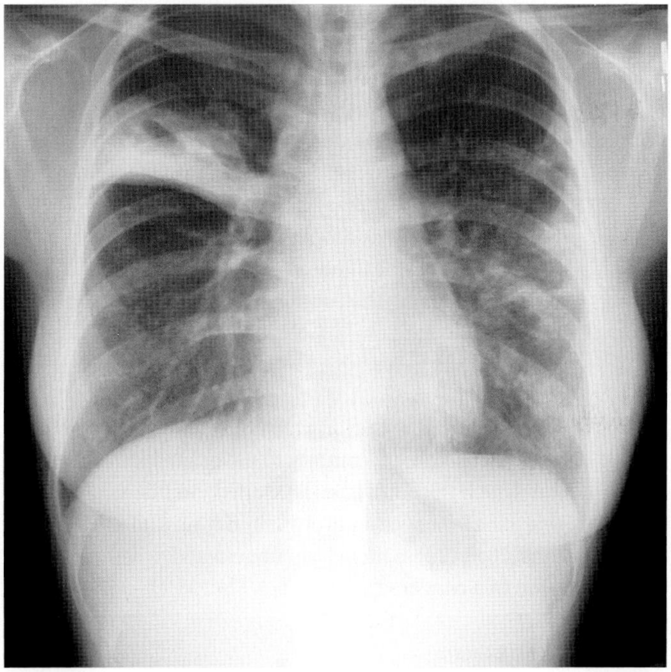

Fig. 77.15. A small lung abscess in an area of consolidation in the right upper lobe (anterior segment).

Empyema

This is defined as purulent pleural effusion. It may arise acutely or may complicate chronic infection. It is a most important problem in infancy and childhood. By far the most common and important cause is an extension of infection from infected lung, whether due to pneumonia, lung abscess tuberculosis, or more rarely bronchiectasis. Empyema may also arise when an amoebic abscess spreads upwards from the liver, when severe trauma to the chest is complicated by infection or when the oesophagus ruptures.

The commonest infecting organisms are *Staphylococcus aureus, Strep. pneumoniae* (adults), *Strep. pyogenes*, and anaerobic streptococci.

Clinical features

In many patients with pneumonia a purulent pleural effusion is not suspected until the patient fails to improve, his temperature rises again, or signs of fluid are detected at the base of the lung. A radiograph may help if the empyema is large, but it is often indecisive if the lung is consolidated beneath it. It is essential to aspirate fluid, examine it for cells and organisms, and to culture it. In patients with amoebic empyema the fluid may show high serum alanine amino transferase and alkaline phosphatase.

Treatment

Antibiotics

Penicillin or chloramphenicol should always be tried first if no laboratory help is available.

Removal of pus

This is essential. Aspirate as much as possible daily. If pus does not flow through the needle, a chest drainage tube should be put into an intercostal space, connected to an underwater seal. Loculation of empyema cavities often prevents adequate drainage: streptokinase can be instilled to help break down fibrin and aid drainage. Measure the volume of pus every day. Thereafter it is a matter of watching the volume of the pus and its systemic effects on the patient.

Pyopneumothorax

This indicates that the lung has broken down and perforated, presumably secondary to the original infection from which the empyema developed. An intercostal drain is essential: most cases eventually dry up and the air is reabsorbed unless there is an undetected tuberculous lesion or a cancer.

Decortication

In some patients surgical decortication of thick fibrinous empyema wall is needed.

Bronchiectasis

Bronchiectasis is an anatomical or morphological term which means stretching or dilatation of bronchi. It is proved by bronchography, CT scanning or by morbid anatomical examination. The abnormality is not only dilatation, but there is considerable distortion and stenosis of involved bronchi.

Bronchiectasis is important and common all over Africa: it follows childhood respiratory infections – particularly measles and pertussis; chronic collapse of a lobe whose bronchus is compressed by hilar nodes; and lobar pneumonia.

Pathogenesis

Two factors are responsible for bronchial dilatation:

(i) Obstruction of bronchus. This causes collapse of surrounding alveoli, and the negative intrapleural pressure pulls directly on the bronchial wall so that it dilates.

(ii) Infection of bronchial wall with destruction of elastic tissue and muscle. If infected secretions are retained in the bronchi, an inflammatory reaction takes place throughout the bronchial wall, damaging the muscle and elastic tissue so that the bronchus must inevitably dilate. Children are susceptible to the effects of obstruction and infection because:
   - The small bronchus of a child makes obstruction more likely.
   - The interalveolar pores of a child are few and, therefore, collateral circulation of ventilation is poor and lung collapse more likely.
   - The bronchus of a child is softer and more easily damaged.

Common causes

Bacterial pneumonias following measles and whooping cough are important causes of bronchial obstruction and infection. In Africa, tuberculosis is also a frequent cause of bronchiectasis, chiefly when tuberculous glands obstruct the middle-lobe bronchus and cause collapse, or rupture into the bronchus to cause endobronchitis of the middle and lower lobes.

Clinical features

These are due to:

- local inflammation within the bronchi – cough with purulent sputum, worst in the morning, and haemoptysis from time to time, with signs of persistent coarse crepitations over the affected lobe and patchy or cystic shadows in the chest radiograph.
- loss of normal drainage and defective epithelium in bronchi – recurrent infections.
- chronic pulmonary suppuration – clubbing of the fingers.
- metastatic abscesses – chiefly cerebral.

Diagnosis

Before the advent of CT scanning, this was by bronchography. This invasive and unpleasant test has now been superseded completely by CT scanning, which provides precise visualization of the site and extent of bronchiectatic disease (Fig. 77.16).

Treatment

The principles of treatment are shown in the Box.

> **Principles of treatment in chronic bronchiectasis**
>
> To promote drainage of infected secretions; this is best done every morning. The patient should bend over a chair and get someone to percuss over bases of the lungs until no more sputum is produced.
>
> To give the appropriate antibiotic as soon as a secondary infection lung occurs.
>
> Only rarely is surgical treatment advisable – if the patient has much pus which cannot be dried up, and the disease is strictly limited to one lobe.

Pulmonary manifestations of tropical diseases

In this section the pulmonary manifestations or complications of the classical tropical diseases are discussed. HIV-associated parasitic pulmonary conditions such as pulmonary toxoplasmosis and cryptosporidiosis are not discussed here.

Helminthic infection

Some helminthic infections can have pulmonary manifestations. The best known is the *Löffler syndrome.* This is a syndrome of non-productive cough, low grade fever, chest pain, urticaria and asthma. There is a marked eosinophilia and transient, recurrent infiltrates on chest X-ray (Fig. 77.17). The syndrome can be idiopathic, but in Africa it is mostly secondary to the passage through the lungs of the larvae of *Ascaris lumbricoides* or in a lesser extent of *Necator americanus, Ankylostoma duodenale* or *Strongyloides stercoralis.* The course of the syndrome is normally a spontaneous resolution within 8–10 days. The treatment is with anthelminthic drugs such as mebendazole. In severe cases with systemic illness a course of oral steroids (for example, prednisolone 30 mg daily for 2 weeks, reducing rapidly afterwards) can be highly effective.

Strongyloides stercoralis

Strongyloides infections can be very persistent with recurrent re-infections and larva migrans (see Chapters 21–31). The recurrent lung passages can cause chronic respiratory symptoms like cough and asthma. Immune suppression, for example in AIDS, can cause hyperinfection

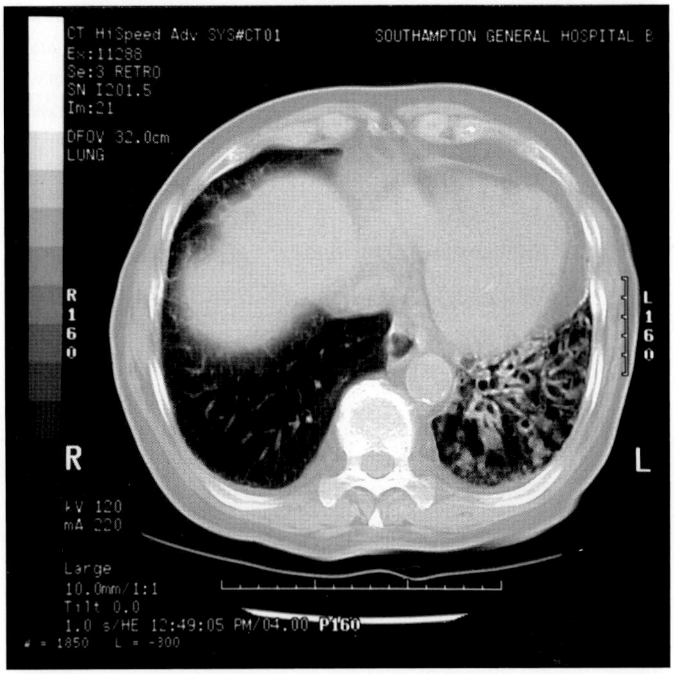

Fig. 77.16. CT scan showing bronchiectasis of the left lower lobe.

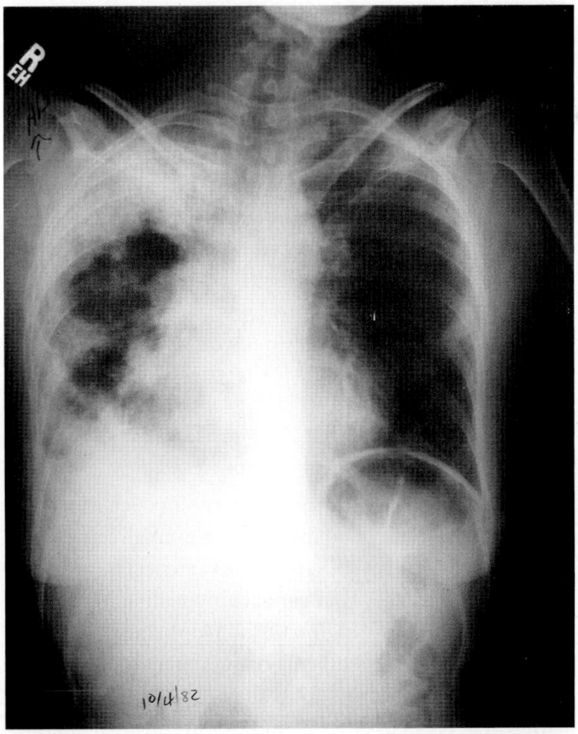

Fig. 77.17. Widespread infiltrates due to pulmonary eosinophilia.

(*hyper-strongyloidosis*) with migrating skin lesions, diarrhoea, Acute Respiratory Distress syndrome (ARDS) and meningoencephalitis. Treatment of strongyloidosis is with ivermectin 150 micrograms/kg (single dose), albendazole 400 mg twice daily for 3–6 days or thiabendazole 25 mg twice daily for 3 days.

Schistosomal infections

Schistosoma mansoni and rarely *S. haematobium* can cause respiratory symptoms 3 to 8 weeks after the first infection of the larvae through the skin. This phenomenon of acute schistosomiasis (Katayama fever) is not due to worms, but to an immunological reaction with immune complexes, and elevated IgE, IgM and IgA immunoglobulins. It consists of fever, dry cough or wheezing, especially at night, and flu-like symptoms. If untreated, it can persist for weeks to months and then spontaneously resolve. Treatment is difficult. Praziquantel has little effect at this stage, because it works against the mature worms. Steroids have been used to suppress the symptoms. Rarely, chronic schistosomiasis can cause granulomatous lesions in the lung eventually leading to interstitial fibrosis, pulmonary hypertension and cor pulmonale (Bethlem et al., 1997).

Tropical pulmonary eosinophilia

Filariasis caused by *Wucheria bancrofti* can cause a chronic asthma-like syndrome with cough, expiratory bronchial obstruction, especially at night, and sometimes chest pains and fever. This syndrome is called tropical pulmonary eosinophilia and is a hypersensitivity reaction against the microfilaria. A spectacular improvement of symptoms can be reached with treatment with diethylcarbamazine 6 mg/kg per day for 3 weeks.

In infections with *Loa loa* similar respiratory complications are described.

Hydatid disease

Echinococcus granulosus can cause echinococcosis or hydatosis. After infection the eggs of the small tape worm develop in hydatid cysts. These cysts can nest in several organs of which 15–30 per cent are in the lung. The cysts grow and can be asymptomatic for a long time, but will eventually cause mechanical obstruction or atelectasis, with cough and shortness of breath. A cyst may rupture, with severe consequences. Rupture can cause an anaphylactic reaction with urticaria, bronchospasm and shock. It can lead to an acute and severe cough where the content of the large cyst is expectorated, which can even lead to acute suffocation. If the cyst ruptures into the pleura, it can cause a hydropneumothorax. After rupture, metastatic cysts throughout the lung can develop. Lastly, a secondary bacterial infection can lead to the development of a lung abscess.

The medical treatment of choice is albendazole 10–20 mg/kg per day for 6 to 8 weeks. In rare cases where surgery is required to relieve pressure on surrounding structures, albendazole is given post-operatively to prevent recurrence from spillage.

The lung in malaria

The Adult Respiratory Distress syndrome (ARDS), particularly in tropical malaria in non-immune adults, can complicate malaria. This is a condition of massive non-cardiogenic pulmonary oedema, with many neutrophils in the pulmonary capillaries and alveoli. It manifests with tachypnoea and hypoxia. In a short time there is 80 per cent mortality when untreated. The only effective treatment is mechanical ventilation with positive end expiratory pressure. However, even with good intensive care facilities the mortality is still high (30%). Other organs also fail in complicated malaria, causing coma, acute renal failure and jaundice, although ARDS can occur in isolation (Taylor & White, 2002).

Amoebiasis

Entamoeba histolytica causes invasive amoebiasis. A liver abscess can break through into the lungs and cause a lung abscess or an empyema. Consecutively, it can break into the bronchus causing multiple metastatic abscesses. This condition has a high mortality. Metronidazole 750 mg three times daily for 10 days is the treatment of choice. Amoebic empyemas must be drained urgently.

Leishmaniasis

Leishmaniasis or kala azar can cause an interstitial pneumonitis. Intercurrent bacterial infections or reactivation of tuberculosis can be a complication.

Fungal infections

Most fungal infections of the lung are opportunistic (see ealier section on HIV associated conditions). Two fungal infections are not known to be related to HIV:

Actinomyces israel and *Aspergillus fumigatus* (with other *Aspergillus* species).

The uncommon actinomycosis occurs in 15 per cent of infections with *Actinomyces.* This gram-positive anaerobic rod-shaped fungus is a commensal organism mainly living in the mouth. The inflammation in the lung is severe, destructive and invasive, sometimes even outside the lungs into the chest wall and the ribs. Treatment is initially with benzylpenicillin i.v. for 4–6 weeks and should be continued for 6–12 months with oral penicillin or with doxycycline.

Aspergillus is a ubiquitous environmental organism. Pulmonary aspergillosis has four different patterns.

1. Asymptomatic colonization.
2. Allergic bronchopulmonary aspergillosis (ABPA) is an asthmatic syndrome with a combined allergic response (IgE, IgG and cellular mediated) to colonizing fungus. Clinically, the asthma is hard to treat and the chest X-ray may show infiltrates. Sputum may show *Aspergillus* and eosinophilia is common. The infiltrates do not persist. Exacerbations respond well to steroid treatment. Proximal bronchiectasis frequently occurs.
3. An aspergilloma is a tumour-like structure in damaged lungs, especially in cavities. It is due to growth of Aspergillus. The radiological presentation is sometimes very typical with air surrounding the dense ball of fungus in a pre-existing cavity (Fig. 77.18). This density may change position in the cavity if an X-ray is taken in consecutive erect and supine position. The condition may cause massive haemoptysis but is usually asymptomic.
4. Invasive aspergillosis is a serious condition mainly observed in patients with severe immune suppression such as advanced HIV or neutropenia. The acute fungaemia is life threatening and has a very high mortality. Chronic necrotizing aspergillosis is less aggressive. It can be found in immune competent patients with damaged lungs, e.g. after bronchocavitary tuberculosis. Treatment is with anti-fungal drugs such as amphotericin B or itraconazole.

Moniliasis (candidiasis, thrush)

The thrush fungus, *Candida albicans,* is found frequently in normal mouth, respiratory tract, vagina, and intestinal tract. Bronchopulmonary infection may follow prolonged antibiotic therapy, and is manifest as fever, cough, and shortness of breath. Diagnosis is made by demonstration of fungi in large numbers from sputum. Treatment is by inhalation of nystatin.

Table 77.13. Main causes of occupational lung disease

Inorganic (mineral) dusts	
Asbestos, silica, kaolin, coal dust, copper, tin, aluminium, uranium, and beryllium	
Organic dusts	
Cotton (byssinosis); sugar-cane bagasse (bagassosis); cocoa, coffee bean, and grain dusts; saw dusts from all sorts of timber; mouldy hay (farmers' lung), and pigeon droppings or feathers (bird-fanciers' disease)	
Gases or fumes	
Ammonia, chlorine, sulphur dioxide, and phosgene, petrochemicals	

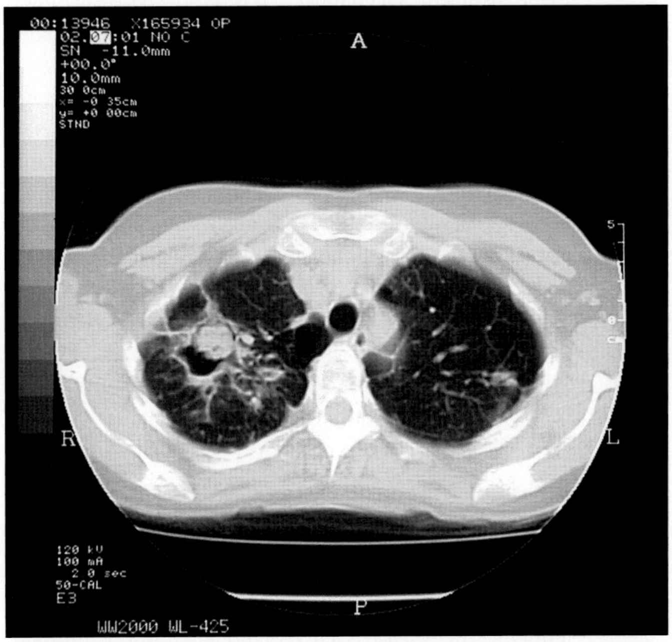

Fig. 77.18. An aspergilloma in a pre-existing tuberculous cavity.

Occupational lung diseases (Table 77.13)

As industry increases in Africa, so too do the occupational diseases. Many involve the lung, with occupational asthma and industrial pneumoconioses heading the list. In industrialized countries, there is much litigation and financial compensation in relation to industrial disease. Proper action and legislation are needed now in Africa, where there are numerous permanently disabled patients from these diseases (Asuza, 1996).

Occupational asthma can be caused by almost any industrial pollution, ranging from simple irritants such as concrete dust to highly specific asthmogenic agents such as toluene di-isocyante, enzymes, and platinum salts. From a clinical point of view, a high index of suspicion is needed whenever a worker complains of cough, wheeze and breathlessness at work, but not on holiday or at weekends (see Chapter 71).

The pneumoconioses are pulmonary disease caused by inhalation of mineral or organic dusts. The clinical picture varies from simple cough and dyspnoea to extreme respiratory disability and death. Characteristically, these conditions produce a diffuse or patchy type of pulmonary infiltrate and restrictive ventilatory disturbance.

Pathogenesis

The deposition of particulate matter in the lungs and the mechanisms by which most of it is removed by the lung is complicated. More of the aerosols or dusts are ingested than are inhaled. The toxic effects of inhaled particles, deposited anywhere from the nose to the alveoli, depend on their site. Mucociliary clearance of particles (aerosols) is fairly constant in the same individual but different from person to person. The integrity of the respiratory epithelium, for example, the presence of chronic bronchitis, affects the mucociliary action significantly. The larger particles (> 5 microns) are cleared more quickly than the smaller ones: the smaller the particle, the more distal it is deposited. These particles initiate immunological or inflammatory processes which lead to airways disease, either restrictive or obstructive, or both.

Inorganic (mineral) dusts

Miners' pneumoconiosis (CWP)

Coal is still important as a source of industrial energy in Africa, although it is gradually being replaced by petroleum oil. The disease is a useful model for understanding the other pneumoconioses. Coal-mining in Nigeria has not been associated with pneumoconiosis, because the silica content of the coal bed is low and the mines are so damp that very little dust is raised.

Dust particles between one and 10 microns diameter settle in the alveoli. Reactions occur in the interstitial tissue as a result of dust particles only or dust particle – protein complexes (the protein is released from ingesting macrophages). The resulting fibrosis affects all elements of lung tissue – the bronchi, arterioles, veins, and lymphatics.

The chest radiograph shows punctiform (up to 1.5 mm), micronodular or miliary (between 1.5 and 3 mm), and nodular (3–10 mm) opacities: severe cases have massive fibrosis, especially in the upper zones which may be difficult to distinguish from tuberculosis and bronchial carcinoma (Fig. 77.19).

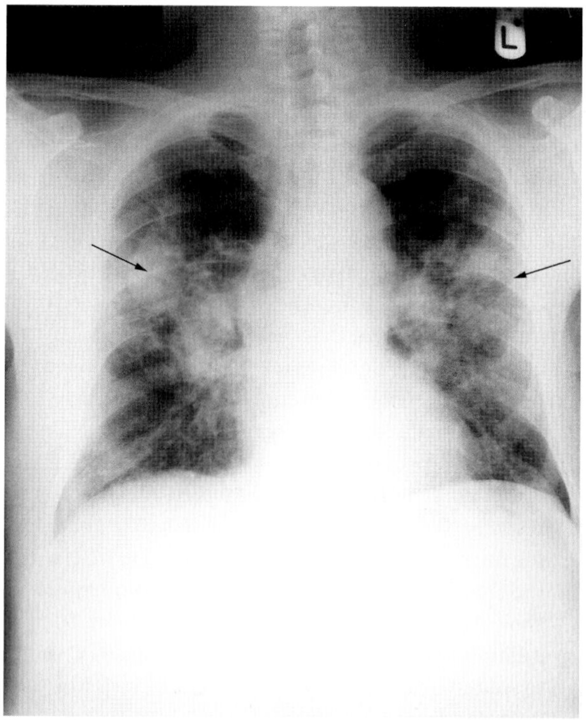

Fig. 77.19. X-ray of a coal miner showing multiple nodules and areas of progressive massive fibrosis (arrowed).

Those with normal radiographs or those with minimal changes have no symptoms, but others have effort dyspnoea, cough, chest pain, and sometimes haemoptysis, especially if there is Progressive Massive Fibrosis (PMF).

The functional abnormality depends on the anatomical change. PMF destroys large areas of lung so that there are reduced areas for diffusion and gas exchange. Arterial oxygen desaturation, pulmonary hypertension, and cor pulmonale may result. Extensive bronchial damage leads to compensatory emphysema and bronchiectasis. Pulmonary function tests are normal in miners with no demonstrable radiological damage; the most sensitive test of disturbed function is to measure blood gas tensions after exercise, when arterial oxygen tension will be found to be reduced.

Asbestos

Asbestos is a fibrous mineral found in certain types of rocks in many parts of the world. The Republic of South Africa is the third country in the world in asbestos production but the first in blue asbestos (crocidolite). The use of asbestos increased to over four million tonnes per year in the 1970s, but is now declining rapidly due to the imposition of health and safety regulations in most countries. Four types of asbestos fibres exist: chrysolite (this accounts for 95 per cent of asbestos used), crocidolite (blue asbestos, the most dangerous), amosite and anthophylite.

Risk of exposure includes work in rock mines, spraying insulators, handling asbestos in textile and vehicle manufacturing industries, and those engaged in construction. Those who live near asbestos mines or in places where asbestos is plentiful may be inadvertently exposed to dust. There is a steady increase in the incidence of asbestos-related disease at present, not predicted to decrease until 2020 due to the long 'incubation period' following exposure (up to 50 years).

The long filaments of asbestos, 50 microns long and 0.5 microns in diameter, are inhaled and fall perpendicularly to penetrate the alveoli and even reach the pleura, pericardium, and peritoneum. They produce damage to all these structures through an unknown mechanism.

Radiological changes

- Hazy infiltrates with irregular or linear opacities limited to the lung bases
- Benign pleural plaques, which may calcify along the diaphragm and pericardium (Fig. 77.20)
- Pleural effusions (due to active asbestos-related pleuritis)
- Diffuse pleural thickening on the lateral chest wall, or typical 'tear-drop' or 'candle-wax'-shaped pleural thickenings
- Diffuse fibrotic changes affecting predominantly the lung bases (the term asbestosis should be reserved for this pathology)
- Changes suggesting mesothelioma (lumpy unilateral pleural thickening with contraction of the affected hemi-thorax, Fig. 77.19).

Sputum

Asbestos bodies consisting of an asbestos fibre covered with a proteinaceous material with a drumstick appearance at both ends may be seen, but they are not diagnostic.

Diseases

The range of disease caused by asbestos exposure is wide:

- benign pleural plaques without any serious sequelae
- extensive pleural plaques and active pleuritis, leading to restrictive lung function
- asbestosis – pulmonary fibrosis, with restrictive lung function
- malignant mesothelioma – untreatable pleural tumour with mean survival time of 12 months from diagnosis
- bronchial carcinoma – the commonest cause of death, particularly if the asbestos exposure has been combined with cigarette smoking (100 times increase in incidence compared with non-smoking, non-exposed population)

Silicosis

Inhalation of silica dust occurs in the mining of several metals – gold, copper, tin, and during quarrying for granite. Silica dusts cause a more intensive fibrous reaction in the lungs than in coal-workers' pneumoconiosis. The radiological patterns are similar and progressive massive fibrosis is common. The pathology and functional derangements are similar to those of coal-workers' pneumoconiosis. Silicosis is associated with increased incidence of pulmonary tuberculosis, which must always be considered particularly if a patient gets quickly worse. Silicosis is a progressive disease. Withdrawal from further exposure does not halt the process.

Because silica occurs widely in nature and is used extensively in industry, silicosis is one of the oldest and most important pneumoconioses. Silicosis results from the inhalation of crystalline free silica or silicon dioxide.

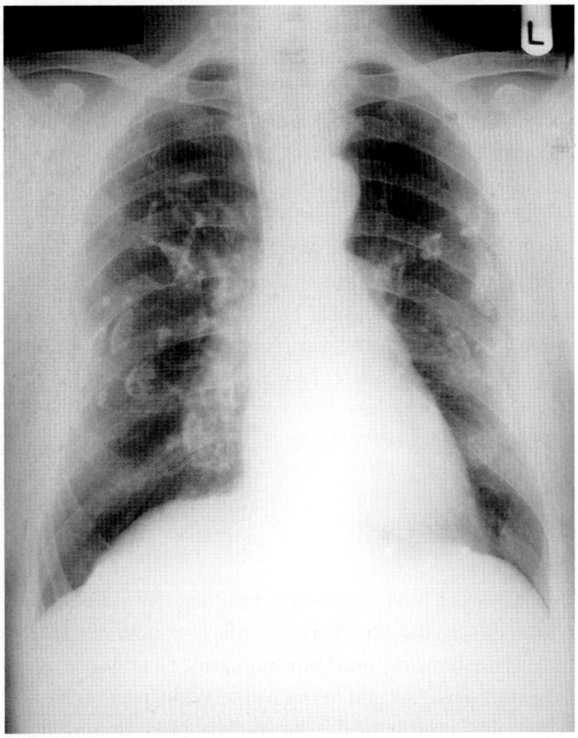

Fig. 77.20. Calcified pleural plaques in a patient exposed to asbestos 30 years previously.

Inhalation of 0.3 to 5.0 micron particles starts the destructive inexorable process.

Some of the types of occupational exposure to silica which occur in Africa are:

- mining, quarrying and tunnelling for metals such as gold in Zimbabwe and South Africa, copper in Zambia, and tin in Nigeria
- open-cast sandstone quarrying in northern Nigeria
- foundry working in Egypt
- domestic use of silica-containing grindstones inside huts in Transkei and Ciskei regions of South Africa.

The situation in the gold mines of South Africa is particularly serious. Post-mortem studies have shown a steady increase in silicosis in gold workers between 1975 and 1991 (Murray et al., 1996). A rapid rise in tuberculosis incidence has been found in miners who have both HIV infection and silicosis, risk factors for TB which appear to combine multiplicatively. Current figures give a TB incidence in HIV-positive silicotic miners of 16.1 per 100 person-years, raising the spectre of a TB epidemic of rapidly developing disease (Corbett et al., 2000).

Pathogenesis

Silica particles penetrate to the peripheral airways and are then ingested by suicidal macrophages whose residue form the acellular silicotic nodule surrounded by 'onion peel'-like layers of collagen. These nodules are responsible for the radiological mottling which is seen throughout the lung fields, but mostly in the middle and upper zones. Silica in hilar nodes is deposited at the periphery ('egg-shell' calcification). This stage is known as simple silicosis, with minimal or no symptoms.

The disease can, however, progress to pulmonary fibrosis (including PMF). Because of the killing of macrophages in the initial stage, these patients become highly susceptible to tuberculosis. For example, amongst grindstone cutters near Dambatta, Nigeria, the prevalence of active pulmonary tuberculosis was 7 per cent compared with the estimated case prevalence of 2 per cent in tropical Africa.

Organic dusts

Byssinosis

Byssinosis is a pneumoconiosis produced by inhalation of cotton dust in the early part of textile production, namely in carding, blowing, and spinning areas. The disease also occurs in sisal, flax and hemp workers. The part of the cotton dust producing the disease is not known and the mechanism by which it produces disease is unclear. Affected persons feel tightening chest, shortness of breath and wheezing 1 to 6 hours after exposure on a Monday morning after a free weekend. At first, symptoms clear by the end of the day, but gradually get prolonged until finally the patient has symptoms throughout the week. As the disease progresses, symptoms worsen and the patient becomes a cripple with chronic byssinosis, clinically indistinguishable from chronic bronchitis and emphysema. The disease is preventable but there is no specific treatment.

Extrinsic allergic alveolitis

Farmers' lung, which results from inhalation of thermophylic actinomycetes in mouldy hay, is an example of this group of diseases. Cocoa bean handlers may develop the same syndrome. The mechanism here is well worked out – a type 3 allergic reaction results in the formation of immune complexes in the walls of the exposed alveoli. Specific IgG antibodies to the allergen can be detected as serum precipitins (precipitating antibodies).

Bagassosis is an example of extrinsic allergic alveolitis induced in workers employed in the sugar industry, typically in parts of Kenya and Uganda surrounding Lake Victoria. After crushing and shredding, sugar cane (bagasse) is stored in large heaps, where the high temperature and humidity provide ideal conditions for thermophilic actinomyces. Vast concentrations of spores are released when the bagasse is handled (Tanimowo, 1996).

Sometimes, poorly characterized organic dusts produce a variety of problems in workers, such as the seafood processors of South Africa who suffer rashes, asthma and probable extrinsic alveolitis (Jeebhay et al., 2000).

Gases or fumes

Ammonia, hydrochloric acid, chlorine, sulphur dioxide, nitrous oxide, and phosgene can cause upper respiratory tract damage or pulmonary oedema.

Pulmonary fibrosis

Fibrosis of the lungs occurs secondarily to infections or as a response to various pulmonary stimuli, but frequently its cause is unknown. Fibrosis may be interstitial or peribronchial and perivascular, and may involve the alveoli. There are many causes, which broadly fall into the following groups.

Infections

Fibrosis occurs following necrotizing pneumonias caused by *Staphylococcus aureus*, *Klebsiella*, *M. tuberculosis*, or fungi. Viruses (such as influenza) and parasitic diseases (for example, schistosomiasis) may also be responsible for some cases. In Africa tuberculosis is the most important cause of fibrosis associated with destruction of alveolar walls and accumulation of exudate. It also produces peribronchial fibrosis, bronchiectasis, and emphysema secondary to destruction of bronchi. In schistosomiasis, ova arrive through the pulmonary artery and initiate a granulomatous reaction and perivascular fibrosis.

Drugs
Nitrofurantoin, hydralazine, hexamethonium, methysergide, busulphan, chlorambucil, bleomycin, and cyclophosphamide can all cause pulmonary fibrosis.

Radiation
Following radiotherapy for intrathoracic cancer severe fibrosis may occur in adjacent lung.

Oxygen toxicity
If 100 per cent oxygen is administered continuously over several hours, there will be type II alveolar cell proliferation and oedema. If oxygen is continued, irreversible pulmonary fibrosis will result.

Sarcoidosis
This is a non-caseating granulomatous systemic disease of unknown cause, which, until recently, was thought to be very rare in Africa, despite its high prevalence among black Africans living in the UK. There are now well-validated reports of many clinical cases throughout Africa.

Clinical features
Typical symptoms are progressive dyspnoea on exertion, with or without cough. Many patients are asymptomatic. The majority have a subacute course, with complete resolution over a period of months or years. However, a minority of patients develop progressive pulmonary fibrosis, with pulmonary hypertension and eventual death from right heart failure and respiratory failure.

Chest radiograph
Typically, in benign subacute sarcoidosis the chest X-ray shows bilateral hilar lymphadenopathy, which may or may not resolve. The minority of patients with pulmonary fibrosis show typical X-ray patterns, including honeycombing in advanced disease. The X-ray may show evidence of pulmonary hypertension (large pulmonary arteries and dilated right ventricle).

Pulmonary function tests
Spirometry shows a restrictive pattern: the FEV1 and VC are both reduced, but FEV1/VC ratio is normal or increased. Transfer factor (measured with carbon monoxide) becomes abnormal early on, and there is hypoxia on exertion.

Diagnostic problems
Tuberculosis must be excluded by sputum examination: the tuberculin test is negative in sarcoidosis. The diagnosis is confirmed by skin, lymph node, lung or liver biopsy.

Treatment
There is no specific treatment, but pulmonary fibrosis in sarcoidosis may respond to prednisolone.

Idiopathic pulmonary fibrosis (synonyms: Hamman–Rich syndrome, cryptogenic fibrosing alveolitis, diffuse pulmonary fibrosis)
This is rare in Africa. It occurs mainly in older persons (male: female ratio 2: 1), begins insidiously, and leads to progressive dyspnoea on exertion, cyanosis and finger clubbing with basal crepitations. No cause is identified, and the fibrosis seldom responds to corticosteroids. It is usually fatal within 5 years.

Fibrosis in association with connective tissue disorders
Patients suffering from a variety of connective disorders (rheumatoid arthritis, systemic lupus erythematosus, overlap syndromes, ankylosing spondylitis) may develop lung fibrosis. The fibrosis tends to respond to corticosteroids and other immunosuppressant treatment more convincingly than in idiopathic fibrosis, and the prognosis is better.

Tobacco and health

Since the 1984 edition of this book, the relentless increasing in smoking across Africa has continued. In the absence of recent figures, a passage from the earlier edition is reproduced here.

General comment

There is plenty of evidence to prove that cigarette smoking is hazardous to health. Although the degree of harm is directly proportional to the duration and amount of cigarettes consumed, there is no absolutely safe dosage of cigarettes. Cigarette smoking is associated with increased mortality in general and cancer of the lung, chronic obstructive pulmonary disease, and myocardial infarction in particular. Cancer of the larynx, oral cavity, oesophagus, and urinary bladder are more common in smokers than non-smokers. Smoking is also associated with increased incidence of peripheral vascular disease, peptic ulcer, spontaneous abortion, small babies, stillbirths: more will doubtless follow. Cigarette smoking is associated with frequent upper and lower respiratory tract infections, and small airways function is significantly reduced even in those who are chronically exposed passively to tobacco smoke.

The constituents of cigarettes that are harmful to health are tar, nicotine, and carbon monoxide. Tar is responsible for the proliferative and destructive effects which may result in chronic obstructive lung disease and bronchgenic carcinoma. Nicotine is associated with increased heart disease and hypertension. Carbon monoxide increases oxygen consumption in coronary disease and worsens angina pectoris.

African scene (1980 figures quoted)

Whilst cigarette smoking is declining in industrialized countries, it is dismaying that it is increasing alarmingly in Africa. Smoking is more prevalent in urban than in rural areas. In Lagos 42 per cent of men and 2.4 per cent of women smoke cigarettes. Sixty-two per cent of black workers in a Johannesburg factory smoke cigarettes. Smoking has also increased among African teenagers. Forty per cent of boys and 8.4 per cent of girls from a Nigerian secondary school smoke. In Uganda 33.4 per cent of male and 7 per cent of female students smoke. In South Africa 16 per cent of 1505 high-school pupils smoke regularly. In an Ethiopian high school of 538 pupils, 27.5 per cent of boys and 2.8 per cent of girls smoke.

Several factors are responsible for this tragic state of affairs. Many African countries are encouraged to grow tobacco because of the large revenue it brings. Tanzania increased its output seven-fold between 1962 and 1974, and plans to increase its production further thanks to misguided international aid. Zaire and Nigeria have also increased their tobacco growth significantly. Tobacco is the number one export crop for Zimbabwe and Malawi. Cigarette sale advertising is uncontrolled and heavy. The tobacco companies shamelessly tell people all over Africa that smoking is the key to success in college, business, and farming, and claim that it is a sign of high social status, and that it makes women more attractive and glamorous. The cigarette packages exported to Africa do not carry any warning labels, as opposed to those in most industrialized countries, whence the same brand of cigarette has a higher content of tar and nicotine when it is exported to Africa. In other words, the African is not given the choice between smoking and health. It is no surprise that diseases related to smoking have started to emerge in Africa. This is a major disaster when infectious and nutritional disease control is not yet in sight, but governments hide behind economic expediencies!

By 2000 at last some African governments were recognizing the immense damage caused by smoking (Mzileni et al., 1999). By 2001 smoking was being banned in public places in the Republic of South Africa, and restrictions were being placed on cigarette advertising (Holzman, 2001).

The two rapidly emerging respiratory diseases directly related to smoking in Africa are chronic obstructive pulmonary disease and bronchial carcinoma. Figure 77.22 shows a patient suffering from both these deadly diseases.

Chronic obstructive pulmonary disease (COPD)

The spectrum of COPD embraces patients with predominantly chronic bronchitis at one end, and patients with predominantly emphysema at the other. All share the element of more-or-less fixed and progressive airway obstruction, and all have at least some degree of both bronchitis and emphysema.

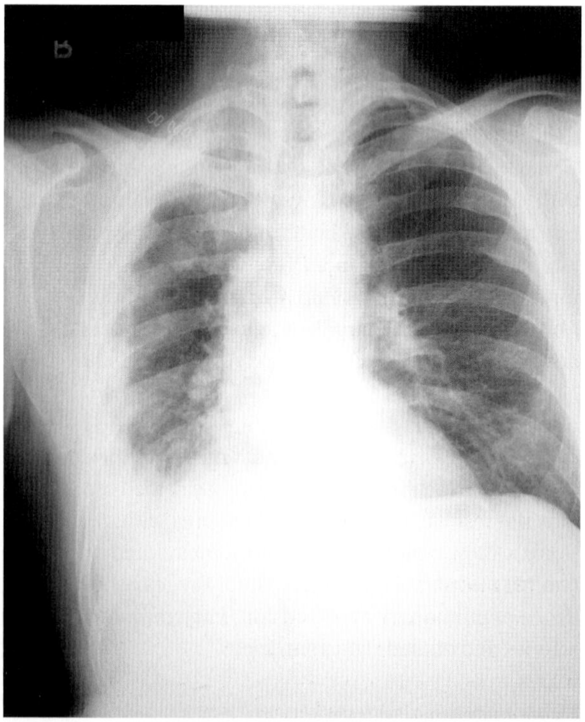

Fig. 77.21. Malignant mesothelioma of the right pleura. Note the mediastinal involvement and contraction of the right thorax.

Definition of chronic bronchitis

The patient has had cough productive of sputum for at least 3 consecutive months in each of at least 2 consecutive years.

Causes

Tobacco smoking, atmospheric pollution, and repeated respiratory infections have been implicated. Hereditary alpha1-antitrypsin deficiency has been recognized in 5–10 per cent of severely emphysematous patients in Europe, but there are few data from Africa. In women, cooking over a smoky fire in a poorly ventilated hut may be responsible for a heavy burden of chronic lung disease.

Pathophysiology

Hypertrophy of mucous glands and increased numbers of goblet cells, particularly in large bronchi, explain the excessive sputum. Blockage by mucus and swelling of the airway wall contributes to obstruction and to underventilation of affected regions of the lung. Infection superimposes inflammatory oedema with cellular exudate, and eventually leads to obstruction and distortion of the airways and adjacent blood vessels.

Some areas of emphysema (enlargement of the gas-exchanging air spaces distal to the terminal bronchiole caused by destruction of their walls) are usual in the lungs. Emphysema further distorts the anatomy of the airway and so contributes to airways obstruction and to maldistribution of ventilation and perfusion.

When airways resistance is increased, greater transpulmonary pressure gradients are required to force air through the airways. These high pressures acting around the intrathoracic airways may make them collapse. One way of preventing this collapse is to increase the lung volume so that airways are held open by connective tissue ultimately connected to the pleural surface of the lung. This explains the hyperinflated lungs of patients with severe airways obstruction. Another way of preventing airway collapse is to increase pressure inside the airways by breathing out against an external resistance, for example through half-closed lips. This type of 'pursed lip' breathing is seen in some patients with severe chronic airways obstruction.

Clinical features

Cough with sputum, at first in the early morning but later throughout the day and night, is typical. Episodes of infection make symptoms worse, and the sputum becomes purulent. Breathlessness gets steadily worse, and may be accompanied by wheeze.

In severe cases, the development of oedema, cor

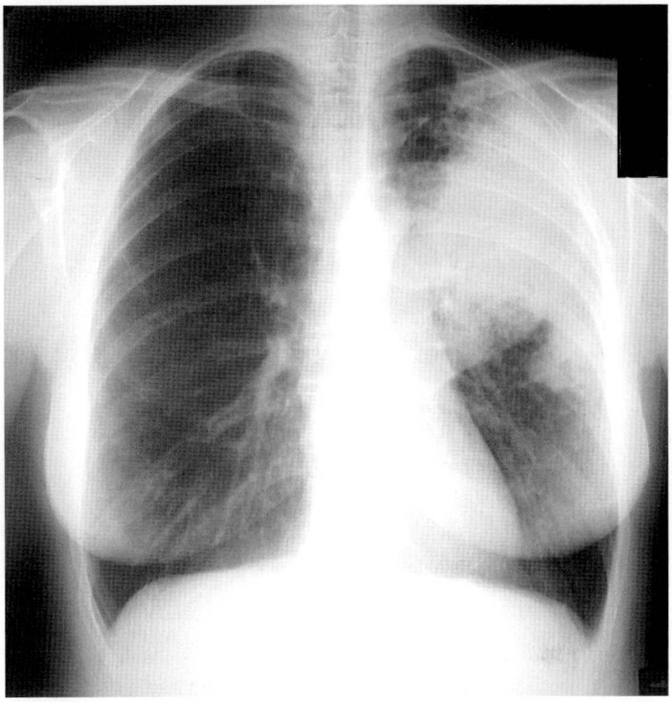

Fig. 77.22. Large bronchial carcinoma in a patient with pre-existing emphysema. Note the hyperinflated right lung with sparse lung markings.

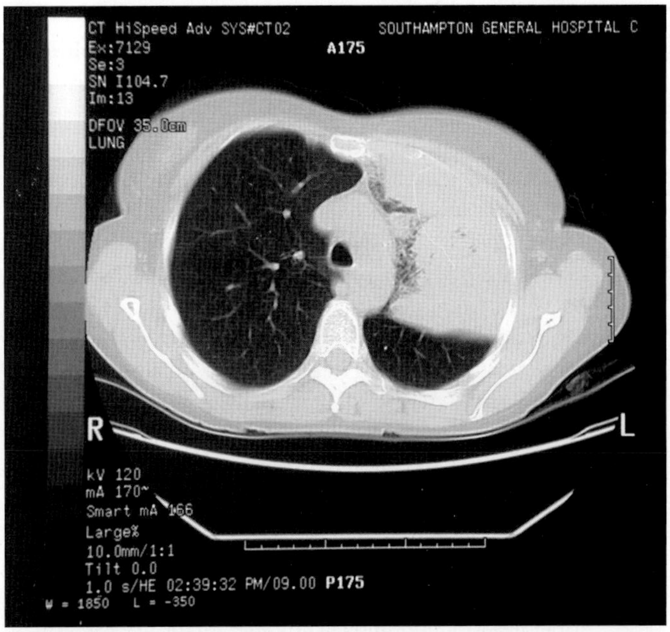

Fig. 77.23. CT scan of the same patient showing the extent of a large peripheral bronchial carcinoma.

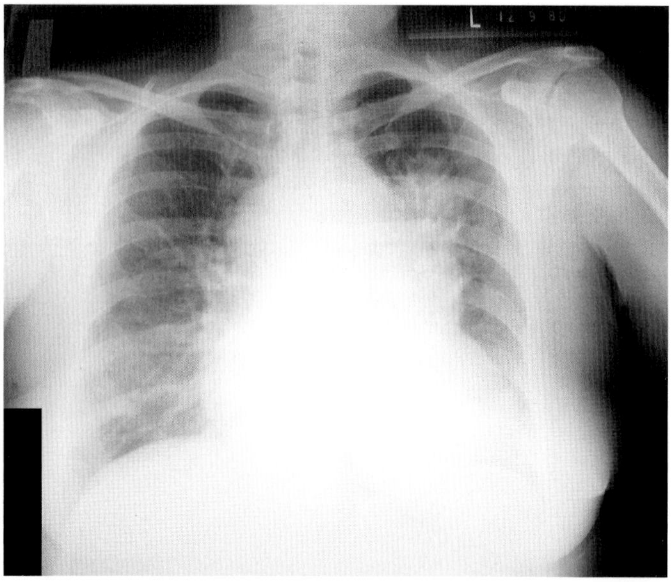

Fig. 77.24. Small cell bronchial carcinoma presenting with left hilar mass and massive mediastinal lymphadenopathy.

pulmonale, and polycythaemia indicates chronic respiratory failure (hypoventilation) with persistent hypoxaemia and hypercapnia. These patients (sometimes called 'blue bloaters') depend on their hypoxaemic drive for ventilation, and must be treated with caution when giving oxygen (initially no more than 24 per cent inspired O_2 is advised).

Investigations

The diagnosis is based on the patient's history of chronic productive cough, and on measurement of airflow obstruction. The earliest changes, which are in the smallest to medium diameter airways, are detectable by special tests many years before dyspnoea develops. Later, low FEV1, and low FEV/VC ratio with increased TLC (total lung capacity) and RV (residual volume) are found. Arterial blood gases should be measured, if possible.

Chest radiographs may be normal in the early stages of the disease. Later there may be areas of lung with attenuated vascular markings (emphysema), enlarged heart and pulmonary arteries (cor pulmonale) and hyperinflation of the lungs (airways obstruction). Mixed respiratory tract flora are usually cultured from the sputum, and not one dominant pathogen.

Treatment

The patient should be encouraged to stop smoking, for this slows deterioration at any stage of the disease. Bronchodilator drugs may produce some response, but should be prescribed long term only if tests show a response of 15 per cent or more on simple pulmonary function measurement (peak flow rate or FEV1). In industrialized countries there tends to be much over-prescription of bronchodilator drugs, which are sometimes taken in excessive dose by nebulizer. Severe side effects, particularly tachycardia and anxiety, are not infrequent.

All patients with severe airflow obstruction should be given a controlled trial of corticosteroid, e.g. prednisolone 30 mg/day for 2 weeks. If this produces an increase of 15 per cent or more in pulmonary function it is reasonable to give inhaled steroids long-term. Antibiotics, e.g. ampicillin, tetracycline, should be prescribed promptly if there is obvious infection, together with a short course of oral prednisolone.

Table 77.14. Histological classification of bronchial carcinoma

Small cell lung carcinoma (SCLC)
Non-small cell lung carcinoma (NSCLC):
Squamous cell carcinoma
Adenocarcinoma
Alveolar cell carcinoma

Bronchial carcinoma

The prevalence of carcinoma of the lung is increasing in Africa. The main cause is undoubtedly tobacco smoking, but there are also contributions from industrial and domestic pollution, plus specific risks such as asbestos exposure and uranium mining.

Bronchial cancers are classified by their histology. Biopsy is an essential part of the diagnosis in every case, because histological type increasingly dictates therapy. Currently the classification is in Table 77.14.

Clinical features and diagnosis

As with any cancer, these can be local, systemic, metastatic, or due to an association peculiar to the tumour. Most commonly, symptoms and signs are local, and in Africa where pneumococcal pneumonia is so common, the problem is usually persistent radiological and clinical signs after an acute infection.

The disease must be suspected in any heavy smoker who has systemic or local symptoms and persistent chest signs with an abnormal radiograph. Some typical presentations are in the Box, and Figs. Figures 77.22, 77.23 and 77.24 show examples of typical radiology in bronchial carcinoma.

Typical presentations of bronchial carcinoma

- Persistent or recurrent pneumonia
- Persistent cough
- Scanty intermittent haemoptysis
- Bone pain from metastatic disease
- Symptoms due to biochemical change:
  - hypercalcaemia in metastatic disease and squamous cell tumours
  - hyponatraemia (small cell tumours producing ectopic anti-diuretic hormone)
  - hypernatraemia and hypokalaemia (small cell tumours producing ectopic ACTH)
- Neurological symptoms (metastatic disease or paraneoplastic syndromes)
- General weakness and weight loss

Despite this impressive list, the clinician in most parts of Africa must remember that infections (especially tuberculosis) are still much more common than bronchial cancer.

Treatment of bronchial carcinoma

The principles of treatment are as follows.

1. Make an accurate histological diagnosis.
2. Stage the tumour as accurately as possible. In practice this means having access to CT scanning, which alone can provide the detail necessary to determine the extent of tumour, particularly when it invades the mediastinum.
3. Small cell tumours must be referred to the nearest oncology centre for chemotherapy.
4. Non-small cell operable tumours must be referred to a thoracic surgical centre (surgical excision offers the only prospect of permanent cure).
5. Palliative treatment must include adequate pain relief. Radiotherapy has a useful place in treating haemoptysis and sometimes pain.

References

Aboulafia DM. (2000). The epidemiologic, pathologic, and clinical features of AIDS-associated Kaposi's sarcoma. *Chest*; **117**: 1128–1145.

Asuza MC. (1996). The development and state of health and safety in the workplace in West Africa: perspectives from Nigeria. *W Afr J Med*; **15**: 36–44.

Bethlem EP, Schettino Gde P, Carvalho CR. (1997). Pulmonary schistosomiasis. *Curr Opin Pulm Med*; **3**: 361–365.

Buvé A, Bishikwabo-Nsarhaza K, Mutangadura G. (2002). The spread and effect of HIV-1 infection in sub-Saharan Africa. *Lancet*; **359**: 2011–2017.

Corbett EL, Churchyard GL, Clayton TC et al. (2000). HIV infection and silicosis: the impact of two potent risk factors on the incidence of mycobacterial disease in South African miners. *AIDS*; **14**: 2759–2768.

Garrison MM, Christiakis DA, Harvey E et al. (2000). Systemic corticosteroids in infant bronchiolitis: a meta-analysis. *Pediatrics*; **105**: 1–6.

Gebremedhin A, Shamebo M. (1998). Deep venous thrombosis in a university teaching hospital, Addis Ababa. *E Afr Med J*; **75**: 432–435.

Graham SM, Coulter JB, Gilks CF. (2001). Pulmonary disease in HIV-infected African children. *Int J Tuberc Lung Dis*; **5**: 12–23.

Hargreaves NJ, Kadzakumanja O, Phiri S et al. (2001). *Pneumocytis carinii* pneumonia in patients being registered for smear negative pulmonary tuberculosis in Malawi. *Trans Roy Soc Trop Med Hyg*; **95**: 402–408.

Hirschtick RE, Glassroth J, Jordan MC et al. (1995). Bacterial pneumonia in persons infected with the human immunodeficiency virus. *N Engl J Med*; **333**: 845–851.

Holzman DC. (2001). Tobacco in Africa. *Environ Health Perspect*; **109**: 113.

Jeebhay MF, Lopata AL, Robins TG. (2000). Seafood processing in South Africa: a study of working practices, occupational health services and allergic health problems in the industry. *Occup Med, Lond*; **50**: 406–413.

Mito K, Maruyama R, Uenishi Y et al. (2001). Hypertrophic pulmonary osteoarthropathy associated with non-small cell lung cancer demonstrated growth hormone-relaeasing factor by histiochemical analysis. *Intern Med*; **40**: 532–535.

Murray J, Kielkowski D, Reid P. (1996). Occupational disease trends in black South African gold miners. *Am J Respir Crit Care Med*; **153**: 706–710.

Mzileni O, Sitas F, Steyn et al. (1999). Lung cancer, tobacco, and environmental factors in the African population of the Northern Province, South Africa. *Tob Contr*; **8**: 398–401.

Pasterkamp H, Kraman SS, Wodicka GR. (1997). Respiratory sounds. Advances beyond the stethoscope. *Am J Respir Crit Care Med*; **156**: 974–987.

Ruffini DD, Madhi SA. (2002). The high burden of *Pneumocystis carinii* pneumonia in African HIV-1 infected children hospitalised for severe pneumonia. *AIDS*; **16**: 105–112.

Tanimowo MO. (1996). Respiratory disease among Nigerians working in the sugar industry. *E Afr Med J*; **73**: 556–559.

Taylor WR, White NJ. (2002). Malaria and the lung. *Clin Chest Med*; **23**: 457–468.

West JB. (2000). *Respiratory Physiology: The Essentials*. 6th edn. Philadelphia: Lippincott Williams & Wilkins.

78 Blood

The problem in Africa

Throughout sub-Saharan Africa, anaemia is highly prevalent, due to infection, malnutrition and genetic polymorphisms. The haemoglobin (Hb) concentration of the blood, in both sexes and at all ages, is about 2.0 g/dl lower on average than that found in rural communities in the temperate zones: this is usual but not normal.

Anaemia is particularly relevant in the following groups.

Infants and children

The average prevalence of anaemia in African preschool children is 56 per cent. Anaemia delays growth and development, reduces learning abilities (particularly with iron deficiency) and increases morbidity and mortality.

Pregnant women

It is estimated that 63 per cent of pregnant African women are anaemic from malaria and malnutrition: their entire family suffers, particularly the younger children: the fetus is handicapped, and may die. The mother herself may die.

Working men and women

About 44 per cent of non-pregnant women and 20 per cent of men in Africa are anaemic so that their work suffers and their dependent families can be crippled.

Anaemia

Anaemia is defined as a Hb concentration lower than normal for the age and sex of the individual (Table 78.1).

Table 78.1. Normal range of haemoglobin concentrations throughout life.

	Hb g/dl
Newborn	14–20
2–3 months	10.5–12.5
4 months–6 years	11–13
6–14 years	12–15
Adult females non-pregnant	12–16
Adult females, pregnant	11–15
Adult males	13–17

Source: Modified with permission from various sources, including World Health Organization (1968)

Blood volume in health and disease

More accurately, anaemia is said to be present when the total red cell volume is lower than normal, but in practice the Hb concentration is used. The peripheral blood Hb may not always reflect the total red cell mass. For example, in pregnancy both the plasma volume and the red cell volume increase, but the increase of plasma volume is greater (Table 78.1; Fig. 78.1(*b*)(*c*)), in splenomegaly when red blood cells (RBC), granulocytes, and platelets are pooled in very large spleens, and plasma volume expands (Fig. 78.1(*d*)), and after acute haemorrhage (Fig. 78.1(*e*)(*f*)).

Pathophysiology of anaemia

Anaemia has three stages of severity:

(i) compensated anaemia
(ii) decompensated anaemia
(iii) anaemia which is life-threatening from (a) tissue hypoxia, or (b) cardiac failure.

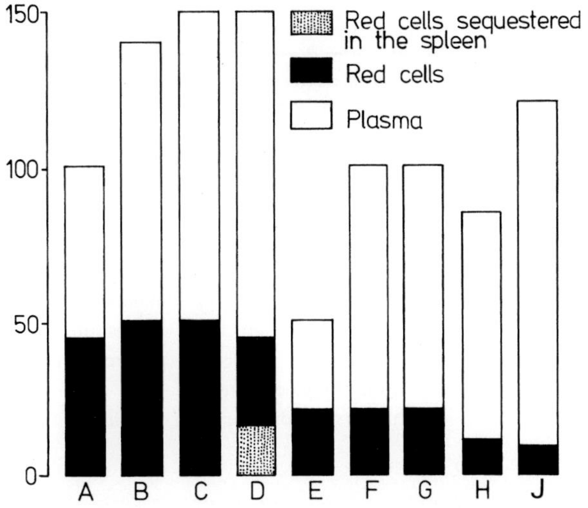

Fig. 78.1. Blood volume changes in health and disease. (*a*) Normal adult. (*b*) Normal single pregnancy. (*c*) normal twin pregnancy. (*d*) Hypersplenism, not anaemic. (*e*) Acute haemorrhage. (*f*) Acute haemorrhage, 48 hours later. (*g*) Moderate anaemia. (*h*) Severe anaemia. (*j*) Severe anaemia with circulatory congestion. Note that two or more of these conditions may be present in the same patient; in particular *e* to *j* are variations on *a* (non-pregnant), but could be shown again as variants on *b* (pregnant), *c* (multiple pregnancy) or *d* (hypersplenism), or the combination of pregnancy and hypersplenism.

The staging of anaemia is defined in clinical and pathophysiological terms, as the severity of anaemia depends not only on the Hb concentration, but also on age, as the young can compensate better than the elderly; on cardiac and respiratory function; on the speed of onset of anaemia; and on plasma volume (Fig. 78.1(*b*)(*c*)(*d*)).

Compensated anaemia (Hb>7.0 g/dl approximately)

Patients are breathless on effort and have pallor of the mucous membranes – not a reliable sign in diagnosis. The plasma volume expands to keep the total blood volume normal (Fig. 78.1(*g*)).

Decompensated anaemia (Hb<7.0 g/dl approximately)

Patients are breathless even at rest, so that they cannot perform usual daily tasks. The cardiac output, stroke volume and cardiac rate rise. The blood volume is reduced (Fig. 78.1(*h*)). Vasodilation and increased peripheral blood flow dominate clinical signs (see the Box).

Clinical signs of anaemia

Compensated anaemia
- pallor

Decompensated (severe) anaemia
- warm hands
- collapsing pulse
- wide pulse pressure
- ejection systolic murmur
- pulsating retinal veins

Life-threating anaemia

Respiratory distress
- nasal flaring
- indrawing of chest wall
- grunting or deep breathing

Circulatory congestion
- pulmonary oedema
- peripheral oedema
- raised jugular venous pressure

Life-threatening anaemia (Hb<5.0 g/dl approximately)

Lactic acidosis

Children with profound malarial anaemia develop respiratory distress, are hypovolaemic (Fig. 78.1), acidotic and have lactic acidaemia (English, 2000).

Severe anaemia with circulatory congestion

Cardiac output increases in proportion to the degree of anaemia over the range Hb 7.0–4.0 g/dl, but there is no further increase below about Hb 4.0 g/dl; symptoms of tissue hypoxia (for example cardiac pain) and signs of heart failure appear (Fig. 78.1(*j*)). The patient is often pregnant or recently delivered, or has splenomegaly.

Treat the cause of the anaemia. Only give blood transfusion, which can be fatal as it further increases the plasma and total blood volume, for anaemic cardiac failure, before imminent obstetric delivery and Hb< 7.0 g/dl, or before urgent surgery.

Transfuse slowly (>3 h per unit) packed red cells (not whole blood) 10 ml per kg body weight, or 2 units of packed cells for an adult: give i.m. or i.v. frusemide 40 mg, or 1 mg/kg.

Aetiology of anaemia

There are three mechanisms of anaemia (Table 78.2):

(i) blood loss
(ii) increased red cell destruction
(iii) decreased red cell production.

Table 78.2. Anaemia classified by its causes

Blood loss		Increased red cell destruction		Decreased red cell production		
Acute	Chronic	Abnormal haemolysis	Abnormal red cells	Nutritional deficiency	Hypoplasia	Aplasia
	Leading	Infection	Haemoglobin	Iron	Infection	Primary
	to iron	malaria	HbS	Folate	HIV	Secondary
	deficiency	others	HbC,etc	Vitamin B_{12}	TB	drugs
		Hypersplenism	Enzyme	Vitamin A	parvovirus B19	chemicals
		Immune mechanisms	G6PD deficiency	Others	others	irradiation
		feto-maternal	Membrane	protein	Malignancy	pancreatic fibrosis
		incompatibility	elliptocytosis	ascorbic acid	Chronic hepatic disease	
		mismatched transfusion	spherocytosis		Chronic renal disease	
		autoimmune				
		Others				
		burns				

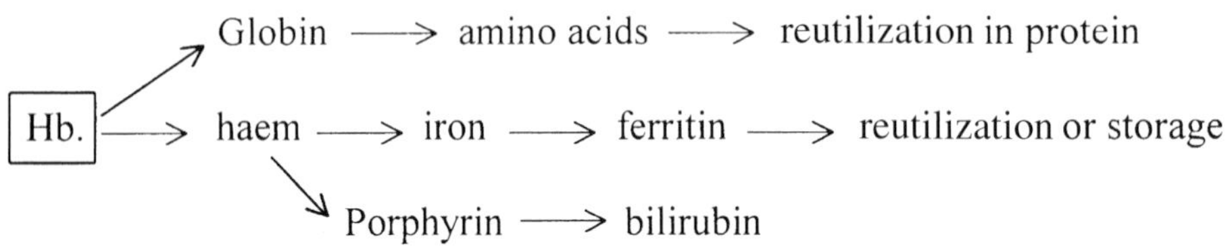

Fig. 78.2. The products of extravascular haemolysis.

Blood loss

Acute blood loss

This results in an immediate decrease of red cell volume and plasma volume (Fig. 78.1(*e*)). Lost plasma is replaced from tissue fluid and the blood volume is restored within 24 hours (Fig. 78.1(*f*)), but the red cell volume does not begin to increase for about seven days and is not restored to normal until 4–8 weeks after severe haemorrhage.

Chronic blood loss (e.g. hookworm, menorrhagia or bleeding peptic ulcer)

Both plasma and red cell volumes are maintained because the marrow can increase red cell production up to eight times normal. RBC contain approximately 1 mg of iron per 1 ml, so that chronic blood loss can deplete the total body iron (normally about 4 g) and thus impede haemoglobin synthesis.

Increased red cell destruction (haemolysis)

Haemolytic anaemia may be the result of abnormal RBC or abnormal destruction of normal cells. Haemolysis may be extravascular in the reticuloendothelial system (RES) including the liver and spleen, or more rarely intravascular.

Extravascular haemolysis

Haemoglobin is degraded in the cells of the RES to amino acids and iron, which are reutilized, and to bilirubin which is carried in plasma bound to albumin (Fig. 78.2); bilirubin is conjugated with glucuronic acid by the liver and excreted in bile; in the small intestine, it is converted into urobilinogen, some of which is reabsorbed; urobilinogen in the plasma is either re-excreted by the liver or excreted in urine (Fig. 78.3).

Intravascular haemolysis

Haemoglobin is first bound to the haptoglobins in plasma and removed by the RES. Further haemoglobin will be free in plasma and some will be degraded to methaemalbumin. Haemoglobin passes the glomerular filter and appears in the urine, where much of it is oxidized to the brown–black pigment methaemoglobin (blackwater fever); some haemoglobin is absorbed by the renal tubular cells and degraded to haemosiderin, which appears in urine several days after an acute haemolytic crisis (Fig. 78.4).

Recognition of extravascular haemolysis

Increase of haemoglobin breakdown products

(i) Clinical jaundice, if haemolysis is severe.
(ii) Plasma unconjugated bilirubin increased.
(iii) Urinary urobilinogen is in excess.

Compensatory increase of red blood cell production

(i) Release into the blood of young red cells, which show anisocytosis (variation of size) and polychromasia (basophilic or blue-staining RNA with eosinophilic or red-staining haemoglobin), and a raised reticulocyte count; in severe anaemia, nucleated red cells may be seen.
(ii) Erythroid hyperplasia in the bone marrow.

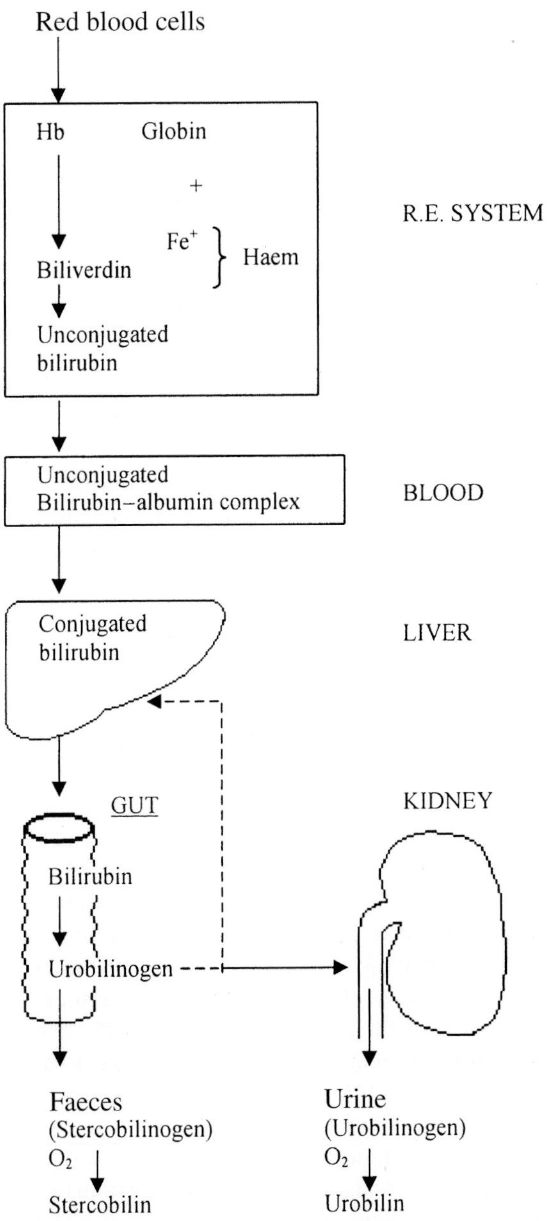

Fig. 78.3. The metabolism of bilirubin.

Shortened red cell survival

This is measured by labelling RBC with radioactive chromium (^{51}Cr).

Recognition of intravascular haemolysis

Features of extravascular haemolysis, with:

- red cell fragmentation – poikilocytosis (variation of shape): schistocytes (fragmented cells).
- haemoglobin and products in plasma: haemoglobinaemia (shown by the spectroscope): methaemoglobinaemia (shown by the Schumm's test).
- haemoglobin and products in urine: haemoglobin in urine without the presence of red blood cells: methaemoglobinuria, haemosiderinuria.

Acquired haemolytic anaemias

Malarial anaemia

Plasmodium falciparum causes the most severe and potentially fatal anaemia (Menendez et al., 2000; World Health Organization, 2000).

Definition

WHO defines severe malarial anaemia as Hb < 5.0 g/dl or a haematocrit (Hct) < 0.15 in the presence of a *P. falciparum* parasitaemia > 10 000 parasites/μl with a normocytic thin blood film. This strict definition, however, is met by only a small proportion of patients, especially of children. Although in general the degree of anaemia correlates with the density of parasitaemia, many patients with severe anaemia present with low or subpatent parasite densities, or with anaemia from multiple aetiology.

Pathophysiology

There is both an increased destruction and decreased production of RBC (Menendez et al., 2000), but the pathogenesis of anaemia is poorly understood.

Increased RBC destruction

- Direct rupture of parasitized red blood cells (PRBC).
- Phagocytosis of parasitized and unparasitized RBC. Hyperactive macrophages remove not only PRBC but also unparasitized RBC, both of which have reduced deformability.
- Hypersplenism.

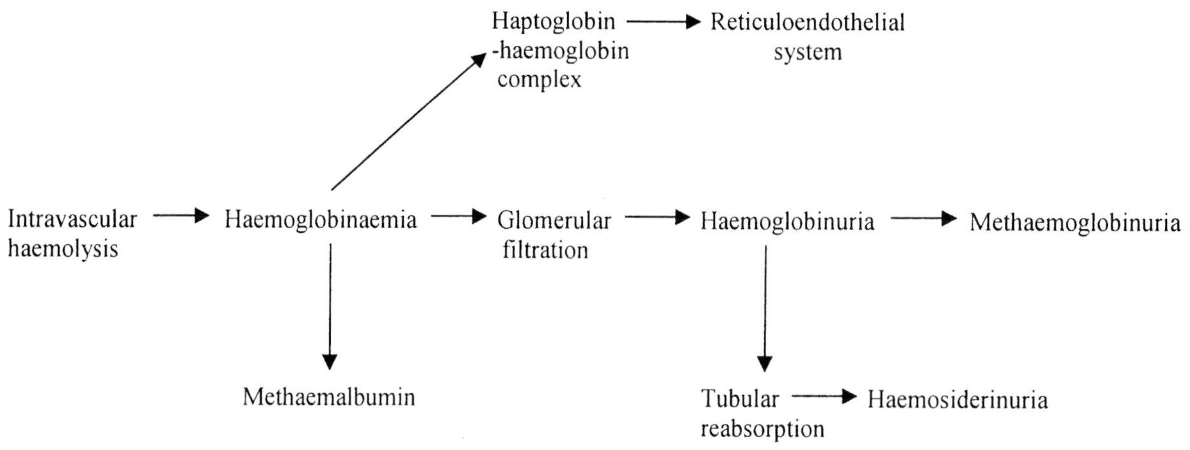

Fig. 78.4. The products of intravascular haemolysis in plasma and urine.

- Autoimmune haemolysis. The evidence of autoimmune haemolysis in the anaemia of *P. falciparum* malaria is conflicting. Many positive direct anti-globulin (DAT) reactions are non-specific but strong reactions are associated with more severe anaemia.
- Blackwater fever. Most patients with haemoglobinuria in the tropics have been exposed to oxidant drugs and are glucose-6-phosphate dehydrogenase (G6PD) deficient.

Decreased RBC production

Erythroid hypoplasia

The reticulocytosis in response to anaemia is delayed by malarial parasitaemia.

Suppression of erythropoietin synthesis

Serum EPO levels are markedly raised in African children with severe malarial anaemia, but are inappropriately low for the severity of anaemia in adults with malaria.

Dyserythropoiesis

Disturbed marrow cell division causing severe anaemia is observed mainly in persons after repeated episodes of *P. falciparum* malaria.

Cytokine imbalance

Concomitant infections Anaemia is more severe in children with malaria and secondary infections.

Epidemiology

In Tanzania, malaria accounted for at least 60 per cent of anaemic episodes in infants exposed to intense and perennial malaria transmission (Menendez et al., 1997). Life-threatening anaemia with dense parasitaemia affects mainly infants and children less than 3 years of age. Where transmission is less intense, older children tend to have severe anaemia with low parasitaemia and dyserythropoiesis.

Haematology

The peripheral blood during acute malaria shows the red cell changes and biochemistry characteristic of extravascular and intravascular haemolysis (p. 927). The neutrophil count is raised initially, but after about 2 days there is usually a neutropenia due to the margination of neutrophils to the endothelium. During the second week, a neutrophil leukocytosis occurs, with a shift to the left (excess of young neutrophils), vacuolation of the cytoplasm and toxic granulation (presence of excess large blue-staining primary granules). The presence of malarial pigment in neutrophils indicates severe disease and a poor prognosis. With secondary infections, the leukocytosis and shift to the left may be greatly exaggerated with release of early granulocyte precursors from the marrow to give a blood picture resembling a chronic myeloid leukaemia (CML) (Table 78.13). The eosinophil count is lowered by acute malaria, but there may be an eosinophilia during recovery. From about the third day of acute malaria, activated B-lymphocytes are present in the peripheral blood; they have dark blue-staining cytoplasm and large nuclei with nucleoli (plasmacytoid cells): the blood picture may mimic an acute lymphoblastic leukaemia (ALL) (Table 78.13).

The monocyte count is raised; the cells are typically vacuolated, often showing erythrophagocytosis and malarial pigment. Malarial pigment persists for up to 5 days after the clearance of parasites and so is useful in diagnosis.

Haemostasis
The platelet count is moderately lowered by acute malaria but in about 5 per cent of patients it is $<50 \times 10^9$/l. Activation of coagulation and anti-coagulant factors occurs, but only rarely in severe malaria does this progress to disseminated intra-vascular coagulation (DIC).

Management

Chemotherapy
Give anti-malarial treatment even in the absence of parasitaemia to patients with severe anaemia, especially those at high risk for malaria, such as children, pregnant women and individuals with sickle-cell disease, and anti-malarial prophylaxis for 3 weeks.

Blood transfusion
Transfusion of blood may be life-saving but there is risk of HIV transmission even with screened blood (1 in 2000 HIV-negative blood units may be infectious for HIV in sub-Saharan Africa).

Haematinics
Give oral iron 3–6 mg/kg/day in children and 120 mg day in adults for 28 days: this does not cause malaria to recur (van Hensbroek et al., 1995). Ideally, continue iron for 3 months to replace iron stores.

Give pregnant women and patients with sickle-cell disease an anti-malarial drug (preferably not an anti-folate) and folic acid, 5 mg per day for 3 weeks and then 50 μg per day, until obstetric delivery or 1 mg per day for life for patients with sickle-cell disease. Give infants 50 μg per day for 28 days; increase the dose for each year of life to 500 μg for those 5 years or over.

Malaria during pregnancy

Pathophysiology
Parasite frequency, parasite density and severity of malaria are increased in pregnant women (Menendez, 1995).The mechanisms may be related to pregnancy-related general immune-depression, local synthesis of immune-suppressive factors, cytoadherence of parasites in the placenta, or increased biting by mosquitoes.

Importance of severe malaria in pregancy (Menendez, 1995)
The level of pre-pregnancy immunity, which depends largely on the intensity and stability of malaria transmission, determines the severity of clinical malaria (Fleming, 1989; Menendez, 1995).

Areas of low transmission
Pregnant women with no or low levels of acquired immunity to *P. falciparum*, present with acute severe malaria. Anaemia is inevitable, is often severe, and may be complicated by blackwater fever or DIC. Women of all parities are affected equally. Severe maternal malaria is associated with high rates of abortion, premature delivery, fetal distress, still birth, low birthweight and increased infant mortality.

Areas of high transmission
In primigravidae especially, clinical malaria and the frequency and density of *P. falciparum* parasitaemia increase to reach a plateau in the second trimester, after which they decline. The incidence of clinical malaria is increased, but much less in multigravidae until the fifth pregnancy, and in the post-partum period compared to the pre- or post-pregnancy rates (Diagne et al., 2000) (see the Box).

Diagnosis of malarial anaemia during pregnancy (see the Box)
Pregnant women with parasitaemia have few or no symptoms: their main morbidity is anaemia in mid-pregnancy, complicated by folate deficiency (Fig. 78.5) (Fleming, 1989).

Diagnosis of malaria in pregnancy
- *Blood films underestimate the number of infected women*

Reason
- The placenta is packed with parasitized RBC

Action
- Treat for malaria all severely anaemic pregnant women exposed to malaria (Shulman et al., 2002).

Without appropriate treatment, maternal mortality rises rapidly when the Hct falls below 0.20 (Fig. 78.6), and the incidences of low birthweight and perinatal mortality rise rapidly when the maternal Hct falls below 0.30 (Fig. 78.7) (Harrison, 1985; Hoestermann et al., 1996; Shulman et al., 2002).

Low birthweight is the consequence of premature delivery and intrauterine growth retardation. Surviving infants are at high risk of infection, malnutrition and anaemia (Fig. 78.5) (Cornet et al., 1998).

HIV and malaria in pregnant women
HIV infection increases susceptibility to clinical malaria and anaemia in women of all parities and decreases effectiveness of prophylactic anti-malarials (van Eijk et al., 2001).

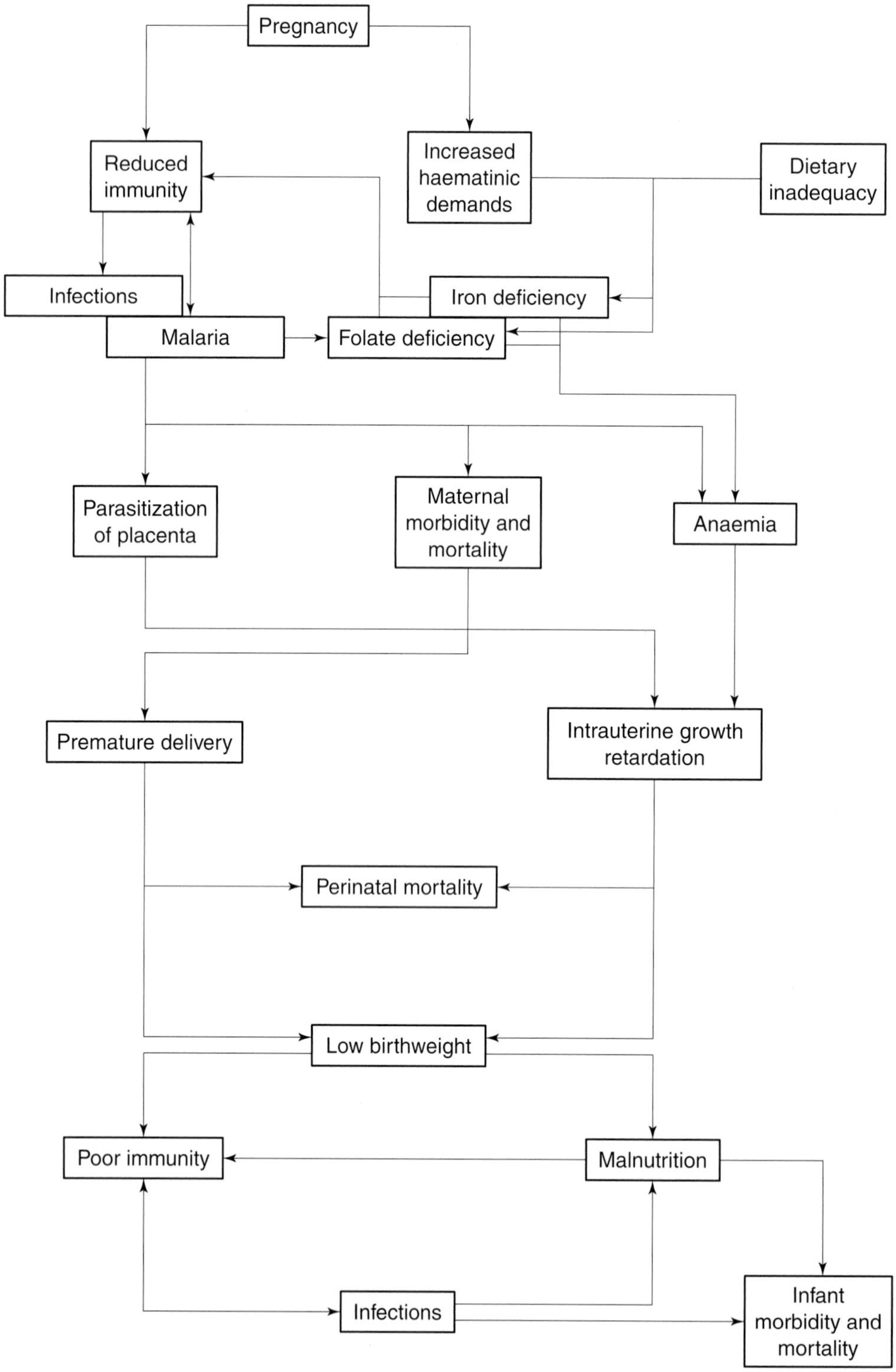

Fig. 78.5. Aetiology and consequence of anaemia in pregnancy in malaria-endemic areas of Africa. (Reproduced with permission of A.F. Fleming, 1991.)

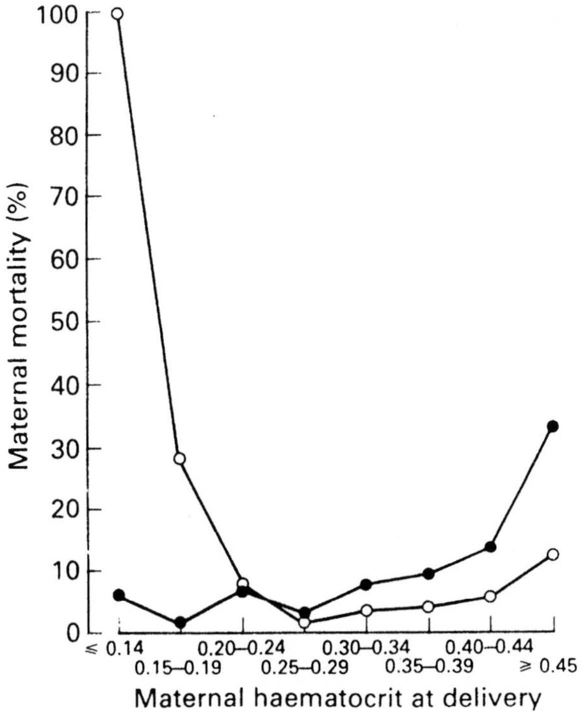

Fig. 78.6. Maternal haematocrit at delivery, blood transfusion and maternal mortality.
● Transfused; ○ not transfused. Severe anaemia was caused predominately by malaria in Zaria, northern Nigeria. (Reproduced with permission from Harrison, 1985.)

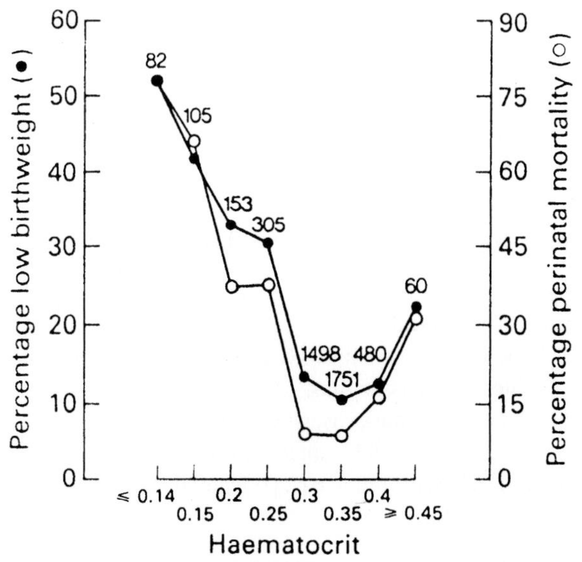

Fig. 78.7. Maternal haematocrit at delivery, low fetal birthweight and perinatal mortality in singleton births. Severe anaemia was caused predominately by malaria in Zaria, northern Nigeria. (Reproduced with permission from Harrison, 1985.)

Treatment of severe malarial anaemia during pregnancy

Give blood only when appropriate (see p. 925).

Give folic acid 5 mg per day by mouth, ferrous sulfate 200 mg per day, or twice per day if iron deficiency is suspected or diagnosed, and an appropriate anti-malarial prophyletic (see above). In most patients the Hb and Hct rise rapidly after about 5 days of treatment with HMS (see below). The few patients with immune haemolysis have a constantly falling Hct and require repeated transfusions: treat them with prednisolone 60 mg per day orally, reduced stepwise each week to 30 mg, and tailed off and stopped preferably before the 36th week of gestation.

If maternal malarial anaemia is corrected and the pregnancy continues for 6 weeks or more before delivery, there is an almost complete recovery of intrauterine growth and birthweight, and low perinatal mortality (Fleming, 1989).

Prevention of malarial anaemia during pregnancy

- Give prophylactics to all pregnant women(Menendez et al., 1995).
- Because HIV reduces the ability of women of all parities to limit *P. falciparum*, give prophylactics to all pregnant women, not primigravidae only (van Eijk, 2001) (see the Box).

Prevention of malarial anaemia during pregnancy

Chemoprophylaxis
- Curative anti-malarials at first attendance
- Regular chemoprophylaxis

or
- Intermittment sulfadoxine/pyrimethamine

Reduction of mother–vector contact
- Insecticide impregnated bed-nets

Haematinic supplements
- Ferrous sulfate 200 mg/folic acid 500 μg daily

Hyper-reactive malarial splenomegaly (HMS)

Children (and non-immune immigrants) exposed to endemic malaria have varying degrees of splenomegaly which regresses as they acquire partial immunity. In a few subjects, however, the spleen continues to enlarge progressively with age: this is known as hyper-reactive malarial splenomegaly (HMS) (previously called the tropical splenomegaly syndrome (TSS)) (Bedu-Addo & Bates, 2002; Fleming & de Silva, 2003).

Pathophysiology (Fig. 78.8)

HMS is an unusual response to recurrent infection by *P. falciparum* or *P. vivax*; *P. malariae* may also contribute. During acute malaria IgM lymphocytoxic antibodies with specificity for activated suppressor T-(CD8+ve) lymphocytes are produced transiently: the CD8+ve cells down-regulate the synthesis of IgM by B-lymphocytes, so that antibodies against these suppressor cells enhance the humoral response to acute malaria. Persistence of the lymphocytoxic antibodies has been demonstrated in Indonesians with HMS, so that inhibition of B-cell activity fails (Piessens et al., 1985). Recurrent malaria stimulates B-cell hyperplasia and there is gross overproduction of polyclonal IgM, only some of which has anti-malarial specificity. IgM forms immune complexes and aggregates which precipitate when plasma is cooled (cryoglobulins). The immune complexes and aggregates are phagocytosed by macrophages, and there is a hyperplasia of macrophages and T-cells. This leads to hepatomegaly and massive splenomegaly, complicated by the pancytopenia of hypersplenism (Fig. 78.1(*d*)). Red cells are sensitized by immune complexes, with resulting erythrophagocytosis. Anaemia may be severe: haemolytic crises occur with infection and in pregnancy. Patients are liable to infection if severely neutropenic. Thrombocytopenia is usually moderate and without clinical consequence.

Epidemiology

HMS is seen where falciparum or vivax malaria are endemic, most commonly in people who have migrated from a non-malarious area to an endemic area within a few generations – Fulani in northern Nigeria and Rwandans in Uganda. Women outnumber men, probably owing to the reduced resistance to malaria in pregnancy.

Clinical presentation

Patients, usually young to middle-aged adults – age range 8–>60 years, have abdominal swelling and an ache from the large spleen; they may present with a haemolytic crisis associated with infection or pregnancy, or because of recurrent infections. Lymphadenopathy is not seen (see the Box).

Laboratory diagnosis

The diagnosis of HMS depends on an abnormally high serum IgM. There are high titres of anti-malarial antibodies (malaria parasites are not usually detected), pancytopenia with a hyperactive bone marrow, lymphocytosis in hepatic sinusoids, spleen, bone marrow and peripheral blood, which may mimic chronic lymphocytic leukaemia (CLL): estimation of serum IgM (high in HMS but low in CLL) usually differentiates between HMS and CLL, but a few patients with intermediate results are probably in transition from HMS to a malignant lymphoproliferative disease.

Hyper-reactive malarial splenomegaly (HMS):

- Residence in a malarious area.
- Chronic splenomegaly greater than 10 cm below the costal margin without other cause.
- Serum IgM elevated to more than 2 SD above the local reference mean.
- High titres of malarial antibodies.
- Lymphocytic infiltration of hepatic sinusoids.
- Clinical and immunological regression with long-term anti-malarial prophylaxis.

(Bryceson et al., 1983)

Prognosis

In Papua New Guinea there was a mortality of 46 per cent over 15 years, mostly from acute bacterial or other overwhelming infection. Progression to malignant lymphoproliferative disease is discussed under *Chronic lymphocytic leukaemia* (p. 962).

Treatment

- A curative anti-malarial course followed by effective anti-malarial prophylaxis for life. Immunological measurements return slowly to normal and the spleen shrinks over 6 months to 2 years.
- If prophylaxis is stopped, HMS relapses.
- Do not do a splenectomy: it carries a high operative, and later, mortality.

Inherited abnormalities of red cells

There are high frequencies of genes for inherited abnormalities in tropical Africa:

(i) haemoglobin synthesis (Fig. 78.9); haemoglobinopathies or thalassaemias,
(ii) red cell enzymes, e.g., glucose-6 phosphate dehydrogenase (G6PD) deficiency (Fig. 78.15),
(iii) red cell membranes, e.g., congenital elliptocytosis (Fig. 78.16).

Homozygous inheritance of the abnormalities may be associated with severe disease, e.g. sickle-cell anaemia, whereas heterozygous inheritance confers survival advantage and hence genetic advantage through providing partial protection against malaria.

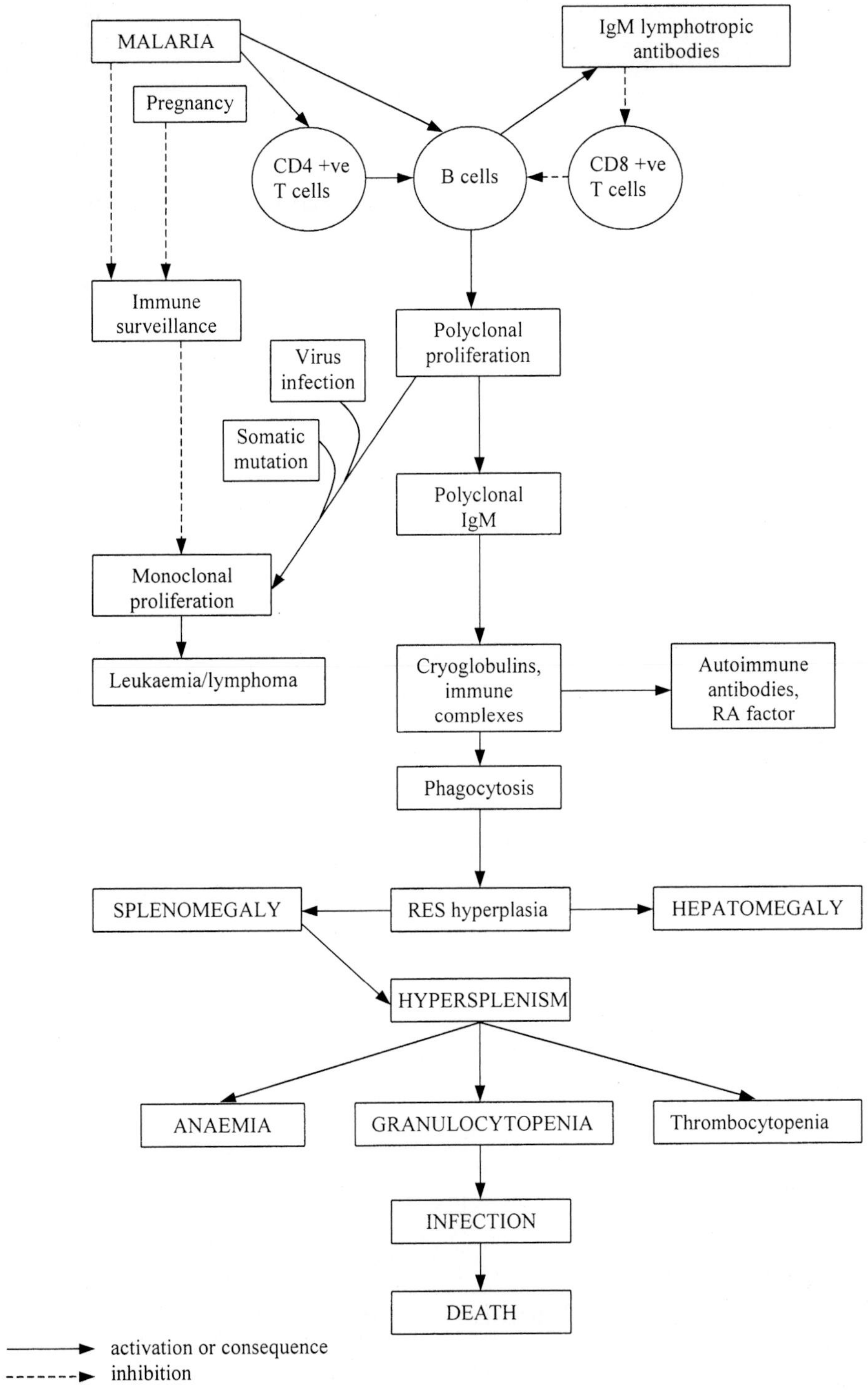

Fig. 78.8. Pathophysiology of hyper-reactive malarial splenomegaly (HMS).

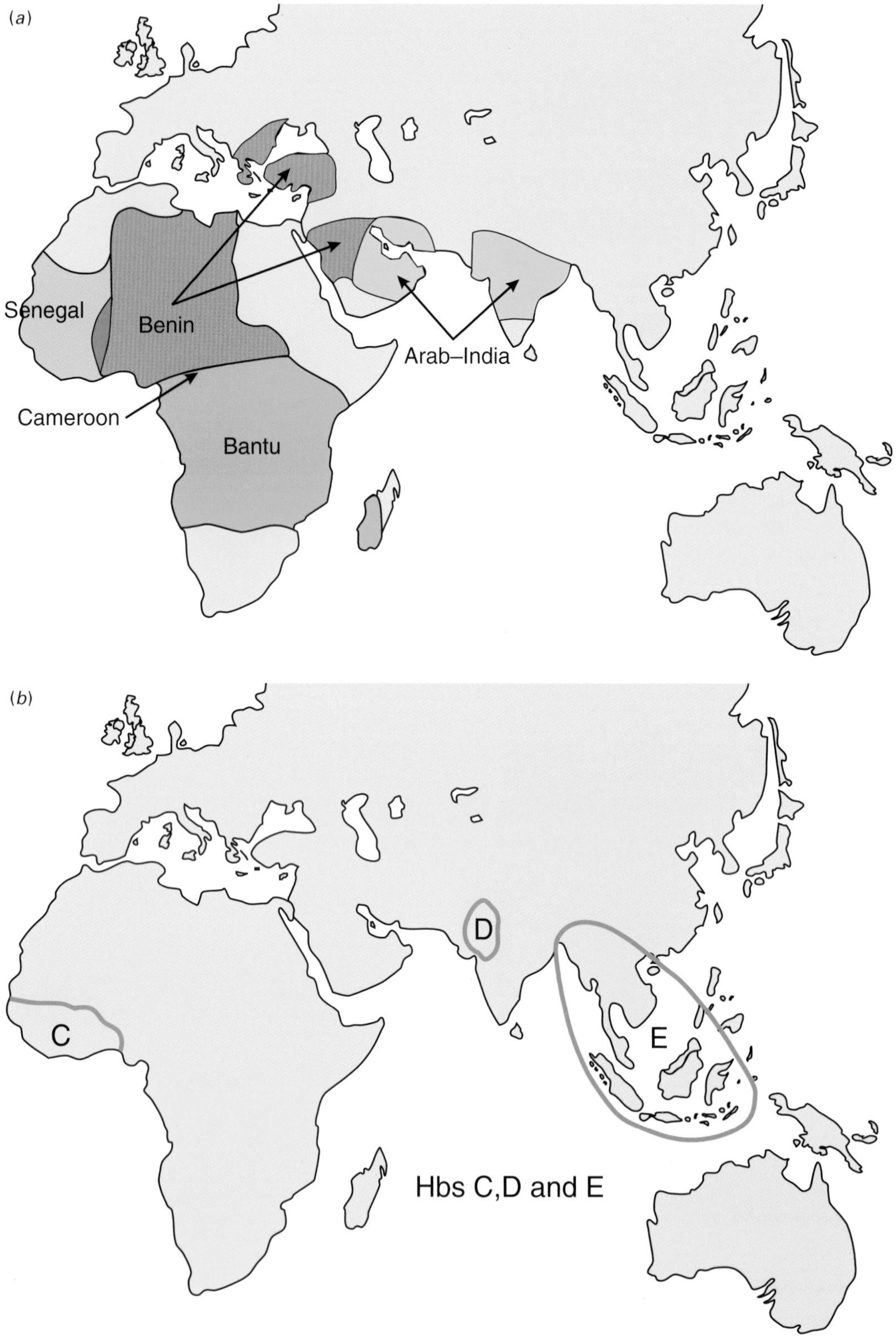

Fig. 78.9. (*a*) Distribution of haemoglobin S. (*b*) Distribution of haemoglobins C, D, and E. (*c*) Distribution of β-thalassaemia. (*d*) Distribution of α-thalassaemia. (Reproduced with permission from Fleming & de Silva, 2003.)

(*c*)

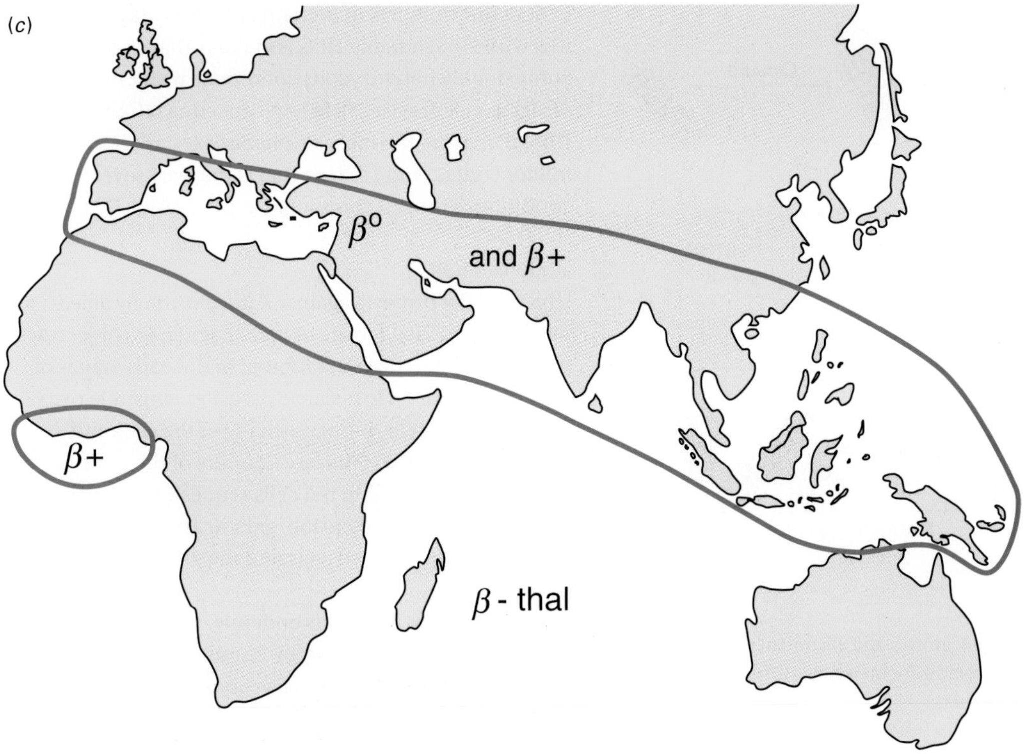

(*d*)

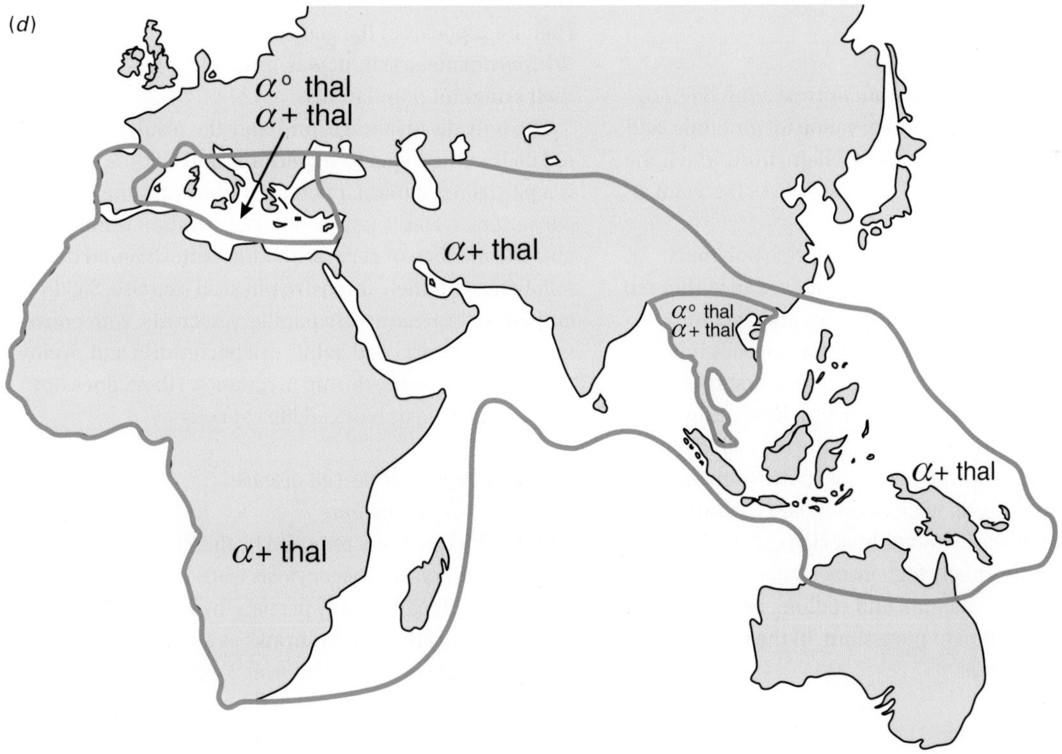

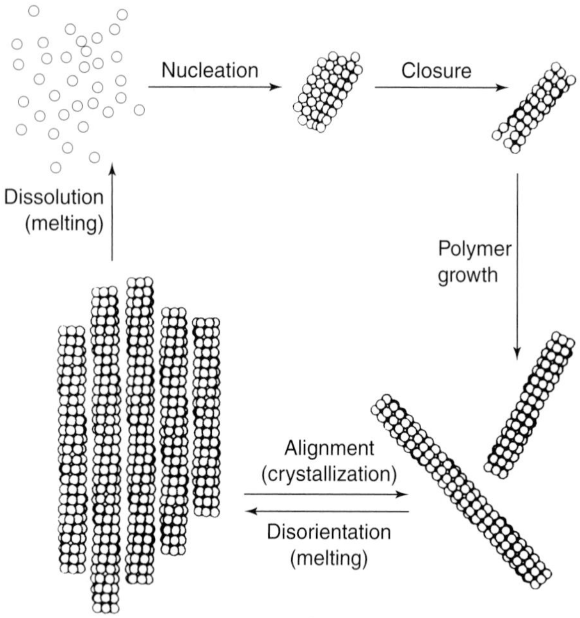

Fig. 78.10. The nucleation, growth and alignment of polymers of deoxyhaemoglobin S. (From Hofrichten et al., 1976, with permission of the publishers.)

Sickle-cell disease

The abnormal haemoglobin

Haemoglobin-S (HbS) differs from normal adult haemoglobin (HbA) by the substitution of valine for glutamic acid in the sixth position of the β-globin chain, from which the whole pathology of sickle-cell disease derives (Serjeant & Sergeant, 2001).

At high concentrations, deoxy-HbS forms polymers; polymerization in solution leads to gelling, and within red cells the polymers act as long stiff fibres and become aligned in parallel (Fig. 78.10), distorting the cells into elongated or sickle-cell forms. Sickling is at first reversible with reoxygenation of haemoglobin and dissolution of the gel, but changes in the membrane of the red cell follow from repeated sickling and unsickling; potassium and water leak out of the cell, while sodium and calcium enter. The result is the irreversibly sickled cell, with a rigid membrane, an abnormally high intracellular concentration of haemoglobin, calcium, and sodium, and a relatively low concentration of potassium. In the homozygous state (HbSS) this causes:

(i) infarction
(ii) haemolytic anaemia;

which lead to:

- increased susceptibility to infection
- disturbance of growth and development
- chronic organ damage.

Other abnormalities of β-chain synthesis may be inherited with HbS, notably HbC and the β-thalassaemias. Some doubly heterozygous conditions result in variants of sickle-cell disease. Sickle-cell anaemia (HbSS) and HbS/β^{o} thal are the most severe diseases. HbSC has a milder course, and HbS/β^{+} thal is the least severe: both conditions are seen commonly in west Africa (Fig. 78.9).

Sickle-cell trait

HbS partially protects against *P. falciparum* by at least two mechanisms. The density of parasitaemia in subjects with sickle-cell trait (Hb AS)) is limited in the early stages of the erythrocyte cycle because parasites consume oxygen within the red cells, induce sickling of the cells and are removed by the RES. The last 12 hours of the cycle of *P. falciparum* are spent in red cells sequestered in deep tissues at low oxygen tension: gelation of HbS inhibits both the invasion of red cells and the growth of parasites within them.

In areas where malaria is endemic, children with HbAS who are non-immune or semi-immune (that is, those aged between 6 months and 5 years) have less intense *P. falciparum* parasitaemia than children with HbAA, so they have a survival advantage, which maintains a population prevalence of sickle-cell trait of up to 30 per cent. High frequencies of the gene for HbS are found where *P. falciparum* malaria is, or was, endemic (Fig. 78.9), and in their emigrant populations.

The only disadvantage, probably the result of sickling of red cells in the hypoxic, hypertonic and acidotic medulla, is a partial renal tubular defect in concentrating urine and conserving water (Chapter 83). Dehydration is the probable mechanism of very rare sudden unexplained death following extremely intensive physical exercise. Sickling and infarction may cause papillary necrosis, with consequent haematuria and liability of bacteriuria and pyelonephritis, especially during pregnancy. Hb AS does not lead to anaemia or reduced life expectancy.

The pathology of sickle-cell disease

Haemolysis and anaemia

Abnormal red cells are removed by the RES: in early childhood, active erythrophagocytosis leads to an enlarged liver and spleen. Hepatomegaly persists invariably into adult life, but usually the spleen shrinks as a result of infarction. A palpable spleen in children over 2 years of age is more common (about 35 per cent) in those with HbSC than in those with HbSS (less than 10 per cent). In occasional patients with HbSS and up to 10 per cent of children aged about 10 years with HbSC, splenomegaly leads to hypersplenism, causing more severe anaemia, a low white cell count and thrombocytopenia (platelets $<150\times10^9$/l).

Chronic anaemia leads to erythroid hyperplasia and expansion of the bone-marrow cavities: the facies is characteristic, with swelling of the forehead which causes an exaggerated supraorbital sulcus, and bossing of the maxilla which results in the bridge of the nose appearing sunken, and forward protrusion of the upper incisor teeth (gnathopathy). The heart is enlarged invariably after about 6 years of age. Moderate jaundice and a raised serum bilirubin are the result of both haemolysis and liver dysfunction with abnormal liver function tests and fatty degeneration of the liver leading to liver failure. Pigment-stones in the gall bladder are found in about 10 per cent of adult Nigerians, but do not usually cause symptoms: in an abdominal crisis, do not assume that stones are the cause of the pain. In the steady state there is a moderate anaemia (Hb 6.0–10.0 g/dl in HbSS and HbS/β^{o}thal; Hb 9.5–14.0 g/dl in HbSC).

There are four types of anaemic crisis, during which the Hb concentration falls catastrophically.

Haemolytic crisis. These cause severe anaemia and jaundice; they may follow infection, for example malaria (Ibidapo & Akinyanju, 2000), but often no trigger is defined.

Sequestration crisis. The properties of the membrane of red cells may be altered during infection, sensitizing them for phagocytosis. When the spleen is intact, for example in young children (about 5 years of age) or pregnant women with HbSC, the spleen enlarges dramatically and the Hb falls precipitously.

Aplastic crisis. If the marrow is depressed by infection – particularly by parvovirus B19 – severe anaemia develops quickly.

Megaloblastic anaemia. Almost all untreated African children with sickle cell disease are folate deficient and more than 10 per cent of Africans with sickle-cell disease have megaloblastic erythropoiesis due to folate deficiency, as a result of poor nutrition, high demands for folate secondary to chronic haemolysis and erythroid hyperplasia, and the effects of intercurrent infections (p. 952).

Types of sickle-cell crises

Anaemic
- Haemolytic
- Sequestration
- Aplastic
- Megaloblastic

Infarctive

Infarction

Deoxygenation of haemoglobin in the capillaries favours polymerization of HbS and sickling. Sickled red cells are rigid and unable to distort within the capillaries. They adhere to each other and to endothelium, block the capillaries and cause infarction, with further endothelial damage and thrombosis. Necrosis of infarcted tissue leads to sudden swelling, severe pain, and fever, which lasts about 5 days with gradual recovery.

Crises are precipitated by infections, dehydration, exposure to cold, fatigue and stasis, which promote the deoxygenation of haemoglobin in the capillaries, but in many instances no trigger is identified (Ibidapo & Akinyanju, 2000). In children aged between 6 months and 2 years, infarcts occur typically in the small bones of the hands and feet (Fig. 78.11), but in older children or adults, the long bones are affected. Chest pain due to pulmonary infarction, pneumonia, infarction in the thoracic cage or rarely myocardial ischaemia, and abdominal pain due to mesenteric or splenic infarction, or infarction in the lumbar spine, or any other coincidental abdominal crisis, are common. Any tissue of the body may be the site of infarction (Table 78.3).

The brain. Children are at risk of stroke, but strokes are less frequent in Africa than America, for reasons that are obscure. Infarctive strokes are more common in children while haemorrhagic strokes are more common in adults. Mortality is about 10 per cent. Most patients recover reasonable function, but permanent loss of neuropsychometric performance is common. Education and development may be impaired also through loss of schooling due to ill-health, but some patients in Africa are now following full professional and family lives.

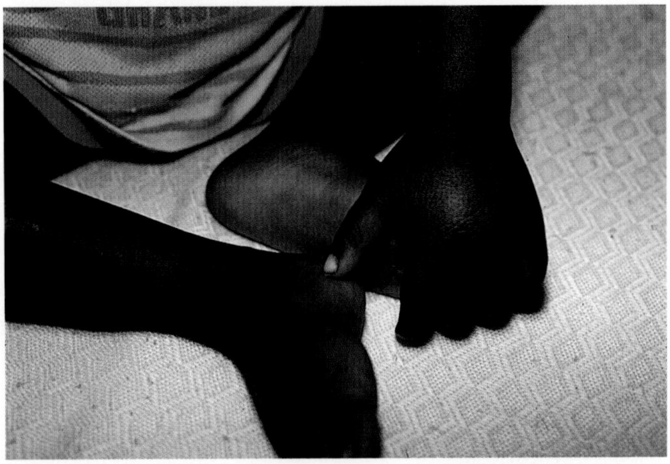

Fig. 78.11. The hand–foot syndrome in a 2-year-old girl. (With kind permission of Professor David Mabey.)

Table 78.3. Sickle-cell infarctive crises

System/organ involved (presumed pathogenesis in brackets)	Clinical manifestations		
	Symptoms	Specific signs	General signs
Musculo-skeletal system (infarcts of bone, synovium) *Note*: osteomyelitis or septic arthritis must be considered	Boring, severe, deep-seated bone pain or joint pain. Lumbro-sacral backache. Patient often crying and writhing in agony	Localized warmth, tenderness Hot swelling with acute osteomyelitis. Joint effusion. Limitations of joint movement	Pyrexia Leukocytosis
Respiratory system			
Lungs (numerous pulmonary micro-infarcts) *Note*: consider bacterial pneumonia, especially in children.	Dyspnoea: painful inspiration and expiration	Signs consistent with pneumonia	Pyrexia Leukocytosis Chest X-rays: patchy shadowing
Nervous system			
Encephalopathy (microinfarcts) *Note*: consider meningitis	Fits, drowsiness, coma	Fits, altered consciousness level. Neck stiffness	Pyrexia Leukocytosis
Cerebral hemisphere infarction	Hemiparesis/plegia	Flaccid hemiparesis/plegia	
Nerve palsies	e.g. foot drop		
Abdomen			
Spleen (splenic infarct)	Pain, generalized or localized to L. hypochondrium	Generalized or localized tenderness and guarding; splenomegaly. Absent bowel sounds sometimes	Pyrexia Leukocytosis
Liver (hepatic infarcts or sinusoidal occlusion by sickled cells) *Note*: splenic and heptatic crises frequently occur simultaneously	Pain, generalized or localized to R. hypochondrium	Generalized or localized tenderness and guarding; hepatomegaly	Pyrexia Leukocytosis Jaundice (increased conjugated bilirubin)
Intestine (local mesenteric infarct)	Generalized abdominal pain	Generalized abdominal tenderness and guarding. Absent bowel sounds	Pyrexia Leukocytosis
Genito-urinary system			
Kidneys (cortical or papillary infarcts and necrosis) *Note*: consider urinary tract infection	Generalized abdominal or loin pain, haematuria	Abdominal tenderness and guarding, haematuria	Pyrexia Leukocytosis Haematuria
Penis	Painful priapism	Priapism	

Infection

Subjects with HbSS have:

(i) partial protection against both *P. falciparum* and *P. malariae*, but even moderate parasitaemia can be followed by haemolytic and infarctive crises. Malaria is still probably the most frequent cause of death in infants and young children with sickle-cell disease.

(ii) an impaired resistance to bacterial infections because of:

- defective complement activation by the alternative pathway, so that opsonization is inadequate
- Hyposplenism
- Lesions of skin and mucous membranes following infarction
- Tissue necrosis following infarction (Figs. 78.12(*a*),(*b*)).
- Diminished cell-mediated immunity (CMI).

Strep. pneumoniae and *Salmonella* spp. are the most common organisms, and, without prophylaxis, *Strep.*

pneumoniae is the commonest cause of infectious death in non-malarious areas, and is second only to malaria in tropical Africa. Acute viral infections are particularly severe, and commonly precipitate infarctive crises.

HIV and AIDS. Patients with sickle-cell disease are at risk of infection by HIV through blood transfusion. In 1985/6, when it was first possible to test for HIV-antibodies, up to 20 per cent of patients in east and central Africa were found to be anti-HIV-positive. There appears to be a shorter asymptomatic period (as little as three months), a more rapid course and greater adenopathy than in HIV-negative people with sickle-cell disease.

Sickle-cell habitus

Growth and development are delayed: maturation of the skeleton is less than expected after the age of about 11 years and fusion of epiphyses is delayed, so that growth may continue until after 20 years of age. Puberty is about 1 year later in both sexes. Body-build is typically slender with long thin limbs, hands, and feet. Zinc deficiency is common. It contributes to retarded growth, male hypogonadism, abnormal dark adaptation, depressed CMI and more frequent vaso-occlusive crises (Prasad, 2002).

Degenerative changes

Late consequences of infarction, infection and anaemia (Serjeant & Serjeant, 2001) include:

- avascular necrosis of bones, in the head of the femur or vertebrae
- chronic leg ulcers
- duodenal ulcers
- retinopathy with loss of vision
- progressive bone marrow failure.

Conditions commonly causing death in adults are hepatic failure, renal failure, stroke and chronic lung disease with cor pulmonale secondary to multiple pulmonary arteriolar thrombi.

Laboratory diagnosis

The diagnosis of sickle-cell disease in confirmed by the characteristic peripheral blood picture (sickle-cells, target cells, macrocytes, polychromasia, nucleated red cells and Howell Jolly bodies), haemoglobin electrophoresis (Fig. 78.13) and the precipitation of HbS in the solubility test.

Prognosis

In tropical Africa, environmental factors are over-riding in determining the course of disease and lifespan of individuals with sickle-cell disease. Disease is less severe if a high

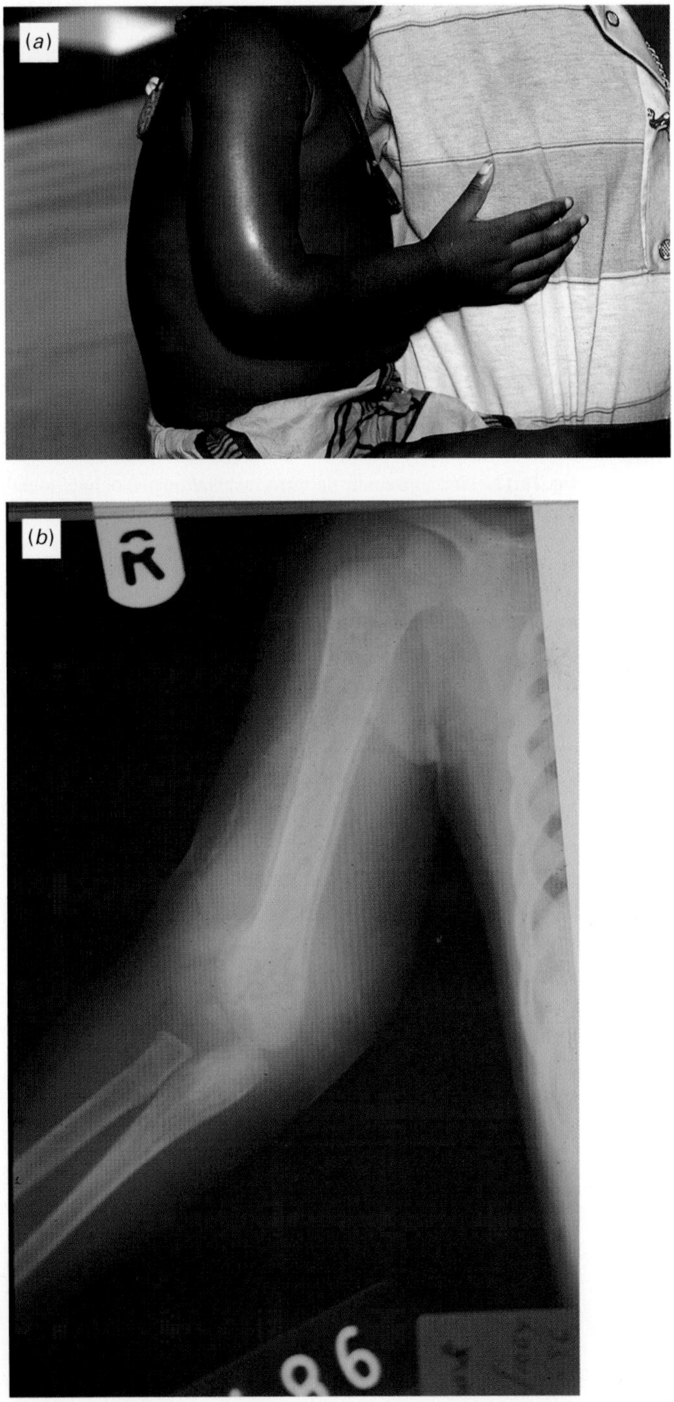

Fig. 78.12. (*a*) Salmonella osteomyelitis of the right arm of a 3-year-old boy.
(*b*) X-ray of the right arm showing osteomyelitis of the humerus; this is the same patient. (With kind permission of Professor David Mabey.)

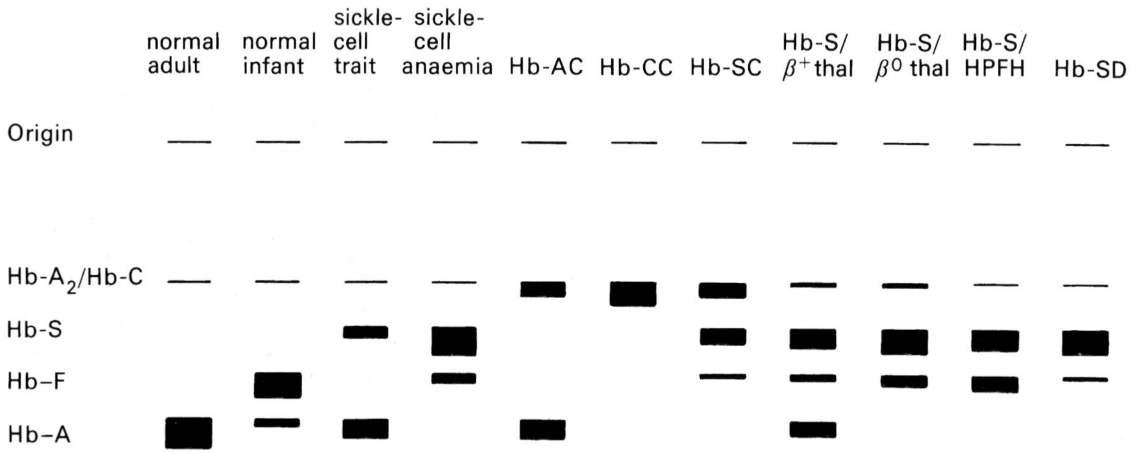

Fig. 78.13. Electrophoretic patterns (at alkaline pH) of haemoglobins from normal individuals and those with haemoglobinopathies. (Reproduced with permission from A.F. Fleming, 1982.)

level of HbF persists beyond infancy. High levels of HbF and milder disease are associated with the Senegal (Hb 8–9%) and Arab–Indian (Hb 15–20%) beta haplotypes, whereas the Benin and Bantu haplotypes are associated with low HbF (6–7% or as low as 1–2%) and severe sickle cell disease (Fig. 78.9(*a*)). (Beta haplotypes are the background DNA sequences on which the Hb S-mutation has occurred.)

Homozygous α^+-thalassaemia (p. 944), when inherited with HbSS, results in a better balance of alpha to beta globin chains and is associated with milder anaemia, more splenomegaly, decreased prevalence of stroke and leg ulces; the higher Hb and blood viscosity, however, may cause increased prevalence of avascular necrosis and of retinopathy.

Maintenance of health

Motivation – political, managerial and professional (Table 78.4) – can achieve much in assisting families to reduce the impact of the environment on the course of sickle-cell disease. This discussion is focused on what is achievable with limited resources.

Early diagnosis will enable advice and treatment to be given before progression to irreversible pathology. Protocols for the recognition of sickle-cell disease in the newborn have been established successfully in the Caribbean, Brazil and in at least one centre in West Africa.

Be alert to the possible diagnosis – do the appropriate laboratory investigations in those you suspect have sickle-cell disease, including all severely anaemic children – as up to one-quarter may be found to have sickle-cell disease.

- Try to identify members of the family who are also affected.
- Make certain that the laboratory worker at the primary health care clinic is able to interpret a thin blood film and has the materials for the HbS-solubility test.
- Make certain, too, that haemoglobin electrophoresis is available at the nearest District Hospital.
- Work with the local community and nationally to raise awareness and understanding of sickle-cell disease in the whole community.
- Educate the families of patients, the patients themselves and health professionals.
- Establish networks of Sickle-Cell Clinics with functions of education and maintaining health.

Prevention of infection

- Ensure an uninterrupted supply of appropriate antimalarial prophylactics and/or by the supply of IIBNs.
- Prevent pneumococcal infection by giving oral penicillin 125 mg twice daily from about two to three months of age until five years of age.
- Vaccinate against *Strep. pneumoniae* and *H. influenzae*.
- Vaccinate against hepatitis B virus (HBV) so as to reduce the risk of transmission of HBV by blood transfusion.
- Ensure that children with sickle-cell disease receive all the routine vaccinations of the Expanded Programme of Immunization (EPI). As vaccinators are taught not vaccinate children when they are ill, and as sickle-cell children are often ill, they can miss all or many of their immunizations.

Table 78.4. Maintaining health with sickle-cell disease (SCD)

Early diagnosis
Neonatal diagnosis
screening of pregnant women
testing newborn infants of mothers carrying HbS

Clinical awareness, laboratory testing of patients
with symptoms of SCD
with anaemia
with siblings known to have SCD

Appropriate laboratory
reporting on thin blood films
HbS solubility test (replacing sickling test) for screening
Hb electrophoresis

Education
General public
Media
Pamphlets
Posters
School and community visits

Parents, guardians, patients
One-to-one or one-to-group counselling
Pamphlets in language of choice
Reinforcement at subsequent clinic visits
Sickle-Cell Societies

Health professionals
Medical students
Postgraduates
Nurses
Laboratory staff
Paramedicals.

Sickle-cell Clinics
Prevention of infection
Anti-malarial prophylactics
Insecticide-impregnated bed-nets
Prophylactic oral pencillin

Sickle-cell Clinics (*cont.*)
Prevention of infection (*cont.*)
Pneumococcal vaccination
Haemophilus influenza vaccination
All routine vaccinations

Nutrition
Folic acid supplements (1mg/day)
General nutritional advice

Self-treatment
Paracetamol

Advice
Avoid cold, fatigue, dehydration, excessive alcohol, useless treatments
Attend clinic regularly
Report when ill
Report when pregnant

Specific treatments
Hydroxyurea
Isobutyramide (under trial)
Clotrimazole (under trial)

Obstetric care
Supervision of pregnancy
Anti-malarial prophylaxis
Folic acid supplements
Monitoring blood pressure, urinary protein
Monitoring Hb

Delivery in hospital
Trial of labour
Caesarean section for pelvic disproportion

Supervision of puerperium
Monitor for infection

Family limitation
Advise not more than two viable children

Nutrition and routine medications

Provide (i) an anti-malarial prophylactic, (ii) folic supplements, 1 mg per day, but 5 mg tablets are also acceptable and (iii) paracetamol for the self-treatment of mild to moderate pain.

Oral zinc supplementation

We recommend that 10 mg per day should be tried in Africa, as it has been shown to enhance CMI, to reduce the incidence of bacterial infections, admissions to hospital and vaso-occlusive crises. The number of irreversibly sickled cells is decreased and red cell survival is prolonged; growth is enhanced and sexual development improved (Prasad, 2002).

Hydroxyurea (specialist units)

The myelosuppressive agent, hydroxyurea, increases the proportion of HbF in the peripheral blood, prolongs the red cell survival, reduces the neutrophil count and function, and reduces the adhesion of red cells to endothelium so that there are fewer painful episodes, including acute chest syndrome. It reduces the need for blood transfusion. Experience in tropical Africa is confined at present to those few patients who can purchase the drug (current price in UK is £2.39 per 20 tablets of 500 mg).

Obstetric care and family limitation

Girls with milder forms of sickle-cell disease, e.g., HbSC, HbS/β^+ thal are likely to survive childhood and enter reproductive life, and an increasing number of women with HbSS are becoming pregnant (Harrison, 2001). Pregnant women with sickle-cell disease are particularly liable to malaria, folate deficiency and consequent severe anaemia, sequestration crises especially in HbSC individuals who have retained their spleens, infarctive crises during late pregnancy, labour and the early puerperium, infections, obstructed labour, abortion, premature delivery, and infants with intrauterine growth retardation.

Practical management

Essential steps to reduce 10 per cent maternal mortality and 30 per cent fetal loss per pregnancy:

- antenatal care – early, regular, meticulous: monitor urinary protein and blood pressure (as indicators of impending crisis), and be alert for infection, including puerperal, give anti-malarial prophylaxis and folic acid supplements.
- delivery in hospital.
- do not give a blood transfusion unless indicated clinically; get the Hb above 8.0 g/dl when delivery is imminent.

Birth control

Advise women with sickle-cell disease to have no more than two viable children, because (i) the risk to the mother increases with rising parity, and (ii) the care they can give to children may be limited through ill-health.

Treatment of crises

Patients must carry sickle-cell identity cards so that they can be treated promptly, at a designated point in the hospital.

- Do Hb, white cell count and reticulocyte count, thick and thin blood films for malaria, examine the urine and do other tests as indicated
- Give a course of curative anti-malarials and continue anti-malarial prophylaxis and folic acid.

Anaemic crisis

Many patients whose Hb has fallen from their usual steady state level will recover with no more than anti-malarial therapy, folic acid and antibiotics if indicated by clinical and laboratory findings.

Blood transfusion is indicated only if:

- the patient has respiratory distress
- the patient is in incipient or actual cardiac failure (but transfuse cautiously) (p. 925)
- there is a sequestration crisis, the Hb is <6.0 g/dl and falling
- obstetric delivery is imminent and the Hb is <8.0 g/dl
- major surgery is indicated and the Hb is <8.0 g/dl.

Donor blood should be Hb AA: blood from sickle-cell trait donors can be identified by performing the Hb–S solubility test; positive blood should not be selected for crossmatching for sickle-cell disease patients, except in urgent cases and the absence of Hb–S negative blood. *Note:* patients with sickle-cell disease may have life-threatening haemolytic transfusion reactions which are not related to any detected antibody. With many repeated transfusions, iron overload (up to total body iron 20 g) occurs, but few develop symptoms of haemosiderosis.

Infarctive crisis

There is no specific treatment.

- Treat the cause if known; give appropriate antibiotics if infected.
- Manage pain.
- Maintain hydration and acid–base balance; replace fluid liberally, either orally if possible or intravenously (see Emergencies).
- Give oxygen to patients with severe chest pain or pneumonia.

Management of pain

Patients with extremely severe pain have few or even no clinical signs. Do not think of them as either drug seekers or drug addicts.

- For severe pain, give morphine in full therapeutic doses at 2 to 4-hour intervals, with additional small doses if the pain breaks through (see Palliative care, Chapter 91).
- For less severe pain give dihydrocodeine or codeine. For mild to moderate pain give paracetamol (see the Box).
- Assess the severity of the pain regularly: adjust doses accordingly.

- Never prescribe analgesics 'as required': the doses will then be determined by the insistence of the patient and the reluctance of the nursing staff to administer addictive treatment.
- Adjunctive treatment can include promethazine and a non-steroidal anti-inflammatory drug.

Pain in sickle-cell crisis
Assess pain. Titrate doses of drugs

Severe pain
- Morphine
- Additional NSAID or promethazine

Less severe pain
- Dihydrocodeine

Mild pain
- Paracetamol

Give a supply of paracetamol to patients for self-treatment. Fentanyl patches are excellent for prolonged moderate to severe pain, if they can be purchased.

Stroke
Management of stroke includes rehydration and red cell transfusion, preferably exchange transfusion with the target of reducing HbS to less than 30 per cent of total haemoglobin and maintaining it subsequently by repeated transfusion to reduce the 67 per cent chance of repeat stroke to 10 per cent within 3 years. Do not embark on such a regimen unless there is a reliable supply of safe blood.

Future prospects

Five out of six infants born with sickle-cell disease are African: most lack basic care. Sickle-cell disease may be prevented through (i) the education of populations, (ii) pre-marital and post-marital screening and counselling.

Haemoglobin C

The substitution of lysine for glutamic acid at the sixth position on the β-globin chain gives rise to HbC: the mutation is at the same point as that causing HbS. HbC occurs at high frequency in the population of central West Africa (Fig. 78.9(*b*)). Over 20 per cent of the population carry the genotypes HbAC in Burkina Faso and northern Ghana: frequency declines to 8–10 per cent in southern Ghana and Mali, and to 5–7 per cent in south western Nigeria. It is found only rarely east of the River Niger.

Haemoglobin AC

The trait is harmless and not a cause of anaemia. HbC contributes about 33 per cent of the total haemoglobin (Fig. 78.13). No treatment is required.

Hb AC does not protect against *P. falciparum* parasitaemia, but is reported to offer significant protection against clinical malaria, severe malarial anaemia and cerebral malaria (Modiano et al., 2001; Argarwal et al., 2002).

Haemoglobin CC

The homozygous inheritance of HbC causes a mild haemolytic anaemia (Hb about 11 g/dl unless complicated by other causes of anaemia), which is generally well tolerated. Palpable splenomegaly is found in about one-third, with hepatomegaly in about half of subjects.

In uncomplicated pregnancy the Hb is 9.0–10.0 g/dl, but folate deficiency often develops; megaloblastic and iron deficiency anaemia can be profound.

The peripheral blood shows numerous target cells and microspherocytes: in some cells the insoluble haemoglobin has been precipitated as a dense elongated mass: there is polychromasia and occasional nucleated RBC. Almost all the haemoglobin is HbC which moves on electrophoresis in the same position as Hb A_2 (Fig. 78.13).

Management
Give folic acid supplements, especially during pregnancy, and throughout reproductive life. If malaria and deficiencies of folate or iron are prevented, pregnancy and delivery are generally uneventful.

In vitro, HbCC cells do not support the growth of *P. falciparum*. The risk of clinical malaria in children in Burkina Faso is reported to be reduced by 93 per cent in those with HbCC (Modiano et al., 2001).

Alpha-thalassaemia

The inherited reduction of synthesis of α-globin is called α-thalassaemia. There are normally two α-globin genes on chromosome 16, so that a normal individual has four genes ($\alpha\alpha/\alpha\alpha$) synthesizing the α-chains of haemoglobin. The α thalassaemias are the result usually of deletions of genes and rarely of point mutations. Deletion of one gene is called α^+-thalassaemia, and deletion of two genes is α°-thalassaemia (Hill, 1992). Only α^+-thalassaemia genes occur in sub-Saharan Africa, resulting in asymptomatic heterozygous ($-\alpha/\alpha\alpha$) and homozygous ($-\alpha/-\alpha$) states. The conditions resulting from inheritence of α°-thalassaemia, HbH disease($-\alpha/-$) and Hb Barts hydrops fetalis (-/-), do not occur in Africa, as they do in Asia (Fig. 78.9(*d*)).

Gene frequency of α^+-thalassaemia in tropical Africa is 0.05–0.27, that is up to 39 per cent are heterozygous and up to 7 per cent are homozygous, making this the most common inherited abnormality of haemoglobin synthesis (Mukwala et al., 1989). The geographical distribution, both on macro-and micromapping, gives strong support to the supposition that α-thalassaemia has been selected through it conferring protection against malaria (Hill, 1992). There are four clinical or laboratory consequences of α-thalassaemia in Africa (Mukwala et al., 1989; Chidoori et al., 1989): (i) At birth, Hb Barts (γ_4) can be detected at <2 per cent of Hb; (ii) After infancy, there are slight microcytosis (MCV 75–80 fl) and hypochromia (MCH at low normal), but insignificant anaemia; (iii) α^+-thalassaemia inherited with sickle-cell trait, lowers the proportion of HbS; and (iv) Homozygous α^+-thalassaemia, and probably heterozygous inheritance to a lesser extent, ameliorates the course of sickle-cell disease (p. 939).

Diagnosis of α^+-thalassaemia can be made at birth by the detection of traces of the Hb Barts (Mukwala et al., 1989). Later in life, the condition cannot be diagnosed by routine haematological methods, but a presumptive diagnosis of homozygous α^+-thalassaemia may be made in a patient with (i) microcytosis, hypochromia, low MCV and MCH, (ii) normal iron status, (iii) high red cell count, and (iv) minimal or no anaemia (Chidoori et al., 1989).

Beta-thalassaemia

The inherited reduction of synthesis of β-globin is called β-thalassaemia. In Africa the condition is confined to west and north Africa and to those of Asian or Mediterranean descent (Fig. 78.9(*c*)). The frequency of β^+-thalassaemia genes is highest in Liberia, where 9 per cent are carriers. Frequency declines eastward along the west African coast, reaching 0.5 per cent in south west Nigeria.

β-thalassaemia minor and malaria

Heterozygous inheritance of either β°- or β^+-thalassaemia results in asymptomatic thalassaemia minor. There is a moderate hypochromic, microcytic anaemia (Hb 9, 11 g/dl or Hb 7, 9 g/dl in pregnancy).

A relative resistance to *P. falciparum* has been described (Willcox et al., 1983), but the mechanism is not fully understood.

β-thalassaemia intermedia

The different mutations found commonly in west Africans and Afro-Americans are all mild β^+-thalassaemia alleles, so that homozygous inheritance of β^+-thalassaemia in west Africa causes a disease of intermediate severity (Hill, 1992). HbC/β^+ thal is another West African thalassaemia intermediate. Co-inheritance of α-thalassaemia trait with homozygous β-thalassaemia reduces the imbalance between α- and β-chains and results in a less severe β-thalassaemia disease.

Anaemia is usually moderate, but may be complicated by haemolytic crises precipitated by infection or pregnancy, splenomegaly and folate deficiency. Skeletal deformities from marrow hyperplasia, iron overload, leg ulcers, gallstones and an increased susceptibility to infection complicate the course of disease in older patients.

Blood films show typical thalassaemic pictures; electrophoresis shows high levels of Hb F with some Hb A (and Hb C in the case of HbC/β^+ thal).

Manage patients as if they have sickle-cell disease.

β-thalassaemia major

The most common genotypes are homozygous inheritance of β°-thalassaemia. In Africa, it is seen only in North Africa and amongst persons of Asian or Mediterranean ancestry.

Anaemia is profound (Hb 2.0–8.0 g/dl) and without treatment, there is death in early childhood from hypoxia, haemorrhage from thrombocytopenia or infection. The blood film is grossly abnormal, with microcytosis, target cells, hypochromia and nucleated red cells. Patients with homozygous β°-thalassaemia have only Hb F and Hb A_2, with no Hb A.

Treatment depends on a hypertransfusion regimen to maintain Hb above 12.0 g/dl, iron chelation to delay haemosiderosis, splenectomy, penicillin and anti-malarial prophylaxis, folic acid supplements and other supportive measures.

Glucose 6-phosphate dehydrogenase deficiency

About 90 per cent of red cell glucose is degraded to lactic acid via the Embden–Meyerhof pathway, adenosine triphosphate (ATP) is produced and energy released. About 10 per cent is degraded by the hexose-monophosphate shunt (pentose shunt) with reduction of nicotinamide adenosine dinucleotide phosphate (NADP) to NADPH (Fig. 78.14). This, in turn, maintains glutathione (GSSG) in the reduced form (GSH), which is essential for red cell integrity. GSH protects red cells from auto-oxidation, and its deficiency results in oxidation of (i) – SH groups of several enzymes, (ii) β-chains of haemoglobin with precipitation of haemoglobin as Heinz bodies, (iii) haem to form methaemoglobin, and (iv) red cell membrane lipids and proteins, with consequent haemolysis. A common cause of failure of GSH production is the inherited deficiency of activity of G6PD, the first enzyme of the hexose – monophosphate shunt (Fig. 78.14) (WHO Working Group, 1989; Sodeinde, 1992).

The enzyme

Genetics

The gene controlling production is carried on the X-chromosome. The hemizygous male inheriting the abnormal gene ($\bar{x}$Y) will have all his red cells deficient in G6PD activity, as will the homozygous female ($\bar{x}\bar{x}$); the heterozygous female ($\bar{x}$X) will have approximately half her red cells deficient, as either the $\bar{x}$ or the X-chromosome is suppressed in every female somatic cell in a random manner (lyonization).

G6PD variants

There are over 400 variants of the enzyme known and classified according to their activity (Table 78.5). In sub-Saharan Africa, there are three common enzyme variants (Ruwende & Hill, 1998).

(i) *G6PD B*, the normal variant, has a frequency 60–80 per cent.
(ii) *G6PD A+* occurs at a frequency 15–40 per cent, has about 90 per cent of normal activity, and has not been shown to confer either disadvantage or advantage.
(iii) *G6PD A−* has moderately reduced activity (Table 78.5): frequency is highest among the Luo of Kenya (32 per cent of males). G6PD A− confers both advantage (partial protection against malaria) and disadvantage (haemolysis). Other variants include G6PD Mali (severe deficiency) and G6PD Gambia (normal activity). G6PD Mediterranean (severe deficiency) is seen in Africa only north of the Sahara and among people of Asian or Mediterranean ancestry (Fig. 78.15).

G6PD deficiency and malaria

The evidence that G6PD deficiency protects against malaria is as follows.

Geographical

G6PD deficiency is seen commonly only where *P. falciparum* malaria is or was endemic, and in emigrant populations from those areas (Fig. 78.15). Within malarial areas, G6PD deficiency and the intensity of transmission of *P. falciparum* are strongly correlated.

Table 78.5. Variants of G6PD

Class	Enzyme activity	Clinical consequences	Some polymorphic variants
I	Near absent	Congenital non-spherocytic haemolytic anaemia	
II	Severe deficiency <10% normal	Intermittent haemolysis	Mediterranean, Mali
III	Moderate deficiency 10–60% normal	Less severe intermittent haemolysis	A−
IV	Normal 60–150%	None	B,A+, The Gambia
V	Increased >150% normal	None	

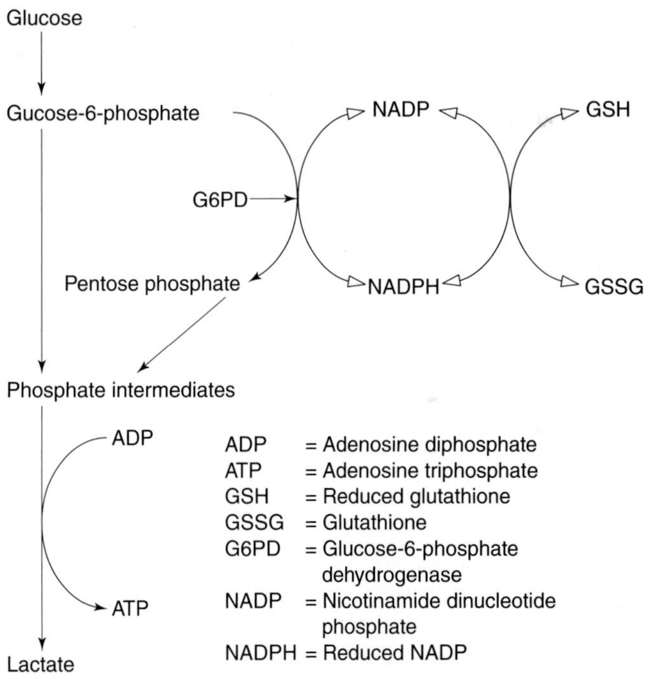

Fig. 78.14. Glucose 6-phosphate dehydrogenase, the hexose-monophosphate shunt and the Embden-Meyerhof pathway.

Clinical

Nigerian girls, heterozygous for G6PD B/G6PD A–,who had *P. falciparum* parasitaemia, had fewer parasites in the deficient than in the normal red cells.

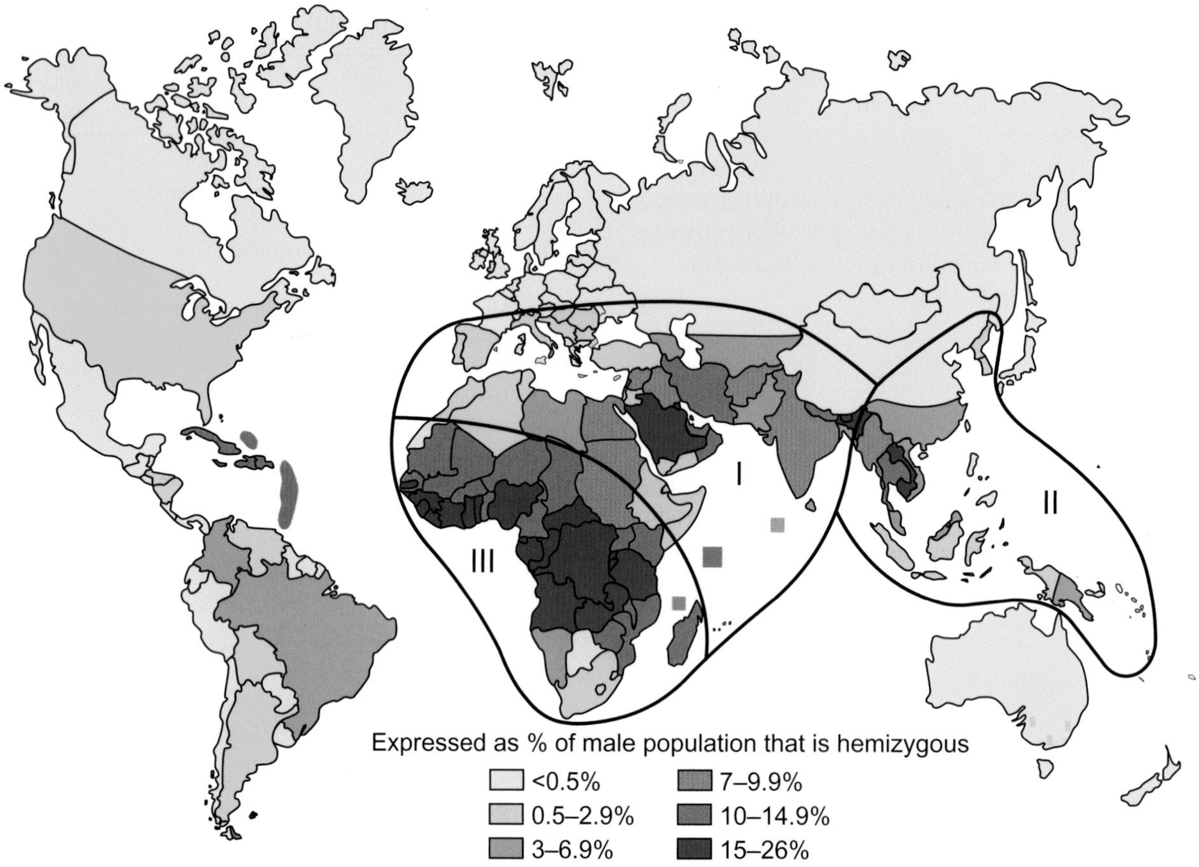

Fig. 78.15. World distribution of G6PD deficiency. Superimposed are three zones where different G6PD variants reach polymorphic frequency.
Zone I. G6PD Mediterranean.
Zone II. G6PD Mediterranean, Canton, Union, Mahidol.
Zone III. G6PD A−.
(Reproduced with permission of the publishers from WHO Working Group (1989) and Fleming & de Silva, 2003.)

Field observations

Male hemizygotes and female heterozygotes were lower in frequency in children with severe malaria than in controls (Ruwende & Hill, 1998).

In vitro observations

P. falciparum can invade equally both G6PD deficient and normal red cells (Cappadoro et al., 1998). During the ring stage of the erythrocyte cycle, the parasite has not started its own G6PD production, and if the host cells are deficient, there is a depletion of GSH making the deficient and parasitized red cell vulnerable to oxidative damage and highly susceptible to phagocytosis. This limits the level of parasitaemia and is probably the main mechanism of protection against severe malaria in G6PD deficient persons.

Clinical manifestations

When in the steady state and not exposed to excessive oxidative stress, red cell survival and Hb concentration are normal with G6PD A–. With class II enzymes, such as G6PD Mediterranean, there may be a constant low grade haemolysis. G6PD deficiency is clinically important in four situations:

- neonatal jaundice
- infection-induced haemolysis
- drug-induced haemolysis
- food-induced haemolysis.

Neonatal jaundice

Severe jaundice (serum bilirubin above 250 μmol/l (15 mg/dl)) on about the fourth day of life is seen at high but unmeasured frequency in sub-Saharan Africa.In west Africa, 33–80 per cent of jaundiced infants are G6PD deficient, and in northern Nigeria, sepsis, prematurity and G6PD deficiency alone or in combination accounted for 85 per cent of jaundice in the newborn.

Anaemia is usually moderate. Total and unconjugated bilirubin levels are high. When the bilirubin rises above 300 μmol/l, the pigment crosses the blood–brain barrier, accumulates in the basal ganglia (kernicterus) and causes severe and permanent brain damage.

Treatment
Ultraviolet light converts bilirubin to substances which are excreted effectively by the liver without conjugation. Phototherapy is the treatment of choice in mature and otherwise healthy infants when the bilirubin is in the range 250–300 μmol/l. A locally made unit or exposure to morning sunlight is also effective: the infant must be cooled and the eyes shielded. If the bilirubin rises above 300 μmol/l, a double volume exchange blood transfusion, with G6PD normal blood, is indicated. With low birthweight or sick infants, start both phototherapy and exchange transfusion at lower bilirubin levels.

Prevention
Prevention is through campaigns of health education; excellent antenatal and obstetric care; screening of neonates for G6PD and follow-up of those found deficient; and, finally, issue of identity cards to patients.

Infection-induced haemolysis
Both haemolysis and liver failure contribute to the jaundice which complicates infection in G6PD deficient patients: anaemia may be severe, as erythropoiesis is suppressed and oxidant drugs worsen the haemolysis. In Africa, infection – whether viral or bacterial – induces haemolysis more commonly and more severely than drug-induced haemolysis (Sodeinde, 1992).

- Treat the primary cause and avoid oxidant drugs.

Drug-induced haemolysis
The range of drugs and chemicals which induce haemolysis (Table 78.6) is smaller and the haemolysis is less severe with G6PD A− than with G6PD Mediterranean. Jaundice appears about three days after the drug is taken. If the haemolysis is severe and intravascular, there will be haemoglobinuria: most blackwater fever without quinine administration is seen in G6PD-deficient subjects. The Hb is lowest after about 8 days, but erythroid hyperplasia, leads to an increase in reticulocytes and Hb. With G6PD A− haemolysis is confined to the oldest red cells. There is erythroid hyperplasia, which compensates for the haemolysis. Treatment with the precipitating drug can continue but any increase in dose may lead to a further episode of haemolysis. Treatment, if necessary, is by withdrawal of the drug. Prevention is by avoiding oxidative drugs and chemicals (Table 78.6).

Table 78.6. Drugs and chemicals which should be avoided by persons with G6PD deficiency

Anti-malarials	primaquine, pamaquine
Sulphonamides	co-trimoxazole (trimethoprim-sulphamethoxazole), sulphacetamide, sulphanilamide, sulphapyridine
Sulphones	dapsone, Maloprim (pyrimethamine-dapsone)
Nitrofurans	nitrofurantoin
Quinolones	ciprofloxacin, nalidixic acid, norfloxacin, oxofloxacin
Schistosomicide	niridazole
Miscellaneous	naphthalene, methylene blue

Food-induced haemolysis
Favism is the acute and often severe haemolytic crisis precipitated by eating the fava bean (*Vicia faba*) or by inhaling its pollen. G6PD A− can cause favism (Galiano et al., 1990), but the fava bean is not eaten generally in sub-Saharan Africa.

Outbreaks of food-related haemolytic anaemia have occurred in Nigeria: the precipitating food was identified as kebab meat coloured by Orange RN (Williams et al., 1988).

Diagnosis

The Hb and red cell indices are normal during the steady state, until a typical haemolytic crisis occurs (p. 926). The peripheral blood film shows Heinz bodies with supravital staining. Routine staining shows blister cells (cells with a pale area immediately below the 'skin' of the red cell) and bite cells (ruptured blisters): both represent the space occupied by Heinz bodies.

Screening can be done with simple kits, which depend on the detection of NADPH production. Kits are not reliable following a haemolytic episode, when there is a population of young red cells and the G6PD activity of the blood is raised. Confirm the diagnosis either by centrifuging the blood and testing the older cells which are at the bottom of the column, or by repeating the test after 6 weeks free of haemolytic episodes.

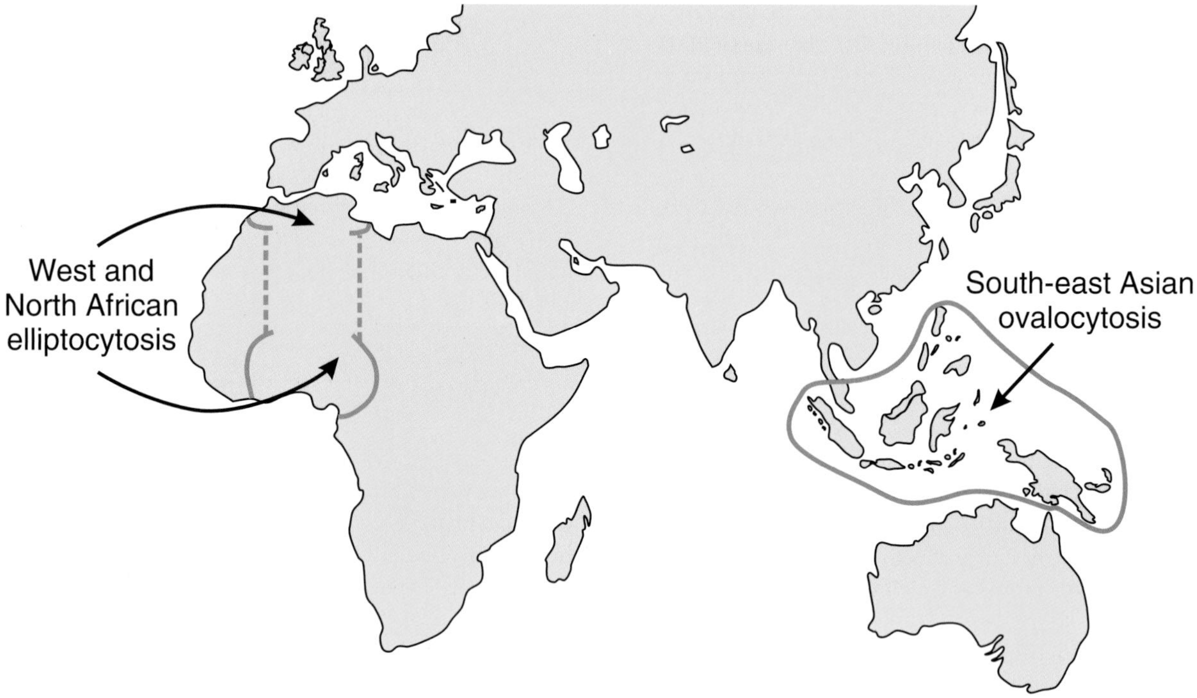

Fig. 78.16. Areas of the Old World where congenital ovalocytosis and elliptocytosis reach polymorphic frequency. (Reproduced with permission of the publishers from Fleming & de Silva, 2003.)

Elliptocytosis and ovalocytosis

Elliptical red cells are seen frequently, in up to 2–3 per cent of the population, in west Africa, the Maghreb (Tunisia, Algeria and Morocco) and the western Sahara amongst the Tuaregs, but not in other parts of Africa (Fig. 78.16) (Nurse et al., 1992). Polymorphic frequency suggests that the condition confers advantage.

Elliptocytosis is usually symptomless. Intercurrent infection can precipitate moderate haemolysis with moderate splenomegaly, but anaemia can be profound with intense *P. falciparum* parasitaemia.

Southeast Asian ovalocytosis is an inherited defect of red cell membrane band 3 commonly seen in people of Malay and Melanesian descent (Fig. 78.16). It has been observed in the population of the highlands of Madagascar (0.8 per cent of children) and in families of mixed race in Cape Town, presumably reflecting Indonesian and Malay ancestry (Coetzer et al., 1996; Rabe et al., 2002). The heterozygous condition is harmless, except that malarial anaemia is exacerbated by ovalocytosis. Ovalocytosis does not protect against *P. falciparum* and *P. vivax* parasitaemia (as was thought previously because the rigid ovalocytes were not invaded in vitro), but gives powerful protection against cerebral malaria, probably through reducing sequestration of parasitized erythrocytes in the cerebral vasculature, a process which involves normal membrane band 3.

Decreased red cell production

Nutritional anaemias

A deficiency of iron can result in a failure of synthesis of haemoglobin, and an anaemia which is characterized by small (microcytic) and under-haemoglobinized (hypochromic) red cells. Deficiencies of either folic acid or vitamin B12 result in a failure of synthesis of DNA, and hence of division of blood precursor (and other) cells, and an anaemia characterized by large red cells (macrocytes) and large precursor cells in the bone marrow (megaloblasts).

Iron deficiency

The problem in Africa

In Africa about 50 per cent of children and pregnant women and 25 per cent of men are affected, compared with 7–12 per cent of children and women in high-income countries. Infants, young children and pregnant women are at highest risk, although adolescent girls also have a high prevalence.

Aetiology

More than one cause may operate in the same individual (Fig. 78.17).

Reduced iron intake

Haem iron from animal food is readily absorbed but this food is regularly eaten only by few people. Most eat a grain staple, containing high amounts of non-haem iron which is poorly absorbed (1–2 per cent of dietary iron), inhibited chiefly by phytates in cereals and tannins in tea. Ascorbic acid from fruit or vegetables and amino acids from animal protein digestion enhance the absorption of non-haem iron, but they are often too costly for poor people. Cooking or brewing in iron pots adds absorbable organic iron to the food (Saungweme et al., 1999). Vitamin A plays a vital role in the utilization of both food and supplemental iron (p. 956).

Increased demand

Iron balance varies throughout different stages of life. The demands for iron are high during infancy, adolescence, menstruation and pregnancy and in babies born with low birthweight and/or gestational age. Numerous and closely spaced pregnancies cause severe iron deficiency but, because of amenorrhoea, breast-feeding is a time of low demands for iron, although milk contains iron.

Increased iron loss

Hookworm infection is the most frequent cause of iron deficiency, from loss of blood, in developing countries (Stoltzfus et al., 1997). The haematuria of *Schistosoma haematobium* (Chapter 25) can lead to an iron loss of 30–40 mg per day, as in the iron deficiency in adolescent boys in Somalia and coastal Kenya (Stephenson et al., 1989). *S. mansoni* also causes iron deficiency through chronic haemorrhage from colonic ulcers, polyps and oesophageal varices. Heavy infections by *Trichuris trichuria* (Chapters 21 and 22) may contribute to iron deficiency in children. Heavy menstrual loss and loss of blood at delivery where the fertility rate is high are important causes in women.

Manifestations of iron deficiency

Symptoms depend on the speed at which anaemia develops. In chronic deficiency, most patients complain of lethargy, dizziness, weakness, dysphagia and dyspnoea,

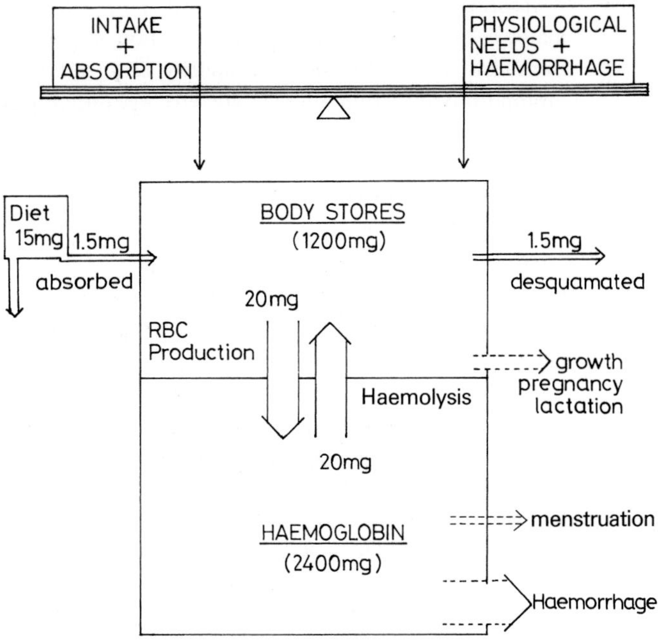

Fig. 78.17. Factors governing iron status.

and have epithelial atrophy with spoon-shaped nails (koilonychia), papillary atrophy of the tongue, and angular stomatitis.

Behavioural changes

Iron deficiency causes changes in behaviour (irritability, short attention) and lower developmental scores in infants and children, while iron supplementation improves cognitive functions of iron deficient adolescent girls (Bruner et al., 1996).

Pica, a common manifestation of IDA, when patients eat earth, chew furniture, ice or other objects, disappears soon after iron therapy is started. Geophagia (earth-eating) is very common among pregnant women in East Caprivi, Namibia (Thomson, 1997).

Growth impairment

Iron deficiency may impair growth in infants and children: children whose food was cooked in iron pots had a better rate of growth (Adish et al., 1999).

Diagnosis

Assessment of iron stores

In any health facility: haemoglobin concentration.

In a district hospital: blood film microcytosis and hypochromia; low MCHC; bone marrow aspirate stained for iron.

In specialized centres: low MCV and MCH on automated cell counter; serum ferritin; serum iron; serum transferrin (as total iron binding capacity, TIBC; red cell protoporphyrin; serum soluble transferrin receptor (sTfR) assay (see the Box below).

Stages of iron deficiency

- *Latent:* macrophages depleted of iron: serum ferritin reduced: all other parameters are normal.
- *Patent:* Serum iron falls (iron stores are depleted): TIBC and, later, red cell protoporphyrin levels rise. Hb levels and red cell indices are normal.
- *Iron deficiency anaemia:* Hb reduced: red cells hypochromic and microcytic.

A lower than normal serum ferritin indicates iron deficiency, but serum ferritin is an acute phase protein and may rise in infections, whereas serum iron and TIBC are lowered in inflammation and infection. Serum ferritin levels are frequently raised (sometimes remarkably) in individuals living in malaria endemic areas, while serum iron may be either reduced or raised (due to haemolysis) and TIBC is usually raised.

Confirm iron deficiency by the absence of stainable iron in a bone marrow aspirate and by a rise of Hb after oral iron therapy.

Iron and malaria interactions

Sound evidence is the basis of the practice outlined here:

(i) Infants and children: oral prophylactic iron is safe in low doses for 4 months during the first year of life; this decreases the incidence of anaemia without increasing the risk of malaria (Menendez et al., 1997; Verhoef et al., 2002).

(ii) Pregnant women exposed to malaria: oral prophylactic iron is safe, but in women with Hb AS, prophylactic iron is of no benefit, increases the prevalence of placental malaria infection and decreases mean birthweight (Menendez et al., 1995).

(iii) Cover or precede oral iron by effective anti-malarial therapy. Parenteral iron increases the risk of malaria in pregnant women and infants, and of sepsis in neonates. If possible do not use it, but if your patient does not respond to oral iron, cover intramuscular iron or total dose iron infusion by a curative anti-malarial course, followed by 3 weeks of prophylaxis and folic acid.

Management

- Ferrous sulphate (200 mg tablet = 60 mg elemental iron), or ferrous gluconate/ferrous fumarate. Side effects are dose related – nausea, constipation and diarrhoea.
- Continue for 3 months after Hb is normal: explain the need for this to patients.
- If Hb does not rise, 0.1 to 0. 2 g/dl per day (2.0 g/dl over 3 to 4 weeks), it is probable that they are not taking their tablets.
- Reticulocytosis is maximal at 7 to 10 days. The red blood cell count becomes normal in about 8 weeks, but epithelial recovery takes considerably longer.

Laboratory findings in iron deficiency anaemia and anaemia of chronic disorders

	Iron deficiency anaemia	Anaemia of chronic disorders
Red cells	Microcytic, hypochromic	Normocytic, normochromic In advanced disease; microcytic, hypochromic
Serum		
Iron	Reduced	Reduced
Transferrin	Raised	Moderately reduced
Transferrin saturation	Reduced	Moderately reduced
Ferritin	Reduced	Raised
Marrow		
Erythroblasts	Micronormoblastic	Hypoplastic, normoblastic Sometimes dyserythropoietic
Macrophage iron	Absent	Increased
Sideroblasts	Absent	Reduced or absent

Dosage of oral iron

Depending on the severity of the anaemia:

1. Adolescents and adults including pregnant women.
   - 1 tablet of 200 mg ferrous sulphate twice or three times daily.
2. Children from 2 to 12 years of age.
   - 1 tablet of 200 mg ferrous sulphate once daily.
3. Children less than 2 years of age.
   - 3 to 6 mg elemental iron /kg body weight per day in fluid preparation.

Prevention

Iron supplementation

(i) *Pregnant women.* Give 200 mg ferrous sulphate daily, combined with folic acid 500 μg, for at least 6 months and for 3 months post-partum. Develop a locally effective method, as for example in the Gambia where community health workers and traditional birth attendants delivered iron supplements effectively to pregnant women in rural areas(Menendez et al., 1994).

(ii) *Infants and children between 2 and 24 months of age.* Give oral iron, 2 mg/kg per day, where there is a high prevalence of anaemia. It is probably too late to start iron supplements in infants aged 6 months, who are at high risk of iron deficiency. Mothers may not give iron for more than 3 months and supply and delivery may be ineliable (Menendez et al., 1997). Iron supplements have been successfully integrated into the EPI in Tanzania (Schellenberg et al., 2001).

(iii) *Older children,* where iron deficiency is common:
2–5 years: iron preparation to deliver 2 mg/kg pelemental iron per day.
6–11 years: iron II sulphate 100–200 mg daily.

(iv) *Adolescence.* No system developed to deliver the needed 200 mg iron(II) sulphate daily.

Iron fortification of food

The mean Hb will rise slowly in the entire population,

Dietary modification

Difficult – those in real need are often too poor and so have no choice. The ideal is shown in the Box.

Prevention of hookworm infection (see Chapter 22)

Dietary modification to increase bioavailable iron

(but these foods are often too expensive and some are seasonally unavailable)

- Increase intake of haem-containing foods – red meat, poultry, fish
- Increase intake of enhancers of absorption of non-haem iron – animal protein, but not eggs: ascorbic acid-rich fruit and vegetables, raw or lightly cooked
- decrease intake or effects of inhibitors of non-haem iron absorption – tea or coffee; not to be drunk with meals; germination and fermentation of grains
- increase intake of absorbable inorganic iron – cooking and brewing in iron pots (Adish et al., 1995)

Folic acid deficiency

Chemistry of folic acid

The basic molecule of folic acid is pteroyl-glutamic acid (PGA) (Fig. 78.18). Active folates are formed when PGA is reduced to dihydro or tetrahydro forms by the action of dihydrofolate reductase, condensed with one-carbon radicals (methyl, etc.), and conjugated with further glutamic acid radicals. Folates are:

- essential co-enzymes in the transfer of one-carbon radicals, and take part in pyrimidine and purine synthesis
- needed for the conversion of uridine to thymidine, required for the synthesis DNA essential for all cell division, and
- involved in amino acid interconversions, notably homocysteine to methionine.

Dietary sources and daily needs

Many common vegetable and animal foods are good sources of folate, although staples are poor. Much of the folate in raw food is lost in storage and prolonged cooking. Approximately one-third of the surviving folate in food is absorbed. Body stores can be depleted in only 3 weeks by a wholly folate-free diet (see the Box at the top of the next page).

Causes of folate deficiency and those at risk

There are five groups of causes: low intake, malabsorption, high physiological requirements, pathologically high demands and disturbed metabolism (Tables 78.7, 78.8).

Nutritional

Diets in many parts of Africa contain little folate, and deficiency is widespread and common, except in Uganda and other areas where matoke/plantain is a staple, and seasonal, as fresh food gets scarce and expensive towards the late dry season and the early rains, as in Nigeria

Sources of folate in food commonly eaten in Africa

- *Rich sources*
  Liver, kidney, yeast
- *Good sources*
  Green leaf vegetables, yam, sweet potatoes, young Irish potatoes, bananas, plantains, fresh beans, red and green peppers (fresh or dried), melon seeds, nuts, chocolate, cocoa.
- *Moderately good sources*
  Red meat, poultry, fish, eggs, milk and milk products, cowpeas, carrots, tomatoes, okra (fresh or dried), some fruit (e.g., mangoes), cabbage, beer.
- *Poor sources*
  Rice, maize, sorghum, millet, tef, cassava, non-green vegetables, alcoholic spirits.

Table 78.7. Daily requirements of folic acid and vitamin B_{12} throughout life

	Food folate (μg per day)	Vitamin B_{12} (μg per day)
0–6 months	50	0.3
7–12 months	120	0.3
1–12 years	200	1.5
13 years and over	400	2.0
Pregnancy	800	3.0
Lactation	600	2.5

Source: Modified with permission from WHO (1972).

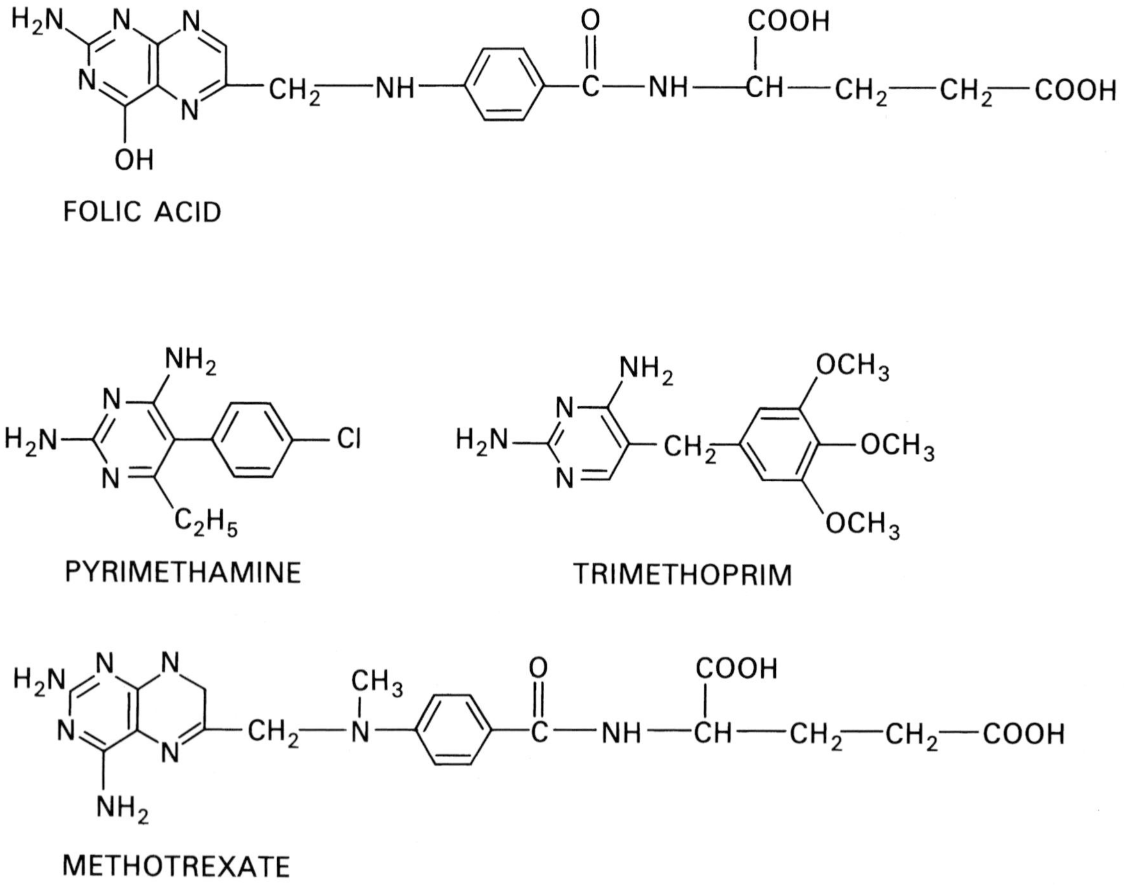

Fig. 78.18. Formulae of folic acid (pteroyl-glutamic acid (PGA), and the folate antagonists pyrimethamine, trimethoprim and methotrexate.

Table 78.8. Causes of folate and vitamin B_{12} deficiency

	Folate	Vitamin B_{12}
Inadequate intake	Overcooking	Breast-feeding by B_{12} deficient mother
	Seasonal food shortage	
	Famine	
	Prolonged storage of food	
	Goat's milk feeding of infants	
	Inappropriate weaning foods	
	Anorexia (recurrent infection, old age)	Starvation – imprisonment
	Taboos and food fads	Veganism
	Alcoholism	Food fads
Malabsorption	Diarrhoea in infancy	Pernicious anaemia
	Acute enteric infections	Gastrectomy
	Acute *Giardia lamblia*	Chronic *Giardia lamblia*
	Systemic infection (pneumonia, TB)	*Diphyllobothrium latum*
	Ileocaecal TB	
	Coeliac disease	Stagnant loop syndrome
	Acute tropical sprue	Chronic tropical sprue
	AIDS	Congenital (rare)
	Drugs (barbiturates, nitrofurantoin)	
High physiological demands	Growth – prematurity	
	– infancy	
	– adolescence	
	Pregnancy	
	Lactation	
Pathologically high demands	Haemolysis – sickle-cell disease	
	– thalassaemias	
	– recurrent malaria in pregnancy	
	Malignant disease – Burkitt's lymphoma	
	– choriocarcinoma	
Disturbed metabolism	Pyrexia	Nitrous oxide
	Overdosage – pyrimethamine	Chronic cyanide poisoning – cassava
	– trimethoprim	
	– methotrexate	
	Congenital disorders – MTHFR variant	

Notes:
MTHFR, methylene tetrahydrofolate reductase.

(Fleming, 1970), Malawi (Paul, 1981), Zimbabwe (Mukiibi et al., 1989) and Kenya (Foster, 1989).

Malabsorption

Absorption is reduced in acute enteric infections, especially in infancy; systemic infections; HIV-enteropathy, intestinal tuberculosis and subclinical sprue, seen chiefly in coastal areas of Africa.

Increased requirements

(i) *Growth.* Premature infants, particularly, and children.
(ii) *Pregnancy,* most commonly in the third trimester or post-partum, but there is usually evidence of deficiency from early pregnancy.
(iii) *Prolonged lactation* (Ingram et al., 1999).
(iv) *Haemolysis,* e.g. malaria, sickle-cell disease.
(v) *Neoplasms,* e.g. megaloblastic erythropoiesis in Burkitt's lymphoma or leukaemia.

Disturbed metabolism – drugs

Antifolates

Dihydrofolate reductase inhibitors – pyrimethamine (in the combinations *Maloprim* and *Fansidar*), trimethoprim which is a constituent of co-trimoxazole, and the cytotoxic drug methotrexate (Fig. 78.18).

Infection
Dihydrofolate reductase is inactive at 39 °C: this is the probable mechanism of acute megaloblastic arrest of erythropoiesis in some pyrexial patients.

Consequences of folate deficiency

The body stores are quickly depleted when intake is low and demands are high.

Megaloblastic anaemia
As DNA synthesis of red cell precursors is disturbed, cell division is delayed: marrow cells are larger than normal (megaloblasts) and anaemia follows with characteristic peripheral blood changes (see below).

Pregnancy
Folate deficiency at conception, possibly a consequence of prolonged lactation, may cause congenital abnormalities, in particular neural tube defects, whose incidence can be reduced by pre-conceptual folic acid supplements. In later pregnancy maternal folate deficiency is associated with impaired cellular growth in the fetus and the placenta, fetal growth retardation, premature delivery and low birthweight. Fetal loss with severe megaloblastic anaemia in pregnancy is over 30 per cent.

Growth
Deficiency impairs growth – children with sickle-cell disease may resemble pituitary dwarfs. Nigerian primigravidae, aged less than 16 years, who received folic acid supplements, grew well, had good pelvic development and had less operative delivery (Harrison, 1985).

Laboratory findings
Peripheral blood: macrocytes, hypersegmented neutrophils, and the occasional megaloblast or giant metamyelocyte in severe anaemia. Both the lymphocyte count and immunoglobulin concentration are reduced moderately in severe megaloblastic anaemia. When anaemia is severe the hypoxic bone marrow releases primitive white cells, causing leukocytosis and sometimes mimicking leukaemia (leukaemoid reaction) (Table 78.13). Platelet production is diminished, leading to thrombocytopenia which responds rapidly to treatment: this may cause purpura or haemorrhage, notably retinal haemorrhages, either following acute disturbances of folate metabolism (folate-antagonist overdose) or with long-standing deficiencies.

Bone marrow: giant metamyelocytes, megaloblasts, and frequently excess intracellular iron.

Megakaryocytes are larger than normal. If possible, measure serum and red cell folate and serum viatamin B_{12}.

Treatment
Give folic acid, 5 mg tablet daily: treatment for 3 weeks will replace the body's stores. Continue for as long as the cause of folate deficiency remains, for example until after obstetric delivery or for life in those with sickle-cell disease. In every patient the cause of the deficiency must be tackled also.

Strategies for prevention
Supplementation
- *Premature infants*: give folic acid 50 μg per day: infants with diarrhoea need 50 μg per day, which can be additional to the supplement for prematurity.
- *Pregnant women*: give 500 μg per day, combined in one tablet with ferrous sulphate 200 mg per day.
- *Chronic haemolytic anaemia (for example, sickle-cell disease)*: give folic acid 1 mg per day, or the readily available 5 mg tablets.

Fortification
In South Africa, central milling allows fortification of maize flour to be done simply and inexpensively.

Diet and health education
'Cook carefully and eat folate-rich foods.'

Vitamin B_{12} deficiency

In subtropical South Africa, it has accounted for 52 per cent of all megaloblastic anaemias in Soweto (Ingram et al., 1999) and in Zimbabwe, 86 per cent of megaloblastic anaemias not associated with pregnancy were due to pernicious anaemia (PA) (Savage et al., 1994). PA is rare in tropical Africa (Akinyanju & Okany, 1992).

The cobalamins, which are generally referred to as vitamin B_{12}, are linked closely with folate in one-carbon radical transfer, including pyrimidine synthesis so that the haematological and some other consequences are identical in the two deficiencies.

Vitamin B_{12} is found in liver, kidney, meat, fish, eggs and milk. It is released in the stomach from its protein binding and combined with the mucoprotein, intrinsic factor (IF), which is secreted by the parietal cells. The IF–B_{12} complex is adsorbed onto the microvillous membranes of the ileum, where ileal factors are required for release from IF and active absorption. The normal serum vitamin B_{12} level in symptom-free Africans (160–2250 ng/l) is much higher than the levels in Europeans (150–800 ng/l). Vitamin B_{12} is transported in plasma combined to proteins called transcobalamins (TC); TCI is derived from neutrophils and TCII from the liver. TCII-bound vitamin is metabolically active: the function of TCI-bound vitamin is not known. The serum unsaturated vitamin B_{12} binding is commonly higher in Africans (900–2350 ng/l) than in Europeans (560–1430ng/l). The higher serum vitamin B_{12} and unsaturated vitamin B_{12} binding are the consequences of TCII alleles in Africans having high vitamin B_{12} affinity (Carmel, 1999). Raised serum vitamin B_{12} is also seen in advanced protein malnutrition, liver disease, and intrahepatic infections, and myeloproliferative disorders, including chronic myeloid leukaemia. Stores of vitamin B_{12} are chiefly in the liver and are sufficient for 2 to 3 years.

Causes of vitamin B_{12} deficiency

Malabsorption

Disease of the stomach and lack of IF, or disease of the terminal ileum. Addisonian PA is an autoimmune disease, with antibody production against IF and/or parietal cells, with consequent failure of IF production.

Occasionally, patients in Africa cannot absorb vitamin B_{12} from an otherwise normal intestinal tract and their disease is related to a long-past severe diarrhoea. Chronic *Giardia lamblia* infection also depresses vitamin B_{12} absorption but the mechanism is not clear.

Low serum vitamin B_{12} is found in up to 40 per cent of patients with AIDS. This seems to be primarily the result of a progressive decline of TCI binding protein derived from neutrophils and does not necessarily represent tissue deficiency.

Food

Dietary vitamin B_{12} deficiency is rare.

Consequences of vitamin B_{12} deficiency

Body stores of vitamin B_{12} are sufficient for 2 or more years, so that any deficiency develops insidiously.

Megaloblastic anaemia

The haematology of vitamin B_{12} deficiency is indistinguishable from folate deficiency. PA is seen at a relatively younger age in Africans, up to 30 per cent are below the age of 40 (Carmel 1999).

Nervous system

Subacute combined degeneration of the cord, peripheral neuropathy, and optic atrophy are prominent in vitamin B_{12}-deficient Africans (Savage et al., 1994).

Skin

Excess melanin in unpigmented skin, most obvious on the palms, soles and knuckles, is seen with vitamin B_{12} deficiency or *prolonged* folate deficiency.

Laboratory diagnosis

The peripheral blood pictures and bone marrow appearances are identical to those of folate deficiency. Measure serum vitamin B_{12} (if possible) when the deficiency is suspected. A therapeutic trial of hydroxocobalamin 1 μg per day intramuscularly causes a reticulocyte and Hb increase within 7 days if the patient is Vitamin B_{12} deficient. If there is no response, give a therapeutic trial of folic acid 50 μg/day. A test for anti-IF antibodies has a high sensitivity in South Africa and is a technique which could be established in referral laboratories in Africa (Carmel, 1999).

Treatment

> Give hydroxocobalamin 1 mg i.m. six times over 2 weeks in order to replace stores, and then 1 mg every 3 months for life to patients with vitamin B_{12} malabsorption. Where only cyanocobalamin is licensed, it has to be given monthly for maintenance.

Hydroxocobalamin has the additional advantage of being a cyanide antagonist (which cyanocobalamin obviously is not) in the treatment of cyanide intoxication from cassava or other sources.

Vitamin A and anaemia

The association between vitamin A, iron parameters and anaemia are not well understood. Several hypotheses have been proposed:

- Vitamin A enhances the release of iron from the RES.
- Vitamin A deficiency is associated with an increase in susceptibility to infectious diseases, including malaria (Serghides et al., 2002).
- Vitamin A enhances the differentation of the red cells.

The anaemia associated with vitamin A deficiency resembles hypochromic iron deficiency anaemia except that ferritin levels are normal. Vitamin A greatly enhances the haemopoietic effect of iron.

Riboflavin and anaemia

Riboflavin or vitamin B_2. In West Africa riboflavin deficiency is common in pregnant and lactating women and children, and is associated with anaemia, raised plasma iron and bone marrow hypoplasia. Sub-clinical riboflavin deficiency has been related to abnormal red blood cells indices. In west Africa, riboflavin enhanced the haematological benefits of iron (Powers et al., 1984). In areas with high prevalence of riboflavin micronutrient deficiency, give riboflavin 5 to 10 mg/day orally to children, pregnant and non-pregnant women, and to men with evidence of deficiency.

Bone marrow depression

Acute infections

Any significant acute infection depresses erythropoiesis, but usually without clinical consequence. Anaemia complicates acute infection when:

- it causes haemolysis directly, e.g., malaria, *Clostridia*
- an autoimmune haemolysis is triggered, e.g., *Mycoplasma pneumoniae*
- septicaemia or viraemia leads to DIC, which then causes microangiopathic haemolysis
- the patient has an idiosyncratic haemolysis, e.g., G6PD deficiency
- it precipitates an aplastic crisis, as in sickle-cell disease.

Anaemia of chronic disorders (ACD)

Erythropoiesis is depressed by many chronic disorders, including infections, malignancy and non-infectious inflammations. Mechanisms of the anaemia are complex, but include:

- depression of erythropoiesis with a loss of sensitivity to erythropoietin
- inadequate erythropoietin production in response to the anaemia
- a moderate shortening of red cell lifespan
- the sequestration of iron in the RES. This may have advantage to the host as it makes iron unavailable to invading organisms.

The anaemia of ACD is usually moderate, but may be profound (see the Box, p. 950). It is normochromic and normocytic, but with time becomes hypochromic and microcytic due to the unavailability of iron. Serum iron is low (<12 μmol/l). Serum transferrin is moderately reduced, as is its percentage saturation by iron (15–25 per cent, which is higher than with iron deficiency). Serum ferritin is raised as an acute reactive protein, often to above 200 μg/l. In the bone marrow, erythropoiesis appears hypoplastic, while the granulocyte precursors are typically hyperactive and the plasma cells are numerous. Megakaryocytes are increased when there is a reactive thrombocytosis. Iron is present in macrophages but normoblasts contain few or no iron granules.

Tuberculosis

ACD complicates TB (Knox-Macaulay, 1992). In disseminated TB, profound anaemia and a leukoerythroblastic or leukaemoid blood picture may be seen. Pancytopenia can be the result of HIV infection or hypersplenism. Platelet counts are sometimes raised to around 1000×10^9/l. Anti-TB treatment can also contribute to anaemia.

HIV and AIDS

HIV/AIDS is the most common cause of severe anaemia in adults in hospital in some areas (Malyangu et al., 2000) and HIV-seropositivity is strongly associated with anaemia, especially in pregnancy (Zucker et al., 1994; van Eijk et al., 2001).

Primary infection

At seroconversion, an initial lymphopenia of a few days is followed by lymphocytosis with atypical lymphocytes in the peripheral blood (Bain, 1997). There may also be a transient neutropenia, thrombocytopenia or anaemia.

Latent period of HIV

Between seroconversion and AIDS, thrombocytopenia is seen in up to 12 per cent of infected persons.

AIDS

Lymphocytes

Lymphopenia is seen commonly and is part of the fundamental pathology leading to AIDS. Atypical lymphocytes, some with lobulated nuclei, are common.

Granulocytes

About half of patients with AIDS have neutropenia. Neutrophils show either toxic changes or dysplastic features.

Red cells

Anaemia becomes increasingly common and severe as AIDS progresses, until it affects 70 to 95 per cent of patients with advanced disease: the Hb may be <5 g/dl in the terminal stages of disease. Red cells are generally normochromic and normocytic but there can be macrocytosis.

Some patients have a thrombotic thrombocytopenic purpura (TTP)-like syndrome complicated by microangiopathic haemolysis. The direct Coombs' test is often positive, but autoimmune haemolysis is rare.

Platelets

Thrombocytopenia is seen in up to 70 per cent of patients with advanced disease.

Bone marrow

The bone marrow progresses from hypercellularity (early) to hypocellularity (late), and becomes increasingly dysplastic. Plasma cells are increased.

Treatment

Treat any cause. Be alert to drug-induced pancytopenia or megaloblastic erythropoiesis as a result of self-medication with folate antagonists (p. 952).

Parvovirus B19

The virus infects most children in Africa in the first 2 years of life: about 90 per cent of adults have protective antibodies. It has a tropism for early red cell precursors, causing erythroid hypoplasia. This usually passes unnoticed, but can cause severe anaemia in (i) patients with severe chronic haemolytic anaemias including sickle-cell disease (p. 937), (ii) immunocompromised patients (Bain, 1997): HIV-infected adults, infants and children co-infected by parvovirus B19 develop severe pancytopenia, and (iii) infants born to non-immune pregnant women are infected transplacentally, and anaemia leads to abortion or hydrops fetalis.

Disorders of white cells

Reference ranges and characteristics

The reference ranges of peripheral blood WBC counts vary with age, pregnancy state, genetic factors and environmental factors.

Neutrophils (Table 78.9) are the front line of defence against bacterial infections. Their largest pool is in the bone marrow (reserve pool), the rest circulate in the peripheral blood (circulating pool) or are in tissues (tissue pool). The circulating pool has two compartments – a marginated pool of cells adherent to the vascular endothelium, and a freely circulating pool, which is the only one counted. The neutrophil count varies with age (Table 78.9). During pregnancy, the mean count rises by the second trimester to a plateau about 3.5×10^9/l higher than in non-pregnant levels. There is normally a neutrophil leukocytosis ($<40 \times 10^9$/l) at the time of delivery.

Table 78.9. Normal leukocyte counts (mean and 95 per cent confidence limits $\times 10^9$/l) in children and adults

	Total WBC		Neutrophils		Lymphocytes	
Age	Mean	Range	Mean	Range	Mean	Range
Birth	18.1	9.0–30.0	11.0	6.0–26.0	5.5	2.0–11.0
12 hours	22.8	13.0–38.0	15.5	6.0–28.0	5.5	2.0–11.0
2 weeks	11.4	5.0–20.0	4.5	1.0–9.5	5.5	2.0–17.0
6 months	11.9	6.0–17.5	3.8	1.0–8.5	7.3	4.0–13.5
6 years	8.5	5.0–14.5	4.3	1.5–8.0	3.5	1.5–7.0
16 years	7.8	4.5–13.0	4.4	1.8–8.0	2.8	1.2–5.2
21 years	7.4	4.5–11.0	4.4	1.8–7.7	2.5	1.0–4.8

Notes:
WBC: white blood cells.
Source: Data from Dallman (1977).

Table 78.10. Leukocyte counts (mean and 95 per cent confidence limits $\times 10^9$/l) in non-elite male northern Nigerian blood donors

	Mean	Range
Total WBC	5.1	2.6–10.2
Neutrophils	2.8	1.1–7.1
Eosinophils	0.11	0–2.0
Basophils	0.002	0–0.02
Lymphocytes	2.1	0.7–3.1
Monocytes	0.13	0–1.3

African adults have an apparently genetically determined neutropenia when compared to standard reference ranges (Table 78.10).

Eosinophils make up about 3 per cent of circulating WBC and are important in the defence against helminths, and in the pathogenesis of allergic and neoplastic processes. Eosinophils decline during pregnancy, and tend to disappear from the blood during obstetric delivery even when the count was initially high.

Basophils are extremely scanty in the blood.

Monocytes make up about 3–8 per cent of circulating white blood cells. They migrate to extravascular tissues where they increase in size and are named macrophages. Both macrophages and monocytes are important in phagocytosis of foreign particles and in the regulation of the immune system. The monocyte count may be raised in symptom-free people with undiagnosed infections, or low due to hypersplenism (Table 78.10).

Lymphocytes: In the peripheral blood two-thirds are T-cells, which participate in cell-mediated immune

Table 78.11. Some causes of reactive leukocytosis in African medical practice

Neutrophilia	Acute bacterial infections
	Chronic bacterial infections (e.g. TB)
	Acute viral infections
	Tissue damage
	Haemorrhage
	Haemolysis
	Malignancy
	Cigarette smoking
	Pregnancy and delivery
	Hyposplenism
Eosinophilia	Helminthic infections
	Recovery from malaria, viral and other infections
	Malignancy
	Systemic fungal infection (e.g., pulmonary aspergillosis)
	Splenectomy
	Allergic disorders
Lymphocytosis	Infections in childhood
	Malaria
	Other protozoal infections
	Viral infections
	Hyperreactive malarial splenomegaly
Monocytosis	Malaria
	Other protozoal infections
	Rickettsial infections
	Subacute or chronic bacterial infection (e.g. TB, brucellosis)

responses: one-third are B-cells which produce antibodies. About 10 per cent of lymphocytes are large granular lymphocytes named natural killer (NK) cells because of their ability to kill virus-infected and HLA-incompatible target cells.

The lymphocyte count is high at birth, rises to a peak at 6 months of life, and then declines slowly during childhood (Table 78.9). There is a slight decline of numbers during pregnancy, but of more importance are the changes of function and immune responses during pregnancy (p. 929).

Leukocytosis and leukopenia

Neutrophilia

The most common causes of neutrophilia are infections (Table 78.11). Total counts may rise to 40×10^9/l. There is often a 'shift to the left', when

1. young non-segmented neutrophils are released, their cytoplasm showing toxic granulation (an excess of large dark blue staining primary granules) and phagocytic vacuoles: the cells frequently appear ragged;
2. myelocytes, promyelocytes, and even blasts, appear – a leukaemoid reaction (Table 78.13).

The neutrophil count is chronically raised in smokers.

Eosinophilia

Helminthic infection of tissue and the larval migration of nematodes are the common causes of eosinophilia, but it may be seen also during convalescence from viral or other infections. Symptom-free people in rural Africa often have raised eosinophil counts, presumably due to exposure to helminths. Patients with hypersplenism and a helminthic infection (e.g. *S. mansoni*) can have an intense eosinophilia in the bone marrow, but low counts in the peripheral blood because of sequestration in the spleen. In people with AIDS, eosinophilia may indicate fungal infection.

Lymphocytosis

The characteristic response to infection in childhood is a lymphocytosis (Table 78.11). In acute malaria, many activated lymphocytes (plasmacytoid cells) with large nuclei containing nucleoli and dark blue staining cytoplasm are seen, and in acute viral infections, atypical lymphocytes with grey or light blue cytoplasm, so that the peripheral blood can be mistaken for ALL (Table 78.13). Adult rural Nigerians have more B-cells in their circulating lymphocytes (about 30 per cent) than Europeans (10 to 15 per cent).

Neutropenia

The usual definition of neutropenia is a neutrophil count $<2.0 \times 10^9$/l, but counts in the range $1.1–2.0 \times 10^9$/l are usual in Africa, related to genetic factors and splenomegaly (Table 78.10). The most important cause of neutropenia in Africa today is AIDS (Table 78.12).

Lymphopenia

AIDS is the commonest cause of severe lymphopenia in Africans (Table 78.12): an absolute reduction of CD4 positive T-lymphocytes is one of the earliest immunological consequences of HIV-infection.

Malignant disorders

The leukaemias are a group of malignant diseases characterized by the proliferation of leukocytes or their precursors in the bone marrow and peripheral blood. There are four main types shown in the Box (next page).

Table 78.12. Some causes of leukopenia in African medical practice

***Neutropenia*: <2.0 × 10⁹/l**
Racial (see Table 78.10)
AIDS
Acute malaria
Acute viral infections
Typhoid
Brucellosis
Overwhelming bacterial infections
Hypersplenism
Megaloblastic anaemia
Chemicals (e.g. benzene in petrol-vendors)
Drugs, herbal remedies
Acute leukaemia
Aplastic anaemia
***Lymphopenia*: <1.5 × 10⁹/l**
AIDS
Viral infection in prodromal phase
Corticosteroids
Lymphoma
Acute leukaemia

Categories of leukaemia

Leukaemia type	Predominant cells
• Acute lymphoblastic leukaemia (ALL)	Lymphoblasts
• Acute myeloid leukaemia (AML)	Myeloblasts
• Chronic myeloid leukaemia (CML)	Whole myeloid series with mature forms predominating
• Chronic lymphocytic leukaemia (CLL)	Mature lymphocytes

The four main types are further classified by light microscopy, cytochemistry, immunophenotyping of surface or cytoplasmic markers, cytogenetically and by molecular biology. The leukaemias are more common in Africa than was once thought, but there are distinct and important epidemiological differences between Africa and the industrialized countries (Fleming et al., 1999).

Acute lymphoblastic leukaemia

ALL is characterized firstly by viewing Romanovsky stained blood and bone marrow under light microscopy: immunophenotyping classifies ALL according to the maturity of the probable cell of origin.

Table 78.13. Conditions which can give blood pictures resembling leukaemias (leukaemoid reactions)

Acute lymphoblastic L R	**Acute malaria.** Miliary TB. Measles. Pertussis. Chickenpox. Syphilis. Infectious mononucleosis.
Acute myeloid or monocytic L R	Severe pulmonary or extrapulmonary TB
Chronic myeloid L R	TB. Meningococcal meningitis. Septicaemia. Megaloblastic anaemia in pregnancy. Eclampsia. Acute liver necrosis. Amoebic liver abscess. Severe haemorrhage. Mercury poisoning (from skin-lightening creams). Severe burns.
Chronic eosinophilic L R	*Ancylostoma duodenale* in infancy.
Chronic lymphocytic L R	Hyperreactive malarial splenomegaly

Notes:
L R, leukaemoid reaction. TB, tuberculosis.

Epidemiology

ALL is very rarely diagnosed where laboratory services are limited: in parts of Africa with good referral hospitals, the incidence of ALL is <1 in 10^5 per year which is much lower than in the industrialized countries. Although genetic factors are involved in leukaemogenesis, the deficit of c(common)-ALL in childhood in Africa is unlikely to be genetically determined, as the condition is now emerging in the black population of America, South Africa and Zimbabwe but not in Zambia (Fleming et al., 1999).

Clinical features

The symptoms and signs of ALL are due to malignant infiltration (lymphadenopathy, hepatosplenomegaly, bone pain and tenderness), loss of immunity and infection, haemorrhage and thrombosis, and anaemia.

Diagnosis

The total white cell count is 20.0–200.0 × 10^9/l in about 70 per cent of patients on presentation, but others have normal or low counts. The most common condition to be mistaken for ALL in Africa is an intense lymphocytic response to malaria, but other infections may also give leukaemoid blood pictures (Table 78.13). The sudan black or myeloperoxidase stains are negative with ALL but positive with AML.

Treatment and prognosis

As supportive treatment, give curative, followed by prophylactic, anti-malarials and antibiotics for any associated infection, red cell transfusions for severe anaemia and platelet transfusions (if available) for profound or symptomatic thrombocytopenia. Average survival is about 20 weeks from diagnosis with these measures.

Cytotoxic drugs – the dilemma

Long-term remissions that are probably cures can be achieved in up to 90 per cent of children with ALL in specialist centres, but such highly effective treatment with cytotoxic drugs, which have transformed the prognosis for patients with ALL, especially children, are rarely available in tropical Africa, unless perhaps twinning with hospitals in the richer northern countries can be developed (Fleming et al., 1999).

Acute myeloid leukaemia

Epidemiology and aetiology

AML is diagnosed as frequently as ALL in children in sub-Saharan Africa, whereas in industrialized countries ALL is seen about four times more often than AML. This is due not only to a low incidence of ALL, but also to a high incidence of AML in African boys, aged 5–14, from poor families, but it occurs in all age groups (Paul et al., 1992; Fleming et al., 1999). Recognized aetiological factors for AML include:

1. Exposure to benzene: cigarette smoke accounts for over 20 per cent of cases in some populations. A rising incidence of AML in Africa is a predictable consequence of the irresponsible activities of international tobacco companies. Unofficial vendors of petroleum and mechanics in roadside repair workshops have high exposure to benzene and a high prevalence of blood dyscrasias which are known to be pre-malignant (Niazi & Fleming, 1989).
2. Myelodysplastic syndromes (Mukiibi & Paul, 1994)
3. Alkylating agents.

Clinical presentation

Symptoms and signs are similar to those of ALL. *Chloroma* is a tumour of leukaemic tissue, greenish in colour on its cut surface; it is exceedingly rare in other populations, but 10–25 per cent of African children with AML present with a chloroma, most commonly in the orbit.

Laboratory diagnosis

Severe TB, especially extrapulmonary disease, may be accompanied by a leukaemoid reaction, which can fluctuate between a predominantly myeloid and a predominantly monocytic appearance (Knox-Macaulay, 1992) (Table 78.13). The AML blasts are myeloperoxidase/Sudan black positive.

Treatment and prognosis

Average survival from time of diagnosis is only 2 months. This can be prolonged to 9 months with cytotoxic therapy.

Chronic myeloid leukaemia

CML is a haemopoietic stem cell disorder, although the predominant cells seen in marrow and peripheral blood are later granulocytes. Chromosome 22 has lost much of its long arm (the remaining chromosome being the characteristic Philadelphia chromosome, seen in over 90 per cent of patients) in a recipocal translocation with chromosome 9.

Epidemiology

Incidence is about 1 in 10^5/year throughout the world: the M:F is 1.5:1, with a slightly higher rate in black males. Age-specific incidence rises with age from childhood. In Africa more patients are seen under 40 years than over; 10–20 per cent of African cases occur in childhood, contributing in Nigeria 15 per cent of all childhood leukaemias: this reflects the age distribution of the African populations rather than any significant difference of epidemiology from industrialized countries. Exposure to irradiation is a risk factor.

Clinical presentation

Patients present with gross hepatosplenomegaly: spleens are on average larger and anaemia more severe in African than European patients.

Diagnosis

The total white cell count may be as high as 500×10^9/l. Many inflammatory or infective conditions may sometimes give rise to high white cell counts and be mistaken for CML (Table 78.13). Leukaemoid reactions may be distinguished from CML by the leukocyte alkaline phosphatase reaction which is strongly positive with reactive neutrophils but negative with the granulocytes of CML.

Treatment and prognosis

Tumour mass can be reduced and the quality of life improved by oral hydroxyurea: median survival is 4 years. Treatment with oral busulphan gives a slightly shorter survival, but, as it is easier to control the white cell count with busulphan than with hydroxyurea, busulphan still has a place in the management of patients for whom attendance at a specialist clinic is difficult. The aim of treatment is to adjust dosage to maintain the total white cell count below $20 \times 10^9/l$. Transformation to AML or ALL is the usual terminal event. Imatinib inhibits *bcr-abl* tyrosine kinase (produced as a result of the chromosome 22/9 translocation), selectively blocks CML cell proliferation, and induces complete remission in the majority of patients. Its administration and monitoring are very simple, but it costs $2000 per month.

Chronic lymphocytic leukaemia

Between 90 and 95 per cent of CLL arises from mature B-cells.

Epidemiology and aetiology

In Africa, CLL is seen in subjects as young as 15 years, and the overall M: F ratio is 1:1. There is a bimodal distribution over 45, men predominate 2:1. Below the age of 45, women predominate 2:1: the frequency peaks toward the end of reproductive life; poor rural people are affected. Exposure to malaria and other intercurrent infections may stimulate, both antigenically and mitogenically, a polyclonal proliferation of B-cells (Fleming, 1990). The poorest people living in rural areas and women, because of the physiological depression of resistance to malaria and of cell-mediated immunity during pregnancy, are particularly liable to B-cell proliferation, which in an extreme form becomes HMS (p. 931). Polyclonal expansion of B-cells provides targets for neoplastic transformation, which could follow infection by an unidentified leukaemogenic virus or some other agent (Fig. 78.9). The human T-cell lymphotropic virus (HTLV-I) (see below) has a weak and non-causative association with CLL in Africa and the Caribbean, but more research is needed before 'African CLL' or 'tropical splenic lymphoma', are understood (Fleming et al., 1999; Beddo-Addo & Bates, 2002).

Clinical presentation

The course of CLL is insidious. Splenomegaly, which may be massive, is present in 90 per cent, usually with hepatomegaly. Lymphadenopathy is found in two-thirds of Africans with CLL, but not in the younger patients with 'African CLL'. Anaemia is moderate unless there is autoimmune haemolysis and thrombocytopenia is usually moderate, but some patients have bruising or purpura. Patients are immunodepressed and may have neutropenia from hypersplenism or marrow infiltration; opportunistic infections are common.

Laboratory diagnosis

The lymphocyte count is above $5 \times 10^9/l$ and up to $400 \times 10^9/l$. The bone marrow is infiltrated by lymphocytes. CLL must be distinguished from HMS with a high lymphocytosis (p. 931).

Treatment and prognosis

Patients may not require specific treatment, but antimalarial prophylaxis can reduce the size of the spleen and increase the Hb of patients with early CLL (Fleming, 1990). Specific treatment aims to reduce the total white cell count to below $20 \times 10^9/l$ by intermittent courses of oral chlorambucil. Prednisolone can help control the lymphocyte count or manage autoimmune haemolysis. Average survival is 4 years.

Adult T-cell leukaemia/lymphoma

Epidemiology of HTLV-I in Africa

The highest seroprevalence rates of 10–15 per cent have been reported from the rain forests of west central Africa (Cameroon to the DRC), in both Bantu-speakers and Pygmies, and lower rates (<6%) in other countries of West Africa. There are low prevalences in North, East and Central Africa. There is a geographical cluster, prevalence up to 3.5 per cent, in KwaZulu/Natal and neighbouring Transkei and Free State (Bhigjee et al., 1994). Seroprevalence increases with age and women are up to twice as often infected as men: high rates of prevalence have been reported in female sex-workers and there is an association with HIV-1 and HIV-2 positivity (Weber et al., 1992).

Transmission and means of prevention

Vertical transmission from mother-to-child occurs in 15–20 per cent of breast-fed infants of mothers carrying HTLV-I: transplacental transmission is less important. Transmission is also by sexual contact, by blood transfusion or through contaminated needles shared by intravenous drug users.

Pathogenesis

HTLV-1 invades CD4+ve T-lymphocytes predominantly, which are transformed and immortalized.

The lifetime risk of developing adult T-cell leukaemia lymphoma (ATLL) is approximately 5 per cent in individuals infected before 20 years of age. The incubation period between infection and the development of ATLL is decades and longer than that of tropical, spastic paraperisis (TSP).

T-cell mediated immunity is defective in carriers of HTLV-1 and patients with ATLL, so that opportunistic infections, such as *Strongyloides*, are common.

Clinical presentation

ATLL is classified as *leukaemic* acute, chronic or smouldering or as *lymphoma*. In Africa acute ATLL is commonest (47%) and lymphoma is second (27%).

Lymphadenopathy, hepatosplenomegaly, hypercalcaemia and skin lesions are seen commonly: osteolytic lesions and CNS involvement are less common. Hypercalcaemia can lead to coma and death.

Diagnosis

Patients are seropositive for HTLV-I on ELISA (confirmed by western blotting). The white cell count is $30–130 \times 10^9/l$ in patients with acute ATLL. Peripheral blood and bone marrow lymphocytes have polylobulated nuclei. Lymph node histology is of a diffuse non-Hodgkin's lymphoma, with CD4+ve and CD 8−ve T-cells. ATLL is seriously underdiagnosed in Africa, and probably contributes at least 15 per cent of all non-Burkitt's NHL (Williams et al., 1993).

Prognosis and treatment

The disease is aggressive and treatment is disappointing. Prevention and treatment of infections improve the quality of life.

Prevention

Transmission from mother-to-child can be reduced to less than 5 per cent by avoidance of breast-feeding: where this is not advisable, as in much of tropical Africa, stopping breast-feeding before 6 months reduces the risk of transmission to about 5 per cent.

Testing of blood donors for antibodies to HTLV-I should be mandatory wherever prevalent.

Haemostasis and its disorders

Reference ranges

The range of results of several laboratory measurements of haemostatic factors in healthy adult inhabitants of sub-Saharan Africa differ from the standard reference ranges.

Platelets

The internationally accepted reference range of the peripheral blood platelet count is $150–400 \times 10^9/l$. Lower counts, for example in Nigerians – $70–370 \times 10^9/l$ (Essien, 1992) could be explained as follows. The total body's platelets are in the expected range but a greater proportion of the platelets are pooled in the enlarged spleen secondary to recurrent malaria. As there are no geographical or ethnic differences in the platelet count of neonates, lower ranges in later life are probably environmentally determined.

Platelet adhesion to subendothelial tissues, and platelet aggregation in Africans are often less than in Europeans: these are probably the consequences of high plasma concentrations of macroglobulins secondary to recurrent infections (Dupuy et al., 1978; Essien, 1992).

Coagulation and anti-coagulation

Fibrinogen levels tend to be high in non-elite Africans compared to elite Africans and Europeans, probably in response to frequent and intense muscular exercise.

The ranges for thrombin time (TT), prothrombin time (PT) and activated partial thromboplastin time (APTT) do not show ethnic or geographical variation. Factor VII coagulant activity is around 25 per cent lower in Black than in White South Africans: in contrast, factor VIII coagulant activity and factor VIII related antigen are both considerably higher in Africans (Dupuy et al., 1978).

Activity of the natural anticoagulant antithrombin III is the same in healthy Africans as in Europeans. Patients with hepatic disease may have prolonged PT and TT and low levels of antithrombin III.

Fibrinolysis

Rural and poorer Africans have higher plasminogen-activator levels and higher spontaneous fibrinolytic activity than privileged urban Africans and Europeans (Dupuy et al., 1978). Fibrinolytic activity declines with urbanization and rising social class, showing that the high activity is a consequence most likely of frequent muscular exercise.

Thrombosis

The reasons for difference in prevalence of thrombotic disease have been discussed in Chapter 73.

Purpuras

This group of diseases results from (i) disorders of endothelium, (ii) defects of platelet function (thrombopathies), (iii) a low platelet count (thrombocytopenia) (Tables 78.14–78.16).

They present with:

Petechiae: pin-point purple-red spots from intradermal or submucosal haemorrhages.

Ecchymoses: haemorrhagic spots in the skin or mucous membranes, larger than petechiae.

Purpura: diffuse haemorrhage into skin or mucous membranes.

Table 78.14. Causes of purpura arising from endothelial disorders encountered in Africa

Infections	direct toxicity – viraemia: yellow fever, the haemorrhagic fevers – bacteraemia: mengingococcal septicaemia, typhoid, gram-negative septicaemias
	early immune damage: measles, scarlet fever, chicken pox, rubella, tuberculosis
	late immune damage: Henoch–Schönlein purpura, purpura fulminans
Drugs	idiosyncratic reactions: streptomycin, isoniazid, penicillins, sulphonamides
Metabolic	uraemia, scurvy, dysproteinaemia – myeloma
Fat embolism	sickle-cell disease marrow infarction, fracture of long bones
Miscellaneous	purpura simplex in young women, senile purpura, factitious purpura in psychiatrically disturbed
Congenital (rare)	Ehlers–Danlos, Osler–Rendu–Weber, others

Table 78.15. Some causes of purpura arising from disorders of platelet function encountered in Africa

Infections: Lassa fever, Marburg, Ebola

Metabolic: alcoholism, hepatic cirrhosis, uraemia, paraproteinaemia

Drugs: aspirin, indomethacin, others

Haematological disorders: acute leukaemias, myeloproliferative disorders – chronic myeloid leukaemia, polycythaemia, essential thrombocythaemia, myelofibrosis

Congenital: rarities

The bleeding time is a simple but highly sensitive test of disorders of endothelial integrity, platelet function and platelet numbers.

Vascular purpuras

Acute infections are by far the most important causes (Table 78.14): for example, the viral haemorrhagic fevers, and gram-negative, including meningococcal, and gram-positive septicaemias. Damage to endothelium can lead secondarily to consumption of platelets and thrombocytopenia (which is unusual with Lassa fever) and DIC. Ebola and Marburg virus infections cause hepatic failure and severe depression of production of clotting factors in addition to the consumption of clotting factors of DIC (p. 965).

Table 78.16. Some causes of thrombocytopenia encountered in Africa

Primarily increased consumption or destruction of platelets

Infections: acute malaria, trypanosomiasis, secondary to endothelial damage (Table 78.14)

Hypersplenism: hyper-reactive malarial splenomegaly, *Schistosomiasis mansoni*, hepatic cirrhosis with portal hypertension

Immune: AIDS, acute viral infections, idiopathic thrombocytopenia, onyalai, drug-induced – quinine, mefloquine, penicillins, disseminated tuberculosis, lymphomas and chronic lymphocytic leukaemia

Disseminated intravascular coagulation (Table 78.17)

Primarily low production of platelets

Infections: typhoid, brucellosis, parvovirus B19

Megaloblastic anaemias

Alcoholism

Aplastic anaemia

Marrow infiltration: acute leukaemias, disseminated carcinoma

Drugs: overdosage – pyrimethamine, trimethoprim, cytotoxic drugs
idiosyncratic – sulphonamides, others

Chemicals: benzene

Miscellaneous: cyclic, congenital

Thrombopathies (disturbances of platelet function)

Lassa, Marburg and Ebola infections also disturb platelet function. Other causes of thrombopathies seen in sub-Saharan African are alcoholism, hepatic disease, renal disease and overdosage with aspirin (Table 78.15).

Thrombocytopenia

Spontaneous purpura and haemorrhage rarely occur until the platelet count is less than $20 \times 10^9/l$, but an injury may bleed excessively if the platelet count is less than $50 \times 10^9/l$ and their function is impaired. In sub-Saharan Africa, the conditions which commonly progress to purpura include:

- acute viral and bacterial infections
- AIDS (p. 957)
- immune thrombocytopenic purpura (ITP) (Mukiibi, 1989; Essien, 1992)

- onyalai
- the ingestion of drugs or herbal remedies (Table 78.16).

The diagnosis of thrombocytopenia depends on the platelet count, but the experienced microscopist can recognize the near-absence of platelets on a well-spread and stained peripheral blood film.

Onyalai

The condition derives its name from the word for a blood blister in the Kimbundu language of western Angola. Since the first description at the beginning of the twentieth century, many Africans with purpura from ITP or other causes were said to have onyalai, and the diagnosis fell into disrepute. It is now clear, however, that onyalai is distinct epidemiologically, immunologically and clinically from ITP (Hesseling, 1992).

Epidemiology and aetiology

Onyalai has been described only in Africa south of the Equator. The area in which it is found has shrunk, possibly due to more strict criteria for diagnosis but also because of undefined changes in lifestyle. It occurs commonly now in rural Okavango valley and neighbouring southern Angola and northern Namibia (Ovambo and Kavango). In Kavango, the minimum incidence is calculated to be 151 in 10^5 per year, and it accounts for 1 per cent of all hospital admissions. Over half of patients are aged less than 20 years, and the male to female ratio is 1:1.5.

The aetiology of onyalai remains unknown: fungal contamination of millet is suspected. Both IgG and IgM autoantibodies with specificity for platelet membrane glycoprotein (Gp) IIb/IIIa are present in most patients, whereas anti Gp IIb//IIIa, mainly IgG, is found in only about one-third of patients with ITP.

Clinical presentation and haematology

Patients present with haemorrhagic bullae, commonly in the mouth but also in the skin including the soles of the feet. Epistaxis is frequent and may be severe. The median duration of haemorrhage is 8 days, but the condition may last for months, and it tends to recur. Mortality in the acute phase without appropriate treatment is about 10 per cent.

There is profound thrombocytopenia with normal platelet morphology and erythroid and megakaryocytic hyperplasia in the bone marrow.

Treatment

Specialist hospital care is essential. Transfusion of whole blood for haemorrhagic shock, and platelet-rich plasma for profound thrombocytopenia, with excellent general nursing care, have reduced mortality to 3 per cent. Steroids are not effective. Splenectomy is followed by a rise of platelet count to normal, and is indicated when bleeding cannot be controlled, but in the long term onyalai may return and be fatal.

Onyalai is locally a common cause of morbidity and mortality: further research is required into its aetiology, management and prevention.

Coagulopathies

The acquired disorders of coagulation, DIC (including snake envenoming) and hypoprothrombinaemia, are met much more often in clinical practice in Africa than the congenital disorders, such as the haemophilias and von Willebrand's disease.

Disseminated intravascular coagulation

Aetiology

The precipitating factors of DIC are (i) damage to endothelium, which is often from infection in Africa, (ii) release of tissue factor (thromboplastin) from traumatized or dead tissue or cells, or (iii) injection of snake venoms which contain procoagulants (Table 78.17). Pregnant women are susceptible to DIC because of enhanced coagulability and fibrinolytic activity of blood, which remain latent until activated either normally by delivery or pathologically by obstetric accidents.

Pathogenesis

IL6 and TNF are principal mediators of the activation of coagulation. There is widespread deposition of fibrin in small blood vessels, consumption of coagulation factor and platelets, and activation of the fibrinolytic system (Fig. 78.19).

Haemorrhage

The consumption of coagulation factors and platelets causes the blood to become incoagulable, and leads to uncontrolled haemorrhage, which is the dominant complication of acute DIC. Activation of fibrinolysis is usually insufficient to clear the fibrin depositions, but in some circumstances, for example acute promyelocytic leukaemia, excessive fibrinolysis is a feature and contributes to the haemorrhagic state: activated plasmin digests fibrin, fibrinogen and coagulation factors, while the fibrin degradation products (FDPs) interfere with normal fibrin polymerization and act as antithrombins. Natural antithrombin systems (antithrombin III, protein C and protein S) are all depressed.

Tissue necrosis

Obstruction of blood vessels leads to tissue necrosis and increases the risk of organ failure, circulatory collapse, renal failure and death. Tissue necrosis causes the release of tissue factor, further DIC and a vicious circle.

Haemolysis

In sub-acute or chronic forms of DIC (Table 78.17), red cells are ruptured by being forced through the fibrin network, causing microangiopathic haemolytic anaemia. The blood film shows small fragmented red cell of bizarre shape (schistocytes).

Diagnosis

Acute DIC is often diagnosed when the blood is noticed to fail to clot. The TT, PT and APTT are all prolonged, and the platelet count is low. Fibrinolysis is demonstrated by the presence of FDPs or D-dimers. Subacute or chronic DIC is characterized by thrombocytopenia, products of fibrinolysis in plasma, moderate decrease of coagulation factors and schistocytes in the peripheral blood film.

Treatment

The first principle of treatment is to treat the primary cause. Other measures are to treat hypovolaemic shock, and to transfuse whole blood when the Hb is <7.0 g/dl. In specialized hospitals, factors can be replaced by platelet transfusion, fresh frozen plasma (FFP) or cryoprecipitate.

Snake bite and haemorrhage

There are two African snakes whose venoms act primarily by activation of coagulation, *Echis ocellatus* (previously called *E. carinatus*) found north of the equator, and *Dispholidus typus* south of the Equator: *Naja nigrocollis* and *Bitus* species have venoms which do not have their main effects on coagulation, but secondarily may disturb haemostasis.

Hypoprothrombinaemia

Vitamin K is essential for the post-translational carboxylation of the precursor proteins of coagulation factors II, VII, IX, and X, and the antithrombotic factors protein C and protein S, all of which are synthesized in the liver. Acquired deficiencies of these factors result from either vitamin K deficiency, hepatocellular failure or the ingestion of coumarin anticoagulants, of which warfarin is the most commonly used in clinical practice or as a rat poison (Table 78.18). The deficiencies are multiple involving all the vitamin K dependent factors, not just

Table 78.17. Causes of disseminated intravascular coagulation (DIC) encountered in Africa

Acute DIC	Subacute DIC	Chronic DIC
Infections	*Obstetric disorders*	*Metabolic*
Viraemia	Pre-eclampsia	Liver disease
Septicaemias	Eclampsia	Renal disease
Trypanosomiasis	Retained dead fetus	*Malignancies*
Rarely malaria	Hydatidiform mole	Prostatic carcinoma
Obstetric disorders	*Malignancies*	
Septic abortion	Acute promyelocytic leukaemia	
Abruptio placentae		
Ruptured uterus	Others	
Amniotic fluid embolus	*Cytotoxic therapy*	
Shock	*Miscellaneous*	
Accidental trauma	Purpura fulminans	
birth trauma or anoxia		
head injuries		
thoracic crush injuries		
fractured femur		
Surgical trauma		
thoracic		
Burns		
Heatstroke		
Snake envenomation		
Miscellaneous		
Incompatible blood transfusion		
Acute hepatic necrosis		
Cytotoxic therapy		

Source: Modified from Fleming & de Silva (2003).

Table 78.18. Acquired causes of hypoprothrombinaemia (deficiencies of vitamin K dependent coagulation factors)

Vitamin K deficiency: haemorrhagic disease of the newborn, sterilization of the gut – with broad spectrum antibiotics, fat-free diet, fat malabsorption – coeliac disease, pancreatic insufficiency, obstruction of common bile duct

Hepatocellular failure: acute hepatitis, chronic hepatic disease, cirrhosis

Warfarin poisoning: accidental overdosage (adults or children), potentiation by other medication (e.g., co-trimoxazole), rat poison (accidental in children, suicide in adults)

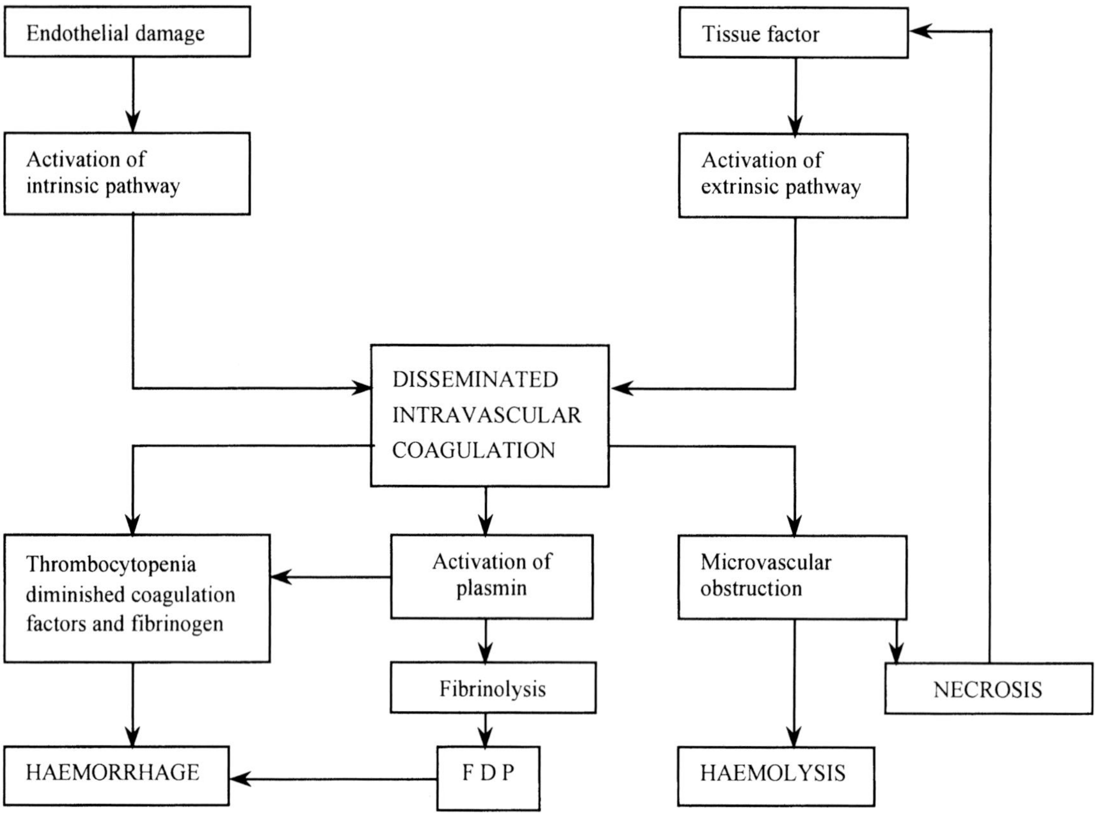

Fig. 78.19. The pathogenesis of disseminated intravascular haemolysis.

prothrombin (factor II), but are referred to as 'hypoprothrombinaemias'.

Haemorrhagic disease of the newborn

The normal newborn infant is deficient of vitamin K because the vitamin is poorly transported across the placenta, breast milk is a poor source and the gut is sterile initially. The vitamin K-dependent factors are at about 50 per cent of the adult levels. Colonization of the infant's gut is followed by a rise of vitamin K within 72 to 120 hours after birth. Haemorrhagic disease of the newborn (HDN) may occur during the critical first days of life: risk factors include prematurity, maternal anti-tuberculosis or anti-convulsant treatment. It is more common in breast-fed than in bottle-fed infants. Incidence in Africa is not known, but, because of ubiquitous breast-feeding and the frequent need for anti-tuberculosis treatment, it is likely to be higher than the 1 in 2500 reported from industrialized countries before the routine administration of prophylactic vitamin K.

Late HDN occurs at 1 to 3 months of age, exclusively in breast-fed infants who have been treated with antibiotics.

Clinical features

The infant bleeds spontaneously into skin, mucous membranes, the gastrointestinal tract or umbilical stump, or bleeds heavily after circumcision. Intracranial haemorrhage can cause brain damage and death. HDN needs to be differentiated from other causes of haemorrhage in the newborn, including DIC and hereditary defects such as haemophilia or factor XIII deficiency. Diagnosis is confirmed by the prolongation of the PT with all other tests of coagulation and the platelet count being normal.

Treatment and prevention

HDN is reversed by a single intramuscular injection of vitamin K 10 mg, or 5 mg if the infant weighs less than 2500 g.

HDN is prevented by the routine administration of vitamin K 1.0 mg intramuscularly to all newborn. Oral prophylaxis at birth prevents early HDN but not late HDN. Natural lipid-soluble vitamin K_1 must be used. Water-soluble vitamin K is no longer available as it triggered oxidative haemolysis, leading to neonatal jaundice and kernicterus: G6PD-deficient infants were at greatest risk. The belief that prophylactic vitamin K increases the incidence of leukaemia or other malignancies has not been substantiated.

Hepatic disease

Liver disease is an important cause of bleeding tendency. Mechanisms include (i) failure of synthesis of the vitamin K-dependent factors, (ii) decreased synthesis of fibrinogen, (iii) increased fibrinolysis due to failure to inactivate plasmin, (iv) thrombocytopenia secondary to hypersplenism from portal hypertension, and (v) DIC.

The laboratory findings reflect these mechanisms: a prolonged PT is usual; a long TT demonstrates hypofibrinogenaemia; a prolonged APTT is evidence of DIC; the presence of FDPs or D-dimers indicates excessive fibrinolysis; thrombocytopenia is a measure of hypersplenism.

When the PT is four times normal, excessive haemorrhage will follow accidental or surgery trauma, which could be a percutaneous liver biopsy. Spontaneous haemorrhages occur with more deranged haemostasis.

Vitamin K may be given, but has partial action only or none. Bleeding can be controlled with the transfusion of cryo-poor plasma (CPP: the plasma from which cryoprecipitate has been extracted) or FFP. Cryoprecipitate is indicated if there is hypofibrinogenaemia (World Health Organization, Global Programme on AIDS, Global Blood Safety Initiative, 1989).

The haemophilias

The problem in Africa

Frequencies in Africa do not differ significantly from other continents, but rates of diagnosis are low: for example, of the expected 500 haemophilics in the Zimbabwean population, only 190 had been diagnosed and registered in 1993 (Adewuyi et al., 1996). Haemophilia A (congenital factor VIII deficiency) occurs in about 1 in 5000 male births; haemophilia B (congenital factor IX deficiency, sometimes called Christmas disease) in about 1 in 25 000 male births. Haemophilia A and haemophilia B are sex-linked. Disease is expressed fully in males, but female carriers may have a mild bleeding tendency.

Clinical presentation

Patients with severe haemophilia have frequent spontaneous haemorrhages, haemarthrosis and joint deformities. Others have moderate (occasional spontaneous haemorrhage) or mild (post-traumatic or post-surgical bleeding only) disease.

Haemorrhage after circumcision, and cerebral haemorrhage precipitated by raised intracranial pressure from coughing, are common presentations in Africa. Severe disease is complicated by repeated haemarthroses and subsequently deformed joints.

Diagnosis

Suspect haemophilia in a male child who bleeds excessively; there may be a history of bleeding in male relations of the mother, but about one-third of affected families have new mutations.

The clotting time is not a sensitive test, and may be normal or only slightly prolonged. The bleeding time, TT and PT are normal but the APTT is prolonged. This profile of results is sufficient for a working diagnosis of haemophilia, but differentiation between haemophilia A and haemophilia B requires assays of factor VIII and factor IX.

Comprehensive haemophilia care

Eighty per cent of haemophilics are born in developing countries and do not benefit from the major advances in diagnosis and management which have occurred during the last 25 years (World Health Organization, 1998). National programmes for haemophilia care are feasible, including health education, training of staff and identification and registration of people with haemophilia, as has been shown in Zimbabwe (Adewuyi et al., 1996). But strong political will is needed.

Management

Blood transfusion services could produce cryoprecipitate if they had a refrigerated centrifuge and a deep freeze unit (Lloyd, 1997). The transfusion of cryoprecipitate is a crude but effective method of replacement of factor VIII in the treatment or prevention of haemorrhage. FFP and CCP are used in the treatment of haemophilia B. These blood products can transmit HIV, HBV, HCV and other agents, so it is essential to screen donors and to immunize haemophiliacs against HBV. Newly developed methods of inactivating virus in cryoprecipitate and FFP should be introduced. The World Federation of Haemophilia advocates the introduction of virus inactivated and recombinant factors VIII and IX into the developing world. Mild haemophilia A responds to desmopressin, which releases factor VIII into the circulation.

von Willebrand's disease

von Willebrand's disease is the commonest congenital coagulopathy. The disease is mild, however, in many subjects and the diagnosis is often missed. It is inherited most often as an autosomal dominant. von Willebrand factor deficiency has features of both a platelet disorder and a coagulopathy. Patients present with epistaxis, menorrhagia and excessive bleeding from any wound. Bleeding time and APTT are prolonged. Factor VIII and vWF concentrations or activities are low. In advanced centres, control of haemorrhage is with desmopressin in most patients. Tranexamic acid, an antifibrinolytic agent, is useful in topical application. Cryoprecipitate or factor VIII are indicated for severe bleeds.

References

Adewuyi JO, Coutts AM, Levy L, Lloyd SE. (1996). Haemophilia care in Zimbabwe. *Centr Afr J Med*; **42**: 153–156.

Adish AA, Esray SA, Gyorkos TW, Jean-Baptiste J, Rojhani AA. (1999). Effect of consumption of food cooked in iron pots on iron status and growth of young children: a randomised trial. *Lancet*; **353**: 712–716.

Akinyanju OO, Okany CC. (1992). Pernicious anaemia in Africans. *Clin Laborat Haematol*; **14**: 33–40.

Argarwal A, Guindo A, Cissoko Y et al. (2002). Hemoglobin C associated with protection from severe malaria in the Dogon of Mali, a West African population with a low prevalence of hemoglobin S. *Blood*; **96**: 2358–2363.

Bain BJ. (1997). The haematological features of HIV infection. *Br J Haematol*; **99**: 1–8.

Bedu-Addo G, Bates I. (2002). Causes of massive tropical splenomegaly in Ghana. *Lancet*, **360**, 449–454

Bhigjee AI, Thaler D, Madurai S et al. (1994). Seroprevalence of HTLV-1 in Natal/KwaZulu. *S Afr Med J*; **84**: 368.

Bruner AB, Joffe A, Duggan AK et al. (1996). Randomised study of cognitive effects of iron supplementation in non-anaemic iron deficient adolescent girls. *Lancet*; **348:** 992–996.

Bryceson ADM, Fakunle YM, Fleming AF et al. (1983). Malaria and splenomegaly. *Trans Roy Soc Med Hyg*; **77**: 879.

Cappadoro M, Giribaldi G, O'Brien E. et al. (1998). Early phagocytosis of glucose-6-phosphate dehydrogenase (G6PD)- deficient erythrocytes parasitized by *Plasmodium falciparum* may explain malaria protection in G6PD deficiency. *Blood*; **92**: 2527–2534.

Carmel R. (1999). Ethnic and racial factors in cobalamin metabolism and its disorders. *Seminars in Hematology*; **36**: 88–100.

Chidoori C, Paul B, Gordeuk VR. (1989). Homozygous $\alpha+$ thalassaemia in Zimbabwe: an unrecognized cause of hypochromia and microcytosis. *Centr Afr J Med*; **35**: 472–476.

Coetzer TL, Beeton L, van Zyl D, Field SP (1996). Southeast Asian ovalocytosis in a South African kindred with hemolytic anemia. *Blood*; **87**: 1656–1657.

Cornet M, Le Hesran J-Y, Fievet N et al. (1998). Prevalence of and risk factors for anemia in young children in southern Cameroon. *Am J Trop Med Hyg*; **58**: 606–611.

Dallman PR. (1977). In *Pediatrics*, 16th edn., ed. AM Rudolph, p1178. New York: Appleton Century.

Diagne N, Rogier C, Sokhna CS et al. (2000). Increased susceptibility to malaria during the early postpartum period. *N Engl J of Med*; **343**: 598–603.

Dupuy E, Fleming AF, Caen JP. (1978). Platelet function, factor VIII, fibrinogen, and fibrinolysis in Nigerians and Europeans in relation to atheroma and thrombosis. *J Clin Pathol*; **31**: 1094–1101.

English M. (2000). Life-threatening severe malarial anaemia. *Trans Roy Soc Trop Med Hyg*; **94**: 585–588.

Essien EM. (1992). Platelets and platelet disorders in Africa. *Baillière's Clin Haematol*; **5**: 441–456.

Fleming AF. (1970). Seasonal incidence of anemia in pregnancy in Ibadan. *Am J Clin Nutrit*; **23**: 224–230.

Fleming AF. (1982). *Sickle-cell Disease: A Handbook for the General Physician*. Edinburgh: Churchill-Livingstone.

Fleming AF. (1989). Tropical obstetrics and gynaecology. 1. Anaemia in pregnancy in tropical Africa. *Trans Roy Soc Trop Med Hyg*; **83**: 441–448.

Fleming AF. (1990). Chronic lymphocytic leukaemia in tropical Africa: a review. *Leukemia Lymphoma*; **1**: 169–173.

Fleming AF. (1991). Anaemia in pregnancy; part 1. *Postgraduate Doctor Middle East*; **14**, 278–282.

Fleming AF, Terunuma H, Tembo C, Mantini H. (1999). Leukaemias in Zambia. *Leukemia*; **13**: 1292–1293.

Fleming AF, de Silva PS. (2003). Haematological diseases in the tropics. In *Mansons's Tropical Diseases*, 21st edn. ed. GC Cook, A Zumla, pp. 169–243. London: W.B. Saunders.

Foster RM. (1989). The seasonal incidence of megaloblastic anaemia in Mombasa. *E Afr Med J*; **45**: 673–676.

Harrison KA. (1985). Child-bearing, health and social priorities: a survey of 22 774 consecutive hospital births in Zaria, northern Nigera. *Brit Journal of Obstetrics and Gynaecology*, **92** (suppl. 5), 32–39, 86–99, 100–115.

Harrison KA. (2001). Haemoglobinopathies in pregnancy. In *Maternity Care in Developing Countries*, eds. JB Lawson, KA Harrison, S Bergström, pp. 129–45. London: Royal College of Obstetricians and Gynaecologists.

Hesseling PB. (1992). Onyalai. *Baillière's Clin Haematol*; **5**: 457–473.

Hill AVS. (1992). Molecular epidemiology of the thalassaemias (including haemoglobin E). *Baillière's Clin Haematol*; **5**: 209–238.

Hofrichten J et al. (1976). A physical description of hemoglobin S gelation. In *Proceedings of the Symposium on Molecular and Cellular Aspects of Sickle Cell Disease.* ed JI Hercules, GL Cottam, MR Waterman, AN Schechter, pp. 185–223. Bethesda, MD: US Department of Health, Education and Welfare.

Ibidapo MO, Akinyanju OO. (2000). Acute sickle cell syndromes in Nigerian adults. *Clin Laborat Haematol*; **22**: 151–155.

Ingram CF, Fleming AF, Patel M, Galpin JS. (1999). Pregnancy – and lactation-related folate deficiency in South Africa: a case for folate food fortification. *S Afr Med J*; **89**: 1279–1284.

Knox-Macaulay HHM. (1992). Tuberculosis and the haemopoietic system. *Baillière's Clin Haematol*; **5**: 101–129.

Lloyd S. (1997). The preparation of single donor cryoprecipitate.

Facts and Figures. (Available from the World Federation of Hemophilia).

Malyangu E, Abayomi EA, Adeqayi J, Coutts AM. (2000). AIDS is now the commonest clinical condition associated with multilineage blood cytopenia in a central referral hospital in Zimbabwe. *Centr Afr J Med*; **46**: 59–61.

Menendez C. (1995). Malaria during pregnancy: a priority area of malaria research and control. *Parasitol Today*; **11**: 178–183.

Menendez C, Todd J, Pedro A et al. (1994). The effects of iron supplementation during pregnancy, given by traditional birth attendants, on the prevalence of anaemia and malaria. *Trans Roy Soc Trop Med Hyg*; **88**: 590–593.

Menendez C, Todd J, Alsonso PL. et al. (1995). The response to iron supplementation of pregnant women with haemoglobin genotype AA or AS. *Trans Roy Soc Trop Med Hyg*; **89**: 289–292.

Menendez C, Kahigwa E, Hirt R et al. (1997). Randomized placebo-controlled trial of iron supplementation and malaria chemoprophylaxis for prevention of severe anaemia and malaria in Tanzanian infants. *Lancet*; **350**: 844–850.

Menendez C, Fleming AF, Alonso PL. (2000). Malaria-related anaemia. *Parasitol Today*; **16**: 469–476.

Modiano D, Luoni G, Sirima BS et al. (2001). Hemoglobin C protects against clinical falciparum malaria. *Nature*; **44**: 305–308.

Mukiibi JM. (1989). Autoimmune thrombocytopenic purpura (AITP) in Zimbabwe. *Trop Geog Med*; **41**: 326–330.

Mukiibi JM, Paul B. (1994). Myelodysplastic syndromes (MDS) in central Africans. *Trop Geog Med*; **46**: 17–19.

Mukiibi JM, Paul B, Mandisodza A.(1989). Megaloblastic anaemia in Zimbabwe. 1: Seasonal variation. *Centr Afr J Med*; **35**: 310–313.

Mukwala EC, Banda J, Siziya S et al. (1989). Alpha thalassaemia in Zambian newborn. *Clin Laborat Haematol*; **11**: 1–6.

Niazi GA, Fleming AF. (1989). Blood dyscrasia in unofficial vendors of petrol and heavy oil and motor mechanics in Nigeria. *Tropical Doctor*; **19**: 55–58.

Nurse GT, Coetzer TL, Palek J. (1992). The elliptocytoses, ovalocytosis and related disorders. *Baillière's Clin Haematol*; **5**: 187–207.

Paul B, (1981). Rain and anaemia: the seasonal variation of malaria and megaloblastosis. *Journal of Medical Association of Malawi*; **8**: 19–20.

Paul B, Mukiibi JM, Mandisodza A et al. (1992). A three-year prospective study of 137 cases of acute leukaemia in Zimbabwe. *Centr Afr J Med*; **38**: 95–99.

Piessens WF, Hoffman SL, Wadee AA et al. (1985). Antibody-mediated killing of suppressor T lymphocytes as a possible cause of macroglobulinemia in the tropical splenomegaly syndrome. *J Clin Invest*; **75**: 1821–1827.

Powers JJ, Bates CJ, Lamb WH. (1984). Haematological response to supplements of iron and riboflavin to pregnant and lactating women in rural Gambia. *Hum Nutrit: Clin Nutrit*; **39C**: 117–129.

Prasad AS. (2002). Zinc deficiency in patients with sickle cell disease. *Am J Clin Nutrit*; **75**: 181–112.

Rabe T, Jambou R, Rabarijaona L et al. (2002). South-East Asian ovalocytosis among the population of the Highlands of Madagascar: a vestige of the island's settlement. *Trans Roy Soc Trop Med Hyg*; **96**: 143–144.

Ruwende C, Hill A. (1998). Glucose-6-phosphate dehydrogenase deficiency and malaria. *J Mol Med*; **76**: 581–588.

Saungweme T, Khumalo H, Mvundura E et al. (1999). Iron and alcohol content of traditional beers in rural Zimbabwe. *Centr Afr J Med*; **45**: 136–140.

Savage D, Gangaidzo I, Lindenbaum J et al. (1994). Vitamin B_{12} deficiency is the primary cause of megaloblastic anaemia in Zimbabwe. *Br J Haematol*; **86**: 844–850.

Schellenberg D, Mendendez C, Kahigwa E et al. (2001). Intermittent treatment for malaria and anaemia control at time of routine vaccination in Tanzanian infants: a randomized, placebo-controlled trial. *Lancet*; **357**: 1471–1477.

Serghides L, Kain KC. (2002). Mechanism of protection induced by vitamin A in falciparum malaria. *Lancet*; **359**: 1404–1406.

Serjeant GR, Serjeant BE. (2001). *Sickle Cell Disease*, 3rd edn. Oxford: Oxford University Press.

Shulman CE, Dorman EK, Bulmer JN. (2002) Malaria as a cause of severe anaemia in pregnancy. *Lancet*; **360**: 494.

Sodeinde O. (1992). Glucose-6-phosphate dehydrogenase deficiency. *Baillière's Clin Haematol*; **5**: 367–382.

Stephenson LS, Kinoti SN, Latham MC et al. (1989). Single dose metrifonate and praziquantel treatment in Kenyan children. I. Effects on *Schistosoma haematobium*, hookworm, hemoglobin levels, splenomegaly, and hepatomegaly. *Am J Trop Med Hyg*; **41**: 436–444.

Stoltzfus RJ, Chwaya HM, Tielsch JM et al. (1997). Epidemiology of iron deficiency anemia in Zanzibari schoolchildren: the importance of hookworms. *Am J Clin Nutrit*; **65**: 153–159.

Thomson J. (1997). Anaemia in pregnant women in eastern Caprivi, Namibia. *S Afr Med J*; **87**: 1544–1547.

van Eijk AM, Ayisi JG, ter Kuile FO et al. (2001). Human immunodeficiency virus seropositivity and malaria as risk factors for third-trimester anemia in asymptomatic pregnant women in western Kenya. *Am J Trop Med Hyg*; **66**: 623–630.

van Hensbroek MB, Morris-Jones S, Meisner S et al. (1995). Iron, but not folic acid, combined with effective antimalarial therapy promotes haematological recovery in African children after acute falciparum malaria. *Trans Roy Soc Tropi Med Hyg*; **89**: 672–676.

Verhoef H, West CE, Nzyuko SM et al. (2002). Intermittent administration of iron and sulfadoxine – pyrimethazine to control anaemia in Kenyan children: a randomised controlled trial. *Lancet*; **360**: 908–914.

Weber T, Hunsmann G, Stevens W et al. (1992). Human retroviruses. *Baillière's Clinical Haemotology*; **5**: 273–314.

Willcox MC, Bjorkman A, Brohult J. (1983). Falciparum malaria and β-thalassaemia trait in northern Liberia. *Ann Trop Med Parasitol*; **77**: 335–347.

Williams CKO, Osotimehin BO, Ogunmola GB et al. (1988). Haemolytic anaemia associated with Nigerial barbecued meat (Red Suya). *African Journal of Medicine and Medical Sciences*; **17**: 71–75.

Williams CKO, Alexander SS, Bodner A et al. (1993). Frequency of adult T-cell leukaemia/lymphoma and HTLV-I in Ibadan, Nigeria. *Br J Cancer*, **67**: 783–786.

WHO (1968). *Nutritional Anemias.* Technical Report Series, **405**, 9. Geneva: World Health Organization.

WHO (1972). Nutritional Anemias. Technical Report Series, **503**. Geneva: World Health Organization.

World Health Organization, Global Programme on AIDS, Global Blood Safety Initiative (1989). *Guidelines on the Appropriate Use of Blood.* WHO/GPA/Inf/89: 18. Geneva: WHO.

World Health Organization Working Group (1989). Glucose-6-phosphate dehydrogenase deficiency. *Bulletin of the World Health Organization*, **67**: 601–611.

World Health Organization (1998). *Control of haemophilia: haemophilia care in developing countries.* WHO/HGN/WFH/WG/98.3. Geneva: World Health Organization.

World Health Organization (2000). Severe falciparum malaria. *Trans Roy Soc Trop Med Hyg*, **94**.

Zucker JR, Lackritz EM, Ruebush TK et al. (1994). Anaemia, blood transfusion practices, HIV and mortality among women of reproductive age in western Kenya. *Trans Roy Soc Trop Med Hyg*, **88**: 173–176.

79

The gut

The problem in Africa

Gastrointestinal disease accounts for a major proportion of the workload of health care workers throughout the world, and this is especially true in Africa. Unfortunately, there is little published information on the prevalence of many important diseases, which makes it difficult to analyse time trends and geographical differences around the continent. There are many challenges for the twenty-first century physician, and in Africa the shortage of information is one of them. In particular, the epidemiology of those diseases which require diagnosis by endoscopy or radiology (for example, inflammatory bowel disease and cancer) is not well characterized.

We begin with the epidemiology of selected important disorders of the digestive tract, then describe the spectrum of disease by anatomical location and symptom. We will try to point out what is firmly established and what is less clear. There are specific chapters on several gastrointestinal infectious diseases elsewhere in the book, which complement, and so need to be read together with, this chapter. These include acute diarrhoea, cholera, shigellosis, salmonellosis, amoebiasis and other intestinal protozoa.

Epidemiology of selected diseases

Peptic ulceration and *Helicobacter pylori*

The cause of peptic ulceration remained unexplained for many years, and even now there are many unanswered questions. In the early 1980s it was discovered that the great majority of peptic ulceration is related to infection with a recently discovered bacterium which colonizes the gastric mucosa of a large proportion of the world's population: *Helicobacter pylori.* However, it is not understood why *H. pylori* infection only causes gastroduodenal disease at certain points in time in a small proportion of those individuals infected. *Helicobacter* is one of the commonest chronic bacterial infections of humans, affecting more than 50 per cent of the world's population; the majority of those infected develop histological chronic gastritis but remain asymptomatic throughout life. About 20 per cent of infected adults manifest one of several different outcomes, such as:

- duodenal ulcer
- gastric ulcer disease
- gastric cancers
- lymphoma.

In industrialized countries there is generally a low prevalence of *Helicobacter* and gastric cancer, yet a relatively high prevalence for peptic ulcer disease.

In sub-Saharan Africa *Helicobacter pylori* infection is common but some studies have indicated a low incidence of peptic ulceration. Serological studies have shown that the infection is acquired early by children (50% by 10 years): around 80 per cent of adults are infected. This apparent discrepancy between the high frequency of infection and the low frequency of disease has been termed the 'African enigma', but our experience in Zambia is that peptic ulceration is just as common as elsewhere in the world (Fernando et al., 2001). There do seem to be geographical variations across the continent: a high prevalence of gastroduodenal mucosal lesions was reported from Sudan (El-Mahdi et al., 1998) and Nigeria but there is older evidence that prevalence may be low in some other countries, and there may be differences between rural and urban populations.

Cancer of the digestive system

The epidemiology of digestive cancer in Africa provides a dramatic contrast with industrialized countries with lower incidence rates overall and especially low rates of colorectal carcinoma. The pattern is not clear because published data are few but there is also significant evidence of variation across Africa. For example, a comparison of cancer data from The Gambia, Mali and South Africa with data from black people in the USA showed lower incidence rates in Africa, but a high incidence of gastric cancer in Mali (Walker et al., 1993). Cancer of the oesophagus was the commonest digestive cancer in the other countries. By contrast, a smaller study from Jos, Nigeria, found the commonest digestive cancer to be rectal carcinoma, followed by stomach, colon and oesophagus in that order (Obafunwa, 1990). In Zimbabwe, the commonest was oesophagus in men, while in both sexes hepatocellular carcinoma was common (Parkin et al., 1994). In Senegal, gastric cancer was commonest, followed by colorectal and oesophageal (Peghini et al., 1990). In Malawi, oesophageal cancer was more than ten times commoner than other digestive cancers (Banda et al., 2001).

To summarize, there are three major points of interest in the epidemiology of digestive cancer in Africa.

- Overall incidence rates appear to be lower than in industrialized countries.
- Oesophageal cancer (and probably gastric cancer) is common in some areas, but it is not yet possible to make generalizations about the overall pattern or to speculate as to reasons. Even within South Africa there is considerable variation in incidence (Gamieldien et al., 1998).
- Colorectal cancer, at least in South Africa, is uncommon and may not follow the same pathway as in industrialized countries. In Soweto, Johannesburg, adenomas are very rare (Segal, 1998) despite dietary risk factors, which would be thought to pre-dispose to colorectal adenoma and carcinoma formation.

The commonest oesophageal cancer is squamous cell carcinoma, and there is no published evidence yet of the emerging world-wide trend towards increasing adenocarcinoma. Again, there is regional variation in epidemiology, with men much more susceptible in a Zimbabwean series (Vizcaino et al., 1995), equal risk in men and women in a Nigerian series (Pindiga et al., 1997) and an Ethiopian series intermediate (Ali et al., 1998). The reason for this variation is unknown. Smoking is clearly a risk factor for this cancer, and this may contribute to such variation. Much more work needs to be done to understand the emerging trends in cancer incidence, which are probably changing all over the continent, at least in cities.

Inflammatory bowel disease

Inflammatory bowel disease refers to two diseases which are caused by spontaneous inflammation in the gut. Ulcerative colitis (UC) is a disease of the large intestine, which is characterized by mucosal inflammation. Crohn's disease, by contrast, may occur anywhere in the digestive tract, from mouth to anus, and the inflammation typically affects all layers of the gut wall.

Both diseases may be associated with inflammation elsewhere, such as joints, skin or eyes. There is a significant genetic predisposition to these diseases, but there is no satisfactory explanation for what triggers the inflammation.

These diseases are uncommon in Africa, but again there is a shortage of information from most of the continent. Most relevant information comes from South Africa, and indicates that incidence in different racial groups differs (Wright et al., 1986). The incidence of UC in coloured, white and black patients in Cape Town was 1.9, 5.0 and 0.6 per 100 000 per year, respectively. Data from Johannesburg suggest that black patients with UC had more extensive, severe disease (Segal, 1988), but the long delay in diagnosis may mean that only the most severe cases are being seen in hospital, owing to unequal access to health care in different ethnic groups in the past. UC has also been recorded, albeit infrequently, in Ethiopia (Mengesha & Tsega, 1989) and Zimbabwe (Muguti, 1989).

Crohn's disease is commoner in South African whites than in coloured or blacks (incidence 2.6 compared to 1.8 and 0.3 per 100 000 per year, respectively (Wright et al., 1986). Crohn's disease has also been reported from Ethiopia (Mengesha et al., 1997). As the diagnosis is hard to establish in countries where intestinal infectious disease is common, few data regarding frequency are available. The most important disease that can be confused with Crohn's disease is intestinal tuberculosis. Although this is rare (Segal, 1984), it is important to stress that radiological diagnosis is usually insufficient: histology and culture should be applied to biopsy material if possible to ensure that intestinal TB is not treated with steroids. If there is still doubt, give a trial of anti-tuberculosis chemotherapy.

Digestive disease by anatomical location

The mouth

Disease of the mouth presents with local pain, swellings, altered taste, or visible lesions, and there is a wide variety of pathology which can underlie these symptoms. A full description of the whole range of oral pathology is beyond the scope of this book, but we will discuss some important disorders which present to physicians.

Oral ulcers

There are many causes, many of which do not require specific treatment.

Herpes simplex stomatitis

This occurs in childhood and presents as diffuse oral ulceration. The virus may then lie dormant on the dorsal root ganglion of the trigeminal nerve and presents occasionally throughout life as a 'cold sore', usually around the lips at times of psychological or immunological, e.g. pneumonia, stress.

Aphthous ulceration

This is idiopathic and presents with tiny scattered ulceration which, although painful, resolves spontaneously and harmlessly. Frequent aphthous ulcers may indicate Crohn's disease, but this is rare.

Stevens–Johnson syndrome

The oral ulceration is recognizable as it is associated with erythema multiforme and usually follows ingestion of drugs, particularly sulphur-containing antibiotics such as co-trimoxazole or thiacetazone.

Behçet's disease

The oral ulceration is usually associated with characteristic joint and skin lesions.

Drugs

Oral ulceration may also be due to drugs, for example, carbimazole and proguanil.

Syphilis

Ulcers in the mouth are seen in secondary syphilis, and may be associated with a hoarse voice. Such unexplained lesions should prompt testing with RPR and TPHA tests. Gummata are rare.

Cancer

This is a well-recognized cause of oral ulcer (see below).

Oral candidiasis

Infection with *Candida* is commonly, but not always, associated with AIDS. The oral mucosa may be covered with white furry patches, or the infection may be confined to a few strands inside the lower lip or the hard palate. It may be associated with oesophageal infection which requires endoscopy or barium swallow for confirmation. Treatment depends on severity: gentian violet may suffice for mild cases but more severe infection will require nystatin suspension (0.5 ml rinsed around the mouth 2-hourly), ketoconazole or fluconazole.

Examine the mouth

Look for

Kaposi's sarcoma on hard palate
Hairy leukoplakia
Oral candidiasis

Mucosal irregularity

This may be due to leukoplakia (idiopathic) or hairy leukoplakia (on the side of the tongue and associated with HIV).

Kaposi's sarcoma (KS)

The typical appearance is purplish plaques best seen on the hard palate. We cannot over-emphasize the importance of looking in the mouth as part of the general examination in parts of Africa where HIV prevalence is high. Very commonly, a clinical problem that appears to be confusing is solved by identification of KS, hairy leukoplakia or oral candidiasis in the mouth, and the first two of these are virtually diagnostic of HIV infection (Fig. 79.1(*a*) and (*b*)). This can then be followed by appropriate counselling and testing.

Pyogenic infections

These may arise in dental or gingival disease and lead to suppuration or abscess requiring treatment with broad-spectrum antibiotics including metronidazole.

Vincent's angina is a pyogenic infection of the floor of the mouth. On palpation of the neck below the mandible there is a tender and firm induration. Treat with benzylpenicillin and metronidazole.

Occasionally, there are patients who complain of halitosis or a painful tongue in whom no pathology can be seen on inspection. If no lumps or mucosal irregularity

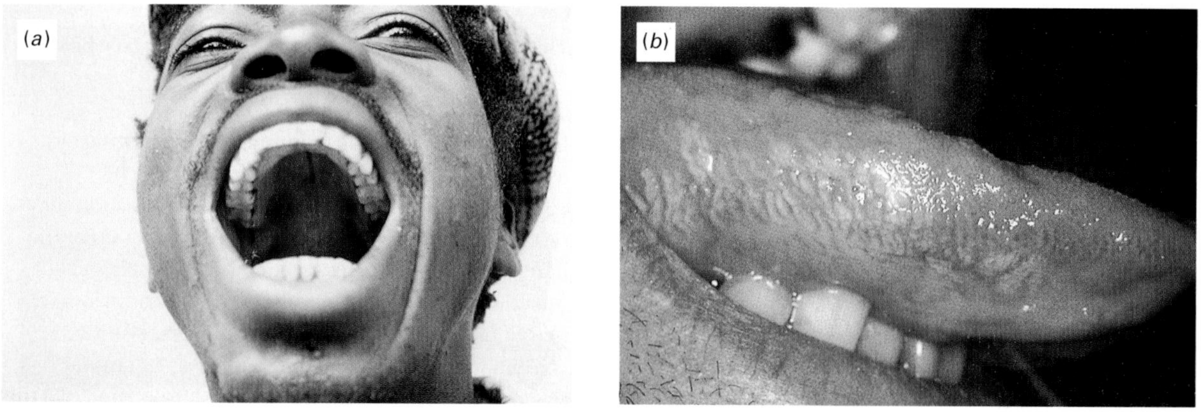

Fig. 79.1. (*a*) Oral Kaposi's sarcoma: dark purple plaques on the hard palate. A few strands of *Candida* are also seen in the midline. Palatal KS is virtually pathognomonic of AIDS. (*b*) Oral hairy leukoplakia.

can be felt by an experienced physician or surgeon, the problem may well be psychogenic.

Oral cancer

Cancer is an important cause of ulceration and swelling in the mouth: the ulcer commonly bleeds and the patient may first be seen when lymph nodes are involved. Smoking and use of chewed tobacco and related stimulants are important risk factors (Idris et al., 1994). Suitably trained surgeons must manage such cases.

Oesophagus

Oesophageal disease presents with heartburn (a hot feeling behind the sternum due to reflux of acid up the oesophagus), dysphagia (difficulty in swallowing), odynophagia (pain on swallowing) or regurgitation (effortless regurgitation of food, which is distinct from true vomiting).

Gastro-oesophageal reflux disease (GORD)

Heartburn is due to GORD, but the condition may also be asymptomatic until complications arise, for example peptic stricture or haematemesis. Symptoms attributable to GORD may be present with or without oesophagitis, which can only be reliably diagnosed endoscopically.

- Note that GORD and reflux oesophagitis are not synonymous.

Treatment

Give liquid antacids, particularly those containing alginates such as Gaviscon, which control symptoms well in many cases. Some patients may get benefit from H_2 receptor antagonists such as cimetidine or ranitidine, but the most reliable results are obtained with proton pump inhibitors such as omeprazole (20–40 mg once or twice daily) or lansoprazole (30–60 mg once or twice daily). These are expensive. Very difficult cases may require surgery, with fundoplication the best option. This is difficult and should not be attempted outside very specialized centres with access to pre-operative physiological assessment, but fortunately GORD of this severity is very rare in our experience in Lusaka. Minor degrees of reflux oesophagitis are quite commonly seen in our practice.

Dysphagia and its causes

Causes of dysphagia are summarized in Table 79.1.

Strictures may be benign (following trauma, reflux oesophagitis, or ingestion of acids or alkalis commonly used in suicide attempts) or malignant. If swallowing becomes difficult or impossible, the best treatment is endoscopic or surgical dilatation, irrespective of whether the stricture is benign or malignant. Local expertise should be taken into account when deciding management.

Cancer of the oesophagus is the commonest cause of dysphagia in older people. The onset of dysphagia is gradual, and the difficulty begins with solid food, in contrast to achalasia in which the initial difficulty is often with liquids. The commonest oesophageal cancer in Africa by far is squamous carcinoma. Diagnosis is best made by endoscopy as this permits biopsies to be taken for histology, but barium swallow also gives very useful information (Fig. 79.2). Unfortunately, cure of this cancer is almost impossible and treatment is palliative (see below).

Achalasia is a disorder of the oesophageal neural network which leads to failure of relaxation of the lower oesophageal sphincter during swallowing. It is progressive and of unknown aetiology. Diagnosis is made by barium swallow or physiological studies; endoscopy is of no diagnostic value but is useful in older patients to exclude a small cancer mimicking achalasia (so-called pseudo-achalasia).

Endoscopic dilatation or surgery (Heller's myotomy) is standard. Oral long-acting nitrates, in the doses used for angina pectoris cardiac pain, are sometimes useful while awaiting definitive treatment.

Infection of the oesophagus gives rise to two major problems.

- Candidiasis, which is seen very commonly in AIDS and in patients immunocompromised for other reasons such as cancer chemotherapy. Treat with nystatin oral suspension (taken 2-hourly), ketoconazole or fluconazole; older remedies such as gentian violet are useful in the mouth but sadly ineffective in oesophageal infection (Fig. 79.3).
- Solitary ulcers, which may be due to CMV, herpes simplex, or other as yet unidentified aetiologies. Solitary ulcers are very difficult to treat and in our experience even acyclovir is not usually successful.

Stomach and duodenum

Gastroduodenal disease most commonly presents with epigastric pain. Vomiting is also a symptom, but persistent nausea alone is not usually due to gastroduodenal disease and the cause of hiccups may be difficult to find. Gastric cancer may cause profound weight loss.

Peptic ulcer

Gastric ulcer and duodenal ulcer cannot reliably be distinguished clinically. They typically present with epigastric (not generalized abdominal) pain before or after food, often at night. Gastric carcinoma also presents with similar pain and often a substantial weight loss. Although gastric cancer seems to us to present in younger patients in Africa than in industrialized countries, it is generally safe to treat younger patients with suspected ulcers with a course of ulcer-healing drugs without further investigation. Ideally, all patients over the age of 50 years presenting for the first time with epigastric pain should be investigated promptly with barium studies or endoscopy to detect gastric cancer before it is too late to offer gastrectomy (Fig. 79.4).

Table 79.1. Causes of dysphagia

	Common	Rare	Treatment
HIV-unrelated	Oesophageal cancer		Surgery/palliation
	Benign stricture		Endoscopic dilatation
		Achalasia	
		Scleroderma	None
		Dysmotility	Trial of nitrates
HIV-related	Candidiasis		Anti-fungals
		Solitary ulcer	Trial of acyclovir

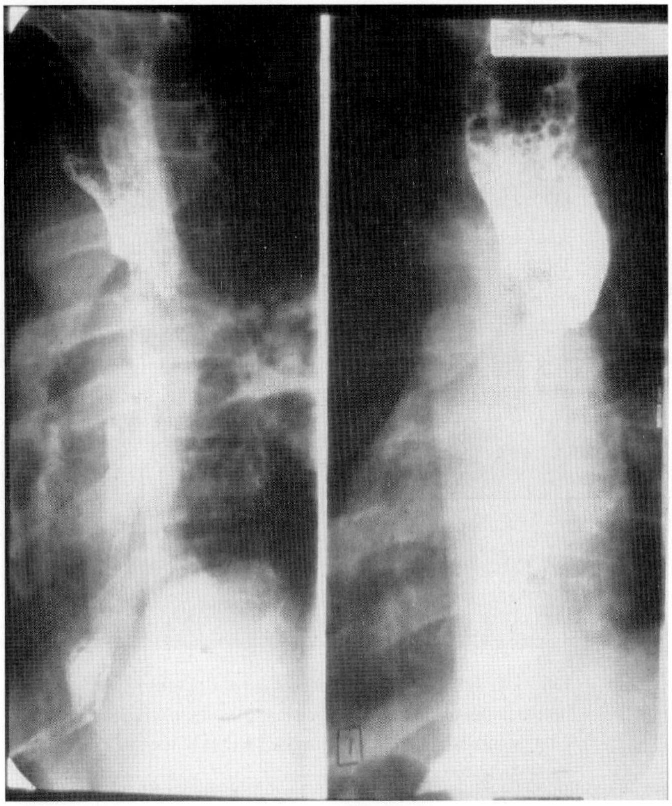

Fig. 79.2. Oesophageal carcinoma. Barium swallow to show barium retarded in the middle third of the oesophagus (By courtesy of the physicians of the Hospital for Tropical Diseases, London, and the Wellcome Trust.)

Treatment

The treatment of peptic ulceration was complex in the past, but is now simpler since the importance of *H. pylori* has been recognized. Ulcers can be healed by H_2 receptor antagonists (for example, cimetidine 400 mg twice daily for 8 weeks, ranitidine 300 mg twice daily for 6 weeks) or proton pump inhibitors (for example, omeprazole 20 mg nocte for 4 weeks, lansoprazole 30 mg nocte for 4 weeks).

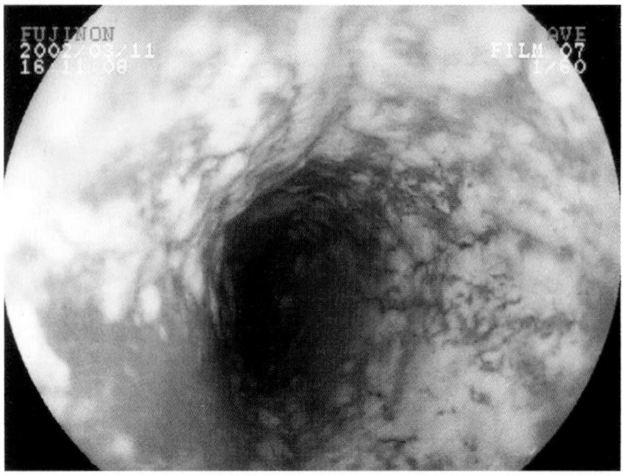

Fig. 79.3. Oesophageal candidiasis in a patient with AIDS. Note the confluent plaques of fungal growth.

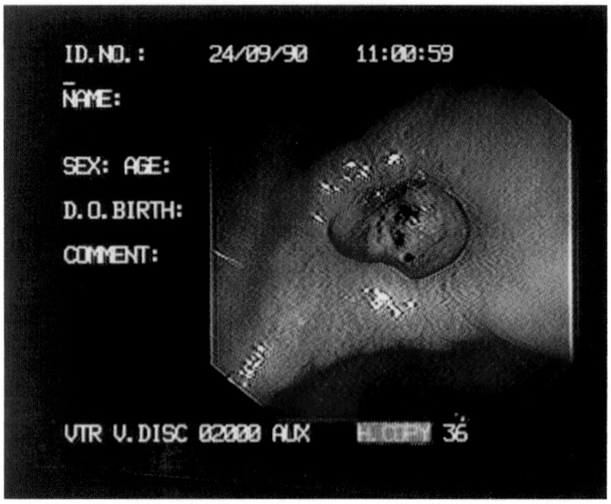

Fig. 79.4. Gastric ulcer. This is seen at endoscopy on the angle between the antrum and body of the stomach: it is deep and the edge is smooth, indicating that it is benign (if it were a cancerous ulcer, the edge would be irregular).

Healing can also be achieved solely by eradication of *H. pylori*. Suggested eradication regimes are shown in Table 79.2; the choice made will depend on the drugs that are locally available, and inevitably on whether the patient is able to afford the needed drugs. We find in Lusaka that metronidazole-based regimes seem to be less effective and we suspect that antibiotic resistance is the reason.

Gastritis

The clinical significance of gastritis is a contentious issue. During endoscopy it is common to see minor degrees of reddening, and gastric biopsies often show gastritis, which is related to the high prevalence of *H. pylori* infection. These are not responsible for dyspepsia. As the gastric mucosa is not sensitive to pain (for example, taking endoscopic biopsies in unsedated patients is not painful), it is difficult to believe that gastritis causes symptoms unless sufficiently severe to induce the release of submucosal inflammatory mediators. This relationship between gastritis and pain is therefore in doubt. Functional pain relating to disturbed gastric motility is a common cause of dyspeptic symptoms, and is common in patients with bloating and belching, often from upper socio-economic urban groups. Often, however, doctors find it easier to label the patient as having 'gastritis' rather than explain such nebulous ideas to anxious patients. We believe, however, that when there is no demonstrable pathology it is better to tell this to the patient. Functional dyspepsia is analogous to the irritable bowel syndrome and is common in our patients in Lusaka.

Table 79.2. Commonly used regimes available for eradication of *H. pylori*

Drug	Dose	Duration	Efficacy
Bismuth subcitrate	120 mg ×4	28	91
Tetracycline	500 mg ×4	28	
Metronidazole	400 mg ×4	28	
Omeprazole	40 mg	14	96
Amoxycillin	500 mg ×3	14	
Metronidazole	400 mg ×3	14	
Omeprazole	20 mg	28	85
Tetracycline	500 mg ×3	7	
Metronidazole	400 mg ×3	7	
Omeprazole	20 mg	7	95
Clarithromycin	250 mg ×2	7	
Tinidazole	500 mg ×2	7	
Ranitidine	300 mg	56	88
Amoxycillin	750 mg ×3	12	
Metronidazole	500 mg ×3	12	

Pyloric stenosis

Pyloric stenosis is an important complication of peptic ulcer disease and presents with profuse and intractable vomiting which may be projectile. Many reports from west Africa stress that it is a common complication of chronic peptic ulcer (Sabo & Ameh, 1999).

Diagnosis is often made clinically as the patient has a succussion splash (best heard by shaking the patient from side to side while listening to the abdomen). Endoscopy gives a reliable diagnosis and treatment is by surgical pyloroplasty or partial gastrectomy. Perforated ulcers present with an acute abdomen, and peptic ulcers also bleed (see below).

Small intestine

Digestion and absorption

The function of the gut is nutrition. Three processes are involved: digestion, absorption and elimination of waste. Digestion begins in the mouth when food is broken down by mastication and salivary amylase is mixed into it. Further breakdown takes place in the stomach leading to emulsification of fats and dispersion and solubilization of other components. The function of the duodenum is to mix the gastric chyme with bile and pancreatic secretions, thus neutralizing pH and rendering the luminal stream isotonic. The major site of absorption is the jejunum and ileum. Fermentation of undigested complex carbohydrates occurs in the caecum and the resulting short-chain fatty acids, together with water, are absorbed in the colon. The formed stool is stored by the rectum and expelled when appropriate.

Nutrients can be divided into macronutrients and micronutrients. Macronutrients are the building blocks required for molecular synthesis and the substrate for energy metabolism. They include carbohydrates, proteins, fats and nucleic acid precursors. Their digestion/absorption is outlined in Figs. 79.5, 79.6 and 79.7. Micronutrients include vitamins and minerals, including retinol, B vitamins, zinc, folic acid and many others. Their absorption is often mediated by specific carriers and may be localized to specific regions of the intestine. For example, iron is taken up by the divalent metal cation transporter; efficient absorption requires gastric acid to achieve the optimal redox state and is largely achieved in the duodenum and proximal jejunum. B_{12} absorption requires gastric intrinsic factor (IF) but absorption of the B_{12}-IF complex takes place in the terminal ileum and resection or disease of a significant length of the terminal ileum runs the risk of precipitating B_{12} deficiency.

Small intestinal defence

The large surface are of the small intestine is a consequence of the villi, which project into the lumen so that

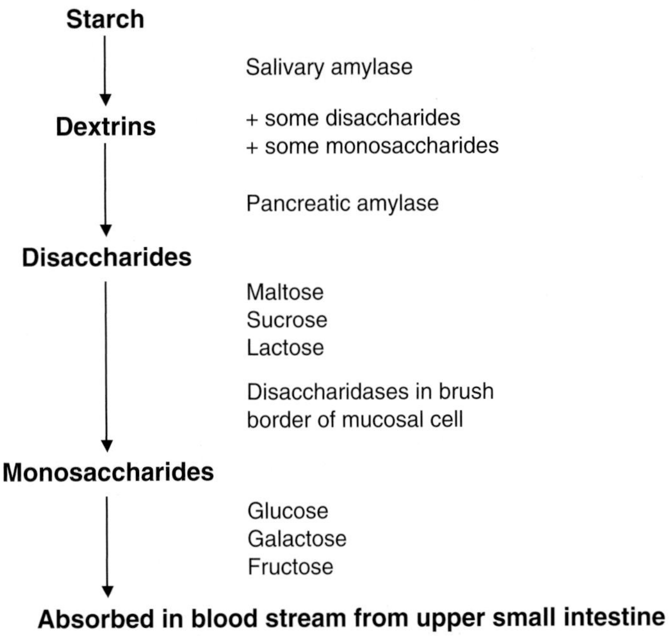

Fig. 79.5. Digestion and absorption of carbohydrates.

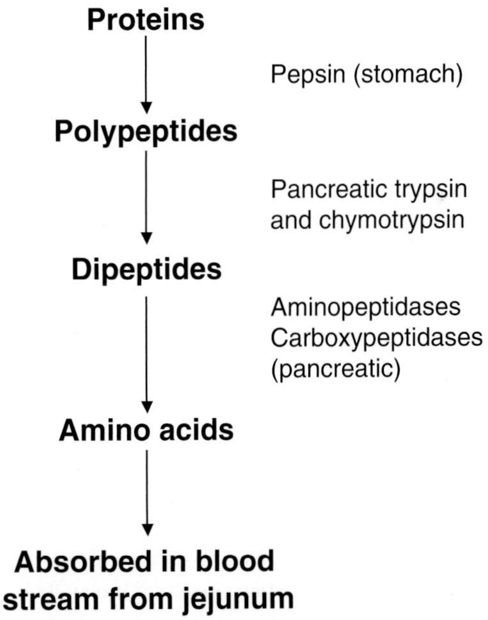

Fig. 79.6. Digestion and absorption of proteins.

enterocytes can absorb nutrients. This is a large, nutrient-rich area, which potential pathogens could easily colonize. There is consequently a need for a diversity of robust mechanisms for host defence, and this is a very exciting area of current research. Host defence mechanisms are of three types: the physical and mucus

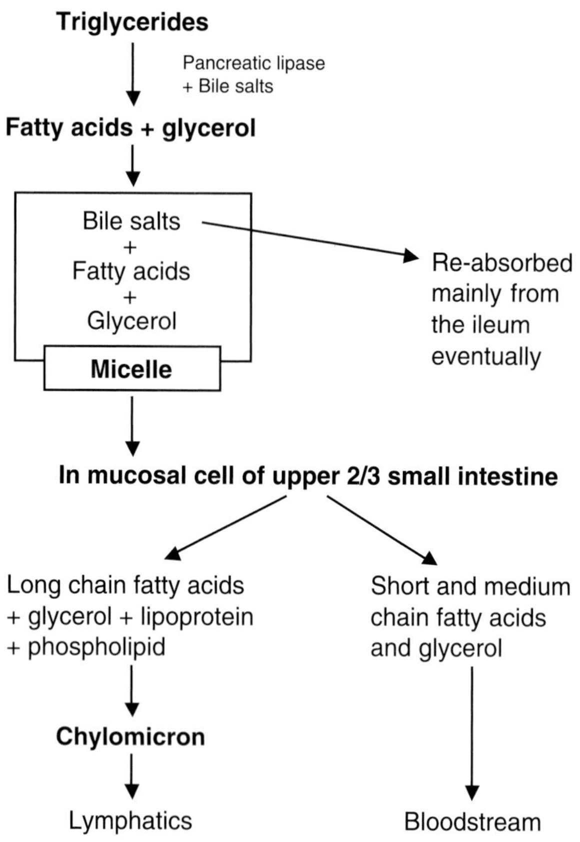

Fig. 79.7. Digestion and absorption of fats.

barrier providing mechanical protection, the adaptive immune system of T- and B-cells which kill pathogens directly and secrete antibodies, and the innate immune system, which secretes anti-microbial peptides and other defence molecules. These systems interact in a way that is just beginning to be understood. The consequences for our understanding of human disease are not yet clear.

Loss of weight and the small bowel

Diarrhoea is the commonest presenting symptom of small intestinal disease, and when persistent is usually associated with malnutrition. The cause of the weight loss, which in AIDS patients is often dramatic, is predominantly anorexia leading to reduced food intake. Although malabsorption causes some wastage of calories, this is easily overcome by slight increases in food intake. A surgical example illustrates the point. In patients who have undergone massive intestinal resection, intestinal failure is unlikely unless the remaining length of small intestine is 1 metre or less, so minor changes in villous architecture alone can not explain weight loss. Anorexia, probably mediated by inflammatory messengers such as cytokines, explains the weight loss related to intestinal disease.

Malabsorption

Malabsorption is a confusing problem. It means impaired absorption of one or more nutrients, and it describes a pathophysiological process. It is not a diagnosis. Its contribution to symptoms varies with the disease underlying it. For example, lactose malabsorption is normal in most Africans unless their ancestral origins were in tribes which drank appreciable quantities of milk. It is exacerbated during recovery from intestinal disease. It is not a significant clinical problem in adults unless an individual habituated to milk drinking develops a degree of enteropathy, i.e. diffuse small intestinal disease with reduced villous height, and then develops secondary lactose malabsorption. It usually either recovers spontaneously or the individual affected learns to avoid milk products.

There are three major categories of malabsorption:

- *global malabsorption* associated with small intestinal disease such as rotavirus infection, cryptosporidiosis or coeliac disease; this makes a contribution to diarrhoea and is often associated with anorexia.
- *specific malabsorption* of single nutrients such as vitamin B_{12} (as in pernicious anaemia), iron, lactose or bile salts; the first two lead to anaemia (but see below) and the latter two lead to diarrhoea.
- *maldigestion* due to achlorhydria (lack of gastric acid, often asymptomatic) or biliary obstruction or pancreatic disease leading to steatorrhoea.

Distinctive tropical conditions

Before going on to discuss important small intestinal disease, it is important to clarify two more terms.

Tropical enteropathy

A poor term applied to the normal small intestinal mucosa in healthy adults in under-resourced countries. Villi are fused, shortened and broadened compared to adults in temperate countries, crypt depth and permeability are increased (Figs. 79.8 and 79.9). This has no known implications for human health and probably represents an adaptive response to a contaminated environment.

Tropical sprue

In contrast to tropical enteropathy, tropical sprue is a serious disease of unknown aetiology, characterized by

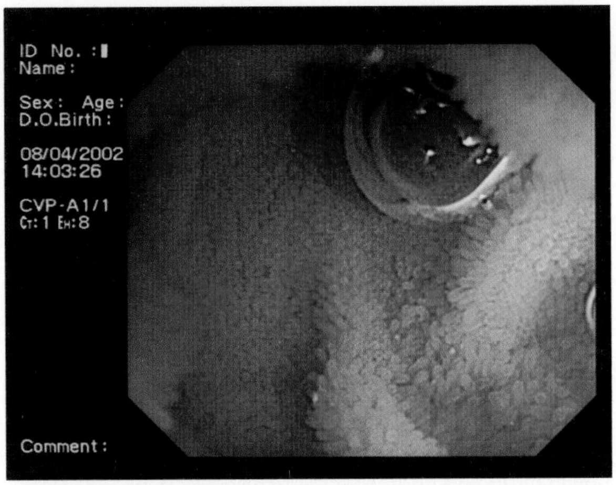

Fig. 79.8. Normal small intestinal villi seen through an endoscope at high magnification. The villi are finger shaped.

persistent diarrhoea and severe weight loss; it is very rare indeed in Africa.

Coeliac disease

It was thought that coeliac disease does not occur in Africa, but a recent report (Catassi et al., 1999) shows that it may occur at least in some tribes in the Sahel. It is an autoimmune disease resulting from a sensitivity to gliadin (in gluten, a cereal component) which is processed by, and probably cross-reacts to, small intestinal tissue transglutaminase and leads to an enteropathy. It is associated with the HLA DQ2 genotype. Patients present at any age with persistent diarrhoea, weight loss and evidence of malabsorption of micronutrients (folic acid and iron in particular). Diagnosis is made by small intestinal biopsy (usually done at endoscopy) which shows villous atrophy and crypt hyperplasia. Treatment is by adopting a diet free of wheat or related cereals.

Bacterial overgrowth

Bacterial overgrowth of the small intestine may lead to diarrhoea due to malabsorption. It occurs in people with a structurally abnormal gut, for example, jejunal diverticulosis or a post-surgical blind loop. Occasionally, it complicates diabetes mellitus. Treatment is with antibiotics such as tetracycline for 4 weeks.

Rare disorders

Malabsorption may also be associated with enteropathy due to radiation, amyloidosis, lymphangiectasia, systemic

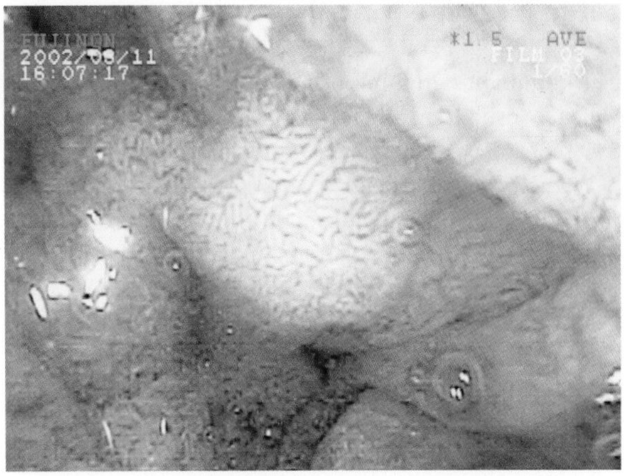

Fig. 79.9. Enteropatic mucosa: the villi are partly blunted, shortened and have a ridge like appearance. In coeliac disease, the villi almost disappear, leaving a very flattened mucosa, referred to as 'sub-total villous atrophy'.

sclerosis and eosinophilic gastroenteritis, but these are all very rare in Africa.

Tuberculosis

Tuberculosis of the small intestine most frequently affects the terminal ileum and caecum. It presents with diarrhoea, weight loss, fevers and vague right lower quadrant abdominal pain. It is difficult to diagnose and hard to distinguish from Crohn's disease; the best confirmation is to identify acid-fast bacilli in endoscopic or surgical biopsy sections or to succeed with mycobacterial culture from biopsies. Treatment is with standard rifampicin-based anti-tuberculosis regimens.

Crohn's disease

Crohn's disease (see p. 972) is a rare transmural inflammation of the intestinal wall. Suspect the disease in patients with persistent diarrhoea and weight loss, particularly if there is a suggestion of an abdominal mass or if there is post-operative or perianal fistulation. Initial treatment is with steroids (such as prednisolone 40 mg daily) but management must be done in a specialist centre.

Cancer

Cancers of the small intestine are very rare. When non-infectious growths are discovered, the commonest diagnoses are carcinoid tumours and lymphomas.

Large intestine (colon)

The dominant symptoms of colonic disease are diarrhoea, constipation and rectal bleeding (also called haematochezia) (see Chapter 20, Acute diarrhoea).

When the left side of the colon is involved in inflammatory processes, the patient usually has bloody diarrhoea; if this is due to infection (with or without an accompanying fever) it is referred to as dysentery. Dysentery is commonly due to *Shigella* spp., *Entamoeba histolytica*, *Campylobacter* spp., and occasionally to *Schistosoma mansoni*. Bacillary dysentery is usually of abrupt onset and requires treatment with antibiotics, depending on local sensitivity patterns.

Ulcerative colitis (see above) presents in the same way, usually less acutely. It may present with acute severe colitis, with very frequent diarrhoea, fever, tachycardia and abdominal tenderness, leukocytosis and sometimes with colonic dilatation, when it may be confused with severe amoebic dysentery (but no amoebic trophozoites are found in the stool or in biopsies). This may require surgery if colonic perforation is impending.

Constipation

Constipation (often defined as frequency of defaecation less than every 3 days) may be a minor nuisance or may result from severe bowel disease such as idiopathic megarectum (which follows from disordered rectal innervation). Constipation as a presenting symptom of colonic disease is uncommon in our practice and most cases require simple advice (a diet adequate in fresh fruit and vegetables, generous water intake, regular exercise) and sometimes simple laxatives such as lactulose and magnesium compounds. Avoid prescribing stimulant laxatives such as docusate and senna in the long term, as increasing doses will be required and the over-stimulated colon will become increasingly refractory and unresponsive in some cases. If constipation is very severe, for example in a few neurologically disabled people and women with obstetric-related perineal damage, it is important to establish if a finger has to be used to aid evacuation. If this is found, refer the patient to a specialized surgical coloproctology unit. Management can be difficult.

Diverticular disease

Diverticular disease (diverticulosis) is common in industrialized countries, but is still uncommon in South African black populations despite the reduction of fibre in the diet of urban adults (Walker & Segal, 1997). The mere presence of diverticula (diverticulosis) in a patient in Africa, as in any other population, does not imply that the diverticula are responsible for symptoms such as vague abdominal pain or irregular bowel habit. Diverticulosis may lead to diverticulitis, overt rectal bleeding or to formation of a diverticular mass.

Colorectal cancer

Colorectal cancer is uncommon in Africa (see above) but we do see cases in Lusaka. It is commoner in older age groups. Important clinical features include iron deficiency anaemia and rectal bleeding (see below), which should always be investigated in older people: altered bowel habit and abdominal pain also occur, but are less strongly indicative of cancer. Diagnosis is by colonoscopy or barium enema and the objective of effective management should be to detect cancers as early as possible so as to offer surgical resection while there is still a possibility of cure.

Anorectal disease

Most anorectal disorders are treated by those with surgical expertise but not all require surgery.

Haemorrhoids

The commonest cause of perianal lumps and often give rise to bleeding which occurs at the end of defaecation and may streak the outside of the stool or may only be seen on the paper. Haemorrhoids are painless unless thrombosed. It is important to ensure that there is no constipation which forces the patient to strain at defaecation.

Anal fissure

Presents with severe pain and bleeding occurs as with haemorrhoids. Management is as above, but if either of these problems persists, surgical referral is advisable.

Incontinence

Usually related to obstetric trauma when the anal sphincters have been damaged. This may also lead to recto-vaginal fistula. With expert surgical management, as is so supremely practised at the Addis Ababa Fistula Hospital, women with either of these very distressing complaints can usually be cured completely.

Table 79.3. Factors that indicate poor prognosis in acute pancreatitis

Age	>55 years
Leukocyte count	$>15\times10^9$/l
Blood urea	>16 mmol/l
Blood glucose	>10 mmol/l
Serum albumin	<30 g/l
Serum ALT	>200 U/l
Serum calcium	<2 mmol/l
Serum LDH	>600 U/l
Arterial PaO_2	<8 kPa (<60 mmHg)

Pruritus ani

A persistent itching, which is usually of psychogenic origin and does not require surgical management. It is important to offer advice about perianal hygiene, avoiding perfumed or coloured soaps or disinfectants, and encouraging careful drying. It is important to reassure the patient also.

The pancreas

Consider pancreatic disease in patients who present with generalized abdominal pain associated with pain in the middle of the back. Vomiting is often prominent, especially in acute pancreatitis. For unknown reasons, the incidence of pancreatitis varies greatly around Africa, being common in South Africa but rare in Zambia. In South Africa, the aetiology was alcohol-related in 83 per cent, and the consequences were serious with mortality in 8 per cent and recurrent problems in two-thirds (John et al., 1997).

Acute pancreatitis

Acute pancreatitis presents with pain and vomiting. Predisposing factors include high alcohol intake, passage of gallstones down the common bile duct, instrumentation of the sphincter of Oddi (during endoscopic retrograde cholangio-pan creatography (ERCP)), hypertriglyceridaemia and drugs (including antiretroviral drugs).

Diagnosis

This can be difficult; important confirmation is obtained from elevated amylase or lipase concentrations in serum or from typical appearances seen with ultrasound or CT scanning (Fig. 79.10).

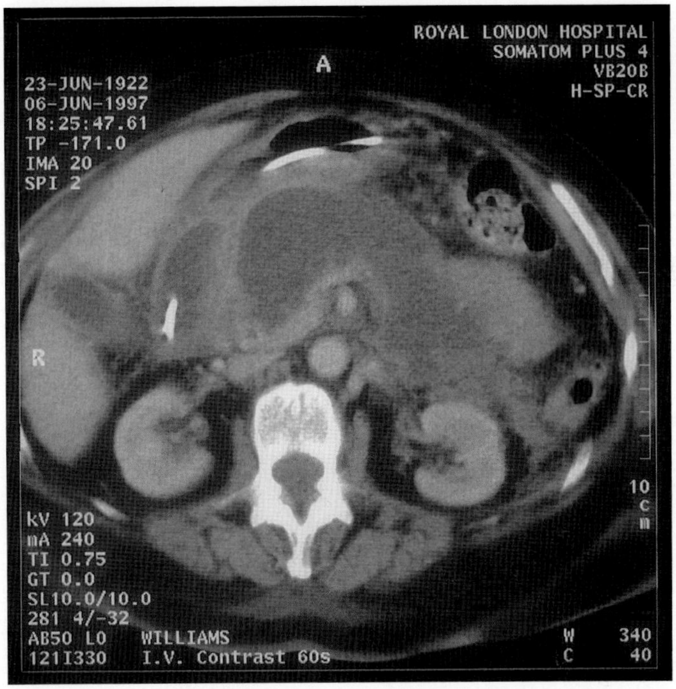

Fig. 79.10. Acute pancreatitis. The CT scan shows the pancreas to be grossly enlarged with a loss of definition between it and the surrounding tissues. The kidneys, liver, gall bladder and aorta all appear normal and the bowel is displaced forward.

Management

Give basic supportive treatment.

- Monitor cardiovascular and respiratory functions.
- Maintain careful fluid balance.
- Treat infections promptly.

Surgery has no place in management except in units engaged in research into pancreatitis. Mortality varies from 1 per cent to 50 per cent depending on the severity of illness. Adverse prognostic factors are shown in Table 79.3.

Chronic pancreatitis

There are two syndromes of chronic pancreatic disease in Africa.

Fibro calculous pancreatitis (of the young and malnourished)

This syndrome is very well recognized in southern India, where it has long been thought to be associated with dietary cassava, and has also been reported from many African countries. The diagnostic criteria are: occurrence in a tropical country, diabetes and pancreatic calculi. An alternative set of criteria are that there should be at least three of the following: demonstrable pancreatic pathology, history of recurrent abdominal pain since childhood, steatorrhoea, abnormal exocrine pancreatic function and exclusion of other causes of chronic pancreatitis.

The patient is typically male, poor, young and malnourished. The pathogenesis of the pancreatic disease is uncertain: it may be the sequel of repeated episodes of dehydrating diarrhoea, which lead to inspissation of pancreatic secretions within the pancreatic ducts so that calculi form and enlarge (Nwokolo & Oli, 1980). The possible causes have been reviewed by Osier and Newton (1999). The pancreatic disease leads to endocrine failure (insulin dependent diabetes mellitus without ketosis), exocrine failure (malabsorption and stunting) and chronic abdominal and back pain.

Chronic pancreatitis strongly associated with alcohol abuse

This disease presents with chronic abdominal and back pain, often with exacerbations which actually represent minor (and sometimes major) episodes of acute pancreatitis. There are no drugs that alter the course of the disease, but total abstinence from alcohol usually stops progression of the disease.

Diagnosis is usually by endoscopic retrograde cholangiopancreatography (ERCP), but plain abdominal radiographs show typical pancreatic calcification in perhaps one-third of cases and sometimes it will be seen on abdominal ultrasound by an experienced radiographer (Fig. 79.11).

Treatment

The pain is difficult to treat and may require opiate analgesics especially during acute exacerbations. This may lead to problems with opiate dependence and the physician will need to balance sympathy with firmness. An important benefit may be obtained with pancreatic enzyme supplements which will help pain and steatorrhoea. Give 2–4 g with each meal, avoid the highest strength capsules as they have been associated with colonic stricturing; cimetidine may be required also to reduce gastric acid secretion.

Carcinoma

Pancreatic carcinoma may present with similar symptoms (although the history is unlikely to be more than a few months), but more usually it presents with painless obstructive jaundice. This cancer is very problematic as it presents late, is difficult to diagnose, and is usually incurable. Late stage cancer spreads around the retroperitoneum and may cause very severe pain indeed. In advanced units, if it is possible, jaundice may be relieved by stenting performed at ERCP.

Endocrine tumours

A small proportion of pancreatic tumours are not carcinoma but endocrine tumours such as carcinoid or even rarer cell types. These may be silent or may present with symptoms attributable to the hormones or growth factors secreted. They are all rare. Carcinoid tumours present with episodic flushing of the face and extremities due to liberation of serotonin from liver metastases. VIPomas present with persistent secretory diarrhoea due to release of VIP (vasoactive intestinal polypeptide). Insulinomas present with hypoglycaemia. Glucagonomas present with hyperglycaemia and a necrotizing rash which is extremely unpleasant. Some of these cancers are resectable, but the surgery is difficult.

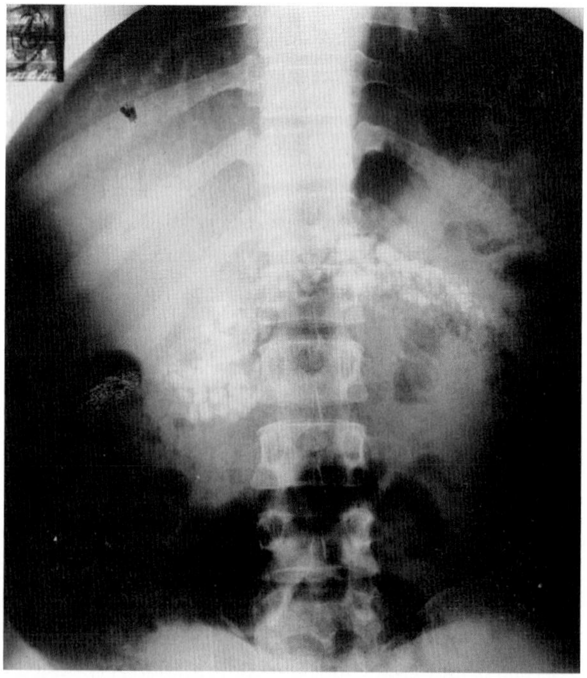

Fig. 79.11. Pancreatic calcification: plain radiograph of abdomen.

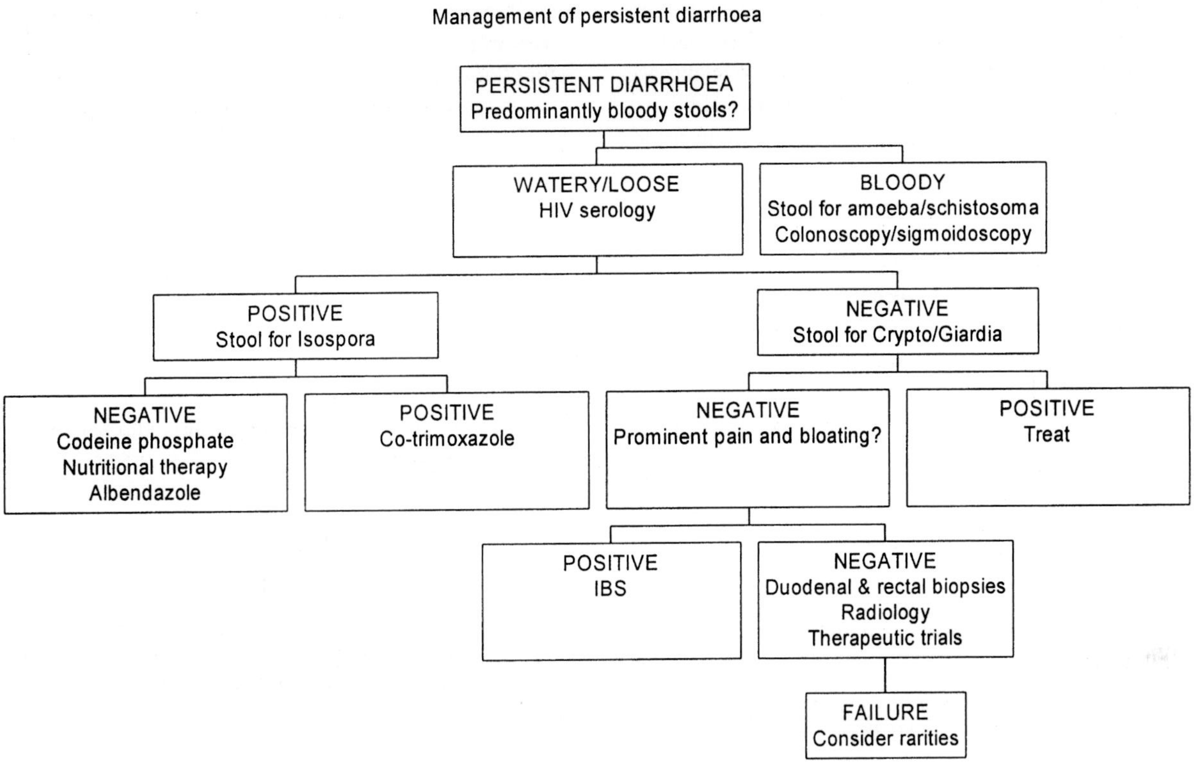

Fig. 79.12. Management of persistent diarrhoea. IBS: irritable bowel syndrome.

Major clinical problems

Persistent diarrhoea

Persistent diarrhoea is a diarrhoeal episode which lasts more than 14 days. Diarrhoea is defined clinically as loose or watery stools three or more times per day, or physiologically as 300 g stool or more per 24 hours.

The problem in Africa

It is important to remember that persistent diarrhoea often has strong socio-cultural connotations in Africa. In certain circumstances in Zambia, persistent diarrhoea traditionally implies a broken taboo or cultural infringement, and in the era of AIDS it is severely stigmatizing to be seen to have persistent diarrhoea and weight loss. Discussion of this clinical problem therefore requires sensitivity and some local cultural understanding as cultural beliefs may explain why patients have very firm ideas about what is, and what is not, good treatment, and will often influence their treatment seeking behaviour.

It is not useful to distinguish between persistent and chronic diarrhoea as the causes are so similar, and we therefore recognize only acute and persistent categories. In our experience the great majority of patients presenting with persistent diarrhoea in Lusaka have HIV-related problems: 97 per cent of inpatients and 85 per cent of outpatients were HIV-seropositive. In other parts of Africa where HIV infection is not so common, this pattern is unlikely but many will have infectious causes, particularly intestinal protozoa and *Schistosoma mansoni.* A minority will have inflammatory bowel disease (see above) and rarely thyrotoxicosis, neuroendocrine tumours or vitamin deficiencies, e.g. niacin deficiency: (see Chapter 3), will be responsible.

Management

The management of persistent diarrhoea is therefore very much dependent on the HIV-seroprevalence in the population being served. HIV-related diarrhoeal disease is described in Chapter 13, intestinal protozoa in Chapter 35 and schistosomiasis in Chapter 25. A flow diagram for management is suggested in Fig. 79.12.

Investigation

The choice of investigation depends on the cause: thus a duodenal biopsy can be used to detect coeliac disease, duodenal and rectal biopsies to detect low-level infection such as giardiasis, cryptosporidiosis or schistosomiasis, and biopsies may also reveal inflammatory bowel disease if that area is affected. Radiology means small bowel follow-through to detect Crohn's disease, tuberculosis or lymphoma.

Therapeutic trials depend also on the suspected diagnosis: for example metronidazole for *Giardia lamblia*, anti-tuberculosis chemotherapy, or gluten withdrawal. Rare causes of persistent diarrhoea include intestinal hormone disorders, primary bile salt malabsorption, which may respond to a therapeutic trial of cholestyramine, or rare osmotic diarrhoeal disorders.

Abdominal pain

Epigastric pain

Epigastric pain has a wide differential diagnosis.

- Ask specifically if the patient experiences a burning behind the sternum.
- Ask about the relationship to eating: a consistent relationship to food may indicate peptic ulceration or functional dyspepsia.
- Ask about night time pain, which indicates GORD or peptic ulceration.
- Establish how long the pain lasts; pain lasting for a few seconds or a minute or two is not due to organic disease.

The single most informative investigation is gastroscopy.

RUQ pain

Right upper quadrant (RUQ) pain is due to biliary disease or functional symptoms. Occasionally biliary disease presents with epigastric pain or gastroduodenal disease presents with RUQ pain. Biliary colic (pain due to gallstones) is pain which comes for several hours at intervals of a few weeks. The single most informative investigation is ultrasound of the biliary tree.

Lower abdominal pain

Lower abdominal pain is the most difficult of all as it may be difficult to distinguish gynaecological and intestinal causes. It is important to establish the relationship of pain to menstruation and intercourse.

Pain – but no demonstrable disease

It has been evident for many years that many patients with abdominal pain and other symptoms of gastrointestinal disorder do not have any demonstrable pathology. It is very important to recognize that these individuals have a functional disturbance not a structural one.

Irritable bowel syndrome

It has been claimed that the irritable bowel syndrome (IBS) is not common in Africa, but this does not appear to be true, according to our experience in our largely urban patients in Lusaka. It certainly is true that the reason why one individual comes to seek medical help at a particular time varies between cultures and with social circumstances, and the frequency with which any condition is seen may vary between town and country and between socio-economic groups.

Clinical features

The dominant feature of IBS is abdominal pain, and it is often accompanied by abdominal bloating and wind. There are three major groups: pain predominant, constipation predominant and diarrhoea predominant, and other symptoms may also be found, such as nausea, rumbling sounds (borborygmi) or a dragging feeling. However, it is important to stress that weight loss, intestinal bleeding or anaemia can never be accepted as attributable to IBS.

Pathophysiology

This is centred on the enteric nervous system (ENS) which controls intestinal motility and secretion. The lifelong, day-by-day process of integration of conscious and subconscious stimuli to maintain nutritional homeostasis is carried out by the ENS, which contains as many neurons as the spinal cord. IBS patients have visceral hypersensitivity, which can be demonstrated by an increased sensitivity to bowel distension. Thus the normal business of digestion and elimination becomes recognizable as painful sensations as if there was intestinal pathology. There is some evidence that IBS may sometimes follow intestinal infectious disease. In a small minority of sufferers there is actual damage to the ENS, often a neuronitis, which can be diagnosed using full thickness biopsies of the intestinal wall. This is still the subject of research.

Diagnosis

Diagnosis is based on clinical symptoms alone, and it may be useful to use a small number of selected investigations (usually including full blood count and stool microscopy) to help avoid missing other diagnoses. Remember, however, that helminth infections of the gut only lead to symptoms when very heavy. A heavy burden of hookworms may lead to pain in the epigastrium or central abdomen. A trial of mebendazole or albendazole may be worthwhile but do not be surprised when the pain persists or recurs after a few weeks.

Treatment

Treatment is difficult in some cases, but most merely require reassurance. Severe spasmodic abdominal pain may be helped by anti-spasmodics such as mebeverine or hyoscine butylbromide. In severe cases, low doses of certain anti-depressants (for example, amitriptyline 25–50 mg nocte) may reduce the sensation of pain.

Weight loss

Weight loss in the absence of other symptoms is a difficult diagnostic problem, but usually accompanying symptoms (fever, cough, diarrhoea, neurological symptoms) assist in establishing the cause. Some systemic infections, such as miliary tuberculosis, may cause real problems in diagnosis. Intestinal disorders usually present with abdominal pain or diarrhoea or evidence of bleeding (iron deficiency anaemia, bleeding per rectum). There is no substitute for disciplined clinical method – a detailed history, a careful and thorough clinical examination and any obviously indicated test, based on cause postulated for the loss of weight.

Inoperable cancer

Palliative care of inoperable cancer is described in Chapter 91, and so we comment here on particular problems in gastrointestinal disease.

In oesophageal cancer, pain relief will usually require opiates but the dysphagia may progress so relentlessly that even saliva cannot be swallowed. This may require oesophageal stenting, if such facilities are available. Anticholinergic drugs may be useful to dry the mouth if stenting proves impossible. In other digestive cancers, palliative surgery may be of great benefit. This may allow relief of jaundice in pancreatic cancer or relief of intestinal obstruction in colorectal cancer. Pain relief is always important. Obstructive jaundice is associated with itching, which can be very unpleasant and this may be helped with a combination of H1 and H2 receptor antagonists. Nausea can be relieved by metoclopramide or domperidone. Major neuroleptics such as chlorpromazine or haloperidol are also useful for nausea. In terminal care, the correct dose and timing is that which controls symptoms (pp. 1235–38). Nothing else matters: long-term toxicity is irrelevant.

Gastrointestinal haemorrhage

A bleed may present with anything from dramatic, life-threatening haematemesis to slow occult haemorrhage leading to iron deficiency anaemia. Overt GI bleeding and iron deficiency anaemia will be discussed separately as the approach to management of these disorders is very different.

Haematemesis and melaena

The clinical syndrome

Rapid bleeding into the stomach or duodenum usually leads to vomiting blood (haematemesis) almost immediately, and the passage of altered (i.e. digested) blood per rectum some hours or days later. Mortality rates during the acute episode vary from one centre to another. There are few data on mortality due to GI bleeding from African centres; but in the UK rates probably range from 1–8 per cent depending on the patient mix, when death usually occurs in patients with co-morbid disorders, such as co-existing cardiac, respiratory or systemic disease. In Africa, three common disorders give rise to this medical emergency:

- peptic ulceration
- oesophageal varices
- the Mallory–Weiss syndrome.

Less common are gastric cancer and erosive gastritis. The suggested management of upper gastrointestinal bleeding is given in Fig. 79.13.

Significant circulatory signs (see also p. 1342)
Circulatory compromise is indicated by clinical features of volume depletion. These features are tachycardia (pulse rate over 100/min), hypotension (or postural hypotension – a fall in systolic pressure of over 10 mm Hg), sweating, restlessness, mental slowing and/or oliguria. Beware the patient already taking beta-adrenoreceptor antagonists such as propranolol or atenolol, in whom the tachycardia may be masked.

Bleeding and liver failure (see Chapter 80)
Liver failure is important to identify as it is important to watch for and treat hypoglycaemia, coagulopathy and encephalopathy. Furthermore, it may indicate that oesophageal varices may be the source of bleeding, when the Sengstaken–Blakemore tube may be life saving

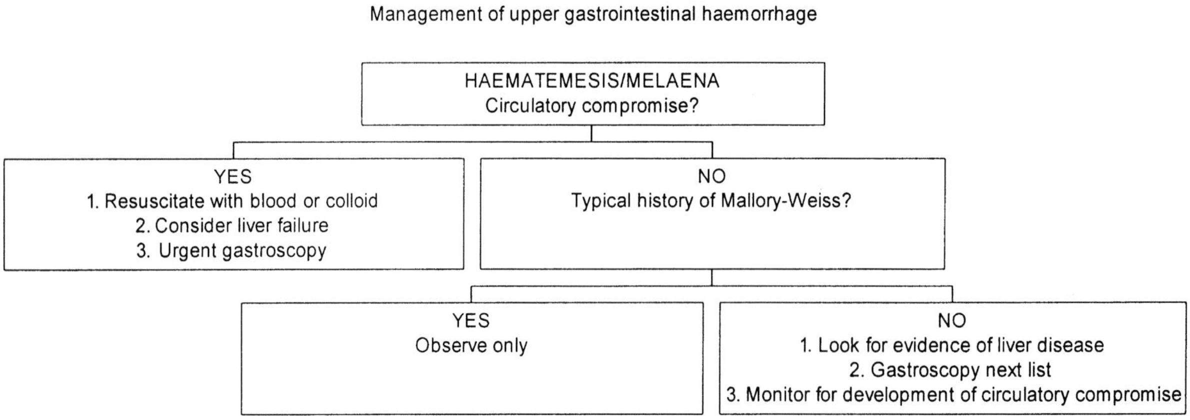

Fig. 79.13. Management of upper gastrointestinal haemorrhage.

(Fig. 79.14). The tube is deployed to control very severe variceal haemorrhage. The tube should be kept refrigerated if possible to increase its stiffness. It is lubricated and introduced through the mouth. The Sengstaken–Blakemore tube can be life-saving, but it requires care. Never leave it in place for more than 12 hours in order to reduce the chance of mucosal necrosis. It is also extremely unpleasant for the patient!

The Mallory–Weiss syndrome

The patient typically describes vomiting for some other reason, for example, infective gastroenteritis or alcohol excess. After one or more vomits, blood suddenly appears in the vomitus, which was not there at the outset. It is due to a tear at the gastro-oesophageal junction. It is very rarely a cause of large volume blood loss and this history therefore identifies a group of patients with a very good prognosis.

Bleeding per rectum

Bright red blood on the paper (or whatever people in a given area use to wipe the anus), or at the end of defaecation, usually signifies perianal disease (see above). If it is heavy or persistent, or mixed in with the stool, it may require investigation, and sigmoidoscopy is the procedure of choice.

Iron deficiency anaemia

Throughout Africa, hookworm disease is the dominant cause of anaemia, which is proved to be due to iron deficiency (Chapter 78). In industrialized countries, however, this anaemia is a strong indication for colonoscopy, as it

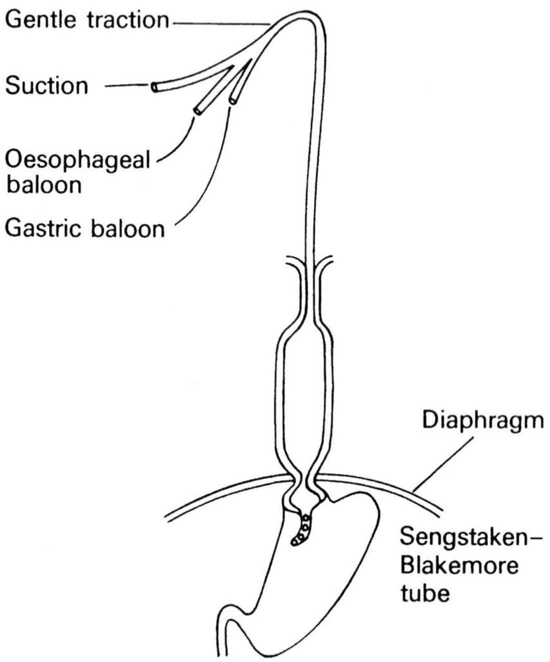

Fig. 79.14. The Sengstaken–Blakemore tube. There are four lumens. The first is the distal (gastric) aspiration port. Air is flushed through while the operator listens over the stomach to hear the bubbles in the stomach and then blood is aspirated. The second port to be used is the gastric balloon which is inflated with 200ml air and pulled up against the cardia of the stomach. This is usually sufficient to control bleeding. The third (oesophageal) lumen should be aspirated regularly to prevent overflow of secretions into the lungs. The fourth lumen (the oesophageal balloon) should only be inflated if bleeding continues as this balloon sometimes perforates the oesophagus.

may indicate cancer of the right side of the colon, which would otherwise remain undiagnosed until it is too late for curative surgery. Treatment begins with mebendazole or albendazole, but older patients and possibly patients from urban environments should be monitored carefully for their response to treatment: if their haemoglobin does not rise, a large bowel cancer is possible.

GI investigations

Investigation of GI disease begins with simple haematology and biochemistry and progresses through immunology, radiology and endoscopy.

Haematology (see Chapter 78, section on anaemia)
Anaemia may indicate digestive disease. Iron deficiency usually indicates occult bleeding, and the commonest site of such bleeding is into the gut. It presents with a microcytic anaemia. A macrocytic anaemia may indicate malabsorption of folic acid or vitamin B_{12}. Leukocytosis may indicate severe inflammation as in amoebic or ulcerative colitis. Leukopenia may occur in AIDS or other immune deficiencies. Thrombocytosis and the ESR are useful markers of inflammatory severity in Crohn's disease.

Biochemistry

Liver function tests are obviously important when it is suspected that hepato-biliary disease may be present (see Chapter 80). There are a few biochemical tests which relate to gastrointestinal disease itself.

Serum albumin concentration may be reduced in a range of disorders, but it is not a useful marker of nutritional status alone. Albumin is reduced in response to severe inflammation when protein synthesis in the liver switches from 'peace-time' proteins like albumin to 'acute phase reaction' proteins, like C-reactive protein (which has a role in innate immunity). These tests usually indicate that there is inflammation present, which is particularly useful for monitoring conditions like inflammatory bowel disease.

Biochemistry can also be useful in assessing the severity of micronutrient deficiencies, for example assessment of iron status or the increased alkaline phosphatase seen in vitamin D malabsorption.

Immunology

Serum immunoglobulin assays may be useful in diagnosis of hypogammaglobulinaemias, for example, IgA deficiency, which is associated with giardiasis. T-cell counts (CD4 and CD8 cells) are useful in assessing the severity of deficiency in AIDS (Chapter 13).

Although auto-antibodies can be found in several digestive diseases, there is only one condition in which they are diagnostically useful. Anti-endomysial antibodies are present in most cases of coeliac disease and have a high positive and negative predictive value. It has recently been found that the target of this antibody in the small intestine is tissue transglutaminase, although it is not yet clear how this relates to the cereal component gliadin which precipitates the auto-immune reaction. As coeliac disease appears to be rare in Africa, and the test is difficult and expensive, it will rarely be used.

Radiology

The plain abdominal radiograph is still an important tool in assessment of the acute abdomen. A supine film will show dilated loops of bowel in intestinal obstruction, and it will show colonic dilatation in acute severe colitis. It is important to remember that when perforation of a viscus is suspected, it is an erect chest radiograph which will reveal the air under the diaphragm (Fig. 79.15).

Ultrasound examination has the advantage that it is completely safe, quick, painless, and running costs are low. It is an important tool in diagnosing hepato-biliary disease. It is also very helpful in assessing the distended abdomen and abdominal masses.

Double-contrast barium studies are not available in many centres as the X-ray imaging required has to be of

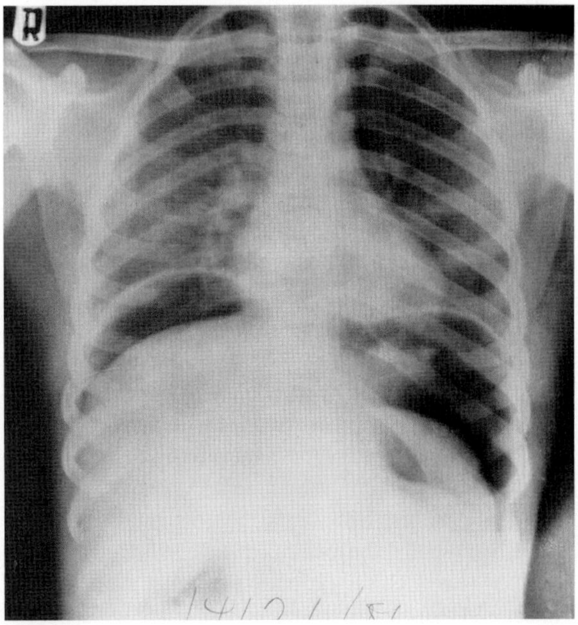

Fig. 79.15. Perforation of the gut: note the clear line of the diaphragm, shown because of the gas under each leaf of the diaphragm.

Table 79.4. Barium contrast studies

Study	Indication	Comments
Barium swallow	Dysphagia, pain	Shows cancer and motility disorders Rapid and easy for patient
Barium meal	Epigastric pain Vomiting	Difficult to interpret Gastroscopy usually preferable
Small bowel follow-through	Persistent diarrhoea, pain	Only way of studying small bowel anatomy
Barium enema	Changed bowel habit	Requires bowel preparation Colonoscopy usually preferable

high quality to be useful, and such equipment is expensive to buy and maintain. The principal features are shown in Table 79.4.

The CT scan provides a series of cross-sectional images of the abdomen. It is an important investigation, but rarely available in Africa. It is useful in the diagnosis of difficult abdominal pain and masses. When performed by skilled radiologists, it can be used to clarify the level of an intestinal obstruction, but otherwise limited information is obtained about the intestine itself.

Endoscopy

The development of fibre-optic endoscopes and then video endoscopes has revolutionized gastroenterology. These scopes allow the investigator to see the inside of most of the hollow organs of the digestive tract: oesophagus, stomach, duodenum, proximal jejunum, terminal ileum, colon and rectum. The only part which is very difficult (though not impossible) to inspect is the mid small bowel.

Oesophagogastroduodenoscopy (OGD) is the most frequently performed procedure as it is relatively easy (usually under sedation but experienced endoscopists can perform it with throat spray alone), gives much useful information, and mucosal biopsies can be obtained painlessly. Complications are rare. It is most useful in the investigation of epigastric pain and GI bleeding.

Sigmoidoscopy can be carried out with rigid or fibre-optic scopes. The rigid scope is warmed and lubricated, introduced gently into the anus angled towards the front, then gently pointed backwards, the trochar taken out and a pipe fixed so that the rectum can be insufflated and the mucosa viewed. This is a good way of looking for colitis or cancer and biopsies can be taken. Using a proctoscope, haemorrhoids can be diagnosed.

Colonoscopy should only be performed by experienced endoscopists as the risk of perforation by inexperienced operators is high. The colon must be cleaned out, usually with a combination of laxatives over 2 days prior to the procedure. The whole of the colon can be inspected, including the terminal ileum where appropriate. Sedation is almost always required.

Endoscopic retrograde cholangio-pancreatography (ERCP) is a very demanding investigation, performed with a side-viewing endoscope, through which a tube is inserted into the bile or pancreatic duct to allow radio-opaque dye to be flushed in. X-rays are then taken of the ducts, usually to look for causes of obstructive jaundice or to confirm chronic pancreatitis, and sometimes to remove duct stones.

Functional tests

In general, these tests are not widely used outside very specialized gastroenterology centres. Anatomical assessments, using radiology and/or endoscopy with biopsy, achieve most diagnostic results.

Motility studies of the oesophagus and rectum have entered clinical practice in the diagnosis of achalasia and defaecatory disorders, respectively. They are not available in most of Africa as these disorders are rare.

Tests of absorption are rarely necessary in Africa. Sometimes, it will be useful to see if diarrhoea is due to lactose malabsorption, by detecting reducing substances in the stool (using Clinitest tablets) which would be present while taking, but not on withholding, milk. A Schilling test can be used to detect B_{12} malabsorption (see Chapter 78). Hydrogen breath tests can be used to test for small bowel bacterial overgrowth. Sugar markers (combinations of lactulose, xylose, rhamnose, 3–*o*-methyl D-glucose or mannitol) can also be given and their excretion over 5 hours in urine used to assess normal and abnormal absorption. This is a research tool. Most other tests of absorption have become obsolete even in highly specialized centres.

Tests of pancreatic function have largely been replaced by ERCP and faecal elastase estimation.

The acute abdomen (see Table 79.5)

While detailed discussion of surgical emergencies is beyond the scope of this book, an outline of some important points may be useful in differential diagnosis.

Pattern of disease

Acute appendicitis, acute diverticulitis and ruptured diverticula are uncommon in rural Africa, but in an urban

Table 79.5. Causes of the acute abdomen

Process	Cause	Clinical features	Management
Inflamed viscus	Cholecystitis Diverticulitis Salpingitis Appendicitis	Severe local pain, local tenderness, fever	Antibiotics; surgery elective if required Urgent surgery
Peritonitis	Ruptured ulcer, appendix, colon, diverticulum	Sudden onset generalized pain, with or without antecedent illness, board-like rigidity, rebound tenderness	Resuscitation, urgent surgery
	Intestinal infarction	Sudden onset pain, shock, generalized tenderness in elderly patients	Resuscitation, urgent surgery
	Ruptured vessel, e.g. aorta, ectopic pregnancy	Shock, vascular collapse	Resuscitation, urgent surgery
Obstruction	Volvulus, cancer adhesions, intussusception, ascariasis	Pain, vomiting, distension, absolute constipation	Resuscitation initially; surgery later if required
Medical	Diabetic ketoacidosis, lower lobar pneumonia, renal colic, lead and other poisoning, IBS, porphyria, zoster pain, myocardial infarction		Careful history always check blood sugar

Note:
In early tetanus, spasm of the abdominal wall muscles may be confused with the rigid abdomen of an acute abdominal emergency.

Accra surgical unit hospital, acute appendicitis was the most common cause of acute abdominal pain emergencies (responsible for 23.5 per cent – Naaeder et al., 1999). Thus there are changing patterns of disease. However, even in South African and Zambian populations, which consume a 'westernized' diet, there seems to be a much lower incidence than expected by comparison with industrialized countries.

Intestinal obstruction

Intestinal obstruction when fully developed presents with a classic tetrad of clinical features: abdominal distension, vomiting, pain and absolute constipation (passage of neither faeces nor flatus). The cause varies across the continent – strangulated hernia and sigmoid volvulus dominate, but, intussusception, a ball of *Ascaris lumbricoides*, colonic cancer and adhesions are also seen. In Libya, incarceration of the bowel in a hernia was the commonest cause, followed by post-operative adhesions. Sigmoid volvulus was rare in that series (Kuruvilla et al., 1987). Sigmoid volvulus is common in many parts of Africa, but appears to be declining in South Africa. It is particularly common in some highland areas of Ethiopia, where males over whelmingly outnumber females, a pattern which Ayalew Tegegne(1995) has attributed to cultural differences in habits of defaecation.

Sigmoid volvulus presents a characteristic radiological appearance, with the gas-filled distended loop of sigmoid colon pushed up out of the left iliac fossa. If the diagnosis can be made before surgery, surgery can be made safer by decompressing the sigmoid by passing a flatus tube or sigmoidoscope gently up the rectum and standing well back. This is a standard initial treatment in Gondar (Ali, 1998).

Ruptured ectopic gestation

The diagnosis of a ruptured ectopic, when there is a sudden massive loss of blood and classical signs of peritonitis, with perhaps a history of amenorrhoea, is not difficult. The early diagnosis, however, is more difficult, particularly if loss of blood is small. Such a woman presents with vague lower abdominal discomfort; but her early peritonitis may be detected by tenderness localized at the umbilicus, or on rectal examination. We have seen a case referred for diagnosis of ascites: a diagnostic tap of peritoneal fluid will reveal blood. In her case, a plain radiograph of the abdomen would not show gas under the diaphragm, as would be expected in most cases of perforation of the gut (Fig. 79.15).

References

Ali A. (1998). Treatment of sigmoid volvulus: experience in Gondar, north-west Ethiopia. *Ethiop Med J*; **36**: 47–52.

Ali A, Ersumo T, Johnson O. (1998). Oesophageal carcinoma in Tikur Anbessa Hospital, Addis Ababa. *E Afr Med J*; **75**: 590–593.

Banda LT, Parkin DM, Dzamalala CP et al. (2001). Cancer incidence in Blantyre, Malawi 1994–1998. *Trop Med Int Health*; **6**: 296–304.

Catassi C, Ratsch I-M, Gandolfi L et al. (1999). Why is coeliac disease endemic in the people of the Sahara? *Lancet*; **354**: 647–648.

El-Mahdi AM, Patchett SE, Char S et al. (1998). Does CagA contribute to ulcer pathogenesis in a developing country such as Sudan? *Eur J Gastroenterol Hepatol*; **10**: 313–316.

Fernando N, Holton J, Zulu I et al. (2001). *Helicobacter pylori* infection in an urban Zambian population. *J Clin Microbiol*; **39**: 1323–1327.

Gamieldien W, Victor TC, Mugwanya D et al. (1998). p53 and p16/CDKN2 gene mutations in esophageal tumors from a high-incidence area in South Africa. *Int J Cancer*; **78**: 544–549.

Idris AM, Prokopczyk B, Hoffman D. (1994). Toombak: a major risk factor for cancer of the oral cavity in Sudan. *Prev Med*; **23**: 832–839.

John KD, Segal I, Hassan H et al. (1997). Acute pancreatitis in Sowetan Africans. A disease with high mortality and morbidity. *Int J Pancreatol*; **21**: 149–155.

Kuruvilla MJ, Chhallani CR, Rajagopal AK et al. (1987). Major causes of intestinal obstruction in Libya. *Br J Surg*; **74**: 314–315.

Mengesha B, Johnson O, Taye M et al. (1997). Crohn's disease: report of seven cases from Ethiopia. *E Afr Med J*; **74**: 397–399.

Mengesha B, Tsega E. (1989). Idiopathic ulcerative colitis among Ethiopian patients with chronic diarrhoea. *Ethiop Med J*; **27**: 63–72.

Muguti GI. (1989). Ulcerative proctocolitis in black Zimbabweans. *Centr Afr Med J*; **35**: 300–303.

Naaeder SB, Archampong EQ. (1999). Clinical spectrum of acute abdominal pain in Accra, Ghana. *W Afr J Med*; **18**: 13–16.

Nwokolo C, Oli J. (1980). Pathogenesis of juvenile tropical pancreatitis syndrome. *Lancet*; **1**: 456–458.

Obafunwa JO. (1990). Pattern of alimentary tract tumours in Plateau State: a middle belt area of Nigeria. *J Trop Med Hyg*; **93**: 351–354.

Osier FHA, Newton CRJC. (1999). Fibrocalculous pancreatic diabetes in a child: case report. *E Afr Med J*; **76**: 703–705.

Parkin DM, Vizcaino AP, Skinner ME et al. (1994). Cancer patterns and risk factors in the African population of southwestern Zimbabwe 1963–1977. *Cancer Epid Biomarkers Prev*; **3**: 537–547.

Peghini M, Barabe P, Touze JE et al. (1990). Epidemiology of cancer of the digestive tract in Senegal. Review of 18,000 endoscopies performed at the principal hospital of Dakar. *Med Trop Mars*; **50**: 205–208. [article in French].

Pindiga HU, Akang EE, Thomas JO et al. (1997). Carcinoma of the oesophagus in Ibadan. *E Afr Med J*; **74**: 307–310.

Sabo SY, Ameh EA. (1999). Obstructing duodenal ulcers in a tropical population. *E Afr Med J*; **76**: 690–692.

Segal I. (1984). Intestinal tuberculosis, Crohn's disease and ulcerative colitis in an urban Black population. *S Afr Med J*; **65**: 37–44.

Segal I. (1988). Ulcerative colitis in a developing country of Africa: the Baragwanath experience of the first 46 patients. *Int J Colorect Dis*; **3**: 222–225.

Segal I. (1998). Rarity of colorectal adenomas in the African black population. *Eur J Cancer Prev*; **7**: 387–391.

Vizcaino AP, Parkin DM, Skinner ME. (1995). Risk factors associated with oesophageal cancer in Bulawayo, Zimbabwe. *Br J Cancer*; **72**: 769–773.

Walker AR, Segal I. (1997). Effects of transition on bowel disease in sub-Saharan Africans. *Eur J Gastroenterol Hepatol*; **9**: 207–210.

Walker AR, Walker BF, Segal I. (1993). Cancer patterns in three African populations compared with the United States black population. *Eur J Cancer Prev*; **2**: 313–320.

Wright JP, Froggatt J, O'Keefe EA et al. (1986). The epidemiology of inflammatory bowel disease in Cape Town 1980–1984. *S Afr Med J*; **70**: 10–15.

The liver

80

The problem in Africa

Liver diseases are common in Africa and account for high morbidity and mortality. Hospital-based analyses indicate that acute viral hepatitis, chronic hepatitis, cirrhosis and hepatocellular carcinoma are responsible for at least 12 per cent of medical admissions and over 20 per cent of hospital mortality in many parts of Africa. Hepatocellular carcinoma remains the commonest cancer but autoimmune-related liver diseases are relatively uncommon.

The dramatic progress in our knowledge of viral hepatitis during the past decade has made it possible to diagnose the various types accurately and has allowed us to understand their clinical and epidemiological aspects. The predominant clinical features of chronic liver disease in African patients, often modified by the human immunodeficiency virus and other endemic infective causes, are different from those commonly observed in Western European and North American patients (Tsega, 1992). This chapter focuses on the liver diseases and related conditions that are relevant in the African continent.

Anatomy

Size and position

The liver is the largest organ in the body and weighs approximately 1.5 kg. On clinical examination, measure the number of centimetres the liver protrudes below the costal margin in the midclavicular line on the right side. Define by percussion its upper border, which is at the level of the fifth rib in the right midclavicular line, and record the total vertical span along the midclavicular line in centimetres in a diagram (a normal range in an adult subject is 12 plus or minus 2 cm) (Fig. 80.1).

The liver, especially the left lobe, is relatively large in the new born and at this age is normally felt 2–3 cm below the costal margin. By the age of 5 the liver is not palpable

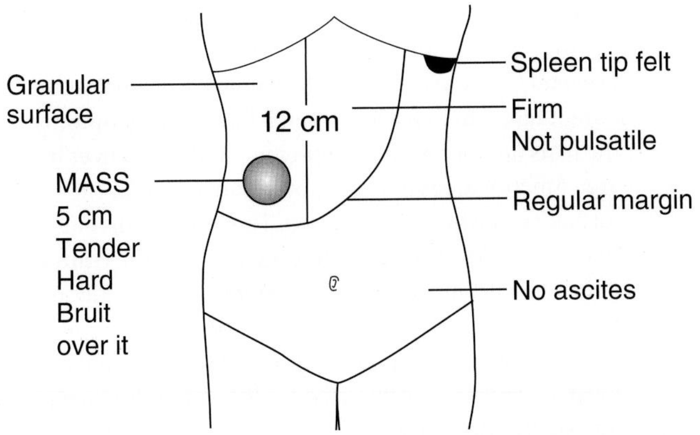

1. Size – in cm below costal margin
2. Edge – regular or irregular
3. Surface – smooth, nodular granular
4. Consistency – hard or soft or firm
5. Tender – or not tender – diffuse or local
6. Pulsatile, or not
7. Bruit, precent or not, and its position

If a mass is found define its margins
– is it fluctuant?

Fig. 80.1. The enlarged liver: record your physical signs clearly in case notes and use a labelled diagram.

except in full inspiration. In parts of Africa, like the tropical west coast where malaria is holoendemic, liver and spleen are normally increased in size due to reticuloendothelial hyperplasia, and both organs are easily palpable in children. These livers are smooth and not tender, so if the liver is tender, enlarged more than 4 cm, and has an irregular surface, it is abnormal.

Riedel's lobe

The right lobe of the liver may be elongated as an extra lobe. It is of no clinical relevance but may be confused with an enlarged liver, a liver mass, or an enlarged right kidney.

Histology

The liver is made of plates or sheets of cells separated by sinusoids lined with reticuloendothelial cells and tunnelled by the portal tracts and the hepatic centrals. These two systems run in perpendicular planes and are separate from each other. The portal tracts contain a small branch of the portal vein, the hepatic arteriole, and a small bile duct. Blood moves from this tract through the sinusoids to the central hepatic canals, which contain radicles of the hepatic vein. Bile is excreted by the hepatic cells into the bile canaliculi, which surround the liver cells, and then flows into the bile-ducts of the portal tract.

The larger structures of these systems can be seen by radiography and the smaller structures by microscopic examination of a liver biopsy.

Needle biopsy of the liver

This is best done with the Menghini needle which sucks up a small core of tissue. (The *Trucut* needle, if available, is an alternative choice.) Do not do a biopsy if:

1. platelet count below 60×10^9/l
2. prothrombin time more than 3 s longer than the control
3. deep jaundice
4. demonstrable ascites.

Although severe bleeding is rare it is desirable to have blood available.

Needle biopsy is useful in patients with unexplained hepatosplenomegaly (often due to cirrhosis); presumed malignant disease affecting the liver, whether primary or secondary; hepatic failure, because viral hepatitis, acute hepatic necrosis, and active chronic hepatitis can be differentiated; and sometimes in pyrexia of undetermined origin when granulomata due to tuberculosis or brucellosis, or neoplastic tissue, may be found; when abnormal liver enzyme are unexplained and in intrahepatic cholestasis.

Liver function and its measurement

The liver is an organ composed of highly specialized parenchymal cells connected to the gut by biliary and portal venous systems and to the systemic circulation by the hepatic arteries and veins.

Major functions of the hepatic parenchymal cells include:

1. metabolism of proteins, carbohydrates, fats, and vitamins
2. storage of glycogen, vitamins, and minerals
3. detoxification and inactivation of endogenous and exogenous substances such as hormones and drugs
4. secretion of bile and excretion of substances removed from the blood into bile. Bile ducts convey bile into the duodenum.

The circulatory system of the liver, via the portal vein, conveys substances absorbed from the gastrointestinal tract directly to the liver. The reticuloendothelial system (RES) of the liver forms part of the general defence mechanism of the body.

Liver function testing is used in the diagnosis and management of patients with liver disease. However, these tests are not specific for liver disease as they may be abnormal in conditions not primarily affecting the liver.

Use of liver function tests

1. To help in establishing the presence of liver disease, either primary or secondary
2. To classify the type of liver disease, e.g. parenchymal damage or extrahepatic biliary obstruction
3. To help assess the progress of liver disease as an aid to prognosis and management.

If several tests are abnormal, it is almost certain that the patient has a diseased liver even if he has no symptoms. The tests do not reveal the aetiology, and as the liver has a large functional reserve, tests of its function may be normal even when it is diseased. The tests mean little, therefore, unless they are interpreted within the context of the overall clinical picture. No single test provides a precise picture of liver function and it is wasteful and often confusing to request a battery of tests. Simple and inexpensive tests of established value, carefully chosen, are usually adequate.

Table 80.1 shows some basic tests.

Tests of parenchymal cell function

Serum proteins

Liver parenchymal cells are the only synthesizers of albumin, as well as of most alpha- and beta-globulins. Gamma-globulins are produced mainly by reticuloendothelial tissues.

Clinical significance

Serum albumin

Because it is synthesized exclusively by the liver, the serum albumin level falls in chronic liver disease. In acute liver disease such as acute hepatitis serum albumin levels may remain normal or fall only gradually because of the relatively long half-life of albumin. Serum albumin level tends to fall in malnutrition, infection and fever, and prolonged cholestasis, but may be normal or low in compensated cirrhosis. Although in cirrhosis failure of synthesis is partly responsible, plasma dilution due to retention of fluid, and altered distribution between body fluid compartments are more important factors.

Serum globulin and immunoglobulin

These are increased in liver disease. A low albumin and raised total globulin suggest chronic liver disease, particularly chronic active hepatitis and cirrhosis. In Africa, lower levels of serum albumin and higher globulin levels are commonly found due to high rates of parasitic infection and subclinical malnutrition.

Prothrombin time (PT) and partial thromboplastin time (PTT)

Most clotting factors, except factor VIII, are synthesized in the liver. Prothrombin time measures the conversion of prothrombin to thrombin in the presence of thromboplastin, calcium, and other activation factors, followed by conversion of fibrinogen to fibrin. Prothrombin and partial thromboplastin times, although primarily tests of coagulation, are very useful especially in acute liver disease.

Indeed, the prothrombin time is probably the best guide to prognosis in acute hepatitis. It is essential in assessment of a patient to decide whether liver biopsy may or may not be dangerous.

The one-stage prothrombin test and thrombo test are simple tests of coagulation. In obstructive jaundice an abnormal prothrombin time can be corrected by parenteral vitamin K therapy.

Table 80.1. Liver function tests

Test	Normal levels	Result	Disorders
1. Total serum bilirubin	2–17 μm/l	Increased	Excess production, e.g. haemolysis, G-6–PD, sickle cell disease. Impaired uptake (cholestasis) or coagulation
2. Urinary bilirubin	Absent	Absent	Unconjugated hyperbilirubinaemia
3. Serum albumin	30–46 g/l	Reduced	Liver disease Nephrotic syndrome Malnutrition Protein-losing enteropathies
4. Serum aspartate amino transferase (AST)	3–24 i.u./l	Increased	Liver cell damage Myocardial infarction Muscle diseases
5. Serum alanine aminotransferase (ALT)	3–18 i.u./l	Increased	Liver cell damage
6. Serum alkaline phosphatase	20–100 i.u./l	Increased	Cholestasis and some other liver diseases Bone diseases, e.g. osteomalacia Pregnancy
7. 5′-nucleotidase	0.3–2.6 u/dl	Increased	Cholestasis
8. Serum γ-glutamyl transpeptidase (GGT)	7–48 i.u./l	Increased	Liver disease Alcoholism Pancreatitis Myocardial infarction Drugs causing enzyme induction

Serum enzymes

When a cell dies or the membrane is damaged, its enzymes are released into the blood. Amino transferase (transaminases) and dehydrogenases are liver enzymes, which are useful for diagnosis of liver cell damage.

Aminotransferases (transaminases)

Serum alanine aminotransferase (ALT) (formerly glutamic pyruvic transaminase – SGPT) and aspartate aminotransferase (AST) (formerly glutamic oxalo acetic acid – SGOT) are the enzymes most frequently used to assess liver cell injury. Very high levels of aminotransferases are of diagnostic value. Alanine aminotransferase (ALT) is found predominantly in the liver and high levels suggest liver cell damage. Aspartate aminotransferase (AST) is present in liver as well as heart, skeletal muscle, kidney, brain, lungs, pancreas, leukocytes and erythrocytes, and its level rises when these organs are acutely damaged.

The aminotransferases are useful for detecting early liver cell damage. In the pre-icteric and early icteric phase of viral hepatitis very high levels are recorded. The levels do not necessarily correlate with the severity of liver cell necrosis, but in any one patient it is useful to do serial estimations to monitor the progress of the disease. In chronic hepatitis and cirrhosis serum aminotransferases may be raised. In cholestatic obstructive jaundice they are usually normal or slightly increased (up to 100 i.u.). An AST: ALT ratio greater than 2: 1 is highly suggestive of alcoholic liver disease.

Alkaline phosphatase

Alkaline phosphatase is a phosphomonoesterase, which is present in various tissues including bone, liver, kidney, and gut. It is excreted by the liver into the bile. In cholestatic jaundice the serum level rises, partly due to lack of excretion and partly due to increased synthesis. In hepatocellular jaundice it rises slightly to about 225 i.u./l (30 K.A. units per 100 ml) but in obstructive jaundice the level is usually above 225 i.u./l; it also rises in hepatic tumours, whether primary or secondary. During the cholestatic phase of viral hepatitis the serum bilirubin and alkaline phosphatase levels may be very high, but may be low in long-standing extrahepatic biliary obstruction (p. 1015). The level is raised in children and when osteoblastic activity is increased, particularly in boys at puberty.

Lipid metabolism

The liver is important in cholesterol synthesis, esterification, and excretion. In parenchymal disease of the liver, the total serum cholesterol is normal or low and the ester fraction is always reduced. In obstructive jaundice total cholesterol may be raised and the ester fraction increased.

Very low values of cholesterol, around 2.5 mmol/l have been recorded in certain tribal groups in Africa.

Tests based on bile pigment metabolism

Bilirubin metabolism

The pathways of bilirubin metabolism are shown in Fig. 78.3. Haemoglobin released from destroyed, aged, and damaged red cells by the reticuloendothelial system (RES) is converted to unconjugated bilirubin, which is water insoluble. The iron fraction is used again in synthesis of haemoglobin. Unconjugated bilirubin is carried in the blood to the liver bound to serum albumin. A small fraction of unconjugated bilirubin is produced from certain haem precursors in marrow and liver, myoglobin precursors, and non-haemoglobin haem proteins. The liver cells conjugate bilirubin to glucuronic acid by the acid glucuronyl transferase. The resulting bilirubin diglucuronide (conjugated bilirubin) is water soluble and is secreted in bile whence it is excreted into the intestine. Conjugated bilirubin is converted by bacterial action in the gut into urobilinogen, stercobilinogen and stercobilin. The intestinal mucosa is relatively impermeable to conjugated bilirubin but permeable to urobilinogen, some of which is reabsorbed and transported via the portal vein to the liver and re-excreted into the bile. A small portion of the reabsorbed urobilinogen escapes hepatic excretion and reaches the systemic circulation and is excreted in the urine as urinary urobilinogen. Stercobilinogen and stercobilin are excreted in faeces, to which they impart the characteristic brown colour.

Serum bilirubin

Total

An increase may arise from:

- over-production of bilirubin
- decreased uptake of bilirubin by liver cells
- decreased conjugation of bilirubin by liver cells.

These will all lead to unconjugated hyperbilirubinaemia, as in haemolytic jaundice, or when conjugating enzymes are immature, as in neonates.

- Spill-over of conjugated bilirubin from liver or bile into circulation.
- Decreased excretion of conjugated bilirubin.

These two will lead to conjugated bilirubinaemia, as in cholestatic jaundice, or hepatocellular jaundice.

Direct and indirect bilirubin

These are based on methods for approximate measurements of conjugated and unconjugated bilirubin levels, respectively.

Urine tests

The presence of bile in the urine gives it a dark colour. If, in a jaundiced patient, no bile is detected in the urine (acholuric jaundice), unconjugated hyperbilirubinaemia is probable.

Urobilinogen

Normally, a small amount of urobilinogen can be detected in the urine. Urinary urobilinogen increases in haemolytic anaemias. In hepatitis, when jaundice is deepest, urobilinogen disappears because excretion of bile into the gut is greatly reduced. Urobilinogen is diminished or absent in cholestatic jaundice, and, much more rarely, after the bowel has been sterilized by antibiotics, or in severe diarrhoea or renal failure.

Faecal bile pigment

In obstructive jaundice fecal stercobilinogen decreases and the stool becomes pale. It is absolutely essential to inspect the stool colour in any jaundiced patient. In haemolytic jaundice the faeces are always dark because there is normal excretion of an increased load of bilirubin.

Other tests

Serum immunological tests

Hepatitis markers

Hepatitis A virus (HAV)

The presence of the IgM class of hepatitis A antibody (anti-HAV-IgM) confirms the presence of acute HAV infection.

Hepatitis B virus (HBV)

Hepatitis B surface antigen (HBsAg) is present in the sera of 20–60 per cent of adult patients in the early phase of viral hepatitis. Among healthy adults in sub-Saharan Africa, Asia, the Middle East and the Mediterranean regions, 5–20 per cent are asymptomatic carriers. The prevalence varies from region to region (p. 712). The presence of the IgM class of antibody to hepatitis B core antigen (anti-HBc – IgM) will identify the patient with acute HBV infection and the concomitant presence of hepatitis Be antigen (HBeAg) and HBsAg indicates high level of viraemia and hence a high risk of transmission. HBsAg is useful to screen blood donors.

Hepatitis C virus (HCV)

Although the test is not widely available yet, hepatitis C virus antibodies (anti-HCV) should, ideally, be looked for in adult African patients with chronic hepatitis, cirrhosis, hepatocellular carcinoma (HCC) and porphyria cutanea tarda (PCT), and in screening blood for transfusion.

Hepatitis D virus (HDV)

Also known as delta virus, HDV is found only in the presence of HBsAg. The IgM class of HDV antibody confirms active infection.

Hepatitis E virus (HEV)

An IgM class of hepatitis E virus antibody (anti-HEV-IgM) indicates the presence of acute HEV infection. This test should be done in all pregnant women with acute hepatitis, and in endemic and epidemic hepatitis.

Mitochondrial antibody test

This is positive in over 90 percent of primary biliary cirrhosis but is uncommon in other liver disorders.

Antinuclear factor and antismooth muscle antibody

These are commonly seen in autoimmune hepatitis.

Alpha-fetoprotein (AFP)

A normal hepatic fetal protein (alpha 1-globulin) which disappears soon after birth. Detection later in life indicates hepatic dedifferentiation, with levels >250 ng/ml occurring as relatively specific markers in most cases of hepatocellular carcinoma and, occasionally in other tumours. Levels <100 ng/ml are non-specific and occur in hepatic regeneration such as in recovering hepatitis, pregnancy and some upper GI malignancies.

Imaging procedures

Radiology

A plain X-ray of the abdomen may show radio-opaque gallstones (15 per cent are radio-opaque), hepatomegaly, splenomegaly, pancreatic calcification and possible gas in the biliary tree. A chest X-ray may show a raised right diaphragm suggestive of amoebic liver abscess, HCC or other malignancy. A barium swallow may reveal oesophageal and gastric varices.

Ultrasonography (US)

This is now the most widely used imaging procedure and it has replaced oral cholecystography. It is reliable in the diagnosis of gallstones (with sensitivity of greater than 95 per cent) but is less sensitive (about 40 per cent) in detecting common bile duct stones. However, it is quite reliable in detecting a dilated biliary tree, which is evidence of mechanical obstruction, and thus is very useful in distinguishing extrahepatic from intrahepatic cholestasis. Ultrasound can detect focal lesions such as abscesses, tumours and cysts, as well as fatty liver (increased echogenicity).

Other imaging procedures

These expensive, not widely available in the African continent, highly technical methods are used in advanced centres: computerized tomography (CT), nuclear magnetic resonance imaging (NMRI), endoscopic retrograde cholangiopancreatography (ERCP), percutaneous transhepatic cholangiography (PTC) and radionuclide scanning using different isotopes.

Simple tests of liver function

These tests can be performed in health centres or hospitals with simple laboratory facilities. The range of what is available varies greatly, from these simple and older tests to the widely used, but expensive, dipsticks.

Urine

Appearance

Dark reddish or 'coca-cola' urine in a jaundiced patient suggests haemolysis. The urine is dark due to haemoglobinuria secondary to intravascular haemolysis: common causes are *P. falciparum* malaria, typhoid and G6PD deficiency.

Bile

1. Shake the urine to produce froth, which is yellow if bile is present. 2. Fouchet's test or *Ictotest.*

Urobilinogen

Ehrlich's test.

Protein

May be detected by 1. Boiling test. 2. Sulpho-salicylic acid test.

Faeces

Pale or 'clay-coloured' stool in a jaundiced patient indicates cholestasis. If the stool is dark, there must be bile pigment in it so that obstruction to excretion of bile cannot be complete.

Acute hepatic failure

The onset of acute liver failure is heralded by an altered mental state, agitation and confusion proceeding to coma, and signs of coagulopathy. Patients with acute liver failure may be categorized on the basis of the rapidity of onset, from the time of first symptoms or the appearance of jaundice. The prognosis partly depends on the speed of the evolution of the clinical presentation – the slower the evolution, the poorer the prognosis. When liver failure occurs with hepatic encephalopathy within 8 weeks of onset of jaundice or symptoms in a previously healthy subject, the evolution is often very rapid. In such cases, the term fulminant hepatitis is used (Lee, 1993). Such patients have a bad prognosis: their only hope would be the rarely available liver transplant.

Aetiology

Viral infections

The main causes of acute hepatic failure are viral infections and drug toxicity. Hepatitis B virus (HBV) and hepatitis E virus (HEV) (in pregnant women) are probably the commonest causative agents in Africa, while other viruses may be implicated in different parts of the world (Tsega et al., 1992).

Drugs

Among the drugs known to cause acute liver failure, paracetamol is more common in the United Kingdom and the United States of America than in Africa. Traditional remedies must be considered in the African patient (see under Drugs, Toxins and the Liver, p. 1020). Beware of the enhanced hepatotoxicity of isoniazid and rifampicin in patients with HIV/AIDS.

Precipitating factors

Infection, gastrointestinal bleeding, hypoxia, drugs such as tranquilizers, sedatives and analgesics, excess protein load, and fluid and electrolyte changes often induced by diuretic therapy, may all cause acute liver failure in patients with pre-existing acute or compensated chronic liver diseases.

Unknown

The cause of acute hepatic failure is not known in over 15 per cent of cases in spite of thorough investigation.

Clinical features

The main clinical features are changes of personality, behaviour, level of consciousness and neuromuscular function. Hepatic encephalopathy is the most dramatic clinical presentation but there may be many other symptoms and signs before this develops.

Hepatic encephalopathy

This is a complex neuropsychiatric condition resulting from acute or chronic liver disease. Though potentially reversible, clinically it can occur as acute, acute recurrent, chronic recurrent and chronic permanent encephalopa-

Table 80.2. A grading system for hepatic encephalopathy[a]

Grade	Level of consciousness	Personality and intellect	Neurological signs	Electroencephalographic abnormalities
0	Normal	Normal	None	None
Subclinical	Normal	Normal	Abnormalities only on psychometric analysis	None
1	Inverted sleep pattern, restlessness	Forgetfulness, mild confusion, agitation, irritability	Tremor, apraxia, incoordination, impaired handwriting	Triphasic waves (5 cycles/s)
2	Lethargy, slow responses	Disorientation as regards time, amnesia, decreased inhibitions, inappropriate behaviour	Flapping tremor, dysarthria, ataxia, hypo-active reflexes	Triphasic waves (5 cycles/s)
3	Somnolence but rousable, confusion	Disorientation as regards place, aggressive behaviour	Flapping tremor, hyperactive reflexes, Babinski signs, muscle rigidity	Triphasic wave (5 cycles/s)
4	Coma	None	Decerebration	Delta activity

Note:
[a] The system is based on clinical and electroencephalographic features suggested by Gitlin.

thy. Hepatic encephalopathy may arise spontaneously but more commonly occurs as a result of precipitating factors in the presence of acute and chronic hepatitis.

Mechanism

The syndrome results from intoxication of the brain with metabolites such as ammonia produced by the action of bacteria on protein in the bowel. These substances reach the brain either because the acutely diseased liver fails to detoxify them or through portosystemic shunts (Fig. 80.2).

Clinical features

1. Early symptoms include irritability, reversal of sleep pattern, personal neglect, intellectual deterioration or failure to orientate in space, best demonstrated by inability to produce simple designs such as five-pointed stars or blocks (constructional apraxia), illegible writing and slurred speech.
2. Later stages present with delirium, coma, seizures, lateralizing signs, increased muscle tone, hyper-reflexia of deep tendon reflexes and ankle clonus, but with a flexor plantar response), rigidity and myoclonus. The level of consciousness in hepatic encephalopathy is graded as shown in Table 80.2.

Flapping tremor is a non-specific neurological sign of hepatic encephalopathy. It may be present in uraemia, respiratory and cardiac failure. To elicit flapping tremor, the hands are dorsiflexed (or hyperextended) at the wrist and the fingers splayed out. The hands or fingers flap intermittently (Fig. 80 3). Flapping tremor can also be

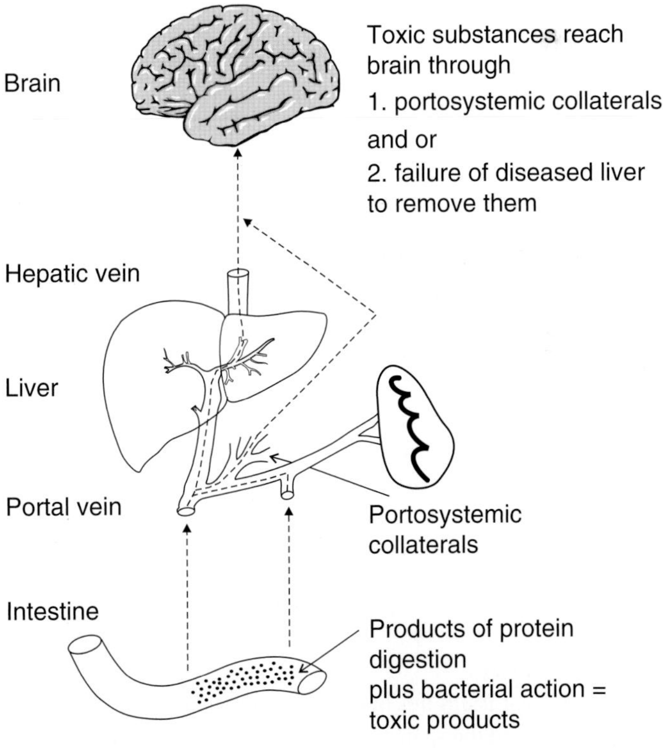

Fig. 80.2. The mechanism of portosystemic encephalopathy.

demonstrated using a dorsiflexed foot. It is frequent in chronic hepatic encephalopathy, but uncommon in acute hepatic failure.

Foetor hepaticus, a sweet and characteristic smell caused by mercaptans excreted in the breath, is easily recognized by the practised observer. Seek it in every patient

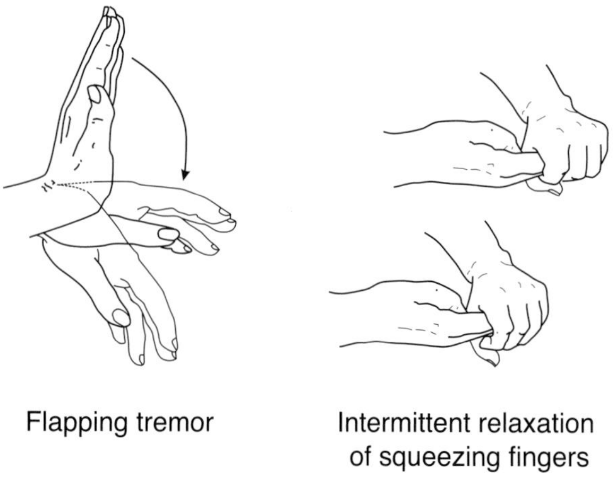

Fig. 80.3. Flapping tremor (also sometimes called asterixis).

with jaundice, a confusional state, or coma. Put your nose very close to the mouth: a distant whiff is valueless.

Jaundice

This is present in most patients. However, the absence of jaundice should not preclude the diagnosis of acute hepatic failure, which should be suspected if a patient becomes aggressive or restless, or if a patient known to have liver disease suddenly develops a change of character.

Gastrointestinal bleeding may occur early in acute hepatic failure and is usually fatal. The liver produces essential coagulation factors II, V, VII, IX, and X; hence a combination of deficiencies, rather than a single deficiency, may be responsible for the bleeding. These include reduced production of coagulation factors, lack of vitamin K, disseminated intravascular coagulation (DIC), and thrombocytopenia due to depressed production of platelets by the marrow or hypersplenism, increased consumption in DIC, and defective platelet function. Sites of bleeding include oesophageal varices, mucosal erosions, and peptic or stress ulceration.

Liver size

Always assess this by palpation and percussion: you will find that the span of the liver has decreased considerably. This is due to the loss of hepatic mass.

Major complications

Renal problems

A syndrome resembling the hepatorenal syndrome and best called hepatic nephropathy is common and causes oliguria and a very low urinary sodium excretion. It may progress to acute tubular necrosis. It is difficult to manage these patients: base their fluid replacement on colloid rather than crystalloid preparations.

Metabolic problems

Hypoglycaemia is common, particularly if the patient has an infection.

Infections

Bacterial infections are very common: take regular blood cultures in anyone with acute hepatic failure. Sample the ascitic fluid for polymorphonuclear count and culture for bacteria.

Cardiovascular changes

Hypotension, tachycardia, high cardiac output, low systemic vascular resistance, with hypoxia leading to lactic acidosis occur in some patients with acute hepatic failure. These changes are associated with poor prognosis. The aetiology is unknown. Cardiac arrhythmias may occur rarely.

Other

Adult respiratory distress syndrome is another rare clinical feature.

Fulminant hepatic failure (FHF)

This is a serious form of acute hepatic failure with a high mortality (up to 90 per cent), especially when there is a deep coma.

Viral causes

The most frequent cause is viral hepatitis: types A, B, B and D, C and E can cause AHF, A and E being the least likely in healthy adults. However, in Africa (and also in South East Asia), hepatitis E virus is a major cause of FHF among pregnant women, often in epidemics and with high fetal and maternal morbidity and mortality (Tsega et al., 1993). Also, FHF is common when hepatitis A virus infection occurs in patients with chronic hepatitis C virus (Vento et al., 1998).

Other causes

1. Traditional remedies and herbs are a recognized cause, but their exact offending chemicals have not been identified.
2. Overdose of paracetamol is not yet common in Africa, but it is a significant problem in Europe.

3. Fatty liver of pregnancy.
4. Surgical shock.

Clinical features

The patient becomes delirious and rapidly comatose. Deep jaundice is invariable but may be preceded by mental disturbances. Flapping tremor may be transient and so it can be overlooked.

Complication

The most serious complication of FHF is cerebral bleeding leading to intracranial hypertension. The pathogenesis is unknown.

Diagnosis

Clinical

As some of the earliest signs of hepatic failure are psychiatric changes and flapping tremor, the diagnosis must be suspected in any person who is jaundiced and who behaves abnormally. A clinical diagnosis is usually reliable although coma in a jaundiced patient must be distinguished from coma due to drugs and renal failure (see the Box).

JAUNDICE with ABNORMAL BEHAVIOUR ?Hepatic encephalopathy

Laboratory

Although tests of liver function are abnormal, they do not necessarily reflect the true extent of hepatic damage and the prognosis. Estimate blood glucose and, when possible, arterial blood gases (pH, pO_2, pCO_2) and paracetamol level.

A liver biopsy in these sick patients with coagulopathy is seldom possible but, where possible, transjugular biopsy will demonstrate massive necrosis with varying degrees of inflammation.

Electroencephalogram (EEG)

This shows characteristic changes (Table 80.2).

Effect of treatment

When investigations are not possible, the effect of treatment for hepatic failure may confirm the diagnosis.

Course and treatment

Although acute hepatic failure has a bad prognosis, the syndrome is reversible if the patient does not have chronic liver disease. The prognosis is poor in patients with advanced coma, renal failure and metabolic acidosis.

Principles and details of treatment

Reducing the production and absorption of ammonia

Food

During acute hepatic failure no protein food should be given.

Purgation

A dose of 30 ml magnesium sulphate and a high enema empty the gut: the enema should be of acid or neutral pH to reduce ammonia and amine absorption.

Reduce bacterial activity

Neomycin 1 g 6-hourly orally (up to 6 g a day for up to 10 days) is effective. Very little neomycin is absorbed from the gut. Use with caution in patients with renal disease to avoid ototoxicity and nephrotoxicity.

Metronidazole in a dose of 200 mg every 6 hours is as effective as neomycin, whether clinical, biochemical (blood ammonia levels) or electro-encephalographic criteria are used, in mild or severe encephalopathy.

Rifaximin, a non-absorbable derivative of rifampicin, is a proven alternative at a dose of 1200 mg per day.

Lactulose

Exogenous protein and endogenous protein (shedding of gut epithelial cells) metabolized by bacteria produce ammoniagenic substances which are removed from the intestinal lumen by osmotic cathartic action of the non-absorbable disaccharide lactulose. It is the mainstay therapy of chronic hepatic encephalopathy, but should also be used in acute hepatic failure. Lactulose also lowers the pH of the colon due to production of organic acids by bacterial fermentation. The low pH creates a hostile environment for the survival of urease-producing intestinal bacteria. In addition, the acidic colonic secretion prevents absorption by anionic diffusion of ammonia as well as it resulting in the net movement of ammonia from the blood into the bowel lumen. Water enema is ineffective, suggesting that acidification is what is working but not bowel cleansing (Uribe et al., 1987). Most patients will require 30–60 g/day to achieve 2–4 loose bowel movements.

Lactitol

Another disaccharide, given in a dose of 30–45 g/day, is as effective as lactulose, produces less flatulence as a side effect and is more palatable (Riordan & Williams, 1997).

Combined antibiotic and lactulose
The combination has an additive effect if one alone fails.

Fluid balance and calories

Nasogastric tube

- Ensure adequate daily fluid together with lactose or dextrose to provide 2000–3000 calories daily.
- Keep an accurate fluid balance because fluid overload is easy.
- Give no protein.

Vitamins

- Give vitamin supplements, including intramuscular vitamin K 10 mg, for 3 days.

Hypokalaemia

Potassium depletion is common:

- Give potassium chloride, either by intravenous infusion in 5 per cent dextrose (at least 80 mmol may be needed), or by mouth in a dose of 1–2 g 6-hourly.
- Stop diuretics.

Infection

- Look often and carefully for any evidence of infection in chest, urine or blood. Blood culture is essential. In the patient with ascites, paracentesis must be done for cell count and culture of the ascitic fluid.

Bleeding

If possible, give 3 units fresh frozen plasma daily. Fresh blood corrects the coagulation defects. Avoid local trauma and arterial punctures. To prevent upper gastrointestinal bleeding, give an intravenous H_2-receptor antagonist, such as ranitidine, 50 mg 8-hourly, or, preferably and if available, an intravenous proton pump inhibitor such as pantoprazole 40 mg daily.

Restlessness

All sedatives are dangerous.

- Do not use opiates of any sort: a small dose of diazepam, 5 mg i.v. or i.m. daily, may be tried and can be repeated if the patient is very restless. Up to 40 per cent of phenobarbitone is directly excreted by the kidney; therefore, phenobarbitone 30–60 mg i.v. 6-hourly can be given.

Comment

Fulminant hepatic failure (FHF) is potentially treatable, despite the very grave prognosis, and normal liver function can be restored, so that the time and toil spent in the care of such patients is thoroughly justified. Be on the alert throughout; watch for hypoxaemia, which may delay recovery of cerebral function, and for a fall in urinary output, which may signal hepatic nephropathy. Death may occur from progressive hepatic failure, cerebral oedema, gastrointestinal bleeding, sepsis and cardiac arrhythmia.

HEPATITIS

Different species of viruses, including cytomegalovirus, Epstein–Barr, herpes simplex, adenovirus, Coxsackie virus, mumps, yellow fever, and others cause parenchymal hepatic inflammation, but the term viral hepatitis generally implies the five hepatotropic viruses: hepatitis A virus (HAV), hepatitis B virus (HBV), hepatitis C virus (HCV), hepatitis D virus (HDV or delta virus) and hepatitis E virus (HEV). These are grouped by their mode of transmission: enteral (HAV and HEV) and parenteral (HBV, HCV, HDV). The former group cause acute viral hepatitis only, while the latter group may cause acute and chronic hepatitis. Hepatitis G virus and TT virus have not been shown to cause hepatitis.

Acute hepatitis is also caused by drugs, toxins, alcohol, ischaemia, and other insults, but the commonest causes of acute and chronic hepatitis in Africa are hepatitis A, B, C, D, and E viruses.

Acute viral hepatitis

The clinical spectrum of acute viral hepatitis ranges from asymptomatic to fulminant infection. The causative virus cannot be distinguished with certainty from the other types of viruses on the basis of clinical presentation. The incubation period varies according to the type of hepatitis virus involved (Chapter 67).

The epidemiological background

This has been fully discussed (p. 709), where the distinctive modes of transmission of each of the hepatitis viruses and their prevalence are considered.

Symptoms

Prodromal – systemic

The prodromal symptoms of acute viral hepatitis are variable and are systemic. Malaise, fatigue, anorexia (with a deep dislike for alcohol and cigarettes), vomiting, headache, photophobia, cough, sore throat, myalgia and arthralgia may precede the onset of jaundice by 5–14 days. Low grade fever is more often present in hepatitis A and E than in hepatitis B or C, and lasts for 2–5 days.

Local – abdominal

The patient may complain of pain over the liver or epigastric region.

Serum sickness-like syndrome

This sometimes occurs during the prodromal phase of icteric or anicteric hepatitis B, but not with hepatitis A or E, and is characterized by fever, urticaria, arthralgia and angioedema

Signs

Mild hepatitis

Asymptomatic and subclinical viral hepatitis is the commonest presentation in Africa. In those patients with mild viral hepatitis, there is no jaundice, they are merely unwell and there may be slight liver tenderness.

Moderate hepatitis

The patient is jaundiced and has an enlarged tender liver and may also rarely have splenomegaly and cervical lymphadenopathy.

Rarely, patients may present with a cholestatic feature, which will clear completely later.

The patient may remain anorexic and may vomit food, resulting in significant weight loss. The stools are pale and the urine dark.

After a week or two, the appetite returns, the stools and urine become normal and jaundice fades.

The posticteric phase is variable in duration (1–4 months), being more prolonged in acute hepatitis B and C. Biochemical recovery may be slow. Simultaneous infection with HBV and HDV may lead to more severe clinical symptoms than with HBV alone, and a superinfection with HDV in the patient who is a chronic carrier of HBV is associated with rapid course and higher morbidity (Craxi et al., 1984). Spontaneous reactivation due to conversion of anti-HBe (non-replicative infection) to HBeAg (replicative infection) in HBV carriers may result in a clinical picture of acute viral hepatitis.

Severe hepatitis

The signs are those of acute hepatic failure, with deep jaundice, foetor hepaticus, flapping tremor, drowsiness, coma, ascites, and signs of coagulapathy.

The liver shrinks: estimate its size daily by percussion.

The patient may die or recover completely, or the illness may progress to a chronic form which may result in cirrhosis and slowly developing hepatocellular failure and/or hepatocellular carcinoma leading to death.

Fulminant viral hepatitis occurs more commonly with HBV infection than with hepatitis C and hepatitis A virus infection. However, fulminant hepatitis is common in pregnant African women infected with HEV during the second and third trimesters (Tsega et al., 1993) and in subjects who are chronic carriers of HCV and develop HAV superinfection (Vento et al., 1998).

Diagnosis

Jaundice is visible when the serum bilirubin level is greater than 2.5 mg/dl (43 μmol/l).

Levels of serum transaminase (which may be significantly raised, often to levels >1,000 i.u./l) do not correlate well with the severity of liver damage.

Haematology

Transient neutropenia and lymphopenia occur. The prothrombin time, which correlates well with the degree of hepatic necrosis, is measured to follow the course of acute viral hepatitis.

Hepatitis markers

The presence of IgM anti-HAV and IgM anti-HEV during the acute illness confirms active HAV and HEV infection, respectively. The clinical interpretation of HBV markers is summarized in Table 80.3. The presence of HBsAg and IgM-anti-HBc in the serum confirms the presence of acute HBV infection. Where facilities permit, determine anti-HCV and anti-HDV for the diagnosis of HCV and HDV infections (p. 712).

Table 80.3. Clinical interpretation of hepatitis B markers

Marker	Interpretation
H BsAg	Active HBV infection: may be acute or chronic
anti-HBs	Immune to HBV; may be natural immunity or following vaccination
anti-HBc-IgM	Acute HBV infection
HBeAg	High infectivity, active viral replication
anti-HBe	Low or no infectivity; need only be measured in chronic HBV
HBV-DNA	Direct measure of infectivity or replicative state

Liver biopsy

This is rarely necessary in acute viral hepatitis except when chronic hepatitis is suspected or the diagnosis is in doubt.

Treatment

Most cases of acute viral hepatitis resolve spontaneously and require no specific treatment. There is no justification for strict bed rest and the patient should be allowed activities which do not cause exacerbation of symptoms. The belief of many African patients that fatty meals aggravate or worsen the illness has no scientific basis although it is true that fatty foods may cause nausea.

Diet

This should be liberal and as high in calorie content as the patient can tolerate.

Alcohol

None, until the patient has complete clinical and biochemical recovery.

Drugs

Avoid drugs, especially sedatives and tranquillizers.

Nausea

An antihistamine, such as promethazine, 25 mg before food, is useful.

Corticosteroids These have no proven benefit in the healing of acute viral hepatitis and may increase the risk of a chronic carrier state.

Health education

Many patients in Africa realize that hospital treatment has little effect on jaundice due to hepatitis and turn to indigenous practitioners for help. Unfortunately, some of their remedies may be hepatotoxic. Thus, there is a need for public education.

Prophylaxis

See pp. 710, 712.

Chronic hepatitis

Definition and classification

Chronic hepatitis is an active, continuing inflammation of the liver persisting for at least six months. The previous classification of chronic persistent hepatitis and chronic lobular hepatitis (mild forms), and chronic active hepatitis (severe form), based on histopathology alone, is no longer accepted. This is now replaced by a classification based on cause, histological activity or grade and degree of progression or stage.

Causes

These include chronic viral hepatitis (B, B plus D, C and possible other unidentified types but A and E never cause chronic hepatitis), autoimmune hepatitis, drug-associated chronic hepatitis, Wilson's disease, alpha 1-antitrypsin deficiency, nonalcoholic steatohepatitis and cryptogenic chronic hepatitis.

Histological activity or grade

This focuses on the following histological features: infiltration of the portal tracts by inflammatory cells, piecemeal necrosis, bridging necrosis, disruption of the limiting plate and fibrosis. These changes are graded as none, mild, moderate and marked, and are scored from 0 to 10 based on the Histological Activity Index proposed by Knodell and Ishak (Ishak et al., 1995). The degree of progression or stage assesses the degree of fibrosis from 0 (no fibrosis) to 4 (cirrhosis).

Aetiology

HBV and HCV are the commonest causes of hepatitis in Africa. There is evidence to suggest that HCV infection is more commonly associated with chronic liver disease than HBV infection (Tsega et al., 1995). It should also be noted that over 90 per cent of acute HCV infections become chronic. Foci of endemic infections with HDV are reported from some parts of Africa and a significant association between this virus and chronic liver disease has been documented (Tsega et al., 1992). Alcohol is not a major cause of chronic hepatitis in most parts of Africa, but a small group of patients presenting with porphyria cutanea tarda consume locally brewed alcoholic beverages resulting in, or associated with, chronic hepatitis and haemosiderosis (Addy, 1974; Tsega et al., 1982). Drugs, especially isoniazid and methyl dopa, known to cause chronic hepatitis, are widely used.

Autoimmune hepatitis such as lupoid hepatitis is uncommon as are most autoimmune conditions in Africa. Wilson's disease (copper deposition in the liver tissue) and alpha 1-antitrypsin deficiency are rare. In many cases, the cause of chronic hepatitis cannot be identified (cryptogenic chronic hepatitis).

Clinical features

Symptoms

Irrespective of the aetiology, patients with chronic hepatitis complain of easy fatigability, post-prandial dyspepsia and poor appetite, though some are asymptomatic until discovered during a routine investigation.

Signs

Patients with chronic viral hepatitis (due to HBV, HBV plus HDV and HCV) are commonly not jaundiced. The liver and spleen may be slightly enlarged but ascites and features of hepatic encephalopathy are uncommon. About 5–20 per cent of people in Africa are healthy carriers (carrier state) of HBV without signs, symptoms or inflammation of the liver (Kiire et al., 1990).

Phases

Chronic hepatitis due to HBV has three phases in its natural course: replicative, inflammatory and inactive.

Replicative

During the replicative phase the AST and ALT are not significantly raised, the HBeAg as well as HBV-DNA are positive, but the liver biopsy is either normal or slightly abnormal.

Inflammatory

The replicative phase, for unexplained reasons, is converted to an inflammatory phase, characterized by the significant rises of AST, ALT and histological changes which worsen severely. By then the HBeAg and HBV-DNA levels are declining.

Inactive

If the immune system successfully clears viral replication, the inflammatory phase enters the inactive phase when the AST and ALT become normal and there is seroconversion of HBeAg to anti-HBe, disappearance of the HBV–DNA and quiescent liver histology. It is the duration and severity of the inflammatory phase that determine progression to cirrhosis (20–30 per cent of all HBV infected patients). It is also the inflammatory phase that responds favourably to therapy.

The course of hepatitis D

Whether HDV infection occurs as co-infection (acute simultaneous HDV and HBV infection) or superinfection (HDV infection of HBV carrier subjects), chronic hepatitis D is often aggressive and severe with rapid progression to cirrhosis.

The course of hepatitis C

Chronic hepatitis C virus infection clinically presents with mild or no symptoms, with normal AST and ALT. Over 90 per cent of acute HCV infections persist to become chronic. A wide range of fluctuation of AST and ALT is more typical of HCV than HBV infection. After several years, about 20 per cent of chronic HCV infection will progress to cirrhosis and a few of these will develop hepatocellular carcinoma.

Porphyria cutanea tarda and the liver

Clinical features

Hyperpigmentation of the face and of the backs of the hands, with or without blisters over the hands and/or hypertrichosis of the face comprises the syndrome of porphyria cutanea tarda or PCT. This is a common feature of chronic liver disease in certain African countries, usually starting with the full picture of PCT at the early stage of chronic hepatitis. This darkening of the face and backs of the hands is so well known to the public in Ethiopia that they often consult physicians on the status of their livers. These patients admit to excessive drinking of locally brewed alcohol (*Tej* in Ethiopia, *Akpeteshie* in Ghana). They have red urine which turns deep red on standing for a few hours in sunlight, markedly elevated levels of AST and ALT, elevated 24-hour urinary uroporphyrin and coproporphyrin and serum iron levels. All these abnormalities are reversed when they stop drinking alcohol and are treated with chloroquine.

Histology of the liver

Percutaneous liver biopsy reveals porphyrin pigments fluorescing under ultra-violet light, hepatic siderosis and variable degrees of inflammation, without steatosis and Mallory bodies, suggestive of mild chronic active hepatitis with or without early cirrhosis. Patients with well advanced cirrhosis with portal hypertension show no more fresh blisters on their hands but only scars and hyperpigmentation of the face and hands (Addy, 1974; Tsega et al., 1982).

What is this syndrome?

Is this common association between overt or latent (without blisters) forms of PCT and chronic hepatitis peculiar to a few African countries or is it a wide-spread problem? Studies are needed from different parts of Africa. During the past 5–10 years, there are increasing numbers of reports from Western Europe and North America indicating that about 70 per cent of sporadic PCT is associated with HCV infection with the rising prevalence of HCV infection (Cribier et al., 1995). Thus, where facilities permit, patients with partial or complete clinical features of PCT should be screened for HCV infection.

Diagnosis

History

A detailed drug history must include questions about the use of drugs such as isoniazid, methyldopa, methotrexate and local herbal remedies.

Hepatitis markers

For hepatitis markers, see p. 1005 and under acute viral hepatitis. Antinuclear, antimitochondrial and antismooth muscle antibodies are uncommon in the African patient with chronic liver disease. Low levels (<100 ng/ml) of alphafetoprotein do occur in chronic hepatitis.

In a referral centre, if Wilson's disease is suspected, determine the serum level of ceruloplasmin: <20 mg/dl is diagnostic especially in the presence of Kayser–Fleischer rings. PCT is confirmed by a significant rise in 24-hour urine uroporphyrin, porphobilinogen and coproporphyrin.

Liver biopsy is essential in all patients suspected to have chronic hepatitis.

Treatment

Most patients with chronic hepatitis are well enough to be investigated and managed without admission to hospital. Alcohol and drugs, including herbal remedies, must be avoided. Specific therapy for chronic hepatitis B, C and D requires expensive drugs (interferon alpha, ribavirin or lamivudine) and advanced laboratory facilities and so treatment can only be offered in very few places in Africa.

Lupoid hepatitis

Systemic corticosteroids with, or without, azathioprine will induce and maintain clinical remission, and improve biochemical and histological abnormalities. A common starting dose of prednisone is 30–40 mg daily by mouth. When azathioprine is indicated, the usual dose is 50–75 mg twice daily by mouth with reduced dose of prednisone.

Porphyria cutanea tarda (PCT)

In the African health care setting, chloroquine 500 mg daily per os for 10 days is more practical than long-term, intermittent phlebotomy. The Jarisch–Herxheimer-like reaction which occurs on the third or fourth day of chloroquine therapy is tolerable but it is vital to warn the patient before the start of treatment (Tsega et al., 1981).

CIRRHOSIS OF THE LIVER

Cirrhosis is a diffuse disease of the liver in which liver cells necrose, the reticulum framework collapses, and fibrous tissue septa form and surround regenerating liver cell nodules. The septa contain anastomoses between branches of the hepatic artery and vein and portal vein. The regenerating nodules compress neighbouring tissues, particularly hepatic vein tributaries, so that intrahepatic circulation is impeded, parenchymal blood flow becomes ineffective, and portal hypertension follows.

The morphology of the liver varies greatly in cirrhosis and can usually be defined accurately from a needle biopsy specimen.

Shunting of blood through sinusoids at the periphery of the nodules leads to impaired perfusion of the nodules. Fibrosis alone does not constitute cirrhosis, neither does nodule formation alone. Therefore, cirrhosis is a chronic diffuse disease characterized by fibrosis and nodule formation, regardless of aetiology.

Pathological types of cirrhosis depend on the size of the regenerating liver cell nodules:

1. Micronodular: typically in alcoholics, but also seen in malnutrition and ischaemia.
2. Macronodular: typically in most viral hepatitis.
3. Mixed: both micronodular and macronodular features exist: this tends to occur in alcoholic cirrhosis when the injury, i.e. alcohol, has stopped.

Diagnosis

A needle biopsy is helpful in the diagnosis of micronodular and macronodular cirrhosis. Laparoscopy may be needed to confirm macronodular and mixed types of cirrhosis.

Clinical features

These features depend on the severity of the disease but not on the aetiology. Fibrosis and distortion of the blood vessels lead to portal hypertension, which will result in gastro-oesophageal varices, splenomegaly, caput medusae and bleeding from inferior haemorrhoidal veins. Destruction and loss of hepatocyte function leads to jaundice, oedema, a bleeding disorder and several metabolic abnormalities. The combination of portal hypertension and hepatocellular insufficiency result in ascites and hepatic encephalopathy.

Causes of cirrhosis

Cirrhosis is the end stage of several disorders affecting the liver. In Africa cirrhosis occurs at a younger age than in Europe and America but is still uncommon under the age of 10. The disease is commoner in males than females, 3:1. Higher rates are found in areas where haemosiderosis and alcoholism are common.

Major causes and some examples of each are:

Infections

Viral hepatitis Hepatitis B, C, or B plus D.

Toxic substances

Alcohol; iron (haemosiderosis); herbs (*Crotolaria* and *Senecio* species); drugs (methotrexate, methyldopa).

Disturbed immunity (autoimmune)

Chronic active hepatitis; primary biliary cirrhosis.

Cardiac

Chronic congestive heart failure, particularly when the right atrial pressure, and thus the hepatic venous pressure, is sustainedly high, as in endomyocardial fibrosis and unrelieved constrictive pericarditis.

Cholestatic

Sclerosing cholangitis.

Cryptogenic

No identifiable cause.

Schistosomiasis

S. mansoni granulomas (*Schistosoma* pseudotubercles) develop as a result of an immune reaction to the eggs; fibrous tissue forms around portal veins (pipe-stem fibrosis), see p. 422 and Fig. 80.4 but this is not a true cirrhosis. Hepatomegaly with portal hypertension, splenomegaly, and oesophageal varices follow. Usually, the liver function tests are normal and hepatic encephalopathy is unusual, but repeated haematemeses may occur.

Metabolic and inherited

Haemochromatosis, Wilson's disease, alpha 1-antitrypsin deficiency, Type IV glycogenosis, galactosaemia, cystic fibrosis.

Other causes

Non-cirrhotic fibrosis is also found in idiopathic portal hypertension (Banti's syndrome) and congenital hepatic fibrosis, which may be associated with hepatic and renal polycystic disease.

Nutrition and herbs

In the past it was thought that cirrhosis was a sequel to infantile malnutrition, but this has not been confirmed. It is not yet known whether hepatotoxins derived from traditional medicines or mycotoxins contaminating badly stored grains and nuts are important in cirrhosis in Africa. Veno-occlusive disease (VOD), usually associated with herbs such as *Crotalaria* and *Senecio* species, may also occur with other herbal medicines.

Clinical presentation

Cirrhosis may cause no symptoms and may only be suspected when an enlarged firm liver or spleen, or a little ascites, is found. This is latent or compensated cirrhosis. More commonly, however, it becomes evident as chronic

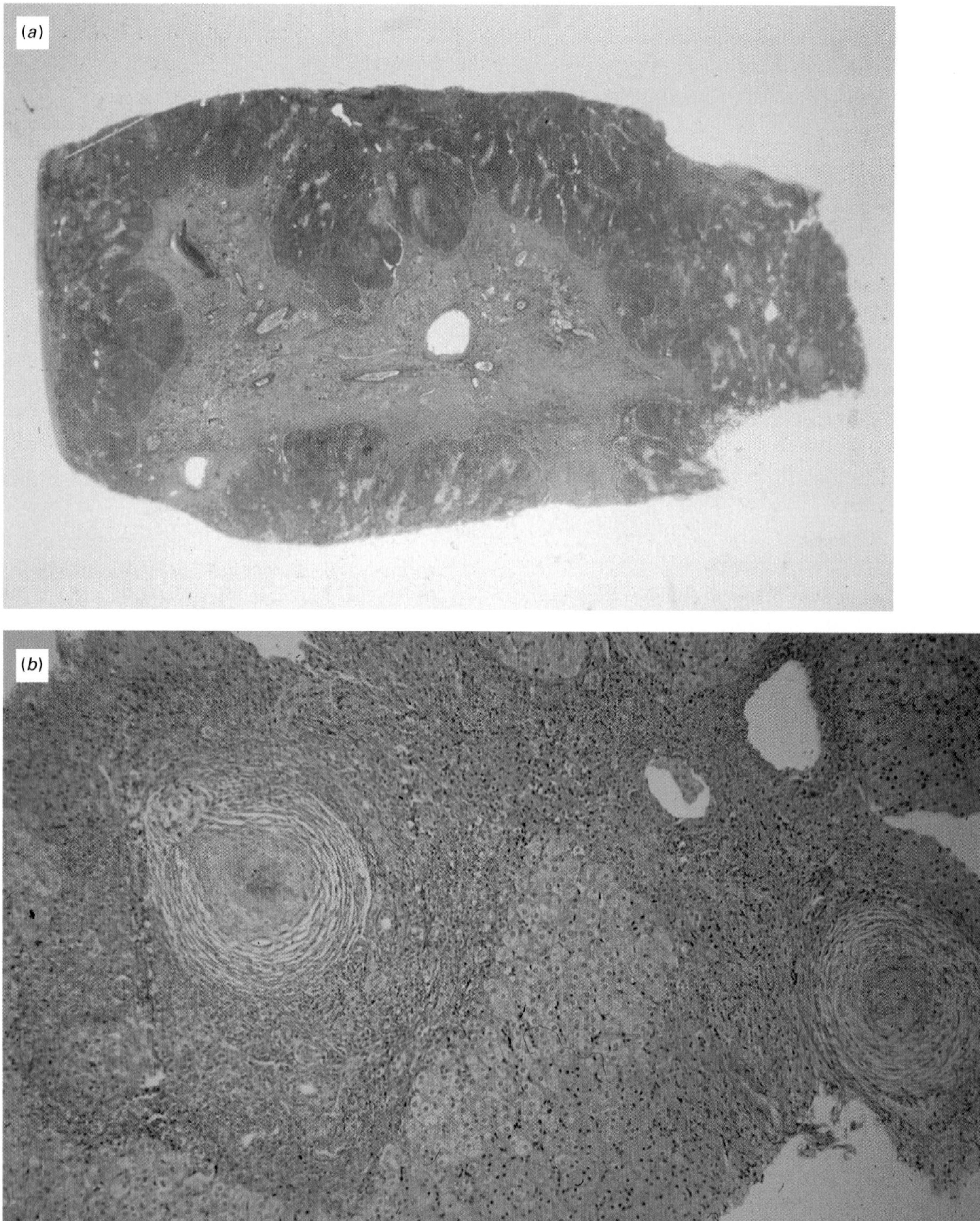

Fig. 80.4. Schistosomal hepatic fibrosis: (*a*) Low power of section of liver with severe periportal fibrosis due to chronic *S.mansoni* infection (MSB stain: fibrous tissue stained blue and liver parenchyma purple). (*b*) Medium power view of active schistosome infection of liver. Two granulomata with concentric rings of fibrosis: portal tracts increased in size (van Gieson stain, fibrous tissue red). (By courtesy of the Wellcome Trust and Professor S.B. Lucas.)

hepatic failure with portal hypertension. This is active, decompensated, and the liver is no longer palpable due to advanced cirrhosis.

Chronic hepatic failure

Symptoms

Patients with hepatocellular failure may complain of weakness, fatigue, poor appetite, dyspepsia often experienced as vague right upper quadrant discomfort, postprandial distension and weight loss.

Signs

Associated with hypoproteinaemia

Water retention with dilution of plasma proteins, leading to an expanded plasma volume and maldistribution of fluid between body fluid compartments, is responsible. Muscle wasting, particularly of the proximal muscles of the arms, is another important sign, and the familiar signs associated with hypoproteinaemia – silken brown hair, and patchily depigmented, hyperpigmented, fissured skin – are also seen in patients with cirrhosis of the liver.

Ascites

This results from both portal hypertension and hepatocellular insufficiency. Ascites rarely occurs from portal hypertension alone. See the pathogenesis of ascites (pp. 1010).

The volume of ascitic fluid varies from very little to many litres. It is a most important sign of cirrhosis. Umbilical hernia, sometimes infected or ruptured, may become a problem in massive ascites. As fluid continuously circulates, any that is removed by tapping re-accumulates, and protein and electrolytes are lost. However, this is no longer a contraindication to repeated therapeutic paracenteses in refractory ascites, which causes severe discomfort. Up to 5 litres of ascitic fluid can safely be removed in patients with peripheral oedema.

Other signs

Neuropsychiatric

Any patient with chronic liver failure due to cirrhosis may have signs of acute liver failure (decompensation) provoked by infection, haemorrhage, excessive protein in food, drugs, or hypokalaemia. Confused or comatose patients may have no signs of liver disease except muscle wasting and possibly a palpable spleen. Foetor hepaticus and flapping tremor are valuable signs.

Skin and nail changes

Look for stigmata such as hyperpigmented skin, with or without blisters, in exposed parts, hypertrichosis, white or clubbed nails, and breast atrophy in women. Dupuytren's contracture, a thickening of the palmar fascia, which is rare in Africa, is a feature of alcoholic cirrhosis, but not of other types.

Infections

Tuberculosis is a common problem in Africa, but abdominal tuberculosis, especially peritonitis, appears to be commoner in cirrhosis. Always remember that any patient who develops pyrexia or deteriorates without obvious cause may have septicaemia. In the patient with ascites, always consider spontaneous bacterial peritonitis and/or tuberculous peritonitis.

Endocrine

In men gynaecomastia, testicular atrophy, and loss of pubic and axillary hair are common. These are also features of alcoholic cirrhosis.

Circulatory

A hyperkinetic circulation, palmar erythema (liver palms) and spider angiomas are seen sometimes – either alone or together.

Bleeding

Defective synthesis of prothrombin, fibrinogen, and factors V, VII, IX, and X may lead to coagulation defects and bleeding.

Pallor and anaemia

Both iron and folate deficiency contribute to the anaemia, which is very common. Anaemia is usually normochronic, normocytic with target cells but occasionally macrocytic. If peripheral morphology shows a microcytic picture, this is almost certainly due to blood loss from gastrointestinal varices or other sites resulting in iron deficiency.

Portal hypertension

The portal venous pressure rises when there is obstruction to the flow of blood along the course of the portal venous system – either in the liver, as in cirrhosis

Table 80.4. Common sites of portal-systemic collateral formation

Location	Portal circulation	Systemic circulation	Clinical consequence
Proximal stomach and distal ooesophagus	Coronary vein of stomach	Azygos vein	Submucosal gastro-oesophageal varices
Anterior abdominal wall	Umbilical vein in falciform ligament	Epigastric abdominal wall veins	Caput medusae
Retroperitoneal	Splenic vein branch Sappey's veins (around liver and diaphragm)	Left renal vein Retzius's vein	Usually none Usually none
Anorectal	Middle and superior haemorrhoidal veins	Inferior haemorrhoidal vein	May be mistaken for haemorrhoids

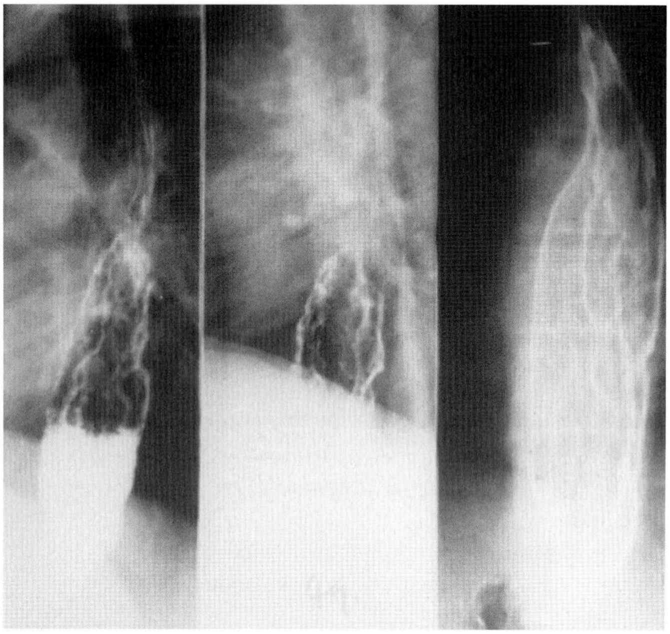

Fig. 80.5. Oesophageal varices, demonstrated as filling defects in a barium swallow in a patient with schistosomal portal hypertension. (By courtesy of the Wellcome Trust and Professor S.B. Lucas.)

(intra-hepatic or sinusoidal), or outside the liver (pre-hepatic or pre-sinusoidal, or post-hepatic or post-sinusoidal).

Portal hypertension leads to the formation of:

Portosystemic anastomotic collaterals (Table 80.4)
These are important for the following reasons.

Bleeding

Gastro-oesophageal varices (Fig. 80.5) may bleed profusely so that the patient presents with haematemesis and melaena. Depending on the degree of hepatic function loss, mortality from such bleeding is high (p. 985) but data are scarce in Africa.

Many cirrhotic patients with portal hypertension also bleed from nonvariceal upper gastrointestinal sources. Cirrhosis of the liver is associated with increased incidence of peptic ulcer disease. A peculiar form of gastropathy causing painless bleeding has also been described in cirrhosis with portal hypertension (Triger & Hosking, 1989).

Shunts

The collaterals act as a shunt to bypass the liver so that the products of protein digestion in the gut reach the brain and cause portosystemic hepatic encephalopathy.

Splenomegaly

This sign is of limited value in Africa, but in portal hypertension the spleen is firm on palpation and quite unlike the soft spleen of acute infection.

Course and treatment

Acute hepatic failure can be precipitated by infections, bleeding from gastro-oesophageal varices and peptic ulcers, and overdose of certain drugs. Ascites and oedema, although uncomfortable and unpleasant, do not threaten life, but if the patient has jaundice, easy bruising, and ascites resistant to treatment, the prognosis is poor.

Assessment of risk

The Child–Pugh classification is commonly used to identify severity or to evaluate the safety of invasive procedures in cirrhotic patients (Table 80.5).

Principles of treatment

1. Manage complications, for example bleeding varices (p. 986).
2. Reverse portosystemic encephalopathy. It is sufficient in most patients to reduce protein in food and to ensure daily bowel movement. Most patients in rural Africa take a low-protein diet, little different from their normal.
3. Control ascites and oedema. This depends on drastic salt restriction (2 g or 100 mmol sodium/day) which is exceedingly difficult to enforce, and often requires continuous and expensive treatment with spironolactone starting with 100 mg per day in a single dose and gradually increased to 400 mg/day. If there is no response, add a loop diuretic such as frusemide, 40 mg daily.
4. Restrict use of drugs to a minimum: if narcotics, hypnotics or tranquillizers have to be used, give a low dose.
5. Avoid alcohol altogether and eat a healthy and adequate diet.

Alcoholic liver disease

Alcoholism is a world-wide problem and alcoholic liver disease has long been recognized. Alcohol is largely (90 per cent) metabolized by the liver, which is therefore the target organ. There is evidence that alcohol has a direct toxic effect on the liver and that the frequency of alcoholic liver cirrhosis is related to the quantity and duration of alcohol consumed, which is itself closely related to available spare cash. The steady daily drinker is more at risk than the occasional heavy drinker, whose liver can probably recover from any acute harmful effect. However, not all alcoholics develop cirrhosis so other factors must be responsible, perhaps inherent susceptibility, or nutrition.

The liver becomes enlarged and fatty: later, alcoholic hepatitis, alcoholic sclerosing hyaline necrosis, and micronodular cirrhosis can develop.

Clinical features

1. The patient with a fatty liver may present with obesity and general ill-health. The liver, mainly the left lobe, is enlarged.
2. Acute alcoholic hepatitis usually follows a bout of heavy drinking and may be precipitated by vomiting, diarrhoea, or infection. Pyrexia and jaundice, sometimes with ascites and polymorphonuclear leukocytosis, are present. The patient looks ill and has a tender palpable liver. Liver function tests reveal both hepatocellular damage and cholestasis. Death may occur from shock or hypoglycaemia.
3. Sclerosing hyaline necrosis presents in a similar fashion to alcoholic hepatitis but the mortality may be higher.
4. Established liver disease. These patients present with portal hypertension, splenomegaly and ascites. In almost all textbooks written in western Europe and North America, however, where liver cirrhosis is most commonly due to alcohol, enlarged parotid glands, Dupuytren's contracture, clubbing of the fingers, gynaecomastia, testicular atrophy, palmar erythema and multiple spider naevi are described as common clinical features of cirrhosis of the liver. These signs are relatively uncommon in the African cirrhotics, except in those with established alcoholic cirrhosis. Hyperpigmentation of the face and hands, with or without blisters and hypertrichosis, are more common in the African patients with cirrhosis. These differences in clinical signs are likely due to the different causes of cirrhosis, alcohol in the western world and viral hepatitis in Africa.

Acute episodes of chronic relapsing pancreatitis, delirium tremens and Wernicke's encephalopathy, and nutritional deficiencies (p. 70) are also seen.

Table 80.5. Criteria for Child – Pugh classification of cirrhosis

Group designation	A	B	C
Serum bilirubin (μmol/l)	Below 34.2	34.2–51.3	Over 51.3
Serum albumin (g/l)	Over 35	30–35	Under 30
Ascites	None	Easily controlled	Poorly controlled
Neurological disorder	None	Minimal	Advanced 'coma'
Nutrition	Excellent	Good	Poor, 'wasting'

Prognosis

The prognosis of alcoholic cirrhosis appears to be better than that of non-alcoholic cirrhosis. It depends on whether the patient stops drinking alcohol completely or not; if he (in Africa this is overwhelmingly a problem in men) stops completely, he can survive for years. Hepatocellular carcinoma may develop in about 15 per cent of patients with alcoholic cirrhosis after the patient gives up drinking, because micronodular cirrhosis is transformed into the macronodular variety.

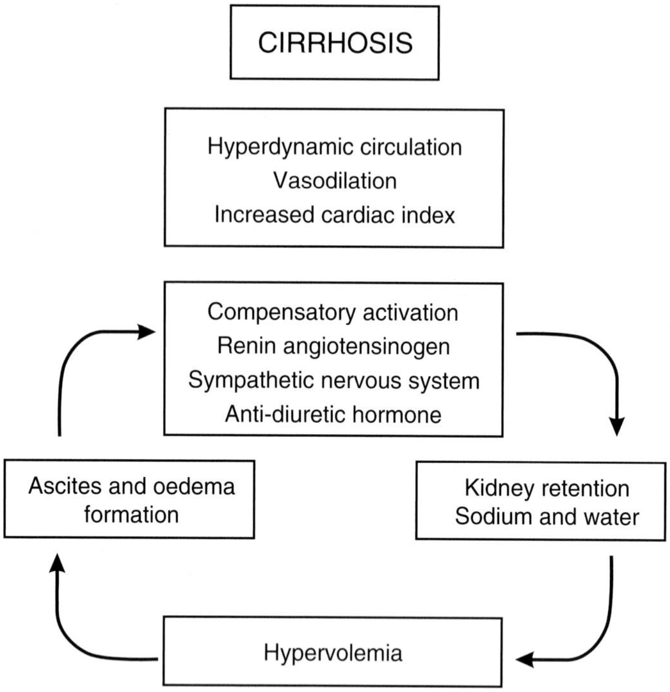

Fig. 80.6. Pathophysiology of ascites formation.

Poor prognostic indicators include encephalopathy, persistent jaundice, a low haemoglobin, low serum albumin, increased INR/PT and azotaemia.

Treatment

Total abstinence from alcohol, vitamin B1, a high-protein diet (except in hepatic failure), and treatment of any intercurrent infection are needed, with the management of complications of cirrhosis. Treat withdrawal symptoms with thiamine and chlordiazepoxide or diazepam. Treat severe alcoholic hepatitis with hepatic encephalopathy with steroids. Hypomagnesaemia, hypokalaemia and metabolic acidosis are common and must be corrected promptly.

Ascites and spontaneous bacterial peritonitis

Ascites is a collection of detectable fluid in the peritoneal cavity. It is the most frequent complication of end-stage cirrhosis, other liver diseases and portal hypertension. Significant ascites causes abdominal discomfort, impairs respiratory function and limits physical activity. Patients with ascites are prone to spontaneous bacterial peritonitis and the hepatorenal syndrome.

Pathophysiology of ascites formation

In the past, reduction of plasma oncotic pressure due to reduced hepatic synthesis of albumin, plasma volume expansion and altered distribution of albumin, as well as intrahepatic vascular obstruction, were widely accepted as factors in the formation of ascites. Other theories included the 'underfilling' and 'overflow' concepts. However, the most current theory, 'the peripheral arterial vasodilation hypothesis', is the most widely accepted since it also unifies the earlier theories.

Typically, patients with cirrhosis have vasodilation with decreased vascular resistance and mean arterial pressure. The cardiac index, plasma volume and splanchnic blood flow are increased resulting in a hyperdynamic circulation. The vasodilation activates the sympathetic nervous system, renin–angiotensin pathway and antidiuretic hormone excretion. These responses lead to secondary vasoconstriction of the renal circulation, with increased renal sodium reabsorption and impaired water excretion: ultimately this results in the formation of ascites (Fig. 80.6).

Evaluation of ascites

Ascites greater than 500 ml can be elicited by shifting dullness, fluid thrill and fullness in the flank with dullness to percussion. Ultrasound can detect ascites as little as 100 ml. Except in the patient with coagulopathy, complications due to paracentesis are uncommon. All patients with ascites of recent onset, who deteriorate while in hospital and develop fever with abdominal tenderness, must have paracentesis.

The serum ascites albumin gradient (SAAG)

This is measured by subtracting the ascitic fluid albumin from the serum albumin, both taken on the same day. It correlates well with causes of ascites. Patients with SAAG >11 g/l have ascites due to cirrhosis and portal hypertension, while those with SAAG <11 g/l have inflammatory, infectious or neoplastic causes (Table 80.6).

The ascitic fluid cell count

This count and its differential is important: an absolute polymorphonuclear (PMN) count greater than 250×10^9/l is diagnostic of spontaneous bacterial peritonitis, or of peritonitis due to a local pyogenic focus, for example a ruptured abscess, and the patient must

Table 80.6. Classification of ascites by serum-ascites albumin gradient

High gradient (>11 g/L) portal hypertension	Low gradient (<11 g/L) non-portal hypertension
Chronic liver disease	**Inflammation**
Cirrhosis	Pancreatitis
Viral hepatitis	Serositis from collagen disease
Autoimmune hepatitis	Bowel obstruction/infarction
Primary biliary cirrhosis	
Primary sclerosing cholangitis	**Infection**
Haemochromatosis	Bacterial peritonitis
Wilson's disease	Tuberculosis
Antitrypsin deficiency	
Alcohol liver disease	**Malignancy**
Massive liver metastases	Ovarian
Fatty liver of pregnancy	Colon
	Gastric
Venous obstruction	Peritoneal carcinomatosis
Budd–Chiari syndrome	
Veno-occlusive disease	**Other**
Portal vein thrombosis	Nephrotic syndrome
Cardiac disease	
Congestive heart failure	
Constrictive pericarditis	
Others	
Myxoedema	

receive empirical antibiotic therapy. If the ascites is haemorrhagic, use the correction factor of 1 PMN for 250 red blood cells.

Culture of ascitic fluid

If infection is suspected, inoculate 10 ml of the ascitic fluid into a blood culture bottle by the bedside (85 per cent positive yield: old methods had 50 per cent yield). If the lymphocyte count is significantly raised, make a smear of the ascitic fluid and culture for acid-fast bacilli. Secondary deposits of cancer on the peritoneum may also cause this cell pattern. An increase in adenosine deaminase activity (ADA) in ascites is diagnostic of tuberculous peritonitis (Voigt et al., 1989; Bhargava et al., 1990).

Management of ascites

Bed rest

There is no proof that bed rest promotes more rapid natriuresis.

Salt restriction

A practical and feasible approach is 'no-added-salt diet' which contains 2 grams (100 mmol) sodium/day.

Fluid restriction

Do not restrict fluid unless the serum sodium concentration drops below 120 mmol/l.

Paracentesis

Tense ascites can be treated by the removal of 5 litres of ascites safely (Kao et al., 1985; Pinto et al., 1988). This will relieve shortness of breath and decrease the feeling of fullness soon after food is eaten, To prevent leakage from the paracentesis site, use simple size16–18 needles and avoid the use of a trocar. Suction may be used. This is now done to relieve symptoms only and is contrary to previous recommendations that paracentesis should be avoided.

Hospital care

If possible, admit the patient and give intensive dietary instructions and counselling against alcohol, and full investigations including monitoring of electrolytes, urea, creatinine, and investigation of the cause(s) of the liver disease.

Diuretics

The current recommendation is a combination of spironolactone and frusemide. Start with spironolactone 100 mg and frusemide 40 mg both together in the morning. Divided doses are not recommended. Keep doubling the dose of each up to 400 mg and 160 mg, respectively, but monitor the response and adjust the doses accordingly. Nearly all (90 per cent) of patients respond and most continue to take this regimen. If painful gynaecomastia develops, replace spironolactone by amiloride or triamterene. Patients with peripheral oedema tolerate aggressive diuresis. Muscle cramps may respond to quinine sulphate 200 mg once or twice daily by mouth.

Refractory ascites

This is ascites which is unresponsive to 400 mg of spironolactone and 160 mg of frusemide daily for 2 weeks. It can be treated with repeated paracentesis, if ascites is intense.

Spontaneous bacterial peritonitis (SBP)

This is a common (up to 25 per cent) complication of cirrhotic ascites, and it is often fatal (30–50 per cent

Table 80.7. Commonly isolated organisms in spontaneous bacterial peritonitis

Gram-negative bacilli (70%)	Anaerobes (5%)	Gram-positive organisms (25%)
Escherichia coli	Bacteroides	*Streptococcus viridans*
Klebsiella	Clostridia	*Group* D *streptococcus*
Citrobacter freundi	Lactobacillus	*Streptococcus pneumoniae*
Proteus enterobacter		*Staphylococcus aureus*

mortality). An apparent rising incidence over the past decade is due to greater awareness. Most cases of SBP occur when patients are in hospital, especially in those who have advanced cirrhosis with jaundice.

Clinical picture

About one-third of patients with SBP have no symptoms; therefore be alert and ready to do an early paracentesis without any hesitation, especially in patients with:

- worsening liver function
- previous episode of SBP
- clinical deterioration or
- early signs of hepatic encephalopathy.

Pathogenesis

Bacteria from the intestinal lumen migrate across the gastrointestinal wall into the lymphatics and then into the peritoneal cavity where they infect susceptible ascitic fluid. Infection is usually due to a single species of microorganism. About 70 per cent of infection is due to gram-negative bacilli, of which *Escherichia coli* (*E. coli*) accounts for 40 per cent: while 25 per cent of infections are due to gram-positive organisms (Table 80.7). Whether there is any geographical variation in the types of organisms involved is not known.

Treatment

1. Treat all patients who have an ascitic fluid polymorphonuclear cell count of more than 2.5×10^9/l or an absolute WBC count of more than 5×10^9/l.
2. The combination of ampicillin and an aminoglycoside, for example gentamicin, were used to good effect in the past. These are effective antibiotics and may well be the only possible combination in many district hospitals, but gentamicin is an aminoglycoside so there is a risk of nephrotoxicity.
3. In advanced centres:
   - the current ideal preferred regimen is a third-generation cephalosporin, cefotaxime 2g, 8-hourly intravenously for 5 days (Runyon et al. 1991). Besides being a broad spectrum antibiotic, it is safe in cirrhosis.
   - In early and less severe SBP, oral floxacin or ofloxacin is as effective as cefotaxime. Avoid aminoglycosides because of risk of nephrotoxicity.

Recurrence

This is common, especially in:

- cirrhotics with serum bilirubin levels greater than 4 mg/dl,
- prothrombin time less than or equal to 45 per cent of control,
- ascitic fluid protein concentration less than or equal to 1g/dl.

Give these patients secondary prophylaxis for SBP: either trimethoprim/sulfamethoxazole 160/800 mg daily, or ciprofloxacin, single weekly dose of 750 mg (Singh et al., 1995; Rolachon et al., 1995). The prognosis of these patients remains poor despite successful treatment of SBP.

INFECTIONS AND THE LIVER

Liver response to infection

The liver is involved in almost all systemic infections. The effects depend on the type and severity of infections and the immune system of the host, and range from elevated serum transaminases and alkaline phosphatase, the formation of granulomas, or of single or multiple abscesses to mild to severe hepatic necrosis, which can lead to hepatic decompensation.

Liver and septicaemia

Role of the liver

In early sepsis, the liver plays a major role in host defence mechanisms: Kupffer cells are responsible for scavenging of bacteria, inactivation of bacterial products, and clearance and production of inflammatory mediators. When this control is not adequate, Kupffer cell-derived proinflammatory cytokines produce hepatocellular dysfunction during early sepsis. However, the exact mechanism for the extensive liver damage, which may result in decompensation and liver failure, remains unknown (Dhainaut et al., 2001; Koo et al., 1999).

Clinical and hepatic changes

Hepatocellular dysfunction occurs early after the onset of sepsis. Liver failure is frequent in seriously ill patients in hospital. Moderate to marked midzonal and peripheral necrosis with acute inflammation and cholestasis are found in the liver histology.

Pneumococcal pneumonia

Patients with early lobar pneumonia in Africa often have a rise in the level of serum aminotransferases, and are sometimes clinically jaundiced with a raised bilirubin.The degree of abnormality depends on the virulence of the *Streptococcus pneumoniae* and the immunity of the host, being worse in patients with HIV/AIDS. The mechanism may be similar to that of early sepsis (Tugwell & Williams, 1977).

Hepatic granulomas

Causes

About 75 per cent of hepatic granulomas occur in relation to systemic processes while the rest have no known cause (Sartin & Walker, 1991).

(i) Major infectious causes of hepatic granulomas include bacteria (tuberculosis, *Mycobacterium avium intracellulare*, brucellosis, listeriosis, tularemia, leprosy, rickettsiae (*Coxiella burnetti* or Q-fever), secondary syphilis, fungi (histoplasmosis, cryptococcosis) and parasites (schistosomiasis, toxocariasis).
(ii) Drugs, including sulphonamides, methyldopa, phenytoin, nitrofurantoin, hydralazine and others.
(iii) Cancer does not lead to granuloma, but Hodgkin's and non-Hodgkin's lymphoma and renal cell carcinoma have histological changes defined by biopsy which may be mistaken for granulomata.
(iv) Miscellaneous conditions: sarcoidosis and inflammatory bowel disease.
(v) Non-microbial causes, not dependent on immunological mechanisms, for example metal salts, and silica.

Formation of a granuloma

Macrophages recruited to the site of inflammation try to get rid of the unwanted antigens. In tuberculosis the antigens are mycobacterial lipids. Schistosomal ova also have similar antigens. If macrophages fail to clear the antigens, monocytes, from the blood stream and bone marrow, aggregate to form tissue epithelioid histiocytes, which then fuse to become multinucleated giant cells. They lose their phagocytic function and become secretory cells. Further activation of the immune system results in necrosis or caseation. In contrast, non-microbial components (such as silica or metal salts) act through non-immunological mechanisms (Williams & Williams, 1983).

Tuberculosis and PUO

The commonest cause of hepatic granulomata worldwide is tuberculosis. As a result of the HIV/AIDS epidemic, atypical mycobacteria are becoming more and more common. Hepatic granulomata occur in almost all cases of miliary tuberculosis, but they do not lead to any sign or symptom, except for fever. Therefore, liver biopsy is a valuable method and is indicated in fever of unknown origin (PUO). The serum alkaline phosphatase is usually elevated. Corticosteroids readily resolve granulomata of non-infectious origin but are contraindicated in granulomata of infectious origin. Therefore, a careful search for the right cause is essential.

Hepatic abscess

Amoebic abscess (p. 492)

These are always preceded by intestinal colonization which is often asymptomatic. Trophozoites invade veins by lysis to reach the liver parenchyma via the portal veins, but without being affected by complement-mediated lysis (non-pathogenic amoebae are lysed and therefore confined to the bowel). Proteinases of amoebae degrade collagen, elastin and parts of extracellular matrix. Other enzymes of the parasite disrupt glycoprotein bonds between cells and lyse neutrophils, neutrophil toxins, monocytes, lymphocytes, colonic and hepatic cell lines. Such cytolytic effects require direct contact between the parasite and target cells. The result is necrosis of hepatocytes and replacement of liver parenchyma by dark brown necrotic material ('anchovy paste') with few or no cells in it. Usually, a single abscess is formed near the dome of the right lobe of the liver. It is not known why amoebic abscess affects mainly males, and, unlike bacterial abscesses, it tends to form solitary lesions. There is no immunity against subsequent infection and antibodies are not protective.

Bacterial abscesses

These are either single or multiple. The sources of infection include an infected umbilical stump in infants, appendicitis, ascending cholangitis due to extrahepatic biliary duct obstruction, inflammatory bowel disease via portal veins, diverticulitis, infections in contiguous structures such as cholecystitis, any distant infection via the arterial route, direct penetrating wounds and cryptogenic (no known cause). *Escherichia coli* and anaerobic bacteria (*Strep milleri*, Bacteroides spp. and Actinomyces spp.) account for the majority of causative agents. *Staphylococcus aureus* and Group A streptococcus cause 20 per cent of all hepatic abscesses. Staphylococcus is more frequent in children and microabscesses are a feature of the systemic effects of a septicaemia due to *Staphylococcus aureus*, in those with an impaired host defence, as in acute leukaemia, or the rare chronic granulomatous disease (Larzarchick et al., 1973).

Rarely *Candida* may cause hepatic abscess as part of systemic infection.

Liver and HIV/AIDS

Abnormal liver function, with raised aminotransferases and alkaline phosphatase, is common in patients with HIV/AIDS. The liver can be affected as:

- hepatocellular necrosis as in viral hepatitis
- granulomatous hepatitis due to mycobacterial or fungal infection
- hepatic masses secondary to tuberculous abscess or AIDS-related Kaposi's sarcoma.

Fatty infiltration has been described in association with nucleoside therapy.

The biliary tree

Papillary stenosis is commonly found, and AIDS cholangiopathy, with features similar to sclerosing cholangitis and with cryptosporidia, microsporidia, and sometimes cytomegalovirus in the biliary tract, is now a recognized entity. The cholangiopathy occurs in the advanced stage of AIDS with markedly reduced CD4 count. The cholestasis associated with this condition is often non-icteric. The prognosis depends on the stage of AIDS (Mahajani & Uzer, 1999).

Microbes and the liver

Patients with HIV/AIDS may have acute or chronic hepatitis and so can be infected with hepatitis A, B, C and D (with B), Epstein–Barr virus, cytomegalovirus, herpes simplex virus, adenovirus, varicella-zoster virus. Mycobacterium (*M. avium* complex, *M. tuberculosis*), fungi (*Histoplasma capsulatum, C. neoformans, Coccidioides immitis, Candida albicans, Pneumocystis carini, Penicillium marneffei*), protozoa (*Toxoplasma gondii, Cryptosporidium parvum, Microsporidia* spp., *Schistosoma* spp.) and bacteria (*Bartonella henselae* – Peliosis hepatitis).

Cancer and the liver

HIV/AIDS-associated malignancies include Kaposi's sarcoma and non-Hodgkin's lymphoma.

Drugs and the liver

The liver is vulnerable in HIV /AIDS patients, so that hepatotoxicity due to isoniazid, rifampicin, trimethoprim-sulfamethoxazole, fluconazole, zidovudine, didanosine and other HIV-1 protease inhibitors is very common in African and other patients with HIV/AIDS (Ungo et al., 1998).

Effects of immunosuppression

1. *Chronic viral carriage* About 20 per cent of HIV-infected patients who acquire acute HBV infection become chronic carriers of HBsAg as compared to only 5 per cent in non-HIV-infected subjects. Also, spontaneous reactivation of HBV replication occurs in patients with anti-HBs due to severe immunosuppression (Hadder et al.,1991; Vento et al., 1989).
2. *Immune-related liver injury* Gilson and associates (1997) have reported that HBV infection is less severe in immunosuppressed subjects with HIV/AIDS due to attenuated immune-mediated liver injury and that HBV does not influence HIV disease progression.
3. *Coinfection* The majority of patients co-infected with HCV and HIV have raised levels of enzymes but are without symptoms. In many of these patients HCV infection leads to fibrosis, cirrhosis and hepatic decompensation. This enhanced HCV replication and accelerated progression of liver disease is due to HIV-related immunosuppression (Thomas et al., 1996). By contrast, chronic HCV infection does not accelerate the clinical or immunological progression of HIV disease (Dorrucci et al., 1995). In general, the morbidity and mortality related to HCV infection in patients with HIV/AIDS are high.

CHOLESTASIS

Definition

A condition which results from impaired or absent flow of bile from the liver to the duodenum. It may be extrahepatic (obstructive or surgical) or intrahepatic.

Causes

The major causes of cholestasis in the adult are listed in Table 80.8.

Gallstones

There are three types: cholesterol, mixed, and pigment stones. In industrialized countries these stones are the main cause of gallbladder and biliary tract disease, which is common, especially in fat, elderly women.

Bile consists of bile salts, cholesterol, phospholipids, lecithin, and bile pigments. The insoluble cholesterol is kept in solution by the formation of micelles. These macromolecular complexes consist of a solvent centre containing cholesterol around which bile salts and phospholipids are so arranged that the whole complex stays in solution. An increase in the amount of cholesterol or decrease in the amount of bile salts or phospholipid may lead to the formation of stones. These variables depend on the diet and other factors such as race, infection in the gallbladder and the amount of bile pigment. Africans have been found to have a higher bile salt: cholesterol ratio than whites and high levels of biliary phospholipids. This may explain the low incidence of gallstones and hence the low incidence of cholecystitis and biliary tract disease. It is surprising that the bile-pigment stones are not seen more often because haemolysis due to malaria and sickle-cell disease is common. It has been suggested that differences in gallbladder motor function may account for the racial difference in prevalence of gallstones (Davion et al., 1989).

Clinical features

These depend on the underlying cause, but the features of jaundice are independent of its cause: its intensity varies but it is usually progressive and is accompanied by pruritus, hepatomegaly, and often splenomegaly.

When the obstruction is due to cancer, the patient may lose weight, have palpable supraclavicular lymph nodes, deepening jaundice, and an enlarged gallbladder. Recurrent fever, pain over the liver, and jaundice suggest recurrent cholangitis (the classically described 'intermittent hepatic fever'). Long-standing cholestasis is associated with xanthelasma, xanthomata, shiny nails, and increased skin pigmentation. The urine is dark and the stools are pale.

Diagnosis

Take a careful history: this must include a detailed list of drugs and an account of any previous surgery. Examine the patient very carefully: look for all possible signs including scratch marks secondary to the pruritus of chronic cholestasis; an enlarged gallbladder, indicating obstruction to flow of bile somewhere in the bile duct; xanthelasma or xanthoma, which appear in chronic cases; hepatosplenomegaly, and advanced wasting, which may suggest a cancer.

Table 80.8. Causes of cholestasis

Infection	Toxins	Cancer
A. Intra-hepatic		
Viral hepatitis (A–E)	Alcohol	Secondary cancer
Hepatitis – other than viral		Primary hepatocellular cancer
Chronic active hepatitis	Herbal preparations	
Septicaemia	Drugs – chlorpromazine, oral contraceptives testosterone	–
Liver abscess		*Miscellaneous*
Cholangitis		Pregnancy
		Cirrhosis
		Sickle cell disease (SS)
		Primary biliary cirrhosis
		Primary sclerosing cholangitis
		Cystic fibrosis
		Benign recurrent cholestasis

B. Extra-hepatic
1. Outside the bile duct:
   Carcinoma of the pancreas
   Pancreatitis, chronic fibrosing/calcific (p. 981)
   Secondary deposits in lymph nodes in primary or secondary liver cell cancer
2. Within the wall of bile duct:
   Stricture (post-cholecystectomy, carcinoma)
   HIV/AIDS-related papillary stenosis and cholangiopathy
3. Within the lumen:
   Gallstones
   Parasitic infections – clump of Ascaris
   – Fascioliasis (rare)

Investigation

Select tests relevant to the context of the patient, the history, and signs. First, it is essential to test urine and examine stool for bile; estimate serum bilirubin, and do a plain radiograph of the abdomen to look for radio-opaque gallstones (about 15 per cent are radio-opaque).

Liver function tests

Liver function tests will not define the cause of cholestasis but merely show typical features of obstructive jaundice.

Stool
Bile pigment is absent and so the stools are pale in colour.

Blood
Raised serum bilirubin, greatly raised serum alkaline phosphatase (three to ten times normal), 5′ nucleotidase, raised serum aminotransferase, raised serum cholesterol, prolonged prothrombin time (correctable with vitamin K).

Urine
The urine contains bilirubin and so is dark: urobilinogen is absent in complete obstruction of the bile duct.

Ultrasonography

Ultrasound of the liver and biliary tree reveal dilated bile ducts in over 90 per cent of cases of extra-hepatic biliary obstruction, but will not reveal undilated bile ducts in cases of intrahepatic obstruction. Mass lesions in the liver, porta hepatis and head of the pancreas are detectable by ultrasonography.

Barium meal

Gastric carcinoma, or distortion of the duodenal loop due to pancreatic or ampullary carcinoma, can be seen, and a linear mass across the duodenal bulb caused by a dilated common bile duct can also sometimes be seen.

More advanced tests

For a definitive diagnosis of biliary obstruction, further techniques, some of which are invasive and potentially hazardous and are practised only in specialized units, may be necessary. These include percutaneous transhepatic cholangiography, endoscopic retrograde cholangiopancreatography (ERCP) and radioisotope tests.

Immunological tests
1. The presence of HBsAg (with or without HDV) and anti-HCV, does not prove that cholestasis is intrahepatic as a result of these infections because they are widespread in the population of tropical Africa.
2. Antimitochondrial antibody is positive in primary biliary cirrhosis.

Liver biopsy
If intrahepatic cholestasis is supported by the history, physical signs, ultrasound and other relevant tests, a liver biopsy is indicated to make a specific diagnosis.

Laparoscopy
The gall bladder and liver can be inspected, and a liver biopsy can be done under direct vision.

Laparotomy
When more sophisticated techniques are not available, laparotomy is possible, and is essential in suspected extrahepatic obstruction.

Complications of biliary obstruction

Complications develop in cholestasis, whatever its cause; they become more severe as the obstruction becomes prolonged.

Liver cell dysfunction

Raised intrabiliary pressure, biliary tract infection, bile duct damage and later parenchymal fibrosis with nodular regeneration lead to liver cell dysfunction and, eventually, after months or years, to cirrhosis and liver cell failure.

Acute renal failure

Patients with intrahepatic or extrahepatic bile duct obstruction are susceptible to acute renal failure especially when undergoing major surgery to relieve the obstruction. The pathogenic mechanism is not well understood but endotoxins, nitric oxide and thromboxane are suggested (Inan et al., 1997; Kossard & Lindor, 2000).

Metabolic bone disease

Both osteoporosis and, less commonly, osteomalacia leading to collapsed vertebrae, develop in chronic biliary obstruction. Defective metabolism of vitamin D by hepatic microsomal enzymes (and kidneys) may be partly responsible, but this is not definite. Cholestyramine (*Questran*), the bile salt chelating agent for treating pruritus, can also aggravate osteomalacia by reducing absorption of dietary vitamin D and 25-hydroxycholecalciferol. Secondary or tertiary hyperparathyroidism may also develop. Vitamin D_2 or 1-hydroxycholecalciferol is used prophylactically but nothing has been found to help osteoporosis.

Septicaemia

Sepsis remains a serious and frequent complication in patients with chronic bile duct obstruction despite broad spectrum antibiotics and improved surgical techniques for biliary decompression. In acute suppurative cholangitis, septic material passes into the circulation as a result of tension in the biliary ducts.

In non-purulent cholangitis, the pathogenesis of sepsis is not completely understood. Gram negative bacterial endotoxins, cytokines and depression of the reticuloendothelial system are partly the cause (Allen et al., 1989).

Sepsis is common in gallstone obstruction with infection, after ERCP and surgery.

The infection has both systemic and local effects with rigors, fever, increasing jaundice and a tender large liver; shock develops in some patients.

Bleeding

As a result of vitamin K malabsorption, and the deficiency of blood clotting factors II, VII, IX and X, prothrombin time is prolonged and a bleeding diathesis develops; therefore give prophylactic vitamin K.

Other complications

Steatorrhoea

In long-standing cholestasis, steatorrhoea may occur with subsequent malabsorption of fat-soluble vitamins (vitamin A, D, E and K). The elevated serum cholesterol is not associated with increased prevalence of ischaemic heart disease. Xanthelasma is also seen in some of these patients.

Management

Give vitamin A and D orally and vitamin K parenterally. Maintain the usual amount of fat taken by the patient.

Pruritus

This is a chronic problem in some patients and some, also, may be aware of darkening skin.

Treatment

Intrahepatic cholestasis

Here again the technical care is not available outside special units.

Treat pruritus with cholestyramine 2–3 grams per day. Ultraviolet light helps. In recent years, ursodeoxycholic acid (Ursodiol) has been found effective in intrahepatic cholestasis: primary biliary cirrhosis, primarily sclerosing cholongitis, intrahepatic cholestasis of pregnancy and cystic fibrosis. It has few side effects and causes a significant fall in all biochemical markers especially in primary biliary cirrhosis. The usual adult dose is 12–15 mg kg^{-1} daily per os. It has cytoprotective, membrane stabilizing, anti-oxidative and immunomodulatory effects. Corticosteroids are contraindicated in most of the above conditions. Granulomata causing cholestasis, as in sarcoidosis, respond to corticosteroids.

Extrahepatic biliary obstruction

Gallstones, strictures and tumours are the commonest diseases affecting the large bile ducts. These are treated surgically and with operative endoscopy, which may include stenting. Use vitamin K intramuscularly to prevent bleeding.

Treat AIDS and opportunistic infections with appropriate agents to prevent AIDS cholangiopathy and papillary stenosis.

HEPATOCELLULAR CARCINOMA

The problem in Africa

Primary hepatocellular carcinoma (HCC) is one of the most common tumours worldwide. It is probably the commonest tumour in sub-Saharan Africa and parts of Asia with an annual incidence of up to 100 cases per 100 000 population. The incidence in Africa varies from country to country (Tsega, 1977; Bijlsma, 1981). In sharp contrast, the annual incidence of HCC in western Europe and North America is 1–3 cases per 100 000 population. The tumour is more commonly seen in males, the male-to-female ratio being 3:1 in the African patients. It occurs at an early age (20–40 years), one to two decades earlier than in western European and North American patients.

Aetiology

The main reason for the high prevalence of HCC in Africa is the high infection rate with hepatitis B virus (HBV) and hepatitis C virus (HCV). The risk of acquiring HCC in HBV carriers is estimated to be 100 times higher than in non-carriers (Kew, 2000; Beasely, 1982). Also, the association between HCC and HCV infection is high. In some African countries this association is higher than with HBV infection (Tsega et al., 1995). Since HCV infection becomes chronic in over 90 per cent of cases compared to 10–15 per cent in HBV infection, HCV is a likely future major cause of HCC in Africa. The HBsAg carrier state is more common in men than in women. This may partly account for the higher incidence of HCC among males.

A significant number of patients with HCC are negative for HBV and HCV markers. Possible causes of HCC in these patients include macronodular cirrhosis of the liver (HCC is more commonly associated with cirrhotic than normal liver), aflatoxin A1 from *Aspergillus fumigatus* (a fungus which commonly contaminates ground nuts and stored grains, also known to cause cancer in animals), traditional herbal medicines, and iron storage disease (HLA-linked haemochromatosis and African iron overload) (Gangaidzo & Gordeuk, 1995).

Pathology

Tumours tend to be multiple, often involving both lobes of the liver. A solitary tumour restricted to one lobe is uncommon because most African patients are seen late in the course of their disease and the tumour is fast growing. The majority of tumours are poorly differentiated HCC which arise from macronodular cirrhosis: this accounts for their rapid course (Kashala et al., 1990). Metastases can develop in bones, lungs, brain, adrenal glands, and the peritoneum.

Clinical features

Symptoms

1. Pain in the right upper quadrant and/or epigastrium is the commonest complaint. The pain arises from the capsule of the liver, stretched and inflamed by the tumour beneath it.
2. Easy fatiguability and anorexia are common. Some patients may have pruritus.
3. Fever may be the only presenting symptom (Chapter 12, p. 191).

Signs

1. Mass in the right upper quadrant. This is often obvious to the patient and the examiner. The mass is palpable, tender, hard and often multi-nodular with gross enlargement of the liver, which may be ballotable.
2. Bruit over the liver. This may be heard in up to 80 per cent of patients (Tsega, 1977). A friction rub may also be heard.
3. Ascites with fullness in the flanks and shifting dullness is common (Fig. 80.7). A sudden increase of abdominal girth should suggest a subcapsular oozing of blood or a sudden rupture of liver due to invasion of the capsule of the liver by the tumour.

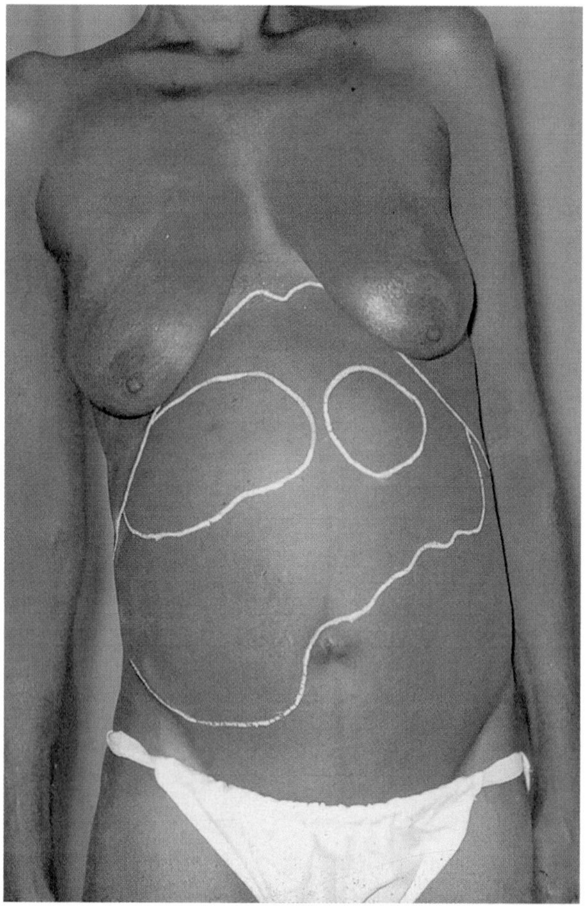

Fig. 80.7. A patient with gross hepatomegaly – proven hepatocellular carcinoma. (Copyright: Dr John Ziegler and Makerere University)

4. Jaundice is also common and may be due to obstruction of the bile duct or hepatocellular failure associated with advancing cirrhosis and the invading and growing tumour.
5. Loss of weight. The patient steadily loses weight and has severe wasting of muscles (Fig. 80.7).
6. Metastases cause local signs in the target organ or tissue, bones, lungs, brain, adrenal glands and the peritoneum. Some patients may present with paraplegia, cholestasis or metastatic lesions only.

Paraneoplastic syndrome

In a few cases, HCC can produce hormone-like substances, but this is uncommon in Africa. Erythropoietin-like sub-

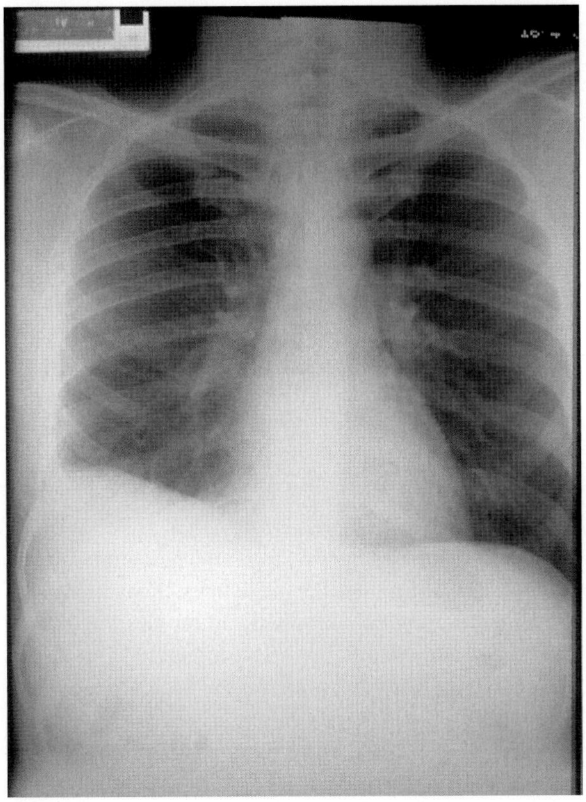

Fig. 80.8. Chest radiograph in a patient with an amoebic liver abscess: note the raised right hemi-diaphragm, the small right pleural effusion and some indefinite lung changes in the right lower zone. (By courtesy of the Wellcome Trust and Dr R. Davidson.)

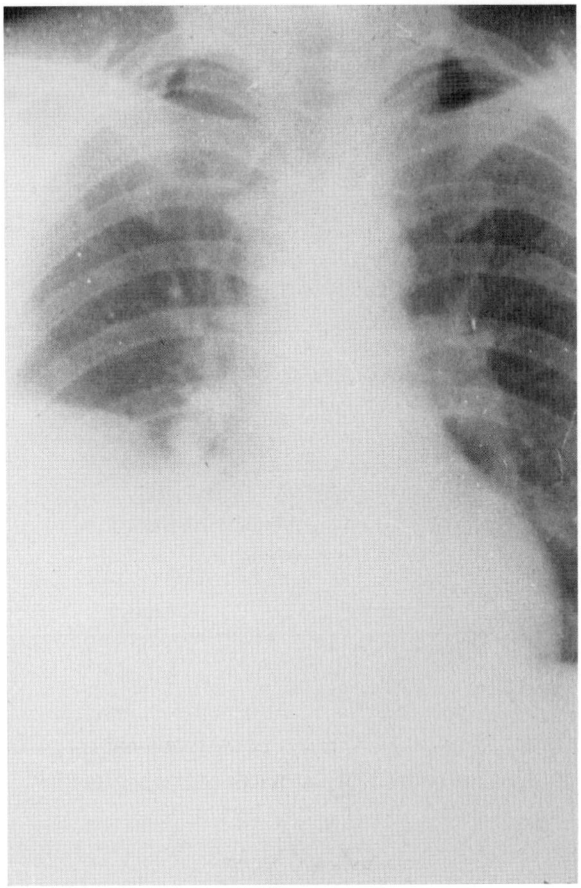

Another example with higher right diaphragm.

stance produces erythrocytosis and a parathyroid-like hormone secretion results in hypercalcaemia. Other manifestations include hypoglycaemia, hypercholesterolaemia and porphyria cutanea tarda (Ndububa et al., 1999).

Investigations

Alphafetoprotein

A level greater than 500 μg/l is present in 70–80 per cent of HCC. Lower levels are found in metastatic tumours of the liver from the colon, stomach and other organs.

Liver function test

As with metastatic tumours and infiltrative disorders, the serum alkaline phosphatase is raised in more than 80 per cent of HCC cases. Therefore, neither the raised alkaline phosphatase nor abnormal levels of aminotransferases and bilirubin are diagnostic of HCC.

Chest radiograph

This may demonstrate an elevated right hemi-diaphragm, blunted costo-phrenic angle and pleural effusion (Fig. 80.8).

Imaging procedures

Where available, the ultrasound and CT-scan will readily identify the mass. Sometimes radionuclear scanning (using gallium) and hepatic artery angiography may define the nature of the tumour.

Liver biopsy

Percutaneous liver biopsy may yield conclusive diagnosis. The yield is much higher if ultrasound- or CT-scan-guided biopsy is performed. Both visual and histological diagnosis are possible where laparoscopic service is available. The procedures will also reveal the presence or absence of cirrhosis.

Table 80.9. The diagnosis of amoebic liver abscess or hepatocellular carcinoma

	Carcinoma	Abscess
Length of history	Months	Weeks
Liver	Tender mass	Tender mass
	Hard	Rarely hard
	Bruit often	Bruit very rare
Ascites	Blood-stained often	Rarely blood-stained
Jaundice	Sometimes	Sometimes
Fever	Sometimes	Almost always
Leukocyte count	Sometimes raised	Leukocytosis common
Chest radiography	R. dome raised	R. dome raised
	Basal collapse rare	Basal collapse common
Aspiration	Blood sometimes	Brown pus
Alphafetoprotein	Positive in over 65%	Negative
Amoebic gel precipitation test	Negative (unless previous attack of amoebiasis)	Positive in 97%
Effect of metronidazole	None	Signs improve quickly
Ultrasound	Mass image	Fluid image

Paracentesis

The ascitic fluid may be blood-stained,but cytological examination of the fluid for tumour cells is negative in most patients.

Diagnosis

The typical picture

Exhaustion, loss of appetite, rapid loss of weight, right upper quadrant and/or epigastric pain, a big, hard, tender and grossly nodular liver with a bruit, signs of portal hypertension, and/or hepatic encephalopathy, in a young man with a rapid downhill course, characterize the African patient with HCC.

Differential diagnosis

Coalescing tuberculomas, secondary tumours of the liver, and the common problem of amoebic liver abscess are all possible. The differences between HCC and amoebic liver abscess are summarized in Table 80.9 (Fig. 80.9).

If a firm diagnosis of HCC from amoebic abscess is impossible, a therapeutic trial with metronidazole 750 mg three times per day intravenously or by mouth for 5 days will cause the fever and tenderness associated with an abscess to regress.

Treatment

This is a dreadful disease to treat. The clinical course is rapid and most patients die within 3–6 months.

Chemotherapeutic trials in different parts of Africa have been disappointing (Kiire et al., 1992). Early detection of focal HCC, restricted to one lobe of the liver and without cirrhosis and distant metastasis, may benefit from surgical resection but such cases are rare.

Different forms of advanced treatment, including liver transplant, have been tried in regions of the world where facilities and expertise permit, but the outcome remains poor.

Prevention

As treatment is so ineffective, by far the best strategy against HCC is to reduce the incidence of hepatitis B by implementing a policy of universal immunization of infants and adolescents, preferably integrated into the national immunization programme of each African country.

DRUGS, TOXINS, AND THE LIVER

The liver is the main organ for drug metabolism. It is located between the splanchnic and systemic circulations and it has numerous enzymes that can change drugs into pharmacologically active compounds or break them down for final clearance.

Drugs administered in their inactive forms are changed by the liver into the active forms, for example prednisone to prednisolone, and azathioprine to 6-mercaptopurine. Some drugs are changed to toxic metabolites, which may become hepatotoxic, for example isoniazid and paracetamol.

The metabolism of drugs will be impaired in patients with significant liver disease. Therefore, choose a safe drug and adjust the dose and interval accordingly.

Several factors will influence drug metabolism by the liver: age, sex, dose, duration, interval and route of administration, drug interaction, tissue oxygenation, underlying disease, genetic factors, nutritional state and hormonal abnormalities.

Drug-induced liver injury

The types of liver injury and examples of drugs causing the abnormality are summarized in Table 80.10.

Subclinical liver injury

Some drugs cause elevated aminotransferases and/or alkaline phosphatase. The level may be two to three times the upper limit of normal. In most cases, this level does not progress and some may return to normal even when the drug is continued.

Follow such patients by periodic liver function tests, and, if the enzymes rise further (three or four times the upper limit of normal), stop the drug to prevent overt liver disease.

Acute hepatocellular injury

Some drugs or their metabolites are directly toxic to the liver cells. The direct toxic effect is exerted on the cell membranes. This type of injury is dose-related and predictable. It is not frequent. Toxic necrosis occurs due to paracetamol, declofenac (non-steroidal anti-inflammatory drug), alcohol, carbon tetrachloride (CCl_4), etc.

Hepatitis-like acute hepatocellular injury occurs, with jaundice and levels of enzymes up to 8-fold to 100-fold.

Table 80.10. Drug-induced liver disease

Type of liver injury	Example
Subclinical liver injury	Erythromycin, rifampicin, nifedipine, nadalol
Acute hepatocellular injury	
Toxic necrosis	Phenacetin, declofenac, CCl_4
Hepatitis-like	Isoniazid, methyldopa, halothane, phenytoin
Acute steatosis	i.v. tetracycline, CCl_4
Cholestasis	
Inflammatory	Chlorpromazine, other phenothiazines
Pure (bland)	Anabolic and contraceptive steroids
Miscellaneous acute/subactute	Amiodarone, sulphonamides
Chronic liver disease	
Chronic hepatitis	Isoniazid, methyldopa
Chronic steatosis	Alcohol, methotrexate, glucocorticoids, valproate
Chronic cholestasis	Chlorpromazine
Fibrosis/cirrhosis	Methotrexate, arsenicals, high dose vitamin A
Vascular lesions	Contraceptives, pyrolizidine alkaloids, azathioprine
Tumours	Oral contraceptives, vinyl chloride

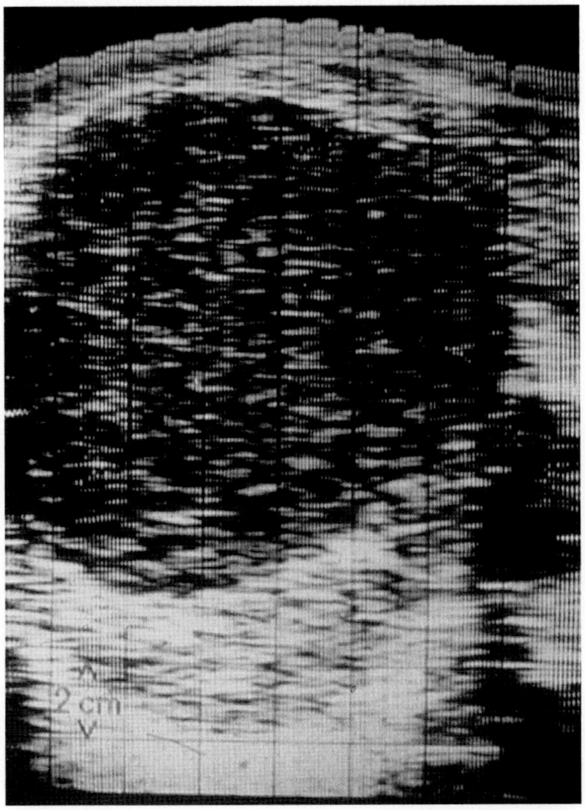

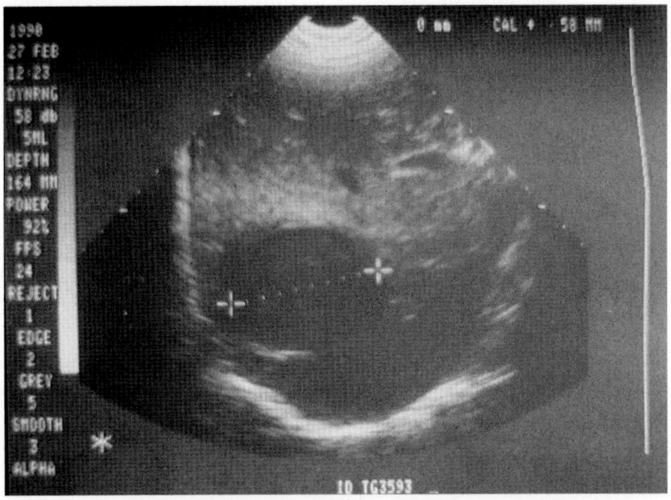

Fig. 80.9. Amoebic liver abscess: Ultrasound to show a large abscess, marked with +..+: a similar picture would be given by a large cancer. (By courtesy of the Wellcome Trust and Dr R. Davidson.)

The clinical picture resembles viral hepatitis and may lead to fulminant hepatic failure. Isoniazid, methyldopa, halothane and phenytoin are frequently implicated in this type of massive hepatocyte necrosis. The pathogenesis may be immunological, metabolic, genetic idiosyncratic and due to genetic predisposition, but in many cases it is not well understood. The occurrence of such drug-induced liver injury is not dose-related and it is unpredictable. In rare cases where immune hypersensitivity is blamed, a skin rash, arthralgia and eosinophilia may occur. Halothane produces damage after repeated exposure and isoniazid hepatitis may develop after several months of treatment. Acute steatosis occurs after high dose of intravenous tetracycline and carbon tetrachloride. The clinical and biochemical features resemble those of acute fatty liver of pregnancy and Reye's syndrome. Jaundice is slight and enzyme levels are not as high as those of hepatitis-like necrosis. However, the illness is serious with poor prognosis.

Cholestasis

Cholestatic injury resembles the clinical and biochemical features of extrahepatic obstructive jaundice. Aminotransferase levels are only modestly elevated. There are two types of cholestatic injury:

- *Inflammatory type cholestasis* is a result of acute periportal necro-inflammatory reaction due to drugs like chlorpromazine and other phenothiazines. There is a minimal degree of hepatocyte injury.
- *Pure type* (also known as bland, canalicular or steroid cholestasis) is exemplified by anabolic or contraceptive steroid jaundice. In this type, impairment of bile flow, with little or no associated hepatocellular injury, occurs and is due to idiosyncratic exaggeration of the physiological effect of sex hormones on bile canalicular transport. It may also have a genetic component. The clinical features include progressive pruritus, dark urine and jaundice without associated systemic symptoms. The alkaline phosphatase is elevated but the enzymes are only minimally increased. Women who develop this kind of reaction while on contraceptives are prone to develop cholestasis of pregnancy with identical pathogenesis.

Miscellaneous acute and subacute reactions

There are many drugs that are associated with mixed hepatocellular and excretory abnormalities. The laboratory and histological changes are never typical or diagnostic. Some drugs like sulphonamides cause granulomatous inflammation and others like amiodarone cause alcoholic hepatitis-like clinical and histological features. The pathogenesis for these variable changes remains unknown.

Chronic liver disease

Most drug-induced liver injury is acute or subacute and rarely proceeds to chronic disease. A few cases of chronic liver injury occur due to long exposure to drugs.

Chronic hepatitis

Chronic active hepatitis, indistinguishable from the clinical, biochemical and histological features of idiopathic or autoimmune chronic active hepatitis, occurs due to long-term ingestion of some drugs. The best examples are isoniazid and methyldopa. The disease is reversed to normal by stopping the offending drugs. The pathogenesis is not clear but idiosyncracy, immunological and metabolic abnormalities are suspected.

Chronic steatosis

This is a milder form of liver injury compared to acute cholestasis. The clinical manifestations are few. Steatosis caused by ethanol, glucocorticoids and methotrexate cause hepatomegaly but steatosis caused by asparaginase, valproate and amiodarone may produce chronic liver failure (Zimmerman & Ishak, 1995).

Chronic cholestasis

Chlorpromazine-induced cholestasis tends to persist even after discontinuing the drug. It mimics primary biliary cirrhosis but the immunological features of the latter do not exist.

Fibrosis and cirrhosis

Slowly progressive fibrosis without any clinical manifestation may proceed to cirrhosis and portal hypertension. Such changes occur in patients on long term treatment with methotrexate, some other cancer treatment agents, arsenicals or vitamin A in big doses. Liver biopsy is the only way to establish the diagnosis. Patients on long term methotrexate treatment for rheumatoid arthritis or psoriasis should have liver biopsy periodically.

Vascular lesions

1. Hepatic vein thrombosis leading to Budd–Chiari syndrome, characterized by a tender, enlarged liver, abdominal pain, ascites and mild to moderate eleva-

tion of enzymes, but rarely jaundice, may be seen in patients taking oral contraceptive agents.

2. Veno-occlusive disease of the central hepatic venules, caused by pyrrolizidine alkaloids, also presents like the Budd–Chiari syndrome. Urethane, azathioprine and other drugs used to treat cancer are known to cause the same condition.

Tumours

Benign liver adenomas occasionally occur following prolonged intake of oral contraceptives. These are usually asymptomatic but may rarely cause an acute abdomen due to rupture and intraperitoneal bleed. Very rarely such adenomas may become malignant. Angiosarcoma may occur from exposure to vinyl chloride.

Liver disease and drugs

Drug clearance is impaired in the presence of significant liver disease. This results in high concentration of the drug in the circulation and may give rise to hepatic encephalopathy – benzodiazepines, such as chlordiazepoxide and diazepam, are not fully degraded by oxidation in hepatitis and cirrhosis, and often precipitate hepatic encephalopathy when administered repeatedly. Some drugs which are cleared by acetylation, such as isoniazid, may have a prolonged high concentration in the blood to give rise to further damage of the liver.

Mechanisms of impaired drug metabolism

Liver

1. The liver cell mass and function may be significantly reduced. Enzymes involved in the clearance of drugs may be reduced in amount or have poor function in the intact hepatocytes.
2. Drug delivery to the liver cells may be impaired due to portosystemic shunting and reduced sinusoidal blood flow. Reduction in arterial blood supply to the liver results in hypoxia which depresses drug metabolism.
3. Reduction of bile flow due to cholestasis may affect drugs that are excreted in bile without undergoing biochemical changes, e.g. nafcillin, piperacillin, ceftriaxone, etc.
4. Reduced drug binding to protein due to hypoproteinaemia secondary to cirrhosis (albumin is formed by liver cells only) results in a high level of unbound drugs in the blood. This is especially significant for highly bound drugs such as naproxin and diazepam. Albumin binds acidic and neutral drugs whereas alpha 1-acid glycoprotein and lipoprotein bind mainly basic drugs.

Kidney

Decreased renal clearance of drugs like morphine, cimetidine, etc. occurs in cirrhotic patients with abnormal kidney function.

Other causes

Malnutrition leads to impaired drug biotransformation by either oxidation or conjugation, and endocrine changes which occur in patients with chronic liver disease may change drug metabolism, e.g. oral contraceptives inhibit the oxidation of drugs such as prednisone, chlordiazepoxide, triazolam, etc.

Toxic hepatitis and traditional remedies

Hepatotoxicity related to herbal remedies occurs in different parts of the world, including Africa. Pyrolizidine alkaloids present in more than 60 different plants account for veno-occlusive disease (first reported from the Caribbean in 1957). The most important of these plants, drunk as herbal tea, are *Senecio, Crotalaria, Heliotropium* and *Symphytum.* Ingestion of akee fruit causes vomiting and hypoglycaemia and is associated with liver steatosis. Scientific information on hepatotoxicity and herbal medicine in Africa is limited. However, it is common knowledge that traditional remedies are widely used. Of 40 different Ethiopian plant materials, 10 species of plants of the genera *Senecio, Crotalaria, Heliotropium* and *Cynoglossum* were reported hepatotoxic in rats (Schoental & Coady, 1968). *Callilepsis laureola* is known to cause fatal liver necrosis in South Africa (Wainwright et al., 1997).

Diagnosis of drug-induced liver diseases

Ask the patient and/or relatives if the patient has taken any kind of drug, toxin or herbal medicine, including drugs obtained 'over the counter'. Be alert to suspect that a drug or toxin is responsible. The clinical and laboratory pattern of hepatic injury may suggest the use of certain types of drugs. Systemic manifestations such as rash, fever, eosinophilia with multisystem involvement may be helpful. Sometimes liver biopsy may be diagnostic, e.g. fibrosis/cirrhosis in patients on long-term treatment with methotrexate. Avoid rechallenge, that is, giving the patient the same suspected drug to reproduce observed clinical features, except when the drug is essential and there is no alternative.

Treatment of drug-induced liver diseases

- Stop the suspected drug immediately.
- Give antidote when indicated, e.g. *N*-acetylcysteine for paracetamol overdose.
- Reduce the doses of drugs known to cause hepatic injury in patients with liver disease.,
- Monitor closely drugs known to cause idiosyncratic (with unpredictable liver injury) hepatotoxicity, even in the absence of liver disease. Corticosteroids may be tried in hepatic injury with hypersensitivity, which does not respond to withdrawal of the offending drug.

References

Addy JA (1974). Pathogenesis and natural history of porphyria cutanea tarda. Letter to the editor. *Lancet*, **i**: 213.

Allen MO, Wilton PB, Barke RA et al. (1989). Effects of biliary obstruction on hepatic clearance of bacteria. *Arch Surg*, **124**: 973–977.

Altemeier WA, Culbertson WR, Fullery WD et al. (1973). Intra-abdominal abscesses. *Am J Surg*, **125**: 70–79.

Beasely RP. (1982). Hepatitis B virus as the etiologic agent in hepatocellular carcinoma – epidemiologic consideration. *Hepatology*, **2**: 215–265.

Bhargava M, Kalvaria I, Trey C et al. (1990). Diagnostic value of ascites adenosine deaminase in tuberculous peritonitis. *Tubercle*, **71**: 121–126.

Bijlsma R. (1981). Malignant tumour in Mozambican Africans with special reference to primary liver carcinoma. *Trans Roy Soc Trop Med Hyg*, **75**: 451–454.

Craxi A, Raimondo G, Longo G et al. (1984). Delta agent infection in acute hepatitis and chronic HbsAg carriers with and without liver disease. *Gut*, **25**: 1288–1290.

Cribier B, Petian P, Keller F et al. (1995). Porphyria cutanea tarda and hepatitis C viral infection. A clinical and virological study. *Arch Dermatol*, **131**: 801–804.

Davidson S, Brock JF, Passmore R. (1972). *Human Nutrition and Dietetics*, 5th edn. Edinburgh: Churchill Livingstone.

Davion T, Tossou H, Delamarre H et al. (1989). Racial differences in gallbladder motor function. Lancet, **i**: 724–725

Dhainaut JF, Marin N, Mignon A et al. (2001). Hepatic response to sepsis: Interaction between coagulation and inflammatory process. *Crit Care Med*, **29**: 542–547.

Dorrucci M, Pezzotti P, Phillips AN et al. (1995). Coinfection of hepatitis C virus with human immunodeficiency virus and progression of AIDS. Italian Seroconversion Study. *J Infect Dis*, **172**: 1503–1508.

Gangaidzo IT, Gordeuk VR. (1995). Hepatocellular carcinoma and African iron overload. *Gut*, **37**: 727–730.

Gilson RJ, Hawkins AE, Beecham MR et al. (1997). Interaction between HIV and hepatitis B in homosexual men: effects on the natural history of infection. *AIDS*, **11**: 597–606.

Hadder SC, Judson SN, O'Malley PM et al. (1991). Outcome of hepatitis B virus infection in homosexual men and its relation to prior human immunodeficiency virus infection. *J Infect Dis* **163**: 454–459.

Inan M, Sayek I, Tel BC et al. (1997). Role of endotoxin and nitric oxide in the pathogenesis of renal failure in obstructive jaundice. *Br J Surg*, **84**: 1747.

Ishak K, Baptisa A, Bianchi L et al. (1995). Histologic grading and staging of chronic hepatitis. *J Hepatol*, **22**: 696.

Kao HW, Rakov NE et al. (1985). The effect of large volume paracentesis on plasma volume – a cause of hypovolemia? *Hepatology*, **5**: 403–407.

Kashala LO, Conne B, Kalengaayi MR et al. (1990). Histopathalogic features of hepatocellular carcinoma in Zaire. *Cancer*, **65**: 130–134.

Kew MC. (2000). Epidemiology of hepatocellular carcinoma and its viral risk factors. *Acta Gastro-Enterol Belg*, **63**: 227–229.

Kiire CF. (1990). Hepatitis B infection in sub-Saharan Africa. *Vaccine*, **8**: S107–S112.

Kiire CF, Gombe-Mbalawa C, Tsega E et al. (1992). Multicentre study of the treatment of primary liver cancer in Africa with two anthracycline drugs. *Centr Afr J Med*, **38**: 428–431.

Koo DJ, Chaudry IH, Wang P. (1999). Kupffer cells are responsible for producing inflammatory cytokines and hepatocellular dysfunction during early sepsis. *J Surg Res*, **83**: 151–157.

Kossard AA. Lindor KD. (2000). Medical management of chronic cholestatic liver diseases. *Can J Gastroenterol*, **14**: 1–98.

Larzarchick J, deSouza E, Silva NA et al. (1973). Pyogenic liver abscess. *Mayo Clinic Proc*, **48**: 349–355.

Lee WM. (1993). Medical progress: acute liver failure. *N Engl J Med*, **329**: 1862–1874.

Mahajani RV, Uzer MF. (1999). Cholangiopathy in HIV-infected patients. *Clin Liver Dis*, **3**: 669–684.

Molinié C, Saliou P, Roué R et al. (1988). Acute epidemic non-A, non-B hepatitis: a clinical study of 38 cases in Chad. In *Viral Hepatitis and Liver Diseases*, pp 154–157, Alan R Liss, Inc.

Ndububa DA, Ojo OS, Adetiloye VA et al. (1999). The incidence and characteristics of some paraneoplastic syndromes of hepatocellular carcinoma in Nigerian patients. *Eur J Gastroenterol Hepatol*, **11**: 140–144.

Okamoto H, Nishizawa T, Ukita M. (1999). A novel unenveloped DNA viruses (TT virus) associated with acute and chronic non-A to G hepatitis. *Interviral*, **42**: 196–204.

Pinto PC, American J, Reynolds JB et al. (1988). Large volume paracentesis in nonedematous patients with tense ascites: its effect on intravascular volume. *Hepatology*, **8**: 207–210.

Riordan SM, Williams R. (1997). Treatment of hepatic encephalopathy. *N Engl J Med*, **337**: 473–479.

Rolachon A, Cardier L, Bacq Y et al. (1995). Ciprofloxacin and long-term prevention of SBP: results of a prospective controlled trial. *Hepatology*, **22**: 1171–1174.

Runyon BA, McHutchison JG, Antillon MR et al. (1991). Short-course vs. long-course antibiotic treatment of spontaneous bacterial peritonitis: a randomized controlled trial of 100 patients. *Gastroenterology*, **100**: 1737–1742.

Sartin JS, Walker RD. (1991). Granulomatous hepatitis: a retrospective review of 88 cases at the Mayo Clinic. *Mayo Clinic Proc*, **66**: 914–918.

Schoental R, Coady A. (1968). The hepatotoxicity of some Ethiopian and East African plants, including some used in traditional medicine. *E Afr Med J*, **45**: 577–800.

Singh N, Gayowksi T, Yu VL et al. (1995). Trimethoprim – sulfamethoxazole for the prevention of spontaneous bacterial peritonitis in cirrhosis: a randomized trial. *Am Intern Med*, **122**: 595–598.

Thomas DL, Shih JW, Alter HJ et al. (1996). Effect of human immunodifficiency virus on hepatitis C virus infection among injection drug users. *J Infect Dis*, **174**: 690–695.

Triger DR, Hosking SW. (1989). The gastric mucosa in portal hypertension. *J Hepatol*, **8**: 267–272.

Tsega E. (1977). Hepatocellular carcinoma in Ethiopia: a prospective clinical study of 100 patients. *E Afr Med J*, **54**: 281–292.

Tsega E. (1992). Chronic liver disease in Ethiopia: A clinical study with emphasis on identifying common causes. *Ethiop Med J*, **30**: 1–33.

Tsega E, Besrat A, Damtew B et al. (1981). Chloroquine in the treatment of porphyria cutanea tarda. *Trans Roy Soc Trop Med Hyg*, **75**: 401–404.

Tsega E, Besrat A, Landells JW et al. (1982). The liver in Ethiopians with porphyria cutanea tarda. *E Afr Med J*, **59**: 682–688.

Tsega E., Hansson BG, Krawczynski K et al. (1992). Acute sporadic viral hepatitis in Ethiopia: causes, risk factors, and effects on pregnancy. *Clin Inf Dis*, **14**: 961–965.

Tsega E, Krawczynksi K, Hansson B-G et al. (1993). Hepatitis E virus infection in pregnancy in Ethiopia. *Ethiop Med J*, **31**: 173–181.

Tsega E, Nordenfelt E, Hansson BG. (1995). Hepatitis C virus infection and chronic liver disease in Ethiopia where hepatitis B infection is hyperendemic. *Trans Roy Soc Trop Med Hyg*, **89**: 171–174.

Tsega E, Nordenfelt E, Mengesha B et al. (1998). Age specific prevalence of hepatitis A virus antibody in Ethiopian children. *Scand J Infect Dis*, **338**: 286–290.

Tugwell P, Williams AD. (1977). Jaundice associated with lobar pneumonia. *Quart J Med*, **46**: 97–118.

Ungo JR, Jones D, Ashkin D et al. (1998). Antituberculosis drug-induced hepatotoxicity. The role of hepatitis C virus and the human immunodeficiency virus. *Am J Respir Crit Care Med*, **157**: 1871–1876.

Uribe M, Campollo O et al. (1987). Acidifying enemas (lactilol and lactulose) vs. non-acidifying enemas (tap water) to treat acute portal systemic encephalopathy: a double blind, randomized clinical trial. *Hepatology*, **7**: 639–643.

Vento S, diPerri G, Luzzati R et al. (1989). Clinical reactivation of hepatitis B in anti-HBs-positive patients with AIDS. *Lancet*, **1**: 323.

Vento S, Garofano T, Renzini C et al. (1998). Fulminant hepatitis associated with hepatitis A virus superinfection in patients with chronic hepatitis C. *N Engl J Med*, **338**: 286–290.

Voigt MD, Gupta M, Nijhawan S et al. (1989). Adenosine deaminase (ADA) in peritoneal tuberculosis: diagnostic value in ascitic fluid and serum. *Lancet*, **1**: 751–753.

Wainwright J, Schonland MM, Candy HA. (1997). Toxicity of Callilepsis laureola. *S Afr Med J*, **52**: 313–315.

Williams GGT, Williams WJ. (1983). Granulomatous inflammation – a review. *J Clin Pathol*, **36**: 723–730.

Zimmerman HJ, Ishak KG. (1995). General aspects of drug-induced liver disease. *Gastroenterol Clin N Am*, **24**: 739–757.

81 The spleen

Function

The spleen serves three main functions:
- to filter damaged cells from the blood
- to produce antibodies
- to provide protection against infections, particularly malaria and capsulated bacteria such as pneumococci.

Structure related to function

The spleen acts primarily as a lymphoid organ and has a complicated structure provided by the capsule and a network of trabeculae. Between the trabeculae is the splenic pulp, made up of various phagocytic and plasma cells. The phagocytic cells act as a filter for invading organisms and damaged red blood cells. Any blood-borne infection such as septicaemia or malaria will ultimately result in hypertrophy of these cells and cause the spleen to enlarge. Splenic plasma cells within the splenic pulp are responsible for antibody production. These cells will hypertrophy in response to any antigenic stimulation – and again cause the spleen to enlarge.

Blood supply and vascular structure

The spleen is one of the areas in the body where the portal system meets the systemic. The splenic pulp derives its blood supply from the terminal arterioles of the systemic splenic artery. Near the end of these arterioles are the Malphigian bodies, areas of lymphoid tissue in which lymphocytes are made. Capillaries then drain blood from the splenic pulp into venous sinuses and, ultimately, into the splenic vein which drains into the portal system. A valvular structure at the end of the splenic arterioles ensures that any increase in pressure as a result of portal hypertension is exerted on the splenic pulp – and therefore results in an increase in the size of the spleen.

Definition of splenomegaly

In a normal individual the spleen is not palpable in the abdomen because it is covered in the left upper quadrant by the lower ribs. Splenomegaly is usually defined as the presence of a palpable spleen in the left upper quadrant of the abdomen – and is therefore subjective, particularly when the spleen is only mildly enlarged. The spleen needs to be swollen to roughly twice its normal size in order for it to be palpable.

The clinical characteristics that help differentiate a palpable spleen from an enlarged left kidney or another palpable mass are as follows.
- The spleen moves downwards and medially with respiration.
- The spleen has a palpable notch on its medial border.
- It is impossible to delineate the upper border which is covered by the lower ribs – as a result, it is not possible for the palpating hand to 'get above it'.
- The enlarged spleen does not have a band of colonic resonance over it, whereas the enlarged kidney has such a band of resonance.
- Percussion of the spleen from behind and forwards reveals a continuous band of dullness to percussion.
- The spleen is not palpable bimanually in the loin: the kidney can be palpated bimanually.

The size of the spleen

Words used to describe the size of the spleen have very limited value. The massive spleen is obvious: at the other

Table 81.1. Causes of splenomegaly

Infections
Common infections associated with splenomegaly Malaria, typhoid and other salmonelloses, any septicaemia, HIV, dengue fever and other arboviral infections, hepatitis, disseminated tuberculosis, infective endocarditis
Infections common in a particular area Brucellosis, leptospirosis, relapsing fever,
Unusual manifestations of common disease Katayama fever in schistosomiasis
Much less common causes Trypanosomiasis, histoplasmosis, lepromatous leprosy/erythema nodosum leprosum,
Local splenic infection Abscess

Non-infectious disease
Blood diseases Haemoglobinopathies, leukaemias
Other diseases Rheumatoid arthritis, systemic lupus erythematosus, amyloidosis
Malignant disease Lymphoma
Liver disease Portal hypertension – (chronic schistosomiasis)

Massive splenomegaly
Visceral leishmaniasis, hyper-reactive malarial splenomegaly, myelofibrosis, chronic myeloid leukaemia, B-cell lymphoma

extreme, when the tip of the spleen is just felt on full inspiration, it is better to state this and no more.

Rather than use an adjective, measure the size of the spleen from the costal margin. This measurement can be very helpful clinically in patients in whom the spleen will shrink with treatment, for example those with hyper-reactive malarial splenomegaly.

A list of the most recognized causes is provided in Table 81.1. This is a list and no more: as infections dominate the list, any list has to be related to the local pattern of disease, because the frequency of any specific infection will vary enormously across different parts of Africa.

Splenomegaly in Africa

Splenomegaly is common in sub-Saharan Africa, particularly in children, but the cause varies considerably between different regions of the continent. Reports from different countries vary according to the patients who were studied and so are often not strictly comparable: these reports may reveal the interests of the investigators or the specialization of the hospital and little more. This is evident from the series described below.

Rural Kenya

In a cross-sectional study involving 2941 people living in a rural area of Kenya in 1991–1992, splenomegaly was found in 60 per cent of children aged between 2 and 9 years, in 52 per cent of adolescents aged 10 to 17 years and in 38 per cent of adults (Schaefer et al., 1995). In that area, endemic for visceral leishmaniasis, kala-azar was associated with massive splenomegaly, while moderate enlargement of the spleen was more predictive of malaria.

Urban Kenya

Among 131 hospital patients with chronic splenomegaly in Nairobi, hyper-reactive malarial splenomegaly accounted for 31 per cent, hepato-splenic schistosomiasis 18 per cent and visceral leishmaniasis 5 per cent (De Cock et al., 1987).

Northern Nigeria

Thirty of 75 patients with large spleens were found to have hyper-reactive malarial splenomegaly, 5 chronic lymphatic leukaemia, 4 gross lymphoid hyperplasia, 23 had miscellaneous conditions but no firm diagnosis could be made in 13, while none had visceral leishmaniasis (Bryceson et al., 1976).

Zambia

Of 344 patients with massive splenomegaly, 40 per cent were attributed to hyper-reactive malarial splenomegaly, 17 per cent portal hypertension (excluding schistosomiasis), 17 per cent haematological malignancies and 12 per cent schistosomiasis (Lowenthal et al., 1980).

Kumasi, Ghana

In a report written by haematologists, the pattern was different again: among 221 patients with a palpable spleen of at least 10 cm, collected over 12 years, B-lymphoproliferative disorders were the second most common diagnosis after hyper-reactive malarial splenomegaly (Bedu-Addo & Bates, 2002).

Causes of splenomegaly

There are four main causes of splenomegaly.

1. Pooling of red blood cells within the spleen – often the result of a blood-borne infection and resulting from hypertrophy of the splenic pulp

2. Proliferation of splenic tissue – particularly the plasma cells and Malphigian bodies and often the result of antigenic stimulation
3. Portal hypertension – in an African context, commonly the result of chronic *Schistosoma mansoni* infection or secondary to cirrhosis resulting from chronic hepatitis B
4. Space-occupying lesions within the splenic capsule – usually an abscess.

Splenomegaly may be acute or chronic.

Acute splenomegaly is usually the result of a febrile illness caused by malaria, septicaemia, in particular salmonelloses, or a viral illness.

Chronic splenomegaly is more likely to be the result of HIV infection, hyper-reactive malarial splenomegaly, malignancy or portal hypertension.

Steps towards a clinical diagnosis

The finding of an enlarged spleen implies the presence of an active inflammatory process and in most patients the cause has to be searched for. One exception is splenomegaly in otherwise healthy African children, which is almost invariably due to chronic, asymptomatic *Plasmodium falciparum* malaria.

Clinical method

Rigorous clinical method is essential in any patient with an enlarged spleen: the clinical features mentioned below are merely examples of what may be found in different diseases.

- Record the spleen in cm from the costal margin.
- Is the spleen tender? This indicates local infection (abscess) or infarction.
- Is the spleen soft (acute enlargement) or firm or hard (chronic splenomegaly)?

Fever is such a common sign among patients throughout Africa that it is of little help in differentiating between the various causes of splenomegaly, but the pattern of fever may sometimes help. A pyogenic septicaemia and visceral leishmaniasis may produce a high swinging fever: do not jump to a hasty diagnosis on the basis of a pattern of fever, as we have emphasized in Chapter 12.

Anaemia

Most patients with chronic splenomegaly will have an associated anaemia but in children, in particular, anaemia may suggest an underlying haemoglobinopathy.

Typical symptoms and signs

1. HIV: wasting, lymphadenopathy and oral candidiasis.
2. Infective endocarditis: a low grade fever, a just palpable spleen, an unexplained normocytic normochromic anaemia, cardiac murmurs and embolic phenomena.
3. Abscess: tenderness – look for other septic foci, and a polymorph leukocytosis:
4. Infarct: tenderness – look for a source of emboli, is this a haemoglobinopathy?
5. Shoulder pain: perisplenitis may be suggested due to abscess or infarct.
6. Portal hypertension: is there a little and so unexpected free ascitic fluid? Are there distended collateral veins on the abdomen?
7. Splenomegaly may be found incidentally in cases of rheumatoid arthritis or systemic lupus erythematosus, but these diseases are dominated by their typical signs.

Investigations

Whatever the investigation, the decision to do it and the result obtained can not be separated from the history and physical signs, and the common diseases of the area.

Blood film

The importance of a blood film examination for malaria parasites cannot be over-emphasized – but interpret the results with caution. A few trophozoites in a high-power field may well represent asymptomatic infection while some other process is responsible for the splenomegaly. The blood film may also reveal the presence of trypanosomes.

White cells and white cell count

In a patient with a pyogenic abscess, or a septicaemia which is not overwhelming – such as staphylococcal septicaemia in an old person – the white cell count is usually raised and has young neutrophils with a shift to the left. Pancytopenia is one of the cardinal features of visceral leishmaniasis. An eosinophilia might suggest Katayama fever, an acute manifestation of schistosomiasis. Lymphopenia is suggestive of an arboviral infection or HIV. Both typhoid and leptospirosis classically present with a normal white cell count.

The morphology of the white cells on a blood film may reveal the abnormal white cells of leukaemia. The commonest cause of splenomegaly among children in a series reported from Lagos (Akinyanju & Lawoyin, 1972) was sickle cell disease, which may be revealed by sickled cells (Chapter 78).

The erythrocyte sedimentation rate (ESR) is often raised in healthy people throughout Africa, the result of a polyclonal gammopathy rather than an acute inflammatory process, which may make a raised ESR difficult to interpret.

Definition of an organism

If the patient with splenomegaly is thought to have an infection, try to define the organism: for example, sputum microscopy for acid fast bacilli, blood and bone marrow cultures for salmonellae, lymph node aspirates for trypanosomes, splenic aspirate for leishmania, or repeated blood cultures for infective endocarditis.

Serological tests, can be very useful, particularly to confirm the diagnosis of HIV, leptospirosis and visceral leishmaniasis. Among immunocompetent individuals, leishmania serology is invariably positive although coexistent HIV infection is becoming increasingly common and makes the test much less sensitive. Hyper-reactive malarial splenomegaly (Chapter 78) has to be considered in any patient with massive enlargement of the spleen. The blood film should be negative for malaria parasites, the immunofluorescent antibody test (IFAT) strongly positive and the total IgM concentration markedly increased (Wallace et al., 1998).

Ultrasound is a useful technique as it may not only confirm the clinical suspicion and exclude, when the signs are difficult to elicit, an enlarged left kidney, but it may also demonstrate splenic abscesses (Tshibwabwa et al., 2000).

References

Akinyanju A, Lawoyin V. (1972). Aetiology of splenomegaly among Africans in Lagos, Nigeria. *Trop Geog Med*; **24**: 49–54.

Bedu-Addo G, Bates I. (2002). Causes of massive tropical splenomegaly in Ghana. *Lancet*; **360**: 449–454.

Bryceson ADM, Fleming AF, Edington GM. (1976). Splenomegaly in Northern Nigeria. *Acta Trop*; **33**: 185–214.

De Cock KM, Hodgen AN, Lucas SB et al. (1987). Chronic splenomegaly in Nairobi, Kenya. I. Epidemiology, malarial antibody and immunoglobulin levels. *Trans Roy Soc Trop Med Hyg*; **81**: 100–106.

Lowenthal MN, Hutt MSR, Jones IG et al. (1980). Massive splenomegaly in Northern Zambia. I. Analysis of 344 cases. *Trans Roy SocTrop Med Hyg*; **74**: 91–98.

Schaefer K-U, Khan B, Gachihi GS et al. (1995). Splenomegaly in Baringo District, Kenya, an area endemic for visceral leishmaniasis and malaria. *Trop Geogr Med*; **47**: 111–114.

Tshibwabwa ET, Mwaba P, Bogle-Taylor J et al. (2000). Four-year study of abdominal ultrasound in 900 Central African adults with AIDS referred for diagnostic imaging. *Abdom Imag*; **25**: 290–296.

Wallace S, Bedu-Addo G, Rutherford TR et al. (1998). Serological similarities between hyper-reactive malarial splenomegaly and splenic lymphoma in West Africa. *Trans Roy Soc Trop Med Hyg*; **92**: 463–467.

82 Body fluids

Water

Steady state

Human beings are approximately 50 per cent water (17–39 years 55%, >60 years 48%), which means that a 70 kg individual carries about 35 litres (=35 kg) of water; of this 16 litres is extra-cellular (tissue fluid and plasma), and 19 litres intracellular.

It is the extra-cellular water, which is effectively sodium chloride solution, that is vulnerable to change in the presence of disease or adverse circumstances. The cells, which contain the intracellular water, are bathed in extra-cellular fluid. It is this extra-cellular fluid therefore that protects the body's cells from damage.

The composition of these two major body 'compartments' are very different from one another (Fig. 82.1). As mentioned above, the extra-cellular fluid is largely sodium chloride solution, whereas the dominant electrolyte inside cells is potassium. It is the cell wall that, by means of its sodium and potassium pumps, maintains this difference.

In a healthy individual, day-to-day body weight remains constant. Water intake and output must therefore be equal. Typical values in a tropical climate are given below.

Water in (ml)		Water out (ml)	
As drinks	1500	Urine	1000
In food	850	Skin	750
Oxidation from food	350	Respiratory tract	750
		Stools	200
Total	2700		2700

Regulation

In the tropics, water losses from the skin and lungs can be as much as 2 litres a day especially in the presence of fever, hyperventilation and low ambient humidity; therefore access to water – clean water – is very important.

There are two important neurophysiological centres for the control of water balance. The thirst centre is in the antero-lateral hypothalamus and, close by, in the neurohypophysis anti-diuretic hormone (ADH) is secreted. There are osmoreceptors in the anterior hypothalamus that stimulate both the thirst centre and the centre in the supra-optic and paraventricular nuclei responsible for ADH release; there are further osmoreceptors in the carotid body that again stimulate the thirst centre and ADH release. There may also be direct sympathetic stimulation of the thirst centre and there is also the stimulus to fluid restriction engendered by hypovolaemia and mediated via the renin–angiotensin system.

Sodium

Steady state

Sodium is the principal cation (140 mmol/l out of a total of 150 mmol/l) in the extra-cellular fluid and with its anions (chloride and bicarbonate) is the most osmotically active constituent. A major function of the body is to retain sodium. Indeed, while mechanisms involved in the retention of sodium are well understood those involved in sodium excretion are only now being elucidated.

Sodium is not a normal constituent of food so individuals without access to salt can have a very low intake. The

!Kung bushmen of northern Botswana live on food that is 70 per cent vegetable by weight. They eat mainly fruit, nuts, roots, bulbs and other vegetables, as well as freshly killed meat. Their urinary sodium output is around 40 mmol/day and their blood pressure remains normal throughout life (Truswell et al., 1972).

In contrast, in industrialized (and some developing) countries the dietary sodium can be as high as 400–500 mmol/day. Such an intake generates thirst so that as much as 2–3 l or more of water may be drunk in 24 h. The requirement of humans, and indeed other mammals, for salt is unknown but it is probably no more than 10 mmol/day.

Since all the salt ingested is absorbed, the most reliable way of estimating sodium intake is by measuring the urinary sodium because other losses of sodium, even in those taking in a lot of salt, are negligible. In people eating little salt, there will be a low urinary sodium, and sweat and saliva that is virtually free of sodium chloride.

Changes in plasma sodium are not a good indicator of sodium status but a much better indicator of water status.

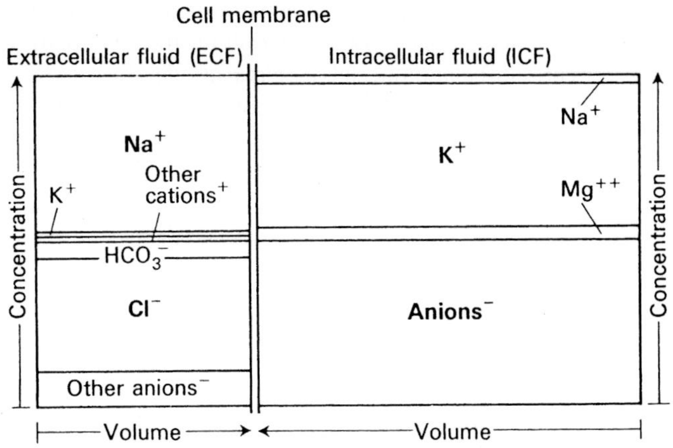

Fig. 82.1. Diagram of fluid compartments in a normal subject in the steady state, and the normal distribution of electrolytes between intra- and extracellular fluid. Heights represent concentrations of substances and widths, volume. The area of each compartment shows the total ionic content. (Modified from Elkinton and Danowski, 1955.)

Regulation

In the steady state, the urinary content of sodium (and a number of other elements including potassium and chloride) is a very accurate measure of intake.

Aldosterone

When conservation of salt is necessary, which is unusual except in disease states, the renin-angiotensin system is activated and as a result of stimulation by angiotensin II, aldosterone, which acts on the distal tubule and collecting ducts of the kidney to retain sodium and excrete potassium, is secreted (see Fig. 82.2, p. 1033). A further mechanism for the retention of sodium, but of lesser importance, is through stimulation of the sympathetic nervous system.

Natriuretic hormone

The search for the mechanisms by which sodium is excreted has occupied the efforts of research workers for at least 40 years. It was thought at one time that the natriuresis following ingestion of salt was simply due to a rise in glomerular filtration rate (GFR) and suppression of aldosterone. However, in rats blood volume expansion experiments in which GFR and plasma sodium were kept constant was still followed by a natriuresis. This occurred even when volume expansion was produced using the rat's own equilibrated blood rather than saline. It was then shown that plasma taken from an 'expanded' rat and injected into a control rat produced a sodium diuresis in the control rat. It was this experiment that demonstrated for the first time that the sodium diuresis was not simply the result of suppression of aldosterone, but the result of secretion of an active natriuretic substance. The search for this 'Third factor' has borne fruit in recent years (Cusi & Taglietti, 2002). It is now known that there are at least four 'natriuretic' hormones, all of which are peptides secreted by the brain, heart and kidney. In the heart the right atrium is one source of peptide and this raises questions as to the role of such peptides in right heart failure; the other cardiac source is probably the ventricular wall.

Potassium

Steady state

Potassium is the body's major intracellular cation just as sodium is the dominant cation in the extracellular fluid. Cell walls actively transport sodium out in exchange for potassium, and when cells die this process stops so sodium leaks in and potassium leaks out. The normal plasma potassium is 3.5–5.0 mmol/l.

A typical daily intake of potassium is 50–150 mmol, which is derived mainly from fruit and vegetables. In the steady state there will be a similar amount of potassium in the urine other than the 5–10 mmol in the stools.

Potassium is important, together with calcium, magnesium and hydrogen ions in determining the excitability of neuromuscular tissue. It is essential also for the activity of some enzymes and for normal renal tubular response to ADH. Unlike plasma sodium, which is minimally affected by cellular shifts, alterations in plasma potassium are considerably influenced by shifts of potassium between the cells and the plasma, and relatively small shifts of potassium from cells (catabolism, fever, etc.) can produce quite significant rises in plasma potassium especially in the presence of reduced renal function.

Regulation

Kidney

Regulation of body potassium is the responsibility of the kidney: most of the potassium filtered at the glomerulus is reabsorbed by the proximal convoluted tubule. It is in the distal convoluted tubule and collecting ducts that hormonal influences (aldosterone) can alter potassium excretion and retention.

Aldosterone

Stimuli to aldosterone secretion and therefore potassium loss in the urine are hyperkalaemia and (in a state of activation of the renin–angiotensin system) angiotensin II. Under the control of aldosterone, potassium can be excreted (in exchange for sodium) according to the needs of the body.

Hydrogen ions (acid–base)

Steady state

Normal body fluid is slightly alkaline with a pH of 7.4. This pH is the optimum to ensure that normal everyday cellular and enzymatic processes within the body are at their most efficient. Small alterations in pH, in either direction, affect metabolism and essential body function and will result in symptoms due to impaired cardiopulmonary and neurological function. More severe alterations can be fatal.

Daily, 80–100 mmol of hydrogen ions ($[H^+]$) and 20 000 mmol of volatile acids in the form of carbon dioxide (CO_2) are added to the body fluids from the metabolism of proteins (H^+) and carbohydrates and fats (CO_2), respectively. The addition of H^+ and CO_2 will tend to make the body fluids less alkaline. Also, certain physiological processes have a similar effect on acid–base status, for example, the secretion of acid by the gastric mucosa and bicarbonate by the pancreas.

Regulation

The body has the task of defending its alkaline environment at all times. There are three lines of defence available. These are:

- buffers
- alterations in respiratory activity
- alterations in kidney handling of hydrogen ions and bicarbonate.

Buffers

Buffering is the first line of defence. Buffers are solutions of a weak acid and its conjugate base. They function by altering their degree of ionization to mop up excess H^+ or, when there is a shortage of H^+, release more. Buffers provide an early defence against acid–base disturbances and limit any potential change in body fluid pH that would otherwise occur from the sudden addition of H^+ or loss of bicarbonate (HCO_3^-).

Extracellular buffers

The most important buffer in the extracellular fluid (ECF) is the H_2CO_3/HCO_3^- system. It is linked to dissolved CO_2, the level of which is regulated by alveolar ventilation. Through this system, H_2CO_3 can be removed or regenerated, by increasing or decreasing alveolar ventilation. The equation is shown below where carbonic anhydrase catalyses the first step:

$$CO_2 + H_2O \rightleftharpoons H_2CO_3 \rightleftharpoons H^+ + HCO_3^-$$

The measurement of blood levels of CO_2 (PCO_2) and HCO_3^- gives an indication of the overall acid–base balance of the body. The Henderson–Hasselbach equation shown below shows the relationship:

$$\frac{PCO_2}{[HCO_3^-]} \propto [H^+]$$

Using this expression, it becomes clear that a rise in PCO_2 will result in a rise in $[H^+]$. In order to restore $[H^+]$ to normal, the kidney must conserve HCO_3^-.

Other important extracellular buffers are plasma proteins.

Intracellular buffers

The most important buffers in the intracellular fluid (ICF) are phosphate and intracellular proteins such as haemoglobin.

Lungs

The lungs provide a means of defence against acid–base disturbances caused by changes in concentration of volatile acids (mainly CO_2). The elimination of CO_2 by the lungs is increased when there is acidosis – for example, the overbreathing that is so familiar in diabetic ketocidosis – and decreased in individuals with alkalosis, by means of a direct effect of pH on the respiratory centre in the medulla.

The ventilatory response to metabolic acidosis starts within minutes of the challenge and reaches a peak in 12 to 24 hours.

Kidneys

To maintain acid–base status, the acids added to the body fluids daily have to be eliminated; the volatile acids by the lungs and the non-volatile acids by the kidneys. The kidneys achieve this by altering the tubular handling of H^+ and HCO_3^-. When the pH is reduced (acidosis), relatively more HCO_3^- is reabsorbed from the renal tubules whilst the secretion of H^+ is increased. By contrast, increased pH (alkalosis) is corrected by increasing the excretion of HCO_3^- and conserving H^+.

Apart from normal metabolic processes, there is gain of H^+ with a tendency to acidosis following episodes of severe diarrhoea as seen in cholera, excessive exercise, salicylate overdose, chronic renal failure and from uncontrolled diabetes mellitus where accumulation of β-hydroxybutyric acid, acetone and aceto-acetic acid occur in body fluids.

Hydrogen ion loss or a net gain of HCO_3^- and hence a tendency to alkalosis results from excessive vomiting as seen in gastritis, hyperemesis gravidarum and vomiting accompanying febrile illnesses, e.g. malaria, urinary tract infection. This can also happen from iatrogenic overadministration of potassium bicarbonate.

Volume (salt and water) depletion

Volume depletion is lack of extracellular fluid involving both plasma and interstitial compartments, in approximately the proportion 1: 11. Usually, there is proportionate loss of water and sodium chloride so the plasma sodium and chloride will be normal.

Hypovolaemia where the plasma sodium is usually normal

Losses from the gastrointestinal tract

Up to 8 litres of fluid daily is either ingested or secreted into the gut. About 97 per cent of this volume is reabsorbed. Failure of reabsorption as a result of pathology leading to diarrhoea and vomiting, nasogastric tube drainage or lack of adequate ingestion, e.g. in disease, is a common cause of volume depletion (Fig. 82.2). Sometimes,

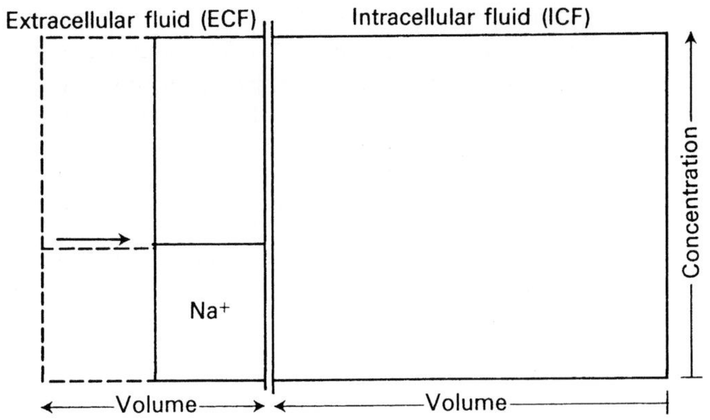

Fig. 82.2. Depletion of water and sodium – since the fluid lost, for example gut secretions, is isotonic and has the same [Na^+] as ECF, the plasma [Na^+] remains normal but there is depletion of ECF volume so the patient is hypovolaemic. The treatment is therefore isotonic fluid until signs of hypovolaemia have gone. ECF: interrupted lines indicate difference between normal state and hypovolaemic state.

there can be increased secretion of fluid and electrolyte into the gastrointestinal tract as occurs in cholera.

Where loss of fluid is mainly from the stomach, large amounts of sodium, chloride and hydrogen ions in addition to water are lost from the body. The result is hypovolaemia, hyponatraemia, hypochloraemia and alkalosis (metabolic). When the bulk of fluid loss is from the lower gut as in diarrhoea or drainage from fistulae, hypokalaemia and low plasma bicarbonate are prominent and the patient becomes acidotic. Additionally, massive bleeding into the gut such as occurs in bleeding oesophageal varices or peptic ulcer can also result in hypovolaemia.

Losses through the kidney

Some causes of polyuria can lead to volume depletion as follows:

- diabetes mellitus – uncontrolled or newly presenting
- excessive use of diuretics
- diuretic phase of acute renal failure
- salt-losing nephropathies.

Losses through the skin

In a tropical climate, especially with low ambient humidity, fluid losses through the skin can be very high: such losses will be exacerbated when there is fever. Remember that patients with burns and certain skin diseases can lose large quantities of fluid and protein by this route, but such patients lose isotonic fluid (plasma), whereas those who lose fluid primarily through sweat lose a hypotonic fluid (sweat), see below.

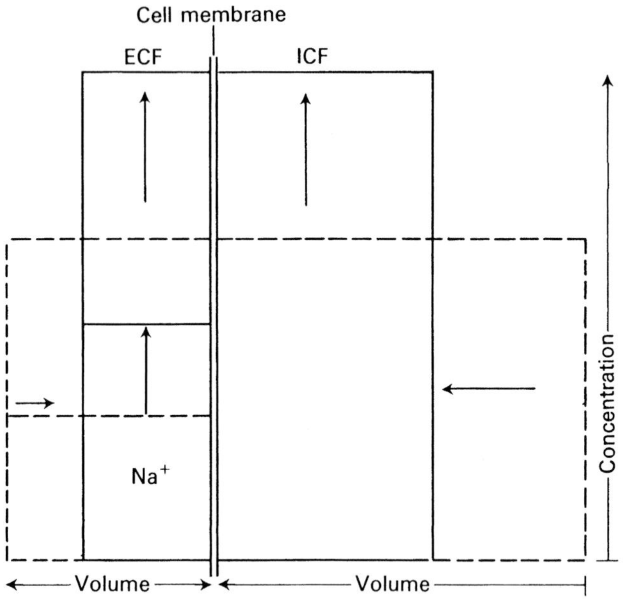

Fig. 82.3. Pure water depletion and hypernatraemia, for example heatstroke, or sweating and tachypnoea in a patient with pneumonia who has had a long and hot journey to hospital without drinking water on the way. Water depletion is dominant, but since there is nearly always also some Na^+ depletion, half-isotonic (0.45%) saline with dextrose can be used in treatment. Both ECF and ICF volumes are reduced and electrolyte concentrations are increased (Elkinton & Danowski, 1995). Normal boundaries shown by the dotted line. Arrows denote direction of change. Note: the volume of water replacement can be calculated as follows:

$$\text{Vol(l)} = 0.05 \times \text{body wt(kg)} \times \frac{\text{plasma Na}^+\text{mmol/l}}{140} - 1$$

'Losses' within the body

Fluid including blood may accumulate in body cavities, within soft tissues, and the gastrointestinal tract. Examples are as follows.

- Body cavities, for example, ascitic fluid especially after drainage
- Soft tissues, for example, at the site of severe trauma including fractures, in snake bites with envenoming and in unrecognized internal bleeding, which in some cases is retroperitoneal.
- Gastrointestinal tract, when much fluid may accumulate in paralytic ileus including post-operative ileus, and in bowel obstruction

Loss of water out of proportion to sodium chloride

Volume depletion can be the result of lack of access to water (in the desert or inability to drink for any reason) or of fever with excessive sweating or heat stroke. In both situations there will be hypovolaemia with high plasma sodium, and the patient will be thirsty (Fig. 82.3).

Loss of sodium and chloride out of proportion to water

This is uncommon but may occur when there is lack of aldosterone (an adrenal hormone responsible for sodium reabsorption in the distal convoluted tubule and collecting ducts of the kidney). Such individuals, who sometimes have complete atrophy of the adrenals, may also be vomiting and thus losing sodium chloride and water additionally through this route.

Correction of volume depletion

Correction of volume (salt and water) depletion must take account of:

- the type of fluid loss
- the severity of depletion of volume
- an estimation of continuing losses, including insensible loss
- the underlying disease condition.

When depletion is mild-to-moderate and the patient is fully conscious and can drink, give fluid by mouth: this is much better than intravenous treatment. Give solutions of oral re-hydration salts liberally until the volume depletion is corrected.

In patients with mild-to-moderate volume depletion who cannot take in oral fluids and in those with severe dehydration, parenteral administration of replacement fluids is necessary. Give the replacement fluid intravenously. Monitor its effects on the signs of volume depletion, blood pressure, the patient's symptoms (including thirst) and urinary output.

Various solutions are available for intravenous administration. Table 82.1 shows the types and composition of solutions available in a typical West African Hospital.

Potassium

Hyperkalaemia

Causes

Hyperkalaemia commonly results from reduced renal excretion of potassium as in renal failure (see Table 82.2). It is also seen when there is altered distribution of potassium between the intracellular and extracellular compart-

Table 82.1. Composition of various solutions available for intravenous infusion in a typical hospital in West Africa

Solution	Constituents	g/l	mEq/l	mM	Cal/l
Isotonic (0.9%) sodium chloride solution	Na^+	3.54	154	154	–
	Cl^-	5.46	154	154	–
5% glucose solution	Dextrose anhydrous	50	–	278	200
10% glucose solution	Dextrose anhydrous	100	–	556	400
50% glucose solution (strong dextrose)	Dextrose anhydrous	500	–	2775	2000
Dextrose 5% + 0.9% sodium chloride solution	Na^+	3.54	154	154	–
	Cl^-	5.46	154	154	–
	Dextrose anhydrous	50	–	278	205
Ringer lactate solution	Na^+	3.0	130.5	130.5	–
	K^+	0.21	5.4	5.4	–
	Ca^{2+}	0.07	3.6	1.8	–
	Cl^-	3.95	111.3	111.3	–
	Lactate	2.51	28.2	28.2	–
Sorbitol 10% in 1/3 Ringer lactate + potassium chloride (Badoe's Solution)	Na^+	0.995	43.3	43.3	–
	K^+	0.634	16.0	16.0	–
	Ca^{2+}	0.026	1.3	0.65	–
	Cl^-	1.835	51.7	51.7	–
	Lactate	0.801	90	90	–
	Sorbitol	100	–	–	390

Table 82.2. Causes of hyperkalaemia

Inadequate excretion
Renal disease
Acute renal failure
Severe chronic renal failure
Addison's disease
Altered distribution between ECF and ICF
Tissue damage
Severe trauma
Massive haemolysis
Severe infections
Acidosis
Drugs
Potassium-sparing diuretics
Angiotensin converting enzyme (ACE) inhibitors
Non-steroidal anti-flammatory drugs (NSAIDS)
Potassium containing drugs
Increased intake
Transfusion of stored blood

ments of body fluids in cell damage, e.g. severe trauma, massive haemolysis, burns, in acidosis and in insulin lack (diabetic ketoacidosis). Patients on potassium-sparing diuretics and those on angiotensin-converting enzyme (ACE) inhibitors can also develop hyperkalaemia. Serum potassium may appear to be raised as a result of haemolysis occurring in the blood sample before laboratory analysis, or when sampling has been slow and difficult.

Clinical features

Cardiac arrythmias such as ventricular fibrillation and asystole precede the neurological effects of hyperkalaemia. They result from abnormalities of cardiac conduction. The ECG will show tall, peaked T waves in mild hyperkalaemia: in more severe hyperkalaemia, flattening of P waves, prolonged PR interval and widening of the QRS complex is seen. The patient may complain of tingling and weakness.

Treatment

- Prompt treatment is essential when the serum potassium exceeds 6.5 mmol/l because of the risk of cardiac arrest. The aim of treatment is to reduce the potential for cardiotoxicity and to remove potassium from the body.
- Give 10 ml of 10 per cent calcium gluconate slowly i.v.; this can be repeated in 30–60 minutes depending on response.
- Drive potassium into the cells by giving insulin plus glucose infusion (50 ml of 50 per cent dextrose with 10 units of soluble insulin slowly over 30 minutes).
- Measure the blood glucose every hour.

Table 82.3. Causes of hypokalaemia

Gastrointestinal	
Increased losses	
Vomiting, diarrhoea	
Fistulas	
Laxative abuse	
Deficient dietary intake (rare)	
Renal	
Potassium-losing diuretics	
Corticosteroid excess	
Hyperaldosteronism	
Altered distribution between ECF and ICF	
Insulin effect	
Alkalosis	
Hypokalaemic periodic paralysis	

- Calcium resonium (polystyrene sulphonate resin) is given orally (15 g four times daily) or rectally (30 g once daily) to remove potassium from the body; this may take up to 6 hours to be effective.

Hypokalaemia

Causes

A low plasma potassium occurs as a result of either increased losses or redistribution between the ECF and ICF as is typical of alkalotic states, where potassium moves into cells. In health, lack of potassium in the diet alone rarely causes a fall in plasma potassium. The causes are shown in Table 82.3.

Clinical features

Mild hypokalaemia (serum potassium 3.0–3.5 mmol/l) may be completely asymptomatic but some patients complain of fatigue, weakness and muscle cramps. More severe hypokalaemia results in cardiac arrhythmias, constipation and hepatic encephalopathy in patients with underlying liver disease. It can also potentiate the unwanted cardiac effects of digoxin and of drugs that prolong the QT interval such as quinine and halofantrine. Patients with a serum potassium below 3 mmol/l will show ECG changes. These include broad flat T waves, ST depression, QT interval prolongation, ventricular arrhythmias, and sometimes a 'U' wave.

Treatment

With the exception of patients with renal failure, give potassium supplements to any patient with serum potassium below 3.0 mmol/l. In those on drugs with arrhythmic side effects enhanced by hypokalaemia supplements must be given when serum potassium is below 3.5 mmol/l.

It is preferable to give supplements by mouth either as dietary supplements (bananas, beans, orange juice, etc.; see Table 76.1) or as slow release potassium chloride tablets (Slow K) at a dose of 40–120 mmol/day. Intravenous replacement is itself dangerous and can only be considered for those with life-threatening depletion and for those who cannot tolerate oral potassium.

Acid–base disorders

Mild disturbances of acid–base status are common in disease and do not require specific management. Occasionally, however, the derangement is more severe and requires active management.

There are two fundamental forms of acid–base disorder:

- a respiratory disorder in which a change in pCO_2 is the primary problem
- a metabolic disorder where the primary problem is a change in the plasma concentration of HCO_3^- or H^+.

Respiratory acidosis

A raised arterial pCO_2, a common feature of a wide variety of respiratory disorders, leads to a change in equilibrium of the Hendersen–Hasselbach equation and the plasma pH tends to fall (acidosis). The causes are given in Table 82.4.

Clinical features

There may be evidence of the underlying cause; these include chronic respiratory disease and chest injury. Typical signs are drowsiness, irritability, flapping tremor and central cyanosis. If the patient is left untreated or given 100 per cent oxygen inappropriately, coma may ensue. Arterial or mixed venous pCO_2 is high with a low arterial pO_2.

Treatment

The treatment is correction of the underlying disorder, assistance with ventilation and administration of the appropriate concentration of oxygen by face mask. It is important not to deprive a patient of oxygen who is in need of it. For most patients, 100 per cent oxygen is suitable but in a patient with chronic respiratory failure it can be dangerous and precipitate worsening drowsiness and eventually coma.

Respiratory alkalosis

This is a common acid–base disorder. It is produced by a decrease in pCO_2 as a result of hyperventilation, either acute or chronic. Important causes are shown in Table 82.4.

Clinical features

Typical symptoms are a feeling of light-headedness and tingling. Signs are tachypnoea and, sometimes, altered consciousness. There may also be signs related to the underlying disorder.

Treatment

Treatment is that of the underlying disorder. Patients with acute hyperventilation and anxiety need appropriate reassurance and sedation. Re-breathing into a bag (preferably not plastic) may reduce the symptoms.

Metabolic acidosis

This is the most important of the acid–base disorders as it tends to occur in very sick patients. The acidosis must be corrected – quickly but cautiously – as death either from the worsening acidosis itself or the underlying condition is common. Usually, the problem is one of overproduction of H^+ such as in the ketoacidosis of diabetes mellitus, where breakdown of fat produces both ketones and H^+. In patients with chronic renal failure the problem is one of lack of excretion of H^+ by the kidney. Sometimes, the condition is a consequence of loss of HCO_3^- into the intestine (cholera) or urine (renal tubular acidosis).

Causes

Important causes are shown in Table 82.4.

Clinical features

When metabolic acidosis is the result of diabetic ketoacidosis, features of the primary condition such as fluid depletion, hypotension and peripheral vasoconstriction are likely to dominate the clinical picture. However, such patients are likely in addition to be overbreathing, which is characteristically slow, deep, 'sighing' ventilation.

Sometimes a clue to the presence of metabolic acidosis is that the patient is apparently 'breathless' yet lying flat, since patients with breathlessness secondary to respiratory disorders, or even more classically cardiac failure with pulmonary venous congestion, are rarely comfortable unless sitting upright.

Table 82.4. Common causes of acid–base disturbances

Acidosis	Alkalosis
Respiratory	**Respiratory**
Alveolar hypoventilation	Hypoxaemia
Opiates, benzodiazepines	Congestive heart failure
Head injuries, encephalitis	Pneumonia
Tetanus	Pulmonary embolism
Massive obesity	Stimulation of respiratory centre
Peripheral nervous system disorder (e.g. Amyotrophic lateral sclerosis)	CNS infections (e.g. encephalitis, meningitis)
Ventilation–Perfusion disturbances	Sepsis
Asthmatic attack	Asthma
Severe pneumonia	Severe anaemia
Pneumothorax	Pregnancy
Aspiration of foreign body	Volitional hyperventilation
Thoracic cage abnormalities	Anxiety-induced
	Hyperventilation syndrome
Metabolic	**Metabolic**
Ketoacidosis	Loss of acid
Diabetic	Vomiting, gastric drainage
Alcoholic	Hyperemesis gravidarum
Starvation	Diuretic usage (e.g. thiazides, frusemide)
Lactic acidosis	Gain of alkali
Excessive exercise	Primary aldosteronism
Generalized convulsions	Liquorice ingestion qu
Chronic renal failure	Excessive alkali ingestion
Salicylate overdose	
Loss of alkaline intestinal secretions	
Diarrhoea	
Fistulae	
Acetazolamide usage	
Renal tubular acidosis	

Treatment

Treatment is directed to both the acidosis itself and the underlying cause.

- Give patients with diabetic ketoacidosis insulin, intravenous fluids and usually (since infection is often the primary problem) antibiotics.
- If the acidosis is severe (pH <7.15 or HCO_3^- <8 mmol/l), give intravenous 1.26 per cent or 1.4 per cent sodium bicarbonate rather than saline (0.9 per cent sodium chloride).

Metabolic alkalosis

Metabolic alkalosis, unlike metabolic acidosis, is not usually life threatening. Typically it occurs in patients with upper gastrointestinal tract disease in whom vomiting is a major feature, or in pregnant women with hyperemesis gravidarum. Important causes are shown in Table 82.4.

Clinical features

The alkalosis itself does not cause any symptoms, but the hypocalcaemia and hypokalaemia that accompany it do produce symptoms. These include tingling around the mouth and in the hands and feet, carpo-pedal spasm, weakness and arrhythmias.

Treatment

Treatment is directed to the underlying cause.

References

Cusi D, Taglietti V. (2002). The time honoured galilean method and genetic association studies: the importance of hypothesis-driven selection of intermediate phenotypes in detecting genes associated to hypertension. *J Hypertens*; **20**: 1703–1705.

Elkinton JR, Danowski TA. (1955). *The Body Fluids. Basic Physiology and Practical Therapeutics*, London: Ballière.

Truswell AS, Kennelly BM, Hansen JDL et al. (1972). Blood pressures of !Kung bushmen in Northern Botswana. *Am Heart J*; **84**: 5–12.

The kidney

83

The problem in Africa

Diseases of the kidneys and urinary tract are seen often in tropical Africa, but the spectrum of disease is very different from that of non-tropical industrialized countries because bacterial, viral and parasitic infections are prevalent and diseases that occur with age and affluence are much less common in Africa.

This chapter brings together the anatomical and physiological basis of renal medicine and the pathological conditions that present whether in health centre or teaching hospital.

Renal function

Glomerular filtration

The waste end products of metabolism, such as urea and creatinine, and the end products of metabolism of many exogenous substances and drugs, are eliminated by the kidney. This function is lost in renal failure so that the action of drugs, for example benzodiazepines, is prolonged (Fig. 83.1).

Tubular function

About 150 litres of glomerular filtrate is formed daily and about 24 000 mmol of sodium is filtered into the nephrons per day. The formation of only about 1–1.5 litres of urine and the reabsorption of up to 99 per cent of the filtered load of sodium per day show the enormous capacity of the kidneys for salt and water conservation.

The kidneys regulate the levels of salt and water in the body. Failure of this will result in salt and water retention with the consequent increase in blood pressure that is seen in most patients with chronic renal failure.

Synthesis

The kidneys are important sites for the production of erythropoietin, which stimulates erythropoiesis, and activation of vitamin D through the 1-α-hydroxylation of 25-hydroxycholecalciferol. Failure of production of erythropoietin is one of the reasons for the normocytic normochromic anaemia that is commonly seen in patients with chronic renal failure. Vitamin D is important in ensuring the proper mineralization of bone and the maintenance of normal calcium levels.

Degradation

The degradation of endogenous substances such as parathyroid hormone and insulin is important and renal failure may lead to the prolongation of the action particularly of insulin. Insulin needs of diabetic patients decrease with the onset of renal failure and such patients will require their dose of insulin modified to avoid the possibility of hypoglycaemia.

Assessment

Glomerular function

The glomerular filtration rate (GFR) is the volume of plasma filtered across the glomerulus per unit time, normally about 80–120 ml/min. In clinical practice the GFR is measured by the clearance of creatinine, formed as a product of normal muscle turnover, that is freely filtered at the glomerulus and is neither absorbed nor secreted by

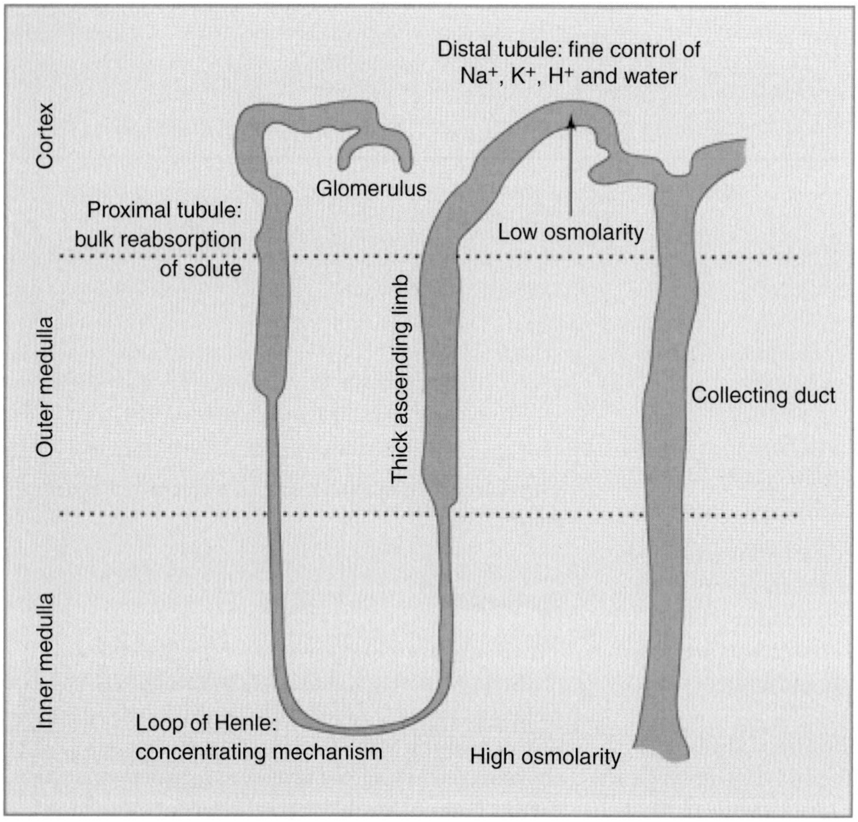

Fig. 83.1. Diagram of a single human nephron.

the renal tubules. Creatinine has another particular advantage in that its plasma level remains relatively constant throughout the 24 hours (Fig. 83.2).

A 24-hour urine collection for urinary creatinine estimation and a single sample of blood for plasma creatinine level are required for the calculation of C_{Cr} using the standard clearance equation thus:

$$\text{GFR (ml/min)} = \text{Creatinine clearance } (C_{Cr}) = \frac{U_{Cr} \times V \times 1000}{P_{Cr} \times 1400}$$

(U_{Cr} = urinary concentration of creatinine; V = 24 h urinary volume; P_{Cr} = plasma creatinine concentration).

24-hour urine collections are unreliable, so a formula directed to predicting C_{Cr} using serum creatinine alone has been developed (Cockroft & Gault, 1976) and been validated in Nigerian patients (Sanusi et al., 2000).

$$C_{Cr}\text{ (ml/min)} = 1.23 \times \frac{(140 - \text{age}) \times \text{weight (kg)}}{\text{Serum creatinine } (\mu\text{mol/l})} \quad \text{(men)}$$

$$C_{Cr}\text{ (ml/min)} = 1.04 \times \frac{(140 - \text{age}) \times \text{weight (kg)}}{\text{Serum creatinine } (\mu\text{mol/l})} \quad \text{(women)}$$

Tubular function

Ability to acidify the urine

The ability of the kidney to acidify the urine within the distal tubule can be tested by the administration of ammonium chloride capsules, the dose being 7 grams (14 ×0.5 gram capsules). It is important to take the capsules with a large volume of water as the capsules can cause gastric irritation. Urine pH is measured every 2 hours for 6 hours; normal subjects can achieve a urine pH of at least 5.1. The test is useful in the detection of renal tubular acidosis but should not be carried out in anyone with plasma bicarbonate $<$20 mmol/l as there is a risk of producing severe acidosis.

Ability to concentrate the urine

The ability to concentrate urine can be demonstrated by overnight water deprivation followed by the parenteral administration of 20 units (1 ml) of pitressin. Normal individuals can achieve a maximal urine osmolality of 1200 milliosmoles/kg. The test is most useful in individuals with unexplained polyuria.

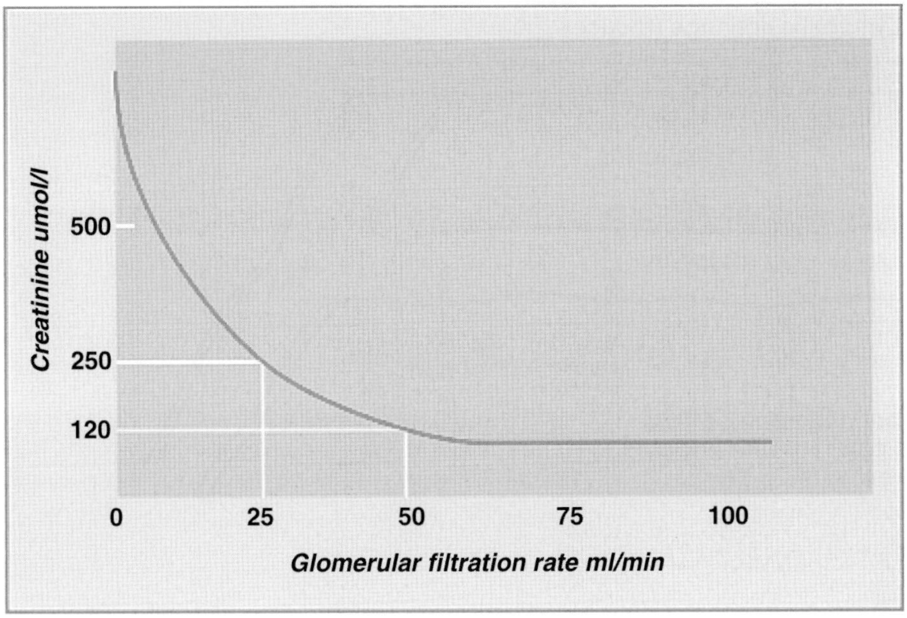

Fig. 83.2. Relationship between serum creatinine and glomerular filtration rate.

Oedema formation

Volume overload is excessive extracellular fluid involving both plasma and interstitial fluid compartments. Usually, there is proportionate retention of water and sodium chloride so there is no change in extracellular (ECF) sodium. The plasma sodium may be low without any explanation, or the consequence of a patient taking a diuretic such as frusemide. Failure of the sodium pump in the cell wall (which is responsible for maintaining the intracellular sodium very low at about 10 mmol/l, compared with a typical plasma sodium of 140 mmol/l) will cause the intracellular sodium to rise. This is called the 'sick cell syndrome'. The prognosis is poor.

Retention of fluid leads to the accumulation of fluid in dependent parts, especially the legs.

Starling's forces

To understand why fluid accumulates in subcutaneous tissues it is necessary to understand the forces operating at the level of the capillary. The principles of the Starling equation are outlined in Fig. 83.3.

Capillary hydrostatic pressure

Capillary hydrostatic pressure is controlled by the pre-capillary sphincter, i.e. at the arterial end of the capillary, so it protects the capillary from increased arterial pressure – as in individuals with high arterial pressure. However, there is no sphincter at the venous end so a rise of pressure in the veins raises intra-capillary pressure.

Plasma oncotic pressure

This is the pressure (negative) exerted by plasma proteins, especially albumin, that holds fluid in the capillary lumen. A fall in plasma albumin disturbs the equilibrium and allows fluid to leak through the capillary wall into the interstitium.

Capillary permeability

Albumin, and if the insult is severe enough larger molecules, will pass into interstitial fluid if the capillary wall becomes more permeable. A common cause is local inflammation, which may be secondary to infection, allergy, burns or toxins; physical damage, such as that caused by stretching, can also be responsible.

Interstitial fluid oncotic pressure

Any protein that leaks out of capillaries is taken away by the lymphatics. Indeed, the lymphatics represent a very efficient system for maintaining the interstitial space relatively free of fluid; they can increase their efficiency considerably. If the lymphatics are obstructed for example by tumour, by secondary deposits from advanced cancer, or by fibrosis, podoconiosis or adult *Wuchereria bancrofti*, the balance will be upset. The

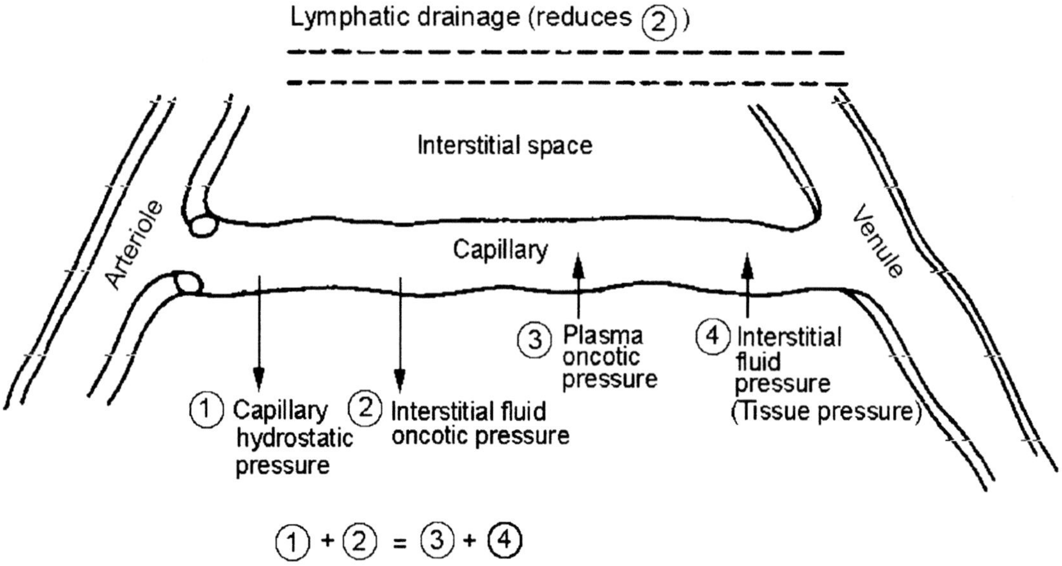

Fig. 83.3. Diagrammatic representation of arteriole, venule and capillary to show the forces involved in the formation of oedema.

woody, grossly swollen leg or scrotum in chronic elephantiasis is an example.

Interstitial fluid hydrostatic pressure or 'tissue pressure'

The hydrostatic pressure is at or slightly below atmospheric pressure, i.e. lower than the capillary hydrostatic pressure. This difference, which on its own might encourage oedema to form, is in health easily outweighed by the oncotic pressure.

Clinical aspects of oedema

Oedema does not form in a normal individual unless the equilibrium described above is disturbed by a change in any of the factors

The site of swelling depends on two influences:

1. *the effect of gravity*, i.e. in the ambulant individual the fluid will be in the feet and legs; in the recumbent position it will be around the buttocks and sacrum;
2. *tissue distensibility*. In some individuals with oedema of the lower legs there may also be peri-orbital or scrotal oedema (Fig. 83.4).

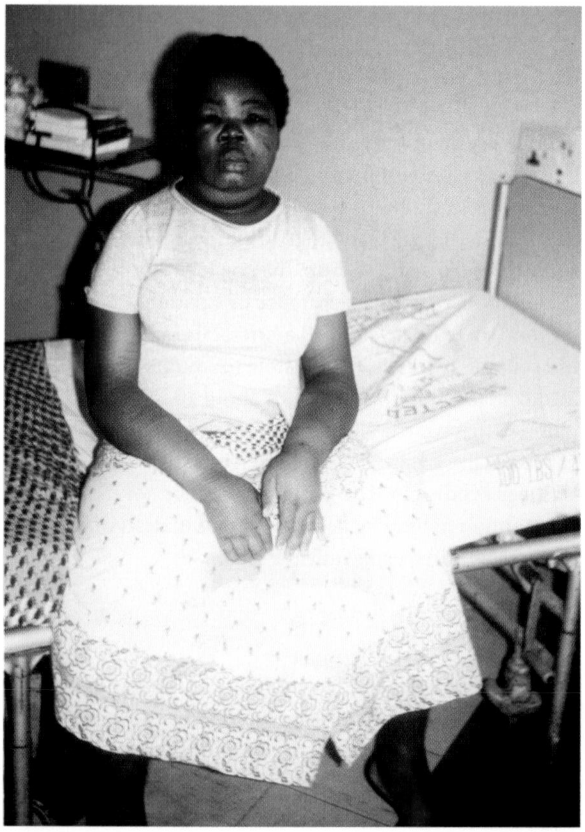

Fig. 83.4. 21-year-old woman with nephrotic syndrome showing oedema of face, arms and legs.

Causes

Hypoproteinaemia

Hypoproteinaemia, especially hypoalbuminaemia, causes a fall in plasma oncotic pressure, which, since the net hydrostatic force does not oppose oedema formation, leads to symmetrical oedema of dependent parts. This fall in plasma volume leads to aldosterone secretion and increased reabsorption of sodium in the distal convoluted tubule and collecting ducts of the kidney.

Cardiac failure

The decreased cardiac output leads to a fall in renal blood flow. This in turn leads to renin secretion by the juxtaglomerular cells in the kidney, and formation of angiotensin I, which is converted to angiotensin II in the lungs. Angiotensin II acts as a direct stimulus to the secretion of aldosterone by the adrenal glands – with consequent retention of sodium. The increase in plasma volume leads to a rise in pressure in the veins, especially of the legs, and this pressure is transmitted via the venules to capillaries. Oedema is the result.

Immobility

Paralysis of a limb – or even immobilization, for example, of a fractured wrist in a plaster cast – leads to loss of the muscle contraction that normally assists flow along veins and lymphatics. The result is accumulation of tissue fluid, and oedema. Other examples are the unilateral swelling of a patient with a hemiplegia, or swelling of the legs of lorry and aeroplane passengers who can be immobile for many hours.

Venous varicosities

Tortuosity and dilatation of leg veins leads to malfunction of the venous valves that normally protect the venules and capillaries from the effects of high pressure. Loss of the protective effect leads to stagnation, dilatation and permanent damage to the skin and subcutaneous tissues.

Lymphatic disease

Disease of the lymphatics is of two types: obstruction and rare inherited conditions. Inherited conditions lead to inadequate lymphatic flow and therefore increasing tissue pressure. In these conditions there are either inadequate numbers of lymphatic vessels or abnormally reduced calibre of lymphatics that are numerically normal.

Symptoms and signs of kidney disease

Symptoms/history

The presentation of renal disease differs from that of other systems; a patient can often be completely unaware that their tiredness and itching, for example, are caused by end-stage renal failure. Many forms of glomerulonephritis are silent, though some produce macroscopic haematuria; others present as swollen feet. Renal involvement in conditions as diverse as diabetes mellitus, hypertension, tuberculosis, sickle cell disease, malaria and leprosy is likely to be silent and only detected by blood or urine testing, or by the finding of high blood pressure.

By contrast, bacterial infection of the kidneys will produce symptoms referable to the urinary tract by causing pain in the loins, frequency, dysuria and sometimes haematuria. Likewise, stone disease is likely to present with loin pain and lower urinary symptoms.

Urine volume

Oliguria and anuria

A common presenting symptom is lack of urine. The so-called 'obligatory' minimum volume of urine is 500 ml/day, which is based on the premise that the body needs to excrete 600 mOsm of solute per day, the maximum urine osmolarity achievable being 1200 mOsm/l. For this reason the term oliguria is applied to a urine volume of <400 ml in 24 hours. Anuria implies no urine at all, a circumstance that may give a clue to the underlying diagnosis.

In the medicine of Africa the most likely cause is hypovolaemia, i.e. the cause is pre-renal (Table 83.1).

Table 83.1. Common causes of oligo-anuria

Pre–renal
Extracellular fluid volume depletion, e.g. diarrhoea, vomiting
Congestive cardiac failure
Haemorrhage, e.g. ante-partum and post-partum haemorrhage
Sepsis
Renal
Rapidly progressive glomerulonephritis, renal vasculitis, etc.
Drugs
Post-renal
Schistosomiasis
Nephrolithiasis
Benign prostatic hypertrophy

Pre-renal oliguria

Clinical history

It is essential to take a focused relevant history.

- Has the patient had a recent or have a current acute febrile illness?
- Has the patient taken any herbs or prescribed drugs?
- Has the patient any urinary tract symptoms?

Clinical signs

The best bedside sign for assessing volume is the jugular venous pressure (JVP). With the patient lying at 45°, and in a good light (preferably daylight), the diffuse distension of the lower neck that occurs with each expiration should be observed carefully. If no rhythmic distension is visible, increase the intra-abdominal pressure by gentle pressure in the centre of the abdomen; you may then be able to see the neck veins. Lying the patient flatter may make the neck veins stand out better, but the reference point remains the manubrio-sternal joint. Once the top of the column of venous blood can be seen, it is possible to make a judgment as to the state of hydration.

Management

In a fluid depleted individual the JVP will usually only be detectable with the patient lying flat, but not at 45°.

Other signs of fluid depletion are a low blood pressure, a small pulse pressure, cold extremities, sunken eyes and facial features, and a decrease in body weight. When these signs are not found a decrease in blood pressure while the patient is seated (or, if safe, standing) should be sought: a fall in either systolic or diastolic blood pressure of 20 mmHg suggests the possibility of volume depletion.

Post-renal oliguria

Symptoms

Loin pain, pain on passing urine, frequency, hesitancy, or urgency suggest possible disease of the ureters or bladder/prostate, or urinary tract obstruction, particularly at the bladder neck.

Signs

Palpate the abdomen and feel for the bladder, which can occasionally be palpable up to the umbilicus. In chronic bladder neck obstruction, the bladder is neither firm and tense, nor tender, because long-standing overdistension of the bladder leads to excessive stretching of, and damage to, the muscle (detrusor) of the bladder wall which therefore becomes very thin. A clinically distended bladder will be dull on percussion. If in doubt pass a sterile bladder catheter. If successful, note the volume of urine passed (residual urine) and keep an hourly record.

Measure urea, creatinine, electrolytes and haemoglobin, and culture the urine. The diagnosis of obstruction can be made unequivocally by ultrasound examination. A plain X-ray of the abdomen might show urinary tract stones, a full bladder or even bony metastases.

Where bladder neck obstruction is possible and a urethral catheter cannot be passed, insert a supra-pubic catheter. Suspicion of ureteric obstruction in the presence of raised urea and creatinine also needs assessment by ultrasound. If not available, nephrostomy may be necessary.

'Renal' causes

If there is no evidence of a pre-renal or post-renal cause, the cause may be renal.

(i) Forms of rapidly progressive glomerulonephritis (microscopic polyangiitis, systemic lupus erythematosus, Goodpasture's syndrome – see below) are uncommon but very important as they are all potentially treatable with corticosteroids.
(ii) Interstitial nephritis may be caused by drug allergy, ascending urinary tract infections and brucellosis.
(iii) A renal biopsy is needed to define the cause precisely.

Polyuria

Polyuria is usually defined as a daily urine volume of more than 3 litres, compared with a usual daily urine volume of 1.0–1.5 litres. In young people about 1 litre is passed during the day, and 0.5 litres at night. In the elderly day and night volumes are roughly equal.

Nocturia

This term is less precise than polyuria and refers to the number of times the bladder is emptied during the night. Increased night time frequency may indicate polyuria but often the problem is one of local lower urinary tract problems and the total volume is not high.

Investigations

Collect a complete 24-hour urine and measure it. If it proves to be >3 litres various possibilities should be considered. There are two main groups of causes:

(a) Solute diuresis, i.e. water is dragged out by the increase in solute.
(b) Water diuresis, i.e. lack of ADH, or psychogenic polydypsia.

Table 83.2 gives the more important causes of polyuria.

Blood pressure

There is an intimate connection between the kidney and blood pressure.

- Many forms of renal disease, especially those affecting the glomeruli, are associated with a high blood pressure.

Table 83.2. Causes of polyuria

Solute-induced	Water-induced
Electrolyte	*Diabetes insipidus*
Sodium chloride	Head trauma
Saline-loading	Surgery
Frusemide	Resection of benign pituitary tumour
Sodium bicarbonate	Post-hypophysectomy
Sodium bicarbonate loss	Idiopathic
	Tuberculosis
	Sarcoidosis
	Post-encephalitis
Non-electrolyte	*Nephrogenic diabetes insipidus*
Glucose	Drugs
Urea	Lithium
Protein-loading	Electrolytes
	Hypokalaemia
	Hypercalcaemia
	Renal interstitial disease
	Sickle cell disease or trait
	Sjögren's syndrome
Both	*Neither*
Post-urinary tract obstruction	Primary polydipsia
Post-acute renal failure	Psychogenic

- Patients with hypertension develop renal damage (Adelekun & Akinsola, 1998; Hussain et al., 1999; Lengani et al., 2000; Veriawa et al., 1990).
- The prognosis of many renal diseases is usually dependent on scrupulous control of blood pressure (Salako et al., 1999).
- Loss of GFR in patients with renal disease is often relatively slow if the blood pressure is well controlled.

Taking the blood pressure

The patient must be sitting comfortably with the arm supported on a flat surface so that the cuff is at the same level as the heart (Fig. 83.5). Squeeze all the air out of the cuff before inflation; apply the cuff to the arm as closely as possible; remove all tight clothing from the arm.

Mercury sphygmomanometers are very accurate and durable but are being replaced in many parts of the world to avoid potential environmental toxicity of the mercury. Measure blood pressure to the nearest 2 mm Hg – not to the nearest 5 mm as has been customary in the past. In research trials three measurements are usually made after the patient has been sitting undisturbed for 5 minutes.

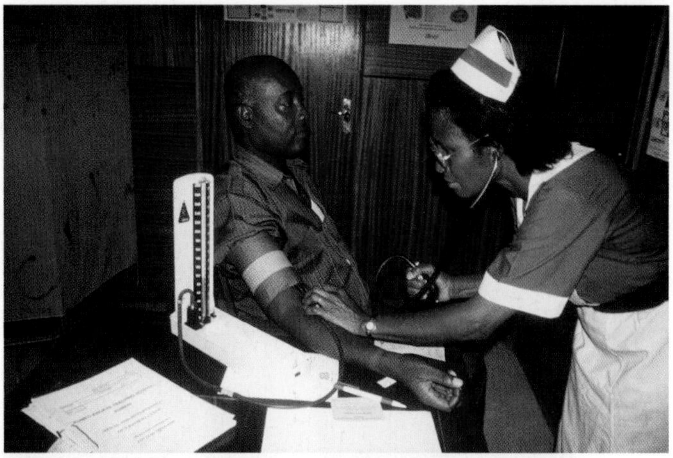

Fig. 83.5. Taking the blood pressure. Note the correct application of the cuff with the arm resting on a flat surface, and at the level of the heart.

The final value is taken as the average of the second and third readings.

Weighing patients

This is fundamental, particularly to assess the effect of treatment (Fig. 83.6). Ordinary 'bathroom' scales are adequate: measure to the nearest 0.5 kg.

- Weigh patients with renal disease and oedema every day, and monitor the effect of their treatment, diuretics or other drugs, by the change in body weight.

Investigation of renal disease

Blood tests

Plasma concentrations of urea and creatinine provide an indication of the state of renal function: plasma creatinine is the more reliable because its plasma level is stable throughout the day, whereas the blood level of urea varies according to protein intake and state of hydration.

In some post-operative patients sometimes the urea is raised out of proportion to the creatinine. The explanation is that under conditions of low urine flow urea leaks back through the renal tubular epithelium and re-enters the circulation. The normal creatinine clearance is 80–120 ml/min whereas the normal urea clearance is only 50–80 ml/min.

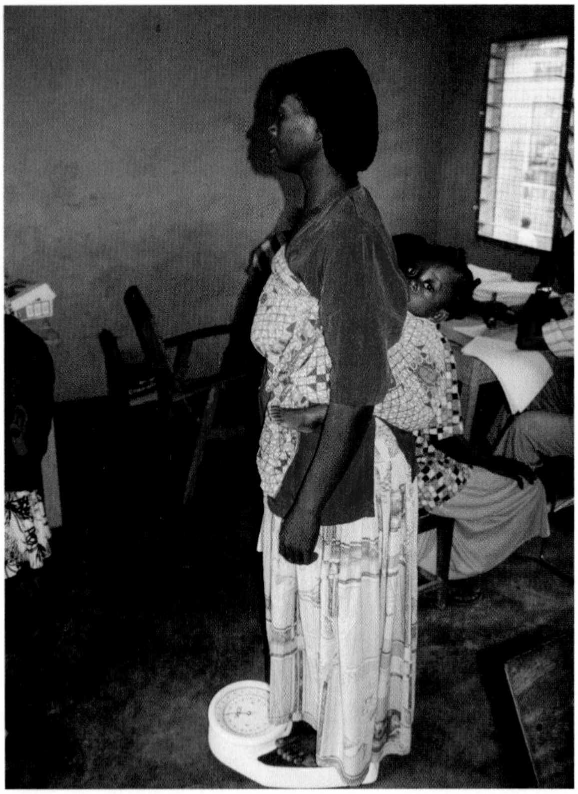

Fig. 83.6. Weighing. Patient being weighed on 'standing' scales; these are widely available and sufficiently accurate for most purposes, but the patient must be without baby or bag.

Causes of a disturbed urea:creatinine ratio

Increased	Decreased
Raised urea	**Reduced urea**
Hypovolaemia	Inadequate intake
Corticosteroids	Reduced liver manufacture
Tetracyclines[a]	
Reduced creatinine	**Raised creatinine**
Muscle mass low	Muscle mass high
	Rhabdomyolysis

[a] All drugs of the tetracycline group other than doxycycline and minocycline raise the blood urea and should be avoided. However, doxycycline and minocycline can be given in normal doses.

Examination of urine

Always examine the urine if you suspect renal/ urinary tract disease and at follow-up of known kidney disease.

Ideally, this is carried out by the attending health worker as part of the routine clinical evaluation of the patient, and preferably in a laboratory attached to the ward or clinic.

Table 83.3. Causes of haematuria

Site of haematuria	Cause
The kidney	Some forms of glomerulonephritis Adult polycystic kidney disease Papillary necrosis Tumours Trauma Tuberculosis Bleeding disorders
The ureter	Stones
The bladder	Infection, e.g. schistosomiasis Tumours Stones

The sample

For most tests, a mid-stream urine (MSU) sample collected into a clean specimen bottle will suffice. In women the external genitalia should be cleaned before the specimen is taken. If possible examine the sample within an hour. If this is not possible, the sample can be stored at 4 °C overnight before examination with very little loss of diagnostic yield.

Appearance

Usually urine is amber in colour and clear. However, the intensity varies according to the patient's state of hydration.

- Deep yellow urine may simply indicate dehydration but may reflect increased bilirubin or urobilinogen in the urine as may be seen in patients with hepatitis or extravascular haemolysis.
- Turbid urine is usually explained by precipitation of phosphate but may indicate pus cells, i.e. infection within the urinary tract.
- 'Smoky' urine is typically seen in patients with acute nephritis when there are red cells in the urine but not enough to cause the urine to be red.
- Red urine

Urine that is red in colour is usually due to macroscopic haematuria as is seen in patients with renal stones, urinary tract infections, schistosomiasis and bladder tumours, or following the ingestion of certain drugs such as rifampicin (Table 83.3). Reddish-brown ('Coca–Cola') urine is seen in patients with intravascular haemolysis and signifies the presence of haemoglobin in urine. Massive muscle destruction with myoglobinuria may also present this way (Fig. 83.7). Centrifugation of a sample of red urine provides an idea of the cause of the colour change. A red sediment with a clear supernatant indicates that the red colour is due to the presence of red blood cells. If the supernatant is red after centrifugation, the red urine is usually due to haemoglobinuria, myoglobinuria or the presence of lysed red cells.

- Frothy urine signifies the presence of large amounts of protein in the urine as in the nephrotic syndrome.
- Milky urine (chyluria) is due to the presence of lymph in the urine and is due to blockage of the efferent lymphatic channels of the renal pelvis: *W.bancrofti* filariasis is one possible cause (Figs. 83.8(a), (b)).

Proteinuria

Normal subjects

In the normal individual, protein enters the urine from three sources:

- plasma proteins which pass through the glomerular filter and are not reabsorbed by the tubules;
- renal tissue proteins secreted by tubular cells or escaping into the urine because of tubular damage;
- bladder and urethral glands.

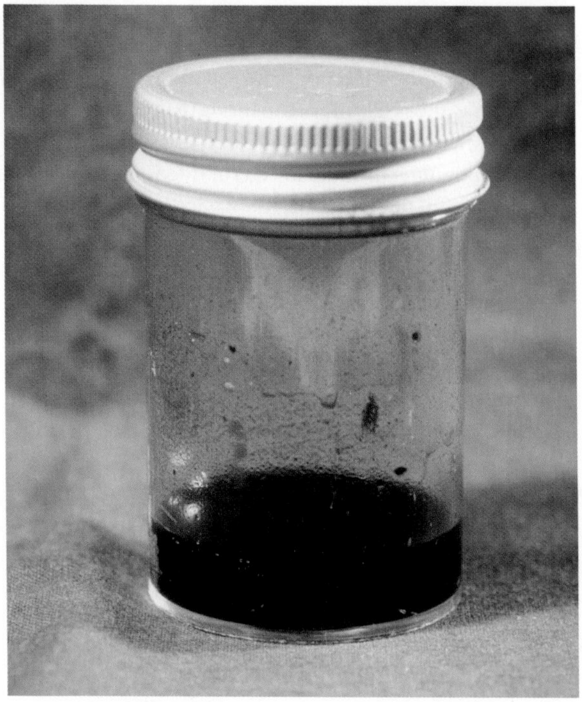

Fig. 83.7. Rhabdomyolysis. Urine taken on presentation from a man with rhabdomyolysis secondary to trauma while intoxicated with alcohol.

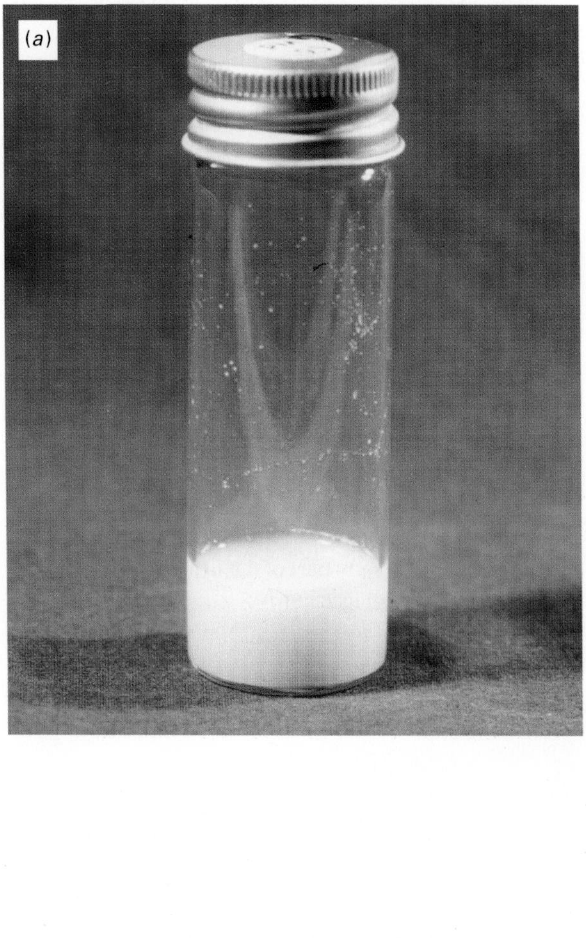

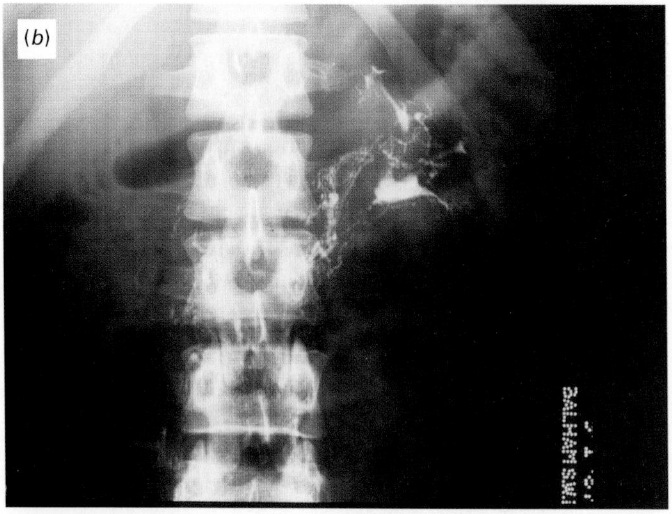

Fig. 83.8. (*a*) Chyluria. Urine passed in out-patients by a man with *Wuchereria bancrofti* infestation. (*b*) Lymphangiogram from same patient. Film shows contrast in para-aortic lymphatics on the left side passing into the adjacent pelvi-calyceal system.

The normal excretion of protein is 80 ± 24 (S.D.) mg/day contributed to more or less equally by plasma and the lining and glands of the urinary tract. About a third of the protein in urine is albumin; the rest is made up of low molecular weight globulins such as β_2 microglobulin, immunoglobulins (principally IgG and IgA) and Tamm–Horsfall mucoprotein.

Pathological proteinuria

There are four types: glomerular, tubular, overflow and 'selective'.

- *Glomerular.* Protein that leaks into the urine through damaged glomerular capillaries. This is typically caused by forms of glomerulonephritis, diabetes mellitus and amyloidosis.
- *Tubular.* Protein that passes into the urine through normal tubular cells, or debris arising because of tubular damage. The usual range is 0.2–2.0 g/24 hours.
- *Overflow.* High levels of low molecular weight substances in the blood overflowing into the urine. The glomerular filtration rate can be normal. Examples are immunoglobulin light chains (in myeloma), haemoglobin and myoglobin.
- *Selective.* In individuals with the form of nephrotic syndrome known as minimal change nephropathy, the urine protein is composed mainly of albumin. In settings where renal biopsy is not possible, and if the laboratory has good resources, calculation of the IgG clearance: transferrin clearance ratio can separate out those whose proteinuria is selective i.e. composed mainly of albumin. If the IgG clearance: transferrin (surrogate for albumin) clearance ratio is <10 per cent, the proteinuria is said to be 'highly selective' and suggests a diagnosis of minimal change nephropathy. This is important for treatment (see below).

Healthy adults excrete no more than 150 mg of protein a day in the urine. This level increases during pregnancy, and transiently during febrile illness, following seizures and after exercise. Amounts up to 1 g a day do not indicate significant disease. Proteinuria of 1–2 g/day is likely to be of tubular origin. Amounts of >3 g/day are likely to have a pathological cause. Apart from overflow proteinuria, significant proteinuria – amounts can range from 2–50 g/day – indicates glomerular damage.

Reagent strips are useful in the evaluation of urinary proteins. The test is based on detecting negatively charged proteins, especially albumin; positively charged proteins including immunoglobulins and Bence-Jones protein (light chains) are not detected. Albumin concentrations below 250 mg/l are not detectable.

Cells

Centrifuge the urine specimen at 3000 r.p.m. for about 5 minutes and make a wet preparation from the sediment for examination.

Three main types of cells are seen on urine microscopy – red blood cells, white blood cells and renal tubular epithelial cells; casts are also seen – hyaline, granular, white cell and red cell casts. Red cell casts are the hallmark of acute glomerulonephritis.

Red blood cells

Count the number of red cells per high power field in the urinary sediment to assess the number of red cells in the urine (Fig. 83.9(*a*)). The normal range is 0–2 cells/high power field (equivalent to1000–5000 red cells/ml). Other causes of red blood cells in urine are urinary tract infection, stone, bladder malignancy, certain types of glomerulonephritis and polycystic kidney disease. Remember, extraneous sources of red cells that may contaminate the urine, such as balanitis, vulvitis and menstrual blood.

Red cells vary in appearance in urine depending on their site of origin. Generally, dysmorphic red cells (acanthocytes of budding yeast-like appearance) are glomerular in origin. In patients with glomerular disease >20 per cent of erythrocytes are dysmorphic (Fig. 83.9(*b*)). Red cells of non-glomerular origin are usually more uniform in size.

White blood cells

White cells in the urine suggest inflammation of the urinary tract and the type of white cells in the urine gives an idea of the type of inflammation. Neutrophil polymorphs (pus cells) are the white cells commonly found in the urine. They are larger than red cells and have a granular cytoplasm and a multi-lobed nucleus. More than four white cells per high power field in spun urine indicates the presence of pyuria, which is the hallmark of bacterial infection of the urinary tract.

Both neutrophil polymorphs and lymphocytes are found in the sterile urine of patients with tuberculosis of the urinary tract. White cells are found in the urine of patients with renal calculi, papillary necrosis and polycystic kidney disease (Fig. 83.9(*c*)).

Epithelial cells

Epithelial cells from any part of the urinary tract may appear in the urine (Fig. 83.9(*d*)).

Other cells

Sediments from spun urine may show malignant cells derived from tumours in the urinary tract.

(a) (b)

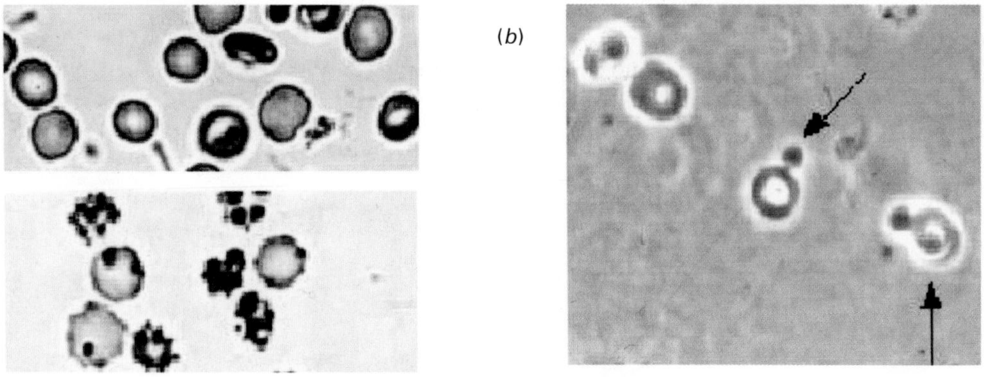

(c) (d)

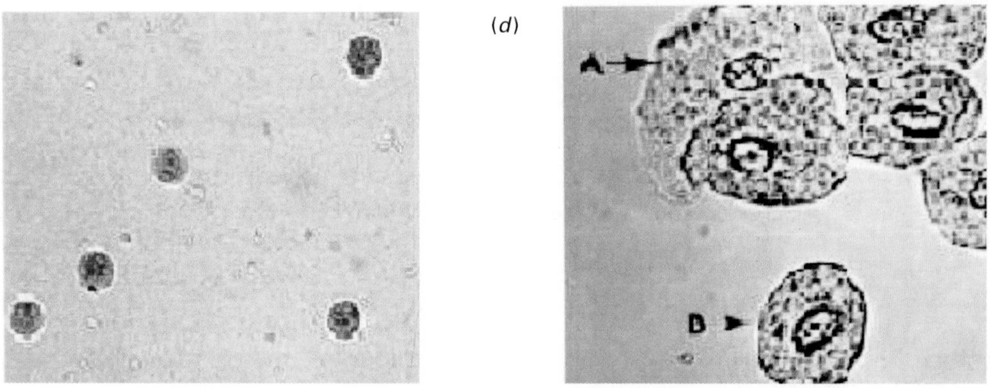

Fig. 83.9. Cells. (*a*) Normal erythrocytes. Note that they may have a crenated appearance (lower panel), often the result of urine with a high osmolality. (*b*) Dysmorphic erythrocytes. (*c*) White blood cells: neutrophil polymorphs with granular-appearance and multi-lobed nuclei. (*d*) Squamous and transitional epithelial cells. Photographs (*a*) and (*d*) reproduced with permission from: Ruthanne Hyduke, MA, University of Iowa from Virtual Hospital (www.vh.org), copyright University of Iowa (*b*) with permission from Hans Kohler, MD and (*c*) Frances Andrus BA. (*b*) and (*c*) were both reproduced from Post, TW, Rose BD. Urinalysis in the diagnosis of renal disease. In: UpToDate, Rose, BD (Ed), UpToDate, Wellesley, MA, 2000. Copyright 2000, UpToDate, Inc (www.uptodate.com).

Casts

Urinary casts are formed from the aggregation of cellular debris and glycoproteins (for example Tamm–Horsfall protein) deposited in the tubule and they may therefore appear in urine. The different types of urinary casts seen provide some idea of the underlying pathology (see Fig. 83.10).

Hyaline casts

These are formed from Tamm–Horsfall protein and are seen in the urine of patients with fever of any cause and sometimes following strenuous exercise.

Red cell casts

Red cell casts indicate glomerular bleeding and are diagnostic of active glomerulonephritis (Fig. 83.10(*a*)).

White cell casts

White cell casts are seen in the urine of patients with acute or chronic inflammation of the renal parenchyma, usually of infectious origin (Fig. 83.10(*b*)).

Epithelial cell casts

Epithelial cells casts are formed from renal tubular epithelial cells. They are usually found in acute tubular necrosis (Fig. 83.10(*c*)).

Granular casts

Granular casts are derived from degenerating cellular casts of all types. Their presence in urine is always pathological. They are seen in glomerular disease with heavy proteinuria but can be a non-specific finding (Fig. 83.10(*d*)).

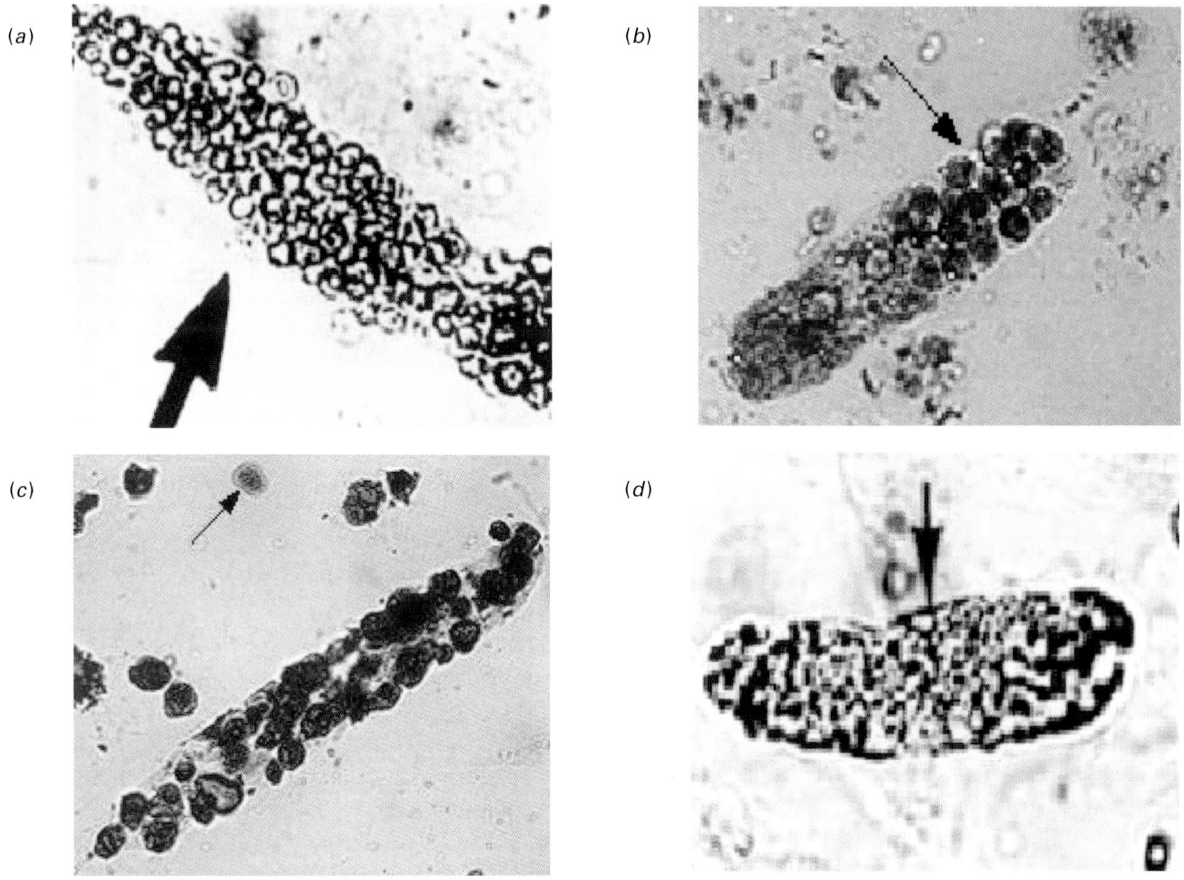

Fig. 83.10. Casts. (*a*) Red cell, (*b*) white cell, (*c*) epithelial cell (note that the epithelial cells are larger than the white blood cell (arrowed)), (*d*) granular. Photographs (*a*) and (*d*) reproduced with permission from: Ruthanne Hyduke, MA, University of Iowa from Virtual Hospital (www.vh.org), copyright University of Iowa and (*b*) and (*c*) with permission from Frances Andrus BA from Post, TW, Rose BD. Urinalysis in the diagnosis of renal disease. In: UpToDate, Rose, BD (Ed), UpToDate, Wellesley, MA, 2000. Copyright 2000, UpToDate, Inc (www.uptodate.com).

Other microscopic findings in urine

Urine microscopy may reveal the presence of crystals, bacteria and the ova of *Schistosoma haematobium* when the patient may report terminal haematuria.

Crystals, which depend on diet, pH and the concentration of the urine, may be seen in the urine of normal individuals and also in those with disease. Typical examples are urate, phosphate and oxalate crystals. Many do not indicate pathology, but cystine crystals are always diagnostic of cystinuria.

Chemical analysis of urine

Several reagent strips exist for the qualitative and semi-quantitative estimation of various chemicals present in urine. These plastic strips, impregnated with chemicals for determining the presence of particular substances, depend on a colour change on contact with urine. It is essential that these reagent strips be read at the time interval specified on the bottle.

Urine pH

Normal urine pH varies between 4.5 and 7.8 depending on the person's diet. It is normally measured using reagent strips during urinalysis or by the use of a pH meter when performing special tests, e.g. for renal tubular acidosis. Clinically, urine pH is important in urinary tract infections with urea-splitting bacteria such as *Proteus mirabilis* when urine of very high pH is produced. It is also important in determining the aetiology of renal stones. Acidic urine is found in patients with metabolic or respiratory acidosis.

Urine specific gravity (SG)

The range is from 1.002 to 1.030. It is useful in:

- determining urinary protein, since a very dilute urine sample may have protein that is too dilute to be detected: use the first urine sample in the morning for determining urine protein.
- determining the cause of polyuria: the SG is low (less than 1.005) in diabetes insipidus where there is loss of urine concentrating ability and also in psychogenic polydipsia. It is increased (greater than 1.020) in diabetes mellitus.

Imaging of the renal tract

Plain film and intravenous urogram

Sometimes one can visualize soft tissues such as liver and kidneys on the plain film and it may be possible to measure the lengths of the kidneys. Urinary tract calculi, if more than 2–3 mm in diameter, can usually be seen as can any bony abnormalities – which, if involving the bony pelvis, may be useful diagnostically.

An intravenous urogram (IVU) (Fig. 83.11) involves the injection of iodinated contrast medium into a vein in the arm. Usually a preliminary film and immediate, 5-, 10- and 20-minute films, and a pre- and post-micturition film are taken; only the preliminary, 20-minute and post-micturition films are full-length. If film is scarce, take only four films (preliminary, 5-minute, 20-minute and one further post-micturition film).

Intravenous urography is very useful for outlining the excretory pathway of the urinary tract (Fig. 83.11) – especially for abnormalities of the calyces (reflux nephropathy, renal tuberculosis, stones, dilatation), pelvis (dilatation, stones), ureters (dilatation, stones, double ureters) and bladder (dilatation, diverticula, stones, anatomical abnormalities, prostatic impression). It is less good for detecting abnormalities of the renal parenchyma.

Ultrasound

The appropriate probe and jelly can be used to define the kidneys, ureters (but only if dilated), and bladder; other abdominal organs can also be imaged.

Ultrasound is useful for the following:

Evaluation of renal anatomy

Renal length and cortical thickness can be measured (Fig. 83.12(*a*)) using a conventional ultrasound machine; also the dimensions of the pelvi-calyceal system. Cysts (simple, or multiple as in polycystic disease, Fig. 83.12(*b*)), solid masses, for example a carcinoma, and calcific densities, such as calculi, which appear 'bright' and cast an 'acoustic' shadow.

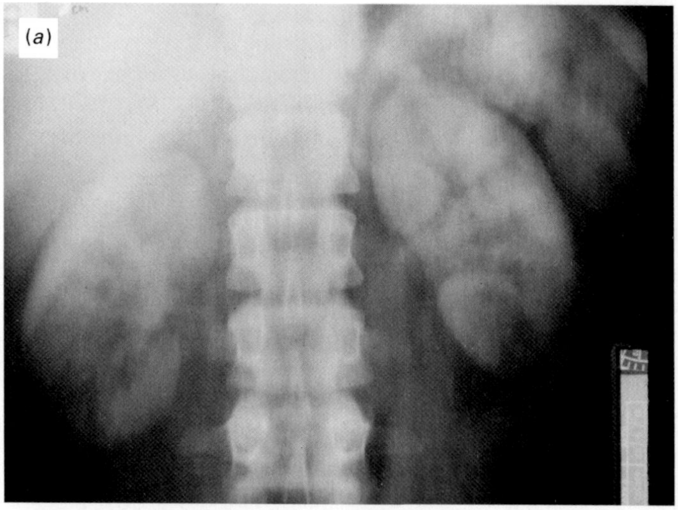

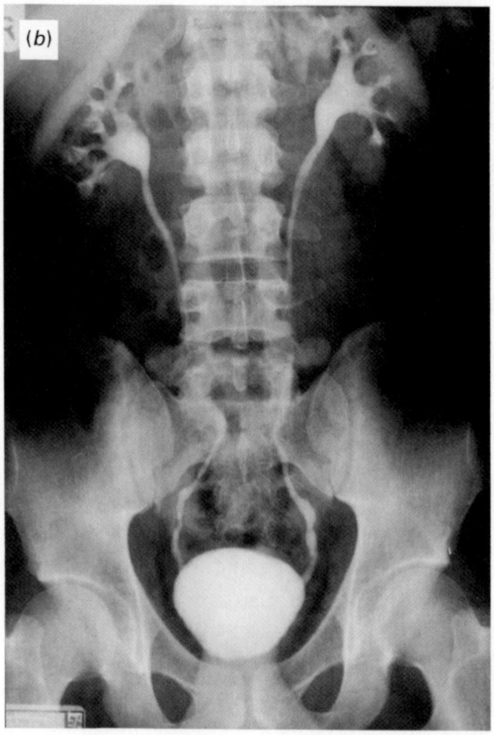

Fig. 83.11. Normal intravenous urogram (IVU).
(*a*) Film taken immediately after contrast given, i.e. 'nephrogram phase' of the IVU. The renal parenchyma becomes diffusely opaque as the contrast reaches the glomerular capillaries.
(*b*) *Same patient.* Full-length IVU film 20 minutes after contrast given. Film demonstrates the fact that the contrast has passed from the parenchyma into the pelvi-calyceal system, ureters and bladder.

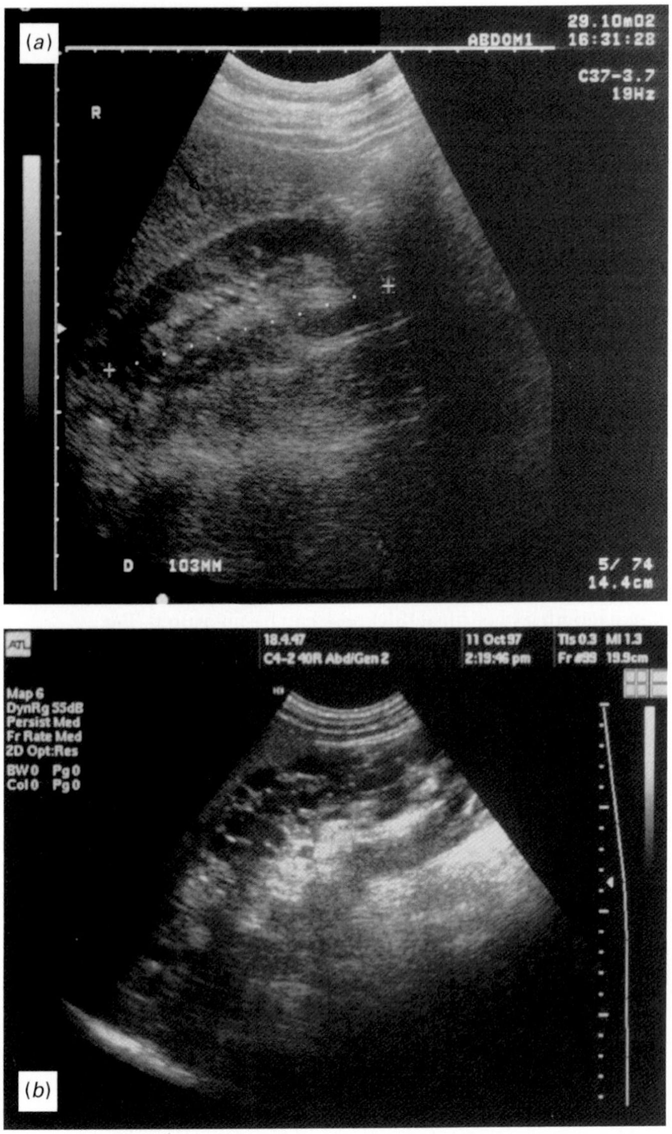

Fig. 83.12. (*a*) Ultrasound scan of normal right kidney, the poles of which are denoted by crosses. Note lack of echogenicity (dark) of renal cortex, which is less echogenic than the normal liver. (*b*) Right kidney shows a number of cysts as circular echo-poor (black) areas.

Evaluation of renal echogenicity

The echo-texture of the normal kidney is less than that of the liver. Increase in renal echogenicity usually indicates an increase in fibrous tissue and often denotes a chronic process.

Evaluation of the bladder

It is important to examine the bladder ultrasonically in any patient with renal impairment. Look for:

- an enlarged bladder, with a thickened wall, or dilated as a consequence of bladder neck obstruction;
- stones or tumour;

Note: The ureters are not normally seen unless they are dilated.

- ability to empty the bladder: this is particularly important in a patient with recurrent urinary infections. Ultrasound before and after micturition will provide approximate volume of urine in the bladder for the two examinations.

Computed tomography (CT)

CT scanning can give important information on renal anatomy. Comparison of images before and, after contrast, can determine the operability of renal tumours, and secondaries in the chest, thereby preventing unnecessary surgery.

Urinary tract masses and other pathology outside the urinary tract can be visualized by CT scanning but not by IVU or with any accuracy by ultrasound.

In patients with acute or chronic renal failure, or in those on dialysis, in whom the level of consciousness is disturbed, a CT scan of the head can be invaluable in distinguishing between sub-arachnoid haemorrhage, subdural haematoma, intracerebral abscess and diffuse inflammatory conditions.

Other investigations

- Renal arteriography can define renal artery stenosis, whether due to idiopathic tropical aortitis or a disorder of the renal artery itself (Fig. 83.13). Very rarely, it will reveal the arteriolar aneurysms of polyangiitis nodosa.
- Radio-isotopes can also be used to define renal function and structure.
- Magnetic resonance imaging (MRI) too can sometimes be useful.
- Doppler ultrasound.

Renal biopsy

Percutaneous renal biopsy is an important investigation, but it is not without risk – chiefly bleeding.

Figure 83.14 shows a slide of normal renal histology. Therefore, only do a biopsy if there are:

- trained operators in a safe hospital environment
- disposable biopsy needles
- access to cross-match and speedy blood transfusion
- assured transport to the laboratory
- specialist renal histopathology.

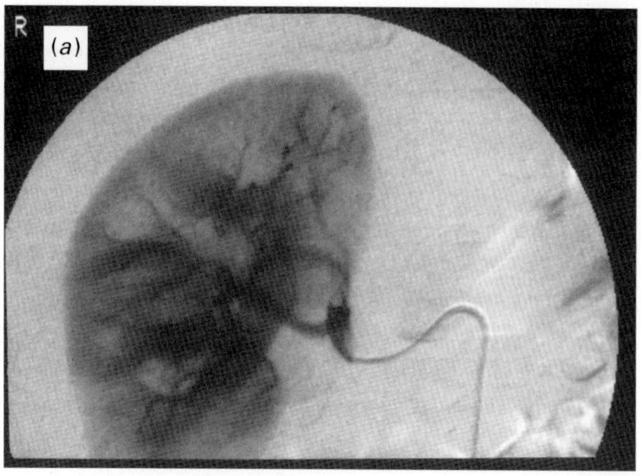

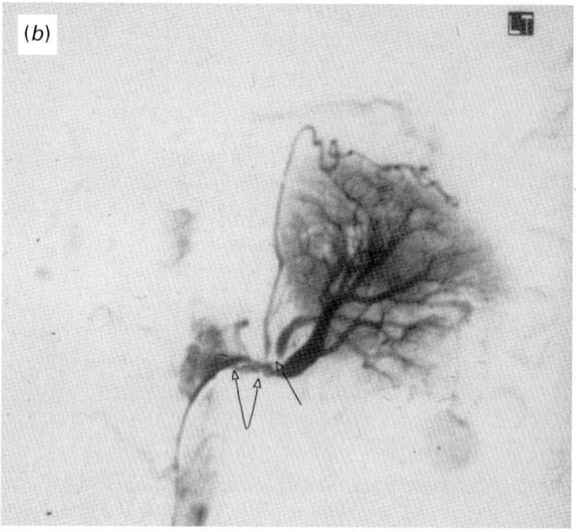

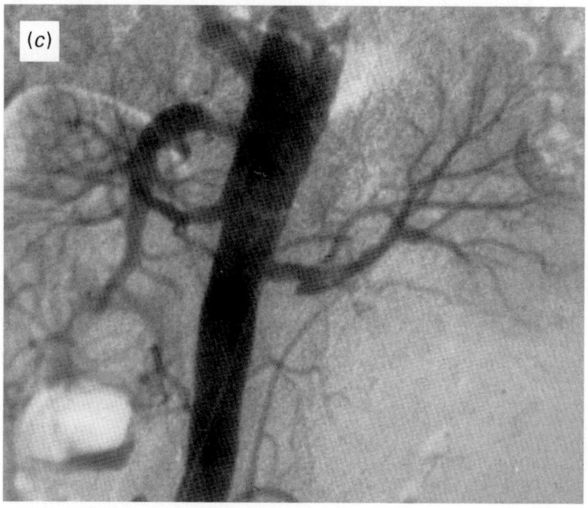

Fig. 83.13. (*a*) Polyarteritis nodosa. Selective right renal arteriogram showing a number of arterial anerysms (black dots) in the upper pole of the right kidney.
(*b*) Renal arteriography shows stenosis of the main artery (pair of arrows) to small left kidney, and stenosis of origin of superior branch (arrow). Both vessels show post-stenotic dilatation. The features are typical of fibromuscular dysplasia (42-year-old Ghanaian man with severe hypertension.)
(*c*) Three weeks after intra-luminal dilatation of both stenoses: the renal vessels now appear normal. Note that the aorta shows no evidence of atheroma.

Indications

Restrict biopsy to patients where knowledge of renal histology will affect management.

Nephrotic syndrome
In adults, in contrast to children, prednisolone-responsive conditions do not predominate. A biopsy should be taken if prednisolone treatment is being considered.

Proteinuric states
Usually, renal biopsy is the only way of making a firm diagnosis, unless there is other evidence of systemic disease as in systemic lupus erythematosus (SLE), or vasculitides. Sometimes, both patient and doctor benefit from a firm diagnosis.

Suspected glomerular pathology in non-nephrotic patients
Patients with possible renal vasculitis respond well to prednisolone.

Acute renal failure
Most patients with acute renal failure have relatively normal kidneys histologically: renal biopsy is only indicated if an acute vasculitis or acute interstitial nephritis is considered and prednisolone treatment contemplated.

CLINICAL RENAL DISEASES

Nephrotic syndrome

The problem in Africa

The spectrum of causes is very different from that of industrialized countries (McLigeyo, 1990; Diallo et al., 1997b).

Cardinal physical signs of the nephrotic syndrome are swelling of the legs and abdomen as well as swelling around the eyes. These signs are seen in other conditions in sub-Saharan Africa also, so the diagnosis of nephrotic syndrome must be confirmed by urine testing for protein.

Definition

The nephrotic syndrome is the presence of heavy proteinuria (>3.5 g/day) in association with generalized oedema, hypoalbuminaemia (<30 g/l) and hyperlipidaemia.

Swelling of the lower extremities is a classical sign of renal disease. Urinary stick testing will reveal protein of '+++' or '++++', depending on the level of proteinuria and the volume of urine. Since plasma volume is not increased, hypertension is uncommon unless there is a mixed nephritic/nephrotic picture.

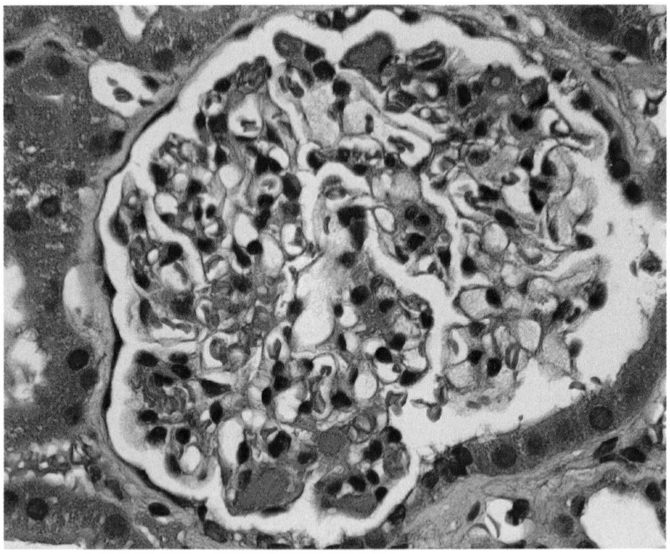

Fig. 83.14. Normal glomerulus. Haematoxylin and eosin stain.

In Africa, post-streptococcal glomerulonephritis is a particularly common cause, but minimal change nephropathy (see below) and membranous nephropathy (Fig. 83.15) are also common. Other causes include diabetes mellitus, leprosy, malaria, drugs (especially NSAIDs) and systemic erythematosus.

There have been a number of reports of renal histology in nephrotic syndrome in Africa. Among 119 adults and children in Zimbabwe with sustained proteinuria, proliferative forms of glomerulonephritis, including IgM nephropathy and membranous glomerulonephritis, were revealed as important causes (Table 83.4). There were 11 cases of minimal change nephropathy but no cases of IgA nephropathy. Interestingly, no patients with HIV nephropathy were identified but we suspect such cases will become more common (Borok et al., 1997).

Pathophysiology

Glomerular damage

The primary problem is glomerular damage with consequent leak of protein through the damaged glomerular capillary walls into the glomerular filtrate and ultimately the urine. Proteinuria of 5–10 g/day can be associated with a very low plasma albumin and oedema and yet the liver can synthesize 25–50 g/day. The reason for this apparent paradox is that in patients with nephrotic syndrome the kidney breaks down albumin; so that much albumin is lost other than as measured albumin in the urine. While the amino acids generated by this albumin

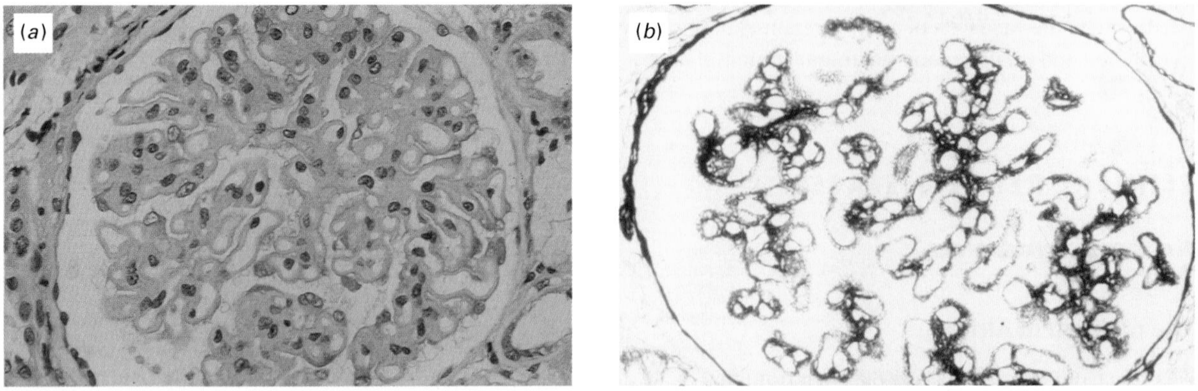

Fig. 83.15. Membranous glomerulonephritis. (*a*) Glomerulus shows thickening of capillary loops; there is no increased cellularity. Haematoxylin and eosin stain. (*b*) Section shows basement membrane. The 'chain-link' effect in the membrane is produced by the contrast between the darkly staining material (basement membrane) and the lucent areas (caused by deposits not taking up the stain). Silver stain.

Table 83.4. Histology in 119 patients with proteinuria in Zimbabwe

Histopathology	Percentage
Glomerulonephritis	
Minimal change	9.2
Membranous	15.1
Focal segmental glomerulosclerosis (FSGS)	15.1
Proliferative	
Diffuse mesangial	21.0
Membrano-proliferative	12.6
Other	17.0

catabolism can be used by the liver, its synthetic capacity is inadequate to maintain a normal plasma albumin.

This leads to a fall in plasma oncotic pressure and leakage of fluid into the interstitial space. The loss of fluid leads to a (potential) fall in circulating blood volume, stimulation of the renin-angiotensin system and secretion of aldosterone. This causes tubular reabsorption of salt and water, and the process continues until equilibrium is reached. Unlike many other forms of renal disease, nephrotic syndrome is not usually associated with hypertension.

Hypercholesterolaemia

This is another typical feature of the nephrotic syndrome. The precise mechanism is unclear but it appears to be a consequence of the hypoalbuminaemia. There is both increased formation of lipoprotein in the liver and decreased clearance by lipoprotein lipase.

Clinical features

The typical patient has:

- oedema of the legs
- periorbital oedema
- ascites
- pleural effusions.

Oedema may involve the thighs, abdomen and face. In individuals whose nephrotic syndrome is of long standing, the typical changes of a low protein state are seen in hair, skin, finger nails and muscles.

Differential diagnosis

In a malnourished population, where hepatitis B and other liver conditions are common, the differential diagnosis is wide, so that a specific diagnosis can be difficult. Indeed, the clinical picture of nephrotic syndrome in Africa may present earlier because of the relative undernutrition and marginal protein status of the population.

Management

There is very often no specific treatment for the underlying condition.

General treatment

The oedematous limbs are prone to infection. It is important, therefore, to try to reduce the oedema by oral diuretics. Thiazides, frusemide and spironolactone are all effective. First, give bendrofluazide 5 mg daily. In unresponsive patients, 40–120 mg of frusemide daily should be given orally. It is important to avoid over-diuresis, especially in individuals (with 'minimal change' nephropathy) about to respond to prednisolone as there may be hypovolaemia and 'pre-renal' renal failure. Hypovolaemia may also predispose to venous thrombosis. Record the patient's body weight daily to assess the response to diuretic therapy. Aim to reduce the weight of the patient by 0.5–1.0 kg per day.

In the absence of uraemia, a high protein diet (1.5–2.0 g/kg body weight) has been reported to be beneficial. It is worth noting, however, that high protein diets do not cause the plasma albumin to rise.

Skin infections must be detected early and treated vigorously with broad-spectrum antibiotics such as ampicillin and flucloxacillin.

Specific treatment

There are two important conditions that respond to specific treatment.

Minimal change nephropathy

Heavy proteinuria, lack of RBC in the urine, normal urea and creatinine, and a normal blood pressure make the diagnosis likely. If, in addition, the proteinuria is of the selective (mainly albumin) type it is highly likely that the condition will respond to corticosteroids such as prednisolone: the aim is to induce remission, i.e. loss of proteinuria, in 10–20 days. The diuresis and loss of oedema may take a further 7–14 days. The usual dose in adults is 60 mg daily. The dose can be halved when there is no longer any proteinuria. The aim is to reduce and stop the prednisolone by 3–6 months. Non-responders are those who do not respond by 2 months, so in such cases reduce the prednisolone over a number of weeks and then stop it. About 50 per cent of patients with minimal change nephropathy relapse, often within a year. It is usual to use the same regimen that induced remission in the first episode.

Table 83.5. Histological classification of the glomerulonephritides

Classification	Clinical association
With glomerular hypercellularity ('proliferative')	
Diffuse proliferative without polymorphs	IgA and other nephropathies
Diffuse proliferative with polymorphs	Acute glomerulonephritis
Membrano-proliferative	SLE, sub-acute bacterial endocarditis
Focal proliferative	
Without glomerular hypercellularity	
Membranous	Hepatitis B
Minimal change	
Focal segmental glomerulosclerosis (FSGS)	Sickle cell anaemia

Lupus nephritis
The diagnosis is made if there are the typical symptoms (symmetrical small joint arthropathy, fever, solar hypersensitivity, skin rashes, hair loss) or signs (butterfly rash on bridge of nose and cheeks, vasculitic skin lesions on fingers) in combination with microscopic haematuria. Like minimal change nephropathy, the treatment of choice is prednisolone, given as described under nephropathy (above).

Use of prednisolone
In Africa, studies of renal histopathology indicate that, while some 80 per cent of nephrotic children will have minimal change disease, in adults the proportion is only about 20 per cent. It is usual to give a 'trial of steroids' in children but in adults it is best practice to give prednisolone only when there is evidence of minimal change nephropathy on renal histology, or at least highly selective proteinuria (<10%). Remember that there are unwanted effects of prednisolone – reactivation of latent tuberculosis and of *Strongyloides*, peptic ulceration, adrenal suppression – so any course of high dose prednisolone should be no longer than 2 months at most. Also, do not stop the drug abruptly!

Prognosis

For African children with the nephrotic syndrome the prognosis is excellent, because individuals with minimal change nephropathy only rarely develop renal failure and then only because of some unforeseen adverse event.

For adults, the prognosis – apart from the 20 per cent with minimal change nephropathy – is likely to be poor. Poor prognostic factors are high blood pressure, raised urea and creatinine, heavy proteinuria and an active urinary sediment (see below).

Glomerulonephritis (Table 83.5)

The problem in Africa

There are a number of reports from sub-Saharan Africa of different forms of glomerulonephritis (Wiggelinkhuizen, 1987; Youmbissi et al., 1999), which may be commoner in Africa than in temperate countries.

Proteinuria is the hallmark of this group of disorders, which are characterized by bilateral renal disease, where diffuse immunological damage is an important aetiological factor; in most types the cause is unknown and there is no specific treatment.

Clinical features

Patients present in several ways:

- chance finding of proteinuria
- recurrent macroscopic haematuria (p. 1058)
- nephritic syndrome as exemplified by acute (post-streptococcal) glomerulonepritis (see below).
- nephrotic syndrome (p. 1053)
- acute renal failure (p. 1060)
- chronic renal failure (p. 1064).

The most consistent feature of glomerulonephritis is proteinuria. Nevertheless, there are forms that may not be associated with proteinuria, for example IgA nephropathy. Other features are hypertension and, in many cases, by the time patients present they may be in early or even more advanced renal failure.

The acute nephritic syndrome

The acute nephritic syndrome is an acute febrile illness, often with upper respiratory symptoms and pharyngitis, in association with oedema, high blood pressure and raised jugular venous pressure. Typically, the urine is darker than normal because it contains large numbers of red blood cells, which can be seen on microscopy.

Pathogenesis

The commonest cause is acute glomerulonephritis (acute nephritis). This typically presents 18–21 days after a sore throat caused by Lancefield group A β-haemolytic Streptococci; Types 12 (throat) and 2, 26 and 49 (skin) are most frequently responsible. Very often the site of infection is not the pharynx but the skin, especially as secondary infection in a child or young adult with scabies. In industrialized countries the condition is much less common than formerly, and when it does occur evidence of recent streptococcal infection, i.e. a positive anti-DNA – B or anti-streptolysin O titre, is usually lacking.

Pathophysiological disturbances

Renal histology shows hypercellularity: the pathognomonic feature is polymorphs stuck to the endothelium of glomerular capillaries (Fig. 83.16). This glomerular damage leads to the passage of protein and red cells into the urine. In some patients the albumin is as low as in patients with the nephrotic syndrome.

Clinical presentation

The child or young adult presents with hypertension, volume overload and sometimes worsening renal function, when hyperkalaemia and acidosis become pressing clinical problems. Oliguria indicates a bad prognosis especially if there is no prospect of dialysis. In this acute illness there is marked salt and water retention leading to hypertension, a raised jugular venous pressure, pulmonary oedema, peripheral oedema and oliguria. Around 50 per cent of patients are nephrotic. It is the most oliguric patients that potentially have the largest gains in fluid volume and highest blood pressures, so are most likely to develop severe pulmonary oedema and hypertensive encephalopathy. Seizures are a poor prognostic sign. Most children recover spontaneously from an attack of acute glomerulonephritis.

Management

Fluid overload

- Assess the degree of fluid overload both clinically and by weighing the patient. If you know the patient's usual weight, a target weight can be calculated with confidence. If you do not know it, try to work out the patient's dry weight but be ready to adjust your calculation as the illness progresses.

A combination of fluid restriction and oral diuretics should effect a satisfactory diuresis.

- Give frusemide 40 mg daily, doubling the dose every day or so until there is a satisfactory response. Sometimes a dose of 200–300 mg a day is required. Remember that 'input-output' charts, even when well kept, can be misleading. They are often only a rough estimate of fluid balance and do not take account of sweating, diarrhoea and other fluid losses, but use them to detect a falling urine output.

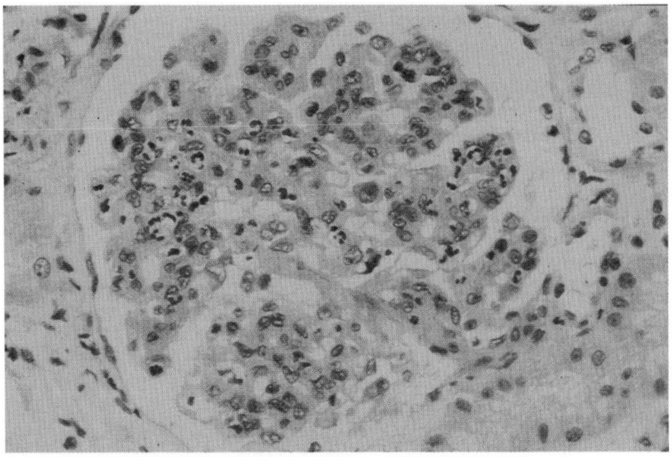

Fig. 83.16. Acute glomerulonephritis.
Glomerulus shows hypercellularity, many of the cells being polymorphonuclear leukocytes. These cells are pathognomonic of acute glomerulonephritis.

- Weigh the patient every day: there is no substitute for this simple procedure.

High blood pressure

A most important aspect of management is lowering the blood pressure to take the strain off the heart as well as to prevent the very serious complication of hypertensive encephalopathy as manifested clinically by confusion, headache, seizures and coma.

- Oral drugs are safe and effective; intravenous and intramuscular administration can lower the blood pressure dangerously quickly and should be avoided.
- Aim to bring the blood pressure down slowly, i.e. step-wise day by day, in patients with a very high blood pressure – above 220 mm Hg systolic or 120 mm Hg diastolic. A blood pressure of 180/110 after 24 hours is a safe and satisfactory response.
- Start with nifedipine tablets 'Adalat Retard' 10 or 20 mg (swallowed) or long-acting formulation 'Adalat LA'. Nifedipine capsules, which are sucked not swallowed, can produce a devastating fall in blood pressure and should on no account be used. Add a beta-blocker, such as atenolol 50 mg, in patients who have a tachycardia or ischaemic heart disease.
- Treat seizures with diazepam 5–10 mg intravenously as a short-term measure; at the same time give phenytoin (if available) in a dose of 200 mg, intravenously. This is important as early administration of phenytoin (which is metabolized in the liver so can be given

Table 83.6. Differential diagnosis of acute glomerulonephritis

Condition	Clinical	Investigation	Potential treatment
Sub-acute bacterial endocarditis	Heart murmurs	Blood cultures	Antibiotics
Systemic lupus erythematosus	Skin, hair, joint symptoms	Anti-nuclear antibodies	Prednisolone
Microscopic polyangiitis (Wegener's granuloma)	Nasal stuffiness, collapse of cartilaginous nasal septum	Anti-neutrophil cytoplasmic antibody	Prednisolone and cyclophosphamide
Anti-glomerular basement membrane (Goodpasture's) disease	Respiratory symptoms, including haemoptysis	Anti-glomerular basement membrane antibody	

in normal dosage) will reduce the need for repeated doses of diazepam, which in patients with impaired renal function tends to accumulate and can lead to extreme drowsiness and hypoventilation producing a most confusing clinical picture.

Eradication of Streptococcus
Penicillin V orally or Procaine penicillin intramuscularly will eradicate the Streptococcus but there is no evidence that there is any effect on the clinical course of the disease or outcome.

Other causes of acute nephritic syndromes (see Table 83.6)

Chronic glomerulonephritis

The group of disorders known as the chronic glomerulonephritides are characterized by:
- proteinuria
- diffuse immune-mediated renal disease
- kidneys that are usually normal on imaging.

Some, such as IgA nephropathy, may not be associated with proteinuria but may present as macroscopic haematuria. Some forms, such as membranous nephropathy, typically present as the nephrotic syndrome. All forms may simply come to notice when proteinuria is detected on urine testing.

Recurrent macroscopic haematuria and related conditions

This is a condition of young adults characterized by recurrent episodes of macroscopic haematuria often in association with an upper respiratory infection or sore throat. Renal biopsy will usually show IgA nephropathy, a condition characterized by deposition of immunoglobulin A in the glomerular mesangium (Swanepoel et al., 1998).

Henoch–Schönlein syndrome is a condition of children and young adults that presents with purpura (often widespread), joint pain, abdominal pain and blood in the urine. The haematuria can sometimes be macroscopic, i.e. the urine is red to the naked eye. Renal biopsy reveals IgA and fibrinogen in glomeruli.

Glomerulonephritis with blood in the urine is usually due to one of these two conditions. The prognosis for both is very good and there is no specific treatment. Occasionally, a patient with IgA nephropathy will develop progressive renal failure and after 5–10 years eventually reach end-stage, and be in need of dialysis.

Mesangial IgA nephropathy, the commonest form of glomerulonephritis worldwide, has hardly been reported in studies from Africa, e.g. Table 83.4.

Renal disease and parasites

Schistosoma haematobium – bilharziasis

Infection of the lower urinary tract with eggs and adults of *S. haematobium* classically causes fibrosis of the ureters and bladder, and so leads to urinary tract obstruction (Subramanian et al., 1999). Plain X-rays may show calcification of the bladder (Fig. 83.17) and radiology with contrast (IVU, antegrade or retrograde pyelography) may show ureteric dilatation (Fig. 83.18). There is now evidence also that the parasite may cause glomerular damage and proteinuria.

Schistosoma mansoni

Patients with hepatosplenic schistosomiasis may show deposits of immune-complexes in the glomeruli.

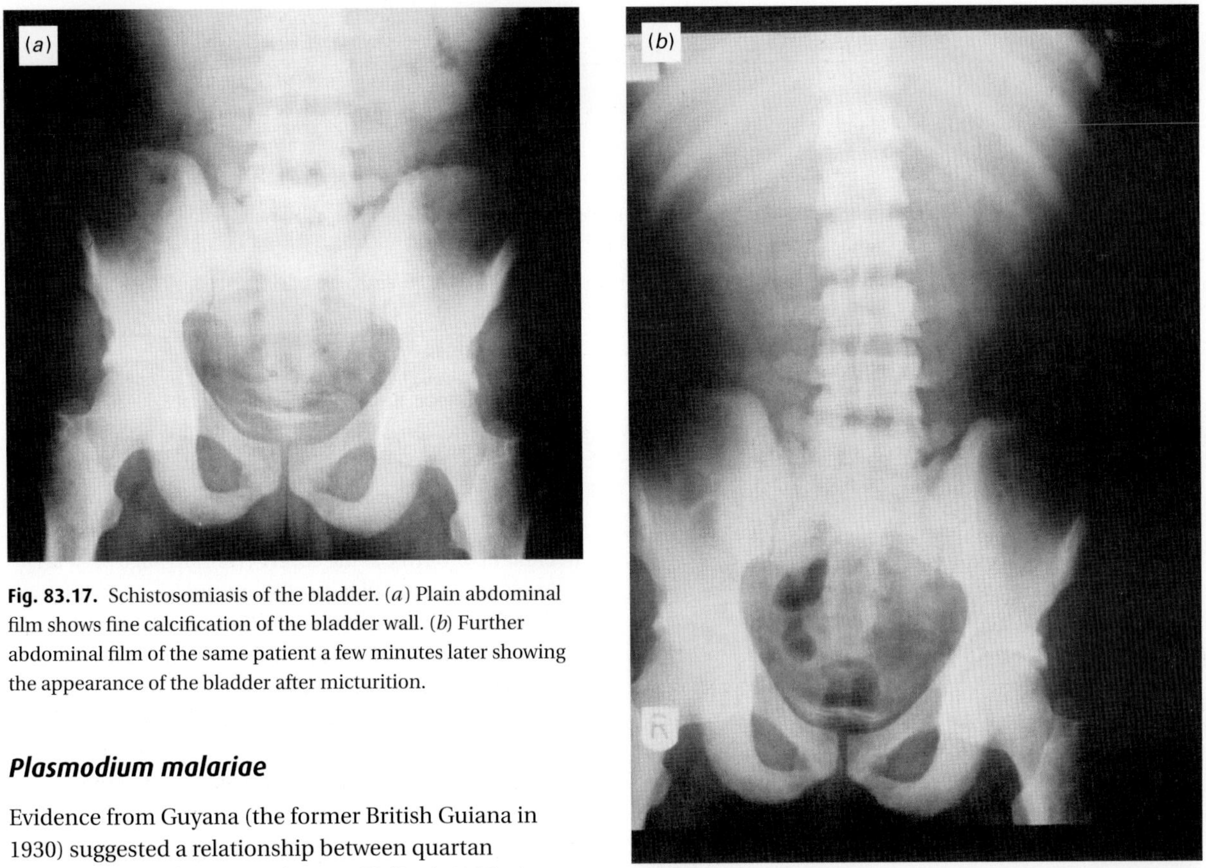

Fig. 83.17. Schistosomiasis of the bladder. (*a*) Plain abdominal film shows fine calcification of the bladder wall. (*b*) Further abdominal film of the same patient a few minutes later showing the appearance of the bladder after micturition.

Plasmodium malariae

Evidence from Guyana (the former British Guiana in 1930) suggested a relationship between quartan malaria and nephrotic syndrome (Giglioni, 1930). A further report by the same author 30 years later, by which time malaria had been eradicated, showed that this form of nephrotic syndrome had disappeared (Giglioni, 1962).

Histologically, the appearances are of thickening of the walls of some of the glomerular capillaries. The distribution is focal (focal segmental glomerulonephritis).

Plasmodium falciparum

P. falciparum malaria, particularly when there is heavy parasitaemia, is a well-known cause of acute renal failure, which results from a combination of hyperpyrexia, hypovolaemia and haemolysis. Unlike *P. malariae, P falciparum* does not seem to induce any form of chronic renal disease.

Renal disease and viruses

Hepatitis B

Hepatitis B is common in sub-Saharan Africa. Usually there is complete recovery and such individuals will be Hepatitis B core antibody positive, i.e. they will be immune. Those who do not clear the antigen will remain Hepatitis B surface antigen positive. It is this group who may develop renal disease, with deposition of immune complexes, a nephropathy of membranous type, and proteinuria (Settie, et al., 1984).

Human immunodeficiency virus (HIV)

Impairment of renal function has been a feature of HIV disease since it first appeared in the early 1980s. Histologically, the lesions are best categorized as focal segmental glomerulosclerosis (Fig. 83.19), and there is proteinuria, sometimes nephrotic syndrome (Attolou et al., 1998; Laradi et al., 1998; Pantanowitz et al., 1999). In the context of untreated HIV, the nephropathy has been of little clinical consequence since the progressive renal failure has been only one of a number of potentially fatal complications, but if drugs for the treatment of HIV disease become available, HIV-infected individuals may develop HIV-related renal disease while otherwise well.

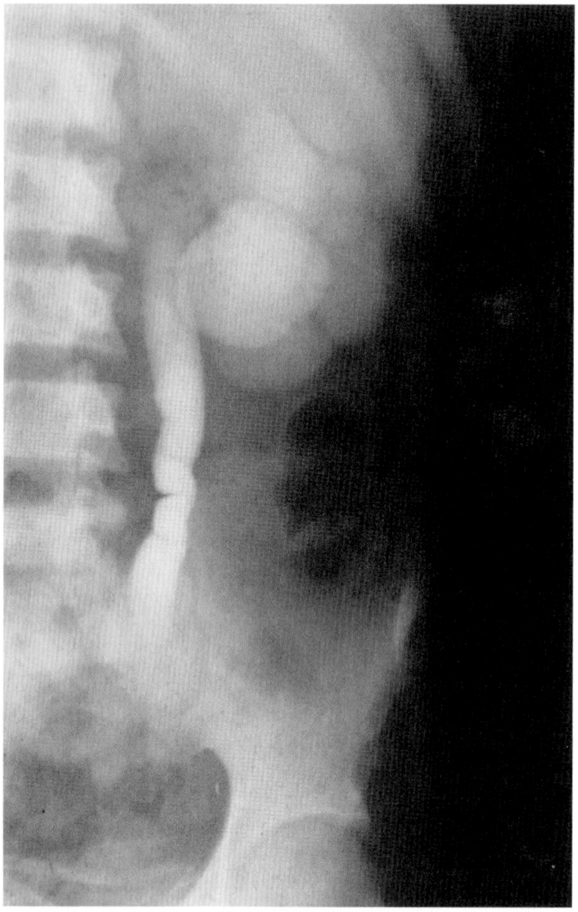

Fig. 83.18. Retrograde ureterography on the left side shows a dilated ureter with irregularity of the wall; the bladder wall calcification is just visible. Same patient as illustrated in Fig. 83.17.

Renal failure

Renal failure is a clinical syndrome resulting from the reduction in glomerular filtration rate (GFR). It involves the loss of nephrons with the failure of the glomerular and/or tubular functions of the kidney. These are mainly the excretory, conservative, regulatory, acid–base balance and secretory functions of the kidney which are aimed at providing the optimum body fluid volume and composition in which normal physiological and metabolic processes can occur efficiently.

Depending on the time course for its development, renal failure is classified as acute, rapidly progressive and chronic failure. Acute renal failure develops over hours to days, rapidly progressive renal failure develops over weeks to months and chronic renal failure develops over months to years.

Acute renal failure

In acute renal failure glomerular filtration rate falls rapidly over hours to days. It is accompanied by abnormalities in electrolyte and water balance.

Clinically, it is characterized by oliguria where the daily production of urine falls below 400 ml or, anuria, in combination with the accumulation of endogenous waste products such as urea and creatinine.

Classification

For convenience, aetiology of renal failure can be classified into pre-renal, renal and post-renal causes.

'Pre-renal' renal failure indicates those causes that lead to a reduction in the effective renal blood flow. They generally result either from massive extracellular fluid loss, as in cholera or burns, acute severe haemorrhage or heart failure with a large fall in cardiac output.

Usually, when body fluid volume and renal blood flow are restored by isotonic fluid or blood, renal function recovers.

'Renal' renal failure indicates disease of the renal parenchyma itself.

'Post-renal' renal failure indicates obstruction to the flow of urine in the lower urinary tract.

Causes

In Africa, the spectrum of causes of acute renal failure is different from that seen in the industrialized world (Ka et al., 1999; Mate-Kole et al., 1998; Randeree et al., 1995; Were & Otieno, 1992; Zewdu, 1994) (Table 83.7). Indeed, acute renal failure may complicate many clinical conditions in Africa. Generally, however, the causes can be classified into three main groups:

- those that are related to changes in systemic haemodynamics in which there are reductions in renal blood flow
- those that result from the effects of nephrotoxins.
- urinary tract obstruction.

Reduction of effective renal blood flow

Acute reduction in effective renal blood flow represents the commonest cause in Africa. It can result from:

- severe diarrhoea, e.g. in cholera
- severe burns
- massive haemorrhage, e.g. following trauma, antepartum and post-partum haemorrhage. *Note*: acute renal failure may also complicate pre-eclampsia and eclampsia

Table 83.7. Causes and histology of acute renal failure

Clinical problem	Histology	Treatment
Diarrhoea Vomiting Burns Post-surgery dehydration Ante-partum haemorrhage Post-partum haemorrhage Sepsis Paracetamol poisoning, NSAIDs	Acute tubular necrosis (glomeruli, vessels, interstitium normal)	Supportive Volume replacement Antibiotic (as indicated)
Drug sensitivity, e.g. Penicillin	Interstitial nephritis	Corticosteroids, etc.
Infections such as brucellosis Vasculitic disorders Goodpasture's syndrome SLE	Glomerular pathology with crescents (vessels abnormal sometimes)	Corticosteroids, etc.
Haemolytic–uraemic syndrome	Obliteration of arteriolar lumina, ischaemic glomeruli	Supportive
Urinary tract obstruction	Not relevant	Relieve obstruction
Other Pre-eclampsia Eclampsia	 Swelling of endothelial cells Fibrin deposition	 Preventive (low dose aspirin) Prompt delivery of baby Treat hypertension

- dehydration in the immediate post-operative period. In surgical patients hypovolaemia is common in the first 48 hours for a number of reasons. Insensible losses in the tropics tend to be high, especially in the hot season. Many patients are on a nothing by mouth ('Nil per os') regimen in both the pre-operative and immediate post-operative period. It is not surprising that when, as can easily happen, fluid replacement does not keep up with losses, patients become seriously fluid deplete. Associated sepsis can be a powerful further precipitant of acute renal failure.
- sepsis

Nephro-urological causes/toxins

(i) Acute deposition of haemoglobin in the renal tubules as a result of intra-vascular haemolysis; this is well recognized because both glucose-6-phosphate-dehydrogenase deficiency and sickle syndromes are common in Africa.

(ii) Drugs and toxins. Acute interstitial nephritis may result from the ingestion of prescribed drugs, and remedies from traditional practitioners (Otieno et al., 1991). The use of non-steroidal anti-inflammatory drugs and the ingestion of naphthalene-containing

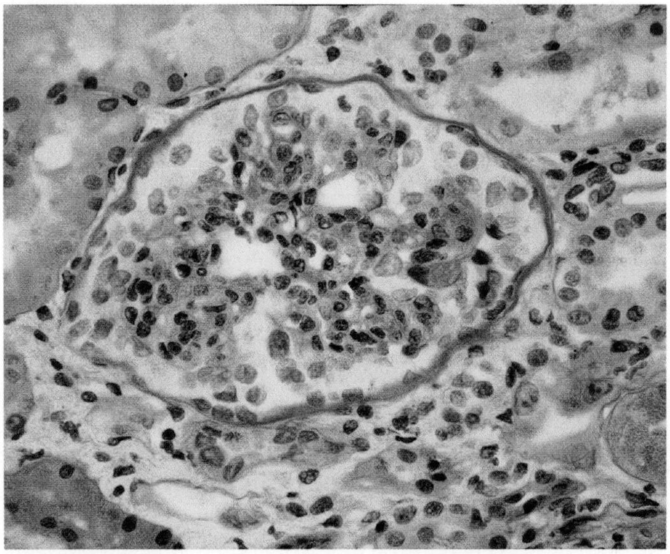

Fig. 83.19. HIV nephropathy.
Section shows typical 'collapsing' glomerulopathy, the glomerular tuft appearing contracted but not hypercellular. There are a number of epithelial cells in Bowman's space. Periodic acid Schiff diastase stain, which stains the basement membrane, shows Bowman's capsule as a distinct line and indicates (more diffusely) the glomerular tuft.

remedies have also resulted in the development of acute renal failure. An uncommon cause of acute renal failure is multiple stings from the African honey bee (Hommel et al., 1998).

(iii) Urinary tract obstruction is not a common cause of acute renal failure in Africa. When it does occur, it is likely to be due to bilateral renal calculi or the involvement of both ureters in carcinoma of the bladder. Advanced carcinoma of the cervix may also be responsible.

Clinical features

Classically in acute renal failure, there is sudden reduction in urine output (oliguria) accompanied by increasing serum levels of urea, creatinine and potassium. Sodium and water retention may result in increased blood pressure and pulmonary oedema.

Management

- Assess the state of the patient's blood volume. Simple clinical assessment may be misleading and the best guide is given by measurement of central venous pressure (CVP). However, in patients who are clearly volume depleted it is probably safest (and technically easier) to go some way to achieving repletion before attempting central venous access.
- Correct hypovolaemia with 0.9 per cent sodium chloride solution to achieve a JVP that is just visible at the base of the neck. If CVP is available aim for a CVP of 8–10 cm above the mid-axillary line, i.e. just visible at the root of the neck if the patient were sitting up at an angle of 45°.
- Measure arterial pH and bicarbonate; if acidotic, use 1.4 per cent sodium bicarbonate solution instead of saline.
- Treat hyperkalaemia if the potassium is >6.5 mmol/l. If the ECG is abnormal give 10 ml of 10 per cent calcium gluconate by slow intravenous injection to stabilize the myocardium. Repeat the dose if necessary 30–60 minutes later. To move potassium into the cells give a dextrose with insulin infusion, 50 ml of 50 per cent dextrose with 10 units of soluble human insulin, over 30 minutes. If the hyperkalaemia persists, the infusion can be repeated. If it is available, start calcium polystyrene sulphonate resin (calcium resonium), in a dose of 15 g four times a day, to remove potassium from the body. This resin, which can be given by mouth or by nasogastric tube, may take up to 6 hours to have an effect. The resin can also be given rectally (in a dose of 30 g a day).
- Stop any drugs that cause potassium to be retained.
- Insert a bladder catheter to monitor urine output. If there is anuria or oliguria (<400 ml/day) it need not remain *in situ*. If the systolic BP is below 100 mm Hg in a patient who has been restored to euvolaemia, consider inotropic drugs.
- If a diuresis does not occur despite achieving optimal intravascular volume, give fluid by mouth hourly to replace measured losses as well as estimated insensible losses.
- If the patient is well enough, measure the body weight daily so that you have a useful guide to maintenance of optimal intra-vascular volume.
- Give all patients an antacid or H_2-blocker to prevent gastric haemorrhage.
- Do a renal ultrasound as early as possible to exclude obstructive uropathy and assess renal size and anatomy. Also do urine analysis, microscopy and culture. In a specialist centre consider renal biopsy if there are atypical features or evidence of multi-system disease.
- Consider haemodialysis or peritoneal dialysis

Indications for dialysis or haemofiltration

- Life-threatening or intractable pulmonary oedema
- Uncontrollably rising plasma potassium
- Severe (arterial pH <7.2) or worsening acidosis
- Uraemia, e.g. uraemic pericarditis.

Guidelines for management of acute renal failure

- Assess and correct circulatory impairment
- Manage life-threatening hyperkalaemia and salt and water overload
- Exclude obstruction to the urinary tract
- Establish underlying cause(s)
- Obtain a drug history.

Renal histology

Acute tubular necrosis

It is likely that in the context of the common acute diarrhoeal illnesses and fevers as are found in sub-Saharan Africa, most patients with acute renal failure will have a histological diagnosis of acute tubular necrosis ('ATN'), i.e. there is normal histology with or without some evidence of tubular damage. This appearance is most likely in patients with sustained acute volume depletion.

Nevertheless, some acute febrile illnesses are accompanied by glomerular and interstitial abnormalities, i.e. immune complex deposition with acute and chronic inflammatory cells in the interstitium. Examples are leptospirosis, meningococcal meningitis and miliary tuberculosis. As can be imagined there is little information on some of the more uncommon conditions.

Acute interstitial nephritis

This is typical of drug hypersensitivity. It also occurs in autoimmune and some bacterial conditions.

Vasculitic and crescentic glomerulonephritis

These conditions sometimes present as an acute uraemic emergency. There may be suggestive clinical indicators of vasculitis, such as purpura, haemoptysis, sinusitis and nasal blockage, but often there are none. The classical histological finding is the epithelial cell 'crescent', the crescent being simply a cross-section of a cap of epithelial cells (Fig. 83.20).

For both these groups of disorders, administration of corticosteroids can be life-saving, especially if dialysis is not available. It is this therapeutic necessity that makes renal biopsy so important in these groups.

Haemolytic–uraemic syndrome

In this condition there is red cell damage and lysis, with uraemia. Sometimes, the cause is one of the causes of outbreaks of diarrhoeal illness. Most common are *E. coli* O157 (which produces a verotoxin) and *Shigella dysenteriae* type 1 (which produces a Shiga toxin) but sporadic cases also occur. Histology reveals severe sub-intimal hyperplasia of small arterioles with (often) complete obliteration of the lumen. The glomeruli reflect the lack of afferent blood supply and look ischaemic.

The haemolytic–uraemic syndrome sometimes occurs during pregnancy without any gastrointestinal illness; occasionally the syndrome occurs in the post-partum period after a completely normal pregnancy.

Vasculitic syndromes

All these disorders may lead to rapidly progressive end-stage renal disease. Unlike most forms of progressive renal disease, treatment can have a major impact on prognosis, but specialist tertiary care is needed.

Systemic lupus erythematosus and microscopic polyangiitis respond well to oral prednisolone (0.75 mg/kg). Once a response has been achieved – clinical improvement and improvement in GFR – introduce a corticosteroid sparing drug such as cyclophosphamide or

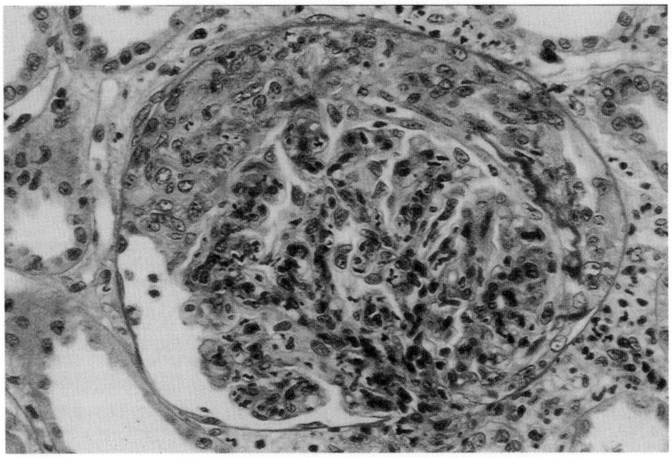

Fig. 83.20. Crescentic glomerulonephritis.
Section shows in the upper part of Bowman's space a 'crescent' of epithelial cells reducing the space available for the glomerulus.

azathioprine. The response of classical polyarteritis nodosa and Goodpasture's syndrome is less predictable.

Chronic renal failure

Chronic renal failure is defined as a diminution in renal function (GFR) of long duration, i.e. for years. The impairment of renal function may be static or progressive, more commonly the latter.

When rising plasma creatinines are plotted against time, the relationship is a curve (see Fig. 83.2) and it is not possible to predict the timing of end-of-shape renal failure. When the creatinine is plotted as the reciprocal, a straight line results and prediction (by extrapolation of the line) is much easier. In Fig. 83.21 imagine the direction of the black dots if treatment had not been given. A steeper than expected decline may be due to intercurrent urinary infection, volume depletion, poor control of blood pressure, drug toxicity; conversely, a less steep decline can reveal better control of blood pressure or treatment of a urinary infection.

Causes of chronic renal failure

There are various reports on the causes of chronic renal failure in Africa (Diallo et al., 1997a; Essamie et al., 1995; Lengani et al., 1997; Nseka & Tshiani, 1989; Seedat et al. 1984). The spectrum of causes and the age of the patients affected differs from those found for the developed world with relatively younger patients being affected. Some of these causes are shown in Table 83.8.

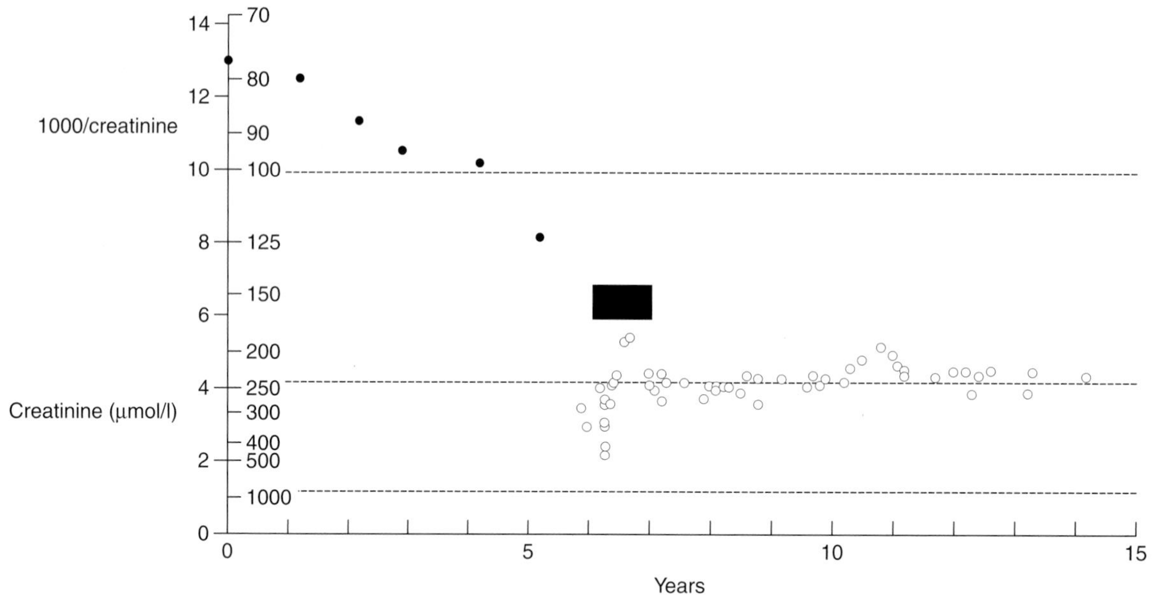

Fig. 83.21. Reciprocal creatinine chart demonstrates the straight line of declining renal function over 6 years until treatment was given. The black rectangle indicates 6 months of anti-tuberculosis treatment following which the plasma creatinine remains stable.

Table 83.8. Causes of chronic renal failure

Pre-renal	Renal	Post-renal
Renal arterial disease	Forms of glomerulonephritis	Schistosomiasis – bladder
Generalized atheroma	Diabetes mellitus	Tuberculosis – ureters, bladder
Renal artery stenosis	Hypertension	Prostatic obstruction
Fibromuscular hyperplasia	Inherited	
	Adult polycystic kidney disease	
	Alport's syndrome	
	HIV infection	

Clinical features

Most patients with progressive chronic renal failure are asymptomatic for all but the last 12 months of declining function. The first symptoms are often thirst and polyuria but this may not be noticed by the patient unless nocturia is prominent. There may also be general malaise induced by the uraemic state and contributed to by the anaemia that is common when the GFR is below 20–30 ml/min.

The health worker may be well aware that the patient has renal disease and chronic renal failure at a time when the patient is feeling perfectly well. Some patients are not seen until their terminal renal failure is manifest with pallor, uraemic frost and deep acidotic breathing. Proteinuria and high blood pressure are markers of chronic renal disease, and plasma creatinine gives very specific information on the level of renal function.

Anaemia

There are a number of factors involved (Akinsola et al., 2000).

- There is impaired incorporation of iron into red cells, so that higher than normal levels of ferritin are needed for blood formation.
- Erythropoietin production falls as the kidneys become smaller and fibrotic.
- Red cell life is shorter than in normals.
- There may be blood loss.

Hypertension

Most patients with chronic renal failure have a raised blood pressure (Plange-Rhule et al., 1999). In some patients renal failure may be the consequence of sustained high blood pressure: it is now clear that effective control of blood pressure influences the rate of decline in GFR.

Bone disease

Loss of renal function has two main consequences.

(i) The decline in GFR leads to retention of phosphate and a rise in plasma phosphate. The rise in phosphate leads to a fall in plasma ionized calcium and release of parathyroid hormone (PTH). The normal effect of a rising PTH is phosphaturia and restoration

Table 83.9. Factors adversely affecting renal function in patients with chronic renal failure

Factor	Problem	Action
Salt and water depletion	Diarrhoea, vomiting, fever, lack of access to water, intercurrent infection, malaria, too much diuretic	Oral fluid, intravenous saline
Inadequately controlled BP	BP not measured, availability of drugs, cost of drugs, compliance	Close attention to BP control
Urinary tract obstruction	Diagnosis not considered, inadequate facilities for diagnosis and treatment	Exclude urinary tract obstruction in all patients
Drugs	Herbal remedies, tetracyclines, aminoglycosides, digoxin, non-steroidal anti-inflammatory drugs, ACE inhibitors (sometimes)	Ask carefully about drug and traditional remedy ingestion in all patients. Check doses of all drugs given to patients with chronic renal failure
Urinary tract infection	Ascending infection causing bacterial interstitial nephritis	History, urine culture, investigate

of the equilibrium but this is not possible in individuals with renal failure so the PTH remains raised.

(ii) The failing kidney fails to synthesize 1,25–$(OH)_2$ vitamin D_3, the most active of the metabolites of vitamin D. This lack of calcitriol has two effects – reduced absorption of calcium from the gut and relative insensitivity of the parathyroid gland to rising levels of ionized calcium, i.e. apparently adequate levels of ionized calcium are not adequate to reduce PTH release.

In practice, however, hyperparathyroidism is an uncommon complication of chronic renal failure in adults and occurs only in those with chronic renal failure of many years' standing; in children it is more common and presents clinically as rickets.

Conservative management of chronic renal failure (Table 83.9)

In many parts of sub-Saharan Africa renal replacement therapy, i.e. haemo- or peritoneal dialysis, and transplantation, is not available so conservative management is the norm.

When the GFR is $<$10 ml/min the patient is likely to have significant symptoms, including nausea, vomiting, itching and fatigue. The patient may also notice 'restless legs' – a form of myoclonus – especially in bed at night. Nearly all patients will be drinking excessive fluid and getting up at night to pass urine, sometimes three or four times.

Blood pressure

Of prime importance is control of blood pressure so that GFR deteriorates as slowly as possible. There is evidence from industrialized countries that before dialysis was used in treatment low protein diets prolonged life and reduced morbidity. As shown in Table 83.9, it is important to prevent acute falls in GFR.

Nausea, vomiting and 'restless legs'

The nausea is helped by oral metoclopramide, 10 mg as required; if the patient is vomiting the drug can be given parenterally. A good drug for itching is hydroxyzine 25 mg taken at night; if this dose does not produce relief it can be increased to 25 mg three times a day. Sometimes the itching is secondary to hyperphosphataemia and oral calcium carbonate may produce relief by lowering the plasma phosphate. The myoclonic jerks can be helped by clonazepam, 1 mg at night, though the dose may need to be increased. Remember that clonazepam can cause respiratory depression so the dose should be increased cautiously.

Polyuria and nocturia

The nocturia may cause the patient some inconvenience; unfortunately, the excessive urine volume is necessary for removal of retained nitrogenous waste products. Fluid restriction at night, therefore, is not an option, and in any case the polyuria will continue even it the patient is fluid deplete.

Anaemia

Fatigue can be a dominant symptom. It is usually due to the anaemia, for which there is no easy answer. Patients are often iron deficient so should be given iron. Oral ferrous sulfate (600 mg daily containing 120 mg of ferrous iron) is a good choice and it is usually well tolerated. If not tolerated, a suitable alternative is ferrous gluconate (600 mg daily, 70 mg ferrous iron).

Erythropoietin will raise the haemoglobin and enhance the quality of life. The starting weekly dose of synthetic human erythropoietin is 25–50 units/kg body weight and it is usually given once or twice a week. The dose should be adjusted to maintain a haemoglobin concentration of 10–12 g/dl. It is advisable to monitor blood pressure regularly in patients on erythropoietin as there is a tendency for it to rise as the haemoglobin rises.

Blood transfusion is not usually an option because, though it produces a good rise in haemoglobin, the haemoglobin falls again within 2–3 weeks to its former level. The occasional patient who presents with a haemoglobin of <5.0 g/l and has severe symptoms, may warrant transfusion of blood to relieve their acute symptoms. Otherwise, restrict blood to patients who are actively bleeding.

Renal replacement therapy

When a patient's level of renal function (GFR) falls to 20 ml/min or below, it is important to consider future options. The full range of peritoneal dialysis (continuous ambulatory peritoneal dialysis = CAPD), haemodialysis and renal transplantation (Arije et al., 1995; Barsoum et al., 2002) is available in very few centres in sub-Saharan Africa. See the Box for indications for renal replacement therapy.

Indications for renal replacement therapy

- Hyperkalaemia uncontrolled by other measures
- Severe salt and water overload unresponsive to diurectics
- Severe uraemia
- Acidaemia.

Haemodialysis and peritoneal dialysis

Haemodialysis is the most appropriate form of dialysis for acute renal failure and for most patients peritoneal dialysis is unsuitable. Indeed, in hypercatabolic patients (who are often septic) peritoneal dialysis is sometimes unable to lower adequately the rapidly rising urea. The factors influencing choice are given in the Box.

Factors affecting choice of dialysis

	Haemodialysis	Peritoneal dialysis
Absolute requirement	Central venous access	Suitable peritoneum
Highly trained staff?	Yes	Less so
Set-up cost of service	High	Low
Maintenance cost	Moderate	High
Suitable for hyperacute renal failure?	Yes	No
Drugs during dialysis?	Heparin	None
Able to remove fluid quickly?	Yes	No
Infection risk?	Line sepsis	Peritonitis

Transplantation

Renal transplantation can only be offered in highly specialized centres in sub-Saharan Africa.

Management of high blood pressure in patients with renal disease

Patients with a minor degree of proteinuria.

Microalbuminuria

A very early sign of kidney disease is 'microalbuminuria'. This is the finding of small amounts of albumin in the urine, defined as either: (a) a concentration of 20–200 μg/l of albumin in the urine, or (b) 30–300mg of albumin in a 24-hour urine collection. In other words, either a random untimed sample (for measuring concentration) or a timed sample (for the quantity excreted in a given time) will give useful information.

Microalbuminuria is important because it is a marker of current, and predictor of future progressive, renal disease – especially in patients with two of the commoner causes of renal failure, namely diabetes mellitus and 'essential' hypertension.

The finding of microalbuminuria gives time for preventive strategies to be implemented. Look for risk factors and correct them. Thus, in diabetes mellitus there is good evidence that scrupulous control of blood pressure will significantly postpone any future loss of renal function, and the magnitude of the benefit is considerably greater than any benefit gained by maintenance of normoglycaemia. This benefit of careful blood pressure management holds true, whatever form of drug treatment is chosen, provided the blood pressure is kept at a level no higher than 135/80 mm Hg.

The benefits of the the 'reno-protective' effects of angiotensin II receptor antagonists, irbesartan and losartan, were found to be greater than could be explained by the level of blood pressure achieved alone (Brenner et al., 2001; Lewis et al., 2001; Parving et al., 2001). There is therefore a good argument for using these drugs if resources allow.

In a major study of patients with hypertensive renal disease who had proteinuria, amlodipine and ramipril produced similar falls of blood pressure, but ramipril produced a more pronounced slowing in the fall in GFR and a significantly greater fall in proteinuria than amlodipine. Thus it is possible that pressure-mediated glomerular injury could contribute to the greater increase in proteinuria and more rapid decline in GFR (Agodoa et al., 2001).

Patients with renal failure with a GFR of <20 ml/min

High blood pressure is the most potentially reversible risk factor for continuing loss of renal function. In patients with poor renal function, thiazide diuretics are generally relatively ineffective and it is of course important to avoid potassium-retaining diuretics. Loop diuretics such as frusemide and bumetanide do work but a higher dose is usually needed.

Salt reduction

It is important to advise patients to reduce their intake of salt. Any reduction in salt intake will make anti-hypertensive drugs more effective, and therefore less expensive. This should be relatively easy in rural people as they eat very little processed food, so virtually all the salt is either added in cooking or derived from salted fish. In practice, advise patients:

- to avoid salted fish and meat, seasoning liquids and cubes,
- not to purchase salt in the market.

Which drugs?

The most appropriate drugs to use are the dihydropyridines, i.e. nifedipine and amlodipine. A usual starting dose of nifedipine (SR, i.e.slow release) is 20 mg by mouth twice or three times a day. On the other hand amlodipine and nifedipine LA (long-acting formulation) only need to be given once a day at a dose of 5–10 mg and 30–60 mg, respectively. Beta-blocking drugs are relatively ineffective on their own but are useful as a second agent in combination with a dihydropyridine. Remember that water soluble beta-blockers (atenolol, celiprolol, nadolol, sotalol) are excreted by the kidney so are retained in patients with poor renal function. The drug of choice is metoprolol in a dose of 100–200 mg twice a day.

Angiotensin-converting enzyme (ACE) inhibitors and angiotensin II receptor antagonists are also effective but hyperkalaemia limits their usefulness.

Figure 83.22 shows renal histology from a patient with a very high blood pressure.

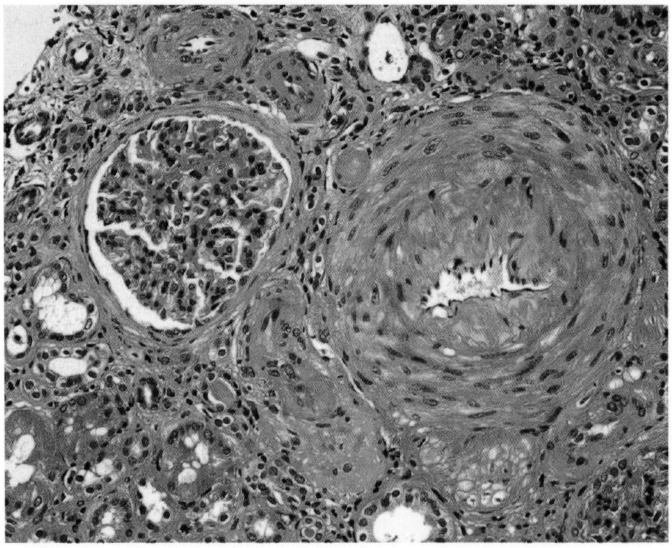

Fig. 83.22. Accelerated hypertension. Section shows marked subintimal thickening of afferent arteriole and some loss of volume of glomerulus (ischaemia).

Urinary tract infections

Clinical syndromes of urinary tract infection

Bacterial infection of the urinary tract may present as acute pyelonephritis, acute cystitis or asymptomatic bacteriuria.

Pathophysiology

The human urinary tract is normally sterile. Urinary tract infection arises when bacteria gain access along the urethra. The shorter urethra in women explains why urinary infections are commoner in women than men. However, even in women, organisms reaching the bladder are unlikely to survive provided that the bladder empties properly so that the anti-bacterial secretions of the bladder wall can exert their effect.

Predisposing factors in men and women

Inadequate bladder-emptying, anatomical abnormalities, urinary tract calculi, instrumentation of the urinary tract, in-dwelling bladder catheter and urinary tract obstruction.

Micro-organisms

The organism most commonly involved is *Escherichia coli* but other bacteria sometimes found are Klebsiella, coagulase-negative Staphylococci and Proteus. Proteus has a particular association with upper urinary tract disease and Pseudomonas with long-term catheters.

Urine collection

Any urine sample collected for reagent strip testing or microbiological diagnosis must be as fresh as possible. Ideally, it should be passed in the vicinity of the health clinic or laboratory. If the sample is not taken cleanly, there may be a mixed growth of organisms. If this happens repeatedly, the only certain way of getting a good sample is by supra-pubic aspiration, when the sample should contain neither bacteria nor white blood cells.

Reagent strips

Chemical test strips usually include leukocyte esterase and nitrite reductase portions. Urine from someone with a classical symptomatic urinary tract infection would be expected to show both tests as positive. Similarly, a strip negative for both elements would make a bacterial urinary infection very unlikely (see the Box). A problem arises when one test is positive and the other negative. For example, some acute bacterial urinary infections are associated with very few leukocytes, when the nitrite test would be positive but the leukocyte test negative. On the other hand, some organisms do not reduce nitrate to nitrite so the test could be positive for leukocytes but negative for organisms, as may also be found in a patient who has received an antibiotic. Leukocytes in the absence of a urinary infection can be caused by inflammation in any part of the urinary tract; for example, balanitis in the male and vulvitis in the female. Sometimes, renal calculi give rise to an increased number of leukocytes but usually there are increased numbers of red blood cells as well. In a patient with a 'sterile pyuria' it is most important to consider tuberculosis of the renal tract – see below.

Urine testing in possible urinary infection

		Leukocytes +	Leukocytes −
Nitrite	+	Urinary tract infection	Infection without WBC. Nitrite from food. Urine left in sunlight.
Nitrite	−	Treated urinary tract infection Non-nitrite producing organism Tuberculosis	Urinary tract infection unlikely.

Classical examination of urine

Microscopy and culture (see p. 1046).

Acute pyelonephritis

Clinical features

Acute pyelonephritis is an acute febrile illness: the patient may present as a case of pyrexia of unknown origin (PUO). It occurs especially in young women who may present with headache, vomiting, malaise, rigors, myalgia and loin pain that is sometimes bilateral. There is marked tenderness in the renal angle especially on the affected side and bimanual palpation of the kidney may not be possible because of pain. These are so-called 'upper' urinary symptoms. There may also be dysuria (painful micturition), frequency of micturition and supra-pubic tenderness.

Investigations

The early diagnosis may be difficult before urinary symptoms and signs appear: hence the great importance of examining the urine. There is usually a polymorph leukocytosis and it may be possible to culture the responsible organism from both urine and blood. Imaging reveals large kidneys and renal biopsy (even of the unaffected side) shows florid infiltration of the interstitium with organisms and leukocytes.

Treatment

In uncomplicated urinary tract infection, give an effective and low cost drug whenever possible: remember the hazard of drugs in those with G6PD deficiency. The following are effective:

nitrofurantoin 50 mg, three times a day, for 5 days, but beware of G6PD deficiency which may lead to haemolysis.

trimethoprim 200 mg, twice daily for 5 days.

In cases when the organism is not eradicated and symptoms persist, a more costly but very effective second-line drug is oral ciprofloxacin 500 mg twice daily for 3–5 days. An alternative is a 5-day course of oral cefuroxime at a dose of 125 mg twice daily. It is useful to have the results of 'dipstick' urine analysis before treatment is given because in patients who are not systemically unwell unnecessary treatment can be avoided by the finding of negative routine urine analysis.

In patients who are acutely ill, start treatment before routine urine analysis and culture results are available. Give intravenous ciprofloxacin (400 mg 12-hourly) or intravenous cefuroxime (750 mg 8-hourly) for 48 hours before changing to oral ciprofloxacin or cefuroxime when the patient is able to tolerate oral medication. In these ill patients repeat the urine culture one week after the course of the antibiotic has been completed.

In all patients, encourage a high oral fluid intake (at least 2 litres daily). In some very ill patients it may initially be necessary to give intravenous fluid.

- If urinary tract infections recur, look diligently for evidence of urinary tract obstruction, for example from renal stones, prostatic hypertrophy, anatomical urinary tract abnormalities and problems with bladder emptying.
- Pre- and post-micturition ultrasound is very helpful as it will reveal whether the bladder fails to empty.
- Do not keep treating urinary infections – look for the cause of the infection.
- Monitor sensitivity of local organisms.

Cystitis

Symptoms include suprapubic pain, frequency, dysuria and, sometimes, macroscopic haematuria. In about 50 per cent of patients an organism is obtainable on culture and the antibiotic treatment shown above is effective. Trials have shown that in uncomplicated urinary infection a 3-day course is adequate.

In the other 50 per cent – so-called 'abacterial cystitis' – the reason for the symptoms is not clear. Possibilities include a bacterial infection with a low count, or possibly infection with Chlamydia, Trichomonas, Mycoplasma or even Candida. This condition is also known as the urethral syndrome.

Asymptomatic bacteriuria

In the group of patients who are found to have a pure growth of $>10^5$ organisms/ml yet neither symptoms nor causal factors no treatment is necessary. It has been suggested that, in such patients, the organisms have simply colonized the bladder without tissue invasion.

Reflux nephropathy – formerly known as pyelonephritis

In the normal subject urine passes from the ureters into the bladder; retrograde flow does not occur. Vesico-ureteric reflux may occur as a result of congenitally abnormal muscle in one or both ureters as they enter the bladder; the condition is detectable by ultrasound scanning in utero and in the neonate. Coexisting bacterial infection (developing because of failure of bladder emptying) may damage the kidneys. The urinary tract sepsis may present as fever, unexplained abdominal pain and failure to thrive; very often the diagnosis of urinary tract infection (and vesico-ureteric flux) is not made. As the child grows, the damaged portions of the kidney and the healthy parts grow differentially, giving rise to the typical focal scarring of reflux nephropathy seen in adult life. The importance of the condition in adults is that, if the vesico-ureteric reflux persists, there may be recurrent urinary infections. If the condition is discovered in pregnancy, be alert to the possibility of the condition in the newborn baby.

Other features are hypertension, the finding of abnormal renal anatomy on imaging and, where it is bilateral, a diminished GFR.

Further management of urinary infection

Any patient with more than a single episode of lower urinary tract infection, and certainly anyone who has had acute pyelonephritis, should be investigated with urine culture and microscopy, routine blood tests, plain abdominal film (for stones) and, when available, renal ultrasound (for anatomical abnormalities and urinary tract obstruction). If all these are normal and there is no proteinuria, no further investigation is necessary.

Renal tuberculosis

The problem in Africa

There are few reports of renal and urinary tract tuberculosis in Africa. Tuberculosis affects the kidneys and urinary tract relatively late in life and its rather indolent presentation is likely to lead to delay in diagnosis (Njeh et al., 1993; Otieno, 1983).

Pathogenesis

Haematogenous spread of *M. tuberculosis* leads to the primary complex in the kidney – cortical granulomas. These heal, but in about 5 per cent they re-activate and seed AFB to the lower urinary tract, and to the epididymis in men.

Clinical features

An adult complains of dysuria, frequency and other urinary symptoms but efforts to culture an organism from the urine are unsuccessful. There may be systemic symptoms such as fever and loss of weight.

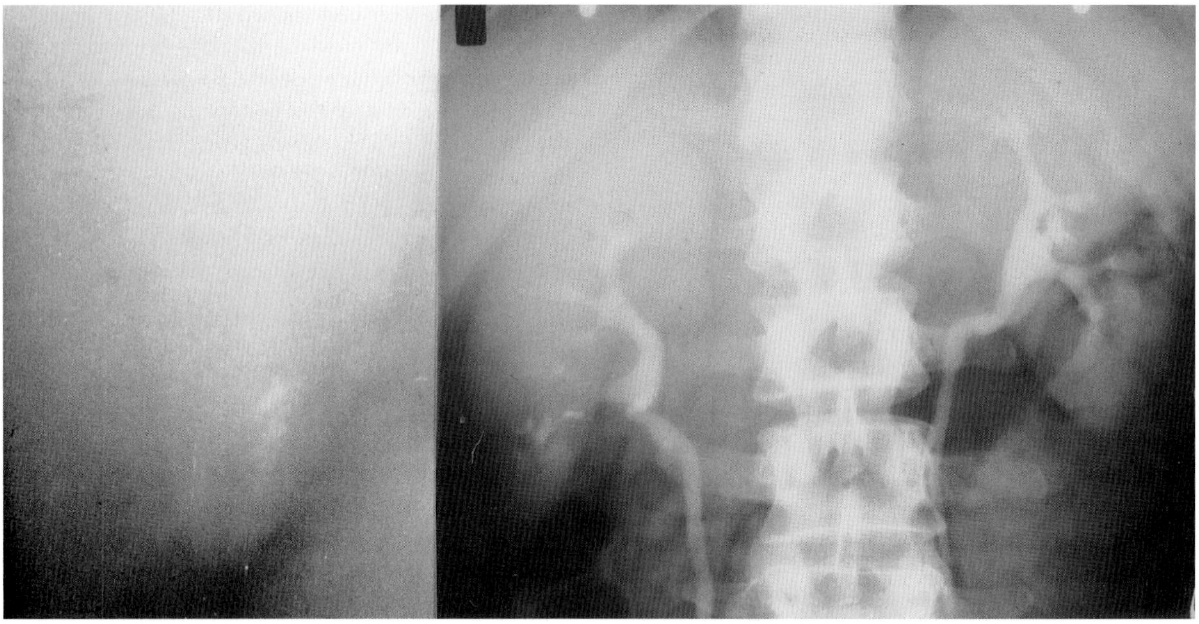

Fig. 83.23. Early focal renal tuberculosis. Plain film shows calcification in the lower pole of the right kidney. The 5-minute IVU film shows the abnormal lower pole calyx with loss of adjacent parenchyma. There was sterile pyuria and *Mycobacterium tuberculosis* was cultured from the urine.

Microbiological diagnosis

There are likely to be polymorphonuclear leukocytes in the urine in numbers well above the upper limit of normal, i.e. $100–200 \times 10^9/l$ as opposed to an upper limit of $<10 \times 10^9/l$, i.e. the patient has a sterile pyuria (see box below).

Causes of a sterile pyuria*

- Tuberculosis of the urinary tract
- *Chlamydia trachomatis* infection
- Chemically induced cystitis
- Renal calculi
- Coliform (or other pathogen) urinary tract infection but antibiotic inhibiting growth

* Remember that white blood cells from the foreskin or vulva may contaminate the urine. If in doubt a supra-pubic sample using a needle of appropriate length will settle the matter.

An individual with proven sterile pyuria should provide complete early morning urine samples on 3 successive days for culture on Löwenstein–Jensen medium. The organism may take 6 weeks to grow.

Radiological features

A plain radiograph sometimes shows calcification in the affected kidney, and an intravenous urogram (IVU) may reveal just one calyx affected (Fig. 83.23) or focal areas of ureteric narrowing and bladder disease. Only one-third of patients have an abnormal chest X-ray.

Treatment

Standard anti-tuberculosis drugs are needed, but they may provoke ureteric obstruction due to inflammatory oedema around dying bacilli.

Leprosy

A significant proportion of individuals with leprosy die of renal failure. A report of autopsy material from 199 patients with leprosy from Sao Paolo, Brazil revealed renal disease in no fewer than 144 (Nakayama et al., 2001). Sixty-one (42.1%) of those with renal disease had amyloidosis, 29 (20.0%) glomerulonephritis and 22(15.2%) nephrosclerosis (Gupta et al., 1977). Amyloid occurs in about one-third of those with lepromatous leprosy but rarely in those with tuberculoid disease. Clinically, 95 per cent of the patients with amyloid had proteinuria and 88 per cent chronic renal failure. Treatment is with standard anti-leprosy drugs.

Amyloidosis

A complex glycoprotein termed amyloid is laid down in a number of tissues including the kidneys (Fig. 83.24). The amyloid material is usually produced in response to infection or inflammation but there are also familial and neoplastic forms. It is a common cause of death in patients with leprosy.

In Africa the most likely causes are tuberculosis, leprosy, osteomyelitis, parasitic infections, HIV/AIDS and other inflammatory conditions. The type of amyloid produced in response to infection is so-called AA amyloid which is deposited especially in the liver, spleen and kidneys. World-wide, the condition is probably becoming less common because in many countries it is possible now to reduce the inflammation associated with the predisposing condition.

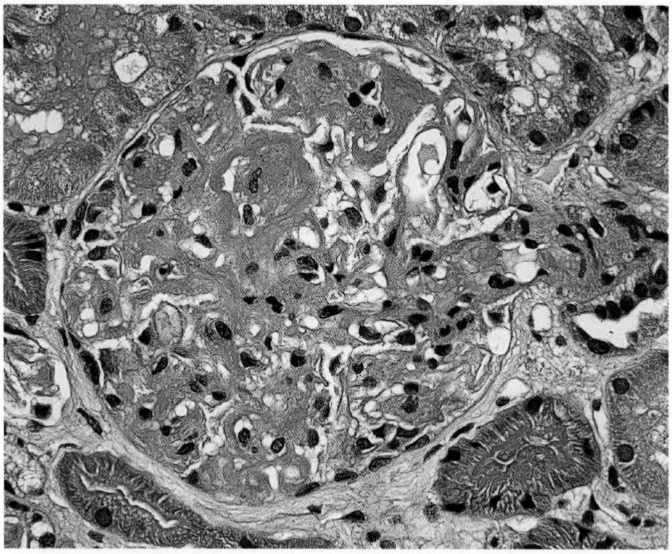

Fig. 83.24. Renal amyloidosis. Section shows deposition of homogeneous acellular pink material in the glomerulus.

Renal involvement in multi-system disease

Systemic lupus erythematosus (SLE) (see Chapter 84)

Patients with SLE commonly have proteinuria and may have a nephrotic syndrome.

Vasculitic syndromes

The prevalence of these conditions in sub-Saharan Africa is unknown. Typically, patients present with malaise, purpura, weakness, fever and weight loss. Importantly, patients with this group of disorders respond to prednisolone and cyclophosphamide

Myelomatosis

Myelomatosis, a plasma cell disorder, is uncommon in sub-Saharan Africa. Patients in whom there are large quantities of immunological 'light' chains in the urine (NB not detectable by urine test strips used for detecting albumin), can develop acute renal failure because of precipitation of protein in renal tubules. The kidney may also be affected by hypercalcaemia, infiltration of the kidney by plasma cells, hyperuricaemia and amyloid.

Sarcoidosis

Sarcoidosis presents often as erythema nodosum on the shins and sometimes with malaise and shortness of breath. Chest X-ray reveals hilar lymphadenopathy or a pattern suggestive of miliary tuberculosis. Indeed, differentiation between tuberculosis and sarcoidosis can sometimes be difficult.

Biopsy of lymph glands reveals non-caseating granulomas. Hypercalcaemia is common, and depends on the quantity of granulomata, the macrophages of which synthesize the active form of vitamin D (1,25-$(OH)_2$ vitamin D_3 or calcitriol) and lead to increased calcium absorption from the gut. In the kidneys granulomata may be widespread, and hypercalcaemia (with hypercalciuria) can lead to renal stone formation.

Diabetes mellitus and the kidney

Diabetic renal disease is becoming increasingly common (Djrolo et al., 2001; Sobngwi et al., 1999). 'Microalbuminuria' is the earliest evidence of renal involvement in diabetes and may precede the development of overt renal failure by many years (see Chapter 70). Renal histology shows nodular glomerulosclerosis (Kimmelstiel–Wilson lesion) (Fig. 83.25).

Sickle cell disorders

Adult sickle cell SC patients lose glomerular function with age. Many patients have proteinuria, 1–2 g/day, and a low plasma albumin is common. Some develop end-stage renal disease, histology showing focal segmental sclerosis.

Table 83.10. Clinical abnormalities in patients with sickle cell syndromes

	Haemoglobin SS	Haemoglobin SC
Focal segmental glomerulosclerosis	Yes	Uncommon
Renal failure	Not common	Unusual
Acute renal failure	Occasionally	No
Renal papillary necrosis	Yes	Yes
Incomplete renal tubular acidosis	Yes	Uncommon
Hyperkalaemia, high plasma urate	Yes	Uncommon

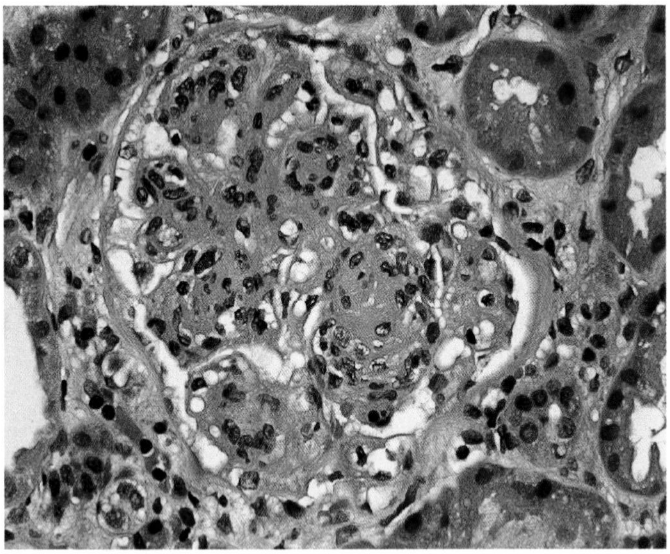

Fig. 83.25. Diabetic glomerulosclerosis. Section shows glomerulus illustrating nodular glomerulosclerosis (Kimmelstiel –Wilson lesion).

Renal papillary necrosis

In parts of West Africa, where SC disease is common, patients may present with the syndrome of acute loin pain associated with red urine. Sometimes, the patient will notice a fragment of tissue, often triangular in shape, in the urine – a sloughed papilla. These symptoms (Table 83.10) may be recurrent and eventually the picture is one of partial or total loss of papillae. Patients with homozygous SC disease may also exhibit papillary necrosis (Fig. 83.26, Table 83.11).

Drugs and the kidney

The kidney is a major excretory route for drugs, so doses may have to be modified in renal disease. A number of drugs have toxic effects on the kidney or affect renal function.

Table 83.11. Conditions associated with necrosis of renal papillae

Diabetes mellitus	Urinary tract obstruction
Sickle cell syndromes	Acute pyelonephritis
Analgesic nephropathy	Infants with dehydration, hypoxia and jaundice

- Find out what drugs – both prescribed and self-prescribed – the patient is currently taking and has taken in the past.
  - Past potentially toxic drugs — Phenacetin, Chinese herbs.
  - Current or recent drugs — Idiosyncratic reactions, toxic effects.

Past drugs

Certain drugs provoke the deposition of immune-complexes in the glomeruli and cause the nephrotic syndrome. Examples are penicillamine and gold (both used in rheumatoid arthritis). Stopping either drug leads to resolution of the renal condition.

Another chemical that led to renal failure was phenacetin. This was a constituent of a common over-the-counter remedy for headache known as 'APC', which contained aspirin, phenacetin and codeine. It caused renal papillary necrosis and a fall in GFR. If the diagnosis was made in time and the drug was stopped any further fall in GFR could be prevented. Even today, it is important to look at the box of any pharmaceutical preparation purchased.

Current drugs

In a patient newly presenting with renal dysfunction it is important to determine what drugs the patient is taking.

Some drugs have toxic effects on the kidney. All types of non-steroidal anti-inflammatory drugs (NSAIDs) can cause abnormal renal pathology and renal dysfunction. In addition they can potentially cause gastrointestinal bleeding and hypovolaemia. This group of drugs is by far the most important in this context.

Other drugs, for example, ranitidine/cimetidine, rifampicin and penicillin can produce an idiosyncratic reaction in which interstitial nephritis and renal dysfunction are important features. Note that these drugs are normally

Characteristic of drug	Examples	Action
Wholly excreted by the kidney	Ethambutol, digoxin, aminoglycosides (streptomycin, gentamicin, vancomycin)	Use alternative drug if possible. If none available, measure blood level of prescribed drug. If in doubt seek suitable advice – pharmacist or physician.
Partially excreted by the kidney	Penicillins, cephalosporins, benzodiazepines (beware of over-sedation)	Modify dose after consulting suitable formulary.
Not reliant on the kidney for excretion	Paracetamol, aspirin[a], clindamycin, erythromycin, most anti-hypertensive drugs, loop diuretics (frusemide, bumetanide)	
Toxic metabolites	Pethidine, morphine, opioid analgesics (codeine and related drugs)[b]	Avoid as much as possible. If there is no satisfactory alternative use with great care.

Notes:

[a] Remember that aspirin causes gastric irritaton. Also the effect on platelet stickiness means that aspirin is best avoided in patients with advanced renal failure.

[b] Avoid if possible as respiratory depression is a very serious unwanted effect.

safe but any patient who has produced an idiosyncratic reaction – sometimes including skin manifestations – should not receive that drug again.

Prescribing in patients known to have renal failure

Many pharmacopoeias have a section devoted to 'Prescribing in renal impairment', an example being the *British National Formulary*, which devotes Appendix 3 to the topic.

- Keep a suitable formulary at hand whenever drugs are prescribed: such a book is a storehouse of important information about drugs and prescribing.

Some drugs are wholly excreted by the kidney so the dose of these needs to be modified in all patients with renal failure. Others are partially excreted by the kidney and some are not dependent on renal excretion at all. Finally there is a group that is metabolized by the liver yet the metabolites – which can be toxic – are dependent on renal excretion (see the Box).

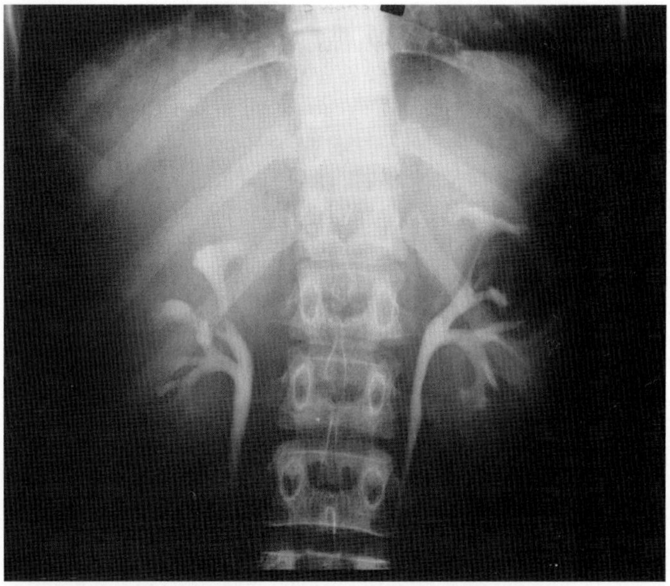

Fig. 83.26. Sickle cell disease. Papillary necrosis of sickle cell anaemia in a 16-year-old girl. Ten-minute IVU film shows lack of the normal cup-shaped calyces because of loss of the papillae. Compare with Fig. 83.11(*b*) (normal).

Potassium and prescribing

In patients with chronic renal failure it s essential to ensure that the potassium is not increased by prescribed drugs. Always avoid potassium-containing compounds (slow K, etc.) and potassium-sparing diuretics (amiloride, spironolactone). NSAIDs, which should in any case be avoided because of toxic effects on the kidney, also cause a rise in plasma potassium. By a similar mechanism – suppression of aldosterone – so do ACE inhibitors and angiotensin II blockers. There are plenty of cheap alternative anti-hypertensive drugs so only use them if potassium can be measured regularly.

Antibiotics

For treating urinary infections in patients with renal failure, use short courses of trimethoprim, ciprofloxacin, a cephalosporin or a penicillin. In patients where the symptoms are atypical or troublesome, it is imperative to confirm the diagnosis by urinary culture, and consider imaging of the urinary tract.

Dialysis patients
The same principles apply as for patients with renal failure not on dialysis.

Inherited renal disease

Adult polycystic kidney disease

This is an autosomal dominant condition resulting from a defect in Chromosome 16 or occasionally Chromosome 4. At birth it is not usually possible to detect cysts by any form of imaging. They develop and enlarge over two of three decades and it is only in the fourth or fifth decade that the disease becomes evident. Typical symptoms are macroscopic haematuria, acute pain in a cyst or a dragging sensation in one or both loins. Often a renal mass is palpable on each side of the abdomen. Abdominal ultrasound reveals the diagnosis: in 20 per cent of cases there are also cysts in the liver. Sometimes the diagnosis will have been made by investigating relatives of a known case, by abdominal ultrasound done during pregnancy, by the finding of a raised blood pressure in a young person or by finding an abdominal mass. An important feature in some families is sub-arachnoid haemorrhage as a result of a ruptured berry aneurysm.

When the plasma creatinine starts to rise, it continues to rise (see reciprocal creatinine chart) and it usually takes 10 years for the patient to reach end-stage renal failure. In the absence of dialysis or transplantation death usually occurs in the fifth to seventh decade.

In industrialized countries the gene frequency in the population is around 1 in 1000–2000 and the condition accounts for 5–10 per cent of all patients entering dialysis programmes. The incidence of, and location of, the gene in sub-Saharan populations is unknown but there are sporadic reports of the condition in Africans (Diouf et al., 1998).

Cystinuria

This is an autosomal recessive condition in which large quantities of four dibasic amino acids (cystine, ornithine, arginine and lysine) leak into the urine. It is only the cystine that is important. It tends to precipitate out of solution when it is in high concentration in acid urine. Stones may be recurrent over many years and their importance is that they are usually radiolucent and therefore difficult to detect. Most patients can be managed by being encouraged to drink large quantities of water especially before retiring at night, i.e. to prevent the very high urine concentrations of cystine that occur at night. It is at night too that the pH tends to be low so precipitation is most likely. High excretors may continue to form stones on a high fluid intake, even when taking sodium bicarbonate as well. Penicillamine chelates cystine, and so prevents stone formation.

Urinary tract obstruction

The problem in Africa

Just as in most patients with acute renal failure (where the kidneys themselves are not primarily diseased but affected secondarily by virtue of overwhelming bacteraemia, hypovolaemia, and low blood pressure), many patients with chronic renal failure do not have primary renal disease at all – but obstruction to urine flow below the kidneys. The problem in Africa is that even when the diagnosis of chronic renal failure has been made, it is not easy to decide to which patients scarce resources should be diverted.

The clinical presentation

Patients with chronic urinary tract obstruction may simply manifest the symptoms and signs of chronic renal failure, or additionally exhibit features of the cause of their obstruction. Individuals with chronic urinary tract schistosomiasis may have a history of macroscopic haematuria with dysuria and frequency. Prostatic (benign hypertrophy especially) and urethral (past trauma, sexually transmitted disease) problems in men is likely to produce chronic symptoms when emptying the bladder. In both men and women renal calculi can sometimes manifest remarkably few symptoms. In the ureter, however, colic is usual.

Management

The diagnosis of urinary tract obstruction should be considered in any patient with renal failure, even in patients where there is a known renal diagnosis. Anyone with upper urinary tract dilatation detected on ultrasound or IVU should be referred to a urologist for cystoscopy and further investigation (Plange-Rhule et al., 2002). Relief of obstruction should prevent further decline in GFR.

Renal tumours

Tumours can occur anywhere in the urinary tract. Renal cell carcinoma often presents with malaise and macroscopic haematuria. In the absence of macroscopic haematuria, the patient may present late when there is already direct spread into the renal vein and metastasis to local lymph nodes, lung and bone. The prognosis even in the best centres is not good. Transitional cell tumours are found in the pelvi-calyceal system and ureters. Carcinoma of the bladder is a late complication of chronic schistosomiasis.

Renal stones

The problem in Africa

Renal stones have been said to be relatively common in the countries of the Sahel but rare further south in sub-Saharan Africa. Surveys in Nigeria, Cameroon, Kenya, Tanzania and South Africa, suggest that there has been an increase in the last 20 years (Ekwere, 1995; Klufio et al., 1996). The estimated incidence in hospital series varies from 19.1 per 100000 hospital admissions in Calabar, Nigeria to 243 per 100000 in Dar-es-Salaam, Tanzania (Mkony et al., 1991). The male:female ratio varies from 2:1 to 5:1. Evidence from Sudan, Zambia and Zaire suggests that causes other than *Schistosoma haematobium* are responsible (Elem, 1984; Ibrahim, 1978).

Clinical presentation

As stones form on the surface of the renal papillae or within the urinary collecting system, they do not give rise to symptoms. Accordingly, asymptomatic stones are often discovered when a plain X-ray of the abdomen is done for unrelated reasons. Sometimes, stones cause macroscopic haematuria alone (Oliech et al., 1998). Often, however, stones break loose and either occlude the pelvi-ureteric junction or, more commonly, enter the ureter causing pain and bleeding.

Renal colic

A stone can pass down the ureter without producing symptoms, but usually there is pain ('renal colic') and bleeding. The pain begins gradually, usually in the flank, and increases over 20–60 min to become very severe, the patient often requiring potent analgesics to gain relief. Later the pain spreads downwards and anteriorly toward the iliac fossa, testicles, penis or vulva, indicating that the stone has passed to the lower third of the ureter (Fig. 83.27).

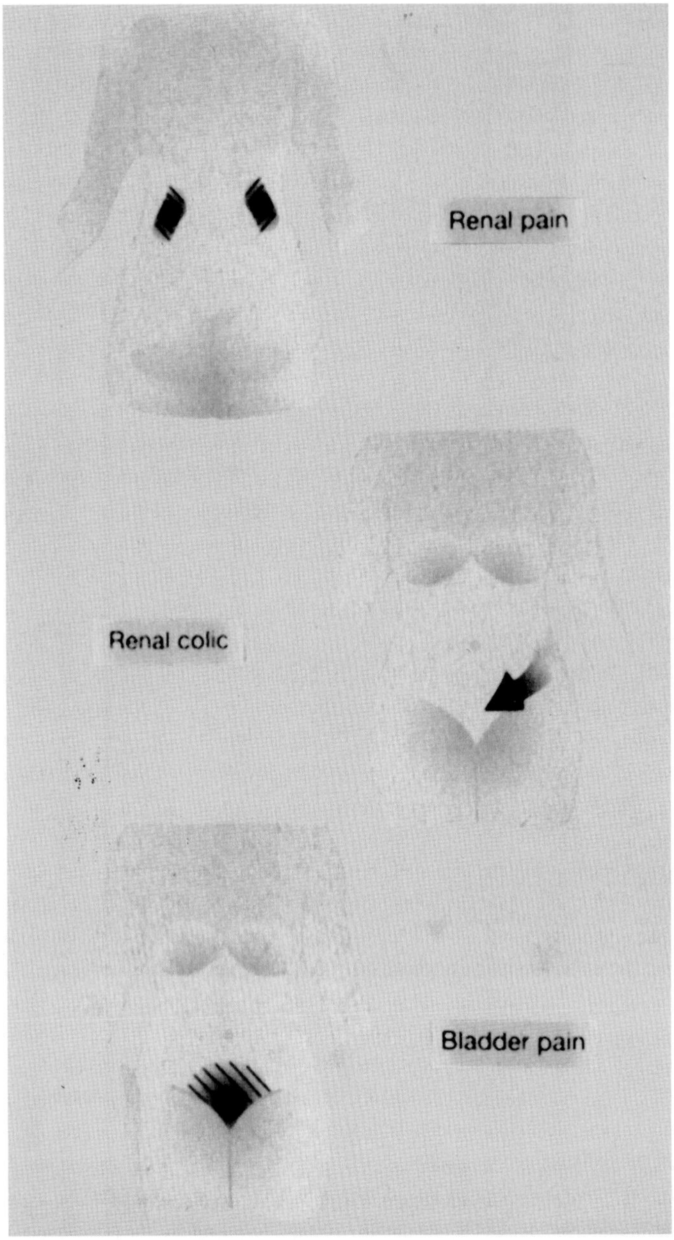

Fig. 83.27. Sites of pain in renal colic.

Frequency, urgency and dysuria develop when the stone reaches the segment of ureter within the bladder wall so that a urinary tract infection rather than a renal stone may be suspected.

Haematuria

When the stone is passed, haematuria is common.

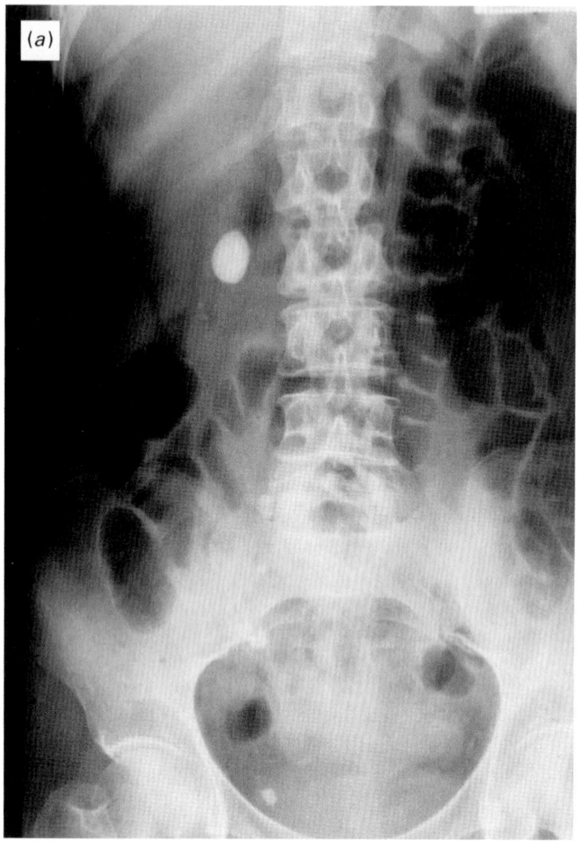

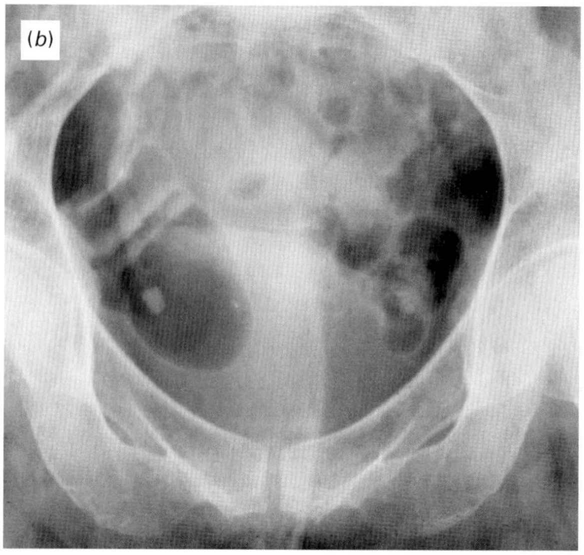

Fig. 83.28. (*a*) Plain film of abdomen showing two radio-opaque urinary tract calculi. One is in the right pelvi-calyceal system; the other is at the lower end of the right ureter. (*b*) 20-min IVU film showing hold-up of contrast in the ureter above the ureteric stone.

Investigations

In any patient presenting with stones in the renal tract:

- Deal first with the urgent clinical problem.
- After the acute episode, search for underlying metabolic abnormalities as it may be possible to prevent formation of further stones.

Acute presentation, i.e. 'surgical' aspects

Renal stone
In any patient presenting with suggestive symptoms, there are three potential problems:
- pain
- infection
- obstruction

(i) The pain is best controlled with diclofenac or pethidine: the place of smooth muscle relaxants is now much less certain.
(ii) Routine urine testing will usually show blood and there will be red blood cells on microscopy.
(iii) Urine culture is essential in all patients as any infection must be identified as soon as possible.
(iv) A plain film will reveal any calcification along the course of the urinary tract; abdominal ultrasound is useful for detecting dilatation, i.e. obstruction. Sometimes, however, in patients with acute ureteric colic, there may be obstruction but as yet no dilatation. It is these patients with an obstructed urinary tract that are at particular risk of developing proximal infection, and if the obstruction is not relieved a pyonephrosis may be the result.
(v) An IVU is still the single most important investigation in the management of patients with renal colic because it provides a precise assessment of renal anatomy. For stones in the pelvi-calyceal system or lower third of the ureter, endoscopic removal is usually possible. It is stones in the upper and middle thirds of the ureter that present the clinician with uncertainties in management. Nevertheless, overall less than 10 per cent of all urinary tract calculi need operative intervention (Fig.83.28).

General management

Many patients with urinary tract calculi, i.e. those without an obstructed urinary tract, can be managed without surgical intervention. The principles are to relieve pain with oral analgesics and to ensure that the patient drinks liberal volumes of fluid, 3–4 litres a day. Later, careful follow-up is essential.

- Remember that some urinary tract calculi are radiolucent. They will not usually be visible on plain X-ray but are detectable on ultrasound. IVU is often very useful as the stones will show up as negative images among the contrast. In the bladder they may become encrusted with a calcific shell and be visible on plain film.

Investigation of the cause of urinary tract calculi

Types of stone

The commonest stones in Africa are composed of calcium oxalate (Dawam et al., 2001) (Fig. 83.29): they are radio-opaque and, if more than 2–3 mm in diameter, can be seen easily on a plain abdominal film. They may be seen in the calyces, renal pelvis, ureter or bladder. Bladder stones in particular are more common in Africa than in industrialized countries and are very much more common in boys than girls. Other radio-opaque stones are calcium phosphate stones and 'struvite' calculi. The latter are formed in the presence of infection with urea-splitting organisms, when the ammonia produced causes the urine to be alkaline, which encourages their formation. A diagnostic problem arises when urinary tract stones are radiolucent; examples include urate and cystine stones, both of which form in acid urine. Staghorn calculi and nephrocalcinosis are relatively unreported in Africa.

Biochemical investigation

Very often it is not possible to identify an underlying metabolic disorder but hypercalcaemia and hypercalciuria are found in some cases: therefore measure plasma calcium, phosphate, urate and bicarbonate. It is useful also to perform 24-hour urine collections for calcium, urate, oxalate and sodium. In any patient with urinary tract calculi it is important to check that the GFR is normal.

Oxalate stones are occasionally found in patients with inflammatory bowel disease where the fat in the intestine becomes esterified with calcium and free oxalate becomes available for absorption. The link with sodium is more complex. There is good evidence that a high salt intake causes hypercalciuria through effects in the kidney. Another reason why salt is best avoided is the prevention of high blood pressure and subsequent stroke. A sustained reduction in salt intake should therefore be advised.

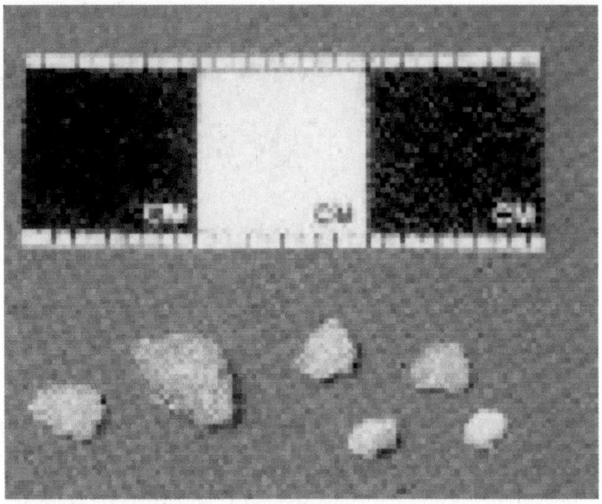

Fig. 83.29. Fragments of renal calculi.

Complications

Sometimes there is considerable pain and bleeding but infection is the greatest threat to life. The obstructed urinary tract may not only be infected when the patient presents, but it may also become infected if the obstruction is not relieved, and surgical intervention may itself lead to infection. Such infections can lead to serious complications including septicaemia and loss of renal function.

References

Adelekun T, Akinsola A. (1998). Hypertension induced chronic renal failure: clinical features, management and prognosis. *W Afr J Med*; **17**: 104–108.

Agodoa LY, Appel L, Bakris GL et al. (2001). Effect of ramipril vs amlodipine on renal outcomes in hypertensive nephrosclerosis. *J Am Med Assoc*; **285**: 2719–2728.

Akinsola A, Durosinmi M, Akinola N. (2000). The haematological profile of Nigerians with Chronic renal failure. *Afr J Med Sci*; **29**: 13–16.

Arije A, Akinlade K, Kadiri S et al. (1995). The problems of peritoneal dialysis in the management of chronic renal failure in Nigeria. *Trop Geographical Med*; **47**: 74–77.

Attolou VG, Bigot A, Ayivi B et al. (1998). Renal complications associated with human acquired immunodeficiency virus infection in a population of hospital patients at the Hospital and University National Center in Cotonou. *Sante*; **8**: 283–286.

Barsoum R, Rihan Z, Ibrahim A et al. (2002). Long term intermittent haemodialysis in Egypt. *Bull Wld Hlth Org*; **51**: 647–654.

Borok M, Nathoo K, Gabriel R, Porter K. (1997). Clinicopathological features of Zimbabwean patients with sustained proteinuria. *Centr Afr J Med*; **43**: 152–158.

Brenner BM, Cooper ME, de Zeeuw D et al. (2001). Effects of losartan on renal and cardiovascular outcomes in patients with type 2 diabetes and nephropathy. *N Engl J Med*; **345**: 861–869.

Cockroft D, Gault MK (1976). Prediction of creatinine clearance from serum creatinine. *Nephron*; **16**: 31–41.

Dawam D, Layaya GD, Osuide LA, Muhammad I, Garg SK (2001). Haematuria in Africa: is the pattern changing? *Br J Urol Int*; **87**: 326–330.

Diallo A, Niamkey E, Beda Yao B. (1997a). Chronic renal insufficiency in Cote d'Ivoire: study of 800 hospital cases. *Bull Soc Pathol Exot*; **90**: 346–348.

Diallo A, Nochy D, Niamkey E. et al. (1997b). Etiologic apects of nephrotic syndrome in Black African adults in a hospital setting in Abidjan. *Bull Soc Pathol Exotique*; **90**: 342–345.

Diouf B, Dia D, Ka MM et al. (1998). Autosomal dominant polycystosis in the hospital milieu in Dakar (Senegal). *Dakar Med*; **43**: 205–208.

Djrolo F, Attolou VG, Avode DG et al. (2001). Diabetic nephropathy: an epidemiological study based on proteinuria in a population of black African diabetics in Cotonou, Benin. *Sante*; **11**: 105–109.

Ekwere PD. (1995). Urinary calculus disease in South-eastern Nigeria. *Afr J Med Med Sci*; **24**: 289–295.

Elem B. (1984). Urinary calculus in Zambia: its incidence and relationship to *Schistosoma haematobium* infection and Vesicovaginal fistula. *Br J Urol*; **56**: 44–47.

Essamie M, Soliman A, Fayad T et al. (1995). Serious renal disease in Egypt. *Int J Artif Org*; **18**: 254–260.

Giglioni G. (1930). *Malaria Nepritis*, London: Churchill.

Giglioni G. (1962). Malaria and renal disease with specific reference to British Guiana. The effect of malaria eradication on the incidence of renal disease in British Guyana. *Ann Trop Med Parasitol*; **56**: 225–241.

Gupta JC, Diwakar R, Singh S, Gupta DK, Panda PK. (1977). A histopathological study of renal biopsies in 50 cases of leprosy. *Int J Leprosy Other Mycobact Dis*; **45**: 167–170.

Hommel D, Bollandard F, Hulin A. (1998). Multiple African honeybee stings and acute renal failure. *Nephron*; **78**: 235–236.

Hussain A, Elzubier A, Ahmed M. (1999). Target organ involvement in hypertensive patients in Eastern Sudan. *J Hum Hypertens*; **13**: 9–12.

Ibrahim A. (1978). The relationship between urinary bilharziasis and urolithiasis in the Sudan. *Br J Urol*; **50**: 294–297.

Ka EF, Diouf B, Ka MM et al. (1999). Evaluation of acute renal insufficiency in Dakar. *Dakar Med*; **44**: 84–87.

Klufio GO, Bentsi IK, Yeboah E et al. (1996). Upper urinary tract stones in Accra, Ghana. *W Afr J Med*; **15**: 173–176.

Laradi A, Mallet A, Beaufils H et al. (1998). HIV-associated nephropathy: outcome and prognostic factors. *J Am Soc Nephrol*; **9**: 2327–2335.

Lengani A, Coulibaly G, Laville M et al. (1997). Epidemiology of severe chronic renal insufficiency in Burkina Faso. *Sante*; **7**: 379–383.

Lengani A, Samadoulougou A, Cisse M. (2000). Characteristics of renal disease in hypertensive morbidities in adults in Burkina Faso. *Arch Mal Coeur Vaisseaux*; **93**: 1053–1057.

Lewis EJ, Hunsicker LG, Clarke WR et al. (2001). Renoprotective effect of the angiotensin-receptor antagonist irbesartan in patients with nephropathy due to type 2 diabetes. *N Engl J Med*; **345**: 851–860.

McLigeyo SO. (1990). Nephrotic syndrome in the tropics. *E Afr Med J*; **67**: 380.

Mate-Kole M, Yeboah E, Affram R et al. (1998). Haemodialysis in the treatment of acute renal failure in tropical Africa: a 20 year review. *Renal Failure*; **18**: 517–524.

Mkony CA, Chuwa LM, Kahamba JF et al. (1991). Urinary stone disease in Dar es Salaam. *E Afr Med J*; **68**: 461–467.

Nakayama EE, Ura S, Fleury RN, Soares V. (2001). Renal lesions in leprosy: a retrospective study of 199 autopsies. *Am J Kidney Dis*; **38**: 26–30.

Njeh M, Jemni M, Abid R et al. (1993). La tuberculose renale a forme pseudo-tumorale. *J d'Urol (Paris)*; **99**: 150–152.

Nsek M, Tshiani K. (1989). Chronic renal failure in tropical Africa. *E Afr Med J*; **66**: 109–114.

Oliech J, Kayima JK, Otieno LS. (1998). Urinary tract stone disease in Nairobi. *E Afr Med J*; **75**: 30–34.

Otieno LS. (1983). Genitourinary tuberculosis at Kenyatta National Hospital. *E Afr Med J*; **60**: 232–237.

Otieno LS, McLigeyo S, Luta M. (1991). Acute renal failure following the use of herbal remedies. *E Afr Med J*; **68**: 993–998.

Pantanowitz L, Goetach S, Butler O, Katz I. (1999). Renal biopsies in HIV positive patients at the Baragwanath Hospital 1989–1997. *Kidney Int (Abst)*; **55**: 2130

Parving HH, Lehnert H, Brochner-Mortensen J et al. (2001). The effect of irbesartan on the development of diabetic nephropathy in patients with type 2 diabetes. *N Engl J Med*; **345**: 870–878.

Plange-Rhule J, Phillips R, Acheempong JW et al. (1999). Hypertension and renal failure in Kumasi, Ghana. *J Hum Hypertens*; **13**: 37–40.

Plange-Rhule J, Micah FB, Eastwood JB (2002). Clinical nephrological problems important to the urologist. *Br J Urol Internat*; **89** (suppl): 44–49.

Randeree I, Cnarnocki A, Moodley J et al. (1995). Acute renal failure in pregnancy in South Africa. *Renal Failure*; **17**: 147–153.

Salako B, Kadiri S, Fehintola F et al. (1999). The effect of antihypertensive therapy on urinary albumin excretion in Nigerian hypertensives. *W Afr J Med*; **18**: 170–174.

Sanusi A, Akinsola A, Ajayi A. (2000). Creatinine clearance estimation from serum creatinine values: evaluation and comparison of five prediction formulae in Nigerian patients. *Afr J Med Med Sci*; **29**: 7–11.

Seedat Y, Naicker S, Rawat R et al. (1984). Racial differences in the causes of end stage renal failure in Natal. *S Afr Med J*; **65**: 956–958.

Seggie J, Nathoo K, Davies PG. (1984) Association of hepatitis B (HBs) antigenaemia and membranous glomerulonephritis in Zimbabwean children. *Nephron*; **38**: 115–119.

Sobngwi E, Mbanya J, Mououri E et al. (1999). Microalbuminuria and retinopathy in a diabetic population of Cameroon. *Diabetes Res Clinical Pract – Suppl*; **44**: 191–196.

Subramanian A, Mungai P, Ouma J et al. (1999). Long-term suppression of adult bladder morbidity and severe hydronephrosis following selective population chemotherapy for Schistosoma haematobium. *Am J Trop Med Hyg*; **61**: 476–481.

Swanepoel C, Madaus S, Cassidy M et al. (1998). IgA nephropathy: Groote Schuur Hospital experience. *Nephron*; **53**: 61–64.

Veriawa Y, du Toit E, Lawley C et al. (1990). Hypertension as a cause of end stage renal failure in South Africa. *J Hum Hypertens*; **4**: 379–383.

Were A, Otieno LS. (1992). Acute renal failure as seen at Kenyatta National Hospital. *E Afr Med J*; **69**: 110–113.

Wiggelinkhuizen J. (1987). Membranous glomerulonephropathy in childhood. *S Afr Med J*; **72**: 184–187.

Youmbissi TJ, Mbakop A, Eloundou (1999). Extramembranous glomerulonephritis: clinico-pathological finding in a group of 45 Cameroonians. *Arch Anat Cytol Pathol*; **47**: 48–52.

Zewdu W. (1994). Acute renal failure in Addis Ababa, Ethiopia: a prospective study of 136 patients. *Ethiop Med J*; **32**: 79–87.

84

Bones and joints

Musculoskeletal disorders encompass a wide range of disorders of bone and joints, including disorders of connective tissue structures in and around joints (Fig. 84.1). There are no data for Africa, but in industrialized countries about a quarter of all consultations to primary care physicians are for musculoskeletal complaints (Wood & MacLeish, 1974), many of which are self-limiting conditions.

Articular cartilage, synovium and bone are key structures in maintaining the integrity of diarthrodial joints. A primary insult to any one of the structures shown in Fig. 84.1 is often followed by secondary involvement of surrounding structures. In rheumatoid arthritis (RA), for example, synovial inflammation is the primary problem, but as the disease progresses there is secondary destruction of cartilage and bone.

Rheumatology in Africa

Limited financial resources and the scarcity of trained rheumatologists in most parts of Africa have meant that many patients with rheumatic diseases do not receive good care. For example, of the 4000 doctors in Kenya, only two are rheumatologists, who serve a population of

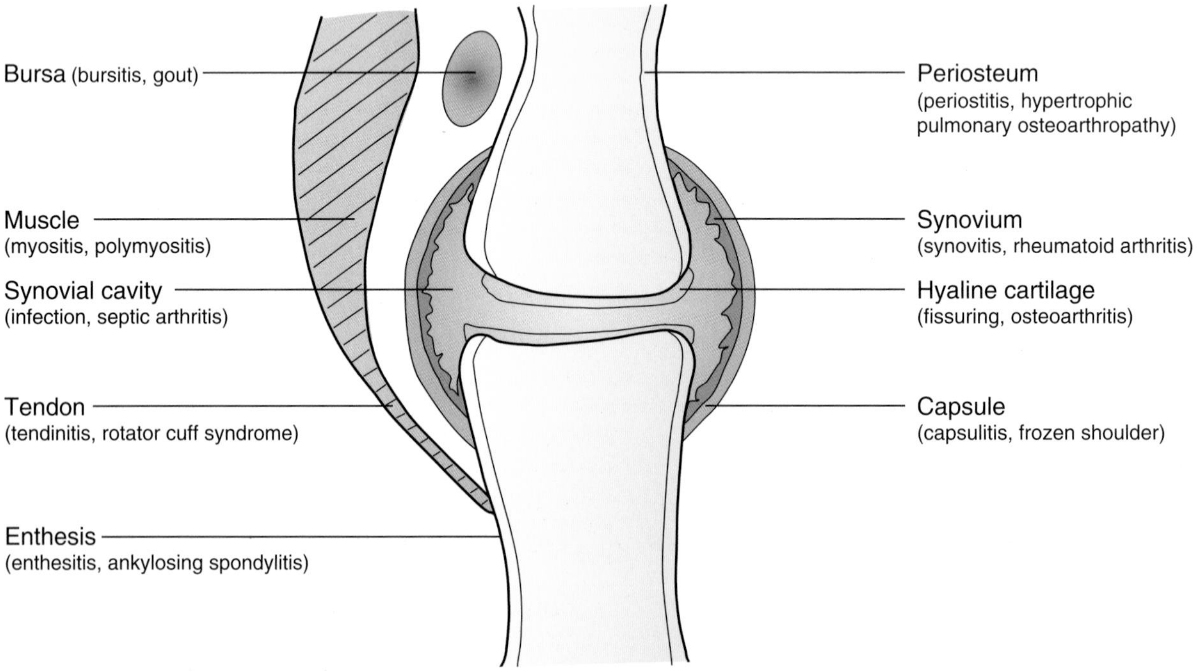

Fig. 84.1. Schematic diagram of key anatomical structures (pathology and disease examples in and around a diarthrodial joint).

Table 84.1. Glossary of rheumatological terminology

Arthralgia: Pain arising from joint (subjective)
Arthritis/arthropathy: Objective signs of joint abnormality
Bursitis: Inflammation of bursa
Monoarthritis: Arthritis affecting a single joint
Oligoarthritis/pauci-articular disease: Arthritis affecting 2–4 joints or small groups of joints
Polyarthritis: Arthritis affecting >4 joints (or groups of joints)
Synovitis: Clinically apparent joint inflammation – swelling + tenderness
Tenosynovitis: inflammation of tendon sheath
Enthesitis: Inflammation of enthesis or site of insertion of tendon ligament to bone

approximately 30 million (Tikly et al., 2000). The African League Against Rheumatism (AFLAR), an umbrella body of national rheumatology associations in Africa, together with the International Leagues of Rheumatology Associations (ILAR), is making a concerted effort to improve skills and training in rheumatology in Africa. The ILAR internet website, *www.ilar.org* has excellent clinical skills training features. From a research perspective, the changing epidemiological patterns of rheumatic diseases resulting from urbanization and the HIV pandemic in Africa, provide unique opportunities to study the role of nature (genetics) and nurture (environment) in the causation of complex rheumatic diseases like RA and the seronegative spondyloarthropathies.

The patterns of rheumatic diseases and their impact on physical function in sub-Saharan Africa are, in many respects, vastly different from that in industrialized countries. For example, monoarthritis is commonly due to an infectious arthritis, including acute septic arthritis and tuberculous arthritis, whereas Reiter's syndrome is rare in sub-Saharan Africa. Chronic inflammatory joint diseases, like RA, although less common and generally milder in Africans, often cause greater physical disability and handicap than in industrialized countries, primarily because optimal medical care and rehabilitation are not available.

Clinical approach to musculoskeletal disorders

A sound knowledge of the functional anatomy and stepwise clinical approach form the basis of a successful diagnosis of musculoskeletal disorders. Laboratory investigations and imaging are helpful in confirming a clinical diagnosis and assessing disease activity and disease progression, but are seldom specific or pathognomonic. Apart from making an accurate diagnosis, it is important to assess the functional disability. A glossary of common terminology in the rheumatic diseases is shown in Table 84.1.

History and examination

The four key elements of the diagnostic process are summarized in the Box.

Steps in the clinical diagnosis of rheumatic disease

1. **Anatomical localization:** articular or non-articular
2. **Mode of onset:** acute or chronic
3. **Extent of joint involvement:** monoarticular/oligoarticular/polyarticular
4. **Determination of underlying pathological process:** inflammatory or non-inflammatory.

Pain is one of the cardinal symptoms of rheumatic diseases. It is characterized in terms of site(s) of involvement, radiation, quality, intensity and aggravating/relieving factors. Pain may arise from within the joint or periarticular structures, e.g. bursitis. Referred pain may be shooting in nature when it arises from nerve root compression in the spine and may, for example, be referred to buttocks or legs. Pain that worsens with use is usually due to mechanical causes, like osteoarthritis. Inflammatory pain is worse at rest and eases with activity and exercise. Stiffness or 'gelling' is another key symptom. Prolonged early morning stiffness and inactivity stiffness are features of inflammatory joint disease. In contrast, stiffness associated with osteoarthritis occurs in the evening and after use. Other symptoms which patients occasionally notice are joint swelling or deformity.

The overall integrity of the musculoskeletal system can be quickly and efficiently assessed using the 'GALS' approach (see the Box).

'GALS' approach to assessing the integrity of the musculoskeletal system

G Gait
A Arms (upper limbs)
L Legs (lower limbs)
S Spine

Individual joint examination involves the three steps of look, feel and move. Inspection at rest may reveal swelling, malalignment or deformity of a joint and periarticular muscle wasting. Erythema of the overlying skin is a feature of inflammation as may be seen in gout and septic arthritis. Warmth and tenderness on palpation also implies joint inflammation. Joint line tenderness occurs in osteoarthritis. Joint swelling results from either excess synovial fluid, synovitis or periarticular bony proliferation.

Both active (initiated by patient) and passive (initiated by clinician) movements need to be elicited. Restriction of active movements only is a feature of periarticular disorders, e.g. supraspinatus tendinitis. In true articular conditions, both active and passive movements are restricted. Fine crepitus occurs with tenosynovitis. Coarse crepitus on movement is indicative of osteoarthritis.

Special investigations

The three main types of investigations in rheumatic diseases are synovial fluid analysis, blood tests and imaging of joints and bones.

(i) Joint aspiration and synovial fluid analysis are mandatory in the diagnosis of an acute monoarthritis (Schumacher & Reginato, 1991). Turbid fluid, which has a white cell count in excess of 75000/ml, is highly suggestive of sepsis or gout. Bacteria can often be detected on microscopy and culture of the fluid. In specialized centres, uric acid and calcium pyrophosphate crystals in synovial fluid are detected under polarized light microscopy.

(ii) Blood tests fall into three categories:
   (a) Acute phase reactants, including the ESR and C-reactive protein, are elevated in inflammatory rheumatic conditions.
   (b) Biochemical tests, of which the serum uric acid is essential in the diagnosis of gout.
   (c) Autoantibody tests are often positive in inflammatory arthropathies. The rheumatoid factor (RF) is an antibody directed against native IgG and is usually present in high titres in RA. The antinuclear antibody test is a generic test for detecting autoantibodies directed against various nuclear proteins. It is frequently positive in high titres in connective tissue diseases. Specific autoantibody tests, which are only necessary if the antinuclear antibody test is positive, help to further define specific connective tissue diseases and their subsets (Table 84.2).

(iii) The plain radiograph is one of the most useful and cost-effective investigations in rheumatology. Many of the rheumatic diseases produce characteristic articular and periarticular X-ray changes (Fig. 84.2). A single view of the affected joint/bone is all that is required in most cases. More specialized imaging modalities such as scintigraphy, ultrasonography, CT and MRI, usually only available in highly specialist centres, are reserved for specific, complex and difficult situations (American College of Rheumatology, 1996).

Table 84.2. Common autoantibody tests in rheumatic diseases

Test	Significance
RF	RA, SLE
ANA	Non-specific generic test; positive in SLE, SSc, RA and inflammatory myopathies; may be positive with chronic infections (e.g. HIV)
Anti-dsDNA	SLE
Anti-RNP	SLE (especially in Africans), SSc, MCTD
Anti-Sm	SLE
Anti-Ro (SSA)	Sjogren's syndrome, SLE, SSc
Anti-La (SSB)	Sjogren's syndrome, SLE, SSc
Anti-topoisomerase I	Diffuse cutaneous SSc
Anti-centromere	Limited cutaneous SSc (rare in Africans)
Anti-Jo-I	Polymyositis with overlap features
Anti-cardiolipin	SLE, primary antiphospholipid syndrome
Lupus anticoagulant	SLE, primary antiphospholipid syndrome
c-ANCA	Wegener's granulomatosis
p-ANCA	Other systemic vasculitides

Notes:
RF: rheumatoid factor, RA: rheumatoid arthritis, SLE: systemic lupus erythematosus, SSc: systemic sclerosis, MCTD: mixed connective tissue disease, ANA: antinuclear antibody, ANCA: anti-neutrophil cyto-plasmic antibody, RNP: ribonuclear protein.

An algorithm outlining the clinical approach to polyarthralgia is shown in Fig. 84.3. A differential diagnosis and key clinical radiological and laboratory features of the more common rheumatic conditions seen in Africa are shown in Table 84.3.

Principles of management

The management of the rheumatic diseases is, wherever possible, directed at the underlying cause, such as treating with antibiotics in the case of septic arthritis and controlling hyperuricaemia in the case of gout. In most chronic inflammatory arthritides, where the aetiology is not clear, management is aimed at reducing the symptoms of pain and stiffness as well as restoring joint function. A multi-disciplinary team approach is often necessary to achieve these objectives.

Bedrest

Brief bedrest may help to relieve pain and inflammation in patients with very active arthritis. Prolonged bedrest is to be discouraged since it may have a negative impact on functional outcome in the long term.

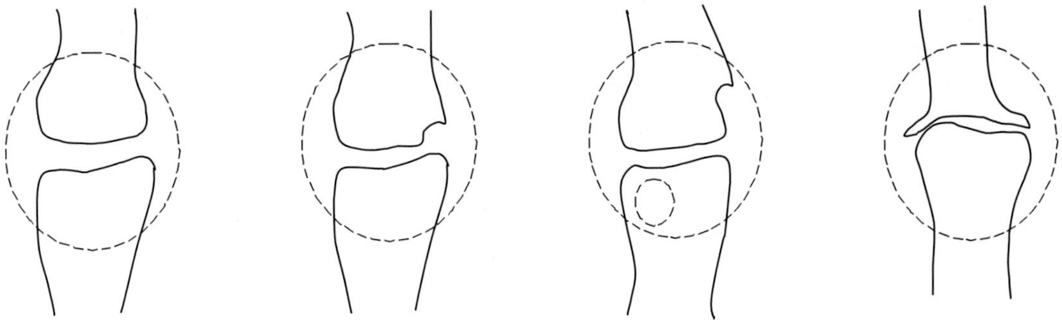

	Normal	Rheumatoid arthritis	Gout	Osteoarthritis
Soft tissue	normal	swelling	swelling (eccentric)	normal
Alignment	normal	malaligned	normal/malaligned	malaligned
Bone density osteopenia	normal	juxta-articular	normal	subchondral sclerosis
Osteophytes	none	none	none	present
Erosions	none	marginal	periarticular	none
Cysts	none	present ('grades')	large	present
Joint space (in early phase)	normal	reduced	normal	reduced

Fig. 84.2. Diagram of radiological features of the common chronic forms of arthritis.

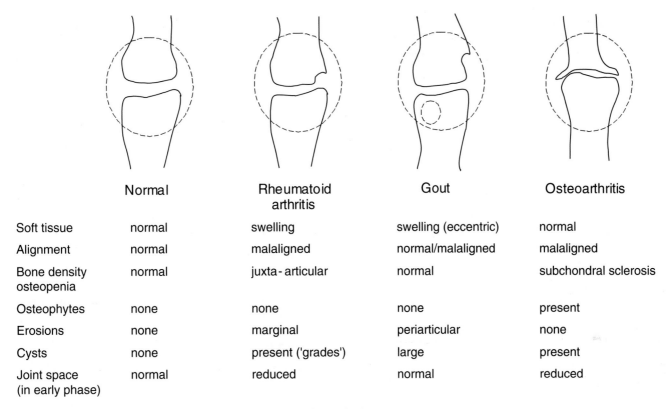

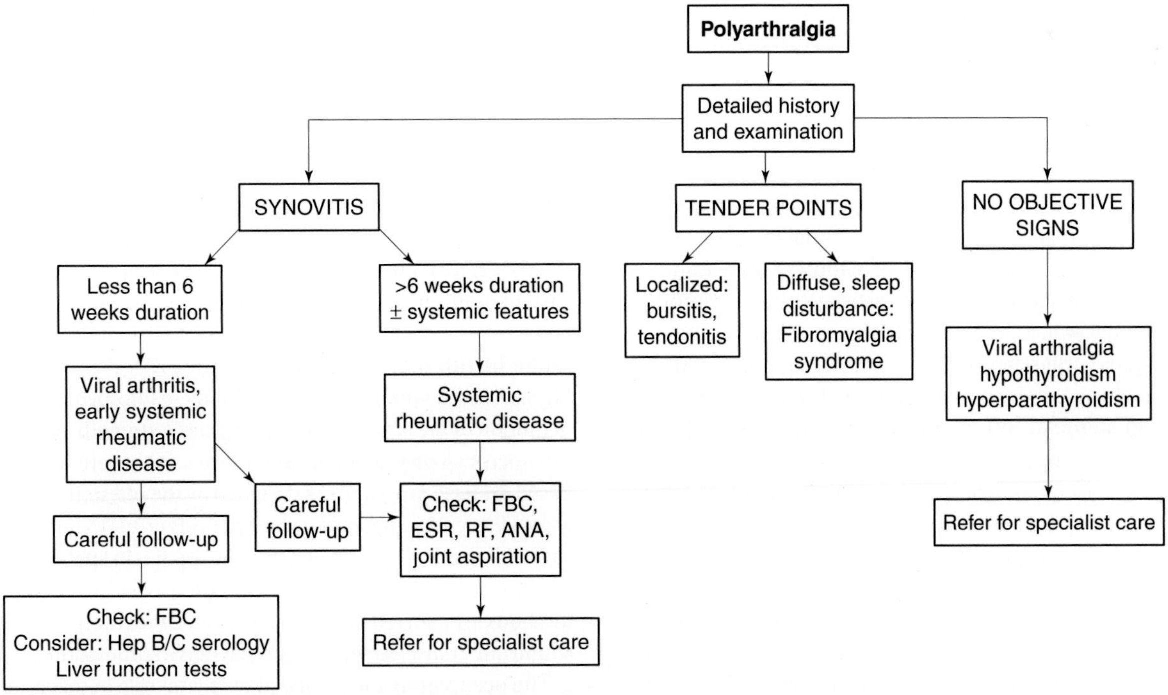

Fig. 84.3. Approach to polyarthralgia (adapted from ACR guidelines, 1996).

Table 84.3. Differential diagnosis of the common arthritides

Condition	Age	Sex	Mode of onset	Joint distribution	Other features	Laboratory features	Radiography
Septic arthritis (non-gonococcal)	Any age	F=M	Acute	Mono/oligoarthritis of large joints	Fever; septic focus elsewhere	↑WCC; organism detected in SF and blood	Soft tissue swelling initially
Gonococcal arthritis	Young adults	F=M	Acute/ subacute	Mono/oligoarthritis of large joints	Fever; skin pustules; urethritis/cervicitis	↑WCC; organism detected in SF and genital tract	Initially normal
Gout	Adults	M>F (post-menopausal)	Acute/ subacute	Mono/oligoarthritis of large joints; occasionally asymmetric polyarticular	Tophi, renal calculi, obesity, hypertension	Urate crystals in SF; ↑ serum uric acid	Periarticular erosions
Reactive arthritis/ Reiter's syndrome	Young adults	M>F	Subacute	Mono/oligoarthritis in lower limbs	Enthesitis, urethritis, conjunctivitis, skin rash	↑ ESR; may be HIV positive	Initially normal
Juvenile idiopathic arthritis	<16 yrs	F=M	Chronic	Oligoarticular/ polyarticular	Uveitis; fever, skin rash, lymphadenopathy with systemic variant	Anaemia, ↑WCC and platelets	Fusion of cervical spine, peripheral erosions rarely
Osteoarthritis	Older adults	F>M	Chronic	Monoarthritis of large joints or asymmetric polyarthritis	None	Normal	Focal joint space narrowing, subchondral sclerosis, osteophytes
Rheumatoid arthritis	Adults	F>M	Chronic	Symmetrical polyarthritis of small and large joints, especially hands	Nodules, sicca syndrome	Anaemia, ↑ platelets and ESR, +ve RF	Periarticular osteopaenia, marginal erosions

Notes:
SF: synovial fluid; WCC: white cell count; RF: Rheumatoid factor

Drugs

Analgesics are important for pain relief in both mechanical and inflammatory disorders. Paracetamol in a dose of up to 1 g four times daily is effective in most cases of non-inflammatory arthritis, such as osteoarthritis. Occasionally, additional pain relief with more potent analgesics including opioid drugs, may be required. Avoid the long-term use of opioid analgesics because of the risk of addiction.

Non-steroidal anti-inflammatory drugs (NSAIDs) have analgesic, antipyretic and anti-inflammatory actions. They are useful for relief of both pain and stiffness associated with joint inflammation. Due to the potential risk of side effects, especially peptic ulcer disease, prescribe NSAIDs for the shortest possible period and at the lowest effective dose, particularly in the elderly (Table 84.4). Selective cyclo-oxygenase-2 inhibitors are a new class of NSAIDs with efficacy similar to that of the older NSAIDs, but cause less serious gastrointestinal side effects.

Disease-modifying anti-rheumatic drugs (DMARDs) and immunosuppressive agents are drugs that appear to slow down the clinical course of the inflammatory arthritides such as rheumatoid arthritis. These drugs need careful monitoring for side effects.

Allied health professionals

Physiotherapy should be instituted early to improve range of motion of the affected joints and muscle strength. Family members can play an important role in carrying out home-based exercise programmes designed by the physiotherapists. Heat packs applied for short periods of 10–15 minutes to the affected joint often help to relieve pain. In specialized centres, physiotherapists also use a variety of electrotherapy methods for pain relief, including infrared radiation, ultrasound and transcutaneous electrical nerve stimulation.

The occupational therapist plays a vital role in teaching new skills and advising patients on making adjustments

Table 84.4. Non-steroidal anti-inflammatory drugs according to risk for gastrointestinal complications

Drug	Dosage	Frequency/day
Low risk		
Ibuprofen	400–600 mg	3
Sulindac	100–200 mg	2
Meloxicam	7.5–15 mg	1
Celoxocib[a]	100–200 mg	2
Rofecoxib[a]	12.5–25 mg	1
Intermediate risk		
Diclofenac	25–50 mg	3
Naproxen	250–500 mg	2
Indomethacin	25–50 mg	3
High risk		
Piroxicam	10–20 mg	1
Azapropazone	600 mg	3

Notes:
[a] selective cyclo-oxygenase-2 ('COX-2') inhibitors

to the home environment, which allows the patient to have greater physical independence. In resource-poor areas, 'home-made' aids can be can be very effective. The traditional African family is also of great importance in helping the patient with chronic rheumatological disease, and they deserve education and support.

Nurses play a vital role in the education of the patient and the family, both about the disease and its therapy. Other important team members ideally include the podiatrist, orthotist and medical social worker.

Surgery

Surgery is indicated for pain and functional disability resulting from local joint problems not responding to medical and rehabilitative measures. Surgical procedures include joint fusion (arthrodesis) and joint replacement (arthroplasty).

Inflammatory joint disorders

Rheumatoid arthritis

Rheumatoid arthritis (RA) is a chronic inflammatory joint disorder of unknown aetiology. The overall prevalence of RA is about 1 per cent in adults with a female:male ratio of 3–4:1. The age of onset peaks in the fifth to sixth decades, but Africans have a younger age of onset compared to Caucasians (Mody, 1995). There is no clear explanation of why RA is so rare in some rural African populations, whereas its prevalence in urban populations approaches that in industrialized countries (Ali-Gombe et al., 1995). RA is associated with the HLA alleles DRB1*0401, DRB1*0404 and DRB1*01.

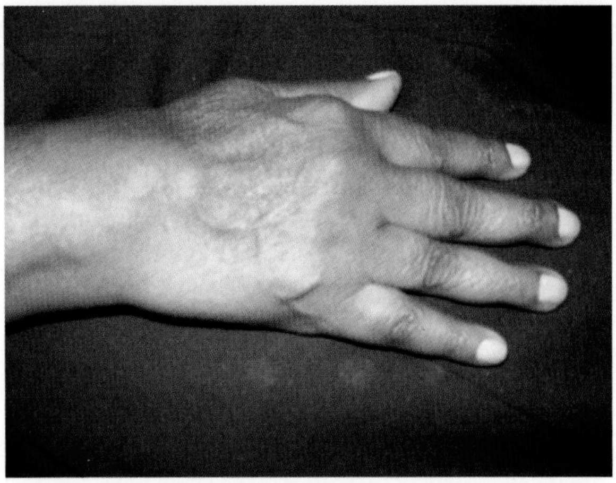

Fig. 84.4. Rheumatoid hand with swelling of wrist, metacarpophalangeal and proximal interphalangeal joints.

Pathology

The synovium in RA is organized into an invasive tissue termed pannus. It consists of T-cells, macrophages and fibroblast-like synovial cells. If left unchecked, pannus, directly and indirectly by secreting cytokines, invades and degrades cartilage and bone.

Clinical manifestations

RA presents as a symmetrical, destructive and deforming arthritis of insidious onset. It commonly affects the proximal interphalangeal (PIP) and metacarpophalangeal (MCP) joints of the hands, wrists, elbows, shoulders, hips, knees, ankles and metatarsophalangeal joints of the feet. In long-standing disease, classical hand deformities include radial deviation at the wrist and ulnar deviation at the metacarpophalangeal joints (Fig. 84.4). Occasionally in Africans, there is ulnar deviation at the wrist and relative sparing of the MCP and PIP joints, changes that are more reminiscent of juvenile idiopathic arthritis. Atlanto-axial subluxation in the cervical spine can be a serious and potentially life-threatening complication when it causes spinal cord compression.

Disease activity (inflammation) is assessed on the basis of the duration of early morning stiffness, severity of pain, number of tender and swollen joints, functional disability, and acute phase response (ESR or C-reactive protein).

Extra-articular features are frequently associated with severe, seropositive joint disease. They include anaemia of chronic disorders, subcutaneous nodules, keratoconjunctivitis sicca, scleritis, serositis, carpal tunnel syndrome, peripheral neuropathy, cutaneous vasculitis and Felty's syndrome. RA varies in severity across the African continent. West Africans have mild disease compared with East and Southern Africans, in whom extra-articular features are also more common (Adebajo & Reid, 1991).

Special investigations

The RF is positive in most patients, but up to one-third of African patients are seronegative. Radiographs of the hands and feet characteristically show juxta-articular osteopenia and/or marginal erosions.

Treatment

A multi-disciplinary team approach combining the skills of the doctor, physiotherapist, occupational therapist, podiatrist and social worker is required. NSAIDs and simple analgesics help to reduce the inflammation and relieve pain. Early intervention with DMARDs is aimed at controlling disease activity and reducing long-term disability (American College of Rheumatology, 2002). The choice of the specific DMARD depends on the severity of the disease, and available facilities and expertise to monitor therapy. Chloroquine (200 mg daily) is a safe and effective agent in mild disease. Sulphasalazine (1 g twice daily) and methotrexate (7.5–20 mg weekly) are indicated in established disease. Severe disease is treated with a combination of DMARDs. The anti-TNF biologic agents, infliximab and etenercept, are effective in refractory cases but are very costly. Intra-articular steroids help to reduce pain and inflammation in individual joints. Oral steroids should be used sparingly and are mainly indicated for serious extra-articular manifestations, like scleritis. Surgery is indicated for intractable pain and functional disability not responding to medical and physical therapy.

Seronegative spondyloarthritides

Seronegative spondyloarthritides are a group of inflammatory joint diseases characterized by (a) absence of RF, (b) sacroiliitis, (c) enthesitis, (d) familial clustering and (e) association with the HLA B27 antigen. Included in this group of disorders are ankylosing spondylitis, Reiter's syndrome/reactive arthritis, psoriatic arthritis, inflammatory bowel disease associated arthritis and Whipples disease. These conditions were, until recently, exceedingly rare in sub-Saharan Africans, primarily because of the low prevalence of the HLA- B27 antigen in the general population. The HIV pandemic has resulted in a dramatic increase of seronegative arthropathies in Africa, particularly Reiter's syndrome and psoriatic arthritis (McGill et al., 1997).

Ankylosing spondylitis

Affects mainly young men, presenting with features of inflammatory backache, i.e. pain and stiffness of the spine that improves with physical activity, and restricted lumbar spine movements. Large peripheral joint involvement, especially of the hip, can occur. Enthesitis can be very troublesome. Anterior uveitis is a common extra-articular manifestation. Cardiorespiratory complications of aortic regurgitation and apical lung fibrosis are very rare.

The presence of sacroiliitis, seen best on plain A–P or prone view radiograph of the pelvis, helps to confirm the diagnosis. A positive HLA B27 is not essential for diagnosis and in fact only a small minority of the cases in sub-Saharan Africa are HLA B27 positive (Mbayo et al., 1998). Most patients respond to NSAIDs and extensor back exercises. Sulphasalazine or methotrexate is used to treat significant peripheral joint involvement.

Reactive arthritis

An arthritis that is distant in place and time to an infection elsewhere in the body. Reiter's syndrome is the triad of reactive arthritis, urethritis, conjunctivitis. It is a disease mainly of young men, following a Chlamydia infection of the urogenital tract or acute diarrhoeal illness due to a Shigella, Salmonella, *Campylobacter* or Yersinia infection. In most cases of HIV-associated reactive arthritis there is no evidence of co-infection with any of these bacteria. The arthritis is usually self-limiting and responds well to NSAIDs. Sulphasalazine may be of benefit in refractory cases.

Psoriatic arthritis

Rare in sub-Saharan Africa but severe cases occur in association with HIV infection. There are five recognized variants, including an oligoarthritis, symmetrical polyarthritis, arthritis of the distal inter-phalangeal joints, arthritis mutilans and spondylitis. Dystrophic nail changes are a feature of psoriatic arthritis. HIV-associated psoriatic arthritis is associated with extensive skin disease and shows a poor response to NSAIDs.

Inflammatory bowel disease associated arthritis

Clinically indistinguishable from ankylosing spondylitis. It is extremely rare due to the fact that ulcerative colitis and Crohn's disease are rare in Africans.

Table 84.5. Clinical features suggestive of a connective tissue disease

Non-specific	
Fatigue, malaise, fever, myalgia, depression, weight loss	
Specific	
Raynaud's phenomenon (episodic vasospasm of digits on exposure to cold)	
Photosensitivity	
Alopecia	
Cutaneous vasculitis	
Dryness of mucosal surfaces (xerophthalmia and xerostomia)	
Oesophageal dysmotility	
Inflammatory arthritis	
Proximal myopathy	
Recurrent abortions	
Stroke in a young patient	

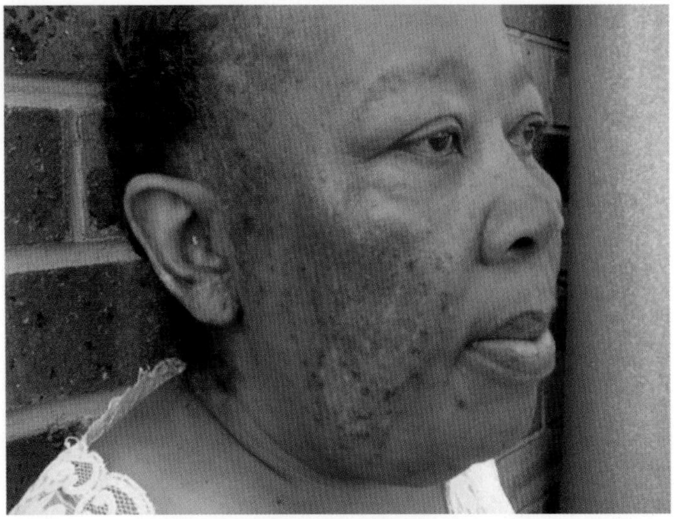

Fig. 84.5. Discoid lupus rash affecting external ear and face.

Juvenile idiopathic arthritis

Juvenile idiopathic arthritis (JIA) is a group of chronic inflammatory arthritides that by definition occurs in children under the age of 16 years (Petty et al., 1998). The three major patterns of JIA are as follows

(i) Systemic-onset arthritis (Still's disease), characterized by fever, an evanescent maculopapular rash, lymphadenopathy, hepatosplenomegaly and arthritis.
(ii) Pauciarticular disease, in which one to four joints are affected, is rare in Africans.
(iii) Polyarticular disease, where more than four joints are affected, is the commonest variant in Africans. It affects mainly the wrist, ankle, knee and hip joints. Micrognathia and associated cervical spine fusion is common. The majority of these children are seronegative for RF but a minority of patients have seropositive disease similar to that seen in adults.

The overall prognosis of JIA, especially the pauciarticular form, is better than adult RA. Pain relief is achieved with simple analgesics and NSAIDs, including aspirin. Oral steroids and DMARDs, particularly methotrexate, are reserved for established cases. Aggressive physiotherapy is essential to prevent joint contractures and deformities.

Connective tissue diseases

Connective tissue diseases are a group of autoimmune multi-system disorders that are characterized by the presence of circulating anti-nuclear antibodies. They occur especially in women in the child-bearing age group. Included in this group are systemic lupus erythematosus (SLE), systemic sclerosis or scleroderma (SSc), Sjogren's syndrome and polymyositis/dermatomyositis. Some patients have overlap features, sometimes referred to as mixed connective tissue disease (MCTD). Clinical features that should alert the clinician of the possibility of a connective tissue disorder are shown Table 84.5.

Systemic lupus erythematosus (SLE)

SLE is mainly a disease of young women. Its prevalence varies across the African continent, being very rare in tropical areas and more common in North and South Africa (Tikly et al., 1996). There are no precise epidemiological studies available, but as an example from South Africa, the rheumatological service at Baragwanath Hospital in Soweto, sees approximately 30 new SLE patients each year. The exact aetiology is not known but it is likely that environmental factors (ultraviolet rays, drugs and infections) trigger the disease in genetically susceptible individuals (Pisetsky et al., 1997). HLA-DR2 is associated with SLE in Africans. The high female:male ratio of 10:1 suggests that sex hormones modulate expression of the disease.

Skin rashes, especially the classical butterfly malar rash and chronic discoid lupus rash (Fig. 84.5), and arthritis occur in more than half the patients. Other less common cutaneous manifestations include cutaneous vasculitis, photosensitivity, Raynaud's phenomenon, alopecia and livedo reticularis. Immune-complex glomerulonephritis, manifesting as asymptomatic proteinuria/haematuria, nephrotic syndrome or renal failure, and neuropsychiatric complications, like psychosis, epilepsy and strokes, are a

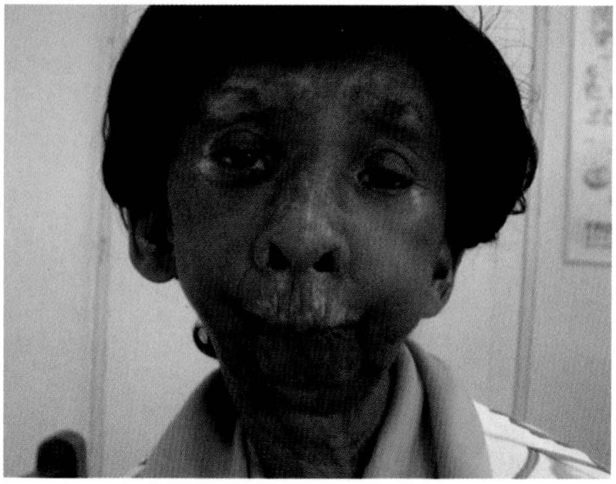

Fig. 84.6. Diffuse cutaneous systemic sclerosis with microstomia and 'salt and pepper' depigmentation.

major cause of morbidity and mortality. Serositis (pericarditis and pleuritis) is sometimes the sole clinical manifestation of SLE and not surprisingly, in the African context, is often initially misdiagnosed as tuberculosis (Taylor & Stein, 1986). Verrucous valvular thickening or 'Libman–Sacks' endocarditis may simulate, and more importantly, predispose to infective endocarditis. Fever in a patient with SLE can pose a major diagnostic problem, resulting from either a disease flare or systemic infection. Infection must therefore be actively excluded especially since infections are one of the leading causes of death in SLE. The antiphospholipid syndrome is a rare complication of SLE and is characterized by arterial/venous thrombosis, recurrent mid-trimester abortions, and presence of antiphospholipid antibodies (anti-cardiolipin antibodies and lupus anticoagulant).

Investigations: Laboratory features include anaemia of chronic disorders or a Coombs' positive haemolytic anaemia, leukopenia/lymphopenia and thrombocytopenia. The ANA is positive in virtually all cases. Anti-dsDNA antibodies and C4 hypocomplementaemia are a feature of active disease.

Treatment: General measures:

- avoid direct sun exposure
- avoid drugs (e.g. high dose oestrogens) that precipitate a disease flare
- discourage women from becoming pregnant during periods of active disease, especially renal disease

Drug therapy is stratified according to the type of organ involvement. Skin and joint features can be effectively treated with topical steroids and sunscreen lotions and NSAIDs and analgesics, respectively. Chloroquine is useful for the skin and joint features and as a steroid-sparing agent. Oral corticosteroids are reserved for more serious complications. Immunosuppressive drugs (cyclophosphamide, azathioprine) are combined with oral steroids in patients with severe renal and neuropsychiatric complications.

Systemic sclerosis or scleroderma (SSc)

SScis characterized by widespread sclerosis and fibrosis of the skin and various internal organs, most commonly the gastrointestinal tract, heart and lungs, are characteristic. Underground goldminers in South Africa are at increased risk of developing SSc from silica dust exposure.

Most patients present with Raynaud's phenomenon or progressive skin thickening. In diffuse cutaneous SSc, which is the predominant subset in Africans, the skin induration extends to involve the trunk, often associated with 'salt and pepper' pigmentary changes of the affected skin (Fig. 84.6) (Tager & Tikly, 1999). Arthralgia, pulmonary fibrosis and anti-nucleolar antibodies are common. In limited cutaneous SSc or CREST syndrome (Calcinosis, Raynaud's phenomenon, Esophageal dysfunction, Sclerodactyly, Telangiectasia), Raynaud's phenomenon occurs invariably and the skin changes are limited to the extremities. This subset, which is associated with anticentromere antibodies, is extremely rare in Africans.

Vasodilators are used to treat Raynaud's phenomenon. There is no effective treatment for the skin changes. Oral steroids should be used with extreme caution because of the risk of precipitating a hypertensive renal crisis. Cyclophosphamide is used to treat the pulmonary fibrosis. Physiotherapy is important for the prevention and treatment of joint contractures

The idiopathic inflammatory myopathies

Polymyositis and dermatomyositis are diffuse connective tissue diseases characterized by proximal muscle weakness, raised muscle enzymes, electromyographic features of muscle inflammation, and histological features of inflammatory cell infiltration and necrosis of skeletal muscle. In dermatomyositis there are additional skin changes of a periorbital heliotrope rash (Fig. 84.7), Gottron's papules over the knuckles, and cutaneous vasculitis in childhood dermatomyositis. In adults, myositis can occur either in isolation or in association with either another connective tissue disease or malignancy. In the anti-Jo-1 syndrome variant of myositis, there are additional features of Raynaud's phenomenon, interstitial lung disease, 'mechanics hands' and antibodies to Jo-1 (histidyl tRNA synthetase). Prednisone (1mg/kg) is used for the myositis. Azathioprine and methotrexate are indi-

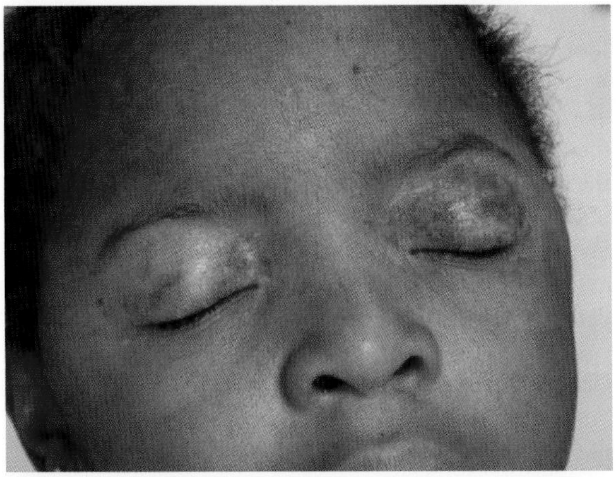

Fig. 84.7. Heliotrope rash of dermatomyositis.

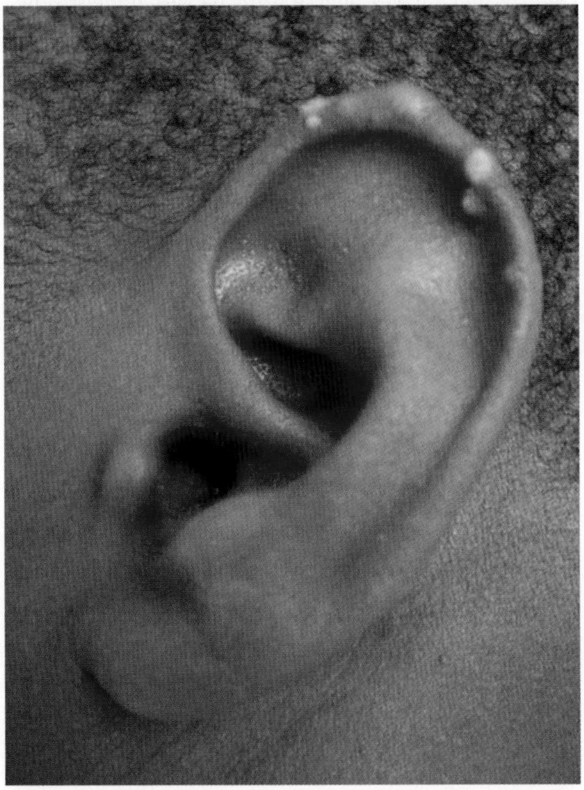

Fig. 84.8. Gouty tophi on pinna of ear.

cated in refractory cases. The skin changes respond to chloroquine and topical steroids.

Sjogren's syndrome

Sjogren's syndrome is a disorder characterized by xerophthalmia (dry eyes) and xerostomia (dry mouth) as a result of inflammation of exocrine glands, especially salivary and lacrimal glands, are characteristic. Primary Sjogren's syndrome is extremely rare in Africans but secondary SS associated with RA or SLE or PSS is not uncommon. Biopsy of a minor lacrimal gland is sometimes necessary to confirm the diagnosis of Sjogren's syndrome and histology shows lymphocytic infiltration and destruction of acinar glands. Regular use of artificial tears helps to relieve the xerophthalmia.

Table 84.6. Causes of hyperuricaemia

Under-excretion of uric acid (90% of cases)
Familial
Intrinsic renal disease
Drugs, e.g. diuretics, low-dose aspirin, pyrazinamide
Lead poisoning
Over-production of uric acid (10% of cases)
Inherited enzyme defects, e.g. Lesch–Nyhan syndrome
Increased cell turnover, e.g. malignancies and psoriasis
Alcohol
High purine diet
Cytotoxic drugs

Crystal arthropathies

Gout

Gout results from hyperuricaemia and deposition of monosodium urate crystals in joints which induce attacks of arthritis. It occurs almost exclusively in adult men and postmenopausal women only. A marked increase in the incidence of gout in Africans has been observed over the last decade, so that in some centres it is now the commonest type of acute arthritis. Rapid urbanization and associated sedentary lifestyle, obesity, hypertension and alcohol intake have contributed to this increased occurrence of gout (Tikly et al., 1998). The common causes of hyperuricaemia are shown in Table 84.6.

Acute gout presents as a monoarthritis or oligoarthritis, most commonly affecting lower limb joints and typically the big toe ('podagra'). Polyarticular tophaceous gout is seen more commonly in Africans of both sexes than in other populations and can be easily mistaken for RA. Tophi over the elbows, hands, and helix of ear (Fig. 84.8) are common. Uric acid renal calculi are rare.

Diagnosis

Best confirmed by the presence of urate crystals in synovial fluid or tophi under polarized light microscopy. Serum uric acid levels are raised but are occasionally normal during acute attacks of gout. Radiographs show periarticular bony erosions.

Treatment

Treat the acute attack initially with high doses of NSAIDs, e.g. indomethacin 50mg four times daily. Colchicine is an effective alternative, especially in patients with an active peptic ulcer or renal disease. In cases where both NSAIDs and colchicine are contraindicated, an intra-articular steroid injection or a short course of oral prednisone is indicated. Prophylactic therapy with allopurinol or a uricosuric agent like probenicid is indicated in patients with (i) frequent acute attacks of >3 per year, (ii) chronic tophaceous gout, and (iii) renal calculi.

Calcium pyrophosphate dihydrate disease

An uncommon crystal arthropathy of the elderly and seldom seen in Africans. It presents either as an acute monoarthritis ('pseudogout') or as a chronic arthritis with features of severe osteoarthritis and associated chondrocalcinosis. Positively birefringent rhomboidal shaped crystals are found in the synovial fluid. Secondary causes include primary hyperparathyroidism and iron overload. Treatment for the acute attacks is the same as for gout and the underlying secondary cause should be treated where possible.

Osteoarthritis

Osteoarthritis (OA) is a degenerative joint disorder characterized by loss of cartilage with secondary osteophyte formation and mild synovitis. The prevalence of primary OA increases with age so that more than half the elderly over 65 years have OA. Trauma, mechanical problems and inflammatory joint diseases can result in secondary OA (see the Box).

Classification of osteoarthritis

Primary
Generalized nodal OA
Primary OA of knee or hip

Secondary
Mechanical, e.g. post-traumatic, malalignment
Inflammatory, e.g. rheumatoid arthritis
Metabolic, e.g. haemachromatosis
Neurological, e.g. Charcot's arthropathy

Primary OA of the knee is common, especially in women (Kouakou et al., 1998). Other sites of primary OA are the hip, distal interphalangeal joints and spine. Mseleni disease is a rare endemic form of OA that manifests during the first decade of life in people living near Lake Sibiya in the north east of South Africa (Adebajo, 1995). It is a crippling disease, most commonly affecting the hip joint, but other large joints like the elbows and knees can be affected. No genetic or environmental factors, including dietary deficiencies, have been identified to date.

Clinical features

The main clinical features of OA are pain aggravated by physical activity, bony swelling of the joint, joint line tenderness, crepitus and restricted range of motion. Effusions occur occasionally in knee OA. Radiographic changes include joint space narrowing, osteophytes and subchondral sclerosis and cysts.

Simple analgesics and NSAIDs provide symptomatic relief. Intra-articular steroid injections are effective in some patients, especially in knee OA when there is an associated synovial effusion. Physiotherapy helps to improve muscle strength and range of motion. Surgical intervention (essentially joint replacement) may be necessary in patients with severe intractable pain and/or severe deformity of the hip or knee joint.

Infections and the musculoskeletal system

Infectious agents cause joint disease by two principal mechanisms: (i) directly by invasion of the synovial cavity, resulting in acute or chronic septic arthritis, or (ii) indirectly by immune-mediated mechanisms as in viral arthritis and reactive arthritis/Reiter's syndrome.

Viral arthritis

Viral infections such as parvovirus B19, hepatitis B and rubella produce a symmetrical inflammatory polyarthritis. The arthritis usually resolves within 4–6 weeks and responds well to symptomatic treatment with analgesics and NSAIDs.

HIV-associated rheumatic syndromes

The human immunodeficiency virus (HIV) pandemic in sub-Saharan Africa has produced a myriad of rheumatic syndromes, some of which were previously rare in Africa (Njobvu et al., 1988). These include non-specific arthralgia, fibromyalgia, inflammatory oligo/polyarthritis,

Table 84.7. Characteristic of gonococcal and non-gonococcal septic arthritis

	Gonococcal	Non-gonococcal
Patient and risk profile	Young, sexually active adults Female > male Recent menses Pregnancy and immediately post-partum	Extremes of age – children and elderly Previously damaged joints (e.g. RA or OA) Prosthetic joint implant Diabetes mellitus Sickle cell anaemia Immunocompromised host IV drug abuse
Organisms	*Neisseria gonorrhoeae*	*Staph aureus* (>50%) *Staph epidermidis* (prosthetic joints) *Streptococci* Gram-negative bacilli: *Salmonella* species (sickle cell disease), *H. influenzae* and *E. coli* Anaerobes (rare)
Clinical presentation	Migratory polyarthralgia, tenosynovitis, dermatitis, multiple joints (40%), urethral discharge	Single hot swollen joint, multiple joints (10%)
Recovery of bacteria	<50% synovial fluid <10% blood, 70–90% genitourinary tract	>90% synovial fluid >50% blood
Outcome	Excellent, response within a few days	Disability in 30–50%, slow response

Reiter's syndrome, psoriatic arthritis and sepsis in muscle, bone and joints. Some manifestations, like diffuse infiltrative lymphocytosis syndrome (a condition that is clinically similar to primary Sjogren's syndrome), cutaneous vasculitis, inflammatory myositis and presence of antinuclear antibodies, closely mimic and may be difficult to distinguish from the primary autoimmune connective tissue diseases.

Septic arthritis

Septic arthritis due to pyogenic bacteria is potentially the most destructive form of acute arthritis. It commonly presents as a monoarthritis, affecting the knee most often, but can affect multiple joints simultaneously. Table 84.7 shows the major differences between gonococcal and non-gonococcal arthritis. Diagnosis is based primarily on the synovial fluid findings of a purulent effusion, a large number of leukocytes and detection of the offending bacteria on microscopy and culture. Prompt and adequate drainage of the joint by needle aspiration, arthroscopy or open arthrotomy, combined with broad-spectrum parenteral antibiotics is essential. Definitive antibiotic therapy will depend on the culture and sensitivity of bacteria from the synovial fluid or blood. Intravenous antibiotics are necessary for at least a week for gonococcal arthritis and 2–4 weeks with non-gonococcal septic arthritis, followed by oral antibiotics in some cases (Goldenberg, 1998).

Tuberculosis

Tuberculosis can affect bone and joints in several ways. Tuberculous arthritis, which is the commonest form of chronic infective arthritis in Africa, presents as a chronic monoarthritis, often affecting the hip, knee or wrist. Radiographs show osteopenia and marginal erosions with joint space narrowing occurring in late disease. Synovial biopsy and histology is needed to confirm the diagnosis.

Tuberculous spondylitis or Pott's disease commonly affects the thoracic spine. It typically produces an angulated 'gibbus' deformity of the spine, often with associated signs of nerve root or spinal cord compression. Radiographic changes include erosion of vertebral bodies and disc space, often with a paravertebral shadow of a cold abscess (Fig. 84.9). Other rare musculoskeletal manifestations are dactylitis in children and Poncet's disease, which is a polyarthritis resulting from a hypersensitivity reaction to *M. tuberculosis*. Atypical mycobacterial joint infections occur in HIV-positive patients with very low CD4 counts of less than 100/ml. Treatment includes at least 18 months of antituberculous therapy and surgical decompression of the spinal cord in some cases of tuberculous spondylitis.

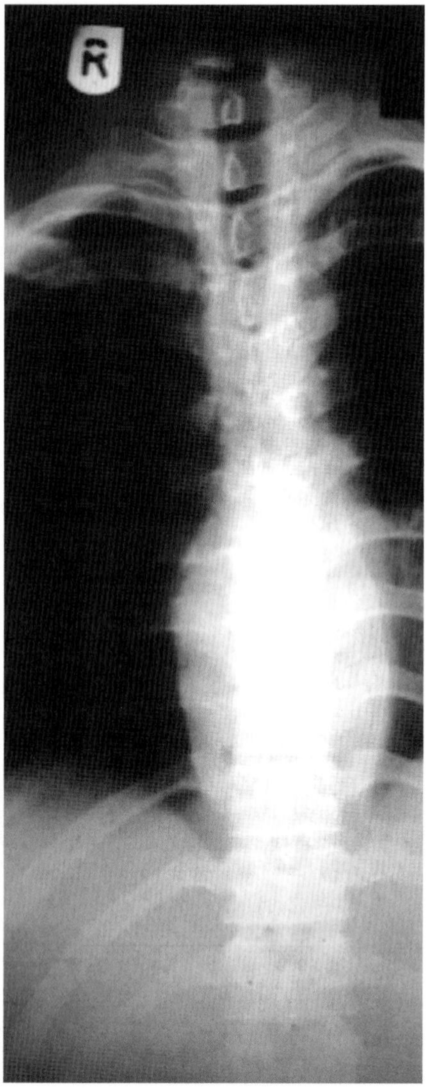

Fig. 84.9. Plain chest x-ray: paravertebral abscess. Tuberculosis of the spine. The plain film shows paraspinal soft tissue swelling which is a good indicator of underlying infection. By courtesy of the Institute of Orthopaedics and the Wellcome Trust.

Fungal infections

Fungal infections, specially sporotrichosis, blastomycosis and histoplasmosis, are rare causes of destructive bone and joint disease. Lyme disease, a chronic arthritis caused by *Borrelia burgdorferi*, has not been reported in Africa.

Osteomyelitis

Osteomyelitis or infection of bone results in progressive inflammatory destruction of the bone, bone necrosis, and new bone formation. In most cases, osteomyelitis follows haematogenous spread from a distant infection, often a urinary tract infection or an infected intravenous line. Rarely it is secondary to a contiguous focus of infection or vascular insufficiency. In children it usually presents as a painful swelling of limb with fever. In adults, vertebral osteomyelitis is more common, manifesting with vague symptoms and signs consisting of dull, constant back pain and spasm of the paravertebral muscles. In acute cases radiographs show soft tissue swelling, bone destruction and periosteal new bone formation. Bone sclerosis and sequestra are features of chronic disease. *Staphylococcus aureus* is the most common causative organism, followed by gram-negative bacilli in about 30 per cent of adult cases. Both antibiotics and surgical debridement (to remove sequestrae) are used for treatment.

Pyomyositis

Pyomyositis or bacterial infection of muscle is a disease mainly seen in tropical Africa (McGill, 1995). It also occurs more often in HIV-infected patients. Transient bacteraemia, in most cases due to *Staphylococcus aureus*, results in localized muscle infection and necrosis. Pyomyositis commonly affects the quadriceps, paraspinal and gluteus muscles and shoulder girdle. It presents with fever and a localized, fluctuant and tender swelling of muscle. Paraspinal muscle involvement may cause muscle spasm, mimicking tetanus and meningitis. The diagnosis is confirmed by aspiration and culture of fluid from fluctuant areas. Surgical drainage and antibiotics are indicated for treatment.

Systemic vasculitis

The systemic vasculitides are a heterogeneous group of disorders characterized by inflammation and necrosis of the wall of blood vessels, resulting in tissue or end-organ damage. The classification of these disorders is based on (a) whether the vasculitis is a primary phenomenon or secondary to another systemic illness and (b) the size of the affected blood vessels (Table 84.8). Small vessel hypersensitivity vasculitis presents as purpura or cutaneous ulceration/gangrene, and is commonly secondary to drugs, systemic infections and connective tissue diseases. The primary medium-vessel vasculitides, Wegener's granulomatosis and polyarteritis nodosa, cause serious renal damage, but are very rare in Africa. Takayasu's arteritis is a common large-vessel vasculitis in Africans affecting mainly teenage and young adult females. Inflammation and occlusion of large vessels of the aorta and vessels of

Table 84.8. Classification of vasculitis

Small-vessel vasculitis
Hypersensitivity or leukocytoclastic vasculitis
Connective tissue diseases, e.g. SLE
Drugs, e.g thiazides
Infections, e.g. Neisseria, mycobacteria, HIV
Mixed essential cryoglobulinaemia (associated with hepatitis C)
Microscopic polyangiitis
Henoch-Schonlein purpura
Medium-vessel vasculitis
Polyarteritis nodosa (associated with hepatitis B in one-third of cases)
Wegener's granulomatosis
Kawasaki disease (mucocutaneous lymph node syndrome)
Rheumatoid systemic vasculitis
Large-vessel vasculitis
Takayasu's arteritis
Giant cell arteritis

aortic arch result in absent peripheral pulses and are sometimes complicated by hypertension and strokes. Myalgias and arthralgias are frequently reported in the early stages of this disease, in which an inflammatory process affects the aorta and its large branches. Tuberculosis has been suggested as a possible cause.

Histology is the gold standard for the diagnosis of vasculitis. In the case of medium- and large-vessel vasculitis it is not always possible to make a histological diagnosis, in which case angiography is useful. In most types of vasculitis, treatment is initiated with prednisolone. Cyclophosphamide is effective in medium-vessel vasculitis and methotrexate is indicated in refractory cases of Takayasu's arteritis.

Rheumatic manifestations of systemic disorders

Rheumatic complications may occur with a variety of systemic disorders. In haemophilia frequent bleeds into joints result in degenerative and erosive joint destruction. Hypothyroidism can be associated with a polyarthritis, carpal tunnel syndrome and myopathy. In type 1 diabetes there may develop pseudoscleroderma of the hands, also known as diabetic cheiroarthropathy (see Chapter 70), Dupuytren's contractures, frozen shoulder, and diffuse idiopathic hypertrophic skeletal ostosis (DISH) syndrome. DISH, which is a form of degenerative spondyloarthropathy, is especially common in the elderly, even in the absence of diabetes (Cassim et al., 1990). Sarcoidosis can cause a symmetrical non-destructive inflammatory state, that has a particular predilection for ankles but can also affect the knees and wrists. A more chronic osseous form of sarcoidosis with cystic bone lesions is especially found in Africans. Malignancy can present as arthralgia in children with acute leukaemia or an explosive seronegative inflammatory arthritis affecting the lower limb joints. Neuropathic arthropathy or Charcot's arthropathy is a destructive/resorptive arthropathy of the small joints of the foot and is usually secondary to a sensory neuropathy associated with diabetes, chronic alcohol abuse or leprosy.

Soft tissue rheumatism

Aches and pains are often due to periarticular soft tissue problems. Conditions such as tennis elbow, plantar fasciitis and rotator cuff syndromes are very common. Fibromyalgia syndrome is a disorder mainly of women and presents as diffuse aches and pains which interfere with sleep. Eliciting specific focal tender points in the absence of objective joint disease is essential for the diagnosis. Treatment includes aerobic exercise and tricyclic antidepressants. Importantly, NSAIDs do not provide much pain relief.

Backache

Lower backache is an extremely common ailment in adults and a major cause of lost days at work (Hart et al., 1995). In most cases, mechanical injury to the paraspinal soft tissues of muscle and ligaments is the cause and patients improve spontaneously. Non-mechanical causes are not common, but should never be overlooked. They include spondyloarthropathies, spinal infections, osteoporotic fractures, metastatic cancer and referred visceral pain, e.g. an abdominal aneurysm. 'Red flags' that suggest serious pathology, are shown in the Box.

Red flags for serious causes of lower backache
Age of onset <20 or >55
Fever, weight loss, night sweats
Intractable pain with no improvement in 4 to 6 weeks
Nocturnal pain or pain of increasing severity
Recent severe trauma
Inflammatory features of early morning/inactivity stiffness
Neurological deficits

Table 84.9. Secondary causes of osteoporosis

Endocrine/metabolic	Thyrotoxicosis, primary hyperparathyroidism, Cushing's syndrome, hypogonadism, iron overload
Gastrointestinal/nutritional	Malabsorption, chronic liver disease, calcium deficiency, scurvy, alcoholism
Rheumatological	Rheumatoid arthritis, ankylosing spondylitis, systemic lupus erythematosus
Malignancy	Multiple myeloma
Drugs	Corticosteroids, heparin (chronic use)

Diseases of bone

Osteoporosis

Osteoporosis is a metabolic bone disease characterized by low bone mass and microarchitectural deterioration of bone tissue, leading to enhanced bone fragility and increased fracture risk. Bone loss, which results from an imbalance between the rates of resorption and formation, occurs at about 1 per cent a year in both sexes after the peak bone mass is achieved at about age 30. Women have an accelerated phase of bone loss after the menopause because of oestrogen deficiency. The incidence of osteoporotic fractures thus rises after the menopause in women and about a decade later in men.

Osteoporotic fractures are not as large a problem in African as in Western populations (Daniels et al., 1997). A higher peak bone mass in Africans is thought to be protective against fractures. However, with an increasingly ageing population and change to a more sedentary urban lifestyle, the incidence of osteoporosis is likely to rise. Risk factors for primary osteoporosis include being female, menopause before 45 years, hypogonadism, smoking, high alcohol intake, low calcium intake, thin body habitus, and physical inactivity. Secondary causes of osteoporosis are shown in Table 84.9. The use of oral corticosteroids, often injudiciously, for inflammatory conditions like asthma and rheumatoid arthritis is a major cause of osteoporosis.

Osteoporosis is asymptomatic, unless complicated by a fracture. The three common sites for osteoporotic fractures are the forearm (Colles' fracture), vertebrae, and hip. Vertebral fractures present as backache, loss of height and kyphosis. Spinal radiographs show osteopenia and wedge fractures in advanced cases of osteoporosis. Osteoporosis is detected earlier and more accurately by instruments that measure bone mineral density. However, these costly densitometry instruments are not readily available in most of Africa.

Since osteoporosis is essentially an irreversible process, prevention is essential. Lifestyle changes are important in reducing the rate of bone loss. They include regular physical exercise, adequate calcium intake (1.5 g/day), and stopping or reducing smoking and alcohol intake. Oestrogen replacement therapy is the treatment of choice for the prevention of osteoporosis in women. Other drugs that are effective include the bisphosphanates (e.g. alendronate), calcitonin, anabolic steroids and vitamin D supplements. Preventative measures aimed at reducing falls that predispose to fractures in the elderly are also very important. They include improving vision by wearing correct prescription glasses, avoidance of sedatives and antidepressants and attending to medical conditions that predispose to dizziness and syncope, such as cardiac arrhythmias and postural hypotension.

Osteomalacia and rickets

Vitamin D deficiency causes osteomalacia in adults and rickets in children. It is most commonly due to reduced dietary intake or less often from lack of sunlight exposure, malabsorption and renal failure. In both osteomalacia and rickets there is increased bone turnover and failure of bone mineralization. Osteomalacia presents as bone pain and proximal muscle weakness and tenderness. Radiographic features include osteopenia and pseudofractures (Looser zones) in the shaft of femur and pubic and ischial rami. The serum calcium and phosphate are typically low and serum alkaline phosphatase is elevated. Symptoms improve with Vitamin D supplementation.

Other bone disorders

Hypertrophic pulmonary osteoarthropathy is the triad of finger clubbing, arthritis and periostitis. Causes include carcinoma of the lung and suppurative lung disease. Osteonecrosis or avascular necrosis of the bone epiphysis usually presents as a monoarthritis. It most often affects the hip, and less commonly the knee or shoulder. Most cases are secondary to chronic oral corticosteroid use, alcohol abuse and sickle cell anaemia (Mijiyawa et al., 1994). Paget's disease of bone (osteitis deformans) is a disease of the elderly characterized by an accelerated rate of bone turnover. It presents with pain and deformity of the affected bone and can cause deafness when it affects the skull.

Conclusions

Rheumatic diseases are a significant cause of disability and morbidity world-wide. This is increasingly being recognized in Africa. There is a great need to understand these diseases so as to enable accurate diagnosis and appropriate treatment, whilst taking into account local circumstances.

References

Adebajo AO. (1995). Osteoarthritis. *Baillières Clin Rheumatol*; **9**: 65–74.

Adebajo AO, Reid DM. (1991). The pattern of rheumatoid arthritis in West Africa and comparison with a cohort of British patients. *Quart J Med*; **80**: 633–640.

Ali-Gombe A, Adebajo A, Silman A. (1995). Methodological problems in comparing the severity of rheumatoid arthritis between populations. *Br J Rheumatol*; **34**: 781–784.

American College of Rheumatology Ad hoc Committee on Clinical Guidelines. (1996). American College of Rheumatology guidelines for the initial evaluation of the adult patient with acute musculoskeletal symptoms. *Arthritis Rheum*; **39**: 1–8.

American College of Rheumatology Subcommittee on Rheumatoid Arthritis Guidelines. (2002). Guidelines for the management of rheumatoid arthritis. *Arthritis Rheum*; **46**: 328–346.

Cassim B, Mody GM, Rubin DL. (1990). The prevalence of diffuse idiopathic skeletal hyperostosis in African blacks. *Br J Rheumatol*; **29**: 131–132.

Daniels ED, Pettifor JM, Schnitzler CM, Moodley GP, Zachen D. (1997). Differences in mineral homeostasis, volumetric bone mass and femoral neck axis length in black and white South African women. *Osteoporos Int*; **7**: 105–112.

Goldenberg DL. (1998). Septic arthritis. *Lancet*; **251**: 197–202.

Hart LG, Deyo RA, Cherkin DC. (1995). Physician office visits for lower back pain: frequency, clinical evaluation and treatment patterns from a U.S. national survey. *Spine*; **20**: 11–19.

Kouakou EE, Daboiko JC, Ouali B, Ouattara B, Gabla KA, Kouakou MN. (1998). Epidemiology and features of knee osteoarthritis in the Ivory Coast. *Rev Rhum Engl Ed*; **65**: 766–770.

Mbayo K, Mbuyi-Muamba JM, Lurhuma AZ, Halle L, Kaplan C, Dequeker J. (1998). Low frequency of HLA-B27 and scarcity of ankylosing spondylitis in a Zairean Bantu population. *Clin Rheumatol*; **17**: 309–310.

McGill PE. (1995). Bacterial infections: pyomyositis. *Baillières Clin Rheumatol*; **9**: 193–200.

McGill P, Adebajo AO, Njobvu PD, Brooks PM. (1997). Tropical rheumatology: challenge of the future. *Br J Rheumatol*; **36**: 781–784.

Mijiyawa M, Segbena A, Vovor A, Nubukpo P, David M, Amedegnato MD. (1994). Rheumatic diseases and hemoglobinopathies in Lome. *Rev Rhum Ed Fr*; **61**: 174–178.

Mody GM. (1995). Rheumatoid arthritis and connective tissue disorders: sub-Saharan Africa. *Baillières Clin Rheumatol*; **9**: 31–44.

Njobvu P, McGill P, Kerr H, Jelis J, Pobee J. (1998). Spondyloarthropathy and human immunodeficiency virus infection in Zambia. *J Rheumatol*; **25**: 1553–1559.

Petty RE, Southwood TR, Baum J, et al. (1998). Revision of the proposed classification criteria for juvenile idiopathic arthritis: Durban, 1997. *J Rheumatol*; **25**: 1991–1994.

Pisetsky DS, Gilkeson G, St Clair EW. (1997). Systemic lupus erythematosus – diagnosis and treatment. *Med Clin North Am*; **81**: 113–118.

Schumacher HRJ, Reginato AJ. (1991). *Atlas of Synovial Fluid Analysis and Crystal Identification*. Philadelphia: Lea & Febiger.

Tager RE, Tikly M. (1999). Clinical and laboratory manifestations of systemic sclerosis (scleroderma) in Black South Africans. *Rheumatology*; **38**: 397–400.

Taylor HG, Stein CM. (1986). Systemic lupus erythematosus in Zimbabwe. *Ann Rheum Dis*; **45**: 645–648.

Tikly M, Burgin S, Mohanlal P, Bellingan A, George J. (1996). Autoantibodies in black South Africans with systemic lupus erythematosus: spectrum and clinical associations. *Clin Rheumatol*; **15**: 261–265.

Tikly M, Kalla AA, Mody GM. (2000). Rheumatology in Africa at the turn of the century: a report on the third Aflar Congress, Stellenbosch, South Africa. *J Clin Rheumatol*; **6**: 103–106.

Tikly M, Lincoln D, Bellingan A,Rusell AJ. (1998). Risk factors for gout: a hospital based study in urban black South Africans. *Rev Rheum Engl Ed*; **65**: 225–231.

Wood PNH, McLeish CL. (1974). Statistical appendix. Digest of data on the rheumatic diseases: recent trends in sickness, absence and mortality. *Ann Rheum Dis*; **29**: 324–329.

85 Endocrine and metabolic disease

Thyroid disorders

The thyroid gland plays a critical role in regulating the growth, development and metabolism of virtually all body tissues. These effects are mediated by the thyroid hormones, of which iodine is an indispensable component. In Africa the commonest thyroid disease is goitre (enlargement of the thyroid gland) and in nearly all cases it develops as a response to insufficient iodine intake. Goitre is one of a wide range of disorders caused by iodine deficiency. Nearly all body systems are vulnerable, particularly the nervous system during fetal life and infancy. The most extreme adverse consequence is cretinism (or neonatal hypothyroidism), but of greater significance is the fact that, in areas of iodine deficiency, milder degrees of mental impairment may affect the whole population (Bleichrodt et al., 1996).

Goitre, cretinism, endemic mental deficiency and all other iodine deficiency disorders (IDD) can be readily prevented by regular consumption of adequate amounts of iodine. This is most effectively delivered by iodizing salt for human consumption. In 1990 the World Health Assembly set the goal of eliminating iodine deficiency worldwide by the year 2000. Since 1990 there has been remarkable progress, especially in Africa, with iodized salt now widely available in most countries on the continent.

If this progress is maintained, the pattern of thyroid disease seen in Africa will change dramatically, with goitre and its complications becoming much less common (although long-standing cases will only resolve slowly, if at all). Meanwhile autoimmune thyroiditis and Graves' disease will increase in occurrence.

Thyroid anatomy and physiology

The thyroid gland is situated at the front of the lower part of the neck, in very close relation to the trachea. It is divided into two lobes, joined by a small isthmus just below the cricoid cartilage. The normal thyroid, which weighs about 15–25 grams, is not usually palpable or visible. The oesophagus lies medial to each lobe, behind the trachea. The recurrent laryngeal nerve lies between the trachea and oesophagus. Blood supply, which is abundant, is from the superior and inferior thyroid arteries. At the microscopic level the thyroid is composed of thousands of spherical follicles, each of which is lined by a single layer of cells with colloid in the central lumen. The function of the thyroid is to produce thyroxine (T4) and tri-iodothryonine (T3). These are composed of an organic component, tyrosine, and iodine. The production and regulation of thyroid hormones is summarized in Fig. 85.1.

The iodine deficiency disorders (IDD)

To ensure normal production of thyroid hormones, an adult must ingest at least 150 µg iodine per day (more in pregnancy and during lactation). Iodine deficiency occurs when iodine intake falls consistently below these levels. The iodine content of food and water reflects levels in the soil and groundwater. The type of food consumed and cooking methods are also important: animal sources are generally much richer in iodine than fruits and vegetables, putting the poor at highest risk. Soil erosion due to clearing of vegetation for agricultural production and overgrazing by livestock and tree-cutting causes loss of iodine from the soil.

Traditionally iodine deficiency was recognized as occurring in inland, mountainous areas with poor soils and high rainfall, and was confirmed by a high prevalence of goitre in the resident population. While IDD tend to be very severe under these conditions, IDD can, and do, occur in many areas where there are none of these features. For example, iodine deficiency has been identified in coastal areas, in large cities and in areas where the prevalence of goitre is normal.

The term iodine deficiency disorders was coined to emphasize that the problem of iodine deficiency extends far beyond goitre (Hetzel, 1983). The major harmful known effects are shown in Table 85.1. The effects on the brain largely result from low levels of maternal thyroxine, and the most critical period is from the beginning of pregnancy to the third year of life when the central nervous system is developing rapidly.

Iodine deficiency reduces the potential of the whole community. There may be low achievement, poor quality of life, and blunted ambition. Iodine deficiency should be regarded as a public health problem and tackled at this level, rather than by treatment for individual patients. Indeed, the main significance of goitre should be as a marker of iodine deficiency (see Fig. 85.2).

The role of goitrogens

Apart from iodine deficiency, in Africa the most important known goitrogen is thiocyanate, derived from

Table 85.1. The spectrum of the iodine deficiency disorders (IDD)

Fetus	Abortions
	Stillbirths
	Congenital anomalies
	Increased perinatal mortality
	Increased infant mortality
	Neurological cretinism (*mental deficiency, deaf mutism, spastic diplegia, squint*)
	Myxoedematous cretinism (*mental deficiency, dwarfism, hypothyroidism*)
	Psychomotor defects
Neonate	Neonatal hypothyroidism
Child and adolescent	Retarded mental and physical development
Adult	Goitre and its complications
	Iodine-induced hyperthyroidism (IIH)
All ages	Goitre
	Hypothyroidism
	Impaired mental function
	Increased susceptibility to nuclear radiation

Source: Modified from Hetzel (1983).

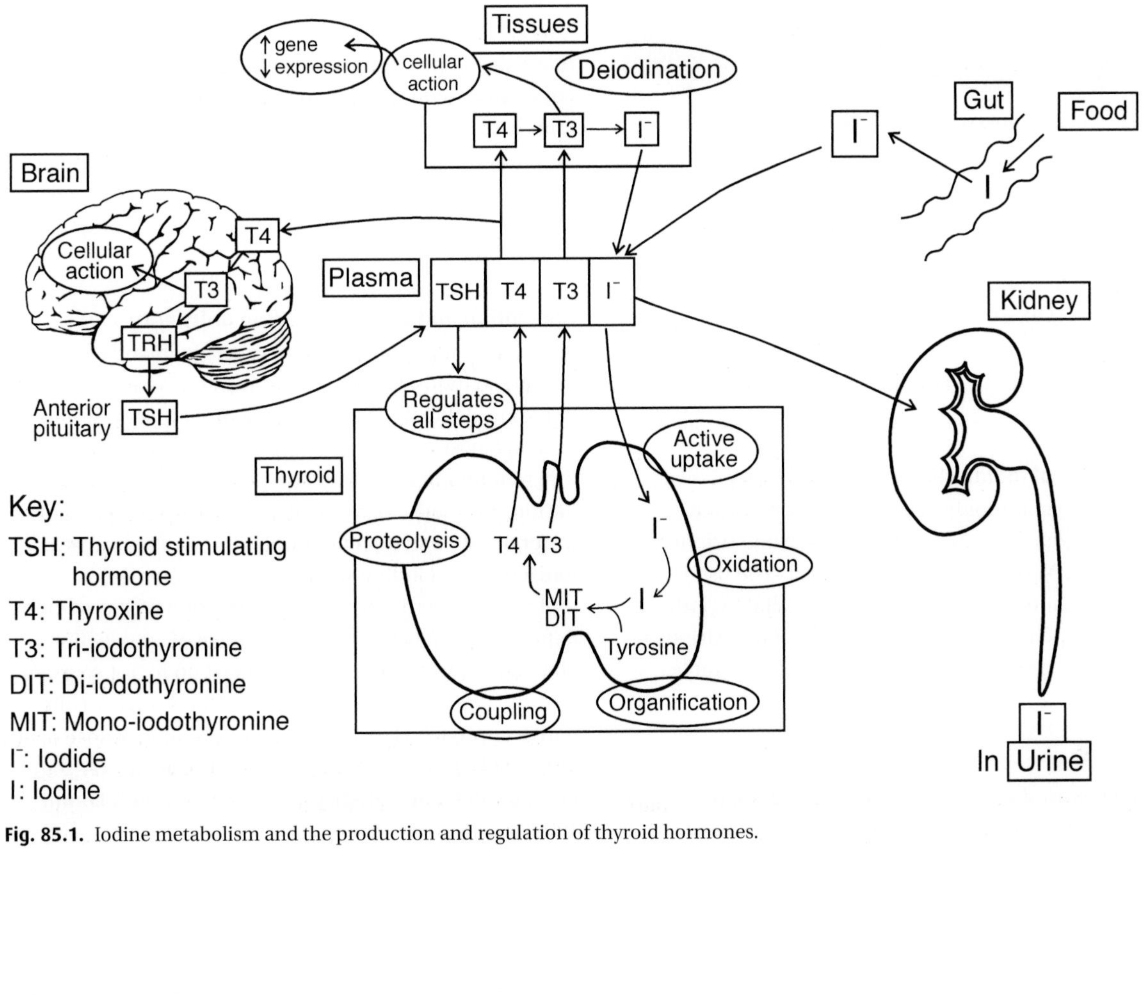

Fig. 85.1. Iodine metabolism and the production and regulation of thyroid hormones.

Table 85.2. Summary of indicators of iodine deficiency disorders

		Severity of IDD		
Indicator	Target population	Mild	Moderate	Severe
Goitre	Schoolchildren	5–19%	20–29%	>30%
Median urinary iodine (μg/l)	Schoolchildren	50–99	20–49	<20
Frequency of TSH >5mU/L	Neonates	3–19%	20–39%	>40%

Source: From WHO (2001).

Fig. 85.2. A patient from rural Congo with a massive goitre.

poorly detoxified cassava. Selenium deficiency may also play a role. Increasing the intake of iodine, however, reverses the harmful effects of thiocyanate on the thyroid. Vegetables from the genus Brassica possess goitrogenic properties. High concentrations of fluoride have also been described in relation to endemic goitre in Africa.

Investigation of iodine status in a community

There are two commonly used indicators of iodine status in a given community: thyroid size and urinary iodine levels. Neonatal TSH levels may also be used where a screening programme for congenital hypothyroidism is in place (WHO, 2001). Details of the various indicators are given below, and summarized in Table 85.2.

Urinary iodine

This is the most useful and reliable indicator of iodine status. The amount of iodine excreted in the urine is related to recent dietary iodine intake. Ideally 24-hour urine collections are required, but the profile of iodine levels in casual urine specimens taken from a sufficient number (at least 30) of randomly selected individuals in a given population, e.g. school children, reflects that population's iodine intake. Median levels of about 100 μg/l are satisfactory.

Thyroid size (goitre surveys)

The traditional method of assessing thyroid size is by simple palpation, although ultrasound examination gives a precise measure of thyroid volume and is much more reliable. Results of surveys are expressed as 'Total Goitre Rate', which is the number with goitre divided by the total examined. The term 'endemic goitre' refers to a total goitre rate of greater than 5 per cent in a given community. Thyroid size responds only slowly to changes in iodine intake, therefore goitre surveys are more useful in assessing IDD severity than evaluating the impact of iodine supplementation. The preferred group for examination is school-aged children because of their easy accessibility and relatively rapid responsiveness to changes in iodine intake.

Thyroid stimulating hormone

TSH screening programmes have been introduced in many developed countries for the early detection of congenital hypothyroidism in neonates. These programmes also give useful epidemiological information on the severity of iodine deficiency in a given population; but it is not cost-effective to establish neonatal screening for the primary purpose of monitoring IDD programmes.

Prevention and control of iodine deficiency

Iodine-rich food, such as sea fish and kelp and certain processed foods, are not available to most people living in iodine-deficient areas, owing to their inaccessibility and high cost. Supplementation programmes are therefore required to ensure an adequate intake of iodine. Various methods are available, including iodization of water or salt, and direct administration of iodine as iodized oil and iodine solutions. The main role for iodized oil is in the short-term correction of severe iodine deficiency. It may be given in the form of an injection (480 mg iodine), when the effects last up to 3–4 years; or by mouth, when the effects last 12–18 months. An alternative approach is to administer a regular oral dose of an iodine solution such as Lugol's iodine, one drop (7 mg) every 2 weeks, or 4 drops every month (Todd & Dunn, 1998).

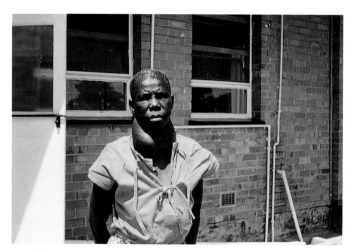

In most countries, the most practical method of iodine supplementation is by iodization of all salt for human consumption. Salt is used by nearly everyone, even in the poorest households, and amounts used are fairly constant. Iodization of salt is sustainable because the cost, which is very low, is borne by the consumer. Potassium iodate is recommended for iodization rather than iodide because it is more stable, especially when the salt is not pure. WHO/UNICEF/ICCIDD (1996) recommend that in order to provide 150 μg/day of iodine via iodized salt, iodine concentration at the point of production should be between 20 and 40 mg of iodine per kilogram of salt. Salt iodization has proved particularly successful in countries with a small number of large salt suppliers. In areas where there are small producers it is generally more difficult to implement. Here, the best approach is for the producers to form co-operatives for communal iodization.

Monitoring of salt iodization programmes is essential, to ensure that salt is adequately iodized and that it is having the desired impact. Successful and sustainable national programmes for ensuring the elimination of iodine deficiency in a country require a number of key elements. These are listed in the Table 85.3.

Table 85.3. Requirements for a successful national IDD control programme

1. An effective, functional national body (council or committee) responsible to the government for the national programme for the elimination of IDD. This council should be multidisciplinary involving the relevant fields of nutrition, medicine, salt industry, education, the media and consumers; with a chairman appointed by the Minister of Health.
2. Evidence of political commitment to universal salt iodization and the elimination of IDD.
3. Appointment of a responsible executive officer for the IDD elimination programme.
4. Legislation or regulations on universal salt iodization. While ideally regulations should cover both human and agricultural salt, if the latter is not covered, this does not necessarily preclude a country from being certified as IDD-free.
5. Commitment to assessment and re-assessment of progress in the elimination of IDD, with access to laboratories able to provide accurate data on salt and urine iodine levels.
6. A programme of public education and social mobilization on the importance of IDD and the consumption of iodized salt.
7. Regular data on salt iodine levels at factory, retail and household level.
8. Regular laboratory data on urinary iodine in school-aged children with appropriate sampling for higher risk areas.
9. Co-operation from the salt industry in maintenance of quality control.
10. Database with recording of results or regular monitoring procedures, particularly for salt iodine, urinary iodine and, if available, neonatal TSH levels with mandatory public reporting.

Source: From WHO (2001).

IDD in Africa

Iodine deficiency has been described in all but two of the 46 countries of the WHO Africa Region (the exceptions are Mauritius and Seychelles.) WHO (1999) estimate that of the total population of 610 million, 48 per cent (or 295 million people) live in areas where the total goitre rate is above 5 per cent and therefore are at risk of iodine deficiency. Most African countries are now developing IDD control programmes along the lines outlined in Table 85.3, and the overall availability of iodized salt at household level has increased markedly from about 30 per cent in 1990 to around 70 per cent now. Despite this success, many problems remain, which are a barrier to achieving sustainable elimination of IDD from the continent. These include: lack of political will; wars and social strife, making programme implementation impossible; numerous small-scale salt producers; poor quality of iodized salt; 'leakage' of non-iodized salt; weak capacity for enforcement, and weak or absent monitoring systems.

Pathophysiology of thyroid disorders other than IDD

Hyperthyroidism

Hyperthyroidism refers to excessive amounts of thyroid hormone in the circulation, and thyrotoxicosis to the clinical effects that result. The most important causes are as follows

Toxic nodular goitre (TNG)

Presently the most common cause in many African countries, TNG is a particular problem when iodine supplementation is rapidly introduced into communities affected by endemic goitre. Affected subjects are usually over 40 years old, with a long-standing nodular goitre. Eye signs, if present, are mild. Spontaneous remission is unlikely. Solitary toxic adenoma is included in the syndrome of TNG.

Graves' disease

Here, stimulatory auto-antibodies to the TSH receptor on the thyroid follicular cell induce excessive thyroid hormone production. It is about ten times more common in women than men; and may occur at any age including childhood, though most cases are between 20 and 40 years old. Most, but not all, affected subjects have an obvious diffuse goitre. Eye signs, such as proptosis, swelling around the eyes and abnormal eye movements are frequently present and may be severe. Spontaneous remission occurs in about 40 per cent of cases.

Iatrogenic hyperthyroidism
This occurs when a subject is over-treated with thyroxine – usually for the treatment of hypothyroidism. A similar condition may occur if someone eats meat or offal containing thyroid glands.

Sub-acute and autoimmune thyroiditis (see below)
There may be a brief period of relatively mild hyperthyroidism in such cases.

Iodine-induced hyperthyroidism
This results from ingestion of iodine-containing compounds. Amiodarone, a drug increasingly used for treating cardiac arrhythmias, is an important example. Two forms of hyperthyroidism occur, one is due to iodine-induced increase of thyroid hormone synthesis, the other involves cytotoxic damage to the thyroid gland.

Other causes
Much rarer causes are factitious (or self-induced) thyrotoxicosis, and tumour-associated hyperthyroidism, e.g. struma ovarii.

Hypothyroidism

Hypothyroidism is defined as insufficient amounts of thyroid hormones in the circulation, and myxoedema is a somewhat outdated term referring to the resulting clinical effects. Important causes are as follows.

Iodine deficiency
Affected subjects are usually goitrous.

Excessive iodine intake
The effect is usually temporary.

Autoimmune thyroiditis (including Hashimoto's disease, atrophic thyroiditis, silent thyroiditis and post-partum thyroiditis) Thyroid cells are destroyed by specially activated CD8 lymphocytes and auto-antibodies directed against thyroglobulin and thyroid peroxidase (Dayan & Daniels, 1996).

Following administration of radioactive iodine or thyroidectomy
Such treatments are usually for hyperthyroidism.

Disease of the pituitary gland (which produces TSH)
An uncommon cause of hypothyroidism sometimes referred to as 'secondary'.

Subacute thyroiditis

This condition, which is caused by a viral infection, is also known as de Quervain's or granulomatous thyroiditis. About 50 per cent of cases are associated with hyperthyroidism due to release of thyroid hormone from damaged thyroid cells.

Thyroid cancer

This is an uncommon cancer in Africa. In areas of iodine deficiency the follicular type is more common than papillary cancer, but there is no good evidence that the incidence is higher than in non-iodine deficient areas.

Clinical approach to thyroid disorders

Thyroid disorders may present to health workers with the problems shown in the Box.

Presentation of thyroid disease

- Swelling in the neck, which may be localized or generalized
- Symptoms resulting from pressure effects (e.g. difficulty in breathing or dysphagia)
- Symptoms of hyper- or hypothyroidism. (See Table 85.4)
- Rarely, symptoms due to distant metastases from thyroid cancer (usually bone pain)
- A combination of some of the above

History and examination

In cases of goitre it is important to know how long it has been present, whether there has been any change in size, and whether any presure symptoms are present. Ask the patient about change in mood, energy, sleep pattern, appetite, bowel habit, menstruation, presence of palpitations, and any preference for hot or cold weather (see Table 85.4). Do a general examination and also specifically of the thyroid gland. The neck should be inspected from the front in both the normal and fully extended position.

Examination of the thyroid

- Palpate from behind, particularly feeling the area between the sterno-mastoid muscles and the trachea.
- A normal thyroid gland is not visible and is rarely palpable.
- Assess the size of any goitre: is it tender, diffusely enlarged, or nodular?
- Ask the patient to swallow – the thyroid will move upwards, confirming that the mass is, indeed, thyroid, and the manoeuvre will also allow more of the gland to be palpated.
- Percussion over the upper sternum can be useful in detecting a retrosternal goitre.
- Auscultate over the gland to listen for a bruit.

In hyperthyroidism the face may appear wasted with staring eyes, and the patient may appear restless or fidgety. Eye signs include lid retraction (rim of white sclera visible around the iris) and lid lag (rim of sclera visible above the iris on looking down), which may be seen in any type of hyperthyroidism. Other eye signs are only seen in patients with Graves' disease, and include soft tissue swelling, conjunctival oedema, proptosis, paralysis of certain eye movements, and corneal damage. Eye signs may be asymmetrical. Tachycardia is often present, and the pulse pressure (on BP recording) wide. The palms are warm and sweaty, and there may be a tremor (placing a piece of paper on the outstretched hands shows this best).

In hypothyroidism there may be a puffy face, and sometimes diffuse hair loss, particularly affecting the outer part of the eyebrow. The skin generally may be thickened and dry, and sweating is rare. The hair is coarse, dry and brittle. Xanthelasmas may be present due to associated hyperlipidaemia. The pulse rate is usually slow (<60 beats per minute), and the heart sounds quiet. The tendon reflexes often show a slow relaxation phase, best shown at the ankle.

Differential diagnosis

The clinician in Africa frequently has to rely on clinical acumen to make a diagnosis. Most patients do not present in a classical textbook manner, and thyroid function testing, if available at all, may take several weeks. Diseases and conditions that are commonly confused with hyperthyroidism are shown in the Box.

Differential diagnosis of thyrotoxicosis

- Anxiety
- HIV/AIDS
- Malignant disease
- Pregnancy
- Alcoholism
- Localized eye disorders
- Septicaemia

Table 85.4. The contrasting clinical effects of hyperthyroidism and hypothyroidism

System	Hyperthyroidism	Hypothyroidism
Central nervous	Nervousness, irritability, insomnia, tremor	Slowing down, poor hearing, fatigue, delayed reflexes
	Anxiety, emotional outbursts	Depression, behaviour change
Musculoskeletal	Fatigue, muscle weakness	Fatigue
Metabolic	Weight loss, increased appetite	Weight gain
	Heat intolerance	Cold intolerance
Gastrointestinal	Frequent loose stools	Constipation
Cardiovascular	Palpitations, shortness of breath	Angina, bradycardia
	Heart failure, atrial fibrillation	Pleural and pericardial effusions
Skin	Hot, sweaty palms	Dry, puffy skin, cold peripheries
Reproductive (female)	Amenorrhea or scanty periods	Menorrhagia

Source: Modified from Todd (1999).

Hyperthyroidism should also always be considered in unexplained cases of heart failure and atrial fibrillation. Hypothyroidism, on the other hand, may also be missed. Uncommon presentations include depression or psychosis (so-called 'myxoedema madness'), syndromes of chronic fatigue, and severe constipation or faecal impaction.

Investigation of the thyroid

Thyroid function testing

Thyroid function testing is costly and should only be carried out on when hormone imbalance is likely on clinical grounds, or as part of a neonatal screening programme. A logical approach to testing to minimize costs is based on an understanding of thyroid physiology. This involves starting with an initial screening test for TSH and proceeding to measure thyroxine levels only if this is abnormal. Additional tests are rarely needed.

Highly sensitive thyroid stimulating hormone (HS-TSH) assays, can reliably discriminate between euthyroid, hypothyroid and hyperthyroid states. If the HS-TSH assay is normal, no further tests need to be carried out unless

Table 85.5. Anti-thyroid drugs: doses and adverse effects

Drug	Total daily dose, with children's doses in brackets (LaFranchi & Mandel, 1996)		Adverse effects
	Initial	Maintenance	
Carbimazole (or methimazole) (5 mg tablet)	20–60 mg/day (0.5–1 mg/kg/day)	5–20 mg/day (0.125–0.5 mg/kg/day)	Nausea, headache, rashes, itching, jaundice, agranulocytosis[a]
Propylthiouracil (50 mg tablet)	200–600 mg/day (5–10 mg/kg/day)	50–150 mg/day (1.25–5 mg/kg/day)	As for carbimazole; also hepatitis

Note:
Anti-thyroid drugs are safe for pregnant and lactating women, but use the lowest possible dose.
[a] If a subject on one of these drugs develops a severe sore throat, check the white cell count. If the neutrophil count is below normal, the drug should be stopped.

there are very compelling clinical reasons to do so. If the HS-TSH result is abnormal, a total (T4) or free (FT4) assay should be done. FT4 is a measure of the tiny fraction of thyroxine that is free in the serum and therefore physiologically active. The assay is not affected by changes in the levels of carrier proteins. In hyperthyroidism, TSH is suppressed below normal and T4 raised. Tri-iodothyronine (T3) assay should only be carried out if the T4 is normal, when 'T3 toxicosis' should be considered. In hypothyroidism, TSH is raised and T4 is low (a T3 assay is not helpful in this situation). Where TSH is abnormal, but other tests normal, a 'sub-clinical' condition may be present. In these cases the patient should be followed, but if symptoms are marked then appropriate treatment may be initiated.

Levels of thyroid hormones may also be non-specifically abnormal in a variety of non-thyroidal conditions. The most common is the 'sick-euthyroid syndrome', which occurs in other medical conditions. Thyroid function testing should therefore not be performed in acutely ill patients unless there is a high suspicion of thyroid disease. A number of drugs may affect thyroid function test results, including heparin, beta-blockers, anti-convulsants, frusemide, corticosteroids and lithium.

Thyroid imaging

Plain X-rays may be helpful to assess the degree of tracheal compression by a large goitre prior to surgery, but otherwise are of little use. A barium swallow allows assessment of oesophageal compression and helps define the position of a retrosternal goitre.

Ultrasound is a valuable non-invasive technique which permits visualization of lesions within the thyroid of as little as 2–3 mm diameter. The normal thyroid gives a fairly homogeneous echo pattern, and while relatively echolucent (dark), it is lighter than surrounding muscle. Ultrasound can differentiate well between cysts and solid nodules, and also shows different patterns from normal thyroid tissue in colloid goitre and thyroiditis. Thyroid malignancies may give complex patterns, but these are not diagnostic. Finally radioactive scintigraphy provides useful information on thyroid structure and function, but accessibility is very limited.

Fine needle aspiration

This is a useful technique whereby thyroid tissue from suspicious areas, e.g. solitary nodules, is aspirated and preserved on a glass slide for subsequent cytological examination. The method requires a competent cytological service, and if this is not available it is unreliable.

Management of hyperthyroidism

Hyperthyroidism is diagnosed on the basis of suspicious clinical features and confirmed by suppressed TSH and raised T4 levels. If untreated up to one-third of affected patients may die – mostly due to heart failure, pneumonia, thyroid storm and complications of atrial fibrillation, e.g. embolic stroke. With early diagnosis and modern therapy, the mortality from hyperthyroidism should be negligible. Accurate diagnosis of the underlying cause is essential to determine the optimal treatment (Franklyn, 1994; Vanderpump et al., 1996).

There are three treatment options: anti-thyroid drugs, surgery and radioiodine. The decision as to which to employ is guided by availability and circumstances. Unless the patient is asthmatic, beta-blocking drugs, e.g. propranolol 20–80 mg three times daily, have a useful role to play in controlling symptoms, and are more effective than digoxin at controlling the heart rate in atrial fibrillation (AF) associated with hyperthyroidism. When AF is present, anticoagulation should be considered. Low dose aspirin (75 mg daily) is a useful option which is reasonably effective, cheap and requires no monitoring.

Anti-thyroid drugs

These act by blocking production of thyroid hormone while awaiting spontaneous remission in Graves' disease, or prior to ablative treatment. Doses and adverse effects of the various anti-thyroid drugs are given in Table 85.5. Important points about drug therapy are as follows.

- Start with carbimazole (or methimazole). Propylthiouracil is used if the patient develops a rash or other side effects that cannot be tolerated.
- Rashes may clear despite continuing with the same drug: only change treatment if severe.
- Monitor response clinically, and if available by measurement of FT4 or T4 (not TSH which may only respond very slowly) every 2–3 months. After the initial period of treatment, the dose is titrated according to the response. Give the lowest possible dose to maintain euthyroidism.
- In Graves' disease anti-thyroid drugs should be continued for 1 year. Follow up subjects after treatment is complete for at least 1 year. Relapse is common – particularly in subjects with a large goitre and when large doses of anti-thyroid drugs were needed.
- In toxic nodular goitre higher doses are generally needed than in Graves' disease.
- Anti-thyroid drugs may be continued indefinitely if surgery and radioiodine are not available, not practical or are refused.
- The most common cause of treatment failure is poor adherence.
- Anti-thyroid drugs are relatively ineffective in treating hyperthyroidism associated with thyroiditis and that due to amiodarone. Beta-blockers may be used as required to control symptoms.

Surgery

Surgery is indicated in Graves' disease after relapse or poor response to treatment, and in large toxic nodular goitres (with no access to radioiodine). Sub-total thyroidectomy, where more than 90 per cent of thyroid tissue is removed, is the operation of choice. However, surgery should only be considered if there are suitably trained staff, and the patient can be rendered euthyroid prior to operation. Large doses of iodine – as aqueous iodine (Lugol's) solution 4 drops three times daily – are frequently given for 1–2 weeks prior to surgery to render the gland less vascular and to assist with control of hyperthyroidism. Complications are summarized in the Box above).

Complications of thyroidectomy

- Death: the risk can be as high as 50% when surgery is carried out under unsuitable conditions
- Haemorrhage
- Nerve injuries – particularly to the recurrent laryngeal nerve
- Hypocalcaemia due to damage to the parathyroid glands
- Recurrent hyperthyroidism
- Hypothyroidism.

Radioiodine

This is aimed at destroying sufficient thyroid tissue with radioactivity by administration of an unstable isotope of iodine (usually ^{131}I). While increasingly the preferred option in developed countries, it is only available in Africa in specialized centres in major cities. Radioiodine is administered as a capsule or a simple drink, and requires no special preparation. Anti-thyroid drugs need not be started prior to treatment. If the patient is already on anti-thyroid drugs, they should be stopped 3–4 days prior to administration and may be restarted a week afterwards. Radioiodine should not be given to pregnant or lactating women, but it is now considered safe for men and women under 40 and even in childhood (Rivkees et al., 1998). Women should avoid pregnancy for at least 6 months. Radioiodine may worsen eye problems in Graves' disease, and should be avoided in those with severe ophthalmopathy (see below). Hypothyroidism commonly results from radioiodine treatment, especially in the treatment of Graves' disease, and in some centres a high dose is deliberately given in order to induce hypothyroidism rapidly. Otherwise, it may not manifest itself for many years.

Graves' ophthalmopathy

In most cases of Graves' disease the eye problems are not severe enough to warrant specific treatment, but artificial tears and taping the eyes shut at night may be helpful. Severe proptosis with inability to close the eyelids, marked paralysis of eye movements, and corneal ulceration are all signs of severe disease and urgent treatment with large doses of corticosteroids should be given, e.g. prednisolone 40–120 mg daily (Larkins, 1993). Treatment should be continued for 1 month then tapered off slowly. If the response is poor, referral should be considered for possible radiotherapy or surgical decompression.

Thyroid storm

This is characterized by fever, delirium, weakness and extreme tachycardia (sometimes with supraventricular tachycardia or atrial fibrillation). An uncommon medical emergency, it may be misdiagnosed as malaria or septicaemia. It occurs as a complication of long-standing untreated hyperthyroidism or can be precipitated by infection, thyroidectomy, iodine or non-thyroid surgery. Treatment should be started immediately with large doses of anti-thyroid drugs (carbimazole 20 mg 4–6-hourly); high dose beta-blockers (e.g. propranolol 40 mg

4 hourly); corticosteroids (intravenous hydrocortisone 100 mg 6 hourly; or oral prednisolone 20 mg 6-hourly); and iodine 1–2 g daily starting one hour after the first dose of carbimazole (e.g. Lugol's solution 2.5 ml four times daily by mouth diluted with water). In severe cases, propranolol may need to be given intravenously, e.g. 1–5 mg very slowly and cautiously – preferably with ECG monitoring.

Management of hyperthyroidism in extremely resource-poor settings

The following points may be helpful where facilities are limited (see the Box).

> **Thyrotoxicosis treatment where resources are poor**
> - Diagnosis is made on clinical grounds alone
> - Give propranolol or other beta-blockers, unless contraindicated (i.e. asthma)
> - In severe hyperthyroidism, administration of large doses of iodine, e.g. Lugol's solution 2.5 ml four times daily by mouth, will temporarily control the condition
> - There is no place for heroic surgery: mortality is likely to be very high
> - If anti-thyroid drugs can be obtained, give the lowest dose that controls symptoms and continue indefinitely.

Management of hypothyroidism

The diagnosis is made on the basis of suspicious clinical features and confirmed by finding high TSH and low T4 levels. Treatment requires a replacement dose of thyroxine – except in iodine deficiency when iodine itself should be given (though if there is no response after 2 months, thyroxine should be used). The initial dose of thyroxine in adults is 50–100 μg daily, adjusting the dose by 25–50 μg every 4–6 weeks according to response (Oppenheimer et al., 1995). If thyroid function testing is available, T4 and TSH should both be normal. The typical adult replacement dose is around 150 μg daily. In subjects with very long-standing disease, the elderly, and those with heart disease, treatment should be started cautiously at 25 μg daily, and increase by 25 μg every 3–4 weeks until symptoms are controlled. Once established, the dose of thyroxine usually remains constant. Thyroxine is safe in pregnancy, but doses may need to be increased by 25 to 50 μg in the later stages.

Infants and children require relatively larger doses of thyroxine. Neonates should be commenced on 10–15 μg/kg per day – an average baby will therefore require around 37.5–50 μg/day. In older children doses are around 4 μg/kg per day. As in adults, doses should be adjusted in the light of clinical response and thyroid function test results.

'Hypothyroid coma' or pre-coma is a rare complication of severe, advanced, and untreated hypothyroidism. Patients are usually elderly and present drowsy or unconscious with marked hypothermia and facial and other features suggestive of hypothyroidism. Biochemical confirmation is never immediately available, and the diagnosis is thus clinical. Patients should be given intravenous fluids and slowly rewarmed. Infection may be a precipitant, and should be treated vigorously. Empirical steroids (intravenous hydrocortisone) are worthwhile in severe and/or unresponsive areas. There is controversy over optimal urgent thyroid replacement in these cases. Standard advice has been to give T_3 (tri-iodothyronine 5–10 μg by slow i.v. injection, repeated each 8 to 12 hours). Parenteral T3, however, may be unavailable, and can have significant cardiac side effects on ill and elderly patients (e.g. arrhythmias and heart failure). A better and safer option is to give a large oral (or nasogastric) bolus of thyroxine (e.g. 500 μg), and allow this to be slowly absorbed over the next few hours or days. More standard daily replacement can commence 3 or 4 days later, when the diagnosis is confirmed and the patient hopefully improved. It should be mentioned however, that the mortality of myxoedema coma – even with adequate treatment – is very high.

Management of other thyroid conditions

Sub-acute thyroiditis

In this condition there is rapid onset of a painful and tender goitre, often with general symptoms such as fever, malaise and myalgia. About 50 per cent of cases are thyrotoxic, but this is usually mild. The ESR is markedly raised. The condition usually lasts from 2–8 weeks. Aspirin or non-steroidal anti-inflammatory drugs should be used to relieve pain. In severe cases steroids, e.g. prednisolone 40 mg daily, may be required. Associated hyperthyroidism rarely requires specific treatment.

Goitre and thyroid nodules

In iodine-deficient areas many goitrous patients are likely to present at hospitals every day, and it is not cost effective to exclude significant thyroid disease in all. Careful clinical assessment usually renders thyroid function or biopsy unnecessary in most cases. In areas of endemic goitre and iodine deficiency, patients with simple, diffuse goitre should be treated with physiological doses of iodine, and not with thyroxine. Thyroid function testing is unnecessary. Supplemental iodine should not be given to subjects with established nodular goitre, even in areas of iodine deficiency, due to the risk of thyrotoxicosis. In areas where iodine deficiency does not exist or was eliminated many years previously, the most likely cause of goitre is chronic auto-immune thyroiditis. Thyroxine should be given if there is evidence of hypothyroidism, of course, but small doses may also reduce goitre size in the euthyroid state, though the effect is not dramatic. Partial thyroidectomy may be necessary for the treatment of subjects with very large goitres, provided surgical facilities are satisfactory and euthyroidism is confirmed on blood testing (Hermus & Huysmans, 1998). In iodine deficient areas, the patient should be advised to take regular iodine after the operation to prevent recurrence.

The main concern in patients with single or multiple thyroid nodules is whether malignancy is present (Jones, 2001). In all cases it is therefore necessary to look for suspicious clinical features, and if present excision biopsy is recommended. Many patients with thyroid cancer, however, do not exhibit these features and unless there is access to fine needle aspiration cytology (Mazzaferri, 1993), the best course of action is watchful waiting (see the Box).

Features of thyroid nodule that suggest malignancy

- Recent growth
- Pain
- Fixation
- Unusual firmness
- Enlarged regional lymph nodes
- Hoarseness of the voice

Thyroid cancer

This most commonly presents as a solitary thyroid nodule, but may also occur in a multinodular goitre. Less commonly, the presentation is rapid enlargement of the whole gland, or the result of local invasion or distant metastases (bone). Affected patients should be referred for specialized treatment. Management relies on a combination of surgery and radioiodine depending on histological type and stage. In the absence of such specialist facilities, total thyroidectomy is advisable, with lifelong thyroxine and vitamin D replacement.

Pituitary disorders

Anatomy and physiology

For the amazingly important life-preserving processes which it performs, the pituitary gland is tiny. It is a

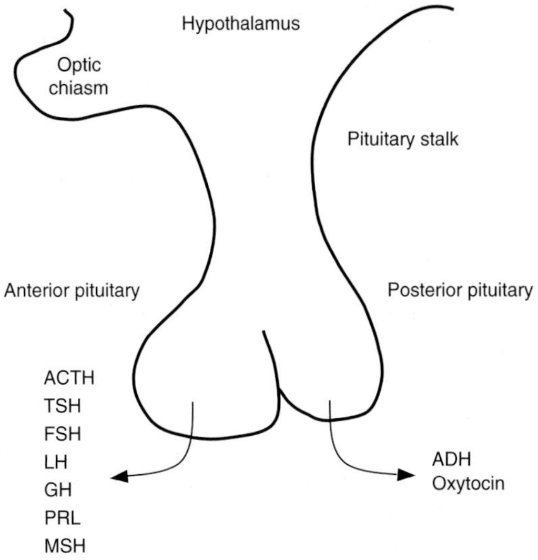

Abbreviations:
ACTH: corticotrophin (adreno-corticotrophic hormone), TSH: thyrotropin (thyroid stimulating hormone), FSH: follicle stimulating hormone, LH: luteinizing hormone, GH: growth hormone, PRL: prolactin, MSH: melanocyte stimulating hormone, ADH: anti-diuretic hormone

Fig. 85.3. Schematic diagram showing the essential structure and function of the pituitary gland.

rounded structure a little less than one centimetre in diameter. It lies deep in the skull, in a recess of the sphenoid bone known as the 'sella turcica'. Its two lobes, the anterior and posterior, are connected to the brain above by the pituitary stalk, but they have quite different embryonic origins and physiological functions. The anterior pituitary (or 'adenohypophysis') is a glandular structure originating from the ectoderm of Rathke's Pouch; whereas the posterior pituitary (or 'neurohypophysis') arises from neural ectoderm of the floor of the forebrain. The anterior pituitary produces many hormones (see Fig. 85.3), but the posterior pituitary few – and only one of clinical importance – ADH or the antidiuretic hormone. The more technical name for this hormone is arginine vasopressin or AVP, and it is actually secreted in the hypothalamus, travels down the neural pituitary stalk and is released from the posterior pituitary. Most anterior pituitary hormones are secreted in response to 'releasing factors' which are produced again in the hypothalamus into the portal microcirculation of the pituitary stalk, and act on the individual hormone-producing cells of the anterior pituitary. These releasing factors include GnRH (gonadotrophin-releasing hormone), and TRH (thyrotropin-releasing hormone); and are substances which can now be synthetically produced, and used as investigative or therapeutic agents.

Pathological processes

The various pathological processes that may affect pituitary hormone release are shown in the Box.

Pathological processes affecting pituitary hormone secretion

- Tumours
- Trauma
- Vascular
- Autoimmune
- Infiltrations
- Idiopathic

Tumours are usually benign adenomas, which may be of secretory cells (which therefore cause syndromes of autonomous over-production of individual hormones), or may be 'non-functioning'. Even these latter tumours may have endocrine effects, however, as they may expand and exert pressure on functioning pituitary cells which then reduce or cease hormone production – leading to hypopituitarism. Trauma is usually a severe head injury, and commonly manifests itself as post-traumatic diabetes insipidus, which may often be transient. Vascular causes include infarction or haemorrhage. The classical cause of pituitary infarction is following severe post-partum haemorrhage (so-called 'Sheehan's syndrome'). Haemorrhage, or 'pituitary apoplexy', can occur as part of a more general cerebral haemorrhage but may be an isolated event, presenting as sudden collapse with severe headache, and later pituitary underfunction. Autoimmune processes are being increasingly recognized as a cause of hypopituitarism (similar to auto-immune thyroid and adrenal insufficiency). Infiltrations of the skull base may involve the pituitary rarely, and these can include sarcoidosis, haemochromatosis, and even sometimes tuberculous meningitis. Finally, a significant proportion of pituitary diseases – particularly those involving hypofunction – often remain of unknown cause. The spectrum of pathological processes seen in Africa is broadly similar to that seen elsewhere, except that Sheehan's syndrome is seen more commonly because of the increased frequency of post-partum haemorrhage. Road traffic accidents also account for an increased load of pituitary disorders of traumatic origin.

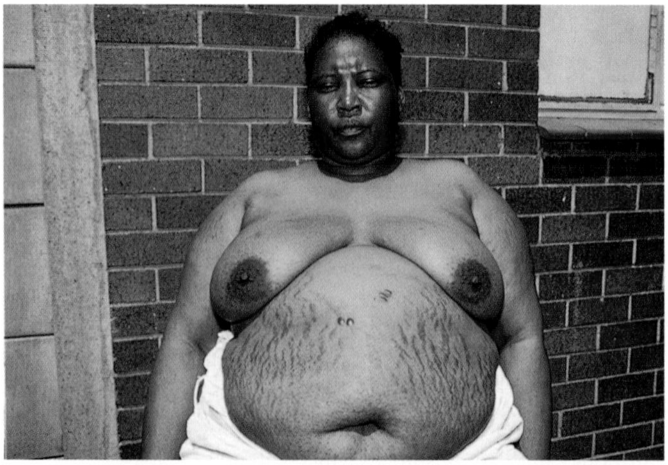

Fig. 85.4. Classical features of Cushing's syndrome in a patient with marked central obesity and striae.

Clinical syndromes of pituitary disease

These will be divided into syndromes of *hyper* and *hypo*-function. Some pituitary disorders may not, of course, affect endocrine function, but these will present very rarely.

Disorders of pituitary overactivity

All hormone-producing cells may potentially become hyperplastic or adenomatous, but in clinical practice there are only three disorders of pituitary hyperfunction, all affecting the anterior pituitary. These are pituitary-driven Cushing's syndrome, acromegaly and prolactinoma.

Cushing's syndrome

Though Cushing's syndrome may be caused by an adrenal adenoma, or an ectopic source of ACTH, the majority of cases are due to an ACTH-producing pituitary adenoma (Cushing's disease). This appears to be also true in African endocrine practice (Shires et al., 1994). The clinical features of Cushing's syndrome in an African patient, with marked central obesity, are shown in Fig. 85.4. In practice, however, the presentation may be very varied, and though the disease is rare, a high index of suspicion is needed. The various manifestations of the disease are shown in Table 85.6, and it can be seen that the presenting features and their variable and multi-system nature, make this often a very difficult diagnosis (Boscaro et al., 2001).

Investigations

Investigations can be divided into two phases – the demonstration of biochemical cortisol excess, and then the 'siting' of the lesion to a pituitary, adrenal or ectopic source (by both biochemical and radiological means). In addition, a useful screening test is the 'short overnight

Table 85.6. Clinical manifestations of Cushing's syndrome

1. Weight increase and fat redistribution
   - central obesity
   - moon face
   - buffalo hump
2. Skin changes
   - striae
   - acne
   - bruising
   - hirsutes
   - plethoric facies
3. Menstrual disturbance
   - amenorrhoea
   - oligomenorrhoea
4. Psychiatric effects
   - depression
   - psychosis
5. Miscellaneous
   - diabetes mellitus
   - hypertension
   - osteoporosis
   - proximal myopathy

dexamethasone suppression test'. The patient is given 1 mg of oral dexamethasone at 12 midnight and a plasma cortisol level is taken at 9 am the following morning. Normal people suppress their cortisol level certainly to below 100 nmol/l, and usually below 50 nmol/l (Wood et al., 1997). Lack of suppression can occur also in marked obesity, depression and sometimes alcoholism. In the latter group, some patients may even have external features suggestive of the disease – so-called 'pseudo-Cushing's syndrome'.

The next step is to demonstrate elevated cortisol secretion. Twenty-four-hour urine collections for cortisol can be helpful, but ideally the patient should be admitted for diurnal cortisol and ACTH levels (9 am and 12 midnight). Cortisol levels are usually high, though in the early stages of the disease they may be relatively normal, though the diurnal rhythm is lost. Plasma ACTH levels are usually high, or certainly not suppressed (as would occur for example in adrenal Cushing's). Further diagnostic confirmation, as well as indication of the site of hormone secretion (adrenal, pituitary or ectopic), can be obtained with a 'long dexamethasone suppression test'. After a 'run-in' period of 2 days of diurnal cortisol and ACTH levels, dexamethasone 0.5 mg q.d.s. orally ('low dose') is given for 2 days, and then 2 mg q.d.s. ('high dose') for a further 2 days, with continued diurnal cortisol and ACTH levels. In pituitary-driven Cushing's there is normally some suppression, but in adrenal or ectopic disease there is usually failure to show significant suppression, even on high dose dexamethasone.

In biochemically confirmed cases, radiological imaging of the pituitary should take place. A lateral skull X-ray may show an expanded pituitary fossa, but this is an insensitive and non-specific procedure. Computerized axial tomography (CT scanning) is much better, though the ideal procedure is the magnetic resonance (MR) scan.

Obviously, these investigations are complicated. Cushing's syndrome can be suspected, but not fully investigated, at primary health care (PHC) and at most district general hospital (DGH) facilities. Patients will therefore need to be fully assessed usually at teaching hospital level, and in some smaller African countries may even need transfer to cities elsewhere if this is possible.

Management

In most cases of definite, biochemical pituitary-driven Cushing's syndrome, an anterior pituitary adenoma will be demonstrated on MR scan, and the ideal treatment is neurosurgical removal by the transphenoidal approach. This is, of course, highly specialized surgery, and is only available in a few African centres. An alternative is bilateral adrenalectomy, followed by lifelong hydrocortisone replacement. There is a small risk of Nelson's syndrome (anterior pituitary hyperplasia with pigmentation), but this is rarely problematic, and bilateral adrenalectomy is in most African cases the most appropriate treatment for pituitary Cushing's. Medical treatment is possible with drugs such as metyrapone or ketoconazole, but it is difficult and requires close monitoring, and should only be considered where surgical options are not possible.

Acromegaly

Acromegaly is over-secretion of growth hormone (GH) by an anterior pituitary adenoma. If it occurs before adolescent fusion of the long-bone epiphyses, then 'gigantism' may occur. Otherwise, it leads to the classical acromegalic facies, as well as an increase in hand and foot size (see Fig. 85.5). Other features may include hypertension, diabetes, sweating and sometimes carpal tunnel syndromes. Biochemical confirmation is with a glucose tolerance test in which GH levels are measured half-hourly for 2 hours. GH levels are high, and fail to suppress following glucose. Associated radiological features include an expanded pituitary fossa, increased heel pad thickness, and 'tufting' of terminal phalanges. Ideally, however, the pituitary should be imaged with a CT or preferably MR scan, and in

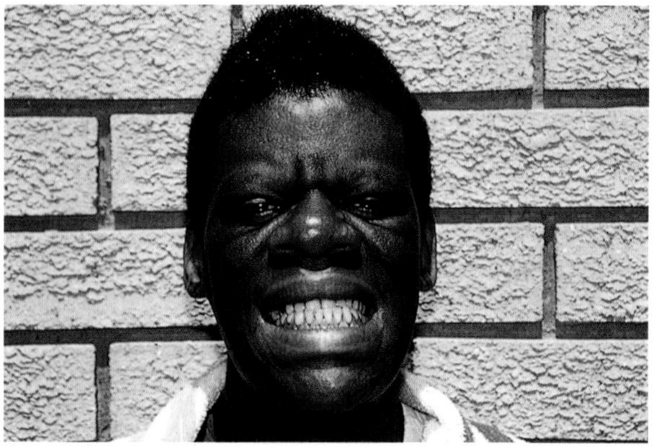

Fig. 85.5. A patient with acromegaly and the typical facial features. There is coarsening of the general facial contours, and prominence of the supra-orbital ridges and protrusion of the chin (prognathism).

definite cases a pituitary tumour is almost invariably found (see Fig. 85.6).

As with pituitary-driven Cushing's syndrome, the ideal treatment is tumour removal via the transphenoidal route. Even with apparently adequate resection, however, biochemical cure is difficult, and post-operative irradiation and/or long-term drug therapy (with bromocriptine, cabergoline, or octreotide) may be needed. Criteria of cure are nowadays strict, with ideally GH levels <5 i.u./l, and normal IgF-1 levels (Clayton, 1993). IgF-1 is a useful measurement – it is one of the somatomedins which mediate the action of GH, and is much more stable in plasma than GH levels.

Diagnosis and treatment of acromegaly in Africa is difficult in all but specialist teaching centres, and as with pituitary Cushing's syndrome referral to other countries may be needed . If neurosurgery is not available, localized irradiation should be given if possible. Bromocriptine may be required long term – relatively high doses are usually needed (up to 20 mg daily), but side effects may be problematic. Starting with low doses (2.5 to 5 mg daily) and slowly working upwards will reduce side effect problems. It is also important to take the drug with meals, as this also reduces side effects.

Prolactinoma

Prolactinoma is the commonest type of hormone-secreting pituitary tumour. However, hyperprolactinaemia may occur physiologically (in pregnancy, for example), and can also be caused by non-pituitary disease. Examples include hypothyroidism, drugs (notably major tranquil-

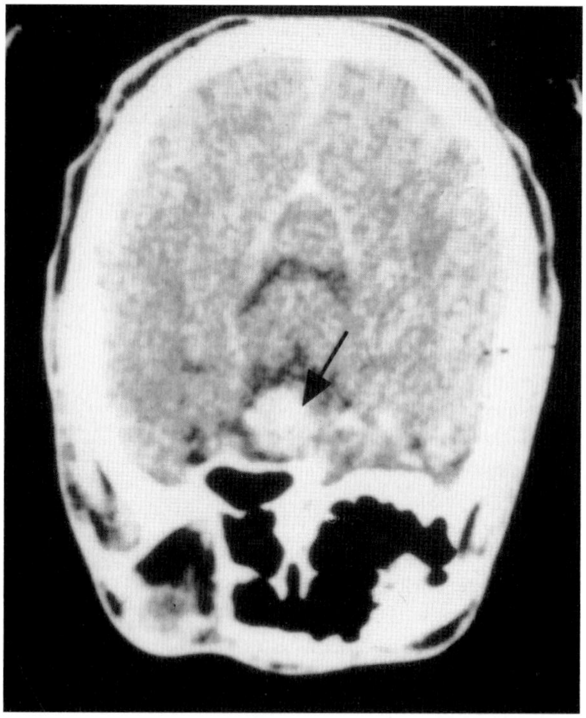

Fig. 85.6. MR scan of the pituitary in a patient with acromegaly, showing a pituitary tumour (arrowed).

lizers), and sometimes chest wall disease or trauma. In women, hyperprolactinaemia may manifest itself by galactorrhoea, amenorrhoea (or oligomenorrhoea) or subfertility. In men, the symptoms are usually of reduced libido and partial or complete erectile impotence. Non-pituitary disease causing hyperprolactinaemia generally leads to only modest elevations, but when an anterior pituitary adenoma of prolactin-secreting cells occurs, elevation of several thousand units per litre are usual. Dynamic pituitary tests are not usually needed, but MR scanning (or at least CT) is needed if available. Prolactinomas can vary enormously in size, from tiny lesions of a millimetre or so ('micro-prolactinoma') to large lesions with suprasellar extensions, which may endanger the optic nerves ('macro-prolactinoma').

Even for large prolactinomas, surgery is rarely needed. Both prolactin levels (with associated symptoms) and tumour size, reduce effectively with drug treatment. Bromocriptine should be used as described above (see under **Acromegaly**). Cabergoline is a more modern alternative, but it is expensive and rarely available in Africa. Treatment should be monitored by symptoms, prolactin levels and intermittent pituitary scans.

Once again, adequate management of prolactinoma in African settings is difficult. However, diagnosis and exclusion of non-pituitary causes may be possible at DGH or tertiary referral centre. Even without imaging facilities, the symptomatic and biochemical response to bromocriptine can be dramatic and highly pleasing both for patient and doctor.

Disorders of pituitary underactivity

There are two major syndromes here. The word 'hypopituitarism' usually refers to anterior pituitary underfunction, which may involve a single hormone ('selective hypopituitarism') or several ('panhypopituitarism'). Under-secretion of ADH from the posterior pituitary leads to the syndrome of diabetes insipidus.

Hypopituitarism

Many pathological processes (see Box, p. 1106) may lead to either selective or pan-hypopituitarism. Some rare genetic conditions can cause selective hormone deficiency – for example, Kallman's syndrome, which is associated with FSH/LH deficiency and anosmia (lack of sense of smell) from birth. It usually presents as delayed puberty and/or adolescent growth retardation. Progressive pituitary disease (for example, an expanding non-functioning adenoma) often impairs hormone release in a recognized 'league table' fashion – FSH/LH first, ACTH next and finally TSH (obviously, this is variable, and exceptions frequently occur). The presentation of hypopituitarism depends on the hormones involved, and will be similar to primary end-organ disease (e.g. TSH – hypothyroidism, ACTH – Addison's disease, etc.). However, the onset is usually more insidious and may be so slow as to be poorly recognized by patients. This is particularly true of ACTH deficiency, where Addisonian symptoms can appear gradually and non-specifically. As already mentioned, a history of significant post-partum haemorrhage in a woman should lead to suspicion of pituitary underfunction, particularly in the presence of oligomenorrhoea or secondary amenorrhoea. Post-partum oligoamenorrhoea with failure to breast-feed are important pointers to Sheehan's syndrome.

Investigation

This should ideally be in a specialized centre, as complex hormone assays will frequently be needed. Dynamic pituitary function testing and MR scanning are also ideally required. To assess pituitary ACTH reserve, the 'gold standard' test is the insulin-stress test (IST) in which hypoglycaemia (blood glucose below 2.2 mmol/l with symptoms) is induced by intravenous soluble insulin 0.1 unit/kg body weight. Blood glucose and plasma cortisol (ACTH does not need measuring) are measured half-hourly for 2 hours. Hypoglycaemia also stimulates GH release. If stimulation of FSH/LH or TSH is needed, synthetic releasing hormones can be used (200 µg/TRH and 100 µg GnRH i.v., respectively, at the start of the test). The IST is labour intensive and potentially dangerous. One-to-one medical care throughout the test is needed, and it is contraindicated in significant heart disease and epilepsy. An alternative stimulus to ACTH and GH secretion is glucagon 1 mg i.m. stat. Sampling needs to be more prolonged (up to 3 hours) and the stimulus provided is not as potent as hypoglycaemia, but the test is easier and safer. There have also been recent suggestions that indirect testing with the 'Short Synacthen Test' (plasma cortisol before and 30 minutes after 250 µg i.m. of tetracosactrin) may be adequate to assess pituitary ACTH reserve (Hurel et al., 1996). In all these tests, a peak plasma cortisol of over 550 nmol/l (and preferably over 600 nmol/l) is required to exclude ACTH deficiency.

Management

Treatment depends on which pituitary hormones are deficient. ACTH deficiency requires hydrocortisone replacement as for Addison's disease (see later). Fludrocortisone should not be needed. FSH/LH cannot be replaced long term, but pre-menopausal deficiency in females requires oestrogen replacement to protect against osteoporosis. In men, pituitary (and testicular) hypogonadism is treated best with parenteral testosterone preparations (e.g. 'Sustanon' or 'Primoteston'), usually given in doses of 250 mg i.m. monthly (sometimes 3- or even 2-weekly injections are needed). Oral testosterone does not work as well and should only be used if parenteral preparations are not available. Testosterone patches, with improved hormone delivery, have recently been introduced. TSH deficiency is treated with thyroxine as for primary hypothyroidism. Adult GH deficiency has been until recently believed to be of no clinical importance. There is possibly some recent evidence that subtle benefits relating to muscle strength and possibly life quality may occur with replacement treatment, and it is being used in some patients in western countries. Treatment is, however, parenteral and expensive, and also still somewhat controversial. Its cost-effectiveness profile makes it inappropriate in an African setting.

Diabetes insipidus

Diabetes insipidus (DI) is rare, and presents with thirst and polyuria (at least 2.5 l/day). In such patients, diabetes

Table 85.7. Water deprivation test for possible diabetes insipidus

1. Patient fasts but is allowed water, and has no alcohol or nicotine for 12 hours before test.
2. Start at 9 am, patient empties bladder, and no more fluid is allowed.
3. Every hour, weigh patient, and measure urine volume and osmolality, and plasma osmolality

Time (h)	Weight (kg)	Urine volume (ml)	Urine osmolality (mOsmol/kg)	Plasma osmolality (mOsmol/kg)
09.00				
10.00				
11.00				
12.00				
13.00				
14.00				
15.00				
16.00				
17.00				

4. If osmolality cannot be measured, measure urine volume and specific gravity only.
5. Stop test if weight falls below 95 per cent of initial weight or if patient becomes ill.
6. Give food and fluids at the end of the test.

mellitus should obviously be first excluded, and if possible hypercalcaemia and chronic renal failure (as they can also cause polyuria). About one-third of cases are related to pituitary tumours (exacting pressure on the hypothalamus, pituitary stalk or posterior pituitary), one-third due to trauma (including neurosurgery), and one-third are idiopathic.

Investigation

The only practical confirmatory test for DI is the water deprivation test, which unfortunately is difficult and often gives confusing results. It must be carried out with care in hot countries, as in true DI patients may become seriously dehydrated. Body weight is therefore closely monitored during the test, and it is stopped and the patient given immediate water if it falls below 95 per cent of the starting weight (e.g. for someone of 60 kg, this would be 57 kg). A suggested protocol is shown in Table 85.7. Ideally, the test ends with i.m. DDAVP (synthetic ADH), and observations are continued less frequently until 9 am the next morning. Parenteral DDAVP, however, may not be available, and this part of the test is only required to differentiate cranial from nephrogenic DI. In true cranial DI, water deprivation is associated with reduced body weight and increased plasma osmolality, but continued excretion of large amounts of relatively dilute urine, with a response to DDAVP (Baylis & Gill, 1984).

Management

DDAVP is given as nasal spray or drops, tablets or injection. In practical terms, nasal drops are likely to be the only available form. They come with a pipette dropper from which doses of, for example, 0.05 ml or 0.1 ml can be given. Most patients will need a dose such as this two or three times daily, though sometimes more. The dose must be adjusted to and governed by the patient's need – and thus the degree of AVP deficiency, ambient temperature and activity. As mentioned above, the results of the water deprivation test are sometimes equivocal, and it may be reasonable at times to give a cautious therapeutic trial of DDAVP, with careful observation. In many neurosurgical units, transient post-operative DI is simply recognized and treated on a clinical basis. Full confirmatory testing is reserved for those in whom DI does not remit with post-surgical recovery.

Adrenal disorders

Anatomy and physiology

The adrenal or 'supra-renal' glands lie above the kidneys, they are roughly pyramidal in shape, and are highly vascular. There is a central medulla and outer cortex. The medulla forms a functional unit with the sympathetic nervous system, and is concerned with the secretion of catecholamines – predominantly adrenaline and noradrenaline. The cortex is divided histologically into three zones – below the outer gland capsule is the *zona glomerulosa*, then comes the *zona fasciculata*, and finally is the inner *zona reticularis* adjacent to the medulla. The adrenal cortex produces and releases a large number of complex steroid hormones which can be broadly divided into glucocorticoids (mainly cortisol in man), mineralocorticoids (mainly aldosterone), and small amounts of androgens and oestrogens. Cortisol is formed by the *zona fasciculata* and *zona reticularis*, and aldosterone by the *zona glomerulosa*. Control of cortisol secretion is, of course, determined by circulating pituitary ACTH. Aldosterone secretion is affected by extracellular fluid electrolyte and volume balance, mainly modulated via renin secretion from the juxta-glomerular cells of the kidney.

Table 85.8. Causes of adrenal cortisol deficiency

Autoimmune adrenalitis
Tuberculosis
Pituitary ACTH deficiency
HIV infection
Histoplasmosis
Adrenal infarction
Adrenal haemorrhage
Carcinomatosis
Infiltrations (sarcoid, haemochromatosis, amyloid, etc.)
Congenital adrenal hyperplasia
Iatrogenic

Pathological processes

The classical disease of the adrenal medulla is, of course, the phaeochromocytoma – a tumour which is usually benign, though in 5–10 per cent of cases can be malignant, and in about 10 per cent may be extra-adrenal. The adrenal cortex may be affected by autoimmune destruction, haemorrhage or infarction, metastatic cancer (because of its high vascularity), tuberculosis, hyperplasia and neoplasia. Especially classical syndromes are Addison's disease (due to autoimmune or tuberculous adrenalitis usually), Conn's syndrome (due to an aldosterone-producing adenoma), adrenal Cushing's syndrome (due to a cortisol-producing adenoma), and the inherited metabolic disorder congenital adrenal hyperplasia (CAH). These will be discussed in more detail from a clinical viewpoint below.

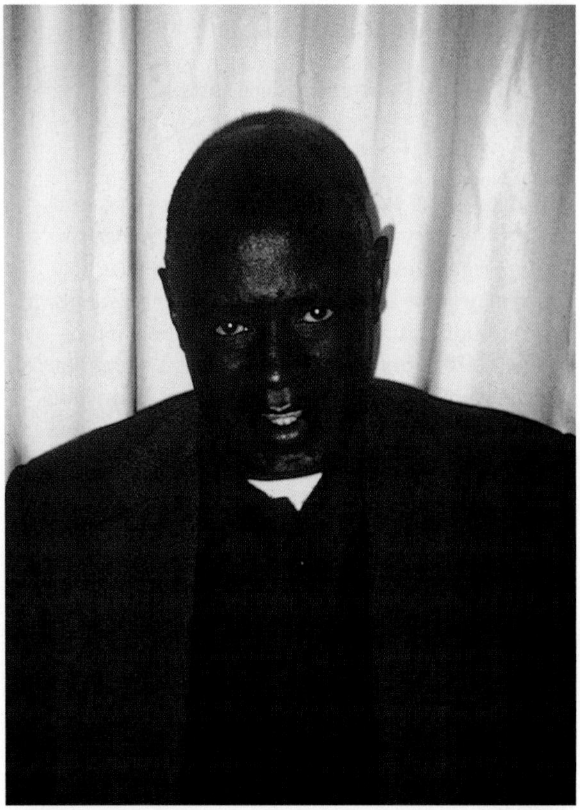

Fig. 85.7. This gentleman from Soweto in South Africa presented complaining of his 'skin going dark'. Compared with his usual skin colour he was quite correct, and investigations showed him to have Addison's disease due to adrenal tuberculosis.

Clinical syndromes of adrenal disease

The most important of these is Addison's disease, or under-secretion of adrenal cortisol. This syndrome, next to thyroid disorders, is probably the commonest endocrine disorder in Africa.

Addison's disease

Causes

The classical cause is autoimmune inflammation, and this is the commonest 'western' cause. In Africa, however, tuberculosis accounts for at least half of cases (Shires et al., 1994), and conversely up to one-third of patients with tuberculosis in Africa may have some evidence of adrenal glucocorticoid hypofunction on careful biochemical testing (Mugusi et al., 1990). Other causes of Addisonian syndromes are shown in Table 85.8. HIV infection is an important and increasingly recognized cause in Africa (Dlughy, 1990). Adrenal haemorrhage may classically occur in children with meningococcal septicaemia (the 'Waterhouse–Frederichsen Syndrome'). Adrenal infarction can occur as part of the 'anticardiolipin' or 'phospholipid' syndrome – an increasingly recognized process in America and Europe, but of uncertain importance in Africa (Hughes, 1998). Iatrogenic hypoadrenalism refers to the syndrome, which may occur on abrupt withdrawal of steroid drugs in a patient who has adrenal suppression from long-term synthetic steroid treatment.

Presenting features

These are notoriously variable (see the Box below), and can be very non-specific (such as weakness, dizziness, weight loss). Patients may initially be thought to be suffering from AIDS, and as Addison's disease is highly treatable, it is very important that the diagnosis is at all times kept in mind. Atypical presentations such as fever and/or vomiting may occur. Also, even in black Africans, increased pigmentation can be a presenting complaint (see Fig. 85.7 and the Box).

Presenting features of hypoadrenalism

• Malaise	• Muscle wasting
• Fatigue	• Postural hypotension
• Weight loss	• Pigmentation
• Fever	• Hyponatraemia
• Dizziness	• Hypoglycaemia
• Weakness	• Anaemia

An important presentation is with 'Addisonian crisis', which may occur at diagnosis, or in a known patient with the condition (usually provoked by cessation of treatment, or intercurrent infection). Patients are typically collapsed, hypotensive and often dehydrated. If available, biochemical investigations may show hyponatraemia and/or hypoglycaemia. The plasma urea is often elevated and there may be modest hyperkalaemia and a mild metabolic acidosis. Treatment is with intravenous hydrocortisone (100–200 mg i.v. stat, followed by 100 mg i.v. 6-hourly), as well as rehydration with appropriate fluids (either 'dextrose/saline' or 0.9 per cent ('normal') saline if blood glucose levels are normal) – usually 1 litre 6-hourly initially. Regular bedside blood glucose monitoring should be done. The response is usually dramatic and patients can be stabilized on oral treatment in 1–2 days.

Diagnosis

In the absence of biochemical facilities, strongly suggestive clinical features may warrant a trial of hydrocortisone replacement treatment. Supportive electrolyte levels, particularly with hypoglycaemia, may be helpful. Ideally, however, low plasma cortisol levels should be demonstrated. As cortisol levels are variable, the ideal diagnostic test is the 'Short Synacthen Test'. Here an i.m. injection of 250 μg of tetracosactrin (synthetic ACTH or 'Synacthen') is given at around 0900 hours, and a plasma cortisol level taken beforehand and 30 minutes later. Normal patients will increase their basal level, usually by at least 200 nmol/l, to a peak of over 550 nmol/l. The post-stimulation value is the most critical, and this test will detect milder degrees of adrenal hypofunction.

Treatment

Standard glucocorticoid replacement is with hydrocortisone tablets, and the traditional adult dose is 20 mg in the morning and 10 mg in the evening, though 10 mg twice daily is probably sufficient. If hydrocortisone is not available, other steroids such as cortisone, or even prednisolone or dexamethasone (in small doses), can be used. Indeed, prednisolone 5 mg (best given at night) daily is a simple and easy way of replacement, especially in resource-poor areas. Treatment should be monitored by well-being, as well as stability of body weight and blood pressure (lying and standing). If available, intermittent plasma cortisol and electrolyte measurements may also be useful (though cortisol levels will be unhelpful if synthetic steroids such as prednisolone or dexamethasone are used). Whatever the treatment, patients should receive appropriate education that their condition is lifelong and that regular treatment is vital. They should also double their replacement doses when intercurrent illnesses occur. Some form of bracelet or medallion identification is ideal. Mineralocorticoid replacement is not always needed, probably because most glucocorticoid preparations have some degree of mineralocorticoid activity. The need for mineralocorticoid may be indicated by persisting malaise, hypotension and/or hyponatraemia despite adequate glucocorticoid treatment. The usual treatment is with fludrocortisone 50–100 μg daily.

Phaeochromocytoma

These tumours arise from chromaffin cells, and 90 per cent are in the adrenal medulla and 10 per cent in sympathetic ganglia. Less than 10 per cent are malignant, and almost all are associated with hypertension. Other symptoms may include palpitations, sweating and headache. Of all hypertensive subjects, only about 1 in 1000 will have a phaeochromocytoma, but the diagnosis should be considered especially in young hypertensive subjects, and those with severe and fluctuating blood pressure levels (Shires et al., 1994; Ross & Griffith, 1989; Huddle et al., 1991). A severe hypertensive crisis during surgery is a classical presentation. Phaeochromocytoma appears as likely to occur in black Africans as in Caucasians (Shires et al., 1994). It may also present as part of the syndrome of multiple endocrine neoplasia (MEN II).

Once suspected, the biochemical diagnosis depends on the demonstration of excess catecholamines or their metabolites in the urine. A 24-hour collection is needed for hydroxy-methyl-mandelic acid (VMA or HMMA) or metanephrines; or ideally directly analysed urinary adrenaline, noradrenaline and dopamine (though this is unlikely to be available in Africa). Imaging is then required, ideally by CT scanning (though ultrasound may also be helpful) or radioisotope (MIBG) scanning. The latter is especially useful when the clinical and biochemical diagnosis seems firm, but adrenal CT imaging is negative. MIBG scans may then help to indicate the site of a possible extra-adrenal phaeochromocytoma.

It can be seen that the diagnosis and localization of phaeochromocytoma tumours is highly specialized, and in Africa is likely to be available only in specialized teaching centres, and referral of patients to these units will be necessary. Once localized, the ideal management is, of course, surgical, and this requires close teamwork between physician, surgeon and anaesthetist. It is vital that the patient is adequately prepared for surgery, or a potentially fatal hypertensive crisis may occur. Alpha blockade (with, for example, phenoxybenzamine) is needed, and patients should be admitted several days before surgery to ensure that this is done adequately. Doses should be gradually increased to give excellent blood pressure control (even with a small degree of postural hypotension). Doses of phenoxybenzamine in the order of 10–20 mg q.d.s. are generally needed. Beta blockade is not usually needed provided alpha blockade is adequate.

If patients are unfit for surgery, or localization and/or surgical facilities are unavailable, then long-term medical treatment is reasonable. Here, combined phenoxybenzamine and propranolol is often very effective.

Conn's syndrome

Conn's syndrome is usually due to an adrenal cortical adenoma which hypersecretes aldosterone. This causes a syndrome of primary hyperaldosteronism characterized by hypertension and hypokalaemia. Accurate diagnosis requires plasma renin and aldosterone levels (lying and standing), as well as adrenal imaging – preferably by CT scan, though ultrasound may be helpful. A significant minority of cases are due to hyperplasia of aldosterone-secreting cells, rather than an isolated adenoma.

The treatment of choice for adenoma is, of course, surgical excision if possible, but medical treatment with spironolactone is often very successful in controlling both hypertension and hypokalaemia.

Adrenal Cushing's syndrome

The clinical features and diagnostic procedures for Cushing's syndrome due to a cortisol-secreting adrenal adenoma are essentially the same as described previously for pituitary-driven Cushing's syndrome. ACTH levels, however, will be suppressed, and during a dexamethasone suppression test, cortisol levels will fail to suppress, even on high doses. Imaging of the adrenal glands is required of course, preferably by CT scanning, and the treatment ideally is adenoma removal.

Other adrenal disorders

'Non-functioning' (i.e. non-hormone secreting) tumours of the adrenal are not uncommon, and may be found incidentally at operation, autopsy, or during scanning procedures for other reasons. They are often referred to as 'adrenal incidentalomas' and present a dilemma for the endocrinologist. If they are small (less than 4 cm diameter) and there are no indications of hormone hypersecretion, they can generally be left alone. Surgery is however indicated for functional and/or large tumours. The concern with a non-functioning tumour of significant size, or of non-uniform appearance on scanning, is that it may be an adrenal carcinoma rather than a benign adenoma (Mantero & Arnaldi, 1999).

Very rarely, genetically determined congenital adrenal hyperplasia (CAH) can present in adult life. These are virtually always 21–OH enzyme deficiencies (usually partial). The presentation is with mild to moderate virilization in adult females, as the enzyme block leads to increased adrenal androgen synthesis. Cortisol production may be reduced, but can also be adequate. Diagnosis is often difficult. Radiological bilateral adrenal hyperplasia (BAH) is generally present, but with no other indications of pituitary-driven Cushing's syndrome. Adrenal androgen levels (e.g. dehydroepiandrostenedione) are raised, as is usually17-α-hydroxy-progesterone (17αOHP). Synacthen stimulation (given as for a short Synacthen test – see under '**Addison's disease**') shows an exaggerated 17αOHP rise. Treatment is with low dose dexamethasone, which suppresses ACTH secretion, thereby reducing adrenal androgen secretion.

Parathyroid disease

Hyperparathyroidism

The hallmark of primary hyperparathyroidism is hypercalcaemia: it is, together with malignant disease, a major cause of elevated plasma calcium levels. Other causes include sarcoidosis, myeloma, excessive vitamin D intake, and the 'milk-alkali syndrome'.

Hyperparathyroidism is almost always due to a benign adenoma of one of the four parathyroid glands, autonomously secreting excessive parathormone (PTH). The clinical features are traditionally of 'bones, stones, moans and abdominal groans'. This refers to the specific bone resorptive syndrome ('osteitis fibrosa cystica' or 'von Recklinghausen's disease of bone'), which can lead to pathological fractures, calcium deposition (causing, for example, renal stones), depression ('moans'), and an increased risk of peptic ulceration and pancreatitits ('abdominal groans'). In addition, polydipsia and polyuria can occur, as well as muscle cramps, myopathy and generalized malaise. Prolonged hypercalcaemia can lead to renal damage.

As well as hypercalcaemia, serum phosphate is usually low, and serum PTH levels inappropriately normal or raised (negative feedback should normally lead to suppression of PTH levels).

If the diagnosis is firm, then the neck should be surgically explored for a parathyroid adenoma. Radiological imaging procedures are generally unhelpful, and it is often said that the 'best localizing system is an experienced surgeon'. There is no effective medical treatment for primary hyperparathyroidism. The disease thus presents considerable diagnostic and therapeutic difficulties in Africa. Fortunately, it appears to be rarer in black Africans than in white Caucasians.

Hypercalcaemic crisis

Primary hyperparathyroidism is (along with metastatic boney malignant disease) an important cause of hypercalcaemic crisis, characterized by:

- serum calcium is usually well in excess of 3.0 mmol/l
- marked dehydration
- muscle pain and weakness.

The most important treatment is intravenous saline, which promotes calciuresis and rehydration. One litre of 0.9 per cent ('normal') saline 4- to 6-hourly is often required initially, and later on small amounts of frusemide may help continue the diuresis. Intravenous pamidronate (a biphosphonate drug) may also be helpful, particularly in severe malignant hypercalcaemia, but it is rarely available in Africa. In the acute situation however, saline is the most effective treatment.

Hypoparathyroidism

In contrast to primary hyperparathyroidsm, idiopathic (possibly autoimmune) hypoparathyroidism appears relatively more common amongst black Africans. Thus, of 146 patients seen at the Endocrine Clinic of Baragwanath Hospital in Soweto, South Africa, only 3 (1%) had primary hyperparathyroidism, but 24 (8%) had hypoparathyroidism (Shires et al., 1994). The hallmark of the condition is, of course hypocalcaemia, which is associated with low or low-normal serum PTH levels, with no other likely causes (e.g. osteomalacia, malabsorption, anticonvulsant treatment, etc.). The condition usually presents in adult life, and common features are tetany and paraesthesia, sometimes with seizures or cataracts (Huddle & Ally, 1989). Less well-recognized features are various neuropsychiatric syndromes, basal ganglia calcification (Fig. 85.8) (Shires et al., 1994; Huddle & Ally,1989) and a reversible cardiomyopathy with congestive heart failure (Huddle, 1988).

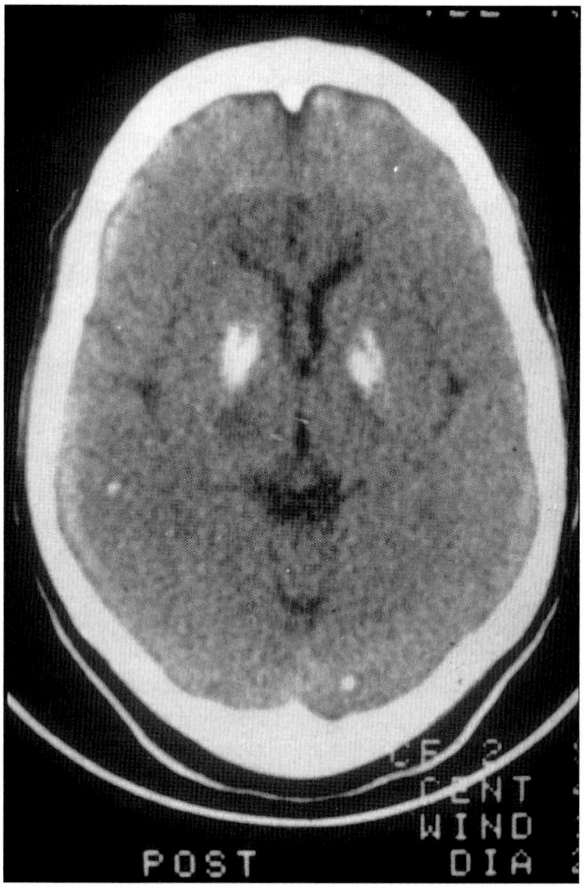

Fig. 85.8. A CT brain scan showing basal ganglia calcification in a South African patient with idiopathic hypoparathyroidism.

Hypoparathyroidism is usually easily treated with vitamin D preparations – preferably the more potent 1-α-hydroxy derivative. If dietary calcium is adequate, then calcium supplements may not be necessary, but in a number of cases these will be needed also.

Other endocrine disorders

Polycystic ovary syndrome (PCOS)

PCOS is a spectrum of endocrine disorder and affects at least 10 per cent of women in western countries. Little is known of its prevalence and characteristics in Africa. Cystic ovaries are a frequent accompaniment rather than a cause of PCOS. The syndrome is characterized by mild to moderate hyperandrogenism, accompanied frequently by obesity, multiple small ovarian cysts and insulin resistance. Clinical manifestations may be oligomenorrhoea or secondary amenorrhoea, hirsutism, subfertility or persistent acne. Biochemical investigations may show a mildly elevated serum testosterone level, and relatively high LH level compared to FSH ('reversed FSH/LH ratio'). The differential diagnosis is usually between an androgen-secreting tumour and adult-onset CAH. Insulin resistance is thought to be a major disorder in PCOS, and patients have a significantly increased risk of hypertension and type 2 diabetes. Treatment is therefore ideally with weight loss and increased exercise. Other treatments are less satisfactory and depend on the clinical manifestations. These include cyclical oesterogens (to increase sex-hormone binding globulin levels and reduce free testosterone), oestrogens combined with the anti-androgen drug cyproterone acetate, and spironolactone (which reduces hair growth). The biguanide oral hypoglycaemic agent metformin has also been recently used, as it increases insulin sensitivity. The recently introduced thiazolidenediones ('glitazones') specifically improve insulin receptor sensitivity and look promising.

Hirsutism

Excess body hair is usually a complaint of young or middle-aged females. It may be familial, ethnic or idiopathic. Other causes include PCOS (see above), some drugs (most notably phenytoin), CAH, and very occasionally androgen-secreting tumours. Investigation is normally only indicated if there are other signs or symptoms of hyperandrogenism (e.g. menstrual disturbance, subfertility, acne, cliteromegaly, etc.). If no specific cause is found, treatment is best with explanation and reassurance; as well as advice on mechanical systems such as shaving, bleaching (only useful with white skins!) or waxing. In very psychologically distressing cases, the use of spironolactone or oestrogen/cyproterone combinations can be considered.

Gynaecomastia

Enlargement of the male breasts is an occasional indication for endocrine referral. Before investigation, it must be ensured that the patient has true gynaecomastia (i.e. breast rather than adipose tissue enlargement). Physiological breast enlargement can also occur normally during male puberty. Unilateral breast enlargement is unlikely to be of endocrine origin: a tumour is possible – breast cancer does occasionally occur in men. Causes of true bilateral gynaecomastia are drugs such as digoxin and spironolactone, abuse of anabolic steroids (increasingly common in 'body-builders' and athletes), hypogonadal states, oestrogen-secreting tumours, and as a paraneoplastic phenomenon. Definite gynaecomastia requires advanced investigation – initial tests include (if possible) plasma levels of testosterone, oestradiol, FSH and LH. A simple chest X-ray is always wise, as well as a careful drug history.

Endocrine subfertility

Much infertility investigation and treatment is now done by gynaecologists, but simple endocrine-based assessment is still helpful. Semen analysis of the male partner is, of course, always a simple and important initial step. Assessing the fertility of a regularly menstruating woman involves checking that ovulation is occurring. This can be done with temperature charts, or better by measuring a luteal phase serum progesterone level (which is raised if ovulation has occurred). If cycles are anovulatory, clomiphene in the first half of the cycle may induce ovulation. If this is not successful, then gynaecological investigation is necessary to check for fallopian tube patency. In subfertile women with oligomenorrhoea or secondary amenorrhoea, hyperandrogenic and hyperprolactinaemic states should be considered, as well as reduced ovarian endocrine function. With primary amenorrhoea, genetic abnormalities such as Turner's syndrome should be considered.

Carcinoid syndrome

Carcinoid tumours are rare, and particularly difficult to diagnose in black populations, as flushing (one of the major symptoms) is very rarely recognized by patients or their friends and relatives. Diarrhoea however can be a prominent feature. Diagnosis requires measurement of 5HIAA (5-hydroxyindole-acetic acid) in a 24-hour urine specimen. When diagnosed, the disease has virtually always metastasized to liver, and treatment is supportive and symptomatic. Some patients may survive however for a great many years. Ocreotide (somatostatin) antagonizes the actions of tumour-released serotonin very effectively, and may also reduce tumour growth. It is very expensive however, and is rarely available in Africa.

Metabolic disorders

Haemosiderosis

In the past, traditional cooking in iron pots sometimes led to dietary iron overload. This particularly occurred when traditional beers were brewed in such iron pots, and was especially seen in South Africa. The common manifestation of such haemosiderosis was often hepatic cirrhosis, and the term 'Bantu siderosis' was used. The condition was, however, recognized elsewhere in Africa. Nowadays, the condition is rarely seen, as such traditional cooking practices have changed, and most pots are now made of steel or aluminium. Nevertheless, occasional cases still occur, most commonly diagnosed on liver biopsy. Treatment is by venesection to deplete the body of iron, as well as appropriate preventive and educational measures aimed at reducing future alcohol and iron ingestion (Bothwell et al., 1979).

African porphyrias

Porphyria cutanea tarda (PCT) occurs particularly in black Africans in the northern part of South Africa. Patients are usually male and almost always abuse alcohol. They usually have hepatomegaly and biochemical liver dysfunction. This, together with a probable genetic susceptibility, leads to reduced activity of hepatic uroporphyrinogen decarboxylase. Clinical features include a photosensitive blistering eruption on light-exposed areas, and sometimes hyperpigmentation and hypertrichosis of the face. The urine contains high levels of uroporphyrin, and may turn red on standing. Abdominal crises are rare, and the disease generally runs a benign course. Alcohol avoidance should, of course, be advised.

'Variegate' prophyria is also found in South Africa, but is found in white Africans of original Dutch origin. It is a genetic defect, inherited dominantly, and dates back to the original settlement times in the Cape colony. Clinically this form of variegate porphyria behaves as a mixture of PCT and acute intermittent porphyria.

References

Baylis PH, Gill GV. (1984). The investigation of polyuria. *Clin Endocrind Metab*; **13**: 295–310.

Bleichrodt N, Shrestha RM, West CE, Hautvast JG, van de Vijver FJ, Born MP. (1996). The benefits of adequate iodine intake. *Nutr Rev*; **54**: S72–S78.

Boscaro M, Barzon L, Fallo F, Sonino N. (2001). Cushing's syndrome. *Lancet*; **357**: 783–791.

Bothwell TH, Charlton RW, Cook JD et al. (1979). *Iron Metabolism in Man*. Oxford: Blackwell Scientific Publications.

Clayton RN. (1993). Modern management of acromegaly. *Quart J Med*; **286**: 285–287.

Dayan CM, Daniels GH. (1996). Chronic autoimmune thyroiditis. *N Engl J Med*; **335**: 99–107.

Dlughy RG. (1990). The growing spectrum of HIV-related endocrine abnormalities. *J Clin Endocrinol Metab*; **70**: 563–565.

Franklyn JA. (1994). The management of hyperthyroidism. *N Engl J Med*; **330**: 1731–1738.

Hermus AR, Huysmans DA. (1998). Treatment of benign nodular thyroid disease. *N Engl J Med*; **338**: 1438–1447.

Hetzel BS. (1983). Iodine deficiency disorders (IDD) and their eradication. *Lancet*; **ii**: 1126–1129.

Huddle KRL. (1988). Cardiac dysfunction in primary hypoparathyroidism. *S Afr Med J*; **73**: 242–244.

Huddle KRL, Ally R. (1989). Idiopathic hypoparathyroidism in black South Africans. *Quart J Med*; **70**: 53–60.

Huddle KRL, Mannell A, James MFM, Plant E. (1991). Phaeochromocytoma. *S Afr Med J*; **79**: 217–220.

Hughes GRV. (1998). Hughes syndrome: the antiphospholipid syndrome. *J Roy Coll Phys Lond*; **32**: 260–264.

Hurel SJ, Thompson CJ, Watson MJ, Harris MM, Baylis PH, Kendall-Taylor P. (1996). The short synacthen test and the insulin stress tests in the assessment of the hypothalamo-pituitary–adrenal axis. *Clin Endocrinol*; **44**: 141–146.

Keston-Jones, M. (2001). Management of nodular thyroid disease. *Br Med J*; **323**: 293–294.

LaFranchi S, Mandel S. (1996). Graves' disease and other forms of hyperthyroidism in infants and children. *Curr Opin Endocrinol Diab*; **3**: 101–109.

Larkins R. (1993). Treatment of Graves' ophthalmopathy. *Lancet*; **342**: 941.

Mantero F, Arnaldi G. (1999). Investigation protocol: adrenal enlargement. *Clin Endrocinol*; **50**: 141–146.

Mazzaferri EL. (1993). Management of a solitary thyroid nodule. *N Engl J Med*; **328**: 553–559.

Mugusi F, Swai ABM, Turner ST, Alberti KGMM, McLarty DG. (1990). Hypoadrenalism in patients with pulmonary tuberculosis in Tanzania: an undiagnosed complication? *Trans Roy Soc Trop Med Hyg*; **84**: 849–851.

Oppenheimer JH, Braverman LE, Toft A, Jackson IM, Laderson PW. (1995). A therapeutic controversy. Thyroid hormone treatment: when and what? *J Clin Endocrinol Metab*; **80**: 2873–2883.

Rivkees SA, Sklar C, Freemark M. (1998). The management of Graves' disease in children with special emphasis on radioiodine treatment. *J Clin Endocrinol Metab*; **83**: 3767–3776.

Ross EJ, Griffith DNW. (1989). The clinical presentation of phaeochromocytoma. *Quart J Med*; **71**: 485–496.

Shires R, Kalk J, Huddle KRL. (1994). Endocrinology. In *Baragwanath Hospital, 50 Years – A Medical Miscellany*, ed. KRL Huddle & A. Dubb, pp. 53–67. Johannesburg: Baragwanath Hospital.

Todd CH, Dunn JT. (1998). Intermittent oral administation of potassium iodide solution for the correction of iodine deficiency. *Am J Clin Nutr*; **67**: 1279–1283.

Todd CH. (1999). *Hyperthyroidism and Other Thyroid Disorders – A Practical Handbook for the Recognition and Management*. WHO/ICCIDD. WHO/NDH/99.1.

Vanderpump MPJ, Ahlquist JAO, Franklyn JA et al. (1996). Consensus statement for good practice and audit measures in the management of hypothyroidism and hyperthyroidism. *Br Med J*; **351**: 539–544.

WHO/UNICEF/ICCIDD. (1996). Recommended iodine levels in salt and guidelines for monitoring their adequacy and effectiveness. Geneva: WHO: WHO/NUT/96.13.

WHO/UNICEF/ICCIDD. (1999). Progress towards the elimination of iodine deficiency disorders (IDD). Geneva: WHO: WHO/NHD/99.4.

WHO/UNICEF/ICCIDD. (2001). Assessment of iodine deficiency diosorders and monitoring their elimination. Geneva: WHO: WHO/NDH/01.1.

Wood PJ, Barth JH, Freedman DB, Perry L, Sheridan B. (1997). Evidence for low dose dexamethasone suppression test to screen for Cushing's syndrome – recommendations for a protocol for biochemistry laboratories. *Ann Clin Biochem*; **34**: 222–229.

Footnote

For those with internet access, an excellent free on-line resource is 'The Thyroid Manager': www.thyroidmanager.org

Note

'ICCIDD' stands for International Council for the Control of Iodine Deficiency Disorders.

86 The nervous system

The problem in Africa

Nervous system diseases in Africa have a spectrum in some ways similar to other parts of the world. Stroke and epilepsy are very common, but dementia or Parkinson's disease are much less so. Obvious questions arise, for example, which of the particular geographical, climatic, social and ethnic factors of the continent govern the pattern of disease? Why is multiple sclerosis almost unknown in tropical Africa, whereas defined local factors account for Burkitt's lymphoma and tropical ataxic neuropathy? While the epidemic of HIV infection is bringing its own range of neurological complications, there are few local data about Parkinson's disease, or even stroke, so that there are exciting opportunities for future research. A comment, which was made about tropical neurology by Spillane in 1973, is still true, '. . . the repeated assertion that many diseases of the nervous system are uncommon or actually rare in certain tropical zones is a premature generalization. . . . We are nowhere near a position to make any broad and confident generalization about the distribution of diseases of the nervous system in the tropics'.

Although epidemiological work in Africa is demanding, some careful studies have already provided valuable data, as the example from Ethiopia demonstrates (Table 86.1).

Table 86.1. Neurological disorders in rural Ethiopia

Diagnosis	Sex M	Sex F	Total	Prevalence (cases/100 000)
Epilepsy	173	143	316	519
Speech disturbance	90	66	156	256
deaf-mutism	38	38	76	125
others	52	28	80	131
Poliomyelitis	82	65	147	241
Mental retardation	71	32	103	169
Peripheral neuropathy	58	36	94	154
leprosy	40	23	63	103
traumatic	11	4	15	24
Bell's palsy	2	6	8	13
hereditary	4	2	6	10
others	1	1	2	3
Hemiparesis	21	17	38	62
early childhood onset	10	8	18	29
cerebrovascular	4	5	9	15
post traumatic	1	1	2	3
unknown aetiology	6	3	9	15
Cerebral palsy	7	5	12	20
Optic atrophy	6	4	10	16
Perceptive deafness	4	3	7	12
Paraparesis	4	2	6	10
Parkinson's disease	4	0	4	7
Motor neurone disease	2	1	3	5
Ataxia	2	1	3	5
Chorea/athetosis	1	2	3	5
Tremors	1	2	3	5
Torticollis	1	0	1	2
Myopathy	0	1	1	2
Hemifacial spasm	1	0	1	2
Total	528	380	908	
Per cent	58.1	41.9	100	

Source: From Tekle-Haimanot et al, (1990).

Clinical method is fundamental

It is an old saying in neurology that '*the history tells you the diagnosis and the examination localizes the lesion*'. Clinical methods therefore remain the most important means for making a neurological diagnosis anywhere in the world – but especially in Africa, because limited resources mean that brain scans or electro-encephalography are possible for only a few.

Most patients who present with neurological symptoms do not have serious disease; for instance, headache is usually caused by stress and only rarely does it indicate a cerebral tumour.

A systematic clinical approach, supported by experience of local disease patterns, should lead to the correct diagnosis and treatment in most cases without recourse to investigations.

The problem of treatment

It is tragic and unacceptable that patients are left languishing in the village with spinal cord disorders or neurological infections which are potentially treatable. Even if a medical assessment can be achieved, it is impractical in many cases for treatment to be provided. Local attitudes also determine whether or not medical attention is sought for a neurological condition (Rwiza et al., 1993).

The example of epilepsy

More than 80 per cent of sufferers in Africa do not have the benefits of seizure control from a regular anti-epileptic drug. This may allow the traditional healer access to medical problems, which should be the responsibility of orthodox practitioners, and lead the villager to part with savings or possessions to pay for futile herbal remedies. If epilepsy is regarded as a form of madness or demonic possession, then a rural or urban individual who is affected will view the local traditional healer as providing the best prospect for a cure. Because some traditional healers are willing to use orthodox medicine alongside their own methods, a temporary solution may be for the traditional healer to dispense phenobarbitone as well as his own prescriptions to a patient with epilepsy.

The neurological history

A good history is fundamental. Listen carefully to your patient, act with sympathy and understanding and guide the reticent, shy or rambling patient with judicious leading questions. An ancient Greek philosopher pointed out that we have two ears and one tongue and should therefore listen twice as much as we talk.

What does the patient mean?

A patient who states that he has weakness of an arm may imply a loss of power in the limb, but some patients use the term to indicate loss of sensation or clumsiness. Thus:

- make certain that it is quite clear what the patient means by each symptom.
- be careful if you do not know the possible meaning of words of the local language
- remember that the patient may feel that you should already know his symptoms, so that the process of history taking may initially seem unnatural.

The environment of the patient

The home, habits and work of the patient must be defined. Why should this particular patient, from this place, fall ill in this way, at this time? The family of the subsistence farmer may develop nutritional neurological disorders in times of shortage. The migrant worker who has tremor, forgetfulness or neuropathy may have sought comfort in alcohol, only to be poisoned by it. Those who distil alcohol may unwittingly poison their customers and cause optic atrophy. The office worker who smokes heavily is liable to develop stroke, transient ischaemic attacks or neurological complications of bronchial carcinoma. The forest worker who complains of drowsiness and headache in the cold or rainy season may have carbon monoxide poisoning from burning charcoal or wood in a closed hut.

Psychological factors

Many neurological symptoms are not due to an organic disorder, but stem from anxiety, depression and a reaction to the stresses or life. These factors need to be carefully considered in patients who present with non-specific headache, dizziness or bizarre symptoms. In many such cases, the doctor is being consulted as a second opinion after visits to a traditional healer, whose interventions may or may not have been helpful. Reassuring the 'worried well' may take up a lot of time, but a few minutes listening to the history and conducting a normal physical examination is essential as it reassures the patient and thus contributes to treatment.

HIV – the new neurological dilemma

In every patient now neurological symptoms may result from HIV infection. The truck driver who has lost weight and has become forgetful could well have developed HIV-associated dementia. The young woman with an acute neuropathy may be sero-converting and the young man with chronic meningitis is more likely than not to be immunosuppressed. Always consider that the clinical picture, however unusual, may be primarily due to HIV infection.

Clinical example

An elderly farmer has been brought to the clinic by his family because he has a right hemiparesis and dysphasia. A history of a sudden onset when he awoke with the symptoms a month earlier leads to a confident diagnosis of a stroke affecting the left anterior cerebral hemisphere. However, if his wife explains that the weakness had been gradually evolving, this would raise suspicion of a cerebral tumour. If more detailed questioning, however, indicated that the farmer had briefly lost consciousness shortly before the onset of the weakness, when his cow had kicked his head, a chronic subdural haematoma is possible and this could potentially be treated.

Common symptoms and their causes

Headache

Most headache is benign. Its nature is almost always evident from a careful history; brain scans and other tests are unnecessary in the great majority of cases.

Prevalence

A survey of headache in a rural district in Ethiopia revealed a prevalence for migraine of 3 per cent and for chronic tension headache of 1.7 per cent (Tekle-Haimanot et al., 1995). These figures are surprisingly low and compare with a study in urban workers and students in Dar es Salaam, where 51 per cent of men and 60 per cent of women admitted to having suffered a headache requiring medication or medical consultation in the past year. The headache in 36 per cent was a combined vascular–tension headache; in 31 per cent it was due to migraine; and in 9 per cent there was an organic cause. Headache patients lost an average of 11.3 work days per year, compared with 5.7 days lost in a control group (Matuja et al., 1995).

Tension headache

This accounts for most of the headaches that are seen in urban or rural patients. The patient may not always recognize or accept that they are under stress, but the wife or husband often has a useful insight. A pressure or tightness is described around the head: this is often bitemporal and is sometimes associated with tension in the neck muscles. Tingling or sharp focal pains over the scalp are common. This type of headache may be increased by bright light or by loud noises, such as quarrelling children. The perceptive patient realises that the headache is worst at times of stress, for example, an imminent examination in a student, or following an argument at work. Tension headache usually responds to reassurance and settles with time, but where treatment is needed, a short course of a tricyclic antidepressant or a beta-blocker is helpful. Unfortunately, some patients have a chronic daily headache syndrome, which is usually resistant to treatment.

Table 86.2. Classification of migraine

Common migraine with headache only, often hemicranial
Classical migraine with visual or sensory aura
Cluster migraine
Ophthalmic migraine
Other migraine variants

Migraine

This is the second most important cause of recurrent headache (Table 86.2). A classification is given above and it should be possible to categorize any patient, although quite commonly migraine and tension headache co-exist in the same patient.

Trigger factors are common in migraine and include diet (especially in children), alcohol, sleep deprivation, missed meals, menstruation and above all else, stress.

Management

Most patients need only reassurance and simple analgesics, but more severe cases respond to prophylactic drugs, such as propranolol, amitriptyline and pizotifen. Treatment of acute attacks which do not respond to standard analgesics is successful with ergotamine preparations or the new and expensive triptan drugs.

Headache in infections

This is very common. Typhoid patients usually have headache, and benign viral infections, such as influenza, may give prominent headache. Meningitis almost always causes acute or sub-acute severe generalized headache, usually with neck stiffness and photophobia. This triad demands urgent CSF examination and appropriate treatment. Para-nasal sinus infection causes focal pain and tenderness over the affected sinuses and is not usually the explanation in cases of recurrent or chronic generalized headache.

Sudden severe headache

The patient who presents with a sudden severe generalized headache, ‘the worst pain I have ever had’, neck stiffness, photophobia and vomiting has probably had a subarachnoid haemorrhage from a bleeding cerebral aneurysm. Lumbar puncture will reveal uniformly blood stained CSF if examined a few hours after the event: the CSF becomes yellow (xanthochromia) later.

Headache in raised intracranial pressure

- Is present on waking in the morning
- Is increased by coughing, straining, sneezing, laughing, bending or by any activity which causes a Valsalva manoeuvre, increases inthrathoracic pressure, and hence limits venous return from the head
- Is often associated with nausea or vomiting.

Note: The patient does not always have papilloedema or focal signs.

Do not do a lumbar puncture in any patient in whom raised intracranial pressure is suspected for fear of causing tentorial coning, unless acute bacterial meningitis is possible (p. 1142).

Giant cell, cranial or temporal arteritis

In patients over the age of 60 years, a relentless temporal headache with scalp tenderness suggests a diagnosis of cranial arteritis, which is confirmed by finding a high ESR or, ideally, by superficial temporal artery biopsy. These patients respond rapidly to steroid treatment using prednisolone 60 mg daily as the starting dose.

Headache in hypertension

Essential hypertension does not cause chronic headache, although accelerated malignant hypertension may cause severe headache.

The great majority of patients who complain of headache do not have a serious condition.

- Always take a careful history: this will lead to a confident diagnosis and appropriate reassurance or treatment.

Blackouts

Blackouts can be due to syncope, epilepsy, cardiac dysrhythmia or psychological disturbance. The patient can tell you how they felt before and after the event, but not what was happening during the period of loss of consciousness. Therefore, in order to evaluate blackouts, it is important to have an eye-witness account from a family member, friend or work mate. There are rarely physical signs in cases of blackout and hence the history is all important.

Syncope

In African medical practice, syncope appears to be relatively uncommon as a presenting condition. Possibly a benign faint is recognized as such and the patient only seeks advice if there are more dramatic features suggesting a seizure, or if the frequency is worrying (Chapter 74).

- *Vaso vagal attack* This often has a trigger such as a sudden pain or cramp, the sight of blood or a sudden shock. The patient often reports dimming of vision and hearing, as well as dizziness before awareness is lost. The witness describes stillness during the unconscious phase and then a fairly quick recovery. The diagnosis may be less clear if a few limb jerks or tremors are present, and in occasional cases the faint may cause emptying of a full bladder. Such features do not necessarily imply an epileptic attack, and these patients can be reassured so that no other intervention is necessary.
- *Cardiac dysrhythmia* Some cases of syncope are due to cardiac dysrhythmia. The patient may have palpitations at the time of the attack or there may be abnormal cardiovascular signs, but these are unlikely in a paroxysmal disorder. The diagnosis may be confirmed by prolonged ECG recording, if this is available.
- *Hyperventilation syncope* This is a form of panic attack when either the patient or an eye witness reports overbreathing before or during the episode. The stertorous respiration of an epileptic fit is quite different. Peripheral and circumoral tingling is often noted and sometimes carpopedal spasm develops. In these patients, there is usually a background of anxiety or other neurotic behaviour.
- *Psychogenic blackout – other types* Suspect these from the context of the patient, for example, the fear of 'witchcraft' in an unsophisticated villager, or work pressures in an office secretary. It is important that these people are not wrongly diagnosed as having epilepsy since their 'seizures' can superficially appear genuine. Do not hurry to make a diagnosis of epilepsy: it is better to allow further time to clarify the cause of the blackouts.
- *Epilepsy* Classification and a full account of epileptic seizures and febrile convulsions is given in Chapter 74. Tonic–clonic seizures with tongue biting and incontinence, and absence seizures, previously known as petit mal in children, are characteristic. Complex partial seizures arising from the temporal lobe or, less commonly, the frontal lobe, may be a difficult diagnosis, especially when accompanied by bizarre automatic behaviour. The attitude of the patient, family or friends to epilepsy also affects the way in which the history is presented.

Dizziness, vertigo and loss of balance

It is important to differentiate between these symptoms as they imply different pathophysiological processes.

Dizziness is a sensation of light-headedness, sometimes with a feeling of disorientation.

Postural hypotension

Dizziness can be due to postural hypotension on standing quickly. Possible causes include:

- Hypovolaemia. A common cause – associated with an acute bleed or loss of fluid from diarrhoea.
- Drugs. It may be due to use of a beta-blocker or other drugs for hypertension. Excessive use of a diuretic causes postural hypotension due to hypovolaemia.
- Autonomic neuropathy, as in diabetes, often causes postural dizziness.
- Vaodilatation of fever, or of lack of acclimatization in an elderly patient, is also a frequent cause.
- A rare cause is Addison's Disease – hypo-adrenalism (p. 1111).

Benign vestibular or labyrinthine disturbance

In most of these cases, dizziness is transient and insignificant, but an underlying disorder is possible if dizziness persists.

Vertigo

This is a sensation of the environment spinning around the head or of spinning within the head. It is most unpleasant and often associated with nausea or vomiting. Vertigo is due most commonly to:

- the syndrome of benign positional or recurrent vertigo:
- acute or chronic labyrinthitis.

Before deciding that the cause is benign, consider:

- Toxicity from streptomycin or other aminoglycoside.
- Menière's disease, where episodic vertigo is associated with tinnitus and progressive deafness. This is rare in African practice.
- Vertebrobasilar ischaemia. This may be responsible in the elderly for acute vertigo, often associated with dysarthria, diplopia or ataxia.
- Cervical spondylosis does not cause vertigo.

Loss of balance or ataxia

This may co-exist with vertigo and does not necessarily imply a more serious cause, but if unsteadiness of the legs and walking persists, dysfunction of the cerebellum or its connections in the brain stem is possible.

History

Ask the patient whether the dizziness, vertigo or loss of balance:

- is sudden and self-limiting
- is induced by head movement or change of posture
- is worse with the eyes closed or in the dark
- is associated with deafness or with symptoms suggesting brain stem dysfunction, and
- is improving or worsening.

Elaborate ENT tests or scans are not necessary in most cases.

Clinical signs

- A peripheral, and hence usually benign, vestibular or labyrinthine dysfunction is probable if vertigo is induced by tilting of the head to the left and right in a recumbent patient (the Barany manoeuvre).
- A sensory ataxia, due to dorsal column dysfunction in the spinal cord, is suggested if the patient becomes unsteady while standing with the eyes closed and the feet together (Romberg's test).

Weakness and sensory disturbance

These symptoms often imply an organic neurological disorder.

Generalized fatigue and tiredness are usually not due to organic disease, except in cases of anaemia. They seldom indicate a rare neurological disease such as myasthenia. Diffuse non-specific sensory symptoms are also likely to have a psychological course.

Focal weakness or sensory symptoms

These symptoms usually have a definable physical explanation.

Terminology – motor

- Monoparesis – weakness of one limb
- Hemiparesis – weakness of arm and leg on one side of the body
- Paraparesis – weakness of both legs
- Tetraparesis – weakness of all four limbs (due to a high cervical or a cerebral disorder).

The terms monoplegia, hemiplegia, paraplegia and tetraplegia are substituted when the limbs are paralysed.

Weakness in a limb can also be described as global (when the entire limb is affected), proximal or distal.

In upper motor neurone lesions the weakness preferentially affects the extensors of the arm and flexors of the leg, this is called a pyramidal pattern.

Terminology – sensory

Numbness – loss of sensation
Paraesthesia – tingling
Hyperaesthesia – abnormal increased sensation
Hyperpathia – abnormal pain sensitivity.

- Always define the pattern of weakness or sensory loss – it gives clues to the cause.

A clinical problem – a patient complains of weakness of extension of the right foot. The cause should be evident from the history and examination.

- Is there sensory loss over the dorsum of the foot corresponding to the territory of the common peroneal nerve?
- Is the sensory loss limited to one (or more) dermatome(s)? If this is associated with absence of the ankle jerk, it suggests an S1 radiculopathy.
- Is spontaneous ankle clonus present and is the plantar response extensor indicating a spinal cord or contralateral cerebral disorder?
- Are the clinical features confined to one leg, so that a spinal cord lesion is less likely?
- Does the patient have symptoms in the arm or face on the same side, which would suggest a contralateral brain lesion?
- Was the onset acute – indicating a vascular or traumatic event?
- Was the onset insidious and is the lesion progressive, so that a tumour is possible?

Localization within the brain

When you approach a neurological patient:

- apply your existing knowledge of neurological anatomy to the diagnostic problem
- focus on simple and basic principles
- learn to define where the neurological lesion is by a careful examination and then by drawing conclusions from the abnormal signs that are present or absent (this may be just as important as signs being present).

Remember that generations of doctors made accurate neurological diagnoses on the basis of a clinical examination long before CT or MR scans were available.

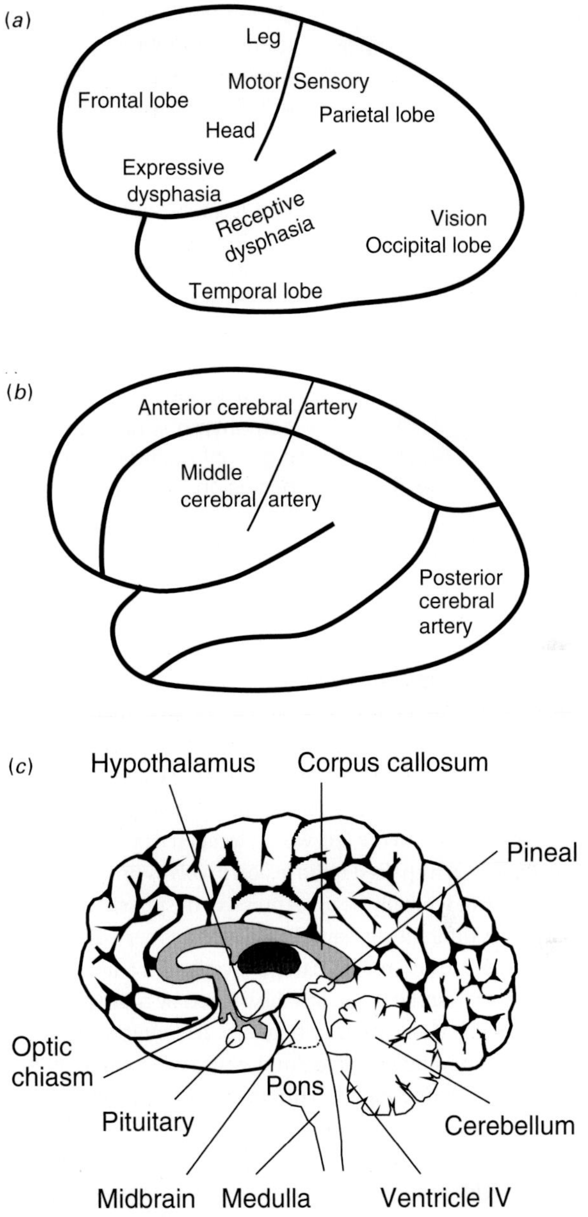

Fig. 86.1. Left cerebral hemisphere to show: (*a*) area representation; (*b*) blood supply; and (*c*) general structure of brain (midline sagittal section).

The frontal lobe

Lesions of the frontal lobe may be relatively 'silent' and there may be few signs, particularly when the anterior portions are involved (Fig. 86.1).

Personality and behaviour

Subtle changes in personality may be seen with impairment of executive functions, or in more extreme cases, there may be disinhibited and inappropriate behaviour, so that, for example, the patient may be unaware or unconcerned about urinary incontinence. A progressive dementia is associated with loss of intellectual drive and thought synthesis. Irritatitive lesions in the frontal lobe cause seizures which can be focal motor, or generalized.

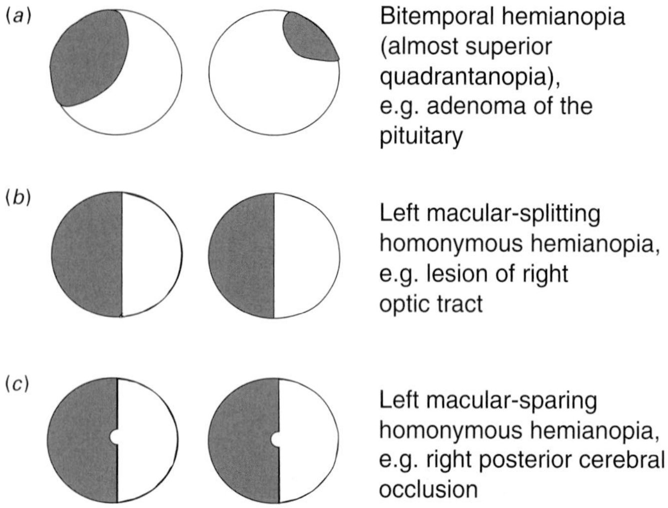
(a)
Bitemporal hemianopia (almost superior quadrantanopia), e.g. adenoma of the pituitary
(b)
Left macular-splitting homonymous hemianopia, e.g. lesion of right optic tract
(c)
Left macular-sparing homonymous hemianopia, e.g. right posterior cerebral occlusion

Fig. 86.2. Visual field defects:

Motor symptoms and speech

Further back in the frontal lobe, a lesion may involve the motor area of the pre-central gyrus. An inferiorly placed lesion such as a stroke or a tumour would cause weakness of the contralateral face or upper limb whereas a lesion higher up closer to the falx would weaken or paralyse the leg. Speech is impaired if the lesion involves Broca's area and this will typically be an expressive dysphasia with particular difficulty in naming objects. It is very difficult to localize a lesion on the basis of dysphasia: a nominal or expressive dysphasia can also be caused by more posteriorly placed lesions. If the patient also has motor, sensory, visual and psychological features, these will help to indicate whether the dysphasia originates from an anterior or more posterior (parietal or temporal) lesion.

Motor signs

Hyper-reflexia is often found on the contralateral side to a frontal lobe lesion and this may be associated with increased tone and an extensor plantar response. Weakness may have a pyramidal distribution, but this pattern is also seen in brain stem and spinal cord disease. Look for a palmomental reflex or grasp reflex on the side opposite the suspected frontal lobe lesion. Where a tumour crosses the midline through the corpus callosum, these signs are bilateral.

The temporal lobe

A lesion of the anterior portion of the temporal lobe, particularly on the non-dominant side, may be relatively silent, but the patient can present with complex partial seizures having periods of loss of awareness (absence), preceded by olfactory hallucinations or déjà vu feelings, and followed by automatic and sometimes bizarre behaviour before recovery. During the episode, there may be smacking of the lips, adversive turning of the head or fumbling with the hands. A lesion on the dominant side not only causes seizures, but also often creates memory dysfunction: there may be impaired speech, classically a dysphasia, which is often of a mixed type, although expressive or receptive components may predominate. If a temporal lobe stroke or tumour involves the inferior fibres of the optic radiation, a superior quadrantic visual field defect results.

The parietal lobe

A large parietal lesion, as in an extensive middle cerebral artery territory infarction or tumour, may give marked hemisensory disturbance which involves all modalities of sensation. More subtle findings include astereognosis (inability to recognize objects such as a coin placed in the hand, when the eyes are closed), dysgraphaesthesia (difficulty in recognizing numbers scratched onto the palm, when the eyes are closed) or impairment of two-point discrimination, which tests the ability to recognize two vs. one prong(s) of an instrument which is allowed to touch the fingers with gaps of a few millimetres between the points).

Sensory inattention may be found contralateral to a parietal lesion, the patient appears to have normal sensation if each side is tested individually, but misses the stimulus to the affected side when simultaneous bilateral stimuli are given. This is often accompanied by visual inattention in which the stimuli are given to the lateral visual fields individually and then simultaneously. In severe cases, a patient may ignore the opposite side of the body (sensory neglect) and be unaware of the deficit (anosognosia). This is usually associated with dense hemiplegia after a stroke.

Visual field defect

Parietal lesions often cause an inferior quadrantic visual field defect due to damage to the upper part of the optic radiation on its way to the occipital lobe.

Visual spatial function

This may be impaired, so that the patient ignores the left side when asked to draw a clock face, house or other simple picture, indicating a non-dominant parietal lesion. Dressing apraxia, an inability to put on clothes normally, is also characteristic of pathology in the non-dominant parietal lobe.

Other features

Dysphasia (speech), dysgraphia (writing), dyslexia (reading), right/left disorientation, dyscalculia (numbers) and dyspraxia (actions) all feature in parietal lobe lesions, particularly when damage arises in the region of the angular gyrus on the dominant side.

Parietal drift

Look for parietal drift, which is a droop of the outstretched arm when a posture is maintained with the eyes closed. This results from a loss of spatial appreciation in a parietal lesion and may sometimes be associated with pseudo-athetotic wriggling movements of the fingers. This should not be confused with a pyramidal drift when the arm is held in an outstretched, but supinated position, and gradually turns over to the pronated position.

Occipital lobe

An infarct or tumour in the occipital lobe will give a contralateral homonymous hemianopia (Fig. 86.2). In bilateral lesions, cortical blindness may be evident. This is sometimes associated with denial and these patients have visual anosognosia. This distressing condition is known as Anton's syndrome. Preservation of the anterior visual pathway and pupillary reactions sometimes causes diagnostic confusion in occipital blindness. Bilateral occipital lesions, which are more limited in their extent, may give a superior or inferior (altitudinous) defect in the upper or lower visual fields (Fig. 86.2).

Thalamus, internal capsule and basal ganglia

Thalamus

The thalamus has a concentration of sensory fibres; a thalamic stroke will therefore cause a dense hemisensory defect in most cases. These patients may later develop the distressing post-thalamic infarction syndrome with intense contralateral hyperpathia and pain.

Internal capsule

There is a similar concentration of corticospinal motor fibres so that a lesion in this area gives a contralateral hemiparesis or hemiplegia. Dysphasia may also occur with lesions of the internal capsule.

Basal ganglia

Acute vascular lesions may cause contralateral involuntary movements of chorea or hemiballismus. Degenerative disorders involving the basal ganglia, such as Huntington's disease, may also cause chorea as well as dementia, but the most classical and common condition is Parkinson's disease where the nigro-striatal pathways are particularly affected and the patient presents with the cardinal symptoms of bradykinesia, rigidity and resting tremor.

Vascular localization in the cerebrum

The cerebral circulation branches into anterior and posterior divisions, supplied via the internal carotid and vertebrobasilar arteries respectively, and connected by the Circle of Willis.

The anterior cerebral branch from the internal carotid supplies the anterior and medial parts of the cerebral hemisphere and small branches also supply the hypothalamus, internal capsule and anterior part of the basal ganglia. A stroke in this territory may preferentially involve the contralateral leg.

The middle cerebral artery supplies the more lateral parts of the cerebral hemisphere so that the patient who has a stroke is likely to have their face and arm affected as well as having sensory loss. Branches of the middle cerebral artery also supply the internal capsule and basal ganglia (Fig. 86.3).

Vertebrobasilar disease may give rise to brainstem signs or, by impairment of the posterior cerebral artery supply, affect the circulation to the occipital lobe, inferior part of the temporal lobe, thalamus or hypothalamus.

When you have evaluated the symptoms and signs in a patient with a stroke, it should be possible in most cases to identify the cerebral artery involved, from this simple guide to the vascular supply of the brain.

The brainstem

The brainstem consists of the midbrain, pons and medulla. It contains descending and ascending long tracts, the origins of the cranial nerves except the olfactory and optic nerves, connections with the cerebellum and important autonomic structures. Thus the brainstem can be regarded as being a very 'busy' area and hence even a small vascular lesion may create a major deficit (Figs. 86.4 and 86.5).

Midbrain lesions

Paralysis of upgaze is the rule in midbrain lesions and there may also be loss of the pupillary constrictor reflex (Parinaud's syndrome).

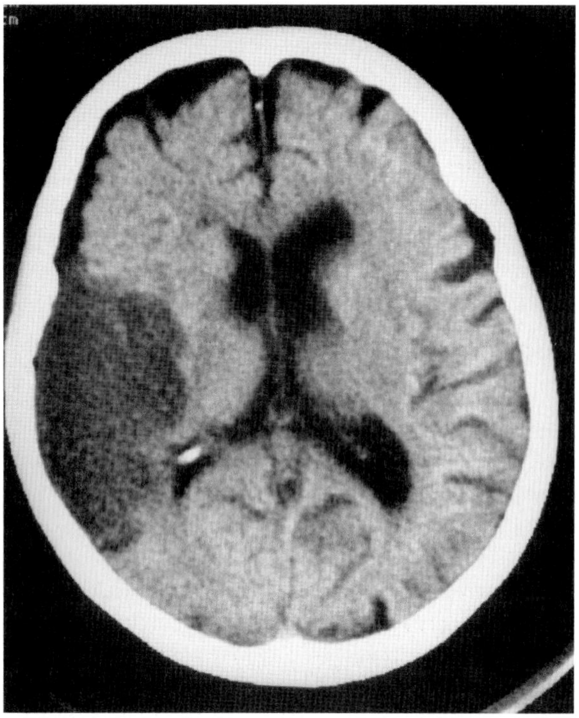

Fig. 86.3. CT scan of brain to show cerebral infarction in right middle cerebral artery territory.

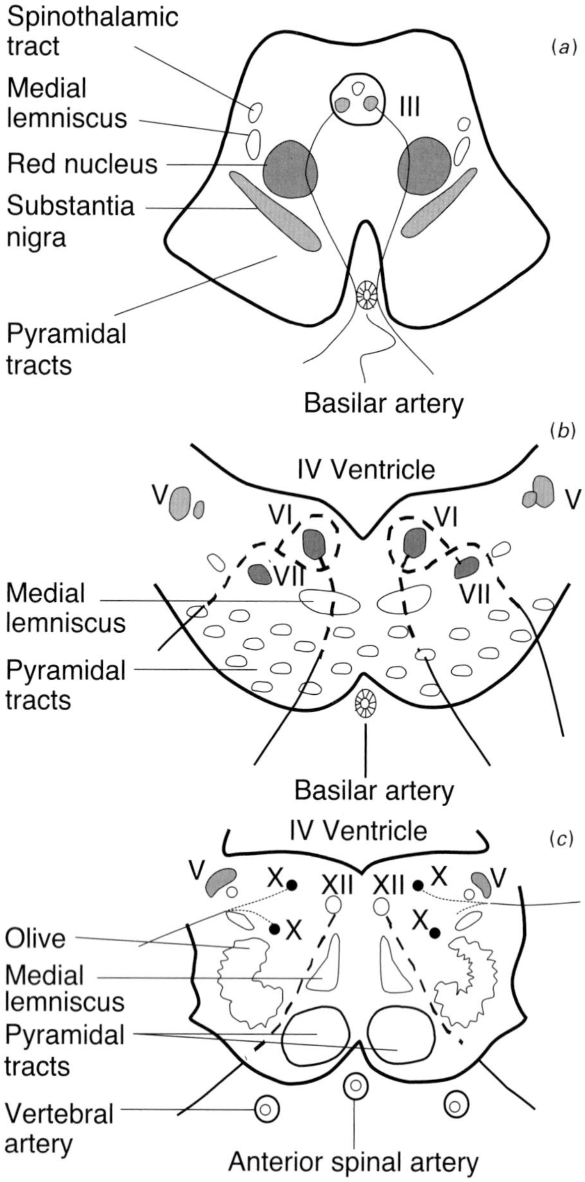

Fig. 86.4. Coronal sections of brainstem at the level of (*a*) mid-brain, (*b*) pons and (*c*) medulla.

Pontine lesions

These commonly cause coma with pinpoint pupils, dysconjugate eye movement, abnormal respiratory pattern, hypertension, tetraparesis and pyrexia. A pontine stroke with these typical characteristics carries a poor prognosis.

Medullary lesions

These often involve the pyramidal tracts and the nuclei of the lower cranial nerves. The lateral medullary syndrome has a characteristic picture of:

- Horner's syndrome
- ipsilateral weakness and incoordination
- contralateral sensory loss in the limbs but ipsilateral in the face
- ipsilateral palatal and tongue paresis
- hoarseness and hiccup.

Bilateral medullary lesions

These are seen in stroke or motor neurone disease and may cause bulbar palsy with impairment of swallowing and speech due to lesions of the tenth and twelfth cranial nerves. More peripheral cranial nerve lesions may also cause bulbar palsy as is seen in poliomyelitis, myasthenia, botulism, organophosphate poisoning and neurotoxic envenoming.

Pseudobulbar palsy

The upper motor neurone supply to the lower cranial nerves is damaged by severe bilateral stroke, motor neurone disease or other diffuse process in the brain stem or cerebral cortex: the patient will also have difficulty with swallowing and speech, although the voice characteristics are different from bulbar palsy and there will usually be spasticity of the tongue, an increased jaw jerk and often emotional lability.

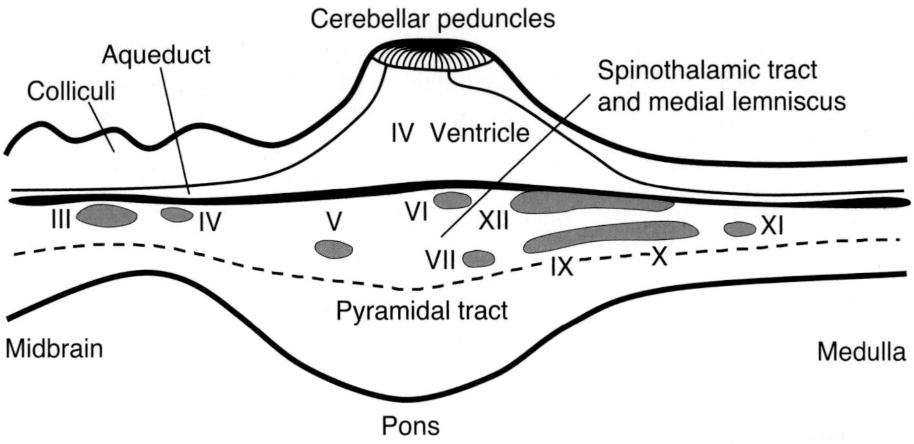

Fig. 86.5. Nuclei of cranial nerves in the brainstem.

Pyramidal lesions

The classical signs of an established pyramidal lesion are those of the upper motor neurone lesion:

- paralysis of voluntary movement
- hypertonia of muscles
- increased tendon reflexes
- extensor plantar response
- absence of muscular wasting; slight wasting may occur as a result of disuse.

The pyramidal tract is a 'long tract' starting from the motor cortex and ending at cranial nerve nuclei in the brain stem, and around anterior horn cells at various levels in the spinal cord. Normally, the site or level of a pyramidal disturbance can be determined with accuracy when there are accompanying neurological signs.

Cortical lesions

The motor area has a wide cortical distribution and so a small lesion in this region may cause only a monoplegia or facial palsy. If there is dysphasia in addition to motor signs, the lesion can be localized in the dominant cerebral hemisphere. Sometimes a superficial cortical lesion causes a flaccid paralysis but this is transient. More often flaccid paralysis is encountered in the early days of a stroke. This is thought to be due to 'cerebral shock', a situation analogous to spinal shock. After a variable period the signs change from flaccidity to typical upper motor neurone features.

Internal capsule, midbrain, pons and medulla

The signs of capsular midbrain, pontine, and medullary lesions involving the corticospinal tract have already been described.

Spinal cord

Pyramidal tract lesions in the cord are discussed below.

Cerebellum

Acute unilateral cerebellar lesions are more likely to produce classical cerebellar signs than chronic lesions in which considerable compensation occurs from the intact side. Pure cerebellar lesions are usually associated with an abnormal posture. Vertigo, if due to a central cause, is the result of disordered cerebellar connections.

The main signs are:

Ataxia

Inco-ordination of the muscles of the limbs leads to:

- a gait which is wide-based, irregular, and staggering even when the eyes are open.
- clumsiness and difficulty in performing rapid alternating repetitive movements of the hands (dysdiadokokinesis).

Intention tremor

Several joints are involved in the act of touching the nose with the finger. In cerebellar disease, synergism is impaired and the movement is consequently broken down into its component parts. The tremor is worse as the finger approaches its target.

Nystagmus

Movement of the eyes is jerky. It is wider and slower when the patient looks to the side of the cerebellar lesion and it has a quick short jerk back. It may also be seen with brainstem lesions.

Dysarthria

This is due to incoordination of muscles of speech and phonation including the diaphragm. The speech is jerky, irregular, and explosive.

Hypotonia

This is usually mild and contributes to the pendular reflexes.

Pendular tendon reflexes

The reflex pattern in cerebellar disorders is often unhelpful but, if the patient sits on the edge of the bed with the knees hanging from the side, there may be a to-and-fro oscillation of the leg following the initial tap of the patellar tendon.

Unilateral cerebellar lesions cause ipsilateral signs of inco-ordination, tremor and clumsiness. Bilateral or midline cerebellar lesions cause gait ataxia and in extreme cases, the patient is unable to sit unsupported. An infarct involving the medial longitudinal fasciculus gives an internuclear ophthalmoplegia, in which there is jerky nystagmus of the abducting eye and failure of adduction of the other eye.

The spinal cord

Lesions in the cervical cord above the fifth spinal segment, i.e. above the brachial plexus outflow, will cause upper motor neurone signs in the limbs. The cranial nerves are not affected.

Cervical spondylosis or upper cervical cord tumour or compression due to a cranial vertebral anomaly commonly cause myelopathy, when there are lower motor neurone signs in the arms, corresponding to the site of the cord lesion, and upper motor neurone signs below the site of the lesion. Typically in spondylotic myelopathy also there are depressed biceps and supinator jerks, and, usually, brisk triceps and finger jerks. A variable degree of sensory loss is found in the arms, and hands, together with a spastic paraparesis. Inversion of the supinator reflex is a common, but not invariable, sign in cervical spondylosis. A cord lesion at the C8–T1 level gives weakness and wasting of the small hand muscles.

Ventilatory failure

Occasionally phrenic nerve paresis occurs in upper cervical cord lesions and, if it is bilateral, respiratory (ventilatory) failure follows. In practice, however, the commonest neurological causes of ventilatory respiratory failure are poliomyelitis, tetanus, and the Guillain–Barré syndrome; myasthenia gravis can also affect respiratory muscles.

Sensory changes

Spinal cord lesions frequently give a mixture of motor and sensory signs. Pain and temperature sensation may be abnormal below a certain level on the trunk due to spinothalamic tract involvement. In a patient with upper motor neurone signs this sensory level must be very carefully defined to localize the level of the lesion. In general, sensory testing is less reliable than motor examination, which demands less co-operation from the patient (Fig. 86.6).

Sensory symptoms and signs result from the damage to sensory fibres illustrated in Fig. 86.7.

Sphincter disturbances or impotence, which are important and common symptoms of a spinal cord lesion, occur late in the disease and may not be readily volunteered by the patient. They imply serious damage to the cord but not necessarily chronicity. If the patient is to be given a chance of reasonable recovery of sphincter function early treatment is essential.

Lower motor neurone lesions

These arise and cause typical signs of a peripheral nerve lesion, whether the anterior horn cell is affected as in poliomyelitis, or the nerve roots are affected within the spinal canal after leaving the cord, for example, in lesions of the cauda equina.

Site of lesion and vertebrae

As the spinal cord is shorter than the vertebral column, the spinal segments do not lie directly under the arches of the numerically similar vertebrae. Since the vertebral spinous processes are useful surgical landmarks it is important to relate the position of a segmental lesion (such as a tumour) to a vertebra if surgical exploration is needed. Only the first four cervical segments correspond to their own vertebrae because there are only seven vertebrae and eight segments. Each of the first six thoracic segments lies two vertebrae higher; seventh to ninth thoracic, three vertebrae higher, while the lumbar and sacral segments lie underneath the last two thoracic and the first lumbar arches.

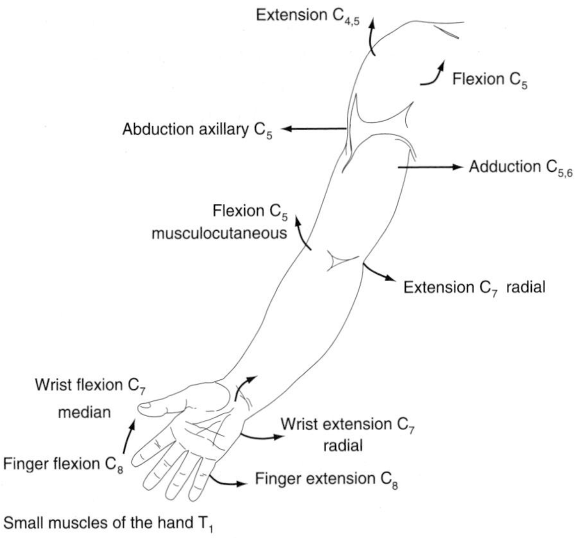

Fig. 86.6. Root values of motor functions of upper limbs.

(*a*)

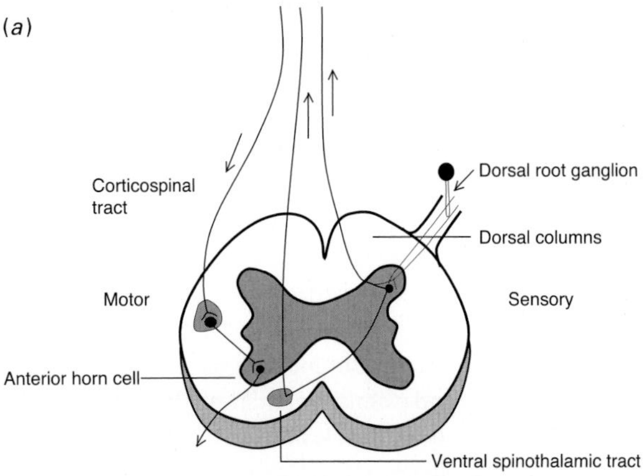

Fig. 86.7. (*a*) (above) The spinal cord and its connections. (*b*) (below) The spinal cord: effects of lesions at different levels.

(*b*)

Lesion	Spinal cord	Tracts affected	Common symptoms	Signs - motor	Signs - sensory
	Right Left		These depend on the speed at which the cord is damaged		
Cervical below C5 Compression : spinal spondylosis, abscess, tumour	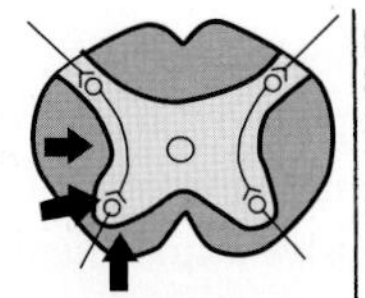	Pyramidal Spinothalamic (pain and temperature) Nerve roots : C7 – T1 (peripheral nerves)	Difficulty in walking Loss of sensation Clumsy weakness of right hand	UMN signs legs (plantars extensor) UMN and LMN signs arms	Loss of sensation below lesion on left side because fibres in right spinothalamic tract have crossed from right to left
Thoracic—acute Transverse myelitis, trauma	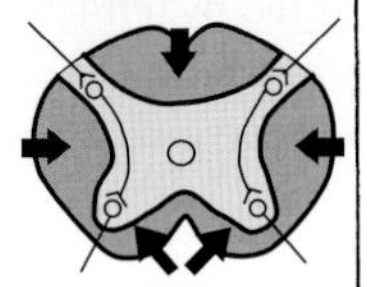		Sudden inability to walk Loss of sensation below lesion Retention of urine	Acute – flaccid paralysis of legs Later – UMN signs legs	Loss of all sensation below lesion
Cauda Equina Compression : trauma, abscess, intervertebral disc	Tumour 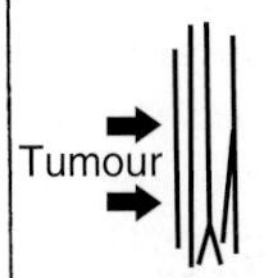	Peripheral nerve roots L2 – S5 (motor and sensory to legs)	Weakness of legs Feet dragged when walking Sciatic pain	LMN signs legs (often a lost ankle jerk) Plantars flexor	Patchy loss of sensation depending on nerves involved (Saddle anaesthesia if lower sacral roots affected)
Posterior columns Compression : trauma, abscess, tumour, rarely tabes dorsalis	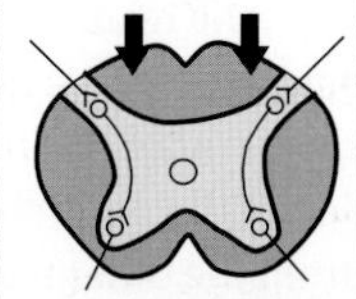	Posterior columns (proprioception, joint position sense, vibration)	Difficulty in walking Loss of balance, particularly at night Lightning pains (tabes)	Absent tendon reflexes and hypotonia if spinal reflex arc is interrupted	Loss of joint position sense vibration sense Romberg's sign positive Argyll Robertson pupil
Intramedullary Tumour : haematomyelia syringomyelia	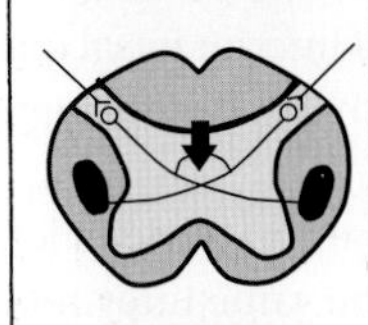	Decussating fibres which ascend in lateral spinothalamic tract (pain and temperature)	Liability to painless burns on hands and feet	(Later – loss of power in muscles, e.g. of hand if lesion involves anterior horn cells of cervical cord)	Dissociated sensory loss : pain and temperature lost below lesion ; touch, joint sense maintained
Anterior horn Poliomyelitis	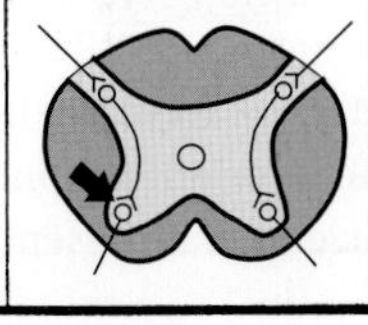	Anterior horn cells (example in lumbar segments r. side)	Acute febrile illness followed by weakness of r. leg	LMN signs in r. leg	None

Defining the level

- If the disease has progressed from arm to ipsilateral leg to contralateral leg and then arm ('clockface march'), this progression suggests a high cervical myelopathy.
- Are there depressed or inverted cervical reflexes with pyramidal signs below? These suggest a midcervical motor level.
- Is there weakness of the arms and legs? This implies a cervical lesion.
- Is there a sensory level or band of pain or dysaesthesia over the trunk? This is typical of a thoracic level.
- Are the ankle reflexes diminished, but with increased knee reflexes and extensor plantar responses? This picture suggests a conus lesion.
- Is there paraparesis, which is often asymmetrical, at least in the early stages? The asymmetry of motor or sensory signs will help to indicate which side of the cord is predominantly affected (pain and temperature sensation reduced in contralateral leg, but pyramidal weakness and posterior column sensation ipsilateral).
- Always examine the thoracic sensory dermatomes to indicate a thoracic sensory level, although the lesion may be above the level detected clinically.
- Is the bladder involved? This is seen at any cord level, but is particularly common as an early feature in conus or cauda equina compression.
- Has the patient had root or localized spinal pains? These are often the first indication of an extradural lesion, due for example to an abscess or a malignant tumour of bone.

The cranial nerves

A cranial nerve may be involved either within the brain and brainstem (central lesion), when other centrally placed structures are also affected, or it may be involved after it has left the brain (peripheral lesion); such lesions are either single or affect more than one nerve. If a cranial nerve lesion is to be accurately localized, a good working knowledge of the anatomical relationships of the nerve throughout its course is necessary.

Olfactory nerve I

Loss of the sense of smell is termed anosmia. Bilateral anosmia is of no localizing value. The commonest causes are:

1. local nasal disease which blocks the air passages, such as inflammation due to a common cold
2. head injuries which sever the fine olfactory filaments as they pass through the cribriform plate of the ethmoid
3. very rarely, a subfrontal tumour may cause unilateral anosmia.

Optic nerve II

Examination of the second cranial nerves is in four parts:
1. assessment of the visual acuity
2. ophthalmoscopic inspection of the ocular fundus and
3. reactions of the pupils
4. testing of the visual fields by simple confrontation perimetry.

The last is important for localizing cerebral disease, because lesions of the various sections of the visual pathway produce characteristic and diagnostic visual field defects.

Visual acuity

The visual acuity is checked at the bedside by asking the patient to read small print or identify other small objects if illiterate. More formally, the acuity is checked with a Snellen chart. Progressive impairment of visual acuity which cannot be corrected by refraction may be due to optic nerve pathology or a lesion of the pituitary gland. Glaucoma is an important cause to consider.

The visual fields

Figure 86.8 shows the anatomy of the visual pathway. The fibres coming from the retina keep the same spatial relationships with each other as do the parent retinal quadrants from which they originate. Thus, in a transverse section of the optic nerve, the relationships are preserved. They are again preserved in the optic tract, except that fibres from the nasal quadrant of one retina have changed places, after decussation at the optic chiasma, with the corresponding fibres from the other retina – the fibres from the superior and inferior nasal quadrants of the left retina exchanging with those of the right retina, respectively.

Within the temporal and parietal lobes, fibres of the radiation maintain the same inter-relationship – superior quadrant fibres being represented in the superior (parietal) lobes while those from the inferior quadrants are represented in the inferior (temporal) lobes. Finally, at the visual cortex level, the representation is preserved.

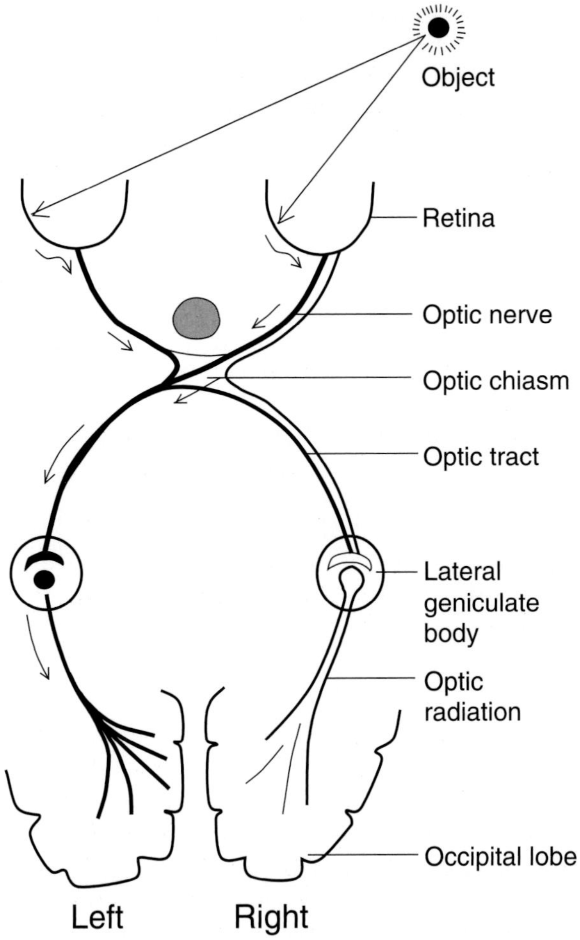

Fig. 86.8. The visual pathway.

Field defects

Some common visual defects resulting from lesions at various levels in the visual pathway are shown in Fig. 86.2.

- Compression of the optic nerve. Commonly an asymmetrical defect is produced.
- Compression of the optic chiasma, producing bitemporal hemianopia. An adenoma of the pituitary would be a common cause.
- Lesion of an optic tract (in this case the right) producing left macula-splitting homonymous hemianopia.
- Posterior cerebral artery occlusion (in this case the right) producing left macula-sparing homonymous hemianopia.

Monocular field defects can only be caused by lesions proximal to the chiasma, i.e. in the optic nerve or retina or by local lesions in the eye itself.

Lesions at, or distal to, the chiasma produce field defects in both eyes: strokes or tumours involving the optic tracts and radiations will cause either a contralateral quadrantanopia or hemianopia depending on whether the temporal, parietal or occipital lobe is affected.

Total blindness in one eye may result from any irreversible optic nerve lesion such as occlusion of the central retinal artery.

The ocular fundus

There is no substitute for regular examination of the normal fundus if any of the major changes are to be recognized.

Raised intracranial pressure

This causes papilloedema: the optic disc is pinker than normal, its margins are blurred, the cup is not seen distinctly and the vessels appear to loop out over its blurred raised margin. The retinal veins are also engorged and broader than normal, and venous pulsation is usually lost. Small haemorrhages are commonly visible on and around the margin of the disc.

The visual acuity is usually normal or minimally reduced until secondary optic atrophy develops, but severe papilloedema in itself may cause visual loss.

Disease of the optic nerve

A patient with acute papillitis complains of blurred vision and has a pink congested nerve head with blurred margins: if the inflammation subsides the disc returns to normal. These changes may simulate those of mild papilloedema. But papilloedema does not usually affect vision whereas acute papillitis or acute optic nerve disease is associated with grossly impaired visual acuity, out of proportion with the apparent 'papilloedema', and direct reaction of the pupils to light is usually impaired.

Acute reversible optic neuritis of unknown but sometimes of viral or demyelinating aetiology is a common cause of such signs. It is usually unilateral but may be bilateral.

Other causes are tropical ataxic neuropathy, arsenical drugs, tobacco and methyl alcohol poisoning. In all these conditions, the optic neuritis is bilateral and the damage is likely to persist and may lead to optic atrophy in some cases.

Optic atrophy

The end result of inflammation of the optic nerve is optic atrophy, where the optic disc is pale and shrunken. Optic atrophy is also caused by long-standing compression of the nerve or optic chiasm, the end stage of untreated glaucoma; and some drugs, neurotoxins, infections and deficiency states also cause optic atrophy.

Disorders of the retinal vessels

The changes of hypertension have already been described. If a patient complains of loss of vision he may have central retinal artery thrombosis or embolism, retinal venous thrombosis, or a large retinal haemorrhage. Retinal venous occlusion has been described as looking 'like a battleground', with unilateral papilloedema, haemorrhages and dilated veins. In retinal arterial thrombosis the retina is pale with narrow empty-looking retinal arteries. Microaneurysms and exudates are common in diabetic retinopathy. Small haemorrhages or exudates, in septicaemia or embolic disease, arise from vascular damage. Retinal haemorrhages are an important sign in cerebral malaria and may be seen in severe folate deficiency or other anaemia.

Choroidal changes

Many disorders may produce choroiditis. In miliary tuberculosis a tubercle may be seen in the choroid: it lies deep to the retinal vessels, whereas an exudate does not and may even displace them laterally.

Oculomotor, trochlear, and abducens nerves III, IV and VI

Anatomy of upper eyelid

- Levator palpebrae superioris: nerve supply – III nerve; function – raises upper eyelid voluntarily.
- Orbicularis oculi: nerve supply – VII nerve; function – closes eye.
- Skin and mucous membrane: nerve supply – ophthalmic division of V nerve; function – common sensation.

Anatomy of pupillary reactions

The dilator pupillae has a sympathetic nerve supply: the sphincter pupillae has a parasympathetic supply via the III nerve. The pathway for the pupillary reflex consists of a sensory limb, a central portion and a motor limb, which are shown in Fig. 86.9.

- *Sensory limb.* The light strikes the retina and the resultant impulse travels through the optic nerve, chiasma, and tract.
- *Central portion.* At the level of the superior colliculus of midbrain the reflex fibres leave the optic tract to descend to the region of the third nerve nucleus (Edinger–Westphal or E–W portion). Some fibres cross the midline to relay with the contralateral E–W nucleus, thus ensuring a pathway for the consensual light reflex.
- *Motor limb.* The motor fibres, originating from the E–W nucleus, travel with the oculomotor nerve and end finally in the sphincter pupillae.

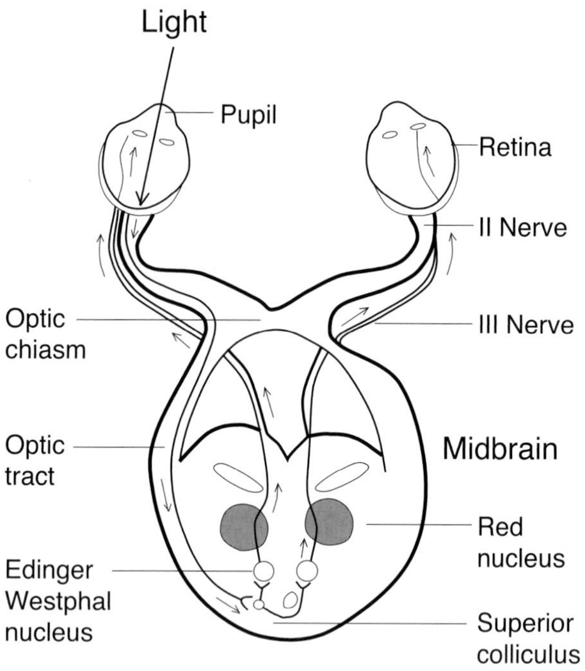

Fig. 86.9. The pupillary reflex.

Two famous abnormalities of the pupillary reflex are the Argyll–Robertson pupil and the Holmes–Adie syndrome. The Argyll–Robertson pupil is small, irregular, and fixed to light, but reacts to accommodation. It is a sign of late (tertiary) syphilis and, more rarely, of other conditions including diabetes mellitus. The Holmes–Adie or tonic pupil is a dilated pupil which reacts slowly but eventually to light, but more rapidly to accommodation. The abnormality is a common explanation for unequal pupils in young women who may also have absent knee jerks and impaired sweating.

Anatomy and actions of external ocular muscles

The external rectus (VI nerve) is a pure abductor, and the internal rectus (III nerve) is a pure adductor in the horizontal plane.

The superior rectus (III nerve) elevates the abducted eye. The inferior oblique (III nerve) elevates the adducted eye, the inferior rectus (III nerve) depresses the abducted eye. The superior oblique (IV nerve) depresses the adducted eye.

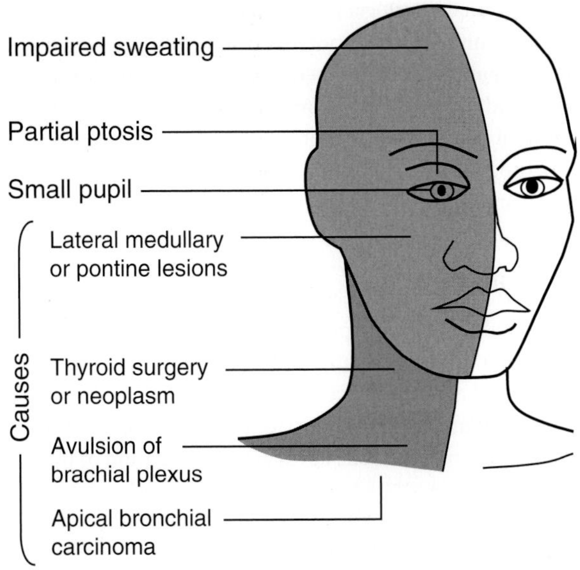

Fig. 86.10. Horner's syndrome as a cause of ptosis.

Clinical signs of III nerve lesions

Ptosis – falling of the upper lid

If complete, and of neurogenic origin, this is always due to third nerve palsy, but partial ptosis may be due to either an incomplete third nerve palsy, or a cervical sympathetic lesion, which leads to Horner's syndrome:

- partial ptosis
- enophthalmos
- constricted pupil and
- diminished sweating (hypohidrosis) of the face on the side of the lesion (Fig. 86.10).

The distinction between ptosis of third nerve and sympathetic origin should be easy if additional signs are sought in the pupils. Partial ptosis makes the patient wrinkle the skin of the forehead in an attempt to raise the upper lid through the VII nerve. Bilateral ptosis may, for example, be due to myasthenia gravis.

Dilated unreactive pupil

It is larger than the other pupil owing to the unopposed action of the sympathetic. It does not react to light because the motor side of the reflex arc is interrupted.

Level of a third nerve lesion

As soon as the palsy is discovered, the site of disease in the course of the nerve must be established.

Midbrain lesions

These were described on pp. 1125–6.

Isolated lesion

If there are no other neurological signs, this is most commonly due to a focal infarction of the third nerve, as in diabetes or hypertension. Where the pupil is dilated, compression of the nerve by an aneurysm of the posterior communicating artery or other lesion is possible.

Cavernous sinus

Lesions here involve the third, fourth, and sixth nerves and may even affect the fifth nerve, especially its upper divisions. Examples are intracavernous carotid aneurysms and cavernous sinus thrombosis.

Incomplete third nerve palsy is often seen due to an intrinsic nerve lesion, such as an infarct, in diabetic arteriosclerotic disease: if the peripherally placed pupillary constrictor fibres are spared, the pupil reaction is not affected. Conversely, the presence of a dilated pupil indicates external compression of the third nerve.

Orbit

Lesions in the orbit tend to cause multiple external ocular palsies.

Trochlear nerve IV

Isolated trochlear nerve palsies are uncommon and are usually due to focal infarction or head injury. The patient will notice diplopia when asked to look inwards and downwards, due to paresis of the superior oblique muscle.

The nerve is more usually involved in lesions affecting the third, sixth and fifth cranial nerves.

Abducens nerve VI

In a sixth nerve lesion, the lateral rectus muscle is paralysed and hence the eye deviates medially. This nerve has a long intracranial course so that an isolated sixth nerve palsy, which is commonly due to increased intracranial pressure, is of little localizing value. The nerve is often transiently affected in pyogenic meningitis, or is trapped in basal meningitis or malignant infiltration at the base of the skull. It can also be affected in diabetes, as is the third nerve.

Trigeminal nerve V

Lesions of the ophthalmic, maxillary, and mandibular divisions of this nerve may cause sensory or reflex abnormalities. Lesions of the mandibular motor component of the V nerve, cause motor disturbances.

Motor–mandibular nerve

The temporalis and masseter muscles on the affected side will be seen and felt to contract less well when the mouth is closed. If opening of the mouth is resisted by the examiner, the jaw will deviate to the affected side due to the unopposed action of the normal pterygoid muscles. In long-standing cases, wasting of the temporalis and the masseter will cause hollowing of the temple and flattening of the angle of the jaw, respectively.

Sensory

There may be blunting of sensation over the face on the affected side, corresponding to the sensory distribution of the three divisions. Lesions within the brain stem or involving the peripheral path of the nerve, may cause sensory loss. If this is associated with deafness, then a tumour in the cerebellopontine angle is suspected.

Corneal reflex

The sensory limb of the corneal reflex is mediated by the ophthalmic division of the V nerve, and the motor limb is mediated by the VII nerve (Fig. 86.11). Normally, the two eyes blink briskly when one cornea is stimulated because the sensory component of the arc relays with the two facial nuclei in the pons. When the sensory limb is damaged, neither eye blinks when the cornea on the affected side is stimulated because the impulse cannot get through. But, if the unaffected side is stimulated, the response is normal and bilateral.

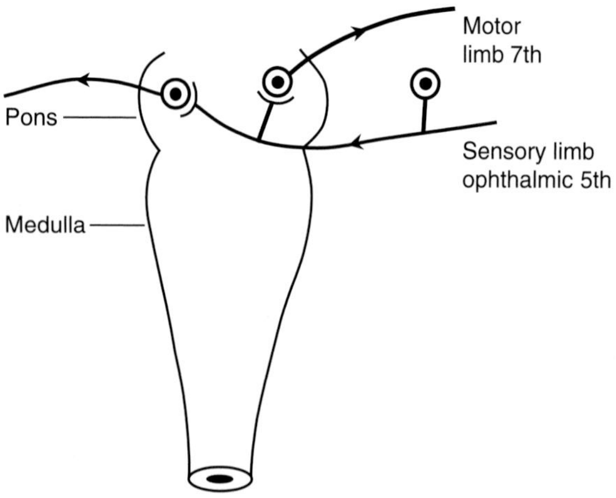

Fig. 86.11. The corneal reflex.

Trigeminal neuralgia is the most common disorder of the trigeminal nerve, is not associated with sensory loss, and is characteristically seen in the elderly who complain of episodic severe pain in one or more branches of the trigeminal nerve, often triggered by chewing, cold wind or touching the face and usually responding to treatment with carbamazepine or phenytoin.

Facial nerve VII

Facial palsy is of two types – upper motor neurone (UMN) and lower motor neurone (LMN). In the former, the muscles of the upper face are relatively spared, especially the orbicularis oculi and the frontalis, as a result of the bilateral (supra-nuclear) cortical representation of this part of the face.

Upper motor neurone facial palsy

The facial nucleus may be thought of as a bilobed nucleus, the upper lobe being responsible for the innervation of the upper face, while the lower lobe represents that of the lower face. Of the two lobes, each receives UMN fibres from the contralateral cerebral cortex. The upper lobe, however, receives additional UMN fibres from the cortex of its own side. A supranuclear lesion at the level of the internal capsule (for example, cerebral infarction) causes a classical hemiplegia with facial palsy on the opposite side, but the upper face is less weak than the lower, since the facial nucleus is still intact and its upper lobe (responsible for the upper face) receives supranuclear fibres from the cerebral cortex on the same side as the lesion (Fig. 86.12).

Lower motor neurone facial palsy

Lesions of the facial nucleus or nerve (LMN; infranuclear) produce facial weakness on the same side. Because the nucleus or its nerve forms the final common path for voluntary movement, both the upper and lower facial muscles are equally weak and the eye hangs open.

If a LMN facial palsy is found, the level of the lesion in the course of the nerve must be defined by looking for additional physical signs.

Pons

Seventh nerve palsy on the affected side may be found with or without contralateral pyramidal signs in the limbs. A tumour, or a stroke, is a possible cause.

Cerebellopontine angle syndrome

If the fifth or eighth or both nerves are affected together with the seventh, then the lesion is at the cerebellopon-

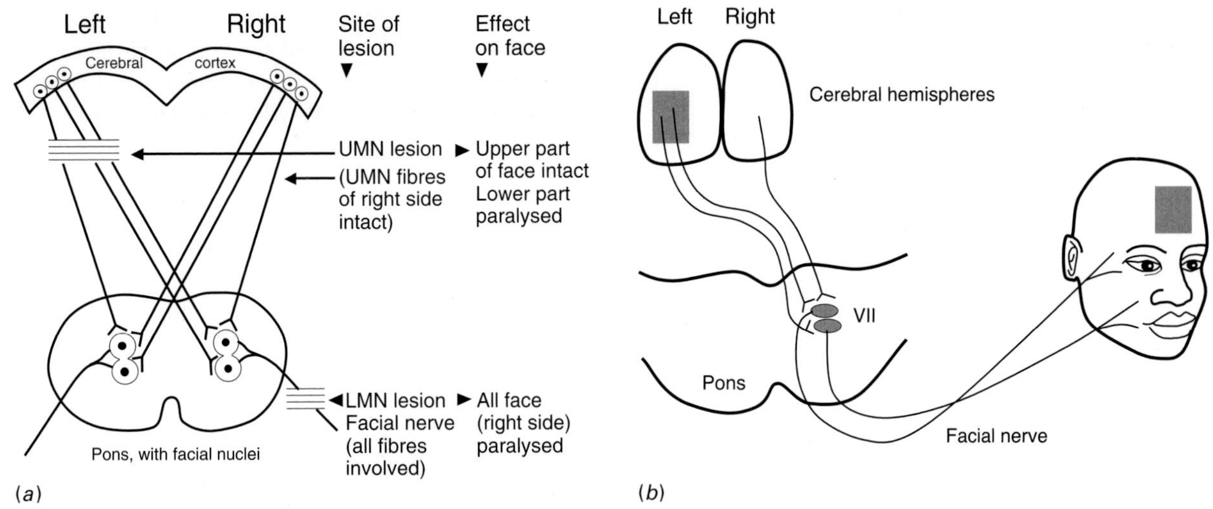

Fig. 86.12. The facial nerve: (*a*) with upper and lower motor neurone lesions and (*b*) with its central connections and cortical representation.

tine angle; the commonest cause is an acoustic neuroma, when the patient notices that he is becoming deaf and later has weakness in his face. The corneal reflex is lost early. Other tumours cause this syndrome, such as meningioma and cholesteatoma and lymphoma.

Facial canal

There are three additional branches of the facial nerve as it passes through the facial canal within the petrous bone:

(i) the greater superficial petrosal nerve to the lachrymal gland
(ii) the nerve to the stapedius muscle
(iii) the chorda tympani carrying taste sensations from the anterior two-thirds of the tongue and also secretor-motor fibres to the salivary glands.

If these branches are affected, a LMN palsy is found together with other signs. Proximal lesions affect hearing, lachrymation, salivation and taste; middle lesions may spare hearing and lachrymation, but not taste, while distal lesions may spare all three branches.

Peripheral lesions

A lesion of the facial nerve at or beyond the stylo-mastoid foramen, where it leaves the skull, causes a LMN palsy without any other neurological signs.

Bell's palsy

A patient without any other symptoms or signs awakes one morning to find his face is misshapen. Most patients think they have had a stroke. A careful neurological examination is essential: there is usually a loss of taste on one side of the tongue due to involvement of the chorda tympani fibres, and there may also be hyperacusis and surprisingly severe occipital pain at the outset due to the sensory branches of the nerve being affected.

It is immensely reassuring for the patient with a Bell's palsy to be informed that the facial weakness has not been caused by a stroke. In most cases, a Bell's palsy will resolve, but there is frequently minor residual weakness or aberrant reinervation leading to synkinesis, in which an intended movement of one part of the face, for example in a smile, may involuntarily cause an ipsilateral wink.

There is no specific treatment except reassurance.

- Cases of acoustic neuroma may be misdiagnosed as Bell's palsy, because signs due to damage of the fifth and eighth cranial nerves were either disregarded or completely missed, with disastrous consequences. Leprosy may also cause facial palsy.

Auditory nerve VIII

The vestibular nerve (from the inner ear) and the cochlear nerve (from the middle ear) join to form the common vestibulocochlear nerve which enters the brain stem at the cerebellopontine angle. Bilateral deafness is of little localizing value, but loss of hearing in one ear is often an invaluable sign.

First, examine the external auditory meatus for wax, and the eardrum for signs of acute or chronic infection. If nothing is found, either middle ear disease (conduction deafness) or a cochlear lesion (perception or nerve deafness) is responsible.

Bone and air conduction

(i) In a normal person, conduction through air is better than through bone.
(ii) In the middle ear disease, conduction through bone is better than through air.
(iii) In nerve deserve, both air and bone conduction are equally depressed but air conduction remains better than bone conduction.

If a tuning fork is made to vibrate and its base is placed on the middle of the forehead (Weber's test), the sound is heard better on the side with middle ear disease. Rinne's test uses the sound of vibrations on the mastoid process (better heard in middle ear disease), compared with those when the fork is held in front of the ear (better heard in nerve deafness.)

Nerve deafness occurring with the fifth and seventh nerve signs has already been described in lesions of the cerebellopontine angle. Nerve deafness is an important sign of the tropical ataxia (p. 1152) syndrome.

Glossopharyngeal, vagus and accessory nerves IX, X and XI

The nuclei of the ninth, tenth and eleventh cranial nerves are so close together within the medulla that isolated nuclear lesions are rare. In bulbar palsy there is dysphagia (pharynx), dysphonia (larynx) and nasal speech and nasal regurgitation of fluids (palate), which patients normally complain of. Direct questions may reveal less severe symptoms, for example how much longer it takes the patient with early bulbar palsy to eat their food.

In practice, we accept the symmetry of palatal contraction as evidence of normal ninth and tenth nerves. Eleventh nerve lesions result in weakness of the sternomastoid and trapezius muscles.

In medullary lesions of these three nerves there may be long tract signs – corticospinal, spinothalamic, and sympathetic. Purely nuclear lesions, like bulbar poliomyelitis, spare the long tracts. Lesions at the level of the jugular foramen involve all three nerves as they leave the skull. The onset and subsequent course will help to indicate whether the patient has had a vascular event, or whether there may be malignant infiltration of the peripheral lower cranial nerves. Neuromuscular junction dysfunction, as in myasthenia, is also possible in such patients. Various eponymous syndromes have been described at this level but are not important.

An isolated accessory nerve palsy is rare, but if present it leads to weakness of the ipsilateral sternomastoid and trapezius muscles, and raises the possibility of a jugular foramen syndrome. Nasopharyngeal carcinoma may present with progressive lower cranial nerve palsies.

Hypoglossal nerve XII

A unilateral hypoglossal palsy causes the protruded tongue to be pushed to the affected side by the normal function of the muscle on the unaffected side. There is usually ipsilateral wasting and fasciculation in the affected half of the tongue. A lesion at the base of the skull or the root of the tongue is suspected. When there is a bilateral hypoglossal palsy, consider more diffuse conditions such as motor neurone disease or neuromuscular disorders.

Neurological investigations

It is essential, before organizing any tests, to carry out a thorough history and examination and establish a differential diagnosis. Neurological tests may not be diagnostic and careful interpretation is needed. Some investigations, such as angiography and lumbar puncture, carry potential risks and these must not outweigh the benefits.

Lumbar puncture

This should be carried out immediately in patients with suspected meningitis or subarachnoid haemorrhage. The only absolute contraindication is local sepsis, when a cisternal puncture may be needed. If papilloedema or focal signs are present a CT scan, if available, should be done, but if this is not possible and meningitis is suspected, a lumbar puncture should still be performed, preferably under cover with intravenous mannitol (1 g per kg as the 20 per cent solution) or dexamethasone (10 mg bolus). Do not do a lumbar puncture in patients with suspected brain tumour or abscess as there is a risk of clinical deterioration from brainstem pressure coning.

Cerebrospinal fluid

Pressure

The normal CSF pressure is 80–200mm of fluid measured at the level of the lumbar theca with the patient lying on their side. There is a free rise and fall on jugular compres-

Table 86.3. CSF in various conditions

	Pressure	Fluid	Polymorphs (per mm^3)	Lymphocytes (per mm^3)	Glucose	Protein (g/l)
Bacterial meningitis	↑↑	Cloudy	10–10000	Post-treatment	↓↓	0.4–10
Viral meningitis	Usually normal	Clear	0	6–1000	Normal	Normal
TB meningitis	↑	Clear Cloudy	0–25	25–500	↓↓	0.4–20
Parasitic or fungal meningitis	↑	Clear Cloudy	Usually 0	0–500 (eosinophils may be present)	Usually low	0.4–1.2
Cerebral abscess (without meningitis)	↑↑	Clear	0–40	Usually 0	Normal	0.4–1.2
Spinal block	↓	Xanthochromic	Raised due to blood in CSF	Not raised	Normal	4–30
Guillain–Barré syndrome	Normal	Clear	0	Not raised	Normal	0.4–3.0
Subarachnoid haemorrhage (12 hours)	↑	Blood stained xanthochromic	Raised due to blood in CSF	Raised due to blood in CSF (1 WBC to every 700 RBCs)	Normal	Elevated due to blood in CSF (1000 RBCs raised protein by 0.01g/l)
Subarachnoid haemorrhage (2 weeks)	Normal or raised	Usually not blood stained. Xanthochromic	0–10	0–100	Normal	0.4–1.2

sion. The pressure is raised in meningitis, subarachnoid haemorrhage and venous sinus thrombosis. It is low in spinal block when the free rise and fall on compression of the jugular vein (Queckenstedt's test) is not seen (Table 86.3).

Cells

The CSF white cell count is raised in any CNS inflammatory disorder. In bacterial meningitis the cells are mainly polymorphonuclear leukocytes while in viral, tuberculous and syphilitic infection they are predominantly lymphocytes. A few days after subarachnoid haemorrhage the white cell count rises as a result of meningeal inflammation, and therefore a greater proportion of white cells is seen in the blood stained CSF. The normal ratio of red blood cells to white blood cells is 700: 1.

Chemistry

Protein

Inflammatory, neoplastic, traumatic, degenerative or metabolic conditions all raise the CSF protein so this is a non-specific change. Very high protein levels are found in spinal block, spinal neurofibroma and in some cases of bacterial and tuberculous meningitis. The CSF in such cases may have a yellow tinge and clot spontaneously. In Guillain–Barré syndrome the protein is often two to three times normal while the cell count is not raised.

Glucose

The CSF glucose level should be more than half of the blood sugar level. It is important therefore to measure blood glucose at the time of CSF examination. A low sugar is typically found in bacterial and tuberculous meningitis, while it is normal in viral meningitis.

Blood stained CSF

Blood staining of the CSF occurs from a traumatic tap or as a result of subarachnoid haemorrhage. The blood staining of a traumatic tap usually diminishes so there is less blood in successive bottles, but this is not always reliable and it is important to centrifuge immediately every blood stained CSF. Six to 12 hours after a subarachnoid haemorrhage enough red cells will have haemolysed to give the supernatant a pink tinge which will not be present if the blood staining is the result of a traumatic tap. Xanthochromia (yellow supernatant) occurs 12 hours after a subarachnoid haemorrhage and may persist for as long as six weeks. It may also be seen

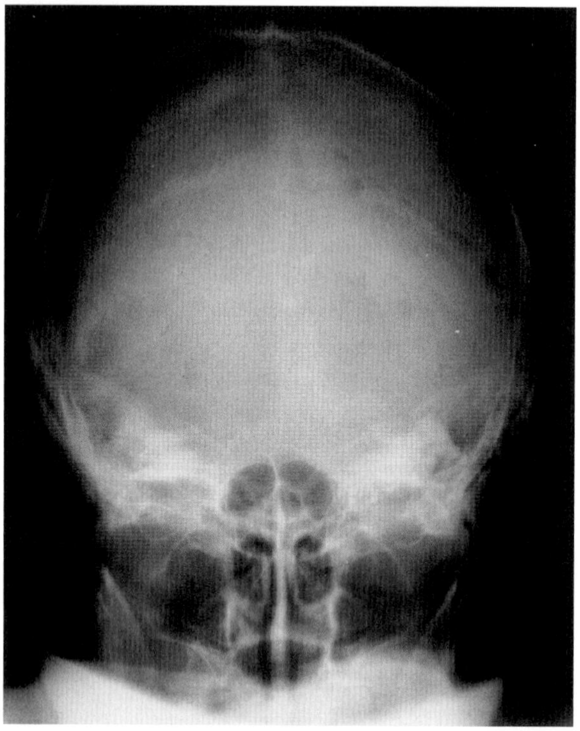

Fig. 86.13. Skull radiograph to show shift of calcified pineal gland and opacified mastoid air cells.

in obstructive jaundice or if the CSF protein is very high.

Radiography

Chest X-ray is helpful in many cases and may show evidence of infection or tumour. Skull X-ray has been largely superseded by the CT scan, but a skull X-ray is still important in the diagnosis of skull fracture. If a CT scan is not available, a skull X-ray may show shift of a calcified pineal indicating a supratentorial space-occupying lesion, evidence of infection such as sinus disease, or raised intracranial pressure which erodes the floor of the pituitary fossa (Fig. 86.13).

Spine

A spine X-ray is needed if there is suspicion of a spinal cord or nerve root syndrome, whether due to tuberculosis of the spine, pyogenic osteomyelitis, metastatic cancer or brucellosis (Fig. 86.14). Normal spinal radiology does not exclude disease.

Myelography

This is being superseded by CT and MR imaging, but is still an important investigation in hospitals where scanning is not available. The presence of spinal cord signs and a sensory level is an indication for myelography or a scan (Fig. 86.15). Myelography is carried out by injection of a water-soluble contrast medium into the subarachnoid space via a lumbar puncture. Flow of contrast up the spinal canal is regulated on a tilt table and the patient is screened during this procedure with X-rays being taken of relevant segments of the spine.

Angiography

This investigation is largely superseded by newer scanning techniques but it is still important for the investigation of subarachnoid haemorrhage. Angiography does not require sophisticated equipment but interpretation of the results can be difficult. Where scanning is not available, angiography can be useful in the diagnosis of subdural haematoma or cerebral tumour by showing the presence of an avascular area or abnormal vascular pattern due to a space-taking effect.

CT and MR Imaging

Computerized tomographic (CT) scanning has revolutionized the investigation of intracranial and to a lesser extent spinal disorders. The technique involves reconstruction of a series of horizontal tomographic images resulting from the passage of X-rays through the body in different directions. Intravenous contrast injection can be given to highlight areas of increased vascularity (Fig. 86.16).

Magnetic resonance (MR) imaging does not depend on X-rays but on the response of protons in a strong magnetic field to the influence of a brief radiofrequency pulse. After the pulse, the protons realign within the magnetic field and the rate of realignment gives information about the physical properties of the tissue. This information can be reconstructed in any plane on a computer. MR scanning gives superior information to CT in most intracranial conditions and, where available, is the investigation of choice in spinal conditions (Fig. 86.17).

Clinical neurophysiology

This comprises electro-encephalography (EEG), evoked potentials, electromyography and nerve conduction studies.

EEG records the spontaneous electrical activity of the brain with recordings taken from electrodes placed on an 8- or 16-channel setting. It is a useful test in the investigation of patients with epilepsy but it is important to remember that the diagnosis of epilepsy is a clinical one. Intracranial lesions may show as focal slow activity while

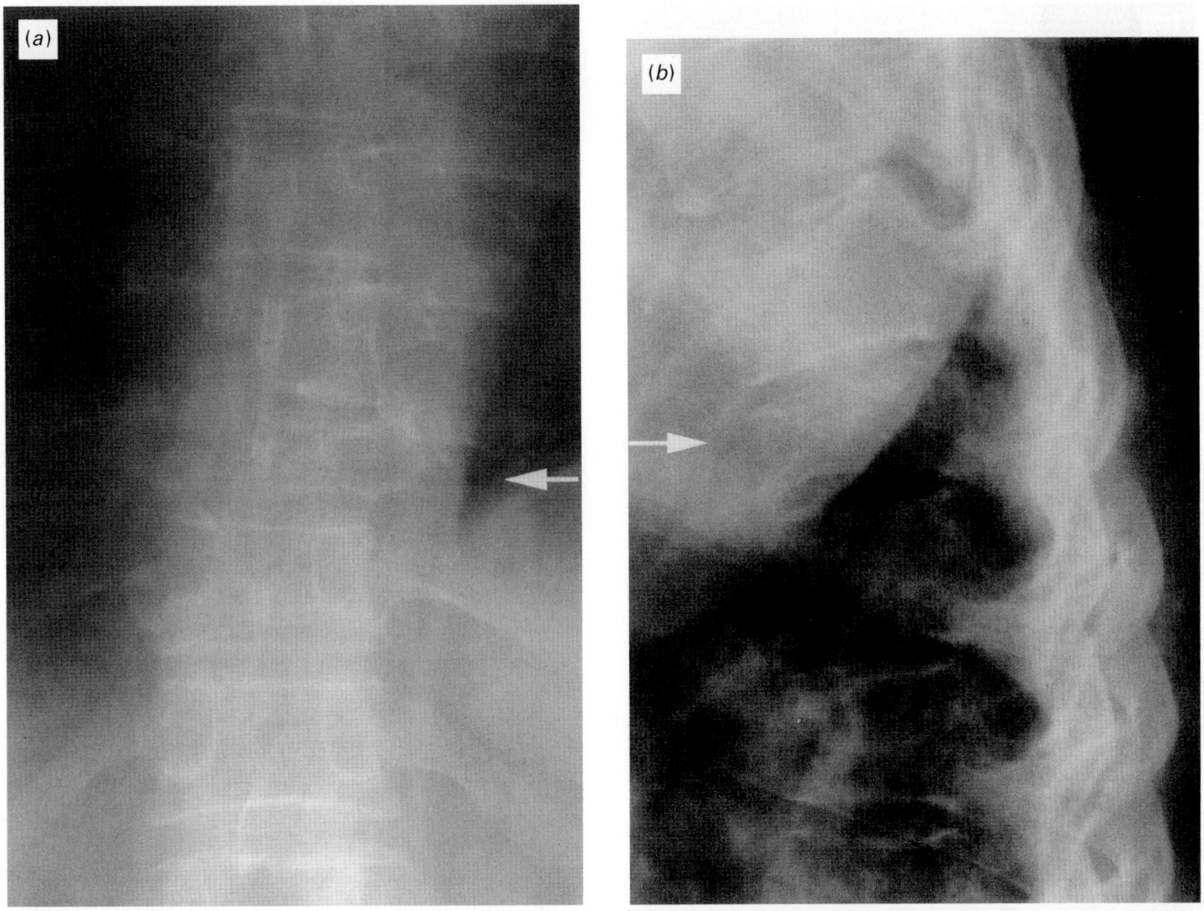

Fig. 86.14. Radiograph of spine to show T10 destruction due to metastatic cancer.

metabolic abnormalities show diffuse slowing of the background rhythm.

Evoked potentials

Visual, brainstem and somatosensory responses rely on sensory stimulation producing electrical signals in the relevant area of the cerebral cortex. This investigation can detect delays in conduction time and may, for example, give evidence of optic nerve dysfunction in patients who are asymptomatic.

Electromyography and nerve conduction studies

These are useful in the investigation of peripheral nerve and muscle disorders. The equipment can be portable and it is therefore possible to carry out this investigation outside hospital.

Electromyography (EMG) involves the insertion of a concentric needle electrode into a muscle to record its electrical activity at rest and on contraction. The main aim is to detect the difference between primary muscle disease (myopathy) and changes secondary to peripheral nerve disorders (denervation).

Nerve conduction studies involve stimulation of the nerve with measurement of the conduction velocity and amplitude of the nerve action potential. Damage to the nerve may be primarily axonal in which case the amplitude is reduced, or demyelinating when the conduction velocity is reduced (Fig. 86.18).

Infections of the nervous system

Infections may involve the nervous system:

- by direct invasion by micro-organisms, resulting in:
  - (i) meningitis with signs of meningeal irritation (headache, neck stiffness and photophobia),
  - (ii) encephalitis (behavioural disturbance, delirium, stupor, fits and focal signs)

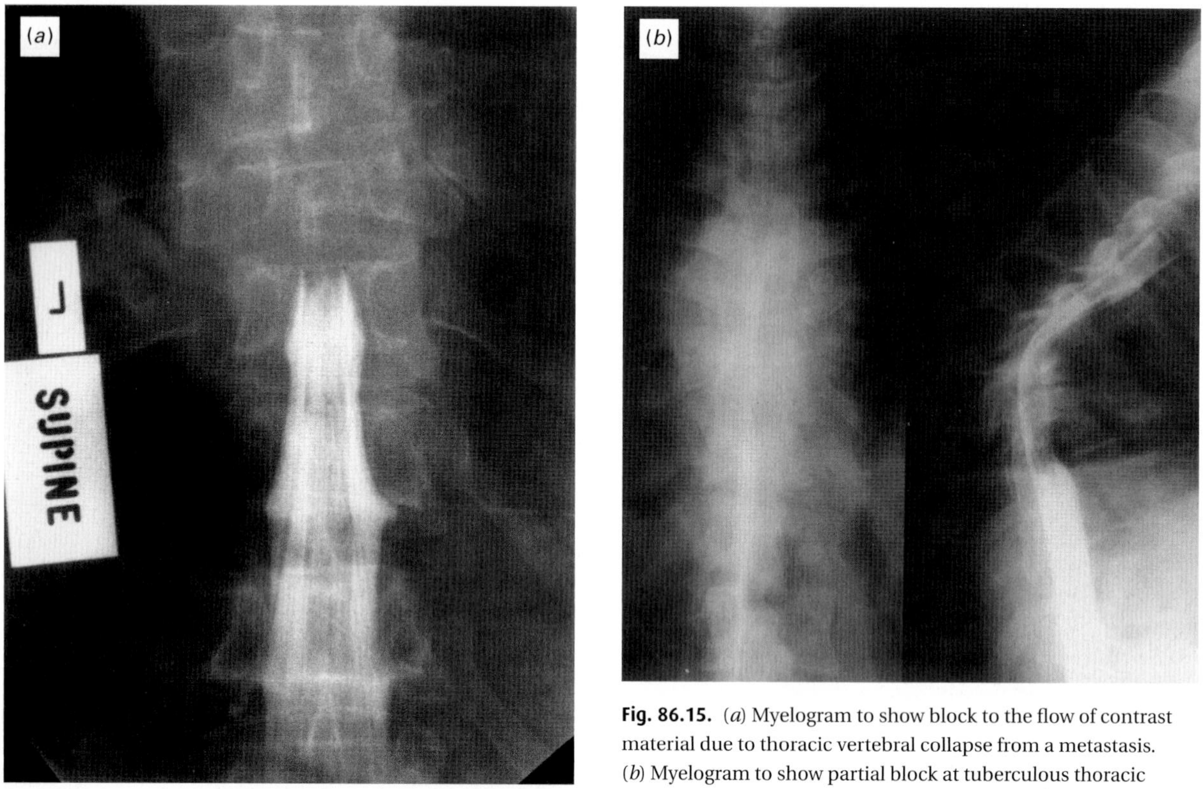

Fig. 86.15. (*a*) Myelogram to show block to the flow of contrast material due to thoracic vertebral collapse from a metastasis. (*b*) Myelogram to show partial block at tuberculous thoracic kyphosis.

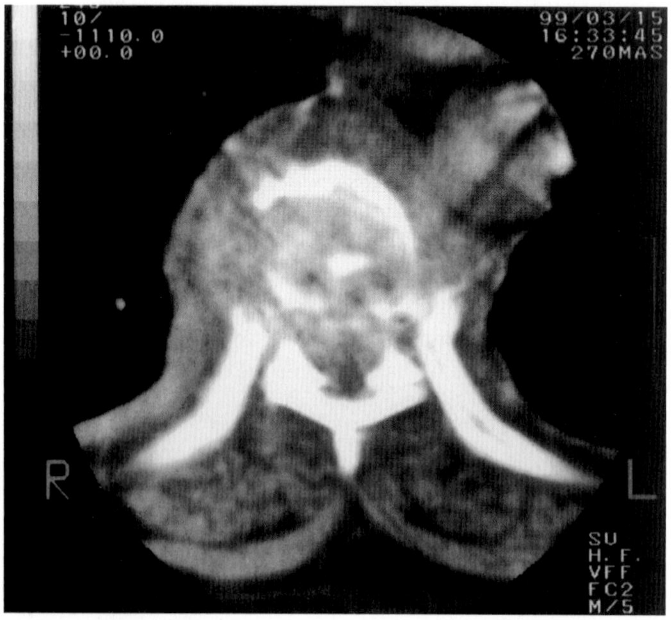

Fig. 86.16. CT scan to show destruction of vertebral body by tuberculosis.

(iii) focal collections of pus (intracerebral abscess and subdural empyema).

- by bacterial toxins, as in diphtheria, tetanus and botulism, or
- as a post-infectious process occurring in the context of a viral illness, for example idiopathic acute disseminated encephalomyelitis and Guillain–Barré syndrome; sub-acute sclerosing panencephalitis following measles; and the post-malaria neurological syndrome; the latter may be mild, with isolated postural tremor or cerebellar ataxia, a diffuse encephalopathy or a severe form with acute confusion, distincitve motor dysphasia, myoclonus, postural tremor and cerebellar ataxia, but responding to corticosteriods (Schnorf et al., 1998).

Infections are usually acute or sub-acute, but may cause chronic, progressive and ultimately fatal disease. In addition, some infections can cause chronic granulomatous inflammation in the brain or spinal cord resulting in epilepsy or cord compression. Bacterial, viral, fungal and parasitic diseases are all common.

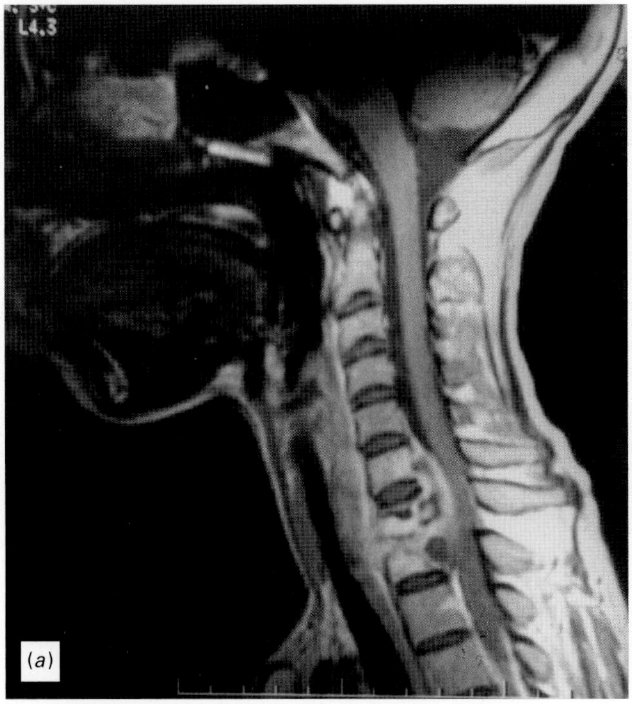

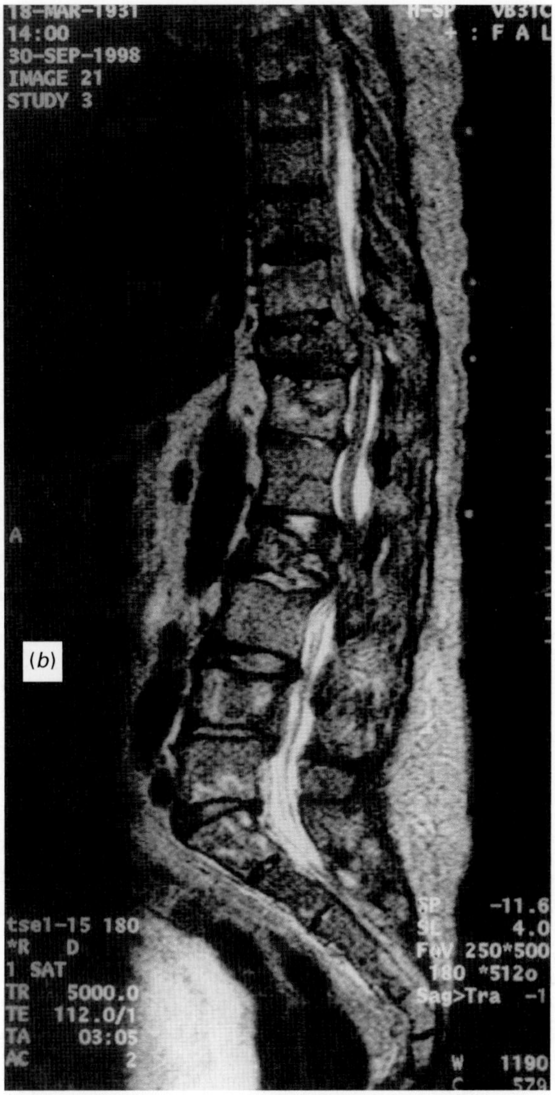

Fig. 86.17. MR imaging of spine to show: (*a*) cervical vertebral destruction with compression of spinal cord due to tuberculosis; (*b*) metastases in thoraco-lumbar vertebrae (T2-weighted technique).

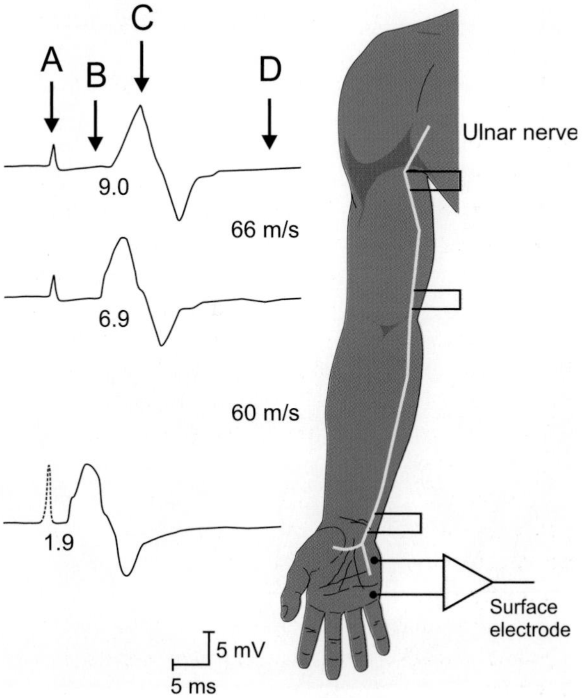

Fig. 86.18. Nerve conduction: sequence of evoked compound muscle action potentials (C) recorded in the hypothenar muscles following stimulation of the ulnar nerve (A=stimulus artefact) at the wrist, elbow and axilla. The latencies to onset of the compound muscle action potentials at each stimulus site are shown (B) together with the calculated conduction velocities (D) in the intervening segments.

Encephalitis

This term implies diffuse inflammation of the brain and describes a clinical state, dominated by disturbed consciousness, often with convulsions and multifocal and sometimes transient neurological signs. The term meningoencephalitis can be used when signs of meningitis and encephalitis occur together.

Causes

Rabies is an important and preventable cause of fatal encephalitis. Encephalitis is associated with pertussis, louse-borne typhus, a variety of viral infections and with the critically important protozoal diseases, cerebral malaria and sleeping sickness. It may also follow yellow fever, rabies and pertussis vaccination. Often, a virus cannot be identified but enterovirus and togavirus (arbovirus) are the most common agents. Other specific virus diseases include herpes simplex, polio, dengue fever, Rift Valley fever as well as Lassa fever, Marburg and Ebola virus disease.

Acute haemorrhagic viral conjunctivitis due to enterovirus EV70 first appeared in West Africa in 1969 and spread to the rest of Africa the following year (Babalola et al., 1990). It occurs in outbreaks, usually in children with an acute haemorrhagic conjunctivitis followed by constitutional features and a polio-like illness. This results in weakness with lower motor neurone features and many patients are left significantly disabled.

The CSF changes depend on the cause, but in viral encephalitis both protein and cells (lymphocytes) are raised and the sugar is normal.

Meningitis

The classical features of bacterial meningitis are fully described in Chapter 16. Remember that meningism (neck stiffness, photophobia and headache) is also seen in subarachnoid haemorrhage. Lumbar puncture can be safely undertaken in patients without focal signs or papilloedema. When these signs are present, a CT scan, if available, should be carried out to exclude a cerebral abscess, but if a CT scan cannot be done and meningitis is suspected then lumbar puncture must be performed with dexamethasone or mannitol cover. If there are signs of herniation (unrousable coma, unilateral or bilateral dilated pupils, abnormal respiratory pattern, abnormal posturing or complete flaccidity) the risk of lumbar puncture outweighs any benefits (Akepede & Ambe, 2000).

In most cases the organism is predicted by gram staining or is cultured from the cerebrospinal fluid (CSF), but sometimes further tests are needed. In viral meningitis, the CSF contains lymphocytes with mildly elevated protein and a normal glucose level. In tuberculous meningitis (TBM) the cell count (usually lymphocytes) and protein are elevated while the CSF glucose is low. Acid-fast bacilli are detected in about 20 per cent of TBM cases by centrifuging 10 to 20 ml of CSF for 30 minutes and preparing a thick smear. Careful examination and X-rays should be undertaken to see if there is any evidence of infection in the teeth, middle ear, mastoid or sinuses. It is important to be aware of less common infections which can cause meningo-encephalitis, but in practice most patients will have pyogenic, tuberculous or cryptococcal disease (Chapter 16).

Parasitic disease

- A schistosomal granuloma may form in the central nervous system and may lead to seizures, focal deficits or spinal cord compression.
- Cysticercosis causes epilepsy in up to 50 per cent of cases of cerebral involvement, and may also present as a space-occupying lesion or as a chronic meningitis (Fig. 86.19).

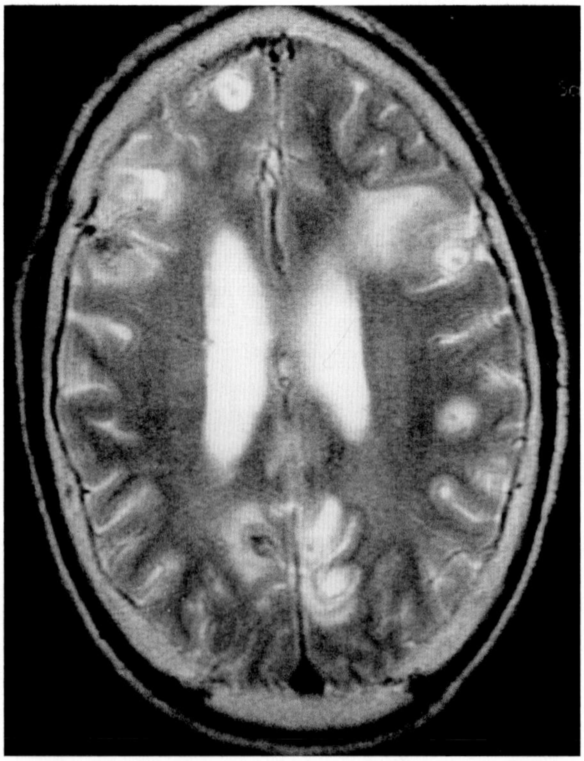

Fig. 86.19. MR brain scan to show foci of neurocysticercosis.

- Hydatid cysts may present as a seizure disorder, as a cerebral space-occupying or rarely a compressive cord lesion. Rupture of a cyst leads to acute meningo-encephalitis.

Cerebral abscess

Pathogenesis

Cerebral abscess develops in an area of suppurative necrosis of the brain parenchyma (Olumide & Adeloye, 1981).

Immuno-suppression predisposes to abscess formation. Most brain abscesses are the result of spread of infection from adjacent areas such as the middle ear, mastoid and sinuses (Samuel et al., 1986). A third of cases are due to metastatic spread, often from the lungs as a result of bronchiectasis or lung abscess. Other sources include the teeth, intra-abdominal or pelvic sepsis, osteomyelitis or infective endocarditis. Penetrating head trauma can result in an abscess. Surprisingly cerebral abscess is unusual in acute meningitis.

Clinical features

A history of less than a month with fever, focal cerebral signs and raised intracranial pressure (headache and papilloedema). Look for evidence of middle ear and dental disease, sinusitis and other potential sources of infection, for example in the chest. Two-thirds of patients have a peripheral blood neutrophil leukocytosis but blood culture is only positive in 10 to 20 per cent. A skull X-ray may show pineal shift, skull fracture or evidence of osteomyelitis or sinusitis. The characteristic CT scan appearance following contrast administration is of a ring-enchancing lesion (Fig. 86.20).

- Do not do a lumbar puncture if you suspect a cerebral abscess as there is a 30 per cent risk of deterioration after it. If the CSF is examined inadvertently, it shows a raised protein and cell count with negative culture.

Organisms responsible

It is usually possible to predict the organism responsible for the abscess when the source of the infection is defined. Frontal abscess is secondary to frontal sinusitis and usually due to *Streptococcus milleri* infection. Temporal lobe abscess secondary to chronic otitis media – aerobic or anaerobic streptococci such as *Bacteroides fragilis*: pulmonary sepsis – actinomycosis and anaerobic streptococci: dog bite – *Pasturella multicoda. Streptococcus viridans* is the most common pathogen.

Treatment

Initially, antibiotics which cover anaerobic organisms, either penicillin plus metronidazole, or chloramphenicol in the doses used to treat meningitis (Chapter 16) and continued for at least 8 weeks.

Surgical treatment is required for any adjacent infection in the middle ear or sinuses, or for drainage of a cerebral abscess.

Subdural empyema

This is usually associated with otitis media, sinusitis or trauma (Glasauer et al., 1978; Nathoo et al., 1999). In children under 3 years, it may occur as a complication of meningitis. Headache, fever and focal cerebral signs develop rapidly in a patient with sinus or middle ear disease. Treatment consists of multiple burr holes, surgical drainage of the underlying infection and 8 weeks of antibiotic treatment.

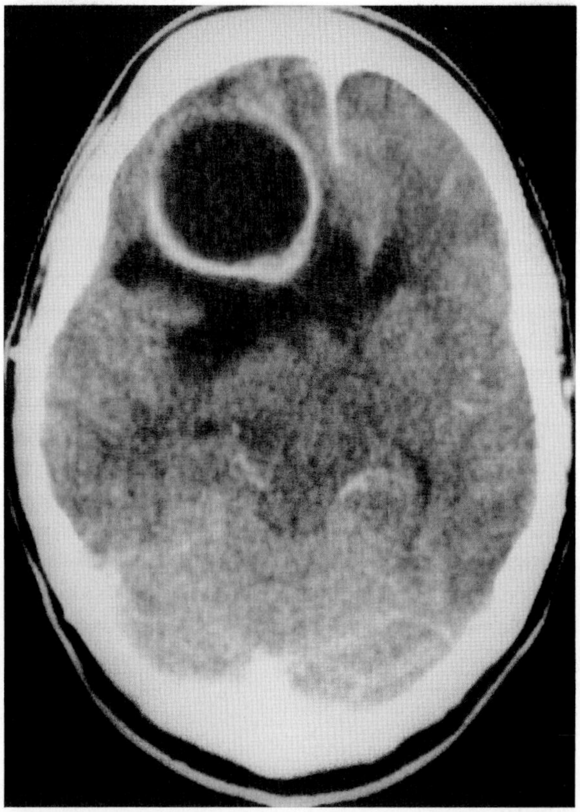

Fig. 86.20. CT brain scan to show right frontal abscess with surrounding oedema and mid-line shift.

Spinal epidural abscess

A spinal epidural abscess presents as a painful acute or sub-acute cord syndrome. One-third of cases are the result of direct spread, one-third from haematogenous spread and the cause is unknown in the rest. Acute epidural abscess is usually caused by *Staphylococcus aureus* but a chronic abscess may be caused by *Mycobacterium tuberculosis*, fungi, syphilis, hydatid disease or guinea worm. The diagnosis of cord compression is made by myelography or a scan. Treatment is surgical decompression and antibiotics.

Brain tumours

The problem in Africa

The increased availability of CT scans has led to a greater understanding of the epidemiology of brain tumours in Africa (Ohaegbulam et al., 1980; Jialal et al., 1986; Abu-Salih & Abdul-Rahman, 1988; Olasode et al., 2000). There is some evidence that meningioma and pituitary tumour are more common in Africa whilst acoustic Schwannoma is rare. Surprisingly, primary cerebral lymphoma appears relatively uncommon despite the high prevalence of HIV infection with which it is associated (Table 86.4).

Table 86.4. Types of cerebral tumour

Metastatic	25 per cent
Meningioma	15–33 per cent
Glioma	20–50 per cent
Lymphoma (including Burkitt's lymphoma)	Uncommon
Pituitary tumour	20 per cent
Craniopharyngioma	Uncommon
Acoustic schwannoma	Uncommon

Source: Percentages amalgamated from Levy and Auchterlonie (1975), Ohaegbulam et al. (1980) and Olasode et al. (2000).

Clinical features

Symptoms begin gradually in most patients but posterior fossa tumours may present sub-acutely when hydrocephalus results from ventricular obstruction. Symptoms are caused by the local effects of the tumour, for example, focal epilepsy, which is common, or the generalized features of headache and vomiting (Figs. 86.21(*a*), (*b*) and (*c*).

Signs will depend on the site of the tumour. A progressive hemiparesis or hemisensory loss is seen in supratentorial tumours. Brainstem signs will develop in posterior fossa lesions. Papilloedema is found in advanced cases where there is mass effect or obstruction of the CSF pathways.

Clinical signs in brain tumour

• Generalized symptoms and signs	Headaches, altered mental status, seizures, papilloedema
• Localizing symptoms and signs	Hemiparesis, visual field defects, deafness, ataxia, hemisensory loss, cranial nerve palsies
• False localizing signs	Sixth nerve palsy

Management

Patients with suspected brain tumours should ideally have a brain scan. Do not do a lumbar puncture. If there is any delay, give steroids, preferably dexamethasone, to reduce oedema and improve symptoms, start with 4 mg four times daily. Always refer patients with suspected brain tumour to a specialist unit, if possible.

Spinal cord disorders

These are disastrous for a working man or woman, or for the education of a child. Some, for example acute spinal trauma or nutritional spinal disease, can be prevented and others, like spinal cord compression or infections, can be effectively treated. The thorough clinician, who takes a good history and makes a careful examination, should be able to identify the nature and cause in most patients and hence decide whether a potentially treatable case should be further evaluated.

In practice in Africa, lesions of the spinal cord are usually due to trauma, spinal infections or a tumour.

Defining the lesion – in time

Spinal cord disorders are:

1. acute – minutes: trauma or vascular occlusion
2. sub-acute – $<$24 h: epidural abscess, transverse myelitis, secondary cancer, intoxication (lathyrism or konzo
3. chronic – weeks: tuberculosis of spine, spinal osteoarthritis.

In examination

The first question, when confronted with a possible spinal cord problem in a patient with weak or paralysed legs, is to confirm that the spinal cord is indeed the site of the pathology.

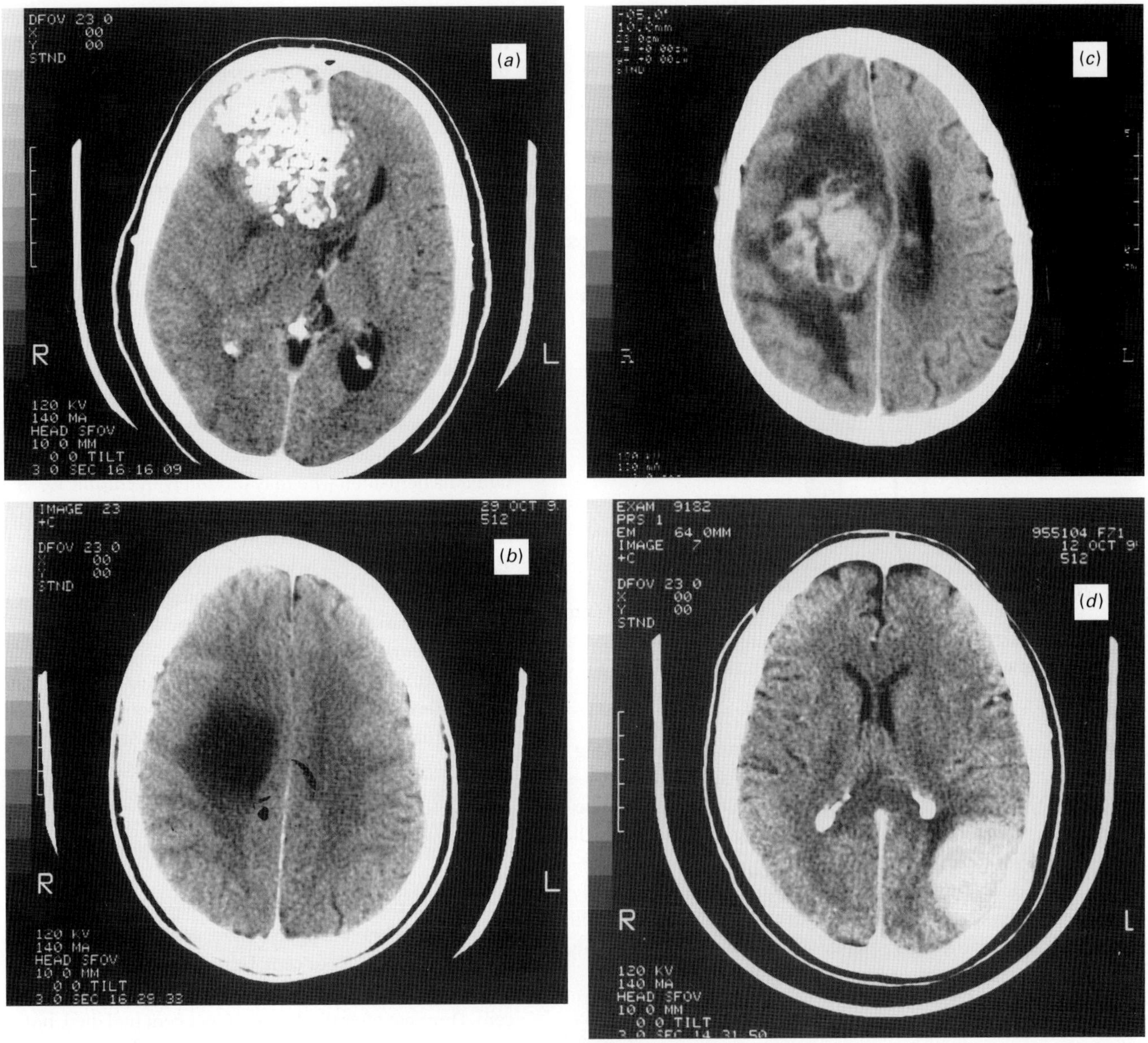

Fig. 86.21. Cerebral tumours. (*a*) CT scan to show calcified right frontal oligodendroglioma: the patient presented with epilepsy and personality change; (*b*) and (*c*) CT scans to show the course of a right parietal glioma in a patient who presented with seizures, was treated with anti-convulsants and, 8 years later, the glioma dedifferentiated and the patient presented with symptoms and signs of raised intracranial pressure; (*d*) CT scan to show left parietal convexity meningioma: the patient presented with right-sided sensory seizures.

The patient may have a lesion of the:

(i) parasagittal area
(ii) brainstem
(iii) spinal cord
(iv) cauda equina (LMN lesion – flaccid legs)
(v) peripheral nerves (LMN lesion)
(vi) muscle.

Note, although the first three lesions cause UMN paralysis with its characteristic pyramidal tract signs (hyperreflexia, clonus, extensor plantar responses, spasticity), there may be a flaccid paralysis in the early stage of spinal shock after injury, or in those with a bad prognosis.

In position

Spinal cord lesions are extradural or intradural.

(i) Intradural – intramedullary, within the cord itself, when root pains are absent, there may be dissociated

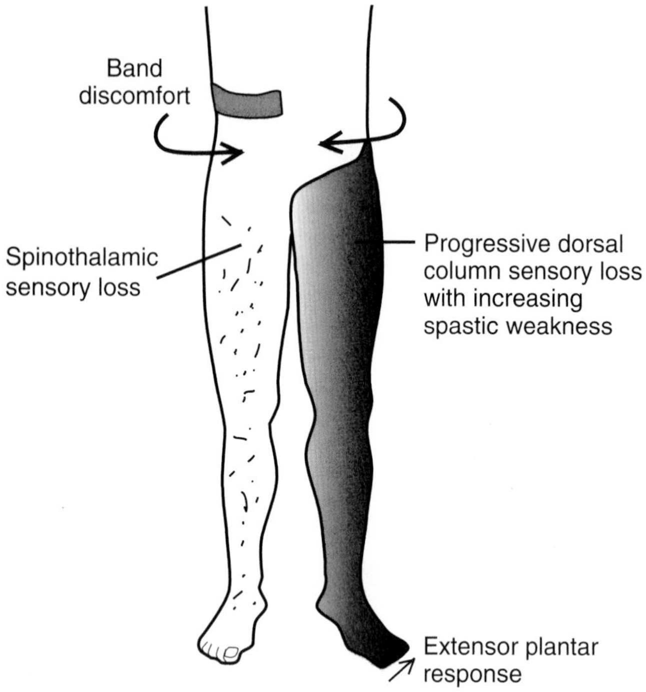

Fig. 86.22. Left lower thoracic spinal cord compression: early symptoms and asymmetrical (dissociated) signs.

sensory loss, sparing of sacral sensation, or sparing of posterior column sensation (if anterior).
– extramedullary: root pains start early, usually due to a tumour related to a posterior nerve root, which produces early pain and then spinal block.

(ii) Extradural – root pains are prominent: local spinal disease, due to infection or tumour is common, with tenderness on percussion – percuss the spine gently: spinal block occurs later (Fig. 86.22).

In its level

(see defining the level – p. 1128–1130)

Investigations

Plain radiographs

Look for vertebral collapse from tuberculosis, metastatic cancer and the effects of spinal trauma. Remember that a man who has the radiological findings of degenerative arthritis in the neck, may have another cause for his spastic paraparesis.

Scanning

The ideal investigation for spinal cord disease is MR scanning.

Myelography

Radiographic dye is injected in a lumbar interspace and is then run up and down the spinal canal to identify the anatomical location of the compression of the cord in the cervical, thoracic or lumbar region.

Causes of spinal cord disease (Table 86.5)

Trauma

Road traffic accidents leading to traumatic paraplegia are the most common non-infective cause of spinal cord damage.

Infections

HIV myelopathy and tuberculous spinal disease account for the majority of non-traumatic cases of spinal cord disease. Brucellosis of the lumbar spine is important in nomadic herdsmen who may present with chronic lower backache. Schistosomal granuloma is a common cause of conus/cauda equina lesions in endemic zones (Chapter 25). Multiple sclerosis, which is so common in temperate zones, is virtually unknown in the indigenous populations of sub-Saharan Africa for reasons associated with genetic and environmental risk (Poser, 1996).

Non-traumatic paraparesis accounted for 18 per cent of all neurological symptoms in patients among 130 paraparetic or quadriparetic admissions in Addis Ababa (Zenebe, 1995). Twenty seven per cent had tuberculous spondylitis and 17 per cent had HIV myelopathy. Metastatic cord compression, tropical spastic paraparesis, cervical spondylosis, primary cord tumours and transverse myelitis were 'not uncommon'. The mortality rate was 11 per cent. In 159 cases of non-traumatic paraplegia in Zimbabwe (Parry et al., 1999) the figures were: neoplasms (only one-third metastatic) 28 per cent; tuberculosis 27 per cent; and transverse myelopathy of unknown aetiology 11 per cent. One year after discharge, 18 per cent had died, but many more were lost to follow-up.

Cervical spondylotic radiculomyelopathy

It is surprising that this is not common as it is postulated that heavy manual work and trauma are implicated in the development of spondylotic compression of the spinal cord and nerve roots.

Clinical features

Cervical cord compression may require surgical decompression. Much more commonly, patients may present with painful cervical radiculopathy which affects the arm and hand. The condition usually settles, helped by rest and by traction or other physical therapy, if available.

Table 86.5. Causes of spinal cord disease

Category	Onset[a]	Pathology	Investigation[b]	Treatment
Trauma	a/sac	*Fracture, dislocation*	XR	Reduction; immobilization
Infective	a	Pyogenic abscess	Myelogram	Surgery; antibiotics
	a	*Viral myelitis, e.g. HIV*	CSF	Steroids
	sac/chronic	*Tuberculosis of spine*	XR; CSF	Anti-TB chemotherapy
	sac/chronic	Other chronic infection	XR; CSF	Appropriate chemotherapy; penicillin for syphilis
	sac/chronic	Schistosomiasis	Myelogram	Praziquantel, steroids
Nutritional	sac/chronic	*Lathyrism, Konzo*	None	Symptomatic
		B_{12} deficiency[c]	B_{12} level	B_{12} injection
Neoplastic	sac/chronic	*Metastatic, (lung, breast, prostate, Burkitt's lymphoma, myeloma)* meningioma, neurofibroma, intramedullary glioma, ependymoma	XR; myelogram	Surgery; radiotherapy plus steroids in metastatic disease
Degenerative	chronic	Spondylosis	Myelogram	Surgery
	chronic	Motor neurone disease	EMG	Symptomatic
Congenital	chronic	Syringomyelia	Myelography	Surgery
Inflammatory	a/sac/chronic	Multiple sclerosis[c] transverse myelitis	CSF	Steroids
Vascular	a	ant.spinal.a. occlusion	none	Symptomatic
		Haematomyelia	CSF	? Surgery
Undiagnosed	a/sac/chronic	Not determined	–	Symptomatic

Notes:
[a] acute (a), subacute (sac) or chronic onset.
[b] assumes MR scanning is unavailable.
[c] virtually unknown in Africa.
Conditions especially common or important in Africa in *italics*.

Thoracic cord disc protrusion is less frequently seen; these patients will have a variable paraparesis with a thoracic sensory level.

Lumbar focal disc protrusion produces the well known features of sharp sciatic pain, down the back of the leg and in the buttock, with loss of sensation usually in the L5 or S1 dermatome, a depressed ankle reflex and sometimes weakness of the foot. Do not confuse this with the much more common mechanical low back pain: this does not have focal signs, is due to facet arthropathy, and responds to active mobilization, whereas rest is the primary treatment for a disc protrusion.

HTLV-1

The human T-cell lymphotropic virus type 1 (HTLV-1) causes a subacute painful spastic paraparesis and is endemic in central, western and southern areas of Africa. This condition may be the cause of some patients with 'unexplained' myelopathy in whom serological testing is unavailable. The condition usually affects adults, more commonly females, and is transmitted sexually, by breast-feeding or via blood products. There is no effective treatment (Vernant, 1996).

Nutritional myelopathies

Myelopathy is a relatively rare feature of nutritional disorders, compared with the much more prevalent nutritional neuropathies. An exception is vitamin B_{12} deficiency, which leads to the classical condition of subacute combined degeneration of the cord. Most physicians in Africa say that they never see pernicious anaemia, but there is some evidence that it is more prevalent than is appreciated (Akinyanju & Okany, 1992). More important are the epidemic parapareses, which follow famine when populations

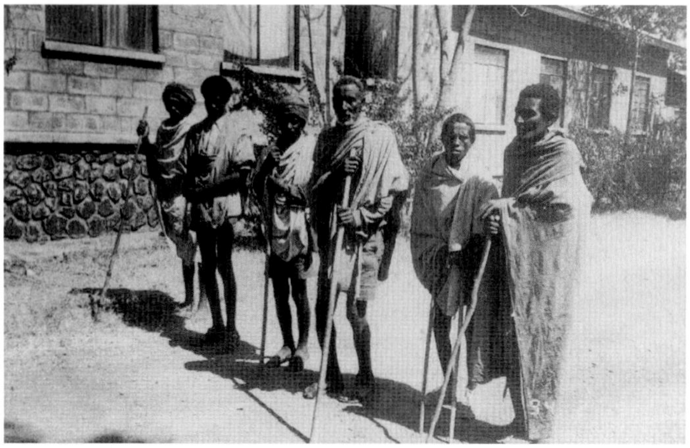

Fig. 86.23. Ethiopian farmers disabled by lathyrism. (By courtesy of Dr. Redda Tekla-Haimanot.)

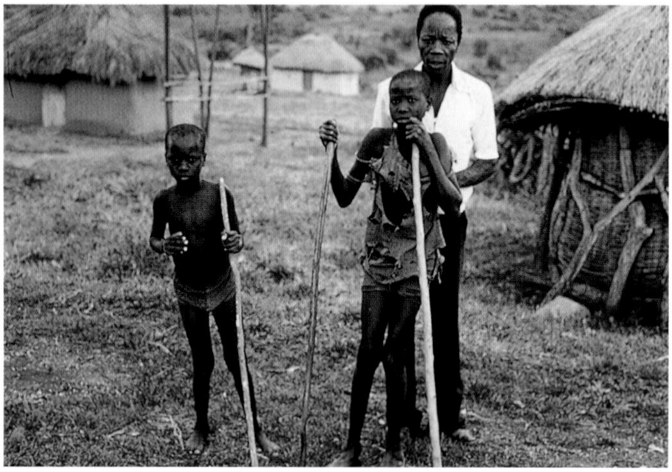

Fig. 86.24. Cassava contains linamarin from which cyanide is formed, which needs -SH groups for detoxification.

turn to chickpea cultivation and consumption (neurolathyrism), or are due to inadequate processing of cassava (konzo).

Neurolathyrism

Lathyrism is an ancient disease. Hippocrates wrote 'all men and women who ate peas continuously became impotent in the legs and that state persisted'.

Pathogenesis

The chickling pea *Lathyrus sativus*, which is a hardy legume, contains a neurotoxic amino acid, beta-*N*-oxalyl-amino-L-alanine (BOAA), which causes axonal degeneration in the pyramidal tracts of the spinal cord.

Epidemiology and prevalence

Lathyrism can be prevented by providing emergency food assistance during times of famine and by educating people that toxicity of the pea can be reduced by soaking or boiling and then discarding the excess water. Epidemics of neurolathyrism have been reported from Ethiopia in 1976–77 and again following the drought of 1995–96 when 2000 patients were identified, most of whom were under 40 years of age, 32 per cent were female and 18 per cent had the most severe crawler stage of the disease (Getahun et al., 1999). Low toxicity seed strains of *Lathyrus sativus* are being sought.

Clinical features

There is a sudden or insidious onset of spastic paraparesis, which, in severe cases, produces immobility and contractures. Men are more often affected, possibly because women eat less in order to save food for their husbands.

Treatment

There is no specific treatment: active rehabilitation is fundamental.

Prognosis

The paraparesis is irreversible (Fig. 86.23).

Konzo (see Chapter 2)

This is a Yaka word meaning 'tied legs' which effectively describes the spastic gait seen in this condition. Konzo mainly affects women and children. Epidemics of this abrupt onset paraparesis are reported from the Central African Republic, Zaire, Tanzania and Mozambique. Up to 40 per cent of cases have a residual moderate to severe disability after the acute development of weakness in the legs, and these patients have spasticity, hyper-reflexia, extensor plantar responses and pyramidal weakness. The cyanide hypothesis of konzo is based on the observations that inadequate preparation of cassava releases cyanogenic activity, which is eventually neurotoxic (Fig. 86.24).

A direct cyanide effect is not plausible, but consequent deranged metabolism creates an over-excitation of upper motor neurones and irreversible damage. A diet deficient in sulphur-containing amino acids provides inadequate sulphydryl groups to detoxify cyanide. Urinary thiocyanate levels are high in cases and affected communities. Prevention of konzo is possible if the cassava root is grated or allowed to ferment to bring linamarin in contact with endogenous glucosidase to break it down to glucose and acetone cyanohydrin, in turn converted by drying or heating to hydrogen cyanide which will evaporate (Tylleskar et al, 1993; Rosling & Tylleskar, 1996).

Spinal tumours

Malignant tumours

A metastatic or locally invading cancer can cause painful spinal cord compression. Lung, breast and prostate are common primary sites of tumours which may metastasize to the vertebral bodies and then cause extradural compression. Myeloma, lymphoma and Burkitt's lymphoma also spread to the spine.

Benign tumours

For example meningioma and neurofibroma, causing extramedullary compression, can be successfully resected, but cancerous compression is best treated with high dose corticosteroids – dexamethasone 16 mg daily, and radiotherapy if available. Intramedullary tumours are rare and often only incompletely treatable, even with the best of neurosurgical facilities.

Motor neurone disease

This relentlessly progressive neurodegenerative disease affects the corticospinal tracts of the spinal cord and the anterior horn cells of the cranial nerves and the spinal nerves.

Clinical features

Patients present with limb or bulbar (speech, swallowing) weakness, and usually have a combination of upper and lower motor neurone signs, with prominent fasciculations in the tongue and limb muscles, but no sensory loss. There is some evidence that the condition as seen in Africa is more likely to present with 'flail arms', but it is an uncommon diagnosis in the Continent (Tomik et al., 2000). Treatment is supportive and symptomatic.

Other spinal cord disorders

There is a large group of myelopathies seen in Africa which are not yet defined. The patients have acute, subacute or chronic spinal cord syndromes, and so present with weakness or paralysis of the legs, sensory loss and often bladder involvement. HIV or other infective conditions are likely to account for many, but these cases are not yet defined and there is a great need for further research.

Peripheral neuropathy

Peripheral neuropathy was common in African populations, even before the grip of HIV was felt. A community study of neurological disorders in Nigeria cited a prevalence ratio for peripheral nerve disorders of 268/100000 (Osuntokun et al., 1987). It is estimated that a third to a half of patients with HIV infection develop a neuropathy (Simpson & Wolfe, 1991), which may have an autoimmune basis similar to Guillain–Barré syndrome (GBS), may be due to a direct viral neurotoxicity, or may be related to the drugs that are used to treat the infection and its complications.

Leprosy is a common cause of neuropathy in much of Africa but diabetes is the most common cause.

Pathological changes

The pathological processes affecting peripheral nerves are:

- Wallerian degeneration (secondary to nerve trauma)
- segmental demyelination
- axonal degeneration.

Nerve conduction studies and electromyography (EMG) help to distinguish demyelinating and axonal patterns. In demyelination there is marked slowing of conduction speeds, whereas in axonal neuropathy, the conduction speeds are relatively preserved, but the amplitude of motor and sensory potentials is reduced; the changes of denervation are detected by EMG needling of affected muscles.

Classification

Neuropathies are classified by:

- pathology, demyelinating or axonal
- distribution (distal polyneuropathy, mononeuropathy)
- duration (acute, subacute, chronic, relapsing)
- clinical features (motor, sensory, mixed, autonomic).

Clinical features

Sensory

Most patients notice sensory symptoms first, with tingling and numbness in the feet and then the hands, classically ascending in a stocking and a glove distribution from the fingers and toes up the limbs. Peripheral loss of pain appreciation is usual, but some neuropathies are painful, for examples, in herpes zoster or in paraneoplastic sensory syndromes. In sensory neuropathies the patient may notice that a burn was not painful or that a small wound on the sole of the foot has become a large ulcer, and yet without pain.

Motor

In motor neuropathy, the weakness characteristically begins in the hands and feet, so that the tailor cannot thread a needle, the mechanic cannot drive home a screw. Wasting of muscles is seen in the more severe cases. The tendon reflexes are diminished or absent in neuropathy. In some mild or early cases of diabetic neuropathy, absent ankle reflexes may be the only sign.

Autonomic

Postural hypotension, cardiac irregularity, diarrhoea, constipation, impotence and anhidrosis are all common features of autonomic neuropathy which is often seen in diabetes or Guillain–Barré Syndrome.

Specific neuropathies

Diabetic neuropathy

Up to 50 per cent of people with diabetes develop peripheral neuropathy. The most common patterns are a distal sensory neuropathy with or without pain, or various mononeuropathies, when only one nerve is affected. This may be a cranial nerve (for example, a pupil-sparing painful third nerve palsy), or a peripheral nerve, such as the femoral, when the patient presents with pain, sensory loss and wasting of the thigh, often referred to as diabetic amyotrophy.

Mononeuropathies are due to infarction of the nerve trunk secondary to diabetic arteriopathy in medium-sized and small vessels, whereas more diffuse neuropathies are caused by a combination of deranged metabolic factors and endoneurial microvascular disease. If the diabetes is more tightly controlled, the peripheral neuropathy sometimes improves, but it can seriously disable the patient and great care has to be taken to avoid trauma to desensitized feet.

Infective neuropathies

These are important and common, particularly the neuropathies associated with leprosy and HIV infection: always think of leprosy and HIV in cases of neuropathy.

The sensory neuropathy of lepromatous leprosy characteristically involves the more exposed extremities; in tuberculoid forms various mononeuropathies may eventually merge into a more diffuse pattern. Disabling deformities result from repeated trauma to anaesthetic extremities.

In HIV, there may be a sensory, motor or mixed neuropathy which develops at seroconversion or at a later stage. After dementia, this is the most common neurological complication of HIV (Chapter 13).

Guillain–Barré syndrome (GBS)

Epidemiology

Studies in Africa (Bahemuka, 1988; Howlett et al., 1996) suggest an annual incidence similar to the figure of 1.8 per 100 000 which is quoted from various Western countries, but this may change as a variant associated with HIV infection is seen (Thornton et al., 1991). Symptoms follow an acute viral infection (upper respiratory tract or gastrointestinal) in about 50 per cent of cases.

Clinical features

The patient presents, characteristically, with weakness that ascends up the limbs over a few days and is associated with truncal aches and pains often with peripheral sensory symptoms, but few sensory signs. Some patients first have proximal weakness, which then spreads distally. The tendon reflexes are depressed or absent, although in some, at the initial presentation, they are still present. Cranial nerves are often affected leading to facial and bulbar weakness. Impairment of swallowing and respiration are potentially life threatening, as can be the associated cardiac autonomic dysfunctions.

Diagnosis

Poliomyelitis, tetanus and botulism are considered in the differential diagnosis. CSF examination usually, but not always, reveals the characteristic 'dissociation cytoalbuminique' with an elevated protein level, but no excess of cells.

Treatment

In advanced centres, intravenous immunoglobulin or plasma exchange are proven treatments. Even where these cannot be given, intensive care and ventilatory support have been very effective in reducing the mortality of GBS from 35 per cent down to 5 per cent. Steroid drugs are ineffective.

Outcome

Most patients survive and gradually regain mobility, but the prognosis depends on the level of care available locally. Residual neurological deficit is common, for example, a foot drop or weakness of a hand.

Table 86.6. Common entrapment neuropathies

Nerve	Site of entrapment	Clinical features
Median	Palmar aspect of wrist (carpal tunnel syndrome)	Sensory loss and pain in thumb, index and middle finger, often worse at night, thenar wasting and weakness.
Anterior interosseous	Compressed in forearm	Loss of thumb–index finger pinch
Ulnar	Elbow (cubital tunnel syndrome) Rarely deep palmar branch	Sensory loss ring and little finger, weakness and wasting, interrossei and hypothenar evidence, clawing Motor features only
Radial	Spiral groove upper arm; axilla	Wrist and finger drop
Posterior interosseous	Compressed in forearm	Weak finger extensors, radial wrist deviation
Long thoracic	Shoulder	Winging of scapula
Sciatic	Sciatic notch (injections)	Posterior thigh pain, weak and numb foot, absent ankle reflex
Femoral	Inguinal ligament	Weak knee extension, absent knee reflex
Lateral cutaneous nerve of thigh	Inguinal ligament	Sensory loss, lateral thigh (meralgia parasthetica)
Common peroneal	Lateral head of fibula	Weak dorsiflexion and eversion of foot with impaired sensation over dorsum

Notes:
(i) These mononeuropathies are distinguished by clinical evidence from the cervical or lumbosacral radiculopathies.
(ii) Entrapment neuropathies not listed here are rarely seen in clinical practice.

Chronic inflammatory demyelinating polyneuropathy (CIDP)

This is regarded as a chronic form of GBS and has a similar prevalence. This condition is sometimes associated with a benign monoclonal gammopathy, or occasionally with myeloma. CIDP is treated by immunomodulation and in some cases, there is a good response to immunosuppression with steroids.

Toxic neuropathies

Farmers and industrial workers are at risk from the toxic effects of organophosphate insecticides, organic solvents, heavy metals and other neurotoxic compounds which create weakness and sensory loss due to an axonal neuropathy. Minor epidemics of toxic neuropathy occur when cooking oils are adulterated by unscrupulous merchants. Numerous drugs cause neuropathy and, of those commonly used, isoniazid, ethambutol (optic neuropathy), dapsone, metronidazole, nitrofurantoin, amiodarone, hydralazine, perhexiline and thalidomide.

Uraemic neuropathy

This is common in patients with chronic renal failure of any cause.

Alcoholic neuropathy

(i) Neuropathy may be a prominent feature of a Wernicke's encephalopathy: it is axonal and has sensory symptoms and signs and reduced tendon reflexes.
(ii) Acute optic neuropathy, sometimes with peripheral neuropathic features, occurs in small epidemics when locally brewed alcohol is drunk or is spiked with toxic raw ethanol, methanol or other adulterants. Local newspapers often carry reports of numbers of people who have gone blind or become disabled following a visit to an illegal drinking den.

Entrapment neuropathy

This term describes the neuropathy when a nerve is trapped in a limited space by bone, fibrous tissue or external pressure. The entrapment neuropathies are common, usually self-limiting and do not demand any action other than correct diagnosis and reassurance. Carpal tunnel syndrome is sometimes resolved by decompression of the median nerve at the wrist, which is a simple procedure. A progressive entrapment syndrome of other nerves may require surgical decompression, as in the rare instances when transposition of the ulnar nerve is necessary (Table 86.6).

Tropical neuropathies

A number of neurological syndromes have been described over the last century in tropical communities with a low standard of nutrition. These syndromes comprise lesions of the skin, mucous membranes and the nervous system in which neuropathy is variably associated with optic atrophy, nerve deafness and sometimes myelopathy. Cinical entities have been recognized and in general terms, the syndromes of spastic paraparesis can be separated from those in which neuropathy predominates (Roman, 1998). Konzo, HTLV-1 associated myelopathy and of course HIV-related disease are identified, as are specific neuropathic disorders such as pellagra, chronic malnutrition and thiamine deficiency in chronic alcoholics. However, a distinct neuropathy has long been recognized and closely studied in poor African communities in which cassava is the staple food, and chronic cyanide intoxication has been implicated – this is tropical ataxic neuropathy (TAN).

Tropical ataxic neuropathy (TAN)

TAN, or a variant in which optic atrophy was prominent, was first noted in Nigeria in the 1930s when boarding school boys who were fed exclusively on cassava during the school term, developed visual failure, skin and mucous membrane lesions. These symptoms improved both during the holidays when they returned home to their mothers' cooking and when the school diet was supplemented (Moore, 1939). In the 1960s a neuropathic syndrome in middle-aged and elderly Nigerians was widely studied in pioneering work by Osuntokun (1968). Cassava-associated TAN is not exclusively found in Nigeria (Njoh, 1990), but contrary to earlier suggestions, it is still commonly seen among the Ijebu people in the south west of the country (Oluwole et al., 2000), with a prevalence of 3.9 per cent in males and 7.7 per cent in females, and age specific prevalence as high as 24 per cent in females aged 60–69 years.

Osuntokun reported that his patients came from the poor socioeconomic classes and had a monotonous diet of cassava derivatives, which was only occasionally supplemented with yam, maize, rice, vegetables or a little animal protein. In two-fifths of cases there is another affected family member.

Clinical features

Symptoms

The disease has an insidious onset and is slowly progressive, often with exacerbations during the rainy season or in pregnancy, lactation and febrile episodes. The initial symptoms are distal lower limb paraesthesiae and dysaesthesiae as well as blurring of vision. Later, patients complain of unsteadiness which is worse in the dark, tinnitus, deafness and weakness with thinning and twitching of the leg muscles. Recurrent sores at the corners of the mouth, a painful tongue and colicky abdominal pain are also common.

Signs

The predominant signs of posterior column sensory loss and bilateral optic atrophy were found respectively in 83 per cent and 81 per cent of Osuntokun's cases, whereas ataxia was present in 60 per cent, perceptive deafness in 41 per cent and mucocutaneous evidence of malnutrition in 40 per cent. Oluwole et al. (2000) have found similar features with sensory polyneuropathy and ataxic gait in 44 per cent of 206 patients, polyneuropathy and optic atrophy in 14 per cent, and all three features of sensory polyneuropathy, ataxia and optic atrophy in a further 21 per cent.

Investigation

Blood tests and CSF examination are normal. Neurogenic atrophy has been found on electromyography and grossly impaired nerve conduction suggests segmental demyelination, a feature also shown on nerve biopsy. The plasma riboflavin level is reduced, but to the same extent as unaffected local controls; other vitamin assays are normal.

The role of cyanide in TAN

Characteristically, the plasma and 24-hour urinary thiocyanate and the plasma cyanide levels are raised in the untreated patient and fall to normal when patients are fed on a balanced diet containing few or no cassava derivatives. The raised levels of thiocyanate and cyanide in TAN are much lower than those found in the outbreaks of konzo (Rosling & Tylleskar, 1996). Possibly different dose rates may determine whether the patient develops the acute spinal cord disease konzo, or the slower onset of a neuropathy. Epidemiological evidence convincingly links both disorders with monotonous ingestion of bitter cassava containing high levels of the cyanogenic glycoside linamarin as the almost exclusive staple food, but the precise pathway of neurological damage in each condition has yet to be fully unravelled. It is possible that cyanide exposure is a contributory, but not essential, factor in one or both conditions.

Course of TAN

Sometimes the symptoms and signs of TAN improve after dietary modifications, but there is no effective treatment for the established condition. Preventative measures include conversion to low-cyanide-yielding varieties of cassava, and education in the correct preparation of the root. It was thought that improved socio-economic standards in Nigeria had led to the disappearance of TAN in the 1980s, but the evidence from rural studies is that the condition is still present in the previous endemic regions and of course, may exist unrecognized elsewhere.

Epidemic optic neuropathy with peripheral neuropathy

Along the coast of Tanzania, there has been an epidemic since 1988 of bilateral visual failure among teenagers and young adults who were found to have symmetrical temporal optic atrophy. Forty-seven per cent of affected patients had evidence of peripheral neuropathy and 42 per cent had impaired hearing (Plant et al., 1997). Low urinary thiocyanate levels make a cyanide cause most improbable. The pathogenesis is unknown but the clinical features resemble a syndrome described by Strachan in the Caribbean and a similar outbreak in Cuba. A micronutrient deficiency may be responsible.

Muscle disease

Although skeletal muscle comprises more than 40 per cent of the body mass, muscle diseases are relatively uncommon except staphylococcal pyomyositis, which is now so much more common because of the immunosuppression of HIV infection.

Muscle investigations
The evaluation of the rarer muscle disorders is complex and will usually require resources which will not be available for most patients. EMG, muscle biopsy, complex biochemical studies and genetic testing help to categorize muscle disease, but a pragmatic approach where these investigations are unavailable will at least allow identification of those patients in whom symptoms or the underlying disease can be treated. This underlines the importance of a sound clinical appraisal.

Pyomyositis (see Chapter 38)

Bacterial infection may cause single or multiple abscesses in the quadriceps or other large muscles, initially with cramping and redness in the affected area, pain and low grade fever. In the later suppurative phase, the muscle is tender and swollen and there is marked oedema: at this stage yellow pus may be aspirated from the lesion; if untreated, systemic features may develop. In a pre-HIV series from Nigeria (Chiedozi, 1979), of 112 cases of tropical pyomyositis seen in one centre over a period of 4 years, 90 per cent of cases were due to *Staphylococcus aureus*. Most cases now are associated with HIV immunosuppression, but the clinical presentation, bacteriology and treatment with surgical drainage and anti-staphylococcal antibiotics are similar (Pallangyo et al., 1992).

Other retroviral-associated muscle disease

HIV-positive people may have a generalized myopathy due to an autoimmune process, or as a reaction to treatment with zidovudine. HTLV-1 infection in some patients is associated with polymyositis in contrast to the more usual spinal cord syndrome (Mora et al., 1988).

Muscle disorders in AIDS
(from Harrison & McArthur, 1995)
- HIV-associated polymyositis
- Zidovudine toxic myopathy
- Pyomyositis
- Cardiomyopathy
- Wasting in advanced AIDS

Myasthenia gravis

Neuro-epidemiological studies in Africa have failed to detect myasthenia, whereas in Europe or the USA the prevalence is approximately 15 per 100 000 population. Sporadic cases are seen.

Pathogenesis
Myasthenia is an autoimmune disorder in which the post-synaptic receptor sites at the neuromuscular junction are damaged by a T-cell-mediated antibody attack.

Clinical features
The characteristic symptom is muscle weakness which increases with use of the muscle (fatigueability) affecting ocular, bulbar or limb musculature, alone or in combination. The 'droopy' face with bilateral ptosis and a transverse smile is typical, but early muscle features are more subtle. Although still useful, the edrophonium ('Tensilon') test is rarely used, and diagnosis relies on single fibre EMG as well as detecting raised levels of acetylcholine receptor antibody. A pragmatic approach is to give a therapeutic trial of pyridostigmine 30–60 mg three times daily or neostigmine.

Treatment

Many patients respond well to corticosteroid treatment, augmented if necessary, with pyridostigmine which can be used as the sole treatment in an uncomplicated case.

In more sophisticated centres, plasma exchange or intravenous immunoglobulin may achieve remissions. As myasthenia is associated with benign thymic hyperplasia, thymectomy is advised in younger patients and in those who are found to have an underlying thymoma. Myasthenia has a good outlook and most patients enjoy reasonably complete remission from symptoms if the disease is carefully managed.

Polymyositis

In Africa, polymyositis is now likely to be triggered by HIV infection but HTLV-1 infection may also be responsible. Uncomplicated polymyositis is less common than myasthenia and presents with a sub-acute or chronic proximal myopathy. Where there is involvement of skin with a characteristic facial and extensor surfaces rash, the term dermatomyositis is used. Patients often have arthralgia and there may be additional collagen vascular disorders or an associated malignancy in a smaller proportion. The ESR and creatine kinase enzyme level are raised in the blood, EMG reveals myopathic changes, and muscle biopsy demonstrates an interstitial inflammatory cell infiltrate with secondary fibre destruction.

The cornerstone of treatment of this autoimmune disorder is high dose prednisolone (60–100 mg) to induce a remission, and then reduction of the dose to a maintenance level of perhaps 15 mg on alternate days which usually continues for several years. Azathioprine or other more potent immunosuppressant drugs are sometimes necessary. Patients can respond well, but the prognosis in polymyositis is often guarded.

Inherited muscle disorders

Duchenne and Becker muscular dystrophies

These X-linked disorders are very rare. Duchenne dystrophy presents in young boys with early lower limb weakness and calf hypertrophy leading to progressive disability and usually death in the teenage years. Becker dystrophy often develops a little later and has a better prognosis, but eventually leads to paralysis. These diseases are associated with dystrophin, an abnormal gene product, but their precise aetiology has yet to be fully worked out. Carrier females can be identified and preconceptual guidance given.

Limb girdle muscular dystrophy

This can be autosomal dominant or recessive. Other patients have fascio-scapulo-humeral, oculo-pharyngeal, scapulo-peroneal or distal phenotypes. These diseases may have a neurogenic or myopathic pathology.

Myotonic dystrophy

This autosomal dominant disorder has a lower prevalence in Africa. The clinical appearance is unmistakable, with frontal baldness, myopathic facies, cataracts and wasting of the neck muscles accompanied by myotonia of the grip and usually a limb myopathy. Some patients also have gonadal atrophy and increased insulin resistance. There is no specific treatment for this or other dystrophies, but symptomatic treatment of the myotonia is achieved with phenytoin or calcium channel blockers.

Benign myotonic disorders

These include Thomsen's disease (myotonica congenita) and the periodic paralyses associated with hyper-, hypo- or normokalaemia, in which episodic attacks of weakness may be associated with myotonia. These conditions are known as channelopathies since in such patients the sodium and chloride channels in the muscles function imperfectly.

Other muscle disorders

Endocrine and metabolic

A proximal myopathy is common in myxoedema (Hoffman's syndrome) and in thyrotoxicosis. Patients with Cushing's syndrome or acromegaly may also have proximal muscle weakness. Osteomalacia causes a proximal myopathy. Alcoholics may have a myopathy as well as the more common neuropathy.

Cancer

A cachectic myopathy associated with malignancy is controversial, but polymyositis is seen as a rare complication in lung, stomach and ovarian cancer.

Drugs

Drug-induced myopathy is seen especially with steroid therapy, and also with chloroquine, zidovudine, amiodarone, colchicine and statins.

Storage disorders

Abnormal storage of glycogen (McCardle's syndrome) and lipids leads to the very rare storage disorders. Mitochondrial disorders may also be a rare cause of myopathy.

Trauma

Local trauma is important. When the damaged muscle is confined within a fascial compartment, for example, vastus lateralis in the thigh, blunt trauma with a significant haematoma may lead to later muscle atrophy. Diffuse crush injury and any widespread muscle injury causes myoglobinuria and renal failure.

Parkinson's disease

Characteristics

Parkinsonism is a syndrome with the cardinal features of tremor, rigidity, bradykinesia and disturbed postural reflexes. The diagnosis is clinical and is made when two of the four cardinal features are present:

(i) The condition is progressive
(ii) The patient responds to dopaminergic medication
(iii) There is no alternative cause
(iv) PD usually presents asymmetrically.

Even in specialist centres, the diagnosis may be incorrect in a fifth of patients: note, not all patients with parkinsonism have Parkinson's disease (PD).

Pathogenesis

In Parkinson's disease there is degeneration of the melanin-containing dopaminergic neurones of the substantia nigra and typical neuroneal inclusions termed Lewy bodies. There is usually a loss of 80 per cent of dopaminergic neurones before symptoms occur. Twin studies have demonstrated that in those rare cases occurring below the age of 50 years there is likely to be a significant hereditary component. In the majority of cases which occur in the older age groups, there may be a hereditary tendency which is triggered by as yet unknown environmental risk factors. In the early 1980s MPTP, an analogue of meperidine, which was injected by i.v. drug abusers in southern California produced a syndrome almost indistinguishable from PD and this has been used since in animal models.

The pattern in Africa

Black African and oriental people have the lowest prevalence of PD, but it is not clear whether this reflects a true difference in susceptibility in these populations. It may be due to low case ascertainment and high selective mortality in populations of African origin (Richards & Chaudhuri, 1996). African Americans in New York have a greater mortality from PD (Mayeux et al., 1996). The prevalence in industrialized countries is about 2 per 1000 population and there is a marked increase with advancing age. The average duration of disease from diagnosis to death is about 13 years. No specific risk factors have been identified to explain the difference in prevalence rates between different populations.

Comparative studies

South Africa

In Durban, South Africa (Cosnett & Bill, 1988), black patients with PD presented much less frequently for neurological consultation than white or Indian patients and those that did tended to be younger. This may be partly due to the reduced life expectancy or the failure of elderly blacks to attend hospital.

Nigeria and USA

In a door-to-door survey of neurological disease in Igbo-Ora (Osuntokun et al., 1987), point prevalence estimates for PD were 10/100 000 for the whole population and 59/100 000 for the population aged 40 years and older but the numbers on which these figures are based were very small. In the USA (Schoenberg et al., 1988), using the same WHO protocol, age-adjusted prevalence rates for PD were similar for African Americans and whites, but when only definite cases were considered a lower age-adjusted prevalence rate was found for the African Americans (196/100 000 and 280/100 000, respectively). When the prevalence ratios were age adjusted the prevalence in African–Americans was five times higher than the Nigerians (Schoenberg et al., 1988).

Clinical features

- Tremor occurs predominantly at rest but may be related to posture. It is usually abated by actions such as writing. (See Table 86.7.)
- Rigidity is classically jerky (cogwheel) and increases when the patient tenses the opposite hand.
- Bradykinesia can lead to an impassive face (hypomimia), breakdown of rapid alternating movements (e.g., foot-tapping), which become irregular on repetition, and difficulty in rising from chairs or rolling over in bed.
- Abnormal posture and righting reflexes are often seen, but less commonly at the initial diagnosis. The patient, when pulled from behind, tends to step backwards (retropulsion) or even fall back, instead of moving their arms forward and swinging the trunk to maintain balance. If gently pushed forwards, the patient appears to be hurrying to catch up with their centre of gravity.
- Abnormal gait, with a stooped posture and reduced arm swing, is common. Later in the disease the length

Table 86.7. Other causes of tremor

The causes of a non-parkinsonian tremor include:	
(a) Essential tremor	The tremor is bilateral, worse with posture and action (e.g. writing) and improved by alcohol. There is a family history in 50 per cent and the other features of parkinsonism are absent.
(b) Wilson's disease	Rare inherited deficiency of a copper-transporting ATPase protein necessary for the incorporation of copper into bile. Leads to accumulation of copper in liver, brain, cornea and kidneys and there is a classical appearance of corneal Kayser–Fleischer rings. There is a low serum caeruloplasmin and raised 24-hour urinary copper excretion. This should be considered in anyone presenting with a movement disorder under the age of 30 years.
(c) Miscellaneous	Thyrotoxicosis, metabolic encephalopathy (flapping tremor), drug-induced (e.g. beta-agonists for obstructive airways disease) and anxiety.

of stride shortens, and festination develops, particularly evident on commencing walking and turning. Freezing episodes occur at imaginary barriers (e.g. doorways).

- Anxiety is common, and depression occurs in a third of PD patients: it is often difficult to diagnose because the disease shares features with depression.
- Dementia occurs in about a third of patients and may have pathology relating to Alzheimer's disease or multi-infarct disease. Lewy-body dementia (LBD) characteristically presents with hallucinations, that may occur in the absence of medication, with the motor features of parkinsonism. Confusion and hallucinations may develop as side effects from any of the anti-parkinsonian medications. Hallucinations are usually visual and non-threatening but patients can develop paranoid delusions.

Treatment

The primary aim of drug treatment of PD is to replace the deficiency of dopamine within the basal ganglia. There are various classes of drugs, all of which have relatively similar side effects, which include nausea (particularly when first commenced), postural hypotension, hallucinations and dyskinesias, which are common later in the disease.

(i) Levodopa with decarboxylase inhibitor: the decarboxylase inhibitor prevents the peripheral breakdown of levodopa, but does not cross the blood–brain barrier. This is still the most effective drug for PD and is standard treatment in the majority of patients.
(ii) Dopamine agonists, e.g. bromocriptine and others: these act directly on the dopamine receptors and have a longer half-life than levodopa.
(iii) Anticholinergics: these may be particularly helpful for tremor and hypersalivation, but their use is limited by their side effects such as dry mouth, urinary retention, confusion and hallucinatons, particularly in the elderly.

Drugs do not alter the natural course of PD: they only control symptoms. As they have significant side effects, prescribe them only as symptoms dictate, and start with the lowest dose possible. When the first drug has reached its maximum total dose, a second agent may be needed. Other features of PD may be as disabling as the motor features, e.g. depression, and require treatment.

Management of confusion associated with Parkinson's disease is by treatment of any potential precipitating factors, e.g. urinary tract infection, decrease of dose of dopaminergic medication where this is practicable, and the use of atypical neuroleptics. These newer drugs do not have the marked Parkinsonian side effects of the older neuroleptics. Postural hypotension results from a combination of the disease and the medication.

Other disorders of movement

Dystonia

This is a sustained muscle contraction leading to abnormal postures or repetitive movements which are often twisting and vary from intermittent task-specific, or action-specific movements, to dystonic movements or postures at rest. The dystonia may be:

- focal, for example, spasmodic torticollis or blepharospasm
- segmental, involving adjacent body regions
- generalized, which usually involves legs and other areas
- hemidystonia.

There are several hereditary causes of primary dystonia including dopa-responsive dystonia which, as its name suggests, responds to small doses of levodopa, and numerous causes of secondary dystonia, some of which, such as Wilson's disease, respond to treatment.

Chorea

This term describes involuntary, abrupt, irregular, purposeless and random movements, usually of the face, hands and arms, and feet.

HIV is now a significant cause of chorea.

Huntington's disease is inherited as an autosomal dominant trait for which the responsible mutation has been identified and can be detected by DNA analysis of blood samples. The prevalence is 5–10/100 000 population. The disease usually presents between the ages of 30 and 50 years, but may start earlier and there is usually associated dementia. The chorea can be treated with a neuroleptic or tetrabenazine.

Sydenham's chorea can follow an acute streptococcal infection and is a major manifestation of rheumatic fever. It usually occurs between the ages of 5 and 15 years, more commonly in girls, and often resolves in time, but may be disabling and require treatment as above. It may also be associated with rheumatic carditis.

Tremor (Table 86.7)

Essential tremor, see p. 1156 above.If necessary it can be treated with propranolol or primidone.

Cerebellar tremor is characteristically worse with action and increases progressively during voluntary movement (intention tremor)

Parkinsonian tremor is reduced by voluntary movement.

Orthostatic tremor is rare, occurs only when the patient is standing still, and may respond to clonazepam.

Tics

These are rapid, brief jerks, usually of the head and arms, which can be suppressed for short periods. They vary from simple localized jerks to complex and elaborate movements. Tics are common, usually self-limiting and require only reassurance. More severe tic syndromes may require suppression with, for example, haloperidol.

Myoclonus

Myoclonic jerks are sudden, brief, shock-like movements caused by active muscular contraction. Cortical focal myoclonus is usually distal and stimulus sensitive and is synonymous with epilepsia partialis continua. Multifocal myoclonus is usually caused by widespread cortical pathology. Generalized myoclonus usually arises from the brain stem. Anti-convulsants may help in treatment.

Physiological myoclonus, especially nocturnal, is common and requires no treatment other than reassurance.

Drug-induced movement disorders

Acute dystonic reactions of the cranial or cervical region, sometimes with oculogyric crisis, can occur following administration of phenothiazines, prochlorperazine or metoclopramide. Treat with an intravenous anticholinergic (e.g. procyclidine 5 mg) or diazepam 5–10 mg.

Tardive dyskinesia affects about 20 per cent of patients on long-term anti-psychotic medication, particularly the elderly, and presents as continuous choreiform involuntary movements of the orobuccolingual and masticatory muscles. It is due to dopamine-receptor hypersensitivity but, paradoxically, increased doses of dopamine antagonists may lead to improvement. Tetrabenazine, baclofen, benzodiazepines and calcium channel blockers are sometimes effective.

Parkinson's disease may be unmasked by the use of phenothiazines and other anti-psychotic drugs. Potentially reversible extrapyramidal syndromes are common in psychiatric patients taking chlorpromazine and other phenothiazines, and can be reduced by concomitant use of an anti-cholinergic drug.

Dementia

The neurological signs of dementia comprise failure of learning, loss of memory and loss of analytical ability. In focal neurological disease there are signs such as aphasia (failure of language) or apraxia (failure to execute learned task). The history from the patient and the family reveals the mode of onset, the speed of progression (if any), drug history and associated illnesses or complaints, while the examination reveals the severity of the cognitive failure, and the presence of other neurological signs which may be clues to the underlying diagnosis.

The pattern in Africa

The few studies of prevalence and incidence of dementia from Africa (Ineichen, 2000) show generally low prevalence figures. These probably underestimate the problem which will become more evident as the numbers of elderly people increase in many parts of the African Continent. A vast reservoir of subclinical or more overt dementia exists in the HIV-infected population.

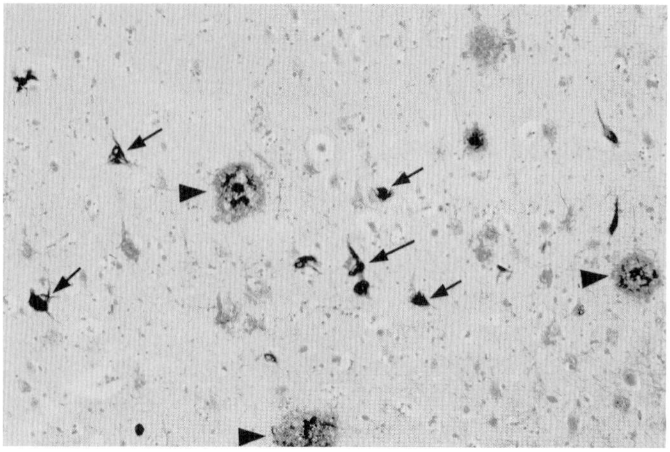

Fig. 86.25. Alzheimer's disease: to show neurofibrillary tangles (arrows) and amyloid plaques (triangles). (By courtesy of Dr D. Hilton.)

Alzheimer's disease (AD) is estimated to have a 6–10 per cent prevalence in patients aged over 65 in developed countries, but is very much less in Africa.

Alzheimer's disease

Pathogenesis

There is degeneration of cortical neurones with shrinkage of white matter and enlargement of the cerebral ventricles. The hallmarks of the disease on microscopy are neurofibrillary tangles and amyloid plaques (Fig. 86.25). Beta-amyloid is toxic to neurones in tissue culture but the exact mechanism of cell death in vivo remains unclear. The cholinergic neurotransmitter system is affected and anti-cholinesterase drugs used in the treatment of AD temporarily improve performance on neuropsychological tests but there is not always an improvement in the patient's performance of activities of daily living.

There is a familial form of AD related to the amyloid protein precursor (APP) gene on chromosome 21 and to another locus (AD3 gene) on chromosome 14. About two-thirds of AD patients have repeats of the apolipoprotein E (APOE) gene located on chromosome 19. Testing for the abnormal gene may predict the risk of AD, but the gene is absent in a third of AD cases and is present in persons without AD. The association of APOE genotype E4 and dementia found in white populations has also been identified in African–Americans (Hendrie et al., 1995), but not among Africans in Ibadan (Osuntokun et al., 1995) or east Africa (Kalaria et al., 1997).

Clinical evolution

The disease progresses slowly, but relentlessly. The patient initially loses short-term memory and has difficulty in analysing information and calculation. In the late stages, myoclonus or seizures occur in about 25 per cent of cases. Neuroleptics may be required to control aggressive behaviour.

Cerebrovascular dementia

Cognitive impairment is common after stroke. Vascular dementia, classically a syndrome of cognitive impairment in conjunction with stroke disease, is characterized by abrupt onset, step-wise deterioration and fluctuating course. Suggestive features include preserved insight, nocturnal confusion, small-stepped gait, focal neurological signs and evidence of vascular disease elsewhere. Vascular dementia may also evolve as a consequence of diffuse small vessel disease with ischaemic lesions in the deep white matter and basal ganglia.

AIDS dementia complex

Direct involvement of the brain by HIV is known under a variety of terms (Brew, 1999), such as HIV encephalopathy, subacute encephalitis, AIDS-related dementia, AIDS dementia complex (ADC) and HIV-1 associated dementia. ADC is a sub-cortical dementia with prominent motor disturbance and an absence of the usual cortical features of aphasia, alexia, and agraphia that characterize dementias such as Alzheimer's disease. Cortical symptoms occur when dementia is advanced and the deficit has become more global. Co-existing disorders and other complications can lead to unusual presentations of ADC such as seizures, myelopathy, tremor, chorea, pseudo-depression, hypomania and transient neurological deficits. Seizures occur in 10 per cent of patients with ADC and may predate other features.

Clinical presentation

The symptoms and the signs of ADC involve motor function and behaviour. Patients become forgetful and have poor concentration. Motor complaints include clumsiness, sloppy handwriting, tremor and poor balance with an unsteady gait. There are primitive reflexes and abnormal tandem gait. Patients often become socially withdrawn and apathetic with a lack of interest in friends and hobbies, but insight is preserved until late in the illness. ADC has a more insidious onset than other HIV complications which may cause cognitive impairment, particularly the opportunistic infections (toxoplasmosis, cytomegalovirus encephalitis, chronic meningitis).

The pathological changes in ADC are predominantly in the deeper parts of the brain, especially the basal ganglia (Nath, 1999). It occurs in 20–30 per cent of patients with advanced HIV disease in developed countries (McArthur et al., 1993), but the incidence has decreased with access to highly active antiretroviral therapy.

Rare causes of dementia

Chronic subdural haematoma and brain tumours may occasionally present with dementia. Pick's disease is similar to AD but is particularly severe in the temporal and frontal lobes. Creutzfeldt–Jakob disease characteristically presents with myoclonus associated with dementia. Recent new variant cases in Europe have been related to cattle infected with bovine spongiform encephalopathy (BSE). Hydrocephalus can cause dementia and is usually associated with wide based gait and urinary incontinence. Systemic lupus erythematosus (SLE) can sometimes cause multiple cerebral infarcts and present with cerebrovascular dementia. CADASIL (cerebral autosomal dominant arteriopathy with subcortical infarcts and leukoencephalopathy) is a rare inherited cause of stroke preceded by migraine and leading to dementia.

Head trauma

The pattern in Africa

Head trauma has become epidemic largely as a result of an ever-increasing number of road traffic accidents. In a study of intracranial haematoma in Jos, Nigeria, 72 per cent were the result of road traffic accidents (Igun, 2000). The additional tragedy is that many victims are young and they are left with long-term disability.

Pathological changes

Head injury causes both focal and diffuse brain damage. Focal injury includes contusion at the impact site and skull fracture which is important to detect because of its association with intracranial haemorrhage.

Diffuse brain damage refers to widespread axonal injury and, in addition, contusion of the frontal and temporal lobes as they impact against the anterior and middle cranial fossa walls.

Table 86.8. Glasgow coma scale

Best motor response	Obeys	M6
	Localizes	5
	Withdraws	4
	Abnormal flexion	3
	Abnormal extension	2
	Nil	1
Verbal response	Orientated	V5
	Confused conversation	4
	Inappropriate words	3
	Incomprehensible sounds	2
	Nil	1
Eye opening	Spontaneous	E4
	To speech	3
	To pain	2
	Nil	1

Assessment of injury

The assessment and management of the unconscious patient is discussed in Chapter 97. Once the patient is stable:

- Monitor the patient and their vital signs very carefully to detect any change in the level of consciousness.
- Use the Glasgow Coma Scale (GCS) (Table 86.8).
- Always examine the pupils.
- Look for any limb weakness when the comatose patient responds to a painful stimulus.
- If the coma score deteriorates, the patient may have an intra-cranial haematoma.

Extradural haematoma

This results from arterial bleeding into the extradural space and is particularly associated with fractures crossing the middle meningeal vessels on the temporal bone. Patients may have a lucid interval after the head injury before becoming rapidly unconscious; they may 'talk and die'. Only if the haematoma is promptly evacuated via a burr hole will the patient survive (Fig. 86.26).

Subdural haematoma

This follows bleeding into the subdural space, usually after an injury in which the head is struck by a broad, hard object.

Acute subdural haematoma

This occurs within 48 hours of injury: the patient deteriorates rapidly due to high pressure arterial bleeding. If

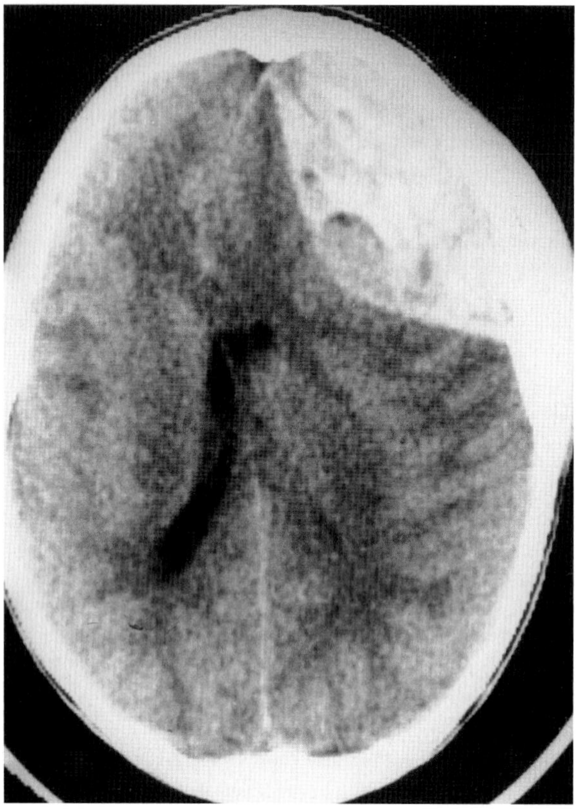

Fig. 86.26. CT scan of brain to show left extradural haemorrhage.

untreated, the patient develops signs of brain herniation, becomes more deeply unconscious and may have signs of ipsilateral third nerve palsy, contralateral hemiparesis and progressive brainstem dysfunction.

- If you suspect a subdural haematoma either do an urgent CT scan or angiogram (if these are available), or do exploratory burr holes.

Chronic subdural haematoma

The symptoms evolve from as short a time as seven days to as long as many months after head injury, when the event itself may have been forgotten. It begins as a small haematoma which expands as a result of clot lysis and further minor bleeding to present as a mass lesion; diagnosis is with CT scan, angiogram or therapeutic burr holes.

- Remember that a patient with a confusional state, for example an alcoholic, may have a second cause of their confusion, that is a chronic subdural haematoma (Table 86.9).

Table 86.9. Other complications of head injury

Hydrocephalus	Early, from aqueduct obstruction due to intraventicular haemorrhage. Late, from failure of CSF absorption leading to communicating hydrocephalus
CSF leaks	Due to dural tears. Leakage of blood stained CSF from nose or ears (test for glucose to confirm it is CSF). Most settle spontaneously; give antibiotic prophylaxis with penicillin
Meningitis	Can follow any injury where the dura has been breached or may be associated with extracranial sepsis
Epilepsy	Early, within a week of head injury, or late. Increased risk with greater severity of head injury, particularly intracranial haematoma, depressed skull fracture and focal neurological signs. Treat with anti-convulsant

Coma

Consciousness is the state of awareness of self and surroundings; coma is defined as 'unrousable unresponsiveness' and is a medical emergency which requires rapid assessment and treatment (Plum & Posner, 1982).

It is crucial to ask any accompanying persons whether the onset was abrupt (suggesting stroke or subarachnoid haemorrhage) or gradual (suggesting conditions such as brain tumour or trypanosomiasis). Preceding fever and headache suggest malaria or meningitis, while a history of middle ear infection, sinusitis or head injury may be relevant. Ask carefully about drug and alcohol abuse and about exposure to toxins such as organophosphates. There may also be clues in a past history of epilepsy, diabetes, or psychiatric disturbance.

Coma is seen most commonly:

- following head injury
- after drug overdose
- as non-traumatic coma caused by anoxia, cerebrovascular disease, infection or metabolic derangement.

Assessment

The ABC of initial assessment

- Assess the patient and ensure that the airway, breathing and circulation are adequate.

The examination should then proceed in two stages.

Preliminary examination

- Define the cause of any associated disease and treat it urgently.
- Look for evidence of head injury, meningitis (fever, neck stiffness, photophobia, conjunctival petechiae).
- Do an immediate lumbar puncture if meningitis is suspected; examine a blood film for malarial parasites. If there are focal signs or papilloedema, and a CT scan is not available, and if meningitis is probable, do a lumbar puncture under steroid or mannitol cover, unless there are signs of cerebral herniation when the risks of lumbar puncture outweigh the benefits.

Detailed examination

- Assess the level of consciousness, pupils, eye movements and reflex ocular movements.
- Assess the response to pain by supra-orbital pressure, nail bed pressure or squeezing the Achilles tendon.
- Measure any asymmetry in motor response.
- Unequal pupils and focal signs suggest structural rather than metabolic brain dysfunction. In metabolic disease the pupils are symmetrical and react normally: an exception is methyl alcohol poisoning which may produce dilated and unreactive pupils. The pupils are small in opiate poisoning.

Reflex eye movements

Assess these by rotating the head from side to side and observing the position of the eyes.

- If the brainstem is intact, the eyes move together (conjugately) in a direction opposite to the head movement (doll's eye movements).
- When the brainstem is depressed, the eyes remain in mid position. In general, patients with drug overdose have a marked depression of brainstem responses yet are in relatively light coma.
- If there is any serious neck injury and the neck cannot be moved, the oculovestibular reflex can be assessed by injecting 50–200 ml of iced water into a clear auditory canal: first make sure that the eardrum is not perforated. The normal response is nystagmus, with a fast phase away from the irrigated ear. Tonic deviation towards the stimulus indicates a supratentorial lesion while no response or a dysconjugate response suggests a brainstem lesion.

Coma scales

The depth of coma can be assessed either using the Glasgow Coma Scale (Table 86.8) or the following simpler scale:

Grade 1 *Confused.* Clouding of consciousness but responds to name and obeys simple commands

Grade 2 *Stupor.* Purposeful movements in response to painful stimuli; easily roused.

Grade 3 *Semi-conscious.* Reacts to pain but does not localize the stimulus.

Grade 4 *Deeply unconscious.* No response to painful stimuli.

Management

- Always assess patients in coma frequently.
- Ensure that nurses and medical staff are capable of doing this. If focal signs associated with increasing coma develop, a focal lesion such as an abscess or haematoma, may be present. Untreated, this may cause tentorial herniation with ipsilateral pupillary dilatation, progressive deterioration in level of consciousness, contralateral hemiparesis, change in respiratory pattern, hypertension, bradycardia, and change in reflex eye movements.
- If these signs develop, urgent treatment can be lifesaving. If a CT scan is not possible, burr holes are needed, the site determined by the focal signs found in the patient. A CT scan could reveal the underlying cause, which has to be dealt with (Table 86.10).

Neurogenetics

One of the most spectacular advances over the last 20 years has been our greater understanding about the genetic causes of neurological diseases. Any progressive neurological condition, particularly in isolated communities, may have a genetic basis. The first clue often comes from a careful family history: enquire about parental consanguinity (for example first and second cousin marriages); and, where possible, examination of other family members. The four main patterns of inheritance are autosomal dominant, autosomal recessive, sex linked and mitochondrial: the rare disorders associated with these patterns are shown in Table 86.11.

Neurological rehabilitation

Rehabilitation can be defined as 'all the steps taken to mitigate the effects of disability and to maximize the

Table 86.10. Evaluation and causes of coma

Clinical examination	Possible diagnoses to be considered
General features	
Fever	Meningitis, cerebral malaria
Jaundice	Malaria, hepatic encephalopathy
Dehydration	Diabetic coma
Ketotic breath	Diabetic ketoacidosis
Acidotic breathing	Diabetic ketoacidosis, renal failure, methanol intoxication
Sweating	Hypoglycaemia
Petechial haemorrhages	Septicaemia, meningococcaemia, louse born typhus
Antecubital needle marks	Opiate drug abuse
Hot dry skin	Heat stroke
Pale skin	Anaemia, haemorrhage
Cyanosis	Hypoxaemia, carbon dioxide poisoning
Cherry red mucous membranes	Carbon monoxide poisoning
Hypersalivation	Organophosphate poisoning
Laceration of the tongue/incontinence	Epileptic seizure
Poor dental hygiene, pustules on face, ear discharge	Intracranial infection
Orbital ecchymosis (racoon eyes)	Anterior basal skull fracture
Haematoma overlying mastoid (Battles sign)	Basilar skull fracture extending into mastoid portion of temporal bone
Neurological signs	
Neck stiffness	Meningitis, subarachnoid haemorrhage, herniation
Papilloedema	Primary brain disorder with raised intracranial pressure
Constricted pupils	Drug overdose (barbiturates, morphine, heroin) organophosphate poisoning, pontine haemorrhage
Hemiparesis	Stroke, subdural haematoma, cerebral abscess
Fluctuating level of consciousness	Subdural haematoma
Muscle fasciculation	Organophosphate poisoning
Cardiovascular signs	
Hypotension	Shock from any cause, septicaemia
Hypertension	Hypertensive encephalopathy, stroke, raised intracranial pressure, organophosphate poisoning
Irregular pulse or heart murmur	Cerebral embolus
Chest signs	
Lung consolidation	Meningitis, brain abscess, brain metastasis
Abdominal signs	
Hepatosplenomegaly	Malaria, cirrhosis with hepatic failure and encephalopathy
Abdominal rigidity	Abdominal injury, peritonitis

potential of the individual'. Disability refers to the restriction or lack of ability to perform an activity considered normal for the individual (Bhattacharji & Saunders, 1996). The estimated prevalence of moderate to severe disability is around 5 per cent. Simple health measures such as improved nutrition, immunization and accident prevention (in particular, the carnage on the roads) can have a significant impact on the disability level in the community. Rehabilitation can be divided into several steps: (a) recognition of the underlying condition with appropriate medical or surgical treatment, (b) prevention of complications, (c) teaching adaptive therapies, and (d) maximizing residual potential.

Prevent complications

The prevention of complications is extremely important since they delay recovery and cause further neurological

Table 86.11. Patterns of inheritance of neurological disorders

Autosomal dominant	Autosomal recessive	X-linked inheritance	Mitochondrial inheritance
Huntington's disease Myotonic dystrophy Neurofibromatosis Tuberous sclerosis Some hereditary ataxias and neuropathies	Friedreich's ataxia Wilson's disease Ataxia telangiectasia Phenylketonuria Some epilepsy syndromes	Duchenne/Becker muscular dystrophy, Fragile X mental retardation syndrome	MERFF MELA Leber's optic atrophy
50 per cent risk to each child	25 per cent risk of homozygosity to children of carriers. Consanguinity increases risk of transmission	Carrier females: 50 per cent risk to sons and 50 per cent risk to daughters. Affected males: No risk to sons. All daughters are carriers.	Transmission via females only. All children at risk.
Males/females Equally affected	Males/females Equally affected	Males affected almost exclusively	Highly variable expression of severity. Cytoplasmic inheritance
Multiple generations affected. Variable severity of disease	Usually single affected generation	Multiple generations affected. Female transmission	

damage. Complications from acute conditions include bedsores, poor hydration and nutrition, chest and urinary tract infections. However, complications may occur later and can be prevented by long-term follow-up. A child, for example, with spasticity due to cerebral palsy can be taught how to walk; if he is untreated, he may develop contractures and secondary deformities which will prevent him ever being able to walk. Patients with chronic neurological conditions may develop scoliosis, which can be minimized by preventive bracing, good posture and seating arrangements and regular physical therapy.

Teach adaptive techniques

Help each individual to adapt to their disability and to make the most of the function that they still have: this can be done if a team works with the patient and with their community and family. In a community-based rehabilitation programme, the local community helps to choose local rehabilitation supervisors to organize the service. The physiotherapist is crucial.

Orthoses (external devices to help movement) can be very helpful; these include callipers or leg braces, upper limb splints and spinal braces, collars and corsets. Often, orthoses are not checked properly and ill-fitting ones are often discarded by the patient.

Drug treatment may be necessary for various long-term complications. Spasticity is a frequent problem following neurological injury and can be treated with baclofen or dantrolene sodium. The aim is to reduce spasticity to a level which improves mobility without causing increased weakness. Botulinum toxin is increasingly used for spasticity and focal dystonias and repeated injections are often necessary. Whereas drug interventions are expensive and unlikely to be available in practice, more pragmatic approaches depend on local enthusiasm and the use of local resources, for example the success in rehabilitation of patients disabled by leprosy.

References

Abu-Salih HS, Abdul-Rahman AM. (1988). Tumours of the brain in the Sudan. *Surg Neurol*; **29**: 94–96.

Akepede GO, Ambe JP. (2000). Cerebral herniation in pyogenic meningitis: prevalence and related dilemmas in emergency room populations in developing countries. *Dev Med Child Neurol*; **42**: 62–69.

Akinyanju OO, Okany CC. (1992). Pernicious anaemia in Africans. *Clin Lab Haematol*; **14**: 33–40.

Babalola OE, Amoni SS, Samaila E, Thaker U, Dargougar S. (1990). An outbreak of acute haemorrhagic conjunctivitis in Kaduna, Nigeria. *Br J Ophth*; **74**: 89–92.

Bahemuka M. (1988). Guillain–Barré syndrome in Kenya: a clinical review of 54 patients. *Neurology*; **235**: 418–421.

Bhattacharji S, Saunders M. (1996). A perspective on neurological rehabilitation. In *Tropical Neurology*, ed. RA Shakir, P Newman, CM Poser, pp. 465–472. London: WB Saunders.

Brew BJ. (1999). AIDS Dementia Complex. *Neurol Clin*; **17**: 861–881.

Chiedozi LC. (1979). Pyomyositis. Review of 205 cases in 112 patients. *Am J Surg*; **137**: 255–259.

Cosnett JE, Bill PLA. (1988). Parkinson's disease in blacks. Observations on epidemiology in Natal. *S Afr Med J*; **73**: 281–283.

Getahun H, Mekonnen A, Tekle-Haimanot R et al. (1999). Epidemic of neurolathyrism in Ethiopia. *Lancet*; **354**: 306–307.

Getahun H, Lambein F, Vanhoome M et al. (2002). Pattern and associated factors of the neurolathyrism epidemic in Ethiopia. *Trop Med Int Hlth*; **7**: 118–124.

Glasauer FE, Coots D, Levy LF, Auchterlonie WC. (1978). Subdural empyema in Africans in Rhodesia. *Neurosurgery*; **3**: 385–391.

Harrison MJ, McArthur JC. (1995). Muscle disease. In *AIDS and Neurology*, pp. 109–117. Edinburgh: Churchill Livingstone.

Hendrie HC, Hall KS, Hui S et al. (1995). Apolipoprotein E genotypes and Alzheimer's disease in a community study of elderly African Americans. *Ann Neurol*; **37**: 118–120.

Howlett WP, Vedeler CA, Nyland H et al. (1996). Guillain–Barré syndrome in Northern Tanzania: a comparison of epidemiological and clinical findings with western Norway. *Acta Neurol Scand*; **93**: 44–49.

Igun GO. (2000). Predictive indices in traumatic intracranial haematomas. *E Afr Med J*; **77**: 9–12.

Ineichen B. (2000). The epidemiology of dementia in Africa: a review. *Soc Sci Med*; **50**: 1673–1677.

Jialal I, Reddi K, Omar MA et al. (1986). Pituitary tumours in African and Indian patients. *Trop Geogr Med*; **38**: 175–179.

Kalaria RN, Ogeng'o JA, Patel NB et al. (1997). Evaluation of risk factors for Alzheimer's disease in elderly east Africans. *Brain Res Bull*; **44**: 573–577.

Levy LF, Auchterlonie WC. (1975). Primary cerebral neoplasia in Rhodesia. *Int Surg*; **50**: 286–92.

Lowe J, Bradley J. (1986). Cerebral and orbital Aspergillus infection due to invasive aspergillosis of ethmoid sinus. *J Clin Pathol*; **39**: 774–778.

Matuja WB, Meteza IB, Rwiza HT. (1995). Headache in a nonclinical population in Dar es Salaam, Tanzania. *Headache*; **35**: 273–276.

Mayeux R, Marder K, Cote LJ et al. (1996). The frequency of idiopathic Parkinson's disease among middle-aged and elderly black, Hispanic and white men and women in Northern Manhattan (1988–1993). *Am J Epidemiol*; **142**: 820–827.

McArthur JC, Hoover DR, Bacellar H et al. (1993). Dementia in AIDS patients: incidence and risk factors. Multicenter AIDS Cohort Study. *Neurology*; **43**: 2245–2252.

Moore D. (1939). Retrobulbar neuritis with pellagra in Nigeria. *J Trop Med Hyg*; **42**: 109–114.

Mora CA, Garruto RM, Brown P et al. (1988). Seroprevalence of antibodies to HTLV-I in patients with chronic neurological disorders other than tropical spastic paraparesis. *Ann Neurol*; **235**: S192–195.

Nath A. (1999). Pathobiology of human immunodeficiency virus dementia. *Semin Neurol*; **19**: 113–127.

Nathoo N, Nadvi SS, van Dellen JR. (1999). Cranial extradural empyema in the era of computed tomography: a review of 82 cases. *Neurosurgery*; **44**: 748–753.

Njoh J. (1990). Tropical ataxic neuropathy in Liberians. *Trop Geogr Med*; **42**: 92–94.

Ohaegbulam SC, Saddegi N, Ikerionwu S. (1980). Intracranial tumours in Enugu, Nigeria. Cancer; **46**: 2322–2324.

Olasode BJ, Shokunbi MT, Aghadiuno PU. (2000). Intracranial neoplasms in Ibadan, Nigeria. *E Afr Med J*; **77**: 4–8.

Olumide AA, Adeloye A. (1981) Intracranial abscess in Ibadan Nigeria. *E Afr Med J*; **58**: 231–239.

Oluwole OS, Onabolu AO, Link H et al. (2000). Persistence of tropical ataxic neuropathy in a Nigerian community. *J Neurol Neurosurg Psychiatry*; **69**: 96–101.

Osuntokun BO. (1968). An ataxic neuropathy in Nigeria: a clinical, biochemical and electro-physiological study. *Brain*; **91**: 215–248.

Osuntokun BO, Adeuja AOG, Schoenberg BS et al. (1987). Neurological disorders in Nigerian Africans: a community-based study. *Acta Neurol Scand*; **75**: 13–21.

Osuntokun BO, Sahota A, Ogunniyi AO et al. (1995). Lack of an association between apolipoprotein E epsilon 4 and Alzheimer's disease in elderly Nigerians. *Ann Neurol*; **38**: 463–465.

Pallangyo K, Hakanson A, Lema L et al. (1992). High HIV seroprevalence and increased HIV-associated mortality among hospitalised patients with deep bacterial infections in Dar es Salaam, Tanzania. *AIDS*; **6**: 971–976.

Parry O, Bhebhe E, Levy LF. (1999). Non-traumatic paraplegia in a Zimbabwean population – a retrospective survey. *Centr Afr J Med*; **45**: 114–119.

Plant GT, Mtanda AT, Arden GB et al. (1997). An epidemic of optic neuropathy in Tanzania: characterization of the visual disorder and associated peripheral neuropathy. *J Neurol Sci*; **145**: 127–140.

Plum F, Posner JB. (1982). *The Diagnosis of Stupor and Coma*. 3rd edn Oxford: Oxford University Press.

Poser CM. (1996). Multiple sclerosis. In *Tropical Neurology*, ed R Shakir, PK Newman, C Poser, pp. 437–455. London: WB Saunders.

Richards M, Chaudhuri KR. (1996). Parkinson's disease in populations of African origin: a review. *Neuroepidemiology*; **15**: 214–221.

Roman G. (1998). Tropical myeloneuropathies revisited. *Curr Opin Neurol*; **11**: 539–544.

Rosling H, Tylleskar T. (1996). Konzo. In *Tropical Neurology*, ed R Shakir, PK Newman, C Poser, pp. 353–374. London: WB Saunders.

Rwiza HT, Matuja WB, Kilonzo GP et al. (1993). Knowledge, attitude and practice towards epilepsy among rural Tanzanian residents. *Epilepsia*; **34**: 1017–1023.

Samuel J, Fernandes CM, Steinberg JL (1986). Intracranial otogenic complication: a persisting problem. *Laryngoscope*; **96**: 272–278.

Schnorf H, Diserens K, Schnyder H et al. (1998). Corticosteroid-

responsive postmalaria encephlopathy characterized by motor aphasia, myoclonus, and postural tremor. *Arch Neurol*; **55**: 417–420.
Schoenberg BS, Osuntokun BO, Adeuja AOG et al. (1988). Comparison of the prevalence of Parkinson's disease in black populations in the rural United States and in rural Nigeria: door-to-door community studies. *Neurology*; **38**: 645–646.
Simpson DM, Wolfe DE. (1991). Neuromuscular complications of HIV infection and its treatment. *AIDS*; **5**: 917–926.
Spillane JD. (1973). *Tropical Neurology*. London: Oxford University Press.
Tekle-Haimanot R, Abebe M, Gebre-Marians A et al. (1990). Community based study of neurological disorders in rural central Ethiopia. *Neuroepidemiology*; **9**: 263–277.
Tekle-Haimanot R, Seraw B, Forsgren L et al. (1995). Migraine, chronic tension-type headache, and cluster headache in an Ethiopian rural community. *Cephalalgia*; **15**: 482–488.
Thornton CA, Latif AS, Emmanuel JC. (1991). Guillain–Barré syndrome associated with human immunodeficiency virus infection in Zimbabwe. *Neurology*; **41**: 812–815.
Tomik B, Nicotra A, Ellis CM. (2000). Phenotypic differences between African and white patients with motor neurone disease: a case control study. *J Neurol Neurosurg Psychiatry*; **69**: 251–253.
Tylleskar T, Howlett W, Rwiza H et al. (1993). Konzo: a distinct disease entity with selective upper motor neurone damage. *J Neurol Neurosurg Psychiatry*; **56**: 638–643.
Vernant JC. (1996). HTLV-1. In *Tropical Neurology*, ed R Shakir, PK Newman, C Poser, pp. 19–36. London: WB Saunders.
Zenebe G. (1995). Myelopathies in Ethiopia. *E Afr Med J*; **72**: 42–45.

Part V

Medical aspects of other important conditions in Africa

87

The pregnant patient

Introduction

Since earlier editions of this book, important changes have affected the management of pregnant women in Africa.

1. Reproductive health has come to mean more than the absence of disease. The modern definition is 'a state of complete physical, mental and social well-being, not merely absence of disease or infirmity in matters relating to the reproductive tract, its functions and processes'. For example, safe motherhood and sexually transmitted infection are now recognized as components of reproductive health.
2. The HIV/AIDS pandemic has profoundly affected management of pregnant women in Africa.
3. Certain cultural practices rife in Africa, such as female genital mutilation, have been recognized to increase morbidity for the pregnant patient.
4. The new global economic order has led to introduction of user fees in health facilities in Africa and other developing nations. Happening in an environment where the health budgets of most African governments are shrinking while the level of poverty is increasing, there has been an attendant deterioration of most maternal health indicators in Africa.

Sub-Saharan Africa reports extremely high maternal mortality rates. Reports show maternal mortality ratios of in excess of 1000/100 000 live births (Ujah et al., 1999; WHO, 2001). The lifetime risk of a maternal death for an average woman in Africa is 1 in 21 – over 400 times higher than for their counterparts in Northern Europe. Haemorrhage, sepsis and eclampsia are the top causes of death, whilst important risk factors include adolescence, multiparity, illiteracy and non-utilization of antenatal care services. The health of the pregnant mother and her fetus is further threatened by co-existing disease, notably HIV infection, malaria, and chronic anaemia.

This chapter deals with medical conditions which may occur in pregnancy and affect its outcome. It does not deal with specific obstetric practice and complications, for which there are many available guides (see recommendations for further reading at the end of this chapter).

To understand the mechanisms by which disease can threaten pregnancy, it is useful to know the physiological changes which accompany normal gestation. These changes prepare the mother to:

- Accommodate the needs of the growing fetus
- Successfully cope with the stress of childbirth
- Initiate and maintain lactation
- Return the body to its pre-pregnancy state.

Physiological changes in pregnancy

Maternal weight gain

Generally, by the end of pregnancy, a primigravida will gain about 12.5 kg, while a multipara is likely to gain up to 1 kilogram less. Although the average weight gain is about 0.45 kg per week, this is likely to be less at both ends of the pregnancy. The weight gain is distributed between maternal and feto-placental components. The maternal weight gain is due to increase in sizes of breasts, uterus, blood volume and extracellular fluid and fat deposition in the thighs, back and abdomen. In total it accounts for about 7.7 kg. The rest of weight gained – about 4.7kg – is accounted for by the feto-placental component (fetus, amniotic fluid and placenta).

Poor weight gain can lead to low birth weight but weight gain varies widely, from nil to up to twice the mean weight gain. There is poor correlation between weight gain and energy intake. In the post-partum period most of the weight is shed – usually in the first week – but commonly the post-partum weight is about 3 kg above the pre-pregnancy weight.

Cardiovascular changes

Cardiovascular changes occur in both cardiac function and the blood vessel reactivity. The majority of these changes are established by 12 weeks of pregnancy. Generally, the pregnant woman's vascular tree is less responsive to the vaso-active agent – angiotensin 2. This is thought to be due to altered prostanoid balance with prostaglandin I2 (prostacyclin) predominating over others like PGF2-alpha. Together, the effects of progesterone on arterial smooth muscles plus the pressure-dissipating effect of fully developed maternal blood lacunae in the placenta lead to:

- reduced arterial blood pressure
- increased venous capacitance, so that more blood pools in dilated peripheral veins.

Arterial blood pressure in pregnancy is sensitive to changes in posture. Sitting blood pressure is higher than supine pressure, which is itself higher than blood pressure with the woman lying on her side. This phenomenon is used in the roll-over test. This is positive if there is a blood pressure rise of more than 15 mmHg on rolling the woman over from the lateral recumbent to the supine position. Done at 12 to 14 weeks gestation, the test predicts those women whose vascular response to angiotensin 2 has not been dampened as expected in normal pregnancy: they are therefore theoretically prone to develop pregnancy-induced hypertension in the second half of pregnancy. Pressure of the pregnant uterus on the vena cava can lead to fainting in the supine position, so called supine hypotensive syndrome.

The cardiac changes include:

- anatomical change such as the upward and lateral shift of the apex beat due to the upward diaphragmatic shift due to the enlarging uterus. Also important is increase in heart volume and the increased myocardial contractility.
- increase in cardiac output by up to 1.5 litres per minute at rest (and 2 litres per minute during a contraction in labour). Increase in heart rate accounts for abut 10–15 per cent of this rise, the rest being contributed by increase in stroke volume.

Haematological changes

Changes occur in blood volume and red cell mass. The plasma volume increases by about 40–50 per cent, reaching maximum levels in the third trimester. The red cell mass also increases, achieving a lesser rise of 33 per cent. On average, the plasma volume increases by about 1250 ml, and the red cell volume by 350 ml. The differential rise in the two components of the blood volume leads to the so-called dilutional anaemia of pregnancy, which accounts for a drop in haemoglobin of up to 2 g/dl, the maximum drop being in weeks 22 to 28 in African women, slightly later in Caucasians. The haematocrit (PCV) falls typically from about 0.4 to 0.34. The mean corpuscular haemoglobin concentration (MCHC) and the mean corpuscular haemoglobin (MCH) do not change significantly. Iron and folate supplements boost the rise in the red cell mass, a phenomenon that may happen naturally in Bantu women with high dietary iron intake.

There is also a rise in the total white cell count, reaching counts of up to 12×10^9/l. Most of this is due to polymorphonuclear leukocytosis. Platelets also rise steadily, and actually peak during the puerperium at about 600×10^9/l.

Respiratory function

Increased ventilation in pregnancy is achieved through deep breathing rather than fast breathing. The changes are as follows.

- The diaphragm rises and becomes progressively splinted by the rising uterine fundus in late pregnancy. This leads to increased reliance on the intercostal muscles for ventilation.
- The inspiratory capacity increases by late pregnancy.
- The vital capacity increases in some women.
- The tidal volume increases by up to 40 per cent thereby increasing minute ventilation. There is a slight decrease in $p\mathrm{CO}_2$, with mild respiratory alkalosis.

Renal function

There are both anatomical and functional changes in the renal system.

- Dilatation of the pelvi-calyceal system and the ureters by end of first trimester. In addition, the ureteric smooth muscle undergoes both hypertrophy and hyperplasia. Vesico-ureteric reflux and dilatation lead to urinary stasis and predispose to urinary tract infections.
- Functionally, there is a 30–50 per cent rise in renal blood flow, with increased glomerular filtration rate. There is also increased tubular reabsorption of sodium and potassium. The effects of these changes include decreased plasma uric acid, creatinine and urea levels. Due to increased GFR, glycosuria is common in pregnancy.

- There is a 2.5-fold rise in plasma renin concentration but there is an accompanying selective loss of vascular response to angiotensin 2 and a gradual increase in aldosterone levels.

Gastrointestinal function

The overriding change is decreased motility of the entire gastrointestinal tract. This is thought to be due to the effect of progesterone on smooth muscle. The net effect is delayed gastric emptying, increased absorption of sodium and water in the colon, and decreased cardiac sphincter tone. The clinical manifestation of all this is heartburn and constipation.

Placental function and endocrine changes

The placenta plays a major endocrine role, together with the fetus, leading to the term, feto-placental unit, especially in the elaboration of steroid hormones. The main placental hormones include the following.

- Human chorionic gonadotrophin, a glycoprotein with beta and alpha subunits. It is detected in pregnancy tests, with levels normally peaking between 7 and 8 weeks gestation. HCG levels are considerably higher than normal in multiple pregnancy and in trophoblastic diseases such as hydatidiform mole, invasive mole and choriocarcinoma. In these diseases it acts as a reliable tumour marker.
- Human placental lactogen, a peptide hormone, thought to be largely responsible for the diabetogenic effect of pregnancy.
- Steroid hormones, derived from plasma cholesterol and synthesized by the feto-placental unit. Examples are:
  - *Progesterone* From the seventeenth week of pregnancy, the feto-placental unit is the major source of this hormone. Up to 350 mg of progesterone is made per day. Plasma progesterone level and urine pregnanediol (the excretory form of progesterone) act as measures of placental function.
  - *Oestrogens* The major oestrogens include estradiol 17-beta, estrone and estriol. The placenta uses fetal adrenal substrate, dehydroepiandrosterone, to make estriol whose levels rise 1000-fold in pregnancy. Estriol is used as a measure of fetal well-being. Estradiol and estrone are made directly by the syncytiotrophoblast.

Other placental functions include gas exchange, fetal nutrition and waste disposal. Other endocrine changes include the following.

- Pituitary gland enlargement, mainly accounted for by anterior lobe prolactin-secreting cell hyperplasia. ACTH levels also rise while gonadotrophin secretion is decreased
- The thyroid gland enlarges as the renal changes lead to increased urinary iodine secretion and relative fall of plasma iodide. The thyroid follicular enlargement enhances iodine uptake. Thyroid binding globulin rises, and therefore total T3 and T4 rise, but unbound (free) T3 and T4 remain essentially unchanged. TSH also remains normal. These hormones do not cross the placental barrier.
- In the adrenal glands, plasma cortisol increases throughout pregnancy due to increase in the binding protein, but the unbound form also rises. Sex hormones, aldosterone and 11– deoxycorticosterone also increase. There is little change in the catecholamines, which are from the adrenal medulla.

Anaemia in pregnancy

Anaemia has been defined as haemoglobin level less than 110 g/l of blood (WHO, 1968). In many African centres a threshold of 100 g/l has been found more realistic.

Pregnancy-associated anaemia is common in Africa. The prevalence ranges between 8 per cent and 30 per cent. A recent Ethiopian study reports a prevalence rate of 18.4 per cent with significant regional differences in the prevalence, even within the same countries (Haidar et al., 1999) – see the Box.

Causes of pregnancy-associated anaemia

Poor nutrition
Secondary to infection
Haemoglobinopathies (HbS and HbC in West Africa)
Thalassaemias (Mediterranean regions)
Malaria
Hookworm

Anaemia in the pregnant patient affects both the mother and the fetus. Fetal effects may be severe, including spontaneous abortion, pre-term delivery, fetal growth restriction, and perinatal fetal death. In the mother even small amounts of blood loss at delivery may lead to heart failure, poor wound healing and burst abdomen where the patient has been delivered abdominally. Anaemia is an indirect cause of maternal mortality.

Clinical evaluation of anaemia

The evaluation of the anaemic pregnant patient has two objectives:

- to assess the severity of the anaemia
- to make an aetiological diagnosis.

Clinical assessment will thus include the presence and severity of pallor, and clinical signs of chronic anaemia, such as angular stomatitis, glossitis, and koilonychia. There may be evidence of haemolysis, such as jaundice or hepatosplenomegaly. Constitutional symptoms such as dizziness, tachycardia and signs of congestive cardiac failure suggest severe anaemia.

The effect of anaemia on the progress of pregnancy is assessed by comparing uterine size with gestational age, as calculated from the last menstrual period.

Investigations

- Full blood count (haemogram) with peripheral blood morphology and red cell indices
- Thick and thin films for malarial parasites
- Stool microscopy for hookworm and other parasites
- Hb electrophoresis and sickling test where appropriate
- Liver function tests
- Bone marrow aspiration and biopsy in appropriate cases.

Treatment

Anaemia is not an indication for termination of pregnancy or induction of labour. Vaginal delivery is allowed unless there are contraindications. However, if pregnancy has reached late third trimester, it is urgent to correct anaemia before the patient goes into labour. Transfusion of packed cells needs to be considered in severe anaemia ($Hb < 70$ g/l). Mild anaemia can be treated with haematinics alone. In the treatment of iron deficiency anaemia, total dose infusion of iron guarantees full treatment. The underlying cause of the anaemia must be treated at the same time (for example, malaria or hookworm).

Severe anaemia where the patient is already in congestive heart failure is very dangerous in pregnancy, with significant risk of maternal death. Exchange transfusion under cover of diuretics such as frusemide should be considered. If the patient goes into labour already in heart failure, management is similar to that of other cases of cardiac disease during labour. This implies labouring in the propped up position, administration of oxygen by facial mask as needed, assisted second stage of labour using vacuum extraction, avoiding ergometrine (using syntocinon only, if needed) and giving loop diuretics in third stage.

A clinical summary of the management of anaemia in pregnancy is presented at the end of this chapter (Table 87.4).

Prevention

Good pre-natal care should prevent anaemia or diagnose it early enough to allow correction before delivery. Haematinic use by pregnant, especially vulnerable target groups such as single mothers, teenage mothers, primigravidae, multiparae, multiple pregnancy, previous history of anaemia, and patients from areas endemic for hookworm and/or malaria infections is to be recommended. The Box summarizes prophylactic measures to be considered.

Prophylaxis of anaemia of pregnancy in African women

- Haematinics (ferrous sulphate, 200mg, or ferrous fumarate giving equivalent of 60 mg elemental –100 mg iron per day, plus folic acid 500 micrograms daily). These are given as supplements to all expectant mothers.
- Anti-malarials in areas of high endemicity (according to local resistance patterns)
- Mebendazole 100 mg or albendazole 400 mg (single doses) where hookworm is prevalent
- Increased dietary fresh fruit (Vitamin C to improve utilization of micronutrients)
- Avoidance of dietary chelators such as tannins in tea and coffee, phytates
- Delay next pregnancy by 3 years to allow replenishment of micronutrient stores.

Malaria in pregnancy

More than 23 million pregnant women in sub-Saharan Africa live in malaria endemic areas. *Plasmodium falciparum* is common in East and Central Africa. *Plasmodium vivax* and *malariae* are commoner in the Western African countries. Mixed infection is not uncommon. Reduced immunity during pregnancy leads to increased susceptibility to malaria. This is particularly pronounced amongst primigravidae for whom malaria may be devastating.

The main complications of malaria in the pregnant patient are anaemia and complications such as cerebral malaria and renal failure. For the fetus, the main sequelae include fetal growth restriction, abortion, pre-term labour and malaria by vertical transmission. Malaria causes up to 30 per cent of preventable low birthweight deliveries and 3–5 per cent of neonatal mortality in endemic regions.

More rigorous prophylactic regimens are recommended in areas with high HIV seroprevalence rates.

Furthermore, drug resistance patterns need to be taken into account and be constantly reviewed by regions. In general, it can be recommended that, in areas with transmission, all gravidas need anti-malarial prophylaxis. Prophylaxis with sulphadoxine–pyrimethamine combinations in an endemic area in Kenya has demonstrated 85 per cent protective efficacy against peripheral parasitaemia and 39 per cent protective efficacy against malaria-related anaemia (Shulman et al., 1999). Similar findings have also been documented in Malawi when the SP combination was administered in second and third trimesters (Steketee et al., 1996). Pregnant women should also be advised to prevent mosquito bites through use of mosquito nets impregnated with pyrethrins. Acute malarial infections require vigorous anti-malarial treatment. Table 87.1 outlines drugs used in management of malaria.

Hypertensive disease in pregnancy

Hypertensive disease in pregnancy is often a silent condition, usually picked up during routine pre-natal care or presents as a life-threatening entity such as imminent or overt eclampsia or as symptoms of related cardiovascular events. Hypertension can be defined in three ways.

- diastolic blood pressure of 90 mmHg and above or systolic blood pressure of 140 mmHg and above on two occasions 6 hours apart after 15 minutes rest
- mean arterial blood pressure (diastolic blood pressure + 1/3 of the pulse pressure) of 105 mmHg on two occasions 6 hours apart after 15 minutes rest
- rise in diastolic blood pressure of 15 mmHg and or in systolic blood pressure of 30 mmHg above the baseline blood pressure.

In Africa, since many pregnant women either do not have pre-natal care or, when they do, make the first visit in the second half of pregnancy, the last definition is seldom used.

In pregnancy, hypertensive disease can be broadly classified into three:

- pregnancy-induced hypertension
- chronic hypertension and
- chronic hypertension with superimposed pregnancy-induced hypertension.

Pregnancy-induced hypertension is unique to pregnancy and, although commonly a progressively deteriorating clinical entity, will often resolve once the pregnancy is terminated. Chronic hypertension, either secondary or essential, is discussed elsewhere in detail.

Table 87.1. Available anti-malarial drugs for use in pregnancy

Drug	Application	Comments on efficacy in Africa and safety in pregnancy
Chloroquine	Prophylaxis/treatment	Widespread resistance, safe
Quinine	Treatment of complicated malaria	Resistance uncommon, watch for pre-term labour and hypoglycaemia
Mefloquine	Treatment/prophylaxis	Resistance increasing, association with still births needs further study
Artemisinin derivatives	Treatment	Efficacious, safe
Mefloquine and artemisinin	Treatment	Use in multi-drug resistance
Pryimethamine	Treatment/prophylaxis	Emerging resistance, safe in pregnancy
Proguanil	Prophylaxis	Resistance, safe
Clindamycin and tetracycline	Treatment	Not for use in pregnancy

The combination of the two often is more rapidly progressing.

For the purpose of clinical management of the patient, hypertension in pregnancy can be divided into:

- mild disease (BP of 140 mmHg systolic and/or 90 mmHg diastolic)
- moderate disease (BP of 140 to 159 mmHg systolic and/or 90 to 109 mmHg diastolic) and
- severe disease (BP of more than 160 mmHg systolic and more than 110 mmHg diastolic).

Public health significance in Africa

Hypertensive disease in pregnancy is a leading cause of both maternal and perinatal morbidity and mortality, as well as being an important cause of pregnancy wastage through fetal deaths. It contributes to about 12 per cent of all maternal mortality in developing countries. Mortality arises from eclampsia and its complications such as pulmonary oedema, stroke and acute renal failure. The fetal and perinatal losses occur through a combination of intrauterine insults leading to growth restriction and eventually abortion, death or through iatrogenic pre-term deliveries which lead to neonatal death in much of Africa. Management of cases of hypertensive disease therefore represents a significant strain on the resources of the fledgling health sectors common in the continent.

Clinical evaluation

Clinical findings are often scant in the mild disease. Normally, the main feature is raised blood pressure fitting one of the above criteria. However, if the first blood pressure reading is in the severe range, then it is assumed significant even without repeat reading. In pregnancy-induced hypertension (PIH), oedema may also be elicited. This is often more clinically significant if it is in the non-dependent areas such as face and hands.

Key features of severe PIH may include:

- headache
- blurring of vision
- right upper quadrant abdominal pain
- palpitations
- dyspnoea
- reduced urinary output
- convulsions in eclampsia
- disease of second half of pregnancy except in multiple, molar pregnancy and sometimes diabetic gravidas.

Evidence of impending or overt cardiac failure may be manifest. Fundoscopy will also be abnormal.

Obstetric evaluation includes the presence of fetal movement, if the gestation is more than 24 weeks, a comparison of the gestational age with the uterine size on abdominal examination, will suggest or rule out fetal growth restriction. Furthermore, the amount of liquor can be assessed clinically, depending on the gestation at presentation. In the eclamptic patient, there is need to perform pelvic examination to exclude or confirm labour. This part of the examination is to assist decision on the mode of delivery, but, it is usually delayed until the convulsions are controlled and blood pressure, if severe, lowered.

Investigations

These can be done to strengthen diagnosis and to assess the severity of disease by laboratory findings:

- albuminuria
- elevated serum uric acid levels
- creatinine clearance
- serum urea
- electrocardiography and echocardiography
- full haematology and biochemistry in severe cases (elevated liver enzymes, except alkaline phosphatase, intravascular haemolysis and thrombocytopenia can all occur).

Obstetric ultrasound, reported as the fetal biophysical profile (see the Box), is useful where clinical parameters suggest fetal compromise, especially in the third trimester. At this stage decisions on pregnancy termination must be weighed against fetal interests.

Fetal biophysical profile (parameters each scored out of 2):

- Fetal cardiac reactivity
- Amniotic fluid volume
- Fetal breathing movements
- Fetal tone
- Fetal movements

Interpretation: score <6 = further evaluation necessary.

Treatment

The obstetric management of a pregnant hypertensive depends on:

- gestation of the pregnancy
- severity of the disease
- level of newborn care services available and
- type of hypertension.

Generally, disease occurring near term often leads to a decision to deliver the patient in the interests of both mother and fetus. Severe disease will weigh the decision in favour of termination of the pregnancy in the interests of the mother, fetal interests usually being secondary. Where the gestation is near extra-uterine viability, depending on the local facilities for neonatal care, then considerable effort is often made to achieve this even among patients with severe disease in the hope of achieving good maternal and neonatal outcome. Careful monitoring of both the mother and fetus then becomes necessary. Adjuvant therapy to hasten fetal lung maturity as with corticosteroid may be considered, but its use in hypertensive patients is controversial.

Chronic hypertension cases may be severe early in the pregnancy leading to poor prognosis for the fetus. Pregnancy-induced hypertension, on the other hand, tends to deteriorate continuously until delivery is achieved, regardless of apparently good hypertensive control. Note that this is a systemic disease and hypertension is only one clinical finding.

Table 87.2 lists commonly available drugs for the treatment of pregnancy-induced hypertension and eclampsia.

In terms of obstetric care, eclamptics need to be delivered by the fastest means possible that is least traumatic to the mother or baby. This reduces the risk of further convulsions which determine the severity of neurological sequelae. Generally, if the patient is already in labour, and there is no contraindication to vaginal delivery, then vaginal delivery with elective vacuum extraction at second stage is allowed. Ergometrine is avoided in the conduct of the third stage of labour. Otherwise, those

Table 87.2. Anti-hypertensive drugs

• α-methyl dopa: 250 mg 8-hourly to maximum of 1 g 12-hourly • hydralazine: 25 mg 8-hourly orally or 20 mg intravenously after test dose followed by 40 mg in 5 per cent dextrose 500 ml titrated against bp in severe disease • nifedipine: 20 mg sublinguinally, followed by 10–20 mg 12-hourly orally
Anti-convulsant drugs • diazepam: 10–20 mg intravenously followed by 20 mg in 5 per cent dextrose given as an infusion titrated against consciousness. Patient kept just rousable • [a]magnesium sulphate: 4 mg intravenously loading dose followed by 1 g hourly, or 5 mg intramuscularly every 4 hours

Notes:
[a] Make certain that your midwives are competent to monitor toxicity through respiratory rate and patellar jerk before putting magnesium sulphate to general use. Serum magnesium assays can also assist in monitoring for toxicity, where the laboratory facility is available.

not in labour are considered for emergency abdominal delivery, unless there is fetal death or the gestation is unlikely to be compatible with extra-uterine life for the neonate and hysterotomy is unacceptable.

In about 20 per cent of eclamptics, the onset of convulsions may be the first 48 hours post-partum.

Prognosis

Hypertension in pregnancy, regardless of the type, carries serious risks for both the fetus and the mother. Possible fetal outcomes include fetal growth restriction, fetal death, iatrogenic pre-term delivery and neonatal death. Maternal sequelae include acute renal shutdown, intracerebral haemorrhage, pulmonary oedema and consumptive coagulopathy. Patients who have had pregnancy-induced hypertension are at higher risk of a similar episode in a subsequent pregnancy.

Prevention

To prevent development of PIH, several strategies have been studied.

- acetyl-salicylic acid – equivocal efficacy
- calcium and vitamin E supplementation useful
- magnesium sulphate: under study in The Magpie Trial.

A further table on clinical mangement is at the end of this chapter (Table 87.5).

HIV and pregnancy

The first case of human immunodeficiency virus infection was described around 1983. Since then the virus has been extensively studied and a large amount of literature about the infection has been and continues to be published. Its toll on humankind, in general, and on the African people specifically, has been similarly heavy.

Epidemiology of HIV infection with specific relevance to Africa

The chief modes of transmission include hetero- and homosexual routes, through exchange of body fluids (for example blood transfusion), and through mother-to-child transmission (MTCT). MTCT can occur antenatally, during labour and in the post-partum period through breast-feeding. It is estimated that globally, 20 to 40 per cent of HIV-positive pregnant women will pass the virus to their babies.

World-wide, the burden of HIV infection is large. At the end of 1998, it was estimated that more than 33 million people were living with HIV and half of these were women in the reproductive age group. There were over 1 million children with HIV acquired through vertical transmission. Sixty-six per cent of infected adults and 90 per cent of the world's HIV-infected children live in Africa (AIDS epidemic Update: December 1998. Joint United Nations Programme on HIV/AIDS, 1998).

HIV infection has become the commonest condition in pregnancy in Africa. It is estimated that 1 million HIV-positive women become pregnant annually leading to approximately 400 000 HIV-positive children annually through mother-to-child transmission.

Two main types of HIV have been identified, namely HIV1, which is the most common, and HIV2 which is mainly found in West Africa and areas of Angola and Mozambique. Dual infection is possible. HIV2 is less virulent and HIV1 is spreading. The most affected areas of Africa are in sub-Saharan Africa. In East, Central and Southern Africa the HIV prevalence rates among pregnant women range between 10 per cent and 40 per cent with pockets of up to 60 per cent. It is known that transmission from the male to female is 2–3 times higher than female to male. In addition to this excessive risk, women in Africa are at further risk due to socio-cultural practices such as dry sex, female genital mutilation and widow cleansing, among others. Other genital tract infections, known to be still quite prevalent in Africa, have also been shown to facilitate the acquisition of the HIV infection. Near universal breast-feeding, together with rampant poverty, lead to a prolonged exposure of the newborn to the possibility of MTCT as alternative baby feeds are commonly beyond the financial reach of the majority.

Effect of HIV infection on pregnancy

Although the available evidence is conflicting, association between HIV infection and several unfavourable pregnancy outcomes has been recorded. Higher rates of spontaneous abortion, ectopic pregnancy, pre-term labour, pre-labour rupture of fetal membranes, abruptio placentae, low birthweight, stillbirths and puerperal sepsis have all been reported. The major weakness in these studies has been the inability to control for confounding factors. These factors include concurrent infection with other sexually transmitted infections such as syphilis; opportunistic infections such as pneumonias, tuberculosis, herpes zoster and urinary tract infections; use of drugs in pregnancy and antenatal care services.

Effect of pregnancy on natural history of HIV infection

Both pregnancy and HIV infection suppress immune function. Cell, antibody and the complement-mediated immune responses are decreased in pregnancy. However, available evidence shows that, in asymptomatic women and in those with early disease, pregnancy does not appear to accelerate the deterioration of the HIV infection, although there seems to be more rapid progression in women with late stage disease.

Factors predisposing to MTCT of HIV

Viral factors

- high viral load
- the viral type – HIV1 more virulent.

Maternal factors

- late disease
- immune deficiency due to vitamin A deficiency
- anaemia, poor nutrition
- rising viral load during pregnancy or breast-feeding due to unprotected sex, multiple partners
- smoking and other substance abuse.

Obstetrical factors

- vaginal delivery (compared to Caesarean delivery)
- rupture of fetal membranes >4 hours
- invasive procedures such as external cephalic version amniocentesis, episiotomy and vacuum extraction.

Fetal/infant factors

- prematurity
- mixed feeding (concurrent breast-feeding and alternative feeding)
- breast disease such as mastitis, cracked nipples.

Maternity care and prevention of MTCT of HIV

In areas of high HIV prevalence, maternity services have three main responsibilities, namely:

- facilitate voluntary testing of women and use the results to help maintain their health
- utilize locally appropriate interventions to reduce MTCT of HIV and
- train staff and provide equipment to prevent hospital transmission of HIV and other infections.

Antenatal care

- voluntary counselling and testing for HIV. Need for more acute services in Africa as follow-up is often difficult.
- For those who are HIV-positive:
  - identify and treat opportunistic infections, e.g. tuberculosis, other respiratory infections, oral/vaginal candidosis, herpes zoster, persistent diarrhoea, skin conditions and other sexually transmitted infections
  - nutritional support with multivitamins and mineral supplements.
  - encouraging lifestyle changes such as safe sex, avoidance of alcohol and substance abuse, stress reduction
  - prophylaxis with tetanus toxoid, anti-malarials according to the parasite drug resistance patterns, and co-trimoxazole (this reduces incidence of chest infections including *Pneumocystis carinii* pneumonia).
  - other routine antenatal care as per level of obstetric risk (similar to the HIV-negative patients).

Labour and delivery care

Some evidence (though not conclusive) is available about the benefit of simple interventions in preventing MTCT of HIV. These include:

- minimizing the number of pelvic examinations
- delaying amniotomy as long as feasible without compromising diagnosis of fetal distress
- vaginal cleansing with 0.25 per cent chlorhexidine solution during first stage of labour.
- avoidance of routine episiotomy
- use of plastic Ventouse caps may be protective

- wiping the baby's mouth and nose is to be preferred to deep suction, unless there is meconium stained liquor
- clamping the cord, tying and cutting immediately, without milking the cord
- washing the baby in warm 0.25 per cent chlorhexidine solution immediately and drying with a towel.
- BCG vaccination, vitamin K injection and 1 per cent tetracycline eye ointment application are also given.

Note that caesarean section, though protective, is unlikely to be a viable public health intervention in Africa.

Post-partum care

In addition to routine post-partum care:

- antibiotic prophylaxis is advised (typically ampicillin 500 mg three times daily, at least 30 minutes before meals)
- use alternative feeds if affordable and available
- if breast-feeding, avoidance of:
  - mixed feeding
  - cracked nipples by proper breast-feeding practices
  - prompt treatment of oral thrush in the baby.

Antiretroviral therapy

Many regimens with demonstrated efficacy exist. However, due to widespread poverty and poorly funded health sector, currently, the only affordable regime is nevirapine 200 mg to the mother once at onset of labour, or first contact in labour, and 2 mg/kg infant weight given within 72 hours of birth.

Preventing health provider occupational exposure

Health workers are expected to be familiar with, and to apply, universal precautions for infection prevention. Where the drugs are affordable, a policy for prophylaxis in response to possible occupational exposure, such as needle-stick injuries, needs to be developed by the various countries and facilities.

Puerperal sepsis

This can be defined as infection occurring at any time between the onset of labour or rupture of membranes and the 42nd day post-partum, in which two or more of the following can be identified: pelvic pain, fever (oral temperature of 38.5 °C or higher on any occasion), abnormal vaginal discharge, usually purulent, foul smelling discharge and sub-involution of the uterus (<2 cm/day in the first week). Note that the term puerperal infection is considered more general and includes extra-genital and incidental infections.

Most of the organisms that cause puerperal sepsis are commensals of the lower genital tract and gut. Eventually, puerperal sepsis is a poly-microbial infection including aerobes, anaerobes and both gram-positive and negative organisms. They gain access to the uterus during labour and through pelvic examination. Prolonged rupture of fetal membranes, prolonged labour, repeated pelvic examinations and retained products of conception have been shown to be independently associated with increased risk of developing puerperal sepsis.

Public health significance and relevance to Africa

Puerperal sepsis and infections are an important cause of maternal morbidity and mortality in the developing countries accounting for as much as 33 per cent of all maternal mortality. In Africa, home deliveries conducted without regard to asepsis, obstructed labour with subsequent operative delivery – either vaginal or abdominal and use of vaginally inserted herbs all contribute to increased risk of puerperal sepsis. Furthermore, genital injuries during labour as a result of previous female genital mutilation scars or pre-existing sexually transmitted infections play a role. Pre-existing genital tract infections are also known to be a etiologically associated with spontaneous rupture of fetal membranes, before onset of labour. Malnutrition and anaemia in the gravida also increase their susceptibility. HIV infection, and especially AIDS, completes the complex picture.

Other important puerperal infections

Important differential diagnoses include:

- malaria
- urinary tract infection
- thrombophlebitis and
- mastitis.

Treatment of puerperal sepsis

Depending on how severely ill the patient is, supportive treatment may be required including intravenous fluids. The choice of antibiotics depends on safety with breast-feeding, availability, and recognition that broad spectrum coverage is mandatory. Antibiotic monotherapy is unlikely to be adequate, commonly combination therapy is called for. New generation cephalosporins, together with aminoglycosides, will commonly suffice.

Complications

These may include:

- endotoxic shock
- pelvic abscess collection (an indication for laparotomy and drainage)
- long-term complications may include ectopic pregnancy, infertility, dysmenorrhoea and chronic pelvic pain.

A further table on the clinical management of puerperal sepsis is at the end of this chapter (Table 87.6).

Other infections in pregnancy

Viral hepatitis

Viral hepatitides are infections by agents whose primary tropism is the liver. At least five hepatitis viruses have been identified to date, designated hepatitis A, B, C, D, and E. Acute hepatitis may occur with human cytomegalovirus, Epstein–Barr virus, herpes simplex virus, yellow fever and rubella viruses.

These infections are both important and common. In parts of Africa, the sero-prevalence for the hepatitis viruses is very high especially in the rural areas. In Zambia, hepatitis B surface antigen has been reported in 6.5 per cent of pregnant women in a region where the range is between 10 and 15 per cent. Concurrent presence of hepatitis B antigen, which is an indicator of vertical transmission of the virus, was reported in 16.1 per cent of pregnant women. It is thought that vertical is less important than horizontal transmission in the region (Oshitani et al., 1995). Clinical features include anorexia, nausea, vomiting, jaundice and right upper quadrant pain. Anicteric infections are much more common and jaundice when it occurs is often a late feature. Liver aminotransferases are usually elevated. Malaria infection with severe haemolysis is also a differential diagnosis. Pregnancy-related liver disease also needs to be considered. Treatment is usually expectant although the immune compromised state that pregnancy confers on the patient could, theoretically, adversely alter the course of the disease. However, there is no evidence that pregnancy alters the course of the hepatitides.

Sexually transmitted infections

These are common and very important because they are known to increase the risk of HIV infection and the risk of vertical transmission to the fetus. They are also known to contribute to pregnancy wastage. Moreover, they are commonly asymptomatic. In many antenatal clinics, screening for syphilis is routinely done, while the first sign of pre-existing gonococcal or chlamydial infection might be ophthalmia neonatorum. Historical risk assessment for sexually transmitted infection – such as single status, not living together, malodorous vaginal discharge and low abdominal pain – may be useful in identifying potential cases. Generally, screening of all pregnant women for sexually transmitted infections is to be strongly recommended. Syndromic approach to management of sexually transmitted infection may then be implemented, using drugs that are relevant to local drug sensitivity patterns (see Chapter 14). Routine prophylactic use of 1 per cent tetracycline eye ointments for all newborns is also recommended. Other sequelae in pregnancy include abortions, low birthweight delivery, pre-labour rupture of fetal membranes and pre-term delivery (Wasserheit & Holmes, 1992) Pre-labour rupture of membranes is an important aetiological association of puerperal sepsis, MTCT of HIV and pre-term delivery and its attendant high neonatal morbidity and mortality.

The use of drugs in pregnancy

Use of drugs in pregnancy must consider the interactions between the maternal, placental and fetal environments. Maternal physiological changes impact drug pharmacokinetics. Some relevant principles in perinatal prescription are outlined in this section. Due to the large number of drugs that could be used in pregnancy, discussion of specific drug indications and contraindications is considered beyond the scope of this section.

Pregnancy

Pregnancy *per se* has little effect on drug absorption. Serum albumin concentration decreases despite increased production. This is due to plasma volume expansion. Consequently, albumin binding capacity to drugs decreases and hence the unbound or free drug available for transplacental transfer is more.

Placenta

The primary drug transfer mechanism is simple diffusion, dependent on drug chemical properties and concentration gradient of the free or unbound drug. Unbound, unionized, lipid soluble drugs of less than 1000 daltons penetrate the placenta. Most drugs have molecular weight of between 250 and 500 daltons. Transplacental transfer is greater in late gestation due to increased free drug availability, increased uteroplacental blood flow, increased placental surface area, decreased thickness of tissue between placental capillaries, greater physical disruption of the placental membrane and the trapping effect on basic drugs by the acidic fetal circulation. Placental drug metabolism is thought to be less than fetal liver metabolism.

Fetus

Fetal plasma levels of drugs that cross the placental barrier are between 50 and 100 per cent of maternal serum concentration. The blood–brain permeability is higher in the fetus than in adults, while the total plasma protein and the protein binding capacity for drugs is lower in the fetus than in the mother. Consequently, there is likely to be higher fetal free drug and higher central nervous system drug levels. Drug excretion is slower in the fetus. The primary excretion route is placental through simple diffusion along the free drug concentration gradient. Fetal urine is the second route, but mainly facilitates the enterohepatic route of metabolism.

In terms of adverse effects, total fetal exposure to drugs is more important than the rate of transplacental transfer. Some drugs have affinity for specific tissue hence the consequences of exposure to them are likely to be tissue specific. Some of the deleterious effects include: no effect, abortions, malformations, altered fetal growth, functional deficit and mutagenesis.

Pregnant women may use drugs for medication, before pregnancy is confirmed, or self-prescribed drugs. Generally, few drugs, if any, are known to be safe for the developing embryo. It is safe practice to assume that most medications are potentially hazardous. The use of drugs in pregnancy, particularly in the first trimester, becomes a delicate balance between benefit to the mother and risk to the fetus.

Gestational diabetes

Pregnancy may be associated with pre-existing diabetes or disease that is first diagnosed during the course of pregnancy or occult glucose intolerance. Diabetes is the commonest metabolic disorder that is compatible with pregnancy. Pregnancy, through the effect of a combination of factors, the most prominent being the human placental lactogen, is diabetogenic. Diabetes discovered for the first time in pregnancy is called gestational diabetes and is the main subject of this section.

Screening

This is usually by a random blood sugar or a 2-hour postprandial blood sugar. Equivocal findings are further evaluated through oral glucose tolerance test. The following clinical findings necessitate screening:

- family history of diabetes
- previous macrosomic baby – >4 kg
- previous unexplained stillbirths
- recurrent glycosuria
- previous major fetal malformations
- polyhydramnios.

Management

The management of any form of diabetes in pregnancy should be a multidisciplinary effort. It should involve obstetricians, neonatologist, diabetologists, nutritionists, at least. The management principles are as follows.

- Soluble insulin or a combination of short- and medium-acting insulin is used. Oral hypoglycemics are not used.
- Tight control is aimed for – blood sugar of below 7 mmol/l.
- In those who are known diabetics, pre-conception care with tight control before conception and in first trimester reduces incidence of fetal malformations.
- Blood sugar is used for monitoring control, urine sugars are misleading.
- Antenatal assessment includes ultrasound to exclude fetal malformation, polyhydramnios and fetal macrosomia.
- Delivery is planned for 38 weeks gestation unless normal blood sugars have been maintained throughout pregnancy, which is rarely the case. Fetal lung maturity should be confirmed before induction of labour. Use of the traditional surfactant test can be misleading. Phosphatidyl glycerol assay is more reliable. Risk of shoulder dystocia is high especially if fetal macrosomia is not diagnosed early. Caesarean section is only indicated for obstetric reasons, not the diabetes *per se*.

Maternal complications

- Hyperglycaemia and ketoacidosis
- Hypoglycaemia leading to fetal death if prolonged.
- Pre-eclampsia
- Recurrent candidiasis, cystitis.

Fetal and neonatal complications

- Malformations are up to five times more common.
- Neonatal hypoglycaemia, babies need to be fed with oral glucose and their blood sugars monitored until lactation is established. Initial feeding must be professionally supervised as there is high risk of gastrointestinal malformations, among others.
- Respiratory distress syndrome especially where lung maturity is not confirmed before induction of labour.

Health services for the pregnant patient in Africa

Discussion of care of the pregnant patient in Africa would be incomplete without a description of the available services. Throughout Africa, there is considerable variation in the type and quality of health care services targeting the pregnant patient. There are regional and rural–urban differentials. Generally, three levels of care can be identified.

Community-based care

This common delivery care occurs at home with the pregnant woman being assisted by either relatives or traditional birth attendants or occasionally delivering without any help at all. Complications occurring during labour and the post-partum period may take time to be recognized leading to severe morbidity and even maternal mortality. Neonatal resuscitation skills are also often deficient or absent leading to perinatal losses.

Health centre-based care

This is commonly a health facility manned by midwives and medical assistants. The facility is supposed to be easily accessible to the communities and to offer basic essential obstetric care such as parenteral antibiotics for cases of puerperal sepsis, parenteral oxytocic drugs for bleeding patients, parenteral sedatives for eclampsia, manual removal of the placenta and uterine evacuation for cases of incomplete abortion. The facility should also be able to refer, promptly, more complicated cases to a facility with comprehensive obstetric care services.

District hospital-based care

This should be manned by both midwives and doctors and should offer all basic or health centre level essential obstetric care, in addition to abdominal surgery – caesarean section and laparotomy for ectopic pregnancy – and should be capable of offering blood transfusion services.

Table 87.3. Antenatal care, place of delivery and delivery assistance: Kenya (based on births 3 years preceding survey)

	Percentage
Antenatal care	
Doctor	28
Nurse/Midwife	64
Traditional birth attendant	2
None	6
Place of delivery	
Health facility	42
Home	57
Delivery assistance	
Doctor	12
Nurse/midwife	32
Traditional birth attendant	21
Relatives/others	24
No one	10

Source: National Council for Population and Development & Central Bureau of Statistic, Office of the Vice President and Ministry of Planning and National Development, Government of Kenya; Kenya Demographic and Health Survey: 1998.

It is estimated that 10 per cent of all pregnancies will become complicated at some stage. These will require care only offered at the health centre or the hospital level. About 90 per cent of pregnant patients have some antenatal care in Africa, but most complications cannot be predicted antenatally. On the other hand, only about 50 per cent of deliveries occur in formal facilities (Table 87.3). Many reasons for not using the formal facilities have been identified, such as physical distance, cost of services and unwelcoming health worker attitudes and practices.

When complications occur, there are likely to be further delays:

- delay in recognizing the complication as potentially life-threatening and hence requiring essential obstetric care
- delay in reaching the health facility with the necessary services
- delay in provision of the actual care once the facility is reached.

An efficient referral system is therefore crucial. The role of maternity waiting homes as an intervention to counter the referral difficulties is not yet fully documented. Any

Table 87.4. Clinical management of anaemia in pregnancy

Suspect	If: tired and or breathless last delivery within a year any history of bleeding, malaria or hookworm disease	
Assess for paleness of tongue, conjunctiva, or palms	Pale	Not pale
Classify as	Clinical anaemia (severe)	Clinically not severe anaemia (mild or moderate)
Treat at: Dispensary	Give higher dose of iron/folate Give malaria prophylaxis and treatment (SP monthly) Refer to health centre If in hookworm endemic area, give broad spectrum anthelminthic	Give standard dose of iron/folate Give malaria prophylaxis and treatment If in hookworm endemic area, give broad spectrum anthelminthic Refer to health centre if has clinical signs of anaemia
Health centre	Estimate severity of anaemia (Hb) If severe: Rx for a month with higher dose If third trimester and no symptoms give i.m. iron (refer to hospital, if no rise in Hb) If very severe or symptomatic refer to hospital If malaria suspected, treat and give prophylaxis If in hookworm endemic area, give broad spectrum anthelminthic	Estimate severity of anaemia (Hb) If moderate give standard dose iron/folate If severe treat as such If malaria suspected, treat and give prophylaxis If in hookworm endemic area, give broad spectrum anthelminthic
Hospital	Treat with total dose infusion of iron, blood (packed cell) infusion according to gestation and severity If malaria suspected, treat and give prophylaxis If in hookworm endemic area, give broad spectrum anthelminthic	As above and: If in hookworm endemic area, give broad spectrum anthelminthic Transfusion as necessary according to gestation and Hb level

Notes:
Anaemia is defined as Hb, 10 g/dl
Anthelminthic treatment 5 single dose albendazole or levamisole or mebendazole or pyrantel (usually not in first trimester)
Severity of anaemia:
moderate 7–10.9 g/dl (PCV = 24–37 per cent)
severe 4–6.9 g/dl (PCV = 13–23 per cent)
very severe <4 g/dl (PCV <13 per cent)
Source: Adapted from Mother – Baby Package: WHO/FHE/MSM/94.11.

health worker looking after pregnant patients in Africa needs to be acutely aware of the level in the referral system at which they are operating and the referral system. The tiered organization of health services for the pregnant patient also offers an opportunity for targeted interventions at various levels to improve the quality of care and reduce both maternal and perinatal mortality.

Antenatal care

Over the years, it has become evident that adequate antenatal care does not necessarily lead to good perinatal and maternal outcomes. Patients who attend antenatal clinic as per the traditional schedule (monthly visits up to 28 weeks followed by fortnightly visits up to 36 weeks and finally, weekly visits until delivered – a total of about 14 visits) still end up with maternal and/or perinatal mortality. Furthermore, the 'risk approach' to antenatal clinic neither consistently predicts poor outcome nor does it significantly improve the maternal survival. Apart from being able to detect medical conditions in pregnancy, identify and treat pre-eclampsia and anaemia (among other co-existent medical conditions), antenatal care, as an intervention package, has little value in predicting many of the known causes of maternal mortality.

Table 87.5. Clinical management of pregnancy-induced hypertension

Suspect	If one or more present: Severe headache Generalized oedema Blurring vision Convulsions	
Assess for		
Blood pressure	Systolic = >140, diastolic = >90 mm Hg	Systolic = <140, diastolic = <90 mm Hg
Proteinuria	Yes	Yes/No
Convulsions	Yes	No
Classify as	Eclampsia	Pregnancy-induced hypertension, PET
Treat at:		
Dispensary	Maintain airway Initiate treatment for convulsions (i.v. diazepam 10 mg stat or i.m. diazepam 20 mg stat) **Refer to hospital** urgently	BP diastolic = 5 90–100 mmHg or systolic = 140–150 and no proteinuria: Bed rest at home BP twice weekly Give phenobarbitone 30–60 mg 8-hourly Instruct mother to monitor fetal movements **Refer to hospital** if: BP rises and/or oedema increases or headache worsens Diastolic 90–100 mmHg or systolic 140–150 mmHg and proteinuria Diastolic >100, systolic >150 mm Hg with or without proteinuria Fetal kicks fewer than 10 in 12 hours
Health centre	Maintain airway Control convulsions: **refer to hospital** urgently If delivery imminent, conduct it and refer to hospital for subsequent management	As above
Hospital	Manage hypertension (i.v. hydralazine 20 mg slowly after a test dose of 5 mg. If BP persists above 140/90 mmHg set up hydralazine infusion of 40 mg in 5% dextrose and titrate with BP. Manage convulsions[a] (i.v. diazepam 20 mg stat. If convulsions persist, set up infusion diazepam 40 mg in 5 per cent dextrose. Aim at maintaining patient just arousable). If in labour, cervix >4 cm dilated and no contraindication to vaginal delivery, do ARM, augment with syntocinon, and do elective vacuum extraction. If not in labour and/or cervix is <4 cm dilated or there is a contraindication to vaginal delivery, do emergency C/S.	Control hypertension Bed rest Methyldopa 250 mg 8-hourly: can be increased to max. 1 g 12-hourly Sublingual nifedipine 10 mg 12-hourly also useful Monitor fetal kicks as above Do urinalysis at least on alternate days Deliver if: Fetal movements persistently reduced and gestation = >32 weeks (baby can survive). Proteinuria >3–4+ persistently Has clinical features of severe disease Gestation >37 weeks Elective vacuum extraction for all cases delivered vaginally.

Notes:
[a] Magnesium sulphate is the ideal drug for controlling convulsions, and should be adopted widely.
Source: Adapted from *Mother – Baby Package*: WHO/FHE/MSM/94.11.

Table 87.6. Clinical management of puerperal sepsis

Anticipate	If there has been: prolonged labour (duration >12 h) prolonged rupture of membranes (duration >6 h) more than four vaginal examinations fetal death or macerated stillbirth	
Suspect	If febrile on the first 10 days post-partum	
Assess for:		
Fever	Yes	Yes
Foul smelling or pus discharge vaginally	Yes	No
Abdominal tenderness	Yes	No
Pelvic pain	Yes	No
Delayed involution of the uterus	Yes	No
Breast pain and tenderness	No	Yes/No
Low blood pressure	Yes/No	Yes/No
Classify as	Puerperal sepsis	Other infections (mastitis, UTI and malaria), deep venous thrombosis
Treat at:		
Dispensary	Give broad spectrum antibiotics **Refer to hospital** if: No improvement in 48 hours Patient very ill	Broad-spectrum antibiotics for mastitis, UTI. Anti-malarials, if malaria suspected **Refer to hospital** if: No improvement in 72 hours Patient very ill DVT suspected
Health centre	Give i.v. fluids if BP low Give antibiotic i.v./i.m **Refer to hospital** if: No improvement in 48 hours Patient very ill	Investigate for malaria Broad spectrum antibiotics for mastitis, UTI Anti-malarials if malaria suspected **Refer to hospital** as in dispensary
Hospital	Give i.v. fluids if BP low Give antibiotic i.v./i.m., combination antibiotics usually applicable for complete coverage Consider pelvic abscess if: No improvement in 48 hours Pelvic fullness or mass detected in the pouch of Douglas Drain abscess by laparotomy or colpotomy as possible – leave a drain	Determine the specific cause Treat appropriately

Notes:
Puerperal sepsis is genital infection from rupture of membranes to 42 days postpartum characterized by fever and one or more of the following: pelvic pain, abnormal vaginal discharge (pus), abnormal/ foul smelling discharge, delayed involution of the uterus (<2 cm/day in first week).
Broad spectrum antibiotics combination of: ampicillin + metronidazole + gentamycin or third generation cephalosporins.
Source: Adapted from *Mother – Baby Package*: WHO/FHE/MSM/94.11.

Moreover, with dwindling resources in the health sectors that are already overburdened with HIV/AIDS, the traditional antenatal care schedule appears to emphasize quantity of visits at the expense of quality. Evidence is now available to show that a new schedule that encourages a minimum of four clinic visits, each with specific value-added content, achieves the same pregnancy outcome as the traditional 14-visit schedule (Mujanja et al., 1996). Key features of the re-focused antenatal care include:

- fewer visits
- improved birth preparedness of the pregnant patient
- increased ability of the gravida to recognize and act on pregnancy complications
- the health workers recognize the possibility of complication in every pregnancy, regardless of risk rating, and prepare the women and immediate relatives accordingly.

The basic content for a suggested re-focused antenatal care is outlined below.

- Encourage voluntary counselling and testing for HIV.
- Detect and manage:
  - anaemia
  - pre-eclampsia
  - sexually transmitted infections
  - asymptomatic bacteriuria
  - medical conditions such as heart disease, diabetes.
- Check blood pressure, urinalysis at every visit.
- Provide appropriate prophylaxis:
  - tetanus toxoid injections
  - haematinic supplementation
  - iodine in areas with deficiency
  - anti-malarial prophylaxis especially for primigravidae.
- Provide information on danger signs of pregnancy:
  - any bleeding
  - severe headaches
  - drainage of liquor
  - swelling of the face or upper limbs
  - reduced fetal movements
  - diet, exercise and rest, sexuality in pregnancy, personal hygiene, breast-feeding and sexually transmitted infections.
- Assist the pregnant patient to develop a 'birth plan': the expected date of delivery, the danger signs in pregnancy, labour and post-partum, who will assist at the delivery – emphasizing the need for a trained attendant, how she will be transported to facility where she will deliver or if she develops any of the complications and post-partum contraception.
- Encourage the pregnant patient to involve and keep informed the spouse and/or mother-in-law about the above 'birth plan'.

References

Haidar J, Nekatibeb H, Urga K. (1999). Iron deficiency anemia in pregnant and lactating mothers in rural Ethiopia. *E Afr Med J*; **76**: 618–623.

Mujanja SP, Lindmark G, Nystrom L. (1996). Randomized controlled trial of a reduced visits program of antenatal care in Harare, Zimbabwe. *Lancet*, **348**: 364–369.

Oshitani H, Kasolo F, Tembo C, et al. (1995). Hepatitis B virus infection among pregnant women in Zambia. *E Afr Med J*; **72**: 813–815.

Shulman CE, Dorman EK, Cutts F et al. (1999). Intermittent sulphadoxine–pyrimethamine to prevent severe anaemia secondary to malaria in pregnancy: a randomized placebo-controlled trial. *Lancet*; **353**: 632–636.

Steketee RW, Wirima JJ, Slutsker WL, Khoromana CO, Breman JG, Heyman DL. (1996). Objectives and Methodology in a study of malaria treatment and prevention in pregnancy in rural Malawi: the Mangochi Malaria Research Project. *Am J Trop Med Hyg*; **55**: 8–16.

Ujah IAO, Uguru VE, Aisen AO et al. (1999). How safe is motherhood in Nigeria? The trend of maternal mortality in a tertiary health institution. *East Afr Med J*; **76**: 436–439.

Wasserheit JN, Holmes KK. (1992). Reproductive tract infections: challenges for international health policy, programs, and research. In *Reproductive Tract Infections: Global Impact and Priorities for Women's Reproductive Health*. ed. Germain A et al, p. 7. New York: Plenum Press.

World Health Organization (1968). *Anaemia*: WHO Technical Report Series No. 405.

WHO (2001). Maternal Mortality in 1995. Estimates developed by WHO, UNICEF, UNFPA: WHO/RHR/ 01.9.

Recommended further reading

Cunningham F et al. (eds.). (2001). *Williams Obstetrics*, 21st edition. New York: McGraw Hill.

Decherney AH. (2002). *Current Obstetric and Gynecologic Diagnosis and Treatment*, 9th edition, Appleton and Lange.

Lees C, Campbell S. (2000). *Obstetrics by Ten Teachers*, 17th edition. London. Arnold.

Rayburn WF, Zuspan FP. (1992). *Drug Therapy in Obstetrics and Gynecology*. Mosby.

UNAIDS (2000). *Report on the Global HIV/AIDS Epidemic*. Geneva, UNAIDS. www.unaids.org/publications.

UNAIDS (1999). *HIV in Pregnancy: A Review*. WHO/CHS/RHR/99.15. UNAIDS/99.35E. Geneva, UNAIDS. www.unaids,org/publications.

WHO (1995). *The Prevention and Management of Puerperal Infections* WHO/FHE/MSM/95.4. Geneva.

The disturbed patient

88

The disturbed patient is the main focus of psychiatry. Psychiatry derives from the Greek words *psyche* (spirit or soul) and *iatreuo* (to heal) and describes that branch of medicine that deals with the 'spirit' rather than the 'body' of a sick person. Even though regarded as one of the newest branches of medicine, psychiatry has its roots in antiquity, for throughout history and in almost all societies, some people have been observed to exhibit disturbed behaviour that has required more than treatment of their bodies to get them well again. Indeed in many parts of Africa maintaining strict tradition, traditional healers including priest–physicians use various methods to treat the sick, among whom are those invariably considered to be sick in 'spirit'.

Psychiatry deals with two main groups of disturbed persons.

(i) People who might be having difficulty in adjusting to society again after an unfortunate event, and who therefore develop problems like insomnia, poor appetite, palpitations and other symptoms. Whilst their reaction to their problems leads to suffering and may reduce their ability to function, most of us can understand their complaints as they are extreme degrees of usual phenomena.

(ii) People who exhibit behaviour more difficult to understand, such as 'a boy in Maiduguri covered with dust, completely naked, who was in the habit of haunting the market roundabout and throwing garbage at cars as they passed by' (Westley, 1993). Such people are very sick; they might lose touch with reality around them and become a problem for themselves, their family and their society. People with psychiatric problems make up approximately 20 per cent of those attending health facilities in Africa (German, 1987).

Psychiatry or mental health

Psychiatry deals with the diagnosis and treatment of problems involving the two groups of persons mentioned above.

Mental health is much broader and should include all those factors that enhance the comfort and happiness or quality of life of the individual – the composition of the family, their relationships with other people, adequate housing, access to schooling, money and ready cash, employment, etc.

Whereas psychiatry has predominantly to do with medicine, mental health involves many disciplines and sectors.

Assessing the patient

The interview

The most important method of assessing the patient with a psychiatric problem is the interview. Nevertheless, since people express themselves not only in words but also by their body language, it is essential to observe the patient's behaviour and bodily expressions during the interview. Through interviewing the patient and his immediate relations, we can obtain the history of his illness or disorder. Where a patient is unwilling or unable to speak, describe in the notes what actually happens in the interview, and how the patient behaves. In either case, it is essential to augment such information with a third party account by relatives, friends and any significant others.

It is also very helpful to assess the patient further through psychological tests e.g. of intelligence and personality, best done by a clinical psychologist, and the study of various relevant documents (certificates, letters, drawings) of the patient. By these means a picture can be built up of the physical, psychological and social aspects of the patient's life, and the way in which the current illness developed.

As resources are scarce in Africa, this ideal assessment often cannot be made. However, even when work is very heavy, this basic framework helps to organize the clinician's thinking while making the best assessment possible.

Attitude to the patient

The encounter between the clinician and the patient is like the host who receives a visitor to his home. In many African homes, there is a pattern with several steps, as illustrated by the Akan of Ghana:

- The visitor is allowed in with a hug or handshake and a word of welcome and is then offered a seat.
- He is offered a drink or some fruit against his presumed tiredness.
- He is asked for the reasons for the visit (even when this is already known by the host).
- After he has given his reasons (uninterrupted by the host), he is welcomed once more and politely asked if he might want to add any more, or alternatively if he might want to emphasize a particular point.
- The host then tells the visitor what has happened to him since the two last met.
- Next, the host might reply to the visitor's point of emphasis.
- Finally, if the host and visitor want to discuss the matters further, a date and place is agreed.

In the first two steps the host wants to make the visitor feel safe and comfortable, and to show his interest in his immediate welfare. The next two steps allow the visitor to say whatever he might have in mind without being interrupted, whilst the next steps allow the host to give his opinion on the matter. The last step is at the heart of the psychiatric interview, when both listen and talk so that they can both derive benefit from the interview.

The interview in practice

Whilst it might be impractical to offer a drink or fruit to our patients, the process outlined above is otherwise easily replicated in the clinic. We greet the patient and introduce ourselves to him.

(i) We offer him a seat or, if he is lying down, ensure he is comfortable. Then we ask him to introduce himself by asking for his personal details such as age, occupation, marital status (see under history below).
(ii) We ask him, 'What has brought you to us?', not 'What is wrong with you?'.
(iii) After he has described his problems, we ask him to emphasize for us what he considers to be his most worrying complaint or problem.
(iv) We attempt to understand his problems better by asking relevant questions on his background (see under history below).
(v) We summarize our views and suggest what measures, including investigations, need to be done.

For those familiar with the techniques of interviewing, it is easy to discern two important phases in the process outlined above – establishment of rapport, which merges smoothly into the phase of fact finding and problem solving. That is to say, we first seek to establish a good working relationship with the patient, who is thus encouraged to participate actively in finding a solution to his problem.

Dispelling stigma

We must remember that, in most societies, the mentally ill are stigmatized by many. The person in front of the clinician may have been laughed at, despised and even abused because of his illness. It is essential that he is treated with respect, dignity and kindness by the person from whom he is seeking help.

The history

Personal details

Record name, age, sex, marital status, job and source of referral.

Reason for referral

Ask about events and symptoms leading to their presentation.

History of present illness

Ask about when the illness started, any events that may have precipitated the illness, clinical symptoms and the course of the illness since it started. Ask about the patient's understanding of the illness.

Family history

Ask about the relationships within the family, and always ask about family history of mental illness.

Personal history

Include childhood experiences (including developmental milestones), schooling, occupational history, marital/relationship history and social circumstances now.

Past medical history

Record any serious illnesses and ask about epilepsy and head injury.

Past psychiatric history

Record previous illnesses, what treatment the patient had, if any, and if the treatment was effective.

Use of drugs and alcohol

If used, record the amount and any harmful effects, including dependence.

Involvement with police or prison

Has the patient been involved in crime and if so, what?

Current medication used

Previous personality before illness

Are the current problems an illness or part of the patient's personality?

Mental state examination

The interview and observations made during it provide data on the mental functioning of the patient. While the patient tells his story, the clinician concerns himself with both what the patient says and how he says it, and asks himself whether and how the patient by his nature and behaviour differs from other people in his environment. The mental state summarizes the impressions gained by the doctor into the mental functioning of the patient before and also throughout the interview. Observe, analyse and record the following areas of mental state: the general nutritional state, posture, dress, self care, facial expression and any abnormal movements.

Behaviour

Observe the attitude towards the doctor, whether relaxed and trusting, guarded and suspicious, or hostile and aggressive. Describe what the patient does and what the clinician sees, including any bizarre behaviour which is difficult to understand.

Speech

Listen to the patient's speech – the tone of voice, volume, continuity and organization.

Emotion

- Let the patient describe his feelings, called mood and affect.
- Note any elation, sadness, irritability, anxiety, agitation tearfulness or fear.
- Does the patient's mood change rapidly and suddenly during the interview (labile mood) or remain the same?
- Is the expressed emotion appropriate or inappropriate, as when a patient laughs when describing the death of his mother? This is called incongruity of affect.
- Always ask about thoughts of suicide and plans and attempts made.

Thought

- Describe the content of the patient's thoughts and delusional beliefs (see the Box).
- Note if the patient's thoughts do not make sense, but the patient is not aware that he cannot be understood: this is termed formal thought disorder.
- Note the flow of the patient's thoughts, e.g. fast or slow, and whether the patient believes that any outside force or person is influencing his thoughts (possession of thought).

Perception

Note the presence of any illusions or hallucinations (see the Box).

Cognition

Identify his level of consciousness, orientation in time and place, attention and concentration, memory, language and viso-spatial awareness.

Insight

Does the patient show an understanding of his situation which is realistic and would be shared by most from his community?

Delusion: a fixed, false belief held with conviction, without appropriate evidence and out of context with one's educational, cultural and social context.

Hallucination: a false perception in the absence of a stimulus.

Illusion: a perception which is a false interpretation of a stimulus (e.g. looking at a belt, but perceiving it to be a snake).

Children

The assessment may be different. Information from parents and family is very important in assessing whether the child's development is similar to that of children of similar age, including intelligence, relationships with siblings and peers, and the way the child plays.

Physical examination

A complete physical examination is essential, especially of the central nervous system: it helps to:
- reinforce the rapport established with the patient and confirm to him that his problem is being taken seriously;
- exclude any underlying medical disorder as a cause of the patient's symptoms.

When a patient is unco-operative or needs emergency treatment, the physical examination may have to be done later.

Laborarory investigations

1. Basic simple tests, for example haemoglobin, white cell count and urinalysis.
2. Specific tests to define any suspected organic disorder: for example, in larger hospitals, EEG, CT scan of the brain and tests for HIV may be available.

Diagnosis

No psychiatric diagnosis can be made on the basis of a single symptom, nor before a thorough physical examination, including investigations, has been done. Detailed operational criteria for diagnosis used in psychiatry are described in the ICD 10 (World Health Organization, 1993) and DSM IV (American Psychiatric Association, 1994).

ORGANIC DISORDERS

Case history:
A 53-year-old woman presents with bed wetting for 4 weeks and poor memory for 2 weeks. Her attention and concentration are poor, and she is more irritable with her children.

The key questions in this case are:
Is this a mental illness with an organic cause?
If organic, is it an acute or chronic organic disorder?
Is the cause reversible or irreversible?

Acute organic reaction (delirium)

Clinical features

These are listed in the Box. The crucial sign which can help to distinguish delirium from dementia is that in delirium there are frequently (but not always) fluctuating levels of consciousness.

Treatment

It is essential to find the cause of the delirium (see the Box) and treat this urgently. Delirium has a high mortality if untreated. If the patient is agitated and needs sedation, give chlorpromazine up to 100 mg every 8 hours or diazepam 2–5 mg every 6 hours. Try to find the cause of the delirium before sedating the patient.

Delirium	**Dementia**
Fluctuating level of consciousness	Consciousness not impaired
Cognitive deficits, especially disorientation	Global cognitive deficits, especially memory
Muddled thinking	Personality/behavioural changes
Labile mood	Labile mood
Anxiety/panic	Developing neurological signs
Vivid delusions and hallucinations (auditory and visual)	Delusions and hallucinations

Causes of delirium
Brain: infections – meningitis, encephalitis, cerebral malaria
space-occupying lesion – tumour, haemorrhage etc.
raised intracranial pressure
injury/trauma
epilepsy – post-ictal, status
Non-brain:
Metabolic – uraemia, liver failure, hypoxia (respiratory/cardiac failure), electrolyte imbalance
Prescribed drugs – anticholinergics, anticonvulsants, opiates, L dopa, digitalis
Alcohol and illegal drug use – including delirium tremens
Endocrine – hypoglycaemia
Infection – including typhoid fever
Nutritional deficiency – deficiencies of thiamine, B_{12}, nicotinic acid, folic acid
Post-operative – notably water intoxication
Poisons – heavy metals

Chronic organic reactions (dementia)

Clinical features: as listed in the Box

Causes

Reversible

Syphilis, thyroid abnormalities, thiamine deficiency. Space-occupying lesion, chronic raised intracranial pressure, normal pressure hydrocephalus, trauma, sarcoid, encephalitis, HIV infection, poisons, and deficiencies of B_{12} or folic acid.

Irreversible

Alzheimer's disease – a progressive neurodegenerative illness resulting in death. Multi-infarct dementia – loss of brain tissue due to vascular insufficiency. Hypertension. Other rare forms of irreversible dementia.

Treatment

Actively treat any reversible cause. If irreversible, give any practical support for the patient and family possible and treat agitation symptomatically with low doses of antipsychotics, e.g. haloperidol 5 mg b.d.

> *Case history follow-up*: The woman continued to deteriorate in her cognitive functioning. Physical examination, blood tests and skull X-ray were all normal. A CT brainscan was performed and a left frontotemporal tumour diagnosed. The patient had surgery to remove the tumour.

PSYCHOSES WITH NO ORGANIC CAUSE

> *Case history 1*: A 33-year-old woman has, for the last year, been assaulting her husband and his relations for no reason. This is not her usual self. She accuses her husband of infidelity and talking about her to their neighbours. She is brought to the clinic and on questioning informs the health worker that she can hear her sisters-in-law talking about her to her husband, even when they are far away from her. She believes her husband is plotting behind her back. Otherwise she is coherent and has no other problems.
>
> *Case history 2*: A 22-year-old man is brought to the clinic by his mother. He says he is ready to become president of the country (he is working in a petrol station). He is preaching strangely on the street, not sleeping or eating properly, and very irritable if challenged about his behaviour. He has been acting like this for 6 weeks, and previously was a popular, level-headed young man.

Both individuals have a psychosis. This term does not have an easy definition, but the following have been used:

(i) The presence of delusions, hallucinations or thought disorder
(ii) A loss of contact with reality
(iii) Bizarre behaviour, difficult to explain.

Psychotic illnesses may have an organic cause, as in dementia and delirium, but often an organic cause is not found. The two most common conditions are schizophrenia and bipolar affective disorder.

Schizophrenia

Clinical presentation

Schizophrenia can present in different ways, but the following symptoms are common.

- Delusions and auditory hallucinations: certain types, known as first-rank symptoms, make a diagnosis of schizophrenia much more likely in the absence of an organic cause (See the Box).
- Bizarre behaviour.
- Negative symptoms: these are social withdrawal, a lack of drive, a lack of expressing normal emotions, general lack of interest in life.
- The delusions and hallucinations are not 'mood congruent'; that is, they do not fit with a high or low mood.
- Symptoms present for at least a month.

First-rank symptoms of schizophrenia

- Delusional perception: a delusional interpretation of a normal perception
- Third-person auditory hallucinations: the patient hears one or more voices referring to the patient in the third person.
- Thoughts echoing: the patients hear their own thoughts spoken aloud.
- Running commentary: there are voices commenting on the patient's behaviour.
- Thought insertion
- Thought withdrawal
- Thought broadcasting or 'thought incontinence': the patient believes that his thoughts can be picked up by those around him.
- Somatic passivity: patients believe that an outside force is interfering with their body.
- Made actions
- Made emotions

Treatment

Antipsychotic medication

Give haloperidol 10 mg daily at night or in divided doses, or, if sedation is required, chlorpromazine 200 mg daily in divided doses, increasing to 300 mg if there is an inadequate response. If the patient has extrapyramidal side effects, give benztropine 2 mg orally or by intramuscular injection.

Depot antipsychotic medication

If the patient cannot use oral medication, a depot intramuscular treatment can be used, after a test dose. A maintenance dose can be fluphenazine 25 mg every 4 weeks.

Psychosocial care

The care of someone suffering from schizophrenia is not only about medication, but also helping their general functioning. Look out for ways to give support for the family, including educating them about the illness. The patient may need help with daily living skills, domestic skills, social activities and getting work. The service provided will depend very much on local resources. In mental health institutions, occupational therapy and psychology skills may be available to organize these treatments. Other organizations may help, such as charities and churches. One charity organization in Kumasi, Ghana, has opened a residential home where many patients with schizophrenia live and work manufacturing clothing, wreaths and shoes for sale. They may stay for up to 3 years.

Bipolar affective disorder

This is also known as manic-depressive illness. Patients are prone to elated or low moods. We shall here describe manic illnesses and describe depressive psychoses later under depression.

Clinical features of mania

There are three main features of manic illnesses

(i) Elation or irritability in mood – if irritable the patient can be aggressive.

(ii) Over-activity – this can result in excessive energy and activity, refusal to eat or sleep, pressure of speech and flight of ideas and disinhibition, e.g. sexual promiscuity or excessive spending not in character with the patient's normal habits.

(iii) Grandiosity – grandiose delusions and hallucinations fitting in with the high mood, e.g. believing oneself to have supernatural powers.

Treatment

Admission into an inpatient unit, if the patient is very unwell. Frequently, patients with a manic illness lack insight and good judgement.

Antipsychotic medication to treat the acute mania

The drug of choice is haloperidol 10 mg daily in divided doses. If unavailable, give chlorpromazine up to 300 mg daily in divided doses.

A mood stabilizer

Give carbamazepine 200 mg daily, if available, as the drug of choice, as lithium also is rarely available and needs monitoring of blood levels, renal and thyroid functions. Ideally, titrate the carbamazepine dose by blood concentration, but if this is not possible, do not increase beyond 600 mg daily. If the patient has had recurrent illnesses, carbamazepine can be maintained as a **prophylactic mood stabilizer** to prevent relapse.

Case outcomes: The 33-year-old woman was diagnosed with schizophrenia and responded well to haloperidol as an outpatient. The 22-year-old man was diagnosed as having a manic illness, admitted and treated with haloperidol and carbamazepine, responding well and ready for discharge in 2 weeks.

COMMON MENTAL DISORDERS

Depression

Depressive illnesses are unusual in that they are broad in their severity. At its most severe depression can involve psychotic symptoms (depressive psychosis). This can be part of a bipolar disorder, or a patient may have depressive psychotic illnesses without ever having a manic episode (unipolar depressive psychosis). At the other end of the spectrum of depression, it may be a mild illness often precipitated by difficult times in someone's life. This kind of depressive illness is very common in all cultures.

Clinical features

These can be divided into psychological, physical and psychotic.

Psychological

These include low mood, hopelessness, negative thoughts about the present and future, inability to enjoy the things one used to enjoy (called anhedonia), a loss of confidence, reduced interest in life, guilt and reduced self worth. The person will often have suicidal thoughts, may have made plans to kill himself or attempted to do so.

Physical

Appetite is reduced with weight loss, sleep is poor with early morning wakening, energy is diminished and physical symptoms trouble the patient. The depressed person often exhibits a slowing down of thought and movement (psychomotor retardation) which, when extreme, can lead to a depressive stupor. At this stage the patient's life is at risk as he will stop eating and drinking. Patients often feel worse in the morning (diurnal mood variation).

Psychotic

Delusions fit the depressed mood. Persecutory delusions are common, as are delusions of guilt. Nihilistic delusions are beliefs that one is dying, or parts of one's body have disappeared. Auditory hallucinations are usually in the second person and often derogatory, fitting in with the low mood.

Patients with depression often get symptoms of anxiety, obsessional thoughts and depersonalization.

Treatment

Only treat depression if there are at least three or more of the symptoms described above, and the patient has had such symptoms for at least two weeks. Normal sadness is part of life, and should not be treated as depression. No health worker can make everyone happy.

Give antidepressants if the depression is severe. Imipramine or amitriptyline are appropriate, starting with 25 mg daily and increasing to at least 75 mg daily. Some pharmacologists suggest the minimum dose should be 100 mg daily. The dose can be increased but not over 200 mg daily.

Depression with psychotic symptoms

Give antipsychotic medication, for example chlorpromazine 200 mg in divided doses, in addition to the antidepressant.

Social support

Arrange as much support as is available in helping the family, and any practical help with house work, etc.

Talking therapies

The availability of talking therapies will vary greatly. In specialist centres, psychotherapy, group therapy, family therapy and counselling may be available. There is some evidence that cognitive therapy is as effective as antidepressants. Anti-depressant medication and cognitive therapy are often used together, but if these therapies are not available, talking with the patient, identifying problems and possible solutions will help. Other sources of help in the community, such as church workers and traditional healers, may be of great benefit to depressed people and may also help with a patient's spiritual needs.

Electroconvulsive therapy (ECT)

This treatment is the most rapid in its effectiveness and can be the best option when the patient is in a depressive stupor, refusing food and water, is dangerously suicidal, or a delay in treatment presents a serious risk to health. Whilst the mode of action is unclear, ECT is remarkably safe and free of side effects. Short-term retrograde amnesia and a temporary defect in new learning can occur but are short lived. ECT should only be given at centres of expertise and where an anaesthetic is safely available. The patient receives the anaesthetic (usually thiopental 125–150 mg) and a muscle relaxant (usually suxamethonium 30–50 mg). An electric current of usually 80 volts for 0.1–0.3 seconds is given across electrodes applied to the anterior temporal areas of the scalp (bilateral) or both electrodes applied to the same side of the scalp (unilateral). A modified convulsion is produced, ideally lasting about 30 seconds. A course of six to eight treatments over 3 weeks is commonly effective. Do not give more than 12 sessions of treatment. ECT should not be used if the patient has raised intracranial pressure, a cerebral aneurysm or a history of cerebral haemorrhage.

Anxiety disorders

> *Case summary*: A 19-year-old student presents to the emergency clinic with palpitations, tachycardia and insomnia. No physical cause is found. He is sweating profusely and has a mild tremor. On closer questioning he is worried about failing exams which he is due to take in 1 month's time.

Anxiety disorders are common in all cultures. We all worry about things in our lives, but an anxiety disorder is when fear, the predominant emotion of this condition, becomes out of proportion to the situation and leads to great suffering.

Symptoms

The symptoms of anxiety disorders can be divided into psychological and physical.

Psychological
Fear (sometimes of impending death), worrying, irritability, insomnia.

Physical
Palpitations, body and muscle pains, headache, hyperventilation and breathlessness, pins and needles, tremor, 'butterflies' in stomach.

Treatment

> The main long-term treatment for anxiety is anxiety management and talking therapies, not medication.

Medication
If necessary, give an anxiolytic such as diazepam 5–10 mg daily. There is a risk of dependence with diazepam and other benzodiazepines, so ideally give for 3 days only. Do not prescribe diazepam for longer than 2–4 weeks or there is a risk of the patient becoming dependent.

Talking treatments
Calm the patient, educate him about the nature of anxiety symptoms and reassure him that no physical cause can be found. Talk about any problems he is facing which may explain his symptoms.

Anxiety management
A behavioural treatment may relieve symptoms in an acute attack: it involves relaxation techniques, such as finding a quiet place to sit down, slow, deep breathing exercises, visualizing, calming down and assuring oneself that this situation has happened before and will end without problems. Teach the patient to feel his heart slow down, his breathing calm down and his muscles relax.

> *Case follow-up*: The patient was admitted for a few days but not given medication. He improved with counselling and anxiety management. The university agreed to postpone his exams for 6 months. He later passed these and his illness did not recur.

Clinical presentations of anxiety

Generalized anxiety
Symptoms are present all the time.

Panic disorder
Symptoms come in sudden, unpredictable bursts.

Phobias
Anxiety is related to specific objects or situations. In agoraphobia (literally, fear of a market-place) symptoms come when the patient fears there is no easy way out especially in crowded situations, such as a busy market or crowded bus. Specific object phobias (called simple phobias) might involve dogs, thunder or height. Social phobia is the fear of embarrassment in social situations. Phobias lead an individual to avoid the situation or object. Treatment is behavioural, by systematic desensitization.

Obsessive–compulsive disorder (OCD)
Obsessional thoughts are unpleasant, intrusive thoughts (recognized as coming from the self), which repeatedly come into the patient's head, despite the patient trying to resist them. Compulsions are acts that the patient feels compelled to do, often checking, cleaning, counting or hoarding, even though he realizes the act is nonsensical. Resisting obsessional thoughts or compulsions results in anxiety. OCD can be treated with behavioural techniques such as exposure and response prevention and also some antidepressants, especially clomipramine at a maintenance dose of 100–200 mg daily, or selective serotonin reuptake inhibitors such as paroxetine 20 mg daily.

Other neuroses

Dissociative disorders

These are the phenomena of mental distress resulting in physical or psychological symptoms. An example is when patients present with loss of voice or paralysis of the legs with no organic cause but psychological problems underly the presentation. Patients can also present with symptoms similar to seizures or altered states of consciousness. These illnesses can occur within groups, all presenting with the same symptoms. But be careful, because symptoms dismissed as psychogenic can be later found to have an organic cause. Also, if symptoms are dissociative in nature, patients should not be dismissed as 'hysterical': instead, they require support and counselling for their distress.

Somatoform disorders

Psychological distress presenting with multiple physical symptoms or fear of having an illness. Such patients are difficult to manage. Ideally, consistent reassuring treatment from one doctor is the best option, as otherwise these patients go from one doctor to another (see the Box).

> **Neurosis**
> This is a commonly used term but it is difficult to define. The neuroses are a group of mental illnesses that:
> - are not explained by organic illness
> - have no psychotic symptoms such as delusions, hallucinations or thought disorder
> - are recognized to be an illness by the patient
> - are usually extreme forms of normal emotions which cause suffering to the patient and which impair functioning

Puerperal disorders

After childbirth, women are vulnerable to mental illness. Such disturbances are divided into maternity blues, postnatal depression and puerperal psychosis. Maternity blues describes the brief episodes of emotional lability, irritability and tearfulness occurring in 65–90 per cent of women 2–3 days post-partum. These resolve within a few days and do not need treatment. Depressive illnesses occur in the first year in 10–20 per cent of mothers and may need treatment. Post-partum psychosis occurs in 0.1–0.5 per cent of mothers and needs active treatment. Most are affective psychoses and usually have their onset in the 2 weeks following birth. Delusions can occur about the child (e.g. the baby is evil) and suicide attempts or harm to the child can occur.

ALCOHOL AND DRUG MISUSE

Alcohol

The consumption of alcohol is common in many cultures, and when it is only moderate, there is no evidence of any harm. However, prolonged excess drinking leads to serious consequences.

How much is too much? A unit of alcohol is 250 ml of normal strength beer, a measure of spirits or a glass of wine (these all contain 8 g of alcohol approximately). Safe drinking for men is a weekly consumption of 21 units or less, for women 14 units or less. It can be very difficult to calculate alcohol consumption as patients may be drinking their own distilled or brewed alcohol, and the health worker needs to use clinical experience.

Effects of alcohol

Physical

Cirrhosis of the liver, gastric ulcer, certain carcinomas (including buccal cavity, larynx, oesophagus and stomach), alcoholic cardiomyopathy, pancreatic disease; and the acute dangers of drunkenness: head injury, injuries from fighting, or lung abscess from aspirated vomit.

Psychological

Depression, anxiety, alcoholic hallucinosis, delirium tremens, alcoholic dementia, Wernicke–Korsakoff syndrome.

Alcohol use can lead to mental illnesses across the spectrum, from organic psychoses (alcoholic dementia, Wernicke–Korsakoff syndrome), to an illness similar to schizophrenia (alcoholic hallucinosis) and depression and anxiety. If a patient presents with depression and/or anxiety, it is essential to ask about alcohol as it is necessary to cut down the alcohol consumption before any other treatment will be effective.

Social

Unemployment, aggression, family breakdown, crime.

Delirium tremens

This is an acute confusional reaction, precipitated by withdrawal from alcohol in a heavy drinker, usually within 48–72 hours of stopping drinking. Seizures and autonomic instability are common. It is life threatening and should therefore be treated carefully in hospital.

Treatment

Sedate with diazepam, initially using a high dose (5–10 mg four times per day) reducing gradually over a week. Give intramuscular or oral thiamine from the beginning to prevent brain damage through Wernicke–Korsakoff syndrome. Nurse the patient closely as he will often be agitated and potentially aggressive.

Alcohol dependence

One or more of the following features: craving alcohol, letting a drink take priority in the patient's life, withdrawal symptoms when stopping drinking, tolerance (gradually needing more alcohol to have the same effect), regular drinking pattern, needing an early morning drink and reinstatement of old drinking habits after a period of abstinence.

The problem of management

People with alcohol problems are often helped by self-help groups such as Alcoholics Anonymous. Other talking treatments will help, although the patient needs to be motivated to attend. Treat any underlying condition, such as depression or anxiety, when the patient has controlled his drinking.

Drugs

Drug use is a problem in Africa as it is in all parts of the world. Cannabis use is frequent, Cha'at or khat is a popular drug in the Horn of Africa, and general drug use is increasing all over Africa (see pp. 1198). Not only are there problems with dependence, especially with opiates, but some drugs, including amphetamines and cannabis, can also cause a psychotic illness.

Another important factor to remember in the mental health clinic is that, if someone is suffering from a mental illness and uses drugs or alcohol (termed 'dual diagnosis'), the illness will get worse and treatment is less likely to be effective. Prescribed drugs can also be abused. For example, steroids can be taken, in women for their appearance and men for body building – steroids can induce psychosis. Local herbs may have an effect on mental health and it is important that health workers are aware of this.

Learning disabilities and child mental health

A learning disability (also known as mental handicap or mental retardation) is an organically caused limitation of intellectual ability from early childhood. Causes include genetic abnormalities, metabolic deficiencies, brain trauma at birth and infections during pregnancy. Brain damage in later childhood, often through infections such as cerebral malaria, lead to similar problems. Parents bringing children to the clinic, who are concerned about a possible learning disability, must be taken seriously, because they are usually correct.

The problem in Africa

Rural

Incapacity may be less for milder forms of learning disability, because the extended family protects the individual throughout daily life and there are always simpler tasks in the household or compound to do.

Urban

In urban society the emphasis is on school education, and this creates a gap between those who can and those who cannot learn. In addition, although urban society offers many jobs, unemployment is high, so that there is strong competition among the educated. The nuclear family, much more prevalent in towns, offers less protection than rural extended families, with both parents often having to work. But a learning-disabled child is more likely to survive in urban areas because health services are better.

Management

The key question for the health worker is 'what can we do for this child?' Whilst the child's condition is usually incurable, there is a lot the health worker can offer, including:

- educating the parents by defining their child's problem
- psychological support for the parents and teachers
- advice on letting the child learn skills even though this takes longer than with the average child. In this way the parents are encouraged to let the child reach his full potential and not do everything for him
- special schools for children with learning disabilities. Where these exist, in some urban areas, health workers should encourage parents to enrol their child
- in an older child or adolescent, if aggressive or disinhibited behaviour occurs, it is important that the diagnosis is considered if there are any criminal justice proceedings

Acute psychotic illnesses are more common in patients with a learning disability and can be successfully treated by a change of environment and management with antipsychotic medication.

Other mental health problems in children

The overactive child

This is a common problem in all cultures, with a plethora of diagnostic terms associated with it, most commonly being called attention deficit hyperactivity disorder (ADHD). Treatment can involve medication, including Ritalin if available. Sometimes low doses of haloperidol can be helpful.

Bedwetting

Children wetting the bed at night is very common but can lead to severe chastisement by the parents and trauma for the child. If presenting to the clinic, a simple behavioural chart is often effective. Ask the child to make a record of each night, whether 'wet' or 'dry', and encourage the parents to praise the child's successes and reassure when there are setbacks.

Psychiatric emergencies

Rapid tranquillization for the very disturbed patient

When a patient presents as very disturbed, or becoming increasingly disturbed, due to his mental illness, swift action is necessary. Take the following steps:

1. Try to calm the patient verbally. The majority of patients can be settled through good communication skills. Adopt a calm body posture, listen to them and speak calmly to them.
2. If the patient cannot be calmed verbally and the safety of the patient or others is at risk, rapid tranquillization is needed. Assess the safety of the situation – if the patient is armed, police help may be necessary. If safe to do so, the first step is controlling and restraining the patient. Ensure an adequate number of trained staff are present. Plan your actions as a team, e.g. if five staff are present, allocate one person for each limb and one to protect the patient's head. The leader should indicate the moment when the team approach the patient so that all move together. Use the minimum force necessary and try to prevent injury to the patient and staff. Remember if the patient is confused or deluded, he will be genuinely terrified. Talk to him explaining what you are doing, even if his understanding is minimal. It is essential for nursing staff on inpatient units to have training in control and restraint techniques.
3. Medication can be given intramuscularly or intravenously.
   - Intramuscular – give either lorazepam 2–4 mg or diazepam 5–10 mg (not both): haloperidol 5 mg is an antipsychotic alternative, and can be combined with one of the above. Intramuscular sedation can be repeated in 30 minutes, but do not exceed 30 mg haloperidol in 24 hours, or exceed recommended 24-hour doses of diazepam or lorazepam.
   - Intravenous – give diazepam 5–10 mg or lorazepam 2–4 mg but beware the risk of respiratory depression and possible death. The injection must be given gradually over 2–4 minutes and never as a bolus. Ensure restraint is adequate for safety of the patient and staff.
   - Use smaller doses and repeat if necessary rather than using large doses. Reduce the doses of sedative drugs as the patient improves.
   - Monitor respiratory rate, pulse and blood pressure after emergency sedation.
   - Rehydrate, patients are frequently dehydrated due to inadequate fluid intake and may need rehydration.

The goal of emergency tranquillization is not somnolence or sedation but to reduce agitated behaviour. Always respect the patient's right to safe, humane treatment.

Extrapyramidal crises

Antipsychotic medication can cause acute dystonic reactions in the muscles of the tongue, orbit (oculogyric crisis), sternomastoid (torticollis) or back (opisthotonus). These episodes are extremely painful and alarming for the patient. Give intramuscular or oral anticholinergics as a matter of urgency, e.g. benztropine 2 mg.

Stupor

Stupor is the state of unawareness of one's surroundings. Severe depression can result in the patient being stuporose, neither eating nor drinking. Dehydration is common and treatment is required urgently. After rehydration, the treatment of choice is electroconvulsive therapy, as response to treatment is rapid.

Patients can also become stuporose if they have schizophrenia (called catatonic stupor) and antipsychotic medication is required.

Medication and mental health

Antipsychotics

These drugs are used to treat psychotic symptoms, manic symptoms and, in certain circumstances, such as severe agitation, for sedation. We have suggested the use of haloperidol and chlorpromazine as oral medication, and fluphenazine as depot intramuscular injection, because these are commonly available in Africa. There are many other antipsychotic drugs, listed in psychopharmacology and psychiatry textbooks. A new group of antipsychotic drugs termed atypical antipsychotics (examples are risperidone, olanzapine and clozapine) are widely used in richer countries as they have fewer side effects, but are rarely available in most of Africa because of cost.

Side effects of antipsychotics

(i) Extrapyramidal effects
- Muscle dystonia – treat with oral or intramuscular anticholinergics, e.g. benztropine 2 mg.
- Parkinsonism – tremor, muscle stiffness, bradykinesis: treat with oral anticholinergic, e.g. benztropine 2 mg up to twice daily.

- Tardive dyskinesia – abnormal movements most commonly of the lips/tongue: resistant to treatment.
- Muscle restlessness (akathisia) – reduce the dose of antipsychotic.

(ii) Postural hypotension
(iii) Sedation
(iv) Jaundice/skin sensitivity to sun – especially with chlorpromazine
(v) Autonomic dysfunction – dry mouth, blurred vision, urinary retention, impotence
(vi) Metabolic effects – weight gain, amenorrhoea, galactorrhoea
(vii) Neuroleptic malignant syndrome – a rare severe reaction characterized by muscle stiffness, autonomic instability and fluctuating consciousness. There is a risk of death and the antipsychotic should be stopped for at least 2 weeks.

Antidepressants

Imipramine and amitryptiline are recommended because they are widely available in Africa. There is now a bewildering choice of different antidepressants available in richer countries, and specialist textbooks will inform the reader of these. However, newer drugs have not been shown to be more effective than amitryptiline or imipramine, but they may have different side effects.

Imipramine is alerting and is the drug of choice in depression with psychomotor retardation.

Amitryptiline is sedating and is the drug of choice in agitated depression.

Side effects

(i) Cardiovascular – risk of arrhythmias, can cause death in overdose
(ii) Anticholinergic – dry mouth, blurred vision, urinary retention, constipation
(iii) Postural hypotension – especially in the elderly
(iv) Drug-induced mania.

Mood stabilizers

These drugs are often unavailable in Africa. Lithium is the most common mood stabilizer used in developed countries but, for safe use, monitoring of blood lithium concentration, and of renal and thyroid function are essential. Additionally, the lithium blood concentration is affected by hot weather as it is excreted renally, hence its use in tropical countries can be problematic.

Carbamazepine is a suitable alternative for Africa. Ideally, its blood concentration should be monitored and kept within the therapeutic range. If blood monitoring is not possible, be cautious, starting with a dose of 200 mg daily, increasing in inadequate response to 600 mg maximum.

HIV and mental illness

HIV and AIDS have devastated Africa, and their effects include mental illness. HIV can cause organic neurological disorders which can have mental health consequences, such as infections, e.g. meningitis, cerebral toxoplasmosis, neuromuscular effects, progressive encephalopathy of childhood and tumours. In addition, people with HIV/AIDS can present to mental health services with delirium, dementia, acute psychoses, mood disorders and adjustment disorders.

Delirium

As with any delirium, patients can present with one or more of the following: altered/fluctuating levels of consciousness, cognitive impairment, hallucinations, delusions and restlessness. The causes of delirium in AIDS include viral meningitis, cryptococcal meningitis, possibly tuberculous meningitis, other infections, brain lesions such as lymphoma or tumour, metabolic disorders and sometimes drug therapy.

Dementia

Signs of AIDS dementia include mental slowing, poor concentration, difficulty in thinking and solving problems and poor memory, apathy and social withdrawal, and neurological symptoms. Patients with AIDS may present for the first time with dementia, but more commonly it occurs towards the end of the illness.

Acute psychosis

If you are confronted with a patient with a psychotic illness similar to schizophrenia, or a bipolar affective disorder accompanied by persistent cognitive impairment, be alert to the possibility of HIV infection.

Mood disorders

Depression and anxiety are common with HIV/AIDS. This may be due to a brain disorder secondary to the infection, or an understandable psychological reaction to the illness. Patients may be at risk of suicide.

Adjustment disorders

Again it is understandable that patients can suffer a psychological reaction to the diagnosis. Certain reactions are common, including shock, denial, fear, anger, guilt and low mood. It can take time for the patient to adjust to the diagnosis, and many of the listed emotions may be experienced before the patient accepts the situation. Counselling and support will often help patients through this process.

Trauma and mental health in Africa

Trauma affects the lives of those who survive it, whether it is personal violence or sexual assault, or the appalling suffering in wars and conflicts. Refugees and post-conflict societies, such as in Rwanda, can have mental health problems resulting from terrible experiences.

The consequences of trauma

(i) Post-traumatic stress disorder (see the Box)
(ii) Depression with suicidal ideas
(iii) Anxiety disorders
(iv) Alcohol and drug misuse
(v) Physical symptoms with no organic cause found.

Management

It is important to treat people with these conditions when they result from trauma in the same way as any other patient would be treated. Many patients who have had terrible experiences are helped if they can talk about them in a supportive, understanding environment. Different cultural forums for support would be appropriate according to local needs.

Fear of revenge

Sometimes, the victims of trauma will be too scared to talk as they fear others, in a refugee camp for example, who they may regard as potential oppressors.

- Be sensitive to local circumstances.
- Respect confidentiality at all times.

Clinical features of PTSD

- Flashbacks and nightmares of the past trauma
- High levels of vigilance and anxiety that the trauma will happen again
- Insomnia
- Often co-morbid depressive illnesses.

Treatment of PTSD

- Give antidepressant medication if the patient has a depressive illness
- Counselling in a safe environment can help
- Help with social needs: housing, finances, work
- A new treatment, eye movement desensitization and reprogramming (EMDR), is rarely available but has been shown to help many.

Epidemiology of mental illness in Africa

The pattern and frequency of mental illness in Africa is similar to that in other parts of the world. Mental illness accounted for 11 per cent of the world disease burden in 1990 and major depression will occupy second place in terms of relative disease burden by 2020 (World Bank, 1993; WHO, 1996).

German (1987) identified some of the difficulties in conducting epidemiological studies in Africa, where qualified personnel are few and are often overwhelmed by clinical demands. Populations can be difficult to reach and population statistics unavailable, so that studies have to be based on populations for whom information is available, such as hospital inpatients, outpatients and students, rather than the general population, although there are some notable exceptions (Orley & Wing, 1979).

Common mental disorders

The anthropologist Field (1960) first questioned the view that Africans are less susceptible to depression and anxiety: this has been shown to be incorrect. The pioneering work of Giel and van Luijk (1969) in a rural Ethiopian town provided early evidence of significant morbidity: 8.6 per cent of the community had significant psychiatric symptoms, and in most health centres, mental disorders were more often diagnosed than infectious diseases. A study using the Present State Examination (PSE) to diagnose depression found rates in rural Uganda to be comparable to London, UK (Orley & Wing, 1979) and in Southern Africa there are similar rates. A large survey of primary care attendees and a sample of women in the community in urban Zimbabwe revealed that 31 per cent of women had been depressed in the previous year and 18 per cent of primary care attendees were currently depressed (Broadhead et al., 1997; Abas & Broadhead, 1997). Another community survey, in which diagnostic criteria were used in rural

South Africa, found rates which may be higher than those in industrialized countries – 24 per cent of the population had depression or anxiety disorders (Bhagbwanjee et al., 1998). In both studies depression was more prevalent than anxiety.

Depression is common in developing countries, especially in women (Patel et al., 2001). Somatic presentations are common, but psychological symptoms are also usually present. Risk factors, so common in Africa, include poverty, disability, lack of support, bereavement and infertility. These findings are similar to those in developed countries.

Psychotic illnesses

The International Pilot Project on Schizophrenia (WHO, 1973) examined the incidence of schizophrenia at eight sites worldwide, including Ibadan, Nigeria. The incidence rates and symptom patterns were similar in all parts of the world, including Nigeria. These data reinforce the view that the features of schizophrenic illnesses are consistent across cultures. Two prevalence studies of schizophrenia in Africa found rates of 1.1 per 1000 population in Ghana (Sikanerty & Eaton, 1984) and 5.3 per 1000 in Botswana (Ben-Tovim & Cushnie, 1986). It is possible that, whilst incidence rates are similar to the developed world, prevalence rates are lower due to under-reporting of cases, better recovery and higher mortality of patients in the developing world (Warner & de Girolamo, 1995). Indeed, the outcome in developing countries has been found to be better than in industrialized countries (WHO, 1979; Jablensky et al., 1992). There is some suggestion that catatonic symptoms, rarely seen in the west, are more common in Africa (Okasha, 1968). There has been little work on bipolar affective disorder in Africa, but Paes et al. (1981) found patients in Morocco presented with similar symptoms as in Europe. Patients on antipsychotic medication can just as easily develop abnormal voluntary movements as those elsewhere (Odejide, 1981).

Suicidal behaviour

In an overview of psychiatry in Africa (Odejide et al., 1989), the authors concluded that suicidal behaviour was less common in Africans than in Caucasians, but higher rates were found in East Africa than in West Africa, while 19 per cent of over 7000 high school students in Cape Province, South Africa, had considered ending their lives in the previous year and 8 per cent actually attempted to do so (Flisher et al., 1993). This high rate of deliberate self harm in South Africa is supported by the findings of Peltzer et al. (2000), who found prevalences of attempted suicide of 11.3 per cent amongst blacks, 13 per cent amongst whites and 13.5 per cent amongst Asians in secondary school pupils.

Alcohol and drug use

The abuse of psychoactive substances – alcohol, cannabis and khat – is growing in Africa according to a WHO report (Nkowane & Jansen, 1999). The common substances misused (other than tobacco) are alcohol, cannabis and khat. Alcohol consumption has risen nine times in twelve years in some African countries, and in one rural community in South Africa, 56 per cent were dependent on alcohol (Claasen, 1999). Obviously, alcohol use rates vary considerably across Africa. Cannabis use is common in young men across the continent: 85 per cent of Egyptian secondary school students were using it in one study (Nkowane & Jansen, 1999). Khat use is common in the horn of Africa and it was used more commonly than cannabis in a Kenyan survey (Othieno et al., 2000). Consumption of opiates and stimulants is less common but is increasing, and this has serious consequences for physical and mental health.

HIV and AIDS

The devastation of HIV/AIDS has also increased psychiatric morbidity, which is higher in HIV/AIDS patients than in the general population: thus,among South African patients, 35 per cent had a major depressive disorder, 37 per cent a panic disorder, 21 per cent a generalized anxiety disorder, 6 per cent a post-traumatic stress disorder and 6 per cent a bipolar disorder (Els et al., 1999). Psychiatric morbidity must be actively treated if the quality of life for those with HIV/AIDS is to improve.

Trauma

Despite the refugee crises in Africa, with massive movements of people, both within country and between countries, few studies have been done on the effects on refugees' mental health. Peltzer (1999) used the Harvard Trauma Questionnaire among Sudanese refugees in Uganda, and found post-traumatic stress disorder (PTSD) in 32 per cent of adults and 20 per cent of children, often with co-morbid depression. Similar findings were reported in refugees in Mozambique (Reeler, 1995) and Gambia (Fox & Tang 2000; Tang & Fox 2001).

Trauma not only affects refugees, but also whole post-conflict societies, including children. For example, many

Rwandan children had experienced post-traumatic reactions after the genocide (Dyregov et al., 2000) – 90 per cent feared they would die and had to hide, 15 per cent under dead bodies. Post-traumatic reactions were associated with loss, exposure to violence and, most importantly, feeling their life was in danger. Children living in shelters were less likely to have reactions despite having experienced more trauma. A rate of PTSD of 15.8 per cent was found amongst randomly selected adults in Ethiopia, a country with recent conflict (de Jong et al., 2001). Risk factors included conflict-related trauma, torture, current and past psychiatric illness.

Cultural aspects of mental health in Africa

The diversity of cultures in a continent as vast and varied as Africa is too great to be summarized in a short space. There are some features of African cultures that are common and have an impact on mental health care.

Local idiom

In assessing, diagnosing and treating mental ill health it is important for the health worker to be understood and to use local language and idioms. For example, in Zimbabwe most depressed individuals think that their symptoms are due to 'thinking too much' – *kufungisisa*. In Botswana 'heart too much' – *pelo y tata* – also can signify depression (Patel et al., 2001). When mental health workers are from a different cultural background from that of the people among whom they work, they must be encouraged to use local cultural ways of understanding and of communicating mental distress.

Traditional healers and religious leaders

Patients will often turn to such people when they are unwell. There are good reasons for this. They have been established in their communities for a lot longer than orthodox health workers. They are more accessible than health services in many parts of Africa and less costly.

Religious organizations, such as Christian churches and Islamic communities, and traditional healers, can address people's spiritual needs, and also provide a beneficial community, in a way that health workers cannot.

It is essential that mental health services have a good relationship with traditional healers and religious organizations in order to work with them, to use their strengths, and to encourage them to refer patients with mental health needs to mental health workers when appropriate.

Legal and ethical aspects of mental healthcare

'The way care is provided to the patients in both the modern and the traditional institutions is not in accordance with the protection of human rights, at least as defined by western culture. Some countries have no mental health legislation except for a few articles in the criminal and civil codes that mention the rights of the mentally ill. . . . The right of a psychiatric patient to receive modern treatment to alleviate suffering is not something within the capacity of most African countries' (Alem, 2000).

The situation that Alem describes in Ethiopia is common. The main tenets of mental health legislation and ethics in the developed world are:

- the right of the mentally ill to receive treatment
- the right not to be abused in any way when receiving treatment
- the right of the general public to be protected from adverse consequences of mental illness.

In order to enact these rights, health and legal services must be available, at a considerable cost. This is clearly not possible for many African countries. The challenge for African mental health services is to set up realistic ethical and legal systems that can monitor mental health services to encourage good, ethical practices while taking into account the limitations in resources.

Delivering mental health care in Africa

Mental illness is as common in Africa as other parts of the world, and because of poverty and other social problems probably more common. However health care resources are scarce. For example in most of Africa there is about one psychiatrist for a million people. There are several important principles of planning future mental health services (Southbank University, 2000):

(i) Mental health care needs to be delivered through primary health care services. The vast majority of people with mental health problems cannot get to hospitals but may see a local health worker. Training these health workers to diagnose and treat mental illnesses, for example by use of diagnostic flow charts, is essential in improving mental health services (Abiodun, 1990).
(ii) Integrating national, district and primary health care systems will enable the few psychiatrists to teach local workers, aid referral of more challenging patients to specialist services and help implement a national policy.

(iii) A positive, co-operative relationship needs to be promoted between health services, traditional healers and religious groups. People will naturally turn to local religious groups and traditional healers, who will have strengths that help people with mental illnesses. If they, in their turn, also refer people to health services, a positive relationship can grow which benefits patients.

(iv) Health promotion and education need to be encouraged at a local level. Local idioms and models of mental illness can be used in helping people to understand mental illness, in encouraging them to accept and continue in treatment and in training health workers.

(v) There are certain problems in Africa that lead to mental illness which need to be emphasized. Refugee populations will have a high rate of PTSD and depression. AIDS has mental health consequences. Health staff working with these groups need to be trained to help patients with mental illnesses.

(vi) An international forum and database would help to inform mental health workers of good practice in similar settings, which can be applied locally.

References

Abas MA, Broadhead JC. (1997). Depression and anxiety among women in an urban setting in Zimbabwe. *Psychol Med*; **27**: 59–71.

Abiodun OA. (1990). Mental health and primary care in Africa. *E Afr Med J*; **67**: 273–278.

Alem A. (2000). Human rights and psychiatric care in Africa with particular reference to the Ethiopian situation. *Acta Psychiat Scand* (suppl); **399**: 93–96.

American Psychiatric Association (1994). ***Diagnostic and Statistical Manual of Mental Disorders, 4th edn.*** Washington DC: American Psychiatric Press.

Ben-Tovim DI, Cushnie JM. (1986). The prevalence of schizophrenia in a remote area of Botswana. *Br J Psychiatry*; **148**: 576–580.

Bhabwanjee A, Parekh A, Paruk Z et al. (1998). Prevalence of minor psychiatric disorder in an adult African rural community in South Africa. *Psychol Medi*; **28**: 1137–1147.

Broadhead J, Acuda SW, Mbape P et al. (1997). Depression in Zimbabwe: a community approach to prevention and treatment. *Centr Afr J Med*; **43**: 75–79.

Claasen JN. (1999). The benefits of the CAGE as a screening tool for alcoholism in a closed rural South African community. *S Afr Med J*; **89**: 976–979.

De Jong JT, Komproe IH, Van Ommeren M et al. (2001). Lifetime events and posttraumatic stress disorder in four postconflict settings. *J Am Med Assoc*; **286**: 584–588.

Dyregov A, Gupta L, Gjestad R et al. (2000). Trauma exposure and psychological reactions to genocide among Rwandan children. *J Trauma Stress*; **13**: 3–21.

Els C, Boshoff W, Scott C et al. (1999). Psychiatric co-morbidity in South African HIV/AIDS patients. *S Afr Med J*; **89**: 992–995.

Field MJ. (1960). *Search for Security: An Ethno-psychiatric Study of Rural Ghana*. London: Faber and Faber.

Flisher AJ, Ziervogel CF, Chalton DO et al. (1993). Risk taking behaviour of Cape peninsular high school students. *S Afr Med J*; **83**: 474–476.

Fox SH, Tang SS. (2000). The Sierra Leonean refugee experience: traumatic events and psychiatric sequelae. *J Nerv Ment Dis*; **188**: 490–495.

German GA. (1987). Mental health in Africa: I The extent of mental health problems in Africa today. *Br J Psychiatry*; **151**: 435–439.

Giel R, Van Luijk JN. (1969). Psychiatric morbidity in a small Ethiopian town. *Br J Psychiatry*; **115**: 149–162.

Jablensky A, Sartorius N, Ernberg G et al. (1992). Schizophrenia: manifestations, incidence and course in different cultures. *Psychological Medicine Monograph* Supplement 20. Cambridge: Cambridge University Press.

Nkowane AM, Jansen MA. (1999). Substance abuse in Africa. *Africa Hlth*; **20**: 15–16.

Odejide AO. (1981). The prevalence of persistent abnormal involuntary movements among patients in a Nigerian long stay psychiatric unit. *Afr J Med Med Sci*; **10**: 39–43.

Odejide AO, Oyewunmi LK, Ohaeri JU. (1989). Psychiatry in Africa: an overview. *Am J Psychiatry*; **146**: 708–716.

Okasha A. (2002). Mental health in Africa: the role of the WPA. *World Psychiatry*; **1**: 32–35.

Okasha A, Kamel M, Hassan AH. (1968). Preliminary psychiatric observations in Egypt. *Br J Psychiatry*; **114**: 949–955.

Orley J, Wing JK. (1979). Psychiatric disorders in two African villages. *Arch Gen Psychiatry*; **36**: 513–520.

Othieno CJ, Kathuku DM, Ndetei DM. (2000). Substance abuse in outpatients attending rural and urban health centres in Kenya. *E Afr Med J*; **77**: 592–594.

Patel V, Abas M, Broadhead J, et al. (2001). Depression in developing countries: lessons from Zimbabwe. *Br Med J*; **322**: 482–484.

Peltzer K. (1999). Trauma and mental health problems of Sudanese refugees in Uganda. *Cent Afr J Med*; **45**: 110–113.

Peltzer K, Cherian VI, Cherian L. (2000). Cross cultural attitudes towards suicide among South African secondary school pupils. *E Afr Med J*; **77**: 165–167.

Paes M, Chkli T, Ktionet J. (1981). Clinical aspects of manic-depressive psychosis in Morocco. *Psychopath Afr*; **17**: 171–189.

Reeler AP. (1995). Trauma in Mozambican refugees. *Torture*; **5**: 18–20.

Sikanerty T, Eaton WW. (1984). Prevalence of schizophrenia in the Labadi district of Ghana. *Acta Psychiat Scand*; **69**: 156–161.

Southbank University (2000). Mental health in sub-saharan Africa. Southbank University, London.

Tang SS, Fox SH. (2001). Traumatic experiences and the mental health of Senegalese refugees. *J Nerv Ment Dis*; **189**: 507–512.

Warner R, de Girolamo G. (1995). *Schizophrenia*. Geneva: WHO.
Westley D (1993). *Mental Health and Psychiatry in Africa*. London: Hans Zell.
Wilkinson M, Mbuluma EL, Masache TG et al. (1990). *A Mental Health Handbook for Malawi*. Malawi: Ministry of Health.
World Bank (1993). *World Development Report: Investing in Health*. New York: Oxford University Press.
WHO (1979). *Schizophrenia: An International Follow-up Study*. Geneva: World Health Organization.
WHO (1993). *The ICD-10 Classification of Mental and Behavioural Disorders*. Geneva: World Health Organization.
WHO (1996). *Investing in Health and Development: Report of the Ad Hoc Committee on Health Research Relating to Future Intervention Options*. Geneva: World Health Organization.

Recommended reading

Sims A. (1996). *Symptoms in the Mind*, 2nd edn. London, Ballière Tindall.
Gelder, Mayou, de Jong et al. (2001). *The Oxford Textbook of Psychiatry*. Oxford: Oxford University Press.
Desjarlais R, Eisenberg L, Good B, Kleinman A. (1995). *World Mental Health*. New York: Oxford University Press.
Patel V. (2003). *Where There is no Psychiatrist*. London: Gaskell.

89 The disabled patient

Introduction

This chapter is different to many others in this book. It is not concerned with specific diseases, their pathology and treatment, but rather with the chronic effect of disabling diseases on patients and their community, and the role that the health worker has in helping those who have disabling conditions.

Most health workers in Africa will be involved in some way with people who have disabilities but, even if their direct professional involvement is minimal, they will always be looked at as role models for the community's relationship with disabled people. Therefore, every health worker must understand the subject of disability and how to promote the rehabilitation and employment of the disabled, if they are to be of help to them. The focus is on the individual person, not on the disability.

If health workers are seen to focus on the disability, and not the person, then the community is likely to do the same, and disabled people may feel labelled by their disability. If, however, the health worker focuses first on the person, rather than on his or her disability, then the community is also likely to adopt the same attitude. People with disabilities may then become more welcomed and integrated into the community, where jobs are often hard to find (Kubheka & Uys, 1999), social and personal difficulties abound (Akesode & Iyang,1981) and benefits may be hard to secure (Muyembe & Muhinga, 1999).

Definition of disability

The word disability has many meanings. Even among health care workers it is often used loosely and interchangeably with 'handicap' or 'impairment', so that an exact definition is important. The World Health Organization (WHO, 1981) has put forward the following progression as a useful framework for understanding terminology in this area:

Disease → Impairment → Disability → Handicap

Disease here means the underlying pathophysiological process that the patient is suffering, or has suffered from.

Impairment is the loss or abnormality of psychological, physiological or anatomical structure or function.

Example: Tuberculosis of the spine

The WHO four-stage progression makes possible a precise description of disability. For example, if a person is paraplegic following a tuberculous infection of the spine, the *disease* is tuberculosis affecting the spine and causing dysfunction of the spinal cord, the *impairment* is a lack of control of lower limbs and bladder. The *disability* is the inability to use the legs for mobility, to void urine when needed, and to control the bladder sphincter when it is inappropriate to pass urine. The *handicap* for this person arises when the disability prevents him or her from leading a normal life within the local community.

Medical management of tuberculosis of the spine can be of value at all stages in the progression from disease to handicap. If the person with paraplegia due to tuberculosis of the spine receives appropriate drug treatment in the early stages of the disease, such treatment may sometimes be able to reverse the paraplegia and thus remove the disability.

In many cases of tuberculosis of the spine the paraplegia is permanent and thus the disability is lifelong. Treatment is, however, still of use in reducing or limiting handicap. For example, the patient can be given a wheelchair and become mobile within the community. He or she can also be trained in intermittent self-catheterization and thus achieve a good level of bladder control. In this case the original disability still exists and is unchanged, but the handicap is significantly reduced and the patient can often fulfil a role that is normal for their culture and community.

Disability is any restriction or lack of ability to perform an activity in the manner or within the range considered normal for a human being.

Handicap is the disadvantage for a given individual, resulting from an impairment or a disability, that limits or prevents the fulfilment of a role that is normal (depending on age, sex, social and cultural factors for that individual) (see the Box).

The range of disabilities

Disease and impairment can affect all systems of the body, for example, visual impairment, hearing impairment, psychological impairment, and mobility or locomotor impairment. This chapter will focus mainly on locomotor impairment as visual or psychological impairment are considered in Chapters 94 and 88. However, the definition of terms above applies to impairment, disability and handicap in all systems of the body.

The clinical problem

Most patients with disability are beyond the initial stage of their disease and already have established impairment and disability. The challenge is thus to minimize the progression to handicap (see the Box).

> **Disability – the challenge**
> to minimize
> the progression to handicap

(*Footnote*: The World Health Organization (WHO) also has a much more complex classification of terms and concepts used in disability. This is called the *International Classification of Functioning, Disability and Health*, and is known as ICIDH-2. It is a section of the WHO family of international classifications and is complementary to the better-known ICD-10 or *International Classification of Diseases, tenth revision*. ICIDH-2 has arisen because of the realization that the progression: *disease → impairment → disability → handicap* is a gross simplification of reality, that the direction of the arrows can be reversed, and that the social and physical environment can have a significant effect on the disablement process. ICIDH-2 is not in common use but is an invaluable tool for research in disablement and in measurement of the effect of disability. Details of this system can be obtained from WHO, see address in further information section.)

The problem in Africa

Prevalence of disability

There are few reliable statistics on the prevalence of disability in Africa and a lot of estimations have been made. For the world as a whole, it is often claimed that 10 per cent of the population is disabled; however, this figure is taken from research in wealthier countries where people live longer and where the majority of disabled people are elderly (BBC, 1998). A survey by Helander et al. (1989) showed that approximately 3 per cent of the population in developing countries would benefit from some type of rehabilitation, but did not estimate the total prevalence of disability. There may be political and economic reasons for governments to over or under report the incidence of disability but a fair figure for all types of disability in Africa is probably between 5 and 10 per cent of the total population (UNESCO, 1995).

Types and causes of disability

UNESCO's 1995 report on types and causes of disability in the developing nations is broadly representative of the situation in Africa (Figs. 89.1, 89.2).

These figures are representative of Africa as a whole, although certain areas may have local causes that are particularly prevalent. For example, in countries where landmines are being used, or have been used, they are a major cause of disability and consequent handicap. In Angola, for example, one person in every 470 has had a limb amputated (Helander et al., 1989).

There may also be foci within a country where a particular type of disability is common, for example, the spastic paraparesis of children with *Konzo* (pp. 37, 1148), in Mozambique, or the blindness of older people with onchocerciasis (p. 434) near the Niger or the Volta river systems in West Africa.

Attitudes to disability

There is a wide range of cultural attitudes to people with disabilities in Africa, just as there is all over the world; from pity to admiration, and from stigma to acceptance. Sadly, in many places, disabled people are perceived to be of less value than able-bodied people as they are less able to work and support the community: thus, disabled children are less likely to go to school, both because of mobility difficulties and because, when money is short, families are less likely to spend what little they have on school fees for a disabled child.

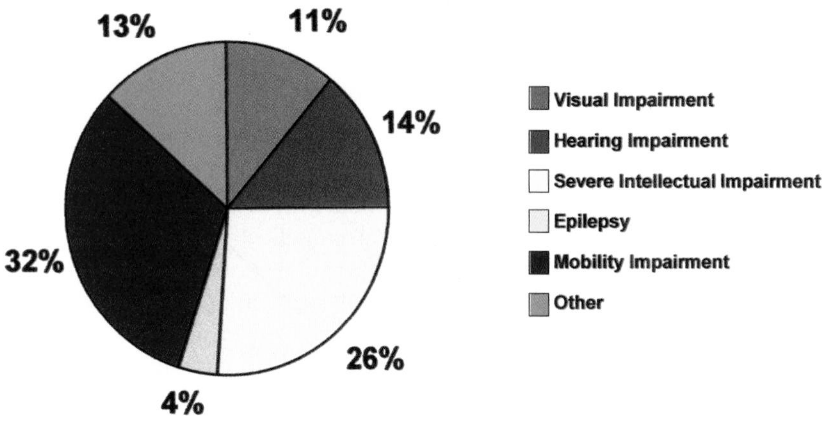

Fig. 89.1. The distribution of impairment by type. It shows that the largest single impairment is mobility, which accounts for almost one in every three people with disabilities.

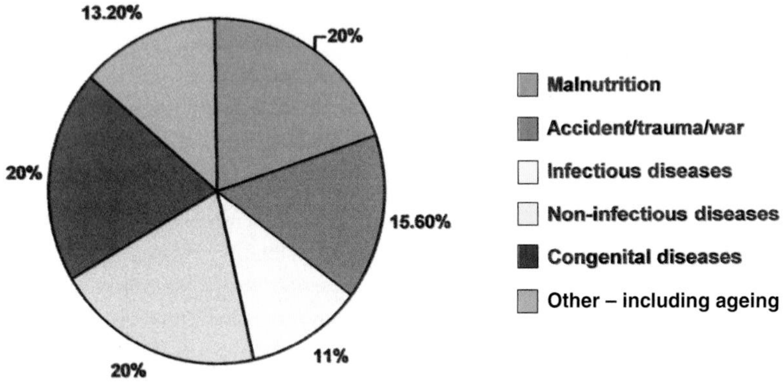

Fig. 89.2. Global causes of impairment (UNESCO, 1995).

Cultural understanding

In some cultures, disability may be thought to be connected in some way with evil spirits. In some areas of Malawi, for example, when a child is born with a club foot, it is thought to be due to bad spirits or an evil spell affecting the mother during the pregnancy (Lavy, 1996). (See the Box).

> **Practical response**
>
> *Awareness* Those who work with disabled people should try to understand the culture in which they are working, so that they can be aware of all the attitudes that may be affecting their disabled patients, their families and communities.
>
> *Action* The health care worker can have an important and a valuable role in the community by encouraging an attitude to the disabled person that involves neither pity nor excessive admiration, but simply an honest respect for the individual as a fellow human being.

Medical aspects of disability

Most of the care given to people with physical disabilities world-wide is given by those with special skills and is not given by doctors. Therapists and other health workers have the dominant and most intensive role. The doctor or medical clinician's role is, however, important as a member of the team, particularly in diagnosis and specialized treatment.

Orthopaedic clinical officers

In Malawi, as there are few doctors with orthopaedic skills, a cadre of non-medically qualified clinicians, called orthopaedic clinical officers, has been trained specially to give appropriate and early treatment to injuries and simple orthopaedic conditions and so to prevent later disability.

Diagnosis

In many African countries a disabled person, particularly a child, can be given a diagnostic label defining his or her disability. This diagnosis may, or may not, be right, and if wrong may lead to false expectations or inappropriate treatment. It is the role of the clinician to make or to clarify the diagnosis and cause of disability at the earliest possible stage.

Basic clinical method is fundamental – a detailed history, a careful clinical examination, and relevant investigations are needed for a precise diagnosis. Some disabilities can appear very similar to the inexperienced observer:

Examples

(i) Congenital absence of the tibia causes the foot to deviate in a varus direction and this may appear like a club foot.
(ii) Congenital kyphosis may cause a prominent gibbus of the spine, which may appear like a TB kyphosis.
(iii) Osteogenesis imperfecta may cause bowing of the tibiae and this may look similar to rickets.

When as clear a diagnosis as possible has been decided, an appropriate plan of management can be worked out.

Treatment of underlying disease

A lot of permanent physical disability in Africa arises because of inadequate treatment of the causative disease. Start adequate treatment of underlying disease as soon as possible and so prevent chronic physical disability.

For example:

- appropriate treatment of open fractures will prevent malunion, non-union, and osteomyelitis
- appropriate treatment of burns will prevent contractures
- appropriate treatment of tuberculosis of the spine will prevent paraplegia
- appropriate treatment of early club foot will prevent severe deformities.

Treatment of intercurrent medical problems

People with physical disabilities are often at particular risk of developing other medical problems. For example, people with paraplegia are likely to get urinary tract infections because of urinary stasis and regular passage of catheters. They are also at risk of developing pressure sores in dependent areas, chest complications and contractures of unexercised joints.

Psychological support

There is often a social stigma and a feeling of inadequacy attached both to the person and to the family of a person with a disability. It is therefore very important for any health worker who has to deal with such people to allay their feelings of inadequacy, for example, by concentrating on and encouraging the other areas in which the patient has no disability. Certain people with disabilities may benefit from professional psychological counselling where this is available, but few African countries have such a service in towns, much less so in remote areas. The health worker should therefore be ready to take the lead in showing the patient, the family and the society, by his or her attitude, that people with disabilities, as indeed all people, have intrinsic value as unique individuals.

Surgery

There are many instances in the field of physical disability where surgery can either remove the disability or at least significantly reduce it. Operations for cataract are an excellent example of simple surgery, which reverses a disability: the examples below are some of the operations commonly performed on people with disabilities in the author's unit in Malawi.

Correction of soft tissue deformity

Release of burn contractures, and surgical release of club foot contracture can often effectively treat the impairment that is causing the disability.

Tendon transfer

Following a radial nerve injury at the level of the humerus, there is no nerve supply remaining to the wrist and finger extensors. Flexor tendons from functioning forearm muscles, supplied by the ulnar and median nerves, can be transferred to the dorsum of the arm and reattached to the extensor tendons of the wrist and fingers to supply the missing extensor functions.

Correction of bony deformity

Osteotomy of the tibia can be used to correct bow legs, and osteotomy of the hindfoot and forefoot can correct late presenting club foot (Figs. 89.3, 89.4).

Fusion of unstable joints

Where a person has lost the power of dorsiflexion of the ankle following a sciatic or common peroneal nerve

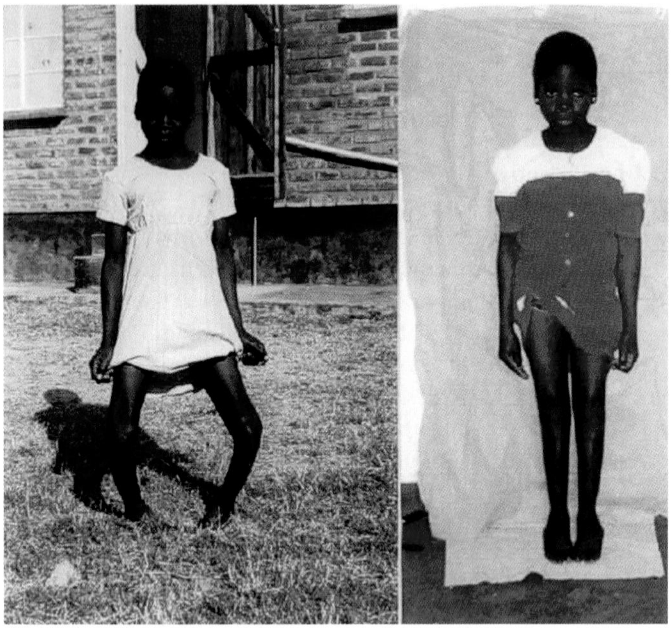

Fig. 89.3. 13-year-old girl from Malawi before and after tibial osteotomy to correct severe genu valgum.

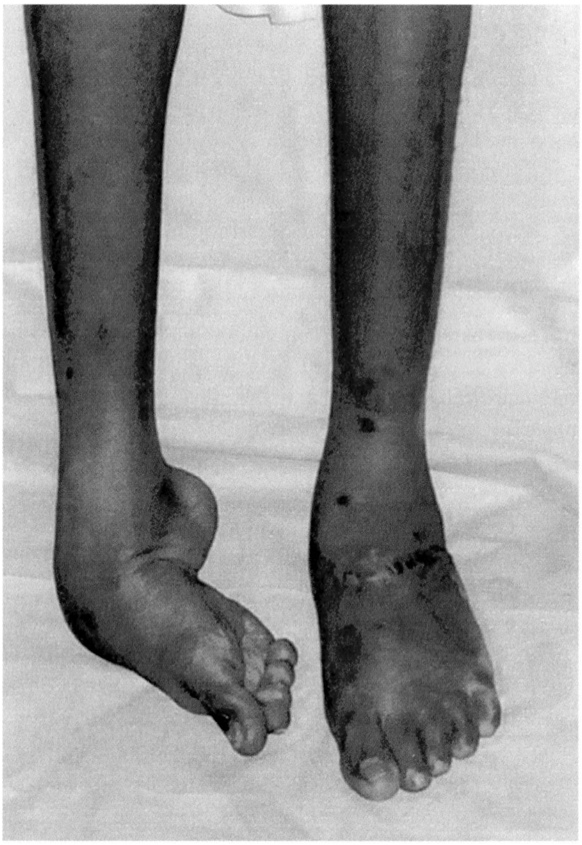

Fig. 89.4. This 16-year-old boy had bilateral untreated club feet and walked on the dorsum of his feet with the soles facing inwards. Following osteotomy to the left side (on the right in the picture) the foot is now in the plantigrade position and he can wear normal shoes. This picture was taken shortly before similar surgery to the right side.

injury, fusion of the ankle can restore stability. It should be noted, however, that surgery is not the only treatment of this common disability and foot drop can also be effectively treated with splints.

Removal of dead bone

Sequestrectomy in chronic osteomyelitis involves the removal of dead and infected bone so that the infection can heal and thus relieve the patient of the disability of chronic pain and discharge.

Prevention of disabilities

Many physical disabilities can easily be prevented by simple measures. One of the best examples is polio. A simple oral vaccine that is administered to all children in an area can effectively eradicate the disease. In Malawi in the 1980s there were hundreds of new cases of polio each year. However, following a very well-organized vaccination programme by the Ministry of Health, there has not been a new case reported since 1995. Other examples of disability prevention include the use of folic acid supplements in women of child-bearing age to reduce the incidence of spina bifida and neural tube defects, and road safety campaigns to reduce speed, overcrowding of vehicles, and accidents on the roads of African countries.

Economic relief and additional income

Many African countries have both governmental and non-governmental agencies that are able to channel relief in the form of extra finances, food and essential services to people with disabilities. Health workers may not be involved with the management of such agencies but they are often the only link that rural people with disabilities have to any official organization, and thus should be aware of what relief is available in their area. Health centres and hospitals are therefore very appropriate places for posters and publicity materials that deal with income and food support for disadvantaged groups, and it is entirely appropriate for health workers to direct people with disabilities and their families to other agencies that can help them. In addition to financial and material support organizations there may be agencies that aim to help in vocational and

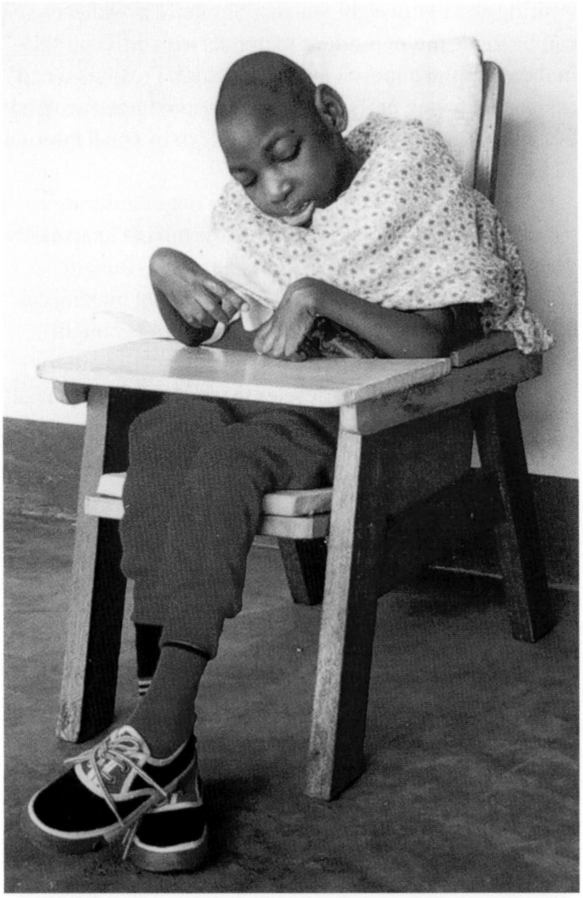

Fig. 89.5. A wooden seat for a child with cerebral palsy, made locally in Uganda. Without the support given by this seat the child would not be able to sit, and might spend his life lying on the floor.

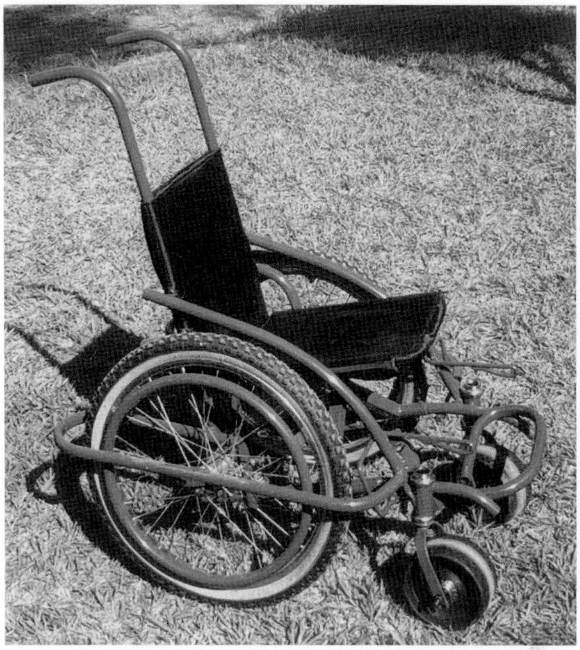

Fig. 89.6. A wheelchair made in Uganda from locally available bicycle parts and steel tubing.

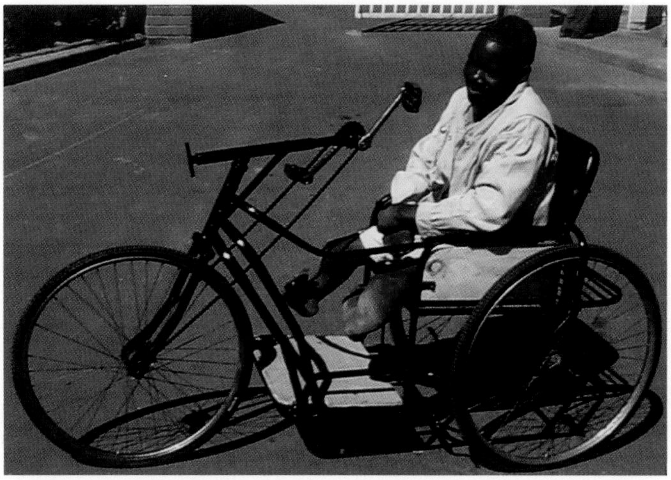

Fig. 89.7. A tricycle made in Malawi out of bicycle parts for a patient with tibial agenesis (absent tibias).

other training of people with disabilities. The health worker's role is again to be aware of what is available locally so that he or she can assist the patient, who may well feel intimidated by official structures, to make the best possible use of all available services.

Appliances for people with disabilities

People with physical disabilities that affect mobility can often be helped by external appliances. These fall into the categories of aids, orthoses and prostheses.

Aids are items such as crutches, chairs (see Fig. 89.5), wheelchairs (see Fig. 89.6), and tricycles (see Fig. 89.7), that can be used by people with disabilities to improve their mobility or independence. Often such aids can markedly reduce the handicap associated with disability and help the disabled person to function normally in society.

Orthoses are items that are attached to the body but are not part of it. They include such items as braces and callipers (see Fig. 89.8) that can support unstable limbs. Many people with polio have some control of their hips but do not have any control of their knees and feet. The use of callipers can give them rigid but stable legs and allow

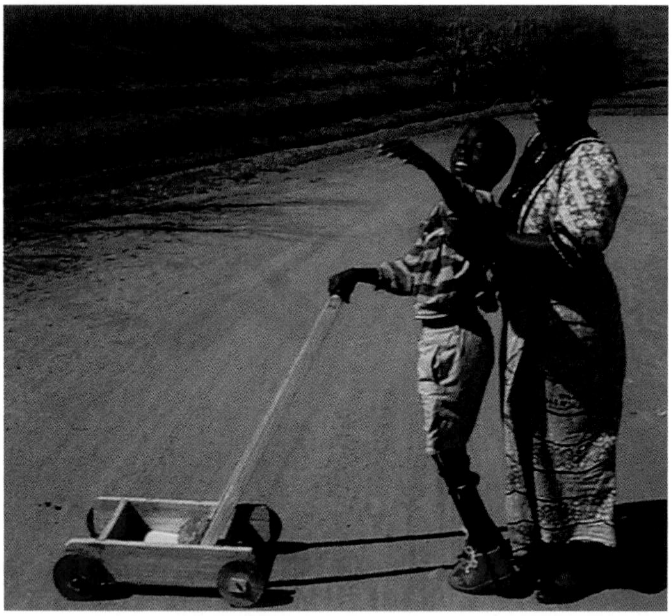

Fig. 89.8. A boy with cerebral palsy learning to walk. He needs the help of callipers to support his knees, a locally made wooden push truck to balance, and at this stage also his mother.

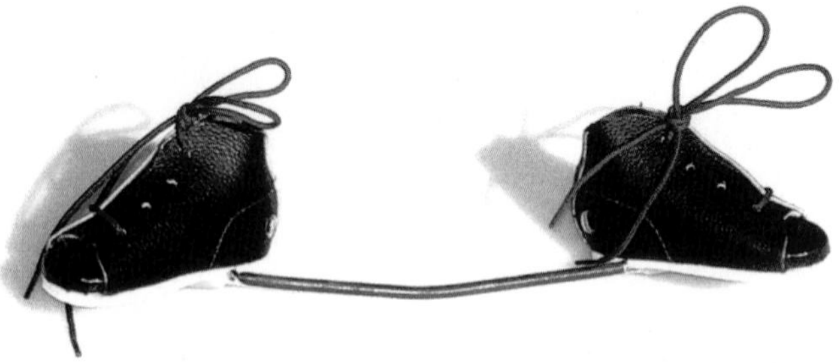

Fig. 89.9. A Steenbeek foot abduction splint made in Malawi from locally available leather, wood, and steel building rods. This splint can be used at night to maintain the position of treated club feet to prevent recurrence.

them to walk upright. Other common orthoses include the foot abduction night splint used in maintaining correction in club foot (see Fig. 89.9), and the ankle foot orthosis used to stop an unstable ankle flopping into an equinus position.

Prostheses are items that replace parts of the body that are missing. The commonest example is the artificial limb. A well-made and well-fitting artificial leg can often restore almost normal mobility.

The technology used in the manufacture of aids, orthoses and prostheses varies greatly throughout the world. In rich countries where cost is not a limiting factor, appliances can be made out of the most modern hard-wearing and lightweight plastics. Similarly, prostheses can be made out of modern materials with artificial skin matched to the patient's own skin colour. Prostheses can also have moving parts such as hands and fingers worked by cables from other parts of the body or by small internal electric motors.

In most countries of Africa cost is a major limiting factor and appliances are locally made out of cheap easily obtainable materials. In the 1960s, Professor Ronald Huckstep in Uganda popularized a system of making callipers out of local wood, leather and iron rods bought from building suppliers. He also introduced the production of wheelchairs and tricycles made out of locally available bicycle parts. The great benefit of the 'Huckstep' system is that all the appliances are locally made and can be locally repaired.

Rehabilitation of the disabled

The need

Many physically disabled need not only appliances, but also a rehabilitation service, which will help them to integrate into their local communities. This is often a long process and may take many years and involve different disciplines within the rehabilitation service. For example, a patient with cerebral palsy would benefit from help by a physiotherapist to gain mobility, an occupational therapist to learn the skills of daily living, an orthopaedic technologist to make splints and a speech therapist to improve verbal communication.

The reality

Rehabilitation services such as outlined above are, however, rare; indeed, it is estimated that only 2 per cent of people with disabilities in Africa have access to appropriate rehabilitation services (Despouy, 1993).

Institutions

Historically, rehabilitation services have been run on an institutional basis, for example, schools for the blind, and homes for physically disabled children with workshops attached.

Community services

Because hospitals and health centres could only care for and serve a limited number of people, community services were developed. These are run in several ways:

Professional rehabilitation workers

One popular method is to send professional rehabilitation workers such as physiotherapists and occupational therapists into the community to provide services where they are needed, rather than requiring people with disabilities to come to an institution.

Community-based rehabilitation or CBR

This aims to keep the person with a disability in their own community, with their rehabilitation needs looked after by someone in their community. There are several models of CBR and all of them involve delegation of rehabilitation responsibilities to the lowest appropriate level. Thus, parents of village children with cerebral palsy may be given supervised exercises by a CBR worker from their own or a neighbouring village who has had a short training course. The local CBR worker would in turn be supervised by the therapist who would cover a whole district. It is estimated that around 70 per cent of rehabilitation needs of a community can be met in this way (Despouy, 1993) (Fig. 89.10).

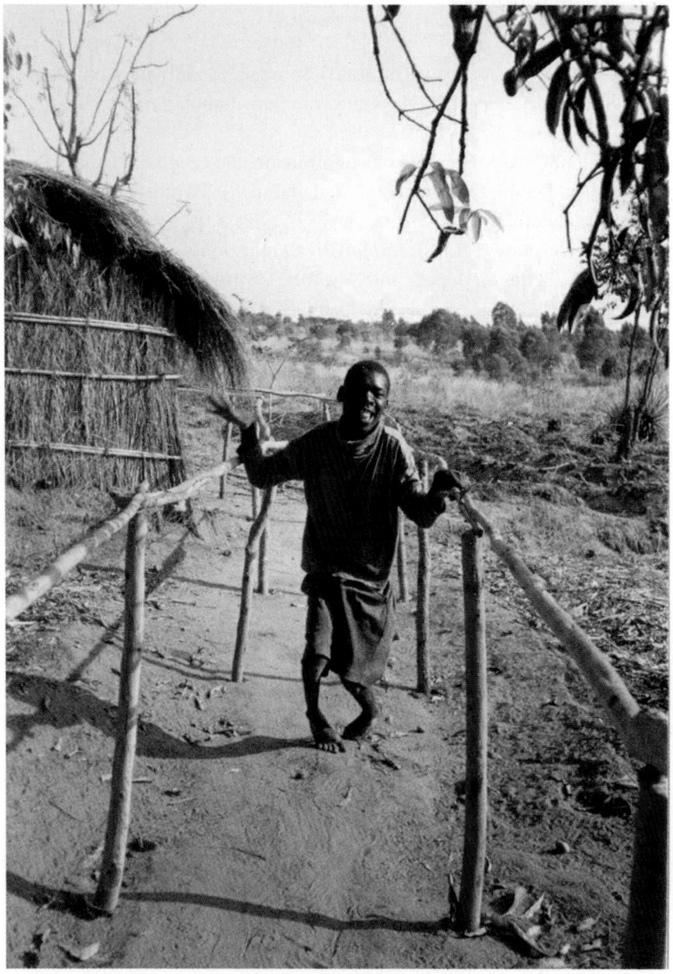

Fig. 89.10. An 8-year-old boy with cerebral palsy whose community rehabilitation worker has enabled the building of locally made parallel bars next to his hut to help him walk.

Referral for rehabilitation

Many patients who would benefit from rehabilitation, either primarily or following surgery, are seen by doctors or clinicians and yet they never receive appropriate rehabilitation. This may be because rehabilitation services do not exist or are overworked. But it may also be because rehabilitation has not become a standard method and principle in the mind of the medical officer. It is important therefore that there are good lines of communication between rehabilitation services and the doctors or clinical officers who refer patients to them.

Community approach to disability issues

This chapter has emphasized the medical approach to disability, which is the first and essential step. But there is much more. People with disabilities have to be fully integrated into society. Therefore, all members of the community have to be willing to play some part in the integration of any person with a disability. The role of doctors and professional rehabilitation workers such as physiotherapists, occupational therapists and their assistants is certainly important, but full integration and thus minimization of handicap will not be achieved without the co-operation of many sectors of society.

- Teachers should be willing to include children with disabilities in their classes, and give them the attention they deserve.
- Town planners and architects should make sure that people with disabilities are not further disadvantaged by problems of access.
- Managers of transport facilities should give consideration to all members of society so that access to, and use of buses, minibuses, taxis, trains, etc. is available to everyone.
- Politicians especially should be aware of the needs and rights of all members of their consitituency, and should be prepared to make a stand in public to support the members of their country with disabilities.

References

Akesode FA, Iyang UE. (1981). Some social and sexual problems experienced by Nigerians with limb amputation. *Trop Geog Med*; **33**: 71–74.

BBC World Service Facts Information and Comment about Disability in Africa. (1998). London: BBC World Service Publications.

Despouy L. (1993). *Human Rights and Disabled Persons* (Study Series 6), Geneva and New York: Centre for Human Rights.

Helander E, Mendis P, Nelson G et al. (1989). *Training in the Community for People with Disabilities*. Geneva: World Health Organization.

Kubheka BA, Uys LR. (1995). Amputation history and rehabilitation of black men living in the greater Durban area who have traumatic amputations of the lower limb. *Curationis*; **18**: 44–48.

Lavy CBD. (1996). Unpublished, Attitudes to disability. PO Box 256, Blantyre Malawi.

Mines Advisory Group Data Bank. 45–27 Newton Street, Manchester M1 1FT, UK.

Muyembe VM, Muhinga MN. (1999). Major limb amputation at a provincial general hospital in Kenya. *E Afr Med J*; **76**: 163–166.

UNESCO. (1995). Overcoming obstacles to the integration of disabled people, DAA, March 1995.

WHO Expert Committee on Disability Prevention and Rehabilitation. (1981). Geneva: World Health Organization.

Further information and reading

Werner D. (1987). Disabled Village Children. The Hesperian Foundation, PO Box 1692, Palo Also, CA 94302, USA. ISBN 0–942364–06–6.

Werner D. (1998). Nothing about us without us. Healthwrights, PO Box 1692, Palo Also, CA 94302, USA. ISBN 0–9655585–3–3.

Vereecken M J. (1996). Cerebral Palsy Children in Africa – early identification and intervention. Wolf-Tool Publications, Postbus 321, 2300 AH Leiden, The Netherlands. ISBN 90–70857–30–8.

Useful address for further information

World Health Organization (WHO),
20 Avenue Appia, CH-1211 Geneva, Switzerland.
Contact the Chief Medical Officer, Rehabilitation.
http://www.who.com

Cancers and lymphomas

90

Introduction

This chapter is an introduction to the subject of cancer in Africa. The diagnosis of malignancy usually, but not always, carries a dire prognosis. Because many cancers are entirely avoidable, their epidemiology, causes and prevention are given first, together with the basic biology of cancer. The clinical problems of the cancers which are particularly prevalent in Africa follow, with the therapeutic dilemmas that they present.

Risk of cancer

Cancer epidemiology

Illness does not occur in a vacuum but as a result of an exposure (such as malarial mosquito, tubercle bacillus or tobacco smoke), a deficiency (vitamin deficiency, malnutrition), or inherited susceptibility (sickle cell disease). Environmental exposures, socio-geographical context, and heritable susceptibility all contribute to a causal web that results in illness.

Epidemiology (from 'epi' – among, 'demos' the people) is the discipline that informs clinicians about disease risk in populations. Thus, epidemiologists help to quantify the contribution of various exposures to the cause and progression of illness. The economic consequences of illness that contribute to the global burden of disease have been expressed numerically by estimating of 'disability adjusted life years' or DALYS (Murray & Lopez, 1997). Basic epidemiological methods must be described if cancer risks are to be understood.

Basic epidemiological method

The mathematical estimation of risk derives from two main types of population research: observational, and interventional. Observational studies examine outcomes (e.g. cancer) in populations in relation to exposures, e.g. smoking, and estimate the risks accordingly.

Cohort studies

A cohort study is the most reliable way to calculate risk in a population. We observe a very large group or 'cohort' of people (say, factory workers, or an entire village) after measuring certain baseline characteristics and exposures (such as HIV infection). Over time, we count diseases of interest (say tuberculosis) and estimate disease incidence by expressing the number of cases of disease per person–years of follow-up. We then calculate the relative risk of disease attributed to a particular exposure by dividing the incidence of disease in exposed persons by the incidence of disease in unexposed persons.

Case control studies

Because cohort studies are expensive and time-consuming, epidemiologists often use the case control method. In this method, cases (persons who already have the disease of interest) are identified in the hospital and are asked to report their lifestyle, occupation, sexual behaviour, etc. from memory. These cases are compared with a concurrent group of controls chosen to be as similar to cases as possible, with the exception that they do not have the disease of interest. Sometimes cases and controls are matched to each other by variables such as age and sex. The relative risk is calculated by dividing the odds of disease in exposed persons by the odds of disease in the unexposed persons. The relative risk is often called the odds ratio in case control studies. In a recent case control study the relative risk of getting Kaposi's sarcoma in HIV-infected persons is 80 times (odds ratio = 80) that in uninfected persons (Sitas et al., 1997).

Descriptive studies

Descriptive studies such as cancer rates in immigrants, or rates of the same cancer in different countries, can also help identify risks such as dietary effects. But such 'ecological' research cannot control for differences in disease rates that are not related to an exposure, for example socioeconomic differences, age structure and reproductive patterns. All epidemiological studies are subject to errors produced by biases (systematic distortions), confounding (an alternative explanation for an effect), and chance (random error, usually due to small sample size). Methodological and analytical techniques can estimate the likelihood of error, and it is always wise to examine the 'confidence interval', or size of estimated error, around the relative risk. The most authoritative study of an effect is a prospective randomized clinical trial, which, by design, helps to eliminate many systematic errors.

Cancer risks in Africa

Table 90.1 shows the rates of selected cancers in Africa by sex, compared with rates in Europe in 1990 (Parkin & Ziegler, 2000). Because population age profiles differ by geographical region, cancer rates are 'standardized' by age to allow more meaningful comparisons. Because they often lack accurate death records, developing countries may have to rely on cancer registries in a defined region to estimate cancer rates. By counting and recording all cancers, a 'population-based' estimate of cancer profiles over time can be inferred (Templeton, 1973; Parkin & Sangli, 1991).

Certain 'endemic' cancers are particularly frequent in Africa: compared with European rates, oesophageal and liver cancer appear in excess, while colon cancer rates are very low. In women, breast cancer rates are about half those in Europe, while cervix carcinoma is more than twice as common. Cancer rates also differ between African regions. Bladder, lung, and laryngeal cancer, for example, are dominant in North Africa. Epidemiologists attribute aetiological risks by region to differences in environment, diet, and lifestyle. Several cancers in Africa, such as carcinoma of the liver (hepatitis viruses) and bladder (*S. haematobium*) have been linked to infectious agents that are more prevalent in certain parts of the continent (See chapters on hepatitis and schistosomiasis.)

Cancer mortality

Cancer deaths in Africa are less than half the rates in Europe and America, owing to competing mortality from perinatal and infectious causes. But as development proceeds with the accompanying hazards of urbanization, patterns of life and illness will change. For example, rates of smoking-related cancers are slowly rising. Dietary changes (more fat, less fibre) could well alter the low rates of colon cancer, and changing reproductive habits (fewer children, delayed pregnancy) may increase breast cancer rates (Parkin & Sangli, 2001).

Causes of cancer

Cancers are derived from one of over 100 different types of cell and are classified according to their embryonal origins, e.g. epithelial cancers are carcinomas, mesenchymal cancers are sarcomas. Each cancer type has its own 'natural history'. Some types, such as skin cancer, are easily cured. Others, such as liver and lung cancer, carry a very high mortality. As the progeny of a single aberrant cell, cancer behaviour and detection depend on the site of origin. For example, liver cancers are often detected late in their natural history while skin cancers can be detected early. Kaposi's sarcoma and breast cancer may have an indolent course, but Burkitt's lymphoma develops very rapidly. Despite their clinical heterogeneity, all cancers have certain common characteristics.

The process of cancer development – oncogenesis – often takes years or decades. In many cancers, the biggest risk factor is age. Some individuals, usually those with strong family history of cancer, inherit a genetic susceptibility to cancer. This may be obvious (as in heritable breast and ovarian cancer caused by mutations in the BRCA genes) or subtle (such as inheritance of variant genes that metabolize carcinogens poorly). In the majority, cancer results from a gradual accumulation of acquired, random accidents to chromosomal DNA, the nuclear instructions that govern cell growth and behaviour.

Basic cancer biology

Structure of DNA

DNA (deoxyribonucleic acid) has a sugar–phosphate backbone, shaped like a twisted ladder or double helix. The rungs of the ladder are 4 bases – cytosine and thymidine (pyrimidines), adenine and guanine (purines). Essential to both the concepts of genetic coding and to cell division is the rule that each base only pairs with one

Table 90.1. Estimated age standardized cancer rates in Africa and Europe, 1990[a]

Region	Mouth/ pharynx		Oesoph-agus		Stomach		Colon/ rectum		Liver		Lung		Melanoma				Corpus			Bladder		Lymphoma		All sites (excl. skin)	
of Africa	M	F	M	F	M	F	M	F	M	F	M	F	M	F	Breast	Cervis	Uteri	Ovary	Prostate	M	F	M	F	M	F
Eastern	16.9	10.4	17.4	4.8	14.1	13.3	6.5	3.9	21.8	9.5	5.5	1.3	5.3	8.3	19.4	49.2	4.8	7.8	27.4	8.0	4.5	7.5	4.5	186.5	180.7
Middle	18.7	10.9	4.7	0.7	20.8	13.3	6.1	6.5	20.7	10.6	9.4	1.7	9.6	9.4	26.3	38.0	9.3	7.1	31.5	9.6	2.3	12.7	7.9	212.1	199.0
Northern	12.4	7.2	5.3	1.7	5.8	3.4	7.9	7.9	5.9	2.7	20.7	5.5	1.3	0.9	57.1	11.4	1.6	3.3	5.0	25.6	6.9	11.1	7.1	157.0	156.4
Southern	13.4	3.4	40.7	12.1	12.9	6.0	11.9	9.3	14.7	4.8	35.5	7.6	2.1	2.0	28.8	46.8	4.1	5.5	20.7	8.4	2.1	3.7	2.1	215.7	166.9
Western	3.5	2.6	1.2	1.6	7.5	4.2	2.5	2.5	22.6	7.7	2.5	1.1	1.1	1.3	11.1	22.0	1.9	6.0	11.5	4.6	1.0	5.1	2.9	82.2	89.9
Europe	16.7	2.6	6.1	1.2	16.7	7.5	33.8	23.7	5.8	2.0	55.6	10.3	4.6	6.5	60.9	10.2	10.7	9.6	28.5	18.8	3.4	16.8	9.5	268.4	196.4

Notes:
[a] Rates are cases per 100 000 population, standardized according to the world population method (Parkin & Sangli, 1991).

other across the ladder rungs (A with T, C with G). This stable pairing ensures that that one strand of DNA, i.e. each half of the ladder, divided vertically, will always be complementary to the other half. The triplet order of bases 'code' for an individual amino acid, one of the building blocks of protein, i.e. TTA is a 'codon' for the amino acid phenylalanine. Because there are only 20 amino acids, but 64 different possible sequences for codon triplets (4×4×4), some of the code sequences are redundant, and some triplets even code for 'STOP!' messages that arrest protein formation. The complementary pairing of bases also ensures faithful replication of DNA during cell division, so that each daughter cell receives an exact copy of the parental DNA.

Function of DNA

Instructions for the manufacture of proteins, the molecular workhorses of cells, are encoded in DNA sequences called 'exons'. A functional gene is composed of several exons. About 95 per cent of the DNA molecules contain non-coding sequences. Some of these sequences help guide gene activity, e.g. promotors, enhancers), but much of the DNA has no known function. The intermediary molecule that manufactures proteins is RNA (ribonucleic acid), similar to DNA with the substitution of uridine for thymidine. With the help of polymerase enzymes, RNA 'transcribes' the DNA code and carries the protein-building information from the nucleus to the cytoplasm as 'messenger RNA'.

Proteins are then manufactured on a cytoplasmic 'ribosome' factory (a large molecule that serves as a scaffold for the amino acid assembly line). Amino acids are brought to the ribosome by a specialized 'transfer RNA' molecule and faithfully linked together on the messenger RNA template in the order originally prescribed by the DNA triplet code. Depending on the order of amino acids, proteins are further processed and folded into a variety of three-dimensional shapes, and perform many housekeeping and specialized jobs. Enzymes are proteins that assist metabolism and provide energy. Receptors are proteins that receive messages at the cell surface. Proteins such as haemoglobin, actinomyosin, and immunoglobulin, provide specialized functions for cell respiration, motion and defence, respectively. Proteins, acting as repressors or activators, also play an important role in regulating gene activity itself.

DNA mutations

DNA is vulnerable to mutation – a stable change in the chemical nature of the molecule. 'Point' or single mutations are usually silent, but a few strategically placed alterations can drastically affect protein production and function. DNA can be also disrupted by loss or gain of chromosomal material or by breakage and rejoining to another chromosome (translocation). The cell is equipped with rescue mechanisms to detect and repair DNA damage, but sometimes these 'checkpoints' are overwhelmed or defective. Mutations occur naturally over time and are usually rare and silent. But prolonged exposure to environmental genotoxic chemicals, e.g. oxidizing agents, tobacco smoke, or physical insults, e.g. solar or gamma radiation, can accelerate the rate of mutations. It is the accumulation of these deleterious changes that can lead to cancer.

What causes DNA mutations?

We now know that chronic, genotoxic exposures are the main causes of cancer. Head and neck cancers, lung, stomach, pancreas, bladder, and cervical cancer are all linked to cigarette smoking. Other environmental exposures include a variety of chemicals (mainly pesticides and petrochemicals), certain heavy metals, and asbestos. Physical agents (X-rays, gamma radiation, ultraviolet solar radiation) are also carcinogenic. A growing list of viruses and other infectious agents are linked to certain cancers. Diet and reproductive habits (that secondarily influence endogenous hormone exposure) also contribute to digestive and gynaecological cancer, respectively (see Vogelstein & Kinzler, 1998).

Cancer-causing genes

Two types of genes are involved in oncogenesis – 'oncogenes', and 'tumour suppressor genes'. Oncogenes are scattered throughout the genome and code for proteins that normally assist in growth and development. The process of mutation, however, may activate them and promote abnormal cell growth. An example of an oncogene is the over-expression of HER-2, a growth factor receptor that promotes cell division in breast cancer cells.

Tumour suppressor genes, on the other hand, normally monitor and repair DNA damage. These genes code for proteins that stop cell division if damage is detected and orchestrate repair of the altered DNA. If damage is severe, a process called 'apoptosis' or programmed cell death sacrifices the defective cell. If tumour suppressor genes are incapacitated, however, cells with damaged DNA can reproduce and undetected mutations are handed down to the next generation of cells. Such cancer cells display 'genomic instability' – a tendency for damaged cells to propagate continuously.

Thus, oncogenes act as growth 'accelerators', and

tumour suppressor genes act as the 'brakes' (Fig. 90.1). In both cases, the result is a renegade cell whose DNA is unguarded and whose division is unchecked. The slow but steady accumulation of DNA defects ultimately confers a growth advantage on some of the cells. A clone of genetically unstable cells then evolves to a more aggressive phenotype, developing properties of invasiveness and metastatic potential, the main characteristics of malignancy. As they develop, malignant cells are able to stimulate their own blood supply (tumour angiogenesis) and to evade detection by the immune system. Some cancers may form and 'die off' because DNA damage is incompatible with survival of the cell. But some cells may proceed autonomously, often forming a pre-cancerous lesion.

The promise of molecular science

The molecular genesis of cancer is now yielding its secrets, thanks to major technological advances in the past few decades. These discoveries promise better means of diagnosis and prevention. They disclose molecular targets for more rational therapy. And they hint at environmental–genetic interactions that may permit prevention and therapy to be designed for the individual.

Cancer precursor lesions

Where cancer of a particular organ or tissue is a significant problem, it may be possible to monitor cellular damage in that tissue and thus detect cancerous change very early. Thus cancer of the cervix can be detected if a smear from a swab of cervical fluid, examined annually, shows microscopic signs of cellular dysplasia. This procedure revolutionized the screening of cervical cancer and lowered mortality in developed countries. Unfortunately, such procedures are not always suitable for use in developing countries because they are expensive and require a centralized, stable medical infrastructure. Colonic adenomatous polyps, oral leukoplakia, unstable melanotic naevi, and actinic keratoses of the skin are other examples of pre-malignant neoplasms. Clinical trials are in progress in many centres in industrialized countries to avert pre-malignant lesions using 'chemoprevention' agents such as vitamin supplements, e.g. folic acid, vitamin E, chemicals that induce cell differentiation, e.g. retinoids, and replacement of deficient nutrients, e.g. selenium. Biologically, these pre-cancers comprise an intermediary stage in the progression from a normal cell to a malignant cell. Clinically, they represent detectable lesions that can be surgically or chemically removed and

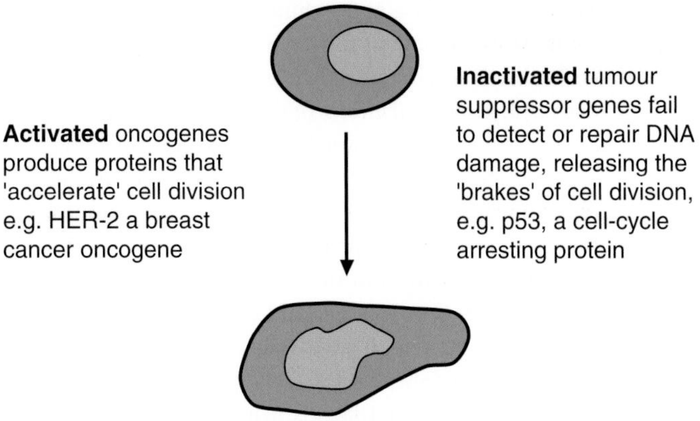

Activated oncogenes produce proteins that 'accelerate' cell division e.g. HER-2 a breast cancer oncogene
Inactivated tumour suppressor genes fail to detect or repair DNA damage, releasing the 'brakes' of cell division, e.g. p53, a cell-cycle arresting protein

Fig. 90.1. Oncogenesis is a consequence of cumulative genomic change that activates oncogenes (whose products drive cell proliferation) and/or inactivates tumour suppressor genes (whose products mitigate cell cycle progression or inhibit cell proliferation).

thus prevent cancer from developing. Cancer can be prevented from advancing to an incurable stage if some of the early warning symptoms and signs of malignancy are recognized (see the Box):

Early warning signs of cancer

Sign or symptom:	*Suspected malignancy:*
Unexplained weight loss or fever	Lymphoma, kidney cancer
Swelling or lump	Breast cancer, lymphoma, sarcoma
Unusual vaginal bleeding or discharge	Carcinoma of the cervix or uterus
Change in bowel habit, blood in stool	Gastrointestinal cancer
Skin lesion that does not heal	Squamous carcinoma, Kaposi's sarcoma, malignant melanoma
Chronic cough	Lung cancer
Difficulty in swallowing	Nasopharyngeal or oesophageal cancer

General approach to the cancer patient

Clinical evaluation

The three main questions that should concern the doctor are:

(i) What is the histological diagnosis of the tumour?
(ii) Where has the tumour spread?
(iii) How does the tumour affect the comfort and well-being of the patient?

Most patients arrive at the clinic or hospital with symptoms attributable to a growing mass. Sometimes this is visible clinically, but often symptoms refer to the anatomical or physiological effects of the mass, e.g. bleeding, obstruction, vomiting, weight loss. A precise histological diagnosis from a biopsy or excision, even if the tumour type appears obvious, provides invaluable guidance for management and prognosis.

In many African countries, cancer patients may present in the later stages of disease and rural health facilities are often ill equipped to diagnose cancer, so that biopsy specimens must be sent to a central laboratory, and treatment is inevitably delayed. Diagnostic imaging is also lacking, although ultrasound in rural hospitals is emerging as an important method (Mindel, 1997). Rapid diagnoses can sometimes be made at the bedside with the use of fine needle aspiration (first Box, p. 1219). In many cases a clinical diagnosis must suffice, and this is always easier when the cancer is superficial.

Clinical staging

The stage of a tumour is related to its local invasiveness and distant spread and is an important management tool. In general, tumours progress from Stage I (localized) to Stage II (regional) to Stage III (metastatic), a common pattern of spread for most malignancies of epithelial origin. Some tumours such as lymphomas and Kaposi's sarcoma are multi-centric, and appear in different anatomical sites simultaneously. Staging procedures involve a careful clinical examination, and selected diagnostic tests to localize tumour deposits. In a tertiary referral hospital these may include laboratory tests (liver and renal function), diagnostic imaging (X-ray, ultrasound, bone scan), biopsy (bone marrow, suspicious lesions), and specialized tests for biological markers, e.g. choriogonadotropin levels for choriocarcinoma, alpha-fetoprotein levels for liver cancer. Accurate staging of a tumour can guide primary treatment, assess response and prognosis, and enable comparisons in different clinical trials.

General management

The principle is to assess how to help the patient cope with tumour-related symptoms and the emotional burden of a cancer diagnosis. Even if a tumour is incurable, much can be done through palliative treatment. Newer drugs alleviate nausea and vomiting from disease or from chemotherapy, and antibiotics can effectively treat complicating infections in immune-compromised patients. The hospice movement has revolutionized pain management, and the hospices in Nairobi and Kampala, for example, are excellent examples of this form of care. The support of the whole family is critical in helping the cancer patient to cope with increasing disability and frailty.

Do not think that you must always 'do something'; in cancer, as in all medicine, do not make the endurance of treatment more grievous than the burden of the disease. It is not always appropriate to give anticancer treatment, but it is absolutely essential to understand how important palliative treatment can be, and how it can transform the life of a patient with metastatic cancer.

Treatment of cancer

Surgery

Over the past century, *surgery* has been the primary means of treating 'operable' – that is localized and resectable – cancer. Palliative surgery can also provide symptomatic relief, such as gastrostomy for feeding purposes, or partial resection of obstructing tumours. In some cases, prognosis may be improved using 'debulking' surgery, and rarely, some cases of metastatic kidney or colon cancer can be cured by the systematic removal of metastatic deposits, in addition to the removal of the primary. Recent research has evaluated treatment first with chemotherapy to 'downstage' the tumour, and surgery is performed following the maximal response. This experimental approach is called 'neoadjuvant chemotherapy'.

Radiation therapy

Radiotherapy is curative in certain tumours that are locoregional in extent. The advent of high voltage equipment, improved dose schedules, and better means to focus gamma radiation exclusively on tumour tissue has brought radiotherapy into prominence in cancer treatment. Unfortunately, modern radiotherapy equipment is very expensive, so that there are few such units in tropical Africa.

Chemotherapy

The medicinal treatment for cancer was developed in the 1940s as an outgrowth of research in anti-malarial treatment and chemical warfare used in World War II. Starting with nitrogen mustard (for malignant lymphoma), methotrexate (for leukaemia) and actinomycin D (for Wilm's tumour), there are now over 100 chemotherapeutic compounds.

Clinical trials have demonstrated better effectiveness with the judicious use of combinations of agents. Hormones or hormone antagonists are also valuable in the treatment of hormone responsive cancers such as leukaemia (corticosteroids), breast cancer (anti-oestrogens) and prostate cancer (anti-androgens).

The main mechanism of action for anticancer drugs is chemical damage to DNA, causing crosslinks, chromosome breaks, and mutations, and inducing cell death. Cytotoxicity works better in cancer cells because of abundant vascular perfusion (from a tumour-induced blood supply), high proliferative rate (more DNA to target), and defective DNA repair mechanisms. Normal tissues (especially the bone marrow, mucosa, and liver) are also damaged by cytotoxic drugs, and empirical doses and schedules try to balance the 'therapeutic ratio' in favour of the host. Sadly, many tumours are resistant to drug therapy or develop resistance during the course of treatment. (Because many drug doses are calculated per m^2 of body surface area, a conversion table is given in the appendix.)

Biotherapy

This is in its infancy, but as the precise DNA sequences of the human genome are discovered, the cause and progression of malignant changes in cells will be more fully understood. Some biologicals, such as interferon, are in clinical use. Molecular strategies that interrupt the tumour blood supply (anti-angiogenesis agents) are in clinical trials. Monoclonal antibodies and 'anti-sense' RNA can specifically inhibit molecular pathways that lead to cancer progression. New data about the mechanism of drug resistance will lead to more effective chemotherapy.

The cancer team

In a specialist hospital, if resources permit, the ideal management is by a team, each member of which brings special skills. The medical oncologist, surgeon, radiotherapist, pathologist, radiologist, and ancillary professionals can decide together on a treatment strategy for each patient. A co-ordinated attack on cancer is more effective than the separate efforts of different specialists.

Alternative and complementary medicine

For centuries, traditional healers, shamans, herbalists and others have been practising the healing arts. For decades, medical science has resisted these approaches, and has labelled them as quacks, charlatans and witch doctors. Ironically, modern medicines have been found to be active ingredients in many of these potions, for example, quinine from willow bark and digitalis from foxglove. The scientific basis for traditional remedies, widely used across the world, is now being examined. In societies where virtually all patients consult a traditional healer before resorting to western medicine, the healers' techniques have become accepted over many centuries because of cultural beliefs in the powers of the healer, the placebo effect, the actual benefit from the administered herbs, or spontaneous improvement from the illness.

Many patients may know something about causes of disease, e.g. malaria, HIV, tuberculosis, food poisoning, but their more fundamental question is why they became ill. Is the sickness due an act of revenge or a spell cast by an enemy? Traditional healers not only treat the illness but will offer advice about why the illness afflicted a particular person at a particular time.

A contemporary example

Relationships between western-trained doctors and traditional healers are slowly improving and can be important in the prevention of disease. In Uganda and other sub-Saharan countries afflicted by HIV, a concerted effort is being made to win the co-operation of traditional healers and to get them to educate patients and their families about HIV transmission, and about safe sexual habits. This is an example of how complementary and alternative medicine practices can be brought within modern medicine. But such practices must be tested more rigorously so that beneficial remedies can be discovered and harmful ones discouraged.

Pain control

Because doctors used to fear drug addiction to powerful analgesics, they prescribed inadequate doses to patients with cancer and so paid little attention to control of pain. This has all changed. The fundamental principle of pain control is to select the appropriate analgesic and to administer the correct dose and schedule, a practice pioneered by the hospice movement (Chapter 91).

Assessment of pain

The aetiology, site, quality, chronicity, aggravating or alleviating features, and effect of medications on pain must be assessed. Cancer pain may result from obstruction, local spread in normal structures, or metastases. Tumour in bone accounts for over half the cases of cancer pain. Chronic pain can often reduce appetite and thus impair nutrition, prevent sleep, and reduce quality of life. The principle of management is to attack the cause of the pain and, as above, to give appropriate analgesia. Often radiotherapy to sites of painful metastases can afford temporary relief.

The support of the family

This is absolutely fundamental and it commonly takes the place of the scanty professional help that may be available. Therefore, make certain that the family understands how best to help their relation with cancer and, where relevant, how and when drugs should be given.

Childhood tumours

Burkitt's lymphoma

This is by far the most common malignant tumour in African children. It was first described by Denis Burkitt in Uganda in 1958. He journeyed all over East Africa, and sent questionnaires by post to ask medical officers in district hospitals whether they had seen cases of the characteristic facial tumour. As a result of this enquiry he described a childhood tumour dependent on climate, which had a distinct geographical distribution across sub-Saharan Africa, in areas where both yellow fever and malaria were endemic (Burkitt, 1983).

The Epstein–Barr virus

The geographical distribution prompted many investigators to favour a viral aetiology. In 1964, Epstein, Barr and Achong discovered a herpes-like virus in cultured Burkitt's lymphoma cells. The Epstein–Barr virus (EBV) has many properties that make it a candidate for oncogenesis (Cohen, 2000).

The virus is found in all cases of African Burkitt's lymphoma and has the ability to immortalize B lymphocytes in culture. EBV was found to have a world-wide distribution and was spread mainly by oral secretions. A prospective study of EBV in Uganda's West Nile District showed that the virus was highly prevalent in children and was present in many children long before Burkitt's lymphoma developed (DeThe et al, 1978). EBV also causes infectious mononucleosis, seen mostly in developed countries where infection occurs during adolescence.

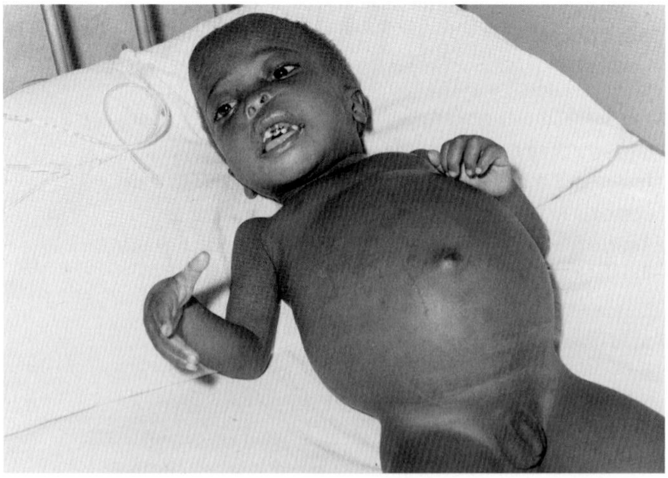

Fig. 90.2. A 5-year-old boy with massive intra-abdominal Burkitt's lymphoma and ascites. Note tumour involvement of the left maxilla as well.

The role of malaria

Because EBV could not be considered as the sole cause of the tumour, Burkitt offered an alternative hypothesis. The geographical distribution, he postulated, could be explained by malaria as a cofactor. The geographical distribution of hyper- and holo-enedemic malaria coincided with that of Burkitt's lymphoma. Many episodes of malaria can lower immune defences, particularly to EBV. The mitogenic effect of EBV on B lymphocytes, combined with impaired immunity induced by malaria, increases the probability of genetic changes that confer a proliferative advantage.

A genetic translocation that moved the growth-promoting *c-myc* gene from chromosome 8 to chromosome 14 (and to a lesser extent chromosome 2 or 22) is a consistent feature of African Burkitt's lymphoma. *C-myc* protein becomes transcriptionally active in these new sites because they are involved in immunoglobulin production. Thus, the confluence of EBV and malarial infection provide a setting where chromosomal translocation in B lymphocytes converts proliferating cells into malignant lymphoma (Magrath, 1989).

Clinical features

This rapidly growing lymphoma develops primarily in the jaws, but it also commonly involves paired abdominal organs – kidneys or ovaries (Figs. 90.2, 90.3).

Lymph node and intra-thoracic involvement are rare. The mean age is about 5 years, and boys are twice as likely to be affected as girls (Ziegler, 1981).

Diagnosis

Burkitt's lymphoma is defined as a small, non-cleaved, high grade lymphoma, and can be diagnosed definitively by biopsy or by cytology (see the Box).

How to make a rapid diagnosis of Burkitt's lymphoma

- *Fine needle aspiration*: Obtain lymphoma cells by inserting a sterile 20 or 22 gauge needle attached to a 10 ml syringe into the tumour. Withdraw the syringe plunger sharply, drawing a small amount of tumour fluid into the needle. Carefully expel a few drops of tumour fluid from the needle (some blood will inevitably be withdrawn as well) onto a clean glass slide. Smear at once, and stain like a blood film.
- *Ascites*: If ascites is present, withdraw a few ml of ascitic fluid, centrifuge, pour off the supernatant, and drop the sedimented cells onto a slide. Smear at once, and stain like a blood film.
- *Touch preparation*: If the biopsy is done, gently touch the cut surface of the tumour to the underside of a slide and air dry. Make a blood smear from the tumour material and stain with Wright–Giemsa stain like a blood film.
- *Diagnosis*: The diagnosis is made by the characteristic appearance of the cells (Fig. 90.4). Typical malignant cells are large, uniform and basophilic; the cytoplasm contains vacuoles and the nucleus has up to 4 prominent nucleoli. Many necrotic cells may be present.

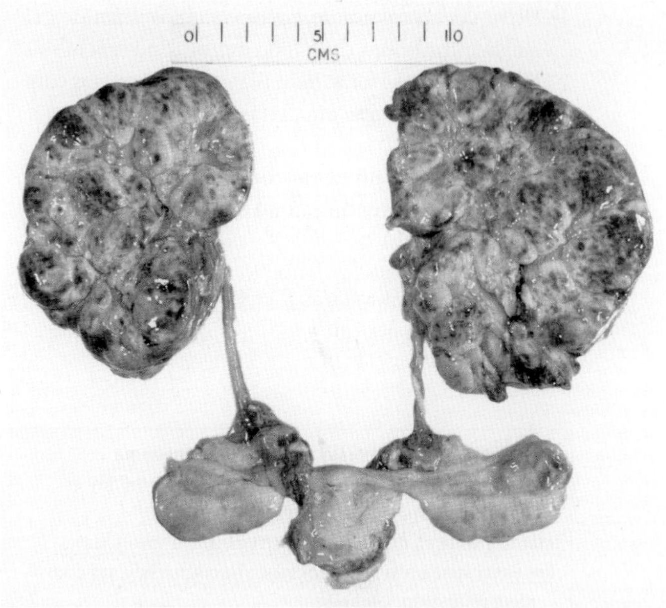

Fig. 90.3. Extensive involvement of the ovaries and kidneys by Burkitt's lymphoma. (Courtesy of Dr D.H. Wright, Dept of Pathology, Makerere University Medical School, Kampala, Uganda.)

A rapid diagnosis is essential because the tumour cells double in number every day. The tumour can spread to the central nervous system. As this is a common site of relapse, be alert for any neurological symptoms (headache, drowsiness) or signs (cranial nerve palsies). If there is doubt, do a lumbar puncture and examine the spinal fluid for Burkitt's lymphoma cells.

Staging

The stage of the tumour can be relatively easily determined by clinical examination and a few selected laboratory tests. The stages currently in use are shown below (see the Box). Prognosis is directly related to stage. Mortality is greater in patients with widespread tumours, and is highest when the central nervous system (CNS) and bone marrow are involved.

Staging of Burkitt's lymphoma

Stage A	Tumour confined to a single site (often the jaw)
Stage B	Tumours in two separate anatomical sites, but excluding the abdomen, thorax, central nervous system (CNS) or bone marrow
Stage C	Tumours in the abdomen or thorax, but excluding the marrow or CNS
Stage D	Tumour involvement of the bone marrow and/or CNS.

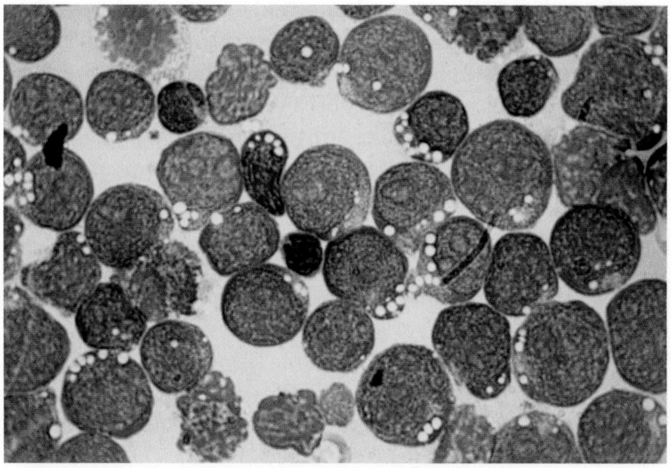

Fig. 90.4. Characteristic Burkitt's lymphoma cells on a tumour imprint (touch preparation). Note the uniformity of cell size, basophilic vacuolated cytoplasm, and granular nucleus containing several prominent nucleoli. (×400, Wright-Giemsa stain).

Chemotherapy and follow-up

At least 50 per cent of patients with Burkitt's lymphoma can be *cured with chemotherapy* (Fig. 90.5).

- Do not delay treatment. Give cyclophosphamide in a single intravenous dose 1000 mg/m^2, and repeat this every 2–3 weeks for at least two courses beyond complete clinical remission, that is after all clinical signs have gone.
- If available, a combination of cyclophosphamide, vincristine and methotrexate is also effective (see the Box).
- If lymphoma cells are found in the central nervous system, give methotrexate, 10 mg diluted in 10 cm^3 of saline, intrathecally with each course of chemotherapy.

Combination chemotherapy for Burkitt's lymphoma
Cyclophosphamide 1000 mg/m^2 intravenously on day 1
Vincristine 1.4 mg/m^2 intravenously on day 1
Methotrexate 15 mg/m^2 by mouth or intravenously, day 1
Repeat course every 2–3 weeks for one course beyond complete remission.

Tumour lysis syndrome

After treatment, large tumours undergo rapid cytolysis and release intracellular contents into the circulation. Patients with any degree of dehydration or renal failure may develop tumour lysis syndrome, a potentially fatal metabolic catastrophe consisting of hyperphosphataemia, hyperkalaemia and hyperuricaemia. This syndrome is a medical emergency because rising potassium levels will cause fatal cardiac arrhythmias. Treat this complication with aggressive intravenous or oral hydration, allopurinol (200 mg orally three times daily), and possibly haemo- or peritoneal dialysis (Cohen et al., 1980).

Effect of treatment

Almost all cases of Burkitt's lymphoma will respond completely to chemotherapy within 2–4 weeks. Chemotherapy will lower white blood counts to a nadir of 1000×10^9–2000×10^9 /l about 10 days after chemotherapy, with full recovery to pre-treatment counts by 2–3 weeks. This level of neutropenia will not lead to opportunistic infection, and patients can be safely discharged from hospital after they become stable. If bone marrow is involved with tumour initially, blood counts may be lower (Fig. 90.5(*a*),(*b*)).

Follow-up and relapse

- Follow patients monthly for the first year after treatment for signs of relapse, especially in the CNS, which may present as a cranial nerve palsy (Fig. 90.6), headache or drowsiness.
- Treat CNS relapse with systemic chemotherapy (see the Box), and weekly doses of intrathecal methotrexate until the cerebrospinal fluid is clear of lymphoma cells.
- If relapse occurs, repeat the initial therapy, especially if several tumour-free months have intervened from the last treatment.
- If relapsing tumours fail to respond, or if relapse occurs within a few weeks of chemotherapy, give doxorubicin (60–75 mg/m^2 in an intravenous infusion over 30 minutes every 3 weeks).
- Drug-resistant relapse carries a poor prognosis.

In specialized cancer centres, bone marrow autografting is a procedure that involves harvesting normal bone marrow, giving high doses of chemotherapy, and then returning the bone marrow by infusion.

Kaposi's sarcoma

Kaposi's' sarcoma in childhood has become increasingly common in Africa (Olweny et al., 1977). In addition, the HIV epidemic has led to a coincident epidemic of Kaposi's sarcoma (Ziegler & Mbidde,1996), which is now the most common malignancy in many African countries (Wabinga et al., 1993). Endemic African Kaposi's sarcoma predated the arrival of HIV, and investigators thought that it might be caused by an infectious agent.

Human herpesvirus 8

In 1994 Chang and Moore discovered a novel herpesvirus, closely related to EBV, in Kaposi's sarcoma tumours (Chang et al., 1994). This virus, now called human herpesvirus 8 (HHV8), is clearly the aetiological agent. It carries a number of genes that transform endothelial cells and stimulate their proliferation. In the immune-suppressed host HHV8 is reactivated (and possibly transmission is augmented). As proof of this concept, in industrialized countries, highly active antiretroviral therapy has controlled HIV viraemia and immune suppression in treated patients, and the rates of Kaposi's sarcoma have declined dramatically (International HIV Collaborative Group, 2000).

Clinical features

Lymphadenopathy is the most characteristic presentation, and classic skin lesions are less common (Figs 90.7, 90.8). Because Kaposi's sarcoma is easily diagnosed histologically, and because lymph nodes may be enlarged in a number of other diseases such as tuberculosis and lymphoma, a biopsy is essential. Kaposi's sarcoma is usually associated with HIV infection, so look for the common complications of AIDS (Chapter 13) – oral can-

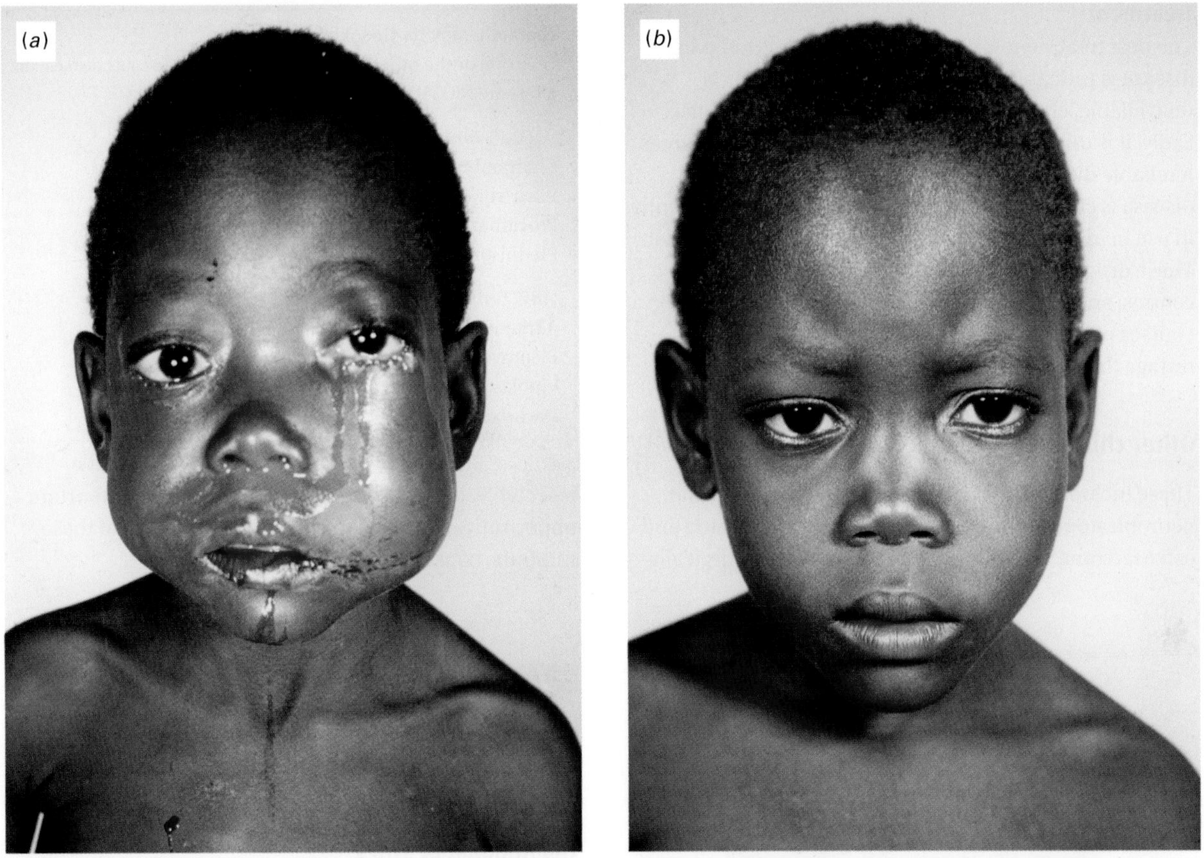

Fig. 90.5. (*a*) An 8-year-old Ugandan girl from Lango District presented to the Uganda Cancer Institute with facial swelling. Burkitt's lymphoma (Fig. 90.3) had invaded both maxillae and left orbit. (*b*) Appearance of the same child several weeks after receiving 1000 mg/m^2 of intravenous cyclophosphamide, representing a complete clinical response. This child went on to become a long-term survivor.

didiasis, a variety of cutaneous infections, e.g. herpes zoster, fungal disease, *Molluscum contagiosum*, pneumonia, tuberculosis, diarrhoea, and severe weight loss.

Treatment

This is the same in childhood Kaposi's sarcoma as it is in the disease in adults.

Hodgkin's disease

After Burkitt's lymphoma and Kaposi's sarcoma, this is the third most common tumour of childhood in Africa. The diagnosis must be established histologically by characteristic atypical mononuclear cells, the pathognomonic Reed–Sternberg cells, in a mixed inflammatory infiltrate, often rich in eosinophils and lymphocytes.

Clinical features

The most common presentation is lymph node swelling, usually in the cervical region. This must be distinguished from tuberculosis or Kaposi's sarcoma. The tumour may grow slowly and the patient may experience fever, loss of weight, and itching all over he body, but without any skin eruption.

Staging of the tumour

This is based on the observation that Hodgkin's disease progresses in a contiguous manner (see the Box).

Staging of Hodgkin's disease

Stage I	Lymph node involvement in a single anatomical area
Stage II	Lymph node involvement of two anatomically separate areas either above or below the diaphragm
Stage III	Tumour in lymph nodes above and below the diaphragm
Stage IV	Tumour in extra-nodal sites.

Treatment

The best treatment for localized or regional Hodgkin's disease is probably radiotherapy, but where this is unavailable, chemotherapy is the treatment of choice. Sadly, it is too costly for countries with limited resources. A reliable diagnosis is important because Hodgkin's disease is curable. A drug combination regimen currently in use in industrialized countries is shown (see the Box). These drugs may only be available in tertiary referral centres, and substitutions will be necessary. At least six courses of combination chemotherapy are needed: restage the patient at the end of treatment.

Chemotherapy for Hodgkin's disease

Give one or the other combination monthly for six courses, or alternate MOPP/ ABVD each month.

'MOPP' combination

Chlorambucil 6 mg/m^2 (max 10 mg) days 1–14
Vincristine 1.4 mg/m^2 (max 2 mg) i.v. day 1 and 8
Procarbazine 100 mg/m^2 orally days 1–14
Prednisone 40 mg/m^2 orally daily days 1–14

'ABVD' combination

Adriamycin 25 mg/m^2 i.v., day 1 and 15
Bleomycin 10 units/m^2 i.v. day 1 and 15
Vinblastine 6 mg/m^2 i.v. day 1 and 15
Dacarbazine 375 mg/m^2 i.v. day 1 and 15

Other childhood tumours

These include Wilms' tumour (renal hypernephroma), neuroblastoma, retinoblastoma, rhabdomysarcoma and osteosarcoma. Sometimes, these tumours are surgically resectable, although chemotherapy offers an important opportunity for cure. For details on treatment of these tumours, consult the references.

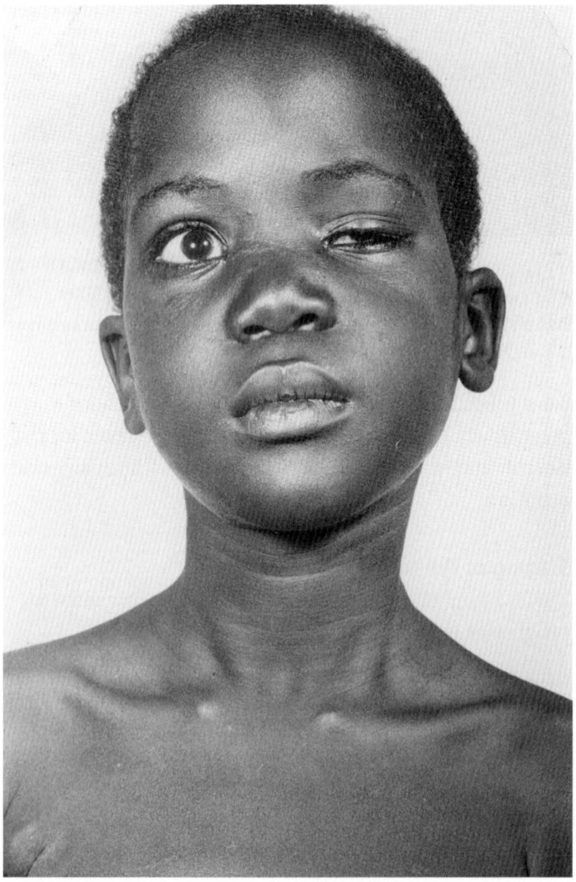

Fig. 90.6. Cranial nerve palsies (left oculomotor, right facial) as a manifestation of relapsing Burkitt's lymphoma in a 9-year-old girl with a previous complete remission. Typical Burkitt's lymphoma cells were found in the cerebrospinal fluid.

COMMON ADULT TUMOURS

Alimentary canal

Oesophageal cancer

The problem in Africa

This is a significant tumour in some parts of the continent and its distribution is unusual, with high concentrations in western Kenya (around Kisumu), the Bale region of Ethiopia (Madebo et al., 1994), Zimbabwe (Parkin., et al 1994), Uganda, Natal, and Transkei. Diet, alcohol and the use of tobacco are important risk factors, but local idiosyncracies (such as nutritional deficiency, tea drinking, spices, and soil composition) may explain the peculiar regional distribution.

Clinical features

The majority of cancers are squamous carcinomas that arise in the lower third of the oesophagus and cause symptoms of dysphagia, first to solids and later to all foods (Sammon & Alderdson, 1998). If you suspect oesophageal cancer, ask the patient 'do you chew your food up small before you try to swallow it?' or 'do you now take much longer than others with you to eat a meal?' Vomiting, weight loss, and aspiration pneumonia are later features.

Diagnosis and treatment

The diagnosis can be established by oesophagoscopy or by barium swallow, but often tumours are inoperable when the patient is first seen. Radiotherapy, if available,

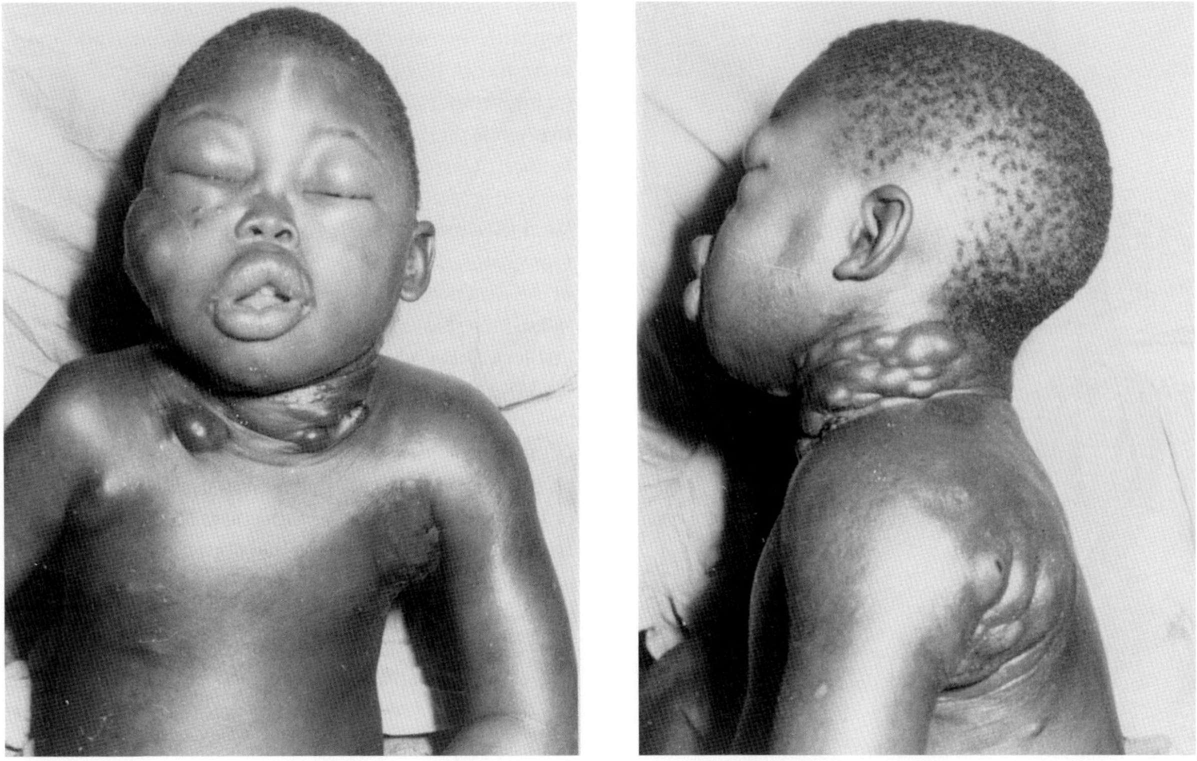

Fig. 90.7. Front and lateral view of a 3-year-old Ugandan boy with extensive Kaposi's sarcoma. Note facial oedema and massive lymphadenopathy, but minimal cutaneous lesions, mainly on the right cheek.

may be temporarily effective, and palliative gastrostomy is helpful to maintain nutrition. Generally, chemotherapy has little to offer in oesophageal cancer and response rates rarely exceed 25 per cent. Survival is poor, and 80 per cent die in the first year.

Hepatocellular carcinoma

The problem in Africa

Cancer of the liver is the most common adult malignancy in some African countries (e.g. Mozambique). The sex ratio in areas where it is common is 3:1 males:females. The most important aetiological agents are the hepatitis viruses, B and C, which are responsible for about 70 per cent and 20 per cent of cases, respectively. The remaining 10 per cent relate to alcohol consumption and iron-storage diseases, but the role of alcohol is small. Chronic hepatitis, usually acquired in childhood, leads to post-necrotic cirrhosis in a significant fraction of sufferers.

Food storage and aflatoxins

Cancer develops in regenerating hepatic nodules as a consequence of diets high in hepato-carcinogens such as aflatoxin (a contaminant of the mould *Aspergillus flavus*) (Linsell & Peers, 1977). If food could be stored dry and ventilated in village and home granaries, it would not become mouldy. Much is lost through contamination with fungi. If resources could be directed to provide better storage, and if traditional methods could be improved, the risk of aflatoxin would be reduced.

Prevention

These two important causes are the basis for prevention. In the Gambia and in Taiwan, hepatitis B vaccination in children has already reduced the burden of infection (Viviani et al., 1999). Education about fungal contamination of foodstuffs (proper dry storage techniques) may lower exposure to aflatoxin. Unfortunately, attempts at early diagnosis, e.g. screening for a raised alpha-fetoprotein level in high-risk populations, are not feasible or cost effective.

Clinical features

Liver cancer usually presents in an advanced stage (Fig. 80.7). Right upper quadrant pain and weight loss are early symptoms, there may be ascites but jaundice is uncommon. A hard mass is palpable in the enlarged liver

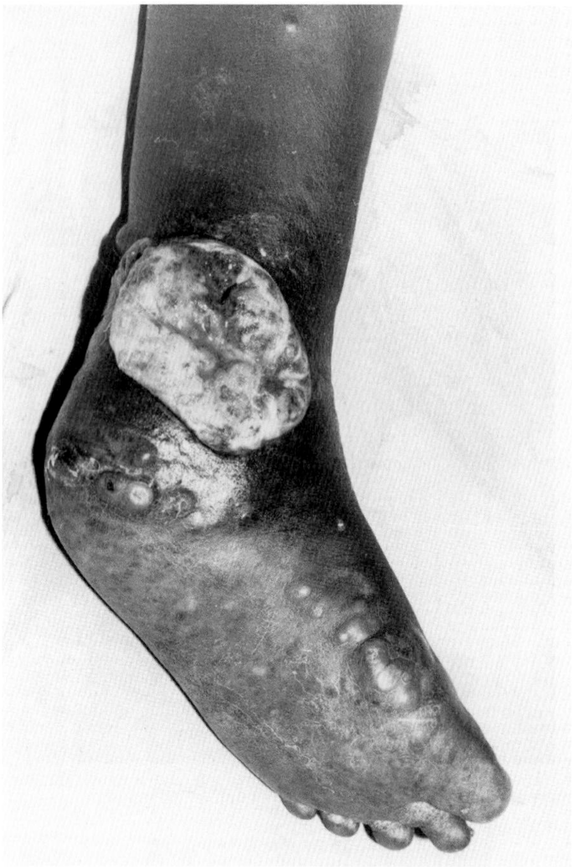

Fig. 90.8. Typical 'endemic' Kaposi's sarcoma in a 55-year-old Ugandan male. Note the multiple nodules on the medial aspect of the soles and the fungating, florid tumour developing on the ankle. There is lymphoedema of the leg.

and a bruit may also be heard over the mass, or over the liver, even if a mass cannot be felt. Ultrasound is valuable as it can detect tumours as small as 1 cm.

Treatment

Partial hepatectomy can be tried if tumours are localized. Hepatic artery ligation provides temporary relief, as does chemotherapy. Adriamycin and flurouracil are the most widely used drugs: they are sometimes given directly into the hepatic artery (Olweny et al., 1975; Venook et al., 1990). The prognosis is poor, however, with 90 per cent mortality within a year from diagnosis.

Stomach cancer

The problem in Africa

Stomach cancer is common in Rwanda, Burundi and in certain highland areas such as Kilimanjaro. Chronic gastritis is a precursor of stomach cancer and chronic infection with *Helicobacter pylori* has received much attention as a contributing cause (Correa, 1992). Dietary factors play an important role. Green vegetables and fruits are protective, while pickled, preserved and salty foods are risk factors. Ingested nitrates are suspected of being carcinogenic in an acid environment. For unknown reasons, stomach cancers tend to aggregate in volcanic areas (Templeton, 1973). Stomach cancer incidence has declined in the west owing to improved hygiene (lower rates of *H. pylori* infection) and better nutrition (more fruits and vegetables). This shows that effective preventive strategies could be used in areas where the tumour is endemic.

Clinical features

Over 80 per cent are adenocarcinomas and usually present when the disease is advanced so that the patient has lost weight, and has also had abdominal pain, vomiting, haematemesis and regurgitation. The diagnosis is established by endoscopy or by contrast studies, and resective surgery is the mainstay of treatment. Overall, survival is poor and rarely exceeds 20 per cent.

Genitourinary tract

Bladder cancer

The problem in Africa

Squamous carcinoma of the bladder is seen most commonly in areas of Africa where *Schistosoma haematobium* is endemic, e.g. Egypt, Uganda. Chronic cystitis (especially in farmers repeatedly exposed to infectious cercariae in irrigation canals) is the main precursor to carcinoma, caused by the presence of highly inflammatory eggs in the bladder wall. Mucosal damage resulting from inflammatory cytokines and oxygen free radicals is responsible for the carcinogenic effect. Early detection and treatment of schistosomiasis, education about avoidance of infection, and awareness of early signs of bladder cancer are among the best preventive measures (Ross & Jones, 1996).

Clinical features

The main symptoms of bladder cancer are haematuria or 'necroturia' (passage of tissue via the urethra).

Treatment

In a specialized hospital, radical cystectomy is the mainstay of treatment. This procedure usually requires diversion of the urine to an external pouch or to an entero-bladder, fashioned in the ileum or rectum (El-Sebai,

1983). Similarly, in sophisticated cancer treatment centres, chemotherapeutic drugs such as cyclophosphamide, etoposide, doxorubicin, bleomycin, *cis*-platinum, and methotrexate, used singly or in combination, produce partial responses in advanced bladder cancer.

Cancer of the prostate

Prostate cancer is a common cancer in men, the largest risk factor being older age. In countries with advanced laboratories, the diagnosis of prostate cancer is rising because cancers are being detected earlier by the increasing use of the PSA (prostate specific antigen) test. A value over 4 ng/dl triggers a prostate biopsy, but the PSA test is not very sensitive, and 25 per cent of prostate cancers have normal PSA values (Garnick, 1993). Prostate cancer is twice as common and more aggressive in men of African descent living in Europe or America. Although genetic factors may account for up to 40 per cent of cases, dietary factors are important. Tomatoes, fruits, vegetables, and diets high in selenium and vitamin E are protective, as is physical exercise. High intake of red meat, animal fat and dairy products increase risk.

Clinical features

Prostate cancer is usually detected because of urinary symptoms (hesitancy, obstruction, nocturia). On rectal examination, the features of cancer are asymmetry of the gland and a stony hard mass. By contrast, in benign prostatic hypertrophy the gland is symmetrically enlarged and is soft. In a cancer centre, staging for prostate cancer involves a PSA test, ultrasound of the pelvis (with rectal probe), magnetic resonance or CT scan imaging. A bone scintigram is necessary to rule out bony metastases. Where these procedures are unavailable, rigorous and careful clinical examination alone can be done.

Treatment

In Africa, radical prostatectomy is the treatment of choice for a localized prostate cancer. If pelvic lymph nodes are involved, further therapy with androgen ablation may be necessary (orchidectomy or diethyl stilboestrol). When radiotherapy is available, either brachytherapy (radioactive seed implantation) or external beam therapy yields an outcome equivalent to surgery, albeit with different side effects.

Cancer of the penis

Penile cancer is common in central Africa, and its aetiology (along with carcinoma of the cervix in women) is linked to infection with human papilloma virus. Poor penile hygiene and lack of circumcision are major risk factors. The best treatment is penectomy (Schmauz, 1995).

Respiratory tract

Nasopharyngeal cancer

The problem in Africa

Nasopharyngeal carcinoma is common in northern and eastern Africa. Like Burkitt's lymphoma, this cancer is aetiologically linked to EBV infection, a situation that undoubtedly reflects the primary infection of EBV in oropharyngeal epithelium. Virtually all of the tumours studied, including *in situ* preneoplastic lesions, contain EBV genomes and express EBV proteins, indicating that EBV infection precedes malignancy (Pathmanathran et al., 1995). In endemic areas, such as southern China, measurement of EBV IgA antibodies is useful for screening and early detection. Heritable influences also contribute to susceptibility, as noted in high rates of nasopharyngeal cancer in migrant populations and an association with certain HLA haplotypes. Dietary factors such as highly salted and spicy foods are also implicated (Fandi et al., 1994).

Clinical features

The expanding mass in the upper nasopharynx causes neck swelling, cranial neuropathy (especially nerves IX–XII), symptoms of regurgitation, difficulty in swallowing and speech, blocked Eustacian tubes, and nasal stuffiness.

Treatment

Radiotherapy offers definitive treatment with 5-year survivals up to 50 per cent. Effective chemotherapy in industrialized country clinics is given by *cis*-platinum, methotrexate, bleomycin and flurouracil (as single agents and in various combinations).

Lung

The problem in Africa

In southern Africa, lung cancer is nearly as frequent as in Europe, owing to high rates of cigarette smoking and exposure to dust and asbestos in the mining industry. More common among men, lung cancer is increasing in other parts of Africa as a result of urbanization and a change of habits. As African cities become more polluted (and diesel fuel is considered carcinogenic), ordinary, non-smoking citizens are at risk. Because of the close association of lung cancer and smoking, this cancer is almost entirely preventable.

Smoking

The revitalized WHO anti-smoking campaign is designed to discourage smoking in Africa's youths, at whom cigarette advertising is primarily aimed. But the inexcusably high-pressure advertising by tobacco companies is a formidable adversary for national prevention strategies. In the meantime, because lung cancer is so deadly, do not forget that, whenever patients come to your clinic, you have an opportunity for health education and advice against smoking.

Treatment

Lung cancer is difficult to detect early, and, with the exception of small cell carcinoma, treatment is primarily surgical. Radiotherapy is palliative.

Chemotherapy is temporarily effective in small cell carcinoma and is also very rarely curative, but response rates in other types rarely exceed 20 per cent.

Tumours of women

Carcinoma of the cervix

The problem in Africa

Squamous carcinoma of the uterine cervix is one of the most common tumours in Africa. It is clearly linked to prior infection with human papilloma virus, a sexually transmitted infection. Epidemiological risk factors include early age at first intercourse, multiple sexual partners, and sexually active partners. The E6 and E7 proteins of human papilloma viruses (types 16 and 18 are especially oncogenic) bind to p53 and Rb proteins, respectively. These tumour suppressor proteins are essential checkpoints for DNA repair; their inactivation through binding and degradation allows damaged cells to undergo malignant change.

Cervix cancer proceeds through stages of 'cervical intra-epithelial dysplasia' (CIN) that can be readily detected by PAP smears of the cervix. Despite a false-negative rate of up to 25 per cent, PAP smear screening is a cost-effective way of reducing cervical cancer morbidity and mortality, but the procedure is not readily available in Africa. Therapy is dependent on the CIN grade, and ranges from colposcopic biopsy for CIN I, cryotherapy or loop excision for CIN II, to conization for CIN III. Management of more invasive disease (chemotherapy, with or without radiotherapy) depends on clinical stage which in turn is determined by pelvic examination under anaesthesia.

Choriocarcinoma

This tumour results from malignant transformation of a hydatidiform mole, a benign neoplasm of the chorionic trophoblastic epithelium, hence of embryonal origin. Although only about 5 per cent of molar pregnancies progress to malignancy, these tumours are routinely treated with methotrexate after evacuation (15 mg/m^2 daily for 5 days) to avert the possibility of choriocarcinoma. Sophisticated treatment depends on a monthly urinary choriogonadotrophic hormone (CGH) level: if this rises above normal, choriocarcinoma must be highly suspect. Obvious tumours, usually indicated by a large pelvic mass, can be readily treated with methotrexate (as above) plus actinomycin D every 2 weeks (1.0 mg/m^2 i.v.) until CGH levels are normal.

Breast cancer

The commonest form of breast cancer is invasive intraductal adenocarcinoma. Risk factors for breast cancer are inversely related to fertility, and indicate that prolonged exposure to unopposed oestrogen is a causal factor. Because birth rates are high in Africa and women start bearing children at an early age, breast cancer is uncommon relative to the industrialized countries.

Diagnosis

Early detection of breast cancer by mammographic screening (usually begun annually at age 50) leads to improved survival in industrialized countries. Diagnosis can be established by open biopsy under local anaesthesia; if available, the laboratory should measure oestrogen receptor (ER) levels in the tumour.

Treatment

Modified radical mastectomy plus axillary lymph node dissection is the treatment of choice in the tropics. (Radical mastectomy has been abandoned.) Where radiation therapy is available, a 'lumpectomy' followed by radiotherapy is preferred by some women and yields equivalent results.

Pre-menopausal women with stage II breast cancer (involvement of axillary lymph nodes or large primary tumours) should receive 6 months of adjuvant chemotherapy, which will reduce recurrences and improve survival. A commonly used regimen is 'CMF' (see the Box).

CMF chemotherapy for breast cancer
Cyclophosphamide 600 mg/m^2, intravenously day 1 and 8
Methotrexate 40 mg/m^2 intravenously day 1 and 8
Fluorouracil 600 mg/m^2 intravenously, days 1 and 8,
Repeat the regimen monthly for six courses.

Post-menopausal patients with stage II, ER positive cancer should receive tamoxifen, an oestrogen antagonist, 10 mg orally, twice a day. Post-menopausal patients with ER-negative tumours will benefit from adjuvant CMF as above. Metastatic breast cancer can be treated with CMF, doxorubicin, and newer drugs such as taxol and *cis*-platinum, if available. Patients with metastatic ER-positive tumours will benefit from ovariectomy or tamoxifen (Margolese et al., 2000).

Skin tumours

Kaposi's sarcoma (KS)

Kaposi's sarcoma was endemic in certain regions of sub-Saharan Africa and comprised up to 10 per cent of adult male malignancies in certain countries. Most common in men, the tumour ranged from 'benign' appearing nodules on the arms and legs, some of which became more florid, ulcerative and malignant (Fig. 90.9 (Taylor et al., 1971), to those occasional tumours which caused an invasive, woody induration with bone involvement. Rare in children, endemic Kaposi's sarcoma appeared in lymph nodes and mucosa (see above).

Clinical features and diagnosis

A clinical diagnosis of Kaposi's sarcoma, in both its endemic and 'epidemic' HIV-associated forms is relatively easy. HIV-associated disease presents with multiple hyperpigmented skin nodules, usually symmetrically distributed on the trunk and limbs (Fig. 90.9). Oral mucosal involvement is frequent, and tumours may appear on the penis, conjunctiva, and lymph nodes. Visceral involvement is also seen, and multiple gastrointestinal lesions may cause diarrhoea and bleeding, while extensive pulmonary Kaposi's sarcoma causes shortness of breath and a range of different patterns in the chest radiograph.

Treatment

In Africa this centres on chemotherapy. The tumour is sensitive to many agents, and treatment choice is designed for each individual. This depends on the extent of the disease and the patient's symptoms and any associated disease, such as tuberculosis. Where available, radiotherapy provides palliative relief, often in a single dose of 800 cGy. Chemotherapy usually starts with single agents (doxorubicin, etoposide, vincristine or vinblastine, bleomycin). Combination treatment is reserved for more advanced lesions (Antman & Chang, 2000).

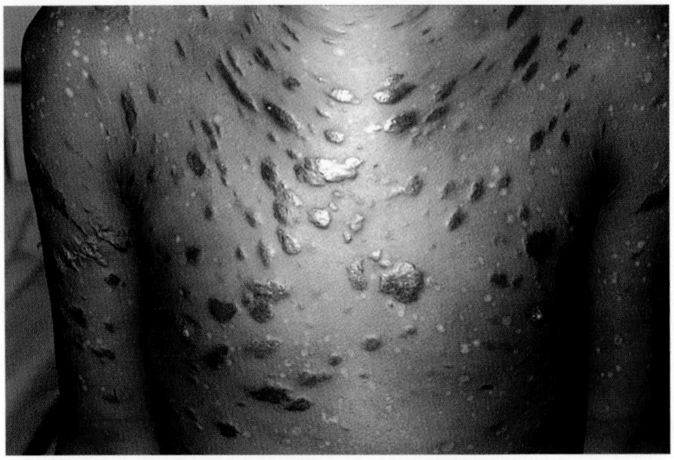
Fig. 90.9. Typical HIV-associated Kaposi's sarcoma, symmetrically distributed on the chest.

Prognosis

The outcome for HIV-related Kaposi's sarcoma depends largely on the morbidity from opportunistic infections (see Chapter 13, HIV).

Melanoma

In temperate zones, skin cancer including melanoma is most common in white-skinned individuals living in low latitudes and exposed to solar ultraviolet radiation. Although pigmented skin protects from cutaneous melanoma, this condition still occurs in black Africans in an acral distribution, i.e. palms of hands and soles of feet, as well as in certain mucosal sites and in the retina, Fig. 90.10). Wide surgical excision is the treatment of choice; the benefit of removing draining lymph nodes in melanoma cases is questionable. Chemotherapy for metastatic melanoma produces marginal response rates, and dacarbazine is the best agent tested.

Epithelial skin cancer

Squamous carcinomas in Africans are infrequent, and usually arise at the margins of tropical ulcers. The main

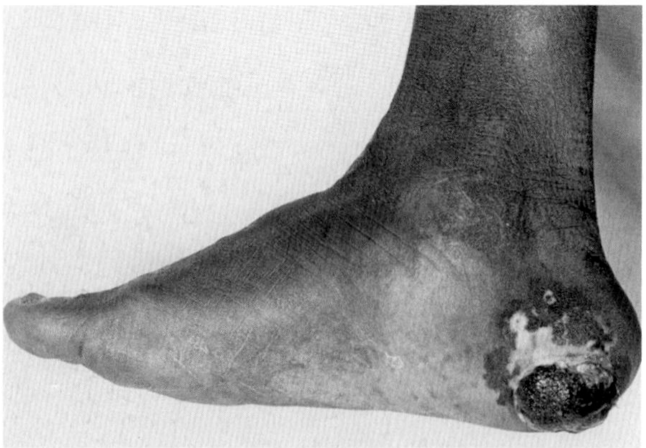

Fig. 90.10. Malignant melanoma of the foot. Note pigmented tumour and border, which easily distinguish this tumour from Kaposi's sarcoma (compare with Figure 90.8).

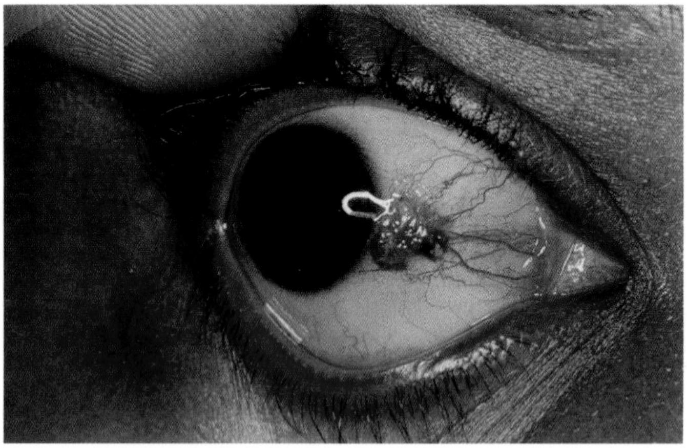

Fig. 90.11. Squamous carcinoma of the conjunctiva, associated with HIV infection. Be alert to the existence of these tumours in young adults who are HIV-infected and exposed to tropical sunlight. The tumours are easily cured with excisional surgery.

treatment of skin cancer is wide local excision. While pigmented skin protects against the damaging effects of ultraviolet radiation, albinos are particularly vulnerable to solar keratosis and squamous cancer at a young age. Thus, albino children must wear protective clothing, sunglasses, and, if they are able to afford it, a sunscreen ointment, and they must try to avoid exposure to the sun between 11: 00 am and 3: 00 pm where possible.

Eye tumours

Retinoblastoma

This is the principal eye cancer of childhood. Cases in infants are due to hereditary mutations in one allele of the RB gene, a tumour suppressor gene that arrests cell division. A second 'hit' of the remaining normal allele disables the RB gene so that cancer results. Retinoblastoma in later childhood results from somatic mutations to both RB alleles. Retinoblastoma is best treated with surgical enucleation and responds to radiation and chemotherapy. Survivors are at risk of second cancers, often sarcomas in previously irradiated sites.

Squamous carcinoma of the conjunctiva

This is a common eye tumour in low latitudes. Epithelial pigmentation is absent in the conjunctiva and intensive UV light becomes more carcinogenic. For unknown reasons, HIV infection has raised the risk of conjunctival cancer about ten-fold (Fig. 90.11). Local excision provides successful treatment, but patients should be advised to wear hats and sunglasses (Waddell et al., 1996).

Malignant lymphoma

Non-Hodgkin's lymphoma is classified histologically, although newer genetic technology now identifies molecular subtypes that vary in natural history and prognosis. From a practical standpoint, lymphomas are grouped into high grade, intermediate grade and low grade according to their clinical aggressiveness. High grade tumours (which include Burkitt's and diffuse large cell lymphoma) comprise rapidly growing tumours, but they paradoxically respond well to chemotherapy and may be cured in at least 50 per cent of cases. By contrast, low grade lymphomas, e.g. follicular, lymphocytic lymphomas, have an indolent natural history, respond to therapy (chlorambucil, cyclophosphamide, prednisone), but are rarely curable.

Diagnosis

Biopsy of pathologically enlarged lymph nodes is essential for an accurate diagnosis of lymphoma. Clinical staging divides cases into local (stage I), regional (stage II), above and below the diaphragm (stage III), and extra nodal (stage IV), although other staging schemes exist. Standard treatment for 'unfavourable grades' (intermediate and high grade) non-Hodgkin's lymphoma consists of a regimen called 'CHOP' (see the Box).

'CHOP' Chemotherapy for non-Hodgkin's lymphoma

Cyclophosphamide	750 mg/m^2 intravenously (i.v.)	Day 1
Doxorubicin	50 mg/m^2 i.v.	Day 1
Prednisone	50 mg/m^2 daily by mouth	Days 1–5
Vincristine	1.4 mg/m^2 (max 2 mg) i.v.	Day 1

Repeat courses monthly for 6 months.

Hodgkin's disease in adults is treated similarly to children (see above).

Conclusions

Essentials for cancer patients and their care

The principles of management are similar in virtually all malignancies:

- Know the risk factors and preventive strategies, together with early warning signs of cancer and precancerous lesions.
- Perform a careful physical examination to determine clinical stage, supplemented with diagnostic imaging if available.
- Establish a histological diagnosis.
- Assess curative or palliative treatment options, whenever possible, in a multidisciplinary Hospital Tumour Team, together with a medical oncologist, surgeon, and radiotherapist if available.
- Refer complex cases to specialized centres, when possible.
- Communicate the diagnosis to the patient with empathy, carefully explaining treatment goals and prognosis, both to the patient and to the family.
- Be aware of hospice care in the region and work with any hospice.
- Master the principles of pain control.

Postscript

Some of the most important advances in modern medicine come from research in developing countries. Such research usually involves partnerships with western universities where the necessary resources can be applied to indigenous research questions. These questions can originate from the inquiring minds of local practitioners. Curiosity, an inquiring habit of mind, and astute observation are the main ingredients of discovery. A large budget and expensive equipment are not necessary.

Acknowledgements

This chapter is based on our work at the Uganda Cancer Institute (initially with Professor Charles Olweny and the splendid staff).

References

Antman K, Chang Y. (2000). Kaposi's sarcoma. *N Engl J Med*; **342**: 1027–1038.

Banda LT, Parkin DM, Dzamalala et al. (2001). Cancer incidence in Blantyre, Malawi 1994–1998. *Trop Med Int Hlth*; **6**: 296–304.

Burkitt DP (1983). The discovery of Burkitt's lymphoma in Africa. *Cancer*; **51**: 1777–1786.

Chang MH, Chen CJ, Lai MS et al. (1997). Universal hepatitis B vaccination in Taiwan and the incidence of hepatocellular carcinoma in children. *N Engl J Med*; **336**: 1855–1859.

Chang Y, Cesarman E, Pessin MS et al. (1994). Identification of herpes-like DNA sequences in AIDS associated Kaposi's sarcoma. *Science*; **266**: 1865–1869.

Clifford P, Linsell CA, Timms GL. eds. (1968). *Cancer in Africa.* New York and London: International Publication Services.

Cohen JI (2000). Epstein–Barr virus infection. *N Engl J Med*; **343**: 481–492.

Cohen LF, Balow JE, Magrath IT et al. (1980). Acute tumor lysis syndrome. A review of 37 patients with Burkitt's lymphoma. *Am J Med*; **68**: 486–491.

Cook-Mozafarri P, Newton R, Beral V, Burkitt DP. (1998). The geographical distribution of Kaposi's sarcoma and of lymphomas in Africa before and after the AIDS epidemic. *Br J Cancer*; **78**: 1521–1528.

Correa P. (1992). Human gastric carcinogenesis. *Cancer Res*; **52**: 6735–6744.

DeThe G, Geser A, Day NE et al. (1978). Epidemiological evidence for a causal relationship between Epstein–Barr virus and Burkitt's lymphoma from Ugandan prospective study. *Nature*; **274**: 756–771.

Doll R, Peto R. (1981). The causes of cancer. Quantitative estimates of avoidable risks of cancer in the United States today. *J Natl Cancer Inst*; **66**: 1191–1308.

El-Sebai I, ed. (1983). *Bladder Cancer*, Vol. II. *Cancer of the Bilharzial Bladder.* Boca Raton: CRC Press.

Fandi A, Altun M, Azli N et al. (1994). Nasopharyngeal carcinoma. Epidemiology, staging and treatment. *Semin Oncol*; **21**: 382–397.

Garnick MB. (1993). Prostate cancer. Screening, diagnosis and management. *Ann Int Med*; **118**: 804–818.

International HIV Collaborative Group (2000). The impact of highly active anti-retroviral therapy on the incidence of cancer in people infected with the human immunodeficiency virus. Collaborative reanalysis of individual data on 47,936 HIV-infected people from 23 cohort studies in 12 developed countries. *J Natl Cancer Inst*; **92**: 1823–1830.

Linsell CA, Peers FG. (1977). Aflatoxin and liver cell cancer. *Trans Roy Soc Trop Med Hyg*; **71**: 471–473.

Madebo T, Lindtjorn B, Henrikson. (1994). The high incidence of oesophagus and stomach cancers in the Bale highlands of South Ethiopia. *Trans Roy Soc Trop Med Hyg*, **88**: 415.

Magrath IT. (1989). Small noncleaved cell lymphomas. In *The non-Hodgkin Lymphomas*, ed. IT Magrath, pp. 256–275. London: Edward Arnold.

Magrath IT, Litvak J. (1993). Cancer in developing countries. Opportunity and challenge. *J Natl Cancer Inst*; 85: 862–874.

Margolese RG, Fisher B, Hortobagyi GN, Bloomer WD. (2000). Neoplasms of the breast. In *Cancer Medicine*; ed.JM Holland, E Frei, pp. 1735–1822. Hamilton: BL Decker.

Mindel S. (1997). Role of imager in the developing world. *Lancet*; **350**: 426–439.

Murray CJL, Lopez AD. (1997). Global mortality, disability, and the contribution of risk factors. Global burden of disease study. *Lancet*; **349**: 1436–1442.

Olweny CLM, Toya T, Katongole-Mbidde E et al. (1975). Treatment of hepatocellular carcinoma with adriamycin. *Cancer*; **36**: 1250–1257.

Olweny CLM, Kaddinmukasa A., Atine I et al. (1977). Childhood Kaposi's sarcoma: clinical features and therapy. *Br J Cancer*; **33**: 555–559.

Parkin DM. (2001). Global cancer statistics in the year 2000. *Lancet Oncol*; **2**: 533–543.

Parkin DM, Sangli LD. (1991). *Cancer Registration in Developing Countries*. IARC Scientific Publication No. 95, Lyon, France.

Parkin DM, Ziegler JL. (2000). Malignant diseases. In *Hunters Tropical Medicine*, ed GT Strickland. Philadelphia: WB Saunders, Philadelphia.

Parkin DM, Vizcaino AP, Skinner MEG, Ndhlovu A. (1994). Cancer patterns and risk factors in the African population of southwestern Zimbabwe, 1963–77. *Cancer Epid Biomark Prevent*; **3**: 537–547.

Pathmanatrhan R, Prasad U, Sadler R. et al. (1995). Clonal proliferation of cells infected with Epstein Barr virus in preinvasive lesions related to nasopharyngeal carcinoma. *N Engl J Med*; **333**: 693–698.

Ross RK, Jones PA. (1996). Bladder cancer: epidemiology and pathogenesis. *Semin Oncol*; **23**: 536–545.

Sammon AM, Alderson D. (1998). Diet, reflux, and the development of squamous cell carcinoma of the oesophagus in Africa. *Br J Surgery*; **85**: 891–896.

Schafer DF, Sorrell MF. (1999). Hepatocellular carcinoma. *Lancet*; **353**: 1253–1257.

Schmauz R. (1995). Cancer of the penis. In *Tropical Surgery*, pp. 113–116. London: The Medicine Group, Ltd.

Schultz TF, Boshoff CH, Weiss RA. (1996). HIV infection and neoplasia. *Lancet*; **348**: 587–591.

Sitas F, Bezwoda WR, Levin V et al. (1997). Association between human immunodeficiency virus type i infection and cancer in the black population of Johannesburg and Soweto, South Africa. *Br J Cancer*; **75**: 1704–1707.

Taylor JF, Templeton AC, Vogel CL et al. (1971). Kaposi's sarcoma in Uganda: a clinicopathological study. *Int J Cancer*; **8**: 122–135.

Templeton, AC., Ed. (1973). *Tumours in a Tropical Country*. Berlin: Springer-Verlag.

Viviani S, Jack A, Hall AJ et al. (1999). Hepatitis B vaccination in infancy in The Gambia: protection against coverage at 9 years of age. *Vaccine*; **17**: 2946–2950.

Volgelstein B, Kinzler KW eds. (1998). *The Genetic Basis of Human Cancer*. New York: WB Saunders.

Venook AP, Stagg R, Lewis BJ et al. (1990). Chemoembolization for hepatocellular carcinoma. *J Clin Oncol*; **8**: 1108–1114.

Wabinga HR, Parkin DM, Wabwire-Mangen F et al. (1993). Cancer in Kampala, Uganda 1989–91. Changes in incidence in the era of AIDS. *Int J Cancer*; **54**: 23–36.

Waddell, KM, Lewallen S, Lucas SB et al. (1996). Carcinoma of the conjunctiva and HIV infection in Uganda Malawi. *Br J Ophthalmol*; **80**: 496–497.

Ziegler JL. (1981). Burkitt's lymphoma. *N Engl J Med*; **305**: 735–745.

Ziegler JL, Mbidde, EK. (1996). Kaposi's sarcoma in childhood. An analysis of 100 cases from Uganda and relationship to HIV infection *Int J Cancer*; **65**:200–203.

APPENDIX: BODY SURFACE AREA OF CHILDREN AND ADULTS

In a child of average size, find the weight and read the corresponding surface area on the boxed scale to the left. If the height is known, lay a straightedge on the correct height and weight for the child, then read the intersecting point on the surface area scale.

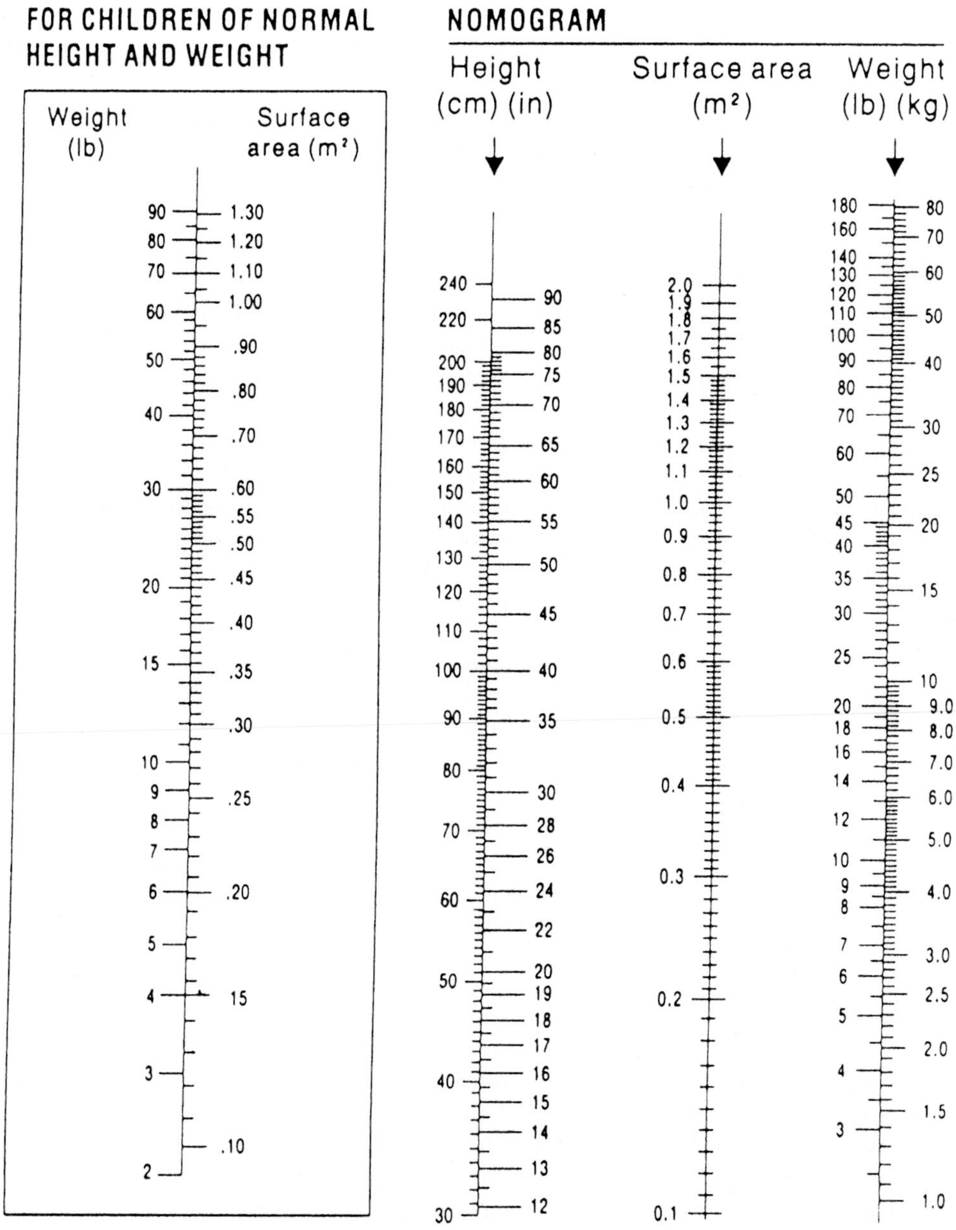

BODY SURFACE AREA FORMULA
(Adult and Pediatric)

$$\text{BSA (m}^2\text{)} = \sqrt{\frac{\text{Ht (in)} \times \text{Wt (lb)}}{3131}} \quad \text{or, in metric: BSA (m}^2\text{)} = \sqrt{\frac{\text{Ht (cm)} \times \text{Wt (kg)}}{3600}}$$

91 Palliative care

Palliative care

The World Health Organization (WHO) defines palliative care as:

the active total care of patients whose disease is not responsive to curative treatment. Control of pain, of other symptoms, and of psychological, social and spiritual problems is paramount. The goal of palliative care is the achievement of the best possible quality of life for patients and their families (WHO, 1990).

What palliative care does

Thus palliative care:

affirms life and regards dying as a normal process, neither hastens nor postpones death, provides relief from pain and distressing symptoms, integrates the psychological and spiritual aspects of patient's care, offers a support system to help patients live as actively as possible until death, offers a support system to help the family cope during the patient's illness and in their own bereavement (WHO, 1990).

The palliative care team

Palliative care is also described as 'total' care: it usually involves a team of carers who work in partnership with the patient and their family and who help them to live as comfortably and fully as possible during the last phase of illness. The patient is viewed as a person with physical, psychological, social and cultural gifts and needs which are specific to them. Each of these aspects needs to be taken into account, together with the patient, in the context of his or her family and community. Teams may consist of a central core of doctors, medical officers and nurses, who may work together with counsellors, religious leaders, social workers, volunteers at a community level, specific therapists such as physiotherapists together with the friends and family of the patient. Different talents within the team are used to assist in various aspects of the patient's care. Good communication between the team and the patient, and within the team itself are essential.

The patient and the team together agree goals and realistic priorities, so enabling the patient to maintain hope. Hope may relate to physical issues or other aspects of life and relationships. Often, towards death, hope may focus on being rather than achieving and on relationships with others or a higher being such as God. Even close to death, hope of a peaceful death or the assurance of not being left alone can remain.

The realities in Africa

Cancer in Africa often presents late, people may not worry about a lump until it becomes painful and stops them working so that tumours present at an advanced stage with less chance of cure even where active treatment is available.

In much of Africa the patients reached by medical services are a fraction of those in need. Many with terminal illness are likely to die in severe pain with uncontrolled symptoms. As health professionals we should be looking at how to take care of the dying, and how to bring pain and symptom control to people in the villages. In Uganda, Hospice Uganda has been training both health and non-health professionals in the principles of palliative care. Non-health professionals can raise community awareness even amongst those with no access to health care. Education of traditional healers and birth attendants can also increase the accessibility of palliative care to terminally ill patients.

Economic adversity

The WHO estimates 9 million new cases of cancer every year, with more than half of them in developing countries (WHO, 1996). WHO acknowledges that chemotherapy and radiotherapy will not be available to the majority of patients suffering from cancer in the developing world, for several generations, because of cost (WHO, 1986). They therefore stress the necessity of bringing pain and symptom relief to these patients by means of the analgesic ladder and other methods of pain and symptom control as researched through the hospice movement. These methods use medicines that are relatively cheap, though often not readily available.

The AIDS epidemic

An increase in both cancer and terminally ill patients suffering from pain is just one of the consequences of the AIDS epidemic. Pain is very common in HIV infection and affects between 30 and 80 per cent of patients. Twenty-five per cent of AIDS patients are said to suffer from severe pain (Katabera, 1998; Moss, 2000). According to the global report released by the United Nations Programme on AIDS in 1999 an estimated 34.3 million people worldwide were infected with Human Immunodeficiency Virus (HIV), the virus responsible for AIDS. More than 95 per cent of all HIV-infected people were living in developing countries and an estimated 67 per cent (24.5 million) of those people living with AIDS globally were thought to be living in sub-Saharan Africa (UNAIDS, 1999), it is likely that these numbers may have increased still further.

The patient at home

Where should the terminally ill patient die in Africa? Most people when questioned wish to die at home, with their loved ones around them. There are exceptions, for example the Kalenjin in Kenya, who believe that death in a house brings misfortune to the occupants. Others may think that hospital with 'experts' around is the best place to die to ensure that everything possible has been done. In a study of 173 terminally ill patients in Kampala, Uganda, 72 per cent of patients said that they preferred to be cared for at home, 14 per cent in hospital, and 14 per cent did not have a preference (Kikule, 2000).

The experience of many who work in palliative care has been that some of the most peaceful and comforting deaths have occurred at home in the centre of the family where family members are involved with the care. Families can easily be shown the simple ways of providing comfort to dying patients in the last hours or days and many draw great comfort themselves from their close involvement with their loved one. The financial burden of supporting a relation to look after and care for a member of the family in hospital many kilometres away, and the costs of transporting a dead body, are avoided by the family who give care at home.

Home-based care has evolved as the main form of palliative care in sub-Saharan Africa because it is the most acceptable especially in the African context of the extended and caring family (Merriman, 2001).

The hospice movement in Africa

The first hospice in sub-Saharan Africa opened in the 1980s in Harare, Zimbabwe: its work has spread throughout Zimbabwe. The second hospice started in Nairobi in 1990 and there are three further hospices in Kenya. Hospice Africa (Uganda) began in 1993, not only to serve Ugandan patients but also to encourage the development of palliative care in other African countries. Now, in 2001, there is a recognized need for palliative care for HIV/AIDS patients, this must include pain and symptom control. The Ugandan Government is the first in Africa to include palliative care as an essential clinical service in their five year health plan (Republic of Uganda, 2000). Palliative care is an expanding discipline now throughout Africa with hospice care spreading to other countries, including Tanzania, Malawi, Zambia and South Africa.

Mobile clinics

The distance and the cost of transport to the nearest health care facility, where palliative care is available, are such major obstacles that poor rural people who need such care may be unable to receive it. In south west Uganda we attempt to overcome this through the provision of mobile clinics. The palliative care team sets off monthly along a particular route, arranging to meet patients at a specific trading centre or sign post. Patients are reviewed in the back of our vehicle, medications adjusted if necessary and supplied for a month. If a patient is too sick to attend, a relation will come and report, and those patients who live close to the road can be seen in their own homes. The mobile clinic ends at a local health centre or hospital where new patients can be referred and old patients reviewed by the team. Mobile clinics can thus extend care to patients outside our immediate area, who could not afford the cost of transportation to the hospice for their care and medications (Fig. 91.1).

Pain control in palliative care

Cancer patients need pain control at all stages of their disease and control of pain is central to palliative care.

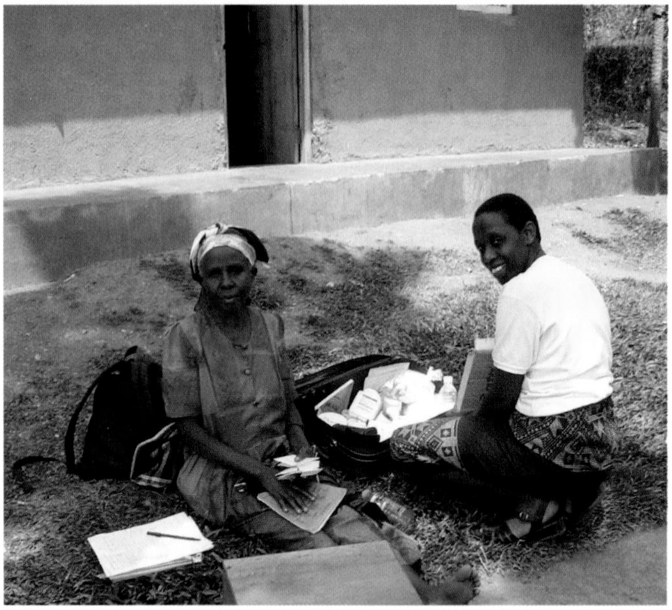

Fig. 91.1. A member of the palliative care team is discussing the use of her morphine solution with a patient who has Kaposi's sarcoma and immune deficiency.

Pain occurs in about one-third of patients undergoing cancer treatment and over two-thirds of those with advanced disease (WHO, 1996) (see the Box). In Uganda, 98 per cent of patients presenting to Hospice Uganda have severe pain. Many terminally ill patients have more than one pain. Pain control, however, is not enough. Attempts to relieve pain without addressing other symptoms and physical concerns are likely to result in failure to relieve pain. Pain control should be part of the holistic approach to the patient.

> **Pain in a cancer patient may be caused by:**
> - the cancer (soft tissue extension, bone, nerve or visceral involvement or raised intracranial pressure)
> - a complication of the cancer (lymphoedema, muscle spasm, constipation
> - treatment (chemotherapy-related mucositis, radiotherapy reactions or post-surgical scar pain)
> - a concurrent disorder (arthritis)
>
> **Pain in the AIDS patient may be caused by:**
> - opportunistic infections (headache due to cryptococcal meningitis, dysphagia due to oesophageal candidiasis)
> - AIDS related cancers (Kaposi's sarcoma, lymphoma)
> - the virus itself (HIV-related painful peripheral neuropathy)
> - treatment (neuropathy due to ARV therapy)
> - a concurrent disorder
>
> (WHO, 1996)

The clinical approach

There is no substitute for a detailed history and a thorough examination, in order to define the likely cause of each pain. Pain is not just physical: psychological, social, spiritual and emotional distress may also manifest as 'pain' and has to be considered and addressed where appropriate. As terminally ill patients often have more than one pain, a body chart can be very useful in describing the characteristics of the different pains. Assess each pain separately (see Fig. 91.2 and the Box).

> **Features in the history useful in the diagnosis of pain**
> **P** Palliating/precipitating factors
> **Q** Quality of pain sharp, colicky, dull
> **R** Radiation of the pain
> **S** Site of the pain
> **T** Time of pain duration, constant/intermittent.

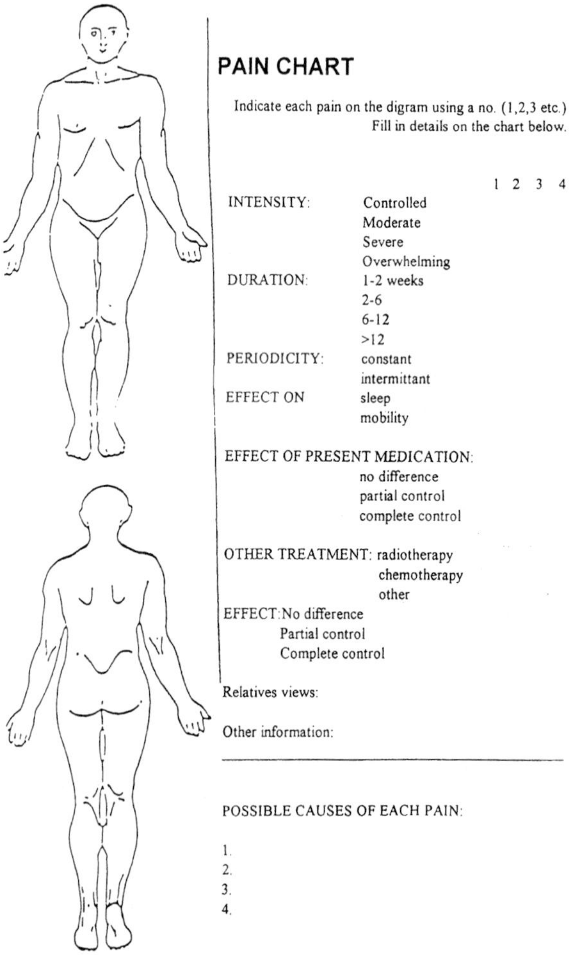

Fig. 91.2. A pain chart.

The types of pain

The diagnosis of the cause of physical pain is important for treatment. Pain can be divided into nociceptive pain and neuropathic pain.

Nociceptive pain

The nerve pathway is intact and the feeling of pain is a normal response to a noxious stimulus. Nociceptive pain usually responds to the analgesic ladder (see below).

Neuropathic pain

The nerve pathway is damaged so that there is an abnormal response to a noxious or normal stimulus. Neuropathic pain is, classically, burning or stabbing in nature, it may be associated with hyperaesthesia or numbness and may have a nerve, a dermatome, or a stocking and glove distribution. Neuropathic pain may be partly or totally resistant to opiates.

The plan of management

When the likely cause of the pain has been defined:

- Give specific treatment, for example, treatment of infection, or treatment of the cancer by whatever means are available. Nerve blocks are rarely indicated in the African context where multiple pains are the norm and most pains can be controlled using affordable medications now available.
- Explain the likely cause of the pain to the patient.
- Address non-physical factors, for example, fears surrounding death or social problems which can affect the perception of pain.

The use of drugs

The WHO has developed a rational method of using analgesics that has been tried and tested world-wide and enables the control of pain in up to 90 per cent of cancer patients (WHO, 1996) (see the Box).

Principles of rational analgesic use
- By mouth
- By the clock
- By the ladder
- By the patient
- Attention to detail/adjuvant treatment.

By mouth

If possible, give analgesics by mouth. In patients with dysphagia, uncontrolled vomiting and bowel obstruction rectal suppositories and subcutaneous infusion pumps can offer an alternative but are seldom available and not always culturally acceptable. Strong solutions (the same dose in a more concentrated solution) of oral morphine (see below) dripped into the mouth and absorbed through the buccal mucosa, or slow release morphine tablets given rectally are successfully used in Uganda.

By the clock

Give analgesics at regular intervals and titrate the dose against pain: give the next dose of analgesic before the effect of the previous one has worn off in order to keep the patient 'pain-free'.

By the ladder

The sequential use of analgesics is shown in Fig. 91.3. The principle of the analgesic ladder is that only one drug from each group should be used at the same time. If a drug ceases to be effective a stronger drug should be prescribed and the ladder climbed another step. Treatment should move stepwise both up and down the ladder as appropriate.

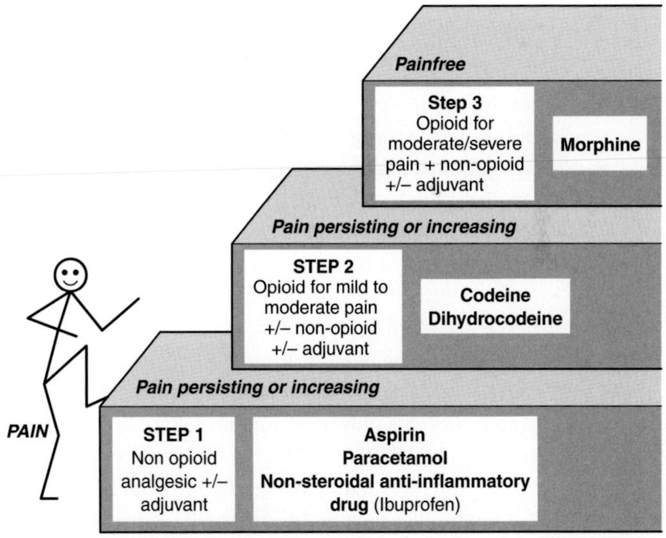

Fig. 91.3. The WHO analgesic ladder.

By the patient

The patient should be in control as long as possible regarding all decisions, especially with medication. He or she knows their body, their circumstances and what they can tolerate. Feedback from the patient on their tolerance and the presence or absence of side effects, is essential for bringing pain relief and comfort. There are no standard doses for opiate drugs, the right dose is the dose that relieves a patient's pain. Doses of morphine may vary from 2.5 mg to more than 1000 mg every 4 hours.

However, in Uganda the most frequent 24-hour requirements are 30 mg. A patient should always be reviewed within 24 hours of starting a strong opiate such as morphine. Too high a dose is diagnosed if the patient is continuously drowsy, although some sleep will be expected when pain has been a long-standing problem interfering with sleep. This side effect is used to good purpose when a double dose is given at night. Other signs of morphine toxicity include confusion (rare), respiratory depression (never seen in our Ugandan patients on oral morphine) and twitching. When these happen, stop the medication for 24 to 48 hours and restart on a lower dose. If a patient on morphine has undergone another pain-relieving procedure such as radiotherapy for bony metastases, the pain stimulus to respiration may be reduced necessitating the opiate dose to be reduced to prevent respiratory depression. Pain is a physiological antagonist to respiratory depression.

Attention to detail/adjuvant treatment

- Adjuvant drugs are often needed.
- Regular laxatives are necessary in all patients who receive opiates except those suffering from resistant diarrhoea, common in severely immunocompromised patients. Most African patients have a favourite laxative, which may be herbal or fruits, and we have recently begun to use paw paw seeds. Prescription laxatives tend to be expensive.
- Anti-emetics are seldom required with initial morphine use in African patients.
- Bone pain often benefits more from the addition of a non-steroidal anti-inflammatory drug than from an opiate. Steroids may be given in resistant bone pain. 16 mg daily for 3 days, reducing by 2 mg every two days, if the pain allows this, and often maintaining on 2–4 mg for life, such as dexamethethasone
- Nerve compression pain may benefit from addition of a steroid.
- Neuropathic pain may respond to small doses of a tricyclic antidepressant (such as amitriptyline which is affordable and available in most African countries) or an anti-convulsant drug (such as phenytoin) in pains with a stabbing element.
- Raised intracranial pressure in brain tumours, or cryptococcal meningitis, often responds to high dose steroids such as dexamethasone 24 mg daily for 3 days, then reduced by 2 mg daily unless pain and symptoms return.
- Right upper quadrant pain due to stretching of the liver capsule in patients with liver metastases may also respond to a reducing dose of steroids. Pain due to muscle spasm often responds to muscle relaxants. Diazepam 5–10 mg at night moving to baclofen 10–20 mg three times a day (skeletal muscle spasm) or hyoscine butyl bromide (*Buscopan*) 20 mg, three or four times a day (smooth muscle spasm, e.g. bowel obstruction).
- Explain to the patient and carer the different medications, and the need for regular doses.
- Give your patient a treatment sheet for them or their family to work from (see Fig. 91.4).
- List the names of each drug, the dose (ml or number of tablets), the reason for use (e.g. for pain) and frequency or time of each dose.
- Warn the patient of possible side effects.
- Review the patient and their medication regularly, as their disease progresses, and they are likely to develop new complications and different pains and symptoms.

In countries where resources are scarce, as in many in Africa, it is absolutely essential to consider whether the medications to be used are affordable, available and need little back up and monitoring with investigations. Economic factors, and for most these are unadorned poverty, prevent patients and families achieving pain relief, and if prescribers use expensive medications then pain control will not be available to the poor.

The use of drugs and the ladder

Step I

The first step is a non-opioid. Non-steroidal anti-inflammatory drugs (NSAIDS) and aspirin have additional anti-inflammatory activity and therefore are useful for bone and soft tissue pain.

- Make certain that the patient takes the drug with food because they can cause gastritis. High doses of NSAIDS can cause renal damage. Paracetamol acts centrally, whereas NSAIDS act peripherally, therefore both can be given together. If one NSAID does not suit the patient, try another. There is usually one that the patient is comfortable with.

Medicine	Reason	Morning		Afternoon		Evening		Night
		On waking	10 am	12 noon	2 pm	6 pm	10 pm	Bedtime
Morphine 5 mg in 5 ml	Pain	2.5 ml	2.5 ml		2.5 ml	2.5 ml		5 ml
Senna	Constipation						2	
Ibuprofen 200 mg	Pain	2		2		2		2

Medication chart for .... Date ....

Fig. 91.4. Medication chart.

Step 2

If a Step 1 analgesic fails to relieve pain, add an opiate for mild to moderate pain, such as codeine phosphate. Weak opiates have a ceiling effect: this means that an increase in dose is associated with increased side effects, but without further relief of pain. Therefore, if this combination fails to relieve pain, substitute a stronger opiate, for moderate to severe pain, for the weaker opiate.

Note: codeine is very expensive in some African countries while morphine made up from powder into solution is very cheap. Therefore, it may be more expedient in the patient with cancer or intractable and worsening pain to omit Step 2 and go to Step 3.

Step 3

Step 3 of the ladder is reached when the stronger opiate has to be given.

Pethidine

We do not recommend pethidine as a Step 3 analgesic because of its short duration of action (3 hours) and the accumulation of its metabolite norpethidine, which can cause convulsions. Pethidine also has to be given by injection so that it is inappropriate except in the management of acute pain at a medical facility.

Morphine

Morphine and codeine are included on the WHO essential drug list. Morphine is a very old drug, very effective, cheap and well suited for control of pain in terminally ill patients world-wide. It does not have a ceiling when titrated against pain and given orally.

Oral morphine is the strong opiate of choice for moderate to severe pain and is best given as morphine solution for oral use in strengths of 5 mg per 5 ml or 50 mg per 5 ml.

Experience in Africa has shown that the African patient is more sensitive to morphine than his western counterpart. It was found in an unpublished study between Kampala (Uganda) and Sheffield (UK) in 1997, that patients in Sheffield under hospice care required three times the average dose of morphine required by Ugandan hospice patients.

- Start patients who have not received opiates, opiate naive patients, on 5 mg 4-hourly and children over 6 months of age on 0.1 mg/kg.
- Reduce the dose for elderly or frail patients, or those with renal impairment, to 2.5 mg 4-hourly.
- Our experience in Africa has led us to use 5 mg 4-hourly initially in patients whose pain is not controlled by codeine 30 mg.
- Give the dose of morphine 4-hourly, with a double dose at night as this will usually enable the patient to sleep right through the night without waking.
- Increase the dose by 30–50 per cent of the previous dose, if the pain is not relieved after the first dose, or it has not been 90 per cent relieved after 24 hours.

Slow release preparations of morphine

Such preparations, for example MST (morphine slow release tablets), are available in some countries, but they are expensive. Start opiate naive patients on 10 mg 12-hourly.

If a patient is already taking liquid morphine, calculate the total daily requirement of morphine from the sum of the doses given in a day and then divide by two to give the twice daily dose.

Morphine for injection

This preparation is available in most African countries (see the Box).

Oral to parenteral morphine has a potency of 1:3.
Converting a patient from oral to parenteral: divide the dose by 3.
Converting from parenteral to oral: multiply the dose by 3.

Pain relief and health care policy

Many patients are dying in severe pain when relief of that pain is possible. Why is this so? The WHO believes that this is partly because health care workers, policy makers, and the public are not aware that most cancer pain can be relieved. Also, governments are concerned lest medical use of opiates will produce drug abuse (WHO, 1996). Oral morphine is not psychologically addictive when properly used to treat pain (Hanks, 1988). Therefore, education of health professionals and the public about palliative care, changing legislation to improve drug availability, administration and prescription, and clear statements by governments on policies to alleviate chronic cancer pain, are needed now (WHO, 2000).

Control of other symptoms in terminal illness

Symptoms in terminally ill patients may be caused by multiple factors. General debility due to the disease can cause malaise, or pressure sores; the disease itself can cause symptoms directly, a cancer may cause bowel obstruction, opportunistic infections in AIDS like *Pneumocystis carinii* cause symptoms like dyspnoea. HIV itself can cause neuropathy. Treatment of the disease may cause symptoms due to its side effects, like mucositis due to chemotherapy. Symptoms may also be due to co-existing pathology, for example arthritis, or concurrent disease such as pneumonia, unrelated to the underlying disease.

Management

Careful evaluation is central to good symptom control. Assessment should include not just physical problems but also psychological, social and spiritual aspects. How the symptom affects the patient's life, and exacerbating and relieving factors need to be considered.

- In order to treat the symptom, the cause should be considered. For example, vomiting may be caused by medication, the smell from a fungating wound, renal failure, bowel obstruction or radiotherapy. The treatments for each of these to control vomiting is different.
- Design an individualized regimen of treatment for each patient, specific to their condition at that particular time.
- Begin by explaining the reason for the symptom, and the possible options for their treatment. Whenever possible, the care team and the patient should decide together on the course of action to take, thus enabling the patient to retain some degree of control over their illness.
- Some symptoms can often be relieved completely, others such as dyspnoea, may only be partly relievable. When full relief is not possible, the aim of treatment is to help the patient move from a sense of helplessness to one of control. Practical advice such as breathing exercises and psychological support are essential parts of symptom control.
- Most symptoms can be improved by non-drug measures such as explanation and reassurance, avoidance of exacerbating factors, promotion of relieving factors, treatment of concurrent disease such as infection, and addressing psychosocial issues.

- Disease-modifying treatment should be considered. If accessible, radiotherapy can be helpful in symptom control even in incurable disease.
- When drugs are used in symptom control give them:
  1. by mouth if possible,
  2. regularly – to ensure continuous relief of symptoms,
  3. carefully – taking into account drug metabolism, the patients likely hepatic and renal function, and interactions with other treatments (WHO, 1998).

Simplicity

Simple treatments that are not costly are able to transform the lives of terminally ill patients. Most drugs used in palliative care are on the essential drug list and much can be done to improve the quality of life for a terminally ill patient and their family if the simple steps and principles in this chapter are followed.

Conclusions

Palliative care is a rapidly evolving and expanding medical specialty as more and more patients with, for example, AIDS, cancer, chronic renal failure and wasting disease are identified and in need of care in Africa, where access to health care is still so limited for so many.

Their care has to be adapted to their physical, social, emotional, psychological and spiritual needs and must be culturally appropriate. The challenge now is to develop the sort of services that can meet their needs. Relief of pain and control of symptoms are possible, they do not require expensive drugs and complicated equipment. The patients require the interest and commitment of individuals who provide their care and of authorities who provide the resources.

As health professionals faced with a terminally ill patient, palliative medicine gives hope to us and the patient and family. Most African patients are aware of the prognosis of cancer and/or AIDS. We may not be able to change the prognosis or ultimate outcome, but we can improve the quality of life, often extending life as well, when the patient and family are at peace. Dame Cicily Saunders, founder of the modern hospice movement, wrote:

You matter because you are,
You matter to the last moment of your life,
We will do all that we can,
Not only to let you die peacefully
but to live until you die.

References

Hanks GW. (1988). Pharmacological treatment of bone pain. *Cancer Surveys*; **7**.

Katabera E. (1998) & Moss V. (2000) Personal Communication from Dr Elly Katabera, Mulago Hospital, Kampala and Dr Veronica Moss, Mildmay International, Kampala to Anne Merriman.

Kikule EMN. (2000). A study to assess the palliative care needs of terminally ill persons and their caregivers in Kampala District, Uganda. Dissertation submitted towards the degree of Master in Medicine in Public Health of Makerere University.

Merriman A. (2001). The Hospice Concept in A Course for Health Professionals Course Notes. pp.6–7. Hospice Uganda, Hospice Africa.

Republic of Uganda (2000). Republic of Uganda, Ministry of Health: Health Sector Strategic Plan, 2000/01–2004/05, p.50.

UNAIDS. (1999). Information taken from UNAIDS website from a report written by UNAIDS estimates about prevalence HIV.

WHO. (1986). *Cancer Pain Relief.* Geneva: World Health Organization.

WHO. (1990). *Cancer Pain Relief and Palliative Care.* Technical Report Series Geneva: World Health Organization.

WHO. (1996). *Cancer Pain Relief.* 2nd edn. Geneva: World Health Organization.

WHO. (1998). *Symptom Relief in Terminal Illness.* Geneva: World Health Organization.

WHO. (2000). *Achieving Balance in Narcotic Control Policies.* Geneva: World Health Organization.

Recommended texts

Doyle D, Hanks WCG, MacDonald N (eds). (1998). *Oxford Textbook of Palliative Medicine.*

Merriman A. (2000). *Pain and Symptom Control in the Cancer and or AIDS patient in Uganda and other African Countries.* 2nd edn. Hospice Africa Uganda.

Twycross R. (1997). *Symptom Management in Advanced Cancer.* 2nd edn. Oxford, UK: Radcliffe Medical Press.

WHO. (1996). *Cancer Pain Relief.* 2nd edn. Geneva: World Health Organization.

WHO. (1998). *Symptom Relief in Terminal Illness.* Geneva: World Health Organization.

Useful Contacts

Hospice Africa Uganda, PO Box 7757, Kampala, Uganda. Email: *hospiceu@africaonline.co.ug*

Hospice Information Service, St Christophers' Hospice London, 51–59, Lawrie Park Road, London SE26 6DZ, UK. Email: *info@his2.freeserve.co.uk* Website: www.hospiceinformation.co.uk

92 Venomous animals

Wounds caused by large animals

Large wild and domestic animals can kill and maim with their teeth, tusks and horns and can crush by kneeling or treading upon the human victim. Large mammals capable of killing or severely mauling humans include hippopotamus, rhinoceros, elephant, the big cats (lions and leopards), hyenas, buffaloes, wild pigs and domestic cattle, camels and dogs. Hippopotamuses are regarded by many as the most dangerous mammals of Africa, while devastating bites by hyenas are not uncommon in several parts of Africa. Nomadic cattle herds, such as the Fulani of West Africa and the Turkana and Masai of Kenya, are sometimes gored by their cattle. Domestic camels are dangerous animals: during a Durbar in Sokoto, northern Nigeria, in 1984, there were nine serious injuries inflicted by camels: four fractures and one dislocation, resulting from kicks or the victim being picked up and then dropped; and four lacerations with crushing injuries of muscles and tendons caused by bites (Tahzib, 1984). Several people have been killed by being trampled upon by domesticated ostriches.

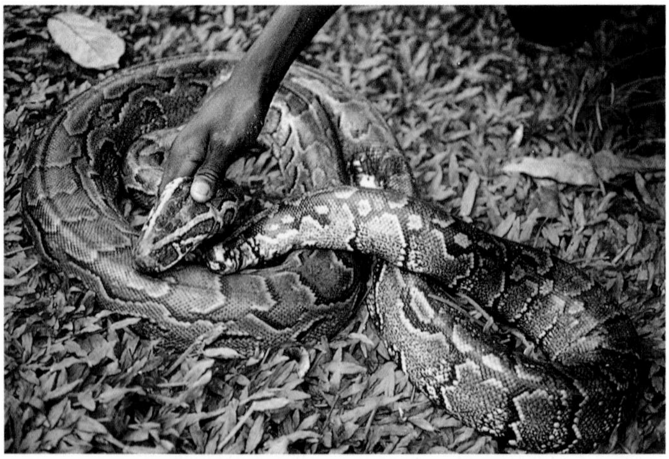

Fig. 92.1. African rock python (*Python sebae*), West Cameroon. Copyright D.A. Warrell.

Sharks

According to *The International Shark Attack File*, there have been 291 confirmed unprovoked shark attacks on humans around the coasts of Africa during the period 1828–2000 with 76 deaths. On South African shores alone, there were 223 confirmed unprovoked attacks from 1920 to 2000 with 44 deaths.

Nile crocodile (*Crocodilus niloticus*)

Fatal attacks have been reported from East, West, Central and Southern Africa and it is estimated that at least 1000 people are killed in Africa each year. Seven deaths per year were reported in Zimbabwe in the 1970s and human remains were found in the stomachs of 1 per cent of crocodiles killed in Central Africa, indicating that they had been killed or scavenged after death. Attacks occur when people walk along paths too close to crocodile-infested rivers or incautiously bathe or collect water from such rivers or pools.

African rock python (*Python sebae*) (Fig. 92.1)

This snake may reach a length of almost 9 metres. It lies in wait beside game tracks, and a large specimen is capable of killing a human by constriction and even swallowing the corpse. Very few deaths have been reliably reported.

Table 92.1. Mammal bite pathogens

Clostridium tetani
Pasteurella multocida
Leptospira species
Anaerobic organisms
Francisella tularensis
Spirillum minus
Streptobacillus monilliformis
Capnocytophaga canimorsus (DF-2)
Bartonella henselae
Rabies virus
Herpes simiae (B) virus

Wounds and complications

Lacerating, penetrating and crushing injuries are inflicted with teeth, tusks, claws or horns. The large cats, cattle and buffaloes often cause severe chest and facial injuries, complicated by pneumothorax, haemothorax, bowel perforation and compound fractures of limbs. There is a high risk of secondary infections with a wide range of micro-organisms including anaerobic bacteria (notably *Clostridium tetani* and *Cl perfringens*) because teeth and claws may be contaminated with decomposing meat (Table 92.1).

Treatment

First-aid

- Containment of the wound with a pressure bandage (for example, in case of evisceration)
- Control of bleeding
- Treatment of pain with injectable opiate analgesics
- Treatment of shock with intravenous fluids.

Safe and rapid transport to the hospital may be difficult as these accidents often occur in remote places. AMREF, the Flying Doctor Service based in Nairobi, rescues some five or six cases of large animal attacks each year.

Hospital

Emergency surgery will be needed, blood loss must be treated with transfusion, fractures fixed or placed in traction, ruptured organs sutured, necrotic tissue debrided and acute life-threatening complications, such as tension pneumothorax and flail chest, dealt with. Delayed primary suturing is the rule except for wounds of the head and neck. Wounds are reviewed in theatre 48–72 hours later for further débridement as necessary and for definitive soft tissue closure either by suture or split skin graft. Prevent infection with broad spectrum antibiotic cover including a penicillin or cephalosporin, an aminoglycoside (such as 48 hours only of gentamicin) and metronidazole for serious contaminated wounds. Tetanus prophylaxis is routine and post-exposure treatment for rabies may be appropriate.

Venomous bites and stings

Snake bites

Among Africa's 400 species of snake, some 40 species have proved capable of causing fatal envenoming or severe physical handicap in humans, while bites by at least another 50 species can cause local pain and swelling and, rarely, more severe symptoms. Hospital returns, which form the basis of the official statistics reported by Ministries of Health, under-estimate the importance of snake bite in Africa. It is largely a rural problem and most patients will seek the help of traditional practitioners rather than travel to busy rural hospitals and dispensaries which, increasingly, lack supplies of anti-venom. Community studies in Malumfashi District, Nigeria; Kilifi District, Kenya and in South East Senegal, emphasize this preference for traditional non-hospital treatment and indicate snake bite mortalities ranging from 1–14 per 100 000 population per year (Table 92.2). Studies of snake bites in several African countries are given in the References: Francophone West Africa (Chippaux & Goyffon, 2002), Congo (Carme et al., 1986); Malawi (Pugh, 1984); South Africa (Wilkinson, 1994) and Zimbabwe (Kasilo & Nhachi, 1993; Muguti et al., 1994; Nhachi & Kasilo, 1994).

Venom-injecting apparatus and venom

Venom glands, situated behind the eye, above the upper lip, secrete venom into a collecting duct which conveys the venom to the base of the fang and, from there, down a groove or, in the case of vipers, through a venom canal, to the tip of the fang which acts like a hypodermic needle. The fangs are enlarged teeth in the snake's upper jaw, modified to conduct venom deep into the tissues of the snake's prey (Fig. 92.2).

Venom composition

Snake venoms are complex secretions which contain:

- high molecular weight enzymes (molecular weight 13–150 kDa) which form 80–90 per cent of viper and 25–70 per cent of elapid venoms

Table 92.2. Snake bite mortality in parts of Africa determined by community studies

	Year	Deaths from snake bite (per 100 000 population per year	Predominant species	Reference
Malumfashi District, Nigeria	1977	1	*Naja nigricollis*	Pugh et al., 1980
Muri District, Nigeria	1961–73	8	*Echis ocellatus*	Warrell & Arnett, 1976
Kilifi District, Kenya	1994	7	*Bitis arietans*	Snow et al., 1994
Bandafassi, Southeast Senegal	1976–99	14	*Echis ocellatus*	Trape et al., 2001

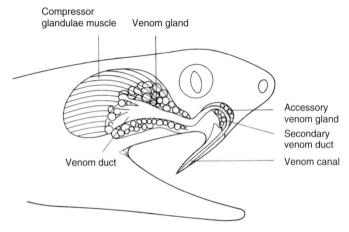

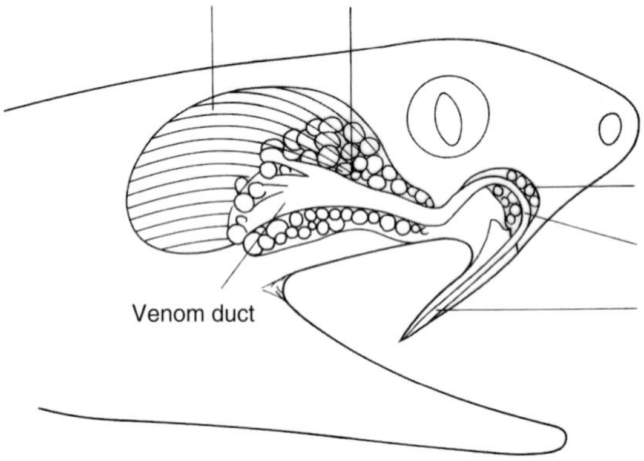

Fig. 92.2. Venom apparatus of a viper.

- polypeptide toxins (molecular weight 5–10 kDa)
- low molecular weight compounds (molecular weight <1.5 kDa).

The enzymes include endopeptidases (to digest the snake's prey), serine proteases (procoagulants of viper venoms) and zinc metalloproteinases (the haemorrhagins of viper venoms). The peptides include polypeptide post-synaptic neurotoxins (for example in the venom of the Egyptian cobra *Naja haje*), cytotoxins and myotoxins which damage tissues and muscles, the endothelin-like sarafotoxins of burrowing asps (Atractaspis).

Echis venoms contain activators of Factor X and prothrombin, while the venoms of two dangerously-venomous colubrid snakes (boomslang *Dispholidus typus*, vine snake *Thelotornis* species) contain prothrombin activators. Venom phospholipases A_2 in sea snake venom damage skeletal muscle and, in the case of the berg adder (*Bitis atropos*) and some other small *Bitis* species, are responsible for pre-synaptic neurotoxic activity. Mamba venoms contain potassium-blocking dendrotoxins and anticholinesterases (fasciculins). The principal activities in humans of the venoms of the medically important African snakes are summarized in Table 92.3.

Classification and characteristics of venomous snakes (Spawls & Branch, 1995)

African venomous snakes belong to four families.

Elapidae (cobras, rinkhals, mambas, African garter snakes, coral and shield-nose snakes and sea snakes)

These have short, fixed, erect front fangs (Fig. 92.3). They are relatively thin and long-tailed and some species can exceed three metres in length (Fig. 92.4). Their scales are usually smooth and shiny. Scales on the top of the head are enlarged. Their colour is more uniform than in vipers with a pale ventral surface.

Cobras

Cobras may have distinctive bands on their throats (pink or red in the case of the black-necked spitting cobra, *Naja nigricollis*) (Fig. 92.5) but, unlike Asian cobras, not on the backs of their necks. Cobras are found around and inside houses, near water but also in rain forest and desert areas. They usually rear up and spread their hoods defensively when threatened (Figs 92.6, 92.7). Unlike vipers, they may not release the bite immediately after striking. The cobra's hood is not visible in a rapidly retreating or dead specimen. Five African species of spitting cobras and the rinkhals can eject their venom forcibly from the tips of the fangs for distances of several metres into the eyes of presumed aggressors.

Mambas

Mambas are very long, thin, agile, alert and active snakes. The three species of green mamba (Fig. 92.8) are found in the branches of trees while the black mamba, coloured greyish or brownish with a black lining to its mouth, lives in more open country, favouring termite mounds. Like cobras, they rear up if threatened, and spread a narrow hood.

Table 92.3. Principal effects of African snake venoms in humans

Venom activity	Clinical manifestations	African snake responsible
Neurotoxicity	Ptosis, external ophthalmoplegia, facial paralysis, paralysis of tongue, inability to open the mouth, bulbar and respiratory paralysis	Elapids (e.g. cobras, rinkhals, mambas); berg adder and Peringuey's adder
Myotoxicity	Trismus, stiff, painful muscles, myoglobinuria	Sea snake
Cardiotoxicity	Hypotension, shock, arrhythmias, ECG abnormalities	Puff adder and other large *Bitis* species, saw-scaled (*Echis*) vipers
Haemorrhagic	Spontaneous systemic haemorrhage (gums, gut, brain, etc.)	Saw-scaled vipers, (puff adder and other large *Bitis* species), boomslang, vine snake
Cytotoxicity	Massive local swelling, blistering, necrosis: extravasation of blood and plasma causing hypovolaemia	Puff adder and other large *Bitis* species, saw-scaled vipers, spitting cobras
Procoagulant	Incoagulable blood, persistent bleeding from trauma and recent wounds	Saw-scaled vipers, boomslang, vine snake

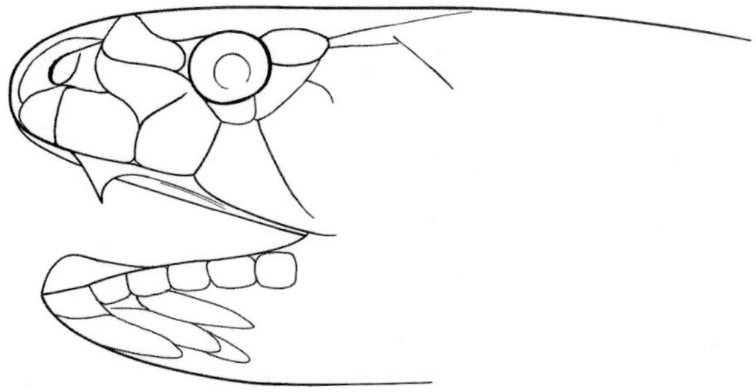

Fig. 92.3. Short fixed anterior fangs of an elapid (black-necked spitting cobra – *Naja nigricollis*).

Venoms

The most characteristic toxins of elapid venoms are polypeptides which are rapidly absorbed into the bloodstream, producing progressive paralysis with little local swelling at the site of the bite. This is true of the mambas and the four 'neurotoxic' cobras; Egyptian cobra (*Naja haje*) (Fig. 92.7), snouted cobra (*N. annulifera*), Cape cobra (*N. nivea*) and forest cobra (*N. melanoleuca*). In contrast, bites by the five species of spitting cobras (*N. nigricollis* – Fig. 92.5, *N. mossambica, N. pallida, N. katiensis* and *N. nigricincta*) cause severe local swelling, blistering and necrosis without neurotoxicity.

Other elapids

The other terrestrial elapids – rinkhals (*Hemachatus haemachatus*), shield-nosed snake (*Aspidelaps scutatus*) (Zaltzman et al., 1984), coral snake (*Aspidelaps lubcricus*), garter snakes (*Elapsoidea*) etc. – rarely cause bites or envenoming.

Sea snake

The only sea snake occurring along the (East) African coast, the yellow bellied sea snake (*Pelamis platurus*), is yellow and black. The body is compressed from side to side like a fish and the tail is flattened. The highly potent venom causes a generalized breakdown of skeletal muscle (rhabdomyolysis), paralysis, myoglobinuria, hyperkalaemia and renal failure. Sightings are uncommon and bites extremely rare.

Viperidae (vipers and adders)

These have long, hinged, front fangs, normally folded back against the upper jaw but, during the strike, erected and plunged into the victim (Fig. 92.9). These snakes are relatively thick and short-tailed (Fig. 92.10). Except for the night adders (Causus), vipers have many small ridged scales of approximately equal size on the top of their heads and a striking and sometimes colourful repeated dorsal pattern (Figs 92.11, 92.12). Apart from the small tree-dwelling bush vipers (Atheris), these are ground-dwelling snakes which appear sluggish but are capable of striking with lightening speed if trodden upon. Puff adders (Fig. 92.11) and night adders inflate their bodies and hiss loudly if disturbed. Saw-scaled vipers (Fig. 92.12) are quick-moving irritable snakes: when threatened they rub their coils together, producing a rasping sound which is sometimes the last thing that the victim hears before being bitten. This sound has given rise to onomatopoeic local names for the species (e.g. in Nigeria: *kurot* – Tangale; *kububuwa* – Hausa; *for'doyri* – Fulani).

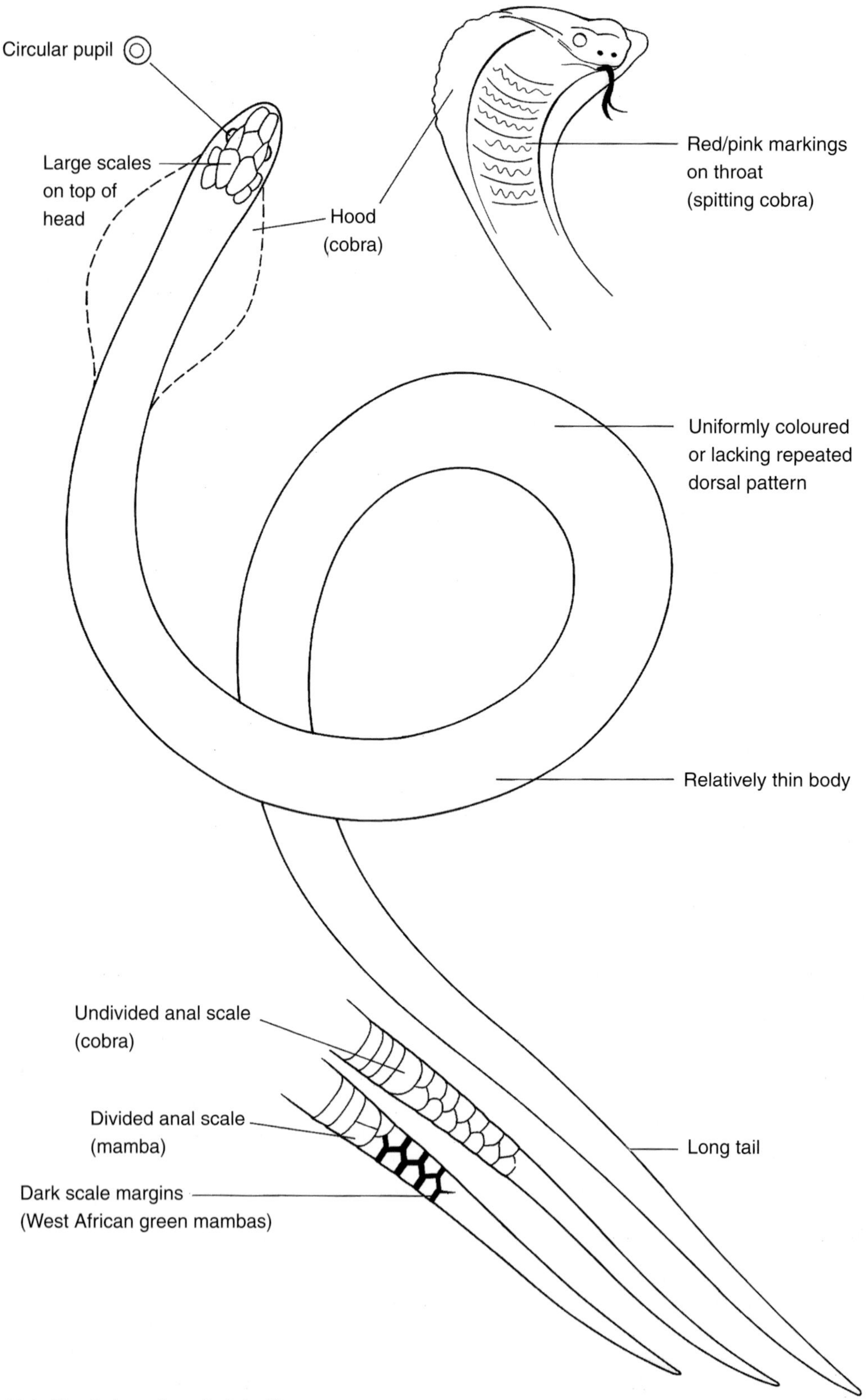

Fig. 92.4. Morphology of a typical elapid.

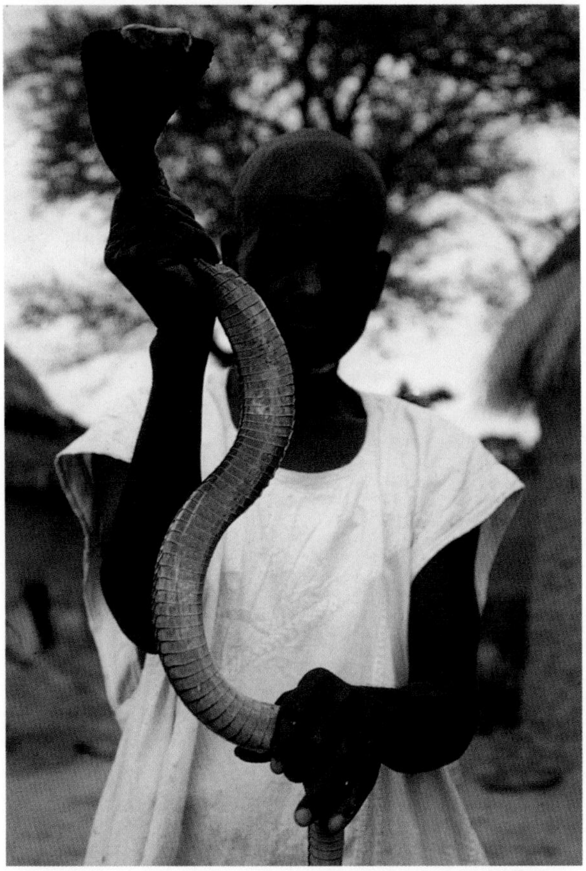

Fig. 92.5. Black-necked spitting cobra (*Naja nigricollis*) showing pinkish neck markings (Nigeria). Copyright D.A. Warrell.

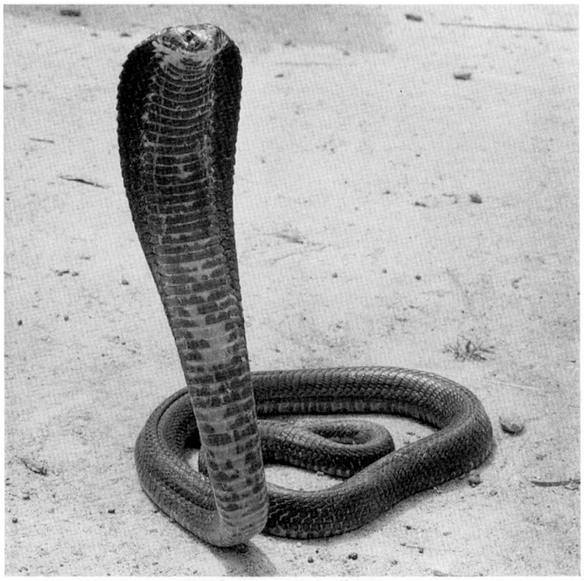

Fig. 92.6. Threatening posture of a cobra (Egyptian cobra – *Naja haje*). Copyright D.A. Warrell.

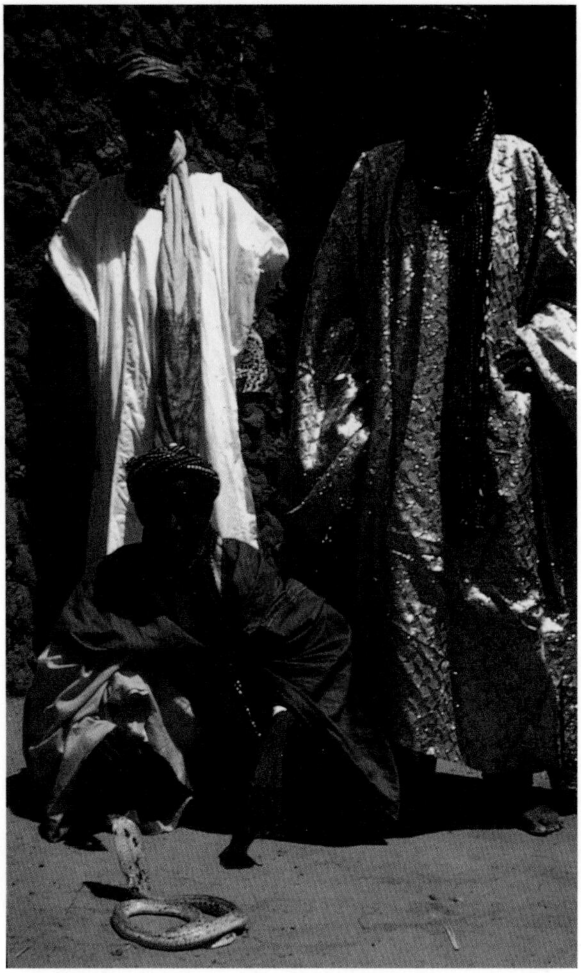

Fig. 92.7. Snake charmers at the Court of the Sultan of Sokoto, Nigeria. Their snake is a pale-coloured Egyptian cobra (*Naja haje*) (Hausa *jan nasuru*). Copyright D.A. Warrell.

Venoms

The relatively large protein molecules of viper venoms are absorbed relatively slowly via lymphatics. Digestive hydrolases and other cytotoxins cause massive local swelling and tissue damage. The venom of saw-scaled vipers contains metalloproteinase haemorrhagins which damage vascular endothelium and procoagulants which cause disseminated intravascular coagulation and consumption coagulopathy. These activities result in incoagulable blood and spontaneous systemic bleeding. A few of the smaller Bitis species, notably the berg adder (*Bitis atropos*), desert mountain adder (*B. xeropaga*) and Peringuey's adder (*B. peringueyi*) of southern Africa, cause neurotoxicity, olfactory dysfunction, as well as local swelling.

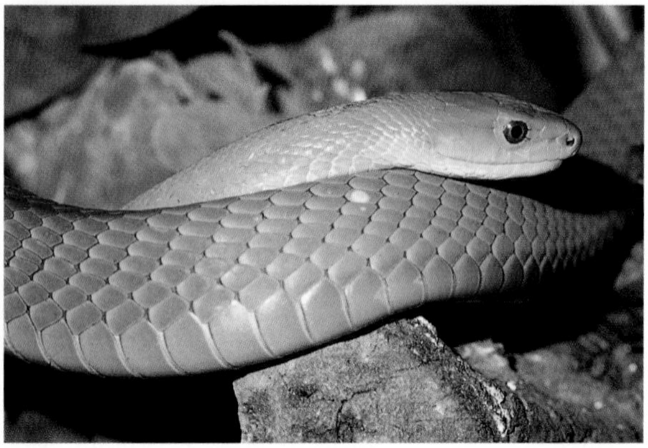

Fig. 92.8. Eastern green mamba (*Dendroaspis angusticeps*) (South Africa). Copyright D.A. Warrell.

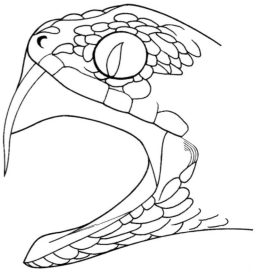

Fig. 92.9. Long erectile anterior fangs of the saw-scaled or carpet viper (*Echis ocellatus*).

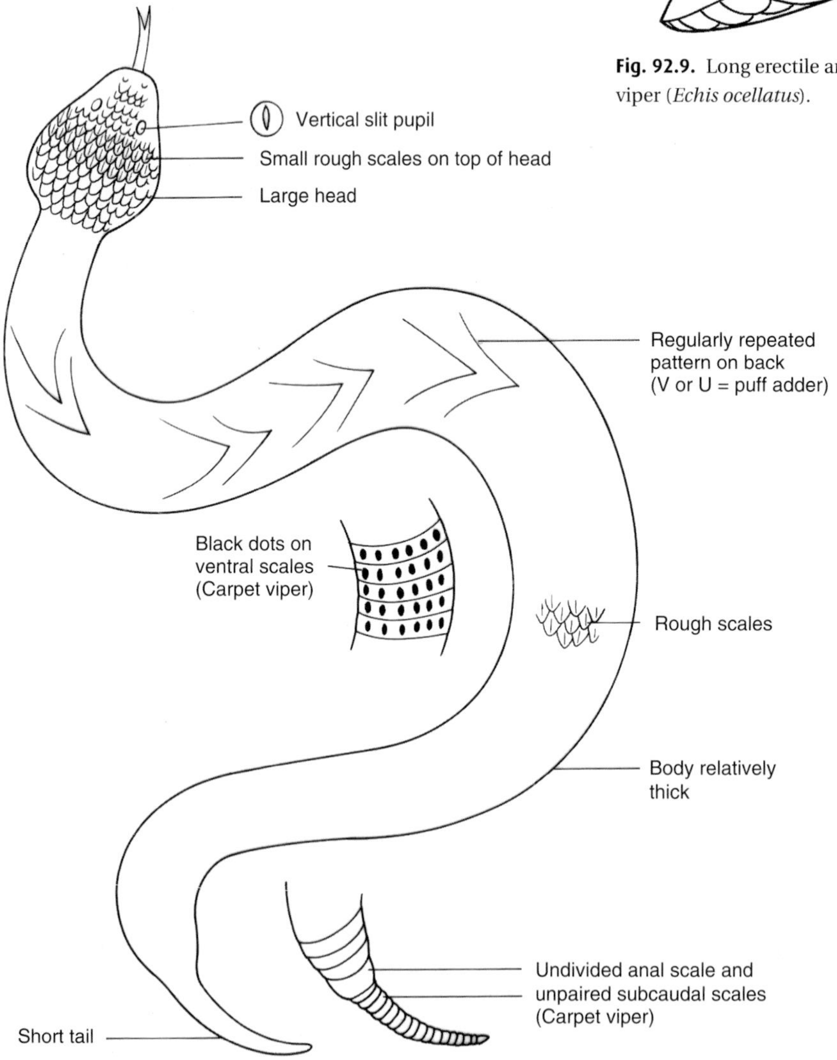

Fig. 92.10. Morphology of a typical viper.

Atractaspididae (burrowing asps, burrowing vipers or stiletto snakes and Natal black snake)

In burrowing asps, the long anterior fang is partially erectile and is protruded from the side of the mouth and used to impale its prey (usually a burrow-dwelling lizard) by a side-swiping motion. The Natal black snake has enlarged grooved maxillary teeth. The venom of *Atractaspis engaddensis* is most unusual, containing 21 amino acid peptides (sarafotoxins), homologues of the endogenous endothelins, which cause vasoconstriction and cardiac conduction abnormalities.

Colubridae (boomslang, vine snake and other back-fanged tree snakes)

Most members of this, the largest family of snakes, are harmless, but three African species – the boomslang (*Dispholidus typus*) and the vine-, tree-, twig-, or bird-snakes (*Thelotornis kirtlandii* and *T capensis*) are potentially dangerous to man. The fangs are enlarged, grooved, maxillary teeth, situated far back in the mouth (Fig. 92.13). These snakes virtually never bite humans unless they are handled. Boomslangs inflate their throats if threatened. The venoms cause spontaneous systemic bleeding, coagulopathy, haemolysis and renal failure.

Epidemiology of snake bite

Distribution of venomous snakes (Spawls & Branch, 1995)

Figure 92.14 shows the areas of Africa where the commonest and most dangerous species are found. The three species responsible for most of the deaths and disabling injuries; saw-scaled viper, spitting cobras and puff adder; all occur in the savannah regions of Africa. Rain forest species such as the forest cobra (*Naja melanoleuca*), western green mambas (*Dendroaspis viridis* and *D jamesoni*) and Gabon and rhinoceros-horned vipers (*Bitis gabonica, B. rhinoceros, B. nasicornis*) cause few bites.

People at risk

Snake bite is most common among farmers, herdsmen and plantation workers who walk and work bare-footed and bare-handed in rural areas of Africa. Snake charmers (Fig. 92.7) are at special risk.

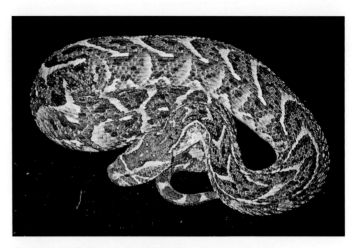

Fig. 92.11. Puff adder (*Bitis arietans*) (Kenya). Copyright D.A. Warrell.

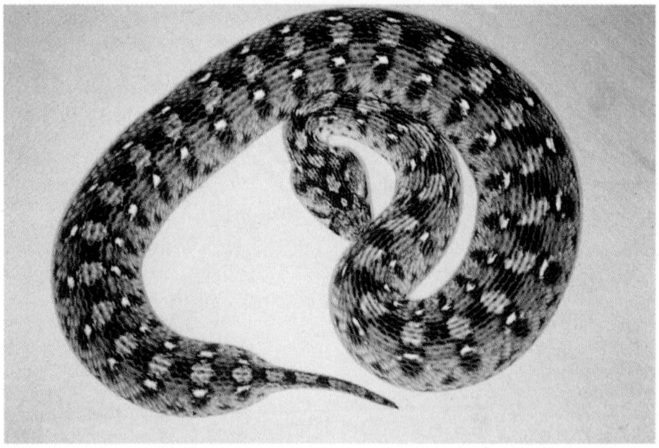

Fig. 92.12. Saw-scaled or carpet viper (*Echis ocellatus*) (Nigeria). Copyright D.A. Warrell.

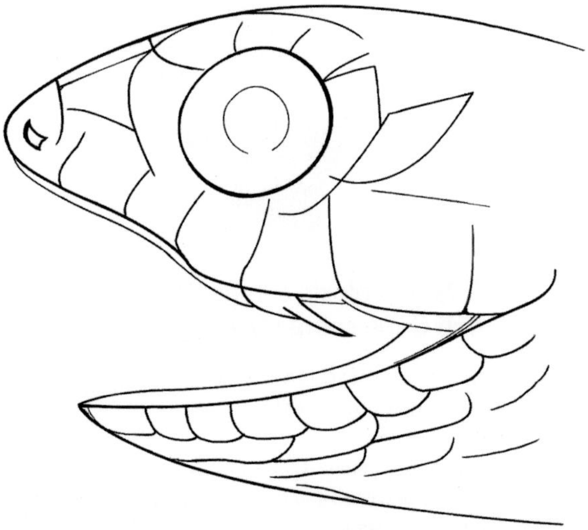

Fig. 92.13. Fixed posterior fangs of a colubrid snake (boomslang – *Dispholidus typus*).

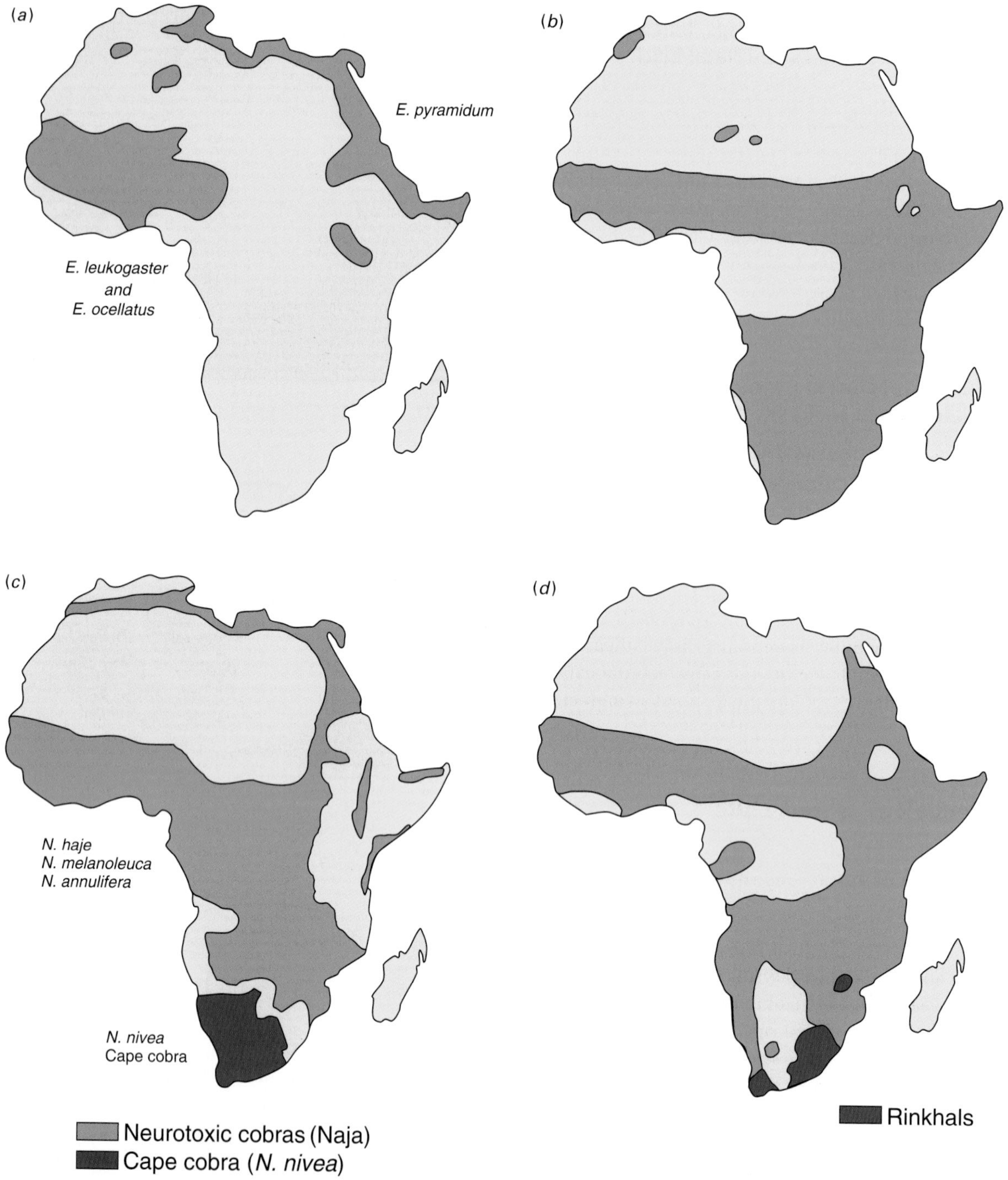

Fig. 92.14. Distribution of venomous snakes in Africa
(*a*) saw-scaled/carpet vipers (*Echis*)
(*b*) puff adder (*Bitis arietans*)
(*c*) neurotoxic cobras: orange – *Naja haje, N. annulifera, N. melanoleuca*; brown – Cape cobra (*N. nivea*))
(*d*) cytotoxic spitting cobras and rinkhals: orange – spitting cobras – *N. nigricollis* etc.; brown – rinkhals (*Hemachatus haemachatus*)
(*e*) mambas (*Dendroaspis*)
(*f*) boomslang (*Dispholidus typus*).

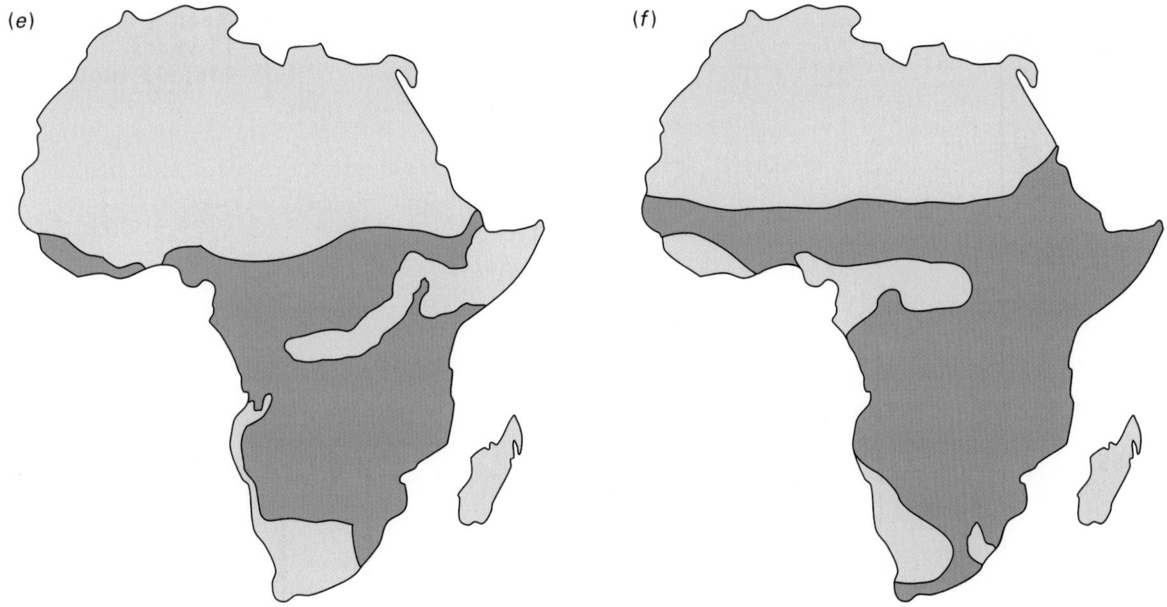

Seasonal changes

Most bites occur just before the rainy season begins (Fig. 92.15), when farmers flock into the fields to till the land and snakes are in the most active phase of their yearly cycle. Heavy rains may flood snakes out of their holes and burrows and so increase the risk of snake bite.

Clinical features of snake bite (Warrell, 1995)

Snake bite is usually a terrifying experience; symptoms and signs attributable to anxiety, fear or even hysteria may confuse the clinical picture. It should be reassuring to snake bite victims to be reminded that up to 50 per cent of bites by venomous snakes, in which skin punctures show penetration of the fangs, are associated with trivial or no envenoming, the so-called 'dry bites'. Even if the patient is envenomed, fatalities are rare. The length of time from bite to death has been reported as up to 16 days (median 24 h) for puff adders; 25 h–41 days (median 5 days) for saw-scaled vipers; 7, 35 and 36 h for black-necked spitting cobras and as early as 6–16 h for Egyptian cobras.

Viper bites

If venom has been injected by the bite, local pain and swelling are likely to develop within two hours.

Puff adder (*Bitis arietans*) (Warrell et al., 1975)

Throughout the whole savanna region of Africa, this species is responsible for the largest number of serious bites. The main problem is massive local swelling, which may spread to involve the whole limb and adjacent areas of the trunk, is associated with hypovolaemic shock in some cases and carries the risk of necrosis. Regional lymph nodes draining the site of the bite become painful, tender and swollen. There is bruising of the swollen tissue and, within 24 hours, bullae filled with bloodstained fluid may erupt around the bite site and up the envenomed limb (Fig. 92.16). Extravasation of blood and plasma into the envenomed limb may deplete the circulating volume sufficiently to cause hypovolaemic shock. Direct effects on the heart are suggested by electrocardiographic abnormalities including cardiac arrhythmias such as sinus bradycardia. Tissue necrosis is primarily the result of digestive hydrolases and other cytotoxic components of the venom; but secondary effects, such as thrombosis of a major artery, compartment syndromes or infection of the gangrenous tissue by anaerobic organisms, will increase the extent of tissue loss. Rarely, vascular damage associated with thrombocytopenia may result in spontaneous bleeding. In fatal cases, serosal surfaces may be found to be studded with petechial haemorrhages. The venom is capable of causing coagulopathy leading to incoagulable blood, but this has rarely been reported in human victims. Bites by the other large *Bitis* species (*B. gabonica, B. rhinoceros, B. nasicornis* and *B. parviocula*)

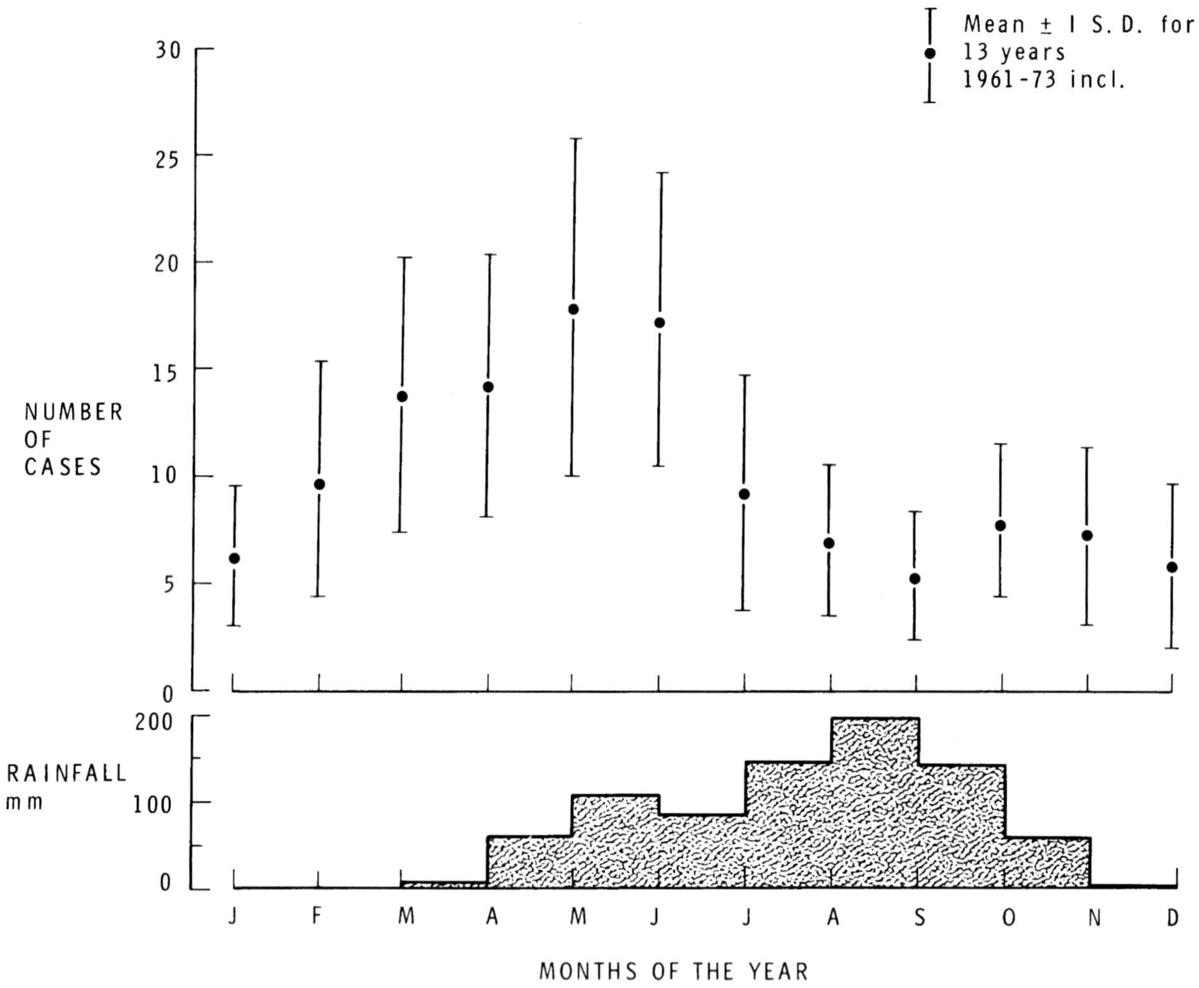

Fig. 92.15. Annual incidence of snake bite admissions to Guinther Memorial Hospital, Bambur, Nigeria (Warrell & Arnett, 1976).

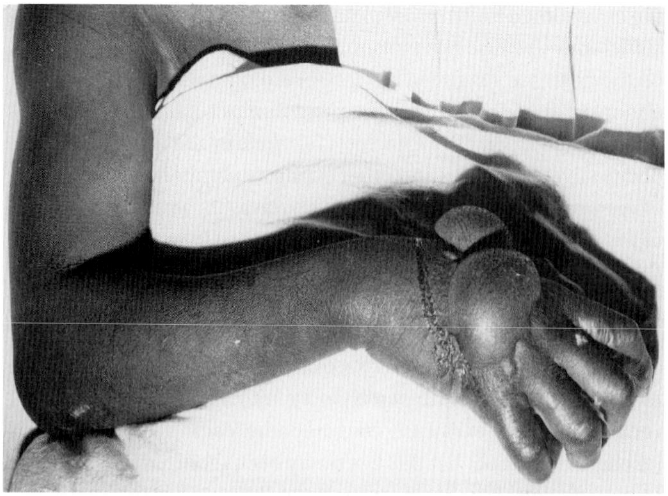

Fig. 92.16. Blistering following a puff adder (*Bitis arietans*) bite in the first interdigital cleft. Copyright D.A. Warrell.

can be expected to produce similar effects. Envenoming by *Bitis gabonica* and *Bitis rhinoceros* can cause profound shock and other cardiovascular effects with coagulopathy and spontaneous systemic haemorrhage.

Saw-scaled or carpet vipers (*Echis ocellatus* and *E. leucogaster* in West Africa, *E. pyramidum* in North and East Africa) (Warrell et al., 1977; Manent et al., 1992; Seignot et al., 1992; Warrell & Arnett, 1976)

Throughout the savannah and semi-desert regions of the northern third of Africa, this species is responsible for most bites and deaths from envenoming. Bites may cause severe local swelling, blistering, bruising and necrosis, but the clinical picture is dominated by spontaneous systemic bleeding with disseminated intravascular coagulation and consumption coagulopathy leading to

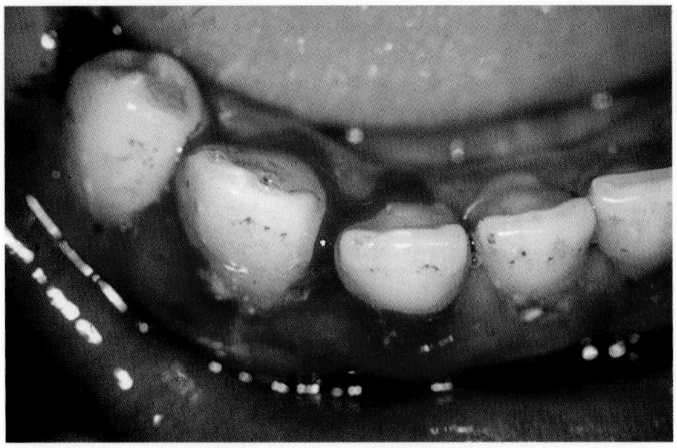

Fig. 92.17. Bleeding from the gums, 90 minutes after a bite by the saw-scaled or carpet viper (*Echis ocellatus*) (Nigeria). Copyright D.A. Warrell.

incoagulable blood. Thrombocytopenia is observed only in the most severely envenomed patients. Early sites of haemorrhage are gingival sulci (Fig. 92.17), nose, sites of trauma or partly-healed wounds and the gastrointestinal and genitourinary tracts. The patient may die within days (rarely later than a week) from intracranial or massive intestinal or retroperitoneal haemorrhage, or, very rarely, after a week or more from bilateral renal cortical necrosis and acute renal failure. Envenoming by the Sahara-desert horned-viper (*Cerastes cerastes*) and the smaller *C. vipera* is less severe, but microangiopathic haemolysis and renal failure have been described.

Night adders (*Causus maculatus, C. rhombeatus, C. resimus,* etc.) (Warrell et al., 1976b)

Bites by these small vipers are common in most parts of Africa. No deaths have reliably been reported. The usual symptoms are local pain and swelling which may spread beyond the bitten segment of limb and enlargement of local lymph nodes. Local necrosis does not occur. Mild systemic features, including fever, hypotension, drowsiness and leukocytosis have been reported.

Burrowing asps (*Atractaspis* species) (Warrell et al., 1976b)

Bites by the numerous species of *Atractaspis* are common in Africa. Usually, they happen in the dark after heavy rain. Local symptoms include pain, swelling, blistering and local necrosis with painful, regional lymphadenopathy. Systemic symptoms include fever, nausea, headache, faintness and generalized weakness. Fatal envenoming has resulted from bites by *A. microlepidota* (and probably the closely related *A. engaddensis*) and *A. irregularis.* There are symptoms resembling anaphylaxis with ECG

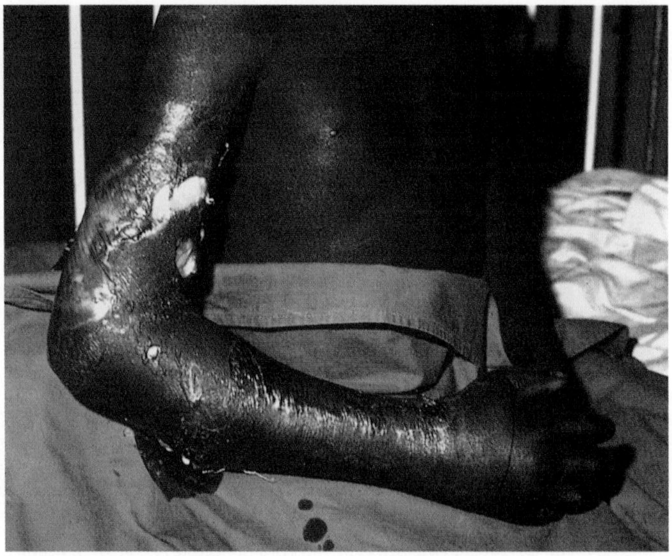

Fig. 92.18. Necrosis 9 days after a bite near the elbow by a black-necked spitting cobra (*Naja nigricollis*) (Nigeria). Copyright D.A. Warrell.

abnormalities resulting in death less than 45 minutes after the bite. Mild disturbances in blood coagulation and liver function have been described.

Elapid (cobra and mamba) bites

Neurotoxic cobra and mamba bites

Mambas are the most feared snakes in Africa, but fortunately bites are uncommon. Venoms of green and black mambas (Dendroaspis) and the 'neurotoxic' cobras (Egyptian cobra – *Naja haje* (Warrell et al., 1976c), snouted cobra – *N. annulifera,* Cape cobra – *N. nivea* (Blaylock et al., 1985) and forest cobra – *N. melanoleuca*) cause relatively mild local envenoming but affect neuromuscular transmission resulting in progressive paralysis. Ptosis, external ophthalmoplegia, dsyphagia, dysarthria and excessive salivation are typical early symptoms. Death, which is usually the result of bulbar and respiratory paralysis, may occur as early as 30 minutes after the bite but is usually delayed for several hours.

Cytotoxic cobra bites

Bites by the spitting cobras (black-necked – *N. nigricollis,* Moçambique – *N. mossambica,* red spitting cobra – *N. pallida,* etc.) are very common throughout the savanna region of Africa (Warrell et al., 1976a; Tilbury, 1982). They cause local swelling, blistering and necrosis which may be mistaken for the effects of a viper bite (Figs 92.18, 92.19). Necrosis develops as an apparently superficial

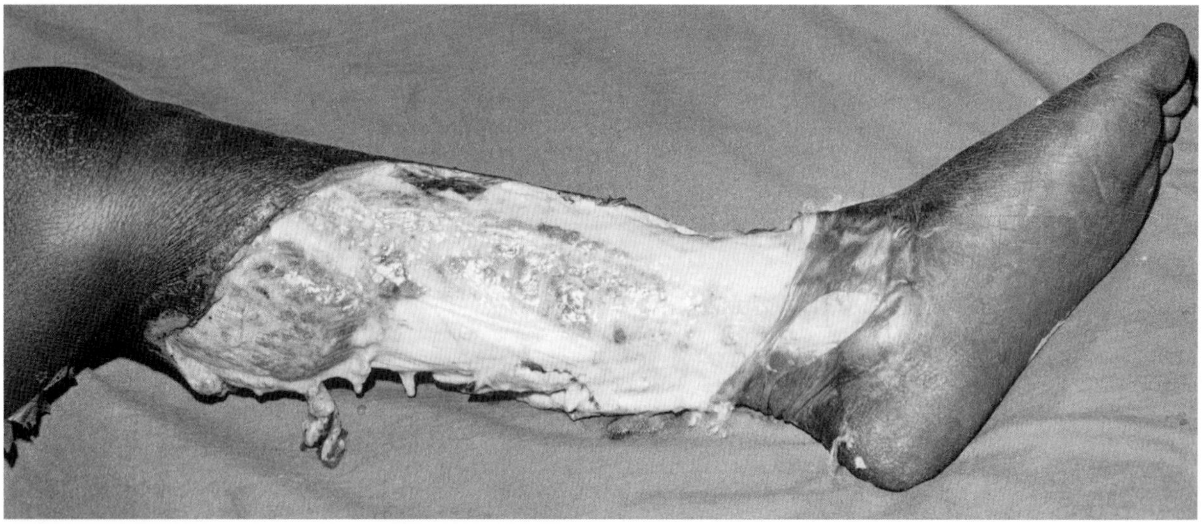

Fig. 92.19. Necrosis of skin and subcutaneous connective tissue following a spitting cobra (*N nigricollis*) bite. Copyright D.A. Warrell.

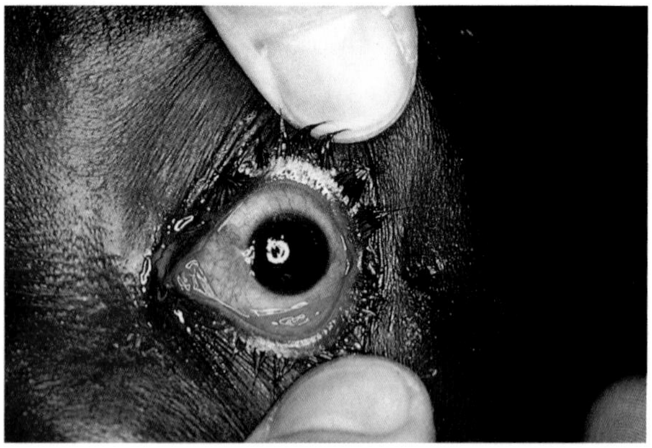

Fig. 92.20. Acute effects of venom spat into the eye by a black-necked spitting cobra (*Naja nigricollis*) (Nigeria). Copyright D.A. Warrell.

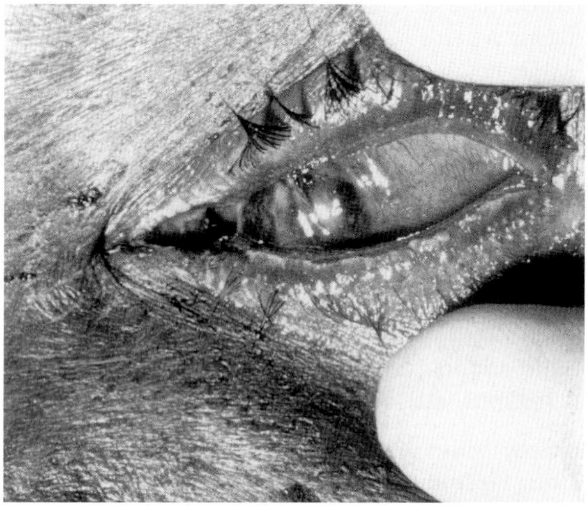

Fig. 92.21. Snake venom ophthalmia complicated by secondary infection. Venom was spat into this patient's eye by a spitting cobra (*N. nigricollis*) but the corneal injury was neglected, panophthalmitis developed and the eye was lost. Copyright D.A. Warrell.

circumscribed area of altered pigmentation, ringed by small blisters and emitting an odour of putrefaction. There are no neurotoxic signs. Venom 'spat' into the eye by these species and by the rinkhals (*Hemachatus haemachatus*) causes intense kerato-conjunctivitis with a risk of corneal ulceration and blindness if secondary infection is not prevented (Fig. 92.20, 92.21) (Warrell & Ormerod, 1976; Pugh et al., 1980).

Diagnosis of snake bite

A distinction must be made between snake bite and envenoming. Fifty per cent or more of bites by venomous snakes may result in trivial or no envenoming, because no venom was injected ('dry bites'). The differential diagnosis includes simple, sharp trauma (such as that incurred by treading on a thorn at night) complicated by cellulitis, insect stings and fish or rodent bites. The diagnosis of envenoming depends on detecting local and systemic signs. In the case of viper bites, the absence of local pain and swelling two hours after the bite suggests that no venom was injected. However, evidence of envenoming may be delayed for many hours in the case of boomslang bites.

- Observe the patient and examine repeatedly for clinical signs of envenoming (Table 92.3) over a period of 24 hours.

Identification of the snake

The victim or witnesses of a snake bite may be able to identify the snake, but, unfortunately, such evidence is frequently misleading. People should not be encouraged to kill the snake as this carries the risk of further bites. However, if, as often happens, the snake has been killed, it is useful clinical evidence.

Classification and characteristics of venomous snakes

Draw a needle from the back of the mouth, forward along the gum of the dead snake's upper jaw. The absence of a pair of enlarged teeth (fangs) suggests that the snake is non-venomous. If the snake was not brought, witnesses of the accident should be asked about the length, thickness, colour, markings, behaviour, habitat and local names of the snake.

Management of snake bite (Warrell, 1995)

First aid

First aid is intended to:

- delay the systemic absorption of venom from the site of the bite
- control distressing or dangerous early symptoms of envenoming
- transport the patient to a place where they can obtain medical care as quickly as possible (see the Box).

> Unfortunately, most of the first-aid methods that are popular, available and affordable in Africa, are:
> - at best – useless and time-wasting
> - at worst – frankly dangerous.

These include local knife/razor cuts at the site of the bite, attempts to suck venom out of the wound, the use of the (black) 'snake stone', tight ligatures or tourniquets, electric shocks (promoted even by some reputable organizations!) and application or ingestion of herbs. Country people often have greater confidence in treatment by traditional healers, 'witch doctors' and snake charmers, than in western medicine.

Recommended first-aid methods

(i) Reassurance: the victim is likely to be very anxious (believing that all snake bites are rapidly fatal). Reassure them.

(ii) Immobilization: encourage the victim to lie still, and immobilize the bitten limb using a splint or sling. Any muscular contraction of the body as a whole, but especially of the bitten part, will increase absorption of venom through the bloodstream and lymphatics.

(iii) Pressure immobilization (neurotoxic cases only!): pressure immobilization (see below and Fig. 92.22) should be used in the case of neurotoxic elapid bites.

(iv) Leave the wound alone! Do not interfere with the bite wound in any way as this may introduce infection, and increase absorption of the venom and of local bleeding.

(v) Do not try to kill the snake: attempts to kill the snake may incur further bites. However, if the snake has already been killed, it should be taken (carefully, not in the bare hands!) to the dispensary or hospital in the hope that it can be identified.

(vi) Transport the patient to hospital/dispensary: snake bite victims should lie as still as possible while they are transported by stretcher, vehicle, boat, bicycle etc to the nearest site of medical care.

Danger of rapid fatal paralysis following neurotoxic elapid bites (mambas, Egyptian, snouted, Cape and forest cobras and sea snake)

Bites by these species may sometimes lead rapidly to life-threatening respiratory paralysis. In an attempt to delay this evolution, pressure-immobilization should be used (Fig. 92.22). A stretchy, crepe or elasticated bandage, approximately 10 cm wide and at least 2 metres long, should be bound firmly around the entire bitten limb, from the fingers or toes up to the arm-pit or groin, incorporating a rigid splint. The bandage is applied as tightly as for a sprained ankle but not so tightly that peripheral pulses are obliterated and the limb becomes painful and ischaemic. Ideally, the bandage should not be released until the patient is under medical care in hospital where facilities for resuscitation and anti-venom treatment are available (see the Box).

> **WARNING!**
> 1. Pressure-immobilization is not recommended after bites by vipers and African spitting cobras as it may increase the local necrotic effects of the venom of these species.
> 2. Tight arterial tourniquets are dangerous and painful and should never be used. They have caused many gangrenous limbs in Africa!

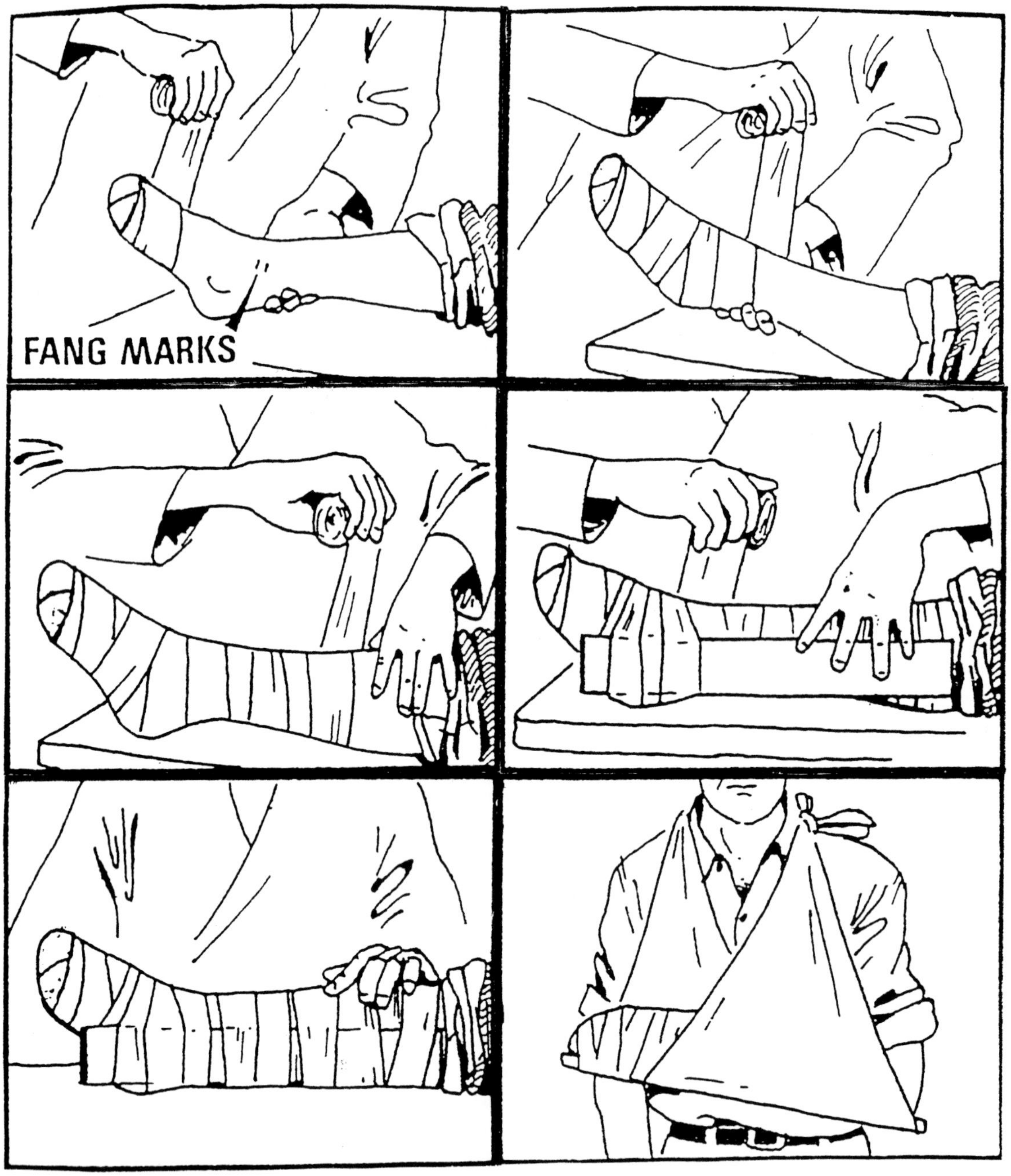

Fig. 92.22. Pressure-immobilization method for neurotoxic elapid bites. By courtesy of Australian Venom Research Unit, Melbourne.

The treatment of snake bite is a medical emergency. When the patient reaches hospital, the following important questions must be answered:

(i) Has the patient been bitten by a snake?
(ii) Is there evidence of envenoming?
(iii) Should the patient be treated with anti-venom? (Table 92.4).

Treatment in dispensary or hospital

(i) *Rapid clinical assessment and resuscitation* may be needed in severely ill patients. Cardiopulmonary resuscitation may be needed. Respiratory failure is treated by endotracheal intubation and assisted ventilation with oxygen if available. Circulatory shock is

Table 92.4. Indications for anti-venom treatment

Systemic envenoming	1. Hypotension, shock, ECG abnormalities 2. Paralysis (ptosis, etc.) 3. Incoagulable blood (20-minute whole blood clotting test) 4. Spontaneous systemic bleeding 5. Black urine
Rapidly evolving local envenoming	1. Progression of local swelling to involve more than half the bitten limb within 24 hours of the bite 2. Bites and swelling of the fingers or toes

treated by urgent intravenous volume replacement and, in some cases, with pressor agents.

(ii) *Detailed clinical assessment and species diagnosis* requires a precise chronological history of the progression of symptoms since the patient was bitten. Three important early questions are:

- 'In what part of your body have you been bitten?' (see how much swelling there is at the site);
- 'At what time were you bitten?' (it may have been too recently for signs of envenoming to have appeared)
- 'Where is the snake that bit you?' (the dead snake is valuable evidence – if it was killed but has not been brought with the patient, send a friend or relation to collect it).

(iii) *Physical examination:*

- Inspect carefully the bitten part for:
  - evidence of fang/tooth marks
  - bruising and persistent bleeding from the punctures
  - extent of local swelling
  - tender and painful enlargement of lymph nodes draining the bite site (an early sign of spreading envenoming).
- Measure blood pressure both lying and sitting up; a postural drop suggests hypovolaemia.
- Record heart rate and rhythm.
- Examine carefully the gums and nose for evidence of spontaneous bleeding, using a torch and tongue depressor.
- Do a full examination: note abdominal tenderness, which may suggest gastrointestinal or retroperitoneal bleeding.

Early neurotoxic envenoming

To detect this:

- Ask the patient to look upwards to reveal evidence of early ptosis.
- Test eye movements and pupillary size and reaction.

If there is evidence of neurotoxicity, examine the patient for:

- early evidence of bulbar paralysis (loss of gag reflex, pooling of secretions in the pharynx);
- respiratory muscle paralysis (paradoxical respiration, reduced peak flow, central cyanosis).

Meningism suggests subarachnoid haemorrhage. Lateralizing motor or sensory signs and dysphonia suggests an intra-cerebral bleed. In pregnant women, check for vaginal bleeding and, in late pregnancy, for fetal distress and threatened abortion.

Species diagnosis

If the dead snake responsible for the bite has been brought, it should be identifiable. Otherwise, the species may be inferred from the circumstances of the bite, the patient's or an onlooker's description of the snake, knowledge of which species occur locally and the pattern of symptoms and signs.

Investigations/laboratory tests (see the Box)

20-minute whole blood clotting test (20WBCT)

This very important bed side test requires a minimum of skill and only one piece of equipment – a new, clean, dry, glass vessel (tube or bottle).

- Place a few ml of freshly sampled venous blood (*without anti-coagulant!*) in the glass vessel.
- Leave upright and undisturbed for 20 minutes at ambient (room) temperature.
- Then tip the vessel once:
- if the blood is still liquid (unclotted) and runs out, the patient has hypofibrinogenaemia (incoagulable blood) as a result of venom-induced consumption coagulopathy.

WARNING!

If the vessel used for the test is not made of ordinary glass, or if it has been used before and cleaned with detergent, it may not activate clotting. If there is any doubt about the result of the test, repeat it, using blood from a healthy person as a control.

Other tests

Haemoglobin concentration/haematocrit will reflect blood loss or haemoconcentration after viper bites.

Table 92.5. Initial dose of anti-venom for patient fulfilling criteria for antivenom treatment (Table 92.4)

Species	Anti-venom	Initial dose
Saw-scaled or carpet vipers (*Echis*)	SAVP Echis monospecific	2 ampoules
Saw-scaled or carpet vipers (*Echis*)	Aventis Pasteur (FAV Afrique polyvalent	4 ampoules
Saw-scaled or carpet vipers (*Echis*)	Therapeutic Antibodies/ MicroPharm EchiTAb monospecific[a]	2 ampoules
Puff adder and other large *Bitis* vipers	SAVP or Aventis Pasteur FAV Afrique polyvalent	8–10 ampoules (within 6 hr to limit local envenoming)
Spitting cobras (*Naja nigricollis* etc)	SAVP or Aventis Pasteur FAV Afrique polyvalent	8–10 ampoules (within 6 hr to limit local envenoming)
Neurotoxic cobras (*Naja haje* etc)	SAVP or Aventis Pasteur FAV Afrique polyvalent	5–10 ampoules (repeat after 30–60 min if neurotoxicity has progressed)
Mambas (*Dendroaspis*)	SAVP or Aventis Pasteur FAV Afrique polyvalent	10 ampoules (repeat after 30–60 min if neurotoxicity has progressed)

Notes:
SAVP = South African Vaccine Producers.
[a] Available only in Nigeria through the Federal Ministry of Health.
[b] Aventis Pasteur FAV Afrique polyvalent anti-venom does not neutralize the venom of the Eastern green mamba (*D. angusticeps*).

Thrombocytopenia may be found in severe cases of envenoming by vipers. Early neutrophil leukocytosis is evidence of systemic envenoming. Raised levels of serum amino-transferases and muscle enzymes, e.g. creatine kinase, may reflect severe local muscle damage. Raised serum creatinine, urea, blood urea nitrogen and potassium indicate acute renal failure. Examine urine by dipsticks for blood/haemoglobin and by microscopy to confirm haematuria.

Anti-venom treatment

Anti-venom is hyperimmune serum from horses or sheep, which have been immunized with the venoms of one or more species of snake. Monovalent (monospecific) anti-venom neutralizes the venom of one species of snake (e.g. SAVP boomslang anti-venom – Table 92.5). Polyvalent (polyspecific) anti-venom neutralizes the venom of several different species of snakes, usually the species identified as being the most important ones in a particular geographical area.

For the following reasons, do not give anti-venoms indiscriminately to all patients who think they have been bitten by snakes:

(i) There is a risk of serious anti-venom reactions which demands an assessment of risk vs. benefit of this treatment.
(ii) Anti-venom may not be necessary, for example, after bites by non-venomous snakes, or even some venomous ones such as night adders – Causus, or if there is no evidence of envenoming.
(iii) No effective anti-venom is available for bites by burrowing asps (Atractaspis) or berg adder (*Bitis atropos*).
(iv) Anti-venom is expensive and scarce. Supplies must be conserved for needy cases.

Indications for anti-venom treatment (Table 92.4)

Anti-venom administration

Anti-venom is most effective when given by the intravenous route. Reconstituted freeze-dried anti-venom or neat liquid anti-venom is given by slow intravenous injection at a rate of not more than 2 ml per minute. Alternatively, these anti-venoms may be diluted in isotonic fluid (5 ml/kg body weight) and infused at a constant rate over a period of 30–60 minutes.

Dose of anti-venom

GIVE CHILDREN
exactly the same dose of anti-venom as adults!

(However, when anti-venom is diluted and given by intravenous infusion, the total volume must not exceed 5 ml per kilogram body weight, to avoid fluid overload.) The initial dose of anti-venom depends on the species of snake involved and the particular anti-venom being used (Table 92.5).

Anti-venoms available for treating envenoming by African snakes (Table 92.6)

Anti-venom reactions

Mechanism

Conjunctival or intradermal test doses of anti-venom do not predict early or late anti-venom reactions and should not be used (Malasit et al., 1986). The reason is that these

Table 92.6. Commercially available anti-venoms for treatment of snake bites in sub-Saharan Africa

(a) *South African Vaccine Producers (Pty) Ltd*
(formerly South African Institute for Medical Research)
Reitfontein, Edenvale, POB 28999, Sandringham 2131, South Africa
Tel ++127118829940; Fax ++27118820812; Telex 4-22211; <savpjhb@global.co.za>
1. *Polyvalent anti-venom* (covers *Bitis* species (except *B atropos*) and *Dendroaspis* species), *Naja* species, *Causus* species, *Pseudohaje goldei*
2. *Echis anti-venom* covers *Echis* species
3. *Boomslang anti-venom* covers *Dispholidus typus* (available by special request only)

(b) *Aventis-Pasteur*
(formerly Pasteur Mérieux Connaught Sérum et Vaccins)
Avenue Général Leclerc, 69007 Lyon, France
Tel ++3372–737707; Fax ++3372-737737
FAV Afrique polyvalent covers *Bitis arietans*, *B. gabonica*, *Echis leucogaster*, *E. ocellatus*, *Dendroaspis* species, *Naja haje*, *N. melanoleuca*, *N. nigricollis*, *Dendroaspis polylepis*, *D. viridis*, *D. jamesoni* (not *D. angusticeps*)

(c) *Vacsera*
51 Wezaret El Zeraa St, Agouza, Giza, Egypt
Polyvalent neutralizes *Naja haje*, *N. nigricollis*, *N. mossambica*, *N. oxiana*, *N. melanoleuca*, *Bitis arietans*, *B gabonica*, *Cerastes cerastes*, *C vipera*, *Walterinnesia aegyptia*, *Vipera palestinae*, *V. ammodytes*, *V. lebetina*, *Pseudocerastes*, *Echis carinatus*, etc.

(d) *Bharat Serum & Vaccines Ltd*
52 Mittal Chambers, Nariman Point, Mumbai 400 021
ASNA Antivenom C (Snake venom antiserum Africa) covers *Bitis arietans*, *N. nigricollis*, *Echis ocellatus*.
Behringwerke Ag (Marburg, Germany) have ceased production of their anti-venoms and have no remaining stocks.

reactions are, in most cases, not the result of IgE medicated type I hypersensitivity to horse/sheep serum but are caused by direct complement activation. Slow, intravenous injection of anti-venom (2 ml/min) is no more likely to provoke an anti-venom reaction than intravenous infusion of anti-venom diluted with 5 ml isotonic fluid per kilogram body weight given over 30 minutes (Malasit et al., 1986).

Early

Most early reactions develop within minutes or up to one hour of starting anti-venom treatment. Symptoms suggest anaphylaxis: itching, urticaria, angio-oedema, vomiting, abdominal pain, diarrhoea, coughing, asthma, fever, tachycardia and hypotensive collapse. They are promptly relieved by adrenaline (epinephrine) (initial dose for adults 0.5 ml of 0.1 per cent solution by intramuscular injection) (see the Box).

Early anti-venom reaction

Relieved promptly by adrenaline (epinephrine)

- Initial dose for adults 0.5 ml of 0.1 per cent solution by intramuscular injection.
- Draw up adrenaline, ready at the bed side, before anti-venom treatment is started.

Late

Late serum sickness reactions may occur a week or more after treatment. Symptoms include fever, urticaria, polyarthralgia, periarticular swellings and lymphadenopathy. The treatment is a short course of anti-histamines or corticosteroid.

Ideally, all patients bitten by snakes should be observed in hospital for at least 24 hours. A flow diagram for hospital management is shown in Fig. 92.23.

Treatment of bites by particular species

Saw-scaled viper and other species causing bleeding and incoagulable blood

The discovery of incoagulable blood (by the 20-minute whole blood clotting test) is the most sensitive indication for anti-venom treatment. Repeat the clotting test 6 hours after the first dose of anti-venom. If the blood is still incoagulable, repeat the initial dose of anti-venom and perform the clotting test again after another 6 hours, and so on (Warrell et al., 1977; Meyer et al., 1997; Chippaux et al., 1998). Once blood coagulability has been restored, repeat the test daily for 3 days in case more venom has been absorbed from the site of the bite. Patients whose circulating volume is seriously depleted by bleeding or extravasation into the swollen limb should be transfused: if this is not possible, a plasma expander, such as Dextran, Haemaccel or Gelofusine, can be used. Prolonged hypotension may lead to acute renal failure.

Puff adder, spitting cobras and other species causing severe local tissue necrosis

There is some evidence that anti-venom, given within a few hours of the bite, may limit the development of tissue necrosis.

- Do not elevate the bitten limb.
- Do not consider fasciotomy until blood coagulability has been restored with anti-venom. In fact, fasciotomy

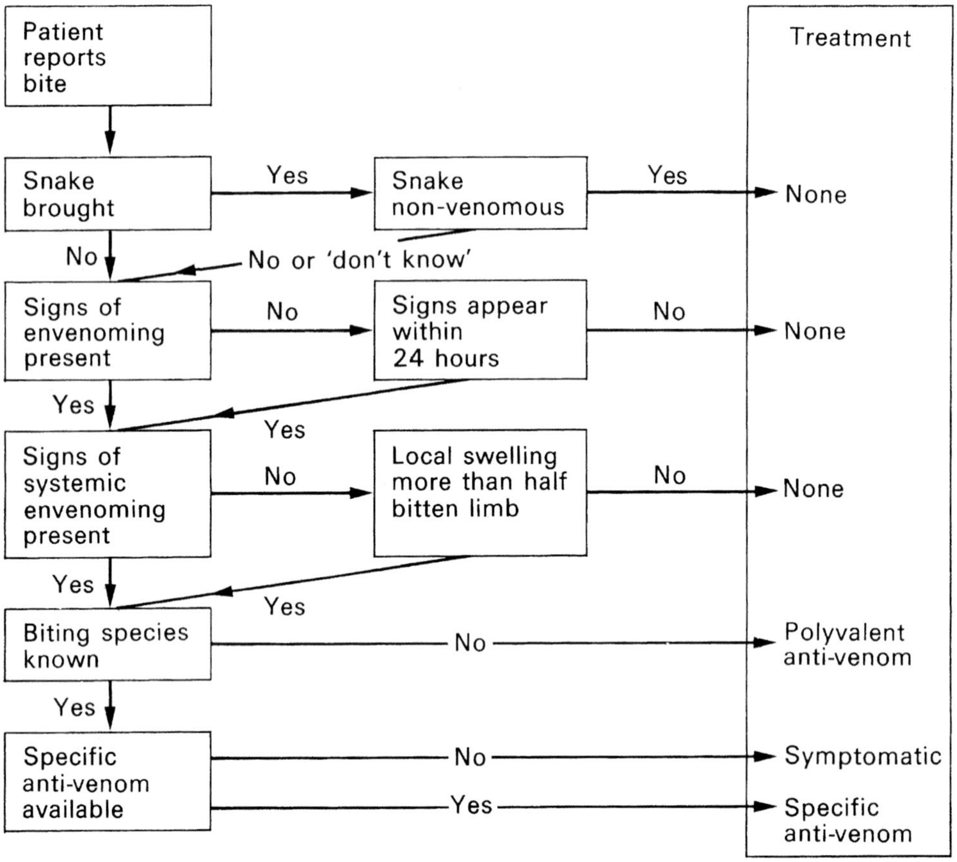

Fig. 92.23. Management of snake bite: algorithm for hospital management.

is rarely, if ever, necessary if anti-venom is given early. The indication for fasciotomy is a dangerously raised intracompartmental pressure (Mars et al., 1991).
- Do not burst bullae but aspirate with a fine needle if they threaten to rupture spontaneously.
- Do not use occlusive dressings, as they conceal important clinical signs and cause maceration of the tissues. Necrotic tissue is discoloured, demarcated, anaesthetic and has a characteristic smell of decomposition.

Once these signs are present, thorough surgical débridement is essential to prevent secondary infection: split skin grafts can be applied immediately. Secondary bacterial infection may complicate snake bites, especially if there is tissue necrosis. Appropriate antibiotics include chloramphenicol, gentamicin (for 24–48 hours only) and metronidazole. Tetanus can complicate snake bite and so appropriate prophylaxis must be used. Hypovolaemic shock is a risk whenever there is massive local swelling.

Neurotoxicity (cobra and mamba bites)

Bulbar and respiratory muscle paralysis present the greatest danger. Once secretions begin to accumulate, the airway must be guarded. Artificial respiration by anaesthetic bag through an endotracheal tube or by mechanical ventilator must be instituted and anti-venom given. The effects of snake neurotoxins are completely reversible with time and so it is well worth maintaining ventilation manually for 12 hours or more, if a mechanical ventilator is not available. In some cases of neurotoxic envenoming, anticholinesterase drugs (edrophonium or neostigmine given with atropine or glycopyrronium) may produce a dramatic improvement in neuromuscular transmission. To test the response, carry out a 'Tensilon test' as is used in suspected myasthenia gravis (p. 1153).

Eye injuries caused by spitting cobras and rinkhals

(Warrell & Ormerod, 1976)

Emergency treatment is the same as for any chemical injury of the eye – generous flushing with large volumes of water or any other bland fluid available (such as milk or even urine). In the hospital or dispensary, examine the surface of the eye after fluorescein staining or by slit lamp to exclude a corneal erosion, and then apply a topical anti-microbial such as chloramphenicol for one week. One per cent epinephrine (adrenaline) drops are said to relieve the pain; otherwise, use conventional analgesics. Topical instillation of anti-venom is not indicated.

Prevention of snake bite

Effective preventive measures may be impracticable for agricultural workers in rural Africa.

1. Snakes never attack without provocation. Avoid snakes: do not attack or disturb them: if you corner one by mistake, keep absolutely still until it has slithered away. Never handle live or dead snakes: many snake charmers and snake collectors have died of snake bite.
2. Avoid walking at night without a light.
3. Avoid walking in undergrowth or in deep sand without boots, socks and long trousers. If you have to walk barefooted, beat the undergrowth in front of you with a stick.
4. Avoid collecting firewood and dislodging rocks, logs, etc. with your bare hands.
5. Never put your hand, or push sticks, into burrows or holes.
6. Avoid climbing trees or rocks which are covered with dense foliage.
7. Avoid swimming in overgrown rivers.
8. Avoid keeping domestic animals, such as chickens, close to the house and keep down the number of rats: these animals attract snakes.

Bites and stings by marine animals
(Halstead, 1988; Williamson et al., 1996)

Fishes

Many species of fish can sting using spines on the gill covers, dorsal fin or tail. The African coast has many venomous fish, but fatal stings are rarely reported.

The most dangerous species is the stonefish (*Synanceja verrucosa*) one of the *Scorpaenidae* which occurs in the Red Sea and round the east and south coasts of Africa. Stings by this species are reported to have killed several fishermen near Pinda, Mozambique: one man who was stung on the toe collapsed and died within an hour (Smith, 1951, 1957).

Clinical features

Fish venoms produce immediate excruciating pain and swelling, which may persist for several days and be complicated by necrosis and secondary infection, particularly if the spine remains in the wound. Systemic effects, such as vomiting, diarrhoea, sweating, bradycardia and hypotension, suggest parasympathetic stimulation. Cardiac arrhythmias, muscle spasms, flaccid paralysis, respiratory distress and convulsions may also occur.

Treatment

The venomous spine, which may be barbed, should be removed as soon as possible and the stung limb immersed in uncomfortably hot, but not scalding, water (not more than 45 °C). Alternatively, 1 per cent lignocaine may be injected, for example as a ring block if a finger has been stung. Specific anti-venom for stonefish stings is difficult to obtain in Africa. In severe cases cardiorespiratory resuscitation may be required. Atropine (0.6 mg by subcutaneous injection) may be tried in patients with signs of cholinergic activity such as bradycardia. Antimicrobials may be required to prevent secondary infection.

Cnidarians (jellyfish) (formerly known as Coelenterates)

Various Portuguese Men-o'-War, hydroids, sea wasps, sea nettles, sea blubbers and sea anemones inhabit African coastal waters. Their tentacles contain millions of stinging nematocysts. Fatal cases have been reported outside the African region (Australia, Asia).

Venoms cause local irritation, inflammation and urticaria. Contact with the tentacles produces lines of painful irritant weals. In severe cases there are systemic effects including rigors, vomiting and diarrhoea, hypotensive collapse, muscle paralysis and convulsions. First-aid treatment involves immediate removal of fragments of tentacles still attached to the skin after coating them with dry sand. Undischarged nematocysts must be inactivated by applying a slurry of baking powder. Avoid using alcoholic solutions, such as sun-tan lotion, which will fire off more nematocysts. NO specific treatment is available. Cardiorespiratory resuscitation may be required for serious cases in whom the application of tourniquets, proximal to the stung area, may produce a useful delay in the absorption of venom.

Echinoderms (sea urchins)

Venomous spines and grapples are used for stinging. They cause local pain and swelling and rarely systemic effects such as cardiac arrhythmias and respiratory paralysis which may be fatal. The spines and grapples (pedicellariae) should be removed from the wound, after softening the skin with 2 per cent salicylic acid ointment. There is no specific treatment.

Bites and stings by arthropods

Bees, wasps and hornets: (Hymenoptera)

The venoms of these insects are combinations of amines, kinins, specific peptides (such as apamin from bee venom), and enzymes such as phospholipase A_2 and hyaluronidase. Stings usually produce only local effects – pain, redness and swelling – due to histamine, 5-hydroxytryptamine and other substances, which are introduced or released. Occasionally, people are attacked by swarms of bees. Several hundred stings may result in dangerous envenoming. A man in Central Africa survived more than 2243 stings, when features of histamine overdose (vasodilatation, hypotension, diarrhoea, headache, coma) may be seen, with haemolysis, skeletal muscle breakdown, myoglobinuria and renal failure.

In contrast, a single sting may cause urticaria, angioneurotic oedema, asthma, hypotensive collapse and death in a patient who has become hypersensitive to the venom through previous stings. This is especially common in bee-keepers. This IgE-mediated, Type I hypersensitivity is confirmed by skin testing with very dilute venom solutions or by radioallergosorbent test (RAST).

Treatment

- Scrape out immediately bee stings embedded in the skin with a finger-nail or a blade.
- Give aspirin – it is an effective analgesic.
- Treat insect sting anaphylaxis with epinephrine (adrenaline). The adult dose is 0.5 ml of a 0.1 per cent solution by intramuscular injection.
- Patients known to be hypersensitive should carry self-injectable epinephrine (e.g. EpiPen, Anapen).

Ants, beetles and caterpillars

Various African species of ants, cantharides or blister beetles (Meloidae) or 'Spanish fly' and some hairy caterpillars (larvae of Lepidoptera) can cause local pain, inflammation, urticaria or blistering on contact (for example, 'Nairobi eye').

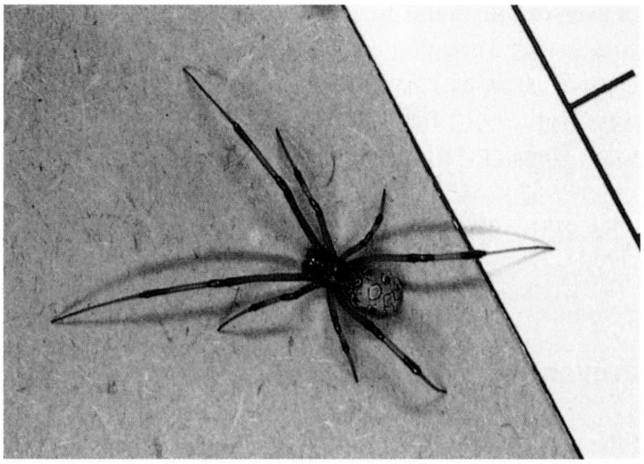

Fig. 92.24. Brown widow spider (*Latrodectus geometricus*) (South Africa). 1 cm scale. Copyright D.A. Warrell.

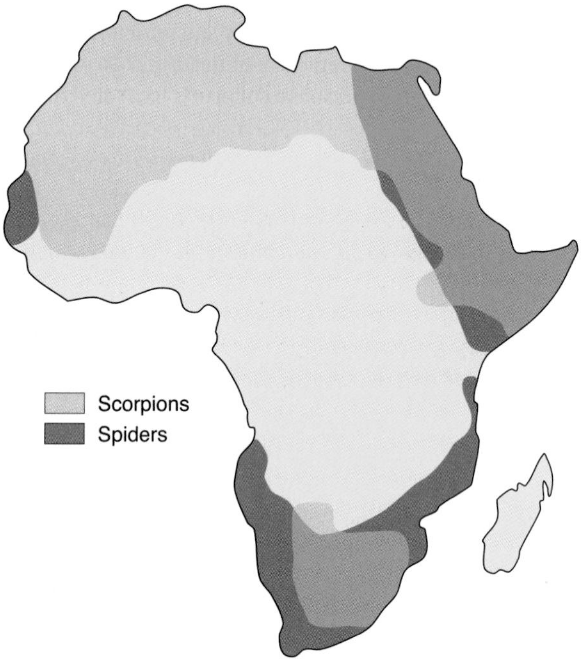

Fig. 92.25. Distribution of dangerous spiders and scorpions in Africa.

Spiders

Representatives of the genera *Latrodectus* (black/brown widow spiders) (Fig. 92.24), *Loxosceles* (brown recluse spiders), and *Harpactirella* (tarantulas) are found in Africa (Fig. 92.25).

Spider bites may prove fatal especially in children. The

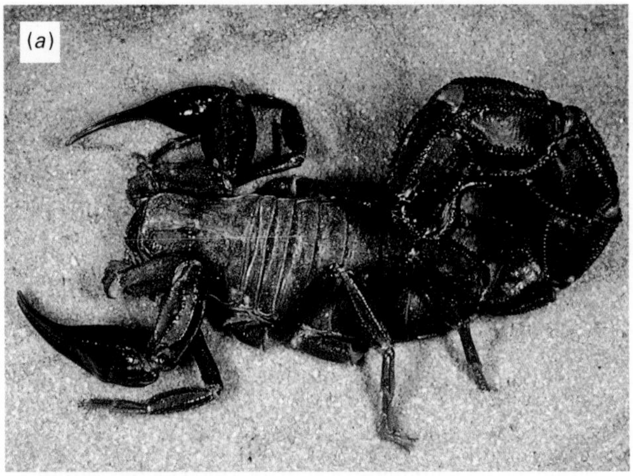

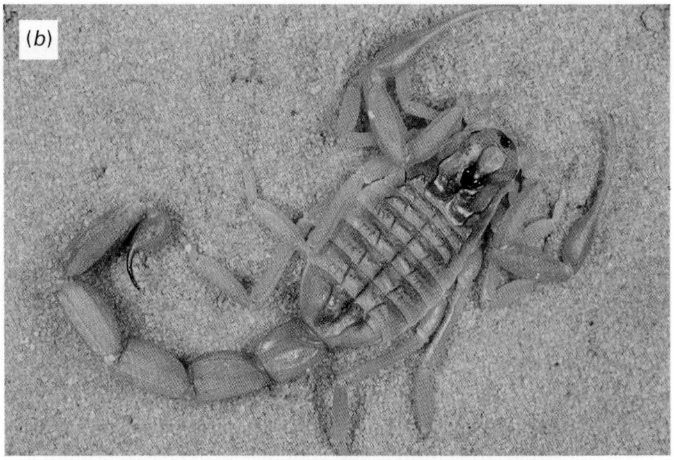

Fig. 92.26. Three dangerous African scorpions.
(*a*) *Androctonus crassicauda*
(*b*) *Leiurus quinquestriatus*
(*c*) *Parabuthus granulatus*
Compare the slender pincers with those of
(*d*) *Pandinus imperator.*
Copyright D.A. Warrell.

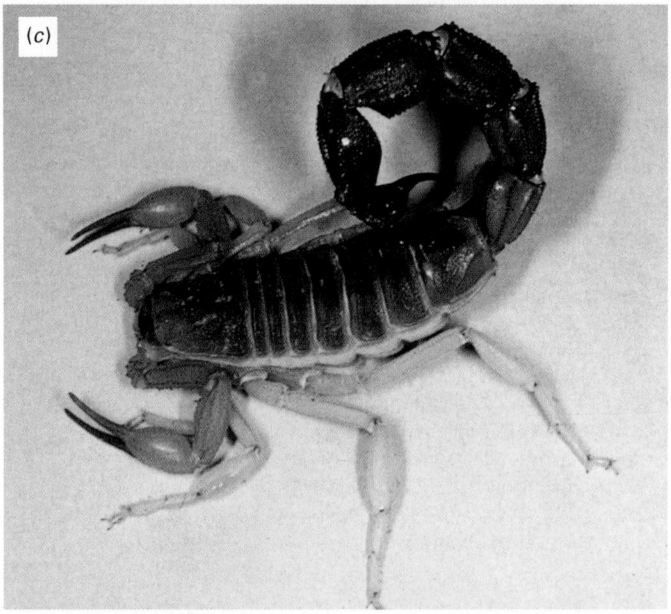

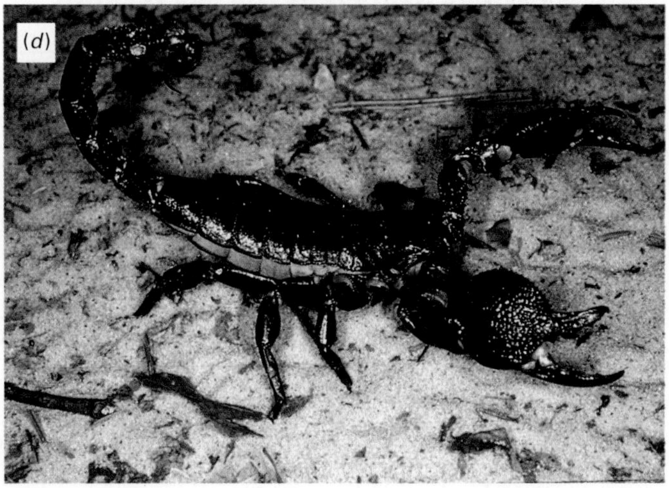

most dangerous genus is Latrodectus. The venom has neurotoxic properties and causes generalized cramp-like pains, weakness, sweating, salivation, fever, nausea, vomiting and convulsions. The bites of other species may cause local necrosis. Bites usually occur when the victim lies on a spider which has crept into their bed.

Treatment

Specific anti-venom for Latrodectus bite is available in South Africa. Consider its use in patients with neurotoxic symptoms, especially in small children.

Scorpions

Dangerous genera occur in parts of Africa (Fig. 92.25) and there are some fatalities. The case-fatality approaches 20 per cent when the victims are children, but most stings in Africa are by non-dangerous species which merely cause severe local pain and minor swelling without systemic effects. Dangerous species have relatively fine pincers (Fig. 92.26).

In addition to causing severe local pain and slight swelling, the venom of dangerous species contains powerful neurotoxins which act on ion channels and release acetylcholine and catecholamines, causing symptoms of autonomic nervous system overactivity (tachycardia, sweating, salivation, gooseflesh, shock). Symptoms may improve after a few hours and then relapse.

Treatment

Severe local pain is usually the main symptom. This can be relieved by injecting 1–2 per cent lignocaine locally (e.g. with a ring block in the case of stung digits). Systemic symptoms indicate the need for specific anti-venom which is manufactured in Algeria (for *Androctonus*), Johannesburg (for *Parabuthus*) and Cairo (for *Leiurus*).

Centipedes

Human deaths have not been reliably documented. The usual result of a sting by its modified front legs is local pain, swelling, inflammation and lymphangitis. Rarely there are generalized effects such as vomiting, headache, cardiac arrhythmias and convulsions. Local treatment is the same as for scorpion stings. No anti-venom is available.

Millipede burns

Some African millipedes (*Spirobelus* etc.) produce irritant defensive secretions which can cause blistering of skin and mucosae, which might be serious if the eye were involved. These have been reported from Nigeria, Tanzania and other parts of Africa. Treatment is the same as for other irritant chemicals: liberal washing with water and analgesics.

Ticks

Many species of soft and hard ticks can inject a toxin which causes ascending flaccid paralysis. Symptoms usually subside after the tick has been detached.

Poisoning from eating fish and shellfish (Halstead, 1988; Williamson et al., 1996)

Eating various species of fish and bivalve molluscs from African waters can cause dramatic symptoms within a few minutes or hours. There are two main syndromes.

Gastrointestinal/neurotoxic syndrome

After acute gastroenteritic symptoms, paraesthesiae spread from the mouth and face and a progressive paralysis may involve the respiratory muscles and so cause death. This syndrome can follow ingestion of molluscs contaminated with toxic protozoa (dinoflagellates, e.g. *Gonyaulax*) and puffer fish containing *tetrodotoxin*. Fish such as groupers, barracudas and Moray eels may contain *ciguatoxin*. After the initial gastrointestinal symptoms, there are persistent paraesthesiae ('electric shock' feelings, reversed hot/cold sensation), rashes and myalgias. Treatment involves elimination of toxic gut contents by promoting vomiting and purging. Assisted ventilation may be required until the respiratory paralysis has worn off. Infusion of mannitol is recommended for ciguatera poisoning.

Histamine-like syndrome (scombrotoxic poisoning)

Decomposition of the flesh of scrombroid fish (tuna, mackerel, etc) by bacteria such as *Morganella morgani* produces a histamine-like activity which causes vasodilatation, headache, urticaria, pruritus, asthma, burning of the mouth and throat, abdominal colic and hypotensive collapse. Treatment includes emetics, purges, antihistamines and bronchodilators.

References

Blaylock RS, Lichtman AR, Potgieter PD et al. (1985). Clinical manifestations of Cape cobra (*Naja nivea*) bites. Two cases. *S Afr Med J*; **68**: 342–344.

Carme B, Trape JF & Lubaki Kumba L. (1986). Les morsures de serpent au Congo. Estimation de la morbidité à Brazzaville et en zone rurale de la région du Pool et du Mayombe. *Ann Soc Belge Méd Trop*; **66**: 183–189.

Chippaux J-P & Goyffon M (eds). (2002). Les envenimations et leur traitement en Afrique. *Bull Soc Path Exot*, **95**: 131–132.

Chippaux J-P, Lang J, Amadi Eddine S et al. (1998). Clinical safety of a polyvalent $F(ab')_2$ equine antivenom in 223 African snake envenomations: a field trial in Cameroon. *Trans Roy Soc Trop Med Hyg*; **92**: 657–662.

Halstead BW. (1988). *Poisonous and Venomous Marine Animals of the World*, 2nd revised edn. Princeton, New Jersey: Darwin Press.

Kasilo OMJ, Nhachi CFB. (1993). A retrospective study of poisoning due to snake venom in Zimbabwe. *Hum Exp Toxicol*; **12**: 15–18.

Malasit P, Warrell DA, Chanthavanich P. et al. (1988). Prediction, prevention and mechanism of early (anaphylactic) antivenom reactions in victims of snake bites. *Br Med J*; **292**: 17–20.

Manent P, Mouchon D, Nicholas P. (1992). Envenimation par *Echis carinatus* en Afrique: etude clinique et evolution indication du serum antivenimeux. *Med Trop*; **52**: 415–421.

Mars M, Hadley GP, Aitchison JM. (1991). Direct intracompartmental pressure measurement in the management of snake bites in children. *S Afr Med J*; **80**: 227–228.

Meyer WP, Habib AG, Onayade AA. et al. (1997). First clinical experiences with a new ovine FAB *Echis ocellatus* snake bite antivenom in Nigeria: randomized comparative trial with Institute Pasteur serum (IPSER) Africa antivenom. *Am J Trop Med Hyg*; **56**: 291–300.

Muguti GI, Maramba A, Washaya CT. et al. (1994). Snake bites in Zimbabwe: a clinical study with emphasis on the need for antivenom. *Centr Afr J Med*; **40**: 83–88.

Nhachi CFB, Kasilo OMJ. (1994). Snake poisoning in rural Zimbabwe – a prospective study. *J Appl Toxicol*; **14**: 191–193.

Pugh RNH. (1984). Venomous snakes of Malawi. *J Med Assoc Malawi*; **17**: 30–33.

Pugh RNH, Theakston RDG, Reid HA, Bhar IS. (1980). Epidemiology of human encounters with the spitting cobra, *Naja nigricollis*, in the Malumfashi area of northern Nigeria. *Ann Trop Med Parasitol*; **74**: 523–530.

Seignot P, Ducourau JP, Ducrot P, Angel G, Roussel L, Aubert M. (1992). Envenimation mortelle par une morsure de vipère africaine (*Echis carinatus*). *Ann Fr Anesth Réanim*; **11**: 105–110.

Smith JLB. (1951). A case of poisoning by the stonefish, *Synanceja verrucosa*. *Copeia*; **3**: 207–210.

Smith JLB. (1957). Two rapid fatalities from stonefish stabs. *Copeia*; **3**: 249.

Snow RW, Bronzan R, Roques T, Nyamawi C, Murphy S, Marsh K. (1994). The prevalence and morbidity of snake bite and treatment-seeking behaviour among a rural Kenyan population. *Ann Trop Med Parasitol*; **88**: 665–671.

Spawls S, Branch B. (1995). The dangerous snakes of Africa. *Natural History: Species Directory: Venoms and Snake Bite.* London: Blandford.

Tahzib F. (1984). Camel injuries. *Trop Doctor*; **14**: 187–188.

Tilbury CR. (1982). Observations on the bite of the Mozambique spitting cobra (*Naja mossambica mossambica*). *S Afr Med J*; **61**: 308–313.

Trape J-F, Pison G, Guyavarch E, Mane Y. (2001). High mortality from snakebite in South-Eastern Senegal. *Trans Roy Soc Trop Med Hyg*; **95**: 420–423.

Warrell DA. (1995). Clinical toxicology of snake bite in Africa and the Middle East/Arabian Peninsula. In *Handbook of Clinical Toxicology of Animal Venoms and Poisons*, ed. Meier J, White J. CRC Press, Boca Raton: 443–492.

Warrell DA, Arnett C. (1976). The importance of bites by the saw-scaled or carpet viper (*Echis carinatus*). Epidemiological studies in Nigeria and a review of the world literature. *Acta Tropica (Basel)*; **33**: 307–341.

Warrell DA, Ormerod LD. (1976). Snake venom ophthalmia and blindness caused by the spitting cobra (*Naja nigricollis*) in Nigeria. *Am J Trop Med Hyg*; **25**: 525–529.

Warrell DA, Ormerod LD, Davidson N McD. (1975). Bites by the puff adder (*Bitis arietans*) in Nigeria and value of antivenom. *Br Med J*; **4**: 697–700.

Warrell DA, Barnes HJ, Piburn MF (1976a). Neurotoxic effects of bites by the Egyptian cobra (*Naja haje*) in Nigeria. *Trans Roy Soc Trop Med Hyg*; **70**: 78–79.

Warrell DA, Greenwood BM, Davidson N McD, Ormerod LD, Prentice CR. (1976b). Necrosis, haemorrhage and complement depletion following bites by the spitting cobra (*Naja nigricollis*). *Quarterly J Med*; **45**: 1–22.

Warrell DA, Ormerod LD, Davidson N McD. (1976c). Bites by the night adder (*Causus maculatus*) and burrowing vipers (genus *Atractaspis*) in Nigeria. *Am J Trop Med Hyg*; **25**: 517–524.

Warrell DA, Davidson N McD, Greenwood BM. (1977). Poisoning by bites of the saw-scaled or carpet viper (*Echis carinatus*) in Nigeria. *Quart J Med*; **46**: 33–62.

Wilkinson D. (1994). Retrospective analysis of snake bite at a rural hospital in Zululand. *S Afr Med J*; **84**: 844–847.

Williamson JA, Fenner RJ, Burnett JW, Rifkin JF. (1996). *Venomous and Poisonous Marine Animals: A Medical and Biological Handbook*. Sydney: University NSW Press.

Zaltzman M, Rumbak M, Rabie M, Zuli S. (1984). Neurotoxicity due to the bite of the shield-nosed snake (*Aspidelaps scutatus*). A case report. *S Afr Med J*; **66**: 111–112.

93 The skin

Introduction

Although skin diseases do not usually threaten life, their unforgiving itching can cause misery and their appearance may be a social stigma (Etemesi, 2001). In sub-Saharan Africa skin diseases are dominated by bacterial and fungal infection and their clinical expression is often modified by HIV-induced immuno-suppression.

Skin diseases constitute up to 15 per cent of all attendances in peripheral health clinics.

Dermatology of the pigmented skin is a distinctive dermatology. Erythema for instance can barely be seen and hypo- and hyper-pigmentation dominate the picture.

Epidemiology

The burden of skin diseases in Africa (Gibbs, 1996; Satimia et al., 1998; Shibeshi, 2000; Smeller & Dzikus, 2001) is summed up by Grossmann (1999) at the Regional Dermatology Training Centre, Moshi, Tanzania, as follows:

- About 30 per cent of disease in urban areas is skin disease; the incidence is even higher in rural areas (industrialized countries ~ 10 per cent).
- Skin diseases are among the top five causes of morbidity.
- There are considerable differences in the pattern of skin diseases between urban and rural areas.
- The 70–80 per cent of the population living in rural areas are, together with the urban poor, at the highest risk of contracting infective-parasitic diseases due to poor environmental conditions, which are the key determinants in the pathogenesis of skin diseases in Africa.
- More than 60 per cent of skin diseases are attributable to infectious-parasitic disorders (industrialized countries 10 per cent).
- Communicable diseases, like scabies, pyoderma and mycotic infections, are common universally and cause a massive morbidity. Onchocerciasis, leishmaniasis and guinea worm are important in some regions.
- Most skin diseases are not only preventable, but are also curable with simple, cheap and effective medication.
- Sixty to ninety per cent of all dermatoses identified in rural areas are caused by only ten conditions.
- More than 80 per cent of the prevailing skin conditions do not need highly specialized expertise for care; an intermediate cadre of health-workers will be able to handle most of the cases.
- Around 90 per cent of skin diseases are first attended to by traditional healers or auxiliary health workers with very little or no training in dermatology.
- Difficult access to dermatological care in remote and under-privileged areas leads to late diagnosis and delayed treatment, which result in disability and incapacity in diseases like leprosy, lymphatic filariasis and others.

Geography and climate

Weather, geology, geography and wildlife influence the type and the severity of skin diseases. Fungal, bacterial and parasitic skin diseases flourish in a hot and humid climate (Kristense, 1991) and insect vectors transmit diseases like leishmaniasis and onchocerciasis. In the savannah (the veldt of South Africa), deep mycoses occur, together with infections like tropical ulcer, veldt sores and cutaneous diphtheria, while Buruli ulcer is found near swamps and podoconiosis (Price's disease) on red volcanic soil (Canizaris, 1982).

Skin diseases like atopic dermatitis and contact dermatitis are more common among town dwellers than among the rural population (Naafs et al., 1986),

Genetics

Racial characteristics (Gowkrodger, 1998) are difficult to dissociate from socioeconomic factors, but it is obvious that whites and albinos are more at risk than blacks of developing sun damage like actinic keratoses, basal and squamous cell carcinomas, whereas blacks are more prone to keloids, ingrowing hairs (pseudofolliculitis barbae) and nuchal acne Keloidalis. In West Africa psoriasis seems less prevalent than in eastern Africa, while in southern Africa and the horn of Africa there is more porphyria cutanea tarda than elsewhere in Africa.

Socioeconomic status

Scabies and the body louse are prevalent in institutions and among the crowded poor (Kristense, 1991). Lepromatous leprosy is relatively more prevalent among the affluent, whereas tuberculoid leprosy occurs more commonly among peasants and the urban poor. Atopic eczema, acne, rosacea, perioral dermatitis and other steroid- or cosmetic-induced dermatitides are more common in the affluent. Skin-lightening creams are a significant cause of disease in urban women (del Giudice & Yves, 2002; Doe et al., 2001) but all social groups spend precious money on ineffective treatment (Figueroa et al., 1998).

Occupations

Farmers and pastoralists risk anthrax, animal mycoses, leishmaniasis and filariasis. Builders are at risk of contact dermatitis to chromate. Cheap rubber footwear can lead to contact dermatitis from the softeners and accelerators used. Barefoot people may be prone to jiggers and fissuring hyperkeratotic feet, whereas people with closed shoes may develop athlete's foot, pitted keratolysis and mycosis pedis.

The HIV epidemic

The prevalence and expression of many infective and non-infective skin diseases is different in HIV-positive patients who may also develop drug eruptions, erythema multiforme and Stevens Johnson syndrome. HIV has added significantly to the burden of skin disease (Mayanja et al., 1999).

Functions of the skin

The skin protects against physical damage and ultraviolet radiation, provides defence against biological invasion, regulates temperature and maintains a proper 'milieu intérieur' and receives sensory stimuli and transmits signals.

The skin produces vitamin D, endorphins and neuroendocrinological mediators and has its own normal 'skin flora', which protects against pathogenic micro-organisms and helps to maintain an effective immune system.

In addition to the specialized cells of the tissues, there are fibroblasts and immune-competent cells like lymphocytes and macrophages, together with mast cells, eosinophils and granulocytes. The specialized cells and immune-competent cells in the epidermis form the skin immune system (SIS), which is responsible for the immune reactivity in the skin and thus for most of the clinical aspects of skin diseases (Bos & Kapsenberg, 1993).

Black versus 'white' skin

Dermatology of the pigmented skin is decidedly different from that of white Caucasian skin. The dermatoses present in a different way. Erythema, redness as a sign of inflammation is difficult to see in a pigmented skin.

Erythema

Because erythema is frequently not visible in a black skin, palpation is important in order to appreciate the other signs of inflammation, calor (warmth), tumor (swelling) and dolor (pain, tenderness).

Cohesion

Lichenification, or thickness, is often particularly striking in black patients who scratch.

Pigmentation

Pigment changes (de-, hypo- and hyper-pigmentation) dominate the clinical picture in the dermatology of the pigmented skin.

Depigmentation

Complete loss of pigment occurs after conditions producing scarring, for example some forms of cutaneous lupus erythematosus, and when melanocyte disappears, for example, in autoimmune diseases such as vitiligo.

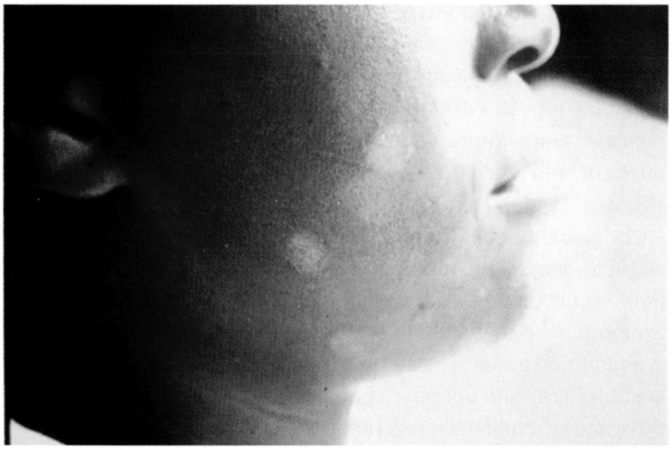

Fig. 93.1. Pityriasis alba – note the depigmentation.

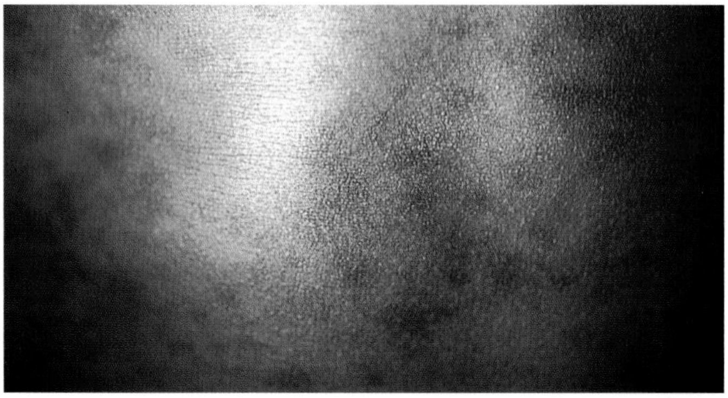

Fig. 93.2. Post-inflammatory hyperpigmentation after secondary syphilis.

Hypo-pigmentation

Reduction in pigment occurs frequently after inflammation, for example in pityriasis alba (an eczema variant) (Fig. 93.1).

It can also occur following suppression of pigment synthesis, for example, in pityriasis versicolor, and in tuberculoid leprosy when synthesis may be inhibited by autoimmunity. Lathogenic hypo-pigmentation following steroids occurs by two mechanisms: the steroid suppresses pigment formation and the epidermis becomes thinner.

Hyper-pigmentation

Hyper-pigmentation can be seen when the epidermis is thickened following scratching which produces thickening or lichenification in eczema, or psoriasis. Pigment incontinence is a third important cause. In many inflammatory conditions, the basement membrane loses its integrity and pigment leaks into the deep dermis where it is phagocytized by phagocytes and melanophages. Such pigment appears to be blue-black and disappears only slowly (Fig. 93.2).

Although dermatoses appear different in different races, their distribution and localization are the same which may be helpful in establishing a diagnosis.

Hair

Hair differs in distribution, colour and form among different races and sub-races. The hair of Afro-Caribbeans is almost always black and thick, and grows in a spiral pattern producing a tightly coiled shaft.

Curly stiff hairs may cause problems, especially after shaving, when the hairs curl inside the skin and cause inflammation as is seen in pseudofolliculitis barbae and nuchal acne keloidalis.

History taking and examination

A careful history is essential. But it is also important to know which diseases are prevalent in the area the patient comes from.

- Ask the patient where and how the disease started, its duration, whether it comes and goes, whether exacerbations are related to seasons, specific work, staying in a specific area, or to stress, and whether or not others in the family or in the surroundings have a similar disease.
- Ask whether the skin itches, is painful or causes any other problems/symptoms. In some African languages a great array of terminology for sensation is used. Good translation is therefore essential; be aware that English is a poor language for a description of sensation.
- Ask about previous treatment – topical, oral or parenteral, orthodox and traditional medications.
- Examine the skin in good light. First, observe the patient from some distance and note the distribution of the lesions, then inspect the lesions close-up (20–30 cm).
- Use a magnifying glass for specific lesions.
- Palpate the lesions for their consistency, signs of inflammation and extent.
- Do not forget to inspect the scalp, hair and hairline, behind the ears, the axillae, groins and submammary region, the feet, between the toes and the mucosae of mouth and genitals.
- Record any signs of systemic diseases.

Distribution of the lesions

Face, trunk, limbs; flexor or extensor side, sun exposed areas.

Is the distribution circumscribed, regional, segmental, generalized or universal?

Are the lesions diffuse, discrete, confluent, follicular.

Are they symmetrical?

The size and shape of individual lesions

Guttate (droplet) 5–10 mm, nummular (coin-like) 2–3 cm or plaques more than 3–5 cm.Round, oval, polygonal (many corners), linear, annular (ring), arciform (bow), circinate (interrupted bow), concentric, the presence of satellite lesions.

Terminology

There are accepted terms to describe the individual lesions:

Macule:	a circumscribed area with colour changes; the lesion is flat.
Papule:	a small raised lesion, less than 1 cm in diameter.
Nodule:	a raised lesion, 1–2 cm in diameter.
Plaque:	a raised lesion, 3 cm or more in diameter.
Weal:	a raised lesion due to dermal or hypodermal oedema (urticaria).
Vesicle:	a small 'blister' filled with fluid.
Bulla:	a blister of more than 5 mm.
Pustule:	a small skin lesion filled with pus.
Ulcer:	a break in the continuity of the epidermis without a clear sign of healing.
Scaling:	excess of keratin that comes off in smaller or larger flakes.
Crusts:	dried serum and cells.
Excoriations:	scratch marks with breaking of the epidermis.
Erythroderma:	more than 90 per cent of body surface red and involved with disease.
Atrophy:	thinning of the skin with loss of skin markings, lines, hairs, etc.
Lichenification:	thickening of the skin, the marking becomes coarse.
Sclerosis:	diffuse or localized induration of dermis and sub-cutis.

ECZEMATOUS DERMATITIS

An eczematous dermatitis means inflammation of the skin. There are many problems which produce skin inflammation, so that eczema accounts for about 25 per cent of childhood skin disease. It occurs when there are small accumulations of fluid in the epidermis (spongiotic dermatitis). This leads to areas with papules and vesicles, excoriations and/or lichenification. There may be scaling and/or crusts. The areas may be wet (Van Hees & Naafs, 2001).

Not all the signs need to be present at the same time. In pigmented skin, because epidermal cells are strongly bound together, the vesicles may not break but look like papules because the fluid content is not visible due to the overlaying pigment. The area may show lichenification. In lighter skin erythema can be seen, but in dark skin this is hardly noticeable, and hyper- and hypo-pigmentation dominate the picture.

The appearance of the eczema depends on whether it is acute, sub-acute or chronic.

- In acute dermatitis the lesions are oozing and wet and show crusts with signs of inflammation. In sub-acute eczema, the lesions become drier and scaly and are frequently hyper- or hypo-pigmented. In chronic dermatitis there is lichenification with some excoriations and cracks/fissures, and there may also be scaling. Lesions usually are hyper-pigmented.

Atopic dermatitis (constitutional eczema)

This dermatitis runs in families with a so-called atopic constitution, a genetic pre-disposition for hypersensitivity reactions such as asthma, hay fever and atopic eczema.

Clinical features

The eczema is easily recognized by its predilection for the flexor sides of knees, elbows, wrists and neck. The eczema comes and goes and can be triggered or worsened by irritants such as detergents (soaps), by allergies or infections, heat and sweating and hairy garments. The lesions itch (Stander & Steinhof, 2002), so scratching is a major feature. Emotional stress may be a trigger (Naafs, 1993).

In general, an atopic person has a dry itchy skin. The disease usually starts in the face during the first months after birth; later it becomes more prevalent elsewhere. Only after 1–2 years does it go to the typical predilection places. In some patients, the whole body is involved and an exfoliative (erythrodermic) dermatitis is seen.

Pompholyx

The hands and feet are affected, alone or together. Sometimes large vesicles, blisters, can be seen. It can also be triggered by contact with allergens or is due to a so-called 'id' reaction (allergic reaction distant from the cause) provoked by an infection elsewhere, notably fungal infections of the feet, or streptococcus in the nose.

The problem in Africa

In the past, atopic eczema was not highly prevalent in Africa, except in some urban centres, probably on account of the pattern of life. In a survey in Zimbabwe in 1985 atopic eczema was hardly seen in the rural areas, though its mild form, pityriasis alba, was highly prevalent. In town clinics, however, atopic dermatitis was the most prevalent condition encountered (Naafs et al., 1986).

In children, during acute exacerbations, the skin is often colonized or super-infected (impetigo) by yeasts and bacteria, especially by staphylococci and sometimes by streptococci. Some authors think these agents act as a 'super-antigen' driving the immunological inflammation that produces eczema (Brockow et al., 1999).

Treatment and prevention

- Avoid soaps and detergents when washing the skin.
- Wash with tepid water and then oil the skin while it is still wet. Coconut oil or other vegetable oil or emulsifying ointment (BP) will do. Rinse clothes well when washing them: retained soap in clothes irritates the skin and provokes itching and consequently eczema.
- Although vaseline is a good moisturiser, in some patients it may clog the skin and worsen infection.

Treatment

Flares of atopic eczema can be treated with mild steroids (hydrocortisone 1 per cent or triamcinolone, 0.05–0.1%). Ointments tend to work better than creams in dry skin conditions. If weaker steroids are not available then stronger steroids, like betamethasone, can be diluted with vegetable oil just before use. Apply the ointment twice daily; when the condition improves, use a weaker steroid; later, once cleared, the steroids can be stopped and emollients (oils, ointments) can be used alone, twice daily to moisturise the skin. If the condition gets worse, start steroids again.

If the skin is infected, wash it first with tepid water containing potassium permanganate (1: 4000). Betadine jodium shampoo can be used as antiseptic soap, and gentian violet as a local antiseptic and anti-irritative (Brockow et al., 1999).

- Do not scrub the skin as this is too aggressive. In severe cases, alternate the steroid ointments with gentian violet.
- Only use antibiotics if there is significant secondary infection, for example, widespread golden crusting, or systemic upset such as temperature.

Coal tar is also useful, especially for lichenified eczema. A 5–10 per cent coal tar solution in ointment is usually used, with or without a mild steroid. When a coal tar solution is not available, tar (asphalt) can be heated and mixed with an ointment; 2–3 per cent is sufficient. Apply tar preparations at night.

When itching is severe, sedating antihistamines such as promethazine and hydroxyzine may help with sleep. Modern non-sedating antihistamines are less effective, because the itch is not histamine-related. UV therapy may sometimes be of help, especially the new modality UVA1, possibly available in specialized centres.

Effect of HIV

HIV infection can simulate or aggravate atopic eczema. It leads to a dry and itchy skin and changes the immunoreactivity. Treat as normal atopic dermatitis but often secondary infection and colonization of the skin demand antiseptics and antibiotics. Simple inexpensive treatments can radically improve the patient's comfort.

Pityriasis alba (Fig. 93.1) mildly scaling guttate or nummular hypopigmented macules, most frequently in the face, does not need any treatment, only reassurance. As it is usually seen in children, advise the parents to keep the skin oiled and to refrain from using detergents.

Is it leprosy?

In areas where leprosy is endemic, the lesion may be thought to be leprosy. Make a careful note and drawing of the lesion and see the patient again after 2–3 months. A leprosy lesion will remain at the same spot and may enlarge. Pityriasis alba may have disappeared or changed place. Testing for loss of sensation, the hallmark of leprosy, is of no use in the face. There are too many nerve endings to detect early loss of sensation (Naafs et al., 1984).

Pompholyx

Strong steroid ointments like betamethasone (0.05–0.1%, twice daily, later once daily) are needed. Occasionally, a short course of oral steroids may be needed to gain control. Search for and treat the cause of the pompholyx – frequently a fungal infection of the feet. Whitfield's ointment or cream is effective (Gooskens et al., 1994). If there is severe itching, betamethasone (0.05–0.1%) or triamcinolone (0.1%) may be added to the Whitfield's.

Discoid eczema

The well-demarcated round or oval eczematous patches of discoid or nummular eczema are common in Africa in patients with an atopic constitution and dry skin, and in HIV-infected patients. Due to its shape, it is often mistaken for a tinea infection but a KOH examination will not reveal fungi.

Treatment is not simple: the condition is chronic. Topical steroid treatment in ointments with antiseptics or alternated with antiseptics like gentian violet may be of help. Sometimes antibiotics induce a remission but recurrences are frequent. As with other causes, detergents should be avoided and, after washing, the skin should be oiled. Alcohol can make this form worse.

Infantile eczema

Infantile eczema may be atopic eczema but it may also have a seborrhoeic component when the lesions are in the nappy area, groins or axillae. It often starts during the first 6 months of life, is chronic and recurrent up to the age of 2–3. It often looks papular (its lesions are, in fact, small vesicles) and it itches severely; scratching causes superinfection. Any part of the body may be involved but specifically face, scalp and neck, frequently also the nappy area when the infant is not bare bottomed (Van Hees & Naafs, 2001).

Treatment with mild topical steroid ointments with or without tar is usually sufficient to achieve a remission. It is important to use oil or an emulsifying ointment on the wet skin after bathing. Since scratching is a major aggravating factor, it is advisable to keep the nails short; a mild sedating antihistamine may be helpful at night.

For seborrhoeic lesions, add sulphur precipitates (5 per cent) to the steroid treatment. To combat superinfection, bathing in potassium permanganate 1: 4000 or bathing with betadine jodium shampoo is useful, though sometimes antibiotics are needed, especially in HIV-infected infants.

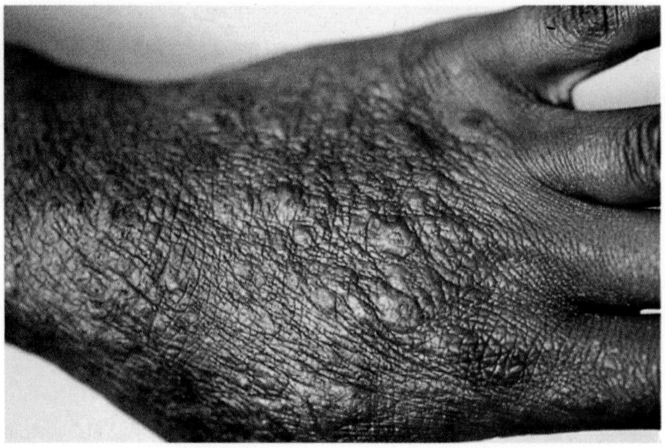

Fig. 93.3. Lichen simplex.

Lichen simplex

Lichen simplex or neurodermatitis circumscripta is common. The direct cause is the recurrent scratching and rubbing of an itchy area by predisposed individuals. The skin shows lichenification (thickening) and hyper-pigmentation, and scratch marks may be present (Fig. 93.3). The areas most involved are the back of the neck, underarms, dorsum of the hands, genitals, knees, shins and instep. Superinfection may occur especially in HIV-infected individuals.

Treatment

Prevent scratching by covering the affected area with zinc oxide adhesive bandaging. Strong steroid ointments, with or without coal tar, help to alleviate the itch and may be used under occlusion. Use gentian violet for infected lesions (alternating with steroids), or antibiotics. Recurrences are frequent.

Contact eczema/dermatitis

Contact eczema is a type IV hypersensitivity to an agent touching the skin. However, detergents may make it worse. Treat with mild steroid ointments and avoid the cause: this may sometimes be difficult.

When an eczema is located on the dorsum of hands or feet, on the ears, the eyelids or any another place not usually involved in atopic or seborrhoeic dermatitis

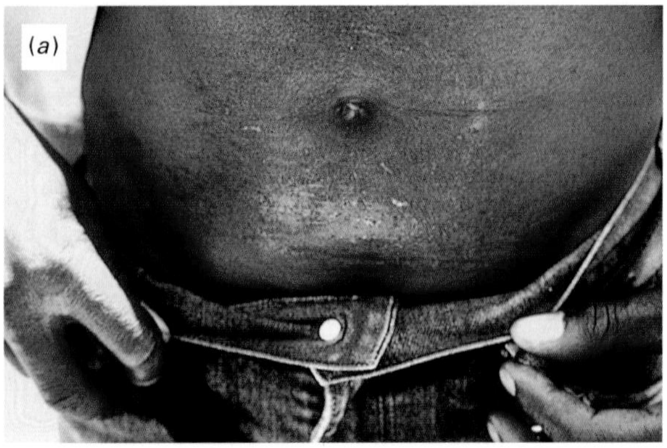

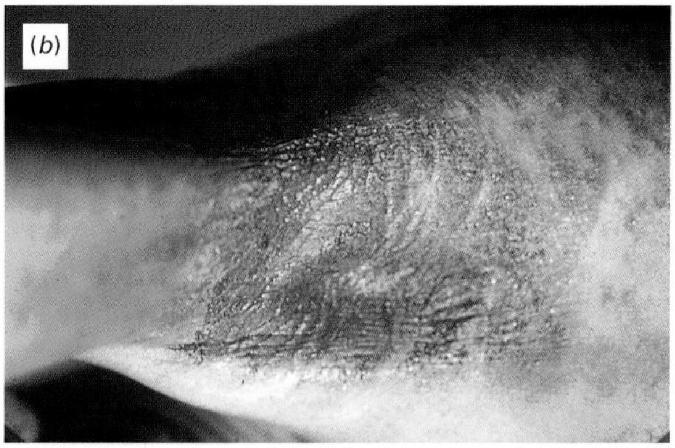

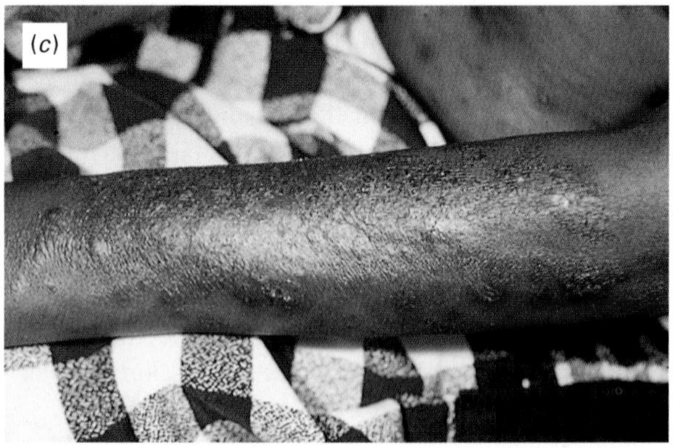

Fig. 93.4. (*a*) Contact eczema. (*b*) Eczema and HIV. (*c*) Prurigo in HIV.

such as the abdomen, hips or shoulders, an allergic component must be suspected. Although the causes in Africa are basically the same as in Europe and America (Soyinka 1978) (Fig. 93.4(*a*), (*b*), (*c*)), economical manufacturing techniques have made allergy to cosmetics, rubber and pesticides more frequent. History and careful observation help to establish the cause. Patch testing – possible in specialized centres – may be helpful.

Common causes

- Domestic: dyes, preservatives, bleach, soaps, shampoos, floor wax, nickel, leather (chromic) and oils.
- Occupational: cement (chromic), oils, diesel, fertiliszers and pesticides.
- Medical, frequently veterinarian: iodide, lanolin, menthol, camphor, local anaesthetics and antibiotics.
- Cosmetics: impure vaseline, perfumes, nail polish, hair chemicals, shampoo, creams and ointments.

The treatment consists of elimination of the offensive agent while the dermatitis is healed with steroids and, when needed, with antibiotics or antiseptics.

Seborrhoeic dermatitis

Seborrhoeic dermatitis is an eczema with typical greasy scales in the seborrhoeic areas: scalp, along the hairline, behind the ears (Fig. 93.5), in the eyebrows, nasolabial fold, chin, axillae, sternum, genital area, between the shoulder blades, lower back and between the buttocks. The areas on face and trunk are usually hypo-pigmented, in the folds hyper-pigmented. Lichenification sometimes occurs. The yeast pityrosporon is thought by some to be a major cause, and by others an opportunistic colonization. The eczema comes and goes; it may be provoked by stress.

Treatment consists of non-greasy topical applications with mild steroids; sulphur precipitates (5 per cent) are a very effective addition.

In HIV

It is frequently seen in HIV-infected patients (Palangyo, 1992), though there are regional differences; for instance, it is more frequent in Zimbabwe than in Tanzania. In HIV-infected patients skin folds, axillae, groins and behind the ears are particularly affected. Superinfection is frequent. In HIV-infected patients pityrosporon is important and eczema in these patients may become very widespread (Van Hees & Naafs, 2001).

For HIV-infected patients an azole-containing topical is more useful (Faergermann, 2000). Oral treatment is sometimes needed. Systemic antibiotics can be of help to combat superinfection, as can local gentian violet (0.5–1 per cent).

Psoriasis

The problem in Africa

Psoriasis is not common in West Africa but is more frequently seen in Ethiopia and East Africa. With the emergence of HIV, the prevalence has increased and the disease is more extensive and severe

Clinical features

In Africa, psoriasis is not an erythemato-papulo-squamous condition, because erythema is virtually absent. The distribution is the same as in the white skin: it affects the glabrous and hairy skin, especially the scalp, extensor sides of the limbs, and sometimes the skin folds (*psoriasis inversa*) or the joints (in psoriatic arthropathy). Clinically the lesions are well demarcated and show small confluent papules with dry silvery scales (Fig. 93.6), unless the skin has been washed and oiled, when they are hyper-pigmented (untreated) or hypo-pigmented (treated). Scratching will reveal the silvery scales, while further scratching leads to pinpoint bleedings (Auspitz sign).

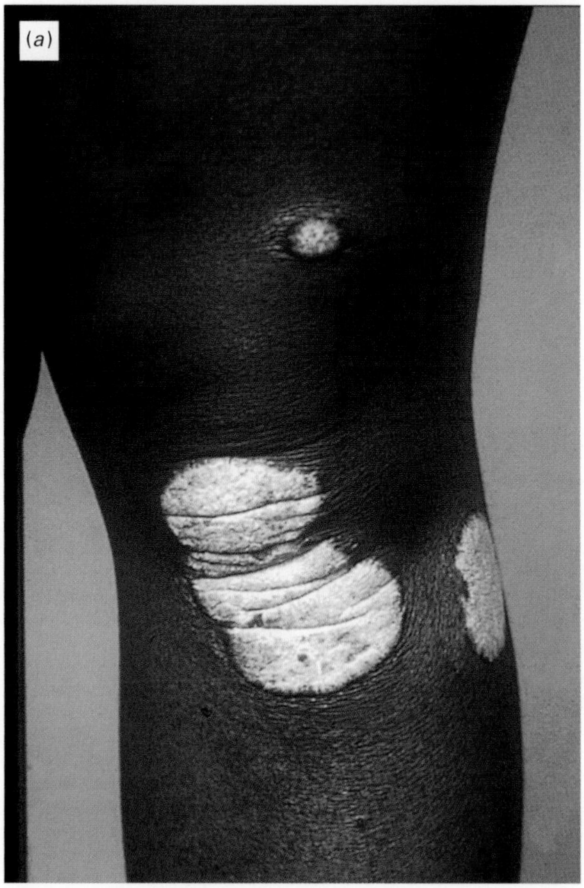

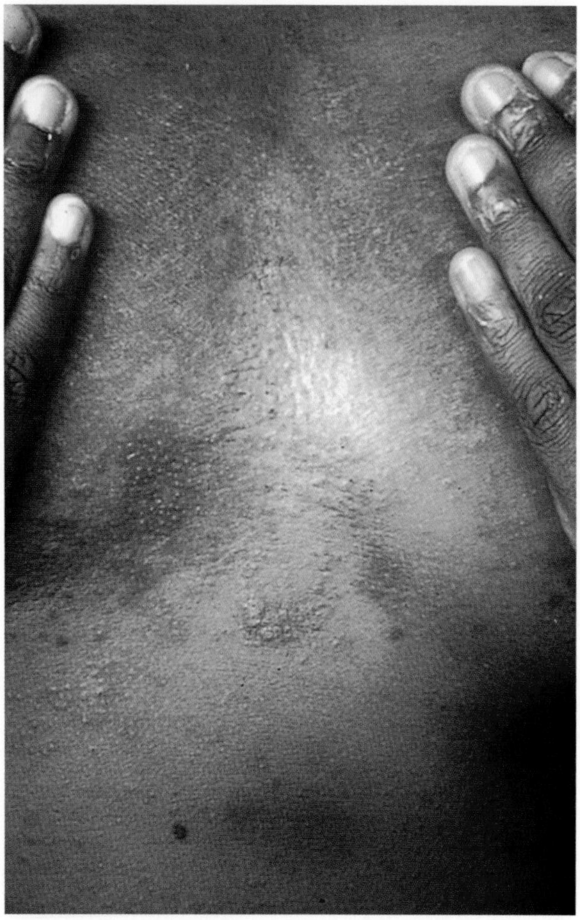

Fig. 93.5. Seborrhoeic dermatitis.

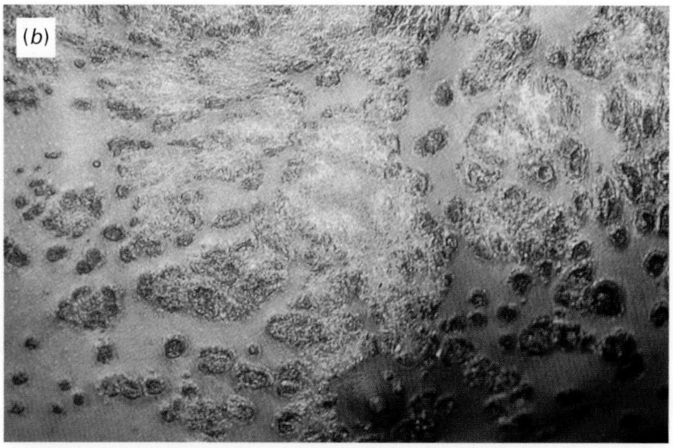

Fig. 93.6. (*a*) Psoriasis (courtesy of Dijkzigt Rotterdam). (*b*) Psoriasis in HIV.

Guttate psoriasis

This is a special subtype of psoriasis, in which droplet lesions are widespread: it often starts after a streptococcal (throat) infection. Here, antibiotic treatment should initially be added to the anti-psoriatic treatment.

Treatment

Treat non HIV-infected patients with tar ointments (Thami & Sarkar, 2002), and sun exposure with or without topical steroids (Mason et al., 2002). HIV-infected patients often need systemic treatment. Methotrexate, 5–15 mg once weekly, has been shown to be very effective; it has very few side effects and improves the quality of life for the sufferer.

FUNGAL AND YEAST INFECTIONS

Yeast infection

Pityriasis versicolor (Fig. 93.7)

The fine powdery (pityriasiform) scaling, different coloured (versicolor) yeast infection is the most prevalent infectious disease in the tropics and sub-tropics and is caused by *Pityrosporon ovale* or *orbiculare.* It produces a significant cosmetic problem, and may itch. In patients with immune suppression it may be very widespread.

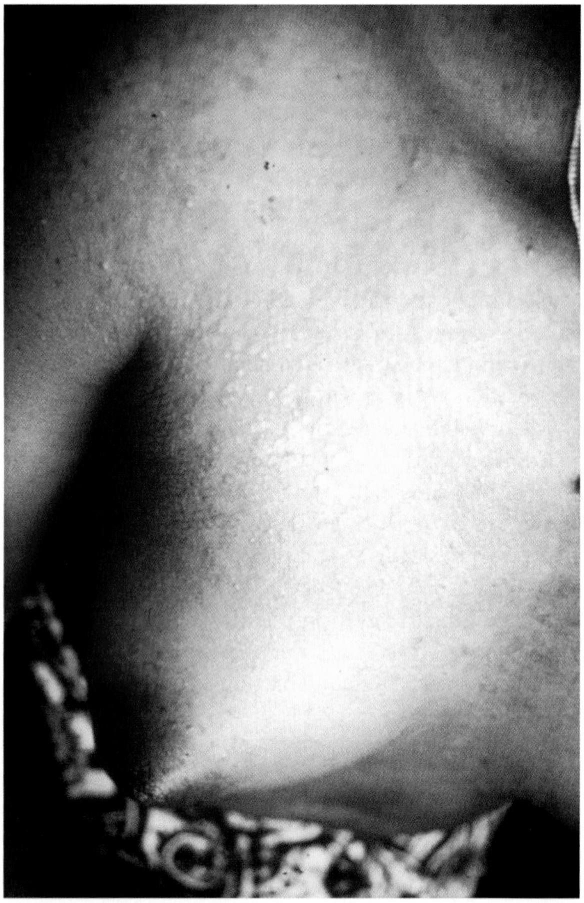

Fig. 93.7. Pityriasis versicolor.

Clinical features

Classically it is limited to the upper trunk, showing hypo- or hyper-pigmented pinpoint to half centimetre large macules with a fine branny scaling when the skin is stretched (stretch-test). It starts in a pinpoint fashion around the hair follicles in which the pityrosporon is a commensal.

Diagnosis

In a KOH preparation stained with Indian ink, the yeast and pseudohyphae look like meat balls and spaghetti.

Treatment

Selenium sulphide shampoo, used at night as a lotion and washed off the next morning, works well. Since the shampoo may irritate the skin, moisturize it afterwards. Avoid olive oil, which may enhance growth of the pityrosporon.

Topical azole preparations are also effective; if it is very widespread, the more expensive systemic ketaconazole and itraconazole may be needed. A 15 per cent sodium thiosulphate solution, applied twice daily, may also help. Griseofulvin does not work! Recurrences are frequent; once monthly treatment with shampoo as body wash may help to prevent relapses.

Pityrosporon folliculitis

In a few patients, especially those with immunosuppression, pityrosporon may cause an itchy folliculitis. Such cases may need systemic treatment.

Candidiasis

Candida albicans is a resident yeast of the mucous membranes. It becomes pathogenic under favourable conditions, including:

- immune suppression due to HIV, malignancies, steroid treatment, cytostatics or radiotherapy

- pregnancy and contraceptive pill use
- heat and moisture (baby's nappy area, under the breasts, in skin folds, etc.)
- use of broad spectrum antibiotics that kill the normal resident flora
- diabetes mellitus.

Clinical features

It presents on the skin with hyper- or hypo-pigmented, sometimes erythematous, macules, which may be shiny wet or scaling. At the periphery small pinpoint pustules are present and some small satellite lesions. A KOH preparation shows budding yeasts.

In oral (Fig. 93.8) and vulvo-vaginal lesions the mucosa is red, and superficial erosions and white adherent plaques may be seen, which are either itchy or painful. Angular stomatitis is frequent, especially in patients with badly fitting dentures. Severe mucosal candidiasis extending into the throat and oesophagus may be seen in HIV.

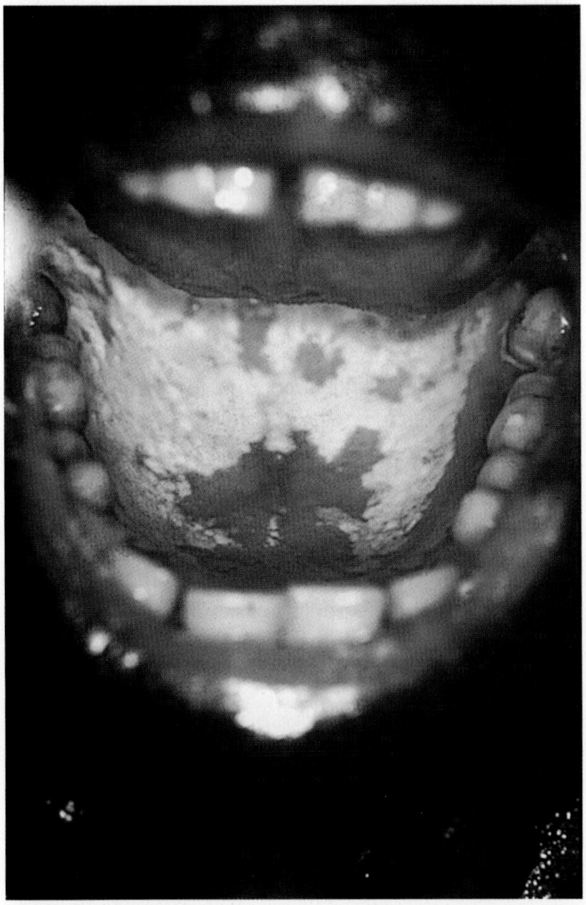

Fig. 93.8. Candida, oral in HIV (courtesy of R.D.T.C. Moshi).

Treatment

- For large oozing lesions, apply potassium permanganate dressings or soaks for 10 minutes twice daily. Thereafter the lesion can be painted with gentian violet (0.5–1 per cent) or an azole-containing cream. Gentian violet is much cheaper and very effective, but it sometimes dries the skin too much, resulting in cracking. A moisturiser may prevent this (Nyst et al., 1992).
- For the mucosae, use gentian violet, or a nystatin solution, ointment or cream. Azole-containing preparations are also very effective, used as pessaries or ovules for vulvo-vaginal infection.
- In severe cases, especially in HIV-infected patients, treatment with an oral azole preparation (ketaconazole, itraconazole, fluconazole) is needed, often for a long time, because the much cheaper griseofulvin is not effective in these cases.

Fungal infection

Superficial fungal infections, ringworm, tinea, may occur at any age. Children easily infect each other or become infected by animals. Treatment needs attention and time, because a fungal infection which is treated incompletely will almost certainly recur. In HIV and other immune-compromised patients infection is more widespread and more difficult to treat.

Diagnosis

Confirm the diagnosis with a 20 per cent potassium hydroxide solution investigation by microscope, and look for hyphae. Culture may confirm the diagnosis. Hypersensitivity reactions to the fungi may give localized eczematous reactions,and as an 'id' reaction on distance, seen on the hand as pompholyx and on the feet as small very itchy blisters (mycids). These disappear when the initial fungus is treated. Fungal infections are usually named after the part of the body which they affect – tinea capitis (head), corporis (body), cruris (groin), pedis (foot), unguium (nail).

Tinea capitis (Fig. 93.9)

Tinea capitis mainly occurs in schoolchildren (Ayaya et al., 2001). Many different dermatophytes are responsible. The organism, as well as host immunity, influences the clinical picture.

The clinical picture varies widely, from areas of hair loss studded with broken off hairs, diffuse scaling, diffuse

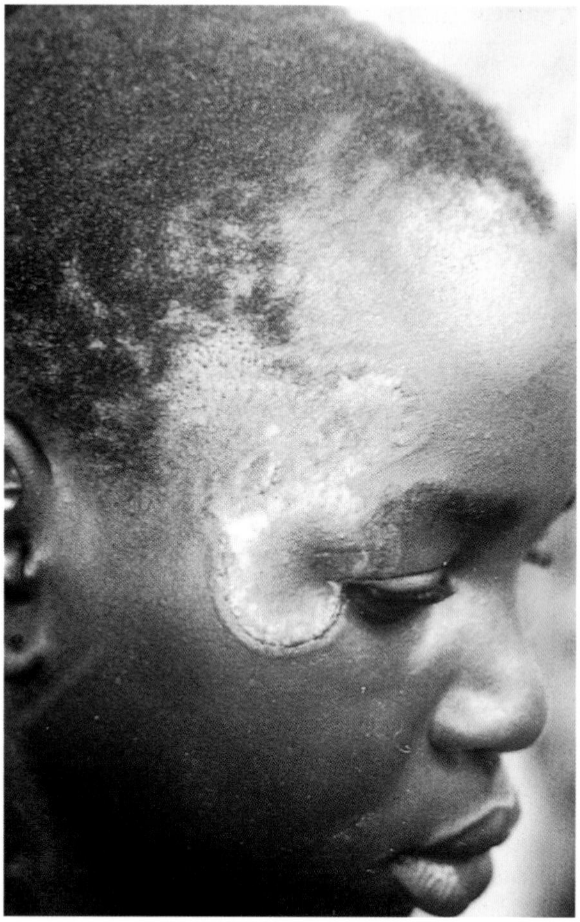

Fig. 93.9. Tinea capitis.

pustules, baggy discrete pustule-studded swellings called lesions. In the inflammatory variant there may be reactive cervical painful lymphadenopathy.

Diagnosis

KOH microscopy of the affected part has shown spores, either on the outside of the shaft (ectotrix) or on the inside (endotrix). Culture also helps to identify the organism.

Treatment

Although some children may resolve spontaneously on entering puberty, untreated tinea capitis may lead to scarring and permanent hair loss.

Treatment is with **oral** antifungals: griseofulvin 10 mg/kg divided dose for 8 weeks. Topical therapy is inadequate.

Tinea corporis

Hypo- and hyper-pigmentated patches and, in lightly pigmented skin, erythema can be seen, with an active scaly or pustular edge. Sometimes concentric active rings can be seen. It can be mistaken for discoid eczema but the KOH preparation shows fungal elements.

Treatment

Whitfield's ointment works well (Gooskens et al., 1994). For some of the animal fungi, this topical treatment may not be sufficient and griseofulvin has to be added orally. Azole derivatives or terbinafine topically or orally are also very effective. Systemic treatment may be needed for HIV-infected patients.

Tinea pedis

In the past, tinea pedis was rare in Africa. However, today it is common because closed shoes and boots are worn. Moisture and maceration provide the right environment in the tropics (Naafs, 2001).

The clinical spectrum is that of hyper-pigmented eczematous patches with scaling and vesicles and pustules.

Athlete's foot

This type of tinea pedis is only caused by dermatophytes in half of the cases; the others are caused by bacteria (diphtheroids). It is an intertrigo of the toe webs, most frequently between the fourth and fifth toe.

HIV patients are particularly prone to a superinfection with *Pseudomonas*.

Tinea cruris

Tinea pedis may lead to tinea cruris when fungal elements are moved by clothing (trousers) from the foot to the groin. This often happens in Islamic society, where athlete's foot is prevalent because of the ritual washing of the feet in communal places.

Treatment

This is the same as for tinea corporis. Gentian violet is very useful, particularly if secondary infection with bacteria has occurred.

Subcutaneous and deep fungal infections

Deep fungal infections, though more common in Mid- and South-America, can also be seen in Africa. Most common, but still rare, are chromomycosis, sporotrichosis, mycetoma and African histoplasmosis (see also Chapters 56–68).

Chromomycosis (see p. 628, Chapter 55)
Chromomycosis, also called chromoblastomycosis, is a localized chronic but progressive fungal infection of cutis and subcutis. It is characterized by warty confluent papules and nodules, sometimes giving it a cauliflower appearance (Fig. 93.10). It occurs in 80 per cent of the cases on the legs especially on the foot and around the ankle. The skin becomes sclerotic and hard; the leg may show elephantiasis. The lesions may become superinfected, start ulcerating and oozing.

It is caused by several species of the pigmented fungi of the Fonsecaea family. In particular peasants who go barefoot are infected. It is most prevalent in Central, East and Southern Africa.

Left untreated it runs a protracted and slowly progressive course. Treatment is extremely difficult: it is described p. 629.

Sporotrichosis (see p. 629)
Sporotrichosis is caused by *Sporothrix schenckii.* The typical pattern in a previously uninfected person is an initial lesion that occurs two weeks after local inoculation. This papule becomes a nodule and breaks down to form a suppurating vegetating papule or plaque with central ulceration. There is also a lymphangitic type, due to spread up lymphatics to lymph nodes, which may suppurate and lead to secondary papular lesions following the lymphatics (sporotrichoid spread) (Fig. 93.11). In patients previously exposed, the lesion may stay localized as a verruceus plaque. In HIV or otherwise immune-suppressed patients, the disease may disseminate.

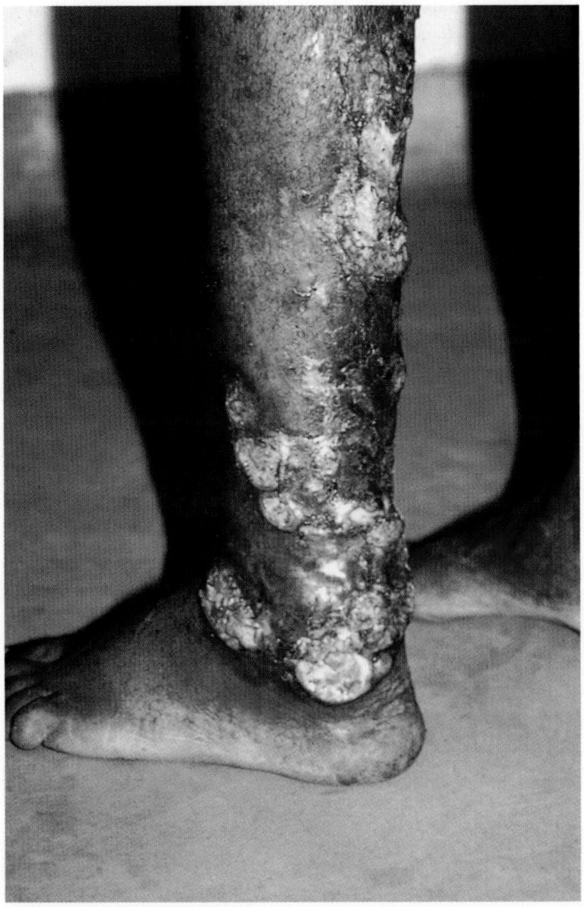

Fig. 93.10. Chromo(blasto)mycosis (see also Fig. 55.3).

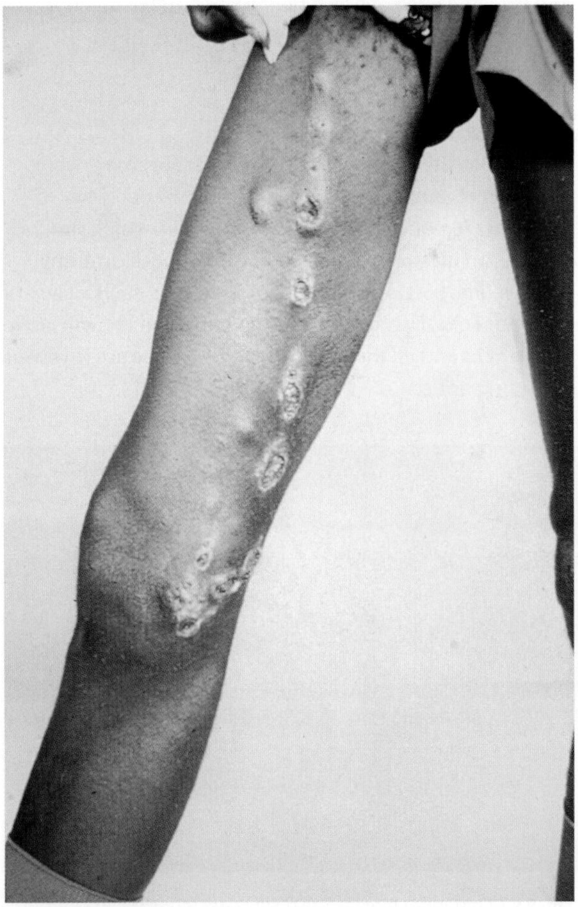

Fig. 93.11. Sporotrichosis.

The fungus seems to live in debris of plants or wood. In some areas cats are infected and pass the fungus to the human.

Treatment is described on p. 629.

African histoplasmosis

The African type of histoplasmosis is caused by *Histoplasma duboisii*. It is a systemic disease involving lungs, bones and lymph nodes but may disseminate to skin and subcutis. The patient may present with skin lesions:

- umbilicated papules or pustules, resembling mollusca contagiosa
- chancriform small ulcers with raised rolled edges
- subcutaneous nodules. These nodules are soft, fluctuate and represent abscesses.

The infection may self-heal, but becomes very widespread if it occurs in an HIV-infected patient.

Treatment

In a specialist centre, give amphotericin B, but flu-, keto- and itraconazole have also been shown to be effective and have fewer side effects (Onwuasoigwe, 1999). Relapses are common.

Mycetoma

Mycetoma (the word means fungal tumour) may occur everywhere, but the foot (ankle) is most frequently involved (70 per cent), hence *Madura foot*, which presents as an indurated, rockhard swelling with draining sinuses (Fig. 93.12). In these sinuses, grains can be seen of different colour and hardness depending on the causative agent. Skin and all the sub-cutaneous tissues are involved including bone.

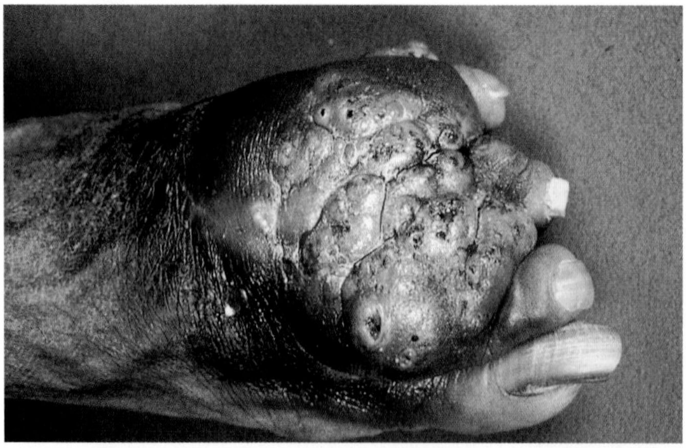

Fig. 93.12. Madura foot (see also Fig. 55(*a*) (courtesy of Dijkzigt Rotterdam).

It can be caused by fungi: eumycetoma, or by bacteria, actinomycetes, streptomyces or nocardia; actinomycetoma. It may slowly disable a nomadic herdsman, who probably became infected after an injury by an acacia thorn, but any penetrating wound can be responsible.

It is important to establish whether it is an eu- or actinomycete. Eumycetes are virtually untreatable except by extensive mutilating surgery. KOH investigations are helpful as well as cultures of the grains.

Treatment for actinomycetoma, described on p. 628, is cotrimoxazole and streptomycin. Amikacin may be used as an alternative for streptomycin. Rifampicin has been used as an alternative for sulphonamides.

Bacterial infections

Bacterial infections are common.

Impetigo (Fig. 93.13)

This is a skin infection often seen in babies, infants and children. It presents with superficial vesicles and pus-

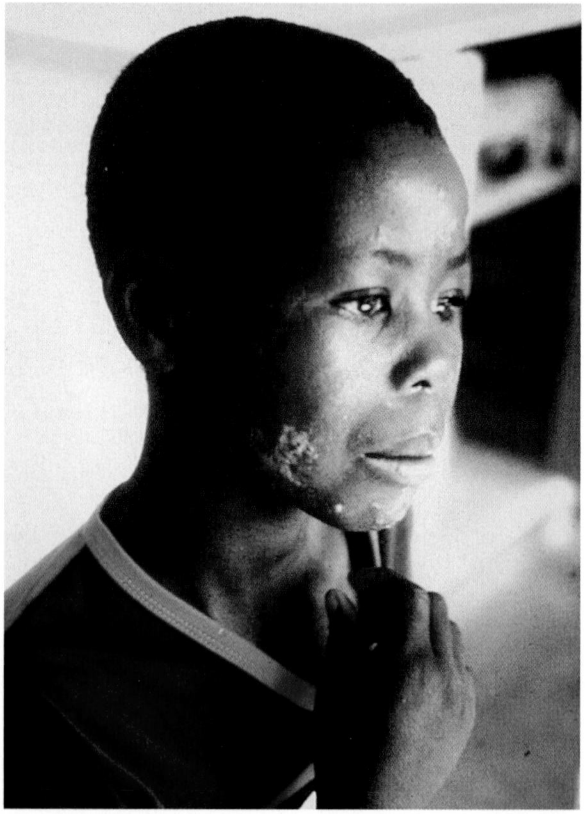

Fig. 93.13. Impetigo.

tules, which leave oozing erosions with yellow crusts (honey crusts).

It is caused by staphylococci and/or streptococci. It is very contagious and may infect small scratch marks due to eczemas, insect bites, pediculosis or scabies. Vaseline, because it is occlusive, makes the condition worse.

Treatment

- Wash with potassium permanganate or a mild antiseptic soap (betadine jodium soap or shampoo), followed by gentian violet (0.5–1per cent) applied to the lesions (Okano et al., 2000).
- Remove old crusts before a new application of gentian violet.
- Antibiotic creams like mupiricin are effective but expensive.
- Do not use neomycin because it easily sensitizes, but tetracycline ointment seems to be effective in many cases.

When severe, or when generalized symptoms are present, with enlarged lymph nodes and fever, systemic antibiotics are advisable.

Staphylococcal scalded skin syndrome (SSSS)

The old name *bullous impetigo of the newborn* characterizes this condition. It is due to specific subtypes of staphylococci that produce an exotoxin that breaks the cohesion between the keratinocytes, in this way causing vesicles and bullae. The condition is potentially life threatening due to large areas of denuded skin left by the blisters. Systemic antibiotics are vital (Machang'u et al., 1997).

Ecthyma

This is a deeper form of impetigo.

Clinical feature

A small blister or pustule appears and enlarges, a hard hyperpigmented crust is formed. When this adherent crust is removed, a shallow irregular punched-out purulent ulcer with surrounding erythema and hyperpigmentation is seen. The legs are most affected and the lesions may persist for weeks.

The causative agents differ, especially in HIV-infected patients, but frequently strepto- or staphylococci are cultured.

Treatment

Remove the crust and apply gentian violet. Systemic antibiotics are also frequently needed.

Erysipelas after cellulitis

This is an acute and serious form of cellulitis of the skin due to haemolytic streptococci which cause a vasculitis of the dermis.

Clinical features

The skin becomes very tender and may be hyperpigmented: erythema, the hallmark in white skin, can sometimes be seen. The lesions are oedematous and well demarcated. Occasionally blisters are seen. The patient is strikingly ill and has systemic symptoms with fever, headache and sometimes vomiting.

Treatment

Penicillin is the treatment of choice. The lesions may be 'cooled' with wet dressings.

Cellulitis

Cellulitis is a diffuse inflammation of the connective tissue of the deep dermis and the subcutaneous fat. It can be caused by an array of bacteria but most frequently staphylococci and streptococci.

Clinical features

The skin is hot and oedematous, hyperpigmentation and erythema may be seen. It is distinguished from erysipelas because the edges are irregular and not well demarcated.

Treatment

Wet dressings and systemic antibiotics.

Botryomycosis (Fig. 93.14)

Botryomycosis is a mycetoma-like condition caused by organisms that usually cause cellulitis or abscesses. Staphylococci, pseudomonas and a number of other micro-organisms have been incriminated.

Exactly why these organisms produce the mycetoma-like condition is unknown. But often there are debilitating conditions such as obesity, diabetes, alcohol misuse or especially HIV. Treatment must be done in specialized centres.

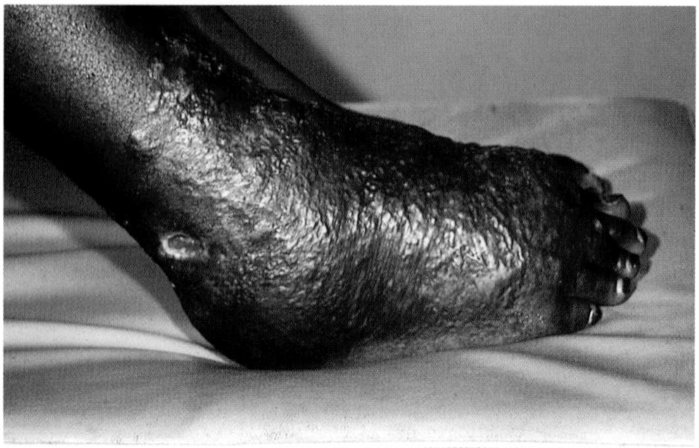

Fig. 93.14. Botryomycosis in HIV.

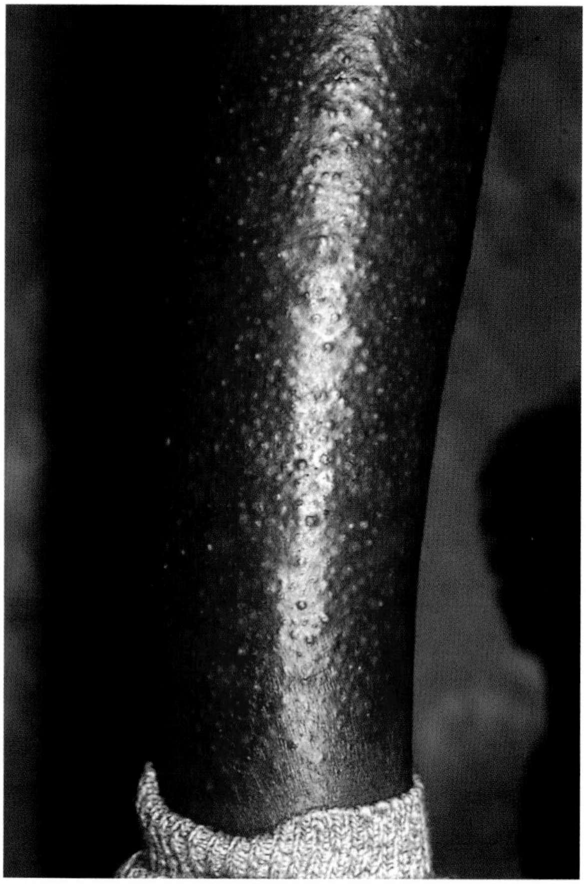

Fig. 93.15. Sycocis cruris. Dermatitis cruris pustulosa et atrophicans (DCPA) (courtesy of Dr C. van Hees).

Folliculitis (Fig. 93.15)

Folliculitis is an inflammation of the hair follicles, papulopustules caused by bacteria, usually staphylococci. Hair follicles everywhere can be affected especially on the face, on the trunk and buttocks. In young girls the typical 'vaseline dermatitis' can be seen on the lower legs.

Folliculitis can be mild and superficial or widespread or deep and then presents with furuncles and carbuncles.

Treatment

- Discontinue vaseline and/or any ointment that is being used.
- Bath with antiseptic soaps (betadine shampoo) or with potassium permanganate or chlorhexidine.
- Sometimes, mild keratolytic creams with salicylic acid and sulphur precipitates may be of use.
- Effective but expensive are lotions with clindamycin or erythromycin or antibiotic creams like mupiricin.

HIV-infected patients

Gram-negative bacteria or pityrosporon may be involved. The folliculitis in these patients is refractory to treatment, so that systemic antibiotics are needed together with an azole.

Furuncles and carbuncles

Initially, treat with heat and moisture: soften the skin with, for instance, diachylon or ichthyol to induce 'ripening' and spontaneous discharge. Sometimes, surgical drainage and removal of the necrotic 'pit' is needed, but antibiotics are seldom necessary.

Nuchal acne keloidalis (Fig. 93.16)

This is common in the African man. The name literally means keloid-forming folliculitis of the neck. Lenticular keloidal papules, small nodules and papulopustules are present at the base of the hair line.

It is induced by the shaving of the hairs in the neck, so that ingrowing hairs lead to inflammation and superinfection with micrococci, staphylococci, corynebacteria and pityrosporon. The result is a chronic fibrosing folliculitis and perifolliculitis with keloid scars. At the rim of the scars new pustules lead to new lesions.

Treatment

No effective treatment is available. Long-term systemic tetracycline (doxycycline or minocycline) treatment together with itra- or ketaconazole and topical strong steroids (betamethasone, clobutasol propionate) may induce a remission. Surgical excision will result in new lesions along a keloidal scar (Glenn et al., 1995).

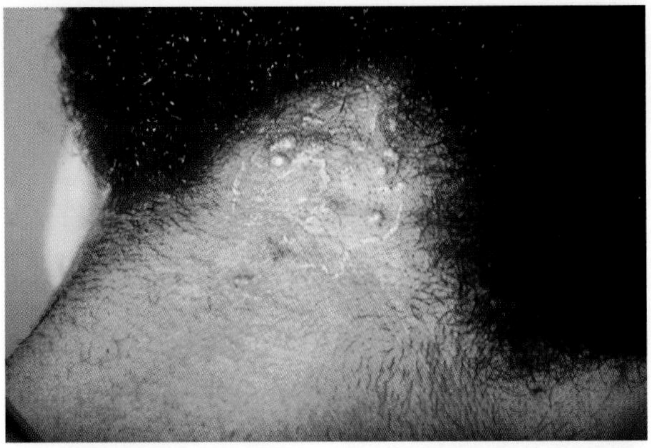

Fig. 93.16. Acne nuchae keloidalis.

Pseudofolliculitis barbae

This has become common since close shaving has been introduced: hairs retract in the dermis after being cut and, being curly when growing, curl in the skin causing inflammation, pustules and scarring.

Treatment

Stop shaving, open all pustules and thus give room to the hairs. Subsequent shaving, followed by the application of a mild keratolytic cream, for example 5 per cent salicylic acid, 5 per cent resorcinol and 5 per cent sulphur precipitate with 1per cent hydrocortisone in aqueous cream, can be useful. An antiseptic aftershave, or use of an electric razor, may help.

Acne vulgaris

Acne is very common in puberty and it usually regresses in early adulthood. It may persist, however, up to the age of 30 or even lifelong. In towns and urban centres, the use of cosmetics, with vaseline and steroids, is a major problem because they induce and maintain acne.

Pathogenesis

Three factors are involved in the pathology of acne:

1. Sebum overproduction, under androgen control.
2. Obstruction, due to hyperkeratinization of the pilosebaceous duct, or a change in the lumen due to pressure or stretch, or simply occlusion by cosmetics.
3. Microbial factors are important, especially *Propionibacterium acnes*. The organisms produce enzymes which form highly irritant-free fatty acids from the sebum triglycerides. On the surface of the skin these products are essential, preventing overgrowth of pathological micro-organisms but, when obstructed, they induce an inflammatory response.

Clinical features

Papules, papulopustules, comedones and sometimes nodules and abscesses occur. Persistent hyperpigmentation may complicate the condition in pigmented skins.

Treatment

The principles are:

(i) to reduce the number of micro-organisms with topical antiseptics, sulphur precipitates, benzoylperoxide or antibiotics like cindamycin or erythromycin, and orally with tetracyclines, cotrimoxazole or macrolides. These treatments sometimes have to be continued for years.

(ii) to keep the sebaceous duct short and open, using a combination of salicylic acid, resorcinol and sulphur or vitamin-A-acid (tretinoin, but this is costly). Even more costly but certainly also effective are the new topical retinoids, adapalene and tazarotene, but these have very little extra to contribute beside being less irritative. Benzoylperoxide or azaleic acid can also be used, being anti-bacterial besides peeling agents.

Note that, especially in more lightly pigmented skin, some topical applications may be too irritant and produce hyperpigmentation. It is therefore useful to add an emollient preparation during the first few months.

(iii) to keep the skin clean to remove occlusive dirt and fat. Most of the cleansing lotions contain alcohol but, since this may be irritant, it should not exceed 35 per cent, or 20 per cent in patients in risk of hyperpigmentation.

(iv) to diminish the sebum production, severe acne can be treated with anti-androgens, cyproteron acetate, or with the vitamin A derivative, isotretinoin, which brings the sebaceous glands into a resting phase, often a permanent involution.

Hiradenitis suppurativa

This is a condition of follicular occlusion, located in axillae and groins.

Treatment is difficult. The ideal is to avoid mechanical trauma and occlusion and to prevent bacterial overgrowth. In addition, topical treatment with antiseptic or antibiotic lotions may be considered. Azaleic acid in

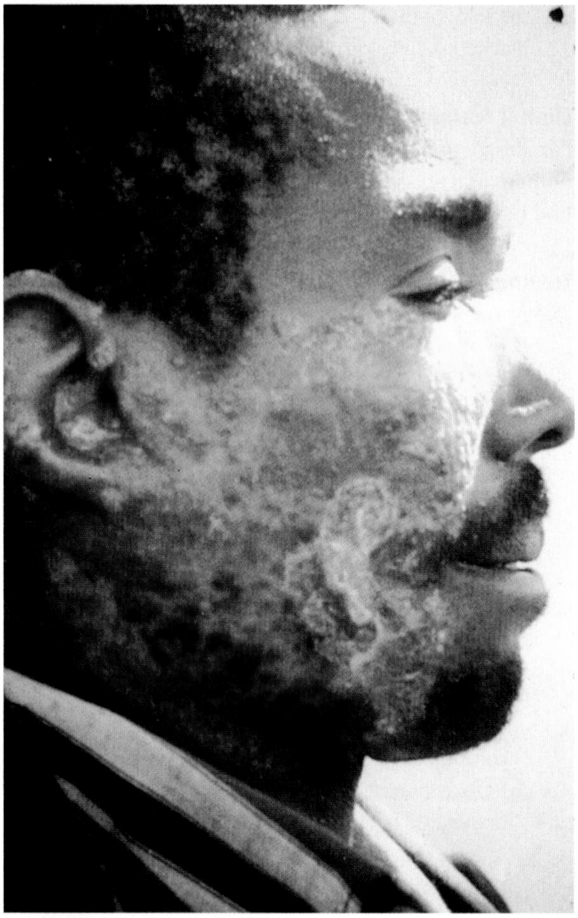

Fig. 93.17. Lupus vulgaris.

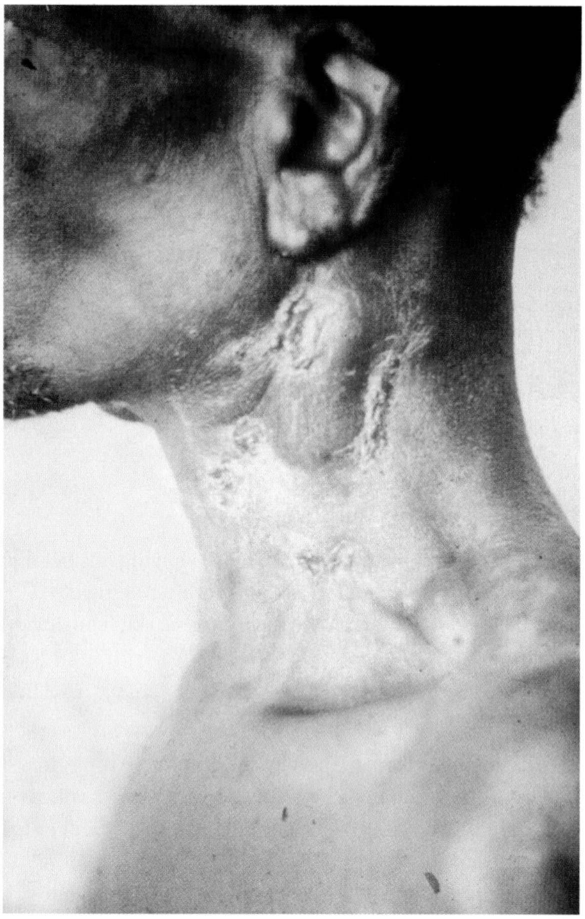

Fig. 93.18. Scrofuloderma (warty or verrucous tuberculosis).

creams (5–20%) have also been shown to be of benefit. Systemic acitretinate may be more effective than isotretinoin, since obstruction is a major cause, and acitretinate makes the epidermis thinner while isotretinoin is mostly sebostatic.

Anthrax

Anthrax may present with its characteristic skin lesion. After inoculation of *B. anthracis* an itch may be noticed: hours or days later a papule can be seen with a dark central vesicle. This enlarges and forms the typical necrotic eschar, which is not painful, surrounded by a rim of vesicles and extensive non-pitting oedema. The treatment is penicillin.

Tuberculosis (Fig. 93.17)

When the primary inoculation occurs in the skin, a small papule forms that ulcerates and extends, it may heal and produce enlarged regional lymph nodes.

Lupus vulgaris

The nodule enlarges and forms a plaque that breaks down and heals with scarring, sclerosis and atrophy, focally hyperpigmented or depigmented. Active new lesions may appear in the scarred areas or at the periphery.

Warty or verrucous tuberculosis

This shows verrucous papules and nodules with crypts in between. It can easily be confused with deep mycotic infections or leishmaniasis. Both lupus vulgaris and warty tuberculosis occur less frequently now, but suppurating lymph nodes, especially in the neck region, are still seen. They heal with characteristic scarring (Fig. 93.18).

Treatment

Give WHO advised MDT+ (p. 339).

Leprosy

Leprosy has been fully described in Chapter 47.

Ulceration and deformity in leprosy

Principles of treatment (Faber et al., 1993) for all ulcers of *the feet.*

- Clean and cover wounds. For superficial wounds, zinc adhesive sticking tape can be applied straight onto the wound and renewed 1–2 weekly. The zinc oxide containing tape is antibacterial, not fully occlusive but protective.
- Trim hyperkeratotic rims.
- Do not use bulky bandages on the feet. They cause local pressure when walked on and the wound will not heal.
- Only use antibiotics when there is cellulitis.

Further deformity can be prevented by daily care provided by the patient himself, daily inspection, soaking and oiling, trimming the sides of cracks, and softening the skin by applying 15 per cent salicylic acid in vaseline.

- Stretch digits of hands and feet regularly, actively and passively to prevent further contractures.

Corynebacteria

Erythrasma

Erythrasma is a chronic superficial infection of the body folds caused by *Corynebacterium minutissimum*. It presents with hyperpigmentation and mild itch. There may be some scaling. It is found in the groins, in the axillae, under the breasts and in the toe webs. The lesions fluoresce coral pink under UV light (Woodd's light). It is frequently mistaken for tinea, however the KOH examination shows no fungi and fluorescence is typical.

Treatment

Oral or topical erythromycin.

Pitted keratolysis

The same bacteria are responsible. It manifests as punched out confluent erosions of the callus of the sole of the foot. It has a 'moth-eaten' appearance

Hyperhidrosis and wet feet due to occlusive footwear are associated with this condition.

Treatment

Open sandals and erythromycin topically.

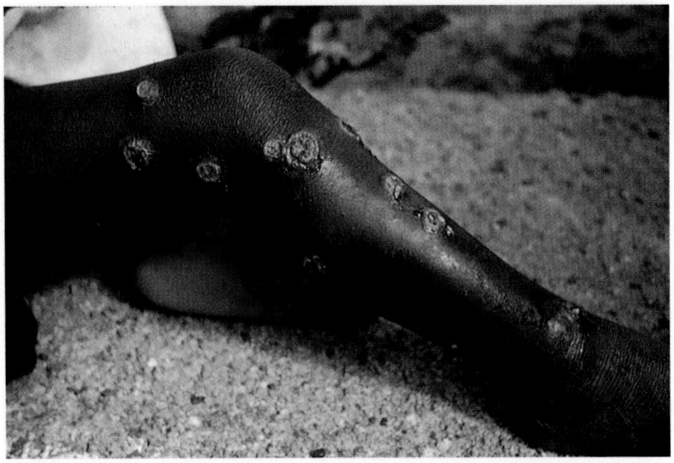

Fig. 93.19. Condylomata of yaws (courtesy of archives Dr D. L. Leiker).

Treponemal infections

Secondary syphilis

It can mimic almost any other skin disease. Classically, it presents with a generalized symmetrical erythematous, hyperpigmented, macular, papular or pustular eruption with or without scaling, but without itching: this is helpful in diagnosis. Palms and soles are usually affected as well as the face. There is usually a history of a primary ulcer on the genital area or elsewhere (lips) 1 to 2 months before the development of the rash (p. 270).

Yaws

The primary lesion of yaws (mother yaws) is a wet, easily bleeding, raspberry-like papule or nodule commonly seen in children, which disappears after a few weeks leaving an atrophic scar. When the primary infection is not treated secondary lesions (daughter yaws) may appear as generalized nodules, ulcerations and condylomata (Fig. 93.19), which are identical to those of secondary syphilis. Late yaws may cause hyperkeratotic areas on the feet interfering with walking (crab yaws).

Noma/cancrum oris

Noma is a form of infectious gangrene of the mouth. It is thought to be caused by fusiform bacteria (Fig. 93.20). It usually affects young, malnourished children after a recent acute infection, particularly measles.

Pathogenesis

The disease generally starts as a peridontitis, followed by an ulcerative stomatitis, always on one side of the mouth,

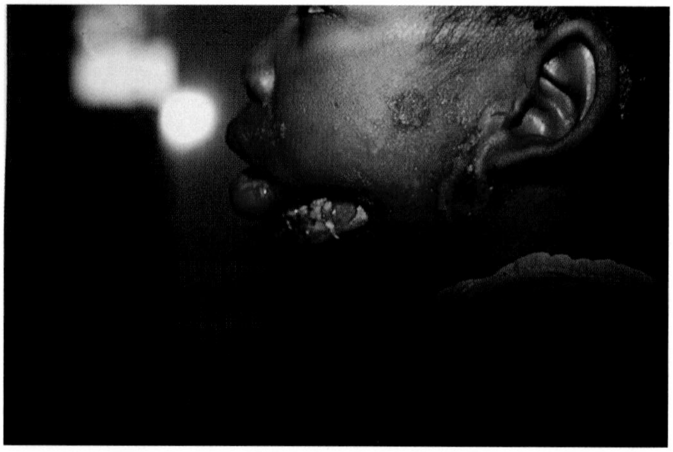

Fig. 93.20. Cancrum oris (noma) in HIV-positive child (courtesy of Dr C. van Hees).

progressing to gangrene with extensive sloughing of adjacent tissue and even necrosis of bone. The area is foul smelling and very painful. Untreated patients may die or survive severely handicapped.

Treatment

- Early treatment transforms outcome.
- When only peridontitis is present, mouth washes with chlorhexidine may prevent development of noma.
- Massive doses of penicillin are very effective, or, in case of penicillin allergy, other broad-spectrum antibiotics, for at least 2 weeks and until all signs of activity have ceased.
- Give a generous mixed diet, with vitamin supplements. Parenteral supplementation may be needed.
- Residual deformities, however, may need skilled reconstructive surgery.

Viral infections

Molluscum contagiosum (Fig. 93.21)

This is caused by a pox virus and is a common disease in children but is also frequently seen in HIV-infected adults.

Clinical features

Small dome-shaped skin-coloured umbilicated papules. In children it occurs anywhere especially around the eyelids, in the genital area and in the elbows, which are a common site in atopic individuals. In healthy children it usually heals spontaneously.

In HIV-infected patients the lesions may be larger and more disseminated.

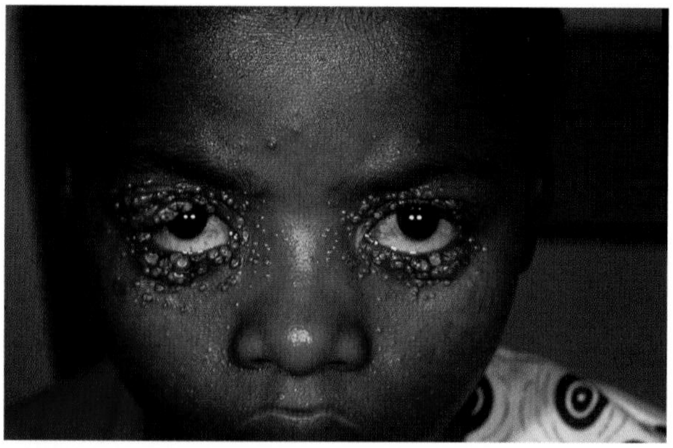

Fig. 93.21. Molluscum contagiosum in HIV (courtesy of Dr D. Verhagen).

Treatment

1. Children: the lesions can be left to resolve spontaneously or, curettage, cauterizing, cryotherapy, or etching with phenol or trichloroacetic acid of a few lesions in healthy children may induce a remission of the other lesions (vaccination).
2. HIV-infected patients: each individual lesion has to be treated.

Warts

These are caused by human papilloma virus (HPV) of which more than 60 are already known. They are designated by number and some are carcinogenic.

Clinical features

Warts are characteristically common on hands and feet in children. In an HIV-infected individual warts can be more disseminated. Warts on the face or on the dorsum of the hand are plane warts: in the genital area and between the buttocks they are termed condylomata accuminata. In HIV-infection these may become huge. The clinical expression of the infection – plane warts, common warts or condylomata – depends on the localization and the type of virus.

Treatment

No treatments are very good but spontaneous resolution occurs. Destruction with cryosurgery, electrosurgery, coagulation, etching or treatment with toxic substances like podophylline or 5-fluorouracil may help.

Warts and cancer

Some of the HPV viruses responsible for condylomata may cause penile or cervical carcinoma. Others, frequently together with co-factors, such as immunosuppression or UV-radiation, may cause Bowen's disease (intraepithelial squamous cell carcinoma) or a frank squamous cell carcinoma of the skin.

Herpes simplex

Herpes simplex may occur as a primary infection, accompanied by fever in children or as a sexually transmitted disease in adults. It may recur. Recurrence may occur during transient immunosuppression accompanying fever, after extensive sun exposure or during and after infections especially viral. The virus remains dormant in the neural ganglia. Herpes simplex virus (HSV) type I and HSV II can both infect lips and genitalia.

Clinical features

Clusters of small vesicles, usually on the lips, the nose, and the face, healing after a crusting phase, without scarring, in 7–10 days. Recurrences become less severe in time. In adults the primary lesions may be on the genitals or buttocks, but can occur elsewhere as well (nose, finger).

In HIV-infected patients

Vesicles are often genital but may occur anywhere: they may break down and ulcerate and sometimes do not heal at all, particularly in children (Fig. 93.22).

When the infection becomes chronic and ulcerative, or is extensive with gingivostomatitis and pharyngitis, systemic anti-viral treatment is needed with acyclovir or one of the newer antivirals. Diagnosis can be supported by means of a Tzank smear.

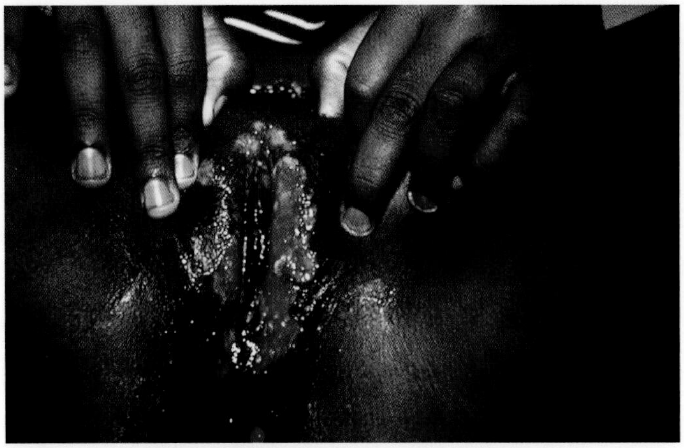

Fig. 93.22. HIV herpes simplex genital ulceration (courtesy of KCMC Moshi, Dr W. Howlett).

Pityriasis rosea

The cause is still debated, but there is some evidence that it is a cutaneous reaction to a generalized viral infection, probably herpes VII (Drago et al., 2002). It occurs usually in young adults and may be confused with secondary syphilis.

Clinical features

The herald patch is the typical first lesion: it is a well-defined slightly erythematous hypo- or hyperpigmented rounded scaly lesion 2–5 cm in diameter, which appears on the trunk or upper arms.

A few days to 2 weeks later, oval erythematous slightly hypo- or hyperpigmented lesions appear with a powdery scaling, hence the name pityriasis, the scaling at the rim may form a collar. The lesions are 10–15 mm along the long axis, which follows the skin lines, so that a fir tree pattern is produced on the back. It is a truncal eruption, confined to the trunk and upper arms and upper thighs. The eruption lasts about 6 weeks but the post-inflammatory hyperpigmentation may last months.

Treatment usually is not necessary unless it is itchy when topical steroids will be needed.

Kaposi's sarcoma

Kaposi's sarcoma caused by HSV VIII can be endemic in older people on the legs or more aggressive and more generalized in children and young adults. Crops of bluish, hyperpigmented papules and nodules appear often associated with severe oedema. Both cutaneous and visceral lesions may occur (Templeton & Viegas, 1970). The latter happens also in the AIDS-related Kaposi's sarcoma (Fig. 93.23(*a*),(*b*),(*c*)) (p. 225). Treatment has to be done in referral hospitals with radiotherapy and chemotherapy.

Varicella zoster virus

Varicella (see Chapter 62)

It is a disease of children but in isolated communities also young adults may show the disease. In most young adults, however, it indicates HIV.

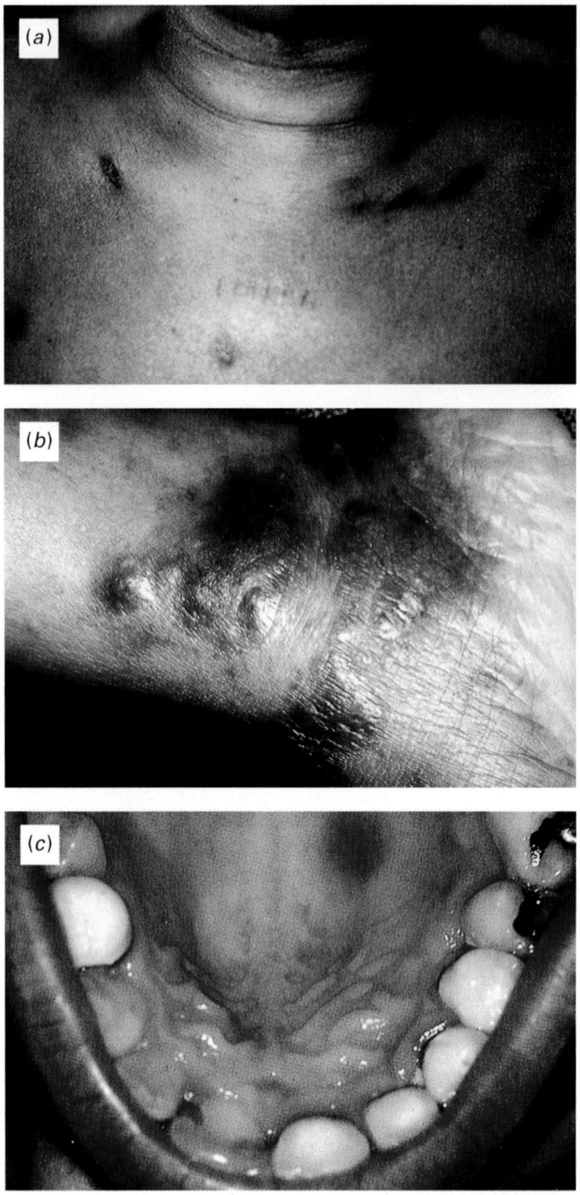

Fig. 93.23. Kaposi's sarcoma in HIV. (*a*) Symmetrical early lesions (courtesy of K.C.M.C. Moshi). (*b*) Later. (*c*) Solitary lesion on the hard palate (courtesy of AMC Amsterdam, Dr H. J. Hulsebosch).

Herpes zoster

The vesicles appear in crops, grouped together, unilaterally in the distribution of a dermatome, because the varicella zoster virus was dormant in the neural ganglia until immunosuppression allowed it to become active. Sometimes the patient has prodromal fever or localized pain and tenderness. In the lighter skin some erythema may be noticed (Fig. 93.24). Later, the vesicles become turbid and after one week crusts form and the lesions heal. Scarring is unusual but, sometimes, extensive scarring and hypo- and depigmentation is seen, especially in HIV-infected individuals. Rarely, keloids form.

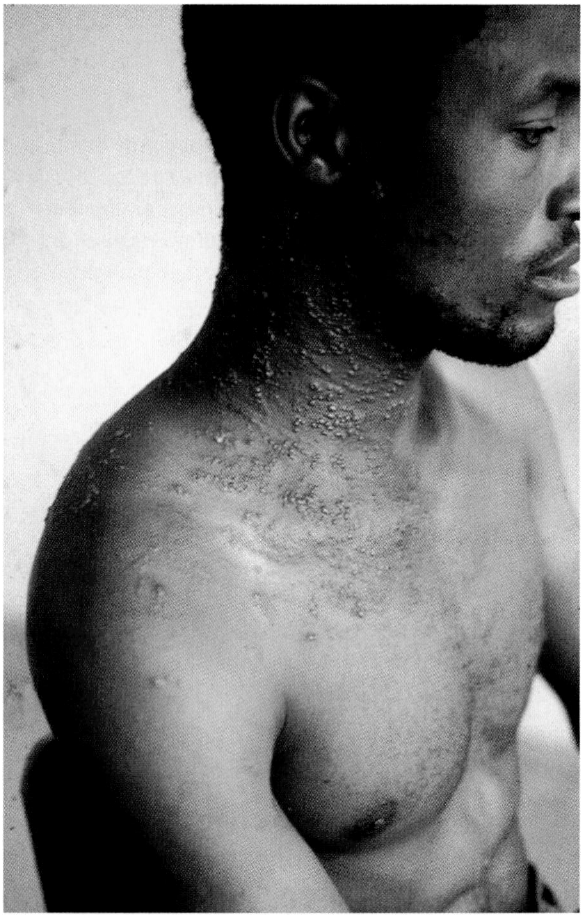

Fig. 93.24. Early herpes zoster with some erythema in HIV.

Herpes zoster is an ominous sign of HIV-infection, in some studies in Africa up to 100 per cent in all age groups have concomitant HIV. It may extend to more than one dermatome or become generalized. The disease may become protracted and become chronic or it may heal, only to relapse again.

Treatment is needed when the eye is involved or when the disease is becoming chronic or relapsing. Modern anti-virals are effective but expensive. Post-herpetic neuralgia can be debilitating and simple analgesics may be inadequate. Standard treatment at present consists of oral amitriptyline or carbamazipine. When these are not effective a 5 per cent phenol containing ointment applied up to five times daily may be useful.

Parasitic infections

Scabies

Scabies is endemic in most of Africa among the poor and overcrowded, prisoners, young recruits of army and police and school children: it is a widespread problem, particularly when complicated by pyoderma (Mahe et al., 1998). It is acquired by close contact with an infected individual and so is often transmitted sexually. It is a significant burden: not only does the itch disturb sleep, but secondary infection with *Streptococcus pyogenes* may lead to an outbreak of acute glomerulonephritis (Dieng et al., 1998).

The parasite

The female of the mite *Sarcoptes scabiei* is fertilized in a small burrow: she then enlarges the burrow and extends it deeper into the epidermis. She lays 40–50 eggs along the way in a 4–6 weeks lifetime. The larva emerges from the egg after 3–4 days, escapes from the burrow by cutting through the roof and then cuts a small burrow and transforms into a nymph. The nymphs later become males and females which can be found all over the body and can be shed. These nymphs are probably responsible for the transmission of the infection. They mate on the new host and copulate in the small burrow made by the female.

Clinical features

The burrow can be found between the fingers, on the side of the hands, the inside of the wrist, around the waist band of trousers, around and in the cleft of the buttocks and on the male genitals. In babies 'and infants' hands and feet, palm and soles are often involved. In adults, persisting itchy papules may be found on the scrotum, umbilicus, axillae and buttocks. A KOH preparation may show the mite and/or the eggs.

Treatment

- The first and most important principle is to treat everyone in contact with the index case at the same time.
- Apply benzylbenzoate 25 per cent emulsion externally especially in infants and children. Other agents include 1 per cent gamma benzene hexachloride (Lindane) cream, a 5 per cent permethrin cream or emulsion, 0.5 per cent malathion or 10–20 per cent sulphur precipitates. They should be applied daily all over the body from neck to the soles, left on for about 10–12 hours and then washed off. Sulphur precipitates are needed for 2 weeks.
- It is advisable to re-treat everyone involved again after 1 week.
- Clothes and bedding should not be used for 48 hours or preferably hot washed or aired. The mites and nymphs do not survive a longer period without 'food'.
- Post-scabetic itch may continue for weeks. If it is very bad, antihistamines and steroids may be needed.

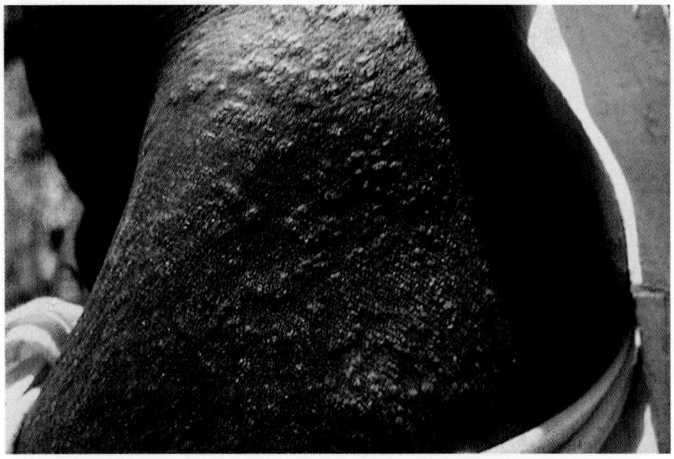

Fig. 93.25. Norwegian or crusted scabies in HIV (courtesy of archives Dr D. L. Leiker).

Norwegian or crusted scabies

Norwegian scabies was described in leprosy patients in Norway in the middle of the nineteenth century. The mite population is enormous and may number hundreds of thousands. In a normal infection usually not more than 12 mites are counted! The whole skin from scalp to soles is involved. The grossly thickened corneal layer is honeycombed with cavities (Fig. 93.25). It may look like a severe erythrodermic psoriasis or eczema, and is often diagnosed as such. It was very rare and was only seen in leprosy patients or severely debilitated patients until the era of HIV/AIDS: it is now frequently seen in HIV-positive patients, when it is often superinfected with pyogenic bacteria. These patients are very infectious!

Treatment

Ivermectin by mouth with sulphur ointment topically.

Papular urticaria

This condition is frequently confused with scabies. The patient is covered with small itchy papules (Fig. 93.26). It

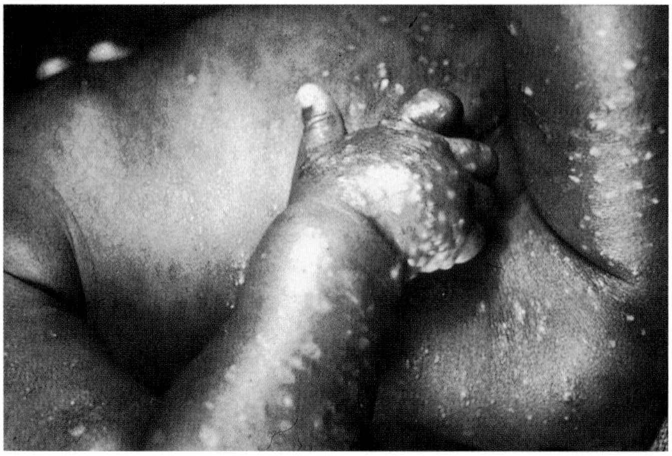

Fig. 93.26. Papular urticaria (courtesy of Dr D. Verhagen).

is a hypersensitivity reaction to insects and is often seen in atopic patients. It can be distinguished from scabies since the patient is the only one in the family with the condition. It is common in atopic families. Treatment consists of antihistamines orally and steroids topically.

Jiggers

Tungiasis, jiggers, is caused by the fertilized female sand-flea (*Tunga penetrans*). After copulation the flea attaches to the skin and penetrates within 5–10 minutes. In the skin she hatches and produces eggs. When the eggs mature, a terrible itch starts and a black dot with surrounding horn can be seen. The areas most involved are the side of the foot, between the toes, under the nails and the area between the toes and the foot sole. When the eggs are 'ripe', the insect can be removed by expression using a needle or a curette. Secondary infection may occur. Since the insect can only jump 1–2 cm, even the use of thick-soled sandals prevents the problem.

Creeping eruption

Larva migrans

Clinical features

The ova of the dog or cat hookworm are deposited in faeces on the soil and under favourable conditions they hatch into infectious larvae that can penetrate the exposed skin (buttocks, feet and hands). Sometimes, the eggs are transferred with clothes or towels.

In the initial phase larva migrans is just an urticarial lesion and can easily be missed. But when the larva (dog or cat hookworms, *Acylostoma caninum* or *A. braziliensis*) starts to migrate and tries to enter the dermis, the characteristic lesion can be seen. As the larva is in the wrong host, it misses the necessary adhesion molecules and enzymes and is confined to the deep epidermis because it is not able to penetrate any deeper. The creeping worm causes a 1–4 mm wide thread-like lesion. The lesions form a bizarre serpentine pattern (Fig. 93.27). Sometimes, the urticarial lesions are obscured by scratch marks.

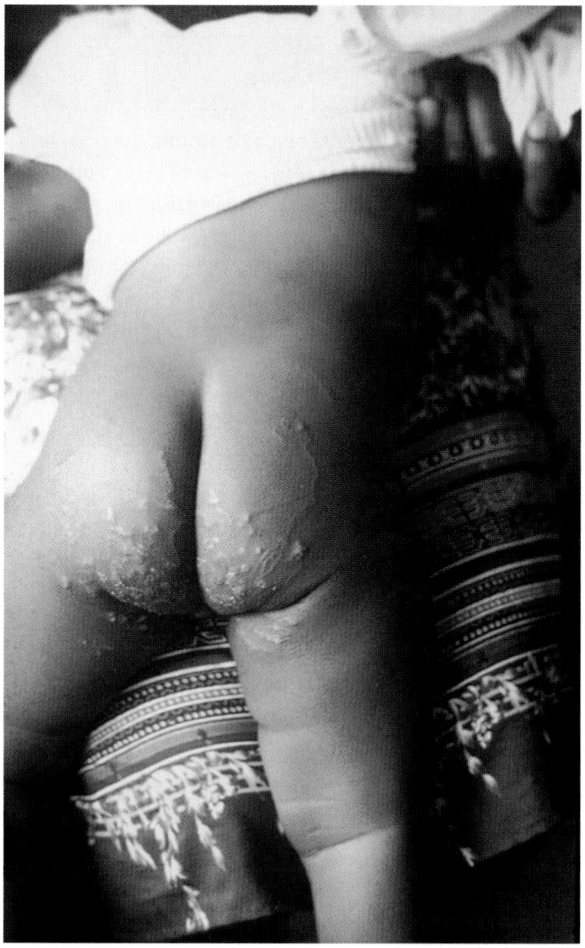

Fig. 93.27. Larva migrans in an infant.

Treatment

Topical 15 per cent thiabendazole cream or oral albendazole or ivermectin.

Larva currens

The larvae of *Strongyloides stercoralis* cause larva currens. They originate from the gut and enter the perianal skin and migrate till they find a blood vessel to enter. The lesion is more or less a straight line and is itchy: it is central – trunk, shoulders, buttocks and thighs. The lesion is shorter and wider than that of the hookworm, and the migration is faster. It can be treated with thiabendazole, albendazole or ivermectin. Repeated courses of treatment may be needed since the adult worms are often not killed (p. 393).

Myiasis

The Tumbu or Putzi fly (*Cordylobia anthropophagus*) may lay its eggs on freshly washed clothes. When the clothes are put on, the larva hatches and penetrates the skin, where it produces an inflamed nodule, which looks like a furuncle but is less painful and may itch. The maggot can often be seen moving. Attempts can be made to extract the maggot.

Treatment

Close the pore of the lesion with vaseline and the larva comes out; alternatively, surgical excision can be undertaken.

Loiasis

The transient non-pitting oedematous areas, which are neither painful nor itchy, are described in Chapter 27.

Dracunculiasis

Guineaworm is described in chapter 29: it may cause itching in people in endemic areas who are infected.

Onchocerciasis (Chapter 28)

Onchocerca volvulus, may cause severe itching, years after the initial infection. At the earliest, between 6 months and 2 years, the patient presents with a severe generalized itch and may initially only show a few erythematous hyperpigmented papules and scratch marks. Microfilariae in a skin-snip settles the diagnosis.

Lymphatic filariasis (Chapter 31)

The presenting features of mild lymphangitis and lymphadenitis may be thought to be due to a skin infection, particularly if there is swelling of a limb, but examination of a night blood film should settle the filarial cause.

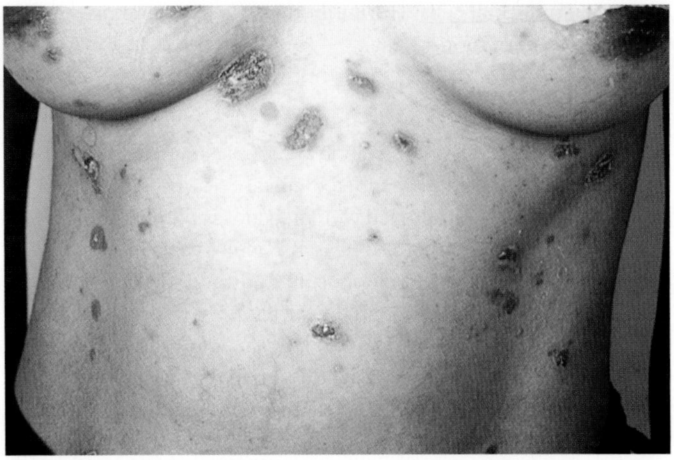

Fig. 93.28. Pemphigus vulgaris (courtesy of Dijkzigt Rotterdam).

Bullous diseases

In these diseases the patient makes antibodies against their own antigenic determinants as a result of internal (malignancies) or external factors (bacteria, drugs) as triggers. The dominant clinical features depend on the site of the involved antigens. These are difficult conditions and are best managed in specialized centres.

Pemphigus vulgaris

Pemphigus vulgaris (Fig. 93.28) is fatal if left untreated. Even with treatment the mortality may be as high as 20 per cent and treatment is often the cause of death.

Pathogenesis

The blisters are located in the lower and middle region of the epidermis. The blister is the result of separation of the epidermal cells, the cohesion is lost.

Clinical features

In 50–70 per cent of patients the first symptoms are blisters and erosions in the mouth and/or genitals. Later the blisters appear all over the body. The blisters are flaccid and when pressed upon enlarge. The roof can easily be rubbed off (Nikolsky sign). A scraping from the erosion shows acantholytic (rounded individual epidermal cells) cells (Tzank test).

Diagnosis

Sophisticated immunohistopathology is needed to demonstrate antibodies in the epidermis of the patients: antibodies from the serum may react with epidermal cells. The antibodies can also be shown in Western blot.

Treatment

Consists of prednisolone at first in a high dosage of 120–180 mg to be tapered off very slowly. The pulse treatment approach with megadoses of methylprednisolon or betamethasone is also effective. Azathioprine can be added. Cyclophosphamide and methotrexate are also used, though the latter may give problems and probably is not very useful. Oral and intramuscular gold have also been tried in addition to the steroids, with some effect. Treatment is prolonged and should only be done in referral centres.

Pemphigus foliaceus and pemphigus erythematosus

In these diseases, which are relatively common in Africa, the blistering is high in the epidermis, in the stratum granulosum or just beneath the stratum corneum, where antibodies can be demonstrated by immunohistopathological studies and immunoblotting. The antibodies are mostly directed against a 160 kDa desmosomal cadherin, desmoglein-1. Complement probably is not involved but most likely proteases are.

Pemphigus foliaceus is less severe than pemphigus vulgaris. As the blisters are very superficial, they are not often seen and leave well-demarcated crusted erosions. The erosion may be painful and extensive; eventually the patient may become 'erythrodermic'. The misdiagnosis of erythrodermic psoriasis may be made.

Pemphigus erythematodes (Senear – Usher) is a variant of pemphigus foliaceus having the lesions mostly on the sun-exposed areas (Fig. 93.29). Patients have immunological features of both pemphigus foliaceus as well as lupus erythematosus, e.g. granular IgG and C_3 at the basement membrane and intercellular IgG high in the epidermis.

Both diseases are sometimes misdiagnosed as impetigo or seborrhoeic dermatitis.

Treatment

Consists of potent topical steroids (clobetasol-propionate) or prednisolone in a dosage of 20–40 mg/day. Azathioprine, cyclophosphamide or methotrexate can be used as additives. Also hydroxychloroquine has been claimed to be effective in pemphigus erythematosus. Dapsone has also been used successfully. Treatment of the more severe cases should be done in referral centres.

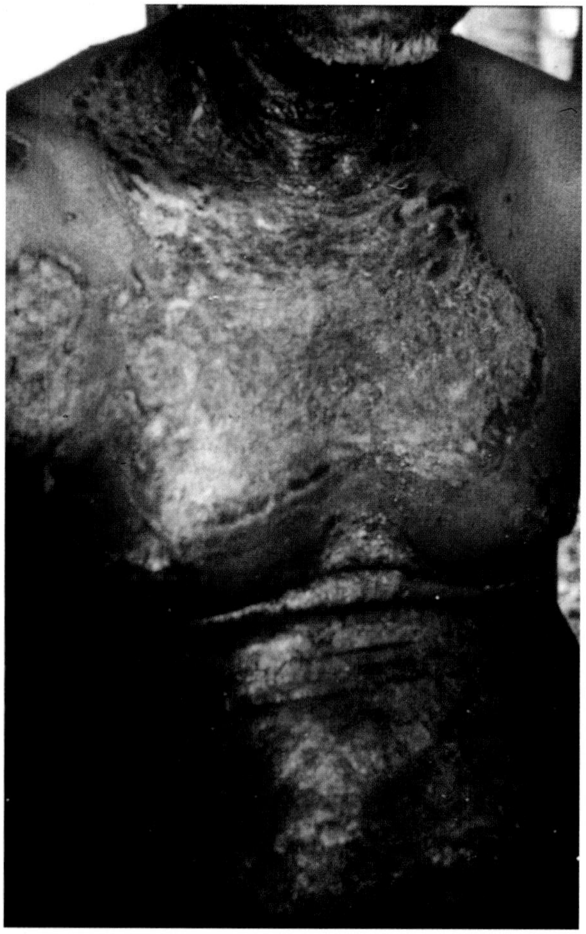

Fig. 93.29. Pemphigus erythematodes (courtesy of Dr P. de Koning).

Bullous pemphigoid

The group of patients with subepidermal blistering is heterogenous.

Pathogenesis

The antibodies are usually IgG, though IgM and IgA are also described. They are found in a line along the basal membrane. Only the IgG antibodies fix complement. Different antigens characterized by their molecular weight have been described, the major one being BP230 and BP180 kDa which seem to be associated with the hemidesmosomes. Lysosomal enzymes from eosinophils may be important for blister formation, as may complement in some patients.

Clinical features

The patients are usually elderly, so that some consider it as a paraneoplastic disease. Generally it starts with an itchy non-specific rash which may be urticarial or eczematous. Later, dome-shaped blisters appear, which are tense and not easily broken. The Nikolsky sign is negative. The blister may appear on erythematous or hyperpigmented areas as well as in clinically normal skin.

Untreated, the disease runs a chronic self-limiting course, the duration in average between 3 and 6 years, however it may be only months. When extended, it may be fatal for the elderly patient.

Treatment

Prednisolone (dosage 60 mg or even less and can be tapered off to 20–40 mg reasonably quickly) with or without adjuvant (azathioprin or cyclophosphamide). In some patients erythomycine or tetracyclines, with or without nicotinamide, have been shown to be effective, as has methotrexate. When IgA is the predominant type of antibody present, dapsone, sulphapyridine or sulphamethoxypyridine may be extremely effective; when IgM is present, thalidomide. Mortality is often treatment related. It can be treated at peripheral level but a specialist treatment is preferable.

Chronic benign bullous disease of childhood

Juvenile dermatitis herpetiformis (syn. chronic benign bullous disease of childhood) is a linear IgA disease (IgA antibody along the basal membrane). This is common in Africa but rare in Europe. The disease again is heterogeneous; antigens described are 285 kDa and 97/120 kDa. These antigens are involved in the anchoring of the epidermis to the dermis (anchoring fibres).

Clinical features

Most of the afflicted are toddlers and pre-school children. The onset is usually acute and the disease may have remissions and exacerbations. Symptoms vary from mild itch to severe burning. In young children the face and genital areas are often involved (Fig. 93.30).

The lesions are erythematous hyperpigmented papules and plaques, annular or polycyclic, arranged with blistering around the edges. New lesions form around the old lesions and thus give the 'strings of pearls' sign. Mucosal involvement is common. The disease is often mistaken for a bullous impetigo.

Treatment

Dapsone is the treatment of choice but sulphamethoxypyridine and sulphapyridine can also be used. Success also has been claimed for erythromycin and tetracycline with or without nicotinamide. In a few patients steroids or azathioprine or cyclosporin is needed.

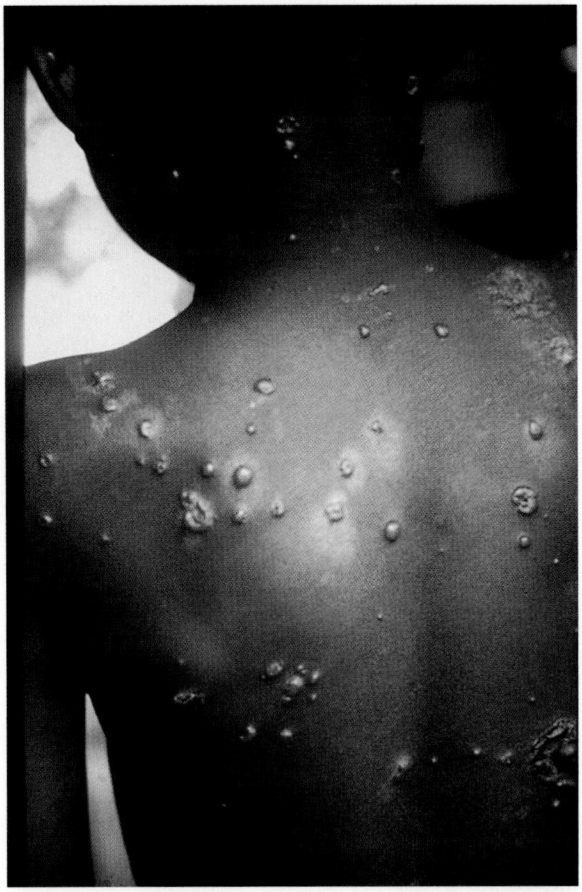

Fig. 93.30. Chronic benign bullous disease of childhood (courtesy of archives Dr D. L. Leiker).

Dermatitis herpetiformis

Dermatitis herpetiformis is well recognized in Africa. The bullae, vesicles, are located in the dermal papillae. A variety of auto-antibodies have been found but antibodies against gluten are nearly always present. The antigen in the skin is not yet identified. Direct immunopathology is always positive, showing granular deposits of IgA in the papillae (Hall, 1992).

Clinical features

The patient has a very severe itching rash which is pleomorphic and may show erythema, hyperpigmentation, urticaria, vesiculae and bullae, often with excoriation and other signs of scratching. The typical lesions are

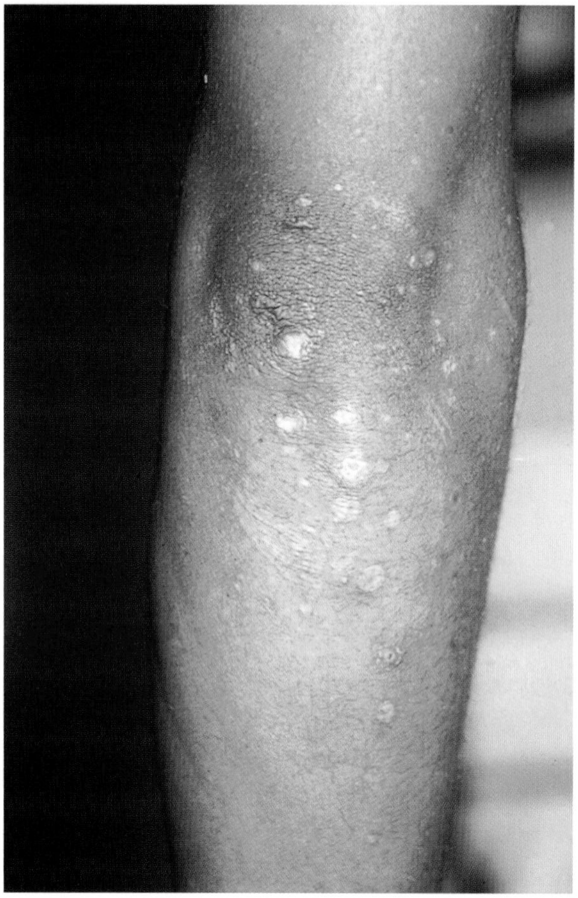

Fig. 93.31. Dermatitis herpetiformis.

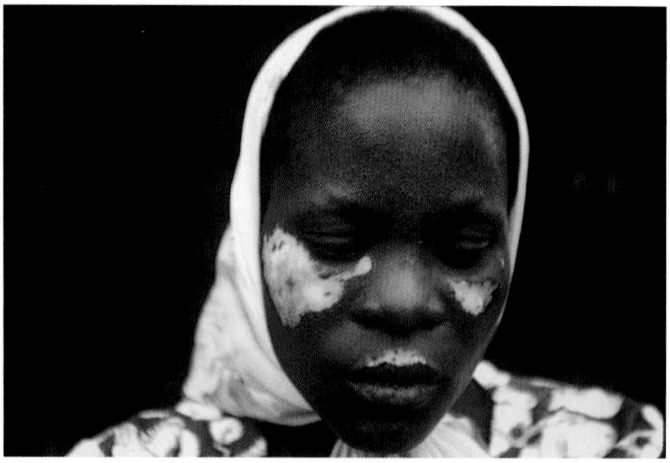

Fig. 93.32. Chronic discoid lupus erythematosus.

herpetiform (grouped) arranged vesicles. The distribution of the lesions is characteristically the extensor sides of the limbs, elbows and knees, the lower back, buttocks, natal cleft and in the nape of the neck. A gluten sensitive enteropathy may be associated (Fig. 93.31).

Treatment

Give dapsone or sulphonamides. Strong topical steroid treatment may also be of help. A gluten-free diet is very effective if it is consistently taken (Leonard & Fry, 1991).

CONNECTIVE TISSUE DISORDERS

Lupus erythematosus

Chronic discoid lupus erythematosus

CDLE is common in Africa and can appear at any age. It is an autoimmune disease in which antibodies against DNA seem to be involved and complement is activated. This causes damage to blood vessels and the dermal–epidermal junction, and secondarily to the epidermis. Immunopathology shows deposition of immunoglobulins and complement along the basal membrane (lupus band) and around blood vessels.

Clinical features (Fig. 93.32)

Lesions are in sun-exposed areas – forehead, nose and cheeks (butterfly pattern), chest and back and extensor surfaces of the arms. They are scaly with follicular plugging and atrophic with hyper- and depigmentation. In lighter skinned patients erythema can be seen and alopecia follows lesions on the head. SLE may develop in from 2–20 per cent. The lesions heal with scarring.

Treatment

Protection from the sun is most important. Topical or intralesional steroids may be helpful, but many patients may need systemic treatment: anti-malarials are most effective, especially hydroxychloroquine or chloroquine in a dose of 200 mg daily or higher. If this fails, dapsone may be added. Cyclophosphamide, methotrexate and azathioprine have also been shown to be effective as has oral prednisolone (Callen 2002).

Systemic lupus erythematosus

SLE in Africa seldom presents as a skin problem – butterfly hyperpigmentation with some depigmentation on

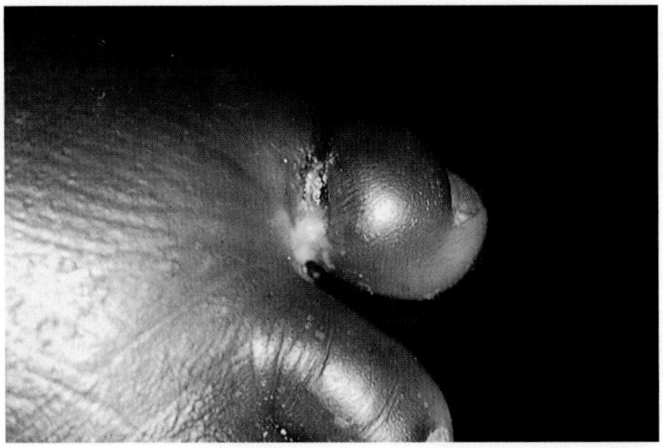

Fig. 93.33. Ainhum courtesy of Dr D. Bruynzeel).

nose and cheeks with a 'mottled' skin on sun-exposed areas. Skin changes due to vasculitis, can be found on the fingers (p. 1087).

Scleroderma

Sclerosis of the skin is seen as a manifestation of morphoea, systemic or acrosclerosis, lichen sclerosis et atrophicans and mixed connective tissue disease.

Morphoea

Morphoea is a circumscribed scleroderma; the dermis is markedly thickened with collagen, there are few recognizable fibroblasts.

Systemic sclerosis

SS is characterized by atrophy and sclerosis of the skin.

Ainhum

A sclerotic band develops around the base of the little toes and leads to spontaneous amputation. Rarely other toes or fingers are involved. The only treatment is to finish the spontaneously started amputation either with a ligature which is gradually tightened or by surgery (Fig. 93.33).

Lichen planus

Lichen planus is common in Africa. Its aetiology is unknown but it may be related to viral infection which others doubt (Daramola et al., 2002). Some may also look lichenoid. It is an immune-mediated disease, with a typical histopathological pattern, a so-called lichenoid infiltrate, a lymphohistiocytic cell infiltrate parallel to the epidermis, with a straight lower border.

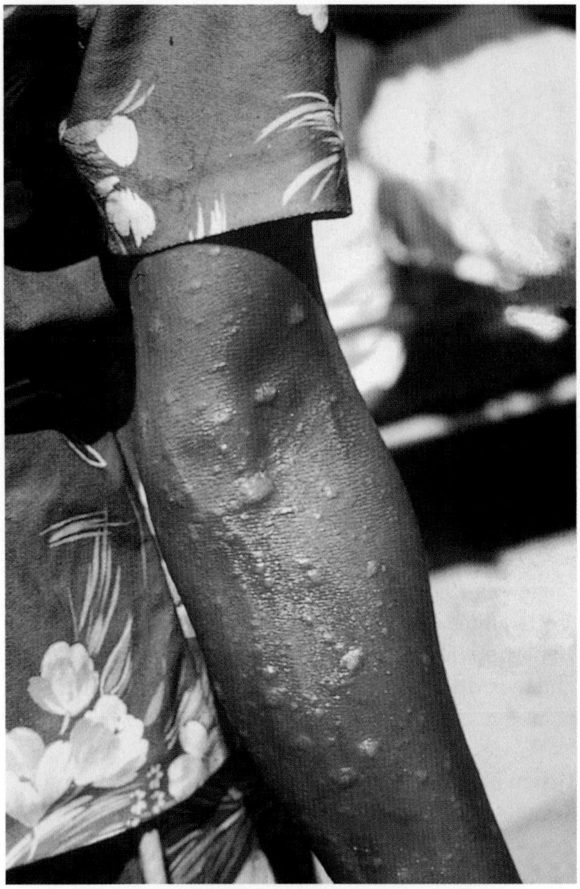

Fig. 93.34. Lichen planus (Wickham's striae).

Clinical features

- The onset may be gradual or abrupt, and
- Itching may be extreme, but the lesions are hardly ever excoriated because the patients usually rub them.The classical lesion is a polygonal flat papule, 2–4 mm across, violaceous in colour. When oil is applied, small white lines become visible (Wickham's striae) (Fig. 93.34).
- When the skin is scratched, new lesions may appear (Köbner phenomenon). The lesions may be grouped.
- The distribution is symmetrical: typically the flexor sides of the wrists, the ankles and the lower back are involved, but no part of the body is exempt. Nails may be affected as well as palms and soles.
- The mucous membranes, particularly in the mouth, are affected and show a reticular pattern of thin white lines with or without focal ulceration. This is seen less in Africa than it is in Europe.

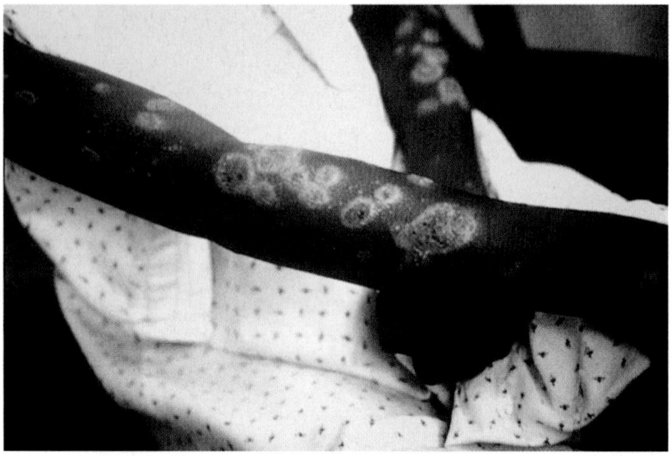

Fig. 93.35. Lichen planus actinicus.

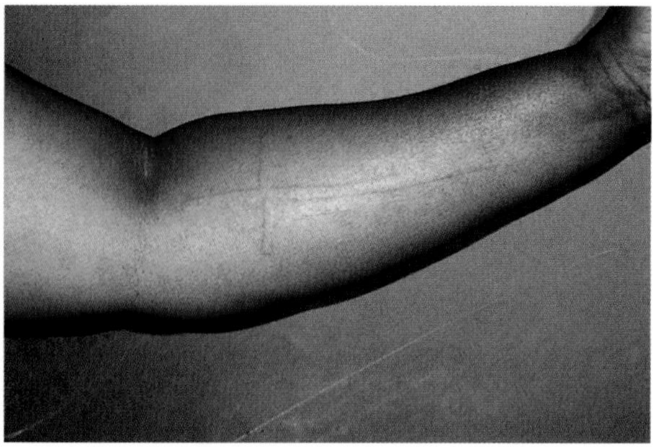

Fig. 93.36. Urticaria after scratching.

- Attacks may continue for weeks, months even years. In a few cases there may be associated liver damage (Daramola et al., 2002).

Hypertrophic lichen planus. This term describes warty and hypertrophic lesions on the lower legs, it is relatively common.

Lichen planus actinicus

Common in Africa, this is typicallly a rounded macula with hyper-pigmentation, often slightly blueish in the centre, surrounded by a hypo-pigmented ring. Frequently, the lesions are mistaken for DLE, because they are not only similar but also located on sun-exposed areas (Fig. 93.35).

Treatment

The condition is resistant to treatment, although corticosteroids orally or topically may alleviate itching. Retinoids and cyclosporin have given some relief for mucosal ulceration. In most cases the disease is self-limiting.

Urticaria

In urticaria (nettle rash, hives) transient itchy weals from half to several centimetres across appear suddenly. They may last for 20 minutes to several hours.

Pathogenesis

The weal is formed by dermal oedema, secondary to an increased permeability of venules and capillaries in response to histamine release and the release of other vaso-active products from mast cells or basophils. The same processes may occur in deeper tissues and then give rise to so-called angio-neurotic oedema.

Classification

Urticaria is traditionally divided into acute, less than 3 months, and chronic. Another classification is related to the triggering factor: physical (urticaria factitia) and cholinergic (exercise, sweating), contact or immune complex mediated.

Acute urticaria

They may be due to a classical type-1 Gell and Coombs hypersensitivity reaction. The antigen is bound to the IgE molecules on the mast cells, which then degranulate. Common antigens are cow's milk, soya, peanuts, fish, egg, penicillins or barbiturates.

Non-allergic mechanisms are also involved and include pseudo-allergy. Traditional medications, NSAIDs (aspirin) and codeine may also lead to mast cell degranulation. Some foods may contain histamine-like vaso-active amines, for example pineapple, fish, meat and blue cheese. Urticaria may be associated with acute intestinal symptoms, vomiting, diarrhoea or serum sickness and anaphylaxis. An attack usually responds to antihistamines.

Chronic urticaria

Lesions may continue to appear for months or years. No definite cause can be found in over 75 per cent of these patients. It may be aggravated by histamine-releasing agents. Rarely, a cancer, systemic illness or a parasitic infection of the gut is responsible.

Physical urticarial lesions that appear after scratching (dermographism) (Fig. 93.36) are sometimes encountered in HIV-infected patients; others are brought upon by heat, cold or even sunlight. Cholinergic urticaria accompanies exercise and sweating. These urticarial lesions are less than 1 cm across and flat, nearly macules. They are thought to be due to the histamine released from mast cells by the acetylcholine from the sympathetic nerve endings.

Treatment

Always look for an underlying cause as avoidance is curative. Careful diary keeping by the patient is more helpful then extensive investigations. Antihistamines relieve itching and swelling. Promethazine and dexchlorofeniramine block not only H1-histamine receptors but some actions of other mediators as well. For urticaria factitia (dermographism) a combination of an H1 (commonly used antihistamines) and an H2 blocker such as cimetidine or ranitidine is most effective.

Drug eruptions

Drug eruptions are common and can occur following orthodox as well as traditional medication.

Pathogenesis

This is broad, from well-understood type I–IV hypersensitivity to poorly understood lichen planus inducing response and fixed drug eruptions. The term drug eruption is really a misnomer.

Drug eruptions and HIV

Since the emergence of HIV, the number of drug eruptions has increased dramatically. The immune system of the HIV patients is in imbalance and hardly any patient escapes an eruption. For example severe Stevens Johnson syndrome, or TEN (toxic epidermal necrolysis) for which thiacetazone, cotrimoxazole, fansidar and anti-epileptics are chiefly responsible, but any drug may cause this reaction.

Clinical features

- Suspect a drug eruption when a previously 'healthy' person develops a more or less symmetrical skin eruption. If food or any other common cause can be excluded, a drug eruption due to medication may be diagnosed.

Any drug eruption may mimic any skin disease from an exantheme, eczema, hand and foot vesicular eczema (pompholyx), exfoliative dermatitis, psoriatiform, lichenoid or acneiform eruptions, urticaria, purpura, photosensitivity or fixed drug eruption, to erythema multiforme or Stevens Johnson syndrome, to TEN.

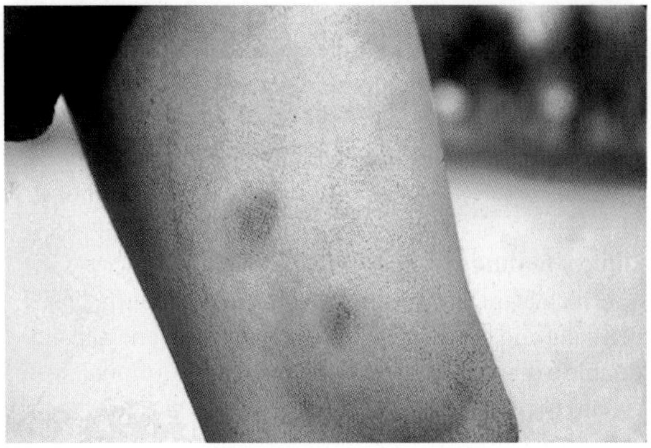

Fig. 93.37. Fixed drug eruption.

Fixed drug eruption

This is a common problem in Africa. At first, erythematous or mildly hyper-pigmented rounded macules, with or without temporary blisters, appear: later, the macules become deep blue-black pigmented (Fig. 93.37).

Each contact with the causative agent results in new activity and more lesions. Usually 2–3 lesions are present when the patient presents in the clinic.

Causes

Fixed drug eruptions may be caused by phenolphthalein in traditional medicines, chloroquine, dapsone and tetracycline, but mineral drinks like tonic water may also be responsible.

Erythema multiforme

In the past, erythema multiforme was thought to be the typical drug eruption. However, now it is known to follow other events, for example herpes infections, vaccinations and bacterial or fungal infections. Traditional medicines, sulphonamides, barbiturates and salicylates may also be responsible.

Clinical features

Papules or round macules, up to 2–3 cm in diameter with or without concentric rings (target lesions), but usually with a hyper-pigmented centre, sometimes with a central blister, appear on the hands and feet especially on palms and soles, knees and elbows, or anywhere on the body, including the genitalia, lips and buccal mucosae.

Stevens Johnson Syndrome

Is the most severe variety of erythema multiforme. The syndrome became common in patients co-infected with HIV and tuberculosis who were treated with thiacetazone, until the association with thiacetazone was identified.

Clinical features

Specifically the mucosae are involved, the mouth, lips, genitalia and eyes. The patient usually is severely ill and unable to eat or drink. The degree of constitutional upset is hard to predict.

Treatment

This consists of withholding the causative agent and general supportive care. Massive and long-term steroids have not been shown to be of benefit, but, if given immediately and only for a short period of time (one week), steroids may improve the prognosis.

- Always refer such patients to a tertiary centre.

Toxic epidermal necrolysis

TEN results in a full thickness damage to the epidermis due to a hypersensitivity reaction of unknown mechanism, although some consider that the condition is within the same spectrum as Stevens Johnson syndrome (Fig. 93.38) (Pichler et al., 2002). The whole epidermis can be stripped off easily and leave erosions which may leak an enormous loss of proteins and electrolytes or become secondarily infected. There may be pulmonary oedema and kidney failure. The overall mortality is high.

Management

- Treat such patients in a tertiary care centre as burn patients, monitor electrolytes, prevent sepsis and minimize secondary infections by the use of silver sulphadiazine or honey.
- Treat infections quickly and carefully.
- Take great care of pressure areas of skin to prevent bed sores.

Steroids may be of benefit but supportive care and withdrawal of the trigger is the key (Criton et al., 1997).

Erythema nodosum

Drugs such as oral contraceptives or sulphonamides may cause erythema nodosum. It is frequently seen in combination with a streptococcal throat infection, a *Yersinia* infection, tuberculosis or, much more rarely in Africa, sarcoidosis. Histopathologically, it is a vasculitis with septal panniculitis.

Clinical features

Tender shiny erythematous hyper-pigmented cutaneous and subcutaneous nodules and plaques, that are often easier palpated than seen, appear typically on the lower legs, especially the shins, but may occur elsewhere. When they subside they leave hyperpigmentation and scaling. Sometimes, there is an arthralgia.

Treatment

If the cause is evident, give specific treatment and alleviate symptoms with NSAIDs or dapsone.

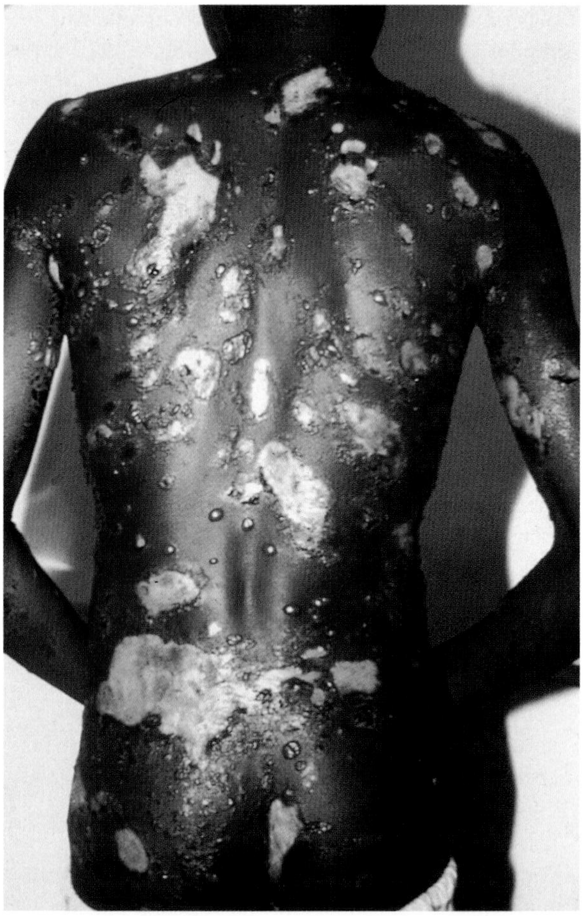

Fig. 93.38. Toxic epidermal necrolysis (courtesy of Dr C. van Hees).

Other immunologically mediated diseases

Vitiligo

Macules of altered pigmentation appear, which vary from white to light brown, sometimes tri-chromic. The macules often start around the orifices: anus, genitalia, mouth and eyes, but also around the umbilicus, in the axillae and groins. However, the whole skin may be involved. A Köbner phenomenon may be present. In some patients it is segmental.

Cutaneous sensation is normal, this distinguishes the lesions from leprosy.

Management

Topical steroids may induce repigmentation. This repigmentation starts at the border and from the remaining melanocytes in the follicles. Narrow band UVB (TL01, 311 nm) and RUVA may have some effect. It is necessary to protect the vitiliginous areas against sun damage.

Alopecia areata

This is an autoimmune disease.

Clinical features

Rounded patches of baldness are characteristic. The patches are shiny and hair follicles are still present. At the border, the hairs can easily be pulled out. 'Exclamation mark' short hairs may be seen in patients with straight hair but usually not in patients with curly hair. The disease may have exacerbations and remissions. In most patients the lesions eventually heal. When one lesion heals, another may appear. Not only the scalp, but all body hair may be involved (universalis).

Treatment

Irritation with dithranol (cignolin) or, for instance, garlic, inducing of a contact allergy (diphencyprone), immunomodulators (cyclosporin) or suppression with intralesional triamcinolone. Or supra-potent topical steroids.

NB It may occur in early HIV disease.

Hereditary diseases

Genetic factors play a role in many dermatoses (psoriasis, atopic dermatitis).

Albinism

This is a recessive inherited disorder in which a normal number of melanocytes is present but fail to produce melanin. The skin is white with or without freckles, the hair is white or reddish, the irises pink or grey/blue.

The incidence of skin cancer is greatly increased, especially squamous cell carcinoma. Most patients die from these aggressive carcinomas.

Management

It is extremely important to start sun protection from birth. Clothes and hats are much more effective than sun protecting creams and lotions, which nevertheless should be used extensively (McBride & Leppard, 2002). Regular control is important and any pre-malignant or malignant lesions should be treated by means of cryosurgery, chemosurgery, electrosurgery or regular surgery.

Some patients have nystagmus due to lack of pigment in the retina.

Protect the eyes; ensure that albino children, who have bad eye sight, sit in the front of the class at school (Kagore & Lund, 1995).

Neurofibromatosis

In this condition, also called von Recklinghausen's disease, there are:

1. 'black coffee spots' in pigmented skin which are called 'café au lait' spots in white skin.
2. Nodules which may be thought to be leprosy. The nodules are soft, a small 'button-hole' can be felt underneath and there may be freckles in the axillae. The nodules are schwannoma. Usually, they are only a cosmetic problem but sometimes, when present on nerves, they may compromise the nerve and cause discomfort and pain. In such cases excision may be tried. The phenotype may vary between generations.

Ichthyosis

Ichthyosis (fish-like scaling) comprises a group of inherited disorders with abnormal keratinization. It also may be acquired (AIDS, malignancies).

Clinical features

Dominant ichthyosis, small scales over the trunk and extensor sides of the extremities, sparing the flexures.

Sex-linked; only males, widespread blackish persistent scaling.

Treatment

With emollients, containing salicylic acid or urea 5–10 per cent the quality of life can be improved. Treatment with systemic retinoids is very helpful in some forms, but is expensive and can only be done in a specialist unit.

Palmo-plantar hyperkeratosis

There are many different kinds: some are very common and may be mistaken for viral warts. For treatment keratolytic agents (20 per cent salicylic acid in vaseline) can be used with or without etretinate.

Dermatosis papulosis nigra

The most common skin condition in elderly Africans (20–30% over the age of 40) (Van Hees & Naafs, 2001). It is probably genetically determined.

Clinical features

Dark brown to black, pinpoint to grain sized, verruceus papules appear in the face, especially on the cheeks and temples, and in the neck (Fig. 93.39). The histopathology is that of a seborrhoeic wart, such as occurs in whites usually on the trunk. It is more common in women then in men.

Treatment

This is not necessary and usually not asked for. Careful cauterization or curetting is possible.

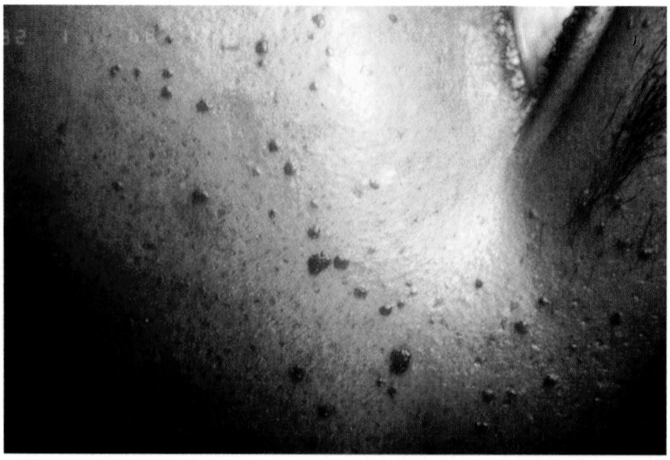

Fig. 93.39. Dermatitis papulosis nigra (courtesy of Dr W. Westerhof).

Malignancies

Malignancies of epidermal origin (see p. 1227) are relatively rare in the black skin (Amir et al., 1992; Yakubu & Mabogunje, 1995), because pigmentation protects against UV radiation.

Malignancies of the lymphocytic cell lines are no longer rare, lymphomas have increased in parallel with the HIV epidemic. The skin signs are discussed in this section.

Epidermal malignancies

BCC

Basal cell carcinoma (BCC), a malignancy of the basal cell line, is rare in the black skin, but is regularly seen in patients with albinism.

Clinical features

In the black skin it is a shiny black papule or a flat papule with a slim raised edge, which grows slowly over 4–5 years and may eventually ulcerate. It can be mistaken for a melanoma. In albinos the lesions are pearly papules with telangiectasia. They also ulcerate when they become larger. The superficial BCC may be scaly, minimal shiny erythematous plaques resembling Bowen's disease (an intra-epithelial SCC) or with nummular eczema.

Treatment

Surgical excision, cryotherapy, curettage and electrocoagulation. In patients with actinic damage regular inspection with cryotreatment of suspected lesions is advisable.

SCC

Squamous cell carcinoma SCCs are common in albinos (Lookingbill et al., 1995), patients with actinic cheilitis and xeroderma pigmentosum. Chronic ulceration may provide a cofactor for the development of a SCC particularly on the lower leg and on the feet following Price's dsease, but also at the margin of a tropical ulcer or other chronic ulceration due to burns or lupus vulgaris.

Clinical features

They are faster growing than BCCs and may present as hyperkeratotic sometimes fungating tumours with or without ulceration or as shiny oozing wet papules and nodules. When not treated early they may metastasize. The intra-epithelial Bowen's disease, a carcinoma in situ, is a slightly scaly black or erythematous macule that may look like nummular eczema but does not react on steroid treatment.

Treatment

Surgical, with radiotherapy as an alternative in specialized centres. Early lesions can be treated effectively with cryotherapy.

The *keratoacanthoma* is a self-healing benign tumour of squamous cell origin. It is a fast-growing slightly shiny nodule with a central keratotic plug. Histopathologically, it looks like a SCC. Although it may self-heal, excision surgically produces a more satisfactory outcome.

Malignant melanoma

This is a malignant growth of the melanocyte (Rampen, 1980; Hudson & Krige, 1995).

Clinical features

Rare in pigmented skin, they are usually on the soles of the feet where they may present as a black macule when superficially spreading, and blueish when growing deep. Sometimes a part or the entire tumour is amelanotic so that it may easily be confused with a SCC. Early diagnosis is essential to avoid metastases, which are found in lymph nodes, liver, lung and brain but may occur anywhere. If diagnosed early and treated immediately, the 5 years' survival is good.

Treatment consists of wide excision. When metastases have occurred, treatment is disappointing, even in specialized centres.

Lymphoma

Lymphomas are neoplasms derived from T- or B-lymphocytes. They are divided in two broad categories Hodgkin's and non-Hodgkin disease. The latter comprise the B-cell cutaneous lymphoma, the mantle cell lymphoma, hairy cell leukaemia, plasmacytoma and Burkitt's lymphoma (all B-cell derived) and the T-cell lymphomas, cutaneous adult T-cell lymphoma, lymphomatoid papulosis, mycosis fungoides (MF), angiocentric lymphoma, anaplastic lymphoma, granular lymphoma and different types of leukaemias (Getachew, 2001; Adelusola et al., 2001).

Hodgkin's disease

If it is found in the skin, it has probably spread from a lymph node.

Non-Hodgkin's disease

Mycosis fungoides

MF is the commonest of the cutaneous T-cell lymphomas. It is thought to consist of a monoclonal subset of T-cells with a specific affinity to the skin: a receptor for a subset of skin associated T-cells (HECA-452) has been identified (Hunger et al., 1999).

It has three stages:

(i) the pre-mycotic phase: non-specific hypo-pigmented macules, or itchy hyper-pigmented eczematous or psoriatiform patches.
(ii) the infiltrative phase: lesions become plaques, exfoliative dermatitis may occur.
(iii) the tumour phase: nodules and plaques which may ulcerate. This stage gives the tumour its name which comes from the mushroom like appearance (both mycosis and fungus stands for mushroom).

Specific manifestations of MF are poikiloderma atrophicans vasculare, a variant with a mottled increase and decrease in pigmentation in an atrophic skin and the Sezary Syndrome, an erythrodermic, hyper-pigmented exfoliative dermatitis with more than 10 per cent Sezary cells (hyper-diploid cells with multiple translocations) in the peripheral blood. These cells are not present in the epidermis but are found in lymphnodes.

The cause is unclear but it is thought to be due to a persistent specific antigenic stimulus with a resulting malignant clonal transformation. Environmental factors have been incriminated, but are not proven. Drugs can induce MF-like syndrome: anti-epileptics (phenytoin, carbamazepine), anti-depressants, NSAIDs, antihistamines, beta-blockers and ACE inhibitors.

The specialized treatment must be in expert hands.

Adult T-cell lymphoma

A lymphoma more prevalent in sub-Saharan Africa, the Caribbean and Japan than in the West is the adult T-cell lymphoma that is caused by the HTLV-1 or HTLV-2 virus, endemic in many regions of sub-Saharan Africa, belonging to the oncovirus group of the retroviruses. It is more prevalent in females than males and is horizontally sexually transmitted: 25 per cent of infants of mothers with the virus are infected vertically from breast milk. After infection it may manifest after a latent period of 20–40 years as a lymphoma in 1 of 80 infected. The role of the virus in the malignant transformation is still unclear.

Clinical features

Single or multiple erythematous or violaceous brown papules, nodules and plaques with or without purpera and ulceration are seen on the trunk > face > extremities. Sometimes, as in MF, poikiloderma is present.

Cutaneous B-cell lymphoma

A clonal proliferation of B-lymphocytes can be confined to the skin but more often is associated with systemic B-cell lymphoma. It is not as rare as originally thought. It seems to be associated with chronic antigenic stimulation, as in Lyme disease (*Borrelia burgdorferi*). It also occurs during immunosuppression and is therefore regularly found in HIV-infected patients. There is also a clear relationship with Epstein–Barr virus (EBV) infection. Neuroleptic drugs may induce a B-cell lymphoma. EBV induces especially the large cell B-cell lymphoma, which is more malignant than the follicular centre cell lymphoma that usually runs an indolent course.

Clinical features

It presents as erythematous hyperpigmented nodules and plaques with a smooth surface, which are firm and not tender.

Burkitt's lymphoma

This is extensively described elsewhere (p. 1218).

Sarcoma

Kaposi's sarcoma

Kaposi's sarcoma (KS) is at present one of the most common malignancies in Africa because it is related to immunosuppression in HIV infection; this is the epidemic KS. It is a tumour of the endothelium of the blood/lymphatic microvasculature, induced by a HSV VIII infection (Fouchard et al., 2000).

Classical KS has its peak after the sixth decade and occurs especially in males chiefly on the legs. It consists of blue–black firm nodules and plaques, which may ulcerate, the evolution is slow.

African endemic KS was common in East and Central Africa, and is still present (Gordon, 1967; Safai, 1984). In Congo, excluding epidemic KS, it constitutes 10 per cent of the malignancies (Bestetti et al., 2000).

Clinical features

Four different patterns are recognized:

1. The nodular type that resembles classic KS and runs a rather benign course in 5–8 years.
2. The florid or vegetating type, which is also nodular but extends deeper in the subcutis, muscle or bone. It is more aggressive.
3. The infiltrative type, which is aggressive with florid mucocutaneous and visceral involvement.
4. The lymphoadenopathic type, especially in children and young adults, which is found in lymph nodes and viscera and occasionally also in skin and mucous membranes.

Treatment

Classic KS responds well to radiotherapy, African endemic KS to systemic chemotherapy, but the response is usually only temporary. The treatment must be in experienced hands.

The epidemic KS is described on p. 1227.

Ulceration of the skin

Ulcers of the skin are very important in the tropics. They may be painful, itchy or nearly indolent and are usually secondary to insect bites or scratches, often on the legs, infected by *Streptococcus pyogenes* or *Stapylococcus aureus*. The lesions are generally shallow ulcerations with or without discharge, surrounded by painful erythema and swelling, and sometimes with satellite lesions.

Treatment with oral antibiotics (flucloxacillin) is often sufficient; however, topical bacteriostatic treatment may be helpful, honey has been found to be effective as are antiseptics. A steroid preparation added to an antibiotic or antiseptic treatment is often useful since, in persistent ulcerations especially those due to insect bites, allergic mechanisms play a role in maintaining the ulceration. When the lesions are present on the lower legs, anti-oedema therapy like non-elastic compression may help to speed up healing.

Tropical ulcer

A tropical ulcer is a phagedenic ulcer possibly caused by a necrotic reaction induced by anaerobic bacteria. Anaerobic fusobacteriae (*F. ulcerans*), together with *Treponema vincenti*, are thought to be the dominant responsible organisms (Adriaans & Drasar, 1987).

The problem in Africa

Disabling pain and an ulcer which refuses to heal may incapacitate farmers, particularly in areas where the legs are repeatedly damaged by Acacia thorns or thick vegetation: in the lowland savannah of western Ethiopia, the prevalence was over 7 per cent (Bulto et al., 1993). The age group 5–14 is however the dominant risk group (Tumwine et al., 1989).

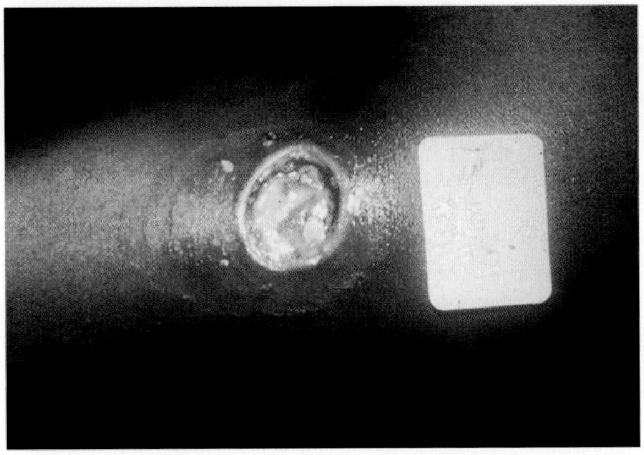

Fig. 93.40. Tropical ulcer (courtesy of Dr P. L. Niemel).

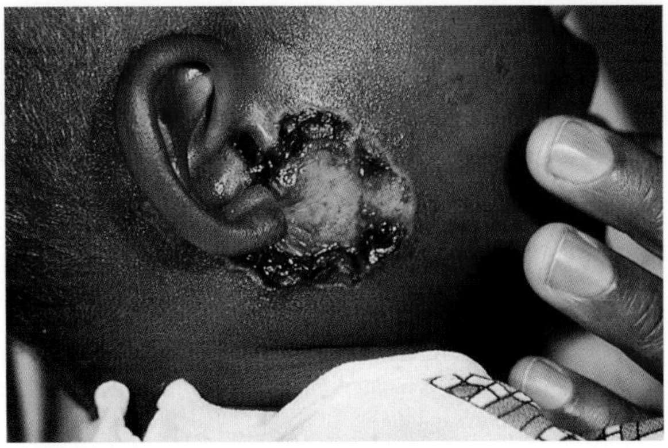

Fig. 93.41. HIV-related herpes simplex ulcer.

Tropical ulcers can be prevented if any small wound is immediately cleaned and dressed: there is no need for anything more. Secondary infection has to be prevented.

The economic burden can be great (p. 1301).

Clinical features

Ulcers may begin as a small papule or vesicle that may be haemorrhagic: this breaks down rapidly to form a sharply defined ulcer with a slightly indurated edge that is usually undermined (Fig. 93.40).

The floor of the ulcer is covered with a foul smelling purulent slough. Most lesions heal spontaneously but some may enlarge quickly.

Treatment

Debridement is essential if there is necrotic tissue. Local treatment is commonly adequate, keeping the ulcer clean and applying local antiseptics. If there are symptoms, oral or parenteral penicillins and/or metronidazole may be needed. Skin grafting may speed up the healing and has been successfully carried out in rural Uganda.

A Buruli ulcer may mimic a tropical ulcer. It is described below (p. 1301).

Diphtheria

In some children a diphtheria ulcer develops. This presents as a ragged ulcer with a clearly defined overhanging edge. The exudate from the ulcer tends to form a tough greyish or brownish adherent membrane. Regional lymph nodes enlarge. The lesions may persist for 2–3 months and then heal with some scarring. However, in HIV-infected persons ulcers may persist. As rates of triple vaccine coverage have fallen, diphtheritic ulcer is being seen more commonly again.

Children and HIV-infected individuals may have general symptoms and even neurological and cardiac manifestations. Treatment especially in children includes a specific antitoxin together with erythromycin and/or penicillin.

Venous leg ulcers

Venous leg ulcers were not common in Africa but as urban lifestyle changes more are being seen in cities. The cause, varicosities, venous stasis, interstitial oedema, capillaritis and vascular cuffing, is not different from that in North America and Europe. Local treatment has to be supplemented with prophylaxis, teaching exercises and non-elastic bandaging. Diuretics as a single measure are useless. Punch and pinch biopsies may accelerate the healing. After healing, elastic stockings or bandages may prevent recurrence.

HIV-related ulcerations

HIV-related ulcerations are common. All types of bacteria may be involved, staphylococci, streptococci, pseudomonas, proteus, *E.coli*, etc., but also candida. Important causes are persistent viral infections, herpes simplex but also the varicella zoster virus. They cause chronic ulceration in children, in adults too the lesions are often anogenital. Anti-viral therapy, when available, will be of great help (Fig. 93.41).

Other causes

Ulcers are also caused by deep mycoses, mycobacteria, spirochaetes and *Leishmania*: these are discussed elsewhere.

References

Adelusola KA, Adeniji KA, Somotun GO. (2001). Lymphoma in adult Nigerian. *W Afr J Med*; **20**: 123–126.

Adriaans B, Drasar BS. (1987). The isolation of fusobacteria from tropical ulcers. *Epidemiol Infect*; **99**: 361–372.

Amir H, Kwesigabo G, Hirji K. (1992). Comparative study of superficial cancer in Tanzania. *E Afr Med J*; **69**: 88–93.

Ayaya SO, Kumar KK, Kakar R. (2001). Aetiology of tinea capitis in school children. *E Afr Med J*; **78**: 531–535.

Bos JD, Kapsenberg ML. (1993). The skin immune system: progress in cutaneous biology. *Immunol Today*; **14**: 75–78.

Brockow K, Grabenhorst P, Abeck D et al. (1999). Effect of gentian violet, corticosteroids and tar preparations in Staphylococcus aureus colonized atopic eczema. *Dermatology*; **199**: 231–236.

Bulto T, Maskel FH, Fisseha G. (1993). Skin lesions in resettled and indigenous populations in Gambela with special emphasis on the epidemiology of tropical ulcer. *Ethiop Med J*; **31**: 75–82.

Canizaris O. (1982). Epidemiology and ecology of skin diseases in the tropics and the subtropics. In *A Manual of Dermatology for Developing Countries*, pp. 21–34. Oxford: Oxford University Press.

Criton S, Devi K, Sridevi PK, Asokan PU. (1997). Toxic epidermal necrolysis – a retrospective study. *Int J Dermatol*; **36**: 923–925.

Daramola OO, George AO, Ogunbigi AO. (2002). Hepatitis C and lichen planus in Nigerians: any relationship? *Int J Dermatol*; **41**: 217–219.

Del Giudici, Yves P. (2002). The widespread use of skin lightning creams in Senegal: a persistent public health problem in West Africa. *Int J Dermatol*; **41**: 137–139.

Dieng MT, Ndiaye B, Ndiaye AM. (1998). Scabies complicated by acute glomerulonephritis in children: 114 cases observed in two years in a pediatric service in Dakar. *Dakar Med*; **43**: 201–204.

Doe PT, Asiedu A, Acheapong JW, Rowland Payne CM. (2001). Skin diseases in Ghana and the UK. *Int J Dermatol*; **40**: 323–326.

Drago F, Malaguti F, Raneiri E, Losi E, Rebora A. (2002). Human herpes virus-like particles in pityriasis rosea lesions: an electron microscopy study. *J Cutan Pathol*; **29**: 359–361.

Etemesi E. (2001). Quality of life affected by skin diseases. M. Med. Dermat. Thesis Tumaini University Moshi Tanzania.

Faergemann J. (2000). Management of seborrhoic dermatitis and pityriasis versicolor. *Am J Clin Dermatol*; **1**: 75–80.

Figueroa JI, Fuller LC, Abraha A, Hay RJ. (1998). Dermatology in Southwestern Ethiopia: rational for a community approach. *Int J Dermatol*; **37**: 752–758.

Fouchard N, Lacoste V, Couppie P et al. (2000). Detection and genetic polymorphism of human herpes virus 8 in endemic or epidemic Kaposi's sarcoma from West and Central Africa, and South America. *Int J Cancer*; **85**: 166–170.

Getachew A. (2001). Malignant lymphoma in western Ethiopia. *E Afr Med J*; **78**: 402–404.

Gibbs S. (1996). Skin diseases and socioeconomic condition in rural Africa: Tanzania household dermatology. *Int J Dermatol*; **35**: 633–639.

Glenn MJ, Bennett RG, Kelly AP. (1995). Acne keloidalis nuchae: treatment with excision and second-intention healing. *J Am Acad Dermatol*; **33**: 243–246.

Gooskens V, Ponninghaus JM, Clayton Y, Mkandawire P, Sterne JA. (1994). Treatment of superficial mycosis in the tropics: Whifield's ointment versus clotrimazole. *Int J Dermatol*; **33**: 738–742.

Gordon JA. (1967). Kaposi's sarcoma: a review of 136 Rhodesian African cases. *Postgrad Med J*; **43**: 513–519.

Gowkrodger DJ. (1998). Racial influences on skin disease. In *Textbook of Dermatology*, 6th edn. ed. Rook, Wilkinson, Ebling, pp. 3239–3258. Oxford: Blackwell Science.

Hudson DA, Krige JE. (1995). Melanoma in black South Africans. *J Am Coll Surg*; **180**: 65–71.

Hunger RE, Yawalkar N, Braathen LR, Brand CU. (1999). The HECA-452 epitope is highly expressed on lymph cells derived from human skin. *Br J Dermatol*; **141**: 465–469.

Jacyk WK. (1999). Xeroderma pigmentosum in black South Africans. *Int J Dermatol*; **38**: 511–514.

Kagore F, Lund PM. (1995). Oculocutaneous albinism among schoolchildren in Harare Zimbabwe. *J Med Genet*; **32**: 859–861.

Kristense JK. (1991). Scabies and pyoderma in Lilonge Malawi. Prevalence and seasonal fluctuation. *Int J Dermatol*; **30**: 699–702.

Leonard JN, Fry L. (1991). Treatment and management of dermatitis herpetiformis. *Clin Dermatol*; **9**: 403–408.

Lookingbill DP, Lookingbill GL, Leppard BP. (1995). Actinic damages and skin cancer in albinos in Northern Tanzania, findings in 164 patients enrolled in an outreach skin care program. *J Am Acad Dermatol*; **32**: 653–658.

McBride SR, Leppard BJ. (2002). Attitudes and beliefs of an albino population towards sun avoidance: advice and services provided by an outreach albino clinic in Tanzania. *Arch Dermatol*; **138**: 629–632.

Machang'u RA, Mgode G, Gisakanyi N. (1997). Recurrent staphylococcal scalded skin syndrome in children, report of two cases. *E Afr Med J*; **74**: 603–604.

Mahe A, Cisse IAH, Faye O, N'Diaye HT, Niamba P. (1998). Skin diseases in Bamako (Mali). *Int J Dermatol*; **37**: 673–676.

Mason J, Mason AR, Cork MJ. (2002). Topical preparations for the treatment of psoriasis: a systematic review. *Br J Dermatol*; **146**: 351–364.

Mayanja B, Margan D, Ross A, Whitworth J. (1999). The burden of mucocutaneous conditions and association with HIV-I infection in a rural community in Uganda. *Trop Med Int Hlth*; **4**: 349–354.

Naafs B. (1993). Atopic dermatitis: a teaching article. *Memisa Med*; **59**: 123–137.

Naafs B. (2001). Health aspects of second hand footwear: comments of a dermatologist. *Memisa Med*; **67**: 88–89.

Naafs B, Matemera BO, Lyons NF, Ellis BPB. (1984). Diagnosis of leprosy. *Centr Afr J Med*; **30**: 86–90.

Naafs B, Matemera BO, Mudarikwa L, Noto S. (1986). Position paper to Ministry of Health, Harare, Zimbabwe.

Nyst MJ, Perriens JH, Kimputu L, Lumbila M, Nelson AM, Piot P.

(1992). Gentian violet, ketaconazole and nystatine in oropharyngeal and esophageal candidiasis in Zairian AIDS patients. *Ann Soc Belg Med Trop*; **72**: 45–52.

Onwuasoigwe O. (1999). Fluconazole in the therapy of multiple osteomyelitis in Africa histoplasmosis. *Int Orthop*; **23**: 82–84.

Palangyo KJ. (1992). Cutaneous findings associated with HIV disease including AIDS: experiences from Sub Saharan Africa. *Trop Doctor*; **1**: S35–S41.

Pichler WJ, Yawalkar N,Britschi M et al. (2002). Cellular and molecular pathophysiology of cutaneous drug reactions. *Am J.Clin Dermatol*; **3**: 229–238.

Rampen F. (1980). Melanoma in Africans. *Arch Dermatol*; **116**: 159–160.

Safai B. (1984). Kaposi's sarcoma: a review of the classical and epidemic form. *Ann NY Acad Sci*; **437**: 373–382.

Satimia FT, McBride SR, Leppard B. (1998). Prevalence of skin disease in rural Tanzania and factors influencing the choice of health care, modern or traditional. *Arch Dermatol*; **134**: 1363–1366.

Shibeshi D. (2000). Pattern of skin diseases at the University teaching hospital Addis Ababa, Ethiopia. *Int J Dermatol*; **39**: 822–825.

Shrum JP, Millikan LE, Batarneh O. (1994). Superficial fungal infection in the tropics. *Dermatol.Clin*; **12**: 687–693.

Smeller W, Dzikus A. (2001). Skin diseases in children in rural Kenya: long term result of a dermatology project within the primary health care system. *Br J Dermatol*; **144**: 118–124.

Soyinka F. (1978). Contact allergic dermatitis 'current topic in tropical dermatology'. *Niger Med J*; **8**: 518–525.

Stander S, Steinhof M. (2002). Pathophysiology of pruritus in atopic dermatitis: an overview. *Exp Dermatol*; **11**: 12–24.

Templeton AC, Viegas OAC. (1970). Racial variation in tumour incidence in Uganda. *Trop Geogr Med*; **22**: 431–438.

Thami GK, Sakar R. (2002). Coaltar: past present and future. *Clin Exp Dermatol*; **27**: 99–103.

Tumwine JK, Dungare PS, Tswana SA, Maoneke WR. (1989). Tropical ulcers in a remote area in Zimbabwe. *Centr Afr J Med*; **35**: 413–416.

Van Hees C, Naafs B. (2001). Eczema. In *Common Skin Diseases in Africa. An Illustrated Guide*, pp.11–21. Voorburg, The Netherlands: Troderma.

Van Hees C. (2000). *Common Skin Diseases in Zimbabwe*. Harare, Zimbabwe.

Yakubu A, Mabogunje OA. (1995). Skin cancer in Zaria Nigeria. *Trop Doct*; **25**: 63–67.

APPENDIX: BURULI ULCER

Buruli ulcer is a necrotizing and ulcerating infection of the skin and the sub-cutaneous fat, caused by *Mycobacterium ulcerans*. Buruli ulcer was named after *Buruli* county, East Mengo district in Uganda, where the disease was common among refugess near the Nile River (Clancey et al., 1961). Children between age 2 and 15 are predominantly affected in endemic areas.

The problem in Africa

Sir Albert Cook described a chronic necrotizing skin ulceration with undermined edges in patients in Uganda in 1897 (1970). The first scientific description of the ulcer and its causative micro-organism, an acid-fast bacillus which was successfully cultured at 32 °C, came from Australia in 1948 (MacCallum et al., 1948). The first report from the African continent dates from 1950 from the Congo (van Oye & Ballion, 1950). In Uganda, a large outbreak occurred among refugees settling near the Nile River (Barker, 1973). Later, patients were reported from Nigeria (Oluwasanmi et al., 1976), and several other West African countries: Cameroon, Gabon and Liberia were later followed by Burkina Faso, Togo and even one case from Angola. Increasing numbers of patients began to be reported from Ghana, Côte d'Ivoire, and Benin in the 1980s and 1990s (van der Werf et al., 1999). Although most researchers believe that this reflects a genuine increase of transmission of the disease, previous under-reporting might also be involved. Some patients with chronic necrotizing, non-healing ulcers may not attend hospital, or only attend dressing rooms of outpatient departments going undiagnosed, with hospital records mentioning 'chronic ulceration, poorly responding to therapy'.

The economic and social burden inflicted by Buruli ulcer disease on patients, their relatives, health budgets and hospitals is daunting (Asiedu & Etuaful, 1998).

Micro-organism

Mycobacterium ulcerans is an environmental mycobacterium that can be cultured on egg-yoke enriched media designed for culture of mycobacteria, e.g. Löwenstein–Jensen media. It does not grow at 37 °C but only at about 32 °C. In vitro growth is difficult and slow. Like all mycobacteria, it can be visualized microscopically after acid- and alcohol-fast staining. Carbol-fuchsin penetrates the thick outer layer which contains the typical lipid structures of mycobacteria. After washing with acid alcohol, the red stain is maintained within. After counterstaining, microscopy reveals red rods in tissue spcimens.

The micro-organism has never been cultured from the environment. With the aid of polymerase chain reaction (PCR) methods, which multiply one of two specific sequences (Stinear et al., 1999) of the genome of *M. ulcerans*, the micro-organism has recently been identified in the water from the environment where infections occurred in Australia (Ross et al., 1997). Genetically, the micro-organism is closely related to *M. tuberculosis*, and even closer to *M. marinum*, which causes fish tank granuloma, an ulcerative skin disease which occurs among swimmers and those who maintain aquariums (Stinear et al., 2000).

M. ulcerans has a unique potential to secrete one or more toxins (George et al., 1998, 1999), which probably cause the extensive vascular necrosis which is typical for Buruli ulcer. The chemical structure of at least one toxin has been elucidated: it appears to be poliketide: mycolactone (George et al., 1999), which blunts the response of TNF-α on a major transcription factor ($NF_{\kappa}B$) in the nucleus of immune cells (Pahlevan et al., 1999). Stimulation of $NF_{\kappa}B$ is an important mechanism in the defence against mycobacterial infection. The inhibition of mycolactone may therefore be important to understand why the local host immune defence is so poor (George et al., 1998).

Epidemiology

In Uganda, ulcers were observed in men after the harvest season; women, who performed farming activities throughout the year, had no seasonal incidence of Buruli ulcers (Revill & Barker, 1972). All of these farming activities were in swampy riverine areas, as has been observed in all other foci where Buruli ulcer is endemic (van der Werf et al., 1999; van Oye & Ballion, 1950).

Most ulcers develop at parts of the skin exposed to vegetation. In adults, most ulcers are seen on the left lower limb; in children, the right hand, as well as the head and neck region appear significantly affected (van der Werf et al., 1989). In Australia, people living near a golf course, that was sprinkled by water pumped from a swamp, developed Buruli ulcers. Water in the swamp was PCR-positive for *M. ulcerans*. Following drainage of the contaminated swamp, PCR-testing became negative, and in the following years, no new cases of Buruli ulcers were detected around the golf course (Veitch et al., 1997).

Mechanical protection helps to prevent Buruli ulcer. In Côte d'Ivoire, men wearing long pants were significantly protected compared to control subjects (Marston et al., 1995).

Transmission

All this evidence suggests that Buruli ulcer develops at sites of trauma to skin (Myers et al., 1974). *M. ulcerans* lives in or near stagnant water (Ross et al., 1997). Transmission is probably by penetrating injuries like thorn pricks, or insect bites, through the skin into the subcutaneous fat tissue, where the bacillus multiplies. *M. ulcerans* appears to be present in various wild animals (Portaels et al., 2001). Certain water insects – notably *Naucoridae*, that live in stagnant water appear to accumulate large number of *M. ulcerans* bacilli (Portaels et al., 1999) and recently, these insects have been shown to be able to transmit Buruli ulcer to experimental animals (Marsollier et al., 2002).

Clinical features

The early, pre-ulcerative lesion is a subcutaneous firm nodule (Fig. 93.42).

In the ulcerative (second) stage, typically undermined ulcer edges can be observed (see Fig. 93.43).

Spontaneous healing may occur after many months or years. Operative treatment helps to salvage affected tissues. Unfortunately, healing is often at the cost of residual impairment and loss of vital tissues and organs, such as an eye. Almost invariably, patients are left with disfiguring scars and considerable contractures in joints (Fig. 93.44).

Multiple synchronous and metachronous ulcers are common. In Benin, osteomyelitis by *M. ulcerans* has been reported (Josse et al., 1995). This suggests that *M. ulcerans* may spread through the blood stream. Multiple local infections might however also cause multiple skin ulcers, and local penetration to bone might explain osteomyelitis.

Diagnosis

In endemic areas, ulcers with undermined edges are easily recognized. Patients do not appear ill or febrile; they are not wasted or anaemic. Pre-ulcerative lesions are more difficult to recognize, and should be differentiated from trauma, insect- and snake bites, tropical ulcers, dracunculosis, onchocercoma, and lipoma. Occasionally, patients present with large pre-ulcerative plaque lesions that are indurated. If patients present with lage pre-ulcerative lesions, they may have systemic signs such as fever. Once the skin breaks down and ulcerates, surgical tissue specimens and smears from the slough or the edge of the ulcer may reveal acid-fast bacilli after Ziehl–Nielsen staining. Pathological examination shows necrosis and numerous acid-fast bacilli (see Fig. 93.45). Culture is difficult, and PCR tech-

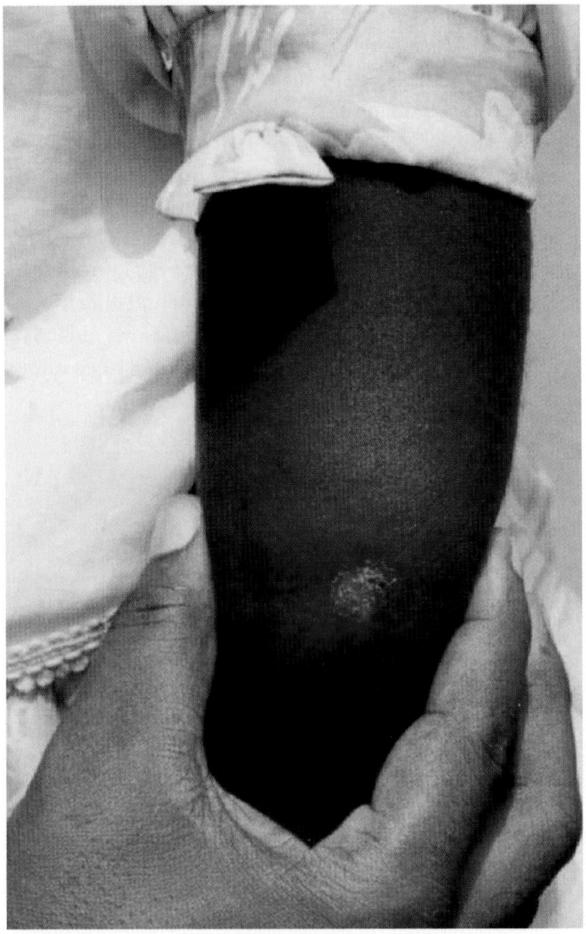

Fig. 93.42. Nodule (pre-ulcerative stage). Pre-ulcerative lesion of Buruli ulcer in a 5-year old girl. Nodulectomy helps to prevent late sequelae and ongoing ulceration. (Courtesy: Dr Kwame Asamoa, Director, Tuberculosis Surveillance Unit and National Buruli ulcer program, Ministry of Health, Accra, Ghana.)

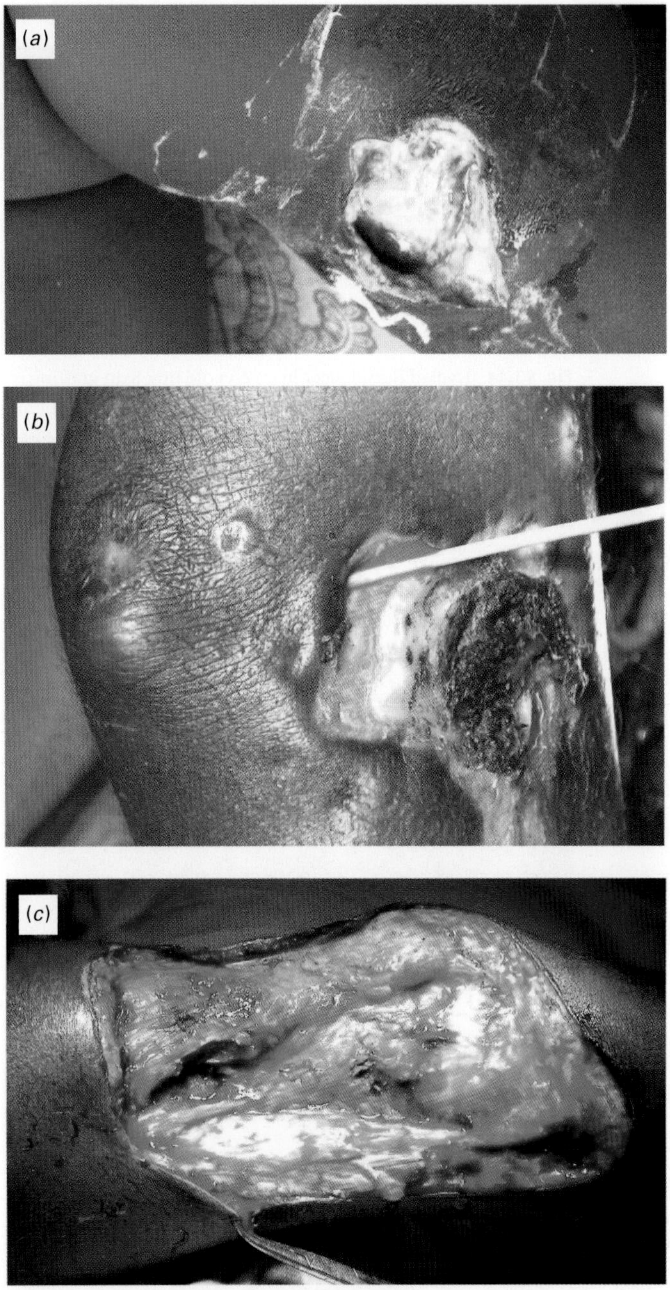

Fig. 93.43. (*a*) Large ulcer with deeply undermined edge on the thigh, just below the right buttock, in a 7-year old girl. (Courtesy Dr Emmanuel Klutse, Dunkwa Hospital, Ashanti Region, Ghana.) (*b*) Large ulcer at the exterior knee in a 14-year old boy. Note the necrotic slough below the swab stick; the tip of the stick can be seen bulging the area of the knee cap (arrow) demonstrating the large area of skin that looks healthy but should be removed for healing to occur. (*c*) Shows the extent of resection necessary to remove all diseased tissue. Skin grafting is usually performed in a second operation. (Courtesy Dr Eric Quarshie Agogo Hospital, Ghana.)

niques (Portaels et al., 1997) are usually not available in Africa.

Treatment

The principle is to excise all affected and diseased tissue. Apparently healthy skin often needs excision because underlying fat tissue may appear to be abnormal and unhealthy. It is often an embarrassing and emotionally distressing dilemma, but, if this diseased tissue is left, the ulcerative disease will be allowed to continue. One to 3 weeks after initial debridement and excision, skin grafting allows fast healing.

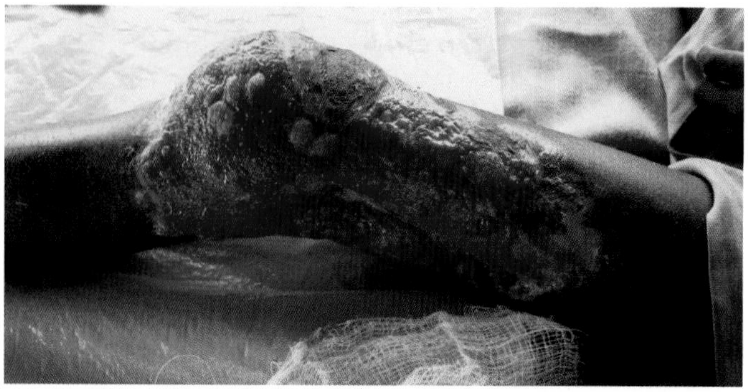

Fig. 93.44. Healed Buruli ulcer in a 12-yr old boy. Skin grafting is now possible as the ulcer is cleaned up after initial debridement. Note severe contracture in the knee joint. (Courtesy Dr Emmanuel Klutse, Dunkwa Hospital, Ghana.)

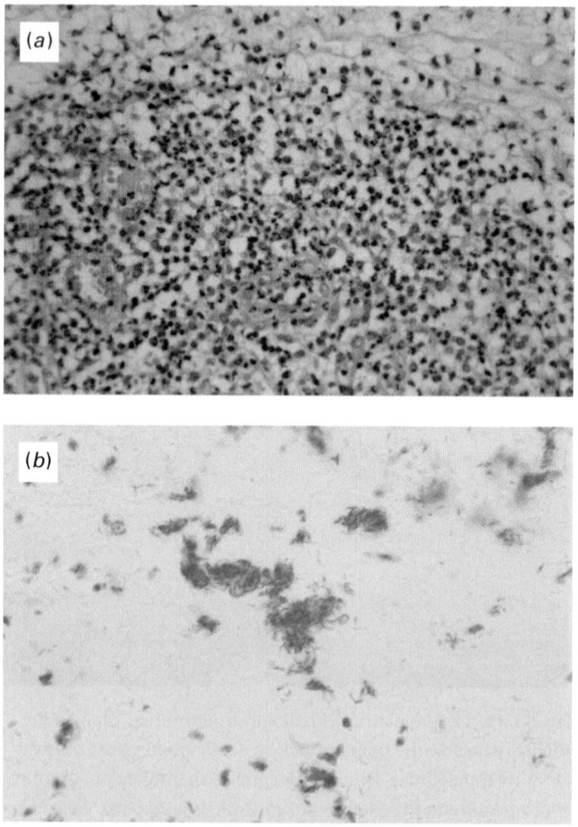

Fig. 93.45. (*a*) Early lesion of Buruli ulcer, with large numbers of inflammatory cells around blood vessels in the subcutis. (*b*) Staining with carbolfuchsin (Ziehl–Nielsen) reveals numerous acid- and alcohol-fast bacilli in clumps in the fat tissue. (Courtesy Dr Jean Knell and Dr Alan Knell, Warwick, UK.)

Occasionally, limb amputation appears inevitable in advanced severe cases, but this is exceptional.

Medical treatment with anti-tuberculosis and anti-leprosy drugs though sensitive in vitro, is ineffective, as reviewed by us (van der Werf et al., 1999). Clofazimine was formally tested in Uganda. Many doctors try rifampicin, ethambutol and other anti-mycobacterial agents, because of their in vitro sensitivity, but presently there is no published evidence that drugs help to heal Buruli ulcer. New hopes based on new experimental data in animal models (Dega et al., 2002) have however fuelled plans to study the use of anti-mycobacterial drug combinations in Buruli ulcer patients.

References

Anonymous. (1970). Buruli Ulcer. *Br Med J*; **2**: 378–379.

Asiedu K, Etuaful S. (1998). Socioeconomic implications of Buruli ulcer in Ghana: a three-year review. *Am J Trop Med Hyg*; **59**: 1015–1022.

Barker DJ. (1973). Epidemiology of *Mycobacterium ulcerans* infection. *Trans Roy Soc Trop Med Hyg*; **67**: 43–50.

Clancey JK, Dodge OG, Lunn HF et al. (1961). Mycobacterial skin ulcers in Uganda. *Lancet*; **ii**: 951–954

Dega H, Bentoucha A, Robert J, Jarlier V, Grosset J. (2002). Bactericidal activity of rifampinamikacin against Mycobacterium ulcerans in mice. *Antimicrob Agents Chemother*; **46**: 3193–3196.

George KM, Barker LIP, Welty DM et al. (1998). Partial Purification and characterization of biological effects of a lipid toxin produced by *Mycobacterium ulcerans. Infect Immun*; **66**: 587–593.

George KM, Chatterjee D, Gunawardana G et al. (1999). Mycolactone: a polyketide toxin from *Mycobacterium ulcerans* required for virulence. *Science*; **283**: 854–857.

Josse R, Guédénon A, Darie H et al. (1995). Les infections cutanées a *Mycobacterium ulcerans*: Ulcères de Buruli. *Med Trop (Mars)*; **55**: 363–373.

MacCallum P, Tolhurst JC, Buckle G et al. (1948). A new mycobacterial infection in man. *J Pathol Bacteriol*; **60**: 93–122.

Marsollier L, Robert R, Aubry J et al. (2002). Aquatic insects as a vector for *Mycobacterium ulcerans. Appl Environ Microbiol*; **6**: 4623–4628.

Marston BJ, Diallo MO, Horsburgh CR Jr et al. (1995). Emergence of Buruli ulcer disease in the Daloa Region of Côte d'Ivoire. *Am J Trop Med Hyg*; **52**: 219–224.

Myers WM, Shelly WM, Connor DH et al. (1974). Human *Mycobacterium ulcerans* infections developing at sites of trauma to skin. *Am J Trop Med Hyg*; **3**: 919–923.

Oluwasanmi JO, Solankee TF, Olurin EO et al. (1976). *Mycobacterium ulcerans* (Buruli) skin ulceration in Nigeria. *Am J Trop Med Hyg*; **25**: 122–128.

Pahlevan AA, Wright DJ, Andrews C et al. (1999). The inhibitory action of *Mycobacterium ulcerans* soluble factor on monocyte/T cell cytokine production and NF-kappa B function. *J Immunol*; **163**: 3928–3935.

Portaels F, Agular J, Fissette K et al. (1997). Direct detection and identification of *Mycobacterium ulcerans* in clinical specimens by PCR and Oligonucleotide-Specific capture plate hybridization. *J Clin Microbiol*; **35**: 1097–1100.

Portaels F, Elsen P, Guimaraes-Peres A et al. (1999). Insects in the transmission of Myhcobacterium ulcerans infection (Letter). *Lancet*; **353**: 986.

Portaels F, Chemlal K, Elsen P et al. (2001). *Mycobacterium ulcerans* in wild animals. *Rev Sci Tech*; **20**: 252–264.

Revill WD, Barker DJ. (1972). Seasonal distribution of mycobacterial skin ulcers. *Br J Prev Soc Med*; **26**: 23–27.

Ross BC, Johnson PD, Oppedisano F et al. (1997). Detection of Mycobacterium ulcerans in environmental samples during an outbreak of ulcerative disease. *Appl Environ Microbiol*; **63**: 4135–4138.

Stinear T, Ross BC, Davies JK et al. (1999). Identification and characterization of US2404 and IS2606: two distinct repeated sequences for detection of *Mycobacterium ulcerans* by PCR. *J Clin Microbiol*; **37**: 1018–1023.

Stinear TP, Jenkin GA, Johnson PD et al. (2000). Comparative genetic analysis of *Mycobacterium ulcerans* and *Mycobacterium marinum* reveals evidence of recent divergence. *J Bacteriol*; **182**: 6322–6330.

van der Werf TS, van der Graaf WTA, Groothuis DG et al. (1989). Mycobacterium Ulcerans infection in Ashanti Region, Ghana. *Trans Roy Soc Trop Med Hyg*; **83**: 410–413.

van der Werf TS, van der Graaf WTA, Tappero JW et al. (1999). *Mycobacterium ulcerans* infection. *Lancet*; **354**: 1013–1018.

van Oye E, Ballion M. (1950). Faudra't il tenir compte d'une nouvelle affection à bacilles acido-résistants en Afrique? *Ann Soc Belg Med Trop*; **30**: 619–627.

Veitch MG, Johnson PD, Flood PE et al. (1997). A large localized outbreak of *Mycobacterium ulcerans* infection on a temperate Southern Australian island. *Epidemiol Infect*; **119**: 313–318.

94 The eye

Patterns of blindness and eye disease

The patterns of eye disease in different parts of the world are determined by genetic factors, the environment, and the availability and quality of preventive and therapeutic eye services. For example, genetic factors result in the high prevalence of open angle glaucoma in some ethnic groups from West Africa, while environmental factors predispose to trachoma in communities living in the dry Sahel and central plains of East Africa. In addition, throughout rural Africa there is a lack of trained staff and facilities to provide adequate preventive and therapeutic eye care. The consequence is that despite relatively inexpensive and very effective interventions being known, over 80 per cent of all blindness in Africa is either preventable or treatable. The awareness of this problem resulted in the launch in 1999 of 'VISION 2020 – the right to sight', a global initiative to eliminate avoidable blindness (WHO/PBL, 1997).

Global blindness

Definition

The term 'blindness' refers to a loss of vision that results in the patient being unable to walk alone without assistance. The World Health Organization classifies visual loss as shown in Table 94.1. (WHO/PBL, 1997).

Table 94.1. WHO categories of visual loss

Visual acuity in the better eye with best correction	
6/6–6/18	Normal
<6/18–6/60	Visual impairment
<6/60–3/60	Severe visual impairment
<3/60–NPL	Blind

Magnitude

Using this definition the number of blind people in the world has increased from 28 million in 1975 to an estimated 45 million in 1995, and is projected to reach 75 million by 2020 if action is not taken. A further 135 million people have visual impairment or severe visual impairment.

The prevalence of blindness varies greatly from country to country and community to community within countries. However, on average it can be said that, in industrialized countries, 2 people per 1000 are blind compared with 5 per 1000 in middle economy settings and more than 10 per 1000 in low economy societies. The incidence of blindness (number of new cases per year) is estimated at 8–10 million per year, with a net annual increase in blindness of 1–2 million people per year. This is due to an increase in the population of the world and increased life expectancy (Thylefors, 1995).

Causes

Nearly half of all blindness is due to cataract and 15 per cent of the world's blindness is due to corneal scarring from eye infections and malnutrition. Other major causes of blindness are glaucoma, diabetic retinopathy and macular/retina degenerations. Details are summarized in Table 94.2.

Cataract occurs in all parts of the world. Environmental risk factors for age-related cataract include nutritional deficiencies, smoking, exposure to ultraviolet B irradiation and severe episodes of dehydration (Brian & Taylor, 2001). Trachoma is particularly a disease of children and their mothers who live in poor areas of the world with inadequate water supply and sanitation (Bailey & Lietman, 2001). Onchocerciasis occurs close to rivers in west and central Africa with some foci of disease in

Table 94.2. Major causes of global blindness

Cataract	20 million
Trachoma/scar	6 million
Glaucoma	7 million
Onchocerciasis	0.3 million
Xerophthalmia	0.5 million
Senile macular degeneration	2 million
Leprosy	0.5 million
Diabetic retinopathy	2.5 million
Others	6.2 million

Ethiopia and East Africa (Chapter 28). Vitamin A deficiency is often associated with measles in Africa, and is most prevalent in children aged 1 to 3 years old, living where there is famine. Eye disease and blindness due to HIV infection is increasing particularly in Southern and East Africa (Kestelyn & Cunningham, 2001).

Control

The priorities in order to reduce blindness and visual loss:
- provision of good quality cataract services aiming at more than 2000 operations per year per million population
- provision of spectacles for significant refractive errors, especially in children aged 10 years and older
- identification and control activities for communities with trachoma, onchocerciasis or vitamin A deficiency.

Blindness in children

Definition

Childhood blindness is defined as a visual acuity of less than 3/60 in the better eye of an individual under the age of 16 years.

Magnitude

There is limited information on the prevalence of childhood blindness, although current estimates suggest a figure of around 3 per 10 000 children in industrialized countries increasing to 10 per 10 000 in lower income countries. This would indicate a total of approximately 1.4 million blind children world-wide, and between 50 and 400 blind children per million total population (Gilbert & Foster, 2001).

Causes

Surveys have shown a wide variation in the causes of childhood blindness. Poorer areas of the world continue to have corneal blindness due to malnutrition and measles, accounting for up to 50 per cent of all childhood blindness in some areas. Cataract is responsible for between 10 and 20 per cent of childhood blindness, with rubella infection in pregnancy being one preventable cause. Retinal diseases including retinopathy of prematurity (ROP) are important causes in more affluent societies.

Table 94.3. Control activities to reduce blindness in children

Primary health care
Nutrition education and measles immunization programmes should result in the virtual eradication of corneal blindness in childhood
Rubella immunization may be feasible in some countries to prevent childhood blindness from congenital cataract
Screening of newborn children for cataract, and glaucoma with appropriate referral to a specialist in neonatal units
School screening for visual loss due to significant refractive error
Specialist child eye care
Screening of low birthweight children for retinopathy of prematurity
Provision of ophthalmological surgical services to treat cataract, glaucoma and ROP
Provision of low vision services as many children with severe visual loss/blindness can be helped to read normal print with low vision aids

Control

The possible control activities are summarized in Table 94.3. They are a combination of interventions as part of primary health care, and interventions in specialist child eye care units (Gilbert et al. 2001).

The causes of childhood blindness are changing. As corneal disease is gradually brought under control, cataract is becoming increasingly important, and ROP is emerging as the most potentially preventable cause of blindness in urban children.

It is important to monitor the changing patterns of childhood blindness in each country so that appropriate preventive and therapeutic measures can be initiated to reduce the number of blind years from avoidable causes of blindness in children.

Blindness in Africa

The prevalence of blindness in Africa varies from less than 0.3 per cent in some urban populations to over 2 per cent in rural communities with hyperendemic trachoma or onchocerciasis. Overall, there are an estimated 8 million blind people in Africa with an average prevalence of over 1 per cent (Whitfield et al., 1990; Zerihun & Mabey, 1997; Faal et al., 2000).

The main causes of blindness vary from place to place. Cataract is responsible for between 30 and 60 per cent of blindness in all countries, and is the number one cause in Africa. Usually, there are between 3000 and 5000 people blind from cataract per million population. Onchocerciasis, endemic in 28 African countries, has its highest prevalence of disease and ocular complications in west and central Africa. Trachoma is a major cause of blindness in the dry semi-arid parts of Africa and is a particular problem in Ethiopia and the Sahel. Chronic glaucoma is responsible for 10–20 per cent of all blindness: the highest prevalence is in west Africa (Johnson & Foster, 1998).

Africa lacks both human and financial resources for eye care. There is an estimated one ophthalmologist per million population and few training programmes for ophthalmologists. The minimum WHO recommended number is four cataract surgeons per million population. For this reason some countries in Africa have developed training programmes for general doctors, medical assistants, or eye nurses in the diagnosis and management of eye diseases, and where appropriate cataract surgery, in an effort to provide a more equitable distribution of eye care services (Foster, 1991).

There is some evidence that onchocerciasis is being brought under control (Chapter 28) and increased efforts are being made to implement the 'SAFE' strategy for trachoma control. The number of operations for cataract is less than 300 000 per year, yet the current target to eliminate cataract blindness in Africa is 1.5 million per year.

Problem-orientated approach to diagnosis and management

History and examination

The examination of a patient with eye problems can be divided into four stages:

- taking the history
- measurement of visual acuity
- basic examination of the external eye with a torch
- further examination of the inner parts of the eye.

Taking a history

Patients attending an eye clinic can be considered according to the main symptom, namely:

- red painful eye(s) – with or without a history of trauma
- cannot see – an inability to see in the distance with one or both eyes
- cannot read – an inability to read small print, or see near objects
- other specific symptoms – e.g. double vision, flashing lights or other specific symptoms.

Measuring the visual acuity

The visual acuity should be assessed in each eye, and can be measured using the Snellen test chart (or the E test type for people who cannot read).

The visual acuity can be usefully divided into four main categories:

satisfactory vision	= 6/6 to 6/18
poor vision	= <6/18 to 6/60 (Counting fingers at 6 metres = CF6 m)
very poor vision	= <6/60 to 3/60 (Counting fingers at 3 metres = CF3 m)
blind	= <3/60 to NPL (No perception of light).

Eye examination with a torch

A simple eye examination can be carried out with a hand torch. If the torch also has a magnifying loupe/lens, then this helps. The important parts of the front of the eye that should be examined are:

- the eyelids – do they look and function normally?
- the conjunctiva – is the white of the eye white?
- the cornea – is the cornea clear?
- the pupil – is the pupil black and does it react to light?

Further eye examination

Besides the basic examination with a torch, there are special examinations which may be required. Some of these are:

- visual acuity with a pin-hole (to check for refractive errors)
- tonometry (to measure intra-ocular pressure)
- ophthalmoscopy (preferably after pupil dilation, to examine the optic nerve head and retina)
- slit-lamp microscopy (to examine the front of the eye in detail)
- ocular movements (to check for strabismus and nerve palsies)
- visual fields.

Often, medical workers may not have the equipment or experience to carry out these detailed examinations. In this chapter emphasis is therefore given to management of common eye conditions at the primary level of health care, based upon a good history, measurement of visual acuity and examination of the anterior part of the eye with a torch (and magnifying lens if available).

Diagnosis and management of eye diseases in Africa

The majority of people with eye complaints have common diseases that are usually straightforward to diagnose and treat. A problem-orientated approach based upon the initial complaint can be used to make a diagnosis and manage the patient.

Acute red eye

Patients with acute red eye are considered as those occurring spontaneously and those due to injuries of the eye. The main causes of acute red eye with no history of injury are:

(i) conjunctivitis
(ii) corneal ulcer
(iii) iritis
(iv) acute glaucoma.

Trachoma is a specific chronic conjunctivitis, which is discussed separately.

Vitamin A deficiency may cause corneal ulcer in infants; it is also discussed in the section on specific diseases.

Clinical method

The differential diagnosis between the common causes of acute red eye can be made by:

- assessing the degree of pain
- assessing the degree of loss of vision
- examination of the cornea
- examination of the pupil
- special diagnostic tests.

Table 94.4 summarizes the symptoms and signs that can lead to a diagnosis.

Table 94.4. Summary of the main causes of acute red eye

	Conjunctivitis	Corneal ulcer	Iritis	Acute glaucoma
Pain	+	+++	++	++++
Vision	Normal	Reduced	Reduced	Reduced ++++
Cornea	Normal	Grey spot	Keratic Precipitates	Hazy due to oedema
Pupil	Normal	Normal	Small and irregular	Dilated and inactive
Special sign	Purulent discharge	Ulcer stains with fluorescein	Irregular pupil after dilation	Raised eye pressure

Acute conjunctivitis

Definition

Inflammation of the conjunctiva.

Causes

There are a variety of causes including bacterial, viral, allergic and chemical agents.

Symptoms

The patient has little pain, good vision and a purulent or mucous discharge.

Signs

- Eyelids may be swollen, but often normal
- Conjunctiva is red, maximal in the fornices, and often with a discharge
- Cornea is clear
- Pupil is normal.

Treatment

It is often not possible to identify the specific infecting micro-organism. Routine treatment is with an antibiotic eye ointment three times a day for 1 week.

Severe allergic conjunctivitis (vernal disease) requires specialist treatment with mast cell inhibitors and the weakest steroid drops used sparingly to relieve severe symptoms.

Ophthalmia neonatorum

Definition

A sticky eye in any baby during the first twenty-eight days of life, (Fig. 94.1). Ophthalmia neonatorum is a special type of conjunctivitis seen in newborn babies due to infection from the mother's vaginal tract during delivery.

Causes

Neisseria gonorrhoea or *Chlamydia trachomatis (serotypes D–K).*

Diagnosis

- Eyelids are usually very swollen
- Conjunctiva is red, oedematous with a purulent discharge

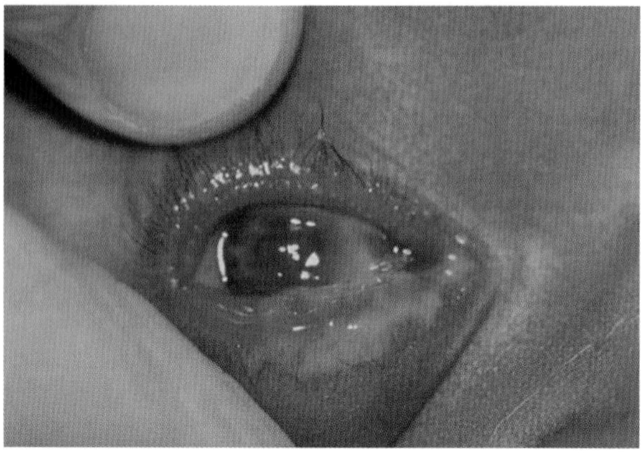

Fig. 94.1. Ophthalmia neonatorum.

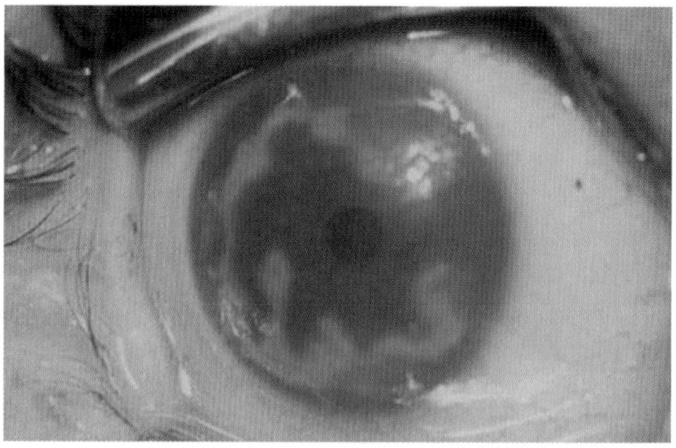

Fig. 94.2. Dendritic ulcer.

- Cornea is usually clear, but may develop a corneal ulcer
- Pupil is normal.

Treatment

- Give systemic antibiotics, e.g. ceftriaxone 50 mg/kg i.m. to a max of 125 mg (or appropriate alternative).
- Clean the eyes with a swab and water
- Apply tetracycline eye ointment hourly for four days and then three times a day for 10 days.
- If there is a corneal ulcer, give gentamicin or chloramphenicol eye drops every 5 minutes for one hour, then every hour for one day, then 3-hourly until there is improvement.

Prevention

Immediately at birth, use a clean swab and water to clean the eyes of each newborn baby and apply 1 per cent tetracycline eye ointment or 1 drop of 5 per cent aqueous povidone iodine to the eyes (Schaller & Klauss, 2001).

Corneal ulceration

Definition

Corneal ulceration usually involves damage to the epithelium and stroma of the cornea. Keratitis is an inflammation of the cornea, usually with no loss of corneal epithelium. Corneal abscess is suppuration within the corneal stroma. The term corneal abrasion or corneal erosion is sometimes used for just epithelial loss of the cornea, with or without minor trauma.

Causes

The common causes of ulceration are summarized in Table 94.6 and include:

(a) bacterial – Staphylococcus, Streptococcus, Gonococcus, Pseudomonas, leprosy
(b) viral – herpes simplex, measles
(c) nutritional – Vitamin A deficiency
(d) others, e.g. harmful eye practices (HEP), trauma.

Symptoms

There is usually moderate to severe pain and marked loss of vision if the ulcer is severe.

Signs

- Eyelids are swollen
- Conjunctiva is red, maximal around the cornea
- Cornea has a white or grey spot
- Pupil is usually normal.

Special test

Fluorescein drops or paper applied to the conjunctiva will show green staining of a corneal ulcer when the epithelium is deficient.

Different types of corneal ulceration

Viral

This is usually due to herpes simplex virus. The ulcer may be branch-like (dendritic) or more like the outline of a map (geographic). The treatment of herpetic ulceration is acyclovir ointment 5× /day for 5–7 days (Fig. 94.2).

Bacterial

Bacterial corneal ulcers may be due to Staphylococcus, Streptococcus, Pseudomonas, or Gonococcus. They usually start as an epithelial defect that involves the corneal stroma (Fig. 94.3).

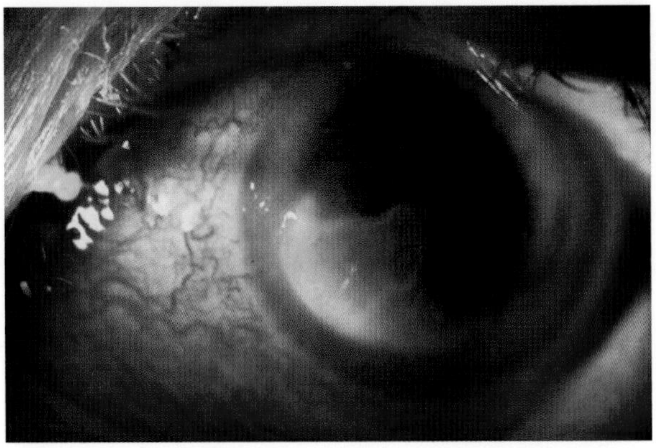

Fig. 94.3. Corneal ulceration with fluorescein staining.

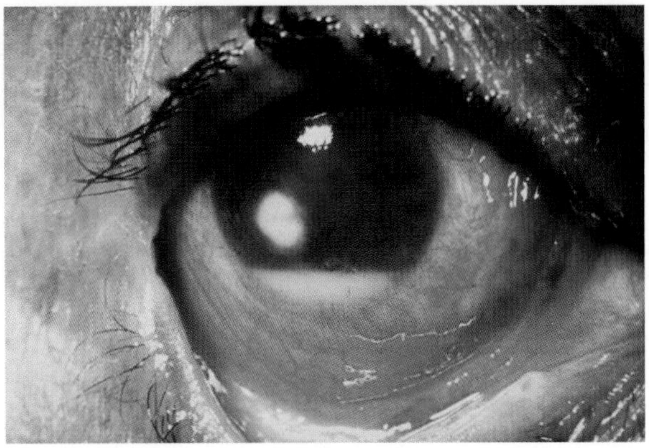

Fig. 94.4. Hypopyon ulcer.

There may be inflammatory cells in the anterior chamber, which can produce an hypopyon (Fig. 94.4).

The treatment is hourly antibiotic drops according to sensitivity and availability. If severe, a sub-conjunctival injection of gentamicin 20 mg may be given (this is useful where compliance to hourly drops cannot be guaranteed).

Nutritional
This is due to vitamin A deficiency and is discussed later.

Fungi
Particularly Fusarium, Aspergillus and occasionally Candida, may also cause an ulcer with hypopyon. A corneal scrape examined by gram stain will often demonstrate fungal hyphae. Treatment is with anti-fungal agents such as natamycin or econazole drops given hourly until the ulcer heals.

Other causes
There are many other causes of corneal ulceration: these include trauma, the use of harmful eye practices, which may cause severe bilateral corneal ulceration with chemical conjunctivitis; and leprosy (Chapter 47), which can cause corneal ulceration from exposure of the cornea due to inability to close the eyelids (lagophthalmos).

Treatment

The treatment of corneal ulcer is that of the cause. It usually involves topical antibiotics and in severe cases mydriatics three times/day to dilate the pupil. An eye pad can be used if it makes the patient more comfortable.

Complications

Corneal ulceration may lead to:

- diffuse scarring of the cornea
- leukoma formation – a dense white scar
- perforation of the cornea with adherent iris – adherent leukoma
- external protrusion of a thin cornea called a staphyloma
- phthisis bulbi (a small shrunken globe), due to loss of intra-ocular contents with or without infection (endophthalmitis).

Iritis

Definition

Inflammation of the iris.

Causes

(a) Leprosy – associated with erythema nodosum leprosum
(b) Onchocerciasis – see Chapter 28
(c) Associated with specific syndromes including some types of arthritis
(d) Trauma or intra-ocular surgery
(e) Idiopathic – the majority of cases.

Symptoms

Pain is moderate and, while loss of vision is usually minimal, it may be severe if the posterior eye is involved. There is often photophobia and lacrimation.

Signs

- Eyelids are normal
- Conjunctiva is red, with ciliary injection around the cornea

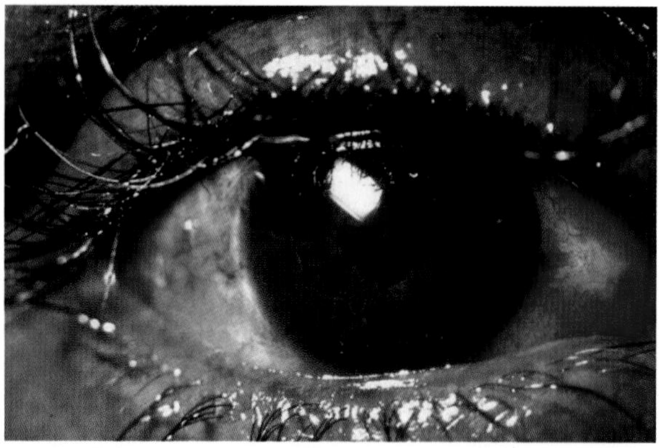

Fig. 94.5. Acute iritis with irregular pupil.

- Cornea may show keratic precipitates (deposits of inflammatory cells) on the endothelium (inside) of the cornea (this requires magnification to visualize)
- Pupil is small, but with dilation it is often seen to be irregular due to posterior synechiae (adhesions between iris and anterior lens surface) (Fig. 94.5).

Special test

Dilate the pupil in the clinic with cyclopentolate 0.5 per cent or phenylephrine 10 per cent and look for an irregularly shaped pupil due to posterior synechiae.

Treatment

- Dilate the pupil immediately with cyclopentolate 0.5 per cent and/or phenylephrine 10 per cent eye drops
- Give atropine ointment or drops daily
- Give topical steroids, e.g. prednisolone drops 0.5 per cent, as required (3–8 times/day) to reduce the redness and inflammation – usually for 1–4 weeks.
- Sub-conjunctival injection of mydriatics and/or steroids may be required for very severe cases of iritis where drops alone are insufficient to break the posterior synechiae.

Complications

If posterior synechiae develop, they may cause secondary opacification of the lens and so lead to a cataract. The posterior synechiae may also occlude the pupil, resulting in a pupil block glaucoma with rise in intra-ocular pressure. Both these complications will result in severe loss of vision.

Acute glaucoma

Definition

Acute rise in intra-ocular pressure.

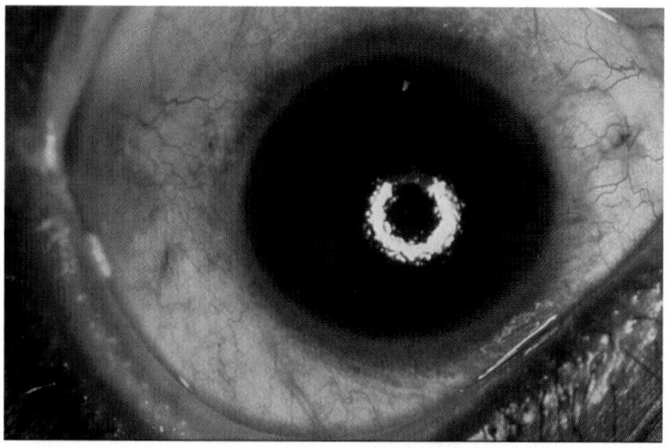

Fig. 94.6. Acute glaucoma with fixed dilated pupil.

Causes

(a) Primary angle closure
(b) Swollen intumescent cataract
(c) Blunt trauma
(d) Iritis.

Symptoms

Severe pain is characteristic, vision is markedly reduced – sometimes to perception of light vision – and the patient may have headache and vomiting.

Signs

- Eyelids may be swollen
- Conjunctiva is red
- Cornea is hazy due to oedema in the cornea
- Pupil is dilated and does not react well to light (Fig. 94.6).

Special test

Measurement of intra-ocular pressure with a tonometer (or digital tonometry), will reveal a pressure in excess of 30 mm of Hg.

Treatment

Give acetazolamide (Diamox) tablets 500 mg by mouth or very slow i.v. injection, followed by 250 mg orally four times a day. Primary angle closure can also be treated with pilocarpine drops, but *do not use* pilocarpine in acute glaucoma due to swollen cataract, trauma or iritis. Refer the patient for treatment of the cause of the glaucoma, e.g. a swollen cataract will require removal.

Complications

Persistent elevation in intra-ocular pressure, even for 1 or 2 days, will damage the optic nerve and cause blindness from optic atrophy.

Injuries to the eye

The main types of ocular injury are:
(a) blunt injuries
(b) perforating injuries
(c) foreign bodies
(d) burns or chemicals in the eye.
Take a careful history to define the type of injury. The visual acuity in each eye should be measured in all patients with ocular injury.

Blunt injury to the eye

Examination

Orbit
There may be a fracture of one of the orbital bones. This most commonly affects the medial bone (ethmoid), or the inferior orbital bone (maxilla). The clinical signs of an orbital fracture are:
- bleeding from the nose – epistaxis
- proptosis of the eye, due to air from a sinus entering the orbit through the fracture
- anaesthesia of the lower eyelid, due to damage of the infra-orbital nerve
- double vision on looking up, due to entrapment of the inferior rectus muscle in an inferior wall fracture; or on looking outwards due to entrapment of the medial rectus in a medial wall fracture.

The management of a fracture of the orbit depends on the signs. If there is air in the orbit, give the patient systemic antibiotics for 7 days. If there is double vision, refer the patient to a specialist for possible surgical exploration of the trapped muscle with a view to releasing the muscle from the fracture.

Cornea
There may be an abrasion of the cornea, which will present as an acutely painful eye. Local anaesthetic drops can relieve the pain and the diagnosis-confirmed by fluorescein staining of the cornea. Treat with antibiotic eye ointment and an eye pad for 24 hours.

Pupil
The pupil may be distorted in shape, and not react to light (traumatic mydriasis); and/or there may be blood in the anterior chamber (hyphaema) (Fig. 94.7).

It is useful to think of hyphaema in two forms, non-painful and painful. Non-painful hyphaema will usually resolve with conservative treatment, i.e. rest, antibiotic eye ointment and an eye pad for 5 days. A painful hyphaema can be due to a rise in intra-ocular pressure (secondary

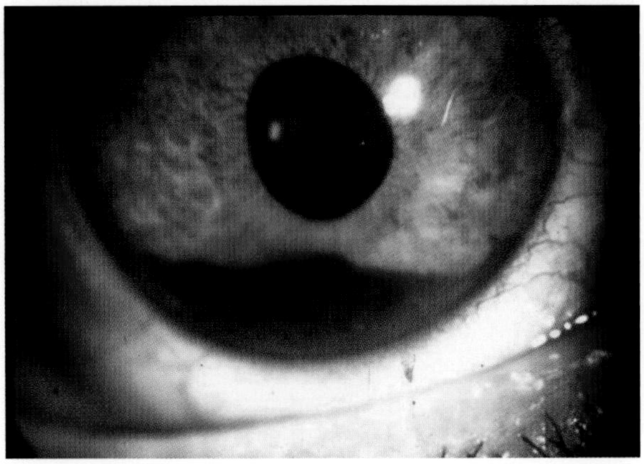

Fig. 94.7. Hyphaema.

glaucoma: treat with acetazolamide (Diamox) 250 mg four times a day. If the hyphaema and glaucoma do not resolve in 48 hours, then surgery may be required to remove the blood from the anterior chamber by paracentesis.

Lens
Occasionally the lens may be damaged by a blunt injury, leading to cataract formation or dislocation of the lens. Dislocation of the lens may also cause a rise in intra-ocular pressure: if this occurs, refer the patient for possible lens extraction.

Retina and optic nerve
Blunt injury can damage the posterior segment of the eye and cause vitreous haemorrhage, retinal oedema and haemorrhage, retinal tears, and even optic nerve damage. These complications are uncommon and not easy to treat.

Perforating injury

If the injury is due to a sharp object, it may result in perforation of the eye.

Examination

Carefully examine the eye without causing any pressure as this may result in further prolapse of intra-ocular contents.

Eyelid
Lacerations that do not involve the lower canaliculus or lid margin can be sutured. If the lid margin is involved, suture carefully ensuring close apposition of the two edges of the lid margin to avoid notching. If the lower canaliculus has been torn, then the patient will require specialist management to avoid a permanently watering eye from canalicular stenosis.

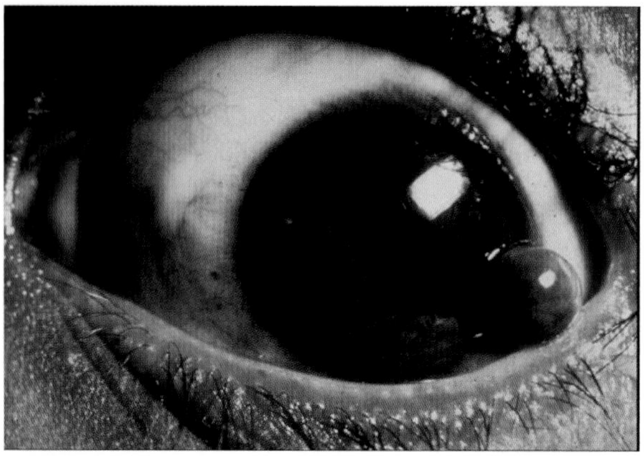

Fig. 94.8. Iris prolapse from a corneal perforation.

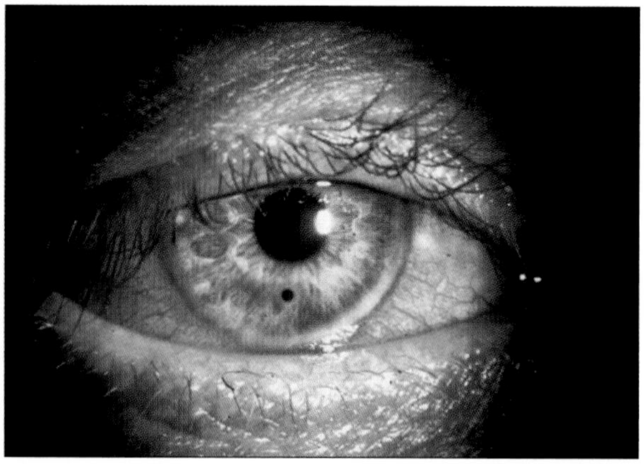

Fig. 94.9. Corneal foreign body.

Conjunctival
Lacerations usually do not require suturing.

Cornea
A perforating injury of the eye that involves the cornea often results in prolapse of iris onto the surface of the eye (Fig. 94.8).

The *pupil* will be distorted and the anterior chamber is likely to be shallow. There may also be hyphaema and damage to the lens with cataract formation.

Treatment
The first aid management of a perforating injury includes:
- antibiotic to the eye (preferably drops)
- atropine to the eye (preferably drops)
- an eye pad
- administration of tetanus toxoid.

When this treatment has been given, refer the patient urgently for specialist treatment. Fresh perforations may be treated surgically by cleaning the wound, excising prolapsed tissue, and re-suturing the wound edges with fine 10/0 nylon sutures followed by reformation of the anterior chamber. With older perforations it may be best initially to treat conservatively with topical antibiotics and atropine.

Foreign bodies

Examination and treatment

Eyelids
Evert the eyelid and look for a sub-tarsal foreign body on the tarsal conjunctiva. This can be simply removed with cotton wool or a piece of paper.

Conjunctiva
Examine the conjunctiva to see if a foreign body is in the conjunctival sac. This again can simply be removed with cotton wool or a piece of paper.

Cornea
Examine the cornea to see if a foreign body is embedded on the cornea. If the foreign body is superficial (Fig. 94.9), then:

- lie the patient flat
- local anaesthetic drops in the eye
- light, to give good illumination of the eye
- loupe magnification to give a good image of the cornea
- lift off the foreign body with the corner of a piece of paper, a matchstick or suitable instrument.

Give the patient antibiotic eye ointment and an eye pad for 24 hours and see them again the next day.

Sometimes the corneal foreign body will be deep, for example a thorn in the cornea. If this is the case, it may be possible to remove the foreign body (as above), using a fine pair of forceps and withdrawing the foreign body in the direction in which it entered the cornea. It is then advisable to give a sub-conjunctival injection of 20 mg of gentamicin. If the foreign body is too deeply embedded, it will be necessary to take the patient to the operating theatre and, under full local anaesthesia, perform an operation to remove the foreign body.

Intra-ocular foreign body
Occasionally following explosive injuries, or an injury where a hammer strikes another piece of metal, a foreign body may penetrate the corneo/scleral protective layer of the eye. The intra-ocular foreign body (IOFB) may be visible in the anterior chamber; or after dilating the pupil, the IOFB may be seen in the lens, vitreous or on the retina. If an IOFB is suspected, refer the patient immediately to a specialist after giving topical antibiotics and atropine. If the IOFB can be located it may be possible to remove it by surgery.

Table 94.5. Differential diagnosis and management of the common causes of loss of vision

Diagnosis	Cornea	Pupil	Examination	Management
Corneal scar	White opacity	Often not clearly visible	Nil specific	Refer for surgery if blind in both eyes
Cataract	Normal	Grey or white; reacts to light	Opacity in pupil after dilation	Refer for surgery if acuity <6/60
Chronic glaucoma	Clear or general haze	Often poor reaction to light	IOP is raised; and cupping of optic disc	Refer for surgery if there is 'travel' vision in either eye
Refractive error (myopia)	Normal	Normal	Visual acuity improves with pin-hole	Spectacles
Retinal and optic nerve diseases	Normal	Often reacts poorly to light	Abnormal optic disc or retina on ophthalmoscopy	As appropriate for specific diagnosis

Burns to the eye

Burns of the eye may affect the eyelids, conjunctiva or cornea. It is important to keep the cornea moist and free from exposure. The first aid management is to apply antibiotic ointment generously all over the conjunctiva, cornea and burned eyelids. An eye pad should not be placed over the eye as this may ulcerate the cornea; instead, antibiotic ointment should be applied every hour to the exposed cornea. The patient may require skin grafting of the eyelids.

Chemicals in the eye

The first aid management of chemicals in the eye is immediate and profuse irrigation with water. Get the patient to lie flat while water is poured into the eye generously for 10–15 minutes. After this time the eye can be examined with fluorescein to see if there is any evidence of corneal ulceration. If there is ulceration, give the patient antibiotics and an eye pad and see daily.

If concentrated sulphuric acid (car battery acid) or caustic soda (lime), have entered the eye then this is much more serious.

- Again, irrigate the eye profusely for 15 minutes, and then refer the patient immediately to hospital for continuous irrigation with a normal saline drip into the eye for 48 hours. Sulphuric acid and lime burns of the eye may lead to permanent corneal scarring and blindness if they are not vigorously treated.

In summary therefore, burns of the eye must be kept lubricated and chemicals in the eye must be thoroughly irrigated.

Loss of vision

Poor vision may occur in one or both eyes, and be sudden or gradual. The common causes of poor vision in both eyes of gradual onset are:
- corneal scar
- cataract
- chronic glaucoma
- refractive errors
- diseases of the retina and optic nerve.

Table 94.5 summarizes the differential diagnosis for the common causes of visual loss.

Emphasis is placed on the common causes, which are treatable, and therefore need to be diagnosed and referred for specialist treatment (often surgery).

Examination with a torch and differential diagnosis

In corneal scar, there is an opacity in front of the pupil; in cataract, the grey–white opacity is in the pupil; and in chronic glaucoma (with loss of visual acuity) the pupil does not react normally to a bright light. If the visual loss is due to a refractive error then the pupil is normal, and the visual acuity should improve if measured with a pinhole in front of the pupil.

Corneal scar

In Africa corneal scarring is responsible for 10–30 per cent of all patients with blindness (Whitcher et al., 2001).

Clinical presentation

There is a grey–white opacity on the cornea, which often obscures the pupil (Fig. 94.10). There are different types of corneal scarring resulting from previous corneal ulceration:

(a) diffuse scar – scar all over the cornea
(b) leukomas – dense white scar in part of the cornea

Table 94.6. Causes of corneal ulceration/scarring in Africa

	Unilateral	Bilateral
Children	Herpes simplex Trauma	Ophthalmia neonatorum Vitamin A deficiency Traditional eye medicines
Adults	Bacterial infection Fungal infection Herpes simplex Trauma	Trachoma Leprosy Traditional eye medicines

(c) staphyloma – bulging out of the cornea
(d) phthisis bulbi – small shrunken eye.

Aetiology

The common causes of corneal ulceration which lead to corneal scarring are given in Table 94.6.

Management

The management of corneal scar in developing countries is difficult. The majority of patients cannot be helped by medical or surgical treatment. An **optical iridectomy** creates an artificial pupil allowing some travel vision (Fig. 94.10). It can be performed on one eye of a blind patient who has a central leukoma. It is a relatively simple operation but the visual results are limited. **Corneal grafting (keratoplasty)**, replaces a corneal scar with a clear cornea from a donor eye. It is difficult to get donor material for corneal grafting and the rejection rate for vascularized corneas is high, unless there is careful follow-up and the use of long-term topical steroids. For these reasons, corneal grafting in developing countries has a limited role.

Staphyloma and endophthalmitis are two of the commonest causes of a painful blind eye which cannot even see light, and for which removal of the eye may be indicated. If the patient consents to this procedure, it can be performed in one of two ways.

Evisceration

The cornea and contents of the eye are removed but the scleral shell and optic nerve are left. This is a relatively straightforward operation and usually produces an acceptable socket that can be fitted with an artificial eye.

Enucleation

The extra-ocular muscles and optic nerve are divided and the whole eye is removed. This is the operation of choice for intra-ocular tumours, e.g. retinoblastoma.

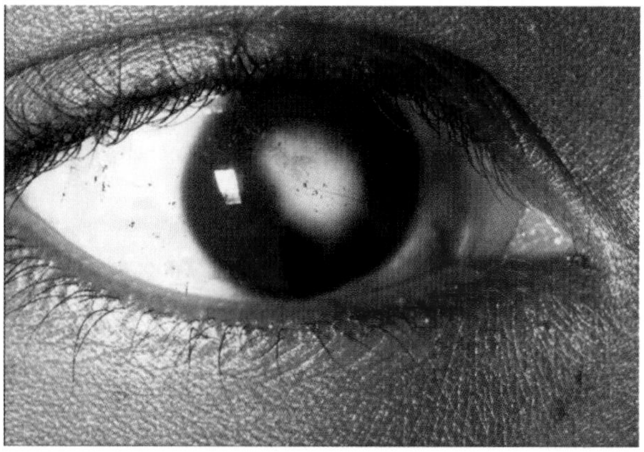

Fig. 94.10. Central corneal scar with an optical iridectomy.

Many patients with unilateral corneal scars, phthisis, or scars that do not cause blindness, may require no treatment.

Corneal scarring is a major cause of blindness, which is difficult to treat. However, the causes of corneal ulcer, which lead to scarring, are relatively easy to prevent (Table 94.6).

Cataract

Cataract is the single most important cause of blindness in the world. There are an estimated 20 million people blind from cataract in the world, of which probably 4 million live in Africa. On average one in every 200 people is blind from cataract in under-privileged communities in the world.

Aetiology

Cataract is defined as an opacity of the lens, which causes visual impairment.

Cataract can be classified as:

- **congenital** – rubella infection in pregnancy and inherited familial cataract
- **traumatic** – perforating and blunt injuries
- **secondary** – eye disease (iritis) and systemic diseases (diabetes)
- **age-related** – represents at least 90 per cent of all cataracts.

The risk factors for age related cataract which are amenable to prevention are smoking, exposure to ultraviolet B irradiation, severe episodes of dehydration and possibly nutritional deficiencies.

Clinical presentation

There is gradual loss of vision usually in both eyes but often asymmetrical. On examination the visual acuity is

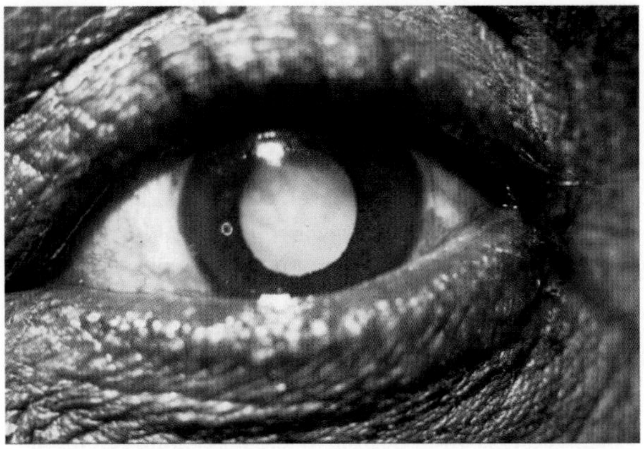

Fig. 94.11. Mature cataract.

reduced, the conjunctiva is white, the cornea is clear, and there is a grey or white opacity in the pupil. Immature cataracts cause a grey opacity in the pupil, while mature, intumescent and hypermature cataracts give a white pupil (Fig. 94.11). If the pupil is dilated the cataract is more obvious to see, and direct ophthalmoscopy will reveal an opacity in the media, which obscures a clear view of the retina.

Assessment of cataract for surgery

In deciding whether to refer a patient for cataract surgery, do the following examination:

- **Visual acuity** – measure in each eye, an acuity of less than 6/60 is a definite indication for surgery if the loss of vision is due to cataract
- **Pupil reaction** – in cataract there is a normal brisk reaction of the pupil. If the pupil does not react to light, diseases of the optic nerve or retina should be suspected as the cause of the loss of vision
- **Tonometry** – measurement of the intra-ocular pressure is important to see if the cause of loss of vision may be due to glaucoma
- **Refraction** – it is advisable to check the patient for refractive error as spectacles may improve the vision, and delay the need for cataract surgery
- **Ophthalmoscopy** – after dilating the pupil, examine the fundus with an ophthalmoscope for the red reflex to assess the density of lens opacity. This is particularly important in immature cataracts. If it is still easily possible to visualize the optic disc and fundus, then the lens opacity may not be the cause of the loss of vision.

Management

The treatment for cataract is lens extraction accompanied by correction of the resultant refractive error with an intra-ocular lens (IOL), or if not available aphakic spectacles. Depending on the individual patient (age and occupation), and upon the available equipment and technology, the visual acuity at which cataract extraction is indicated will vary.

In many parts of Africa there are insufficient ophthalmologists to meet the demands for cataract services so that general duty doctors and ophthalmic assistants are being trained to diagnose and manage eye patients and some are trained to operate on patients who are blind from bilateral, age-related cataracts. A good knowledge of common eye diseases is necessary before starting to learn cataract surgery, so as to ensure that the correct patients are selected for surgery and that the surgeon can manage post-operative complications.

The glaucomas

The glaucomas are a complex group of diseases that are often difficult to diagnose and manage (Johnson, 2001).

Definition

A level of intra-ocular pressure, usually raised, which damages the optic nerve leading to cupping of the disc and loss of visual field.

Classification

(a) Congenital also called buphthalmos, presents with large eyes and corneas in infancy;
(b) Secondary to other causes such as injury, iritis or swollen cataract;
(c) Primary angle closure may present as an acute red eye or gradual bilateral loss of vision in white eyes;
(d) Primary open angle glaucoma is the commonest type of glaucoma seen in Africa.

Clinical presentation

Glaucoma may present as an acute red eye, which has already been discussed; or as gradual loss of vision that is bilateral, but often asymmetrical. It can begin at any age but is more common after the age of 30.

The important signs of chronic glaucoma are as follows.

Cupping of the disc

If the vertical cup: disc ratio is more than 0.6; the disc is pale, and there is asymmetry in size between the two discs, then suspect glaucoma.

Raised intra-ocular pressure

If a Schiotz tonometer with a 5.5 g weight gives a reading of 2 or less, it indicates high pressure (more than 28 mm

Hg). Schiotz tonometry is relatively easy to perform, but not very accurate. Applanation tonometry is more accurate, but difficult to perform.

Loss of vision
This starts as a loss of visual field, followed by a loss of visual acuity, and finally complete loss of light perception.

Abnormal pupil responses
This begins as a relative pupil defect in which one pupil does not react as well as the other to the swinging torch test. Further damage to the optic nerve leads to a partial pupil defect in which there is a sluggish response of the pupil, and finally there is a total pupil defect in which there is no response at all to light (Fig. 94.12).

In summary, chronic glaucoma can be suspected in a patient with loss of vision, who has definite cupping of the disc on ophthalmoscopy, a raised intra-ocular pressure demonstrated by tonometry and possibly an abnormal pupil response.

Management of chronic glaucoma

Glaucoma treatment aims to reduce the IOP in order to avoid further damage to the optic nerve. The pressure may be lowered by medical treatment, which must be taken for the rest of the patient's life, or by surgery.

Medical therapy includes timolol, pilocarpine and other anti-glaucoma drops. The disadvantages are poor patient acceptance and the expense of buying the life-long medication.

Surgery includes trabeculectomy, which is the commonest procedure for chronic glaucoma. It is the recommended treatment for patients who cannot comply with medical treatment and who still have useful vision to save.

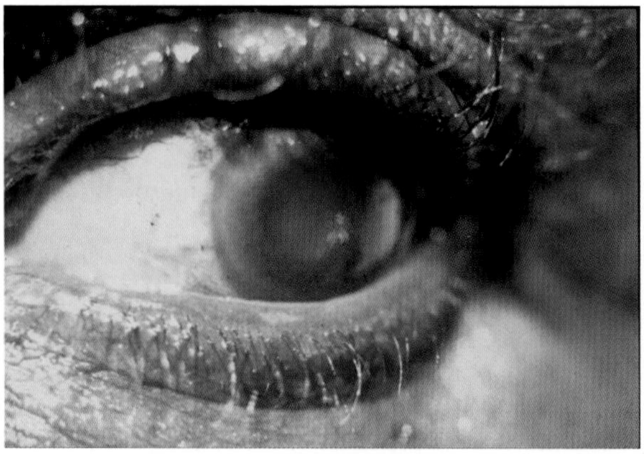

Fig. 94.12. Corneal oedema and poorly reacting pupil due to chronic glaucoma.

Refractive errors

There are different types of refractive error, some which cause loss of distance vision (visual acuity) and some which cause problems with near (reading) vision (Taylor, 2000).

Myopia causes difficulty seeing in the distance (reduced visual acuity). The condition usually starts between ages 5 and 20, and may gradually get worse. It is corrected by *minus spherical lenses.* The spectacles are worn for distance.

Hypermetropia usually occurs in young people. The visual acuity is often normal in early life, although it may deteriorate in middle age if the hypermetropia is not corrected. The treatment is with *plus spherical lenses,* usually worn for distance and reading.

Astigmatism occurs when the refractive error is different in two axes of the eye. Astigmatism causes a reduction in visual acuity for distance as well as headaches and blurring of vision when doing a lot of close work. It is treated with *cylindrical lenses.*

Aphakia is the refractive error, which occurs following cataract extraction when no intra-ocular lens has been inserted. The approximate corrective lens for distance vision is +11 dioptres and for reading +14 dioptres.

Presbyopia is caused by failure of the lens of the eye to focus from distant objects to near ones (accommodation). This difficulty usually begins around the age of 40.

The patient complains of difficulty in seeing near objects, e.g. reading, sewing, which gets worse with increasing age.

The difficulty in reading is treated by giving *plus spherical lenses* (of equal power to both eyes) following these guidelines:

age 45 approximately +1.00
age 50 approximately +1.50
age 55 approximately +2.00
age 60 approximately +2.50
age 65 approximately +3.00.

If the patient wears spectacles for distance vision, the reading correction is given as an addition to the distance correction. Presbyopic glasses are only worn for close work.

Diseases of the retina and optic nerve

Other causes of loss of vision besides corneal scar, cataract, chronic glaucoma and refractive errors include:

- diseases of the retina
- optic atrophy.

Diseases of the retina include age-related macula degeneration, chloroquine maculopathy, and retinitis pigmentosa. The ophthalmoscopic findings of these diseases are diagnostic.

Optic Atrophy may be due onchocerciasis, nutritional deficiencies, toxins, and occasionally tumours of the orbit or optic chiasma.

Occasionally, patients present with sudden loss of vision in one eye. Common causes include the following.

Chorio-retinitis (posterior uveitis) may be unilateral or bilateral. It presents as loss of vision over several days. The causes of posterior uveitis are often unknown, but include toxoplasmosis.

Retinal detachment may present with a flash of light, followed by a black floating 'cobweb' in the vision which gradually gives way to a shadow moving across the vision, eventually causing loss of vision in the eye. After dilation, examination of the retina will reveal an abnormal red reflex in one area of the retina, with elevation and abnormal tortuosity of the vessels and retina. Retinal detachment is more common in people with high myopia, and after cataract surgery. If you suspect a retinal detachment, referred the patient urgently for specialist care.

Optic neuritis presents as sudden loss of vision in one or both eyes. It sometimes follows the use of drugs or methyl alcohol. It may occur in multiple sclerosis, but often there is no known cause. Examination reveals severe loss of vision with a reduced pupil light reflex. Ophthalmoscopy may show a normal optic nerve (retrobulbar neuritis) or a swollen optic disc (papillitis). A trial of systemic steroids is justified in severe bilateral cases.

Central retinal artery or central retinal vein occlusion may be the cause of sudden loss of vision. Central retinal artery occlusion results in a pale oedematous retina with a 'cherry red' spot at the macula. Central retinal vein thrombosis shows a swollen disc with multiple haemorrhages all over the retina. There is no specific eye treatment for these conditions.

Specific diseases

Vitamin A deficiency and xerophthalmia

Definition

Xerophthalmia means dry eyes. The condition is due to vitamin A deficiency and is most commonly seen in infants aged 6 months to 4 years. It may quickly lead to corneal ulceration and blindness, particularly if associated with measles infection.

Risk factors

Conditions that predispose to vitamin A deficiency are:

- malnutrition – insufficient intake of foods rich in vitamin A
- malabsorption – chronic diarrhoea causing malabsorption of vitamin A
- measles – an increased demand for vitamin A during and after measles infection.

As well as occurring in infants vitamin A deficiency is also seen in prisoners, particularly those who have been imprisoned for several years.

Clinical features

Lack of vitamin A results in a deficiency of rhodopsin in the retinal photoreceptors (rods) leading to poor vision in reduced lighting, called night blindness (XN). Treatment with vitamin A reverses the symptom within 72 hours. Other causes of night blindness include retinitis pigmentosa and onchocerciasis.

Deficiency of vitamin A also leads to an absence of goblet cells in the conjunctiva with decrease mucin production leading to drying of the cornea (corneal xerosis X2) and ulceration or melting of the corneal stroma (X3) (Fig. 94.13).

Reduced mucin production over a long period may cause metaplasia of the conjunctival epithelium with keratin formation. The keratin is digested by commensal bacteria producing white foamy spots on the temporal conjunctiva, called Bitot spots (X1B) (Fig. 94.14). Bitot spots are a sign of chronic vitamin A deficiency and even with treatment they may take weeks or months to resolve.

Night blindness and Bitot spots are most prevalent in 3–8-year-old children, while corneal xerosis and ulceration is seen between the ages of 6 months and 4 years.

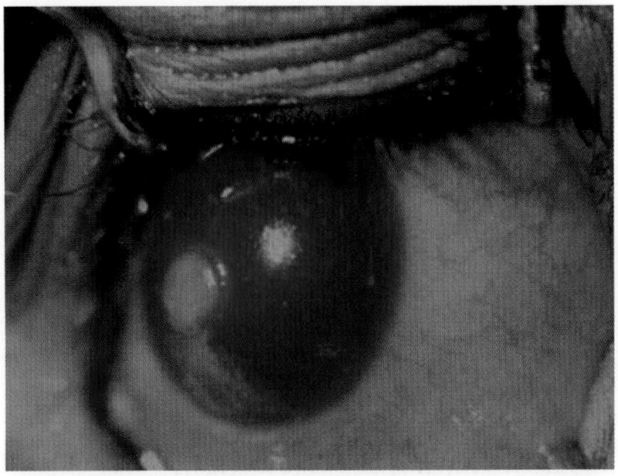

Fig. 94.13. Infant with dry cornea and area of stromal necrosis due to vitamin A deficiency.

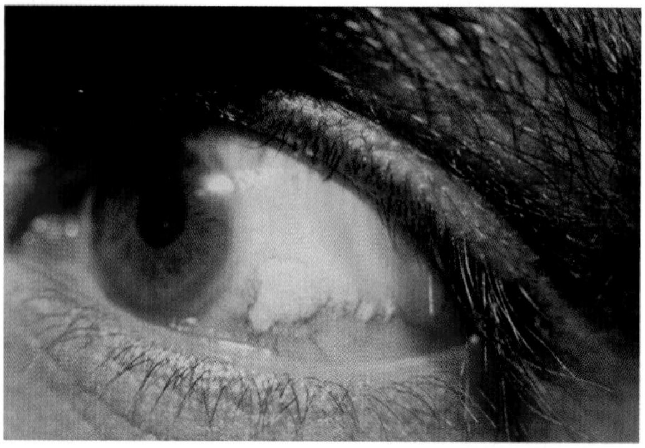

Fig. 94.14. Bitot spots.

Treatment

Large doses of vitamin A by mouth are the recommended treatment. Give the first dose *immediately* xerophthalmia is diagnosed.

The treatment schedule for vitamin A deficiency and/or xerophthalmia in children aged 1 to 6 years is:

- immediately on diagnosis – 200 000 IU vitamin A orally
- the following day – 200 000 IU vitamin A orally
- 4 weeks later – 200 000 IU vitamin A orally

If there is persistent vomiting or profuse diarrhoea, an intramuscular injection of 100 000 IU of water-miscible vitamin A (but not an oil-based preparation) may be substituted for the first dose. Treat children under 1 year of age, or children who weigh less than 8 kg, with half the oral dose (100 000 IU as above).

Children with xerophthalmia are usually suffering from general malnutrition and treatment is required to improve overall nutritional status.

Prevention

A good weaning and pre-school diet rich in vitamin A is the primary prevention, and measles immunization removes an important risk factor. Give children who are obviously malnourished, or who have measles infection, 3 doses of vitamin A, as described above, even in the absence of clinical signs of vitamin A deficiency.

Women at childbirth or in early lactation can also be given 3 doses of vitamin A as above in order to ensure that they and their breast milk have adequate supplies of vitamin A.

When infants less than 6 months old are not being breastfed, give 50 000 IU of vitamin A before they reach 6 months.

Vitamin A deficiency and child mortality

Children living in families/communities, where vitamin A deficiency is prevalent, have an increased mortality, which can be markedly reduced by improving vitamin A nutrition and/or giving vitamin A supplementation.

Table 94.7. Simplified grading of trachoma

Active trachoma	
TF –	Trachoma follicles (five or more follicles on the upper tarsal conjunctiva)
TI –	Trachoma intense inflammation (50% or more of the deep tarsal vessels are obscured by papillary hypertrophy)
Inactive	
TS –	Trachoma scars (conjunctival scars)
Trichiasis – entropion	
TT –	Trachoma trichiasis (at least one lash turns in and touches the globe)
Corneal scar	
CO –	Corneal opacity (an opacity which obscures at least part of the pupil margin)

Trachoma

Definition

Trachoma is a chronic conjunctivitis, which may involve the cornea, due to repeated infection with *Chlamydia trachomatis serotypes A, B, Ba* or *C.*

Risk factors

The disease occurs particularly in poor dry areas of the world in which there is inadequate water supply and poor community sanitation.

The classic trachoma environment is described as:

- dry – lack of water
- dirty – lack of sanitation
- discharge (eyes and nose) – lack of personal hygiene

The transmission of trachoma from child to child and child to mother occurs through:

- flies – flies go from individual to individual
- fingers – direct contact with ocular discharge
- family – within the family.

Clinical signs and assessment of trachoma

The clinical signs of trachoma have been graded into a simple five-point classification by WHO (Thylefors et al., 1987) (Table 94.7). Examination requires eversion of the upper eyelid.

Inflammation from active trachoma infection TF (Fig. 94.15) and TI (Fig. 94.16) are found mainly in pre-school

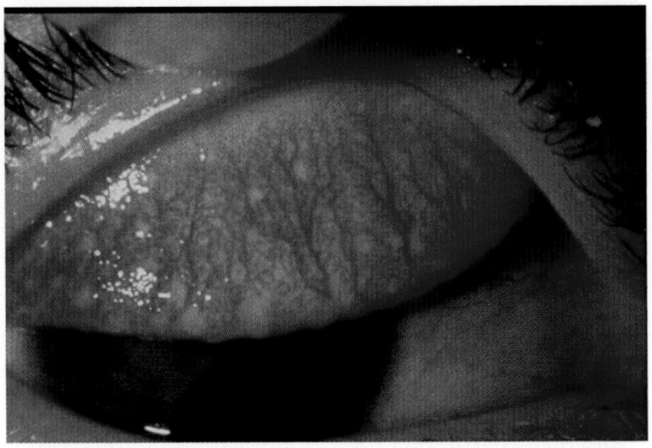

Fig. 94.15. TF – follicles due to active trachoma.

Table 94.8. The SAFE strategy for trachoma control

S	Surgery: lid surgery for all patients with TT, which is threatening vision
A	Antibiotics: tetracycline eye ointment or azithromycin tablets for individuals /communities with active infection (TF and/or TI)
F	Facial cleanliness: health promotion to encourage facial cleanliness through daily washing
E	Environmental improvement: community programmes to improve the water supply and sanitation of the village

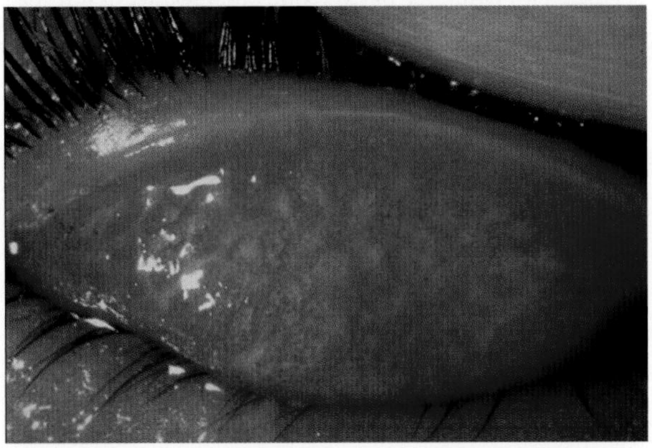

Fig. 94.16. TI – intense inflammation due to active trachoma.

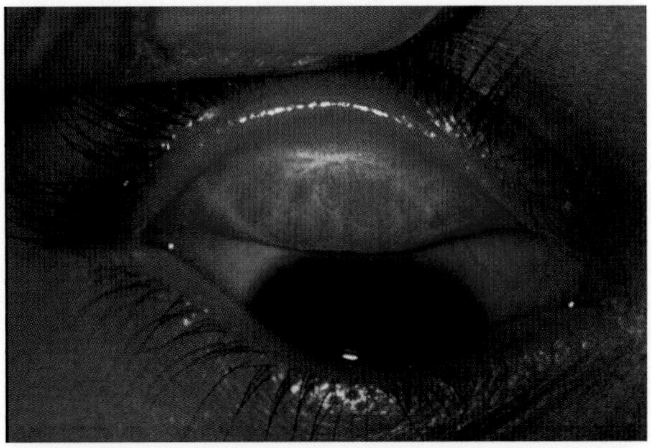

Fig. 94.17. TS – trachoma conjunctival scarring.

children. Repeated infection throughout childhood leads to conjunctival and tarsal plate scarring, TS (Fig. 94.17), starting around the age of 15 and gradually increasing in prevalence. The conjunctival scarring causes the eyelashes to turn in, TT, and the lashes rub on the cornea, producing ulceration, scarring (CO)and blindness (Fig. 94.18) seen more commonly in women than men.

Control of trachoma

The control of trachoma involves first identifying communities with blinding disease. This can be done using the grading scheme. A survey of 1–9-year-old children for TF and TI, and women over the age of 15 years for TT allows communities to be ranked according to the severity of disease. A prevalence of TF in excess of 20 per cent, or TT in excess of 1 per cent identifies a community with severe blinding disease.

The control of trachoma is summarized in Table 94.8 under the acronym SAFE (Bailey & Lietman, 2001).

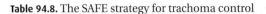

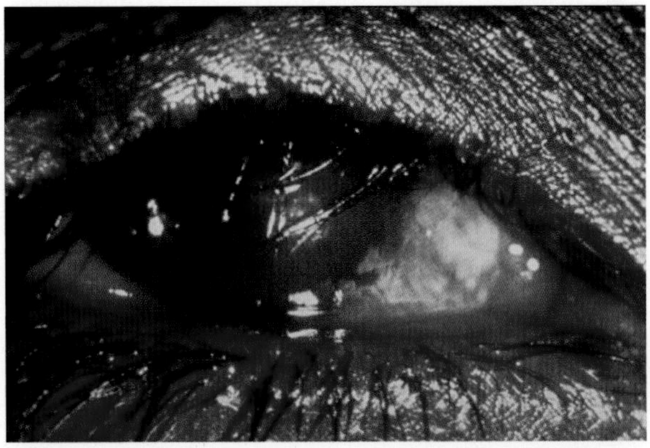

Fig. 94.18. TT and CO – trichiasis and corneal scarring due to trachoma.

Trichiasis

Trichiasis is defined as one or more eyelashes turning in to touch the globe, and entropion is when the eyelid margin turns in so that most or all of the eyelashes touch the eye. One or two lateral inturned eyelashes can be removed by epilation, which may have to be repeated every 6 weeks. If there is any suggestion of corneal damage, then lid surgery is indicated. The recommended procedure is a tarsal plate rotation (Reacher & Foster, 1993). Because trichiasis occurs mainly in women who are poor and live in rural areas, it is good policy to offer trichiasis surgery in the community in order to increase uptake and thereby prevent corneal blindness.

Azithromycin given systemically at least once per year has been shown to be equally effective as 6 weeks tetracycline eye ointment and people adhere to azithromycin treatment better (Bailey & Lietman, 2001). The aim is to treat all members of endemic communities who have the disease, or are at risk of acquiring/transmitting the infection.

A clean face has been shown to be protective for trachoma infection. Flies on faces of children are a definite risk factor. Community measures to reduce flies, improve water supply and sanitation and promote face cleanliness are important in removing the environmental determinants, which encourage the transmission of chlamydial infection.

Leprosy and the eye

See Chapter 47. Leprosy can affect the eyes by damaging the nerves to the eye, or by causing an inflammation in the iris – iritis.

Clinical signs of ocular leprosy

Eyelids

Leprosy can affect the facial (seventh cranial) nerve and cause paralysis of the orbicularis oculi muscle which closes the eye. Inability to close the eye is called lagophthalmos, and can lead to exposure of the cornea and resultant corneal ulceration, scarring and blindness.

Cornea

When the ophthalmic division of the trigeminal (fifth cranial) nerve is affected, the cornea is anaesthetic. The patient does not blink as much as usual and may also be unaware of minor trauma to the cornea. This can cause corneal ulceration, scarring and blindness.

Pupil

In leprosy there may be acute iritis as part of the ENL (erythema nodosum leprosum) reaction, with a red painful eye, and small irregular pupil. Leprosy may also cause a chronic low grade iritis in which the pupil is small and irregular, and will not dilate. The eye is usually white in chronic iritis.

Ocular examination of a patient with leprosy

- Visual acuity – it is important to measure and record the visual acuity in each eye of a leprosy patient.
- Eyelid closure – ask the patient to close the eyes gently and observe whether there is any lagophthalmos with corneal exposure.
- Fluorescein staining – use fluorescein to examine the cornea for evidence of exposure keratopathy or corneal ulcer.
- Dilate the pupil – give short-acting pupil dilators, e.g. cyclopentolate 0.5 per cent, to examine the pupil for evidence of posterior synechiae due to iritis.

Management

Lagophthalmos

If there is evidence of lagophthalmos it is necessary to protect the cornea when the patient is asleep by applying ointment, and strapping the upper eyelid to the cheek at night. If the lagophthalmos is severe and permanent, or if there is any evidence of corneal ulceration, a lateral tarsorrhaphy is indicated. This consists of sewing the upper and lower eyelids together over the lateral third of the eyelid margins.

Corneal anaesthesia

If there is evidence of corneal anaesthesia without ulceration, teach the patient *think-blink*. The patient is asked to think consciously about blinking and so protect the cornea by regular blinking.

Corneal ulcer

If there is a definite corneal ulceration, give the patient topical antibiotics and atropine. If there is lagophthalmos or corneal anaesthesia a lateral tarsorrhaphy is needed.

Iritis

In acute iritis dilate the pupil immediately and give the patient topical atropine and steroids. In chronic iritis it is important to keep the pupil dilated and to maintain the patient on mydriatics for life.

In summary, patients with leprosy can become blind from corneal scarring due to exposure of the cornea from

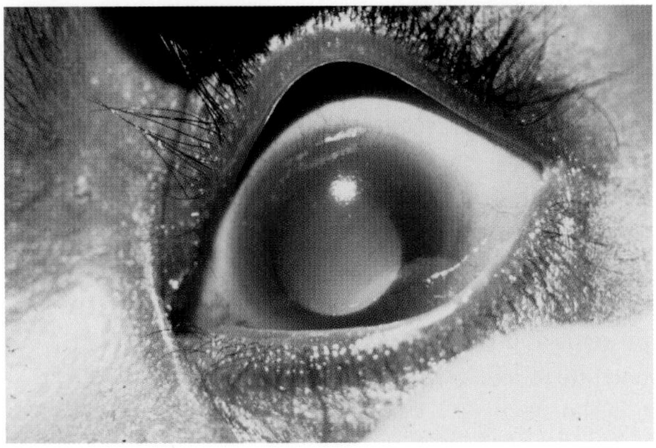

Fig. 94.19. Leukocoria due to retinoblastoma in an infant.

lagophthalmos and corneal anaesthesia. This can be prevented by early recognition of the problem, and educating the patient to protect his cornea during the day by blinking, and at night with ointment and strapping of the eyelid to the cheek. If these measures fail to protect the cornea, then a permanent lateral tarsorrhaphy is required. Leprosy patients can also become blind because of secondary cataract and secondary glaucoma as a consequence of iritis. In a patient with leprosy who has iritis it is important to dilate the pupil immediately and keep the patient on atropine for as long as there is any evidence of iritis.

Proptosis

Proptosis is protrusion of the eye out of the orbit due to a space-occupying lesion in the orbit, in children or adults. It is not common. The history may be of a gradual swelling over many months or years, or rapid over a few days or weeks. A careful history and examination, including palpation of the orbital rim for tumours, can help to identify the cause. Most cases need specialist care. The major causes are summarized in Table 94.9.

Retinoblastoma is a malignant tumour of the retina, which may be familial and can be bilateral. A squint may be the first sign or a white/yellow reflex in the pupil known as leukocoria (Fig. 94.19). Radiotherapy of the eye or enucleation at this stage may save the child's life. Untreated, the tumour spreads along the optic nerve and causes proptosis. The prognosis is poor.

Orbital cellulitis can result from infection entering the orbit from the sinuses or from trauma, with the added risk of spread to the meninges. There is a sudden onset of fever with swollen eyelids and proptosis. Treat with intensive systemic antibiotics.

Table 94.9. Major causes of proptosis in Africa

	Children	Adults
Acute (history of less than 3 months)	Retinoblastoma (0–5 yrs) Orbital cellulitis Burkitt's lymphoma (5–15 yrs)	Orbital cellulitis Pseudotumour Dysthyroid eye disease
Chronic (history of 3 months or more	Optic glioma Vascular abnormalities in the orbit	Lacrimal adenoma Frontal mucocoele Meningioma Hydatid cyst

Burkitt's lymphoma The orbit is one of the common sites. Painless proptosis develops rapidly, but the eye appears relatively normal. Treatment is with cytotoxics. (see Chapter 90).

Optic glioma is a slow growing benign tumour of the optic nerve. There is loss of vision with optic atrophy and then unilateral proptosis.

Vascular abnormalities of the orbit may be present at birth, develop during childhood or appear for the first time in adults. They include cavernous and capillary haemangiomas, arterio-venous fistulae and venous varices.

Pseudotumour The cause is unknown: it typically affects people aged 15–35. Over 1–2 weeks there is proptosis of one or both eyes, with or without paralysis of the extra-ocular muscles. All investigations are normal. High dose systemic steroids, which can be tailed off over 4 weeks, are effective although a maintenance dose of prednisolone 5 mg/day may be required for 3–6 months.

Dysthyroid eye disease may give bilateral or unilateral proptosis with abnormalities of thyroid gland function. It is more common in middle-aged women. Besides signs of thyroid dysfunction there may be lid retraction and limitation of ocular movements. If the proptosis threatens vision then systemic steroids may be used and, if this fails, an operation to decompress the orbit can be performed.

Lacrimal adenoma is a benign but locally invasive tumour of the lacrimal gland. There is gradual proptosis over months or years with a palpable tumour in the superior–temporal quadrant of the orbit. Treatment is total excision of the tumour with the lacrimal gland.

Frontal mucocoele presents as a cystic swelling in the upper medial quadrant of the orbit. There is slowly progressive proptosis. Treatment is by surgical drainage.

Meningioma affecting the sphenoid bone or the optic nerve can present as gradual proptosis, paralysis of eye movements and/or loss of vision. There is no satisfactory treatment. Diagnosis can usually be made on the X-ray, which shows a sclerotic appearance.

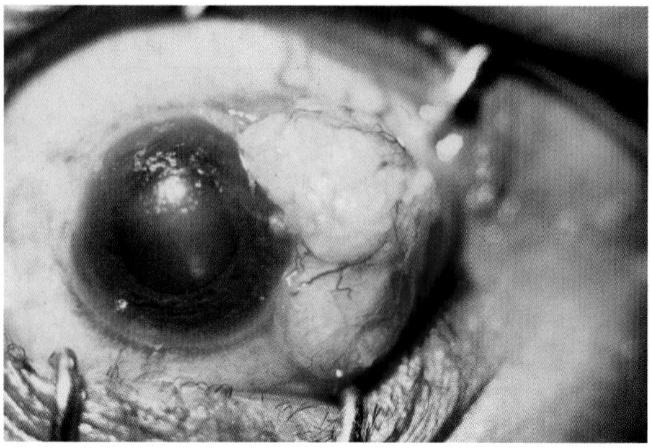

Fig. 94.20. Squamous cell carcinoma of the conjunctiva in a patient with HIV infection.

Hydatid disease (Chapter 24) This present as an orbital cyst and proptosis. Very careful surgical excision can be performed, but it is important not to rupture the cyst.

HIV infection and the eye

The ocular manifestations of HIV infection are varied (Kestelyn & Cunningham, 2001).

Tumours

Squamous cell carcinoma of the conjunctiva appears as a raised irregular lesion on the conjunctiva, which grows to invade the fornices, lids and cornea (Fig. 94.20). Treatment is by wide surgical excision where possible.

Kaposi's sarcoma may occur on the eyelids or conjunctiva. It appears as purple-red nodules on the skin and bright red lesions in the conjunctiva. Radiotherapy is the treatment of choice.

Non-opportunistic infections associated with HIV infection

Certain infectious diseases occur more commonly and are more severe in patients with HIV infection.

Herpes zoster presents initially with pain over one side of the head and face followed by a vesicular rash. The eyelids are always involved and there may be a keratitis and iritis, which can cause a raised intra-ocular pressure. The disease tends to be severe and involves the cornea in HIV-positive patients. Treatment is with oral acyclovir 800 mg × 5/day.

Herpes simplex keratitis with dendritic or geographic ulcers may occur and is sometimes seen in children. Treatment is with acyclovir ointment × 5 per day.

Syphilis may present as uveitis, retinitis or optic neuritis.

Tuberculosis is more common in HIV-positive individuals. Ocular complications include uveitis and choroiditis.

Toxoplasmosis is more severe in patients with HIV. It presents as posterior uveitis in one or both eyes with necrotic retinal lesions and vitreous haze.

Opportunistic infections

Some organisms, which are usually non-pathogenic, may cause intra-ocular infection in patients with HIV infection.

Cytomegalovirus (CMV) infection of the retina is the most common opportunistic infection of the eye and the major cause of blindness in AIDS patients. It is bilateral in 50 per cent of cases. The appearance is one of red haemorrhages and yellow necrotic tissue. It is progressive and can destroy the whole retina. Treatment is with ganciclovir.

Cryptococcus neoformans presents as papilloedema and headaches. There may be fever and neck stiffness indicating meningitis.

HIV retinopathy

Cotton wool spots in the retina are the most common sign of HIV infection. These are similar to those seen in diabetes and hypertension. They may disappear spontaneously.

Other features of HIV infection

HIV infection may be associated with nerve palsies and optic neuritis, in which case opportunistic infections should be suspected such as neurosyphilis.

In summary, infection with HIV is associated with a number of ocular manifestations, herpes zoster ophthalmicus and squamous cell carcinoma of the conjunctiva are particularly important and CMV retinitis is the commonest cause of visual loss due to HIV infection.

References

Bailey R, Leitman T. (2001). The SAFE strategy for the elimination of trachoma by 2020: will it work? *Bull Wld Hlth Org*, **79**: 233–236.

Brian G, Taylor HR. (2001). Cataract blindness – challenges for the 21st century. *Bull Wld Hlth Org*; **79**: 249–256.

Faal H, Minassian DC, Dolin PJ et al. (2000). Evaluation of a national eye care programme: a re-survey after 10 years. *Br J Ophthalmol*; **84**: 948–951.

Foster A. (1991). Who will operate on Africa's 3 million curably blind people? *Lancet*; **337**: 1267–1269.

Gilbert C, Foster A. (2001). Childhood blindness in the context of VISION 2020 – the right to sight. *Bull Wld Hlth Org*; **79**: 227–232.

Johnson GJ. (2001). Editorial: the adult glaucomas. *J Commun Eye Hlth*; **39**: 33–44.

Johnson GJ, Foster A. (2003). *The Epidemiology of Eye Disease. Prevalence, Incidence and Distribution of Visual Impairment.* Arnold.

Kestelyn PG, Cunningham ET. (2001). HIV/AIDS and blindness. *Bull Wld Hlth Org*; **79**: 208–213.

Reacher M, Foster A. (1993). *Trichiasis Surgery for Trachoma. The Bilamellar Tarsal Rotation Procedure.* WHO/PBL 93/29. Geneva: World Health Organization.

Schaller UC, Klauss V. (2001). Is Crede's prophylaxis for ophthalmia neonatorum still valid? *Bull Wld Hlth Org*; **79**: 262–263.

Taylor HR. (2000). Refractive errors: magnitude of the need. *J Commun Eye Hlth:* **33**: 1–12.

Thylefors B. (1995). Global data on blindness. *Bull Wld Hlth Org*; **73**: 115–121.

Thylefors B, Jones BR, Dawson C et al. (1987). A simplified system for the assessment of trachoma and its complications. *Bull Wld Hlth Org*; **65**: 477–483.

Whitchter JP, Srinavasan M, Upadhyay MP. (2001). Corneal blindness: a global perspective. *Bull Wld Hlth Org*; **79**: 214–221.

Whitfield R, Schwab L, Ross-Degnan D et al. (1990). Blindness and eye disease in Kenya: ocular status survey results from the Kenya Rural Blindness Prevention Project. *Br J Ophthalmol*; **74**: 333–340.

WHO/PBL. (1997). *Global Initiative for the Elimination of Avoidable Blindness.* Geneva: WHO, 1997.

Zerihun N, Mabey D. (1997). Blindness and low vision in Jimma zone, Ethiopia: results of a population-based survey. *Ophthal Epidemiol*; **4**: 19–26.

Further Reading

Johnson GJ, Weale R, Minassian D., West SK (2003). *The Epidemiology of Eye Disease.* Arnold.

95 Making the most of the laboratory

The function of a laboratory service

The laboratory service is a core component of any health service (Fig. 95.1). The importance of an efficient and effective laboratory is well recognized by clinicians working on the wards. However, the role of the laboratory is more far-reaching than simply to guide individual patient management. The laboratory can provide information on disease patterns in the hospital and local community and baseline data for research studies and interventions. Laboratories are also in a key position to identify early indications of epidemics and outbreaks.

Organization of laboratory services

Laboratory services are usually available in all but the most basic of health care facilities. In some countries these laboratories are linked to a system of public health or reference laboratories. Although the majority of laboratories are supported by the local government and to a lesser extent, religious organizations, an increasing number of private laboratories are springing up in cities throughout the continent.

In many African countries there is a shortage of qualified technicians and up to 80 per cent of laboratory workers are trained 'on the bench' (Ministry of Health, Ghana, 2000). This means that the smaller laboratories are often 'one-man-stations' with a single, untrained assistant responsible for the laboratory service. These assistants are usually senior or junior secondary school graduates. District hospital laboratories are usually manned by both assistants and technicians. Technicians have received a formal education in medical laboratory technology for 3 years. The central and teaching hospitals are staffed by a combination of scientists (university science graduates), technologists (2 years specialist post-technician training), technicians and assistants.

To ensure that the various laboratories from health posts to teaching hospitals perform well, methods to monitor and measure performance must be in place. This is especially important in countries where the majority of laboratories are in the hands of untrained, single-handed technical staff. Unfortunately most countries in Africa have not been able to establish supervisory systems and as a result the quality and effectiveness of the laboratory services is usually not known. Laboratories are one of the most expensive components of any health system, so poor performance has the potential to result in an enormous waste of resources. The World Health Organization (WHO) and other agencies support schemes for external monitoring of the quality of specific laboratory tests. However, inadequate laboratory networks, poor communications and a lack of senior technicians with the appropriate skills to establish and carry out monitoring and training mean that only a few laboratories in each country take part in the schemes.

What laboratory services should be provided?

Ideally, the services provided by the laboratory should be closely related to the clinical and public health needs and appropriate for the level of health care facility. The range of tests provided by a laboratory will therefore increase in sophistication from the health centre to the central hospital. The WHO has produced recommendations for the type of laboratory services that should be

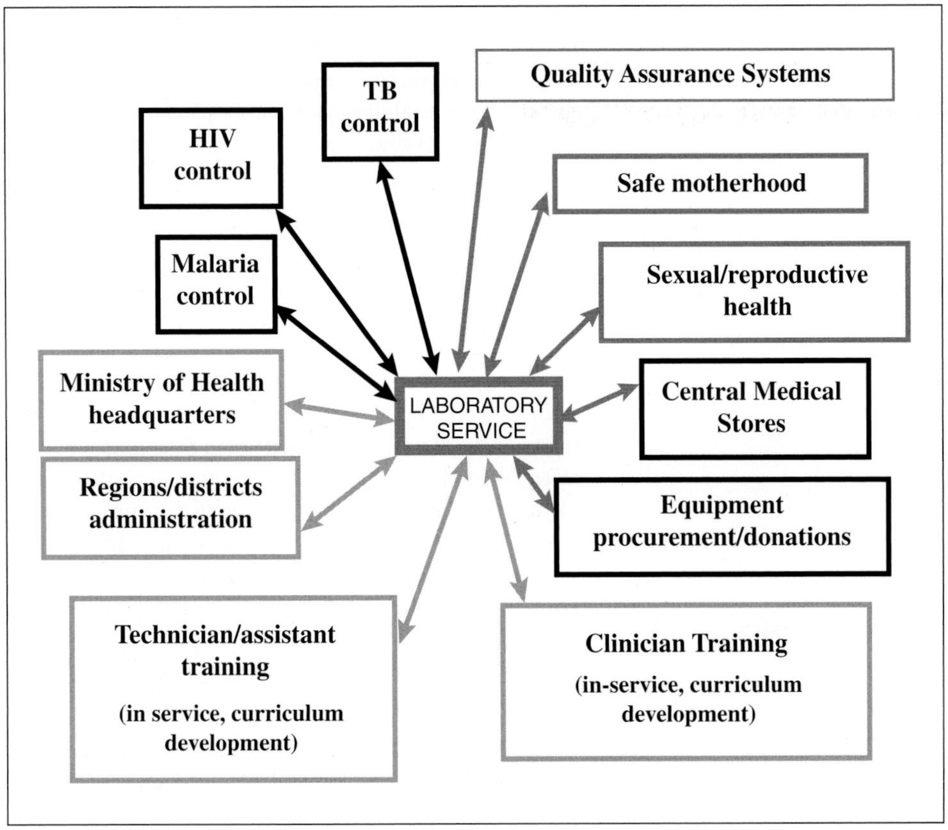

Fig. 95.1. The key role of the laboratory in the health service.

provided at different levels of health care but these may need to be adapted for local circumstances (WHO, 1986 and 1999). An example of the essential tests recommended for district laboratories in Malawi is given in the Box.

Essential laboratory services for district hospitals in Malawi

A: 'Critical' service area:
- Haemoglobin
- Blood transfusion (including donor screening for HIV, HBV and syphillis)
- TB microscopy
- HIV testing

B: 'Important' service areas
- CSF analysis
- Blood glucose
- Urine protein
- Urine and stool microscopy
- Antenatal syphilis screening

C: 'Potential additional services (selected hospitals only)
- Microbiology: blood and CSF culture and sensitivity

Prevalence of disease

Disease prevalence is an important determinant of the range of tests required. In areas where there is high transmission of malaria, the majority of the district hospital laboratory workload will consist of haemoglobin estimation, malaria diagnosis and blood transfusion. If HIV prevalence is high, then tests for tuberculosis and HIV are more important.

Resources

The range of tests to be provided needs to take into account much more than just the clinical demand. It depends critically on factors such as the cost, the skills of the technical staff, equipment maintenance and regular supplies of consumables. Some of the factors that need to be considered are listed in the Box. Laboratories do not usually have their own budget and often have to compete with pharmacy, radiology and other allied services for the same pot of money. Therefore, a balance has to be struck between what tests are needed and what can reasonably be provided with available resources.

Factors which influence choice of essential laboratory tests
- **Tests which are already provided**
- **Clinical and public health needs**
- **Resources**:
  - grades and numbers of staff
  - training requirements for tests
  - state of laboratory premises
  - safety procedures
  - availability and maintenance of equipment
  - regular supply of consumables
  - availability of quality control
  - supervision of requirements
  - transport availability
  - costs of all the above
  - available budget

Maintaining the quality of laboratory results

Why do we need to know the quality of laboratory results?

The drive to improve the quality of health care to reduce costs is a major issue for governments in Africa. Every laboratory should be able to demonstrate that tests are performed to an acceptable and reproducible standard. If laboratory results are poor, the users will lose confidence and either ignore the results or repeat the test elsewhere. This is an enormous waste of resources. In countries where patients bear the cost of tests, cost can deter people from making use of health services. Important budgeting decisions are also made on public health data provided by the laboratory. For example, an iron supplementation programme may be started on the basis of inaccurate haemoglobin results or decisions about the effectiveness of bed-nets may be made on invalid malaria results.

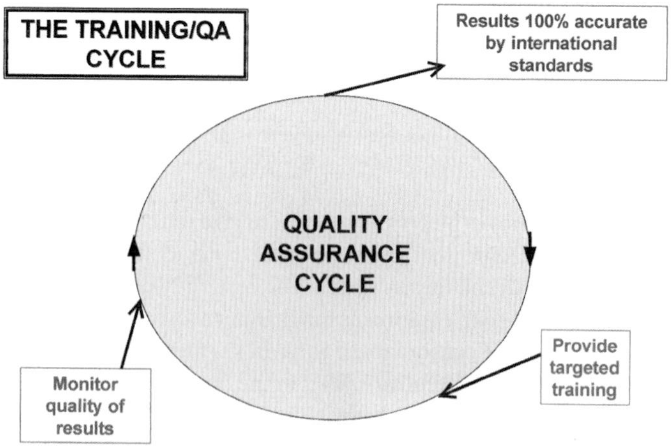

Fig. 95.2. The training/quality assurance cycle for improving the quality of laboratory tests.

Laboratory safety

Laboratory staff are at high risk of acquiring infections through their work, particularly HIV, hepatitis B and tuberculosis. If they are worried about their personal safety, they will not be able to perform their work to the highest standards. Therefore, to ensure that the laboratory is safe is an essential part of providing a high quality service. Laboratory safety guidelines have been published (WHO, 1997) and cover aspects such as personnel protection, adequate space and ventilation, waste disposal, provision of separate eating area and restricting access to the laboratory.

Improving the quality within the laboratory

Improving the performance of the laboratory does not just involve checking that results are accurate but includes the whole process from taking the sample from the patient to using the result to influence patient management (Cheesbrough, 1998; WHO, 1998). Much of this process is the responsibility of the clinician rather than of the laboratory technician.

To assess the quality of the processes within the laboratory, the supervisors need to instigate a cycle of continuous monitoring of quality of results and targeted training (see Fig. 95.2). The details of every method carried out by the laboratory are written down and then followed systematically. These methods may vary depending on the equipment available: several organizations have now produced their own 'Standard Operating Procedures' appropriate for use in African laboratories (Carter & Orgenes, 1994; WHO, 1986). Laboratory supervisors should check that these methods are adhered to, and monitor the quality of a laboratory's results by introducing samples of known value to be processed as part of the day's routine work. In the absence of a national quality assessment scheme it may be difficult for the supervisors to make sure that they have an accurate value for the sample. They may need to check the result with neighbouring laboratories or repeat the sample several times in their own laboratory and take an average value.

When the quality of a test is found to be poor, despite use of the correct method, the problem may lie with the equipment or reagents. For example, the optics of microscopes that are kept on the bench in humid conditions can quickly become covered in fungi. Despite poor visibility, an inexperienced and unsupervised laboratory assistant may continue to report results of malaria or tuberculosis smears (Mundy et al., 2000). The clinician will then make inappropriate treatment decisions based on misleading results, with significant consequences for the patient.

The clinicians' role in improving the quality of the laboratory service

Laboratory staff are responsible for ensuring that results provided by the laboratory are accurate and reach the clinician in time. However, studies of clinical use of the laboratory in Malawi have shown that up to 50 per cent of tests are wasted because clinicians make inappropriate laboratory requests or do not use the results to guide patient management (Ministry of Health and Population, Malawi, 2000). Clinicians interact with the laboratory both before (pre-analytical) and after (post-analytical) the sample has been tested (see Box).

Clinician responsibility – before the test

- Request the appropriate test.
- Provide the laboratory with the correct sample and enough clinical information to process the sample appropriately. (For example, if a request form for transfusion states 'post-partum haemorrhage' rather than just 'anaemia', then the laboratory will be alerted to prepare several units of blood for transfusion instead of just one.)
- indicate the urgency of the test with justification.

Clinical responsibility – results

- Check the result within an appropriate time.
- Interpret the results correctly.
- Use results to make the appropriate clinical decision.

The laboratory may issues correct results that are not useful to the clinician. For example, if the laboratory only reports the sensitivity of an organism to expensive antibiotics, the clinician may not be able to prescribe such costly medicines. Good communication between clinicians and technical staff is therefore critical in ensuring that the laboratory service is used effectively (see the Box).

Improving clinician–laboratory interaction

- Guidelines for urgent and on-call tests
- A booklet outlining the types of samples and bottles for specific tests
- Adaptations to request forms to enable sufficient information to be provided
- Education sessions about provision of emergency blood for transfusion

Making sure that the laboratory service is effective

Clinicians and technicians need to support each other

Technical staff are able to influence the way that clinicians use the laboratory service (Ministry of Health, Ghana, 2001) through a formal education programme such as workshops and clinical meetings. More informal but effective techniques include the preparation and use of guidelines, noticeboards, one-to-one discussions and laboratory staff in local management teams. Technical staff can also identify a local 'laboratory-friendly' clinician with whom they can work in partnership to educate clinicians.

Morale in the laboratory service in Africa is often low due to poor working conditions, low wages, and lack of career structure and professional recognition. Where private laboratories flourish, many technicians move into the private sector where wages can be several-fold higher than in government laboratories.

Clinicians can play a significant role in improving the morale and performance of laboratory staff by making sure that they are involved in making decisions about the practice of the laboratory and encouraging them to acquire higher skills such as management, financial planning and data handling.

The function and goal of the laboratory service is to provide results of an internationally acceptable standard to support individual and public health needs. The clinicians' goal is also to improve the health of patients and the general population. It is only when technical and clinical staff work in partnership that the laboratory service will achieve this goal.

References

Carter J, Orgenes L. (1994). *Practical Laboratory Manual for Health Centres in Eastern Africa.* Nairobi, Kenya: African Medical and Research Foundation.

Cheesbrough M. (1998). District laboratory practice in tropical countries. UK: Tropical Health Technology.

Ministry of Health and Population, Malawi (2000). Report of clinicians' use of district laboratory services in Malawi (available from the HIV Knowledge Programme, Liverpool School of Tropical Medicine, UK)

Ministry of Health, Ghana (2000). Regional in-service laboratory training programme. Workshop 2 report, p35.

Ministry of Health, Ghana (2001). Regional in-service laboratory training programme. Workshop 4 report, p17.

Mundy C, Ngwira M, Kadewele G et al. (2000). Evaluation of microscope condition in Malawi. *Trans Roy Soc Trop Med Hyg*; **94**: 583–584.

WHO. (1986). *Methods Recommended for Essential Clinical Chemical and Haematological Tests for Intermediate Hospital Laboratories.* WHO/LAB/86.3. Geneva: World Health Organization.

WHO. (1997). *Safety in Health-care Laboratories.* WHO/LAB/97.1. Geneva: World Health Organization.

WHO. (1998). *Quality Systems for Medical Laboratories.* Geneva: World Health Organization.

WHO. (1999). *Health Laboratory Services in Support of Primary Health Care in the South-East Asia Region.* Series no. 24. Geneva: World Health Organization.

The approach to treatment

96

The background in Africa

Disease patterns and economic factors

This chapter tries to achieve two goals: (a) practical advice for the hard-pressed clinician supported by too few resources, and (b) a theoretical consideration of the pharmacological principles that underlie therapeutics (with special reference to Africa). It is clear that these goals cannot be comprehensively attained and the reader should thus regard this as a general introduction to the discipline.

Treatment of diseases in Africa must be adapted to existing and fast changing patterns of disease. Infectious diseases currently account for much mortality and morbidity in the developing world, but non-infectious diseases (including psychiatric illness and coronary heart disease) are becoming more prevalent (Table 96.1). In addition, economic realities overshadow health care in Africa. For example:

- Government budgets must balance such essentials as provision of safe water and an appropriate supply of essential drugs.
- High prices often prevent people from buying drugs they need.
- Patients are often unable to reach adequate health facilities because they live too far away.

Late presentation and poor laboratory services

Because many rural people live far from health care and often consult a traditional healer first, they can present late at hospital with severe disease. Furthermore, in many places laboratory services are inadequate, so that a clinical diagnosis must suffice and is not supported by investigative proof. This clinical diagnosis is therefore the basis of treatment, which often becomes a therapeutic trial of the diagnosis.

Table 96.1. The changing pattern of disease burden in developing countries – 'TOP 15' conditions

Estimates for 1990		Projections for 2020	
Rank	Disease	Rank	Disease
1.	Lower respiratory infection	1.	Ischaemic heart disease
2.	Diarrhoeal disease	2.	Unipolar major depression
3.	Perinatal conditions	3.	Road traffic accident
4.	Unipolar major depression	4.	Cerebrovascular disease
5.	Ischaemic heart disease	5.	Chronic obstructive pulmonary disease
6.	Cerebrovascular disease	6.	Lower respiratory infection
7.	TB	7.	TB
8.	Measles	8.	War
9.	Road traffic accidents	9.	Diarrhoeal disease
10.	Congenital anomalies	10.	HIV
11.	Malaria	11.	Perinatal conditions
12.	Chronic obstructive pulmonary disease	12.	Violence
13.	Falls	13.	Congenital anomalies
14.	Iron deficiency anaemia	14.	Self-inflicted injuries
15.	Protein-energy malnutrition	15.	Tracheal, bronchial and lung cancers

Source: Data from Murray & Lopez (1996).

Attitudes towards traditional healing and 'western medicine'

Many people in Africa believe that disease is inevitable and that it may have resulted from supernatural causes. These beliefs are more dominant in unchanged rural societies (especially among the elderly), and apply more to severe or chronic diseases than to simple complaints. The traditional healer has a pivotal role, as it is s/he who is often consulted first, and s/he is the first to treat. Traditional healers are often more readily available than medical workers, and enjoy easy communication with their patients since most share a common language and culture. Until evidence-based health care is available to all, traditional healers will continue to be important. There are, however, many negative aspects to the widespread reliance on traditional healers:

- In an emergency, consultation of the healer may delay critical interventions for life-threatening disease.
- Although many traditional healing methods are harmless, others carry risk (e.g. poisoning or infection).
- Characteristically, traditional healers provide 'once-and-for-all' remedies, and patients usually expect a painful or unpleasant intervention (perhaps scarification or burning) which is not repeated, particularly if it results in an early cure. This may partly explain the popularity of drug administration by injection. These 'once-and-for-all' remedies may make it difficult for some patients to understand that they need the continuous long-term treatment recommended by 'western medicine'.
- Few traditional healers follow up their patients, so patients may move from one healer to another seeking satisfaction (but delaying access to curative intervention and often suffering cumulative risk).

From 'western medicine' (for want of a better term) patients commonly seek the following (see Box):

Common demands on 'western medicine'
- Immediate and dramatic relief of symptoms.
- Administration of drugs by injection.
- Inexpensive treatment.
- Medical facilities that are conveniently placed.

In these expectations they are often disappointed, and may abandon appropriate evidence-based care in favour of the traditional approach. The remedy for this problem lies, as does so much, in the long-term goals of improved education and personal income. In the short term health education campaigns may help target particular problem areas. The doctor ignores these tensions at the risk of disadvantage to his patients.

The aims of treatment

There is no difference here between practice in Africa and other parts of the world: the physician must remember the Hippocratic instruction: 'first do no harm'. In short, the anticipated benefits of an intervention must exceed its predicted risks.

Prevention

At the start of the last century disease burdens in the industrialized nations fell more as a result of improved income, housing and education, than through medical intervention. The same could be expected for Africa – but this is a long-term hope rather than a medium-term goal.

In the short term safe, cost-effective preventive strategies often have clear merit over treatment of established disease. In the case of infectious diseases, vaccination is an established strategy and vector control methods (or personal protection against bites) can be cost-effective but chemoprophylaxis is generally reserved for highly vulnerable groups (e.g. protection of primigravidae against falciparum malaria). Where effective chemoprophylaxis exists, the lack of widespread deployment for populations in disease-endemic areas is usually for one or more of the following reasons:

- high cumulative cost
- supply and distribution difficulties
- non-ending exposure to disease transmission and therefore cumulative risk of drug toxicity
- the risk that drug resistance may develop through extensive exposure.

In the case of the increasingly prevalent non-communicable diseases, lifestyle modification is the goal and health education is the key (although legislation may also have a role). Given that such interventions have had only limited success in industrialized nations (where communications and education standards present a more favourable climate than in Africa), it remains to be seen what impact they might have in Africa.

'Cure' and 'control'

Of the common diseases afflicting developing nations (Table 96.1), cure is the aim for most cases of bacterial/parasitic infection and nutritional deficiency. Conversely, conditions such as hypertension, epilepsy, heart failure, psychiatric illness and diabetes are incurable at present. Maintenance treatment is standard practice, and adherence depends on three principles (see the Box):

Principles of long-term treatment
- The patient must understand the aims of treatment and the risks of interruption of therapy.
- An uninterrupted drug supply must be assured.
- Continuity of medical supervision must be reliable.

In some settings it may be impossible to meet these requirements. Under these circumstances a disease such as type-I diabetes mellitus, which has received successful maintenance treatment for decades in Europe, may prove rapidly fatal in rural Africa. Use of 'highly active anti-retroviral treatment' (HAART) for AIDS, and the infrastructure needed to use these drugs with safety, is another example of this gross North–South imbalance.

Relief of symptoms

Analgesia is the most common example of such symptomatic relief. Unfortunately, potent opiates may not always be freely available in some countries, so that the management of trauma and terminal illness is difficult.

The pharmacological basis of therapeutics

There is no succinct definition of a drug, but it can be taken to mean any molecule used to alter body functions to prevent or treat disease. Although a drug generally produces the same type of effect in different people, there can be wide variation in the degree of that effect. The factors underlying such individual variation in response to drugs have obvious clinical importance.

Most drugs exert their effects on the body by interacting with macromolecules that are usually on the surface of, or within, cells. These 'targets' may be:

- regulatory receptors, e.g., catecholamine receptors to which the asthma drug salbutamol binds
- enzymes, e.g., the mono amine oxidase inhibited by the antiparkinsonian drug selegiline
- structural proteins, e.g., tubulin, to which colchicine binds thereby reducing chemotaxis of inflammatory cells
- molecular 'pumps', e.g., H^+/K^+ ATP-ase which is inhibited by the ulcer-healing drug omeprazole

Variation in these macromolecule 'targets' (such as the number available, mutations and the concentration of other compounds competing for binding to the 'target') is one cause of inter-individual variability in drug response. The processes underlying these concepts are termed pharmacodyamics. Genetic factors also alter pharmacodynamic parameters. At the moment it is often impossible to predict the quantitative response of an individual to a drug, but the human genome project and post-genomic technology are likely to provide a greater degree of precision in the near future.

Clinical response to a drug can sometimes be directly measured with accuracy, like the effect of insulin on blood glucose or warfarin on clotting, and this measurement alone can be enough to predict how much drug is needed and how often. More usually such direct measurements are impossible and an indirect approach (using drug concentrations and their rates of change) can be used to predict the magnitude and duration of action of a drug. Variation in drug concentration (caused by differences in absorption, distribution, metabolism or excretion) is the other major cause of inter-individual variability in drug response: the underlying concepts are termed pharmacokinetics. Genetic factors and disease states alter drug disposition in ways that are relatively well understood, but again the post-genomic era is likely to see enhanced precision in the prediction of pharmacokinetics in individual patients.

Routes of drug administration, absorption and bioavailability

Drugs can be delivered directly to their site of action ('topical' use) as is the case with skin/vaginal/ear preparations and inhaled drugs for asthma. More usually drugs are delivered distant from their site of action ('systemic' use). Systemic routes of administration include the following.

Intravenous injection or infusion

Absorption is not required. Rapid i.v. administration often achieves transient very high blood concentrations, and this can lead to toxicity (for example chloroquine, quinine, phenytoin and aminophylline).

Intramuscular or sub-cutaneous injection

Absorption is required for systemic drug effects (paradoxically, the therapeutic effect of local anaesthetics is, of course, terminated by absorption). The major determinants of the rate of absorption are: (a) blood flow (muscle blood flow falls during shock), and (b) formulation (some drugs, such as some insulin preparations, are formulated to provide a 'slow trickle' of drug for a prolonged period). When given i.m. or s.c., most drugs are rapidly and completely absorbed. However, for physicochemical reasons, some drugs are slowly, incompletely and erratically absorbed from such routes, e.g. phenytoin and diazepam. Local infection (including muscle abscess and tetanus) is a real risk if equipment is re-used but non-sterile.

Rectal suppository

Some drugs are given as suppositories, as topical treatment for the rectal mucosa. In other instances the aim is drug absorption from the rectal site, via the portal system, into the systemic circulation. The rectal route can be useful for patients who cannot take drugs by mouth, and when parenteral administration is impossible, e.g. the use of artesunate suppositories for severe malaria in peripheral health facilities. Retention of suppositories is a real concern when the disease being treated is life-threatening, and staffing levels are sub-optimal: early expulsion of suppositories can easily go undetected, especially in young children.

Oral formulations

This is the commonest route of administration, and usually much safer than parenteral administration. Bioavailability is a quantitative term, that applies to any route of administration (other than i.v.), meaning: 'the proportion of a dose that proceeds unaltered from the site of delivery to the systemic blood'. After oral dosing bioavailability may be incomplete because:

- the drug molecule breaks up in the acid pH of the stomach, e.g. benzyl-penicillin
- the drug molecule is incapable of crossing lipid membranes, e.g. gentamicin
- the drug is metabolized during its first pass through the liver, e.g. glyceryl trinitrate
- disease has changed gut function, e.g. rapid gut transit time or marked reduction in surface area, as in coeliac disease.

Plasma protein binding and tissue distribution

Most drugs travel in the plasma partly in solution in the plasma water and partly bound to plasma proteins, and the ratio of one to the other varies between drugs. Binding is reversible and the bound and unbound drug fractions are always in a state of dynamic equilibrium. Only the unbound drug fraction is available to cross membranes and produce an effect. Acidic drugs mainly bind to albumin, while bases bind more avidly to α_1-acid glycoprotein.

Protein binding can be clinically important when, because of a disease state, plasma protein concentrations fall (e.g. albumin concentrations in liver cirrhosis or nephrotic syndrome) or rise, e.g. α_1-acid glycoprotein in cerebral malaria. Examples of drugs extensively bound to proteins include quinine, warfarin and diazepam. Examples of drugs with less extensive protein binding include: digoxin, penicillin and gentamicin.

Most drugs have their effects in the tissues. The degree to which a given drug is likely to accumulate in a tissue can be predicted (without accuracy) from knowledge of its lipophilicity and the blood flow of the tissue. Highly lipophilic drugs cross membranes readily even in the presence of tight junctions between endothelial cells (e.g. in the central nervous system). The principal determinant of tissue distribution is organ blood flow. For example, the anaesthetic induction-agent thiopentone accumulates to a greater degree in brain than in muscle because of the much higher blood flow in the brain. In contrast, hydrophilic drugs cross membranes poorly. The principal determinant of tissue distribution will, therefore, be the degree of 'leakiness' of the capillary endothelium. For example, gentamicin and penicillin accumulate to a greater degree in muscle than in brain because of the leaky nature of muscle capillaries.

Biotransformation

Most biotransformation takes place in the liver. The chemical processes involved are numerous and are broadly classified into phase I and phase II reactions (which, confusingly, does not mean that phase I necessarily precedes or is followed by phase II).

Phase I processes include oxidation, reduction and hydrolysis. Of these, oxidation reactions are most commonly encountered and are often catalysed by one of the family of cytochrome P450 enzymes (CYP450). Phase I usually results in the introduction or exposure of a polar group, increased water solubility, and abolition of pharmacological activity. However, this abolition of pharmacological activity is not invariable. The phase I products of some drugs have pharmacological activity while the parent compound does not (the so-called *prodrugs*, e.g. proguanil is metabolized to its active form cycloguanil by one of the CYP450s). Furthermore, in other cases the phase I products of a drug are highly toxic (for example the quinoneimine generated in paracetamol poisoning).

Phase II processes (often termed 'conjugation') involve the attachment to the drug (or perhaps a Phase-I product) of an endogenous substance, such as glucuronate, sulphate or acetyl groups. The resulting conjugate is almost invariably polar, water soluble and without pharmacological activity.

Genetic differences have profound effects on the levels of certain drugs in the body. For example, several drugs are eliminated by acetylation, e.g. the TB drug isoniazid. 'Slow acetylators' comprise a group at risk of toxicity from these drugs (and the proportions of fast and slow acetylators vary between ethnic groups). Similarly, disease can also alter the rate of biotransformation: for example, metabolism of opioids is slower in patients with liver disease.

Excretion

The kidney is the main organ for irreversible elimination of parent drugs or their metabolites. Renal blood flow is about 1.5 l/min, and about 10 per cent of this, by volume, appears as glomerular filtrate. Only unbound drug may be filtered since protein molecules are too large. Cells of the proximal convoluted tubule can actively secrete some compounds, mostly relatively strong acids and bases, into the lumen of the nephron (e.g. penicillin). Under these circumstances, and assuming that no reabsorption occurs, the rate of excretion of a drug exceeds its rate of filtration. Active reabsorption has evolved to help conserve nutrients. Certain drugs may also be extensively reabsorbed. Such compounds tend to be lipid soluble and un-ionized at urine pH. This is of most importance in poisoning by drugs, for example aspirin.

Parent drugs and metabolites with molecular weights greater than about 350 may be actively excreted into the bile. Examples include many drug conjugates (products of phase-II metabolism). This process may be followed by loss of the drug in the faeces. However, drug conjugates may be broken down by gut bacteria, releasing the parent drug which may be reabsorbed. The resulting enterohepatic circulation may have important clinical consequences, as it does for oral contraceptive steroids.

Pharmacokinetic parameters

Half-life

This is probably the easiest parameter to envisage and means 'the time taken for concentration to fall to half its original value' in hours. With regular dosing, a drug achieves 50 per cent of its steady-state concentration after one half-life, 75 per cent after two half-lives, 88 per cent after three, 94 per cent after four and 97 per cent after five half-lives. Similarly, if drug treatment is stopped, 97 per cent of the mass in the body has been lost when five half-lives have elapsed.

Clearance

For the majority of drugs the rate of elimination (E) is directly proportional to the drug concentration (c). In other words: $E = kc$, where k is a constant. This constant is termed clearance, and can be envisaged as the volume of plasma that is cleared completely of the drug per unit time. The unit of measurement is, therefore, litres per hour.

Apparent volume of distribution (VD)

Once in the tissue, most drugs bind to macromolecules. Some of this binding mediates drug action, while other binding is 'inert'. Some drugs, like aspirin, mainly stay in the circulation and undergo little tissue binding whereas others, such as the tricyclic antidepressants, are so extensively bound in the tissues (mostly in an 'inert' manner) that plasma concentrations are small. The units of measurement are those of volume, ie. millilitres or litres (often adjusted for body weight). The clinical relevance of VD is most apparent after overdose. The risks of dialysis are worth taking for patients with severe aspirin overdose because most of the drug is in the plasma. In contrast, dialysis is pointless for tricyclic overdose, because most of the drug is in the tissues.

Adverse drug reactions (ADRs)

All drugs cause toxicity, and such ADRs are very common. In Britain it is estimated that ADRs occur in 10–20 per cent of all patients prescribed drugs, and are the cause of up to 10 per cent of all GP consultations, 4 per cent of all hospital admissions and about 1 in 1000 deaths. Such data are unavailable for Africa. There are four types as follows.

Type A

The augmented or attenuated effect, where the ADR is caused by an excessive or inadequate response to the drug. The ADR is predictable from the known effects of the drug and is concentration related. Such effects are very common but are often not severe. Type A ADRs can be managed by dose modification.

Type B

The bizarre effect, which is not predictable from the known effects of the drug and often has an immunological basis. As such, there is often no clear relationship to the dose of drug. Such ADRs are relatively rare but are disproportionately important because of their severity. Some 'special groups' (e.g. HIV-positive individuals) are at particular risk. Withdrawal of the drug is usually necessary.

Type C

Effects of chronic administration of a drug, caused by adaptation, change in receptor sensitivity etc. Examples are rebound angina on withdrawal of beta-blockers, or the 'on-off' phenomenon with L-dopa.

Type D

Delayed effects, such as carcinogenesis or effects on reproduction, for example, stilboestrol (Chapters 32–35).

Pre-marketing testing of a new drug involves its administration to an average of about 1500 people (more usually adults than children, and more commonly men than women; 'special groups' such as the elderly or people with renal impairment, may not be studied at all). Thus type B reactions, which are often infrequent (perhaps 1: 10000 users) are unlikely to be seen in trials. These may only become apparent after the drug is launched and the numbers of humans treated with it rises. Likewise the late type C and D effects are only likely to be seen after the drug has been available for some years. Patients particularly at risk of ADRs include those groups shown in the Box.

Risk groups for adverse drug reactions

- The very young.
- Patients with renal disease.
- Patients with liver disease.
- People predisposed by other diseases, such as HIV.
- Genetically predisposed patients, e.g. with glucose 6-phosphate dehydrogenase deficiency.
- The elderly, who have little physiological reserve and often have unsuspected renal impairment.

Adverse drug interactions

Not all interactions are of clinical importance, and they may not occur in every patient. Constant vigilance is therefore required to spot them when they do occur (and take action). Many lists of possible drug interactions are available (see Appendix 1 in *British National Formulary*, 2000), but rather than memorize these, it is better to consider which patients are at risk, which drugs are most likely to be involved and what the possible mechanisms are. Patients who are at risk of interactions include the following.

- Severely ill patients who often take many medications. In addition, drug interactions may be difficult to distinguish from the natural history of the disease.
- Patients on long-term or lifetime prophylactic therapy, e.g. anti-epileptic, anti-hypertensive and anti-psychotic drugs.
- Patients with liver or renal disease.
- Patients with more than one doctor. Interactions often occur when treatment has been obtained from private practitioners before presentation to the formal health sector.
- Patients who take non-prescribed drugs.
- The elderly because of polypharmacy and poor homeostatic mechanisms.

Some drugs are particularly likely to be involved in serious interactions.

- Drugs with a narrow therapeutic index, e.g. theophylline, quinine, digoxin, cytotoxics, aminoglycosides and warfarin.
- Drugs with a steep dose-response curve, where a minor change in plasma concentration may make a major change in effect, e.g. sulphonylureas.
- Drugs with a major effect on a vital process such as clotting (warfarin).
- Drugs where a loss of effect may lead to disease breakthrough, e.g. anti-epileptics.
- Drugs that may induce or inhibit mixed function oxidase enzymes and so may decrease metabolism of other drugs, and drugs which depend on these enzymes for their metabolism (e.g. theophylline, warfarin, oral contraceptives and many others).

Pharmacokinetic mechanisms of drug interactions include alteration in the following processes.

Absorption

Drugs such as cholestyramine may bind to other drugs, e.g. digoxin, thiazides, in the gastrointestinal tract and prevent their absorption. Some drugs, e.g. opiates, may slow transit time and so may slow absorption. Some drugs depend on enterohepatic circulation to achieve effective drug levels, e.g. oral contraceptive oestrogens. If this is prevented, for example by amoxycillin altering gut flora, the drug may lose its effect.

Metabolism

Some drugs can increase the rate of synthesis of CYP450s and the resulting enzyme induction can enhance the clearance of other drugs. Usually such induction requires exposure to the inducing agent for over a week before effects are seen. Examples of inducing agents are rifampicin, carbamazepine, phenobarbitone and phenytoin.

Other drugs can inhibit CYP450s (usually by competing for the enzyme's active site). This is usually seen rapidly after drug exposure (within a couple of days). Examples of enzyme-inhibiting agents are cimetidine, erythromycin, ciprofloxacin and isoniazid.

Distribution

Only free drug is pharmacologically active, but many drugs are heavily protein bound, e.g. warfarin to albumin. If another drug with a high affinity for protein is prescribed, the result may be a displacement of warfarin from the protein-binding sites, increasing the free drug and its effects (though this is transient). This may cause confusion if therapeutic drug monitoring is used, because this usually measures total rather than free drug.

Excretion

Drugs can interfere with renal excretion, for example quinine reduces digoxin clearance.

Pharmacodynamic drug interactions are common, but are predictable from the known effects of the drug, e.g.

two antihypertensives may be used to lower the blood pressure more than either alone. Alternatively, the actions of diuretics are opposed by NSAIDs, which may cause fluid retention, or the effects of oral hypoglycaemics may be opposed by thiazides.

Effects of disease on drug response

For the majority of drugs, clinically serious interindividual variation in response is not a frequent problem – most have fairly reproducible effects. However, certain diseases alter drug response predictably, so that the dose must be altered to avoid either toxicity or therapeutic failure. Disease may affect (a) pharmacokinetics, and (b) pharmacodynamics.

Pharmacokinetic factors

Absorption

Acute gastrointestinal infections, both viral and bacterial, may increase motility, reducing transit time and hence drug absorption. The severe chronic diarrhoea often seen in AIDS patients may reduce the absorption of anti-TB drugs. Reduced blood flow can have a major effect on the i.m. route. Absorption may also be critically slowed in patients with shock.

Distribution

Diseases which change plasma protein concentrations alter drug effect by increasing or decreasing the drug concentration unbound in the plasma water (see above). Most drugs have their effects in specific tissues, diffusing out of the plasma to reach effective local concentrations: inflammation of membrane barriers and changes in local pH may affect this process, e.g. partition of the penicillins into the brain during meningitis.

Metabolism

Alteration in drug metabolism is among the most commonly encountered causes of disease-induced changes in drug response. Predictably, the drugs concerned (a) are extensively metabolized to inactive derivatives, (b) have serious concentration-dependent toxicity, and (c) have narrow therapeutic indices. Most drugs are metabolised in the liver. This organ has tremendous reserve, and changes in drug effects may not be seen until there is loss of much of the parenchyma, when both first-pass metabolism and systemic metabolism may be reduced. Be cautious in prescribing for patients with acute or chronic liver disease.

Excretion

Drugs that cause concern in patients with renal impairment usually fulfil the following criteria: (a) they are excreted unchanged, (b) they cause serious concentration-dependent toxicity and (c) their therapeutic indices are small. Both acute and chronic renal failure reduce drug excretion rate in proportion to the reduction in glomerular filtration rate. Major examples include, aminoglycosides, digoxin and the sulphonylureas (see Appendix 3 of *British National Formulary*, 2000).

Pharmacodynamic factors

Less responsive 'target'

Disease may compromise the function of target organs or alter their receptor status. For example, type-1 diabetes cannot be treated with sulphonylureas because the disease-state results from the loss of pancreatic β-cells. Since much of the response to sulphonylureas results from increased insulin secretion, their activity is diminished or absent. In contrast, of course, sulphonylureas are routinely used in the treatment of type-2 diabetes.

The presence of endogenous ligands

If the disease allows the accumulation or increased synthesis of endogenous compounds with the opposite effect to that of the drug, it will be rendered less efficacious. For example, phaeochromocytomas present with hypertension (often accelerated), and the use of beta-blockers may cause a rise in blood pressure because the high concentration of circulating catecholamines binds readily to α-receptors causing vasoconstriction (and hence increased peripheral resistance).

More responsive 'target'

Disease may already 'mimic' the desired drug effect, so that addition of the drug causes an unexpectedly marked response. The 'interactions' between chronic liver disease and anticoagulant/antiplatelet drugs are commonly encountered in this regard. Clotting factors are synthesized in the liver, and parenchymal disease often prolongs tests of intrinsic and extrinsic clotting cascades. Thus the effects of warfarin and aspirin are more pronounced than in health.

References

British National Formulary. (2000). London, UK: *British Medical Association and Royal Pharmaceutical Society of Great Britain.*

Murray CJL, Lopez AD (1996). *The Global Burden of Disease (Summary)*, p. 4. Harvard, USA: Harvard School of Public Health.

Part VI

Common life-threatening emergencies

97

Emergencies

Introduction

This chapter covers common emergencies likely to be met in African medical practice. Ideal mangement for the first few hours (until the patient is stable) is covered in each case. Brief summaries are also included to cover emergency management at the front line, in circumstances where resources may be very limited.

While putting together this chapter there has been constant debate about the resources likely to be available in various settings. We are aware of wide variations across the African continent, and of the fact that many health professionals have to cope with emergencies with the barest minimum of resources. For example, recommended managements often depend on high-flow oxygen being available, but in practice there are many hospitals where this is impossible – should oxygen therefore be omitted from the recommendations? Similarly, various blood tests are mentioned, often including electrolyte measurement. Electrolytes can be measured accurately in few African hospitals, but should they therefore be omitted from a management plan?

We have decided to present currently accepted best emergency management, because capital cities and major towns often have centres where there are excellent facilities and well-trained staff. Where it is impossible to put all the recommendations into practice, we know that the resourcefulness and common-sense of local medical teams will adapt the ideal to what is locally possible.

The critically ill patient

This section deals with the emergency management of acutely ill patients, including basic resuscitation and the recognition and management of shock.

Recognizing the patient at risk

The following clinical features often herald a downward spiral into multi-organ failure and death. If recognized early and acted upon, lives can be saved. For ease of memory, the ABCD system is helpful.

Airway	signs of airway obstruction – struggling to breathe, choking, bulging eyes
Breathing	respiratory rate <8 per minute respiratory rate >30 per minute
Circulation	pulse <50 per minute pulse >120 per minute systolic blood pressure <90 mmHg *oxygen saturation <90% on 60% inspired oxygen
Other **D**anger signs	sudden falls in conscious level seizures *hypoglycaemia urine output <30 ml per hour

* = useful measurements when available in the emergency department

Airway

Upper airway obstruction can occur anywhere between the mouth and the trachea. It is always a medical emergency. *The commonest cause of upper airway obstruction is the tongue, which falls back in comatose patients.*

Look for paradoxical movements of the chest and abdomen if the patient is straining to breathe against an obstructed airway (a 'see–saw' pattern between chest and abdomen, instead of the normal expansion of both chest and abdomen as the diaphragm moves down and the lungs inflate).

Look also for contraction of the accessory muscles of ventilation as the patient struggles to breathe.

Open the mouth and look for possible obstructing foreign bodies, blood or vomit. Cyanosis is a very late sign, often accompanied by bulging eyes, protruding tongue and incontinence.

Listen for sounds that may help to localize the obstruction:

- gurgling from liquid in the mouth or upper airway
- snoring when the pharynx is partially obstructed by the tongue, e.g. in the unconscious patient
- crowing (high pitched stridor) when the larynx and vocal cords are affected by spasm, obstruction or oedema
- inspiratory stridor is usually from the larynx or above
- stridor throughout inspiration and expiration is usually from an obstruction in the trachea and main bronchi

Feel for air movement in front of the mouth, and open the patient's mouth to feel for obstructions in the mouth and oropharynx.

Clear an obstructed airway immediately.

- Use back slaps if patient is choking on food, or abdominal thrusts standing behind the patient (Heimlich's manoeuvre). Dangle a small child by the heels and slap the back.
- Explore the mouth and pharynx manually and remove obstructing foreign bodies and vomit.
- Tilt the chin and head up to draw the tongue forward (care if danger of cervical spine instability – if in doubt use the jaw thrust technique, grasping the mandibles at the jaw angles and moving the whole jaw forward).
- If the airway remains obstructed, either perform emergency laryngoscopy or needle tracheostomy followed by 100% oxygen.
- Place unconscious patient in the recovery position.
- Once oxygenation is re-established, seek help and decide on further procedures – laryngoscopy, bronchoscopy, tracheostomy.

Breathing

Look at the depth of respiration and count the respiratory rate. Rates higher than 20 per minute, particularly if rising, often indicate serious illness.

Look at chest movements and note use of accessory muscles. Look for asymmetrical chest movement – reduced movement on one side may mean pleural fluid, pneumonia or pneumothorax.

Feel, percuss, and auscultate the chest. Pneumonia, pleural effusion and pneumothorax all have clear cut physical signs (see section on respiratory emergencies below).

Immediate management of acute breathlessness

- Give all critically breathless patients immediately sufficient oxygen to maintain a saturation of 90%.
- If no oximeter is available to measure saturation, give oxygen at a rate of at least 4 litres/minute. Increase the rate to 10 litres/minute using a mask with reservoir if necessary (filled beforehand and kept full).
- Use high flow oxygen cautiously in patients with a long history of smoking-related chronic obstructive disease (rare in most of Africa). They may have become dependent on their hypoxic ventilatory drive, and giving high flow oxygen could reduce or even stop ventilation.

Circulation

Always remember that hypovolaemia is the commonest primary cause of shock and circulatory failure.

Look and **feel** for cool sweaty hands and underfilled peripheral veins. Is there any evidence of haemorrhage?

Check urine output (oliguria is defined as output below 30 ml/hour).

Feel the arterial pulses, and the apex beat. Weak pulses suggest poor cardiac output, whereas a full pulse may mean sepsis.

Measure the JVP (jugular venous pressure). A raised JVP suggests right heart failure, or gross fluid overload. Peripheral oedema will be present if heart failure is long standing.

Listen to the heart: remember that the combination of distant sounds and a JVP that rises on inspiration may mean acute cadiac tamponade.

Take the blood pressure both lying down and standing (a postural fall of >20 mmHg in systolic pressure is a strong pointer to hypovolaemia). Even in severe shock, the BP may still be normal due to compensatory mechanisms.

Immediate management of circulatory failure

- Give intravenous fluid to patients with sustained tachycardia and cool peripheries, unless there are clear signs of a primary cardiac cause (e.g. cardiac tamponade or congestive cardiac failure)
- Be careful if the patient is already receiving i.v. fluids – there may be overhydration. Look carefully at the JVP.
- Insert a central venous line to monitor CVP accurately. Aim to maintain CVP in the range 5–10 cm H_2O

Rapid neurological assessment

Examine the pupils for size, equality, reaction to light. Then use the AVPU system to assess conscious level:

- **A** **A**lert
- **V** responds to **V**oice
- **P** responds to **P**ain
- **U** **U**nresponsive

At the end of the rapid ABCD assessment, which should be accomplished in a few minutes, seek further information from relatives or other witnesses and look at any charts, letters and other materials relating to the patient.

Record carefully your own findings.

You should now be in a position to plan immediate management, and then to move to the next phases of stabilising, investigating, and treating the patient.

Shock

Definition of shock

Shock is said to be present when inadequate tissue perfusion leads to progressive failure of cellular function.

Types of shock

Hypovolaemic

Blood loss (haemorrhage, trauma, gastrointestinal bleeding)
Plasma loss (burns)
Fluid and electrolyte loss (diarrhoea, vomiting, cholera)
Capillary leak (anaphylaxis, ruptured hydatid cyst, snake bite)

Septic (Widespread capillary and cell damage by microbial toxins)

Abortion, post-partum, infected wounds
Gram-positive or gram-negative septicaemia (including meningitis and pneumonia)
Malaria, dengue fever.

Cardiogenic

Cardiac failure
Cardiac tamponade
Malignant arrhythmias

More than one of these causes may be present at the same time, for example, after an incomplete septic abortion, when both haemorrhage and sepsis may be present simultaneously.

Whatever its cause, failure of tissue perfusion leads to progressive damage in vital organs (heart, lungs, brain, kidneys and liver). All types of shock inevitably lead to profound metabolic acidosis due to release of lactic acid by hypoxic cells as they switch to the anaerobic metabolic pathway. Irreversible damage and death can follow, anything from a few minutes to many hours later. Therefore **be alert – look for the signs – act urgently**.

Clinical recognition of shock

Each vital organ can contribute to the clinical picture:

Myocardium	Cold sweaty skin* Poor pulse volume* Tachycardia (>120 per min, sustained) Low blood pressure (systolic<80 mm Hg) Pulmonary oedema
Lungs	Respiratory failure, cyanosis Shock lung (widespread capillary leakage of protein rich exudate)
Kidneys	Oliguria (<30 ml/hour), anuria Rising creatinine
Liver	Raised liver enzymes Jaundice
Brain	Coma Fits
Blood	Disseminated intravascular coagulation (thrombocytopenia, normocytic anaemia, red cell fragmentation, bruising and bleeding from needle sites and gums)

***Septic shock** characteristically follows a two-phase clinical path. At first the patient may be feverish, warm to the touch, and with a full volume pulse. Disseminated intravascular coagulation (DIC) may be an early complication of sepsis due to widespread damage to leukocytes and endothelial cells, which release pro-coagulant materials. Later there is irreversible hypotension.

Monitoring shock

The following vital signs provide the best clinical guide in treating shock.

- Heart rate – count at the apex
- Pulse volume – the femoral pulse is the most reliable when blood pressure is very low or unrecordable
- Blood pressure – only reliable when systolic pressure is above 60 mmHg
- Urine output – normally over 40 ml/hour
- Respiratory rate – tachypnoea is an early sign of shock
- Central venous pressure

General principles in treating shock

These are:

1. Restore and maintain circulation and breathing.
2. Treat the cause of shock.
3. Watch for development of further complications:
   acute renal failure
   disseminated intravascular coagulation
   acute respiratory failure (ARDS, or 'shock lung')

In practical terms, the following table sets out the first steps in dealing with a shocked patient.

Immediate management of shock

- Set up an intravenous line immediately. Use subclavian, internal jugular or femoral veins if peripheral veins are too collapsed for access.
- Establish a CVP line to allow accurate monitoring of central venous pressure (normally 5–8 cm H_2O).
- Take blood for haemoglobin, electrolytes, blood cultures.
- If hypovolaemia is certain, or strongly suspected, give normal saline at least 1 litre every 4 hours, or a colloid such as dextran solution 500 ml over 4 hours. Be careful not to over-transfuse, especially if cardiac failure is suspected. Auscultate the lung bases to detect fluid overload.
- Transfuse as soon as possible in cases of haemorrhage, using O negative blood in cases of desperate emergency (see below).
- Monitor pulse and blood pressure frequently, at least every 30 minutes in unstable patients.
- Oxygen is mandatory. Aim for 40% inspired oxygen concentration. Monitor by oximetry when available – try to maintain oxygen saturation above 95%.
- In cases of suspected septicaemia, give broad-spectrum antibiotics intravenously. Gram-negative organisms, e.g. from urinary infection, should be covered.
- Consider drug support to maintain adequate cardiac output and renal perfusion.

Massive blood loss

The aims in managing massive blood loss are:

1. to restore the circulation
2. to define and deal with the specific cause of bleeding

Actions in massive blood loss

- Set up an intravenous line and give isotonic saline (1 litre over 4 hours) while cross-matching takes place. In dire emergency use O-negative blood (universal donor blood)
- Haematemesis or melaena demands endoscopy or emergency barium studies when the patient is sufficiently resuscitated. Emergency surgery may be required.
- Patients with splenomegaly may have portal hypertension and bleeding from oesophageal varices. This bleeding may respond to vasopressin (*Pitressin*) 20 units i.v. in 500 ml 5% dextrose over 20 minutes, or to oesophageal tamponade by a Sengstaken–Blakemore tube.
- Massive hemoptysis requires bronchoscopy and sometimes thoracotomy to control bleeding. In advanced centres, pulmonary angiography may reveal a source of bleeding susceptible to artificial embolization.
- Massive epistaxis requires nasal packing.
- Massive vaginal bleeding requires vaginal examination (except in suspected placenta praevia). Following abortion ergometrine 0.5 mg 6-hourly may control bleeding until the uterus can be evacuated.
- Always suspect ruptured ectopic pregnancy in a woman of child-bearing age.

The acutely breathless patient and respiratory emergencies

The common causes of acute breathlessness are

- upper airway obstruction
- severe pneumonia
- pneumothorax
- massive pleural effusion
- acute heart failure
- acute severe asthma
- pulmonary embolism
- respiratory muscle paralysis

Many of these conditions can be accurately diagnosed by physical examination (see Chapter 77).

Acute pneumothorax

Spontaneous pneumothorax may complicate pulmonary tuberculosis or chronic lung disease, especially emphysema in older patients.

Much more dangerous is traumatic pneumothorax, complicating stab wounds, rib fractures and crush injuries, common in road accidents. These pneumothoraces are often of the tension type, requiring immediate (e.g. roadside) pleural drainage to release pressure on the mediastinum and great vessels.

Suspect pneumothorax if there is:

- sudden unilateral chest pain, with or without breathlessness
- a history of trauma, particularly rib fracture
- normal or hyper-resonant percussion note, but distant or absent breath sounds on the affected side
- suspect tension if breathlessness is extreme, with reduced movements on the affected side and evidence of mediastinal shift (trachea deviated away from the affected side).

Management (full resources) of simple pneumothorax

1. Take chest X-ray to assess degree of collapse.
2. If lung less than one-third collapsed, either allow the pneumothorax to resolve spontaneously (with check X-ray in about 10 days), or aspirate pleural air with 50 ml syringe and three-way tap.
3. If lung collapse greater than one-third, and/or there is significant dyspnoea, set up a pleural drain and underwater seal, placing the drain in the second intercostal space 4 cm lateral to the sternal edge.
4. Leave the drain in place for at least 24 hours after air ceases bubbling through the underwater seal and the meniscus stops swinging up and down the tube. Always take a check X-ray before discharging the patient.

Management (full resources) tension pneumothorax

1. Give 60% oxygen.
2. Take a chest X-ray if the facility is immediately available.
3 If there is a suspicion of tension, immediately introduce a large bore needle in the second intercostal space on the affected side to relieve pressure.
4. If air escapes through the needle, set up an intercostal drain and underwater seal.
5. Seek help to deal with other thoracic injuries if present. There may be multiple rib fractures or significant intrapleural bleeding, even requiring thoracotomy.

First-line management of tension pneumothorax with limited resources

- Be aware of the possibility, especially after trauma to the chest.
- In any distressed breathless patient look for the signs of tension: hyper-resonance, absent breath sounds, tracheal and cardiac shift away from the affected side.
- Relieve pressure by introducing any large bore needle through the second interspace, 4 cm from sternal edge. If no needle is available improvise – for example, open the skin with a clean knife and use the outer case of a ball point pen as the cannula.
- Once pressure is relieved withdraw the cannula and cover the site with a dressing or your finger while transporting the patient to hospital. It may be necessary to re-introduce the cannula if respiratory distress develops again.

Massive pleural effusion

Tuberculosis, malignancies and occasionally pneumonia with a large parapneumonic effusion may cause large effusions which collapse the underlying lung, displace the mediastinum from the mid-line and seriously impede venous return.

Suspect massive pleural effusion when:

- the patient is dyspnoeic at rest
- movements are reduced on one side, with a 'stony' dull percussion note throughout
- there is tracheal shift away from the affected side (sometimes a difficult sign)

Management of large pleural effusion

1. Take a chest X-ray to confirm the diagnosis, but do not delay pleural drainage.
2. If there is doubt about the diagnosis try a pleural tap with a 20 ml syringe and green needle. Send fluid for laboratory analysis (cytology, acid-fast bacilli and protein content).
3. Introduce a large bore pleural drain through the eighth or ninth intercostal space on the affected side and allow the fluid to drain via an underwater seal.
4. Control the rate of drainage by a clamp or arterial forceps It is unwise to drain more than about 1.5 litres of fluid suddenly, for fear of severe vasovagal responses and re-expansion pulmonary oedema.
5. If there is doubt about sterility, give penicillin 1 mega unit 6-hourly i.m. during drainage.

Acute severe asthma

These symptoms and signs in a patient with severe asthma demand urgent intervention:

- patient too breathless to speak in sentences
- exhaustion

- dehydration
- persistent tachycardia >110 per minute (>140 in children under 5)
- respiratory rate >25 per minute (>50 in children under 5)
- silent chest on auscultation due to extreme airway obstruction
- mental confusion or agitation
- cyanosis

Note that pulsus paradoxus is often included in this list, but it is a difficult sign.

Aim to maintain adequate oxygen levels, reverse bronchospasm and inflammation, clear sticky bronchial secretions and, if necessary, rescue the exhausted patient whose CO_2 levels are rising, by assisted ventilation.

Management of acute severe asthma

1. Give 60% oxygen and reassure the patient.
2. Set up an intravenous line and give normal saline to restore hydration.
3. Reverse bronchospasm pharmacologically with *any* of the following, depending on availability:
   Subcutaneous adrenaline 0.5–1.0 ml of 1:1000 solution slowly
   Aminophylline 250 mg by slow i.v. infusion (20–30 minutes). Do not give i.v. aminophylline if the patient is already taking the drug orally
   Subcutaneous terbutaline 500 micrograms (child 10 micrograms/kg)
   Nebulised salbutamol 5 mg or terbutaline 10 mg
4. Give corticosteroid, either prednisolone 40–60 mg orally (child 1–2 mg/kg), or hydrocortisone 200 mg i.v.
5. Keep the patient in hospital because bronchospasm may return. Continue oxygen and i.v. fluids, and be ready to repeat step 3 above.
6. If bronchospasm is persistent, aminophylline 500 mg may be given by i.v. infusion over 12 hours in normal saline (not dextrose saline, which degrades the drug).
7. Start a broad spectrum antibiotic (e.g. amoxycillin) if infection is suspected.
8. Watch for signs of exhaustion and worsening respiratory failure. If possible, monitor $PaCO_2$ – a rising level indicates respiratory muscle exhaustion. Intubation and IPPV will then be necessary in the intensive care unit.

When the attack has cleared, the course of steroids is gradually tailed off (usually stepping down by 5 mg each day) and the patient returns to their normal management pattern. Repeated acute attacks require better supervision and careful preventive treatment such as regular inhaled steroids. If inhaled steroids are not available, asthmatic patients may have to depend on a small continous dose of oral prednisolone, say 3 to 5 mg daily.

Pulmonary embolus

Acute pulmonary embolus is a difficult diagnosis, often overlooked but not yet common in tropical rural practice. Long air flights are directly linked to death from pulmonary embolism: other people at risk are those who are bed-ridden, post-operative patients, and women taking the contraceptive pill. Emboli may arise from pelvic veins in pelvic inflammatory disease, or from right heart in dilated cardiomyopathy or infective endocarditis.

Suspect pulmonary embolus when:

- A patient presents with sudden or rapidly increasing breathlessness of no obvious cause, particularly if they have been recently immobilized by surgery or illness.
- There is sustained tachypnoea
- There are signs of acute right heart failure
- The ECG shows acute right ventricular strain (S1, Q3, T3 pattern)
- (Signs of deep venous thrombosis are often absent at the time of an acute embolus to the pulmonary circulation.)

Management of pulmonary embolism (adults)

1. Give 60% oxygen.
2. Set up an intravenous line and give heparin 5000 units loading dose plus continuous infusion 1000 to 2000 units per hour. Alternatively, give 15 000 units subcutaneously every 12 hours. Laboratory monitoring is essential and the dose adjusted accordingly.
3. Consider long-term treatment with warfarin or low molecular weight heparin.

Smoke inhalation

This may be caused by an accident in the home, when a kerosene stove may be overturned or cooking fat ignited. Minor smoke inhalation causes cough and bronchial irritability: major inhalation causes an intense chemical pneumonia.

The aim of management is to support respiration while the intensely inflamed and destroyed bronchial mucosa has time to heal, which can take days or even weeks.

Management of smoke inhalation

1. Give 60% oxygen.
2. Give a broad spectrum antibiotic as prophylaxis against secondary infection.
3. Provide adequate pain relief for the severe discomfort of tracheo-bronchitis.
4. Encourage sputum clearance (the sputum is often deeply coloured, sometimes blood stained, and very copious after smoke inhalation).

Aspiration of gastric contents

Aspiration of vomit is a risk after an alcoholic drinking bout and in comatose patients, who have diminished or absent cough reflex, after head injuries, or a drug overdose. Gastric acid in vomit causes intense chemical bronchitis, whilst particles of food can block bronchi. Bacteria from the oropharynx set up secondary infection which leads to a destructive necrotizing pneumonia.

Management of gastric aspiration

1. Pass a cuffed endotracheal tube and suck out inhaled material. If no endotracheal tube is available, place the patient in the recovery position and aspirate. This will also promote coughing unless the patient is deeply unconscious.
2. Give 60% oxygen.
3. Give broad spectrum antibiotics such as amoxicillin 500 mg 8-hourly and also cover anaerobic bacteria with antibiotics such as metronidazole 400 mg 8-hourly.
4. Ventilation may be required in severe cases.

Flail chest

This follows trauma with fracture of several adjacent ribs, resulting in an unstable segment of chest wall. This unstable area is drawn in as the patient tries to breathe in, resulting in inadequate ventilation of the underlying lung. The condition can be rapidly fatal when bilateral, or when the unstable segment covers many ribs on one side. It is a common complication of road accidents.

Management of flail chest

1. Give 60% oxygen.
2. Relieve pain with appropriate analgesics (non-steroidal agents such as regular ibuprofen are needed)
3. When respiratory distress is evident, maintain ventilation by Ambu bag or mouth to mouth respiration and move patient rapidly to an intensive facility for endotracheal intubation and ventilation, continuing until the ribs unite in 5–10 days.
4. Remember to check for other complications of the injury, especially pneumothorax and pleural haemorrhagic effusion.

Respiratory muscle failure

The respiratory muscles may become suddenly and fatally paralysed in conditions such as cervical injury or neurotoxic cobra bite, or more gradually in Guillain Barré syndrome. In some conditions such as early muscular dystrophy and myasthenia gravis, respiratory muscle power is sufficient to maintain adequate ventilation during the day, but not during sleep – when patients may become profoundly hypoxaemic.

Conditions associated with respiratory muscle weakness or paralysis

Neurotoxic snake bite (cobra, mamba)	Infective polyneuropathy (Guillain–Barré)
Motor neurone disease	Head injury
Cervical cord injury	Tetanus
Botulism	Poliomyelitis
Drug overdose	Muscular dystrophies
Myasthenia gravis	

Management of respiratory muscle failure

1. Monitor the patient in danger. Clinical signs of coma and cyanosis are far too late. It is better to use objective measurements such as the peak flow rate (using a peak flow meter), the minute volume, and oxygen saturation (using a pulse oximeter). The most sensitive monitoring is by blood gas analysis, a rising $PaCO_2$ being the early sign of inadequate ventilation.
2. Protect the airway if the cough reflex is weak or absent. Pass a nasogastric tube to allow safe feeding.
3. If ventilation is inadequate, move the patient early to a facility where endotracheal intubation and ventilation is available.
4. Difficult ethical questions arise when considering long-term ventilation in patients with an underlying slowly progressive cause of respiratory muscle weakness.

Adult respiratory distress syndrome (ARDS)

This term is used to describe widespread alveolar–capillary leakage, which may develop as a consequence of severe sepsis, severe *P. falciparum* malaria, head injury, uraemia, gastric aspiration, fat embolism, and any other cause of severe shock. It is frequently found as part of the syndrome of disseminated intravascular coagulation (DIC). The alveoli are filled with protein rich fluid and blood, and the chest X-ray resembles that of pulmonary oedema due to heart failure.

In every case try to make a precise diagnosis of the cause of ARDS. Without it, no specific tratment can be started, and the patient will almost invariably die. Even with the best facilities the mortality of established ARDS is around 60%.

Management of ARDS

1. Identify the underlying cause of ARDS and treat it.
2. Support the patient by ventilation in an intensive care unit, while waiting for treatment to become effective. Ventilation in these cases should be rapid with small tidal volumes and with as little lung movement as possible.
3. Give oxygen at the maximum rate possible.
4. There is no evidence that corticosteroids are useful in ARDS.

The hypotensive patient and cardiovascular emergencies

Hypotension

Hypotension is a medical emergency. Its cause must be diagnosed by logical application of basic physiology, using the equation:

$$BP = \text{cardiac output} \times \text{systemic vascular resistance}$$

The common causes of a low blood pressure of sudden or recent onset can therefore be explained either by a fall in cardiac output or a fall in systemic vascular resistance.

Reduced cardiac output

1. Reduced preload (central venous pressure) due to hypovolaemia
   Haemorrhage, vomiting, diarrhoea, burns, sepsis, anaphylaxis
2. Reduced contractility
   Cardiomyopathy, arrhythmias, valvular heart disease, cardiac tamponade, myocardial infarction, pulmonary embolism, sepsis
3. Increased afterload (systemic resistance)
   Uncommon, but may occur as a physiological response to falling blood pressure and heart failure

Reduced systemic resistance

Systemic resistance depends primarily on sympathetic nervous activity, but is also influenced by circulating hormones (adrenaline, noradrenaline and vasopressin). Locally produced vasodilatory substances such as nitric oxide and some cytokines also have marked effects in inflammation and sepsis. Common causes of low systemic resistance include: sepsis, high spinal cord damage, drug overdose and epidural anaesthesia

Why is hypotension dangerous?

Most organs require a mean driving arterial systemic pressure of 70 mmHg. Above this pressure blood supply to vital organs such as kidneys and brain is accurately autoregulated. Below this pressure organ failure is inevitable. Therefore monitor by

- regular blood pressure reading
  $$\text{Mean BP} = \text{diastolic BP} + \frac{(\text{systolic} - \text{diastolic})}{3}$$
- urine output (less than 1 ml/kg/per hour warns of renal failure – 70 ml/hour in average adult. An output of <40 ml/hour warrants urgent assessment and correction)
- Conscious level (a fall in Glasgow Coma Scale of >2 points requires immediate action)

Emergency management of acute severe hypotension

1. Ensure a patent airway and give high concentration oxygen.
2. Establish the cause if possible.
3. Give a bolus of i.v. fluid (500–1000 ml normal saline). Monitor the effect.
4. If the blood pressure rises and the patient improves, repeat the i.v. bolus and set up an intravenous line.
5. If available monitor CVP to enable accurate fluid replacement. Aim for a CVP of 7–12 cm water.

NB All cases except those in severe heart failure require i.v. fluid.

Acute pulmonary oedema

Acute pulmonary oedema occurs when pulmonary venous pressure rises to a level at which oedema fluid spills into the alveoli and lung interstium at a rate beyond the capacity of the lung lymphatics to clear it. Common causes of this frightening medical emergency are:

- left ventricular failure
- mitral stenosis
- fluid overload (acute renal failure, careless i.v. fluid administration)

The patient sits up, cannot lie flat, has tachypnoea and coughs: unless immediate treatment is given, terrifying breathlessness, cyanosis, tachycardia, and further cough (sometimes expectorating pink frothy oedema fluid) follow. Crackles at the lung bases are not an entirely reliable sign.

Emergency management of left ventricular failure

1. Relieve acute breathlessness, hypoxia, and anxiety
   - Give high concentration oxygen.
   - Give morphine 15 mg i.m.
   - Ask anxious relations to wait outside the ward.
2. Reduce central venous pressure (thus reducing venous return and pulmonary venous pressure).
   - Sit patient up, with legs down and arms resting on bedside table.
   - Give frusemide 80 mg i.v. or 120 mg orally
   - Consider giving aminophylline 250 mg i.v. over 30 minutes.
3. Correct cardiac arrhythmias if present.
   - Digitalize if atrial fibrillation and fast ventricular response is present (give digoxin 1000–1500 micrograms orally in divided doses over the first 24 hours, then 250 micrograms daily)
   - Consider digitalization in left ventricular failure of any cause, for its inotropic effect.
   - Other arrhythmias may need specialized treatment in a tertiary centre.
4. (Longer term) Reduce salt and fluid intake.
   - Start a low salt diet.
   - Restrict fluids to 1500 ml daily.

Acute cardiac tamponade

This emergency may be seen when there is:

- pericardial infection from local disease, for example tuberculosis, lobar pneumonia, or, much more rarely and seriously, amoebic liver abscess
- malignant involvement from cancers of lung or breast and mediastinal lymphoma.
- bleeding into the pericardium.

Recognition

In acute cardiac tamponade the patient gets rapidly worse, with

- extreme breathlessness
- tachycardia
- pulsus paradoxus – disappearance of the pulse and falling systolic BP during inspiration. In advanced cases, pulse and BP cannot be recorded.
- JVP raised, and rising further during inspiration
- quiet heart sounds and impalpable apex
- chest X-ray is variable: it depends on how much fluid has formed: typically an enlarged globular heart: cardiac ultrasound is diagnostic.

Management

There is no time to lose: aspirate pericardial sac immediately.

Accelerated severe hypertension (Malignant hypertension) – (see Chapter 72)

This is defined as a sustained diastolic BP over 130 mmHg (or 100 mmHg in children under 13 years). At these levels, especially when the pressure has risen rapidly from previously normal levels, there will be widespread damage to small arterioles. In the kidney this can lead to irreversible damage in days, hence the need for urgent treatment. Causes include

- renal disease:
  acute post-streptococcal nephritis (salt and water retention), chronic glomerulonephritis, chronic pyelonephritis and renal artery stenosis (all increased renin–angiotensin levels)
- pre-eclampsia of pregnancy
- amphetamine and cocaine abuse
- idiopathic cases

Management

Whereas 20 years ago it was customary to drop the blood pressure as rapidly as possible, it is now recognized that serious side effects outweigh the benefits. The advice now is to lower the pressure smoothly and gradually over 3 or 4 days. There is no need to use parenteral treatment in every case.

Recommended management in severe hypertension

1. Absolute bed rest
2. Start methyldopa 500 mg three times a day, plus a thiazide diuretic such as bendrofluazide 5 mg daily: a slow fall of BP over 1–3 days is desired.
3. Aim to reduce diastolic BP to 100–110 mmHg within 24 hours, and a normal diastolic pressure within a further 2 days.

4. If absolutely necessary, hydralazine 10 mg i.m., repeated 6-hourly if required.
5. Nifedipine slow release can be used in a dose of 10–20 mg.

Myocardial infarction

Myocardial infarction presents typically with severe crushing central chest pain (sometimes preceded by warning exertional angina), which radiates to the neck, jaws, shoulders and arms. Shock may be present, with sweating and tachycardia. Early complications include arrythmias (including fatal ventricular fibrillation) and heart failure. ECG changes may not appear until several hours after the event. The diagnosis is confirmed by finding raised cardiac enzyme levels (creatine kinase and troponin I) at appropriate times after the onset of pain.

Management

The management of acute myocardial infarction depends on resources, so we outline simple non-specialist management.

Emergency management of myocardial infarction

1. Relieve pain and anxiety with morphine 5–10 mg i.v.
2. Give high concentration oxygen.
3. Give aspirin 300 mg (not slow release) immediately, followed by 75 mg daily, and
4. Give a beta blocker such as atenolol 50–100 mg daily.
5. Treat complications as they arise.

The patient with disordered consciousness and neurological emergencies

Everywhere in Africa patients with reduced consciousness represent a common clinical emergency. They may be confused, drowsy, incoherent, aggressive, or deeply comatose, unresponsive to all external stimuli. Their assessment and management calls for a cool careful approach, taking clues not only from the patient but also from those closest to them. Knowledge of the common causes is essential.

Common causes of reduced consciousness

1. Intra-cerebral causes:
   meningitis/encephalitis, cerebral malaria, cerebral abscess, cerebral haemorrhage or infarction, intracranial haemorrhage (subdural, subarachnoid), head injury, space-occupying lesions (primary and secondary tumours, meningioma), epilepsy
2. Metabolic causes:
   hypoglycaemia, hyperglycaemia, hepatic failure with encephalopathy, renal failure, hyponatraemia, hypothyoidism, hypothermia
3. Respiratory and cardiac causes:
   hypoxia and/or hypercapnia, cardiac failure, hypotension
4. Poisons:
   organophosphates, carbon monoxide, salicylates, barbiturates

Recording reduced consciousness

It is absolutely essential to record accurately the clinical neurological state and progress of an unconscious patient. The rapid AVPU system has been described in section 1 (emergency resuscitation). For more specific monitoring, the 15-point Glasgow Coma Scale (GCS) is valuable.

The Glasgow Coma Scale

See Table 36.8.

As a general principle, a GCS of <9, or a fall in GCS of 2 points, should prompt urgent assessment and transfer to an intensive care unit.

The pupils

Always examine their size, responses and equality.

Sign	*Interpretation*
A unilateral sluggish/ fixed dilated pupil	space-occupying lesion on that side (tumour, haematoma, abscess)
Bilateral dilated pupils	increased sympathetic activity (fear, adrenaline, tricyclic drugs)
Bilateral constricted pupils	brainstem vascular accident opiate drugs

Emergency tests in reduced consciousness

The following tests are *essential*:

Blood glucose	for hypo- or hyperglycaemia
Full blood count	especially Hb and WBC count
Blood film for malaria parasites	always: remember that severe malaria can occur in non-immune migrants from highland areas, and outside endemic areas (e.g. highlands of Kenya).
Biochemistry	If there is clinical suspicion of metabolic cause – urea, electrolytes, liver function.

The following tests are recommended, as indicated:

Lumbar puncture	*Caution.* Only perform if there is no suspicion of raised intracranial pressure (danger of brainstem coning), primarily in suspected meningoencephalitis. (Do a CT scan first, if possible, to exclude space-occupying pathology.)
CT brain scan	If available, this is by far the most useful investigation for intracerebral causes.
Arterial blood gases	When respiratory or cardiac causes seem likely, and when respiration is affected by drugs and poisons.
Toxicology tests	If any suspicion of poisoning.

Emergency care of the unconscious patient

1. Ensure a patent airway and give high concentration oxygen.
2. If ventilation is inadequate, provide support by manual resuscitator.
3. Give i.v. fluids to maintain BP at approx 90 mmHg.
4. Reverse drug-induced unconsciousness if possible (e.g. give naloxone 100–200 micrograms i.v. in opiate overdose. In children the dose of Naloxone is 10 micrograms/kg, repeated at 100 micrograms/kg if necessary).
5. Measure blood sugar and give i.v. dextrose (p. 000) if below 3 mmol/l.
6. Place patient in lateral recovery position.
7. Where possible, transfer to an intensive care unit.

Head injury

Suspect head injury, especially from road accidents and fights. The diagnosis may not be immediately obvious. Look for cuts and bruises on the head, and bleeding from the nose or ears. CSF leaking from the nose or ears means a fracture of the base of the skull. Smell for alcohol.

Diffuse brain injury is typical of blunt trauma and deceleration. There may be raised intracranial pressure with papilloedema and coma.

Focal brain injury is more likely to be associated with motor and sensory signs, often remarkably without changes in conscious level

Emergency management of head injury

1. Careful clinical examination and emergency treatment of wounds and fractures (both to the head and elsewhere)
2. Admit all patients with altered consciousness (even momentary).
3. Monitor and manage level of consciousness (see above). Measure GCS and monitor responses of pupils every 30 minutes.
4. Take X-ray of skull, and CT head if available.
5. If signs suggest rising intracranial pressure, consider emergency burr holes for possible subdural haematoma.
6. If suspicion of skull base fracture, or a penetrating head wound give penicillin 1 mega unit 6 hourly to prevent meningeal infection.
7. Consider giving dexamethasone 10 mg i.m. immediately, followed by 5 mg i.m. 6 hourly if cerebral oedema is likely.

Spinal cord compression

This can be a reversible emergency, even when symptoms and signs have appeared gradually. Tuberculous spinal abscess is an example. After weeks or months of pain, motor signs may herald permanent paralysis unless the abscess if evacuated and the spinal cord decompressed within a few hours.

Clinical evaluation (see p. 000, Neurology, p21 and of typescript).

Emergency management of spinal cord compression

1. Nurse patients very carefully, stabilizing the spine (particularly the cervical region) to avoid worsening the compression. Use sand bags to maintain the patient in slight hyperextension. Prevent bed sores by great care of pressure areas.
2. Take spine X-rays, and CT (or preferably MRI) scans if available to establish level and nature of compression.
3. Refer for urgent decompression.
4. Lumbar puncture is not necessary. It is better to transfer patients to a special centre immediately than to perform LP with Queckenstedt's test, which may be difficult to interpret, and which does not define the level of the compression.

Severe epilepsy (status epilepticus)

Status epilepticus is defined as, 1. the occurrence of serial seizures without recovery of consciousness between them or, 2. a single seizure lasting longer than 30 minutes. Any seizure lasting more than 3 minutes must be regarded as dangerous, and terminated because the risk of death or permanent cerebral damage rises rapidly.

Emergency management of severe epilepsy

1. Ensure a clear airway and prevent tongue biting by inserting an oral airway or mouth gag. Suck out secretions.
2. Give diazepam 10–20 mg intravenously slowly, rectally, if the patient is thrashing about.
3. Set up an i.v. infusion, give either phenytoin 15 mg/kg by slow infusion, not more than 50 mg/min, or diazepam 50 mg in 500 ml normal saline and infuse at a rate sufficient to keep the patient asleep but just rousable.
4. Alternatively use phenobarbitone 100–200 mg i.m. 12 hourly. (Children phenobarbitone 1–2 mg/kg 12 hourly.)

Cerebral malaria (see Chapter 12 for detailed management)

Cerebral malaria is a rapidly progressive potentially fatal complication of *Plasmodium falciparum* infection, which predominates in areas of moderate transmission and in particular where transmission is seasonal. Parasitized red blood cells cause capillary sludging in the brain with resultant petechial cerebral haemorrhages. Even with treatment, there is a 20% mortality.

Clinical presention of cerebral malaria

Depressed conscious level, variable non-focal neurological signs, delirium, convulsions, leading to coma.

Assume that the patient is hypoglycaemic.

Additional complications include lactic acidosis, hypovolaemia, hyperpyrexia, non-cardiogenic pulmonary oedema, renal failure, coagulation disorders and anaemia.

Investigations

- Thick blood film (confirms diagnosis and assesses parasitaemia)
- Thin blood film (identifies *Plasmodium* species)
- Blood glucose
- Haemoglobin
- Blood culture (septicaemia as differential diagnosis in children)
- Arterial blood gases (when available)

Emergency management of cerebral malaria

1. Intubate if Glasgow Coma Score <8.
2. Give oxygen at as high a rate as possible.
3. Set up an intravenous line and give dextrose (2 ml/kg 25% or 5 ml/kg 10%): do not give as a rapid bolus.
4. Give quinine i.v. Start with a loading dose of quinine salt infusion over 4 hours, 20 mg/kg (up to a maximum of 1.4 grams).
5. After 8–12 hours change to quinine salt infusion 10 mg/kg (up to a maximum of 700 mg) infused over 4 hours, every 8–12 hours.
6. Diazepam (0.3 mg/kg) i.v., injected slowly over 5 min, or rectally 0.5 mg/kg, may be required for treatment of uncontrolled seizures, OR
7. Paraldehyde in a dose of 0.2 mg/kg i.m. from a glass syringe.
8. Note that children may appear to be unconscious when they are having seizures, therefore look carefully for subtle signs – they may 'wake up' when given diazepam.

Acute psychiatric states

Patients with severe confusion, shouting and fighting, are alarming to all; urgent measures may be necessary to protect the patient, other patients and staff. Remember that an acute pyschosis may be due to an existing organic illness, potentially reversible, such as subdural haematoma.

- *Always try to establish the underlying cause of the psychosis*

Emergency management of acute psychosis

Clinical state	*Treatment*
Noisy, uncontrollable, confused, schizophrenic, hysterical	Chlorpromazine 100–200 mg i.m., repeat 8-hourly if necessary
Severe anxiety	Diazepam 5–10 mg orally or rectally
Extreme depression	Imiparamine or amitryptiline 50 mg orally 12-hourly. Watch carefully because of danger of suicide.
Alcohol withdrawal (delirium tremens)	Diazepam 20–40 mg orally, followed by 10–20 mg orally 6-hourly.

Delirium

Delirium is an acute generalized, fluctuating impairment of cognitive function – memory, orientation and concentration. Behaviour, mood, thought processes, speech and insight may also be affected: associated psychotic ideas are transient and simple in content. Visual hallucinations may occur. All symptoms are worse at night.

Causes of delirium

Infection Cerebral: cerebral malaria, meningitis, encephalitis, any HIV-associated infection. Systemic, pyogenic bacteraemia, typhoid, typhus, relapsing fever, lobar pneumonia or occult urinary tract infection.

Metabolic Electrolyte disturbances, e.g. hyponatraemia, hypoxia, hypo- and hyperglycaemia, renal failure, liver failure

Drug-related (intoxication/withdrawal) Alcohol, sedatives, anticholinergics

Central nervous system pathology Cerebral infarct/haemorrhage, head injury, primary brain tumours

Endocrine and nutritional Hypo- and hyperthyroidism, primary hyperparathyroidism, adrenal insufficiency, thiamine and Vitamin B_{12} deficiency

Others Shock, heat stroke, heavy metal poisoning (mercury, lead)

Emergency management of delirium

- Assess patient's mental state. The Mini-mental state examination is useful for this purpose.
- Obtain relevant information (medication and drug history) from relatives
- Identify and treat underlying causes. Medical history and clinical findings will guide choice of investigations and specific management.
- Minimize use of sedatives and other centrally-acting drugs, using lowest possible doses, if at all.
- Provide patients with supportive environment:
  - Nurse in single room to aid rest:
  - Reduce unnecessary sensory stimulation
  - Use simple and firm communication.
  - Give repeated reorientation and reassurance (e.g. visible clock)
  - Encourage involvement from family and carers.
- Avoid physical restraint with good nursing care and medication.
- Consider anti-psychotic drugs if agitation and disruptive behaviour poses a danger of injury to the patient and carers. Haloperidol and chlorpromazine are the drugs of choice.
  - Start with a low dose (haloperidol 2.5 mg orally or intramuscularly; smaller doses for elderly patients).
  - Titrate dose to the desired effect (haloperidol maximum 18 mg).
  - Monitor conscious level, respiratory rate and blood pressure.
  - Benzodiazepines such as chlordiazepoxide (30–80 mg daily orally in divided doses) or diazepam (6–30 mg orally in divided doses) are the first-line treatment for delirium associated with excess alcohol intake.

Oliguria and acute renal failure

Normal urine output (>0.5 ml/kg/per hour) is dependent on an adequate blood supply or perfusion, normally functioning kidneys and a patent urinary tract. Oliguria is defined as a reduction in urine output to less than 400 ml per day. This frequently leads to an abrupt rise in creatinine, urea and potassium levels, metabolic acidosis and fluid overload.

See Chapter 83 for causes, assessment and management.

Assessment of patient with oliguria/acute renal failure

Remember that anuria is most often due to obstruction of the urinary tract.

History: Haematuria? Think of bladder or renal tumours: Loin pain? Think of renal stones; Prostatic symptoms (frequency, nocturia, poor stream, etc.)? Drugs (analgesics, diuretics, abortifacients)?

Examination: Hydration (skin turgor, collapsed veins, JVP, pulse, standing and lying BP)

Management of acute renal failure

Stop or avoid nephrotoxic agents.

Exclude renal tract obstruction.
Examine for palpable bladder and enlarged prostate.
Catheterize bladder if in doubt. Record volume of urine.

If available, arrange abdominal ultrasound to exclude renal tract obstruction (hydronephrosis) and determine kidney size.

Correct fluid balance

If hypovolaemia suspected, give 500 ml of normal saline over 30 minutes). Repeat until JVP just visible at root of neck at 45°. Ideally monitor CVP via a central line.

If oliguria persists despite adequate intravascular volume replacement, some physicians give frusemide 250 mg i.v. slowly (maximum 5 mg/min). It does not increase GFR but it does in some patients produce a useful diuresis.

If oliguria persists, refer to a tertiary centre

Recognize and treat life-threatening complications

Hyperkalaemia (see Chapter 82)

If plasma potassium >6.5 mmol/l (with or without ECG signs of hyperkalaemia), give 10% calcium gluconate 10 ml over 60 seconds.

Start insulin/dextrose i.v. infusion (10 units of actrapid insulin in 50 ml of 50% dextrose over 30 min). Check blood glucose regularly for 6 hours to exclude hypoglycaemia.

Measure K^+ regularly and if it rises again repeat calcium gluconate and insulin/dextrose infusion.

Calcium resonium (see Chapter 82).

Pulmonary oedema//fluid overload
Give high flow oxygen (maintain SaO_2>95% if monitoring available).
Give morphine 10 mg, one dose only
Give frusemide 250 mg i.v. over 1 hour.

Metabolic acidosis

Give sodium bicarbonate if pH <7.1 or HCO_3^- <8 mmol/l (500 ml of 1.26% solution over 30 minutes), if no danger of overload.

(Persistent acidosis is an indication for dialysis.)

Sepsis (common cause and complication of renal failure)

Send blood and urine for cultures, if facilities allow. Antibiotic therapy will be guided by suspected focus of infection. Adjust dose of antibiotics for reduced renal function.

Acute gastrointestinal emergencies

'The acute abdomen'

Some causes of acute severe abdominal pain require urgent surgery. Many others are 'medical' and in these surgery can be harmful.

- When confronted by a case of 'acute abdomen', first determine whether or not the cause is surgical.

Remember the following list, plan appropriate tests and avoid unnecessary surgery. The list is not exhaustive, but it includes the causes most likely to be met in African practice. Those needing urgent surgery are marked *.

Primarily intra-abdominal causes

Intestinal
*Intestinal obstruction (strangulated hernia, sigmoid volvulus, intussusception, roundworms), perforation of a viscus (duodenal ulcer, but there is seldom an acute event when a typhoid ulcer perforates), *acute appendicitis (rare in rural Africa), gastroenteritis, inflammatory bowel disease, amoebic colitis, fishbone perforation.

Hepatobiliary tract and pancreas
Acute hepatitis, acute cholecystitis, biliary colic, acute pancreatitis

Vascular
*Mesenteric infarction (sickle cell disease, Henoch–Schonlein purpura), splenic infarction (sickle cell disease), *ischaemic colitis, *ruptured aortic aneurysm

Genitourinary
Acute pyelonephritis, ureteric colic, acute epididymo-orchitis

Gynaecological
*Ruptured ectopic pregnancy, pelvic inflammatory disease, ruptured ovarian cyst

Extra-abdominal causes

These conditions may be diagnostically confusing because they can all present as acute abdominal pain.

Intrathoracic
Lobar pneumonia with pleurisy, pleurisy (from other causes), pericarditis, myocardial infarction

Metabolic causes
Diabetic ketoacidosis, lead poisoning, hypercalcaemia, poryphyria

Skeletal and neurological
Herpes zoster, vertebral collapse (TB, *Brucella* spp., metastases), nerve compression (prolapsed disc).

Vomiting

Nausea and vomiting in adults are non-specific symptoms with a wide variety of causes.

More common causes of acute vomiting in any hospital in Africa are as follows.

Gastrointestinal
Peptic ulcer disease, acute gastroenteritis, gastric outflow obstruction, small and large bowel obstruction, e.g. sigmoid volvulus, paralytic ileus, acute cholecystitis/pancreatitis.

Central nervous system
Raised intracranial pressure (space-occupying lesions), vestibular disorders (motion sickness, viral labyrinthitis).

Metabolic
Renal failure, electrolyte disturbances (hyponatraemia, hypercalcaemia), hyperglycaemia, Addisonian crisis.

Drug-induced
Alcohol, traditional herbal remedies, antibiotics, digitalis, opioids.

Others
Pregnancy, myocardia linfarction, renal colic, post-operative.

Assessment of a patient with acute vomiting

- Obtain a good medical history. Ask about duration, frequency, timing and content of the vomiting.
- Look for signs of dehydration (dry mucosa, loss of skin turgor, tachycardia and postural hypotension).
- Examine abdomen carefully looking specifically for distension, diffuse or localized tenderness, intra-abdominal masses and tinkling or absent sounds.

Management of acute severe vomiting

1. Set up an intravenous line and give normal saline, 1 litre 4-hourly. (Total fluid replacement will be guided by improvement in clinical signs (pulse rate and blood pressure).) Monitor fluid balance. If necessary consider a urinary catheter.
2. Send blood for full blood count, electrolytes, urea, creatinine, calcium, glucose and amylase (when available).
3. Take plain abdominal and chest X-rays.
4. Attempt to identify and treat the underlying cause of the vomiting.
5. Give antiemetic drugs. Metoclopramide orally, intramuscularly or intravenously, 10 mg 8-hourly for an average-sized adult is recommended for gastrointestinal causes (except intestinal obstruction). Prochlorperazine (12.5 mg i.m.) is best for metabolic causes. Cinnarizine 15 mg 8-hourly or promethazine 25–50 mg 12-hourly are anti-emetics of choice for vomiting secondary to vestibular disorders.

Diarrhoea

Please refer to Chapter 20 for the causes, assessment and management of acute diarrhoea.

Acute upper gastrointestinal haemorrhage

Acute upper gastrointestinal haemorrhage can be fatal. Where there are medical and surgical teams, they must work together.

Common causes are oesophageal varices, peptic ulcer, Mallory–Weiss tear: less common, gastric cancer, erosive gastritis.

Haematemesis and melaena may be delayed for hours after bleeding has started. The patient then presents with unexplained shock and hypotension: occult upper gastrointestinal bleeding is the most common cause of hidden haemorrhage. Those with cirrhosis who bleed may present with hepatic encephalopathy.

Emergency management of severe upper gastrointestinal bleeding

1. Give oxygen (5–10 l/min).
2. Insert large-bore intravenous cannulae in each antecubital fossa.
3. Commence i.v. normal saline 1 litre 2–4-hourly.
4. Send blood sample for urgent cross-match and start transfusion as soon as possible.
5. Measure Hb glucose.
6. Arrange erect chest X-ray to look for gas under the diaphragm.
7. Arrange urgent upper GI endoscopy.
8. Correct clotting abnormalities if necessary (Vitamin K 10 mg i.v., fresh frozen plasma 2 units, platelet transfusion).
9. Further treatment will depend upon underlying diagnosis.

Endocrine emergencies

Hypoglycaemia

Hypoglycaemia is one of the most common causes of coma: therefore *measure the blood glucose in every unconscious patient.* Early recognition and treatment are essential in order to avoid prolonged hypoglycaemia and coma, which may be fatal or which may lead to irreversible brain damage.

Common causes of hypoglycaemia include:

- Infection – Malaria, severe infections
- Insulin overdose – accidental, deliberate

- Drugs – oral hypoglycaemics, salicylates (high dose)
- Alcohol
- Tumours – insulinoma (very rare), retroperitoneal sarcoma
- Liver failure

Clinical features of hypoglycaemia

These are caused by two distinct mechanisms. *Adrenergic* stimulation occurs when blood glucose is <3 mmol/l, and causes sweating, tremor, pallor, palpitations, headache and anxiety. *Neuroglycopenia* occurs when glucose is <2.0 mmol/l and causes lethargy, lightheadedness, blurred vision, aggression, confusion, seizures, coma and death.

Emergency management of hypoglycaemia

1. *Conscious patient (able to protect airway):*
   - Treat on suspicion but take blood for laboratory confirmation if available
   - Give oral glucose solution if able to swallow.
   - If necessary set up an intravenous line: give glucose 20–30 g (200–300 ml 10% dextrose: 100–150 ml 20% dextrose: 40–60 ml 50% dextrose) followed by a 10 ml normal saline flush (20% or 10% dextrose is easier to use and more likely to be available). Repeat if response is inadequate.
   - Give a long-acting carbohydrate snack to a diabetic patient on recovery.
   - Patients who are taking oral hypoglycaemic drugs, or who have alcohol-related hypoglycaemia, need prolonged observation with a continuous infusion of 5% or 10% dextrose and regular (2-hourly) glucose monitoring.

Attempt to find cause of hypoglycaemia and offer advice on prevention.

2. *Unconscious patient (see also Table 70.10 in diabetes chapter)*
   - Give 25 ml of 50% dextrose i.v. via a large vein over 60 seconds. Follow with 10 ml of normal saline to flush the vein (or use 20% or 10% dextrose).
   - Repeat if response is inadequate after 3 minutes.
   - If unable to obtain i.v. access give 1 mg of glucagon i.m. (if available). When the patient regains consciousness give oral glucose solution to prevent hypoglycaemic episode later.
   - Consider alternative causes of coma in patients with poor response to 50% dextrose i.e. alcohol intoxication, acute liver failure, septicaemia and drug overdose.
   - Give thiamine one ampoule intravenously to patients suspected of chronic excessive alcohol ingestion before i.v. dextrose to avoid precipitating Wernicke's encephalopathy.

Hyperglycaemia

Diabetic ketoacidosis (DKA) is a significant cause of death in patients with insulin dependent diabetes mellitus. Mortality rates for DKA and hyperosmolar non-ketotic hyperglycaemic coma (HNKH) are similar to Western Europe (7% DKA; 16% HNKH).

Diabetic ketoacidosis (DKA)

DKA is characterized by positive serum or urine ketones, arterial pH ≤7.3 and/or serum bicarbonate <15 mmol/l. Common precipitating factors for DKA are:

- infection
- intercurrent illness, e.g. surgery
- stress
- poor compliance with treatment
- inappropriate reduction in insulin
- newly diagnosed diabetes mellitus

The clinical features, biochemical changes and emergency management of DKA are described in chapter 70.

Hyperosmolar non-ketotic hyperglycaemic coma (HNKH)

HNKH is characterized by comparatively higher blood glucose levels, absence of ketonuria and acidaemia, and a plasma osmolality greater than 350 mosmol/kg. Clinical presentation and management are given in Chapter 70.

Thyroid crisis (thyroid storm)

This is a life-threatening exacerbation of the manifestations of thyrotoxicosis. Patients may present with complications, such as cardiac failure, myopathy and infiltrative ophthalmopathy.

Thyroid crisis may be precipitated by infection, surgery, childbirth, trauma and uncontrolled diabetes.

Emergency management of acute thyroid crisis

1. General supportive measures

Set up an intravenous line and start fluid replacement with normal saline or dextrose saline. Consider central venous pressure monitoring if facilities allow.

Treat hyperthermia with exposure, fans and cold water sponging.

Identify and treat precipitating factor, i.e. infection.

If beta-blockers are not available, chlorpromazine can help with both agitation and hyperpyrexia.

2. Specific measures

Beta-block with propranolol (40 mg every 4 hours orally). This will improve the tachycardia, rate-related cardiac failure, tremors and agitation. In severe cases give slow i.v. propranolol (1.5 mg), preferably with ECG monitoring.

Carbimazole or propylthiouracil can be used. For carbimazole give 20 mg 4–6-hourly, orally or by nasogastric tube.

Give hydrocortisone 100 mg 6-hourly, or prednisolone 20 mg 6-hourly.

Give iodine, e.g. Lugol's Iodine, 2–5ml 6-hourly, diluted in water. Start at least 1 hour after the first dose of carbimazole (to avoid further exacerbation of the thyrotoxicosis).

Acute liver failure

Acute liver failure is described fully in Chapter 80.

Management

The acutely failing liver cannot detoxify ammonia and amines coming from the gut, nor can it synthesize blood clotting factors and glucose. The aim is to counteract these defects and to treat complications (see Chapter 80) and the cause of the failure.

Emergency management of liver failure

General measures:

- ABC with attention to airway, breathing and circulation.
- Set up an intravenous line. Consider central venous monitoring if available.
- Treat and monitor for hypoglycaemia (keep blood glucose >3.5 mmol/l).
- Nurse supine with head tilted up and in a quiet environment. Monitor frequently.
- Give high-flow oxygen.
- Pass a urinary catheter to monitor urine output accurately.
- Pass a nasogastric tube (to prevent aspiration).
- Aim to give 2000–3000 calories daily, with low protein (the subject of nutrition in acute liver failure is controversial – many patients are severely malnourished and need protein).
- Perform a high bowel magnesium sulphate enema 30 ml.
- Reduce bacterial breakdown in the gut by giving neomycin 1 g 6-hourly or metronidazole 200 mg 6-hourly orally or via nasogastric tube.
- If available maintain an empty gut by lactulose 30 ml 6-hourly.
- Monitor creatinine and electrolytes regularly.

Addisonian crisis

A sudden crisis may be precipitated in a patient with known Addison's disease on replacement therapy by acute infection, trauma, surgery and salt loss due to excessive sweating during hot weather.

Think of this as a possible diagnosis in a patient with nausea, vomiting, postural hypotension, weakness, and dehydration. There is a low serum Na^+ and high K^+.

Management of acute adrenal insufficiency

General measures

- Set up an intravenous line and start i.v. normal saline. Rate of fluid replacement will depend on response and clinical signs (heart rate and blood pressure).
- Give high flow oxygen.
- Consider a urinary catheter to monitor urine output accurately.
- If facilities allow, take blood for serum cortisol measurement to confirm the diagnosis but this should not delay specific treatment.
- Monitor blood sugar and treat hypoglycaemia if present.

Specific measures

- Give hydrocortisone 200 mg i.v. immediately and then 100 mg 6-hourly. Normal hydration and the absence of postural hypotension are signs of adequate fluid and corticosteroid replacement.
- Convert to long-term oral hydrocortisone when the patient has stabilized. This may not occur until 72 hours after presentation.

Haematological emergencies

Sickle cell crisis

Sickle cell crisis refers to an episode of acute red cell 'sickling' usually provoked by stress. The most common cause of stress is infection, but others to be kept in mind are surgery, pregnancy and exposure to cold. Even the relative hypoxaemia due to high altitude of air travel can precipitate a crisis.

Sickle cell crises are fully described in Chapter 78.

Emergency management of sickle cell crisis

1. Do Hb, WBC and reticulocyte count, thick and thin blood films for malaria and other tests as indicated by clinical features.
2. Treat for malaria. This is the commonest cause of crisis in endemic malaria areas. Give a curative course of anti-malarials according to local guidelines.
3. Reverse vascular stasis. Give i.v. fluids (normal saline) immediately, at a rate of 10–14 ml/kg/hour to increase hydration. Encourage oral fluids. Continue i.v. fluids for at least 24 hours. Rehydration is the anchor of treatment.
4. Give high flow oxygen, if available, to improve tissue oxgenation in areas of impending infarction
5. Treat pain and titrate doses according to its severity – morphine, or for less severe pain dihydrocodeine, or for mild pain paracetamol.

Treat an anaemic crisis, if present
Always use HbAA, packed cells, and frusemide 40 mg i.v. at the same ti0me.

Poisoning

The problem in Africa

Most poisoning is accidental and occurs at home, commonly from substances in unlabelled containers (often Coca-Cola or soda bottles). Fertilizers, insecticides, disinfectants, pesticides, and herbicides – examples are organophosphates or paraquat or kerosene and methanol for stoves, disguised in tempting bottles. Accidental overdose may occur with barbiturate and iron tablets (especially dangerous in children), and an accidental overdose of aspirin to a febrile child. Alcohol is probably the commonest poison.

Essential management in every case of poisoning

- Terminate the exposure. Remove the patient from fumes. If there are caustic burns, wash the affected part (skin, eyes, mouth) thoroughly with plain water.
- Follow the ABC pathway to maintain the airway, and ensure adequate ventilation and circulation. Remember that the great majority (over 80%) of poisoned patients will recover if they are simply kept alive until the poison has been metabolized or excreted.
- Assess levels of consciousness. The Matthew Lawson Scale is useful for very rapid assessment:
  I Drowsy, responds to verbal command
  II Unconscious, responds to minimal stimulus (e.g. touching hand)
  III Unconcious, responds to maximal stimuli (e.g. rubbing sternum vigorously)
  IV Deeply unconcious: laryngeal reflexes absent
  (Note that bowel sounds are often absent in stage III, and almost always in stage IV). This means that drug absorption is greatly reduced.
- Control seizures with diazepam 10 mg i.v.
- Consider gastric emptying, either by inducing vomiting or by gastric lavage.
  Do not attempt to do this in an unconscious patient because of the danger of aspiration of gastric contents. In unconscious patients, a cuffed endotracheal tube must always be inserted first to protect the airway.
  Vomiting can be induced by mechanical stimulation of the pharynx, or by giving ipecacuanha syrup (10 ml for infants up to 18 months, 15 ml for children up to 5 years, 25 ml for older children and adults – always following with 200 ml of water).
  Gastric lavage is performed with a wide bore Jacques tube in the stomach, and the patient lying in the recovery position. Aliquots of 300 ml of warm water are given and aspirated back until the aspirated fluid is clear. Remember to save a small volume for toxicological analysis.

Specific poisons

Organophosphates

Organophosphates are found in several agricultural insecticides (including Malathion and Parathion). They are readily absorbed through the skin, and are occasionally ingested. They poison by inhibiting the breakdown of ACh by cholinesterase. Excess stimulation by ACh of muscarinic receptors causes bradycardia, heart block, constricted pupils, bronchoconstriction, bladder emptying, nausea, vomiting, diarrhoea, loss of sphincter control, colic, intussusception, sweating, salivation, anxiety, restlessness, convulsions, coma and respiratory arrest. Excess stimulation of nicotinic receptors causes continuous depolarization leading to fasisculation and paralysis of skeletal muscle (including respiratory muscles).

Treatment

- Terminate exposure. If clothes are contaminated, strip patient naked and wash affected parts thoroughly with soap and water.

- If poison has been swallowed, carry out immediate gastric lavage, followed by administration of activated charcoal and purging with sodium sulphate.
- Give atropine sulphate 2 mg i.v. every 15 minutes until secretions dry up and pulse rate reaches at least 80 per minute. Atropinization should continue for at least 48 hours. Some poisoned patients are extremely tolerant of atropine and may require over 100 mg in 24 hours to produce successful atropinization.
- If pulmonary oedema is present, give frusemide.
- The cholinesterase reactivators pralidoxime and obidoxime are useful adjuncts to atropine in some cases, but should never replace it. A single dose of pralidoxime 30 mg/kg slowly i.v. is given after atropinization and repeated if it produces definite increase in muscle strength.
- Sedation may be given with diazepam or barbiturates (not phenothiazines, which have anticholinesterase activity).

Carbon monoxide

Suspicious signs are coma with a cherry red colour to the mucous membranes (due to circulating carboxyhaemoglobin).

Treatment

- Give maximum oxygen possible and provide full supportive care.
- Comatose patients require endotracheal intubation and full artificial ventilation until carboxyhaemoglobin spontaneously dissociates and allows normal oxygen carriage by haemoglobin to return.

Kerosene (paraffin)

This is a common cause of accidental poisoning. Fortunately, kerosene is poorly absorbed by the gastrointestinal tract, but there is nearly always some aspiration, resulting in an intense pneumonitis which can lead to pulmonary oedema and serious hypoxaemia. Nausea and vomiting are common.

Treatment

- Terminate exposure and consider gastric emptying – always with a cuffed endotracheal tube in place to protect the airway.
- Give prophylactic antibiotics (e.g. benzyl penicillin 1 mega-unit 6-hourly).
- Steroids: there is **no** clear evidence that they benefit chemical pneumonitis.

Alcohol (ethanol)

This is by far the most common poisoning in many parts of Africa. Remember that a drunken patient with reduced consciousness may have other serious intracerebral pathology, such as a sub-dural haematoma. Hypoglycaemia may also contribute to altered consciousness.

Treatment

- Put drunken patients on their side to lessen the danger of vomit being aspirated.
- Give a violently disruptive patient minimal sedation with chlorpromazine 50 mg orally or i.m. if absolutely necessary.
- Acute delirium tremens requires diazepam 20–40 mg i.v. immediately, followed by 10–20 mg 6-hourly, gradually withdrawing over about 10 days. Give thiamine, one ampoule by i.m. injection.

Methanol

Methanol is oxidized to formaldehyde and then to formic acid, causing a severe matabolic acidosis. Chronic drinking of methanol causes optic atrophy and blindness.

- In acute intoxication, give ethanol (e.g. as brandy) to compete with the methanol.
- If available, consider haemodialysis urgently to clear methanol rapidly from the blood.

Iron

This is a particular danger to children who may swallow iron tablets in the house. Just five 200 mg tablets can cause fatal cardiac toxicity in a young child. Acute gastric haemorrhage, acute encephalopathy, metabolic acidosis, renal and liver failure can all occur.

- Carry out gastric lavage, if possible using desferrioxamine 2 g/litre of warm water. Leave desferrioxamine 5 g 50 ml water in the stomach after lavage.
- Give desferrioxamine 2000 mg i.m., and further doses i.v. at 15 mg/kg per hour to a maximum of 80 mg/kg in 24 hours.

Salicylates

Initially respiration is stimulated by the increased metabolism caused by uncoupling of oxidative phosphorylation. Hyperventilation results in respiratory alkalosis in adults. However, there is also marked production of lactic acid, and in children the picture tends to be one of metabolic acidosis and reduced ventilation. Salicylate overdose can be rapidly fatal in children.

- Empty the stomach if poisoning occurred less than 24 hours previously.
- Set up an intravenous line and correct dehydration.
- In severe overdose (plasma salicylate level above 700 mg/litre) consider forced alkaline diuresis, or haemodialysis or haemoperfusion if facilities exist.
- Give vitamin K 10 mg slowly to protect against haemorrhage

Paracetamol

- Give i.v. *N*-acetylcysteine to replenish glutathione stores. This may improve survival in patients presenting more than 24 hours after the overdose (for details of indication for treatment and dose, please refer to the manufacturer's instructions). The alternative, away from a well-equipped hospital, is methionine 2.5 g administered orally (1 g in a child under 6 years).

Barbiturates, diazepam, phenothiazines, morphine, pethidine

- Do gastric lavage unless the overdose occurred more than 24 hr previously
- Respiration will often need support, by IPPV in a special care unit.
- For opiates (morphine and pethidine) give naloxone 0.4–1.2 mg i.v. as 0.4 mg boluses until a response occurs. IPPV may still be necessary.

Bites

Animal and human bites

When deciding how to manage a bitten person, the following history is necessary.

- What animal bit the patient?
- What was its appearance and behaviour?
- Recent changes in the animal's appearance and behaviour/bark?
- Has it bitten other animals/humans?
- Has the patient been vaccinated in the past year?
- Has the patient been immunized against tetanus. When was the last booster?
- Is the patient immunocompromised?

NB Take animal to veterinarian for observation and examination of brain for evidence of rabies if possible.

Treatment of bites

- Wash and scrub wound vigorously for at least 5 minutes.
- Remove foreign material, damaged tissue and scabs.
- Irrigate with alcohol, iodine or quaternary ammonium compounds.
- Avoid early suturing, wound closure and dressing.

Antibiotics

- Give amoxycillin/clindamycin which will cover most organisms, for 10–14 days.
- If the patient has penicillin allergy, give clindamycin with trimethoprim-sulphamethoxazole.

Tetanus

- Give human tetanus immunoglobulin if available (3000–5000 units i.v. or i.m.), or equine antiserum 10 000 units by slow intravenous injection (after a test dose)
- Primary immunization is essential also.

Rabies

This subject fully discussed in Chapter 68.

Snake bites

See Chapter 92.

Physical injury

Hyperthermia and hyperpyrexia

When the rate of heat production exceeds the rate of heat dissipation body temperature rises accordingly. This fine balance is regulated by the hypothalamus. In hyperthermia the hypothalamic set point is normal in contrast to hyperpyrexia where the set point is increased by circulating cytokines (IL-1β, TNFα). However, they share similar clinical presentation and basic treatment. There are three basic mechanisms for hyperthermia.

Excessive metabolic production of heat

exertional hyperthermia, malignant neuroleptic syndrome, thyrotoxicosis, tetanus, status epilepticus, hypersensitivity reactions to drugs, malignant hyperthermia of anaesthesia

Prolonged and excessive exposure to environmental heat

heat stroke
dehydration
malignant neuroleptic syndrome

Impaired heat dissipation

cerebrovascular accident
encephalitis
trauma

Note: Heavy exercise in a very high ambient temperature, miners or soldiers, is a well-recognized cause of hyperthermia and heatstroke.

The clinical features of hyperthermia (defined as a core temperature above 40 °C) include headache, nausea, hyperdynamic circulation, muscle rigidity, bleeding, seizures and coma. The patients have not been drinking water and have lost water more than sodium.

Investigations will show evidence of acute renal failure, myoglobinuria and raised creatinine kinase from rhabdomyolysis.

Emergency management of hyperthermia

Primary care:
- Remove all clothing and the subject from the hot environment

In hospital:
- Assess airway, breathing and circulation (ABC).
- Set up an intravenous line and start initial fluid replacement with hypotonic saline. Consider central venous catheter in the elderly and hypotensive patients.
- Insert urinary catheter to monitor urine output and check for myoglobin
- Give high-flow oxygen
- Prescribe diazepam for seizures.
- Regularly monitor pulse, blood pressure and rectal temperature.

External cooling measures. Use any or all of the following
- Sponge with cold water (15 °C)
- Soak sheets with cold water and place over patient (20 °C)
- Use cooling fans
- Avoid immersion in iced water

Stop cooling methods when temperature less than 39 °C.

Hypothermia

Hypothermia is defined as a core body temperature of 35 °C or less. Cases are seen during the winter months particularly in susceptible individuals living in mountainous areas. It is associated with high mortality rates in the elderly (30–75%).

Other causes of hypothermia include inadequate heat production (malnutrition, liver or renal failure) and drugs (alcohol, phenothiazines, opioids). Complications are severe – aspiration pneumonia, renal failure, peptic ulceration, acute pancreatitis, coma and death.

The clinical presentations can be summarized as follows.

Clinical presentation

32–35 °C	28–32 °C	Below 28 °C
shivering	respiratory depression	arrhythmias (VT/VF)
tachypnoea	hypotension	coma
apathy	dehydration	death
confusion	hypertonia	
dysarthria	arrhythmias (AF)	
ataxia	loss of protective reflexes	

Emergency management of hypothermia

Primary care:
- Monitor airway, breathing and circulation (ABC).
- Treat in warm surroundings, remove wet clothes and dry the patient.
- Insulate patient with blankets and bed covers.
- Check core temperature with rectal or low reading thermometer.
- These measures alone may be sufficient in cases of mild hypothermia.

In hospital:
- Set up an intravenous line and give 50% dextrose if hypoglycaemia is present.
- Active external warming is rarely used. Consider immersion in warm water only if hypothermia has been of short duration or rapid onset.
- Active internal rewarming methods:
  heated i.v. fluids (normal saline; up to 40 °C)
  warm humidified O_2 (42 °C) if available
  irrigation of hollow organs, e.g. peritoneal lavage, should only be used in severe hypothermia.

Electric shock and lightning strikes

Injuries result from burns at the site of entry and exit of the current and the direct effects of the electric current on cell membranes and other vital tissues, e.g. myocardial and conduction tissue. The severity of electrical injury is determined by the magnitude of the energy delivered, voltage, type of current (AC or DC), resistance to current flow, duration of contact with the source of electric current and the path taken by the current through the body.

Lightning injuries result from a brief and massive direct current shock. The effects on the cardiovascular system are broad and include tachycardia, hypertension, myocardial ischaemia and life threatening arrhythmias (VF/asystole). Respiratory arrest is due to widespread respiratory muscle spasm or respiratory centre inhibition by the direct current. Nerve tissue is also susceptible and patients may present with delirium and peripheral nerve damage.

Management of electric shocks and lightning strikes

At the accident:

Safety of the rescuer is paramount. Switch off main power source in cases of electric shock and approach the victim only when it is safe to do so.

Begin basic life support as described previously.

Electrical burns of the face and neck may cause soft tissue oedema and airway obstruction.

Remove burnt clothes and shoes to prevent further tissue damage.

Be alert for head and spinal injuries.

In hospital:

Set up an intravenous line and start intravenous fluids. Rhabdomyolysis is a common complication and the result of extensive tissue damage or necrosis. A good urine output (>0.5 ml/kg per hour) should be maintained to excrete excess myoglobin, potassium and phosphate.

Skin burns require early surgical attention.

Patients with electrical injury and loss of consciousness, cardiac arrest, burns or ECG abnormalities should be monitored in hospital.

Submersion and near-drowning

Hypoxia and asphyxiation are the most important consequences of submersion. Outcome is closely related to the duration and severity of hypoxia and the main aim of resuscitation is to restore oxygenation, ventilation and circulation as quickly as possible. Classification by submersion fluid (fresh water or salt water) is irrelevant as they are both managed identically at presentation.

After submersion patients may have severe cough and dyspnoea, and may develop respiratory or cardiac arrest even after successful rescuing. Watch for signs of injury – including neck and spinal injuries in diving accidents, and poisonous stings and bites from jelly fish, stone fish, sea urchins and the like.

The prognosis after near drowning depends on the duration of submersion, the presence of cardiac arrest, age and the existence of other disease.

Management of near-drowning

At the site of rescue

- Attempt resuscitation at the scene unless the victim has a lethal injury or putrefaction and rigor mortis has developed.
- Minimize risks to rescuers when attempting to recover victim from the water.
- Beware of head or spinal injuries. Consider spinal immobilization by keeping the victim's neck in a neutral position (avoid flexion or extension) or use a cervical collar and spine board.
- Remove victim from water in a horizontal position if possible to avoid circulatory collapse.
- Immediate attention to airway, breathing and circulation once the victim is out of the water. Prompt mouth to mouth ventilation is important and correlates with survival.
- Attempts to remove water from the lungs and stomach should be avoided as only a small amount of water is aspirated into the lungs during submersion.
- Vomiting is a common complication after submersion and resuscitation efforts. The victim should be turned onto the side and the vomitus removed by hand or with suction if available.
- Transport all submersed patients to an emergency facility for further management and observation.

In hospital

- Assess airway, breathing and circulation.
- Set up peripheral or central i.v. lines
- Give high-flow oxygen via mask.
- Treat hypothermia as described in the section on hypothermia above.
- Insert nasogastric tube to decompress and empty the stomach.
- Investigations (depending on availability) should include 12-lead ECG, chest X-ray, arterial blood gas analysis, blood glucose, electrolytes and full blood count.
- Patients require close monitoring preferably in a critical care facility.
- Observation for 12 hours and subsequent discharge from hospital is appropriate for asymptomatic patients provided clinical examination, oxygenation and chest radiograph are satisfactory.

Burns

Emergency management of burns

Burns are common in Africa. The risk factors are multiple. They include open fires for heating and cooking, unsafe storage of inflammable liquids, unreliable electric wiring, candles and paraffin lamps, indiscriminate burning of rubbish, and deliberate arson. The victims are often young children (with severe scalds), elderly people, the mentally infirm, and epileptics. This section deals with the emergency management of a burnt patient at presentation.

Emergency treatment at the site of the accident

- Remove the patient to a safe environment (always ensuring that the rescuer is also protected from danger).
- Apply the ABC system of emergency resuscitation (p. 1341). Remember that tracheostomy may be necessary soon after a burn affecting the airway. Look at the nasal hairs to see if they have been burnt by hot gases entering the respiratory tract. Noxious gases such as carbon monoxide may be present in the environment, and the patient needs to be in fresh air as soon as possible, preferably with added high flow oxygen.
- Cool the burnt area quickly with cold water, if necessary straight through the clothing to save time. Keep applying cold water to minimize the spread of heat through surrounding tissue.
- Cover the burn with clean linen to reduce bacterial contamination.
- Transfer the patient, as gently and speedily as possible, to the nearest hospital.

Hospital management

- Continue emergency resuscitation
- Provide adequate pain relief. Mild burns will require paracetamol or non-steroidal analgesics, but more severe burns require morphine, preferably by intravenous route once intravenous access has been established.
- Take a full history of the burn, looking for clues about the depth and extent of the injury. Electric burns and burns sustained while unconscious (e.g. from drunkenness or epilepsy) tend to be deep. Molten metal and hot jam produce deeper burns than tea and boiling water. A serious burn several hours before arrival in hospital will be associated with greater fluid loss.
- Examine the patient, noting particularly signs of shock (cold peripheries, low blood pressure). Monitor urine output closely in any burn case of more than 10% body surface area (these patients must have a urinary catheter).
- Use the Rule of Nines to calculate the percentage of burnt body surface area (Fig. 97.1).

	Percentage of surface area
Head and neck	9
Each arm	9
Each leg	18
Front of trunk	18
Back of trunk	18
Perineum	1

- Estimate the depth of burn by using a sterile needle to see if pain sensation is present. Areas where sensation is absent have full thickness burns. Classify the burn as
  - erythema only
  - superficial partial skin loss
  - deep partial thickness skin loss
  - full thickness skin loss
  - deep burn (involving underlying tendon, muscle, bone, etc.)
- Admit all patients with more than 15% burnt body surface area.
- Start intravenous fluid replacement in all cases with >15% burns (>10% in children). Use a large bore cannula (16- or 17-gauge) with full aseptic technique. The following formula for calculating intravenous fluid replacement allows for the very rapid loss soon after the injury, gradually lessening over 36 hours before stabilizing.
  - First 8 hours (*starting from time of burn*):
    - 1 ml per 1% of burnt surface per kg body weight
  - Next 16 hours:
    - same formula
  - Each subsequent 24 hours
    - same formula
- Transfuse blood to correct haemoglobin to 10 g/dl.
- Cover the burn with sterile dressings, keeping bedclothes off painful areas. Further management needs to be co-ordinated by an experienced surgeon and is outside the scope of this section.

Name .... Age.......
Date of admission .../.../2.....
Date & time of burn ... /.../2..... at ....am/pm

Diagram of the burn:-

Shade in the area of the burn on the appropriate diagram below. Colour in Red the areas that do not feel pin prick

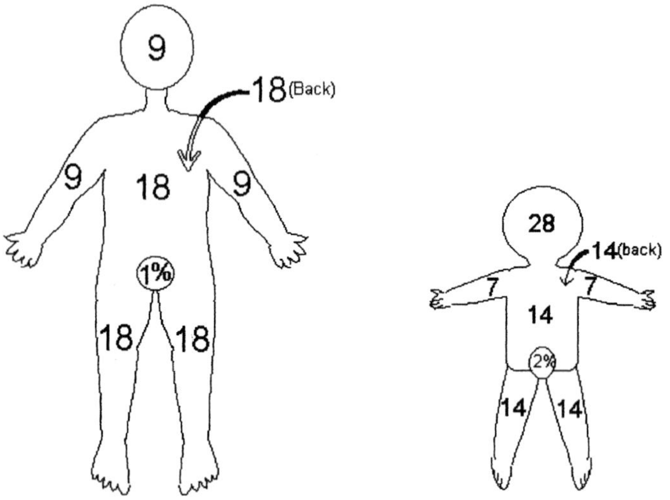

Write your estimate of the percentage of body surface burnt, using the figures in the appropriate chart as a guide:-

Percent body surface Burnt:- | % |

Fig. 97.1. A ward chart for insertion into the notes of burns cases.

The acutely ill child

Many children die in Africa from four major causes – diarrhoeal illness, measles, malaria and pneumonia. A high proportion of these deaths can be prevented by accurate diagnosis and appropriate clinical management during the first few hours of medical care.

This section deals with the initial assessment of the acutely ill child. In many instances the management of children follows the same pathways as in adults, but the initial assessment calls for special skills. Rapid and accurate clinical assessment, followed by calm and decisive initial steps in management are the requirements when faced with a frighteningly ill child and a desperately anxious mother.

A simple plan to follow is

- **primary assessment and resuscitation**
- **secondary assessment (try to make a diagnosis)**
- **definitive diagnosis and management**

Primary assessment

Use the ABCD approach, see table below.

Early essential investigations

If facilities allow, do the following in a very sick child:

- blood glucose
- blood film for malaria parasites
- haematocrit
- blood culture, grouping and cross-match

	Clinical signs	Immediate action
Airway	Stridor, choking, barking cough, agitation, restlessness, cyanosis, intercostal recession, paradoxical abdominal movement	Try to open airway with chin lift. If foreign body suspected, display tongue with spatula or laryngoscope and remove the object with forceps. Do not blindly sweep with a finger – the foreign body may be pushed lower.
Respiration	Raised respiratory rate, intercostal recession, grunting, wheezing, using accessory respiratory muscles, flaring of the alae nasi, tachycardia, cyanosis	Give high flow oxygen by face mask. Use bag and mask if necessary, and consider intubation early. Measure oxygen saturation with pulse oximeter if possible.
Circulation	Tachycardia >150 bpm, capillary refill >2 s, cold hands and feet, low BP (late and sinister sign)	High flow oxygen. Intravenous or intra-osseous fluid (see Fig. 97.2). Give bolus of 20 ml/kg normal saline (use Ringer lactate or half-strength Darrow's solution in cases of diarrhoea. Repeat boluses three times if necessary, and consider blood transfusion.
Disability (neurology)	Coma, convulsions, confusion, lateralizing signs, pupil reactions and size	Use Blantyre coma score, or AVPU to monitor progress. Give high flow oxygen. Check blood glucose, and give 5 ml of 10% glucose solution if <3 mmol/l (or on suspicion). Control seizures with diazepam 0.4 mg/kg i.v. 0.5 mg/kg per rectum. Alternatively paraldehyde 0.5 ml/kg per rectum in arachis oil (paraldehyde 0.2 ml/kg can be given i.m. but do not leave it in contact with plastic for more than 3 minutes).

- serum electrolytes
- blood gases and oxygen saturation
- (consider chest X-ray in respiratory cases)

Secondary assessment

Once the child is stabilized, carry out a full clinical assessment. The following may be useful pointers to an accurate diagnosis:

- fever, diarrhoea or vomiting
- history of epilepsy, asthma, diabetes
- possible accidental ingestion of poison or foreign body
- possible inhalation of foreign body
- medication history
- is the child drinking normally?

Definitive management

It is not always possible to come quickly to a clear diagnosis, therefore treat the treatable (e.g. hypoglycaemia, sepsis, acidosis, hypotension). It is important to be accurate in management so that the child is not made worse by, for example, under ventilating, over transfusing fluids or treating pain and seizures inadequately.

After the full examination and assessment consider the need for a urinary catheter, an intravenous line and a nasogastric tube.

Specific causes of airway obstruction in children

Foreign body

The choking child

- Stand behind a small child standing on a raised surface and do a Heimlich manoeuvre
- Hold infant prone along your forearm with face held in cupped hand and angled towards the floor.
- Hold toddler prone over your knee face down.

1 Give five back blows.

2 Check mouth for foreign body.

If this bring no success, then turn the patient over and with head still angled downwards give five firm chest thrusts.

3 Check mouth for foreign body.

If still no success:

repeat **1–3** above, while shouting for help until the obstruction is dislodged or until equipment is ready and available. Then use a light source and tongue elevator to get a direct view of the back of the throat and upper airway and try to remove any obvious foreign body with McGill forceps or any other suitable instrument to hand.

If a foreign body has passed into a bronchus, there may be reduced air entry to that lung, or localized wheezing. This may be confirmed by chest X-ray. The foreign body should be removed through a bronchoscope under general anaesthesia.

Croup

A viral syndrome of stridor, barking cough and hoarseness, accompanied by low grade fever (see Chapter 77).

In the urgent immediate emergency:

- disturb the child as little as possible.
- give oxygen by face mask or nasal cannulae – oxygen humidified in the dry season.
- inhaled steroids (budesonide 1 mg, repeated if necessary after 30–60 minutes) helps all cases of croup.
- Dexamethasone 0.15–0.6 mg can be given orally or intramuscularly.
- Give nebulized adrenaline (1:1000, 1mg/ml in a dose of 400 μg/kg. Maximum 5 mg.) if there is severe airway obstruction.
- Intubation and ventilation may be required in the worst cases.

Epiglottitis

Inflammation of the epiglottis and supra-glottal tissues due to *Haemophilus influenzae* infection. The child is usually about 3 years old and presents with a short history of high fever, drooling and an unwillingness to swallow. He looks toxic and is afraid to cough as it hurts. He will prefer to sit with his neck bent forward and outstretched to try and keep the swollen epiglottis from obstructing the larynx. It is dangerous to inspect such a child's throat.

- Take the child straight to theatre.
- Examine under anaesthesia.
- If the diagnosis is confirmed, the child will need intubation and ventilation (by a senior anaesthetist as the intubation in an inflamed and distorted upper airway can be very difficult).
- Intravenous antibiotics, chloramphenicol 25 mg/kg 8-hourly, or ceftriaxone 80–100 mg/kg daily should be given (after a blood culture if possible).
- Successful extubation can usually be achieved after 48 hours.

Bacterial tracheitis

Usually due to staphyloccocal, streptococcal or *Haemophilus influenzae* infection secondary to measles or other viral infections.

The child is toxic with fever, hoarseness and stridor but no drooling.

- Consider trachael lavage to remove necrotic tissue and thick secretions. Consider intubation and ventilation.
- Give intravenous antibiotics (chloramphenicol and cloxacillin).

Retropharyngeal abscess

This may follow a partially treated bacterial throat infection. The child has usually been unwell over 5 to 6 days with increasing respiratory distress and stridor. The temperature will be raised but may not be very high. The head is held in extension and sometimes trismus is present.

- Give intravenous antibiotics (chloramphenicol and cloxacillin or ceftriaxone)
- Consider early surgical drainage.

Angio-oedema

Due to allergic reaction to an insect bite or bee sting or peanut allergy, this will cause rapid onset of oral oedema often accompanied by wheezing.

- Give oxygen by face mask.
- Give intramuscular adrenaline.
- Give intravenous hydrocortisone (2 mg/kg) and an antihistamine.
- If the child has circulatory collapse, give a bolus of fluid (20 ml/kg)
- Adrenaline and fluids may have to be repeated after 10–15 minutes
- Intubation may rarely be required

For other acute emergencies in children please refer to the preceding pages on adults. For ease of reference, this section concludes with details of emergency drug doses in children (Box), and some useful practical tips when faced with a desperately ill child (Box). Other boxes give normal values for peak flow rates, heart and respiratory rates.

Table 97.1. Immediate assessment of a critically ill child

Paediatric emergency drug doses

Drug	*Dose*	*Usual concentration of supply*	*Comments*
Adrenaline hydrochloride	0.01 mg/kg	1:10 000 = 0.1 mg/ml	If only 1:1000 available, this must be diluted
Atropine sulphate	0.02 mg/kg 0.2 ml/kg	0.6 mg/ml	Minimum dose 0.1 mg/kg Maximum dose infants/children 1 mg: adolescents 2 mg
Calcium chloride	20 mg/kg	20% solution = 100 mg/ml	Give very slowly. Only use in confirmed hypocalcaemia, or hyperkalaemia/ hypermagnesaemia.
Glucose	0.5–1.0 mg/kg	0.5 mg/ml (50% solution)	Dilute to 10% solution (1 ml 50% glucose + 4 ml saline or sterile water)
Sodium bicarbonate	1 m Eq/ml 1 ml/kg	1 m Eq/ml (8.4% solution)	Only use after correcting fluid needs and having established ventilation.
Naloxone hydrochloride	0.1 mg/kg	0.4 mg/ml or 1.0 mg/ml	Narcotic antagonist Give rapidly.
Flumazenil	25–100 microgram/kg		Benzodiazepine antagonist

Useful tips when faced with an acutely ill child

1. When intubating, hold your breath; when you run out of breath, so does the baby. Go back to bag and mask with oxygen
2. ETT sizes = Age (years) + 4 (internal diameter in mm) OR the diameter of the child's little finger.
3. If blood glucose cannot be checked, give a bolus of glucose.
4. If i.v. burette giving sets, or infusion pumps are unavailable and fluid requirements are small (e.g. neonates) pour away the excess fluid from the bag of i.v. fluid to avoid over-infusion.
5. In malarious areas, if in doubt, treat for malaria in an unconscious or very ill child.
6. Infants lose body heat rapidly when exposed even in hot climates; cover babies as much as management allows.
7. In oedematous or marasmic children it is difficult to assess fluid needs. If i.v. fluids are required give at 10 ml/kg (not 20 ml/kg) boluses and monitor pulse and respiration. If the pulse rate increases by 15 beats/minute or respiratory rate by 5 breaths/minute, slow the infusion or remove it.
   Oral drugs are absorbed unrealiably.
   Hypothermia, hypokalemia and hypoglycaemia are all common.

Predicted values of peak expiratory flow rate in children

Height cm	*Peak flow l/min*
110	150
120	200
130	250
140	300
150	350
160	400
170	450

Normal values for respiratory and cardiac rates and blood pressure

	Respiratory rate/minute	*Cardiac rate/minute*
Infant	40–50	110–160
2–5 yrs	30–40	95–140
5–10 yrs	25–30	80–120
>10 yrs	15–20	60–100

Systolic blood pressure = (80 + age in years × 2)
Diastolic = 2/3 systolic pressure

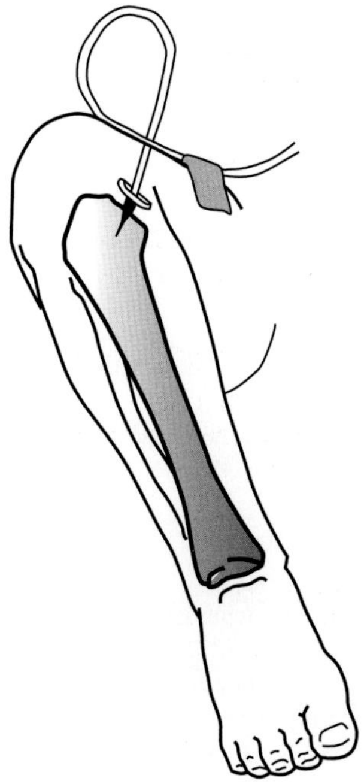

Fig. 97.2. **Site**: antero-medial surface of the upper tibia (infant: 1 finger's breadth below the knee joint line. Child: 2 finger's breadth below the knee joint line). The lower lateral surface of the femur is an alternative site.

Needle: 18G or 16G IO needle. If this is not available use a 21G (green) hypodermic needle.

Technique: Wear gloves, clean the access site with spirit, push the needle through the cortex of the bone with a firm but twisting movement. There is a 'giving' sensation when the marrow is entered which may be aspirated by syringe. Sometimes, and especially with the hypodermic needle, it becomes blocked and may be flushed open with a bolus of fluid. If this fails to function, use the other tibia, or another bony site.

Contraindications: Infection at the injection site, fracture of the tibia.

Uses: Any emergency drugs and fluids (except bretylium tosylate) can be safely given by this route. Aspirate can be tested for glucose and electrolytes; bacterial cultures can be made.

Complications: Do not leave in place for longer than 8 hours as local infection may develop. In infants too much force can fracture the tibia shaft. The needle may be misplaced in the calf muscles and compartment syndrome may develop.

Monitor: Calf size: if there is swelling, the needle is misplaced – remove it. Toe colour: pallor indicated popliteal arterial spasm or compression – remove the needle. Pain in the lower leg may be due to ischaemia – remove the needle.

Index

Note: page numbers in *italics* refer to figures, tables and boxes.